Sanders' Paramedic Textbook

Commissioning Editor: *Robert Edwards*
Development Editor: *Nicola Lally*
Project Manager: *Morven Dean*
Designer/Design Direction: *Stewart Larking*
Illustration Manager: *Bruce Hogarth*

Sanders' Paramedic Textbook

Edited by

Pete Gregory
Aidan Ward

Foreword by **Mick J Sanders**

Adapted from
Mosby's Paramedic Textbook, Third Edition
Written by
Mick J. Sanders, EMT-P, MSA

Contributing Editor
Kim McKenna, RN, BSN, CEN

Physician Advisors
Lawrence M Lewis, MD, FACEP
Gary Quick, MD, FACEP

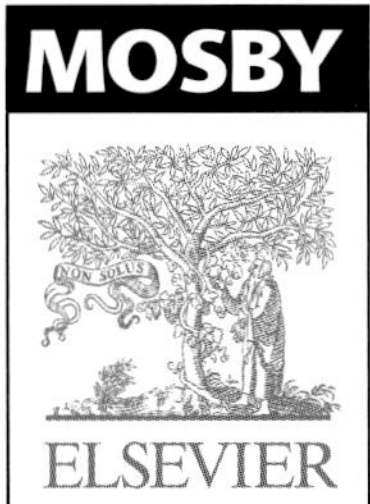

Edinburgh London New York Oxford Philadelphia St Louis Sydney Toronto 2010

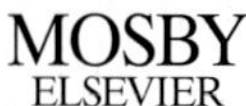

ISBN 978-0-7234-3443-6

British Library Cataloguing in Publication Data
A catalogue record for this book is available from the British Library

Library of Congress Cataloging in Publication Data
A catalog record for this book is available from the Library of Congress

Notice

Knowledge and best practice in this field are constantly changing. As new research and experience broaden our knowledge, changes in practice, treatment and drug therapy may become necessary or appropriate. Readers are advised to check the most current information provided (i) on procedures featured or (ii) by the manufacturer of each product to be administered, to verify the recommended dose or formula, the method and duration of administration, and contraindications. It is the responsibility of the practitioner, relying on their own experience and knowledge of the patient, to make diagnoses, to determine dosages and the best treatment for each individual patient, and to take all appropriate safety precautions. To the fullest extent of the law, neither the Publisher nor the Editors assumes any liability for any injury and/or damage to persons or property arising out of or related to any use of the material contained in this book.

The Publisher

Printed in China

The publisher's policy is to use **paper manufactured from sustainable forests**

Last digit is the print number: 9 8 7 6 5 4 3 2 1

Contents

Foreword

As the author of the US version of Mosby's Paramedic Textbook, I was asked to write this foreword. I am honoured and pleased to do so.

As a paramedic student, you have chosen to work in an exciting and rewarding area of healthcare – prehospital emergency care. Few professions can provide the same type of opportunities that lie before you. Through your training, you will meet the educational demands of a profession that requires knowledge in anatomy and physiology, mathematics, pharmacology, advanced education in the health sciences, and physical skills in using highly technical and sophisticated equipment. You will have an opportunity to play an important role in injury prevention; to participate in research; and to be a role model in your community. And most importantly, you will be entrusted with the lives of the people you serve. This describes today's paramedic – a member of a unique profession composed of highly trained men and women dedicated to making a difference in people's lives.

EMS has experienced rapid changes since its inception in the early 1970s. We have moved from having 'better-than-average' first aid training that focused on *scoop and run* to the nearest hospital, to being recognized as a profession and an important member of the healthcare team. Through advances in training, education, and technology, we are now able to bring many aspects of lifesaving care to the public – a level of care that had only been available inside the confines of a medical center or emergency department. We are not only trained to handle traumatic injuries to help prevent the loss of life or limb … we are also experts in recognizing serious conditions such as stroke, MI, hypoglycaemia, congestive heart failure, and asthma. We have the drugs and technology in our arsenal to initiate therapy at the scene that has proven to save lives.

This edition of the textbook has been adapted specifically for EMS personnel in the UK. The content has been modified for variations in your methods of operations, your scope of practice, your terminology, and pharmacology. Although there may be differences in the way EMS is practised in the UK, I know there is much we have in common across our seas. We are a proud profession that will continue to evolve as we face new demands in our role as protectors of the public. We must be prepared to provide an expanded scope of practice and be committed to continuing education and professional development. And we must remember our important role as caregivers as we adapt to the ever-changing healthcare needs of our society. We must be experts in patient assessment, disease pattern recognition, communications, and infection control. Unheard of only years ago, we now must think of the possibility of facing man-made disasters, terrorist acts, and even weapons of mass destruction. We must be adept at crowd control to ensure personal safety; mass casualty incidents; and medical triage. And we know that we may face these emergencies simultaneously – at any time, amid chaos, where we must be in control. This is a challenging time to be in public service. But it offers a great opportunity, as paramedics, for us to *'show our stuff'*.

As the author of Mosby's Paramedic Textbook, I tried to incorporate the themes of this foreword in every page of the book. I worked to find a happy medium between required book knowledge and they way it affects the emergency care we provide in the streets. I hope reading this foreword reinforces the decision you made to choose this textbook. Welcome to EMS, and good luck with your career.

Mick J. Sanders
Author of Mosby's Paramedic Textbook

Preface

The idea of adapting the well-known, widely used and respected Mosby's Paramedic Textbook was something that the authors of this text considered many times in the past. It was often as a result of conversations and feedback about the availability of material with a focus on the UK paramedic practice environment as the original editions of Mosby's Paramedic Textbook are focused on US practice. Therefore, there is an underlying philosophy behind the adaptation of Mosby's Paramedic Textbook into a text targeted to the UK market.

Firstly that the book reflects the most up-to-date paramedic practice. This is difficult to achieve as the profession evolves and, like all healthcare, revision and refinement of best practice continues unrelentingly. However, it is hoped that this contemporary focus has been achieved.

Secondly, that where parallel material exists these elements are de-emphasized to allow for a more focused content; for example, there are many excellent texts on anatomy and physiology and this element of the original book has been modified to reflect this fact.

Thirdly (but most importantly perhaps) is that the text focuses on UK practice. Whilst some of the practice that is undertaken in the USA mirrors closely that in the UK, other aspects of practice do not and the book seeks to provide a text that clearly recognizes these differences.

Whilst the book is aimed at those working in the UK EMS & ambulance services (such as paramedics, EMTs and ECAs) it will also be of use as a reference to those working in other urgent and unscheduled primary care environments as well as first aiders and those with a responsibility to care for people who are injured or become ill in an out-of-hospital setting. It is aimed at those who are both newly qualified as well as those who are experienced practitioners; this book can be used in initial learning and education as well as an adjunct to continual professional development.

Your feedback in how this book meets your needs and how it might be improved in any further editions would also be valued.

We hope that this book provides you with another 'tool' in your toolbox of learning and we wish you well on that educational journey.

The Authors

Acknowledgements

The authors and contributors wish to thank family, friends and colleagues for their support in undertaking this work. The wise counsel and advice of colleagues and experts is also much appreciated.

Pete Gregory's sincere thanks are extended to Alison and Natalie Gregory for their patience and support during the development of this book.

PART ONE

CHAPTER 1

Emergency Medical Services (EMS) and Ambulance Operations in the UK

Chapter contents

Objectives

Upon completion of this chapter, the paramedic student will be able to:

1. Outline the key historical events that have shaped the development of UK ambulance services and EMS.
2. Identify the key elements that are required for effective ambulance/EMS operations.
3. Differentiate between the different skills levels and roles and responsibilities of providers and the training and education that they undertake.
4. Describe the key national organizations that are involved in the profession.
5. Describe the notion of continual professional development.
6. Describe the concept of clinical governance and quality improvement.
7. List standards that govern ambulance performance and specifications.
8. Discuss the tracking of equipment, supplies, and maintenance on an ambulance.
9. Outline the considerations for appropriate stationing of ambulances.
10. Describe measures that can influence safe operation of an ambulance.
11. Identify air ambulance crew members and training.
12. Describe the appropriate use of air ambulance services in the prehospital setting.

Key terms

advanced life support The provision of care that paramedics or allied health professionals render, including advanced airway management, defibrillation, intravenous therapy, and medication administration.

ambulance A generic term that describes the various land-based emergency vehicles used by emergency medical services (EMS) personnel, including basic and advanced life support units, paramedic units, mobile intensive care units, and others.

basic life support Care provided by persons trained in emergency aid, cardiopulmonary resuscitation, and other non-invasive care. In some cases will include the use of automated external defibrillators.

Clinical Practice Guidelines These are clinical guidelines for use by practitioners in prehospital care, published by the Joint Royal Colleges Ambulance Liaison Committee.

continuous quality improvement A management approach to customer service and organizational performance that includes constant monitoring, evaluation, decisions, and actions.

emergency medical services Ambulance services providing response, assessment, and clinical management of emergencies and unscheduled care; in the UK, relates to a wider service than solely emergency ambulance response and can include the work of emergency care practitioners in 'out of hours' settings, nurse advisors in control rooms, and so on.

paramedic A person who has undertaken an approved programme of education and is registered with the Health Professions Council. Their skills include, amongst other things, patient assessment, cardiac rhythm interpretation, defibrillation, drug therapy, and airway management.

Emergency medical services system development

The role of the emergency medical technician (EMT)/ ambulance technician and paramedic has evolved; the role differs from the ambulance driver of the past. The paramedics of today work in complex EMS systems and take part in an array of professional activities. These activities help paramedics provide quality service in the field and now increasingly also help paramedics to provide state-of-the-art patient care in less traditional healthcare settings.

Assigning a time and place to the birth of organized prehospital emergency care is difficult. To understand EMS system development, one must first consider certain events from ancient times to the present.

Note

In the UK it is worth noting that many different terms are used to describe systems and services in which paramedics and their other colleagues operate. These terms include EMS, ambulance services, paramedic services, NHS trusts and prehospital care, amongst others.

Before the twentieth century

The ancient Egyptians used herbs and drugs as medicine and also splinted fractured bones, and they performed some surgery. The Edwin Smith papyrus (circa the seventeenth century BCE) depicted medical practice in Egypt. This system referred to the beat of the heart, palpation, and abnormal motor functions associated with brain injury. Other ancient texts show that surgery was practiced by the Babylonians of Mesopotamia, an ancient area of Asia, as early as 1700 BCE. At this time Hammurabi, a King of Babylonia, created a set of laws known as the Code of Hammurabi. These laws set forth fees and penalties for surgeons who offered healthcare to some social classes (Box 1-1).

Organized prehospital emergency care has some of its roots in military history. Roman Britain saw the provision of care for the wounded, with eight to ten men solely employed to pick up the wounded. Provided with bandages and water bottles, if a life was saved they were rewarded with a piece of gold. There is reference in Anglo Saxon and medieval England to the use of a horse litter for the wealthy. The seventeenth century saw the use of pest coaches to move those suffering infectious disease, such as the plague, to 'pest houses': Samuel Pepys, in 1665, described a pest coach taking a maid back to a pest house in London from where she had escaped. Indeed it was the prevalence of infectious disease such as cholera and typhoid that spurred many provincial hospitals in the eighteenth and nineteenth centuries in England to provide transport to hospital for those suffering illness or injury.

A covered cart was used by one of Napoleon's surgeons, Jean Larry. He moved injured soldiers to treatment areas

Box 1-1

Code of Hammurabi (1700 BCE)

- If a doctor has treated a freeman with a metal knife for a severe wound, and has cured the freeman, or has opened a freeman's tumour with a metal knife, and cured a freeman's eye, then he shall receive 10 shekels of silver.
- If the son of a plebeian, he shall receive 5 shekels of silver.
- If a man's slave, the owner of the slave shall give 2 shekels of silver to the doctor.
- If a doctor has treated a man with a metal knife for a severe wound, and has caused the man to die, or has opened a man's tumour with a metal knife and destroyed the man's eye, his hands shall be cut off.
- If the doctor has treated the slave of a plebeian with a metal knife for a severe wound and caused him to die, he shall render slave for slave.
- If he has opened his tumour with a metal knife and destroyed his eye, he shall pay half his price in silver.
- If a doctor has healed a freeman's broken bone or has restored diseased flesh, the patient shall give the doctor 5 shekels of silver.
- If he be the son of a plebeian, he shall give 3 shekels of silver.
- If a man's slave, the owner of the slave shall give 2 shekels of silver to the doctor.
- If a doctor of oxen or asses has treated either ox or ass for a severe wound, and cured it, the owner of the ox or ass shall give to the doctor one-sixth of a shekel of silver as his fee.

during the Napoleonic wars in the 1800s. In the United Kingdom, the first organized ambulance services were run by various agencies; in 1831 St John Ambulance commenced providing humanitarian assistance, and the Red Cross was formed (after an international meeting) in 1863 by Durrant. John Furley represented St John Ambulance at the first Red Cross conference and developed the branch in the UK; a canvas stretcher was named after him. Other agencies became involved in ambulance service; mines and other industries experienced a high number of accidents and they often provided a 'works' ambulance and first aid service. Dr James Cantlie helped write the first text on First Aid in 1880. In London, the Metropolitan Asylums Board (MAB) was responsible for conveying patients to its institutions, following the passing of the Metropolitan Poor Law Act in 1867.[1] However, it would be another 15 years before the MAB developed a network of ambulance stations with horse-drawn ambulances. Once established, however, the service provided comprehensive coverage and by the end of the nineteenth century, six ambulance stations were in operation to service the capital, meaning few parts were more than 3 miles from a station. Each station employed housekeepers, drivers, horse keepers, attendants, smallpox nurses, and clerks, as well as having room for 15–20 horses and up to 30 carriages and other wheeled appliances. The United States had some experience of running horse-drawn ambulance carts and a surgeon from Liverpool called Harrison visited New York where a surgeon accompanied the horse-drawn ambulance on calls. He brought his experience back, and this, combined with what was happening in London, meant that hospitals in the UK developed their services and by the turn of the century a number of towns and cities had some form of provision.

Twentieth century

During the first two decades of the twentieth century medical care made rapid progress. Motorized ambulances replaced the horse-drawn vehicles. In the military during World War I wounded soldiers needed urgent care; their injuries often were caused by machine guns and bombs and the military developed battlefield ambulance corps. At this time in the UK many provincial services were run by St John Ambulance, Red Cross, St Andrew's (in Scotland) and other voluntary agencies, as well as local police forces in some areas. Some hospitals ran ambulance services, using voluntary contributions. In London, as in other larger cities, the local council (London County Council) took responsibility for organizational services, using some of the agencies already mentioned.

This level of provision remained until World War II when wartime needs again demanded that ambulances services be provided in a different way; as part of the Air Raid Precautions scheme in 1937, local county and borough councils were required to provide vehicles and equipment to be used for movement of casualties. St John, Red Cross and Civil Defence organizations all provided services, including first aid posts in the towns and many of the larger villages. Ambulances were created, sometimes using delivery vans and even horseboxes mounted on a commercial chassis! At this time a first aid certificate from the voluntary aid societies was generally the highest qualification for an ambulance attendant. In 1936–1937 the '999' system came into being after some larger cities such as London found it hard to cope with the calls placed to operators and police stations for emergency assistance. This (in conjunction with technology that meant small local telephone exchanges were being amalgamated with larger ones) allowed a single point of contact telephone number for use to call any emergency service.

Initially in the first 2 years of World War II, the National Fire Service took control of local authority ambulance services, but in 1941 the Civil Defence Ambulance service was formed, with London being provided with the London County Council Auxiliary Ambulance Service. The National Health Service Act 1946 required all local health authorities to provide ambulance services. In many cases the local borough and county councils provided their own services with others relying partially or totally on services from St John and Red Cross (and St Andrew's in Scotland) on an agency basis; often the staff responded as volunteers (with an annual retainer) from home and work and this contributed sometimes to delays in responding to calls. This continued into the 1950s but gradually the involvement of the voluntary agencies was reduced as local authorities developed and expanded their services. Demand for service, however, was increasing each year and the demand for provision of non-emergency service was significantly increasing as well as the emergency work.

New technologies were being introduced; in many services in the 1950s and early 1960s two-way radio was introduced, for the first time connecting ambulances with a control room. Prior to this time, ambulances were only contacted at the hospitals once crews had delivered their patient or on return to the ambulance station. It was not unknown in some rural areas for a message to be passed from the control room to the crew via a local shop or garage that lay on the route back to the ambulance station, pressing the crew once more into action. Ambulance vehicles were developing and becoming modern in design and new ambulance stations were built to cope with the increasing demands; as often the local authority was also responsible for the Fire Brigade, many stations were joint Fire and Ambulance stations and/or joint Fire and Ambulance Services (examples of which were the City of Birmingham and City of Bath).

At a similar time Dr Ken Easton of Catterick, North Yorkshire was becoming alarmed at the increasing numbers of serious injuries and deaths on the major roads around his home, which included the A1. He started a scheme whereby he responded to support the ambulance service attending road accidents in the locality, often arriving first and providing aid at the scene. His work during the 1950s and 1960s ultimately led to the development in 1977 of BASICS (British Association of Immediate Care Schemes), a network of doctors who give up their time to provide prehospital care. In the 1960s, in the field of coronary care, Drs Pantridge and Geddes created what is considered by many as the first prehospital cardiac care scheme in Belfast, Northern Ireland.

During the 1960s it was recognized by many that the first aid certificate was not sufficient and the Ministry of Health set up a working party in 1966 to consider ambulance staff training and ambulance equipment. The report was published in 1966 under the Chair of E.L.M. Millar and was extremely significant.[2] It made a range of recommendations, including the development of a basic ambulance aid course lasting 6 weeks, as well as providing clear guidance on the minimum equipment to be carried on an ambulance. This, along with a range of other recommendations, transformed ambulance services in the UK and by the end of the 1960s a number of regional ambulance training centres had been set up, to provide the new basic course. Arguably this was the beginning of the modern ambulance service as we know it today.

The 1970s saw various other developments: the upgrading of equipment and skills, and the use of, for example, resuscitation equipment and Entonox, as well as more sophisticated immobilization equipment such as the orthopaedic scoop stretcher.

In 1974 the government of the day undertook a major reorganization of the health service and for the first time ambulance services came under the control of health authorities. This coincided with local authority reorganization and many of the old Borough and County Borough services were amalgamated; additionally the big metropolitan areas brought their many services together to form large metropolitan ambulance services (which included the newly formed counties of West Midlands, Avon, Greater Manchester, South Yorkshire, West Yorkshire and Merseyside). The newly formed area health authorities were charged with responsibility for ambulance service with a Chief Ambulance Officer for each county service and a Regional Ambulance Officer overseeing the newly formed health regions.

In a number of centres around the country, the initial beginnings of advanced care were seen, through local schemes. Ambulance staff and local hospital doctors came together to consider the provision of so-called 'extended training', including coronary care, intravenous fluid replacement and advanced airway management. Centres included Brighton under Dr Douglas Chamberlain and Bristol under Frenchay Hospital's Dr Peter Baskett. Other local schemes existed in a number of other areas of the UK, including Bournemouth and parts of London.

This extended training was finding favour in many quarters and there was a push to emulate the services found in parts of the US, where the term 'paramedic' was coming into everyday use. In 1976, however, the Department of Health and Social Security published a circular that resisted moves to develop these schemes on a national basis and it was not until the following decade that the benefits of such staff were more formally developed, following a report in 1984 by Ken Wright from the University of York which provided evidence of the economical (and clinical) benefits of extended training.

Later in the 1980s the National Health Service Training Authority (NHSTA) took responsibility for drawing together the local ad hoc schemes into a national scheme and those staff previously trained were able to convert to a national qualification.

The late 1980s and early 1990s really saw the proliferation of the UK paramedic, with regional ambulance training centres offering a standard paramedic course, underwritten by the Institute of Health and Care Development (IHCD). At this time the media portrayal of paramedics was much increased through popular TV programmes, and in the early 1990s, services tried to reach the Government's target of a paramedic on every ambulance, which further increased both public acceptance and expectation of paramedics within the ambulance service. The late 1980s and 1990s also saw a change in political landscape of the health service, with the development of NHS Trusts, the first of which in 1992 were Northumbria, Norfolk and Lincolnshire (the first wave). These were quickly followed by most other services over the next 2 or 3 years so that by the mid-1990s all ambulance services were of the new NHS Trusts style, with an executive and non-executive board of directors operating on business principles.

Further changes came about with the development in the early to mid-1990s of university-based higher education courses, the first ones of which were run in conjunction with local ambulance services. This led to the acknowledgement of the need for professional regulation and by year 2000, the Council for Professions Supplementary to Medicine (CPSM) admitted paramedics as the 12th profession, which meant that to be called a paramedic a practitioner had to have undertaken a prescribed and approved training course and meet other requirements. Existing paramedics obtained registration through transitional arrangements and newly qualified paramedics were required to submit an application to the CPSM, which soon after became the Health Professions Council (HPC). This meant that professional accountability and public protection were in place underpinned by recognized educational and practice competence standards.

Twenty-first century

Whilst the HPC is the regulatory (registrant) body, a professional body did not exist (other than the trade unions and some associations). The British Paramedic Association was set up in 2001 and has developed considerably since those early days by working with many different organizations to represent the interests of the paramedic profession in many different ways.

In 2005 the so-called 'Bradley Report' (Taking Healthcare to the Patient: Transforming NHS Ambulance Services) by Peter Bradley and the Department of Health set out a strategic direction for ambulance services to ensure that they were equipped for the rapidly changing environment of emergency care. It provided guidance on improving the effectiveness of emergency call handling (and this led to the development of the 'Call Connect' principle of measuring call answering and response times) as well as improving the pre-arrival advice given to callers (a 'hear and treat' principle). The notion of developing a wider range of services to patients via a mobile healthcare system was supported and this covered urgent as well as emergency care areas ('see and treat').

Current emergency medical services systems

In the UK today, there are 17 ambulance services (including those in the Channel Islands and the Isle of Man). These services are responsible for providing a wide range of emergency, urgent and unscheduled care services to the population, as well as non-emergency transport services. They employ a wide variety of staff types, not only paramedics but also dispatchers, EMTs, emergency care practitioners (ECPs) and non-emergency patient transport staff, as well as the 'behind the scene' staff such as human resources, mechanics, administrators, finance staff and so on.

Call volumes, via the 999 universal emergency call number, have been increasing year on year for a number of years and in 2004–2005 the total number of emergency calls in England to ambulance services reached 5.6 million, with incidents attended reaching around 4.5 million.[3] Each ambulance service has one (or perhaps on occasion more than one) control/communications centre where calls are categorized and prioritized by the call handlers using advanced dispatch systems software, with category A calls being the highest level of urgency. Category B calls are still emergency calls but not deemed to be immediately life threatening and category C calls are lower urgency calls for which alternative responses might be sent.

Emergency medical services system operations

The operations of an effective EMS system include activation by the public and organizations, dispatch, prehospital care, hospital care, and rehabilitation.

Activation

Emergency services are highly visible in the community; however, the public are not always aware of the complex nature of these services. The public expects to have police and fire service provision and they also expect to get a fast response with skilled personnel in an emergency. This is due to years of available emergency service, public relations, press coverage, and national media. The public also expects such service because of public support in the form of taxation/national insurance contributions and donations.

Public involvement in EMS goes beyond funding however; members of the public often are at the scene of an injury or illness and play an important role in recognizing the need for emergency services, giving first aid, help secure the scene and gain access to the patient, and can be instrumental in managing a crisis. Educating the public is fundamental to the development of an effective EMS or paramedic system; paramedics can help prepare the public to respond to a medical emergency and also build support for EMS by helping to develop and present public healthcare education programmes.

Once someone recognizes that an emergency exists, the response is coordinated. Contact is made with communication centres and dispatching services by emergency phone numbers such as 999 (or the European Union emergency number of 112).

Prehospital care

Ill or injured patients may need prehospital intervention and stabilization; interventions may involve basic life support and advanced life support (ALS) skills and depending on the situation (e.g. entrapment, distance to the hospital, and availability of ALS), initial prehospital care may be limited; the care, necessary in some cases, may consist of giving only comfort and reassurance. Care also may require spinal immobilization, airway protection, endotracheal intubation, intravenous therapy, medication administration, defibrillation, and other advanced interventions.

Hospital care

When the patient is brought to the emergency department, patient care resources expand. This care may include doctors, nurse practitioners, nurses, support and diagnostic staff (such as radiographers, laboratory technicians, physiotherapists, social workers, and others), secretaries, and medical record staff. Other resources available beyond the emergency department include surgery, intensive care, pharmacy, nutrition services, and many others.

Rehabilitation

After hospital delivery and definitive care, many patients receive some type of rehabilitation services. Rehabilitation often occurs before and after hospital discharge; services may be in the form of education and physical and occupational therapy that help the patient to recover. Rehabilitation also can help the patient to maintain maximal independence. One example of such therapy is helping patients and families adjust to required changes in lifestyle after a heart attack or retraining in activities of daily living. Job rehabilitation also allows one to adapt to limb impairment or loss.

Emergency medical services provider levels

Various groups of staff come together to make an effective prehospital EMS and paramedic system. These groups include dispatchers/control staff and call handlers, first responders, emergency care assistants (ECAs), EMTs/ambulance technicians, paramedics and emergency care practitioners (ECPs).

Dispatchers/call handlers/control staff

These staff are 'telecommunicators', and serve as the primary contact with the public. The dispatcher directs the proper services to the scene, which may include ground and air ambulances, as well as first responders and other ambulance resources. The term telecommunicator applies to call takers, dispatchers, radio operators, data terminal operators, or any combination of such functions in a control/communications centre. An effective EMS dispatch communications system includes the following functions:

- Receive and process calls for EMS assistance. The call handler receives and records calls for EMS assistance and selects an appropriate course of action for each call. To do this, the call handler must obtain as much information as possible about the emergency event, including name, ring-back number, and address, and may have to deal with distraught callers.
- Dispatch and coordinate EMS resources. The dispatcher directs the proper emergency vehicles to the correct address/location, coordinates the emergency vehicles while en route to the scene, to the receiving unit, and back to the station.
- Relay medical information. The dispatch centre can provide a telecommunications channel among appropriate medical facilities and EMS personnel, via phone, radio, or biomedical telemetry. In most UK services, however, this type of communication will be directly from the ambulance staff to the receiving unit

via mobile phone, telemetry or in some cases by direct CCTV-type real-time links, which some services have piloted.

- Coordinate with other services. The dispatcher aids communications between agencies such as police, fire and rescue, coastguard, mountain rescue and so on as well as with out of hour's services and other health agencies such as GPs etc. The dispatcher must know the location and status of all ambulance vehicles and whether support services are available with the use of computer-aided dispatch (CAD). This provides for one or more of the following abilities:
  - automatic entry of the emergency call (via AMPDS)
  - automatic interface to vehicle location almost always with a map display
  - automatic interface to mobile data terminal (MDT)
  - computer messaging among multiple radio operators, call takers, or both
  - dispatch note taking, reminder aid, or both on the CAD
  - ability to monitor response times, response delays, and on-scene times
  - display of call information
  - emergency medical dispatch review
  - updates of unit status (usually automated)
  - manual entry of call information
  - radio control and display of channel status
  - standard operating procedure review
  - telephone control and display of circuit status.

Many EMS services require specialized training for their dispatch personnel, who can then give directions to the caller while the caller waits for EMS arrival. Many are trained in MPDS or CBD (Medical Priority Dispatch Systems or Criteria Based Dispatch) and the role has become much more specialized over the past few years.

First responder

First responders provide on-call cover as volunteers, and respond at the request of the ambulance/EMS system. These groups may be local Voluntary Aid Societies such as St John Ambulance or Red Cross, other emergency services such as retained firefighters or local police officers, or members of the public in a small community such as a village without local ambulance service presence. Some services also have staff that live in small communities who on their days off are able to respond to pager messages and provide help until their on-duty colleagues arrive.

These First Responder schemes vary across the country according to local need but do contribute to improving response times and in some cases can make a difference in improving some clinical outcomes. The training they receive varies but as a minimum they are First Aid trained with some services providing more in-depth training via the 'First Person on Scene' (FPOS) programme.

Emergency care assistant

This is a relatively new role. The ECA works as a support worker to a paramedic (or EMT) and is trained in skills such as patient assessment, recording of vital signs, ambulance operations/driving, and assisting other staff in preparing drugs and other items for clinical management of patients. The role falls somewhere between that of the first responder and EMT; in some services the training has many components of the EMT training, although services may have slight variances in scope of practice.

EMT (emergency medical technician)/ambulance technician

The EMT has finished training based on the 6-week (or in many cases several weeks longer) initial ambulance aid course/basic ambulance aid course. The EMT is trained in all phases of basic life support, which includes the use of automated external defibrillators, the giving of some emergency medications and airway procedures including laryngeal mask airways. In addition to patient care training, EMTs receive training in emergency ambulance driving, a course based on the 'Roadcraft' system of driving.

Paramedic

The paramedic is an EMT who has completed training or education based on a programme approved by the HPC. Paramedics are trained in all aspects of basic life support and ALS procedures that are relevant to prehospital emergency care. The paramedic has advanced training in patient assessment, cardiac rhythm interpretation, defibrillation, drug therapy, and airway management, and provides emergency care based on advanced assessment skills and the formulation of a working impression. The paramedic works to the HPC's 'Standards of Proficiency' which provide an outline of skill and competence expectations.[4]

National emergency medical services group involvement

A number of organizations are involved in the steering and development of ambulance/EMS provision in the UK.

Health Professions Council (HPC)

The HPC superseded the Council for Professions Supplementary to Medicine (CPSM), in April 2002. The HPC is the profession's regulator and as such has a range of functions which revolve around training and education, standards setting and maintenance, and the publication and implementation of Codes of Conduct (Code of Conduct Performance and Ethics 2008)[5] and Standards of Proficiency (2007),[4] which are profession specific. It holds the register and those who wish to be registered have to meet the requirements of the HPC; the titles of the 13 professions regulated by the HPC are protected, which means, in law, an individual may not call themselves a paramedic unless they are on the HPC register. The HPC produce SET (Standards of Education and Training Guidance – 2007)[6] which give providers of education specific criteria that their programmes must meet; this allows those who successfully complete the programmes to apply to the HPC for registration. The HPC also regulates education in this sense, by requiring providers to be validated and approved, with regular reviews by way of self-assessment and actual visits to ensure high standards are met and maintained.

British Paramedic Association (BPA)

The BPA was set up in 2001 after it became clear that a professional body was vital. At the time, paramedics were the only profession within the CPSM not to have a professional body, and with the paramedic title being protected, it was necessary so that professional standards could be maintained and improved. After a gradual start the association obtained a stronger foothold and is now very much the professional body. Its main aims are related to representing the interest of its members and of the profession at large, ensuring high standards of care, as well as influencing and guiding educational and organizational development, and the development of research that informs the profession and its clinical practice. It provides various services for its members, including Continual Professional Development (CPD), and works closely with other organizations in the day-to-day workings of the profession. It has also produced the Curriculum Guidance document to provide direction for those institutions, such as universities, that develop and provide programmes for education of paramedics.

Joint Royal Colleges Ambulance Liaison Committee (JRCALC)

The Joint Royal Colleges Ambulance Liaison Committee was set up in 1989 with representatives from a number of the Royal Colleges with the aim of providing support to UK ambulance services. Many differing organizations are represented and a variety of functions such as policy, equipment, education and training guidelines writing and audit/research fall under the auspices of this group. The Ambulance Service Clinical Practice Guidelines (CPG)[7] are published by JRCALC and the former Ambulance Service Association (now ASN) in conjunction with the University of Warwick.

Ambulance Service Network (ASN)

The Ambulance Service Network is part of the NHS Confederation and is the successor to the Ambulance Service Association. The ASN represents the ambulance trusts at an organizational level within the wider NHS.

Paramedic education

Initial education

Traditionally, the paramedic was trained after becoming, in the first instance, an ambulance technician or EMT. The training was undertaken in ambulance service housed training centres and was vocationally based, being underwritten by the IHCD (Institute of Health and Care Development) with staff being already employed by the service providing the training. This still occurs to some extent but over the past decade more and more services have been entering partnerships with Higher Education Institutions (HEIs) and have developed university-based programmes of study, which, on successful completion, allow those students to apply to the HPC for registration. These then are pre-registration programmes which often are housed in Schools of Health and in some cases students share generic modules of study with other healthcare students.

The move to Higher Education has been fairly gradual and started with some existing ambulance staff undertaking part-time study at universities that had entered into partnerships with (often) their local ambulance service. This initial move was a result of calls from within the profession to improve on the then existing standards and levels of training and education, which were based on the system first devised in the 1960s and modified in the 1980s. After these early developments the move to Higher Education gained momentum and programmes were offered on a full-time basis and the numbers of both students and institutions offering these programmes began to rise.

Most UK ambulance services now have links with HEIs and many are involved collaboratively in programmes for pre-registration study, which in some circumstances run alongside more traditional programmes still available in vocational settings. This has seen a gradual blurring of the boundaries and most if not all HEIs offering paramedic programmes now employ staff who are paramedics and ambulance tutors, as lecturers and faculty to run and deliver the teaching on the programmes. The HEIs are subject to a range of quality assurance standards such as the SET published by the HPC and the Curriculum Guidance of the BPA.

Continuing education

Continuing education provides a way for all healthcare providers to retain primary technical and professional skills and aids in learning new and advanced skills and knowledge. Some skills learned during the initial course of study may not be used often. However, new data, procedures, and resources are being developed continuously.

Continuing education can take many forms, including the following:

- conferences and seminars
- lectures and workshops
- quality-improvement reviews
- skill laboratories
- certification and recertification programmes
- refresher training programmes
- journal studies
- multimedia presentations
- internet-based learning
- case presentations.

The HPC provides requirements for CPD of all its registrants (HPC 'Your guide to our standards for continual professional development' 2006)[8] and the BPA is heavily involved in helping its members and the profession in developing robust and effective CPD initiatives and opportunities.

Professionalism

Training, education and performance standards, amongst other things, have helped to define EMTs and paramedics as healthcare professionals; the term profession refers to a body of knowledge or expertise, and the profession and its registrants are regulated and have standards to meet. Professionalism refers to the way in which a person follows the standards of a profession and, as described above, includes conduct and performance standards.

Healthcare professional

Healthcare professionals conform to the standards of their profession. They instill pride in the profession. They earn the respect of others by providing quality patient care and striving for high standards. EMS professionals occupy positions of public trust and are highly visible role models. Because EMS professionals are role models, the public has high expectations of EMTs and paramedics while they are on and off duty. Therefore, professional conduct at all times and a commitment to excellence in daily activities complement the image of the EMS professional. Image and behaviour are vital to establishing credibility and instilling confidence. The professional paramedic represents his or her employer, the profession and his or her peers.

Attributes of the professional paramedic

The HPC's Code of Conduct, Performance and Ethics (2008)[5] provides 14 key areas that registrants must maintain or keep. They relate to acting in the best interests of patients and client, maintaining confidentiality and obtaining consent, providing high standards of care, keeping professional competence and expertise up to date and only operating within those boundaries of ability and competence, communication and working in teams as well as more independently and without direct supervision, maintaining accurate records and ensuring that risk and safety policies are followed, as well as acting with honesty and integrity.

Many more general aspects of being professional can be applied to the role of the paramedic and some of these attributes are described below:

1. *Integrity*. Integrity means being honest in all actions. Integrity may be the most important behaviour for EMS professionals. The public assumes EMS professionals have integrity; actions that show integrity include being truthful, not stealing, and providing complete and correct documentation.
2. *Empathy*. Empathy is identifying with and understanding the feelings, situations, and motives of others. EMS professionals always must show empathy to patients, families, and other healthcare professionals. Behaviour that demonstrates empathy includes showing caring, compassion, and respect for others; understanding the feelings of the patient and family; being calm and helpful to those in need; and being supportive and reassuring of others.
3. *Self-motivation*. Self-motivation is the push for merit and self-direction. Self-motivation can mean taking the lead to finish tasks, to improve behaviour, and to follow through without supervision. Self-motivation also includes showing enthusiasm for learning, being committed to providing quality care and accepting constructive feedback.
4. *Appearance and personal hygiene*. Paramedics are aware of how they present themselves as they are representatives of their profession. They must ensure that their clothing and uniforms are clean and in good repair and must be aware of the importance of personal hygiene and good grooming.
5. *Self-confidence*. Paramedics must trust and rely on themselves, often in difficult situations. One key task is to assess personal and professional strengths and weaknesses; the ability to trust personal choices shows self-confidence.
6. *Communications*. An important part of the paramedic's job is communicating. The paramedic must be able to convey key information to others verbally and in writing and be able to speak clearly, write legibly, and listen actively. The paramedic must be able to adjust strategies to various situations as well.
7. *Time management*. Time management refers to organizing and prioritizing tasks to make the best use of time. Examples include being punctual and completing tasks and assignments on time.
8. *Teamwork and diplomacy*. The paramedic must be able to work with others well. In fact, the paramedic must be able to use tact and interpersonal skills to achieve a common goal. As a member of the EMS team, the paramedic must place the success of the team above personal success. A paramedic does this by supporting and respecting other team members, being flexible and open to change, and communicating with coworkers to resolve problems.
9. *Respect*. Respect means having regard for others and showing consideration and appreciation. Paramedics are polite to others and avoid the use of derogatory or demeaning terms. They know that showing respect brings credit to themselves, their service, and their profession.
10. *Patient advocacy*. The paramedic must always act as the patient's advocate, even when the patient disagrees with the care. Paramedics should not attempt to impose their beliefs on patients. They also should not allow biases (religious, ethical, political, social, or cultural) to influence care. The paramedic must always place the needs of the patient above self-interests. The paramedic must protect the patient's confidentiality as well.
11. *Careful delivery of service*. Paramedics deliver the highest quality of patient care. With this care comes attention to detail and proper prioritization of care. Paramedics review their actions and attitude on every call. As part of the careful delivery, paramedics master and refresh their skills; perform full equipment checks; and ensure safe ambulance operations. Paramedics also follow policies, procedures, and protocols and comply with the orders of their supervisors.

Critical Thinking

Which of these professional attributes represent your strengths? Which ones do you think you need to work on?

Roles and responsibilities of the paramedic

The paramedic may practice patient care at an emergency scene, from an emergency scene to the hospital, between healthcare facilities, or in other healthcare settings as permitted by national and local policies and law. The para-

Box 1-2

Roles and responsibilities of the paramedic

Primary responsibilities

- Preparation
- Response
- Scene assessment
- Patient assessment
- Recognition of injury or illness
- Patient management
- Appropriate patient disposition
- Patient transfer
- Documentation
- Returning to service

Additional responsibilities

- Community involvement
- Support of primary care efforts
- Encouragement of public involvement in emergency medical services
- Participation in leadership activities
- Personal and professional development

medic's roles and duties can be divided into two groups: primary responsibilities and additional responsibilities (Box 1-2).

Primary responsibilities

The paramedic must be prepared physically, mentally, and emotionally for the job. Preparation includes being committed daily to positive health practices maintaining own health. In addition, the paramedic must have the proper equipment and supplies, maintain adequate knowledge and skills of the profession and must respond to the scene in a safe and timely manner. During scene assessment, the paramedic must consider his or her own safety; safety of the crew, patients, and bystanders; and the mechanism of injury or probable cause of illness.

The paramedic must perform advanced assessment of the patient at once to determine the injury or illness. At that point, the paramedic can formulate a field impression, and set priorities of care and transportation. Managing an emergency often entails following guidelines. The care provided by the paramedic should minimize secondary injury. After stabilizing the patient in the field, the paramedic should supply proper transport to the receiving unit. The paramedic should comfort the patient and family during transport. Transportation may include ground or air transport and may be based on the patient's condition. The paramedic must know hospital designation and categorization as well, as choosing the correct destination calls for knowing which ones are available and suitable; for instance, transferring a chest pain patient to a unit that has a cardiac catheter laboratory available to direct ambulance admissions. The hospital destination decision should be made carefully with consideration by the paramedic of procedures and unit suitability and ensuring the patient is informed and has consented. Paramedics are also called upon for critical care transport and provide transport and care for patient undergoing inter-hospital transfers.

The paramedic is the patient's advocate as responsibility for care is transferred to the staff at the receiving unit. The paramedic needs to brief the staff about the patient's condition at the scene and during transportation and also needs to provide thorough and accurate documentation in the patient care report. The paramedic should complete required documentation in a timely manner so that the EMS crew can return to service. The crew should prepare the ambulance for return to service by replacing equipment and supplies as per service policy. The crew also should review the call openly; such review helps to identify ways to improve the patient care services that were provided at the scene and during transportation.

Additional responsibilities

Other duties of the paramedic include community involvement, support of primary healthcare efforts, advocating public involvement in the EMS system, participation in leadership activities, and personal and professional development.

A paramedic can be involved in the community and can be a role model for the profession in many ways. The paramedic can advocate accident and injury prevention programmes and can participate as a leader in community activities. A few ways to improve the health of the community include teaching cardiopulmonary resuscitation, first aid, and injury prevention. These activities also help to ensure proper use of EMS resources and help improve the integration of EMS with other healthcare and public safety agencies.

A few communities and their healthcare organizations use paramedics in primary healthcare efforts. These communities also use paramedics to aid in accident and injury prevention and wellness programmes. Paramedics can help to inform the public of the best use of prehospital and other non-EMS healthcare resources and offer options other than ambulance transportation. They can explain non-hospital emergency department clinical providers such as minor injuries units. Programmes on when, where, and how to use EMS and emergency departments promote the best use of the resources.

Getting the public involved in EMS improves the system as a whole as they can help to set the needs parameters for EMS use in the community. They offer an objective view into quality improvement and problem solving. In addition, having involved members of the public creates informed, independent advocates for the EMS system.

Paramedics can take part in leadership activities in their communities in many ways. They can conduct injury prevention initiatives (activities and risk surveys). They can help with media drives to promote EMS issues and can distribute materials about EMS and other health programmes.

A paramedic must work to develop in personal and professional ways. Methods to accomplish this include continuing education, student mentoring, membership in professional organizations, becoming involved in work-related issues that affect career growth, exploring alternative career paths in the EMS profession, conducting and supporting research initiatives, and being actively involved in legislative issues related to EMS.

Clinical direction for emergency medical services

Some of the services that paramedics offer to patients come from practices in medicine and other healthcare professions. This means that paramedics extend the services of these other healthcare providers to patients in the field, which is made possible through clinical guidance and direction. The clinical director or clinical lead acts as the clinical leader for the EMS system and also serves as a resource and patient advocate for the EMS system. The relationship between the clinical director/lead and the service paramedic is critical and allows for the delivery of effective advanced prehospital care.

In most UK services, the clinical director or lead is from a medical background, usually an individual with a keen interest in emergency care or with a prehospital background such as an immediate care scheme. A number of services have now appointed leads or assistant leads from other backgrounds, however, notably paramedics who at this level are operating as Consultant Paramedics; this further shows that the profession is becoming strong and standing, in its own right, alongside other and longer-established professions.

The clinical lead/director may also often be involved in

- EMS system design and operations
- education and training of EMS personnel (by being involved in delivery of teaching and assessment)
- personnel selection
- equipment selection
- development of clinical protocols in cooperation with expert EMS personnel; this might include the development of PGDs (patient group directives)
- quality and standards setting and problem resolution
- direct input into patient care (some clinical directors will undertake on-call roles or be involved in larger or serious incidents)
- interface between EMS systems and other healthcare services and organizations
- advocacy within the medical community
- guidance as the 'clinical conscience' of the EMS system (advocating for quality patient care).

On-scene medical and healthcare professionals

Ambulance services in the UK have a history of working closely with doctors and other healthcare professionals (HCPs), such as local GPs and primary care staff or with doctors working in immediate care systems such as BASICS. At times another HCP may witness the injury or illness and be present on the scene already. When this occurs, careful and clear communication and interaction between the HCP and the EMS crew is essential as another HCP may or may not be familiar with paramedics' roles and abilities and the guidelines and standards that they adhere to.

If a doctor is on the scene, EMS personnel must follow standard practice guidelines (JRCALC CPG and own service procedures) and should work with the doctor in providing care. In most circumstances the EMS/paramedic crew will be able to undertake this care and many doctors will wish to hand over care to the paramedic at this point. There may be occasions when a difference of opinion or misunderstanding occurs between the doctor on scene and the paramedic crew about optimal care; in these cases, the paramedic should ensure clear and considered communication to resolve this variance. Ultimately, if there is a doctor who is insistent that specific care is undertaken that differs from the norm, the paramedic should request they accompany the patient to hospital and the doctor should also complete and sign the patient report form, identifying clearly their name and status and their wish for this non-standard care or intervention to take place. Control should be made aware and it may be prudent to at least request the duty officer is contacted for advice, particularly if the difference in care is significant or could have other consequences.

Improving system quality

A major goal of any EMS system or ambulance service is to evaluate and improve care continually. One way to meet this goal is through a modified form of quality assurance, known as continuous quality improvement (CQI), which is the ongoing study and improvement of a process, system, or organization (Box 1-3). In the UK this process is usually part of clinical governance and initiatives related to clinical effectiveness and clinical audit.

CQI identifies and attempts to improve problems in certain areas such as clinical direction, financing, training, communication, prehospital management and transportation, inter-hospital transportation, receiving facilities, specialty care units, dispatch, public information and education, audit and quality assurance, major incident planning, and

Box 1-3

Quality assurance and continuous quality improvement

Quality assurance (QA) is a system of quality management that by tradition was linked with spotting deviations from a standard (e.g. protocols). Quality assurance also altered these deviations through some type of punitive action. Continuous quality improvement (CQI) is a modified form of QA. Continuous quality improvement focuses on the system and not the individual and thus this removes much of the punitive aspect associated with a QA programme. CQI is less rigid than QA. In addition, CQI considers many factors that often apply to EMS. CQI includes the entire team of staff and involves all health providers in the problem-solving process.

The EMS professional can use input taken from CQI activities to adapt practices and guidelines and educational activities when needed. The goal of CQI is to find and fix problems in a positive manner. CQI also is aimed at improving the overall system. Example CQI activities include a review of the following:

- Outcome measures of prehospital care (e.g. scene times, procedure completion rates, and mortality reviews)
- Care while treatment is ongoing (concurrent reviews)
- Written EMS patient care paperwork (retrospective reviews)
- Random or selected radio communication tapes
- New procedures, equipment, or therapies

mutual aid. CQI is a process that can involve all caregivers in the problem-solving aspect. CQI stresses the value of enabling frontline personnel to perform their jobs well; with this group approach, all parties can be involved in elaborating on the cause of the problem and can work together to develop remedies and can design a course of action to correct the problem. Then they can enforce the plan and re-examine the issue to see whether the problem has been resolved to satisfaction.

Key actions or categories for EMS leaders and manager to improve quality within their organization might include

1. Leadership has to do with the efforts of senior leadership and management. These persons lead by example to add CQI into the strategic planning process and integrate CQI into the entire organization. Such integration promotes quality values and CQI techniques in work practices.
2. Information and analysis deal with managing and using the data needed for effective CQI. Continuous quality improvement is based on management by fact; information and analyses are critical to CQI success.
3. Strategic quality planning has three main parts. The first is developing long- and short-term goals for structural, performance, and outcome quality standards. The second is finding ways to achieve those. The third is measuring the effectiveness of the system in meeting quality standards.
4. Human resource development and management has to do with developing the full potential of the EMS workforce. This effort is guided by the principle that the entire EMS workforce is motivated to achieve new levels of service and value.
5. EMS process management has to do with the creation of high-quality services and with maintaining those services. Within the context of CQI, process management refers to the improvement of work activities. Process management also refers to improving work flow across functional or departmental boundaries.
6. EMS results are related to the assessment of the quality results achieved. These results also have to do with examining the success of the organization at achieving CQI.
7. Satisfaction of patients and other stakeholders involves ensuring ongoing satisfaction. Those internal and external to the EMS system must be satisfied with the services provided.

Benefits gained by applying these seven guidelines and recommendations include improvements in service and patient care delivery, economic efficiency and profitability, patient and community satisfaction and loyalty, and healthful outcomes.

Ambulance standards

The first standards for equipment and training arose from the Millar report (1967) and were further developed in the 1970s when the then Department of Health and Social Security (DHSS) produced additional guidance on specifications for ambulances (such as number of stretchers, length of service before decommissioning and so on).

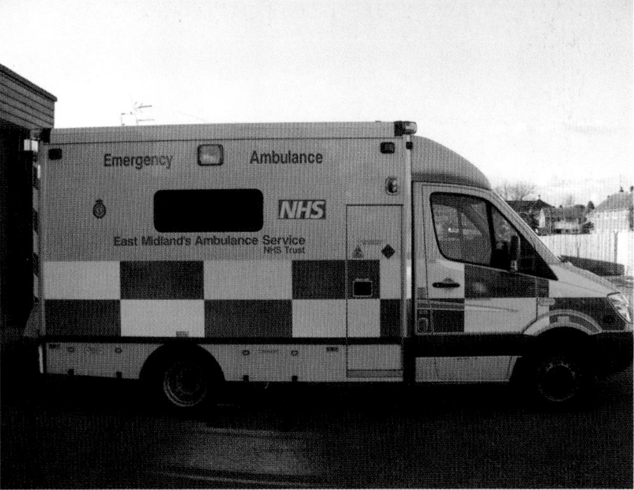

Figure 1-1 Basic ambulance design. Van-based, coachbuilt and modular box type.

In the last 10 or so years, ambulance standards have been further developed with the development of CEN (Comité Européen de Normalization) regulations also known as BS EN 1789:2000. The CEN regulations provide technical criteria for ambulance construction/design (such as the number of stretchers and the equipment carried therein).

Other results of this are the change to the bright yellow colour of ambulances (Euro RAL 1016) and the disappearance some years ago of ambulances with two stretchers; in most services, emergency ambulances are fitted with one stretcher (Figure 1-1).

Checking ambulances

Completing an equipment and supply check at the start of every shift is important and essential for safety, patient care, and risk management. It also helps to ensure proper handling and safekeeping of scheduled medications (Figure 1-2); either paper checklists or special computer software can be used for this purpose. Some equipment (e.g. glucometers and defibrillators) require routine maintenance, testing, and cleaning (Box 1-4) to ensure safe, effective operation.

The procedures for vehicle maintenance vary by service. These procedures are in place to improve the vehicles' reliability and extend their life. The paramedic should follow their service guidelines and procedures for checking vehicles, equipment, and supplies.

Ambulance stationing

In the 1960s and 1970s, the methods for estimating the need for ambulance services and where they should be located in a community were based on population concentrations and on the average response time to the emergency scene and were to some extent arbitrary. Methods for estimating needs have changed and have shifted toward determining the percentage of compliance (standard of reliability) in providing EMS within time frames that meet national guidelines. The first move towards these standards were with ORCON standards (Operational Research and Control) introduced in the 1970s in the UK and this determined that ambulances should reach emergency calls within specific percentile time-

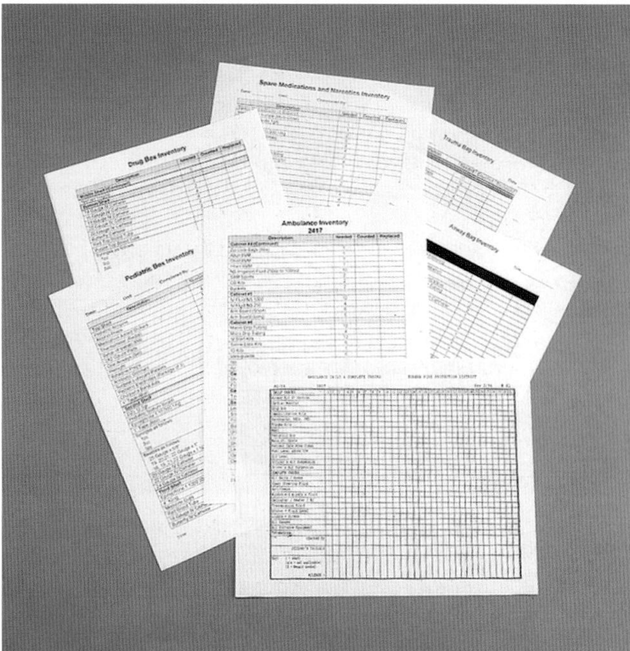

Figure 1-2 Ambulance checklists.

Box 1-4

Examples of equipment checks on an EMS vehicle

General operations

- Airway equipment (basic and advanced)
- Burn supplies
- Drug inventory
- Extrication/rescue supplies
- Infection control supplies
- Immobilization equipment
- Obstetrical/childbirth supplies
- Patient assessment equipment
- Stretchers and related equipment
- Vehicle safety and operations
- Wound care supplies

Specific medical equipment

- Automated transport ventilator (ATV)
- Cardiac monitor/defibrillator
- Glucometer
- Pulse oximetry equipment
- Telemetry equipment

frames (50% of all calls within 7 min, with 95% of all calls reached in 14 min in urban areas and 19 min in rural areas). To this standard was added a maximum of 3 min activation time (from the 999 call being received to the ambulance booking mobile). In 1996, new amended standards were developed and calls were being categorized into one of three categories (A, the highest, B or C), requiring 75% of category A calls to be reached in 8 min, and with 95% of all responses being reached in 14 and 19 min in urban and rural areas respectively. To minimize responses times, the use of response cars as well as other methods have significantly increased over the past few years. Most recently, 'Call Connect', a principle of starting the clock when the call is first connected to the ambulance control centre rather than when the call finishes, has further increased the speed of response needed for category A calls in order to meet the 8-min standard.[9]

Much of this push for better response times has come about due to clinical initiatives such as reducing the time taken to provide thrombolysis or other definitive care for patients with cardiac events; these initiatives are often embedded in Government Health Policy such as the National Service Frameworks.

Some services have varied their skill mixes and vehicles to adapt to these changed practices. Many services used to task their emergency crews with routine work in-between emergency calls. This has changed and services have several tiers of response and crew levels which are deployed to calls and workload in the best possible way.

Factors that may affect an EMS system's standard of reliability include the geographical area, population and patient demand, traffic conditions, time of day, and appropriate placement of emergency vehicles.

Other developments have been related to maximizing the use of the ambulance and its crew: deployment plans mean that crews no longer spend much time in stations but on active deployment where they are sent to areas that, using historical data, are most likely to require ambulance cover. This principle is known as System Status Management, first introduced in the US by Jack Stout in the early 1980s.[10] Strategies for ambulance stationing often are based on areas with the highest volume of calls (peak load); these strategies take into consideration the day of the week and the time of day. Computers and other technological devices may be used to formalize strategic unit deployment and reduce response times but deployment strategies vary by service and can range from simple deployment of one vehicle stationed in the middle of a response area to full automated deployment plans for each hour of the day and each day of the week. The comprehensive plans include 'mini-deployment' plans within each hour, depending on the number of ambulances left in the system; this concept of unit hour utilization (UHU) considers how much work an ambulance will undertake in an hour (productivity) and also is a factor in how ambulance resources are deployed.

Safe ambulance operation

In the UK each year, there are a number of road traffic collisions involving ambulances, including sadly some that lead to serious injury or fatalities; whilst UK national statistics are unclear, some experts have estimated that ambulances are involved in a serious collision on average once per day in the UK. Equally, most ambulance trusts collate data for all ambulance collisions however minor or serious. Safe operation of ambulances is crucial and essential for the safety of patients, the EMS crew, and others in the vicinity of a response. It is standard UK practice for ambulance staff driving under emergency conditions to undertake driver training based on the 'Roadcraft' system.[11] Staff in more enlightened services are required to undergo periodic evaluations of their emergency driving skills (Box 1-5). In addi-

Box 1-5

Guidelines for safe ambulance driving

1. Be tolerant and observant of other motorists and pedestrians.
2. Always use occupant safety restraints (both driver and passenger).
3. Be familiar with the characteristics of the emergency vehicle.
4. Be alert to changes in weather and road conditions.
5. Exercise caution in the use of audible and visual warning devices.
6. Drive within the speed limit except in circumstances allowed by law.
7. Select the quickest and most appropriate route to and from the incident scene.
8. Maintain a safe following distance.
9. Drive with due regard for the safety of all others.
10. Always drive in a manner consistent with managing acceptable levels of risk.

tion to the size and weight of the emergency vehicle and the driver's experience, a number of factors influence safe operation of an ambulance. These include the following:

- appropriate use of escorts
- environmental conditions
- appropriate use of warning devices
- proceeding safely through junctions
- parking at the emergency scene
- operating with due regard for the safety of others
- safely moving a patient into and out of the ambulance.

Critical Thinking

How do you think you would feel if you struck another vehicle while driving an ambulance?

Appropriate use of escorts

Police escorts during an emergency response can be dangerous and should be used sparingly; in the UK it is common practice now not to advocate escorts except under exceptional and unusual circumstances. Collisions can occur as a result of confusion; motorists in the area may wrongly assume that only one emergency vehicle is on the road. In the rare event an escort is used, a clear understanding of how this will work must be agreed between the involved parties before the journey. In some circumstances, multiple responses to a large incident or scene may mean that some emergency vehicles travel close together or though a hazard such as a junction in quick succession; the EMS driver should keep a safe distance between the ambulance and any other emergency vehicles. The use of audible and visual warning devices during escorts should be guided by local policy. If the paramedic uses audible and visual warning devices, it is good practice for the different vehicles to use differing siren tones. This alerts other motorists to the fact that a second emergency vehicle is in the immediate area.

Most UK services use a tiered response system (call categorization), where several units respond to emergency calls. The tiered response system allows for a safer emergency response and helps to ensure that the proper resources and personnel are available during an emergency. For example, a first response unit staffed with a paramedic responds to a collapsed patient (a category A call) with full use of audible and visual warning devices. The paramedic may determine the patient's condition is stable and request an ambulance to respond to the scene in either an emergency or non-emergency mode (at normal speed and without warning devices). The ambulance crew assumes care and provides transport to the hospital. In other cases it may be that the first to arrive on scene is able to stand down other resources that are mobile to the scene as they are not required.

Environmental conditions

Poor weather conditions can create significant dangers when paramedics respond to a call. Factors that can affect safe ambulance operation include road and weather conditions, such as fog and heavy rain that reduce visibility, and slippery road surfaces caused by ice, snow, mud, oil, or water that can cause the ambulance to aquaplane.

When poor environmental conditions are present, the driver of the emergency vehicle should proceed at safe speeds that are appropriate for the road and weather conditions. In adverse weather conditions such as rain or poor light, the driver should use dip beam headlights during all responses. This increases visibility for the EMS crew and also makes it easier for other motorists to recognize the ambulance.

Dry roads and clear weather do not guarantee a safe response; up to two-thirds of all emergency vehicle collisions occur on dry roads, and around three-quarters occur during clear weather.[12]

Appropriate use of warning devices

As noted before, during an emergency response and patient transport, lights and sirens should be used according to standard operating practice. Ambulance services authorize the use of these devices during all responses when the cause or severity of the emergency is such it is deemed a category A or B call, especially for the first responding unit. In these cases, visual warnings should be used, supported by the use of audible warnings. Caution must be exercised when using audible warnings: it is important that they are activated in good time to allow other road users to take appropriate action. A great danger occurs when an emergency vehicle approaches a hazard such as a junction or roundabout, and activates the siren at the last moment, as this can cause panic and confusion amongst other road users. Equally, in urban areas ambulances may become gridlocked in a traffic jam and the use of the siren may actually intimidate drivers to take evasive action that is unsafe and possibly illegal (such as forcing vehicles to 'spill' over into junctions controlled by a red traffic signal). This is poor practice and to be avoided. Ambulance operators must also take into account that the use of sirens and lights may lull them into a false sense of security about their speed and give an unrealistic expectation that other road users will react in the correct way. The use of warning devices during patient transport back to the hospital usually is reserved for patients with significant illness or injury, although on occasions it may be necessary to use warning systems to expedite a route through heavy traffic etc; in this case, it is important to ensure the use can be justified and if service policy requires, control should be notified of the emergency mode of response.

When using lights and sirens, paramedics should keep in mind that motorists who drive with the car windows wound up or who are using a radio or CD player, air conditioning, or the heating system may not be able to hear the sirens; therefore the EMS crew should always proceed with caution. They should never assume that the vehicle's lights or sirens provide an absolute right-of-way to proceed and should never be relied upon. Ambulance staff (and other emergency vehicle operators) in the UK are exempt from certain regulations/laws whilst engaged on emergency calls; these include speed limit exemptions, the ability to treat a red traffic signal as a stop and give way, certain exemptions for parking and use of bus lanes and so on. If claiming exemptions it is important that visual warnings are in use as a minimum and that the claiming of the exemption is both safe and necessary. Paramedics should be familiar with the road traffic laws and the exemptions that cover an emergency response.

Critical Thinking

In what situations do you think the crew member driving an ambulance may be tempted to drive too fast?

Proceeding safely...through intersections and overtaking

Many serious collisions involving ambulances in the UK occur where an ambulance proceeds against a red light at a junction or is overtaking another vehicle(s). It is important that the driver of an emergency vehicle stops at all junctions controlled by a red traffic signal, and makes eye contact with all motorists before going through the junction. Another safety measure for going through a junction is to bring the vehicle to a momentary stop to assess the junction, engaging first (or at least a low) gear before crossing, and crossing the junction at a very low speed (in some cases at walking speed). At least if another road user has failed to notice the emergency vehicle, the ambulance can be brought to a stop quickly. Further safety measures are to treat each lane of a multi-lane junction individually: a large commercial vehicle in a lane nearest the ambulance might obscure another motorist in a lane further away. Some emergency vehicles now have traffic signal pre-empting devices and these devices can change the traffic light at a junction to green (in the ambulance's direction of travel). On approach to junctions and other hazards it is good practice to slow down sufficiently so that adequate time is available to plan the best route through the junction, which in some circumstances may include taking a lane to the right of a keep left sign (one of the allowable exemptions); this may help reduce the tendency for stationary traffic in front of the ambulance to move past the stop line (to get out of the way) when faced with a red traffic signal.

Overtaking, especially queues of slower traffic on single-carriageway roads (either urban or rural), is also another area where collision risk is much increased. Caution must be exercised and the overtake only carried out if it is certain that all other road users are aware of the emergency vehicle. It is not uncommon for one vehicle in a slower moving queue to see the approaching emergency vehicle, but the vehicle behind that one does not and pulls out into the path of the now very close emergency vehicle! Be absolutely sure that all road users are aware of your presence and have taken sufficient steps to slow down and/or move over, before any overtake occurs and that equally, oncoming vehicles are absent or so distant that they will not be forced into sudden evasive action, or that they too have slowed down/stopped and/or moved over sufficiently to allow safe manoeuvres.

Parking at the emergency scene

When parking the ambulance at a scene, the paramedic should make sure that the vehicle's location allows for traffic flow around the area. If police or fire service personnel have arrived on scene, the paramedic should position the ambulance about 30 m past the scene, on the same side of the road or in another suitable location as directed by police officers. It also should be positioned upwind if the presence of hazardous materials is suspected. If the ambulance crew is first on scene consideration must be given to positioning the ambulance about 50 m prior to the scene. This is the 'fend-off' position (Figure 1-3). In this position, the emergency vehicle deflects and averts from the scene other vehicles that may strike the ambulance or providers.

Other safety precautions a paramedic can take when parking an ambulance at an emergency scene include the following:

- Emergency lighting should be used when the vehicle blocks traffic.
- The parking brake should be set.
- Another person should be asked to help guide the vehicle when it is backing up. (This person should be visible in the vehicle mirrors at all times while the ambulance is slowly backing up.)
- High-visibility reflective clothing and other personal protective equipment should be worn when paramedics work near any roadways and also generally at night.

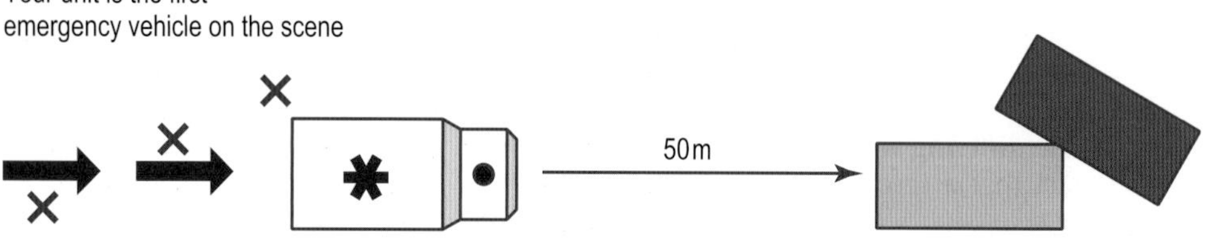

Figure 1-3 The 'fend-off' position.

When choosing a parking area for the ambulance, the paramedic also should consider the possibility of collapsing structures, fires, explosive hazards, and downed electrical wires. Other considerations are ensuring that access and egress are not compromised for any emergency vehicles on site. For instance, in busy urban areas or on narrow rural roads, parking the ambulance in an optimal position to attend the incident may cause inconvenience for other road users, so careful consideration of these competing issues must be undertaken.

Operating with due regard for the safety of all others

As already highlighted, UK road traffic law allows certain exemptions for drivers of emergency vehicles. For instance, they are allowed to exceed posted speed limits, and are allowed to proceed through a junction controlled by red traffic signals during an emergency response (Box 1-6). However, these privileges must take into consideration the safety of all people using the roads. This 'duty of care' for the safety of all others carries legal responsibility. The paramedic and the EMS service can incur liability if damage, injury, or death results from failure to observe this principle. The paramedic must be fully conversant with laws and regulations that cover the operation of an emergency vehicle.

Box 1-6

The 2-second rule

Most rear-end collisions are caused by drivers who follow too closely behind the vehicle in front of them. Therefore it is important that the paramedic keeps enough space (following distance) between the emergency vehicle and the vehicle in front to avoid a crash if the car in front brakes suddenly.

A quick method for gauging the recommended distance is the 2-second rule. It works like this:

1. You (the driver of the emergency vehicle) note an object by the side of the road (e.g. a tree or sign) that the vehicle in front of you will soon pass.
2. Count 'one thousand and one, one thousand and two' or 'only a fool breaks the two-second rule'. If you reach the object before the phrase is complete, you are too close to the vehicle in front of you.
3. This rule applies with good road and weather conditions. If the road and weather conditions are not good, the following distance should be increased to a 4- or 5-second count.

Braking distance is based on average reaction time, average vehicle weight, average road conditions, and average brakes. Wet roadways, poor brakes, poor tyres, heavy vehicle weight, and poor reaction times lengthen the braking distance.

Note

Larger emergency vehicles (e.g. those mounted on a larger commercial chassis) have different handling characteristics and longer braking and stopping distances than conventional vehicles such as cars or smaller van-based ambulances.

Safely moving a patient into and out of an ambulance

After initial stabilization at the scene, the patient must be packaged and safely placed in the emergency vehicle for transport. The paramedic crew should use safe lifting practices (these techniques help to prevent personal injury) and also ensure that the patient is positioned securely on the ambulance stretcher. The patient compartment of the ambulance is equipped with locking devices. These prevent the stretcher from moving while the ambulance is in motion. Unnecessary equipment should be stowed before transport. Also, objects such as monitors should be secured in a locking device; this minimizes the risk of injuries in a collision. All those travelling in the ambulance should have their seatbelts securely fastened (except on some occasions for the paramedic providing patient care as this may hinder their ability to do this). Before the vehicle leaves the scene, the driver of the ambulance should be advised that it is safe to leave scene.

Note

Whenever possible, children should be transported secured in a proper child safety seat. Except in the most critical cases, care can be delivered effectively when the child is restrained in this way.

During transport, the patient should be closely monitored for any changes in status. If emergency care is required while the ambulance is in motion (e.g. intubation, defibrillation), the driver of the vehicle should be advised to slow/stop the vehicle. When possible, the driver should safely park the vehicle and stay parked until the procedure has been successfully performed.

Upon arrival at the hospital, the ambulance should come to a full stop; at that point, personal restraints can be removed and the vehicle can be exited. All patient care equipment must be secured before the stretcher is released from the locking device; this includes, for example, immobilization devices, intravenous (IV) lines, and airway adjuncts. Also make sure that the patient is disconnected from any other vehicle-based equipment and that all lines and cables are clear. Using safe lifting techniques, the patient's stretcher should be removed from the ambulance. The patient should be appropriately transferred to healthcare personnel at the facility.

Aeromedical transportation and helicopter emergency medical services (HEMS)/air ambulances

Like many other aspects of prehospital emergency care, air evacuation is rooted in military history. During the Prussian siege of Paris in 1870, soldiers and civilians were evacuated by a hot-air balloon. In 1928 a Marine pilot used an engine-powered aircraft to evacuate the wounded in Nicaragua. However, the first full-scale use of aircraft for medical evacuation did not occur until 1950, during the Korean conflict;

the experience gained in Korea formed the basis for helicopter rescue in Vietnam. In Vietnam, nearly 1 million casualties were transported by air. In the more recent military confrontations involving the US in Panama, Grenada and the Middle East, massive advanced aeromedical support capabilities and plans were on site before the conflicts began. Response times of 25 min were achieved for air evacuation of wounded soldiers in the Iraq War. Field surgical units were set up to handle the 1500 to 3000 casualties estimated to occur within the first 24 h of the war; most of the injured soldiers arrived by air transportation. In the UK the first air services commenced in the West Country in the late 1980s and gradually developed in other areas of the country. Now, a number of air ambulance services exist with coverage over much of the population. These services do not receive financial support of Government and mostly rely on charitable donations and sponsorship.

Aeromedical crew members and training

The staffing of air ambulances includes a pilot and paramedic(s) and/or a doctor. Air ambulance crews undergo specialized training in flight physiology, aircraft components and construction, safety regulations, aviation and navigation terminology, and operational safety

Use of HEMS/air ambulances

Most ambulance services/EMS systems develop the criteria for requesting helicopter services to the scene of an emergency. The paramedic generally should consider air transport when emergency personnel have determined that one or more of the following is a factor:

- The time needed to transport a patient by ground to an appropriate facility would pose a threat to the patient's survival and recovery. Air ambulances can take a patient to a more distant specialist facility (such as trauma, neurology or burns), bypassing the local hospitals that do not have those facilities.
- Weather, road, or traffic conditions would seriously delay the patient's access to advanced life support.
- Critical care personnel and specialized equipment are needed to care for the patient adequately on scene or during transport (Box 1-7).

Some UK air ambulances have a doctor on board at all times as well as paramedic(s), others do so when staffing availability allows and others are solely paramedic staffed without a doctor. Each service varies but all the staff are well versed in helicopter emergency care and are experts in that form of response.

It should be borne in mind that there are limitations to air ambulances; in the majority of cases aircraft cannot fly at night or in adverse weather. They may actually prolong transfer of the patient to hospital if the scene is close by (for example less than a few miles) as in some cases a land ambulance is required to meet the aircraft at the landing site near the hospital and transfer the patient the short distance by road (some hospitals do have a landing pad on or close to the emergency department so that an ambulance is not required to meet the aircraft). It can also take a few minutes to load a patient onto the aircraft and this can delay removal from the scene, especially if the aircraft has shut down its engines.

Box 1-7

Advantages and disadvantages of air medical services

Advantages

- Transports are rapid and usually smooth.
- Access to accident sites is quick.
- Traffic, trains, mountains, ship canals, and other barriers can be avoided.
- Travel is still possible when road conditions are poor.
- Sophisticated communication equipment is available.
- Some systems have doctors on board which may in some circumstances allow further interventions to be undertaken
- Ground ambulances are not detained for long periods.
- Quality of care is improved in rural areas where reduced resources may be available and patients can be taken to specialist centres if required.
- Fewer air ambulance crashes occur than ground ambulance crashes.

Disadvantages

- In urban settings, ground ambulances are faster in the immediate local area.
- If the helicopter is on another flight, no other aircraft may be available.
- Inclement weather may prevent the aircraft from travelling.
- The high noise level may limit or prevent communication with the patient or crew.
- Space and weight restrictions may limit access to the patient and restrict the crew, patients, and equipment that can be carried.
- Helicopter transports are more expensive than transports by ground ambulance.

Activation of helicopter services

Most helicopter services are requested via the control/communications centre and may be activated by them at the time of the call or once the first EMS crew arrives on scene. Most air ambulance services are airborne within a matter of minutes but some military responses such as Search and Rescue may take longer, dependent on the aircrew being available and the aircraft being tasked/configured into a specific role. However, if paramedics determine that the situation does not require a helicopter response, control should be notified as soon as possible to make the aircraft available for other calls.

If paramedics require air ambulance attendance, they should advise the flight crew (usually via control) of the type of emergency response, the number of patients, the location of a possible landing zone (although the aircraft pilot will make that decision) and any prominent landmarks and hazards (e.g. vertical structures or power lines). Direct ground to aircraft communication may occasionally be available. Other emergency services on scene should be notified of the aircraft's imminent arrival so that the scene is suitably prepared.

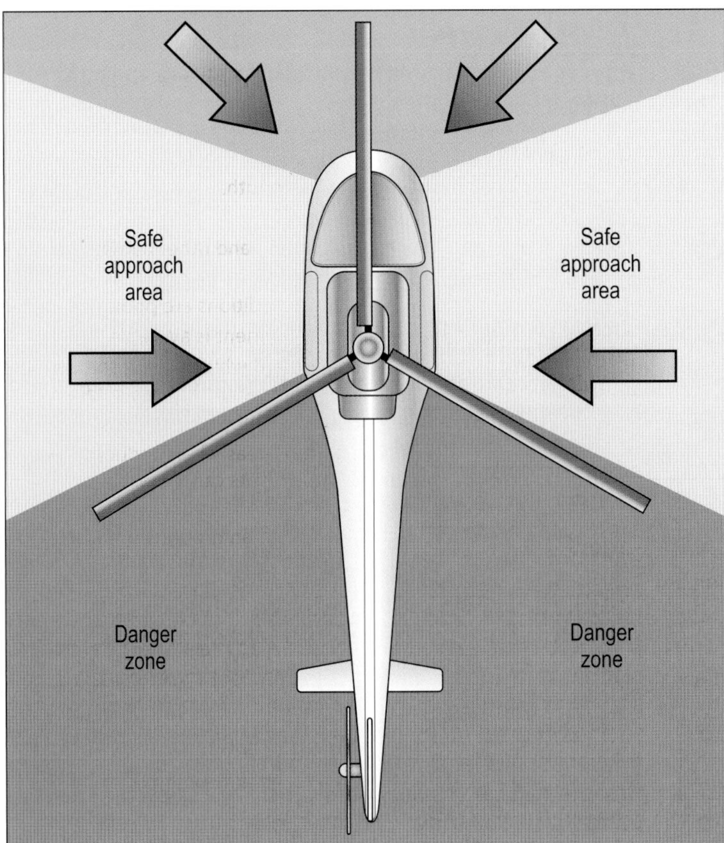

Figure 1-4 Safe-approach zones.

Landing site preparation

The space requirement for a helicopter varies and it is the responsibility of the pilot, not the crews on the ground, to find an appropriate place for the aircraft to land. Air ambulance pilots will self-select a site that is suitable, one that has no vertical structures that can hamper takeoff or landing and is often relatively flat. It is also likely to be free of high grass, crops, or other factors that can conceal uneven terrain or hinder access and, where possible, free of debris that can injure people or damage structures or the helicopter. The landing site will be away from patients and others but it may be prudent to provide protection to any patients on scene and ensure that there are no loose items on site that might be displaced by the downwash of the rotor blades. Rescue personnel close to the landing site should wear protective equipment such as helmets with lowered face shields and safety glasses.

Safety precautions

Everyone should be clear of the landing area during takeoffs and landings (Figure 1-4). A distance of at least 50 m and preferably 100 m is recommended. In addition, paramedics should take the following precautions:

- Never allow ground personnel to approach the helicopter unless the pilot or flight crew asks them to do so.
- Allow only necessary personnel to help load or unload patients; it is better to leave this to the aircraft crew who have experience of the aircraft and any key safety issues.
- Secure any loose objects or clothing that could be blown by rotor downwash (e.g. stretcher, sheets, or blankets).
- Do not allow smoking.
- After the aircraft is parked, move to the front beyond the perimeter of the rotor blades and wait for a signal from the pilot to approach.
- Approach the helicopter in a crouched position, staying in view of the pilot or other crew members.
- Never approach the rear of the aircraft from any direction. The tail rotors on most aircraft are near the ground and spin at 3400 revolutions per minute making them virtually invisible. Tail rotor injuries are likely to be fatal.
- Carry long objects horizontally and no higher than waist high.
- Depart from the helicopter from the front and within view of the pilot.

Patient preparation

Preparing a patient for air transport requires special measures; some medical procedures must be done before the patient is loaded into the aircraft. For example, the patient's airway must be established and secured, or application of a traction splint must be done, before loading. Special equipment (e.g. automated chest compression devices) must be positioned according to the aircraft's configuration. Most aircrews perform a brief patient assessment before lift-off, to verify the patient's condition.

Reassurance of the patient and any family members is also important. Liaise closely with the aircrew about the destination of the aircraft as often different hospitals will be used according to the patient's condition.

Critical Thinking

How do you think an alert patient would feel while waiting for helicopter transportation?

Summary

- The roots of prehospital emergency care may date back to the military.
- In the early twentieth century through the mid-1960s, prehospital care in the UK was provided in a few different ways. Care was provided mostly by hospital-based systems, industry and the voluntary aid societies. These systems later developed into professional services.
- The operations of an effective EMS system include activation, dispatch, prehospital care, hospital care, and rehabilitation.
- The various levels of providers have their own distinct roles and duties. These roles include telecommunicators (dispatchers), first responders, emergency care assistants, EMT/ambulance technicians, paramedics and Emergency Care practitioners. These levels combine to make an effective prehospital EMS system.
- Many professional groups and organizations help to set the standards of EMS. These groups exist at the national and local levels. The groups take part in development, education, and implementation. Being active in such a group helps to promote the status of the paramedic.
- Continuing education is crucial. It provides a way for all healthcare providers to maintain basic technical and professional skills.
- Professionalism refers to the way in which a person conducts himself or herself. Professionalism also refers to how one follows the standards of conduct and performance established by the profession.
- The roles and duties of the paramedic can be divided into two categories. These groups are primary and additional duties.
- The clinical direction that is provided in EMS helps to ensure that the components of quality medical care are in place in the system.
- A CQI programme identifies and attempts to resolve problems in areas such as medical direction, financing, training, communication, prehospital management and transportation, inter-hospital transfer, receiving facilities, specialty care units, dispatch, public information and education, audit and quality assurance, major incident planning, and mutual aid.
- CEN regulations are an example of the systems in place that ensure ambulances and equipment are fit for purpose.
- Completing an equipment and supply checklist at the start of every work shift is important. It is essential for safety, patient care, and risk management. It also helps to ensure proper handling and safekeeping of scheduled medications.
- The methods for estimating ambulance service needs and placement in a community have changed. Compliance in providing EMS services within time frames (response times) that meet national standards is the method that now is commonly used.
- Factors that influence safe ambulance operation include proper use of escorts, environmental conditions, proper use of warning devices, proceeding safely through junctions and whilst overtaking, parking at the emergency scene, and operating with due regard for the safety of all others.
- The staffing of air ambulances includes a pilot and other healthcare professionals. These individuals undergo specialized training in flight physiology and the use of special medical equipment and procedures.
- When paramedics request air ambulance service, the flight crew should be advised of the type of emergency response, the number of patients, and any prominent landmarks and hazards. Paramedics should always follow strict safety measures during helicopter landings. This helps to prevent injury to air medical crews, ground crews, the patient, and bystanders.

References

1. http://www.workhouses.org.uk/index.html?MAB/MAB.shtml accessed January 2009
2. Millar ELM 1966 The Report by the Working Party on Ambulance Training and Equipment. Part 1: Training. Part 2: Equipment and vehicles. Ministry of Health Scottish Home and Health Department. HMSO, London
3. Department of Health/Health and Social Care Information Centre 2005 Ambulance Services 2004–2005 England Bulletin 2005/01/HSCIC
4. Health Professions Council 2007 Standards proficiency – paramedics. HPC, London
5. Health Professions Council 2008 Standards of conduct, performance and ethics. HPC, London
6. Health Professions Council 2007 Standards of education and training guidance. HPC, London
7. JRCALC/ASA/University of Warwick 2006 UK Ambulance Service clinical practice guidelines (2006). Online. Available http://www2.warwick.ac.uk/fac/med/research/hsri/emergencycare/prehospitalcare/jrcalcstakeholderwebsite/guidelines 2 July 2009

8. Health Professions Council 2006 Your guide to our standards for continuing professional development. HPC, London
9. Department of Health 2007 Improving ambulance response times: high impact changes and response times algorithms for NHS Ambulance Trusts. Department of Health, London
10. Stout J 1989 System status management, the fact is it's everywhere. JEMS 14(4)
11. Coyne P, Mayres P, MacDonald B 2007 Roadcraft: the Police Driver's Handbook. Police Foundation/The Stationery Office, London
12. National Safety Council 2002 Injury Facts. National Safety Council, Itasca, IL

Further reading

Ambulance Service Network website http://www.nhsconfed.org/ambulance-trusts/index.cfm

British Paramedic Association website http://www.britishparamedic.org/

Department of Health 2005 Taking healthcare to the patient: transforming NHS ambulance services. DOH, London

CHAPTER 2

Ethics and Law in Paramedic Practice

Chapter contents

Objectives

Upon completion of this chapter, the paramedic student will be able to:

1. Define ethics and bioethics.
2. Distinguish between professional, legal, and moral accountability.
3. Outline strategies to use to resolve ethical conflicts.
4. Describe the role of ethical tests in resolving ethical dilemmas in healthcare.
5. Discuss specific prehospital ethical issues including allocation of resources, decisions surrounding resuscitation, confidentiality, and consent.
6. Identify ethical dilemmas that may occur related to care in futile situations, obligation to provide care, patient advocacy, and the paramedic's role.
7. Describe the basic legal structure in place in the UK.
8. Describe the principles of accountability.
9. Define negligence and the elements necessary for a charge of negligence to be successful.
10. Describe the principle of consent and the elements required when consent is sought.
11. Identify the principle of confidentiality and the paramedic's responsibilities in maintaining patient confidentiality.
12. Detail the differing forms of advance directive and the legal perspectives that might influence paramedic practice.
13. Discuss the role of the coroner.

Key terms

assault Creating apprehension, or unauthorized handling and treatment of a patient.

battery Physical contact with a person without consent and without legal justification.

bioethics The systematic study of moral dimensions, including moral vision, decisions, conduct, and policies of the life sciences and healthcare.

ethics The discipline relating to right and wrong, moral duty and obligation, moral principles and values, and moral character; a standard for honourable behaviour designed by a group with expected conformity.

expressed consent Verbal or written consent to the treatment.

implied consent The presumption that an unconscious or incompetent person would consent to lifesaving care.

informed consent Consent obtained from a patient after explaining all facts necessary for the patient to make a reasonable decision.

morals Social standards or customs; dealing with what is right or wrong in a practical sense.

negligence Failure to use such care as a reasonably prudent emergency medical services provider would use in similar circumstances.

unethical Conduct that fails to conform to moral principles, values, or standards.

ETHICS

Ethical aspects of paramedic practice

Ethics is the field relating to right and wrong, duty and obligation, principles and values, and character. Ethics is a basis for honourable actions designed by a group with expected conformity. Morals refer to social standards or customs, or dealing with what is right or wrong in a practical sense. The term unethical refers to conduct that fails to conform and it is accepted that unethical conduct does not meet moral principles, values or standards. Ethical decisions are based on an appraisal of moral judgements; this idea places the responsibility on individuals.

The notion of ethics dates back to the ancient Greek philosophers, including Hippocrates, Socrates, Plato and Aristotle. These philosophers turned the Greek focus toward questions of ethics and virtue (how should one live?) for moral accountability and away from choice and fate that traditionally had been guided by astrology (Box 2-1). These philosophers laid the basis for a science of medical ethics (bioethics), the analysis of choice in medicine.

Bioethics is the systematic study of moral dimensions. Bioethics includes moral vision, decisions, conduct, and policies of the life sciences and healthcare. Bioethics uses a variety of ethical methodologies in an interdisciplinary setting.

One can make many ethical and other value choices instinctively. One makes these choices by drawing on long-standing personal beliefs, commitments, and habits. For example, most people believe it is wrong to steal, to be deceitful, or to commit murder. In healthcare, however, paramedics are faced with life issues that involve a patient. The patient may have beliefs, commitments, and habits that are different from the paramedic's personal experience. Throughout history, guidance in these situations has been provided through a variety of professional codes. These codes represent the collective wisdom of a group. The HPC Standards of Conduct, Performance and Ethics (2008)[1] is an example.

As with professional codes, a person's personal code of ethics is made up of principles of proper conduct. These values can assist one in making moral choices. A personal code is a critical reflection on one's life. For the paramedic, this code must take into account professional, legal, and moral responsibility (Boxes 2-2 and 2-3).

Critical Thinking

Which of the quotes in Box 2-2 of ethical living best speaks for your personal philosophy?

Ethical principles

There are a number of ethical principles on which ethical healthcare is based. These 'generic' principles guide and provide a context for practice by paramedics; in other

Box 2-1

The Hippocratic Oath (fourth century BCE)

The Oath of Hippocrates is a brief statement of principles. The oath is thought to have been conceived during the fourth century BCE. The oath protected the rights of the patient. The oath also addressed the moral character of the physician as a healer. The Hippocratic Oath was modified in the tenth or eleventh century to eliminate reference to pagan gods. The oath remains an expression of ideal conduct for the physician.

I swear by Apollo Physician and Asclepius and Hygieia and Panaceia and all the gods and goddesses, making them my witnesses, that I will fulfil according to my ability and judgement this oath and this covenant:

To hold him who has taught me this art as equal to my parents and to live my life in partnership with him, and if he is in need of money to give him a share of mine, and to regard his offspring as equal to my brothers in male lineage and to teach them this art – if they desire to learn it – without fee and covenant; to give a share of precepts and oral instruction and all the other learning to my sons and to the sons of him who has instructed me and to pupils who have signed the covenant and have taken an oath according to the medical law, but to no one else.

I will apply dietetic measures for the benefit of the sick according to my ability and judgement; I will keep them from harm and injustice.

I will neither give a deadly drug to anybody if asked for it, nor will I make a suggestion to this effect. Similarly I will not give to a woman an abortive remedy. In purity and holiness I will guard my life and my art.

I will not use the knife, not even on sufferers from stone, but will withdraw in favour of such men as are engaged in this work.

Whatever houses I may visit, I will come for the benefit of the sick, remaining free of all intentional injustice, of all mischief and in particular of sexual relations with both female and male persons, be they free or slaves.

What I may see or hear in the course of treatment or even outside of the treatment in regard to the life of men, which on no account one must spread abroad, I will keep to myself, holding such things shameful to be spoken about.

If I fulfil this oath and do not violate it, may it be granted to me to enjoy life and art, being honored with fame among all men for all time to come; if I transgress it and swear falsely, may the opposite of all this be my lot.

Box 2-2

HPC Standards of Conduct, Performance and Ethics[1]

Your duties as a registrant

The standards of conduct, performance and ethics you must keep to:

1 You must act in the best interests of service users.
2 You must respect the confidentiality of service users.
3 You must keep high standards of personal conduct.
4 You must provide (to us and any other relevant regulators) any important information about your conduct and competence.
5 You must keep your professional knowledge and skills up to date.
6 You must act within the limits of your knowledge, skills and experience and, if necessary, refer the matter to another practitioner.
7 You must communicate properly and effectively with service users and other practitioners.
8 You must effectively supervise tasks that you have asked other people to carry out.
9 You must get informed consent to give treatment (except in an emergency).
10 You must keep accurate records.
11 You must deal fairly and safely with the risks of infection.
12 You must limit your work or stop practising if your performance or judgement is affected by your health.
13 You must behave with honesty and integrity and make sure that your behaviour does not damage the public's confidence in you or your profession.
14 You must make sure that any advertising you do is accurate.

Box 2-3

Statements for ethical living

Socrates: The unexamined life is not worth living. Know thyself. Morality is the necessity of the heart. The soul is that which is.

Plato: Justice is the harmony of all virtues. Truth belongs to the mind.

Aristotle: Sense reveals only individual existence. The universal is immanent in the individual. Man finds his ethic only in his natural self-realization.

Zoroastrianism and Parsis: Good thoughts, good words, good deeds. The Reality is one, the wise by many men call it.

Buddhism: Let a man lift himself up by his own self; let him not depress himself; for he himself is his friend and he himself is his enemy.

Confucianism: Seek to be in harmony with all your neighbours.

Taoism: Being in one's inmost heart in kindly sympathy with all things.

Christianity: Love thy neighbour as thyself.

Judaism: Perform righteousness on earth that ye may find treasures in heaven.

Islam: Do what God likes, and avoid what He dislikes.

words, these principles provide us with a platform on which to build our care and develop our professional practice.

These principles are: beneficence, non-maleficence, self-determination/respect for autonomy, justice, as well as principles connected with professional–patient relationships such as confidentiality, advocacy, veracity and fidelity.

Beneficence

Beneficence is the notion of always to 'do good'. In practical terms the paramedic should strive to do the very best for the patient and to put the patient's interests before one's own needs. It suggests acts of kindness, mercy and is seen to be altruistic. This ethical obligation is well embedded into healthcare and is reflected in the various professional codes that exist for healthcare workers. However, one might question how what is best for the patient is determined (who decides what is 'good' for them) as this might lead to a paternalistic type of paramedic/patient relationship. Furthermore, to what extent must paramedics strive to do good?; is there an 'end point'? Lastly, beneficence for one patient may lead to disadvantageous care for another; certainly it may be difficult to apply the notion of beneficence in its entirety.

Non-maleficence

Non-maleficence is the principle of doing no harm (*primum non nocere*). This is related to the principle found in the Hippocratic Oath, 'I will keep them from harm or injustice'. This tends to be a more stringent principle in that it is less open to interpretation; and the aim is that foreseeable harm is avoided by any action (or omission) of the paramedic. However, what is the definition of harm? In placing an intravenous cannula, puncturing the skin, harm (injury) has occurred, yet the aim of the cannulation is to provide, for example, drugs or fluids that will do the patient good. This is the notion of double effect.

Autonomy and self-determination

Autonomy originates from the Greek: *auto* (self) *nomos* (rule). It is considered to be the principle of self-determination, which is a patient's ability to make decisions for themselves. It is related to the capacity to think, decide and act freely and without adverse influence or coercion; the freedom to choose. Respect for this self-determination, is, therefore, respect for their autonomy. A number of elements are required for effective self-determination; capacity, information and voluntariness.

Capacity is the ability of the patient to think through and reason a decision; many things might influence this ability, such as age, cognitive development, a value or belief system, the patient's comprehension of any consequences as well as the influence of physical changes caused by disease or medications for example. Definitions of capacity are difficult to establish but guidance about the Mental Capacity Act (2005) provides some information for healthcare professionals.[2]

Information giving: in order for an autonomous choice or decision to be made it is necessary for information to be provided that has a number of characteristics associated with it. The paramedic must ensure the quality of the information and that the information is accurate and relevant. This is why paramedics must always be up to date in their knowledge about the role and the professional competences they undertake. It is also important that the patient has an appreciation of the consequences of their decision making; this must be accurate and the consequences must be in context; this is sometimes difficult as emergency care is unpredictable and patient outcomes vary according to a range of differing factors. It is also important that the patient has a true and accurate understanding of the information; this is related to capacity and the paramedic must judge if the information provided is being comprehended; again, this can be very difficult in normal circumstances and even more so in stressful or unusual emergency situations. The timing needs to be considered; there may be a more optimum time to provide this information for the patient and it may also be about repetition to ensure the factors discussed above are reliably in place. Finally, the information giver must have an in-depth understanding of the situation; they cannot give information to a patient fulfilling the criteria if their knowledge and understanding of the situation is weak or limited; again, this implores the paramedic to maintain a broad and up-to-date knowledge base and range of competences.

Finally, the third aspect that must be in place is the notion of voluntariness. This is the sense that the patient is not coerced or persuaded into making a decision that they would otherwise have not made. This, again, is difficult and is a very subjective area, as paramedics might disagree about what actions constitute coercion and what actions do not. However, this means that the paramedic must not overtly exert undue pressure on the patient to follow a specific course of action. In practice, however, this is difficult as there may be situations where the notion of 'duty of care' is in the paramedic's mind and concern about the consequences of the patient's action (or non-action) weigh heavily. Equally, pressure for a patient to follow a course of action can be found from other sources, such as family and friends who may, unbeknown to the paramedic, have a 'hidden agenda' although this is perhaps not common. Mostly, coercion and persuasion occur when the 'best interests' of the patient are being considered and are being done for arguably noble reasons. This is considered in many cases to be 'paternalistic' and when it occurs with good intent is known as 'beneficent paternalism'. However, this can limit free choice and therefore limit to some extent autonomy. This puts the paramedic in a difficult position as the notion of 'patient advocacy' (discussed shortly) and the paramedic being the patient's advocate are also key in professional practice. The components described are also significant factors in the issue of consent, which is discussed later in the chapter.

Justice

Justice is a principle that dictates actions by paramedics should be fair and just. Fairness is sometimes confused with a principle of equality, but in many cases what is fair may not always be equal; as the principle of fairness applies not only to the individual patient but to a wider community as well. When giving thought to whether an action is fair or not, the notion of 'best interests' comes into play, a beneficent notion that may have to accept that the fair action may be about doing the greatest good for the greatest number.

Confidentiality

Confidentiality is both an ethical and legal element and has been deeply embedded into healthcare ethics, tracing its origins in the Hippocratic Oath. More detailed information about confidentiality is found later on in this chapter.

Advocacy

Advocacy relates to the paramedic being focused to the needs of the patient and being, as the term suggests, their 'advocate'. This means that the paramedic might have to support a patient in making a decision or taking a course of action that may be unexpected or making a decision that may be against professional advice. It also relates to the paramedic ensuring that they are accountable and provide care to the very highest standards possible.

Veracity and fidelity

Veracity and fidelity are principles of integrity and truth telling. These are ethical principles which relate to personal and professional integrity and the ability to be honest and truthful beyond any doubt.

A rapid approach to emergency ethical problems

A method of ethical case analysis has been designed which works as a way to deal with emergency ethical problems rapidly. This rule of thumb process involves the following steps:

1. Ask yourself if you have experienced a similar ethical problem in the past. If so, use that experience as a precedent for this problem and follow the rule. (Periodically the paramedic must evaluate these rules.)
2. If you have not experienced a similar ethical problem in the past, buy time for deliberation and for consulting with coworkers and possibly other healthcare professionals.
3. If there is no option to buy time for deliberation, use a set of three tests to help you make a decision (Figure 2-1):
   - Test 1: *impartiality test* – would you accept the action if you were in the patient's place?
   - Test 2: *universalizability test* – would you feel comfortable having this action performed in all relevantly similar circumstances?
   - Test 3: *interpersonal justifiability test* – are you able to provide good reasons to justify and defend your actions to others?

The first test is a good way to correct one's personal bias, the second test helps to do away with moral decision difficulty, and the final test makes sure that the paramedic has reasons for proceeding. The final test also requires that others would approve of the reasons. If the paramedic can answer all three tests in the affirmative, then the paramedic has a fair probability that the action falls within the scope of being ethically acceptable. Even though there may be disagreement about a specific set of values, there often is general agreement over what may comprise wrong actions.

Ethical tests in healthcare

The most basic question of ethical tests in healthcare is, 'What is in the patient's best interest?' However, doing what is best, or what one thinks is best, is not enough to justify

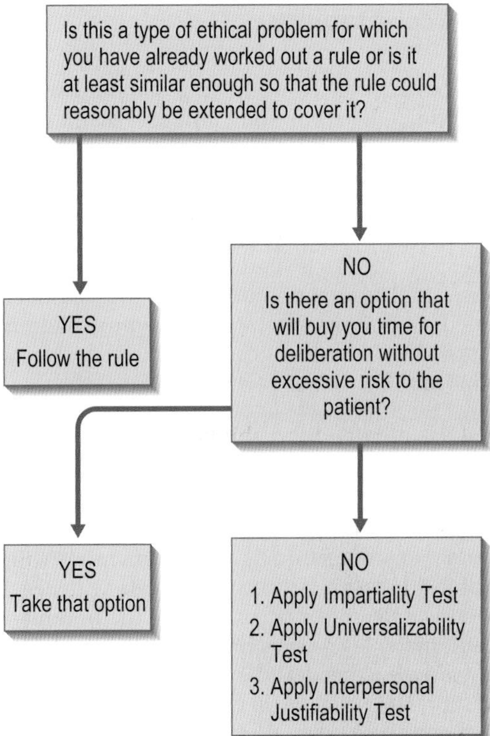

Figure 2-1 A rapid approach to emergency ethical problems.

actions. One must determine what the patient wants. The paramedic can do this using statements by the patient (if the patient is mentally competent) and written statements. Family input is also helpful (if the patient shows altered mental status or incompetence). The role of 'good faith' in making ethical decisions ('Am I doing my best to help and not harm my patient?') should be balanced with the wishes of the patient and the family. The global concept of healthcare (providing patient benefit and avoiding harm) recognizes and respects the patient's autonomy. The concept also recognizes the various legal issues that affect the delivery of healthcare (Box 2-4).

Resolving ethical dilemmas

At times, resolving ethical dilemmas can be difficult. This may be the case when global concepts of healthcare are in conflict. Thus the resolution can be guided by the healthcare community and by the public. The role of the healthcare community in resolving these conflicts is to set standards of care. The healthcare community also must provide research and treatment protocols. Finally, the healthcare community must make prospective and retrospective reviews of decisions and policies. Reviews are done with the intent of educating the paramedic and improving the quality of patient care. The role of the public in managing ethical conflicts in medicine includes creating laws and setting public policy. This role also includes allocating resources to protect patient rights. Lastly, the role of the public includes participating in the use of advance directives and other self-determination documents to make the patients' wishes known.

Box 2-4

Global concepts of ethical healthcare

Therapeutic activity of the Greek doctor was subject to the following rules:

- To help the patient, or at least to do no harm
- To refrain from interfering if the illness were incurable and inevitably mortal
- Insofar as possible, to attack the cause of the disease therapeutically

Today, these global concepts of ethical healthcare can be stated as follows:

- Provide patient benefit
- Do no harm

Box 2-5

Commonly accepted bioethical values

Allocation of resources: The consistent access to quality medical services; distributing health-related services among various persons and uses.

Autonomy: Self-determination; a person's ability to make moral decisions, including those affecting personal medical care. The three components of autonomy are agency (awareness of oneself as having desires and intentions and acting on them); independence (absence of influences that so control what a person does that it cannot be said the person wants to do it); and rationality (rational decision making).

Beneficence: A duty to confer benefits; the practice of good deeds; obligation to benefit others or seek their good.

Confidentiality: The presumption that confidential information will not be revealed to others without the patient's permission. Confidentiality, like privacy, is valued because it protects individual preferences and rights.

Non-maleficence: The prevention of harm, from Hippocratic tradition that established primum non nocere ('Above all, do no harm'); a prohibition on actions with foreseeable harmful effects.

Personal integrity: Adhering to a personal set of values and moral standards.

Ethical issues in contemporary paramedic practice

Paramedics will face some ethical issues during the span of their careers. Most issues deal with the patient's right to self-determination and the paramedic's duty to provide patient care (Box 2-5). These are known as autonomy and beneficence (described earlier). Some of the more common issues (and sample case studies) are described in this section. For each case study, the paramedic should apply the rapid approach to emergency medical problems (described previously in this chapter) and should answer the following ethical questions:

1. What is in the patient's best interest?
2. What are the patient's rights?
3. Does the patient understand the issues at hand?
4. What is the paramedic's professional, legal, and moral accountability?

Allocation of resources

Fairness in the allocation of resources and obligations is a commonly accepted bioethical value. Fairness is integrated into society-wide healthcare policies. This perceived right to universal access to an adequate level of healthcare is a complex economic issue. The issue is affected by the need to contain healthcare costs. Two factors affect true parity in the allocation of resources. The first is a person's ability to access healthcare. This may define what medical services are covered or excluded. The second is treatment decisions made when resources are inadequate to meet patient care needs. This may occur, for example, during a major incident or multi-casualty emergency. When rationing of care is required, it should be based on ethically oriented criteria.

The allocation of resources is more of a policy than a clinical concept. However, allocation can pose ethical dilemmas in prehospital care, as illustrated in the following case study:

Case Study 1

A paramedic crew has been dispatched to the home of a 74-year-old man. The man is complaining of chest pain and shortness of breath. The patient is in obvious distress and provides a significant cardiac history. He asks to be taken to the more distant hospital, 30 miles away. This is a specialist cardiac centre and where he had heart surgery several years ago. Based on the patient's history, physical exam, and electrocardiogram findings, the paramedic crew elect to take the patient to a closer hospital to be stabilized. The patient becomes anxious and complains of increasing chest pain. He tells the paramedic crew that he wishes to be taken to the more distant hospital.

Decisions surrounding resuscitation

Advance directives/decisions, so-called 'living wills', and other self-determination documents can help the paramedic. The paramedic can use these documents to make decisions about the appropriateness of resuscitation in the prehospital setting. The presence of the proper document often makes resuscitation decisions much easier. Having knowledgeable family members also makes such decisions easier. In other cases, however, the decision to initiate or withhold resuscitation measures is not so clear, as illustrated in the following case study:

Case Study 2

The paramedic crew has been dispatched to a restaurant where an elderly woman has collapsed. She has suffered cardiac arrest, and a waiter is performing cardiopulmonary resuscitation. The electrocardiogram monitor reveals ventricular fibrillation. Defibrillation shocks are delivered, but the rhythm remains unchanged. As resuscitation measures are continued, the woman's husband says to the paramedics: 'She said she didn't want this. Her paperwork documenting her advanced directive is at home. Please stop what you're doing and let her go.'

Professional accountability

As professionals, paramedics conform to a standard set by their level of training/education and professional practice. Paramedics are accountable to the patient, their registrant body (HPC) as well as their employing ambulance service for meeting the required standards of care. Duties include commitment to high-quality patient care; continuing education; skill proficiency; and registration. The paramedic is accountable by law to that level of training and that standard of care. A paramedic who is accountable to the profession is more likely to provide good patient care and make decisions that are ethically sound.

Legal accountability

Through patient care the paramedic also assumes a role in the healthcare legal system. Legal issues often are entwined with ethical issues. However, ethics is not synonymous with law. (Ethics deals with moral actions; law deals with legal actions.) Many ethical decisions occur outside the boundaries of the law, and many legal decisions may not be ethical. The paramedic should consider the importance of legal accountability as it relates to medical ethics and abide by the law when ethical conflicts occur.

Moral accountability

Moral accountability refers to personal ethics, that is, personal values and beliefs. Combining moral, legal, and professional accountability may be difficult in an emergency. At times, the paramedic will have to draw on personal ethics to resolve conflicts among these roles and duties. Moreover, the paramedic will have to decide on a course of action. When dealing with ethical questions, the paramedic should remember the following key points:

1. Emotion may not be a reliable determinant for ethical decision making. One should monitor the conscience. The conscience can be a good guide if one's conscience is well informed concerning right or wrong. Rational decision making is making decisions that rely on research and prudence regarding what is right. However, some knowledge deficit may permit the paramedic to come to a flawed decision.
2. Decisions must not be based solely on the opinions of others. The decisions also must not be based on global protocols that were meant to guide, not dictate (e.g. codes of the profession). If paramedics come across a situation that they have never dealt with before, it is possible they might make a poor, or even unethical, decision. In these cases, paramedics should consult with other (more senior) colleagues, a supervisor, other healthcare professionals, or a set of guidelines or other resources. Consultation is better than limiting oneself to one's own knowledge base or principles. At times, input from patients and their loved ones can be a key source of information and can lead to a better decision.
3. Once the ethical question has been answered, the answer becomes a 'rule' to guide behaviour, at least in the particular setting. Once the rule has been identified, it should become a barrier to acting in opposition to

the rule. Paramedics are expected not to break the rule without a strong reason for their actions.

In reference to answering ethical questions, no one knows all the answers. In addition, none of the tools or techniques will work in every case to arrive at the 'right' decision. Nonetheless, healthcare providers are accountable for personal and professional actions and decisions. Seeking counsel and guidance with such decisions is always wise.

Most persons are seen as having a basic right to privacy. The principle of confidentiality refers to one's private and personal information. This information should not be disclosed by a healthcare worker to other persons without the patient's consent.

In some cases, the release of such information is required by law. Conflict between ethics and confidentiality may arise, however, particularly if the public health would benefit from the disclosure of confidential information, as described in the following case study:

Case Study 3

The paramedic crew has been dispatched to a motor vehicle crash. A young man has struck another car head-on, killing the driver of the other car. The patient is shaken but has only minor injuries. While preparing the patient for transport, the patient confides to the paramedic that he had used cocaine shortly before the crash occurred. The patient asks the paramedic, however, to keep the information confidential and not to tell the police officers at the scene.

Critical Thinking

Your partner contacts a former patient to ask for a date using the phone number from the patient care report. Do you think that action violates any ethical principles? If so, which ones?

As explained later in this chapter, competent patients have a legal right to decide on the healthcare they will receive. This right is a basic element of the relationship between the patient and healthcare professionals. Cases in which patients refuse lifesaving care can produce legal and ethical conflicts, as illustrated in the following case study:

Case Study 4

The paramedic crew has been dispatched to an office building. A 55-year-old woman collapsed at a business meeting. She is alert and oriented, complains of chest pain, and is pale and diaphoretic. The paramedics advise the patient of the possibility of a heart attack and the need for immediate care and transport for further evaluation. The patient insists on waiting until after the meeting has concluded to seek medical care on her own, and she asks the EMS crew to leave.

Other ethical principles for patient care situations

Other ethical principles for patient care situations relate to care in futile situations, legal obligations to provide care, patient advocacy and paramedic accountability, and the paramedic's role undertaking advanced skills.

Care in futile situations

An action is seen as futile if it serves no purpose or is totally ineffective. When a paramedic is providing care in a case that may be futile, the paramedic should follow current guidelines. Consultation can help the paramedic to decide on a course of action. An example of a futile situation in healthcare is continuing resuscitation initiated by bystanders when the patient clearly has expired. Another example is providing life support measures for a patient who has fatal injuries. The definition of futility may pose an ethical dilemma. This may be especially true when a dispute or lack of agreement exists about the goals of treatment. Not all futility judgements are controversial. For example, cardiopulmonary resuscitation is futile and should not be provided to patients with obvious signs of death. Some obvious signs are decapitation, rigor mortis, tissue decompensation or extreme dependent lividity.

Critical Thinking

You arrive at a home where you find a 3-month-old baby who obviously has been dead for several hours. The mother is screaming, 'Help her, help her'. Your partner decides to proceed with advanced life support care even though it is clearly futile. Is this decision ethical?

Obligation to provide care

In the prehospital arena the paramedic's duty to provide care seldom is an issue; the patient's request for emergency service presents a legal duty to act to the paramedic and the service as an organization. There is no specific obligation to provide care when off duty, but if the paramedic did undertake care he or she would be covered by the principle of 'Good Samaritan' laws as long as the care given was in keeping with levels of skills and competence and did not fall outside of any other policies or procedures. Individual ambulance services may have a specific policy guiding staff about their actions when off duty in an emergency situation.

Patient advocacy and paramedic accountability

While providing care, the paramedic serves as the patient's advocate. This advocacy may conflict at times with the paramedic's accountability to the patient and, for example, clinical practice guidelines. In such a case, the paramedic should follow the guidelines but may need to consult with others for advice and support. As a rule, it is prudent and ethical to err on the side of providing for the needs of the patient when conflict arises. Examples of ways in which a paramedic can serve as the patient's advocate include the following:

- Educating patients on the delivery of healthcare and the role that they can play to affect change in the nation's healthcare system.
- Ensuring that healthcare decisions are made by patients and their doctors and are based on the medical needs of patients, not financial considerations.

- Informing patients of national healthcare reform initiatives.
- Promoting patient access to reliable information about state-of-the-art medical technologies and treatments.
- Promoting fairness and equality in the UK's NHS and healthcare system.

Role undertaking advanced skills

As a practitioner of advanced skills the paramedic has a role to fulfil. For the most part, the paramedic is to follow guidance that is provided, yet there may be times when these guidelines may not seem appropriate. For example, the paramedic may believe that a drug is contraindicated for the patient or a drug may be medically acceptable but not in the patient's best interest at that time.

The converse can also occur. For example, a paramedic might commence treatment for a case in which the field impression is unsure. When a conflict occurs between normal practice and the individual circumstances of the case, the use of the ethical test described earlier may help. Additionally, as previously stated, the advice of other more senior colleagues and other healthcare professionals may be indicated.

Ethical dilemmas will always be a part of prehospital care. At times paramedics will have to perform duties that may involve conflicts in moral judgement. An example includes issues of patient confidentiality or patient rights or honouring a do not resuscitate order. Such ethical issues are dynamic. The ethical dilemmas of today may be decided by law tomorrow.

Summary

- Ethics is the discipline relating to right and wrong, moral duty and obligation, moral principles and values, and moral character. Bioethics is the science of medical ethics. 'Morals' refers to social standards or customs.
- Paramedics must meet a standard established by their level of training and regional practice.
- Paramedics must abide by the law when ethical conflicts occur.
- A paramedic must act in a way that is seen as morally acceptable.
- The rapid approach to ethical issues is a process. The process involves reviewing past experiences; deliberation (if possible); and performing the impartiality test, universalizability test, and interpersonal justifiability test to reach an acceptable decision.
- Two concepts of ethical healthcare are to provide patient benefit and to do no harm.
- All resources must be allocated fairly. This is an accepted bioethical value.
- Advance directives, living wills, and other self-determination documents can help the paramedic to make decisions about the appropriateness of resuscitation in the prehospital setting.
- A healthcare professional is not allowed to reveal details supplied by the patient to others without the patient's consent. This is the principle of confidentiality.
- In some cases, patients refuse lifesaving care. These cases can produce legal and ethical conflicts.
- Other areas that are likely to raise ethical questions in the prehospital setting include providing care in futile situations, the paramedic's obligation to provide care, patient advocacy, and the paramedic's role providing advanced life support skills.

LEGAL ASPECTS OF PARAMEDIC PRACTICE

Legal duties and ethical responsibilities

The paramedic's legal duties are to the patient, the employer, and the public. These duties are defined by statutes and regulation and based on commonly accepted standards of medical care. Like other healthcare professionals, in addition to legal duties, paramedics have ethical responsibilities that include the following:

- responding with respect to the physical and emotional needs of every patient
- maintaining mastery of skills and competence
- participating in continuing education/refresher training
- critically reviewing performance and seeking improvement
- reporting honestly
- respecting confidentiality
- working cooperatively and with respect for other emergency workers and healthcare professionals
- staying current with new concepts and modalities.

Note

Failing to perform emergency medical services (EMS) duties in a proper way can result in civil, professional or in some cases criminal liability and is related to accountability. As described in this chapter, the best legal protection is providing proper assessment and care to the patient, coupled with correct and full written documentation.

In the UK the legal system is based upon two main elements: civil law and criminal law. However, one has to consider other 'laws' such as health and safety law, employment law, professional law and regulations and so on. These may or may not fall under the remit of civil or criminal laws but nonetheless are influential in shaping paramedic practice and again are related to accountability.

Criminal law considers actions that are against established laws in force at the time and are tried in a criminal court; for instance, the touching, such as actual bodily harm or wounding of a person against their will (without consent) is a criminal offence. However, it could be considered in a civil action where the claimant has brought a civil case against the defendant and this is tried in a civil court. In this case no custodial or similar sentence can be brought (unlike a criminal case) but, if successful, financial compensation (damages) might be awarded. Some examples of civil actions might include negligence, trespass to property or against the person, false imprisonment or defamation of character.

Laws of the land come into being in several different ways: legislation as a result of Acts of Parliament (statute law) or secondary legislation such as statutory instruments. Legal precedents can be set in the form of judge-made law and decisions arising out of specific cases in court. The European Union has its own legal system and therefore some European law is automatically in force in the UK.

Acts of Parliament arise as a result of a bill which itself is predetermined by Green and White Papers, produced by the Government in the early stages of bill writing. The bill then is presented at both Houses of Parliament (first the Commons then the Lords) through readings and different stages such as a committee stage and report stage, before obtaining Royal Assent and becoming an Act.

In terms of civil and criminal law, there are a range of courts through which cases are heard, most of which do not get beyond the first stages. In criminal law, magistrates' courts are the first tier, leading to Crown Courts, then the High Court, which has several different sections, the Court of Appeal (Criminal or Civil Divisions) and ultimately the House of Lords. Civil cases may be heard at tribunals and County Courts, then follow the same process as criminal cases proceeding to the High Court and beyond.

Paramedic–patient relationships

The relationship formed between the paramedic and the patient during a patient care encounter is a legal one and therefore legal issues may arise from providing patient care. These issues include accountability, consent, confidentiality and those related to transportation.

Accountability and negligence, duty of care

Accountability

What is accountability? Definitions might include the notions of responsibility, answerability, culpability, liability, obligation and duty. There are many factors that especially in recent years have brought about changes to paramedic practice in the UK, which it might be argued have contributed to the issue of accountability becoming much more considered. One of the key elements is that of regulation; the Health Professions Council (HPC) is a regulator of 13 professions, which include paramedics. Other reasons that have brought accountability into the spotlight include political developments/agendas and policy by the Department of Health (such as National Service Frameworks), technology/clinical practice development (emergency care practitioners), changes in medical contracts and out of hours provision, the educational developments for paramedics with moves into higher education, financial issues and perhaps an increase in expectations and awareness due to the influence of the media. Organizations that are part of the Clinical Governance umbrella such as the National Institute for Health and Clinical Excellence and the Healthcare Commission also have influenced the need for increased accountability.

Paramedics are no different from other health care professionals in having codes of conduct that explicitly refer to the issues around accountability.

Scope of practice

Scope of practice refers to the range of duties and skills that a paramedic is allowed and expected to perform when needed. These duties are set by national law or regulation. Scope of practice defines the boundaries between the paramedic and the lay person. It also defines the boundaries between different professionals' skills levels. For example, the scope of practice for paramedics would include endotracheal intubation, administration of medications, and other basic and advanced life support procedures.

The four main arenas through which paramedics face accountability for their actions are criminal law, civil law, employment law and through professional registration. In *criminal law* the paramedic would answer to courts if an offence was committed. In this scenario the case would be heard in either a magistrates' court or Crown Court and punishment if found guilty might include a fine or a custodial sentence for example. This would result in a criminal record.

Civil law: this is where an action is taken by a claimant, as described above, against a defendant, which, if successful, may result in civil damages and compensation being paid. In most cases the civil action would be against the employer if a paramedic was the subject of a civil action whilst in employed time and therefore the case is against the employer for harm or negligence.

Employment law: paramedics may also face issues around accountability in employment law; in other words they may be held accountable for a failing that is part of their employment contract. The contract of employment provides the legal substance for this and there is an implied duty.

Finally, in terms of *professional registration*, paramedics are accountable to their regulatory body and should they fall foul of the standards that the body sets may be subject to disciplinary actions which ultimately could see them struck off the register and unable to practise. These cases are heard by professional conduct committees.

Most failures in care most often result in civil action rather than criminal action, and in a sense the idea of 'where there's blame there's a claim' is still prevalent, due to the increasingly litigious society. In this case negligence has to be proven and for this to occur a number of elements have to be determined:

- There is a *duty of care...*
- there has been a *breach of that duty of care...*
- this was *reasonably foreseeable...*
- and that it resulted in *harm*.

Duty of care

A duty of care is the principle that a paramedic has a responsibility to be careful and to avoid harm occurring by acts or omissions. This has been well established for many decades (Donoghue v. Stevenson 1932).[3]

A duty of care can be said to have been established when the paramedic in any way is employed or has responded to an emergency call but it is not universally owed. However, clarification can be sought in the Court of Appeal decision that once an ambulance service has answered a 999 call, it has a duty of care and obligation to provide a service for a named individual at a specified address (Kent v. Griffiths and others, Times Law Report, 23 December 1998). Does an off-duty paramedic have a duty to volunteer help? Morally and ethically perhaps, but strictly in law, not unless a pre-existing relationship exists. However, once a paramedic gives care (undertakes duty of care), they are bound to a standard expected of a reasonable person. The standard of that duty of care is another difficult question to answer; if a duty of care exists, to what level is care deemed to be acceptable? The answer to this is found in what is commonly known as the Bolam test. This case was summarized:

> *When you get to a situation that involves the use of some special skill or competence, the test as to whether there has been negligence or not is... the standard of the ordinary skilled man exercising and professing to have that special skill. If a surgeon failed to measure up to that in any respect (clinical judgement or otherwise) he had been negligent should be so adjudged.*[4]

However, there is debate about what a standard of care might be and in some circumstances paramedics might have to deviate from normal practice due to specific circumstances of a call; this is especially true with the move from protocol-based care to guidelines-driven care. Therefore, it does not follow that failure to follow approved practice is necessarily negligent and this was supported in the House of Lords, which held that there was room for differences of opinion or practice (in the medical profession) (Maynard v. W. Midlands RHA [1984] 1 WLR 634). Importantly, the Bolam test applies where different courses of action have been thoughtfully pre-considered and does not apply where the alleged neglect (negligence) arises out of an oversight or unconsidered action. To determine what a reasonable standard of care might be, courts rely on expert opinion (expert witnesses) to enable decision to be reached. In the case of Bolitho, the House of Lords have stated that such expert opinion must flow logically and reasonably from the specific circumstances.

Foreseeability and causation of harm

For the tort of negligence to be successful a degree of foreseeability has to be in place; this means that the result of the alleged negligence was predictable. It depends on the risks or consequences of an action being known or anticipated. Equally, for negligence to be proved there has to be causation; a link between cause and effect is established.

Defence against negligence

Inexperience of the practitioner is usually no defence against negligence as all patients have a right to an accepted standard of care. However, a probationary member of staff might be mentored by a more experienced member of staff and in that case there may be more shared liability. Contributory negligence may occur where the complainant may be found to have contributed to his or her own injury and compensation or damages awarded may be reduced or eliminated based on the complainant's contribution to the injury.

Protection against negligence claims

Paramedics must be aware of how caring for a patient can pose a threat of litigation for negligence. The best protections against such claims are the following:

- education/training/continuing education and skills retention
- appropriate quality improvement
- appropriate medical direction, online and off-line
- accurate, thorough documentation (see Chapter 11)
- professional attitude and demeanour.

Think back to a call you took as a paramedic or EMT that did not go well and the patient did not do well. Did that call meet any of the elements of negligence? What measures could you take to prevent the recurrence of that type of situation?

Vicarious liability and Clinical Negligence Scheme for Trusts (CNST)

Historically, the NHS as a public body could not be prosecuted and was protected against civil actions from instances of alleged clinical negligence; this was the notion of Crown Immunity. However, this changed in 1990 and Crown Immunity was changed to Crown Indemnity. In 1996 the Clinical Negligence Scheme for Trusts (CNST) was established which is part of the NHS Litigation Authority (NHSLA). The CNST members are the NHS trusts who pay an annual contribution; the risks associated with that NHS trust are projected by actuaries who look at a range of factors. Any claims that arise and are proven are paid out from this scheme; those trusts with good risk management practices or those who make few or no claims are subject to lower contributions, much in the same way motor insurance and a no claims discount is calculated. The NHS trust is still the legal defendant but the NHSLA will handle the processes involved with any claim and its associated costs. Vicarious liability is where the employer is responsible for faults of others; in other words, the employer will be held responsible for the actions of staff such as paramedics it employs if they are the subject of a civil claim. The claimant needs to establish that the employee was negligent or was liable for a civil wrong (as determined above), that the individual concerned was an employee of that organization, and that at the time of the incident that the claim refers to the employee was acting in course of their employment.

Pressure from inadequate resources may on occasions be used as a defence against a claim for negligence. However, even if short staffed a practitioner may still be liable and questions around whether notification of the situation that has occurred was made to senior managers will be asked. However, employers have certain responsibilities and whilst resource deficiency may not be a defence for negligence, they do have to respond to concerns raised by staff. The Public Interest Disclosure Act 1998 requires all NHS trusts to set up procedure for staff to raise concerns and to be able to enjoy protection from victimization and this route would be one used by staff to highlight areas of concern. Indeed it is incumbent on healthcare professionals to bring areas of poor practice or care to the employer's attention and this is embedded in some Professional Codes of Conduct.

Critical Thinking

Certain advanced life support interventions have an increased risk of causing harm to the patient compared with basic life support skills. As a paramedic, what advanced life support interventions do you think that you will perform that have this increased risk?

Paramedic medical defence and liability insurance

Many paramedics and other health practitioners elect to hold additional indemnity insurance, especially those who are self-employed or work outside of their normal employment as a paramedic. Many professional associations and trade unions have as part of their fees some degree of indemnity insurance. This will provide for legal representation and support should an action be taken and an individual practitioner named.

Consent

The legal principle of consent is central to any encounter with a patient in the day-to-day work of a paramedic. To avoid a charge of 'trespass to the person' paramedics need to obtain consent prior to patient contact such as examination or clinical care of a patient. This will then avoid the risk of being accused of battery or assault. It embodies the principles of self-determination described earlier, and in law, a patient has a right to refuse the touching of his or her body. In 1914, in the US, Justice Cardoza asserted:

> *Every human being of adult years and sound mind has a right to determine what shall be done with his own body; and a surgeon who performs an operation without the patient's consent commits an assault, for which he is liable in damages.*[5]

Consent may be given in two forms, expressed or implied. Expressed consent may be given in writing or verbally and implied suggests that it might be by non-verbal communication or action. Consent in writing is less common in prehospital care; one example of its use might be prior to thrombolytic therapy. Most commonly, expressed consent is obtained verbally; often this is due to the difficult nature of prehospital work and also because some interventions carry less risk.

In terms of implied consent, some believe that by calling for an ambulance, the patient consents to any action or intervention. This is not so and is not supported in law. Implied consent might be, for example, where a patient rolls up their sleeve ready for blood pressure to be taken. There are weaknesses in implied consent; for instance, the patient may assume that one intervention is to be undertaken but the paramedic assumes the patient is consenting to the intervention the paramedic has in mind (e.g. blood pressure recording versus cannulation). Therefore, it is preferable for spoken explanation and agreement to be achieved. Once consent is given, an action of trespass cannot succeed except where insufficient information has been given. What about a situation with an unconscious patient? It might be thought that where a patient is unconscious and treated by paramedics, implied consent is given. However, this is not so: paramedics care for patients as part of their duty of care for the patient out of necessity in an emergency (doctrine of necessity) and any defence would be on that basis.

Consent must be valid. As previously described when looking at the ethical principle of autonomy and respect for self-determination, a number of (similar) components need to be in place for consent to be valid. (In fact, consent can only ever be valid; if it is not, it is not consent!) These are capacity/competence, information, and consent must be given in an environment free of coercion, duress or fraud ('voluntariness').

The patient must be able to comprehend the information, especially any consequences, and be able to use information in the decision-making process. The paramedic must assess the patient's capacity, which might be affected by, for example, pain, panic, confusion, medication or fatigue. However, incapacity must not be confused with an informed choice to decline treatment. Such decisions may be based on the patient's own beliefs and values, even if they appear irrational to us. Equally, it is important that the patient understands what the consequences are; for instance, it might be considered that if there is a misperception of reality that exists, then the patient may not have capacity to make a decision (e.g. a patient who says his foot is uninjured even though it is partially amputated).

There are different types of incapacity, including temporary and fluctuating. In this situation, unless a valid advance refusal exists, the law permits interventions which are necessary but no more than reasonably required in the patient's best interests. If the incapacity is longstanding it is lawful to carry out procedures in the patient's best interest, which might include wider care not just lifesaving interventions. However, in prehospital care this scenario is uncommon.

Another component for valid consent is sufficient information (information giving). This would include the nature and purpose of the procedure or action, in a way which is clear, unambiguous, balanced and free of jargon. This is considered to be 'disclosure' and is based on the ethical perspective of veracity (truth telling). The ability of the paramedic to provide accurate information is key: in other words the knowledge regarding the risks and benefits of any proposed procedure must be present. Additionally the paramedic should have the ability to convey information to patients both clearly and concisely, to be able to ensure patients have understood the information and be prepared to support the patient's decisions. So, a person's consent must be based on appropriate understanding and the patient must be intentionally giving permission for the intervention.

Voluntariness

This is the principle that consent must be voluntary and freely given, without pressure or coercion to either agree to or refuse treatment. Coercion may arise from various sources, for example, from practitioners or family. However, coercion must not be confused with information giving and ensuring benefit/risk aspects are clear. Arguably there is a fine line between coercion and encouragement/explanation and the paramedic needs to be able to differentiate between the two.

There are difficulties that are peculiar to the prehospital environment that can influence the obtaining of consent; patients, as well as relatives and others, are likely to be stressed or anxious. There may be a lack of understanding or forgetfulness, particularly in certain groups of patients. Paramedics operate in all sorts of environments and a possible lack of privacy may affect the initial paramedic/patient relationship until rectified. Whilst not unique to the prehospital situation, the patient may feel helpless and unable to assert themselves. Often, the patient's health history is unknown, and, to compound this, paramedics are, in some senses, isolated practitioners: senior help is very often difficult to obtain immediately. Finally, other issues such as practitioner knowledge and on-scene time pressures may also provide difficulties.

Persons aged 18 years and over who have capacity are deemed in law to have the right to refuse treatment and assessment. The Mental Capacity Act 2005 makes it clear that a person is assumed to have capacity unless it is established that they have not; this might be determined by their behaviour or other factors that become apparent. Those aged 16 and 17 years may also give consent to assessment and treatment and the presumption is that they are capable of giving consent unless again there are factors that suggest their capacity is compromised, and they are in reality treated as adults. Those under 16 years should ordinarily have parental or legal guardian consent provided before assessment or treatment, but in an emergency or urgent situation this may not be practicable and the doctrine of necessity (which can be applied to any person of any age) is that some interventions may be necessary to save life or limb. It may also be deemed that a child under 16 is 'Gillick competent' (Box 2-6) and able to consent if they have understanding and capacity; indeed it is good practice to seek the consent of children and ensure their understanding and voluntary cooperation anyway.[6] Refusal of assessment or treatment in the under 16s is not recognized in law and may pose occasional difficulties when dealing with this age group.

Those who are detained under the Mental Health Act 1983 (on a 'section' rather than a voluntary admission) also form another group of patients in whom special consideration should be made. The Act provides that assessment and treatment can be given against the patient's will (in other words, without their consent) only in relation to their mental health illness. Those who have capacity would be in a position to refuse assessment or treatment if it was for a condition unrelated to the metal illness they are detained for under the Mental Health Act. In other words, they have the same power of refusal as any other competent adult.

> **Box 2-6**
>
> **'Gillick competent'**
>
> Gillick competence arose out of a case where, ultimately, a mother took the local health authority to court after it refused to give assurance that none of her children would be given contraceptive advice without parental consent. This came about after a Health Service Circular regarding contraception for under 16-year-olds was published. The action failed in the House of Lords and Lord Fraser stated the exceptional circumstances set out in this case.

Full documentation must be undertaken in all situations whether a patient refuses assessment or treatment. Where possible, obtain the patient's signature and those of witnesses. It is very important that the patient understands the consequences of their decision and also that it is emphasized that they are perfectly entitled to change their mind; if so then the offer of care will remain. In some cases, there may be concerns that the patient actually lacks capacity to make the decision to refuse care and in this case additional help through the patient's GP, the police or others may be necessary. Great care should be exercised not to abandon the patient without appropriate 'safety netting'; the provision and signposting of alternative pathways of care and advice. If any doubt remains, the paramedic should take advice of a more senior colleague such as an on-call or duty officer.

Equally, consent may be withdrawn at any time by the patient and the paramedic must respect the patient's wishes. Withdrawal of consent carries the same weight in law as initial refusal to consent.

Confidentiality

Maintaining the confidentiality of patient health information is a fundamental duty not only from a legal perspective but also an ethical one. Much sensitive information can be obtained by paramedics and extreme care must be taken to uphold the principles of confidentiality.

The need to maintain confidentiality arises from several different areas: it is a legal obligation, a duty under the law; it is also embedded into professional codes of conduct for all health professionals and there is a contractual duty under employment terms and conditions, which are underpinned by the NHS Code of Practice on Confidentiality.[7] Patients and the public have a right and an expectation that information about themselves will be held in an appropriate way and that respect for privacy will be upheld.

The Data Protection Act 1998 and Human Rights Act 1998 are both Acts of Parliament that have a direct relationship on the upholding of confidentiality.

The transfer of information is considered disclosure and this disclosure should only be undertaken when it is correct to do so. Patients have a right to object to disclosure and in this case the healthcare professional has an obligation to uphold this wish. There are some exceptions to this rule, but, in general, patient consent to disclose information must be obtained. Clearly, when paramedics care for patients, there will be a requirement that the patient be handed over to other healthcare professionals and that a patient report form or other health record be completed and again handed over (this would form a duty of care and an actual obligation on the part of the paramedic). Patients will expect however, that those who receive that information will be only those who are caring for the patient and have a right to that information, for that purpose.

Paramedics work in public areas and care must be careful that confidentiality is maintained at all times; taking a history in front of bystanders or even family could put practitioners in a difficult position. Care must be taken that copies of patient report forms are not left in public view or where they could be accessed by unauthorized persons; this is especially true of copies of completed patient report forms kept on ambulances before the crew returns to base.

The Department of Health proposes the confidentiality model, which describes the elements of protect, inform, provide choice and improve. Protect relates to caring for the patient's information, inform relates to the patients being advised how other information will be used, and providing choice is allowing the patient to determine how and if disclosure of information is undertaken. The fourth element supports the first three in that improvements require healthcare professionals to look for the best possible ways of protecting, informing and providing choice.

Caldicott Guardianship principles were developed after the Caldicott Committee review of 1997 relating to patient-identifiable information. Guidelines for handling patient-identifiable data relate to justification of the purpose, ensuring that access is on an as-needs basis, that everyone involved understands their obligations to the law and that use of this information is at no more than the minimum level required. Each NHS trust has an individual charged with ensuring that the principles of Caldicott Guardianship are upheld (they are known as Caldicott Guardians).[8]

There are exceptions to the principle of confidentiality, where disclosure without consent might be made. These include certain circumstances covered by statute such as the Children Act 1989, Road Traffic Act 1988, Prevention of Terrorism Act 1988, Health Act 1999 and the Children Act 2004. Obviously, if a patient consents to information being released, then disclosure may occur. In difficult circumstances or if there is any doubt, it is better not to disclose to another party and seek advice from more senior colleagues or managers.

Advanced directives

Living wills, advanced statements, advanced refusals (sometimes known as advanced decisions) and do not resuscitate orders are collectively known as advanced directives. These are (usually) written documents that identify the patient's wishes in the event of their death or incapacity. Originally, these had no firm legal basis in statute law but were recognized in common law in the UK; the Mental Capacity Act 2005, which came into force in April 2007, now forms the legal basis for these advanced decisions in relation to the patient's capacity. Most ambulance trusts have policies for staff to follow should they be faced with some form of advanced directive from a patient or their family. A lasting power of attorney (previously called enduring power of attorney) is also a form of advanced directive; one form relates to financial and property matters and another to decisions regards healthcare and treatment. It comes into force after the maker of the power (the patient in question) is deemed to have lost capacity to handle their affairs. It can relate to all matters (a general power) or to specific matters only. It is only valid once registered with the Office of the Public Guardian.

Many advance refusals/decisions relate to withholding resuscitation attempts in the event of cardiac or respiratory arrest. To be valid, they must be made by the patient when they have full capacity, and must be very specific about the intervention(s) being refused. The refusal should be in writing. They may be part of a broader document that covers the wishes of the patient but the advice is that as they are effectively refusals of care or treatment they are separated clearly for people to see. Certain criteria need to be in place: the patient has to be 18 years or older, has to specify the treatment to be refused, specify when this refusal would take place and confirm that the decision is made of their own free will without coercion or influence of others. However, if there is any doubt about the validity of the decisions, then paramedics should commence normal care and seek advice, for example, from the patient's GP or from more senior colleagues.

Recognition of life extinct (ROLE)/futile resuscitation

In the past it was commonplace for patients to be resuscitated in cardiac arrest situations when it was clear that the outcome for success was poor or non-existent. This practice led to a call for a more considered approach to managing these situations; in some cases families were given false hope that their loved one might survive, the risks involved in an emergency transfer from scene to hospital with ongoing resuscitation in the back of the ambulance could not be underestimated, and the attempt often consumed vital resources being committed to that call for a period of time.

In the 1990s the ambulance service made the first steps in 'recognizing the fact of adult death' and, in conjunction with local coroners, produced guidelines for stopping resuscitation attempts in some cases. These included patients in asystole for prolonged periods of time and similar scenarios where survival was unlikely (Box 2-7).

These policies were adapted into the 'recognition of life extinct' (ROLE) guidelines, which are part of the clinical practice guidelines of JRCALC. Some ambulance services have specific polices for ROLE in their own areas, often due to slight variations in local practice. As previously mentioned, ambulance services also produce polices for staff that refer to the correct action to take in the event that a patient is transported who has a do not attempt resuscitation (DNAR) order in place. Paramedics should familiarize themselves with the practice in their own area but most DNARs are limited by time (for instance, in some cases 7 days before they require review). In most services the policy requires that ambulance staff have a copy of the DNAR order or a proforma that is completed specifically for the ambulance crew. This type of proforma tends to cover non-emergency and planned journeys, for instance the transfer of a terminally ill patient to a hospice from their home address.

In the event of ROLE being declared, it is important that paramedics follow their service requirements for document

Box 2-7

Physiological changes that occur after death

Within minutes after death, postmortem changes begin to occur in the body. The surface of the skin becomes pale and yellowish; body temperature falls and reaches that of the environment within 24 h; blood pressure and muscle tension decrease; and the pupils become dilated. Blood and fluids begin to drain away from the face, nose, and chin as gravity causes blood to settle in the most dependent, lowest tissues. This drainage results in a bluish-purple discoloration in the tissues known as dependent lividity.

Within 6 h after death, muscle stiffening develops from chemical changes in the body. This is known as rigor mortis. Smaller muscles in the face usually are affected first. This is followed by a stiffening of the entire body within 12–14 h. Signs of tissue decay are usually obvious within 24–48 h after death, depending on environmental temperatures. The rigor mortis diminishes and the body becomes flaccid within 12–14 h after completion of rigor mortis (i.e. 24–48 h after death) but this time frame is variable on a number of factors, such as environmental temperature and chemical content within the muscles. As the body decays, the skin loosens from the underlying tissues, and swelling and bloating may become evident.

completion and that the time of death is noted. Staff may be required to liaise with the coroner's officer, depending on the nature of the case, and if there are any suspicious circumstances or the death is sudden and unexpected then the police will normally become involved anyway.

As discussed previously, if there are any factors that suggest staff should commence or continue resuscitation, then this is what should happen; if doubt exists about the validity of a DNAR order or the criteria for ROLE are not clearly applicable, then it is more appropriate to undertake resuscitation attempts. These are difficult situations to deal with, especially with a distraught family present, but paramedics must be very clear about what the policies and procedures are and try to avoid any on-scene disagreements with the patient's family.

Emergency Workers (Obstruction) Act 2006

This act makes it an offence to obstruct or hinder an emergency service worker in the course of their duty. It applies not only to ambulance staff but also to others such as firefighters, members of the coastguard, RNLI and NHS Blood Transfusion Service. It is in place to ensure that staff from emergency services can be left to undertake their work without being prevented from doing so by members of the public.

The coroner

HM Coroner holds office under the Crown although the post is paid for by the local authority. Appointees are usually from a legal background such as a lawyer but in some cases may also be a medical practitioner. Their role is to establish the facts related to the death of a person in certain circumstances; deaths are reported to the coroner when, for instance, the death was through an accident, during surgery or before recovery from an anaesthetic or where the death is unnatural, sudden and unexplained, or from a violent cause.

The coroner may require a postmortem examination and depending on the results of this may order an inquest. The inquest is likely to be called where the death was unnatural or violent, or if it occurred in prison or in police custody, or where after the postmortem the cause is still unclear.

Ambulance staff may be called to give evidence at a coroner's inquest. The purpose of the inquest is to establish the identity of the deceased, and the time and circumstances of the death. The coroner will examine under oath all those who provide evidence in relation to the case. Documentation and statements may be called upon. The witnesses may be questioned by legal representatives appointed by the family, for instance, or certain other interested persons who the coroner may notify to attend the inquest. It is important to remember that unlike a criminal or civil case, the court is not adversarial; in other words it is only to establish the facts surrounding the death of the person. Where there is a public interest or concern, on occasions a jury may be summoned. The coroner is in charge of the proceedings and determines the order of appearance of witnesses, etc.

Summary

- The structure of the legal system in the UK is composed of differing types of law.
- To safeguard against litigation, the paramedic must be knowledgeable of legal issues. The paramedic also must know about the effects of these issues.
- Paramedics and healthcare workers may be required by law to report some cases. This is known as disclosure and the rules relating to confidentiality allow for this.
- Legal claims that are related to patient care usually result from civil claims of negligence. This refers to the failure to act as a reasonable, prudent paramedic would act in such circumstances.
- Most legal authorities stress that protection against claims of negligence has three elements. The first is training. The second is competent patient care skills. The third is full documentation of all patient care activities.
- Confidential information is threefold. For the most part, confidential information includes any details about a patient that are related to the patient's history. Any assessment findings also are included. Any treatment

Summary—cont'd

given is included as well. Rules exist surrounding disclosure.

- A mentally competent adult (an adult with capacity) has the right to refuse medical care; this is the case even if the decision could result in death or permanent disability.
- A patient with capacity has certain rights. The patient has the right to decide what medical care (and transportation) to receive. This is a basic concept of law and medical practice.
- Legal responsibilities for the patient continue until patient care is transferred to another member of the healthcare system (or it is clear that the patient no longer requires care).
- Resuscitation issues that relate directly to EMS include withholding or stopping resuscitation, advance directives and recognition of life extinct.

References

1. Health Professions Council 2008 Standards of Conduct, Performance and Ethics. HPC, London
2. Office of the Public Guardian 2009 Making decisions: a guide for people who work in health and social care, 4th edition. OPG, London
3. Donoghue v. Stevenson [1932] AC 562
4. Bolam v Friern Barnet HMC [1957] 2 All ER 118
5. Cardoza B 1914 cited in Rumbold G 1999 Ethics in nursing practice, 3rd edition. Bailliere Tindall, Edinburgh
6. Dimond B 2005 Legal aspects of nursing, 4th edition. Pearson, Harlow
7. Department of Health 2003 Confidentiality; NHS Code of Practice. Department of Health, London
8. Department of Health 2006 The Caldicott Guardian Manual 2006. Department of Health, London

Further reading

British Medical Association, the Resuscitation Council (UK) and the Royal College of Nursing 2007 Decisions relating to cardiopulmonary resuscitation: a joint statement. Online. Available http://www.resus.org.uk/pages/dnar.pdf 16 January 2009

Department of Health 2001 Reference guide to consent for examination or treatment. Department of Health, London

Department of Health 2003 The NHS Confidentiality Code of Practice. Online. Available http://www.dh.gov.uk/en/Publicationsandstatistics/Publications/PublicationsPolicyAndGuidance/DH_4069253 16 January 2009

Department of Health 2008 NHS Caldicott Guardians. Online. Available http://www.dh.gov.uk/en/Managingyourorganisation/Informationpolicy/Patientconfidentialityandcaldicott guardians/DH_4100563 16 January 2009

Bolitho v. City and Hackney Health Authority [1997] 3 WLR 115.

Fitch J, Keller R, Raynor D et al 1993 JEMS management beyond the street, 2nd edition. JEMS, Carlsbad, CA

Health Professions Council 2007 Standards of Proficiency: Paramedics. HPC, London

Iserson K et al 1995 Ethics in emergency medicine, 2nd edition. Galen Press, Tucson, AZ

National Health Service Litigation Authority: Clinical Negligence Scheme for Trusts. Online. Available http://www.nhsla.com/Claims/Schemes/CNST/ 16 January 2009

Sanderson B 2002 History of ethics to 30 BC: ancient wisdom and folly. World Peace Communications, Santa Barbara, CA

Veatch R 1997 Medical ethics, 2nd edition. Jones and Bartlett, Sudbury, MA

CHAPTER 3

The Well-Being of the Paramedic, Health Promotion and Injury Prevention

Chapter contents

THE WELL-BEING OF THE PARAMEDIC

Objectives

Upon completion of this section, the paramedic student will be able to:

1. Describe the components of wellness and associated benefits.
2. Discuss the paramedic's role in promoting wellness.
3. Outline the benefits of specific lifestyle choices that promote wellness, including proper nutrition, weight control, exercise, sleep, and smoking cessation.
4. Identify risk factors and warning signs of cancer and cardiovascular disease.
5. Identify preventive measures to minimize the risk of work-related illness or injury associated with exposure, lifting and moving patients, hostile environments, vehicle operations, and rescue situations.
6. List signs and symptoms of addiction and addictive behaviour.
7. Distinguish between normal and abnormal anxiety and stress reactions.
8. Give examples of stress-reduction techniques.
9. Outline the 10 components of critical incident stress management.
10. Given a scenario involving death or dying, identify therapeutic actions you may take based on your knowledge of the dynamics of this process.
11. List measures to take to reduce the risk of infectious disease exposure.

12. Outline actions to be taken following a significant exposure to a patient's blood or other body fluids.

Key terms

addiction A compulsive, uncontrollable dependence on a substance, habit, or practice to such a degree that cessation causes severe emotional, mental, or physiological reactions.

adrenaline An endogenous adrenal hormone that helps prepare the body for energetic action.

anxiety A state or feeling of apprehension, uneasiness, agitation, uncertainty, or fear resulting from the anticipation of some threat or danger.

autonomic nervous system The part of the nervous system that regulates involuntary vital functions, including the activity of cardiac muscle, smooth muscle, and glands.

circadian rhythm A pattern based on a 24-hour cycle, especially repetition of certain physiological phenomena, such as sleeping and eating.

distress Negative, debilitating, or harmful stress.

eustress Positive, performance-enhancing stress.

stress A non-specific mental or physical strain caused by any emotional, physical, social, economic, or other factor that initiates a physiological response.

universal precautions Infection control practices in healthcare that are observed with every patient and procedure and that prevent exposure to blood-borne pathogens.

Wellness components

Wellness has two main aspects: physical well-being and mental and emotional health. Both aspects are key to the paramedic's ability to deliver emergency care safely and help the paramedic to manage stressful events that are a natural part of the profession.

Physical well-being

Several factors play a major role in maintaining physical health. These factors include good nutrition, physical fitness, ample sleep, and the prevention of disease and injury.

Nutrition

Nutrients are foods that hold the elements necessary for body function. The six categories of nutrients are carbohydrates, fats, proteins, vitamins, minerals, and water.

Carbohydrates are composed of carbon, hydrogen, and oxygen and are derived primarily from plant foods. The only important source of animal carbohydrates is lactose (milk sugar). Plants store carbohydrates as starch. All dietary fats contain a mixture of saturated and unsaturated fatty acids. Saturated fats are found mainly in meat and dairy products and in some vegetable fats. These fats raise the cholesterol levels in the blood by shutting down the process that normally removes excess cholesterol from the body. Unsaturated fats are subdivided further into polyunsaturated and monounsaturated fats. Polyunsaturated fats are found in safflower, sunflower, corn, soybean, and cottonseed oils and in some fish. These fats help rid the body of newly formed cholesterol. Omega-3 fatty acids are a form of polyunsaturated fats that are found mainly in cold-water fish such as tuna, salmon, and mackerel. All polyunsaturated fats, including the omega-3 fats, are considered important to human health. Monounsaturated fats are liquid vegetable oils such as olive oil. Like polyunsaturated fats, these may also decrease blood cholesterol levels (Box 3-1). Trans fats are unsaturated fatty acids formed when vegetable oils are processed and made more solid or into a more stable liquid. Trans fats are present in a wide range of foods, including most foods made

Box 3-1

Fat and cholesterol control

Tips for a healthy eating plan

- Select lean cuts of meat, such as loin and round cuts, and trim all visible fat.
- Buy lower-fat versions of your favourite dairy products, such as skim milk and skim milk–based cheeses.
- For added flavour, use herbs and spices in place of high-fat flavourings or sauces on vegetables, meats, poultry, and fish.
- Chill soups and stews and skim off the fat that collects on the surface.
- Choose low-fat or non-fat versions of your favourite salad dressings, mayonnaise, yogurt, and sour cream.
- Use low-fat or fat-free marinades to tenderize and add flavour to leaner cuts of meat.

Tips to reduce saturated fats

- Use polyunsaturated or monounsaturated oil when a recipe calls for melted shortening or butter.
- Use vegetable oil margarine in place of butter or lard. Look for whipped, lower-fat tub margarine.

Tips to be 'fat' smart

- Saturated fats usually are solid at room temperature. They mainly come from animal foods such as meat, poultry, butter, and whole milk. Coconut, palm, and palm kernel oils are also high in saturated fat. Saturated fat is responsible for raising blood cholesterol levels.
- Polyunsaturated fats usually are liquid at room temperature. They are found in vegetable oils. Safflower, sunflower, corn, and soybean oils contain the highest amounts of these polyunsaturated fats. Polyunsaturated fats can help decrease high blood cholesterol levels when part of a good diet.
- Monounsaturated fats also are liquid at room temperature. They are found in vegetable oils, such as canola and olive oil. Monounsaturated fats can help to decrease high blood cholesterol levels if they are part of a lower-fat diet.
- Dietary cholesterol comes only from animal sources such as the fat in dairy products, egg yolks, meats, poultry, and seafood. Vegetables, fruits, and grains do not contain cholesterol.
- Hydrogenation is a process that makes oil more solid at room temperature. Hydrogenated vegetable oils give some processed foods a longer shelf life. Examples of those foods include margarine and crackers.

From American Dietetic Association, National Center for Nutrition and Dietetics 1994 The ABCs of fats, oils, and cholesterol. American Dietetic Association, Chicago.

with partially hydrogenated oils, such as baked goods and fried foods, and some margarine products. Trans fats also occur naturally in low amounts in meats and dairy products. Although trans fats are unsaturated, they appear similar to saturated fats in terms of their effect on blood cholesterol levels.

Note

Cholesterol is present in all foods of animal origin and is concentrated heavily in fat and in poultry skin. Cholesterol is a white, waxy substance found in every cell and is needed by the body for normal functioning. Not all cholesterol is harmful; an adequate amount of cholesterol is needed for body functions. Cholesterol is manufactured in the liver and is carried through the bloodstream. Adding cholesterol to the diet can raise blood cholesterol levels and increase the risk of heart disease and stroke.

Proteins are made of hydrogen, oxygen, carbon, and nitrogen (and most contain sulphur and phosphorus). Proteins are vital to building body tissue during growth, maintenance, and repair. When proteins are digested, they break down into amino acids (classified as *essential* or *non-essential*). Essential amino acids are needed for body growth and cellular life and must be obtained in food because they are not made in the body. Non-essential amino acids are *not* needed for body health and growth and can be made in the body. Proteins that contain all the essential amino acids are complete proteins and are found in meats and dairy products. Proteins that are missing one or more essential amino acids are incomplete proteins (e.g. those in grains and vegetables). Proteins can be used as a source of energy but should be spared for their more important role in body health by the sufficient intake of carbohydrates.

Vitamins are organic substances that are present in minute amounts in foods. Because vitamins are crucial for metabolism and cannot be made in adequate amounts by the body, they must be gained through food or vitamin supplements. (An ample intake of vitamins through a balanced diet should make vitamin supplements unnecessary in healthy individuals.) Vitamins are water soluble or fat soluble. Vitamins C and B complex contain eight water-soluble vitamins; these water-soluble vitamins cannot be stored in the body so must come from the daily diet. Fat-soluble vitamins (vitamins A, D, E and K) can be stored in the body so a daily dietary intake of these vitamins is not required (Box 3-2).

Minerals are inorganic elements that occur naturally in the earth and play a key role in biochemical reactions in the body. Minerals include calcium, chromium, iron, magnesium, potassium, selenium, sodium, and zinc, and, like vitamins, minerals come from the diet (Table 3-1).

Note

Diseases caused by vitamin deficiency (e.g. scurvy, rickets or beriberi) are rare in the UK. Making proper food choices can help to prevent them.

Water is the most important nutrient because cellular function depends on a fluid environment. Water composes 50–60% of the total body weight. (Infants have the greatest percentage of body water; older adults have the least.) Water is obtained through consumption of liquids and fresh fruits and vegetables and is also produced when food is oxidized during digestion.

Box 3-2

Free radicals and antioxidants

Free radicals are natural by-products of chemical reactions in the body that can produce cellular injury. The build-up of these free radicals increases with age. The build-up is thought to be the cause of many diseases, including heart disease, diabetes, and some cancers. Substances that can generate free radicals can be found in fried foods, alcohol, tobacco smoke, pesticides, and air pollution. There are many other commonly encountered substances that may create oxygen free radicals.

Antioxidants are known as free-radical scavengers. They are compounds that reduce the formation of free radicals or react with and neutralize them, making them non-toxic to cells. Antioxidants occur naturally in the body. They also occur naturally in certain foods such as fruits, vegetables, and whole grains. Beta carotene (a form of vitamin A), and vitamins C and E are popular antioxidant supplements. These may benefit a person's health.

Dietary recommendations

Various healthcare groups make recommendations for a healthy diet. These groups include the Department of Health, the British Heart Foundation, and the Food Standards Agency. Further information can be found at http://www.eatwell.gov.uk/healthydiet/eatwellplate/

Critical Thinking

Does your average diet meet these guidelines? If not, in what areas do you need to make changes?

Principles of weight control

People who are overweight tend to be at higher risk for developing certain illnesses, including high blood pressure, diabetes mellitus, heart disease, and some cancers. The tenets of weight control are to eat the right balance of foods in moderation, limit fat consumption, and exercise regularly (Box 3-3).

Anyone committed to weight control for a healthier life should set realistic goals. For example, the general recommendation is a steady weight loss goal of 0.25–0.5 kg (½ to 1 lb) per week. A healthy lifestyle is balanced with proper nutrition and exercise. A healthy diet includes a variety of foods that are low in fat, saturated fat, and cholesterol, and plenty of grain products, vegetables, and fruit (Box 3-4). A diet should also be moderate in simple sugars, salt, and sodium. Alcoholic beverages should be avoided or consumed only in moderation. Finally, a system for checking weight control progress is essential. Adjustments and professional advice may sometimes be needed to achieve weight-control goals.

Table 3-1 The ABCs of nutrition

	Function	Source
VITAMINS		
A	Proper eye function; keeps skin, hair, and nails healthy; helps maintain healthy gums, glands, bones, teeth; helps ward off infection; may protect against lung cancer	Liver,* dairy products,* fish, carrots, yellow squash, dark-green leafy vegetables, corn, tomatoes, papaya
B_1 (thiamine)	Helps convert carbohydrates into biological energy; promotes proper nerve function	Pork,* unrefined and enriched cereals, organ meats,* legumes, nuts*
B_2 (riboflavin)	Crucial in the production of body energy	Milk,* cheese,* yogurt,* green leafy vegetables, fruits, bread, cereals, meats*
B_3 (niacin)	Lowers cholesterol levels in blood only in very high doses; may protect against cardiovascular disease	Yeast, meats* including liver,* cereals, legumes, seeds*
B_6	Essential for protein breakdown and absorption	Beef,* poultry,* fish, pork,* bananas, nuts,* whole grains, vegetables
B_{12}	Essential for the healthy function of nerve tissue	Meats,* meat products,* shellfish, fish, poultry,* eggs*
Biotin	Needed for breakdown of glucose (a type of sugar) and formation of certain fatty acids necessary for several important body functions	Meats,* poultry,* fish, eggs,* nuts,* seeds,* legumes, vegetables
C (ascorbic acid)	Strengthens blood vessel walls; keeps gums healthy; promotes healing of cuts and wounds	Strawberries, citrus fruits, tomatoes, cabbage, cauliflower, broccoli, greens
D	Helps build and maintain teeth and bones; needed for body to absorb calcium	Egg yolks,* fish and cod liver oil,* fortified milk and butter*
E	Helps form red blood cells, muscle tissue, and other tissues; may protect against heart disease	Poultry,* seafood, seeds,* nuts,* cooked greens, wheat germ, fortified cereals, eggs*
K†	Needed for normal clotting of blood	Spinach, broccoli, Brussels sprouts, kale, turnip greens
MINERALS		
Calcium	Helps build strong bones and teeth; promotes proper muscle and nerve function; helps blood to clot; helps activate enzymes needed to convert food to energy; may protect against the development of fragile, porous bones	Milk,* cheese,* yogurt,* buttermilk, other dairy products,* green leafy vegetables
Chromium	Works with insulin to maintain normal blood sugar	Whole-grain cereals, condiments (black pepper, thyme), meat products,* cheeses*
Iron	Essential to make haemoglobin, the oxygen-carrying component of red blood cells	Red meat* and liver,* shellfish and fish, legumes, dried apricots, fortified breads and cereals
Magnesium	Activates enzymes needed to release energy in body; promotes bone growth; needed to make cells and genetic material	Green leafy vegetables, beans, nuts,* fortified whole-grain cereals and breads, oysters, scallops
Potassium	With sodium, helps to regulate body's fluid balance; plays a major role in muscle contraction, nerve conduction, beating of the heart	Bananas, citrus fruits, dried fruits, deep yellow vegetables, potatoes, legumes, milk,* bran cereal
Selenium	Interacts with vitamin E to prevent breakdown of cells in body	Organ meats,* seafood, meats,* cereals and grains, egg yolks,* mushrooms, onions, garlic
Sodium	Helps maintain body fluid balance	Salt, processed foods, foods in brine, salted crackers and chips, cured meats, soy sauce (Note: sodium is so prevalent that low intake is very rare. The problem is avoiding excessive intake of sodium.)
Zinc	Boosts the immune system and helps fight disease; element in more than 100 enzymes—proteins that are essential to digestion and other functions	Red meats,* some seafood, grains

US Department of Agriculture's Center for Nutrition Policy and Promotion, Washington, DC www.usda.gov.
*These foods are high in fat and/or cholesterol. Use sparingly or substitute low-fat versions, where possible.
†Green leafy vegetables and other foods rich in vitamin K can contribute to blood clotting. If you take a drug that prevents blood clotting, talk to your physician before changing your diet.

Box 3-3

Getting a handle on fat

Eat foods that are less than 30% fat. Try to aim for no more than 3 g of fat per 100 calories, which provides about 27% of the total calories from fat. This is important for the following reasons:

- Each gram of fat has more than double the calories of a gram of protein or carbohydrates.
- The body uses fewer calories to store the fat as excess weight.
- In complex carbohydrates, 23% of the calories are burned to make them into a usable form in the body; only 3% of fat calories are burned before they are 'worn' on the hips or abdomen.
- Decreasing fat intake to less than 30% of daily calories helps reduce cholesterol, decreases risk of heart disease, helps with weight loss, and reduces risk of diabetes.

Fat content of various foods

- More than 90% fat: whipped cream, pork sausage, cooking oils, margarine, butter, gravy, mayonnaise
- More than 80% fat: spare ribs, cream cheese, salad dressing, high-fat steaks (T-bone, porterhouse, tenderloin, filet mignon)
- More than 70% fat: peanuts, hot dogs, pork chops, most cheeses and nuts, sirloin steak, bacon, lamb chops
- More than 60% fat: potato crisps, regular ground beef, ham, eggs
- More than 50% fat: round steak, pot roast, creamed soup, ice cream, sweet rolls
- More than 40% fat: whole milk, cake, doughnuts, French fries
- More than 30% fat: muffins, biscuits, fruit pies, low-fat milk, cottage cheese, tuna, chicken, turkey
- More than 20% fat: lean fish, beef liver, ice milk
- More than 10% fat: bread, pretzels, whole grains, legumes
- Less than 10% fat: sherbet, non-fat milk, most fruits and vegetables, baked potato

Box 3-4

Fibre

The human body requires fibre to maintain good health and to fight disease. Fibre (found only in plant foods) may be soluble or insoluble. Examples of soluble fibre include fibre obtained from peas, beans, oats, barley, and some fruits and vegetables. This type of fibre helps control the level of blood sugar. Soluble fibre may also lower the level of blood cholesterol. Insoluble fibre (found in whole grains and many vegetables) helps hold water in the colon and can reduce or prevent constipation. This type of fibre may also help prevent intestinal disease (e.g. diverticulosis, haemorrhoids and certain cancers). Many authorities recommend a dietary intake of 20–35 g of fibre each day.

Physical fitness

Physical fitness varies from person to person and may be described as a condition that helps persons look, feel, and do their best. Physical fitness is influenced by age, sex, heredity, personal habits, exercise and eating habits. Being physically fit offers many benefits, which include the following:

- decreased resting heart rate and blood pressure
- increased oxygen-carrying capacity
- enhanced quality of life
- increased muscle mass and metabolism
- increased resistance to injury

Box 3-5

The body mass index

The body mass index (BMI) is a widely used measurement of body fat that corrects for height. The BMI is the only body fat index that conveys the risk of disease or death. A healthy BMI is 19 to 25. A BMI of 25 to 29 indicates 'moderately overweight.' A BMI of 30 or more indicates 'severely overweight.' To calculate your BMI, use the following formula:

$$\text{BMI} = \frac{\text{Weight in kilograms}}{(\text{height in metres})^2}$$

For example: a person weighing 70 kg with a height of 1.70 m

$$\text{BMI} = \frac{70}{(1.7 \times 1.7)} = \frac{70}{2.89}$$

BMI = 24.2 so fall within the normal category

A BMI calculator is available online at http://www.nhs.uk/Tools/Pages/Healthyweightcalculator.aspx?r=18rtitle=Interactive+tools+-+BMI+tool

- improved personal appearance and self-image
- maintenance of motor skills throughout life.

Cardiovascular endurance

A physical examination or fitness assessment should be carried out before undertaking an exercise regimen for the first time. These can be carried out by a physician or a certified physical trainer respectively. The purpose of these assessments is to evaluate a person's present physical condition and to create baseline assessments for weight, including body mass index (Box 3-5); high blood pressure; heart trouble (including family history); arthritis or other bone problems; muscular, ligament, or tendon problems; and other known or suspected diseases. These assessments help to establish a heart rate target zone as well. This is a measure used to improve cardiovascular endurance through exercise. Ideally, the heart rate target zone should be maintained during exercise for 20 minutes to increase cardiovascular endurance.

Critical Thinking

Calculate your body mass index. Does it fall within the recommendations?

Note

There is a simple way to determine the heart rate target zone. First, calculate the maximum heart rate by subtracting the person's age in years from 220. Then, calculate the lower and upper limits of the target heart rate by multiplying this number by 60% and 80%, respectively.

Example for a 25-year-old:

Maximum heart rate (220 − 25) = 195 beats/min
Lower limit = 195 × 60% = 117 beats/min
Upper limit = 195 × 80% = 156 beats/min

Muscle strength

Another part of the fitness assessment tests muscular strength and endurance. Muscular strength is the ability of a muscle to exert force for a brief period, whilst muscle endurance is the ability of a muscle or a group of muscles to sustain repeated contractions or to continue applying force against a fixed object. Many exercises improve muscle strength and endurance.

The tenets of training for muscle strength and endurance should consider isometric and isotonic exercises, resistance, repetitions, sets, and frequency. *Isometric* exercises are those that do not result in any movement of a joint. An example of this is a contraction performed against an immovable object such as a wall or door frame. These exercises do not increase muscle bulk very much. However, they do strengthen the muscle at the joint angle at which the contraction is performed. *Isotonic* exercises move a joint through a range of motion against resistance of a fixed weight. An example of this is lifting a barbell. These exercises add muscle bulk by creating tension within the muscle. *Resistance* refers to the amount of weight moved or lifted during isotonic exercises. A *repetition* ('rep') refers to the full execution of an exercise from start to finish. A *set* is the number of times an exercise (rep) is done start to finish, one after another, without any rest time. *Frequency* refers to the least number of workouts that will have a positive effect on muscle strength and endurance.

Muscular flexibility

Flexibility refers to the ability to move joints and use muscles through their full range of motion. The fitness assessment tests flexibility in several ways. A lack of normal flexibility may lead to muscle strains and other injuries.

Muscular flexibility can be improved by stretching exercises. These exercises must be done slowly, without a bouncing motion and the intensity should be mild. A person should not strain or hold the breath and should feel no pain or discomfort. How often these exercises are done should match an individual's specific level of activity. For example, if daily work on an ambulance requires lifting patients, then regular stretching exercises specific to the paramedic's arms, back, thighs, calves, and hips would help.

Critical Thinking

How many minutes per week do you perform physical activities that raise your heart rate? What benefits does a paramedic gain by maintaining a high level of personal fitness?

The importance of sleep

Sleep plays an important role in being physically fit because it helps to rejuvenate a tired body. The average adult needs 7 to 8 hours of sleep each day. In emergency medical services (EMS), where rotating shifts and 24-hour work shifts are common, sleep deprivation may occur and interrupt the normal circadian rhythm.

Circadian is Latin for 'about a day'. The circadian rhythm is the physiological ebb and flow of the body as it relates to the rotation of the earth. This timing system is based roughly on the solar day as the earth rotates in its course around the sun. For example, a person gets hungry or tired, energetic or moody, at fairly set times each day as the body systems change. The level of melatonin and cortisol affects the periods of sleepiness and wakefulness. Release of these hormones is stimulated by the dark and is suppressed by light. Thus when the line between night and day is disrupted on an ongoing basis (e.g. working rotating work shifts or responding to emergency calls in the early morning hours during a 24-hour shift), irritability, depression, and illness can result (Box 3-6). Research is under way to help shift workers and their employers modify work schedules so that changes in normal biorhythms will have the least adverse effects on employee health and productivity.

Box 3-6

Getting your Zs

Working nights, 24-hour shifts, and rotating shifts can inhibit getting enough rest. The following are some helpful tips:

- Allow some time to unwind and relax before trying to go to sleep.
- Consider exercise before sleeping as a way to reduce stress.
- Avoid stimulants (e.g. caffeine in coffee, fizzy pop, tea, and chocolate) during the last few hours of your work shift.
- Eat simple carbohydrates (e.g. biscuits or candy bar) to release serotonin (a hormone that may help induce sleep).
- Keep your sleeping area cool and dark so that your body will think it is night-time.
- Make sure your family and friends know about your work shifts and your sleeping schedule to minimize interruptions.
- Try to maintain a 'normal' period of dedicated sleep time each day.
- Consult a physician about your sleep difficulties when needed.

Critical Thinking

Do you get enough sleep? If not, which of the above strategies should you try in an attempt to increase your hours of sleep?

Note

The circadian rhythm causes the jet lag that occurs during air travel to a distant time zone. Studies suggest that the symptoms of jet lag may be relieved by the administration of melatonin.

Disease prevention

A paramedic can do a lot to help prevent serious personal illness. As healthcare professionals, paramedics must serve as role models in helping to prevent disease.

Cardiovascular disease

This disease accounts for more than 110 000 deaths each year in the UK.[1] For most people, cardiovascular disease can be altered through living a healthy life. Boosting cardiovascular endurance can help to prevent this disease but other steps also are needed in the fight. These steps include the following:

Box 3-7

Understanding the cholesterol numbers

Cholesterol moves through the body attached to various sizes of fat-carrying proteins called lipoproteins. Low-density lipoproteins (LDLs) are more common and are thought to carry cholesterol to the cells where they can promote blood vessel disease. Smaller high-density lipoproteins (HDLs) are thought to carry cholesterol to the liver. They may help prevent or slow down blood vessel disease. Very low-density lipoproteins are made mostly of triglycerides (the main fatty substance in the fluid portion of blood) that are absorbed by the intestines and therefore are affected by fasting.

Total cholesterol

Low risk:	less than 5.18 mmol/L
Borderline high:	5.18–6.19 mmol/L
Higher risk:	6.20 mmol/L and above

LDL cholesterol: the 'bad' cholesterol

Optimal:	less than 2.59 mmol/L
Near optimal:	2.60–3.34 mmol/L
Borderline high:	3.35–4.11 mmol/L
High:	4.12–4.89 mmol/L
Very high:	4.90 mmol/L and above

HDL cholesterol: the 'good' cholesterol

At risk:	less than 1.03 mmol/L
Borderline:	1.03–1.52 mmol/L
Optimal:	1.53 mmol/L and above

Triglycerides

Normal:	less than 1.69 mmol/L
Borderline high:	1.70–2.24 mmol/L
High:	2.25–5.63 mmol/L
Very high:	5.64 mmol/L and above

- eliminating cigarette smoking
- controlling high blood pressure
- maintaining a favourable body fat composition through regular exercise
- maintaining a good total cholesterol/high-density lipoprotein ratio (Box 3-7)
- monitoring triglyceride levels
- controlling diabetes
- avoiding excessive alcohol intake
- eating healthy foods
- reducing stress
- obtaining risk assessments periodically.

Cancer

The term *cancer* includes more than 100 diseases affecting nearly every part of the body. All these diseases are potentially life threatening. The main cause of all cancer is a change or mutation in the nucleus of a cell. Most common cancers are linked to one of three environmental risk factors: smoking, sunlight or diet. Dietary factors are associated with some cancers of the gastrointestinal tract and may be linked to others, such as cancer of the breast, prostate, or uterus. A lack of dietary fibre is believed to be a risk factor for these cancers. Steps in preventing cancer include the following:

Box 3-8

The seven warning signs of cancer (CAUTION) as designated by the American Cancer Society

- *C*hange in bowel or bladder habits
- *A* sore throat that does not heal
- *U*nusual bleeding or discharge
- *T*hickening or lump in the breast or elsewhere
- *I*ndigestion or difficulty swallowing
- *O*bvious change in a wart or mole
- *N*agging cough or hoarseness

See also http://info.cancerresearchuk.org/

- elimination of smoking
- dietary changes
- limitation of sun exposure; use of sunscreen
- regular physical examinations
- attention to the warning signs (Box 3-8)
- periodic risk assessment.

Infectious disease

Most infectious diseases can be avoided by doing two things. The first is practising good personal hygiene, including hand washing. The second is following universal precautions and other guidelines in the workplace. These guidelines are established by the Health Protection Agency, the Health and Safety Executive, the Ambulance Trust, and others.

At a minimum, personal protective equipment to guard against the spread of infectious diseases should include the following:

- disposable gloves when contact with blood or other body fluids is likely
- masks and protective eye wear when blood splashing is likely to occur
- gowns to protect clothing from spurting blood (e.g. during emergency childbirth)
- HEPA (high-efficiency particulate air filter) and N-95 respirators when tuberculosis is confirmed or suspected.

A potential exposure to an infectious disease may occur. When exposure occurs, the paramedic should report it as soon as possible to the receiving hospital and to the designated officer in the employing Trust (or private company). That way, an exchange between the hospital and the ambulance service can be set up (see Chapter 24). To defend against such diseases, the Occupational Health Department may have provisions that require that a periodic risk assessment be offered to staff. This may include regular testing for diseases such as tuberculosis and also testing for vaccinations for diseases such as hepatitis B.

Injury prevention

The number of injuries that occur whilst at work can be reduced by knowledge of proper body mechanics during lifting and moving, and by staying alert for hostile settings. A paramedic must prioritize personal safety during rescue situations. Finally, one must practise safe vehicle operations and use safety equipment and supplies.

Box 3-9

Prevention and rehabilitation of low back pain

The back is a complex system of ligaments, muscles, bones, nerves, and intervertebral disks. All of these parts can be injured by improper lifting techniques. Emergency medical services workers are highly vulnerable to low back pain and injury. An area of the back that is often a source of low back pain and injury is lordosis (an inward curvature in the lumbar spine that is normally present to some degree). Abnormal curvature in this area can result from poor posture and from being overweight with associated weak abdominal muscles. Back injury can be prevented or lessened to a significant degree by being physically fit, performing regular stretching exercises, and following some general rules of lifting:

1. Know the weight (ask the patient's weight if you can, and add the weight of the equipment). Two persons should work together to lift objects that weigh more than 27 kg (60 lb).
2. Know your physical ability and limitations.
3. Keep your back positioned with a normal curvature.
4. Use your legs and abdominal muscles to support the weight; use your back muscles to maintain balance.
5. Keep the weight close to your body.
6. Communicate clearly and frequently with your partner.

If back pain or injury occurs when lifting, pushing, pulling, or stretching, tell a supervisor as soon as possible. Treatment for back pain usually begins with rest and ice or cold packs to lessen swelling. Treatment can also include analgesia and muscle relaxants. A rehabilitation programme will usually follow the injury and may include exercises to improve abdominal muscle strength. The exercises also help to improve the control of the pelvis and flexibility of the lower back.

From EMT 1991 Injury free. Ferno-Washington, Wilmington, OH, with permission.

Body mechanics during lifting and moving

Proper body mechanics during lifting and moving are crucial. They help to avoid personal injury and to avoid injury to a partner or patient (Box 3-9). The paramedic should consider the following guidelines when lifting and moving patients or equipment:

- Only move patients that you can handle safely; get additional help if needed.
- Look where you are walking or crawling.
- Move forward rather than backward when possible.
- Take short steps, if walking.
- Bend at the hips and knees.
- Lift with the legs, not the back.
- Keep the load close to the body.
- Keep the patient's body in line when moving.

Hostile environments

Paramedics may not be able to avoid being placed in hostile situations, which may threaten one's personal safety. When these situations occur, paramedics should do the following:

- Carefully check the scene for safety concerns and do not enter the scene until it is safe.
- Coordinate all actions with law enforcement personnel.
- Follow protocols for establishing a medical incident command.
- Plan entrance and escape routes.
- Above all, stay alert and be prepared for the unexpected.

Safely managing a violent scene requires special training and calls for unity among many emergency response agencies. As members of the response team, paramedics should take part in planning, training and practice sessions. These sessions help to ensure provider safety in hostile settings (see Chapter 44).

Rescue situations

Many personal safety issues arise in the case of rescue. Examples include exposure to hazardous materials, bad weather, extremes in temperature, fire, toxic gases, unstable structures, heavy equipment, road hazards, and sharp edges and fragments. For every rescue response the key is to assess the scene for hazards first and to take personal protective measures. In addition, the scene should be monitored constantly during the operation. A safe rescue requires proper use of protective gear, special training, and safe rescue practices (see Chapter 43).

Safe vehicle operation

Safe operation of all vehicles is essential. Many factors affect safe vehicle operations, including the following:

- safe driving of the vehicle
- safe and appropriate use of escorts to and from emergency scenes
- adverse environmental conditions (e.g. inclement weather)
- appropriate use of audible and visual warning devices
- proceeding through junctions safely
- parking at the emergency scene
- maintaining due regard for the safety of all others.

Critical Thinking

Is there any patient situation that would call for using unsafe vehicle operations? Keep in mind that this could risk the safety of those in the ambulance or in other vehicles.

All UK ambulance services require their employees to take a specialized driver training programme, which allows EMS providers to implement a systematic approach to driving in a safe and controlled setting.

Safety equipment and supplies

Correct use of safety equipment and supplies is key to injury prevention for EMS providers. Standards for protective clothing and equipment are required by the Health and Safety Executive. These standards help to ensure employee safety (see Chapter 43). Safety equipment and supplies include the following:

- body substance isolation equipment
- head protection
- eye protection

- hearing protection
- respiratory protection
- gloves
- boots
- coveralls
- turnout coat and pants
- specialty equipment
- reflective clothing.

Mental and emotional health

Many factors play a role in mental and emotional health. An important factor is to be aware of warning signs that could signal a potential problem (e.g. signs of substance misuse and health disorders caused by anxiety and stress). Also key to maintaining good emotional health is realizing the value of having personal time; being connected with family, peers, and the community; and accepting the personal differences that make individuals unique.

Substance misuse and abuse control

The misuse and abuse of drugs and other substances may lead to chemical dependency (addiction). Such dependency may have a wide range of effects on physical and mental health (Box 3-10). Warning signs of addiction and addictive behaviour include the following:

- using a substance to relieve tension
- using an increasing amount of the substance
- lying about using the substance
- experiencing guilt about using the substance
- avoiding discussion about using the substance
- experiencing interference with daily activities as a result of substance abuse.

Box 3-10

Common drugs and substances that are misused or abused

- Alcohol
- Central nervous system stimulants (e.g. cocaine and amphetamines)
- Cigarettes and other tobacco products
- Hallucinogens
- Inhalants
- Marijuana
- Narcotics and related drugs
- Sedative-hypnotics
- Tranquillzers
- Sedatives
- Appetite suppressants
- Laxatives
- Cough and cold preparations
- Nasal sprays
- Analgesics

Critical Thinking

Do you know anyone with these behaviours?

Methods used to manage substance abuse depend on the type of substance being misused. Substance misuse or abuse control may call for professional counselling. Physician-controlled drug therapy and support programmes may also be necessary.

Smoking cessation

Cigarette smoking is a major health hazard. Smoking is responsible for more than 106 000 deaths each year in the UK.[2] The health ramifications of cigarette smoking are numerous, including an increased risk of:

- coronary heart disease
- myocardial infarction
- chronic obstructive pulmonary disease
- sudden death
- dying from a variety of diseases
- miscarriage, premature birth, and birth defects.

Smokers may name many reasons for continuing to smoke, including peer pressure, relief of stress, weight control, and others. Regardless, most people continue to smoke because of the addictive nature of nicotine. Nicotine is the stimulant in tobacco, but there are other harmful chemicals including hydrocarbons (tar) and carbon monoxide. Exposure to these chemicals is also considered a health hazard for non-smokers. Non-smokers have an increased risk of developing smoking-related illnesses through 'passive smoking'.

Many resources and smoking cessation programmes are available to those who want to quit smoking. Support groups and quit smoking campaigns are sponsored by the National Health Service and UK charities, Government health agencies, and local healthcare organizations. Other methods that may be used alone or with these programmes include the use of prescription and non-prescription drugs such as dermal patches and nicotine chewing gum. These products decrease the physical effects of smoking cessation. In a sense, they help to wean the smoker off nicotine (Box 3-11).

Anxiety and stress

Anxiety can be defined as the worry or dread about future uncertainties. *Stress* can result from the interaction of events that cause anxiety and the coping abilities of the person. Stress can be positive (described later in this chapter) although is usually thought of as having a negative effect (e.g. fear, depression, and guilt). Recognizing and coping with anxiety and stress is important for a lasting career in the EMS profession.

Personal time for meditation and contemplation

Setting aside some personal time can boost mental and perhaps even physical health. This time can be spent meditating or contemplating. *Meditation* is a form of relaxation. To meditate, a person limits his or her awareness to a

Box 3-11

Body changes when you stop smoking

Within 20 minutes of your last cigarette

- Pulse and blood pressure drop to normal.
- Body temperature of hands and feet increases to normal.

Within 8 hours of your last cigarette

- Carbon monoxide level in blood drops to normal.
- Oxygen level in blood increases to normal.

Within 24 hours of your last cigarette

- Chance of heart attack decreases.

Within 48 hours of your last cigarette

- Nerve endings begin to regenerate.
- Ability to smell and taste is enhanced.

Within 72 hours of your last cigarette

- Bronchial tubes relax, making breathing easier.
- Lung capacity increases.

Within 2 weeks to 3 months after your last cigarette

- Circulation improves.
- Walking becomes easier.
- Lung function increases up to 30%.

Within 1–9 months after your last cigarette

- Coughing, sinus congestion, fatigue, and shortness of breath decrease.
- Cilia re-grow in lungs, increasing the ability to handle mucus, clean the lungs, and reduce infection.

Within 5 years of your last cigarette

- Lung cancer death rate for the average smoker (one pack per day) decreases.

Within 10 years of your last cigarette

- Lung cancer death rate drops to 12 deaths per 100 000 – almost the rate of non-smokers.
- Precancerous cells are replaced.
- Risk for other cancers – such as those of the mouth, larynx, oesophagus, bladder, kidney, and pancreas – decreases (20 chemicals in tobacco smoke cause cancer).

From http://www.cancer.org/docroot/SPC_1 when smokers_quit.asp

repeated or constant focus. The person may focus on something that holds some attraction (e.g. controlled breathing, a pleasant site, fragrance, or a mantra). This quiet time provides an uninterrupted period for thoughtful introspection (contemplation) of important things in a person's life. Most who practise meditation do so once or twice a day for 10 to 20 minutes.

Note

Spirituality is a unique quality of human existence. Spirituality should not be overlooked as a means for some to achieve mental and physical well-being.

Family, peer and community connections

Belonging to a group can affect a person's motivation and performance in a positive way. People tend to associate with others most like themselves such as family members, coworkers, and members of community and religious organizations. These groups provide a connection with others who share similar values and interests. As a rule, these bonds are healthy and raise self-esteem, and provide a way for one to contribute to group activities and goals. They also allow people to interact in decision making, communication, and cooperative work.

Freedom from prejudice

Accepting cultural differences gives people the chance to learn about other cultures. Such acceptance also helps them to see cultural variations in a positive light. Moreover, one affirms the values of these differences. Of the British population 7.9% are from an ethnic minority group.[3] The major ethnic minority groups are Asian or Asian British (Indian, Pakistani and Bangladeshi), Black or Black British (Black Caribbean and Black African), and Chinese. Many Europeans have also settled in the UK, especially members of the Polish community, although numbers tend to fluctuate. Providing healthcare to patients of some cultures may call for special communication skills and may require some further education to understand the customs and beliefs of that culture. Getting this education can be fulfilling and worthwhile, and it allows the paramedic to see life from another viewpoint.

Stress

As previously stated, stress can be positive and negative. The responses to stress may be physical, emotional, or both. 'Good' stress (eustress) is a positive response to stimuli and is considered protective. 'Bad' stress (distress) is a negative response to environmental stimuli and provides the source of anxiety and stress-related disorders.

Phases of the stress response

Hans Selye was an Austrian-born professor at the University of Montreal. He coined the term *stress* in its medical usage in 1950. The three stages of the stress response he found are the alarm reaction, resistance, and exhaustion (Figure 3-1).[4] Selye called these phases the general adaption syndrome. He gave them this name to describe the attempt of body and mind to deal with stressful events.

Alarm reaction

The human body can prepare itself quickly to do battle or run from danger. This fight-or-flight reaction occurs when a situation threatens one's safety or comfort. This reaction is considered positive (eustress). The stress prepares individuals to be alert and to defend themselves. At first, the response of the body to stress is unaffected by the type of situation. The body reacts equally to events that are pleasant or unpleasant, dangerous or exciting, happy or sad. The purpose of the response is to rapidly achieve top physical preparedness to cope with the event. Examples would be an

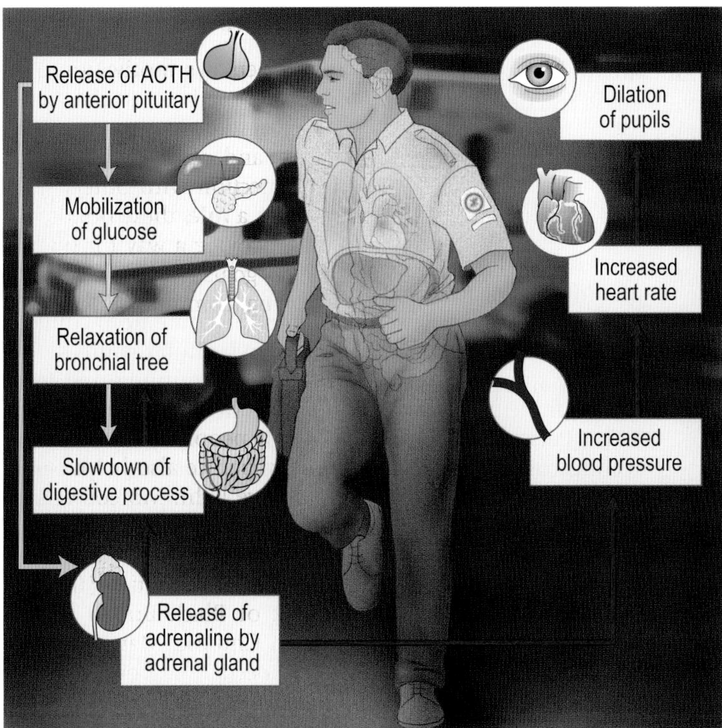

Figure 3-1 Physiological response to stress. During the alarm reaction, the release of adrenocorticotropic hormone (yellow) results in a sympathetic discharge of adrenaline (red). These stress hormones stimulate glucose production and cause the heart rate to increase, blood pressure to rise, and pupils to dilate. The bronchial tree relaxes for deep breathing, the digestive process slows, and the blood supply shifts to accommodate clotting mechanisms in case the body is wounded.

argument with a coworker, performing an unfamiliar patient care procedure, and taking part in the delivery of a healthy infant.

The alarm reaction is set off by the autonomic nervous system. This reaction is coordinated by the hypothalamus, which triggers the pituitary gland to release adrenocorticotropic hormone into the bloodstream. This stress hormone stimulates the production of glucose. The hormone also increases the concentration of nutrients in the blood that provide energy. Adrenocorticotropic hormone also activates the adrenal glands for an intense sympathetic discharge of adrenaline and noradrenaline. These hormones cause the heart rate to increase, blood pressure to rise, and the pupils of the eyes to dilate, which improves vision. Together these hormones relax the bronchial tree for deeper breathing, increase blood sugar for total energy, slow the digestive process, and shift blood supply to accommodate the clotting mechanism in case the body is wounded. After these physiological events, the body is ready for an emergency (fight or flight). The body can perform feats of strength and endurance far beyond its normal capacity. The alarm reaction takes only seconds. The reaction occurs to some extent at the first exposure of the body to a stressor. When the body realizes that an event is not dangerous or does not require the alarm reaction, the response stops. The individual begins to adapt to the situation and bodily functions return to normal.

Resistance

The stress response raises the level of resistance to the agent that provoked it and others like it. That is, if a particular stress persists long enough, a person's reactions change. For example, a paramedic becomes accustomed to responding to emergency scenes in an ambulance using audible and visual warning devices. Thus the alarm reaction that once occurred is no longer elicited. Therefore reactions to stressors may change over time.

Exhaustion

As stress continues, coping mechanisms weaken and resistance fails. For example, paramedics may appear to be unaffected by the stress of life-threatening emergencies yet all of their adaptive resources have been used to reach this stage of resistance. When any reservoir of adaptive resources no longer exists, resistance to other types of stress tends to decline as well. At that point, the body may become at risk for physical and psychological ills. Rest and recovery are usually needed before a person is ready for another emergency.

Factors that trigger the stress response

Each person has unique means to deal with stressful situations. Individual reactions to stress are customized based on previous exposure to a specific type of stress, perception of the stressful event, and personal coping skills. Many factors can trigger the stress response. Examples include the following:

- loss of something that is of value
- injury or threat of injury
- poor health or nutrition
- frustration
- ineffective coping skills.

Physiological and psychological effects of stress

Anxiety is a common symptom of stress. Feeling anxious in certain situations or unusual circumstances is normal and healthy and provides a warning system that protects people from being overwhelmed by a sudden stimulation. Anxiety also prepares persons for action in critical situations. This adaptive response to stress prepares the paramedic to make quick, correct decisions regarding the emergency. Anxiety also allows the paramedic to perform at maximal efficiency.

Sometimes stress is not reduced by a solution to the conflict or emergency, which may lead to an ongoing state of vigilance and alertness beyond the initial event. The paramedic may then begin to feel chronic anxiety. This kind of anxiety fails to stimulate effective coping. In addition, a person may respond to conflict or stress by anxious behaviour alone. Anxiety interferes with thought processes and with relationships and work performance. A person may develop problems concentrating, lose the ability to trust others, or become isolated or withdrawn.

Individuals who are often exposed to stressful situations or who are unable to cope with stressful events may experience a chronic state of anxiety. This state may lead to physical, emotional, cognitive, and behavioural effects (Box 3-12). Some warning signs, such as chest pain and difficulty breathing, may call for immediate evaluation and medical care. Others call for less immediate action. The presence of one or more warning signs is an indicator of distress although absence of warning signs does not preclude the chance of a stress reaction.

Box 3-12

Warning signs and symptoms of stress

Physical

- Cardiac rhythm disturbances
- Chest pain
- Difficulty breathing
- Nausea
- Profuse sweating
- Sleep disturbances
- Vomiting

Emotional

- Anger
- Denial
- Fear
- Feeling of being overwhelmed
- Inappropriate emotions
- Panic reactions

Cognitive

- Confusion
- Decreased level of awareness
- Difficulty making decisions
- Disorientation
- Distressing dreams
- Memory problems
- Poor concentration

Behavioural

- Changes in eating habits
- Crying spells
- Excessive silence
- Hyperactivity
- Increased alcohol consumption
- Increased smoking
- Withdrawal

Causes of stress in EMS

A variety of sources can produce stress in EMS work. Environmental stress includes noise, bad weather, confined spaces, poor lighting, spectators, rapid response to the scene, and life-and-death decision making. Psychosocial stress may arise from family relationships and can come from conflicts with coworkers, abusive patients, and similar sources. Personality stress relates to the way a person thinks and feels. For example, this kind of stress can include the need to be liked. Personality stress can include one's expectations and feelings of guilt and anxiety as well. Choosing a career in EMS requires developing an understanding of job-related stress and effective stress management.

Reactions to stress

Certain types of people may be attracted to certain types of careers. For example, some believe that EMS providers, firefighters, police officers, and others in public safety are inclined to stressful and demanding jobs.[5] However, no one is free from all conflict in managing stress.

Adaptation

Adaptation is a process that involves learning ways to deal with stressful situations. This process usually begins with using defence mechanisms. Next, adaptation focuses on developing coping skills, followed by problem solving. Finally, adaptation concludes with mastery.

Defence mechanisms are adaptive functions of the personality that assist a person to adjust to stressful situations. They also help a person to avoid dealing with problems. *Denial,* for example, is a defence mechanism that might be used to separate a person from the event long enough to deal with a problem that normally would be overwhelming.

Coping is an active process of confronting. Coping involves gathering information and using the information to change or adjust to a new situation. Taking part in regular physical activity is a great way to cope. Finding humour in personal crises and talking though stressful events with family, friends, and coworkers can be helpful.

People may also use harmful or negative coping mechanisms. An individual may become withdrawn or use alcohol or other drugs. Some may have angry outbursts toward family members and coworkers whilst others become silent. These negative coping mechanisms threaten interpersonal relationships with coworkers and loved ones, and should be seen as signs that an individual is having trouble dealing with stress.

Note

Burnout can be the result of cumulative stress. Burnout is defined by physical and emotional exhaustion and negative attitudes. It can develop when one is exposed to chronic stress that cannot be managed with usual coping mechanisms.

Problem solving involves analysing a problem and finding options to deal with the issue now and in the future. Problem solving allows a person to identify the problem clearly and come up with a course of action. This is a healthy approach to everyday concerns.

Mastery refers to the ability to see many options and solutions for problem situations. Mastery results from extensive experience and the use of effective coping mechanisms with situations that are similar. Mastery may be difficult to achieve.

Stress management techniques

To manage stress well, a person must recognize the early warning signs of anxiety. Some of the physical effects of anxiety an individual may notice include the following:

- heart palpitations
- difficult or rapid breathing
- dry mouth
- chest tightness or pain
- anorexia (lack of appetite), nausea, vomiting, diarrhoea, abdominal cramps, flatulence, 'butterflies'
- flushing, diaphoresis (profuse sweating), body temperature fluctuation
- urgency and frequency in urination
- dysmenorrhoea (painful menstruation), decreased sexual drive or performance
- aching muscles, joints.

Physical effects that may not be as noticeable include the following:

- increased blood pressure and heart rate
- blood shunting (diversion of the flow) to muscles
- increased blood glucose levels
- increased adrenaline production by adrenal glands
- reduced gastrointestinal peristalsis
- pupillary dilation.

Many warning signs appear during the emergency response or within 24 hours after the event. Some responses may be delayed for some time and may not appear for months or years after the event. If signs and symptoms of stress-related illness appear, the person should seek appropriate medical or psychological help.

Intervening to relieve stress is as key as recognizing the warning signals. Methods one may initially use to manage stress include reframing, controlled breathing, progressive relaxation, and guided imagery. All of these methods require practice to perform them properly. Reframing involves first looking at the situation from a different emotional viewpoint and then placing it in a different 'frame' that fits the facts of another situation equally well. This acts to change the meaning of the situation. Controlled breathing is a natural stress control technique whereby a person concentrates on depth and rate of breathing to achieve a calming effect. Controlled breathing may begin with deep breathing, followed by less deep breathing, and finally normal breathing. Progressive relaxation is a stress reduction strategy in which the person systematically tightens and relaxes particular muscle groups (from head to toe or toe to head). This fools the brain into initiating muscle relaxation throughout the body. Guided imagery is used with meditation. Another person familiar with the technique acts as a guide during a stress response. The person experiencing stress can then focus on an image that helps relieve stress. (Once guided imagery is learned, a person can use the technique without prompting.)

Other ways to fight stress include being aware of personal limitations, peer counselling, and group discussions. Proper diet, sleep, and rest also help to relieve stress. In addition, pursuing positive activities outside of EMS can balance work and recreation. Ultimately, the individual must maintain personal health and well-being. However, intervention programmes may be available through EMS agencies, hospitals, and other groups.

Critical incident debrief

Most ambulance services will have facility for critical incident debriefing. This aims to help emergency workers to understand their reactions and reassures them that what they are feeling is normal. It also reassures them that what they are feeling may be common to others involved in the emergency. The debrief may involve individuals, various members of the emergency team, or multidisciplinary agencies – e.g. firefighters, police and emergency department staff (Boxes 3-13 and 3-14).

Box 3-13

Potential situations for critical incident debriefing

- Line-of-duty injury or death
- Disaster
- Emergency worker suicide
- Infant/child death
- Extreme threat to emergency worker
- Prolonged incident that ends in loss or success
- Victims known to operations personnel
- Death/injury of civilian caused by operations
- Other significant event

Box 3-14

Techniques for reducing crisis-induced stress

- Allow adequate rest for emergency workers
- Provide food and fluid replacement
- Limit exposure to the incident
- Change assignments
- Provide post-event defusing/debriefing

Note

Defusing usually takes place within 8 hours after an event to allow an initial release of feelings. This also provides an opportunity for people to share their experiences. Defusing is an informal gathering of the people involved in the event and two-person teams trained in critical incident debrief management who are also peers. Defusing usually lasts less than 1 hour.

Debriefing is more formal than defusing. Debriefing is conducted in a private setting and usually takes place 24 to 72 hours after the event. The debriefing is conducted by a specially trained critical incident stress management team of other emergency services personnel and mental health workers. Only those present at the incident are allowed to attend a debriefing.

Critical Thinking

Imagine which type of call would be a critical incident for you personally.

Dealing with death, dying, grief and loss

Death and dying will always be part of healthcare delivery. Medical science has given society the ability to postpone death in some instances and perhaps lessen its physical pain but the fight for self-preservation is still inevitably lost.

Patient and family needs

In the delivery of EMS, paramedics will inevitably provide care to a dying person surrounded by loved ones. In such cases, the emotional needs of the dying patient, family, and loved ones should be of utmost importance. The patient and significant others will need to be comforted, given privacy, and treated with respect and dignity. Loved ones may need to express feelings of rage, anger, despair, and guilt. They may need the paramedic to provide control and direction for this solemn event. The paramedic's role in these cases is important and may be a determining factor in the way survivors adjust to their loss.

Stages of the grieving process

In 1968 Elizabeth Kübler-Ross began her work on the psychological aspects of death and dying. Her studies identified five predictable stages of dying: denial, anger, bargaining, depression, and acceptance. Kübler-Ross found that patients and loved ones dealing with the death process generally experience the following five stages:[6]

1. *Denial* is characterized by the feeling 'No, not me'. Denial is an expected response to news of a life-threatening illness or situation. The patient seeks other opinions, verifies the accuracy of medical reports, or simply seems to ignore what he or she has been told. It is a valuable defence mechanism and is troubling only when no indication exists that the patient understands the seriousness of the situation. Most patients, families, and friends deny death to some degree to continue with the daily business of living.
2. *Anger* can be viewed as the 'Why me?' phase. Anger is probably the most difficult for those who care about or who are trying to help the dying person. In this phase, the person rejects all efforts to help or console. This anger is really the anger of the dying person toward all the people who continue to live or anger towards a 'God' because He does not appear to have acted fairly or justly with the dying person.
3. *Bargaining* is reflected in a 'Yes, me, but…' frame of mind. The person admits the reality of being sick and of probably dying, but the person tries to bargain for extension or quality of life. These bargains are usually secret, frequently are made with God, and are rarely kept. For example, a father promises to be a 'perfect patient' if only he can live to see his son's wedding.
4. *Depression* is the 'Yes, me' reaction to anticipated death. Depression involves preparing to say and saying good-bye to everything and everyone a person has known and loved. The inherent sadness of this phase is appropriate and should be respected.
5. *Acceptance*, the simple and quiet 'Yes,' grows out of individuals' convictions that they have done what they could to be ready to die. Personal energy and interpersonal interests decrease significantly. During this phase, relatives and friends usually need more help than the dying person. The dying person's most important wish at this point is not to die alone.

Note

Dying patients and their loved ones may fluctuate between these stages and may or may not experience all five stages.

Paramedics are only rarely involved in a patient's process of coming to terms with death. However, they often see the reactions of patients and families going through the death process. For example, denial may be obvious in some family members. These people may not appear to see or acknowledge the seriousness of a situation in which decisions about resuscitation must be made. Anger may be directed at the paramedic crew or other healthcare workers. Bargaining may occur in the form of a mother who says, 'Please save my child, and I promise that I'll always make her wear her seat belt!' The paramedic must realize the psychological aspects of the stages of grief (Box 3-15).

When it is necessary to give news of a sudden death to a family, the paramedic's initial contact can influence the grief response greatly. The paramedic should gather the family in a private area and advise them of the patient's death, with a brief account of the situation causing the death. The paramedic should use the words *death* or *dead* and should avoid euphemisms such as 'he's passed on' or 'she's no longer with us'. The paramedic should be compassionate and allow time for the news to be absorbed and for questions to be asked. The family members should be allowed to see the relative if they choose but they should be told in advance if resuscitation equipment is still connected to the patient. These efforts,

Box 3-15

Recommended communication strategies

A situation involving death and dying is uncomfortable. Communication with the patient and loved ones may be difficult. The following recommendations for communications and activities may help a paramedic deal with dying patients and their families:

- Answer questions honestly for the patient and family and explain all activities.
- Do not initiate the subject of dying; let it come from the patient or family.
- If the patient or family asks you whether the patient is going to die, advise that you are doing everything you possibly can but that the situation is critical. This allows a brief time for the patient and family to prepare themselves.
- Do not falsely reassure the patient or family (e.g. 'everything's going to be okay').
- Use compassionate, non-verbal communication (facial expression, touching).
- Offer to contact someone if the patient is alone.
- If family is not present, assure the patient that emergency department personnel will notify them. If they are nearby, encourage the family to come to the patient immediately or to meet the patient at the emergency department.
- Allow the family to stay with the patient when appropriate.

along with empathic interaction with the family, help relatives deal with the loss of a loved one.

Common needs of the paramedic when dealing with death and dying

Dealing with death is difficult for everyone, thus the paramedic's feelings and emotions must also be considered. The paramedic may experience some of the same stages of grief described earlier. These reactions are normal. In fact, the paramedic may expend a great deal of effort to disguise or suppress these emotions at the scene or while rendering care. However, the paramedic should discuss these feelings as soon as possible with friends, coworkers, and family. The paramedic should discuss these emotions in a constructive way that will lessen the emotional burden. Like others, the paramedic will need a chance to process the incident and obtain closure. Available resources, such as employee assistance programmes and counselling and pastoral services, help avoid the effects of cumulative stress.

Critical Thinking

What personal experiences have you had with death? How did you or others who were close to the deceased react to the initial news of the death?

Developmental considerations when dealing with death and dying

The way people cope with their own death or the death of a loved one depends on their age, maturity, and understanding of death. The paramedic should be sensitive to the emotional needs of all age groups during this crisis. The following guidelines may be helpful when offering advice to family members who will be helping the young or elderly cope with the death of a loved one.[7]

- *Children up to age 3* probably will sense that something has happened in the family. They will realize that others are sad and crying and may be aware of increased activity in the household. The family should be urged to watch for changes in eating or sleeping patterns and for an increase in irritability. In addition, the family should be sensitive to the child's needs and try to maintain consistency in the child's routines and with significant persons in the child's life.
- *Children 3–6 years of age* do not have a concept of the finality of death. They may believe that the person will return and may ask 'when' continually. This age group believes in magical thinking and may feel that they are responsible for the death. They may also believe that everyone else they love will die too. The family should watch for changes in the child's behaviour patterns with friends and at school, for difficulty sleeping, and for changes in eating habits. The family should emphasize that the child is not responsible for the death. The family should reinforce the fact that crying is normal when people are sad and should encourage children to talk about their feelings.
- *Children 6–9 years of age* are beginning to understand the finality of death. They want detailed explanations for the death and can differentiate fatal illness from just 'being sick'. Like the 3–6-year-olds, these children may be afraid that other loved ones will die too. This age group may be uncomfortable with expressing their feelings and may act silly or embarrassed when talking about death. The paramedic should suggest to the family that they talk about the normal feelings of anger, sadness, and guilt and that they share their own feelings about death with the child. The family members should not hesitate to cry because crying will let the child know that expression of feelings is acceptable.
- *Children 9–12 years of age* are aware of the finality of death. They may want to know the details surrounding the event. They will be concerned with practical matters involving their lifestyle and may try to 'act like an adult'. (Most of these children, however, will show regression to an earlier stage of emotional response.) The paramedic should suggest to the family that they set aside time to talk to the child about feelings and encourage the sharing of memories to aid in the grief response.
- *Older adults* usually show concern for other family members. In addition, they may be worried about their further loss of independence and about financial matters at hand. Family members should be sensitive and understanding about these issues because they are real for this age group.

Prevention of disease transmission

Emergency workers often manage ill and injured patients; thus, prevention of disease transmission must be a priority in daily practice. Chapter 24 deals with prevention of disease transmission.

Summary

- Wellness has two main aspects: physical well-being and mental and emotional health.
- As healthcare professionals, paramedics have a responsibility to serve as role models in disease prevention.
- Physical fitness can be described as a condition that helps individuals look, feel, and do their best.
- Sleep helps to rejuvenate a tired body.
- Steps to reduce cardiovascular disease include the following: improving cardiovascular endurance, eliminating cigarette smoking, controlling high blood pressure, maintaining a normal body-fat composition, maintaining good total cholesterol/high-density lipoprotein ratio, monitoring triglyceride levels, controlling diabetes, avoiding excessive alcohol, eating healthy foods, reducing stress, and making a periodic risk assessment.
- Most common cancers are linked to one of three environmental risk factors: smoking, sunlight, and diet.
- Injuries whilst at work can be minimized. Knowledge of body mechanics during lifting and moving, and being alert for hostile settings are key. Prioritization of personal safety during rescue situations is wise. In addition, paramedics must practise safe vehicle operation and correctly use all equipment and supplies.
- The misuse and abuse of drugs and other substances may lead to chemical dependency (addiction). This may have a wide range of effects on physical and mental health.
- 'Good' stress (eustress) is a positive response to stimuli and is considered protective. 'Bad' stress (distress) is a negative response to environmental stimuli and is the source of anxiety and stress-related disorders.
- Adaptation is a process by which people learn effective ways to deal with stressful situations. This dynamic process usually begins with using defence mechanisms. Next, one develops coping skills, followed by problem solving, and culminating in mastery.
- Critical incident debriefing is designed to help emergency personnel understand their reactions. The process reassures them that what they are experiencing is normal and may be common to others involved in the incident.
- Often, news of a sudden death must be given to a family. The paramedic's initial contact can influence the grief process greatly.

HEALTH PROMOTION AND INJURY PREVENTION

Objectives

Upon completion of this section, the paramedic student will be able to:

1. Identify roles of the emergency medical services community in injury prevention.
2. Describe the epidemiology of trauma in the UK.
3. Outline the aspects of the emergency medical services system that make it a desirable resource for involvement in community health activities.
4. Describe community leadership activities that are essential to enable the active participation of emergency medical services in community wellness activities.
5. List areas with which paramedics should be familiar to participate in injury prevention.
6. Evaluate a situation to determine opportunities for injury prevention.
7. Identify resources necessary to conduct a community health assessment.
8. Relate how alterations in the epidemiological triangle can influence injury and disease patterns.
9. Differentiate among primary, secondary, and tertiary health prevention activities.
10. Describe strategies to implement a successful injury prevention programme.

Key terms

community health assessment An assessment of a target community to identify needs and resources required to provide prevention and wellness promotion activities.

injury risk Real or potentially hazardous situations that put individuals at increased risk for sustaining an injury.

injury surveillance The ongoing systematic collection, analysis, and interpretation of injury data essential to the planning, implementation, and evaluation of public health practice.

primary injury prevention The practice of preventing an injury from occurring.

teachable moment The time after an injury has occurred when the patient and observers remain acutely aware of what has happened and may be more receptive to being taught ways that the event or illness could have been prevented.

Injury epidemiology

Trauma remains the fourth leading cause of death in western countries and the leading cause of death in those under the age of 40. It is a major cause of debilitating long-term injuries. For each trauma fatality there are two survivors with serious or permanent disability.[8] The socioeconomic burden of trauma is also significant. In 1998, the estimated cost to the NHS, of treating all injuries, was £1.2 billion per annum.[9] Reducing injuries is a key government objective and the Department of Health has set targets to reduce the incidence of accidents by at least 20% from the baseline that was set in 1996 by 2010.[10] Paramedics have a potentially significant role to play in achieving these targets.

Over a third of all deaths due to injury occur as a result of road traffic collisions,[11] with an average of 2946 traffic-related fatalities in Great Britain in 2007.[12] The incidence of severe trauma (Injury Severity Score [ISS] of 16 or greater) is estimated to be four per million per week.[13] In mid-2003 the UK population was around 59.5 million,[14] so this equates to approximately 240 severely injured patients in the UK each week.[15]

Overview of injury prevention

For the most part, emergency medical services (EMS) have been a reactionary medical discipline. This means that EMS is not used until after patients are injured or ill (the so-called tertiary phase of injury prevention). Although EMS excels in acute care, a full system of injury control comprises several facets of which acute care is only one. The injury control strategy of preventing rather than simply treating an injury is known as primary injury prevention.

Preventive strategies yield better outcomes than treatment strategies in terms of lives saved and money spent. The success of these strategies depends on giving injury prevention information to patients. Paramedics are respected in the community and are generally welcomed into homes and businesses; thus, paramedics have a unique chance to find injury patterns and intervene on behalf of persons at risk. Box 3-16 defines terminology related to injury prevention.

> **Box 3-16**
>
> **Injury and illness prevention terminology**
>
> *Injury*: Intentional or unintentional damage to the person resulting from acute exposure to thermal, mechanical, electrical, or chemical energy or the absence of essentials such as heat and oxygen
>
> *Injury risk*: Real or potentially hazardous situations that put individuals at increased risk for sustaining an injury
>
> *Injury surveillance*: The ongoing collection, analysis, and interpretation of injury data essential to the planning, implementation, and evaluation of public health practice, closely integrated with the timely dissemination of these data to those who need to know, with the final link in the chain being the application of these data to prevention and control
>
> *Primary injury prevention*: The practice of preventing an injury from occurring
>
> *Secondary and tertiary prevention*: The care and rehabilitation activities, respectively, that are intended to prevent further problems from an event that has occurred already
>
> *Teachable moment*: The time after an injury has occurred when the patient and observers remain acutely aware of what has happened and may be more receptive to being taught ways that the event or illness could be prevented
>
> *Years of productive life*: The calculation obtained by subtracting the age of the victim's death from 65 (the average age of retirement)

Injury concepts

Definition of injury

A puzzling factor that hindered the study of injury and therefore injury prevention was the seeming unrelatedness of injuries. On the surface, no relationship seemed to exist between a vehicle crash and a poisoning or a gunshot wound and a drowning. However, it now is known that all injuries are the result of either of two things. One is tissue damage caused by the transfer of energy to the human body (mechanical, thermal, electrical, chemical, or radiation energy). The second is tissue damage caused by the absence of needed energy elements such as heat or oxygen (see Chapter 26).

The injury triangle and Haddon's matrix

Injury is also a disease process. Three factors are necessary to cause a disease: host, agent, and environment. Together these three factors are known as the injury triangle. In the injury triangle the host is the victim, the agent of injury is energy, and the environment provides a place for the agent and host to come together over time. The actual injury event may take only a fraction of a second, but the events that lead up to an injury and the events that occur as a result of an injury may take place over seconds, months, or even years.

In the mid-1960s, William Haddon (the 'father' of injury prevention) came up with a tool to aid in understanding the entire injury sequence. This analytical tool is now known as Haddon's matrix. The three factors of the injury triangle are placed in a table on a timeline that is divided into three phases. These phases are pre-event, event, and post-event. For example, the Haddon's matrix in Table 3-2 charts the events that may occur before, during, and after a car crash. The table helps one to see that injuries often result from a predictable and therefore preventable chain of events. The matrix also affirms that most injuries are linked with many causes.

The pre-event phase is the period before the release of injury-causing energy. During this time the person's performance is greater than the task demands and energy is under control. Events in this phase tend to influence the likelihood that an injury will occur. Because the injury has yet to occur, primary injury prevention can take place in this phase. The time frame can be seconds to years, depending on what events come into play to cause the injury.

The event phase is the period during which the person's performance falls below the demands of the task. The result is the release of uncontrolled energy. The time frame is usually a fraction of a second to a few minutes. Events in this phase affect the transmission of energy. Secondary injury prevention recognizes that injuries are going to occur and

Table 3-2 Haddon's matrix for automobile crashes

Phase	Host	Agent	Environment
Pre-event	Impaired capabilities, age, fatigue, alcohol/drug use, driving experience, adherence to driving laws	Defective equipment, dirty windows, improper maintenance, equipment design	Road shoulder too narrow, poor lighting, weather conditions, highway not divided, inadequate notification signs, road design, and construction
Event	Injury threshold due to aging, chronic disease, alcohol, use of restraints, ejection	Failure of doors, impact with sharp objects in the vehicle, vehicle size	Lack of guardrails, large trees near roadside, oncoming traffic
Post-event	Type or extent of injury, knowledge of first aid, alcohol	Bursting gas tanks, entrapment	Quality of rescue, EMS, hospitals, rehabilitation

is centred on reducing the severity of the injury as it is occurring.

The post-event phase is the period after the injury has occurred. This phase can last from a few seconds to years. In this time frame, tertiary injury prevention takes place and traditional EMS exists. The focus of tertiary injury prevention is to lessen the long-term adverse effects of the injury.

The three Es of injury prevention

Three broad practices have typically been used to establish injury prevention programmes. The first E of injury prevention is education; the second E is enforcement; the third E is engineering. A proactive, prevention-oriented EMS professional can play a key role in all three strategies.

Education

The purpose of education is to persuade high-risk persons or groups to change risky behaviour. Education is also meant to teach these persons to adopt safety precautions such as using personal restraints or wearing crash helmets. Education requires the person to do something to take advantage of knowledge learned and often requires the person to make a behavioural change. Education is the most often used approach in injury prevention and is most effective when used with enforcement and engineering.

Enforcement

Enforcement occurs through force of law and requires that persons adopt certain behaviours that reduce risk. Mandatory personal restraint (e.g. seat belts) and compulsory motorcycle helmet laws are examples of this approach. Like education, enforcement is seen as an active countermeasure. Enforcement requires the person to adhere to the law to benefit from it. The success of this approach depends on compliance of individuals and the ability to enforce these laws. Even so, enforcement is more effective than education alone.

Engineering

Engineering refers to product or environmental design. This design automatically provides protection or decreases the likelihood that an injury-producing incident will occur. This approach builds safety into a product such as air bags in cars and sprinkler systems in buildings. Engineering has proved to be the most effective of the three Es but is also the most expensive approach to undertake.

Feasibility of EMS involvement

The following points support the feasibility of EMS involvement in community health and injury prevention:

- EMS providers are often the most medically educated persons in rural settings.
- EMS providers are role models with high profiles.
- EMS providers are often seen as the champions of the customer.
- EMS providers are welcome in homes, schools, and other settings.
- EMS providers are seen as authorities on injury and prevention.
- EMS providers are often the first to spot situations that pose a risk for illness or injury (e.g. unsanitary conditions and unsafe home environments).

Critical Thinking

Can you remember any programme that a firefighter or paramedic taught you when you were a child? How did you feel about the firefighters and paramedics?

Note

As many sicker patients are now cared for in the community, a demand on emergency medical services for supportive care and intervention will increase. Paramedics and EMS agencies must adapt to their new role in the healthcare delivery system (Box 3-17).

Box 3-17

Effects of healthcare reform on EMS

Intermediate care treatment models, such as *'Hospital at home,'* see active treatment provided by healthcare professionals in the patient's home for a condition that would otherwise require hospital care. Because sicker patients are treated at home or released from hospitals earlier, the chance for repeat EMS calls to the same homes or sites is increased. These calls are for emergencies and non-emergency transportations to convalescent care and for readmission to or follow-up services at hospitals. The need to provide some supportive medical care and intervention in the patient's home is also growing (see Chapter 41). Examples of services that paramedics and other healthcare workers provide to patients in their homes include the following:

- caring for patients on monitors, ventilators, infusion pumps, and other complex medical equipment
- drawing blood samples
- providing wound care
- measuring blood pressure
- performing 12-lead electrocardiograms
- performing other duties traditionally done before patients were released from the hospital.

Many patients now take their own intravenous antibiotics and other intravenous medications at home. Premature infants often go home with advanced monitoring and life support equipment. Paramedics must be ready to help these patients with their special needs.

Box 3-18

Personal injury prevention strategies

- Appropriate use of audible and visual warning devices
- Availability and use of police services
- Exercise and conditioning
- Practice of on-scene survival techniques
- Proper driving techniques
- Recognition of health hazards and high-profile crime areas
- Restraint use (self, patient, passengers)
- Safe approach to, parking at, and exiting the scene
- Safe driving
- Scene safety precautions
- Stress management (personal, family, work)
- Traffic control (vehicles, bystanders)
- Use of on-scene survival resources
- Use of personal protective equipment (reflective clothing, helmets)
- Use of proper lifting and moving techniques
- Wellness

Essential community leadership activities

Paramedics should play an active role in community health and injury prevention programmes. Other personnel in public service, such as the fire service, also need to have active roles.

Protect the EMS provider from injury

Policies should help to ensure the paramedic's safety during an emergency response, whilst at the scene, and during patient transportation. Protection can be accomplished with traffic safety laws and public education. Protection can also be enhanced with the help of police, fire service personnel, and other public service agencies.

All EMS workers must have access to personal protective equipment to help lessen eye, back, and skin injury as well as the problems created by exposure to communicable diseases.

Provide education to EMS providers

Primary injury prevention should be included in initial and continuing professional development programmes for paramedics. Community leaders should help to create links between paramedic programmes and public and private specialty groups. These groups may include hospitals, other public health and safety agencies, safety councils, social services, religious organizations, colleges and universities. This link will help with specific education and training. Cooperation among these groups can help to find targets for prevention activities and encourages sharing the tasks of establishing programmes.

Essential paramedic activities

Activities that are essential for paramedics are based on education. These activities include knowing and practising the personal injury prevention strategies. Box 3-18 lists these strategies. The EMS provider also needs to know about illnesses and injuries common to various age groups, recreational activities, workplaces, and other facilities in their community (Box 3-19).

Implementation and prevention strategies

In addition to the primary personal injury prevention strategies described in Box 3-18, other key strategies need to be applied. The recognition of signs and symptoms of exposure to danger and the need for outside assistance; the documentation of primary care and injury data; and on-scene education are discussed below.

Recognition of dangerous situations

A priority for the paramedic is personal safety, thus the EMS worker must stay alert for signs of dangerous situations. This includes recognizing general and specific environmental parameters. These parameters will help the paramedic to assess a patient's need for preventive information. Examples include the following:

- safety hazards in the home
- inadequate housing conditions
- inadequate food and clothing

Box 3-19

Other essential provider activities

Other essential provider activities include review of illness and injuries common to the following:

- infancy (low birth weight; mortality and morbidity)
- childhood (intentional, unintentional, or alleged intentional events; childhood violence to self and others)
- adults
- older patients
- recreation activities
- work hazards
- day care centres (licensed and non-licensed)
- early release from hospital
- discharge from urgent care or other outpatient facilities
- signs of emotional stress that can lead to intentional, unintentional, or alleged events
- self-medication
- dangers of non-compliance (borrowing, not taking medicines on time or finishing the regimen)
- overmedication and polypharmacy

- absence of protective devices (e.g. smoke detectors)
- hazardous materials (e.g. lead-based paint and dangerous chemicals)
- communicable disease (and potential for transmission)
- signs of abuse or neglect.

Critical Thinking

Do you know an EMS provider who was injured on the job? How did the injury occur? Can you identify any measures that could have prevented it?

Recognition of the need for outside resources

Most communities have outside resources that can be helpful. The providers of these resources and services are usually eager to work with the community to develop injury prevention strategies.

Documentation

Taking precise notes of patient care and primary injury data is crucial. This documentation offers a record of the events of the encounter and is helpful to others who will be taking part in the patient's care (see Chapter 11). Gathering primary injury data can be useful in designing injury prevention strategies. For example, one might study a large number of patients who received head injuries whilst riding a horse. This study may help one to observe that helmet use was notably absent in all seriously injured patients. Primary injury data include the following:

- scene conditions
- mechanism of injury
- use of protective devices
- absence of protective devices
- risks at the scene
- other factors as noted by the EMS agency.

On-scene education

The EMS response to an injury or near-injury may provide for a teachable moment. This is a moment in which the patient and the family may be open to injury prevention tips and strategies. The paramedic can use this opportunity to assess hazards in an environment. The paramedic also can provide on-scene, one-on-one injury prevention education. The teachable moment involves a three-step process:

1. *Observe the scene*: The first step is to look for contributing factors or hazards at the scene that may have caused or could cause an injury event. Examples include floor rugs without a non-slip backing and smoke detectors that are not working.
2. *Gather information*: The next step is to gather information from individuals and observers. What did they see? Why do they think the injury occurred? Has this been a common occurrence? Patients, family members or bystanders, and first responders may have valuable insight about a situation that caused an injury event.
3. *Make assessments*: The final step is to make decisions from the information that has been gathered. The first assessment is to decide whether the situation is critical or non-critical. If the situation is critical, the focus must be on patient care. If the situation is non-critical, a teachable moment exists. This is the opportunity to conduct one-on-one injury prevention counselling that may help to prevent another injury. Another assessment uses the information gathered through observation and history taking. The paramedic uses this step to decide whether high-risk persons, high-risk behaviours, or a high-risk setting exists. Based on the assessment of risks, the paramedic can create a remedy.

Three common on-scene remedies are discussion, demonstration, and documentation. Discussion involves talking about proper behaviour or action with the person at risk. Injury prevention discussions are a 30–60-s process. The message must be offered in a patient-appropriate manner. This manner depends on age, education, and socioeconomic status. The message should be conveyed in a non-judgemental, 'here are the facts' tone of voice. Although discussion may not always work, the paramedic should attempt it.

It may be possible to demonstrate proper behaviour as an injury prevention strategy. For example, a paramedic could replace a safety cap on a pill bottle and explain the importance of doing so. The paramedic could put a fresh battery in a smoke detector or could move a throw rug on a slippery floor to a safer location. These demonstrations on the scene draw attention to likely hazards and can work to prevent future injury.

The paramedic should document what was seen, heard, and done at the scene. Written histories allow for follow-up by the receiving personnel. Other injury prevention groups can also use these histories in their data-gathering efforts. Finally, histories make it easier for review in the EMS organization to improve injury prevention.

Critical Thinking

At some point, you will probably visit an older adult family member or friend. Can you identify any potential hazards that exist in that person's home?

Critical Thinking

What method of health education is most likely to change your personal behaviours? Would that same method be equally effective for a 5-year-old or a 70-year-old person?

Summary

- EMS providers are members of the community healthcare system. They can be an important resource in injury prevention.
- Unintentional injuries are the fourth leading cause of death and the leading cause of death in those under 40 years of age.
- For EMS workers to play an active role in the health of a community is crucial. Thus the community must protect the EMS worker from injury. The community also needs to provide education to EMS workers. The community should supply support and promote the collection and use of injury data as well. In addition, the community must obtain resources for primary injury prevention activities. Lastly, the community needs to empower EMS providers to conduct primary injury prevention.
- All EMS workers must have a basic knowledge of personal injury prevention. They should also know about maladies and injuries common to various age groups, recreation activities, workplaces, and other facilities in the community.
- The paramedic needs to spot the signs and symptoms of abuse and abusive situations. In addition, the paramedic should notice exposure to danger.
- Paramedics should identify and use outside community resources. Plus they should document primary injury data properly. Moreover, they should identify and properly use the teachable moment.
- The EMS provider must maximize time and resources. Thus the EMS provider should identify targets for community health education. The EMS provider can do this by performing a community health assessment.
- To identify community education goals, the paramedic must understand several factors: (1) illness or injury is related to the extent of exposure to an agent; (2) illness or injury is also related to the strength of the agent; (3) illness or injury is linked to the susceptibility of the individual (host); and (4) illness or injury is related to the biological, social, and physical environment.
- Primary injury prevention involves preventing an injury from occurring. Secondary and tertiary prevention help to prevent further problems from an event that has already occurred.
- A good injury prevention programme must serve the whole target population in a community. An effective programme also takes into account reading level and age. These aspects are the mark of a successful programme. The EMS provider can provide community health education in diverse ways, such as verbal, written/static material, and dynamic visual.

References

1. Department of Health 2000 National service framework for coronary heart disease. DoH, London
2. HM Government 1998 Smoking Kills; a White Paper on tobacco. HMSO, London
3. Office for National Statistics 2001 Population size; ethnicity. Online. Available http://www.statistics.gov.uk/cci/nugget.asp?id=273 21 September 2008
4. Selye H 1956 The stress of life. McGraw-Hill, New York
5. Mitchell J, Bray G 1990 Emergency services stress: guidelines for preserving the health and careers of emergency services personnel. Brady, Englewood Cliffs, NJ
6. Bassuk EL, Fox SS, Prendergast KJ 1983 Behavioral emergencies. Little, Brown, Boston
7. US Department of Transportation, National Highway Traffic Safety Administration 1998 EMT-Paramedic national standard curriculum. Department of Transportation, Washington, DC
8. Chaira O, Cimbanissi S 2003 Organized trauma care: does volume matter and do trauma centers save lives? Curr Opin Crit Care 9:510–514
9. The Trauma Audit & Research Network. An overview. 2006. Online. Available http://www.tarn.ac.uk/content/images/53/overview%2006.pdf 19 January 2009
10. Department of Health 1998 Our healthier nation – a contract for health. DoH, London
11. The Royal College of Surgeons of England and the British Orthopaedic Society 2000 Better care for the severely injured. RCS, London
12. Department for Transport. Transport statistics bulletin. Road casualties in Great Britain main results: 2007. Department for Transport, London.
13. Gorman DF, Teanby DN, Sinha MP, Wotherspoon J, Boot DA, Molokhia A 1995 The epidemiology of major injuries in Mersey and North Wales. Injury 26(1):51–54
14. Office for National Statistics. Online. Available http://www.statistics.gov.uk/ 19 January 2009
15. NCEPOD 2007 Trauma: who cares. A report of the National Confidential Enquiry into Patient Outcome and Death. NCEPOD, London

Further reading

American Academy of Pediatrics, Committee on Injury and Poison Prevention 1997 Injury prevention and control for children and youth, 3rd edition. AAP, Elk Grove Village, IL

Christoffel T, Gallagher SS 1999 Injury prevention and public health: practical knowledge, skills, and strategies. Aspen, Gaithersburg, MD

Garrison HG, Foltin GL, Becker LR, et al 1997 The role of emergency medical services in primary injury prevention. Ann Emerg Med 30:80–91

Institute of Medicine, Division of Health Promotion and Disease Prevention, Committee on Injury Prevention and Control 1999 Reducing the burden of injury. National Academy Press, Washington, DC

Kellerman AL, Todd KH 1999 Injury control. In Tintinalli JE, Kelen GD, Stapczynski JS, eds Emergency medicine: a comprehensive study guide. McGraw-Hill, New York

Kinnane JM, Garrison HG, Coben JH, et al 1997 Injury prevention: is there a role for out-of-hospital emergency medical services? Acad Emerg Med 4:306–312

PART TWO

CHAPTER 4

Approaches to Assessment

Chapter contents

Objectives

Upon completion of this chapter, the paramedic student will be able to:

1. Discuss how approaches to assessment contribute to effective patient and scene assessment.
2. Describe factors that affect assessment and decision making in the prehospital setting.
3. Outline effective techniques for scene and patient assessment and choreography.
4. Identify essential take-in equipment for general and selected patient situations.
5. Outline strategies for patient approach that promote an effective patient encounter.

Key terms

action plan A plan of action based on the patient's condition and the environment.

pattern recognition The process of comparing gathered information with the paramedic's knowledge base of medical illness and disease.

working impression An impression of the patient's condition that the paramedic makes from pattern recognition and 'gut instinct' that results from experience.

The approach to the assessment of a patient is a very important skill that paramedics must ensure is undertaken correctly. As assessment provides the basis for decision making about patient care, the approach to the assessment should provide a firm base for the appropriate and comprehensive patient assessment that follows. The purpose of this chapter is to 'set the scene' so that the paramedic can give some thought to how he or she might approach the very different and diverse patient populations that are seen in practice.

There are many factors that can impact upon how effective an assessment might be. Some of the common issues are discussed below but there are many possible challenges to assessment and by considering these, in advance of any possible scenario where they might occur, the paramedic is likely to be in a better position to undertake an effective and comprehensive assessment.

Factors that affect assessment and decision making

Many factors can affect the quality of assessment and decision making by the paramedic. The following factors are discussed in this section:

- paramedic's attitude
- patient's willingness to cooperate
- distracting injuries
- labelling and tunnel vision
- environment
- patient compliance
- considerations of personnel availability.

Critical Thinking

Have you ever seen any of these factors affect patient care?

Paramedic's attitude

In order for the paramedic to perform an effective assessment, specific qualities such as a professional attitude and a non-judgemental approach are vital. Inappropriate attitudes may cause difficulties in achieving an adequate assessment of the patient, which may lead the paramedic to miskey pieces of information. For example, a paramedic may assume that an uncooperative patient is intoxicated and in doing this the paramedic may not consider underlying conditions such as hypoglycaemia, hypoxia or hypovolaemia.

Patient's willingness to cooperate

Patients who do not cooperate can complicate the patient assessment, which is required for the paramedic to formulate an action plan. As discussed in later chapters, the paramedic should carefully evaluate patients who are uncooperative, restless, or aggressive for the following conditions:

- alcohol or other drug intoxication
- head injury or concussion
- hypoglycaemia
- hypothermia
- hypovolaemia
- hypoxia
- mental health problems
- stroke.

Distracting injuries

Obvious but non-life-threatening injuries such as open fractures or facial wounds can distract the paramedic and prevent a thorough assessment for more serious problems taking place. The paramedic must focus on the priorities in assessment.

Labelling and 'tunnel vision'

Labelling and tunnel vision can lead to an incorrect assessment and working impression; labelling a patient as 'just another drunk' can lead to a biased and inaccurate assessment. The same can happen by labelling someone who has been transported by ambulance many times for an imagined illness as a 'frequent flyer'. Likewise, tunnel vision is assuming an incorrect working impression based on 'gut instinct' alone or by focusing on a small portion of the presenting illness and thereby missing the bigger picture, which can result in a rushed judgment early in the patient assessment, which in turn may lead to an improper action plan.

Environment

Factors in the environment can have a significant impact and adversely affect assessment techniques and decision making at the scene. Examples include scene chaos, violent or dangerous situations, crowds of bystanders or other emergency workers, adverse weather, and high noise levels. First, the paramedic must ensure personal safety and then establish control of the environment quickly. This can include requesting the help of the police who will work to control the scene and allow the paramedic to deliver appropriate assessment and care without distraction.

Patient concordance

The patient is not always cooperative and their willingness to cooperate with the assessment may depend on his or her trust in the paramedic crew. For example, the patient who sees the paramedic as competent and professional is more likely to give consent to history taking and physical examination. Other aspects that can affect cooperation include cultural and ethnic factors.

Considerations of personnel availability

Depending on the emergency medical service (EMS), crews may consist of combinations of paramedics, emergency medical technicians (EMTs) and increasingly the use of A&E support crews and emergency care assistants (ECA). In the UK there have been moves recently to re-align the skill mix of ambulance crews and many services are beginning to use ECAs crewed with a paramedic or EMT. Additionally, in some circumstances EMS crews will work alongside ECPs (emergency care practitioners) whose focus is often to care for patients with unscheduled healthcare needs in the community. Other agencies such as Fire and Rescue, Police, BASICS (British Association of Immediate Care Schemes) and other healthcare professionals may also be present. In cases in which only EMS is involved and only one paramedic is at the scene, the paramedic will work with their colleague and develop a proper sequence for gathering information and providing care. If additional EMS staff are available, they can all undertake specific roles, under the direction of the first paramedic on scene. This requires coordination and teamwork. A duty officer may also be involved and they will lead the EMS response as required. The Fire and Rescue members may be in charge of extrication and gathering equipment and police officers may be in charge of securing the scene safety.

Critical Thinking

How can too many paramedics on the scene have a negative influence on patient assessment and care?

Assessment and management choreography

In cases where many responders are at the scene of an emergency, a coherent assessment can be difficult. A large emergency response may occur with multiple-tier response systems (e.g. EMS, fire and police). The situation often is made more complex if the responders are trained at the same level (e.g. paramedic) without a clear direction for individual duties. Therefore, members of the response team must have a pre-plan for deciding roles. The team can assign these pre-designated roles by shift or crew or can rotate them among team members.

An example of a pre-plan for two paramedics is to assign one as the team leader (the attendant) and one as a team member, although this type of plan must be flexible in rapidly changing situations. However, the basic plan allows others to participate and is important in preventing confusion at the scene. The following are sample responsibilities for each of the paramedics in this type of pre-plan:

1. Team leader responsibilities (the attendant or first paramedic on scene)
   a. Accompanies the patient through to definitive care.
   b. Establishes contact and a dialogue with the patient.
   c. Obtains the history.
   d. Performs the physical examination.
   e. Presents the patient and gives verbal reports over the radio or at definitive care.
   f. Completes all documentation.

g. Tries to maintain the overall patient perspective and provides leadership to the team by designating tasks and coordinating transportation.
h. Designates and actively participates in critical interventions during the resuscitative phase of initial assessment.
i. Acts as initial incident officer in multiple-casualty or major incident situations (see Chapter 36).
j. Interprets the electrocardiogram, controls access to the drug box, and documents drug administration and effects during advanced life support.

2. Team member responsibilities
   a. Provides scene cover (watches the team leader's back).
   b. Gathers scene information and talks to family members and bystanders.
   c. Obtains vital signs as requested by the team leader.
   d. Assists and performs skills and interventions as requested by the team leader (e.g. attaches monitor leads, provides oxygen, initiates intravenous access, administers drugs, and obtains transportation equipment).
   e. Administers drugs, monitors endotracheal tube placement, and monitors basic life support interventions during advanced life support.

The correct equipment

This means carrying the right equipment to the patient's side; not having the correct equipment can compromise care and can also cause confusion. The paramedic crew should always be prepared for the worst-case scenario and carry essential equipment to manage every aspect of patient care, including initial airway management and C-spine immobilization and items to support breathing and circulation, including cardiac monitoring and defibrillation (Box 4-1). Most services use a first response bag which has the key items of equipment needed.

Note

The concept of having the correct equipment can be compared with backpacking. A person who is backpacking must have essential items that are downsized to facilitate rapid movement with minimum weight and bulk.

Optional take-in equipment

In addition to essential equipment for the EMS crew, the paramedic can also carry other equipment to the patient's side, such as drug bags, equipment for IV access, other immobilization equipment and so on. Other factors that can affect what equipment the paramedic carries to the patient's side depend on the following:

- service practices and procedures
- information with regards to nature of call
- number of paramedic responders
- difficulty in accessing patients and distance to patient.

Box 4-1

Essential items for all aspects of patient care

Personal protection
- Eye shields
- Gowns
- Gloves
- Masks
- High-visibility clothing

Airway control
- Endotracheal tubes, stylettes, gum elastic bougie, 50 mL syringe, catheter mount connector
- Tape, ties or ET tube securing device
- Laryngoscope and blades
- Laryngeal mask airways
- Nasopharyngeal airways
- Oropharyngeal airways
- Rigid tonsil tip (Yankauer) and flexible suction catheters
- Suction (electrical or manual)

Breathing
- Large-bore intravenous cannulae for thoracic decompression
- Manual ventilation bag–valve–mask
- Mouth-powered ventilation device (pocket mask)
- Occlusive dressings
- Oxygen masks (high flow with reservoir and medium flow), and oxygen nasal prongs
- Low/controlled flow oxygen masks
- Oxygen cylinder and regulator
- Monitors for $EtCO_2$ and oxygen saturation
- Peak flow meter

Circulation
- Bandages and tape
- Blood pressure cuff and stethoscope
- Dressings
- Cling film
- Infection-control supplies (gloves and eye shields)
- Intravenous fluids, cannulae, and tubing
- IV tourniquet/IV cannula dressings/alcohol swabs
- IO needles
- Syringes and needles (various)
- Notepad and pen or pencil

Disability and dysrhythmia
- 12-lead ECG/cardiac monitor and defibrillator
- Blood glucose monitor
- Pen-torch
- Cervical collar

Exposure
- Scissors/sharps bin
- Space blanket or other device to cover and protect the patient
- Immobilization and splinting equipment

Other items that are essential on every call include patient report forms, pens, personal wristwatches, flashlights/pen-torches and portable radios or mobile phones. Personal protective equipment also should be readily available.

General approach to the patient

A calm and orderly manner is important for the paramedic when approaching a patient; to gain the patient's trust and cooperation, the paramedic must look and act the part of a professional and show a caring and confident bedside manner (see Chapter 6). Patients may not be able to rate medical performance; however, they generally rate people skills and service.

As described before, a pre-plan should be in place; this plan will help to prevent confusion at the scene and will improve the accuracy of the assessment. Ideally, one team member should be in charge of talking to the patient, using an active and concerned dialogue that allows for careful listening. Taking notes when acquiring the history demonstrates a thorough assessment of the patient and prevents the paramedic from asking repetitive questions, although the need for note taking should be explained to the patient. All essential equipment should be at the patient's side and the crew should be ready to provide resuscitative care if needed. An initial survey of the scene can offer important clues to help the paramedic formulate an impression.

Setting the tone for the patient encounter

It is necessary in the early stages of patient assessment to consider whether the patient is stable or not. This is sometimes known as 'big sick' or 'little sick'; a small proportion of patients will require rapid and involved resuscitative interventions, with the remainder requiring appropriate care given in a less time-critical fashion (sometimes known as a contemplative approach). Patients that require urgent and/or resuscitative measures would include those with conditions such as:

- cardiorespiratory arrest
- coma or altered level of consciousness
- major trauma
- probable cervical spine injury
- respiratory distress or failure
- seizures
- shock or hypotension
- unstable cardiac rhythms.

Where there is a life-threatening problem the paramedic crew must take urgent resuscitative action and should delay history taking and other details; these must wait until the paramedic has performed immediate resuscitation measures.

If immediate intervention is not needed, the paramedic can use the contemplative approach. With this approach, the paramedic obtains a patient history and performs a physical examination before providing patient care.

In any patient care encounter, the paramedic may need to move the patient immediately to the emergency vehicle if any of the following occur:

- The paramedic cannot provide lifesaving interventions at the patient's side.
- The scene is too unstable or unsafe.
- The scene is too chaotic to allow for thorough assessment.
- Inclement weather hinders assessment and care.

Looking to find

Paramedics must find something before they can treat or report it; to find something, the paramedic must suspect it. Therefore, during the initial assessment, the paramedic must look actively for any problems that pose a threat to life. The paramedic must be systematic in the assessment, rapidly determining the patient's presenting complaint and then must assess the degree of distress. Next the paramedic must obtain baseline vital signs. The paramedic must stay focused on the patient's history and physical findings. A mental rule-out list often is a good approach in looking to find; this is a list that considers the most serious problems that could cause the patient's signs and symptoms first.

Experience assists the paramedic in developing the ability for multitasking; this is being able to ask questions, take notes, and perform tasks while listening to the patient's answers. In time the paramedic will gain the level of experience for multitasking, but until then it is best to ask questions and then carefully listen to the patient's response, otherwise crucial clues may be lost by not listening. If a particular task is called for while the paramedic is obtaining a patient history, a colleague should provide the patient care interventions. The patient's ability to describe symptoms and the paramedic's ability to listen may influence the assessment greatly; for instance, the severity and location of the patient's pain may not always correlate well with some potentially life-threatening conditions and a patient with myocardial infarction, for example, may at first complain of pain only in the arm or shoulder. The paramedic's role is to assess and treat rapidly for the worst-case scenario.

Summary

- Assessment-based management 'puts it all together'. This means that the paramedic gathers, evaluates, and synthesizes information. The paramedic makes proper decisions based on the information and then takes appropriate actions required for the patient's care.
- Factors that can affect the quality of assessment and decision making include the paramedic's attitude, the patient's willingness to cooperate, distracting injuries, labelling and tunnel vision, the environment, patient compliance, and considerations of personnel availability.
- Promoting a coherent assessment is the goal; members of the response team should have a 'pre-plan' for determining roles and responsibilities.
- The paramedic crew should always be prepared for the worst event and carry essential equipment to manage every aspect of patient care.
- A calm and orderly manner is essential for the paramedic, especially when approaching a patient. During the initial assessment the paramedic must look actively for problems that pose a threat to life.

Further reading

Bell R, Krivich M 2000 How to use patient satisfaction data to improve healthcare quality. American Society of Quality/ Quality Press, Milwaukee

Elling B, Elling K 2002 Principles of patient assessment in EMS. Delmar Learning, Clifton Park, NY

Gilles A 1997 Improving the quality of patient care. John Wiley & Son, New York

JRCALC 2006 Clinical practice guidelines. Joint Royal Colleges Ambulance Liaison Committee, London

CHAPTER 5

Communication Systems in EMS

Chapter contents

Objectives

Upon completion of this chapter, the paramedic student will be able to:

1. Outline the phases of communications that occur during a typical emergency medical services (EMS) event.
2. Describe the role of communications in EMS.
3. Define common EMS communications terms.
4. Describe the primary modes of EMS communications.
5. Describe the role of dispatching as it applies to prehospital emergency medical care.
6. Outline techniques for relaying EMS communications clearly and effectively.

Key terms

ACCOLC Access Overload Control. The ability of the phone network to be controlled so that only specific numbers have access to the network; this is used when only absolutely necessary to maintain emergency service mobile phone systems, such as in a major emergency or incident.

duplex mode A communications mode with the ability to transmit and receive traffic simultaneously through two different frequencies, one to transmit and one to receive.

EMS communications The delivery of patient and scene information (either in person, in writing, or through communications technology) to other members of the emergency response team.

MDT Mobile data terminal: systems whereby the call details and other dispatch data are passed to a touch screen or similar data screen in the ambulance. Often linked to a satellite navigation system.

multiplex mode A communications mode with the ability to transmit two or more different types of information simultaneously, in either or both directions, over the same frequency.

simplex mode A communications mode with the ability to transmit or receive in one direction at a time. Simultaneous transmission cannot occur.

SOAP format A memory aid used to organize written and verbal patient reports; it includes subjective data, objective data, assessment data, and plan of patient management.

telecommunicator A person trained to work in a call handling/dispatch/control room function. The term applies widely to call handlers, radio operators, dispatchers or any combination of the roles.

telemedicine Technological communications that allow for the transmission of photographs, video, and other information to be sent directly from the scene to a hospital for physician evaluation and consultation.

Emergency medical services (EMS) communications refers to the delivery of information. This information relates to the patient and the scene. The information may be delivered in person, in writing, or through various devices. The information is delivered to other members of the emergency response team. These members include telecommunicators, EMS providers, emergency response workers, EMS system control and administration staff, and medical direction. This chapter focuses on the complexities of communications that are vital aspects of the EMS system.

Phases of communications during a typical EMS event

Several phases of communications occur during a typical EMS event; including the occurrence of the event, detection of the need for emergency services, the notification and emergency response, EMS arrival, treatment, and preparation for transport and preparation of EMS for the next response.

In many urban areas the public requests help via a phone call which goes via a 999 call centre to the relevant emergency service. Communications specialists (telecommunicators) receive the call; in most modern systems, details about the origin of the call and history of the response to that locale are displayed automatically on a console. The call taker then sends these details via digital technology to the dispatcher; this person sends a response unit to the scene. With the development of AMPDS or CBD, pre-arrival instructions are given to the caller, for instance where the patient may require resuscitation measures or action to control bleeding. Emergency medical dispatchers or other qualified personnel give these instructions; the communication with the caller continues until the first EMS unit arrives at the scene.

Note

A telecommunicator is a person trained in public safety telecommunications. The term applies to call takers, dispatchers, radio operators, data terminal operators, or any combination of such functions in a control room such as a fire, police, or EMS communications centre.

The EMS unit is dispatched to the scene and the paramedic crew advises the communications centre of response and arrival status via an MDT (mobile data terminal) or sometimes radio or mobile phone. The paramedics render care at the emergency scene and will package the patient for transport. The crew may contact the receiving hospital to provide pre-alert reports and the patient is delivered to the receiving facility. Following the completion of the reporting, the paramedics make the EMS vehicle ready for the next emergency call.

Role of communications in EMS

Verbal, written, and electronic communications allow the delivery of information between the person requesting help and the telecommunicator and between the telecommunicator and the paramedic. Communications occur between the paramedic, patient, hospital, and between the paramedic and hospital personnel who receive the patient on arrival at the emergency department (Figure 5-1). Good communications can occur only when key elements are in place. These elements make up the basic model of communications.

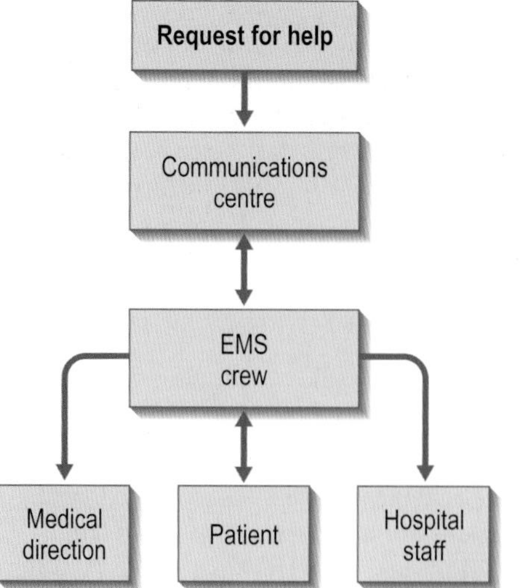

Figure 5-1 Emergency medical services communications.

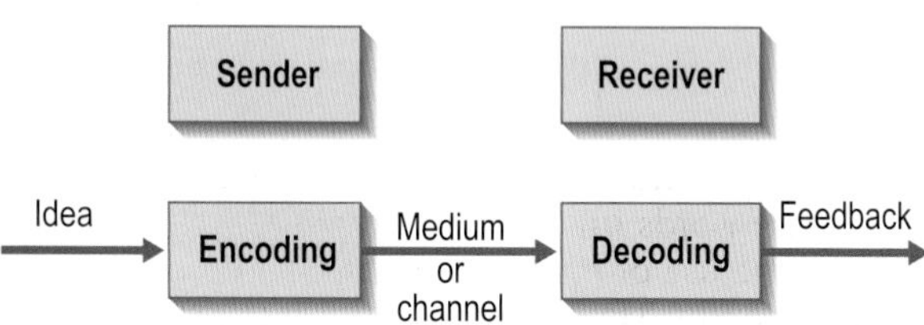

Figure 5-2 Basic model of communications.

Basic model of communications

Communications can be verbal, non-verbal, or written. Communications serves a vital information function for decision making. Communications is the process by which one individual or group transmits meaning to others. The basic model of communications describes the relationships between an idea, encoding, a sender, a medium or channel, a receiver, decoding, and feedback (Figure 5-2).

The idea is the meaning that is intended in the communications. Conveying the idea requires two things: first, it requires the sender to organize the intended meaning through a medium or channel and this is called encoding. The medium or channel may be, for example, written or oral, facial or body expression, or voice modulation. Second, it requires interpretation by the receiver; this is called decoding. The receiver provides feedback that the initial idea was received. If communications are fully successful, there will be an overlap between the idea intended by the sender and the feedback provided by the receiver. (For instance, the receiver would interpret the decoding of the idea in a way identical to that intended by the sender.) Four common barriers to successful communications are as follows:

1. Attributes of the receiver. Different persons react in different ways to the same message or idea. A variety of personal reasons may affect the interpretations of the message. These reasons may include cultural differences or language barriers. For example, a patient from one culture may find personal touch to be comforting, but a patient from another culture may be offended by touch.
2. Selective perception. Persons tend to listen to only part of an idea or message and may block out other information. They do this for a variety of reasons (e.g. values, mood, and motives of the sender). They may block out an idea when new information conflicts with established values, beliefs, or expectations. For example, the input of a newly registered paramedic is not welcomed or respected by a more experienced paramedic.

Critical Thinking

What tends to happen to you when you are talking with someone who continually interrupts you?

3. Semantic problems. Words that are used commonly may carry different meanings for different persons. One common issue is the use of vague or abstract words or phases; these words invite varying interpretation. Another is the use of medical terms and technical language ('lingo'). The receiver may not be able to understand these. For example, a paramedic refers to a patient as 'comatose' during a radio report to the hospital and the hospital staff ask for further clarification using the AVPU (alert, verbal, painful, unresponsive) scale.
4. Time pressures. Time pressures can lead to distortions in communications. A major temptation when pressed for time is to short circuit channels; in these cases the immediate demands of the situation are met. However, a number of unintended consequences can result. For example, the paramedic did not document medications administered in the field to a patient with cardiac arrest; this causes confusion about the next appropriate drug.

The paramedic should consider this basic model and also should take into account the common barriers. These barriers block good communications. These are key to recalling when conveying information to or receiving information from telecommunicators, coworkers, patients, bystanders and other healthcare professionals.

Proper verbal communications during an EMS event

The role of proper verbal communications during an EMS event is to exchange system and patient information; this information is exchanged with other members of the response team. Communications must be done according to approved guidelines and standards regarding confidentiality and consent.

The terms used in EMS communications should be clear; the message should be conveyed in short narrative form and difficult words or phrases may be spelled out using the phonetic alphabet (Table 5-1). Technical or semantic jargon that cannot be understood clearly by all parties should be avoided. Some EMS services use a code to shorten radio transmissions; however, the English language usually is preferred for written and verbal messages. The paramedic should recall that many radio and phone communications are recorded; they may be replayed – for example during patient care audits, disciplinary hearings, and during legal proceedings. Professional conduct is important in all communications. The paramedic should preserve patient confidentiality and EMS staff should avoid giving any patient-identifiable information over unsecured airwaves that might be overheard or scanned; most systems are now digital and the security is now much greater.

Verbal communications can be affected by the terms used. Likewise, the effectiveness of written documentation can be impeded by the use of technical terms. Semantic jargon also can hinder the message. These types of terms often cannot be understood clearly by all parties.

Table 5-1 Phonetic alphabet (international or NATO)

A	alpha
B	bravo
C	charlie
D	delta
E	echo
F	foxtrot
G	golf
H	hotel
I	india
J	juliet
K	kilo
L	lima
M	mike
N	november
O	oscar
P	papa
Q	quebec
R	romeo
S	sierra
T	tango
U	uniform
V	victor
W	whiskey
X	X-ray
Y	yankee
Z	zulu

Proper written communications during an EMS event

Written documentation during an EMS event serves several key roles; it provides a written and legal record of the event as well as conveying key clinical information from one component of the healthcare system (EMS) to the next (emergency department). In addition, documentation is expected as part of professional work. Written documentation of patient care activities also becomes part of the patient's medical record. Other important ways in which written data can be used within the EMS system include the following:

- clinical effectiveness and audit
- quality improvement/quality management
- accounts
- data collection
- research.

In addition to the patient care report, other types of documentation that may be required by an EMS agency include the following:

- Personnel records documenting training and work assignments.
- Call records that list or log dates, times, and other specifics of a call.
- Vehicle maintenance records documenting vehicle service at regular intervals.
- Vehicle and equipment cleaning records documenting procedures used to disinfect vehicle and emergency equipment.
- Drug and equipment inventory records verifying daily checks of drug and fluid expiration, security measures of controlled substances as required by national and service regulations, and monitor–defibrillator, radio, and other equipment checks.
- Incident reports that document problem calls or unusual circumstances (adverse or critical incident reporting) which might include records of significant exposures to communicable disease or biological hazard or exposure to possible hazardous substances.

Technological advances in the collection and exchange of information

As technology evolves, it alters the way EMS gathers information; technology also affects the way in which EMS exchanges information. Technology reduces the reliance on more traditional means of verbal and written communications. Examples of such advances include portable wireless voice and data devices, satellite terminals, global positioning systems for tracking emergency vehicles, diagnostic devices, and handheld tablet computers. These and other devices can allow for real-time capture of EMS events and data. They can provide for advanced notification and reduce the time to in-hospital diagnosis and therapy.

Tablet computers are also known as electronic clipboards. These computers can send out patient information from a scene to a receiving hospital or a host computer. Then the data can be transferred electronically into a final report and patient record. This electronic information has the same legal status as a written document. The data take the place of the paper record of the incident.

Communications systems

The terms used to describe emergency communications technology are specific to the industry (Box 5-1). Some of the information in this chapter refers to the older analogue systems and may not be relevant in the newest digital systems but is retained as some non-NHS ambulance services and other providers of paramedic/ambulance services use some elements of these systems.

The following is an overview of the simple and complex communications systems.

Box 5-1

Communications terminology

999: A three-digit telephone number to facilitate the reporting of an emergency requiring response (the caller is connected to the required emergency service by the 999 call centre)

112: The European Union emergency number will work in the UK in the same way a 999 call will

999 call centre: There are a number of call centres in the UK that operate with the sole function of answering calls made via 999

Abandoned call: A call placed to 999 in which the caller disconnects before the call can be answered

AMPDS: Advanced Medical Priority Dispatch System; a system for EMS call handling and dispatching

Amplitude modulated: The encoding of a carrier wave by variation of its amplitude in accordance with an input signal

Automatic alarm and automatic alerting device: Any automated device that will access the 999 system for emergency services upon activation and does not provide for two-way communication. Automatic fire alarms are one example

Automatic location identification: The automatic display at the call centre of the caller's telephone number, the address or location of the telephone, and supplementary emergency services information

Automatic number identification (ANI): Telephone number associated with the access line from which a call originates

CBD: Criteria-based dispatch: a system for EMS call handling and dispatching

Cell: The wireless telecommunications (cellular or PCS) antenna serving a specific geographical area

Circuit route: The physical path between two terminal locations

Computer-aided dispatch: A computer-based system that aids control room and call centre staff by automating selected dispatching and record-keeping activities

Emergency call: A telephone request for emergency services that requires immediate action to save a life, report a fire, or stop a crime; it may include other situations as determined locally

Global positioning system: A satellite-based location determination technology

Motorway telephone box: A telephone enclosed in a box and placed along a motorway (or similar road) that allows a motorist to summon emergency assistance

Management information system: A program that collects, stores, and collates data into reports to enable interpretation and evaluation of information such as performance, trends, and traffic capacities

Box 5-2

UK Ambulance Digital Radio Programme

In the UK the development of the Ambulance Radio Programme has seen the development of a sophisticated digital system that allows a more robust operating structure; TETRA (Terrestrial Trunked Radio) is the standard that is being used. The older analogue systems historically used by ambulance services are becoming obsolete and are currently being phased out.

Some of the benefits of the new digital system are said to be better geographical coverage, greater clarity in transmission, greater capacity, ability to transmit voice and data simultaneously and the ability to develop so-called 'talk groups' whereby groups of users can be put together in the system to communicate with each other. The new system operates in a TMO (trunked mode operation) whereby the base stations are interconnected and allow greater usability. On occasions where the coverage might be limited, the operation become DMO (direct mode operation) which means individual units can link directly. Other benefits of the system are that there is a tracking facility and the ability to use the system in a similar way to mobile phones with text and normal phone communication being possible if the system is so configured.

Simple systems

The minimum requirements for radio equipment used by an ambulance service include a self-contained desktop transceiver with a speaker, microphone, antenna, and mobile unit, and a two-way radio with multiple-frequency capability in the vehicle. Most EMS services also use handheld portable radios. (These often are called portables.) These radios are capable of communications contact with the base station and data recording. The portable radio protects the crew and aids in optimal patient care. The radio does this by allowing continued contact with the communications centre. The data-recording part of the device offers medical and legal protection for the service and can verify the transmissions when contact is disrupted. The vast majority of services in the UK utilize the more complex systems described below (and are moving to the digital system described in Box 5-2), although some voluntary and private agencies may use more straightforward simple systems.

Complex systems

More advanced radio communications systems exist; these include remote consoles, high-power transmitters, repeaters, satellite receivers, and high-power multifrequency vehicle radios. Services also use mobile transmitter steering, vehicular repeaters, mobile encode–decode capabilities, mobile data terminals, microwave links, and other sophisticated communications devices.

Base stations

Base stations usually are located on a high spot such as a hill, mountain, or tall building; this location ensures optimal transmission and reception. Base stations generally are connected via telephone lines to dispatch centres, where all elements of the EMS response are coordinated. Base station transmitters usually are equipped with an antenna to boost their signal.

Mobile transceivers

Vehicle-mounted transmitters usually operate at lower outputs than base stations and provide a range of 10 to 15 miles over average terrain. Transmission over flat land or water increases this range. However, transmission over mountainous terrain, dense foliage, or urban areas with tall buildings decreases the range. Transmitters with higher outputs are available; these transmitters may offer greater ranges for transmission.

Portable transceivers

Portable transceivers are handheld or hand-carried devices; a paramedic uses these when working away from the emergency vehicle. These devices usually have a limited range. Many systems boost the signal through a mobile or vehicular repeater; portable transceivers may be single-channel or multichannel units.

Repeaters

Repeaters act as a special type of long-range transceiver; they receive transmissions from a low-power portable or mobile radio on one frequency. At the same time, they retransmit it at a higher power on another frequency. Repeaters may be fixed or vehicle mounted; EMS systems often use both. Repeaters are needed for large geographical areas; they are used to increase coverage from portable/mobile to portable/mobile units. They allow low-power units to receive other radio messages and they also allow two or more low-power units to communicate with each other when distances or obstructions normally would hinder this.

Remote console

Most EMS systems use dispatch services located away from base stations; these remote centres control all base station functions. They are connected via dedicated telephone lines, microwave, or other radio means. Hospitals may also be equipped with a terminal that receives and displays telemetry transmissions and provide communication with the paramedic crews in the field. Consoles for these systems may include an amplifier, a speaker, a microphone, receiving capabilities, and remote control circuits.

Satellite receivers and terminals

Satellite receivers sometimes are used depending on the area and the terrain; they are used to ensure that low-power units are always within coverage. The satellite receivers are strategically located and connected to the base station or repeater by dedicated phone lines, radio, or microwave relay. 'Voting systems' automatically select the best audio signal. These systems pick up the signal from among multiple satellite receivers and the main base station receiver. These also are used in other types of communications systems.

Commonly available satellite terminals incorporate ground stations and transportable stations; they provide voice, data, and video communications. Portable satellite terminals are useful when other systems are not available; for example, they may be used during major disasters.

Mobile (cellular) telephones

Many EMS services use mobile phones, primarily digital. Mobile phones are an alternative to dedicated EMS communications systems. One benefit is that they have more channels and in addition, a mobile phone offers a fairly secure link between EMS workers and local hospitals. The mobile phone also allows, for example, a GP or other healthcare professional to speak directly with the patient. Mobile phone use for emergency services has disadvantages, however, including network usage that might limit channel access. High network usage might create problems in maintaining continuous communications in some areas. Another issue is lack of priority access although this can be overcome with the use of ACCOLC. Yet another issue is the inability of calls to be monitored by other members of an emergency response team and therefore many EMS agencies that use mobile phones have a backup option, such as backup radio communications capabilities (Box 5-3).

Digital

Digital modes of communications include digital phones, telemetry, fax transmissions, and digital signals used in some wireless phone, paging and alerting systems. Telemetry and facsimiles are transmitted using electronic signals; these signals are converted into audio tones and then are converted back into electronic signals by the receiver decoder. The signals then can be displayed or printed. An example of telemetry is the transmission of a patient's electrocardiogram.

Computer

Computer technology (e.g. that used with automated external defibrillators and other devices) has the potential to 'save' at every step of data entry. Computers allow for (1) documentation in near real time; (2) sorting information in many categories; (3) creation of multiple reporting formats; and (4) quick online and retrieval system data access. Computer terminals also are used by some communications centres to dispatch units automatically to a scene. As with most technologies, computer devices are subject to human error and other limitations and need regular upgrades. Moreover, the users have to obtain the proper education.

Box 5-3

Mobile phone technology

An analogue cell phone is really a radio that allows two persons to communicate on one frequency. The analogue signal fluctuates with the rise and fall of the caller's voice. This produces a wildly oscillating electrical wave (a 'copy' of speech). The signal can be heard at the receiver's end. Digital cell phones use the same radio technology. They, however, use different frequencies. Moreover, they compress the caller's voice into digital 1s and 0s that remain stable for the length of their travel. Then the digital information is converted back to voice at the receiver's end. The digital signal generally is thought to provide better sound quality. A digital signal also is thought to provide a more secure method of transmission than using analogue. Finally, digital technology provides the platform for wireless services such as data transmission and interactive computers. Analogue communications are generally obsolete and the vast majority of mobile phone and other mobile communications in use now in the UK are digital.

Note

Advances in EMS communications technology and telemedicine continue to evolve at a rapid pace. Video cameras, fax machines, cellular networks and the internet now allow photographs, videos (including movie-type imaging), and other information to be sent directly from the scene to a hospital for evaluation and consultation.

Operation modes used for EMS communications

The operation modes commonly used in EMS communications include simplex, multiplex, duplex and trunked.

Simplex mode

The simplex mode (Figure 5-3) requires a transmitter and receiver at each end of the communications path. Both elements operate on the same frequency. However, only one end may operate at a time. This mode allows speakers to send a message without interruption, although it slows the communications process and takes away the ability to discuss a case.

Duplex mode

The duplex mode (Figure 5-4) uses two frequencies that allow both parties to communicate at the same time. The

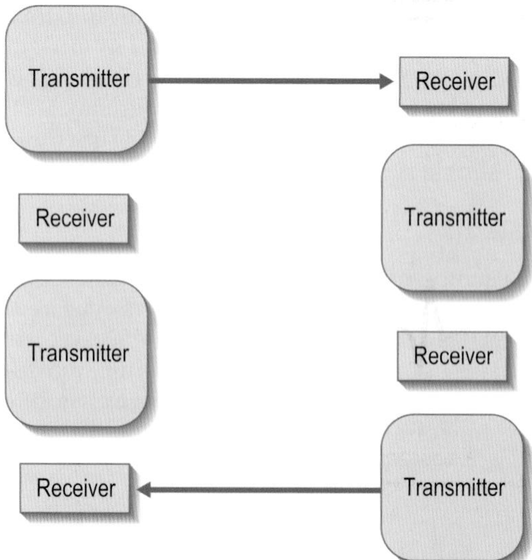

Figure 5-3 Required equipment for simplex mode includes a transmitter and a receiver at each end of the communications path, both operating on the same frequency. In the simplex mode, only one end may operate at a time. Adapted from National Emergency Number Association Technical Committee and PSAP Operational Standards Committee: NENA master glossary of 911 terminology. National Emergency Number Association, Arlington, VA, 1998.

advantage of this mode is that either party can interrupt the other to facilitate discussion. However, a tendency exists for each end to interrupt the other.

Multiplex mode

The multiplex mode (Figure 5-5) has the advantage of transmitting telemetry and voice simultaneously from a field unit. With this mode, either party can interrupt as needed, thereby facilitating discussion. As with the duplex mode, each party tends to interrupt the other. In addition, voice transmission may interfere with the transmission of data.

Trunked system

Trunking refers to systems that have many repeaters that work as a group. Each repeater is on a different channel. The trunking system may belong to a single user, for example a specific EMS service, or may be shared by a number of different public service agencies. When radio transmissions originate, computerized scanning automatically finds an available repeater in the system. Then the computer switches that transmission to the chosen repeater. As one fleet captures an open channel, it locks out all other users who share the system; this bars interference from other services. The trunked system is advantageous in major metropolitan operations where radio frequencies are used heavily.

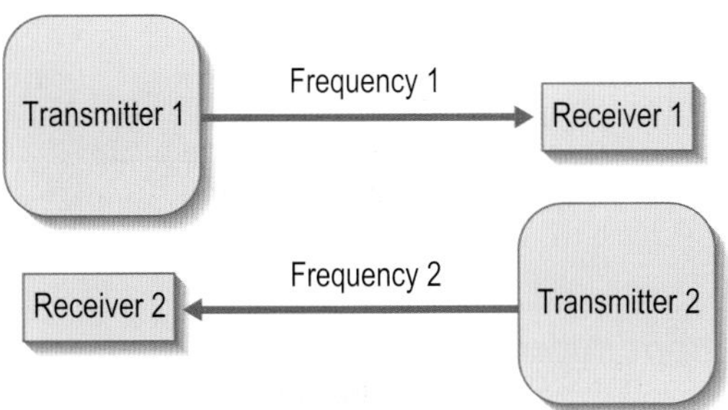

Figure 5-4 Duplex mode requires two frequencies so that both ends can communicate simultaneously.

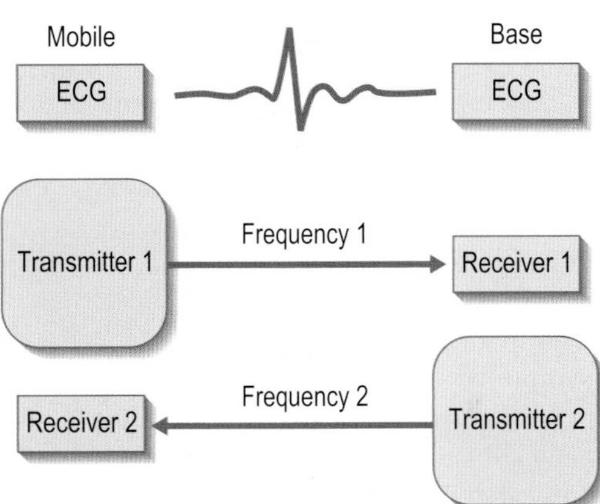

Figure 5-5 Multiplex mode operates similarly to duplex mode with added capabilities, such as simultaneous electrocardiogram and voice transmission.

Components and functions of dispatch communications systems

Some functions of an effective EMS dispatch communications system include the following (Box 5.4)

1. Receive and process calls for EMS assistance. The dispatcher receives and records calls for EMS assistance then selects an appropriate course of action for each call. This function involves obtaining as much information as possible about the emergency event, including name, callback number, and address, and it may include dealing with distraught callers. Emergency care instructions also may be provided while the incident is being dispatched.
2. Dispatch and coordinate the EMS resources. The dispatcher directs the proper emergency vehicles to the correct address and coordinates the movements of emergency vehicles while en route to the scene, to the medical facility, and back to the operations base.
3. Relay medical information. The dispatcher may provide a telecommunications channel between appropriate medical facilities and EMS personnel, fire, police, rescue workers, and the public. The channel may consist of telephone, radio, or biomedical telemetry.
4. Coordinate with other emergency services. The dispatcher provides for communications between public safety units (fire, police, and other emergency services and agencies) and elements of the EMS system. This helps to facilitate coordination of services such as traffic control, escort, fire suppression, and extrication. The dispatcher ensures an integrated, well-coordinated system. To do so, the dispatcher must know the location and status of all EMS vehicles and the availability of support services. CAD (computer-aided dispatching) such as CBD (criteria based dispatch) or AMPDS (advanced medical priority dispatch system) is used; this advanced technology allows one or more of the following capabilities or functions:
   - automatic emergency medical dispatch
   - automatic entry of 999

Box 5-4

999 system and computer-aided dispatch systems

999 was designated in 1937 as the universal emergency phone number. This came about after delays in getting help to a fire in London in which several people died. The system was quickly put in place so that by the following year it was universally accessible.

Most EMS call centres and control rooms use a computer-aided dispatch system. This monitors the available resources. The system makes an assignment based on access and routes for the ambulance closest to the map grid shown on the terminal. Global positioning systems tell the telecommunicator or system status controller which unit is closest to the origin of the call by air miles, or road miles if an intelligent map is used, to automatically route the unit that is closest to the scene. That unit then is sent to the scene. The telecommunicator monitors the call from beginning to end. The telecommunicator records status changes by digital media (e.g. tapes, CDs or DVDs).

- automatic call notification/request for assistance
- automatic interface to automatic vehicle location with or without map display
- automatic interface to mobile data terminal
- computer messaging among multiple radio operators, call takers, or both
- dispatch note taking, reminder aid, or both
- emergency medical dispatch review
- manual or automatic updates of unit status
- manual entry of call information
- radio control and display of channel status
- standard operating procedure review
- telephone control and display of circuit status.

Dispatcher training

EMS services require specialized medical training for their dispatch personnel; this will include training in using systems such as CBD and AMPDS. Emergency medical dispatchers are trained to do the following:

- use approved emergency medical dispatch guide cards (which may be customized to local needs and EMS response priorities)
- quickly and properly determine the nature of the call
- determine the priority of the call
- dispatch the appropriate response
- provide the caller with instructions to help treat the patient until the responding EMS unit arrives.

A base of training in EMS helps the telecommunicator understand functions of the EMS system, personnel capabilities, and equipment limitations; the training also arms the dispatcher with the protocols to give pre-arrival instructions. Examples include CPR instruction and aspirin administration for a patient with a possible acute coronary event. These protocols might mitigate the event before the arrival of an EMS unit.

Call prioritization – pre-arrival instructions systems

In a call screening–pre-arrival instructions system, an emergency medical dispatcher, paramedic or nurse determines what type of assistance is needed for an emergency call. This may include referring the caller to other services such as an out of hours primary care service or the referral to a minor injuries/illness unit or walk-in centre, choosing basic life support or advanced life support response, selecting the appropriate level or category of EMS response and therefore, by default, determining if the call is responded to as an emergency or under normal driving conditions. While dispatching the proper response, dispatchers can give the caller pre-arrival instructions. These instructions are crucial for these reasons:

- They provide instant help to the caller.
- They complement the call prioritization process.[1]
- They allow the dispatchers to give updated information to responding units.
- They may be lifesaving in critical incidents.[2,3]
- They provide emotional support for the caller, bystander or victim.

Critical Thinking

What are some potential consequences of a dispatching error?

Procedures for EMS communications

Most EMS systems use a standard radio communications protocol which includes the desired format for message transmission and key words and phrases. Following this format aids in professional and efficient radio communications within the system. General guidelines for radio communications include the following:

- Think before you speak (formulate the message) to ensure that communications will be effective.
- Speak at close range (5–7 cm; 2–3 inches) when talking into a microphone.
- Speak slowly and clearly. Enunciate each word distinctly and avoid words that are difficult to hear.
- Speak in a normal pitch without emotion.
- Be brief and concise. Break up long messages into shorter ones.
- Avoid codes unless they are systems approved. Avoid dialect or slang.
- Advise the receiving party when the transmission has been completed.
- Confirm the receiving party has received the message.
- Always be professional, polite, and calm.

Critical Thinking

Can you think of three reasons why a concise emergency medical services radio report is essential?

Relaying patient information

A standard format of transmission may be developed as a protocol for some EMS services. This format allows the best use of communications systems; it limits time taken to pass the message. In addition, healthcare professionals can receive details quickly regarding the patient's condition and the chance of omitting any critical details is lessened.

Patient information can be reported to the hospital or dispatcher by radio or phone. Although the order of information delivery may vary by EMS system and scenario, the report should be brief and concise and would include some or all of the following:

- unit and provider identification
- description of the scene or incident
- patient's age and gender
- patient's presenting complaint
- associated symptoms
- brief, pertinent history of present illness or injury
- pertinent medical history, medications, and allergies
- pertinent physical examination findings
  - level of consciousness
  - vital signs

   - neurological examination
   - general appearance and degree of distress
   - electrocardiogram results (if applicable)
   - trauma index or Glasgow Coma Scale score (if applicable)
   - other pertinent observations and significant findings
- any treatment given
- estimated time of arrival.

The ASHICE format

This format is used widely in the UK and is a more simplified version of the above; it does provide a range of data that the receiving staff can use to prepare for the patient's arrival:

Age: the patient's age
Sex: the patient's sex (gender)
History: a brief account of what has occurred
Injuries or illness: the main problems the patient is currently experiencing
Condition: vital signs and other diagnostic findings
Estimated time of arrival: the time the crew estimate their arrival at the hospital, given as the 24-hour clock time not in numbers of minutes to arrive (it the message is passed on to several others the time can be distorted if it is given as, for example, 10 minutes time).

Note

The use of telemetry to transmit a patient's electrocardiogram usually is reserved for the patient who requires diagnosis of a 12-lead electrocardiogram before the administration of some drugs. Telemetry transmission uses excessive air time. If warranted, 15–30 s of electrocardiogram transmission are usually adequate.

The SOAP format

The SOAP format (or a similar method) is used by many paramedics as a memory aid to organize written and verbal patient reports. SOAP is an acronym for the following:

- *Subjective data*: All patient symptoms including chief complaint, associated symptoms, history, current medications and allergies, and information provided by bystanders and family
- *Objective data*: Pertinent physical examination information including vital signs, level of consciousness, physical examination findings, electrocardiogram, pulse oximetry readings, and blood glucose determinations
- *Assessment data*: The paramedic's clinical impression of the patient based on subjective and objective data
- *Plan of patient management*: Treatment that has been provided and any requests for additional treatment.

Summary

- Communications regarding EMS refers to the delivery of information. The patient and scene information is delivered to other key members of the emergency response team.
- Verbal, written, and electronic communications allow the delivery of information between the party requesting help and the dispatcher, between the dispatcher and paramedic, and between the paramedic, hospital, and other healthcare providers.
- Emergency communications technology has industry-specific terminology.
- The primary modes of EMS communications include simplex mode, duplex mode, multiplex mode, trunking system, digital and computer.
- The functions of an effective dispatch communications system include receiving and processing calls for EMS assistance, dispatching and coordinating EMS resources, relaying medical information, and coordinating with public and emergency services.
- A standard format of transmission of patient information is a wise idea. The standard allows for the best use of communications systems. The standard also allows physicians to receive details quickly about the patient. In addition, the standard decreases the chance of omitting any critical details.

References

1. Flynn J, Archer F, Morgans A 2006 Sensitivity and specificity of the medical priority dispatch system in detecting cardiac arrest emergency calls in Melbourne. Prehospital Disaster Medicine 21 (2 Suppl 2): 72–76
2. Clawson J, Olola C, Heward A, Patterson B, Scott G 2008 The Medical Priority Dispatch System's ability to predict cardiac arrest outcomes and high acuity pre-hospital alerts in chest pain patients presenting to 9-9-9. Resuscitation 78(3):298–306
3. Heward A, Damiani M, Hartley-Sharpe C 2004 Does the use of the Advanced Medical Priority Dispatch System affect cardiac arrest detection? Emerg Med J 21:115–118

CHAPTER 6

Therapeutic Communication

Chapter contents

Objectives

Upon completion of this chapter, the paramedic student will be able to:

1. Define therapeutic communication.
2. List the elements of effective therapeutic communication.
3. Identify internal factors that influence effective communication.
4. Identify external factors that influence effective communication.
5. Explain the elements of an effective patient interview.
6. Summarize strategies for gathering appropriate patient information.
7. Discuss methods of assessing the individual's mental status during the patient interview.
8. Describe ways the paramedic can improve communication with a variety of patients. Such patients include (1) those who are unmotivated to talk; (2) hostile patients; (3) children; (4) older adults; (5) hearing-impaired patients; (6) blind patients; (7) patients under the influence of drugs or alcohol; (8) sexually aggressive patients; and (9) patients whose cultural traditions are different from those of the paramedic.

Key terms

decoding The act of interpreting symbols and format.

encoding The act of placing a message in an understandable format (either written or verbal).

therapeutic communication A planned, deliberate, professional act that involves the use of communications techniques to achieve two purposes: (1) a positive relationship with the patient and (2) a shared understanding of information between the patient and the paramedic. These two factors aid in the attainment of the desired patient care goals.

Therapeutic communication can have several important effects. It can improve the paramedic's interaction with the patient, ensure better patient care, defuse potentially violent situations or prevent them from escalating, and reduce the risk of lawsuits.

Communication

Communication is the main element of human interaction. It involves both verbal and non-verbal behaviour and includes all the symbols and clues people use to convey and

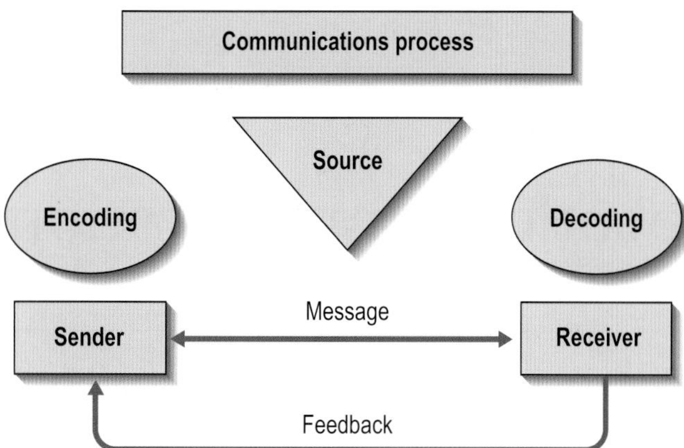

Figure 6-1 The process of communication. Adapted with permission from Legal Advocates for Abused Women, St. Louis.

receive meaning.[1] The process of communication has several elements. The paramedic must be aware of each element to interact well with a patient as every element is crucial. In fact, information and meaning can be gained or lost if any one element is changed (Figure 6-1). To achieve good communication, all participants must take equal responsibility for their part in the process. Communication is successful only when each person clearly gets the message.

Note

This chapter deals with communication between paramedics and their patients. However, these suggestions and techniques can also be used to improve communication between healthcare providers. This may include crew members, nurses, doctors, dispatchers, and other emergency providers.

Elements of the communication process

Communication is a dynamic process that has six elements: the source, encoding, the message, decoding, the receiver and feedback.

Source

Verbal communication uses spoken or written words (common symbols) to express ideas or feelings. These common symbols should be simple, short, and direct so that confusion can be avoided (Box 6-1).

Critical Thinking

Think about the last time you had a misunderstanding with someone. Would any of the techniques listed in Box 6-1 have improved the situation?

Encoding

Encoding involves putting a message in a format that, when translated, is understood by both the sender and the receiver. The format may be either written or verbal. Encoding is the responsibility of the sender (encoder), because the sender defines the content and emotional tone of the message. In the process of communication, the sender role passes from one person to another as information is exchanged. For example, at first the paramedic may act as the sender of the message by asking a patient for information. When the patient responds, that person assumes the role of the sender.

Box 6-1

Techniques for verbal communication

- Use fewer words to avoid confusion.
- Use words that express an idea simply.
- Do not use vague phrases.
- Use examples (including demonstrations) if they will make the message easier to understand.
- Repeat the important parts of a message.
- Do not use technical jargon.
- Speak at an appropriate speed or pace.
- Do not pause for long periods or quickly change the subject.

Message

The message is the information that is sent or expressed by the sender. It should be clear, organized and communicated in a manner familiar to the person receiving it. The message may include verbal and non-verbal symbols (e.g. spoken words, facial expressions, gestures). As a rule, the more ways (or formats) in which a message is communicated, the more likely the receiver is to understand it. For example, combining soothing words and a reassuring touch for a patient in pain communicates the message of compassion better than spoken words alone.

Not all symbols have universal meaning. For example, a reassuring touch might be welcome to persons of certain cultures, whilst those of other cultures may find it offensive. Paramedics must take into account the cultural differences of people and also consider how they will deal with a language barrier before attempting to send a message.

Decoding

Decoding is the interpretation of symbols and formats. It prompts the receiver to respond to the sender's message. The decoding process can fail if symbols or words sent in the message are unfamiliar to both parties. It can also fail if interpretation of the message is based on different understandings of symbols or format. For example, the word pain may mean horrific discomfort to one person but it may mean a mild annoyance to another. Therefore, when communicating with a patient, the paramedic must carefully select words that cannot easily be misinterpreted.

Note

Some medical conditions, such as a stroke, can make it more difficult for a person to encode or decode a message.

Receiver

The receiver is essentially the decoder. This is the person intended to understand the message. As with the role of sender, the role of receiver switches back and forth between participants during the communication process.

Critical Thinking

Have you ever attended a class in which nothing made sense? Think back on the reason you didn't understand the content. Was it an encoding problem or a decoding problem?

Feedback

Feedback is the receiver's response to the sender's message. The quality of the feedback reveals whether the message's intended meaning was received. If the intended meaning was not received, the sender must clarify the message by changing its content. The sender then assesses the new feedback. Like the message, feedback may be verbal or non-verbal.

Internal factors in effective communication

To communicate well with patients, paramedics must genuinely like people and they must be able to empathize with others. They must also have the ability to listen (Box 6-2). Each of these internal factors plays an important role in therapeutic communication.

Liking others

As a helping profession, healthcare depends on the relationships forged between patients and healthcare providers. These relationships are based on trust and caring. In fact, they cannot be achieved without a genuine concern for others and an understanding of human strengths and weaknesses. Patients must trust and believe that a paramedic wants to care for their needs. Paramedics can convey this trust to patients by accepting them as individuals.

Empathy

Empathy is the ability to see a situation from the viewpoint of the person experiencing it and is widely accepted as a clinical aspect of a helping profession. Sympathy, on the other hand, is the expression of one's feelings about another person's problem. Unlike sympathy, empathy uses sensitive and objective communication. This helps patients explain and explore their feelings so that problems can be solved (Box 6-3).

Ability to listen

Listening is an active process that requires complete attention and practice. To be an effective listener, the paramedic should:[2]

1. Face patients while they speak.
2. Maintain natural eye contact to show a willingness to listen.
3. Assume an attentive posture (avoid crossing the legs and arms, because this may convey a defensive attitude).
4. Avoid distracting body movements (e.g. wringing the hands, tapping the feet or fidgeting with an object).
5. Nod in acknowledgment when patients talk about important points or look for feedback.
6. Lean toward the speaker to communicate involvement.

One device for remembering ways to improve communication is the listening ladder (Figure 6-2). This device has six steps to listening. They can easily be remembered from the acronym LADDER.[3]

Box 6-2

Active listening attitudes and guidelines

1. Listen to understand, not to ready yourself to reply, contradict, or argue back. This attitude is extremely important.
2. Remember that understanding involves more than simply knowing the dictionary meaning of the words used. It involves paying attention to the patient's tone of voice, facial expressions, and overall behaviour.
3. Look for clues to what the individual is trying to say. As best you can, put yourself in the patient's position. Try to see the world as the patient sees it. Accept the patient's feelings as facts that must be taken into account, whether you share them or not.
4. Put aside your own views and opinions for the time being. Realize that you cannot listen to yourself inwardly and at the same time truly listen to the patient.
5. Control your impatience. Listening is faster than talking. The average person speaks about 120 words a minute but people can listen to about 400 words a minute. Do not jump ahead of the patient. Give the person time to tell the story. A patient doesn't always say what the paramedic expects to hear.
6. Do not prepare an answer while you listen. Get the whole message before deciding what to say. The patient's last sentence may put a whole new slant on what was said before.
7. Show the patient that you are alert and interested. This encourages the patient and improves communication.
8. Do not interrupt. Ask questions only to obtain more information. Do not try to trap the patient or force the individual into a corner.
9. Expect the patient's use of words to differ from yours. Do not quibble about terms – try to get at what was meant.
10. Your purpose is the opposite of a debater's goal. Look for areas of agreement, not for weak spots to attack with a barrage of counterarguments.
11. Before giving an answer in a particularly difficult discussion, summarize what you understand the patient to have said. If the patient disagrees with this version, clear up the contested points before giving your own views.
12. Let patients describe themselves and their interests, position, and opinions.

External factors in effective communication

Good communication requires a suitable setting. The paramedic has control over a number of the external factors that affect the setting, such as privacy, interruptions, eye contact,

Box 6-3

Empathy versus sympathy

The case below shows the difference between empathy and sympathy. It also shows how empathy can help the paramedic soothe the patient and gain his trust.

Your paramedic crew is sent to the home of a 60-year-old man with substernal chest pain. When you arrive, the patient is sitting on the living room sofa with his wife. They are upset and afraid that he might die. Your crew begins standard procedures for a possible heart attack and prepares to transport the patient to the emergency department. On the way to the hospital, the paramedic and the patient, who is accompanied by his wife, have the following conversation:

Paramedic: Even though you're feeling better, I can tell you're worried and afraid.

Patient: Yes, I am. I'm afraid I'm going to die.

Paramedic: Would you like me to explain to you and your wife what will happen after we arrive in the emergency department? I can also explain what the doctors and nurses will do to make sure you get the best possible care.

Patient: Yes, we would like that very much.

The use of empathy, shown in this conversation, allows the paramedic to accomplish three things: (1) calm the patient and his wife; (2) provide the couple with useful information; and (3) partly address their concerns. If the paramedic had used sympathy alone (e.g. 'I understand how you feel, but don't worry, everything will be OK'), the patient's fears would have been ignored. Also, the problem of the couple's agitation would not have been solved.

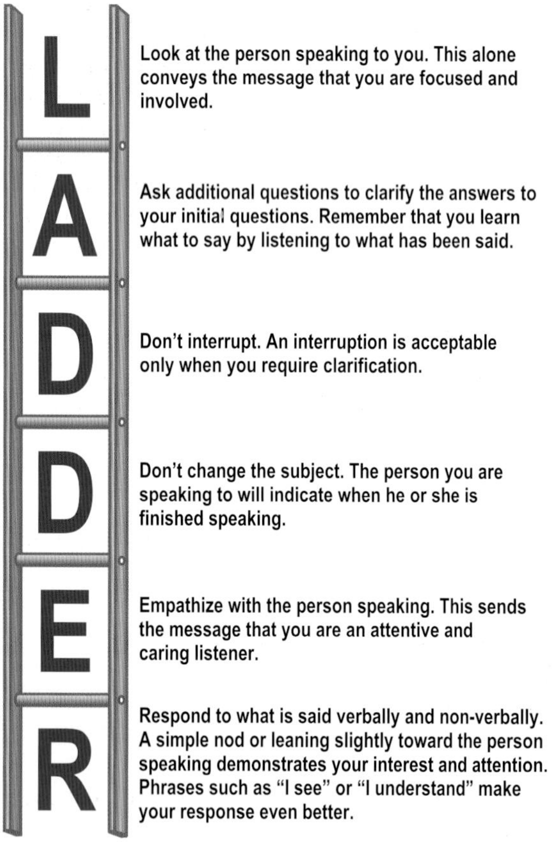

L Look at the person speaking to you. This alone conveys the message that you are focused and involved.

A Ask additional questions to clarify the answers to your initial questions. Remember that you learn what to say by listening to what has been said.

D Don't interrupt. An interruption is acceptable only when you require clarification.

D Don't change the subject. The person you are speaking to will indicate when he or she is finished speaking.

E Empathize with the person speaking. This sends the message that you are an attentive and caring listener.

R Respond to what is said verbally and non-verbally. A simple nod or leaning slightly toward the person speaking demonstrates your interest and attention. Phrases such as "I see" or "I understand" make your response even better.

Figure 6-2 The ladder of listening.

and personal dress. Control of these factors results in a better interaction between the paramedic and the patient.

Privacy, interruptions and the physical environment

When possible, the paramedic should ensure privacy during the encounter. This helps to eliminate distractions and to reduce any inhibitions the patient may feel. Interruptions should be kept to a minimum. Obviously, this is impossible if the paramedic is receiving critical patient care information from crew members. When possible, the lighting should be adequate whilst noise and interference should be minimized. In addition, the patient interview should be started away from distracting equipment.

The paramedic should be aware of the patient's private space. This is a comfortable distance from the patient's body, usually about 1.25 to 1.5 m (4 to 5 feet),[4] or twice the patient's arm length away. Private space is a form of subconscious personal protection that varies by individual and by culture. Some patients may become defensive if this space is invaded. Entering this space usually causes the patient to back away.

Eye contact

The paramedic should maintain eye contact with the patient as much as possible, even when taking notes. Eye contact is a type of non-verbal communication. It can help express gentleness, sincerity, and authority and can help make the patient feel safe and secure. If possible, the paramedic should be positioned at eye level (equal seating) with the patient.

Personal dress

Communication with a patient begins with first impressions. Paramedics' appearance should be professional. Their clothing should be clean and should meet professional standards (e.g. uniforms provided by the ambulance service). These standards help the patient instantly identify an emergency medical services (EMS) provider and help to set the tone of the paramedic–patient encounter.

Patient interview

The ability to conduct a successful patient interview may be as important as physical assessment skills. The information gathered often helps to decide the direction of the physical examination. The patient interview should be started early and should continue throughout the patient encounter.

Because of the emergency nature of their work, paramedics often think in terms of specific illnesses and injuries. They often need to categorize patients into general groups, such as trauma or medical cases. However, good emergency care requires the paramedic to view each patient as an individual and it requires paramedics to attend to a patient's needs in a caring, concerned, and receptive manner.

Communication techniques

The paramedic should approach the conscious patient and make a personal introduction by name and title: 'Hello. My name is [name], and I am a paramedic with [name of ambulance service]. What's your name?' Talking with the patient allows the paramedic to evaluate the person's level of consciousness and sensorium and may also provide information on any hearing or speech impediments and language barriers. During the introduction, the paramedic should maintain eye contact with the patient.

Non-verbal communication can send a message of negative feelings and can also convey the insecurities of both the patient and the paramedic. Voice inflection, facial expression, and body position are examples of these non-verbal cues. They may reflect anger, fear or impatience. Similarly, starting intravenous therapy with trembling, sweaty hands may make the patient question the paramedic's skills. Non-verbal cues should be used to gain the patient's trust and cooperation.

Touch is a form of communication that shows compassion and reassurance. Small gestures can help comfort a person in distress. A few examples are holding a patient's hand, squeezing a shoulder, or wiping tears from a patient's eyes. Experience and familiarity with patient care activities help determine the appropriateness of these gestures.

In talking with patients, the paramedic must listen to what is said and interpret what is said. Patients may say they feel fine. Yet their appearance and tone of voice may indicate that they are ill and afraid. If paramedics are unsure of the message in a patient's response, they should ask additional questions that will help them better understand what the patient is trying to communicate.

Most patients do not understand medical terminology and many have only a vague understanding of the way their bodies work. For these reasons, the paramedic should use common words and phrases that are easy to understand. The paramedic should guide and direct the patient interview without manipulating the patient's response. In other words, the paramedic should avoid asking leading questions (questions that attempt to guide the respondent's answer). Open-ended questions encourage a free-form response and should generally be used in preference to closed questions. For example, the paramedic should ask, 'When did this pain begin?' rather than 'Did the pain begin this morning?'

Note

Open-ended questions:
Are asked in a narrative form
Encourage the patient to talk
Do not restrict the areas of response

The paramedic should ask only one question at a time and allow the patient ample time to answer before asking another question. If the patient's response does not seem relevant to the question, the response should be clarified. Paramedics should be flexible and should not discount the patient's experiences or information.

Paramedics should try to answer all of the patient's questions. However, this does not mean that they must provide a full explanation for each inquiry. Rather, a sensitive response that addresses the question is adequate. Paramedics should choose an answer carefully and should try to make sure that their answer does not upset the patient further.

Box 6-4

Helpful techniques for the patient interview

- Silence – gives patients more time to gather their thoughts.
- Reflection – echoing (i.e. paraphrasing) patients' words allow them to clarify or expand on the information provided.
- Empathy – encourages patients to talk more openly.
- Clarification – lets patients rephrase a word or thought that is confusing to the paramedic.
- Limitation – focuses patients' attention on one specific factor of the interview.
- Interpretation – links events; makes associations or implies a cause; is based on observation or conclusion.
- Explanation – provides information to patients; encourages sharing of facts or objective information.
- Summary – provides a review of the interview; the paramedic can ask open-ended questions that allow patients to clarify details.

Responses

The paramedic can use a number of tactics or responses to conduct a successful patient interview (Box 6-4). For example, the paramedic may use silence, which gives a patient more time to gather his or her thoughts. The paramedic may also paraphrase the patient's words (echoing), allowing the paramedic to clear up or expand on the information provided. Empathy can be used to get a patient to talk more openly. Other tactics include asking a patient to clarify confusing statements and limiting the patient's focus to one factor of the interview (limitation). At times the paramedic may need to interpret information by linking events, making associations, or inferring a cause based on what can be seen or concluded. The paramedic can also give the patient information to persuade the person to share facts or objective information. Finally, paramedics can summarize information by asking the patient open-ended questions that can be used to review and to clear up key details.

Traps in interviewing

Paramedics must be aware of some traps that can be damaging to the patient interview. These include the following:

- providing false reassurance
- offering poor or unwanted advice
- showing approval or disapproval
- giving an opinion that takes away the patient's part in decision making
- changing the subject inappropriately
- stereotyping the patient or complaint
- using professional jargon
- talking too much
- asking leading or biased questions
- interrupting the patient
- asking the patient 'Why' questions (these can be viewed as accusations)
- being defensive in response to criticism.

Developing a good rapport with the patient

Skill in developing good rapport with a patient takes experience and practice. In most patient encounters, paramedics can follow some general guidelines to help establish good rapport:

1. Put patients at ease by letting them know you are 'on their side'; that is, that you respect their comments, and you are there to help them.
2. Be alert for and respond to visual clues that a patient needs help.
3. Show compassion.
4. Assess the patient's level of understanding and insight. Use words and explanations at their level.
5. Show expertise.

Box 6-5

Approaching sensitive issues

Discussing sensitive issues can be awkward for both the patient and the paramedic. Such issues might include alcohol use, sexual subjects, and suicide risk. However, these issues must not be avoided when the information is needed to ensure good patient care. The paramedic should use the following guidelines when sensitive issues are discussed with patients:

- Make sure privacy is maintained.
- Be confident, direct, and firm with your questions.
- Do not apologize for asking a sensitive question.
- Do not be judgemental.
- Use words that are understandable, but do not be patronising.
- Be patient and proceed slowly.

Critical Thinking

A suicidal patient keeps telling you that you don't care about him. What communications techniques could you use to persuade this patient that you are concerned about him?

Strategies for obtaining information

For the most part, patients communicate with healthcare providers in three ways. The first is by pouring out the information in the form of complaints. The second is by revealing some problems while hiding others they think are embarrassing. The third is by hiding the most embarrassing parts of their problem from the paramedic (and personally denying the issue). The best way to obtain information from the patient is to use techniques for open-ended and closed (direct) questions. These techniques include resistance, shifting focus, recognizing defence mechanisms and distraction.

Note

Closed questions allow the paramedic to obtain specific information that focuses on a certain aspect of the patient's condition. 'What part of your back hurts?' and 'When was your last meal?' are two examples of closed questions.

Resistance

Often a patient is reluctant to give information for one of two reasons. First, the patient may want to maintain a personal image and is afraid of losing that image. Second, the patient may fear that the paramedic will respond with rejection and ridicule. Paramedics, therefore, should be non-judgemental. This helps them to obtain information from patients (Box 6-5). To develop a trusting relationship, the paramedic must be willing to talk to the patient about any condition in a professional manner.

Shifting focus

A patient may seem unwilling to discuss an obvious problem. In this situation, the paramedic may have to shift the focus of the questions away from that problem. For example, a man with groin pain at first may describe the pain (especially to a female paramedic) as being in his 'lower back'. By shifting the focus of questioning to low back pain, the paramedic can use another angle. The questions can focus on the presence or absence of radiating pain. This new line of questioning can make patients feel more comfortable when describing their condition.

Defence mechanisms

Paramedics should recognize common defence mechanisms (see Chapter 3). If possible, they should try to anticipate them. For example, an upset parent with a seriously ill child may show regression or denial. The parent may be unable to provide needed information at the emergency scene. Confrontation may be required in these and similar situations to force the parent to deal with key issues. Confrontation can clarify roles and may help others identify problems and goals. However, this technique should be used only to obtain information critical for medical care and must be performed in a professional way. This allows the patient to become aware of inconsistencies in interfering behaviour or thoughts.

Distraction

Paramedics may use distraction to help patients recognize irrational thoughts or behaviour. This type of behaviour may be seen in hostile situations in which patients 'act out'. In such cases, paramedics need to point out the unacceptable behaviour and let patients know the self-defeating nature of the behaviour. Often, this distraction prompts patients to let the paramedic handle the situation until they can gain self-control. When dealing with an angry or hostile patient, paramedics should:

- avoid raising their voices to match the angry person's tone
- have the person identify and describe the cause of anger
- restate the cause of the anger
- offer a solution (if possible) or empathize and acknowledge the person's feelings.

Methods of assessing mental status during the interview

Three methods can be used to assess a patient's mental status: observation, conversation and exploration. (Assessment of the level of consciousness is discussed in more detail in other chapters.)

Observation

The first step in assessing mental status is to observe the patient. Paramedics should note the patient's appearance, level of consciousness, and body movements. Physical characteristics, dress and grooming can provide clues and may even indicate the patient's well-being, social status, religion, culture and self-concept. Conscious patients for the most part are alert and able to speak intelligently. Body movements (e.g. gestures, facial expressions) should be appropriate for the situation. Abnormal body movements may indicate an unstable situation and may include unusual posture or gait or clenched fists.

Conversation

Conversation with patients should reveal whether they know who they are, where they are, and the day or date (i.e. whether they are oriented to person, place and time). If the patient knows these things, the remote, recent and intermediate facets of memory probably are intact. The patient should be able to speak at a normal pace and with even flow. Responses should not have long pauses or rapid shifts (although such nuances vary by geographical location). During normal conversation, the patient should be able to show clear thinking, a normal attention span, and the ability to concentrate on and understand the discussion.

A patient's responses to the setting (affect) should match the situation. Normal reactions to stress may include autonomic responses such as sweating, trembling and odd facial movements (e.g. muscle twitching around the mouth, nose, and eyes). Reactive movements, such as not holding eye contact during conversation, should be noted. Other actions may indicate that a patient is uncomfortable or anxious. These include grooming movements, such as fixing the hair and straightening the clothes.

Exploration

Exploration offers a way to assess the patient's emotions. For example, by observing that the patient's mood is anxious, excited, or depressed and by noting the individual's energy level, the paramedic can gauge the mental status. Exploration can be done simply by interacting with the patient. This allows the paramedic to see whether actions and ideas are appropriate. An objective assessment must weigh the patient's culture and education as well as taking into account the person's values, beliefs, and previous experiences.

Critical Thinking

The mental status examination is critical, both for medical reasons and for legal reasons. Why do you think this is so?

Special interview situations

At times paramedics may have to use special skills to interact successfully with a patient who is uncooperative or frightened or who has a disability (also see Chapter 8).

Patients who don't want to talk

Although most patients are more than willing to talk, some need more time and varying techniques to participate in a successful interview. Tough interviews generally stem from four factors:

1. The patient's condition may affect the ability to speak.
2. The patient may fear talking because of psychological problems, cultural differences, or age.
3. The patient may have a cognitive impairment.
4. The patient may want to deceive the paramedic.

Helpful techniques

The following techniques may be useful for communicating with a patient who is unmotivated to talk:

- Start the interview in the normal way. If the patient does not talk, review the nature of the call as received from the dispatch centre. Take time to develop a rapport with the patient.
- Use open-ended questions to get a response. If this is unsuccessful, try direct questions.
- Provide positive feedback to appropriate responses from the patient.
- Make sure the patient understands the question. (Consider whether a language barrier or a hearing difficulty is a factor.)
- Continue asking questions to obtain critical information needed to provide treatment. (Non-essential information may be difficult to obtain.)
- Question family members or others at the scene. If the patient has been uncommunicative for a long period, try to rule out a disease or disorder as the reason.
- Use summary and interpretation of events or conditions. Also, ask the patient if your summary and version are correct.
- Try to start a conversation by asking the patient questions about your care, equipment, or profession. If the patient responds, answer all questions fully (not with one-word answers).
- Realize that all the information needed may not be obtained.
- Observe the patient's responses to the setting and surroundings and record what you see. This sets a mental status baseline for later evaluations.
- Consider asking questions for which answers are known. This helps to gauge the patient's credibility.

Note

Patients who are unconscious or unresponsive may be able to receive stimuli. Hearing is thought to be the last sensation lost with unconsciousness and is also thought to be the first regained with consciousness.[4] The paramedic must not say anything near an unconscious patient that would not be said if the patient were fully conscious.

Box 6-6

Tips for communicating with children of various ages

- Infants respond best to firm, gentle handling and a quiet, calm voice. Older infants may have stranger anxiety. If possible, the parent should remain in view of the child.
- Pre-school children see the world only from their perspective and base everything on past experience. Use short sentences and give concrete explanations (e.g. you will need to hold still so that I can splint your arm and make you feel better).
- Adolescents want to be adults. Treat them with respect and use age-appropriate words. Do not talk to or treat them as if they were small children.

Hostile patients

Paramedics should be alert for signs that a situation may turn violent. This is part of ensuring personal safety. Such signs may include clenched fists, a rising voice level, a threatening facial expression, or a history of violence toward others. If such a situation exists or is expected, the EMS crew should leave the scene and request the help of the police. If safe retreat is not an option, the paramedics should stay far enough away from the patient to ensure their personal safety (see Chapter 25). Some guidelines that can be used in interviewing a hostile patient are:

- Try to use normal interviewing techniques.
- Never leave the patient alone without adequate assistance.
- Set limits and boundaries with the patient.
- Explain the advantages of cooperation to the patient.
- Follow local protocol for dealing with hostile patients, including the use of physical restraints.

Patients with age-related factors

Communicating with children and older adults should not be difficult or a challenge. It works best when the paramedic takes into account the common developmental characteristics of a particular age group.

Communicating with children

When communicating with children, the paramedic may need to establish rapport with two people – the child and the parent. With children 1 to 6 years old, most conversation should be directed first to the parent. (Offering a toy may distract the child while the parent is interviewed.) The paramedic should be aware that information from the parent is that person's point of view, and the parent might be feeling defensive. Paramedics should not be judgemental if the parents had not provided proper care or safety for the child before the crew arrived. (Paramedics should be observant but not confrontational.)

The paramedic should gradually begin to make contact with the child during the parent interview. This can be done by moving to eye level to speak with the child and by using a quiet, calm voice. The paramedic should keep in mind that children are especially responsive to non-verbal cues. Box 6-6 lists special considerations for communicating with children of various ages (also see Chapter 38).

Communicating with older adults

Many older adults are dealing with age-related diseases and the inevitability of death. Interviewing older adults may take longer than interviewing younger persons. Older patients may tire more easily and may have physical disabilities that distort speech. Touch is generally important to older adults. When interviewing an older person, the paramedic should always use the individual's last name and Mr, Mrs or Ms unless the patient says otherwise. In addition, the patient should be able to see the paramedic's face easily. The paramedic should keep eye contact and speak clearly and slowly. He or she should be willing to take extra time to get the required information. Using short, open-ended questions and talking with family members may be the best approaches for the patient interview (also see Chapter 39).

Hearing-impaired patients

When dealing with a patient with a hearing impairment, the paramedic should determine the patient's preferred method of communicating. It may be lip-reading, signing or writing. Writing is often the best out-of-hospital method for communicating with a deaf patient. If the patient prefers lip-reading, the paramedic should: (1) face the patient squarely; (2) make sure the light is adequate; (3) speak slowly using short words and phrases; and (4) enunciate clearly. Because many deaf patients lip-read, paramedics must speak clearly in full view of these patients. They must also realize that some deaf patients may nod 'Yes' even if they do not understand the question.

If a patient is thought to be hearing-impaired or deaf, the paramedic should try to gain the person's attention. This can be done by a gentle touch or by slowly waving the hands in front of the patient. The paramedic may also try speaking a little louder or speaking into the patient's ear if the person is not wearing a hearing aid. If a hearing-impaired patient needs to be taken to a medical facility, the paramedic should inform the emergency department staff as soon as possible about the impairment. This allows arrangements to be made for someone to help the staff members communicate with patient. (This is also a good practice with patients who do not speak English.)

Paramedics might consider learning finger spelling and simple sign language to aid them in their work. These are both easily learned.

Blind patients

When communicating with a blind patient, paramedics should determine or ascertain whether the patient also has a hearing impairment (even though this is not common). Paramedics should identify themselves in a normal voice and should answer all the patient's questions about the emergency scene and the surroundings. They should also explain all examination and treatment procedures in detail before they touch the patient.

Most patients who have disabilities are very independent and may even resent unsolicited help. If a sightless person has a guide dog and the situation permits, the two should not be separated. If the dog was injured during the emergency, the paramedic should quickly advise the dispatch centre to make special arrangements for care for the dog.

Patients under the influence of street drugs or alcohol

If street drugs or alcohol play a part in an emergency, paramedics should ensure their personal safety. They should also be ready for unpredictable patient behaviour. (The help of the police may be needed to ensure scene safety.) During the patient interview, paramedics should ask simple or direct questions and should avoid any action the patient might see as a threat or confrontation (see Chapters 21 and 45).

Sexually aggressive patients

Paramedics should confront male or female patients who make improper sexual advances. This ensures that the patient is aware of the professional role of the caregiver. Paramedics should document any unusual incidents and also the observations of any witnesses to any of the actions. Sexually aggressive patients should be cared for by paramedics of the same gender and a chaperone or witness should be present during the care and transportation of the patient.

Transcultural considerations

When speaking with a patient from another culture, paramedics should introduce themselves and then ask the patient to do the same. Paramedics must be aware that they may be seen as a stereotype by the patient and family. For this reason, the roles of everyone involved in the care (paramedics, patient and family members) must be clear.

Two pitfalls that paramedics must avoid when speaking with patients of a different culture are ethnocentrism and cultural imposition. Ethnocentrism is seeing one's own life as the most acceptable or best. It includes acting in a superior manner toward another culture's way of life. Cultural imposition is forcing one's beliefs, values, and patterns of behaviour on people from another culture. Paramedics do not generally fall into these pitfalls deliberately but they must be sensitive to how their actions and words may be seen by those of another culture. Other factors to consider in communicating with patients of another culture are:

- Some cultures expect healthcare workers to have all the answers to their illness.
- Different cultures accept illness or injury in different ways.
- Non-verbal cues (e.g. handshaking and touching) are seen differently in different cultures.
- Some cultures consider direct eye contact to be impolite or aggressive; patients may avert their eyes during an interview.
- Paramedics should not use touch as a means of reassurance with members of different cultural groups because touch may be easily misunderstood.
- Language barriers may present difficulties (Box 6-7).
- Personal space is often defined by culture. It also varies by individual (Box 6-8).

Critical Thinking

Do you know anyone whose personal space requirements are much greater or much less than those listed in Box 6-8? How would this affect your interview with that person?

Box 6-7

General guidelines for working with an interpreter

As a paramedic, you will sometimes be called to assist a patient who does not speak English. Often someone in the home or at the scene can help you communicate with the person. When working with an interpreter, use the following guidelines:

1. Explain to the interpreter the key information you are trying to get before you begin the interview.
2. Ask a child to interpret only if no adult interpreter is available.
3. Speak directly to the patient or to a family member when asking questions. This establishes the primary relationship with that individual (not the interpreter). It also allows you to observe non-verbal clues.
4. Ask questions that call for one response at a time. For example, ask, 'Do you have pain?' rather than 'Do you have any pain, trouble breathing or nausea?'
5. Try not to interrupt the patient, family member or interpreter when that person is speaking.
6. Do not make comments about the patient or family to the interpreter; the patient or family may know some English.
7. Use simple language. Do not use medical terms for which other languages may have no similar words.
8. After the interview, if time permits, ask for the interpreter's impressions and observations of the interview.

Modified from Wong D 1995 Whaley and Wong's nursing care of infants and children, 5th edition. Mosby, St Louis.

Box 6-8

General guidelines on personal space

Intimate zone

0–50 cm (1½ feet)
Visual distortion occurs
Best for assessing breath and other body odours

Personal distance

50 cm to 1.25 m (1½ to 4 feet)
Perceived as an extension of self
Speaker's voice is moderate
Body odours are not apparent
Much of the physical assessment occurs at this distance

Social distance

1.25–3.75 m (4–12 feet)
Used for impersonal business transactions
Perceptual information is much less detailed
Much of the patient interview occurs at this distance

Public distance

3.75 m (12 feet) or farther
Interaction with others is impersonal
Speaker's voice must be projected
Subtle facial expressions are imperceptible

These are only general guidelines. Some cultures are more comfortable at a variety of distances when communicating

Summary

- Therapeutic communication is a planned act. It is also a professional act. The paramedic, working with the patient, obtains information that is used to meet patient care goals.
- Communication is a dynamic process. It has six elements: the source, encoding, the message, decoding, the receiver and feedback.
- To effectively communicate with patients, paramedics must genuinely like people. They must be able to empathize with others. They also must have the ability to listen.
- Good communication calls for a favourable physical environment. Factors such as privacy, interruption, eye contact, and personal dress are external influences. These factors can be controlled and allow the paramedic to better communicate with the patient.
- The patient interview often decides the direction of the physical examination. Good care means that the paramedic sees each patient as an individual. It also means that the patient's needs are met in a caring, concerned, and receptive way.
- Open-ended and closed (direct) questions can be used to get information from the patient. Techniques include resistance, shifting focus, recognizing defence mechanisms, and distraction.
- The first step with any patient is to assess mental status. This can be done by observing the patient's appearance and level of consciousness. The paramedic can also look for normal or abnormal body movements. During normal conversation, the patient should be able to show clear thinking, a normal attention span, and the ability to concentrate on and understand the discussion. The patient's responses to the environment (i.e. affect) should be appropriate to the situation.
- Difficult interviews generally arise from four situations: (1) the patient's condition may affect the ability to speak; (2) the patient may fear talking because of psychological disorders, cultural differences, or age; (3) a cognitive impairment may be present; or (4) the patient may want to deceive the paramedic.

References

1. Satir V 1988 The new peoplemaking. Science & Behavior Books, Palo Alto, CA
2. Potter PA, Perry AG 2001 Fundamentals of nursing: concepts, process, and practice, 5th edition. Mosby, St Louis
3. Moore M 1999 Embracing the mystery. MJM Publishing, Madison, WI
4. Rathus S 1987 Psychology, 3rd edition. Holt, Rinehart & Winston, New York

CHAPTER 7

Patient Assessment

Chapter contents

Objectives

Upon completion of this chapter, the paramedic student will be able to:

1. Identify the components of the scene size-up.
2. Identify the priorities in each component of patient assessment.
3. Outline the critical steps in initial patient assessment.
4. Describe findings in the initial assessment that may indicate a life-threatening condition.
5. Discuss interventions for life-threatening conditions that are identified in the initial assessment.
6. Identify the components of the patient history and physical examination for medical patients.
7. Identify the components of the patient history and physical examination for trauma patients.
8. Describe the ongoing assessment.
9. Distinguish priorities in the care of the medical versus trauma patient.

Key terms

general impression An immediate assessment of the environment and the patient's presenting complaint used to determine whether the patient is ill or injured and the nature of the illness or the mechanism of injury.

initial assessment A component of the patient assessment to recognize and manage all immediate life-threatening conditions.

ongoing assessment A repeat of the initial assessment that is performed throughout the paramedic–patient encounter.

patient history A component of patient assessment to ascertain the patient's presenting complaint, history of present illness, medical history and current health status.

priority patients Patients who need immediate care and transport.

scene size-up An assessment of the scene to ensure scene safety for the paramedic crew, patient(s), and bystanders; a quick assessment to determine the resources needed to manage the scene adequately.

Scene assessment

Scene assessment is the first assessment taken during every emergency medical services (EMS) response. These steps ensure scene safety for the paramedic crew, patient(s), and bystanders. The assessment of the scene and setting offer key information to the paramedic. The priorities in scene size-up and assessment include the following:

- Determine the nature of the incident.
- Determine the maximum potential number of persons already ill or injured and needing care.
- Assess for hazards at the scene.
- Initiate a mass casualty or major incident plan if called for (see Chapter 42).
- Notify the ambulance control room to request more resources (e.g. police, fire and rescue, utility companies) and to alert local hospitals (as needed).
- Determine the best access routes and holding areas for responders.
- Secure the area as rapidly as possible, clearing unneeded persons from the scene.
- Begin triage (if needed).

Even scenes that seem safe may not be; paramedics should never enter a potentially unsafe scene until they know it is safe to approach the patient. Examples of unsafe scenes include road traffic collisions, scenes where rescue will be required, areas with toxic substances and low oxygen, patients and others under the influence of intoxicating substances, crime or other scenes where violence or patient/ bystander aggressive behaviour is likely, and scenes that have unstable surfaces (e.g. slope, ice or water). It is important not to have a 'blinkered' or narrow focus on approach; paramedics should be prepared to take in all the information that a scene assessment provides. Personal safety is the first priority of the paramedic.

> **Critical Thinking**
>
> Do you know a paramedic who has been injured on a scene? What caused the injury? Could the injury have been prevented?

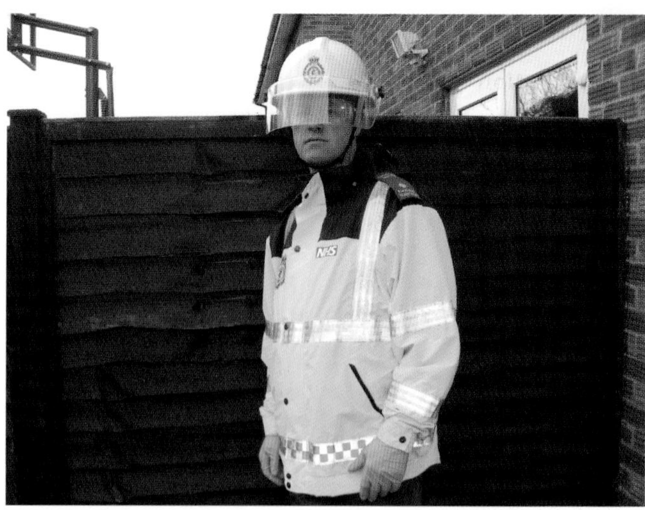

Figure 7-1 Personal protective equipment.

Protective clothing

Health and Safety principles and legislation require that EMS staff should be suitably equipped with protective clothing (Figure 7-1). In the UK, EMS staff should be equipped as a minimum with:

- impact-resistant protective helmet and visor (to BS EN 443)
- safety goggles with vents to prevent fogging (to BS EN 166)
- high-visibility reflective jacket (to BS EN 471 class 3 standard)
- safety shoes or boots with protective toe caps, etc.

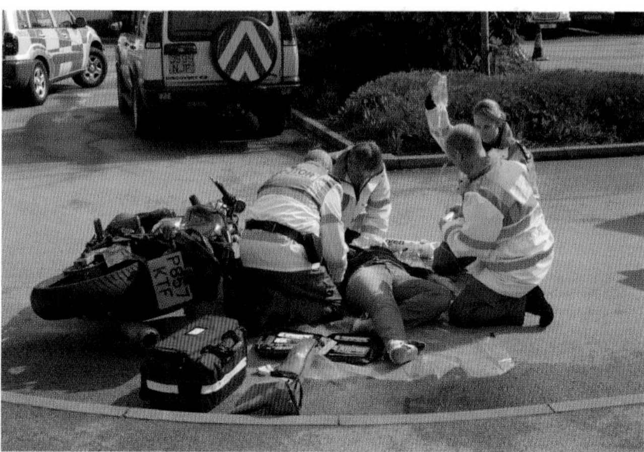

Figure 7-2 Many resources may be needed at an emergency scene.

Personal protection from blood-borne pathogens

Personal protection from blood-borne pathogens should be implemented by all EMS staff. Known as 'universal precautions' these techniques have been adopted by health professionals working in emergency care settings. These precautions are intended to be used in all cases in which the risk of exposure to blood or body fluids is increased and also when the infection status of the patient is unknown. The paramedic should wash his or her hands before (if practicable) and after patient contact to reduce the risk of communicable disease infection. In addition, items of personal protection from blood-borne pathogens should include disposable gloves and masks, eye protection, and gowns when necessary. Personal protection from blood-borne pathogens is addressed further in Chapter 3.

Patient assessment priorities

First, the emergency team must determine that the scene is safe; the team also must ensure that the needed resources are available or have been requested (Figure 7-2). Then the emergency team can begin patient assessment. Patient assessment involves a number of priorities:

1. Initial assessment: to recognize and manage all immediate life-threatening conditions. Resuscitation may be necessary for critical patients (Box 7-1).
2. Patient history: to establish details about the presenting complaint as well as past medical details and drug history.
3. Physical examination: to obtain vital signs, reassess changes in the patient's condition, and perform appropriate physical examination for trauma and medical patients.
4. Ongoing assessment: to continue monitoring the patient's status en route to the hospital and to provide treatment as necessary.

Initial assessment

An initial assessment known as the primary survey is performed on all patients; this assessment establishes priorities of care. The initial assessment consists of the paramedic's general impression of the patients as well as finding conditions that threaten life and identifying priority patients (patients who are 'primary survey positive').[1] These patients

Box 7-1

Resuscitation

Resuscitation may be called for during the initial assessment. The paramedic begins resuscitative measures such as airway maintenance, ventilatory assistance, and cardiopulmonary resuscitation immediately as needed after recognizing a life-threatening condition. Several emergency care procedures generally are required in situations involving seriously ill or injured patients. Nearly all medical and trauma patients, for example, may need some form of supplemental oxygen. Other resuscitation procedures for medical and trauma patients are as follows:

Resuscitation procedures for medical patients

- oxygen and airway management
- insertion of an intravenous line to administer drugs or intravenous fluids
- administration of resuscitation medications
- administration of electrical therapy (defibrillation, cardioversion, external pacing).

Resuscitation procedures for trauma patients

- oxygen and airway management
- cervical spine immobilization
- insertion of intravenous lines for intravenous fluids
- administration of resuscitation medications
- interventions such as chest needle decompression.

need immediate care and transport. The primary survey should be repeated particularly in unstable and time-critical patients or in initially stable patients who appear to deteriorate.

General impression of the patient

The general impression is the paramedic's immediate assessment of the setting and the patient's presenting complaint. The paramedic uses the general impression to determine whether the patient is ill or injured; the nature of illness (NOI) or the mechanism of injury (MOI), although don't forget a medical emergency can have a trauma aspect to it and vice versa. As part of the general impression, the paramedic should identify the patient's general age, sex and ethnicity. There may be clues found in the surroundings that give a sense of what has happened; for instance the patient may have bracelets or cards with medical information available or clues may be provided by the presence of medication or home oxygen supplies. In a trauma scenario the damage to a vehicle or the height from which the patient fell may provide some sense of potential severity and what occurred. Much of this initial impression is undertaken using intuition as well as overt assessment; the patient who appears scared and gasping for breath is clearly more critical than one who is talking in full sentences and smiling.

Assessment for life-threatening conditions

To assess for life-threatening conditions, the paramedic should conduct a systematic evaluation of the patient's response, airway, breathing, circulation and disability. Exposure and a rapid examination of the patient and of the environment are then undertaken and provide an overview of any life threats as well as providing an entry point into the much more detailed secondary survey and assessment. This is generally known as a primary survey.

Response

A priority with any patient is to assess the level of consciousness and can usually be done with an initial exchange with the patient. An example of such is 'My name is …and I'm a paramedic. How can I help you?' If the patient appears unconscious, gentle tactile stimulation (e.g. rubbing the patient's shoulder), along with questions such as 'Are you okay?' and 'Can you hear me?' may get a response. If the patient is unconscious or if spinal injury is suspected, the paramedic should immobilize the patient's cervical spine (see Chapter 32). The paramedic can assess the patient's level of consciousness quickly using the mnemonic evaluation AVPU (alert, verbal, painful, unresponsive). Whilst the Glasgow Coma Score is more specific, it may be better left until a more detailed assessment is undertaken at the end of the initial assessment.

Critical Thinking

What does a patient's level of consciousness tell you about the patient's oxygenation and circulation?

Airway

The paramedic should assess the airway for patency and can use one of three methods. The paramedic can see whether the patient can speak and can note signs of airway obstruction or respiratory insufficiency; these signs could include stridor, gurgling, bubbling or snoring. Moreover, the paramedic can assess for patency by visualizing the oral cavity for foreign objects. Any condition that compromises the delivery of oxygen to body tissues is potentially life threatening; the paramedic must manage such a condition immediately. Factors that may compromise the airway include the following:

- tongue obstructing the airway in an unconscious patient
- loose teeth or foreign objects in the patient's airway
- epiglottitis
- upper airway obstruction from any cause (for example burns, anaphylaxis)
- facial and oral bleeding
- vomitus
- soft-tissue trauma to the patient's face and neck
- facial fractures.

The paramedic must secure a compromised airway manually or with adjunct equipment (e.g. using a jaw thrust in trauma patients, head tilt/chin lift in non-trauma patients, oral or nasal airways, suction, laryngeal mask airway (LMA) or endotracheal intubation described in Chapter 13). When performing an airway procedure for patients who may have a cervical spine injury, the paramedic must keep manipulation of the cervical spine to a minimum. The paramedic must stabilize the head and neck in a neutral position ('in line stabilization'). All patients must have an airway established and maintained during the initial assessment.

> **Critical Thinking**
>
> Securing a patent airway should always receive priority over spinal immobilization. However, both are crucial tasks in the initial assessment.

> **Note**
>
> The patient whose airway is obstructed by a foreign object should be managed using the guidelines currently recommended by the Resuscitation Council UK (www.resus.org.uk). If these manoeuvres fail, direct laryngoscopy or cricothyrotomy may be required (see Chapter 13).

Breathing

The paramedic can assess breathing by evaluating the rate, depth, pattern, tidal volume, and symmetry of chest movement and should expose the chest wall and palpate it for structural integrity, tenderness, and crepitus, observing for use of accessory muscles of respiration in the neck, chest, and abdomen. The paramedic should auscultate for the presence of bilateral breath sounds and should also listen to the patient's speech. A patient who has difficulty speaking without pain or who cannot talk without gasping for air may need ventilatory support. Respiratory abnormalities discovered during the physical examination may indicate a potentially life-threatening condition including the following:

- cyanosis and/or poor oxygen saturation (<93% on air)
- respiratory distress with dyspnoea or hypoxia and/or respiratory rate <10 or >28
- asymmetrical chest wall movement
- chest injury (e.g. tension pneumothorax, flail segment, open chest wound)
- tracheal deviation
- distended neck veins.

Ill or injured patients with ineffective respirations (which can lead to hypoventilation) need ventilatory support. These patients require supplemental high-concentration oxygen. If the respiratory rate of a critically ill or injured patient is less than 10 or more than 28 respirations per minute, ventilatory assistance may be needed. The paramedic may coordinate assisted ventilation with the patient's respiratory efforts or the paramedic may intersperse assisted ventilation between the patient's own respiratory efforts as needed to maintain adequate oxygenation.

> **Critical Thinking**
>
> Some patients with respirations between 10 and 28 per minute may require assisted ventilation. Can you think of any such situations?

If respirations are absent, the paramedic should initiate rescue breathing. The paramedic can initially provide rescue breathing via a pocket mask but positive-pressure ventilation, provided via a bag–valve–mask device, should follow. The use of airway adjuncts such as oropharyngeal or nasopharyngeal airways or an LMA or endotracheal intubation may be indicated. The paramedic also should consider spinal and universal precautions and take these precautions into account during all airway procedures (see Chapter 13).

Circulation

The paramedic evaluates the patient's circulatory status after assessing airway and breathing. For trauma patients, this assessment includes a quick global assessment to find and control severe bleeding. Consideration is given to other evidence of bleeding such as vomiting blood or bleeding per rectum as well as the risk of hidden (internal) bleeding. The paramedic should assess the patient's skin colour, moisture, and temperature quickly as well as evaluate the pulse for quality, rate, and regularity.

Pulse

A quick evaluation of the patient's pulse may reveal a normal heart rate, tachycardia, bradycardia, asystole, or an irregular heart rate. The site of an obtainable pulse also may offer critical details about a patient's systolic blood pressure and tissue perfusion. For example, a radial pulse may not be palpable in an uninjured extremity; the patient is likely to be in a decompensated state of shock (hypoperfusion). A patient may lack a palpable femoral or carotid pulse and the patient is in cardiopulmonary arrest.

Capillary refill

The capillary filling time may offer crucial details about the patient's cardiovascular status. The capillary refill test is thought to be most reliable in children younger than 12 years of age. The paramedic performs this test by blanching the patient's nail bed or the fleshy eminence at the base of the thumb for 5 seconds, with the part being used at or above the level of the heart. Then the paramedic observes the time it takes for normal colour to return. A filling time of more than 2 seconds is caused by shunting and capillary closure to peripheral capillary beds. This indicates inadequate circulation and impaired cardiovascular function. Factors such as the patient's age, gender, existing medical conditions and cold environments may prolong the filling time and the paramedic should use this test only as a possible indicator of circulatory status.[2]

Consideration must be given to acute coronary syndrome, heart failure and sepsis, all of which can affect the circulatory system.

Other signs and symptoms of inadequate circulation and impaired cardiovascular function include the following:

- altered or decreased level of consciousness
- distended neck veins
- increased respiratory rate
- pale, cool, diaphoretic skin
- distant heart sounds
- restlessness and anxiety
- thirst.

> **Critical Thinking**
>
> How do age, gender, and the environment affect capillary refill?

An unconscious person may lack a palpable carotid pulse. If this is the case, the paramedic should implement chest compressions and cardiac arrest protocols (see Chapter 15).

In cases of severe external haemorrhage, the paramedic should control the bleeding using direct pressure, elevation and pressure points (see Chapter 28). In most cases, these procedures to control bleeding also are effective during transport. Regardless of the cause, all patients with circulatory compromise need rapid stabilization. This may include intravenous administration of fluids, drug therapy, and rapid transportation to an appropriate receiving hospital.

Disability

Assessment of level of consciousness is by use of 'AVPU' within the primary survey. The use of the Glasgow Coma Score is reserved for a more detailed assessment of the patient in the secondary survey and is not normally undertaken in the primary survey. At this stage it is often prudent to consider the cause of the reduced level of consciousness if this exists; evaluation of blood glucose should be undertaken as hypoglycaemia is an easily reversible cause. Equally, intoxication with drugs or other substances may also be reversible and consideration of this should take place. Other key assessments that should be considered are looking for signs of meningism, evidence or history of fitting, as well as localizing signs such as pupil abnormalities (the pupils should be assessed for size and reactivity), cranial nerve abnormalities and limbs.

Expose and examine (environment and events)

This is a rapid global overview of the patient from head to toe; looking for a range of probably obvious problems that need to be managed early on. For instance, in medical patients rashes (urticaric or purpuric) may indicate a serious systemic problem such as anaphylaxis or sepsis. The patient's temperature should be gauged as to whether they are hypothermic or hot and feverish. At the circulation stage described earlier any severe haemorrhage should be noted and managed but at this stage that and other obvious injuries and abnormalities might become apparent. In a trauma patient, consideration is given to the mechanism of injury (this is likely to have been considered on the initial scene assessment but is considered again in 'E' in more detail). Significant mechanisms of injury that identify priority patients include the following:

- ejection from a vehicle
- death in same passenger compartment
- falls from greater than 6 m
- vehicle rollover
- high-speed vehicle collision (>40 mph)
- significant intrusion into passenger cell or major damage/deformity
- vehicle–pedestrian collision
- motorcycle crash
- equestrian accidents
- sports, especially contact sports or shallow water diving
- blast or penetrating trauma.

Critical Thinking

A patient may have a mechanism of injury other than those listed here. Does that mean the patient has no life-threatening injuries?

Box 7-2

DCAP-BTLS (used in rapid head-to-toe assessment of trauma patient)

D: Deformities
C: Contusions
A: Abrasions
P: Punctures/penetrations
B: Burns
T: Tenderness
L: Lacerations
S: Swelling

Box 7-3

TRIP-DOCS (used in rapid head-to-toe assessment of medical patient)

T: Temperature/fever
R: Rash
I: Injection marks
P: Pulses
D: Diaphoresis (sweating/clammy)
O: Oedema or swelling
C: Colour
S: Smells

Mechanisms of injury considered significant with infants and children include falls greater than 3 m, bicycle collision, and medium-speed vehicle collision (see Chapter 26).

Vital signs

The point at which basic vital signs and observations such as blood pressure, pulse, respiratory rate and temperature, along with other monitoring such as ECG, $ETCO_2$ and oxygen saturation are recorded will vary according to the patient and call circumstances, personnel and equipment availability. Some elements may have been assessed in the primary survey (for example the respiratory rate). However, it is important that a set of baseline observations are obtained as soon as practicable. For clarity, vital signs/observations are considered here prior to the rapid head-to-toe survey.

In patients who appear to be primary survey positive, a rapid head-to-toe assessment (for both medical and trauma patients) should be undertaken. The use of the mnemonic DCAP-BTLS (Box 7-2) for trauma patients and TRIP-DOCS (Box 7-3) for medical patients may help the paramedic consider some signs of medical emergency. Additional signs to consider are mentioned below in each body area:

- *Head*: consider facial paralysis or weakness.
- *Neck*: tracheal deviation is considered, assessing for jugular vein distension should be undertaken.
- *Chest*: both the front (anterior) and back (posterior) of the thorax are assessed. Look for signs of pneumothorax.

- *Abdomen*: palpation of all four quadrants is important (posterior assessment is also required).*
- *Pelvis*: pelvic integrity was historically assessed by the 'springing' of the pelvis, which might indicate a fracture if found to be unstable, but some advise against this in the pre-hospital phase as it often causes intense pain and there is a risk of worsening blood loss.[3] Any haematuria or blood from the urinary system may indicate pelvic injury.
- *Extremities*: the assessment of motor, sensory and circulation (MSC) ×4; assess the active movements of limbs (motor), ability to feel light touch (sensory), and normal skin temperature and pulses (circulation) in all four limbs.

Identification of priority patients (medical and trauma)

The paramedic uses the findings from the initial assessment above to identify priority patients. These are patients who need immediate interventions and prompt transport and are considered to be 'primary survey positive'. Examples of priority patients may include those with:

- poor general impression
- decreased level of consciousness (depressed or absent gag or cough reflex)
- no response to commands (unresponsiveness)
- difficulty breathing
- shock (hypoperfusion)
- complicated childbirth
- chest pain with a systolic pressure less than 100 mmHg
- uncontrolled bleeding
- severe unmanageable pain anywhere
- multiple injuries or limb-threatening injuries.

Primary survey negative patients

Those patients whose primary survey is intact (so-called 'primary survey negative'), who are not considered to be priority patients and who do not have an immediately life-threatening problem can then be assessed via a secondary survey where a more detailed assessment is undertaken and includes patient history taking and physical assessment/ examination. These patients will be fully alert and coherent, and able to talk normally, completing full sentences, with a respiratory and heart rate in the normal range for their age and not displaying signs of shock or hypovolaemia. In time-critical and unstable patients (the 'primary survey positive' patient) it is likely that the paramedic will not be able to undertake this secondary survey in any great detail as they are likely to be managing this priority patient within the primary survey stage as detailed above (Figure 7-3).

History

Irrespective of whether the patient is a trauma or non-trauma patient, the ability to obtain a patient history will depend

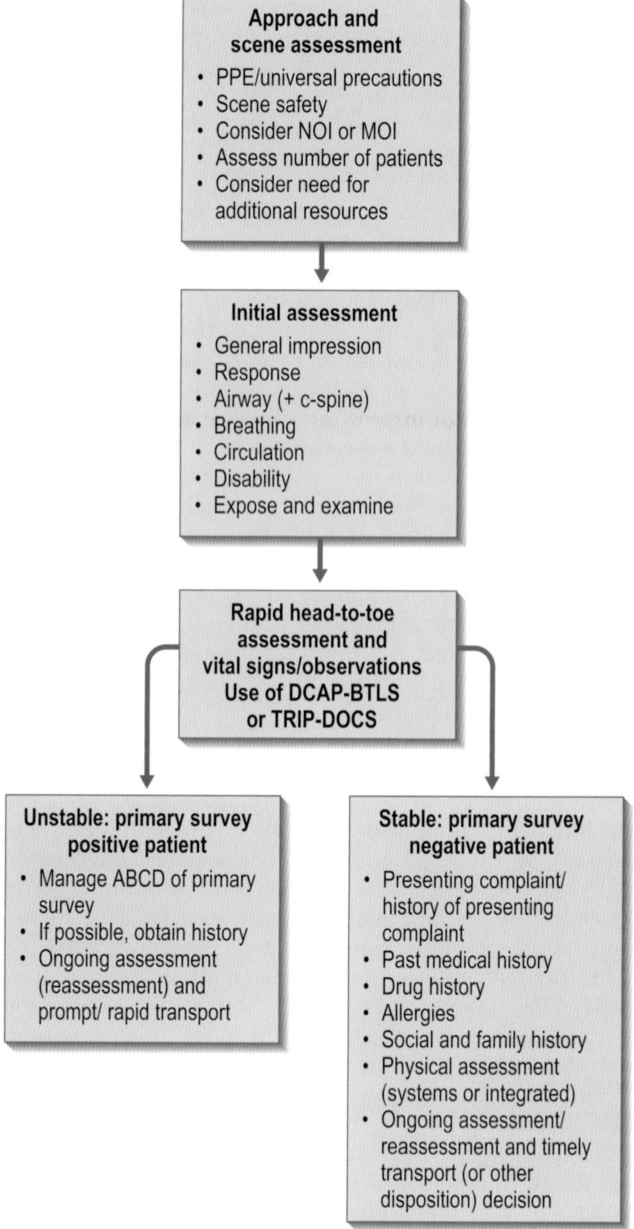

Figure 7-3 Components of patient assessment.

on the level of consciousness and cognition of the patient, although, if reduced, bystanders and family members may be able to give information. If the patient is responsive, the paramedic should assess the patient's history as detailed in Chapter 8; this includes identifying the presenting complaint along with the NOI or MOI, and obtaining the history of the presenting complaint with a review of systems, along with past medical history, the drug history, any allergies and the social and family history. The paramedic then performs a detailed physical examination using the methods from Chapter 9. At some stage during the history taking and the physical examination, a set of observations (vital signs) should be recorded. Patients who are primary survey positive will have had a rapid head-to-toe assessment undertaken as described previously and additional assessment should be undertaken if the patient's condition allows.

*In trauma, the posterior thorax and abdomen may be assessed when log rolling the patient

Note

Many emergency services in the UK and other parts of the world are recommending that 'ICE' be programmed into personal mobile phones. ICE is an acronym for 'In Case of Emergency'. ICE is aimed at giving emergency providers and hospital personnel a fast way to contact friends or family members when an ill or injured patient cannot provide that information. ICE entries are made in the contact list of a mobile phone and the ICE entry is tied to phone numbers of 'ICE partners'. The partners are friends or family members who are easy to reach by phone.

Physical examination

The detailed physical examination should be specific to the patient and injury or illness. A patient with a minor injury such as a sprained ankle should not require a complete physical examination. However, an older patient who is having difficulty breathing is different and should receive a detailed physical examination. A comprehensive and detailed physical examination (described in more detail in Chapter 9) normally includes the following:

- Mental status assessment
  - appearance and behaviour
  - posture and motor activity
  - speech and language
  - mood
  - thought and perceptions
  - insight and judgement
  - memory and attention
- General survey
  - level of consciousness
  - signs of distress
  - apparent state of health
  - skin colour and obvious lesions
  - height and build
  - sexual development
  - weight
  - posture, gait, and motor activity
  - dress, grooming, and personal hygiene
  - odours on breath or body
  - facial expression
- Examination of relevant systems as appropriate (for example):
  - skin (integumentary) system
  - head, eyes, ears, nose and throat (HEENT)
  - respiratory system
  - cardiovascular system
  - gastrointestinal system
  - genitourinary system
  - musculoskeletal system
  - nervous system
- Baseline vital signs (if not already undertaken).

Whilst the physical assessment may be systems focused, in some patients with multiple conditions or complex presentations it may be more appropriate to undertake an integrated assessment, which considers specific elements from each system assessment but starts at the same part of the body and follows a body part sequence/pattern starting with the patient's hand, upper limbs, head, neck, thorax and abdomen (not forgetting the posterior aspects) and then the pelvis and legs. This is also described in Chapter 9.

Ongoing assessment

The ongoing assessment is a repeat of the assessment process, with a focus towards the primary survey (although other assessment components, such as the history, might be repeated to ensure nothing has been missed and to ensure completeness). As the name implies, this assessment should be performed throughout the encounter with the patient. Stable (primary survey negative) patients are lower-priority patients and the paramedic should repeat the ongoing assessment and record it every 15 minutes. Unstable (primary survey positive) patients are high-priority patients and for these patients, the paramedic should perform the ongoing assessment every 5 minutes wherever possible. The purpose of the ongoing assessment is to reassess the key components of the primary survey and compare with the first (baseline) assessment findings; this determines whether the patient is improving or deteriorating and the effectiveness of any interventions. The paramedic must be aware of subtle changes in patient condition as early warning signs of change may be quite slight. The purpose of the ongoing assessment is:

- to reassess response (mental status and disability)
- to reassess airway
- to reassess breathing
- to reassess circulation
- to re-establish patient priorities.

Critical Thinking

The ongoing assessment can identify trends in the patient's condition. What does that mean?

During the ongoing assessment, the paramedic also should reassess and record vital signs and further investigate the patient complaint or injury. Importantly the paramedic should assess the success of any interventions by assessing the patient's response to patient care activities and determining the need to maintain or alter the care plan.

An ongoing assessment of the patient may help the paramedic to notice a trend and full documentation of findings also may help the paramedic to see this trend in the assessment components. For example, a patient may have been cyanotic, hypotensive, and disoriented at the scene. After administering intravenous fluid therapy and high-concentration oxygen, this patient may have improved colour and blood pressure and appear to be more alert during transport. The documenting and reporting of trends in the assessment is crucial. Documentation helps other healthcare workers who are to assume care of the patient on arrival at the hospital.

Care of medical versus trauma patients

Much of the definitive care for medical patients often can be initiated in the prehospital setting. For some patients with cardiac problems and patients with respiratory difficulties and other medical emergencies, paramedic crews can institute definitive care. Because of this, the time spent on scene with these medical patients may be slightly longer.

By contrast, unstable and time-critical trauma patients require rapid transport. These patients should be taken to a proper medical facility for definitive care. Patients with internal bleeding, major fractures, head injury, and multiple-system trauma need specific interventions, many of which are not achievable outside of hospital. Minimal time should be spent at the scene with these patients; most trauma life-support training programmes recommend that patients needing immediate transport be stabilized and prepared for transport ('packaged') within 10 minutes after arrival of emergency medical services. Field management should be limited to airway control and ventilatory support, spinal immobilization, and major fracture stabilization. Intravenous fluid therapy should be initiated en route to the hospital. (Trauma management is addressed further in Chapter 26.)

Note

Due to the unique nature of prehospital care, priorities must be based on good patient assessment. These priorities include scene safety, recognition and management of life-threatening conditions, and identification of patients who require rapid stabilization and transport for definitive care. This chapter provides an overview of patient assessment.

Summary

- Scene assessment consists of the initial steps performed on every EMS response; these steps help to ensure scene safety and provide valuable information to the paramedic.
- Patient assessment comprises five priorities: initial assessment, resuscitation, patient history taking, physical assessment and ongoing assessment.
- The initial assessment includes the paramedic's general impression of the patient, the nature of illness (NOI) or mechanism of injury (MOI), the assessment for life-threatening conditions, and the identification of priority patients requiring immediate care and transport.
- Assessment of life-threatening conditions entails a systematic evaluation of the patient's response, airway, breathing, and circulation.
- The paramedic begins resuscitative measures such as airway management, ventilatory assistance, and cardiopulmonary resuscitation immediately after recognizing the life-threatening condition that necessitates each respective manoeuvre.
- A rapid head-to-toe assessment is undertaken for all primary survey positive patients whether medical or trauma in origin.
- The history and physical examination for medical patients are dictated by the patient's overall condition and level of consciousness.
- The ongoing assessment is a repeat of the initial assessment.

References

1. Wardrope J, Mackenzie R 2004 The ABC of emergency community care. 2. The system of assessment and care of the primary survey positive patient. Emerg Med J 21:216–225
2. Lewin J, Maconochie I 2008 Capillary refill time in adults. Emerg Med J 25:325–326
3. Lee C, Porter K 2007 The prehospital management of pelvic fractures. Emerg Med J 24:130–133

Further reading

Health and Safety Executive website: http://www.hse.gov.uk/index.htm

CHAPTER 8

History Taking

Chapter contents

Objectives

Upon completion of this chapter, the paramedic student will be able to:

1. Describe the purpose of effective history taking in prehospital patient care.
2. List components of the patient history.
3. Outline effective patient interviewing techniques to facilitate history taking.
4. Identify strategies to manage special challenges in obtaining a patient history.

Key terms

clinical reasoning Use of the results of questions to think about associated problems and body system changes related to the patient's complaint.

family history Illness or disease in a patient's family or family's background that may be relevant to the patient complaint.

history of presenting complaint A full, clear, chronological account of the symptoms related to the presenting complaint.

history taking Information gathered during the patient interview.

past medical history A patient's medical and health background (that may offer insight into the patient's current problem).

presenting complaint A patient's primary complaint (the reason they called EMS).

Content of the patient history

The patient history is made up of several parts, each of which has a specific purpose, which offers a 'snapshot' of patients and their condition. Box 8-1 lists the parts of a patient history.

The patient history should include the date and time that the history was obtained, using relevant sections on the patient report form (PRF). The history may contain any identifying information of the patient (e.g. age, gender, ethnicity, birthplace and occupation). Identifying information can be key, as illustrated in the following scenario:

Your crew has been dispatched to a 'unwell female'. On your arrival you find a woman who is ill with flu-like symptoms. The symptoms include nausea, vomiting, and diarrhoea. During your history take, she tells you that she is a 49-year-old businesswoman and has just returned to the UK from an extended visit to her native home in Southeast Asia. In addition to the chance of gastrointestinal illness or food poisoning, you now suspect that she could be ill from an endemic disease (that is, a disease prevalent in a population or geographical region).

Documentation should include the source of the referral and patient history. For example, did the patient request emergency medical services (EMS) help, or did a family member, friend, police officer, or bystander initiate the EMS response?

The paramedic also must decide whether the source of the referral and patient history is reliable, as illustrated in the following scenario:

Box 8-1

Structure of the patient history

Date and time

Identifying data
- Age
- Gender
- Ethnicity
- Birthplace
- Occupation

Source of referral
- Patient referral
- Referral by others

Source of history
- Patient
- Family
- Friends
- Police
- Others

Reliability
- Variable (memory, trust, motivation)
- Determined at the end of the evaluation

Presenting complaint
- The one or more symptoms for which the patient is seeking healthcare

History of presenting complaint
- Provides a chronological account of the patient's symptoms

Review of systems (functional enquiry/systematic enquiry)

Past medical history (current health status)
- Includes: illnesses, surgical procedures, accidents, long-term healthcare conditions, visits to GP or other primary care provider
- Drug history
- Allergies
- Family history, social history

Your crew has been dispatched to an RTC. The driver of the car is a 17-year-old who has minor injuries but is slurring his speech and his breath smells of alcohol. He denies alcohol or other drug use to you and the police officers at the scene. Is this patient history reliable?

The presenting complaint (explained later in this chapter) is the main part of the patient history. The presenting complaint is the reason why EMS assistance was summoned. After identifying the presenting complaint, the paramedic obtains a history of the presenting complaint (HPC). This history provides a chronological account of the patient's symptoms. The paramedic then questions the patient about their past medical history and alongside this undertakes a review of body systems appropriate to the patient's symptoms or complaint (see Chapter 9 physical assessment).

Techniques of history taking

As emphasized in Chapter 6, the paramedic should 'set the stage' for a good paramedic–patient encounter. The paramedic can do this by making a good first impression and make the environment conducive to free-flowing communication. The paramedic should do the following:

- establish a professional demeanour with the patient
- ensure patient comfort and provide a safe environment
- greet the patient by name or surname and avoid demeaning terms (e.g. 'sweetheart' or 'mate')
- avoid entering the patient's personal space
- enquire about the patient's feelings
- be sensitive to the patient's feelings and experiences
- watch for signs of uneasiness
- use language that is appropriate and easily understood
- ask open-ended questions and direct questions (if needed)
- use therapeutic communications techniques.

Opening questions may incorporate facilitation, reflection, clarification, empathetic responses, confrontation, interpretation, and asking patients about their feelings. These methods should use the techniques of communications described in Chapter 6:

Facilitation: Use positive actions or words to encourage the patient to say more. Maintain eye contact and use phrases such as 'go on' and 'I'm listening'. These phrases encourage the patient to continue talking.

Reflection: Repeat or 'echo' what the patient tells you. This encourages additional responses. Reflection will not usually bias the patient's story or interrupt the patient's train of thought.

Clarification: Ask questions to better grasp vague statements or words.

Empathy: Ask about the patient's feelings and show empathy to interpret the patient's feelings. This will help to gain your patient's trust.

Confrontation: Some issues may mean that you confront patients about their feelings. For example, one may ask a patient who is severely depressed, 'Have you ever thought about killing yourself?'

Interpretation: When appropriate, go beyond confrontation and make an inference from the patient's response. For example, draw an inference from the patient who says, 'I think I'm going to die'. One may infer that the patient may be gravely ill.

Presenting complaint

As previously stated, the presenting complaint is the main part of the patient's health history and is usually the reason for the EMS response. The complaint may be verbal (e.g. complaint of chest pain) or non-verbal (e.g. pain or distress expressed by a facial grimace). Most presenting complaints are characterized by pain, abnormal function, a change in the patient's normal state, or an unusual observation made by the patient (e.g. heart palpitations).

The paramedic should be aware that a presenting complaint may be misleading; it may be a problem more serious than the complaint indicates. For example, the patient who has fallen down a flight of steps may complain of an injured ankle. However, physical examination may reveal possible internal injuries. In addition, patients often modify or substitute their presenting complaint, in order to hide a problem they find embarrassing or hard to discuss. For example, a presenting complaint of vaginal bleeding may be modified as 'heavy periods' but actually the bleeding was an abrupt haemorrhage that occurred during intercourse. Likewise, a presenting complaint of 'frequent headaches' may be substituted for feelings of depression with suicidal ideation. Therefore, determining the true reason for the patient's concern is one of the skills of history taking, and the true need may not be the stated presenting complaint. First, the paramedic should determine the presenting complaint and immediately manage any life-threatening situations, and once managed, obtain a history of the presenting complaint and any relevant medical history.

Critical Thinking

What illnesses or injuries could cause a presenting complaint of confusion?

History of presenting complaint

The history of the presenting complaint also provides a full, clear, and chronological account of the symptoms; obtaining a full history of the presenting complaint takes skill in asking proper questions related to the presenting complaint and interpreting the patient's response. For example, a patient's complaint of low back pain suggests a muscle strain. During direct questioning in the interview, however, the patient reveals a history of a burning sensation with urination and a low-grade fever for the past several days, which suggests a urinary tract infection or renal colic. Thus the history of the presenting complaint may be more crucial than the obvious presenting complaint. The mnemonic OPQRST AS-PN helps define the patient's complaint by focusing on essential elements of assessment (Box 8-2). Use of this or another memory device, such as OLD CARTS or SOCRATES PEN (Box 8-2), will help lead the paramedic through a thorough series of questions to better grasp the history of the presenting complaint. The paramedic should take notes while obtaining the health history, and when explained most patients realize that it is hard to remember all details and accept note taking.

Onset/origin

Onset and origin identify what the patient was doing when the presenting complaint began. The paramedic also notes whether there is any history of a similar episode. Questions to ask to obtain this information may include the following:

- 'Did the presenting complaint begin suddenly, or did it occur gradually over time?'
- 'When did you last feel well?'
- 'What were you doing when the presenting complaint started?'
- 'Did the presenting complaint begin during a period of activity or while at rest?'
- 'Have you ever had this type of problem before? If so, is it the same or is it different from what you're experiencing now?'

Box 8-2

History of presenting complaint: various mnemonics can be used

OPQRST AS-PN

O (onset/origin): What were you doing when the symptom started? Do you have a history of this problem?

P (provocation/palliation): What provokes the symptoms? What makes the symptoms better? What makes them worse?

Q (quality): What does the symptom feel like? What is its character? How would you describe it?

R (region): Where is the symptom? Where does it go? Is it in one or more areas?

S (severity): On a scale of 1 to 10, with 1 being the least and 10 being the worst, what number would you give your symptom, pain or discomfort?

T (time): How long have you had this symptom? When did it start? When did it end? How long did it last?

AS: associated symptoms: symptoms that are present other than the presenting complaint

PN: pertinent negatives; symptoms that might be present given the presenting complaint but are not

OLD CARTS*

O: Onset
L: Location
D: Duration
C: Character
A: Aggravating/associated factors
R: Relieving factors
T: Temporal factors
S: Severity

SOCRATES PEN

S: Site
O: Onset
C: Character
R: Radiation
A: Associated symptoms
T: Timing
E: Exacerbating and relieving factors
S: Severity 1–10
P: Previous episodes
E: Effect on daily living
N: Now (is it present now?)

*Taken from Seidel et al 2006 Mosby's guide to physical examination, 6th edition. Elsevier/Mosby.

Provocation/palliation

Provocation and palliation refer to precipitating factors associated with the patient's presenting complaint. Questions to ask to identify precipitating factors may include the following:

- 'What makes the presenting complaint better?'
- 'What makes the presenting complaint worse?'
- 'Does the presenting complaint increase or decrease when you take a breath?'
- 'Does lying down or sitting up affect the presenting complaint's severity?'

- 'Have you taken any medications for your symptoms? If so, did the medications make you feel better?'

Quality

Quality refers to how the patient perceives the presenting complaint. Questions to ask to obtain quality of the pain include the following:

- 'What does the presenting complaint feel like?'
- 'Can you describe the presenting complaint to me?'

If pain:

- 'Is the pain sharp or dull?'
- 'Is the pain constant, or does it come and go?'

Region/radiation

Region and radiation refer to the location of the presenting complaint (if applicable) and if it is pain whether it is localized or associated with pain elsewhere in the body. Questions to ask to identify region and radiation include the following:

- 'Where is the presenting complaint located?'

If pain:

- 'Can you point with one finger to the exact location?'
- 'Does the pain stay in the same place or does it move?'
- 'If the pain moves, where does it go? Does the pain go to more than one area?'

Severity

Severity refers to how the patient rates the level of the presenting complaint. Severity also provides a baseline for future evaluation of the patient's presenting complaint. Questions to ask the patient include the following:

- 'On a scale of 1 to 10, with 1 being the least and 10 being the worst/most severe, how would you rate your presenting complaint?'
- 'How bad is the presenting complaint?'
- 'Does the intensity of the presenting complaint vary or does it stay the same?'
- 'Have you had this type of presenting complaint before? If so, how is this presenting complaint different, or is it exactly the same?'

During the assessment of the severity, the paramedic should make an assessment of the patient's pain. Whilst this is, arguably, very subjective, it nevertheless provides the paramedic with some information about how severe the presenting complaint is (and perhaps can be compared with similar like episodes) as well as providing a measure of whether pain relief and other interventions have reduced the pain and discomfort being experienced. Various pain scoring tools are available, which can be modified for use in children. In the prehospital arena, the simplest tools are most easily utilized (Figs 8.1–8.3).

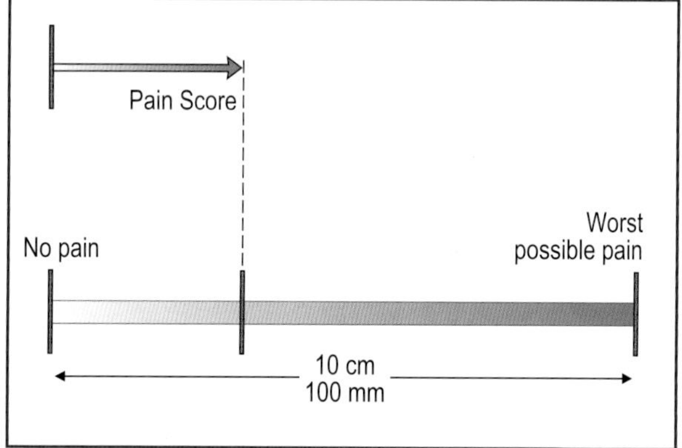

Figure 8-1 Visual Analogue Scale. From Bond and Simpson (2006): Pain: Its Nature and Treatment. Elsevier Ltd.

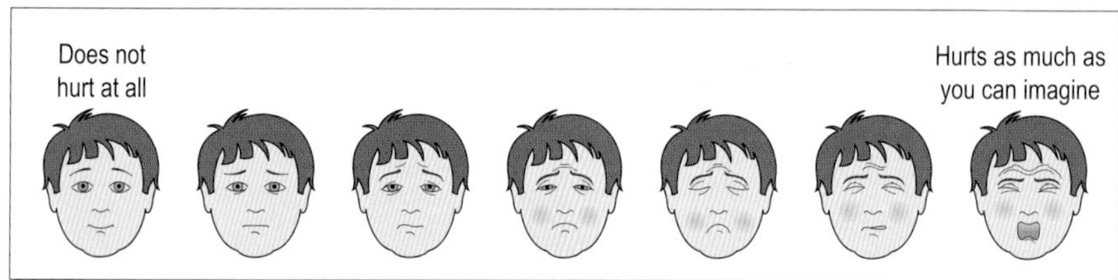

Figure 8-2 Faces Rating Scale. The use of neutral no pain face and the lack of tears on the worst pain possible face avoid the possibility of confusing pain severity with happiness/sadness. The nurse must explain to the child that the first face represents no hurt at all and that the last face represents as much hurt as they can possibly imagine. From Bond and Simpson (2006): Pain: Its Nature and Treatment. Elsevier Ltd.

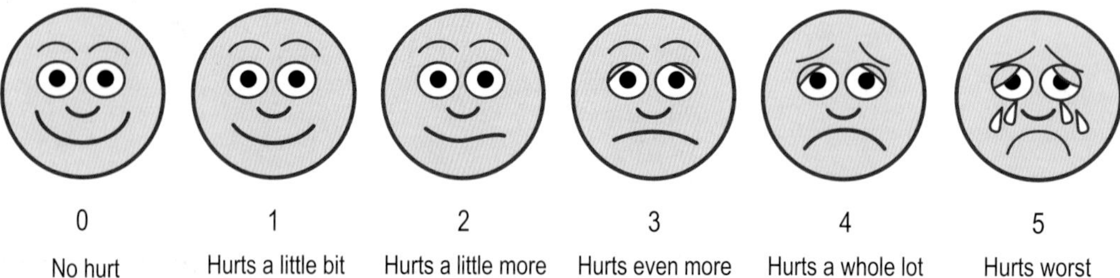

Figure 8-3 Faces pain scales have been developed using cartoon faces. These are popular with children and parents but have been shown to be less accurate. From Wong and Hess (2000): Clinical Manual of Paediatric Nursing, 5e. Elsevier Ltd.

Box 8-3

Review of systems

(may also be known as systemic enquiry or functional enquiry); associated symptoms and pertinent negatives

General

Orientation and communication ability
Appearance (well/unwell)

Respiratory system

Cough (productive, non-productive)
Haemoptysis
Chest pain
Breathlessness
Wheeziness
Fever/night sweats

Cardiovascular and circulatory

Chest pain
Palpitations
Intermittent claudication (pain in legs on walking)
Ankle oedema
Orthopnoea
Dyspnoea (may be constant/exercise related/nocturnal)
Blackouts

Nervous system

Headaches
Dizziness
Disturbances of vision, taste, smell, hearing, speech
Faints/fits, unexplained collapse or losses of consciousness
Falls
Weakness/loss of muscle power
Abnormal or altered sensations
Memory or concentration changes

Musculoskeletal system

Altered mobility
Muscle weakness/loss of power or function
Joint pain, swelling or stiffness
Muscle pain

Gastrointestinal system

Changes in appetite or thirst
Vomiting/nausea
Bowels: diarrhoea, constipation, changes in frequency, consistency of stools, bowel habit
Rectal bleeding or melaena
Jaundice
Dysphagia
Indigestion/heartburn ('reflux')
Significant losses or gain in weight
Abdominal pain

Genitourinary

Dysuria
Haematuria
Frequency
Incontinence
Menstrual cycle/LMP
Sexual history if relevant
Pain/discomfort/itching
Discharge
Unusual bleeding

Time

Time refers to the duration of the presenting complaint. Questions to ask to clarify the duration of the patient's presenting complaint include the following:

- 'How long have you been feeling this way?'
- 'Have you had this same type of presenting complaint before, and if so, how long did it last?'
- 'When did the presenting complaint start?'
- 'How long did the presenting complaint last?'
- 'When did the presenting complaint end?'

Associated symptoms (AS) and pertinent negatives (PN)

By considering any associated symptoms related to the presenting complaint, the paramedic explores symptoms that are commonly associated with the presenting complaint and are either present (associated symptoms) or are not present (pertinent negatives). These specific symptoms are related to specific body systems and establishing their presence or absence is know as a 'review of systems' or a 'functional enquiry/ systemic enquiry'. Box 8-3 identifies the key systems and the possible associated symptoms.

A variety of memory devices are used to recall key questions for gathering medical history. One example is the AMPLE Survey (Box 8-4). The depth and focus of the patient interview are based on the case at hand. However, the paramedic should gather as much information as possible at the scene and during transport to the hospital and use the answers to think about associated problems and body system changes related to the patient's complaint. This is known as clinical reasoning.

Box 8-4

Elements of the AMPLE Survey

A: Allergies
M: Medications/drug history
P: Past medical history
L: Last meal or oral intake
E: Events before the emergency

Current health status

The current health status focuses on a patient's current state of health. It also considers the social history, which incorporates personal habits and environmental conditions

Box 8-5

Social history

- Alcohol
- Smoking
- Family
- Relationships and sexual health (if appropriate to situation)
- Abuse or domestic violence
- Social conditions/domestic support
- Housing/accommodation
- Religious beliefs
- Occupation/work
- Stress and mental health
- Hobbies
- Exercise and recreation
- Immunizations/diet/health screening/health promotion
- Travel

(Box 8-5). Details regarding drug history, allergies, last oral intake, and family and social history can be critical to the patient's current health status. Paramedics should ask female patients who have abdominal pain about their last menstrual period; this is relevant for female patients of childbearing age. Finally, the paramedic should identify any events that occurred before the emergency.

Past medical history

A key for history taking is for the paramedic to gather the past medical history and occurs after the paramedic gains a good grasp of the patient's presenting complaint. The past medical history may include, for example, diabetes, cardiac, or respiratory disorders and may add insight into the patient's current health state. Important past medical history information may include the following:

- general state of health
- childhood illnesses
- adult illnesses
- mental health/illnesses
- previous injuries
- previous surgical procedures
- admissions to hospital.

Drug history

The paramedic should ask whether the patient takes any medications regularly as well as whether the patient has used any medications that the patient does not take regularly. In addition to information about prescribed medicines, obtain information about the use of over-the-counter medicines as well as use of herbs, naturopathic and homeopathic medicines. This line of questioning should include the reason and frequency of use. If possible, the paramedic should determine whether the patient adheres to a medication regimen; this is known as concordance. The medication history may offer clues to the presenting complaint; for example, a diabetic patient may have taken insulin but may have eaten at variable intervals. Other examples include a patient with chest pain who takes various cardiac drugs, an irrational patient who takes prescribed sedatives, and a trauma patient who takes blood-thinning drugs. The patient's medication history may not always be relevant to the problem at hand; however, the history can point to potential problems that may be seen during the patient care episode.

Critical Thinking

What would you do if you could not recognize the names or indications for the patient's home medicines?

Allergies

Few emergency medications cause an allergic reaction. Still, details regarding allergies can be critical and can also be useful to others involved in the patient's care. For example, the patient may be sensitive to tetanus prophylaxis, antibiotics, radiographic contrast medium, and other drugs administered during treatment. Allergies to food and other substances may offer insight into the patient's state. If the patient is unconscious or unable to talk, the paramedic should look for medical alert information or ask family members or friends about the patient's allergies. (Allergic reactions are addressed further in Chapter 18.)

Note

Some people have a life-threatening allergy to latex. Latex may be found in emergency medical services care equipment.

Last oral intake

The time of the last meal or fluid intake is important when considering potential airway problems in a patient who loses consciousness or whose condition begins to deteriorate. Determining the patient's last oral intake also may help establish specific problems, such as food poisoning and food allergies. For example, symptoms of certain types of food poisoning do not usually appear for several hours. In contrast, patients who are sensitive to certain foods would develop an allergic reaction immediately after eating the foods such as peanuts and shellfish.

Note

The time of the patient's last oral intake is crucial. The time can help to determine the appropriateness of surgery, as if a patient has eaten or drunk within the previous 6–8 h, surgery may have to be delayed. The delay is to prevent the patient from aspirating the stomach contents, which may occur during the induction of anaesthesia. However, immediate surgery may be indicated after recent oral intake, and, if so, a nasogastric tube is inserted to evacuate the stomach.

Events before the emergency

The paramedic should ask the patient and bystanders about events or actions that occurred before the emergency. For example, was a fainting episode preceded by exertion or straining? Did a loss of consciousness occur before or after a fall? The paramedic should attempt to correlate any event with the progression of an illness or injury.

Family history

Establishing the presence or absence of diseases and health problems in close family members can provide a useful backdrop to the acquisition of the history. Some diseases are directly inherited (such as haemophilia or sickle cell anaemia) whereas others tend to run in families. Therefore, a family history of illness or disease may be relevant to the presenting complaint. In general, ask first about the health of the patient's parents, then about siblings and finally other family members. Key diseases to enquire about include: heart disease, high blood pressure, cancer, tuberculosis, stroke, diabetes, kidney disease or current infectious illness. It is also important to establish which family members are still alive and those who have died; of particular importance is to consider any premature death, noting the age at which that person died. For instance, in a 55-year-old patient presenting with cardiac chest pain, the fact that their father died at 60 years old from cardiac disease is directly relevant.

Note

In time, the paramedic will develop a 'personal line' of questioning and although some of the history taking can explore sensitive information this personal approach will help the paramedic to analyse a patient's symptoms further.

Social history

It is often very helpful to explore the social history of the patient; this aspect of history taking can be very broad and there are many elements to consider, so it is important to focus on those that are most relevant to the situation at hand but the following are examples of keys areas to ask.

Alcohol

This can be a sensitive issue to explore but it is important to establish the possibility of alcohol-related ill health. Questions to ask are: How many units a day and a week does the patient consume and do they 'binge' drink? What type of alcohol do they drink? Do they drink on their own or with others, and where do they drink? Are they reliant on alcohol? Does alcohol create difficulties in terms of relationships or their work life? The CAGE questionnaire (Box 8-6) is helpful, and positive responses to two or more of the questions suggest a problem with alcohol.

Box 8-6

CAGE questionnaire

C: Have you ever felt you should CUT DOWN on your drinking?
A: Have people ANNOYED you by criticizing your drinking?
G: Have you ever felt uncomfortable or GUILTY about your drinking?
E: Do you feel the need to have a drink first thing in the morning to steady you or relieve your hangover? (EYE OPENER)

Smoking

Use of tobacco is accepted as a significant contributor to ill health. Establishing smoking habits is important; what does the patient smoke, how many times a day and for how many years? It is important to ask ex-smokers about when they gave up. The use of the 'pack years' formula (Box 8-7) can give a estimation of the degree of smoking and therefore of the possible health-related risks that the patient may be exposed to.

Box 8-7

Pack years calculation

The pack years calculation can provide an indication of the risk of disease from smoking; the greater the pack years the higher the possible health complications:

20 cigarettes = 1 packet

(No. of cigarettes smoked per day × no. of years smoking)/20

e.g. 20 cigarettes a day for 10 years would be (20 × 10)/20 = 10 pack years

Family

It is important to establish whom the patient lives with, and what the home circumstances are.

Relationships/sexual health

Equally, finding out about the patient's personal relationships may indicate whether the patient has social support or whether they are vulnerable. Sexual health history is a very sensitive issue and in most cases will not be required in an EMS setting but on occasions careful lines of questioning may need to be used if the presenting complaint is related to the genitourinary system.

Abuse or domestic violence

When asking about relationships another very sensitive issue to consider is the possibility of abuse or harm. This applies not only to the child but also to older adults, those with mental health problems or learning disabilities or indeed anyone who is in a difficult relationship. The abuse may be non-physical and signs are often subtle.

Social conditions/domestic support

Does the patient enjoy a social network of friends and family or are they socially isolated? If they are dependent, is the care and help they require given in a timely fashion and in sufficient quantity?

Housing/accommodation

Is the patient homeless, are they transiently in their current address or do they have their own home? Is the house well lit, heated and do they have sufficient food and necessities for a safe existence? If the patient is older, consider the home's suitability and presence or need for adaptations such as stair lifts.

Religious beliefs

It is helpful to establish the patient's religious beliefs, if they have any.

Occupation/work

Asking about the patient's work not only relates to finding out if they have an income and can support themselves but also gives insight into their social network. Equally, some occupations have direct associations with certain diseases and may give a clue as to the cause of a presenting complaint.

Stress and mental health

This may be related to occupation or to social and home circumstances but asking about whether the patient is coping and if they feel overwhelmed is important. Depression is another common presentation that should be considered. More specific mental health assessment (Chapter 25) should be considered if the patient presents with a complaint that is directly related.

Exercise and recreation/hobbies

Does the patient exercise, do they enjoy non-work-related activities and pastimes?

Immunizations/diet/health screening/health promotion

This may have been considered in the past medical history but ensuring that the patient is up to date with immunizations and health screening with give a sense of general health and wellbeing, as will information related to exercise and a healthy diet.

Travel

With global travel increasing, health-related problems such as infectious disease may be relevant, as will any recent history of a long journey where the patient was not mobile (such as a long aircraft flight).

Getting more information

With experience, paramedics learn to communicate with more skill. They learn to get a fuller picture of a patient's illness or injury and are able to obtain more information about a symptom or complaint whilst using clinical reasoning to evaluate associated problems and possible effects on body systems. With this skill the paramedic is better able to ask direct questions, in a way 'funnelling' down the questions to a more specific focus. The paramedic also may have to obtain a history on sensitive topics; such topics may include alcohol or other drug use, physical abuse or violence, and sexual issues. When questioning a patient about sensitive issues, the paramedic should follow these guidelines:

1. Remember that privacy is essential with all patients, regardless of age or sex.
2. Be direct and firm and explain the reason for asking a question.
3. Avoid confrontation.
4. Be non-judgemental.
5. Use language that is easily understood but not patronizing.
6. Encourage the patient to ask any relevant questions.
7. Document carefully and use the patient's words (noted by quotation marks) when possible.

Special challenges

History taking often presents special challenges and each patient is unique, so each patient encounter is slightly different from all others. The paramedic must be able to adapt quickly to the special requirements of each encounter so that the required information is obtained quickly. Some challenges that commonly affect history taking follow.

Silence

Silence is often uncomfortable and may have many meanings and uses. For example, patients may use silence to collect thoughts, recall details, or decide whether they trust the paramedic. Silence also can defuse an emotionally tense event effectively. The paramedic should stay alert for non-verbal clues of distress or anxiety. These clues may include a worried expression or loss of eye contact which often precede a silent period during the patient encounter. As a rule, when patients are ready to talk again, they will express feelings more clearly. A patient's silence also may result from a paramedic's lack of sensitivity, understanding, or compassion, so an appropriate and caring 'bedside manner' is key to good patient care.

Overly talkative patients

Interviewing talkative patients can be frustrating, especially when the paramedic has a limited amount of time to obtain a health history. Although there are no perfect solutions in these situations, the following techniques may be helpful:

- accept a less comprehensive history
- give the patient free rein for the first several minutes
- ask questions that invite brief 'yes' or 'no' answers when appropriate
- summarize the patient's comments frequently
- refocus the discussion as needed.

Patients with multiple symptoms

Some patients (often older patients) have a longer medical history because of age, chronic illness, and medication use and are likely to suffer from more than one illness. The paramedic should expect a longer interview and use the techniques presented in Chapter 6. These techniques will help patients with multiple symptoms focus on the most relevant aspects of the presenting complaint.

Critical Thinking

Often patients give you a list of multiple problems. You have to identify the presenting complaint. What single question would you ask?

Anxious patients

For the patient, family and bystanders to be anxious in an emergency is normal. The paramedic must be sensitive to the non-verbal clues of anxiety and should be supportive in a calm and confident way. The professional and caring attitude of the paramedic often helps to reduce the patient's anxiety. The paramedic should be aware that the anxiety may not be related directly to the illness or injury; for example, an older patient on a fixed income may worry about increased costs and living expenses and a victim of a road traffic collision may worry about liability and losing car insurance.

False reassurance

The paramedic may be tempted to provide false reassurance in certain cases by saying 'it's all right' or 'everything's going to be OK.' This may be tempting as a way to comfort an ill or injured patient but the paramedic should avoid early reassurance or over-reassurance until such can be given with confidence; false reassurances may block open dialogue between the paramedic and the patient. The paramedic should reassure the patient that the patient's medical condition is understood and that good patient care is available. Patients also will be comforted to know that the outcome is hopeful (if appropriate) and that they will be treated with dignity and respect during their care; these verbal reassurances generally work well in most patient care situations.

Anger and hostility

Anger and hostility are not too different from anxious behaviour in that they are natural responses in some emergency situations. The paramedic should expect these reactions at times to be directed toward the crew and must always ensure personal and scene safety. However, anger and hostility toward the patient is never appropriate. A much more effective approach includes maintaining a calm, confident manner and the paramedic should try to calm the patient as well; this approach also includes setting limits on acceptable behaviour.

Intoxication

The paramedic should manage patients who are intoxicated with alcohol or other drugs with caution as their behaviour may be difficult to predict. The paramedic should not challenge or aggravate intoxicated patients and must ensure personal and scene safety. The paramedic also must set limits for acceptable behaviour. To ensure scene safety, the paramedic should call for police assistance when needed.

Crying

Crying can reduce tension and may help re-establish the patient's emotional stability during an emergency. If crying is excessive or uncontrollable, the paramedic should be patient, show compassion and use direct eye contact to help control the crying. Reducing exhaustive crying conserves energy and promotes comfort.

Depression

Communicating with a depressed patient can be difficult as the types and causes of depression are many (see Chapter 25). The depression seen in an emergency often is due to moderate to high anxiety. Depression also may be enhanced by alcohol or substance use. The paramedic should use the communication techniques described previously for anxious patients. If possible, the paramedic should identify the seriousness of the patient's state and a medical evaluation is encouraged.

Sexually attractive or seductive patients

Paramedics and patients may be sexually attracted to each other and the paramedic should accept these feelings as normal. However, the feelings should not affect the paramedic's behaviour and if a patient becomes seductive or makes sexual advances, the paramedic should firmly set limits of what is acceptable. The paramedic also must make it clear that the relationship is a professional one. As discussed in Chapter 6, providing same-sex care is often the best practice. If this is not possible, an extra caregiver (or a chaperone) should stay with the patient.

Confusing behaviour or histories

Emergency situations are often intense and emotions can run high, leading to confusing histories. The paramedic also must expect to see abnormal behaviour. Factors that may contribute to these situations include mental illness, delirium, dementia, drug use, illness and injury. Although identifying a pattern of patient behaviour may be difficult the paramedic should try to identify one (e.g. signs and symptoms consistent with a certain disorder). In addition, the paramedic should attempt to lead the patient in an appropriate line of questioning.

Developmental disabilities

The paramedic should not overlook the aptitude of patients with developmental disabilities as they are usually able to offer adequate information. The paramedic should interview them just like other patients, using easily understood words and phrases. An obvious omission in the patient's answers reveals the need for more questioning and questions may need to be stated more clearly. If the patient has severe learning disability, the paramedic may need to get information from family or friends.

Communication barriers

As discussed in Chapter 6, barriers to communication may result from social or cultural differences or due to sight, speech or hearing impairments. The paramedic should seek assistance if possible from family members, translators, and those with special training in communicating with the blind or the deaf, who may be helpful in these situations.

Talking with family and friends

Friends and family are often at the scene of an emergency and they are often a good source of information. This is especially the case when the patient cannot provide all of the necessary information because of illness or injury. Sometimes family or friends are unavailable and more patient information is needed; in these cases, the paramedic should try to locate a third party (e.g. a neighbour) who can help supply the missing details.

Note

History taking refers to details that are gathered during an interview with a patient. History taking provides an account of medical and social events in a patient's life. The history also indicates environmental factors that may have an impact on the patient's condition. Obtaining a patient history gives structure to patient assessment. History taking is often crucial to establish priorities in patient care.

Summary

- Obtaining a patient history offers structure to the patient assessment. The history often sets priorities in patient care as well.
- Content of the patient history includes date and time, identifying data, source of referral, history, reliability, presenting complaint, history of presenting complaint, past medical history, and a review of body systems.
- The paramedic should ensure patient comfort. Several methods are available to accomplish this. The paramedic should avoid entering the patient's personal space. Sensitivity to the patient's feelings and watching for signs of uneasiness also are important. The paramedic should use appropriate language and ask open-ended and direct questions. The paramedic should use therapeutic communications techniques as well.
- Many challenges can affect history taking. One of these challenges is silent or talkative patients. Another is patients with multiple symptoms. Then there are anxious, angry, or hostile patients. The paramedic also may see intoxication, crying, depression, and sexually attractive or seductive patients. False reassurance is a major issue to consider. Patients may present confusing behaviours and histories. Two other issues are developmental disabilities and communication barriers. With these last two, the issue of talking with family and friends can be complex as well.

Further reading

Bond M, Simpson K 2006 Pain: its nature and treatment. Churchill Livingstone/Elsevier, Edinburgh

Carpenito L (ed.) 2002 Nursing diagnosis: application to clinical practice, 9th edition. Lippincott Williams & Wilkins, Philadelphia

Douglas G, Nicol F, Robertson C 2005 Macleod's clinical examination, 11th edition. Elsevier/Churchill Livingstone, Edinburgh

Jarvis C 2004 Physical examination and health assessment, 4th edition. Elsevier/Saunders, St Louis

Monahan F et al 1994 Nursing care of adults. WB Saunders, Philadelphia

Seidel H et al 2006 Mosby's guide to physical examination, 6th edition. Mosby, St Louis

Swartz M 2002 Textbook of physical diagnosis: history and examination, 4th edition. Elsevier/Saunders, Philadelphia

Welsby P 2002 Clinical history taking and examination, 2nd edition. Elsevier/Churchill Livingstone, Edinburgh

CHAPTER 9

Techniques of Physical Examination

Chapter contents

Objectives

Upon completion of this chapter, the paramedic student will be able to:

1. Describe physical examination techniques commonly used in the prehospital setting.
2. Describe the examination equipment commonly used in the prehospital setting.
3. Describe the general approach to physical examination.
4. Outline the steps of a comprehensive physical examination.
5. Detail the components of the mental status examination.
6. Distinguish between normal and abnormal findings in the mental status examination.
7. Outline the steps in the general patient survey.
8. Distinguish between normal and abnormal findings in the general patient survey.
9. Describe physical examination techniques used for assessment of specific body regions.
10. Distinguish between normal and abnormal findings when assessing specific body regions.
11. State modifications to the physical examination that are necessary when assessing children.
12. State modifications to the physical examination that are necessary when assessing the older adult.

Key terms

auscultation A technique that requires the use of a stethoscope and is used to assess body sounds produced by the movement of various fluids or gases in organs or tissues.

inspection A visual assessment of the patient and surroundings.

IPPA inspection, palpation, percussion, auscultation.

palpation A technique in which an examiner uses the hands and fingers to gather information from a patient by touch.

percussion A technique used to evaluate the presence of air or fluid in body tissues.

physical examination An assessment of a patient that includes examination techniques, measurement of vital signs, an assessment of height and weight, and the skilful use of examination equipment.

tidal volume The volume of gas inhaled or exhaled during a normal breath.

Physical examination: approach and overview

The physical examination consists of examination techniques, measurement of vital signs, an assessment (or at least estimation) of height and weight, and the skilful use of examination equipment (Box 9-1).

Examination techniques

Four techniques are commonly used in the physical examination. These are inspection (look), palpation (feel), percussion (listen), and auscultation (listen) (often known as an 'IPPA' format). These terms are referred to often in this text because they relate to the evaluation of specific body systems. Alternative formats might include look, feel, move for assessment of, for example, the musculoskeletal system. The order of these might also vary; one common difference is in assessment of the abdomen where auscultation may be undertaken before palpation. Depending on the situation, these techniques may be the sole method for evaluating a patient; for example, this may be the case with an unconscious trauma patient. In other cases, these techniques will be integrated with the history taking and the paramedic should explain each technique that requires touching of the patient before performing it. It is also vital that the patient's consent is obtained.

Inspection (look)

Inspection is the visual assessment of the patient (and the surroundings). This technique can alert the paramedic to the patient's mental status as well as possible injury or underlying illness. Patient hygiene, clothing, eye gaze, body language and position, skin colour, and odour are significant inspection findings. The emergency medical services (EMS) response may be to the patient's home; in this case, the paramedic should make a visual inspection for social factors of self care, prescription medicines, illegal drug paraphernalia, weapons, and signs of alcohol use. These and other items one sees can play a key role in determining the patient care activities.

Palpation (feel)

Palpation is a technique in which the paramedic uses the hands and fingers to gather information by touch. Generally, the paramedic uses the palmar surface of the fingers and the finger pads to palpate for texture, masses, fluid, and crepitus and to assess skin temperature (Figure 9-1). Palpation may be either superficial or deep; the applications for each are addressed throughout this chapter. Examining a patient by palpation is a form of invasion of the patient's body and the approach should be gentle and should be initiated with respect; consent must be obtained.

Percussion (listen)

Percussion is used to evaluate the presence of air or fluid in body tissues. This technique is performed by the paramedic striking one finger against another to produce vibrations and sound waves of underlying tissue. Sound waves are heard as percussion tones (resonance) and are determined by the density of the tissue being examined. The denser the body area, the lower the pitch of the percussion tone. To percuss, the paramedic places the first joint of the middle finger of the non-dominant hand on the patient, keeping the rest of the hand poised above the skin. The fingers of the other hand should be flexed and the wrist action loose. The paramedic then snaps the wrist of the dominant hand downward with the tip of the middle finger tapping the middle phalanx of the finger that is on the body surface. The tap should be sharp and rigid, percussing the same area several times to interpret the tone (Figure 9-2). Box 9-2 describes percussion tones and examples of each. As with any other examination technique, percussion requires practice to obtain the skill needed for the physical examination.

Auscultation (listen)

Auscultation calls for the use of a stethoscope and is used to assess body sounds made by the movement of various fluids or gases in the patient's organs or tissues. Auscultation is best performed in a quiet environment so the paramedic can

Box 9-1

Components of the physical examination

Examination techniques

- Inspection
- Palpation
- Percussion
- Auscultation

Measurement of vital signs

- Pulse
- Respirations
- Blood pressure
- Temperature (especially in children)

Assessment of height and weight

Equipment

- Blood pressure cuff
- Ophthalmoscope*
- Otoscope*
- Stethoscope

*Used less commonly in paramedic practice in the UK.

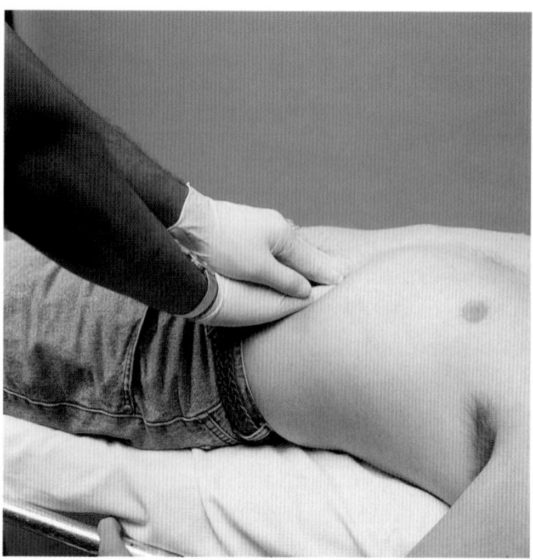

Figure 9-1 Deep bimanual palpation.

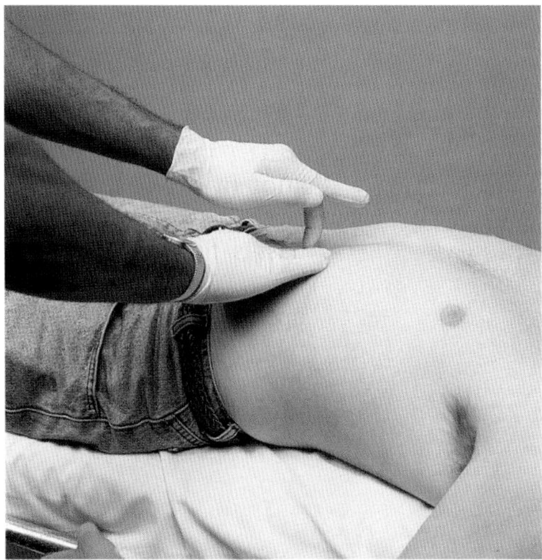

Figure 9-2 Percussion technique.

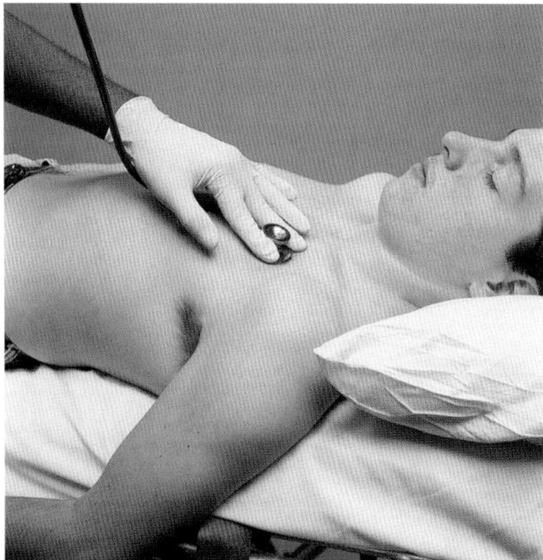

Figure 9-3 Position of the stethoscope between the index and middle fingers.

Box 9-2

Percussion tones and examples

Percussion tone	Example
Tympany (the loudest)	Gastric bubble
Hyperresonance	Air-filled lungs (e.g. chronic obstructive pulmonary disease and pneumothorax)
Resonance	Healthy lungs
Dullness	Liver
Flat (the quietest)	Muscle

focus on each body sound being assessed. The paramedic should isolate a particular area to note characteristics of intensity, pitch, duration and quality. In the prehospital setting, auscultation most often is used to assess blood pressure and to evaluate breath sounds, heart sounds, and bowel sounds. To auscultate, the paramedic should place the diaphragm of the stethoscope firmly against the patient's skin for stabilization (Figure 9-3). If a bell end piece is used, it should be positioned lightly on the body surface, to prevent damping of vibrations.

Note

The bell and diaphragm end pieces of a stethoscope selectively emphasize sounds of different frequencies. The bell is central for listening to low-pitched sounds (e.g. certain heart sounds). In contrast, the diaphragm filters out low-pitched sounds and therefore emphasizes high-pitched ones. Examples of high-pitched sounds include breath sounds and bowel sounds. Some stethoscopes have a single head which combines both the diaphragm and bell head functions.

Examination equipment

Equipment used during the comprehensive physical examination includes the stethoscope, blood pressure cuff (sphygmomanometer), thermometer, pen-torch, and pulse oximetry and capnography devices. In some settings an ophthalmoscope and otoscope might be used; these are non-traditional EMS tools and are being introduced to the paramedic with an expanded scope of practice, such as an emergency care practitioner, and will not be used very often with patients in the prehospital setting.

Stethoscope

The stethoscope is used to evaluate sounds created by the cardiovascular, respiratory, and gastrointestinal systems. The three major types of stethoscopes are acoustic stethoscopes, magnetic stethoscopes and electronic stethoscopes (Figure 9-4a,b).

Acoustic stethoscopes transmit sound waves from the source to the paramedic's ears and most have a rigid diaphragm that transmits high-pitched sounds. The bell end piece transmits low-pitched sounds.

Magnetic stethoscopes have a single diaphragm end piece; the end piece contains an iron disc and a permanent magnet. The air column of the diaphragm is activated as magnetic attraction is established between the iron disc and the magnet. A frequency dial adjusts for high-, low- and full-frequency sounds.

Electronic stethoscopes convert sound vibrations into electrical impulses which are amplified and transmitted to a speaker where they are converted to sound. These devices can compensate for environmental noise and may be beneficial for use in the prehospital setting.

Blood pressure cuff (sphygmomanometer)

The blood pressure cuff is the sphygmomanometer and is most commonly used (along with the stethoscope) to measure systolic and diastolic blood pressure. The common blood pressure cuff used in the prehospital setting consists of a pressure gauge that registers millimeter calibrations, a synthetic cuff with Velcro closures that encloses an inflatable rubber bladder, and a pressure bulb with a release valve. Blood pressure cuffs are available in a number of sizes; adult widths should be one-third to one-half the circumference of the limb. For children, the width should cover about two

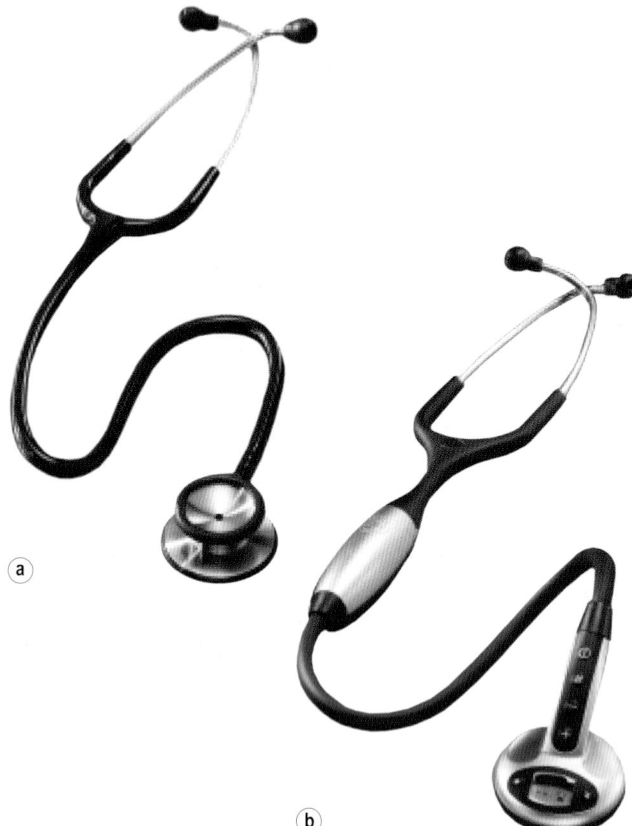

Figure 9-4 Stethoscope types. (a) Acoustic. (b) Electronic.

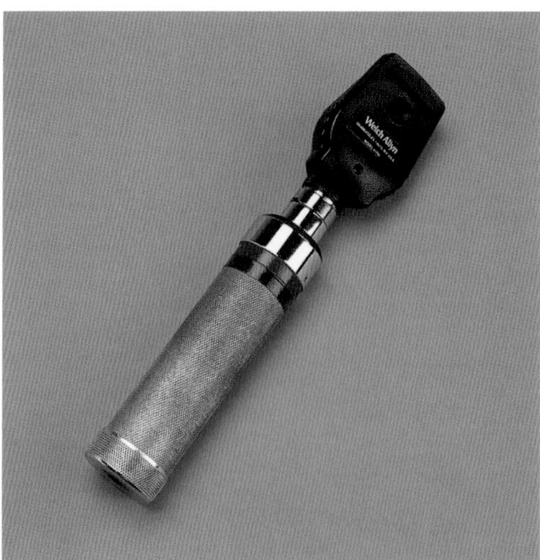

Figure 9-5 Ophthalmoscope.

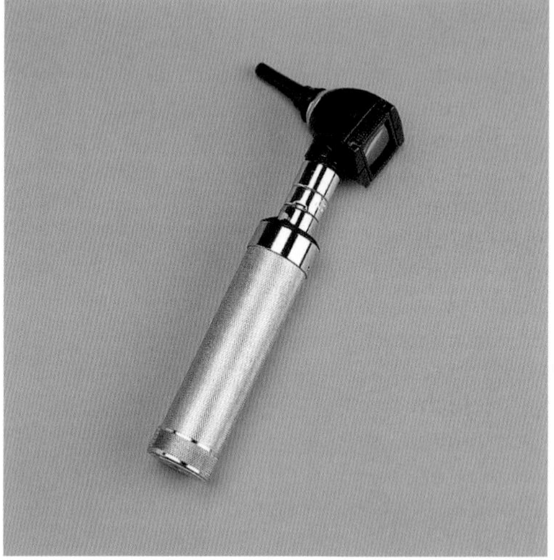

Figure 9-6 Otoscope.

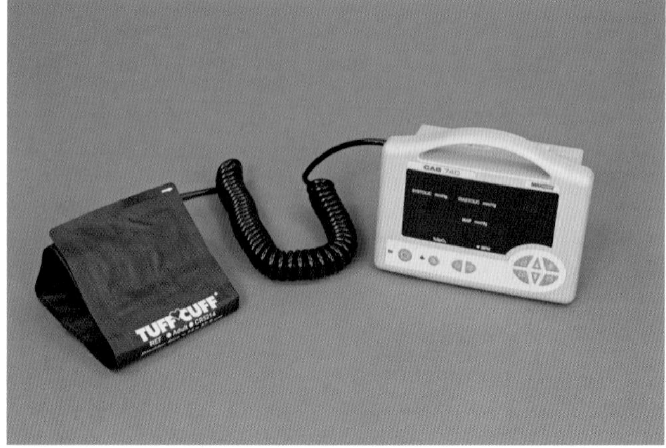

Figure 9-7 Electronic blood pressure device. Modified from Thompson, Wilson, 1995.

thirds of the upper arm or thigh. (Blood pressure cuffs that are too large give a falsely low reading; cuffs that are too small give a falsely high reading.)

Ophthalmoscope

The ophthalmoscope is used to inspect structures of the eye, including the retina, choroid, optic nerve disc, macula (an oval, yellow spot at the centre of the retina) and retinal vessels. This device has a battery light source, two dials, and a viewer (Figure 9-5). The dial at the top of the battery changes the light image and the dial at the top of the viewer allows for the selection of lenses. (Five lenses are available, but the large white light generally is used.)

Otoscope

The otoscope is used to examine deep structures of the external and middle ear and is an ophthalmoscope with a special ear speculum attached to the battery tube (Figure 9-6). Ear specula come in a number of sizes to conform to various ear canals. (The paramedic should choose the largest one that fits comfortably in the patient's ear.) The light from the otoscope allows one to visualize the tympanic membrane.

Electronic devices

Electronic devices that automatically measure a patient's vital signs are available (Figure 9-7). They are used by hospitals and some EMS agencies to monitor the patient's blood pressure, pulse rate, body temperature, end-tidal carbon dioxide (capnography), and oxygen saturation at regular intervals.

General approach to the physical examination

The physical examination is performed as a step-by-step process and special emphasis is placed on the patient's presenting complaint and history of the presenting complaint. The paramedic should know that most patients view a physical examination with some anxiety and often initially feel vulnerable and exposed; establishing a professional trust early in the encounter and ensuring the patient's privacy when possible are important.

Overview of a comprehensive physical examination

Systems-based or integrated physical assessment

There are differing ways of undertaking a physical examination. One is to undertake a system-by-system approach, focusing first on the systems affected by the presenting complaint; the systems are assessed independently. Therefore, in a patient presenting with chest pain the systems assessed might include, for example, the respiratory, cardiovascular and gastrointestinal systems, as causes of chest pain can be found within any of those systems. Many texts on physical and clinical examination and assessment focus on this systems-based approach.[1–3] Another variation commonly used in practice is the integrated physical assessment approach, which follows a body part sequence/pattern starting with the patient's hand, upper limbs, head, neck, thorax and abdomen (not forgetting the posterior aspects) and then the pelvis and legs.[4] With experience and an understanding of the systems-based approach, a paramedic can adapt the assessment into the integrated assessment method. However, the method used in this chapter is to take a systems-based approach so that each component of a system can be considered. However, whichever method is used, it is vitally important that adequate assessment takes place so that no element is omitted.

Note

Universal precautions: This text assumes that all paramedics are gloved for certain care activities. Personal protective measures are dealt with further in Chapter 24.

General impression

Appearance and behaviour

The first step in any encounter with a patient is to note the patient's appearance and behaviour and one also should assess for level of consciousness. A healthy patient is expected to be alert and responsive to touch, verbal instruction, and painful stimuli.

Mental status

As mentioned before, a visual assessment of the patient can yield key information. Abnormal findings may include drowsiness, obtundation (inability to respond), stupor or coma; a patient who is obtunded is insensitive to unpleasant or painful stimuli because of a reduced level of consciousness. Stupor is a state of lethargy and unresponsiveness and patients are usually unaware of their surroundings. Coma is a state of profound unconsciousness; a patient in coma has no spontaneous eye movements and does not respond to verbal or painful stimuli and cannot be aroused.

Note

Some experts discourage the use of these terms to describe a patient's mental status. Because these terms are vague, they may be open to interpretation. Instead, one may describe the patient's reactions and verbal and motor responses with indexes such as the AVPU (alert, verbal, painful, unresponsive) scale or Glasgow Coma Scale (described in Chapters 7 and 31). These measurements often are considered to provide better patient information.

Posture, gait and motor activity

The paramedic should observe the patient's posture, gait, and motor activity and can do this by assessing pace, range, character, and appropriateness of movement. For example, most patients without physical disabilities can walk with good balance and without a limp, discomfort, or fear of falling. Abnormal findings may include ataxia (uncoordinated movement), paralysis, restlessness, agitation, bizarre body posture, immobility, and involuntary movements.

Dress, grooming, personal hygiene, and breath or body odours

Dress, grooming, and personal hygiene should be appropriate for the patient's age, lifestyle, occupation, and socioeconomic group and should match the temperature and weather conditions. (Older adults and children who are improperly dressed for temperatures or who have poor hygiene may be victims of neglect.) Medical jewellery (e.g. copper bracelets for arthritis, medical insignias) should be noted. Hair, fingernails, and cosmetics may reflect the patient's lifestyle, mood and personality and these findings can point to a decreased interest in appearance (e.g. grown-out hair or faded nail polish). This may help to estimate the duration of ill health.

Breath or body odours can point to underlying conditions or illness; odours include alcohol, acetone (seen with some diabetic conditions), faeces (seen with bowel obstruction), and halitosis from throat infections and poor dental and oral hygiene. Renal and liver disease and poor hygiene also may result in body odour.

Facial expression

Facial expressions may reveal anxiety, depression, elation, anger, or withdrawal. The paramedic should be alert to changes in facial expression and should observe these while the patient is at rest, during conversation, during the examination, and when asking questions; facial expressions should match the situation.

Mood, affect, and relation to person and things

The patient's mood and affect also should match the situation and describe the patient's emotional state and the outward display of feelings and emotions; they are expressed verbally and non-verbally. Examples of abnormal findings include an unusual happiness in the presence of major illness, indifference, responses to imaginary persons or objects, and unpredictable mood swings.

Critical Thinking

What physical clues do you look for in your friends or your partner that tell you about their mood?

Speech and language

The patient's speech should be understandable and of a moderate pace. The paramedic should assess the quantity, rate, loudness, and fluency of the patient's speech patterns. Abnormal findings include aphasia (loss of speech), dysphonia (abnormal speaking voice), dysarthria (poorly articulated speech), and speech and language that changes with mood.

Thought and perceptions

A healthy person's thoughts and perceptions are logical, relevant, organized and coherent. Patients should have an insight into their illness or injury and show a level of judgement in making decisions or plans about their situation and their care. Although accurately assessing a person's thoughts and perceptions is difficult, the following usually are considered abnormal findings:

- abnormal thought processes
  - flight of ideas
  - incoherence
  - confabulation
- abnormal thought content
  - obsessions
  - compulsions
  - delusions
  - feelings of unreality
- abnormal perceptions
  - illusions
  - hallucinations.

Memory and attention

Healthy persons normally are orientated to person, place and time ('orientated times 3'). The paramedic can use several other methods to assess a patient's memory and attention; one method is to ask the patient to count from 1 to 10 using only even or odd numbers (digit span). Another is to multiply by sevens (serial sevens). A third method is to spell simple words backward. The paramedic also should assess the patient's remote memory (e.g. birthdays), recent memory (e.g. events of the day), and the patient's new learning ability; this can be evaluated by giving the patient new information (e.g. the year and model of the ambulance) and later the paramedic asks the patient to recall that information.

General survey

The paramedic assesses the patient's level of consciousness and mental status first and then performs a general survey of the patient. In addition to the assessments described previously, the paramedic should evaluate the patient for signs of distress, apparent state of health, skin colour and obvious lesions, height and build, sexual development, and weight. The paramedic also should assess vital signs during the general survey.

Signs of distress

Obvious signs of distress include those that result from cardiorespiratory insufficiency, pain and anxiety. Examples of these signs and symptoms are as follows:

- cardiorespiratory insufficiency
  - laboured breathing
  - wheezing
  - cough
- pain
  - wincing
  - sweating
  - protectiveness of a painful body part or area
- anxiety
  - restlessness
  - anxious expression
  - fidgety movement
  - cold, moist palms.

Critical Thinking

Combine one symptom from each of the groups of distress, and imagine how a patient with these symptoms might look and act.

Apparent state of health

A patient's apparent state of health can be assessed by observation and the paramedic should note the patient's basic appearance as being acutely or chronically ill, frail, feeble, robust or vigorous.

Skin colour and obvious lesions

Skin colour can vary by body part and from person to person and depends on ethnic origin and can range from pink or ivory to deep brown, yellow or olive. Skin colour is best assessed by evaluating skin that usually is not exposed to the sun (e.g. the palms) or skin that has less pigmentation (e.g. lips and nail beds). Box 9-3 describes abnormal skin colours and their possible causes. Obvious skin lesions that can indicate illness or injury include rashes, bruises, scars and discoloration.

Height and build

Patients generally can be described as average, tall or short, with a slender, lanky, muscular or stocky build and these factors can reflect overall health. For example, a patient can be excessively thin (as seen with some eating disorders) or trim and muscular. Age and lifestyle also may affect height and body build.

Weight

Ideally a patient's body weight should be proportional to height. Weight conditions that are easily observed in the general survey include patients who are emaciated (extremely lean from lack of nutrition), plump or obese (body weight

Box 9-3

Abnormal skin colour and possible causes

Colour	Possible causes
Pallor (decrease in colour)	Shock, dehydration, fright
Cyanosis (bluish colour)	Cardiorespiratory insufficiency, cold environment
Jaundice (yellow–orange colour)	Liver disease, red blood cell destruction
Red	Fever, inflammation, carbon monoxide poisoning

Table 9-1 Average vital signs by age

Age	Pulse (beats/min)	Respirations (breaths/min)	Blood pressure (mmHg)
Newborn	120–160	40–60	80/40
1 year	80–140	30–40	82/44
3 years	80–120	25–30	86/50
5 years	70–115	20–25	90/52
7 years	70–115	20–25	94/54
10 years	70–115	15–20	100/60
15 years	70–90	15–20	110/64
Adult	60–100	12–20	120/80

that is 20% greater than desirable body weight for a person's age, sex, height and body fluid). A recent gain or loss is a key finding and may be clinically important. Like body height and build, body weight can reflect the patient's health, age, and lifestyle.

Critical Thinking

Think about three medical conditions that might result in significant weight loss. Now, think about three that might cause a significant weight gain.

Sexual development

The paramedic will assess sexual development and should decide whether the sexual characteristics are appropriate for the patient's age and sex. Normal changes associated with puberty include facial hair and deepening of the voice in men, increased breast size in women, and hair growth in the axillary and groin areas in both sexes.

Vital signs

Vital signs are pulse, blood pressure, respirations, skin condition, temperature, and pupil size and reactivity, as well as measuring parameters such as oxygen saturation and blood glucose.

Pulse

A normal resting pulse rate for an adult is usually between 60 and 100 beats per minute; it may be affected by the patient's age and physical condition (Table 9-1). For example, a child's pulse rate may be 80–100 beats per minute. A well-trained athlete's pulse rate may be 50–60 beats per minute. Factors such as pregnancy, anxiety, and fear also may produce a higher-than-normal pulse rate in healthy individuals.

Pulse rates may be obtained at the carotid artery in the neck, radial artery in the wrist, and femoral artery in the groin, as well as at any sites where the artery lies close to the skin surface. To evaluate the radial pulse, the paramedic places the pads of the index and middle fingers at the distal end of the patient's wrist, just medial to the radial styloid. If pulsations are regular, the paramedic should count them for 30 s and then multiply the number of pulses by 2 to determine the number of beats per minute. In addition to the number of times the heart beats per minute, the paramedic should assess the regularity and strength of the pulse; for example, the pulse can be regular or irregular, weak or strong. Application of an electrocardiogram monitor also may be useful in evaluating cardiovascular status after initial assessment of the pulse.

Blood pressure

The systolic blood pressure is the pressure against the arterial walls when the heart contracts, whilst the diastolic blood pressure is the pressure against the arterial walls when the heart relaxes. For all age groups,[1] systolic blood pressure ideally should be less than 120 mmHg; diastolic pressure should be less than 80 mmHg.

Blood pressure is best measured by auscultation. The blood pressure cuff is placed on the patient's arm with the lower end of the cuff positioned 2–5 cm above the antecubital space. The cuff is inflated to a point about 30 mmHg above where the brachial pulse can no longer be palpated. The stethoscope is placed over the brachial artery, and the cuff is slowly deflated at a rate of 2–3 mmHg per second. As the pressure falls, the paramedic should observe the gauge and note where the first sound or pulsation is heard; this is the patient's systolic pressure. The point at which the sounds change in quality or become notably muffled is the patient's diastolic pressure.

Note

At times, determining the correct diastolic pressure is difficult. The difference between the point of muffled tones and the complete disappearance of pulsations varies by person. In some persons, the difference is a few millimetres of mercury; however, in some people, pulsations never totally disappear. The ability to measure accurate diastolic pressures comes from experience and requires careful listening in a quiet setting.

Blood pressure may be estimated by palpation when vascular sounds are hard to hear with a stethoscope because of environmental noise; however, this method is less accurate than auscultation and can only estimate systolic pressure. To estimate blood pressure by palpation, the paramedic should locate the brachial or radial pulse and apply the blood pressure cuff as described before. The paramedic maintains finger contact at the pulse site as the cuff slowly deflates; when the pulse becomes palpable, the gauge reading denotes the systolic pressure. Like pulse rates, a patient's blood pressure may be unusually high because of fear or anxiety. Other factors, such as a patient's age and normal level of physical activity, may be the cause of unusual blood pressure readings.

Alternative sites may be used to assess blood pressure when use of the patient's upper arm is not possible. Blood pressure readings in these alternative sites vary from those taken in the arm (Figure 9-8).

Respirations

The normal respiratory rate for adults is between 12 and 20 breaths per minute. The respiratory rate is found by watching the patient breathe, by feeling for chest movement, or by auscultating the lungs. The paramedic counts the respirations for 30 s, then multiplies by 2 to get breaths per minute. Rhythm and depth of respirations are assessed by visualization and auscultation of the thorax. Abnormal findings include shallow, rapid, noisy or deep breathing; asymmetrical chest wall movement; use of accessory muscles of respiration; or congested, unequal, or diminished breath sounds.

Skin

The skin can reveal a great deal about a patient's status. Skin colour, temperature and moisture provide valuable details. As discussed before, a patient's skin colour and the presence of bruises, lesions or rashes may indicate serious illness or injury. Skin temperature may be normal (warm), hot or cold.

Temperature

More specific evaluations of temperature may have specific applications in some patient situations. Examples of such are febrile seizures and hyperthermic and hypothermic emergencies. Skin that is hot to the touch points to a possible fever or heat-related illness or injury, whilst cold skin may point to decreased tissue perfusion and cold-related illness or injury. The dorsal surface of the hand is more sensitive than the palmar surface and should be used to estimate body temperature. Normal body temperature is 37 °C (98.6 °F). Various types of thermometer exist but mercury thermometers are now very uncommon and tympanic or electronic oral devices are now used almost exclusively (Figure 9-9a–d). The temperature probe must be covered by a disposable cover which helps to prevent cross-contamination.

Oral measurement Oral temperature is usually measured in patients over the age of 6. The readings may be affected by crying, eating, drinking, smoking, oxygen administration by mask, nebulizer treatments, and by the position of the thermometer in the patient's mouth. If using a traditional glass thermometer to assess oral temperature, the bulb of the thermometer should be placed in the sublingual area of the patient's mouth and should be left in place for several minutes; however, these are very much out of use. Electronic device times are much shorter; a brief tone will alert the paramedic when the measurement is complete. The paramedic should tell the patient to keep the mouth closed tightly around the thermometer. The paramedic can tell children to hold the thermometer in a 'kiss' position and should caution children not to bite on the probe.

Axillary measurement The axillary site often is used to take the temperature in children and is used in children less than 6 years of age as well as those who are uncooperative, have

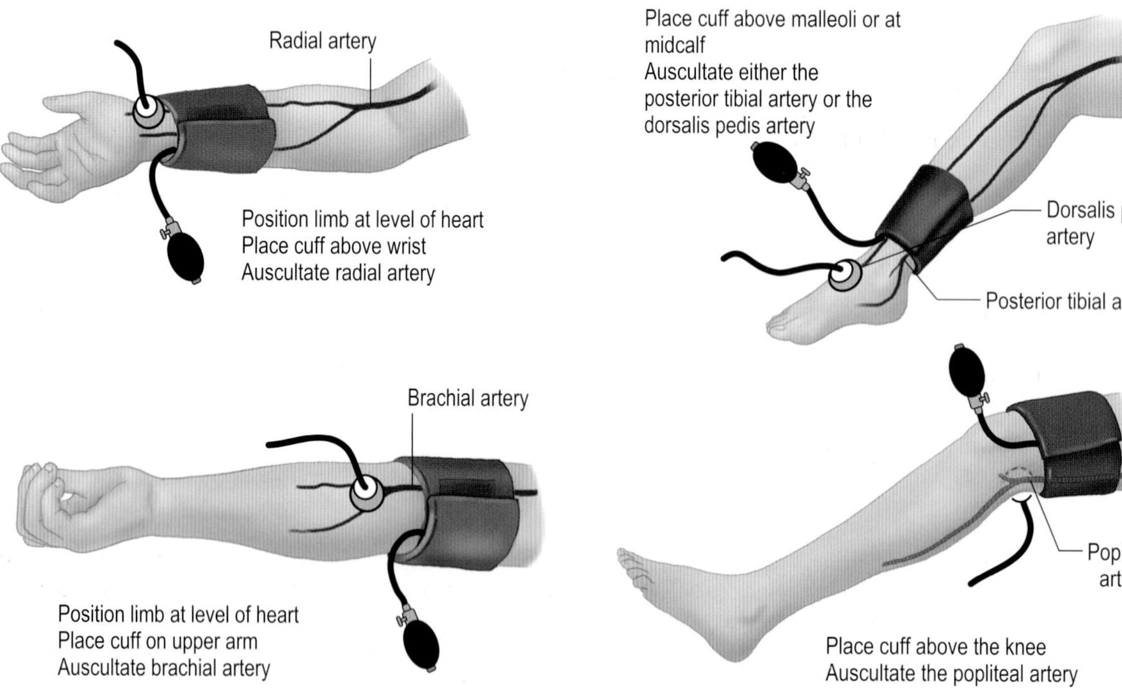

Figure 9-8 Blood pressure measurement sites.

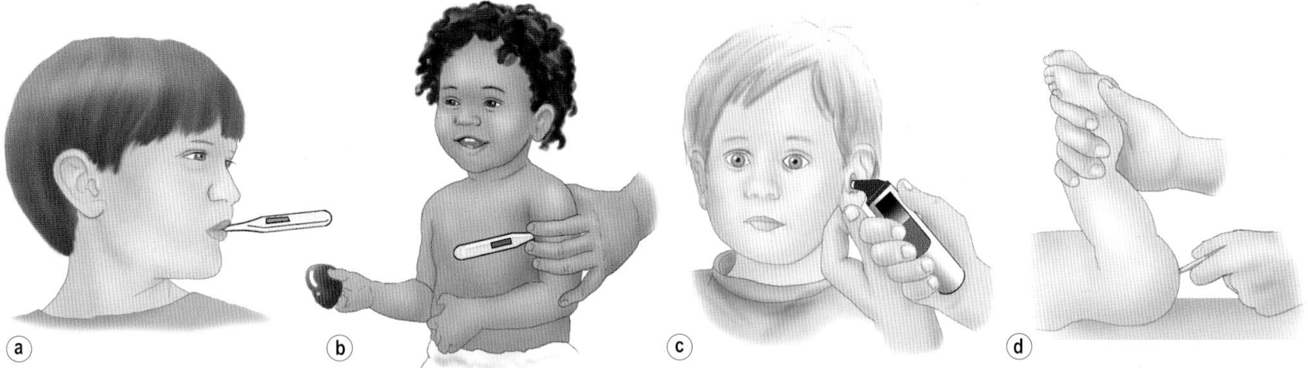

Figure 9-9 Temperature assessment. (a) Oral temperature measurement. (b) Axillary temperature measurement. (c) Tympanic temperature measurement. (d) Rectal temperature measurement.

diseases that suppress the immune system, and in those who have an altered level of consciousness. The paramedic measures axillary temperature by placing the thermometer probe firmly in the centre of the patient's axillary space; the patient's arm should be held against the side of the chest. When an electronic device is used, the paramedic should read it when the alert indicates; the temperature assessed at this site is usually 1 °F (0.6 °C) lower than the core temperature of the body.

Tympanic measurement The tympanic membrane is close to the hypothalamus, which makes the tympanic membrane an ideal place to measure core temperature. The paramedic takes this measurement by placing the tip of the probe into the patient's ear canal, then straightens the ear canal by gently pulling the pinna of the ear down and back in children less than 3 years of age or up and back in patients 3 years of age or older. When the thermometer is in the correct position and is activated per the manufacturer's instructions, a temperature reading is obtained within seconds.

Rectal measurement Measuring a patient's temperature by the rectal route poses a risk of perforation, can be distressing for the patient, and issues about dignity arise. This route generally is reserved for young children and patients who have an altered level of consciousness. When measuring rectal temperature, the paramedic should place the patient in the supine position (infants) or in the left lateral recumbent position with the legs raised. This position exposes the anus. The paramedic inserts a lubricated probe no more than 2.5 cm (1 inch) into the rectum and holds the probe securely in place until the electronic device sounds the alert. Rectal readings provide the most accurate assessment but in many cases are impractical for prehospital use.

Skin moisture

Skin usually is classified as dry or wet; dry skin is normal. Wet skin is clammy or diaphoretic; diaphoretic skin may point to a drop in circulating blood volume called a haemodynamic deficit (for example hypovolaemia). Diaphoretic skin also may point to another illness or injury that results in decreased tissue perfusion or increased sweat gland activity; examples are cardiovascular and heat-related emergencies, respectively.

Table 9-2 Abnormal pupil reactions

Pupil size	Possible cause
EQUAL	
Dilated or unresponsive	Cardiac arrest, central nervous system injury, hypoxia or anoxia, drug use (LSD [lysergic acid diethylamide], atropine, amphetamines)
Constricted or unresponsive	Central nervous system injury or disease, narcotic drug use (heroin, morphine), eye medications
UNEQUAL	
One dilated or unresponsive	Cerebrovascular accident, head injury, direct trauma to the eye, eye medications

Pupils

Examining the pupils for response to light may yield information on the neurological status of some patients. Unequal pupils (anisocoria) may be a normal finding in some patients. However, the pupils usually are equal and constrict when exposed to light; the acronym PERRL indicates that the pupils are equal, round and react to light. When testing the pupils for light response, the paramedic shines a penlight directly into one eye; the normal reaction is for the pupil exposed to the light to constrict and occurs with a consensual constriction of the opposite eye. Table 9-2 lists abnormal pupillary reactions and possible causes.

Pulse oximetry

This is a useful tool that can give an estimation of the percentage oxygen saturation of haemoglobin. However, it is not without its limitations, and a number of factors such as hypotension and poor perfusion, cold extremities, patient movement and poor probe placement can affect the reliability of readings. Readings are also skewed in cases of carbon monoxide poisoning or where there is abnormal haemoglobin such as in sickle cell patients.

Blood glucose

Compact blood glucose machines are commonly used to assess blood glucose levels. The normal range for blood glucose is 4–8 mmol/L, with a low being generally defined as <4 mmol/L. Machines vary but a 'LO' reading will usually be <1.2 mmol/L. 'HI' readings are usually >32 mmol/L. Blood glucose levels may be abnormal not only in diabetic patients but in a number of other conditions where the body reacts to injury or illness by altering the blood glucose levels and therefore, readings may be taken on patients with altered levels of consciousness or those who have, for example, suspected acute coronary syndrome, fever or infection, convulsions, alcohol intoxication or dependency, liver or kidney disease, pancreatitis, and so on.

Systems assessment

The rest of this chapter deals with techniques of the physical examination as they relate to the systems of the body. The paramedic should recall that anatomical and physiological aspects of the human body are age-related and vary by person as well. An examination of the systems should be guided by a patient's presenting complaint.

Skin (integumentary) system

The general assessment of the skin was described previously. In addition, the comprehensive physical examination should include an evaluation of the texture and turgor of the skin, hair, and fingernails and toenails; all of these are part of the integumentary system.

Texture and turgor

The texture of the skin normally is smooth, soft, and flexible, though in older adults the skin may be wrinkled and leathery from decreases in collagen, subcutaneous fat and sweat glands. Abnormal skin texture may result from lesions, rashes, tumours and localized trauma.

Turgor refers to the elasticity of the skin (which normally decreases with age). To test skin turgor, the paramedic should pinch ('tent') a fold of skin and assess the ease and speed at which the skin returns to its normal position. Skin on the back of the patient's hand or over the sternum is good for testing for turgor; tented skin that does not quickly return to its normal position may indicate dehydration.

Hair

As part of the examination, the paramedic should inspect and palpate the patient's hair, noting the quantity, distribution, and texture. Key findings include a recent change in the growth or loss of hair, which may result from chemotherapy or hormone and endocrine disorders (e.g. menopause and diabetes). Thinning hair is common in older men and women.

Fingernails and toenails

The paramedic should note the colour, shape, and the presence or absence of lesions when assessing the patient's fingernails and toenails; uncoloured nails usually are transparent. Healthy nails are smooth and firm on palpation. Box 9-4 describes abnormal findings in the nails; with age, nails often develop longitudinal striations and may have a yellow tint because of insufficient calcium.

Box 9-4

Abnormal nail findings

Beau's lines: Transverse depressions in the nail that inhibit nail growth; associated with systemic illness, severe infection and nail injury.

Clubbing: A change in the angle between the nail and nail base that approaches or exceeds 180 degrees; associated with flattening and often enlargement of the fingertips; may indicate chronic cardiac or respiratory disease.

Onycholysis: The separation of a nail from its bed; associated with psoriasis, dermatitis, fungal infection and other conditions.

Paronychia: Inflammation of the skin at the base of the nail; may result from local infection or trauma.

Psoriasis: Pitting, discoloration and subungual thickening of the nail plate; may lead to splinter haemorrhages.

Splinter haemorrhages: Red or brown linear streaks in the nail bed; associated with minor nail trauma, bacterial endocarditis and trichinosis.

Terry's nails: The presence of transverse white bands that cover the nail except for a narrow zone at the distal tip; associated with cirrhosis.

Transverse white lines: Longitudinal white streaks in the nail plate; may indicate a systemic disorder.

White spots: The presence of white spots that appear in the nail plate; usually result from minor injury or cuticle manipulation.

Head, ears, eyes, nose and throat (HEENT) system

An examination of the structures of the head and neck involves inspection, palpation, and auscultation.

Head and face

To examine the head, the paramedic should inspect the skull for shape and symmetry. The paramedic should keep in mind that hair can hide abnormalities. The paramedic should part the hair in several places to assess for scaliness, lumps, or other lesions; the assessment should use a systematic palpation, moving from front to back, noting any swelling, tenderness, indentations or depressions. The scalp should move freely over the skull, and the patient should not complain of pain or discomfort during the examination.

The paramedic should inspect the face for symmetry, expression, and contour, as well as looking for discoloration or bruising, noting pigmentation, texture, thickness, hair distribution and any lesions. The paramedic should note any asymmetry, involuntary movements, masses, or oedema and palpate for facial bone stability. The temporomandibular joint (TMJ) should be evaluated by placing the index finger in each depression behind the TMJ and in front of the tragus; palpate for tenderness and assess range of motion.

Eyes

The paramedic should verify that both eyes can see. The paramedic can do this by first soliciting the patient's history regarding visual disturbances and then can ask the patient

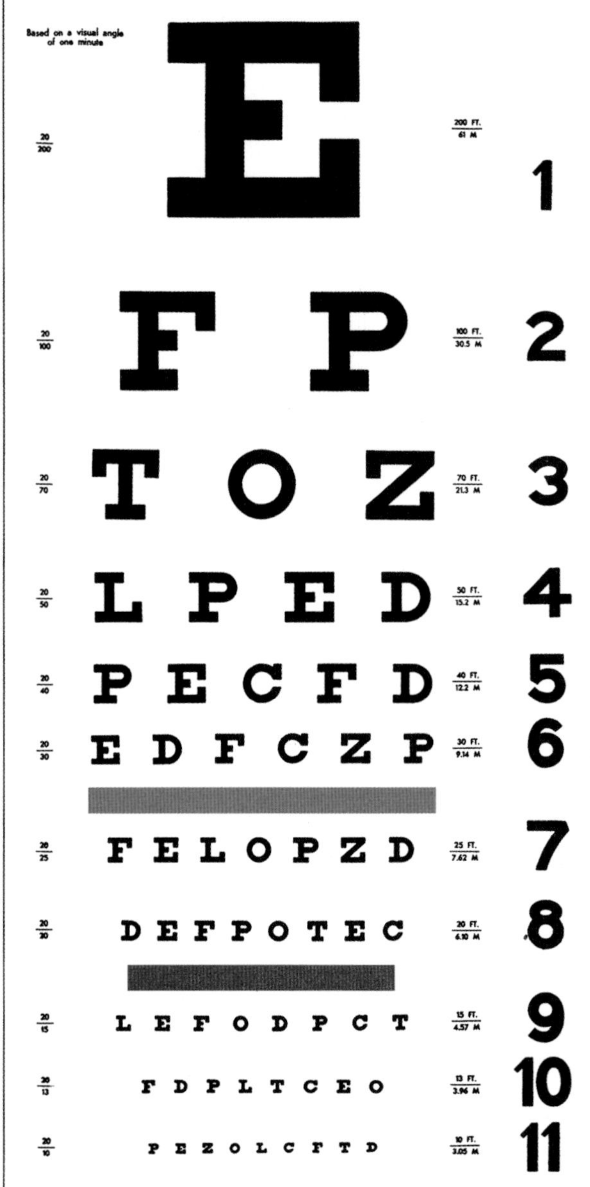

Figure 9-10 Six cardinal fields of gaze. Cranial nerves and extraocular muscles associated with the six cardinal fields of gaze.

to demonstrate visual acuity. The paramedic can assess visual acuity by asking the patient to read printed material, count fingers at a distance, and demonstrate the ability to distinguish light from dark. The use of various eye charts (e.g. a Snellen chart) is less common in prehospital care.

Both eyes should move equally well in the six cardinal fields of gaze (Figure 9-10). To evaluate a patient's gaze, the paramedic should hold the patient's chin and then watch the eyes as they track a penlight or finger (or a toy, in the case of a child) when it moves through the six visual fields in an H pattern. The paramedic should note any nystagmus (involuntary jerking movements of the eyes). Another method to check visual fields is to ask the patient to look at his or her nose. The paramedic then extends his or her arms with elbows at right angles and wiggles both index fingers at the same time to test peripheral vision. By asking the patient to identify finger movement and to track a moving object (e.g. a pencil, finger or penlight), the paramedic can decide whether visual fields are grossly normal. This test should be done in four quadrants (up, down, right and left). The paramedic should also check the eyes for normal position and alignment.

The paramedic should inspect the orbital area for oedema and puffiness. The eyebrows should be free of scaliness. Inspection of the eyelids consists of noting the width of palpebral fissures (the elliptical opening between the upper and lower lids), oedema, colour, lesions, condition and direction of the eyelashes, adequacy of lid closure, and drainage. The paramedic also briefly should inspect the regions of the lacrimal gland and lacrimal sac for swelling and note excessive tearing or dryness of the eye.

The paramedic examines the conjunctiva and sclera by asking the patient to look up while the paramedic depresses both lower lids with the thumbs (Figure 9-11). The sclera should be white; the cornea and the iris should be clearly visible; and the pupils should be of equal size, round, and reactive to light. The paramedic should palpate the lower orbital rim to determine structural integrity. The paramedic should be alert to the presence of contact lenses and ocular prostheses when examining a patient's eyes.

Ears

The paramedic should inspect the external ear and surrounding tissues for signs of bruising, deformity, or discoloration; no discharge should come from either ear canal and pulling gently on the ear lobes (lobules) should not produce pain or discomfort. The paramedic should palpate the skull and facial bones surrounding the ear and inspect the mastoid area for tenderness or discoloration. An alert, hearing patient who speaks the same language as the paramedic should be able to respond to questions without many requests for repetition. The paramedic should note hearing aids. An assessment of gross auditory keenness can be made by covering one ear at a time; the paramedic should ask the patient to repeat short test words spoken by the paramedic in soft and loud tones.

Nose

The paramedic should inspect the nose for shape, size, colour and stability. The column of the nose should be midline with the face and the nares should be positioned symmetrically; slight asymmetry of nares can be considered normal. The paramedic should palpate the column of the nose and surrounding soft tissues for pain, tenderness or deformity and inspect the frontal and maxillary sinuses for the presence of swelling and should palpate for tenderness along the bony brow on each side of the nose and the zygomatic processes.

Discharge from the nose can have a number of causes. For example, cerebrospinal fluid may be present as a result of head trauma; a bloody discharge (epistaxis) may result from trauma or from mucosal erosions involving blood vessels, hypertension or bleeding disorders. A mucous discharge commonly results from allergy, upper respiratory tract infection, sinusitis or cold exposure.

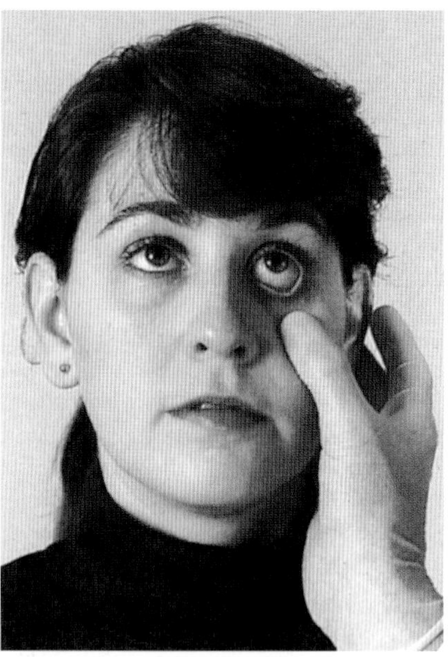

Figure 9-11 Examining the conjunctiva and sclera.

Mouth and pharynx

The paramedic should inspect the lips for symmetry, colour, oedema and skin surface irregularities. The lips should be pink; pallor of the lips is linked with anaemia whilst cyanosis is linked with cardiorespiratory insufficiency and red lips sometimes are a late finding in carbon monoxide poisoning. The lips should show no swelling, deformity or pain on palpation.

Healthy gums in the oral cavity are pink and free of lesions and swelling. Patchy areas of pigmentation in the mouths of Afro-Caribbean patients are not uncommon. Enlarged gums may indicate pregnancy, leukaemia, poor oral hygiene, puberty, or use of some medications (e.g. phenytoin). The mouth should be free of loose or broken teeth. Dental appliances may be present.

The paramedic should inspect the tongue for size and colour; it should be positioned in the midline of the oral cavity and appear non-swollen, dull red, moist and glistening. To inspect the oropharynx, the paramedic can use a tongue blade to depress the tongue. The normal palate is white or pink. If the oral cavity is inflamed or covered with exudate, an infection may be present. Specific breath odours may indicate alcohol or other drug consumption or illness. The tonsils normally are pink and smooth without oedema, ulceration or inflammation. A patient with a typical sore throat often has a reddened and oedematous uvula and tonsillar pillars and a yellow exudate sometimes is present.

Neck

The paramedic should inspect the neck in the patient's normal anatomical position. If the paramedic suspects trauma, the paramedic should use spinal precautions. The trachea should be midline and no use of accessory muscles or tracheal tugging should occur during respiration. To palpate the neck, the paramedic places both thumbs along the sides of the distal trachea and systematically moves the hands toward the head (Figure 9-12). The paramedic should take care not to apply bilateral pressure to the carotid arteries as syncope or bradycardia may result.

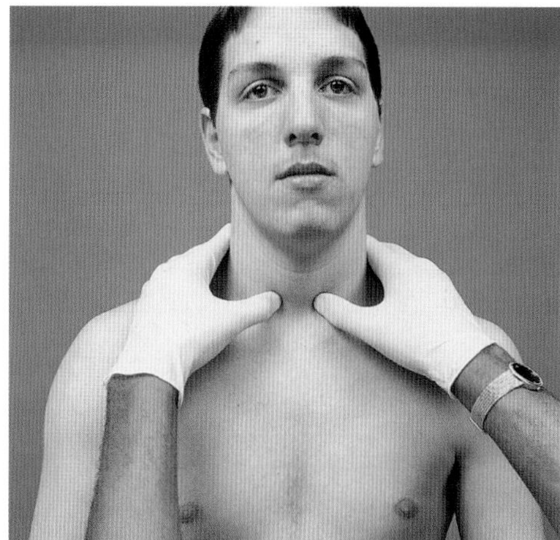

Figure 9-12 Position of the thumbs to evaluate the midline position of the trachea.

The lymph nodes should not be tender; tender or swollen lymph nodes usually are the result of inflammation. The thyroid and cricoid cartilages should be free of pain and should move when the patient swallows. Bubbling or crackling sensations that can be palpated in the soft tissues of the neck may indicate the presence of subcutaneous emphysema. The paramedic should note distended neck veins or prominent carotid arteries (see Chapter 15).

Head and cervical spine

The temporomandibular joint (TMJ) connects the mandible of the jaw to the temporal bone of the skull and can sometimes become painful or dislocated. Normally the patient should be able to open and close the mouth without pain or limitation in movement. TMJ dysfunction is a common complaint.

For the patient who has not undergone trauma and who would meet the rule-out criteria for C-spine immobilization, the paramedic should inspect the cervical spine, palpating for tenderness or deformities. Range of motion can be tested in the following manner:

- flexion: touching the chin to the chest
- rotation: touching the chin to each shoulder
- lateral bending: touching each ear to each shoulder
- extension: tilting the head backward.

The trauma patient may need to be moved for a general or neurological examination. Any such movement must be accompanied by the application of continuous manual protection and stabilization techniques for suspected cervical spine injury (see Chapter 32).

Respiratory system

A paramedic must have a full knowledge of the structure of the thoracic cage, in order to perform a good respiratory assessment. The ribs protect the vital organs within the thorax and offer support for respiratory movements of the diaphragm and intercostal muscles. Damage to the actual bony structure of the thoracic cavity, such as a flail chest, can prevent or limit respiratory function. The ribs of the thorax also are used as anatomical landmarks and help in finding certain areas for examination; Figure 9-13 shows the landmarks of the chest. The paramedic can evaluate the thorax by using the imaginary lines to note examination findings (Figure 9-14a–c). The paramedic should evaluate the chest using inspection, palpation, percussion and auscultation.

Inspection

Part of respiratory assessment is undertaken away from the thoracic area. Inspection of the hands should be made to look for clubbing, cyanosis, tobacco staining and CO_2 retention flap. Assessment of the neck should be made for jugular vein distension (JVD) and accessory muscle use and the tongue for central cyanosis. The paramedic should inspect the chest wall for symmetry on the anterior and posterior surfaces. The thorax is not completely symmetrical. However, a visual inspection of one side should offer a reasonable comparison to the other. Chest wall diameter is often increased in patients with obstructive pulmonary disease and may result in a barrel-shaped appearance of the thorax. Other chest wall deformities or asymmetry include a funnel chest (an indentation of the lower sternum above the xiphoid process known as pectus excavatum), 'pigeon' chest (a prominent sternal protrusion known as pectus carinatum), thoracic kyphosis (a posterior deviation of the spine that results in increased convexity of the chest), and scoliosis (a lateral deviation of the spine that results in an abnormal curvature) (Figure 9-15).

The paramedic should inspect the skin and nipples for cyanosis and pallor as well as look for the presence of suture lines from chest wall surgery, skin pockets enclosing implanted pacemaker devices, implanted central venous lines and dermal medication patches (e.g. nitroglycerin and contraceptives). The paramedic should note the pattern or rhythm of respirations as well as the use of accessory respiratory muscles (e.g. intercostal or supraclavicular retractions or both). Depth of breathing should be assessed as well as the rate.

Palpation

The paramedic should palpate the thorax for pulsations, tenderness, bulges, depressions, crepitus, subcutaneous emphysema, and unusual movement and position. The examination begins with the paramedic noting the position of the trachea, which should be midline and directly above the sternal notch. Starting with the patient's clavicles, the paramedic firmly palpates both sides of the patient's chest wall at the same time, front to back and right side to left side; the examination should proceed systematically and the patient should have no pain or discomfort.

To evaluate the anterior chest wall for equal expansion during inspiration, the paramedic places both thumbs along the patient's costal margin and the xiphoid process, with the palms lying flat on the chest wall. The paramedic should note equal movement as the patient inhales and exhales. The paramedic checks the posterior chest wall for

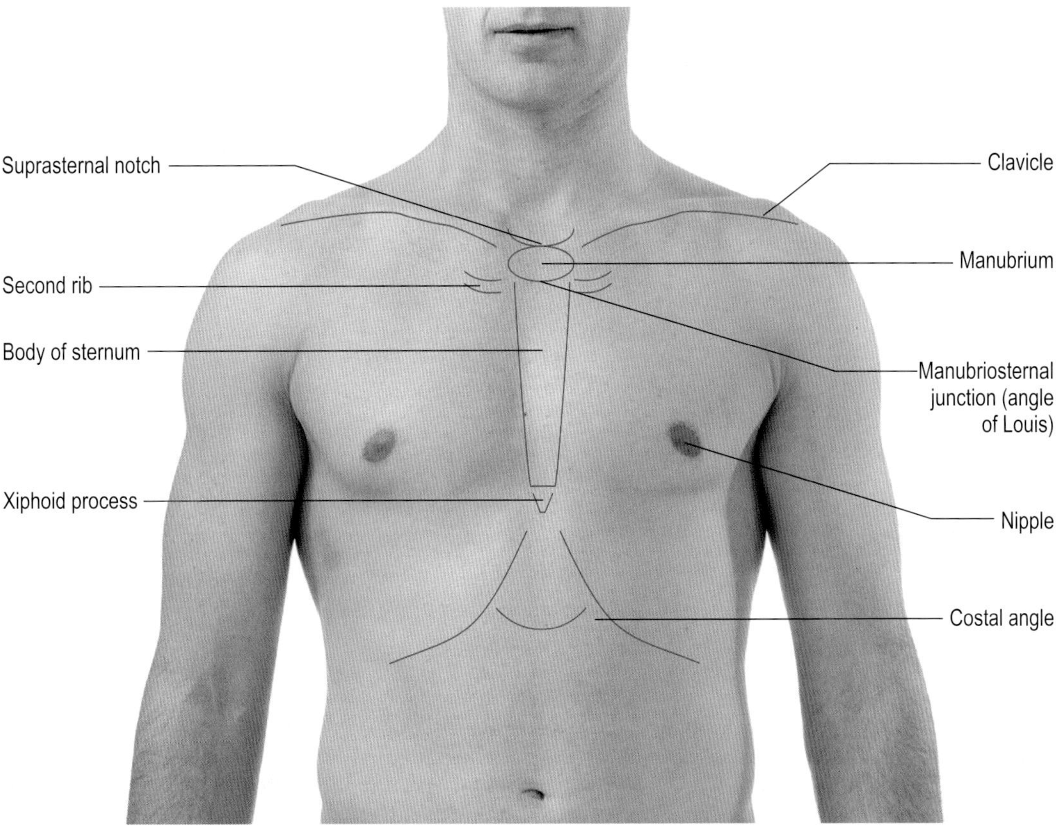

Figure 9-13 Topographical landmarks of the chest.

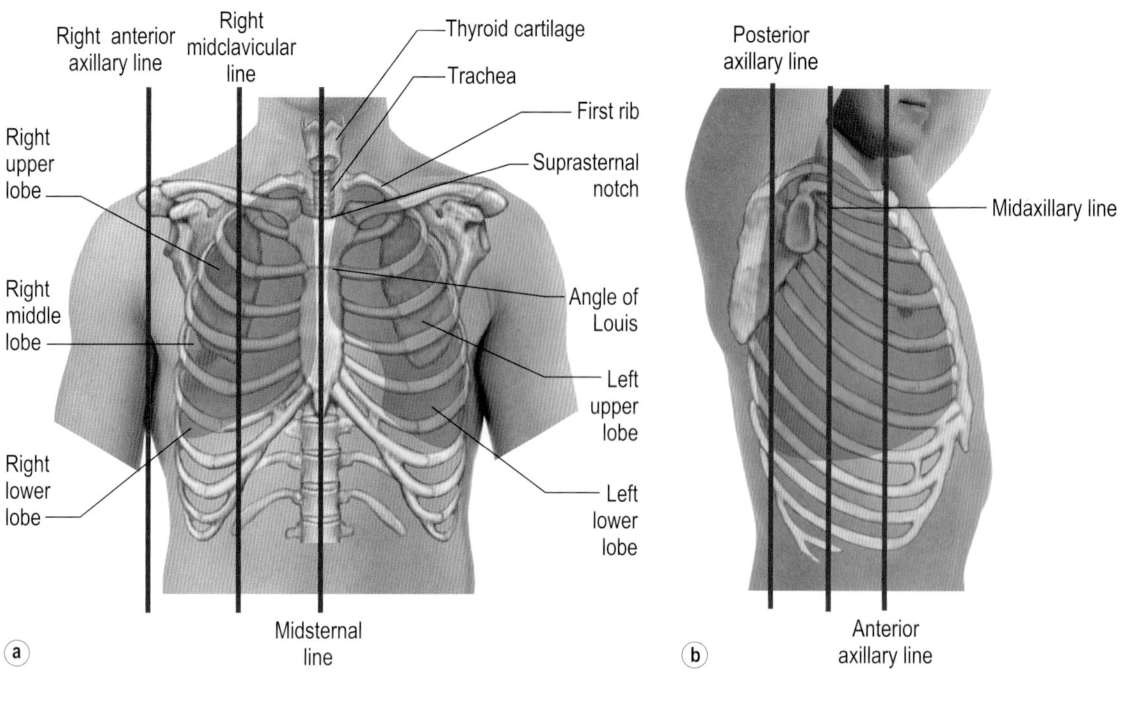

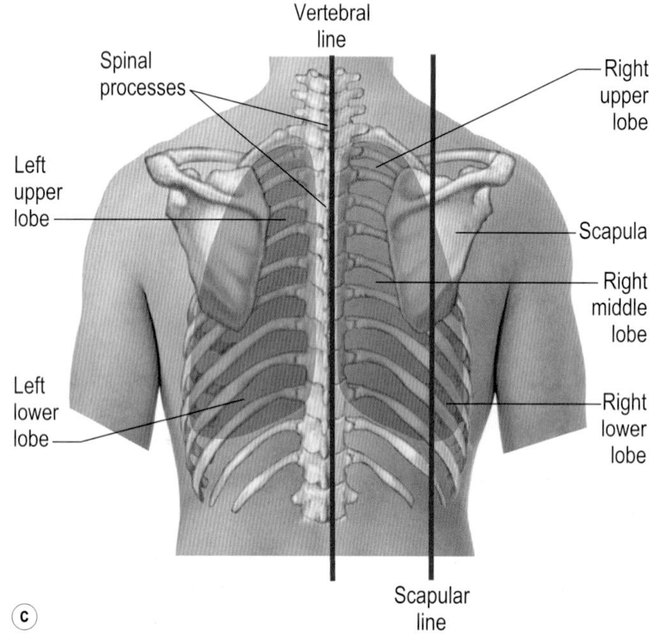

Figure 9-14 Thoracic landmarks. (a) Anterior thorax. (b) Right lateral thorax. (c) Posterior thorax.

symmetrical respiratory movement by placing the thumbs along the spinous processes at the level of the tenth rib (Figure 9-16).

Percussion

The paramedic should perform percussion in symmetrical locations from side to side to compare the percussion note (Figure 9-17a–d). Resonance usually is heard over all areas of healthy lungs. Hyperresonance is associated with over-inflation, or hyperinflation, of the lungs and may indicate pulmonary disease, pneumothorax, or asthma. Dullness or flatness suggests the presence of fluid or pulmonary congestion. The level and movement of the diaphragm during breathing (diaphragmatic excursion) may be limited by disease (such as emphysema or tumour) or pain (such as rib fracture).

Auscultation

The thorax is auscultated best with the patient sitting upright (if possible). The patient should breathe deeply and slowly through an open mouth during the examination but the paramedic should be alert to the chance of resulting hyper-ventilation and fatigue, especially in very ill and older patients.

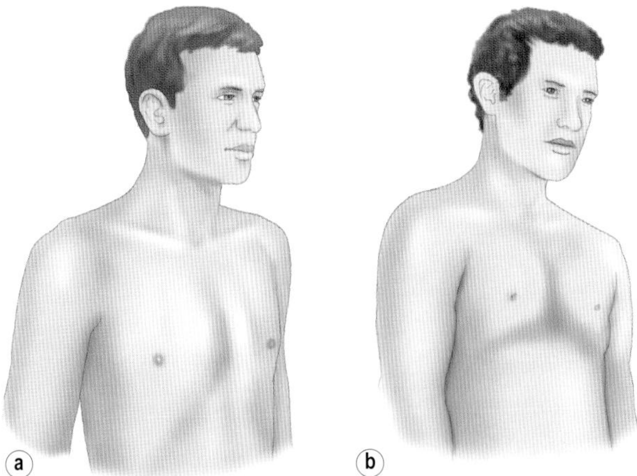

Figure 9-15 (a) Pigeon chest. (b) Funnel chest.

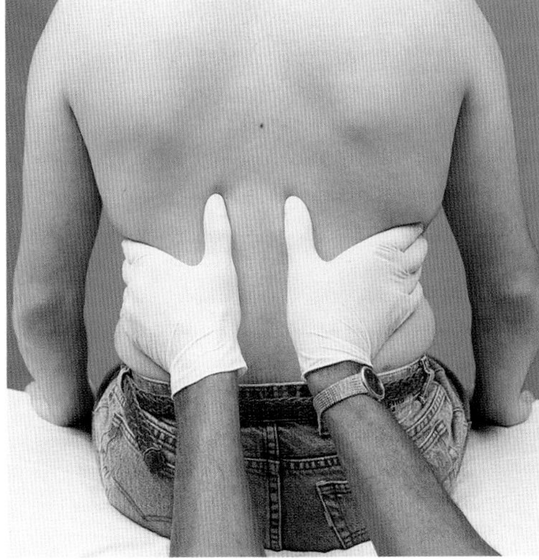
Figure 9-16 Palpating the thoracic expansion. The thumbs are at the level of the tenth ribs.

The paramedic uses the diaphragm of the stethoscope to auscultate the high-pitched sounds of the patient's lungs. The paramedic holds the stethoscope firmly on the patient's skin and should listen carefully as the patient inhales and exhales. The chest auscultation should be systematic and thorough and allow evaluation of both the anterior and the posterior lung fields.

Breath sounds

Air movement creates turbulence as it passes through the respiratory tree. Air produces breath sounds during inhalation and exhalation; during inhalation, air moves first into the trachea and major bronchi, then moves into progressively smaller airways and finally to its final destination, the alveoli. During exhalation, the air flows from small airways to larger ones; this creates less turbulence, therefore normal breath sounds are generally louder during inspiration.

Normal breath sounds

Normal breath sounds are classified as vesicular, bronchovesicular, and bronchial (Figure 9-18a, b). Vesicular breath sounds are heard over most of the lung fields and are the major normal breath sound; lungs considered 'clear' make normal vesicular breath sounds which are low pitched and soft and have a long inspiratory phase and a shorter expiratory phase.

Vesicular breath sounds are classified further as harsh or diminished. Harsh vesicular sounds may result from vigorous exercise. With vigorous exercise, ventilations are rapid and deep. These harsh sounds also occur in children, who have thin and elastic chest walls in which breath sounds are more easily audible. Vesicular breath sounds may be diminished in older persons; these persons have less ventilation volume. Vesicular breath sounds also may be diminished in obese or muscular persons, whose additional overlying tissue muffles the sound.

Bronchovesicular breath sounds are heard over the major bronchi and over the upper right posterior lung field and are louder and harsher than vesicular breath sounds. Bronchovesicular breath sounds are considered to be of medium pitch, have equal inspiration and expiration phases and are heard throughout respiration.

Bronchial breath sounds are heard only over the trachea and are the highest in pitch. They are coarse, harsh, loud sounds with a short inspiratory phase and a long expiration. A bronchial sound heard anywhere but over the trachea is considered an abnormal breath sound.

Abnormal breath sounds

Abnormal breath sounds are classified as absent, diminished, and incorrectly located bronchial sounds and as adventitious breath sounds. Absent breath sounds may indicate total cessation of the breathing process in, for example, complete airway obstruction. Breath sounds may also be absent only in a specific area. Causes of localized absent breath sounds include endotracheal tube misplacement, pneumothorax, and haemothorax. (See Chapters 13 and 27.)

Diminished breath sounds may result from any condition that lessens the airflow. Examples include endotracheal tube misplacement, pneumothorax, partial airway obstruction, and pulmonary disease. Whilst some airflow is present, diminished breath sounds usually indicate that some portion of the alveolar tissue is not being ventilated.

Bronchial breath sounds auscultated in the peripheral lung field indicate the presence of fluid or exudate in the alveoli; either of these problems may block airflow. Diseases that contribute to this condition include tumours, pneumonia and pulmonary oedema.

Adventitious breath sounds

Adventitious breath sounds are abnormal sounds. They are heard in addition to normal breath sounds and may be divided into two categories: discontinuous and continuous. Adventitious breath sounds result from obstruction of the large or small airways and are most commonly heard during inspiration. Adventitious breath sounds are classified as crackles (formerly known as rales or crepitations), wheezes and rhonchi (Figure 9-19).

Discontinuous breath sounds Crackles are the high-pitched, discontinuous sounds that usually are heard during the end of inspiration; the sound is similar to the sound of hair being rubbed between the fingers. Crackles are caused by the disruptive passage of air in the small airways or alveoli or

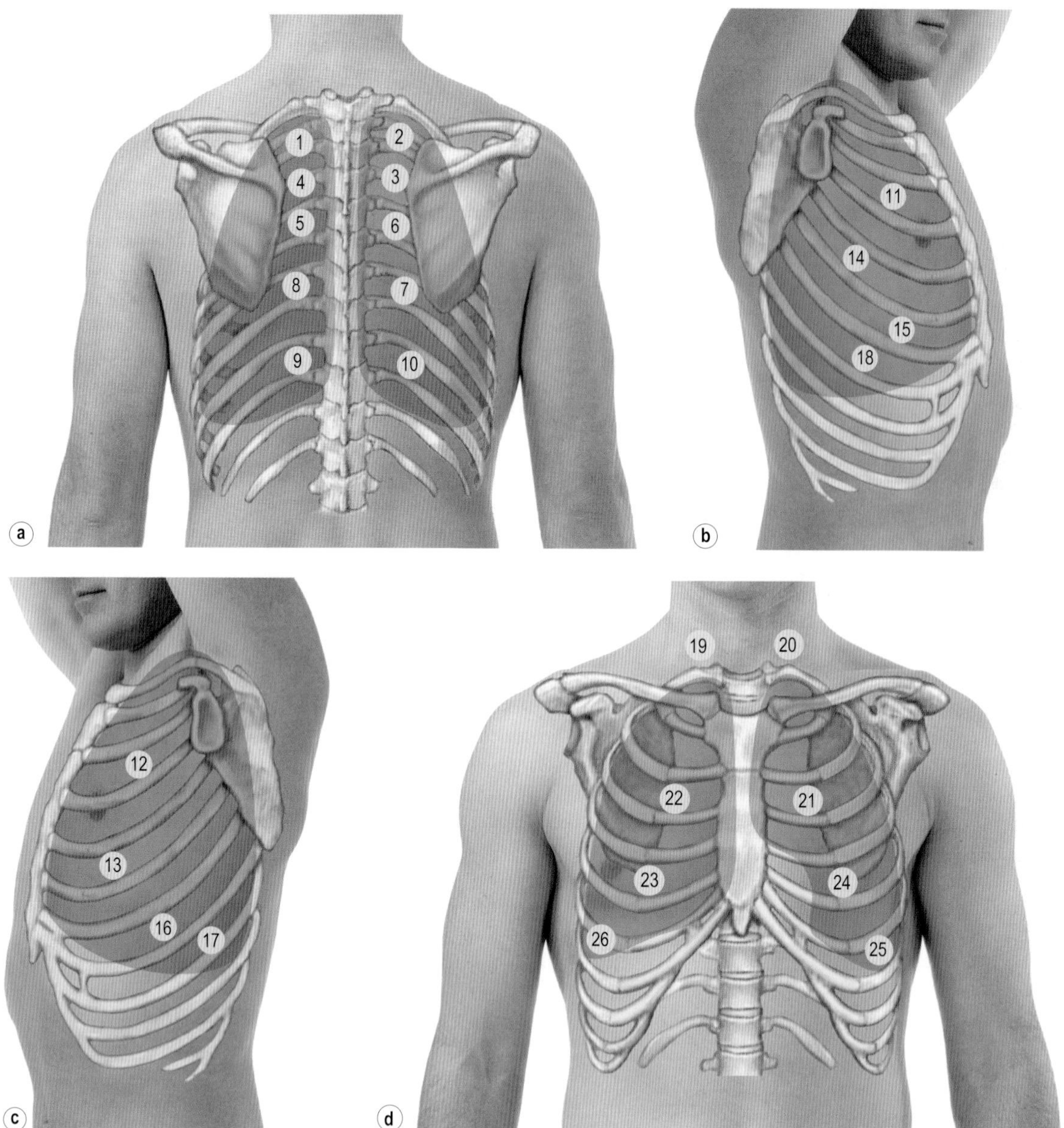

Figure 9-17 Suggested sequence for systematic percussion and auscultation of the thorax. (a) Posterior thorax. (b) Right lateral thorax. (c) Left lateral thorax. (d) Anterior thorax.

both. Crackles may be heard anywhere in the peripheral lung field.

The most typical causes of crackles are pulmonary oedema and pneumonia in its early stages. Because gravity draws fluid downward, crackles often start in the bases of the lungs. Crackles may be classified further as coarse crackles (wet, low-pitched sounds) and fine crackles (dry, high-pitched sounds). Crackles are discrete and sometimes difficult to hear and may be overridden by louder respiratory sounds. If the paramedic suspects crackles when auscultating the chest, the paramedic should ask the patient to cough; a cough may clear secretions and make crackles more audible.

Continuous breath sounds Wheezes are also known as sibilant wheezes which are high-pitched musical noises, usually louder during expiration. Wheezes are caused by high-velocity air travelling through narrowed airways and may occur because of asthma and other constrictive diseases and congestive heart failure. When wheezing occurs in a localized area, the paramedic should suspect a foreign body obstruction, tumour, or mucous plug. Wheezes are classified as mild, moderate and severe and should be described as occurring on inspiration or expiration or both.

Rhonchi are also known as sonorous wheezes. They are continuous, low-pitched, rumbling sounds, usually heard on expiration. Although rhonchi sound similar to wheezes, they do not involve the small airways. Rhonchi are less discrete than crackles and are auscultated easily. Rhonchi are caused by the passage of air through an airway obstructed by thick secretions, muscular spasm, new tissue growth, or external pressure collapsing the airway lumen. Rhonchi may result from any condition that increases secretions such as

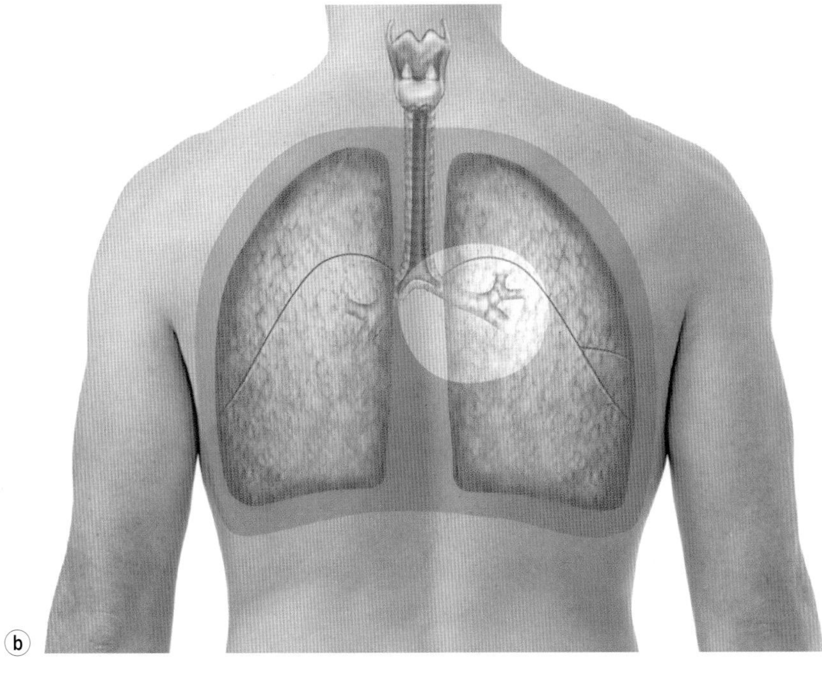

Figure 9-18 Expected auscultatory sounds. (a) Anterior view. (b) Posterior view.

pneumonia, drug overdose, and long-term postoperative recovery.

Stridor usually is an inspiratory, crowing-type sound, which can be heard without the aid of a stethoscope. Stridor indicates significant narrowing or obstruction of the larynx or trachea and may be caused by epiglottitis, viral croup, foreign body aspiration, or more than one of these factors. Stridor is heard best over the site of origin, which is usually the larynx or trachea. Stridor often points to a problem that is life threatening, especially in children; its presence calls for careful observation for ventilatory failure and hypoxia.

Pleural friction rub Although occurring outside the respiratory tree, a pleural friction rub also may be considered an adventitious breath sound. Pleural friction rub is a low-pitched, dry, rubbing or grating sound, caused by the movement of inflamed pleural surfaces as they slide on one another during breathing. The friction rub may be auscultated on inspiration and expiration. Pleural friction rub usually is loudest over the lower lateral anterior surface of the chest wall. Presence of a pleural friction rub may indicate pleurisy, viral infection, tuberculosis, or pulmonary embolism (see Chapter 14). Figure 9-20 shows a schema of breath sounds in ill and well patients.

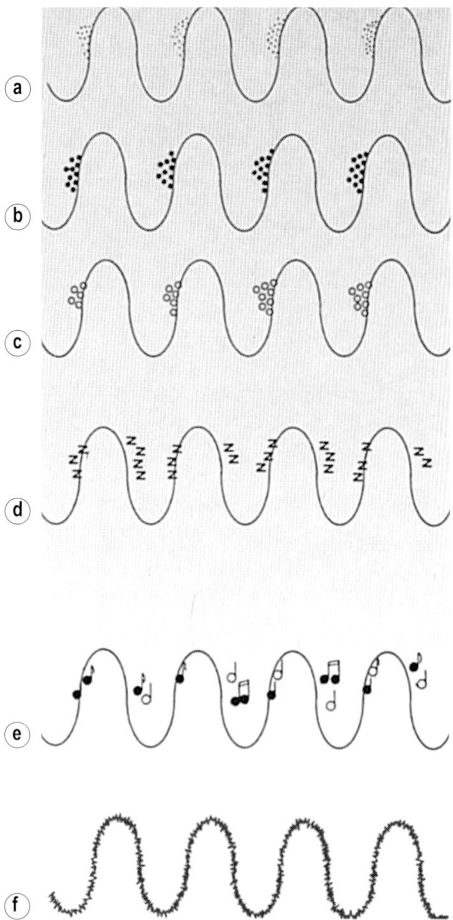

Figure 9-19 Adventitious breath sounds. (a) Fine crackles. (b) Medium crackles. (c) Coarse crackles. (d) Rhonchi. (e) Wheeze. (f) Pleural friction rub.

Cardiovascular (and circulatory) system

In the prehospital setting one must examine the heart indirectly. In spite of this, certain information can be obtained; details about the size and effectiveness of pumping action are obtained through a skilled assessment which includes inspection, palpation and auscultation.

Inspection

Again, as in the assessment of the respiratory system, the paramedic should inspect the chest wall for symmetry on the anterior and posterior surfaces and should look for chest wall deformities again.

The paramedic should inspect the skin and nipples for cyanosis and pallor, being alert to the presence of suture lines from chest wall surgery, skin pockets enclosing implanted pacemaker devices, implanted central venous lines and dermal medication patches (e.g. nitroglycerin and contraceptives).

Palpation

The apical impulse is a potentially visible and palpable force, produced by the contraction of the left ventricle. Palpation of this impulse may be useful to compare the relationship of peripheral pulses with the pulse produced by ventricular contraction. The hearts of some patients with cardiac irregularities, for example, do not always produce a peripheral pulse with every ventricular contraction. By palpating or auscultating the apical impulse and the carotid pulse at the same time, the paramedic can note these pulse deficits (Figure 9-21); however, obesity, large breasts, and muscularity may make this landmark hard to see or palpate.

Auscultation

Heart sounds may be auscultated for frequency (pitch), intensity (loudness), duration and timing in the cardiac cycle (Figure 9-22). A full evaluation of heart sounds calls for a high level of skill and experience, a quiet environment, and ample time to listen closely; however, the paramedic may assess two basic heart sounds quickly that may help to improve understanding of the patient's condition. The basic heart sounds S_1 and S_2 are normal sounds that occur when the myocardium contracts. They are best heard toward the apex of the heart at the fifth intercostal space over the bicuspid valve. For evaluation of heart sounds, the patient should be sitting up and leaning slightly forward (Figure 9-23a), supine (Figure 9-23b), or in a left lateral recumbent position (Figure 9-23c). These positions bring the heart closer to the left anterior chest wall. To listen for S_1, the paramedic should ask the patient to breathe normally and hold the breath in expiration. To listen for S_2, the paramedic should ask the patient to breathe normally again and hold the breath in inspiration.

Heart sounds may be muffled or diminished by obesity or obstructive lung disease. Muffling also may occur as a result of the presence of fluid in the pericardial sac surrounding the heart muscle due to penetrating or severe blunt chest trauma, cardiac tamponade, or cardiac rupture, and is considered a true emergency. Other causes of muffled or diminished heart sounds include infectious uraemic pericarditis and malignancy. (See Chapters 15 and 27 for further discussion of abnormal heart sounds.)

Inflammation of the pericardial sac may cause a rubbing sound that is audible with a stethoscope, known as a pericardial friction rub, resulting from infectious pericarditis, myocardial infarction, uraemia, trauma and autoimmune pericarditis. These rubs have a scratching, grating, or squeaking quality, tend to be louder on inspiration, and can be differentiated from pleural friction rubs by their continued presence when the patient holds the breath.

Extra sounds

Extra sounds that sometimes can be heard during auscultation or can be felt by palpation include heart murmurs, bruits, and thrills. Heart murmurs are prolonged sounds caused by a disruption in the flow of blood into, through, or out of the heart. Most murmurs are caused by valvular defects; some heart murmurs are serious, but others (e.g. some that occur in children and adolescents) are benign and have no apparent cause. Heart murmurs can be detected during auscultation of the heart.

A bruit is an abnormal sound or murmur that may be heard during auscultation of the carotid artery or another organ or gland and may indicate local obstruction. Bruits usually are low pitched and hard to hear. To assess blood flow in the carotid artery, the paramedic should place the

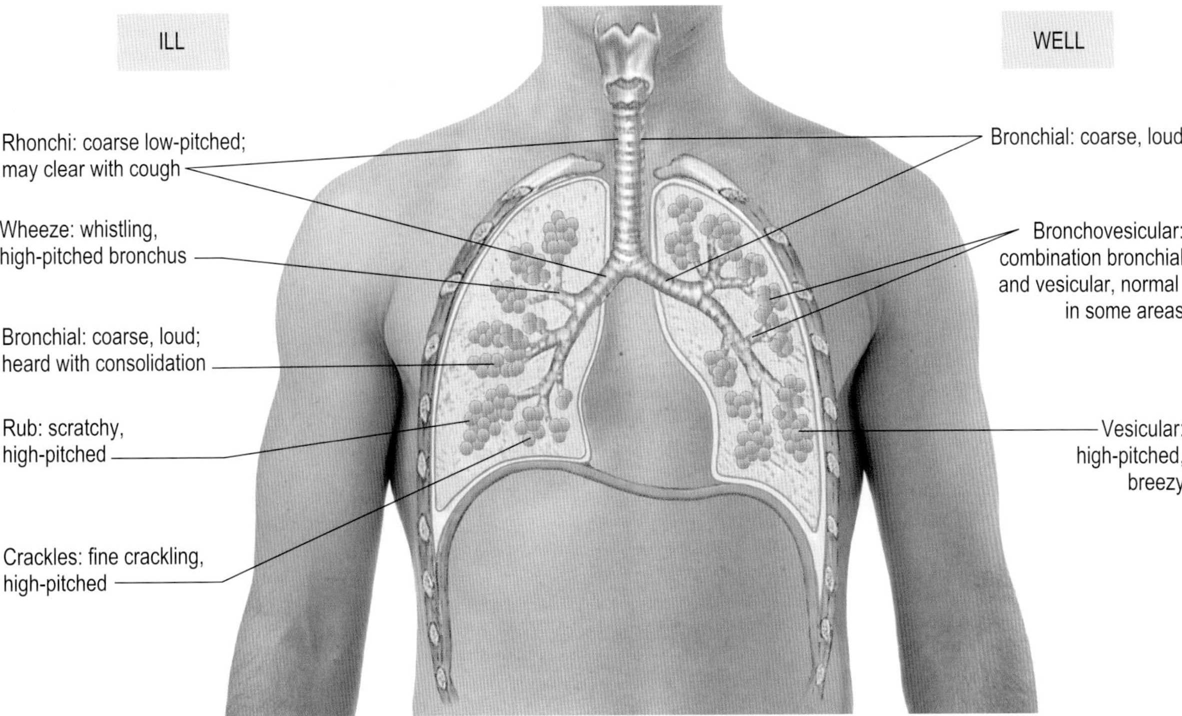

Figure 9-20 Schema of breath sounds in ill and well patients.

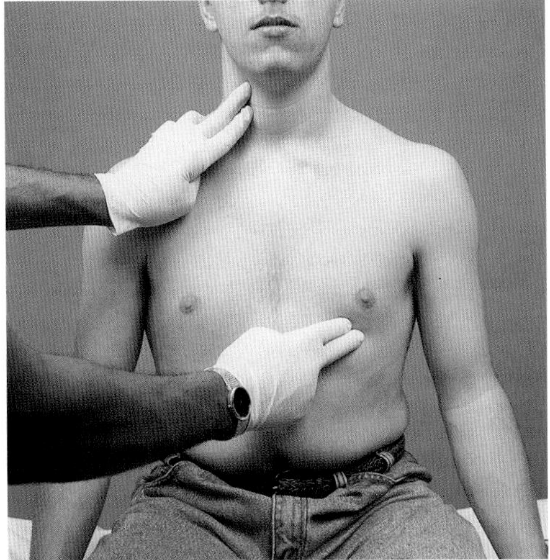

Figure 9-21 Simultaneous palpation of the carotid artery and apical impulse.

bell of the stethoscope over the carotid artery at the medial end of the clavicle. Then the paramedic should ask the patient to hold his or her breath (Figure 9-24).

Thrills are similar to bruits but are described as fine vibrations or tremors that may indicate blood flow obstruction. Thrills may be palpable over the site of an aneurysm or on the precordium (the area of the chest wall that overlays the heart and epigastrium). Like murmurs and bruits, thrills may be serious or benign.

Peripheral vascular system

The peripheral vascular system includes arteries, veins, the lymphatic system and lymph nodes, and the fluids exchanged in the capillary bed, which can be evaluated during the physical examination of the upper and lower extremities.

Arms

When evaluating the arms, the paramedic should inspect from fingertips to shoulders. The paramedic should note size and symmetry as well as swelling, venous pattern, colour of the skin and nail beds, and texture of the skin. If the paramedic notes arterial insufficiency because of a weak radial pulse, the paramedic should palpate the brachial pulse. Epitrochlear nodes and brachial nodes should be non-swollen and non-tender (Figure 9-25). A fine venous network on upper and lower extremities often is visible. The paramedic should be alert for enlargement of superficial veins during the examination.

Legs

During examination of the lower extremities, the patient should be supine and covered properly but shoes, socks, and hosiery should be removed for a full examination. The paramedic should inspect visually from the groin and buttocks to the feet, noting the following:

- size and symmetry
- swelling
- venous pattern and venous enlargement
- pigmentation
- rashes, scars or ulcers
- colour and texture of the skin

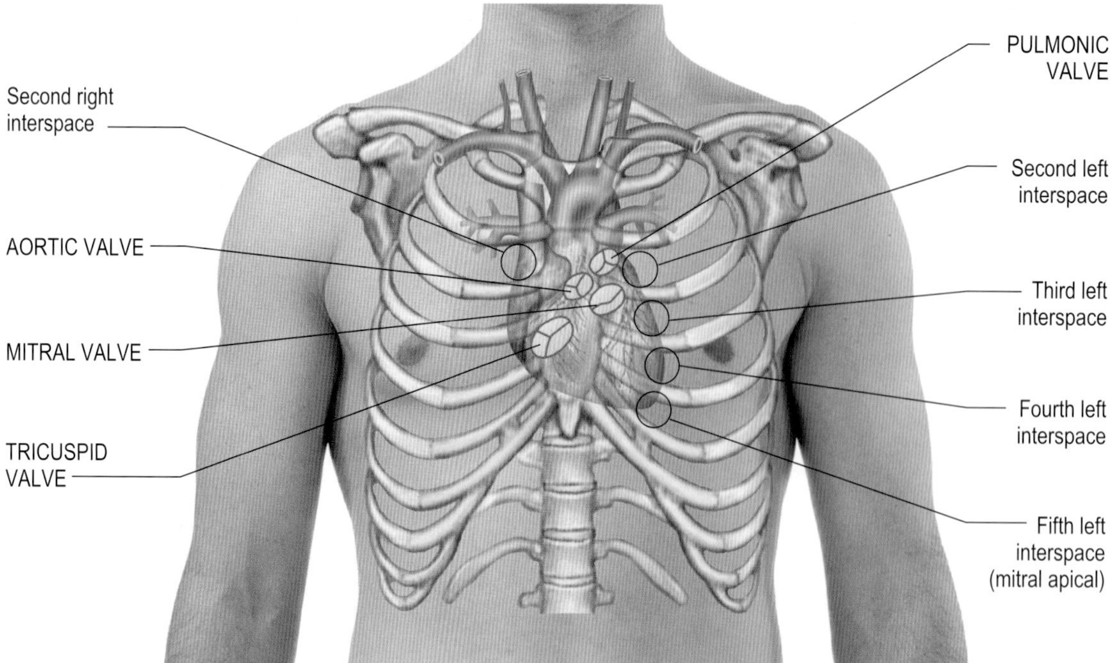

Figure 9-22 Areas for auscultation of the heart.

- presence or absence of hair growth (indicating compromised arterial circulation).

The paramedic should palpate the superficial inguinal nodes in the groin to assess for swelling and tenderness, and assess all lower extremity pulse sites for circulation, strength, and regularity; these sites include the femoral pulse, the popliteal pulse, the dorsalis pedis pulse, and the posterior tibial pulse. The temperature of the feet and legs should be warm, which indicates adequate circulation. The paramedic can evaluate for pitting oedema over the dorsum of each foot, behind each medial malleolus, and over the shins by pressing firmly on the skin with the thumb for at least 5 s; oedema is said to be pitting when depression of the tissue remains after removal of pressure.

Abnormal findings

Findings that are considered abnormal during a peripheral vascular assessment include the following:

- swollen or asymmetrical extremities
- pale or cyanotic skin
- weak or diminished pulses
- skin that is cold to the touch
- absence of hair growth
- pitting oedema.

Gastrointestinal system

The abdomen is divided by two imaginary lines that separate the abdominal region into four quadrants. The quadrants are the upper right, lower right, upper left and lower left (Figure 9-26). These quadrants and their contents provide the basis for inspection, auscultation, percussion and palpation (Box 9-5). Whilst this more simplified version is used, a more detailed nine-regions format is also considered in some circumstances.

When examining a patient's abdomen, the paramedic should make sure that the patient is comfortable (with an empty bladder, if possible) and also make sure the patient is in a supine position. The paramedic's hands and stethoscope should be warm and the paramedic should approach the patient slowly and respectfully. Any painful area should be examined last.

Inspection

The paramedic should inspect the abdomen visually for signs of cyanosis, pallor, jaundice, bruising, discoloration, swelling (ascites), masses and aortic pulsations, as well as to look for surgical scars and implanted devices such as automatic implanted cardioverter defibrillators. The abdomen should be evenly round and symmetrical (Figure 9-27). Symmetrical distension of the abdomen may result from obesity, enlarged organs, fluid or gas, and asymmetrical distension may result from hernias, tumour, bowel obstruction or enlarged abdominal organs. A flat abdomen is common in adults who are athletic, whereas convex abdomens are common in children and in adults who have poor exercise habits. The umbilicus should be free of swelling, bulges and signs of inflammation. The normal umbilicus is usually inverted, or it may protrude slightly. Discoloration around the umbilicus is called Cullen's sign, which may indicate peritoneal bleeding, whilst discoloration found in the flank, called Grey Turner's sign, may indicate possible kidney injury.

Abdominal movement during respiration should be smooth and even. As a rule, males have more abdominal involvement than females during respiration, so limited abdominal movement in the male patients with symptoms may indicate a pathological abdominal condition. Visible pulsations produced by blood flow through the aorta in the upper abdomen may be normal in thin adults; however, marked pulsations may indicate an abdominal aortic aneurysm.

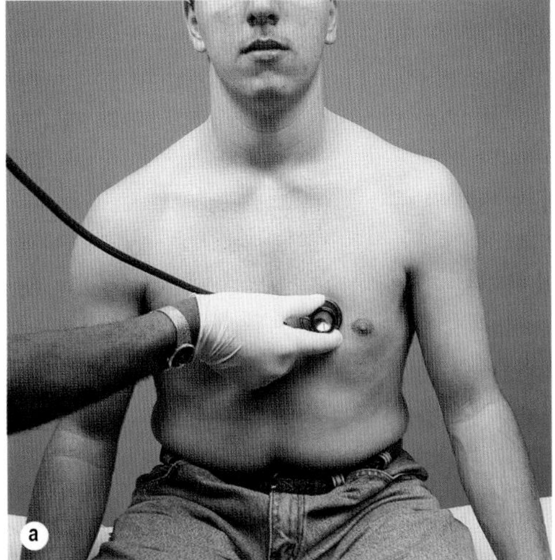

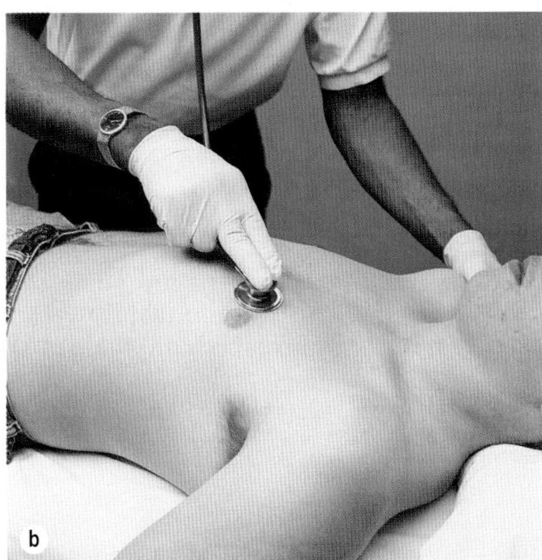

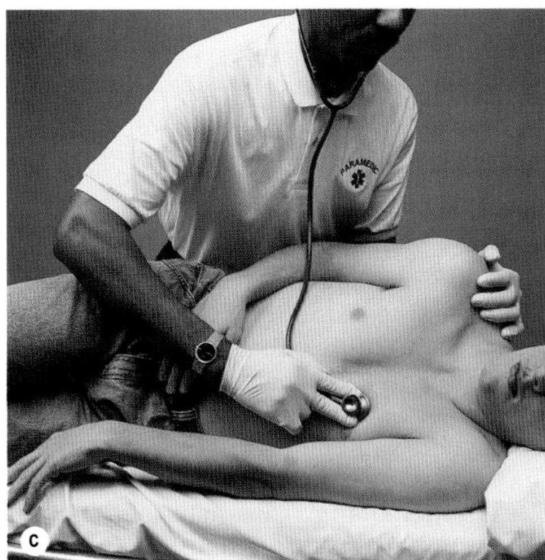

Figure 9-23 Patient positions for auscultation. (a) Sitting up, leaning slightly forward. (b) Supine. (c) Left lateral recumbent.

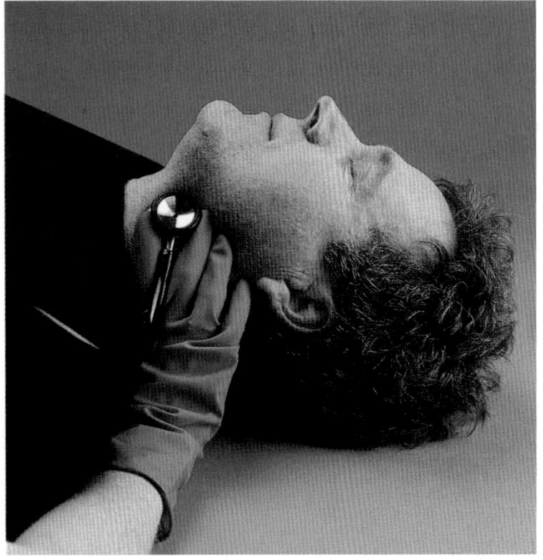

Figure 9-24 Evaluation of carotid bruit.

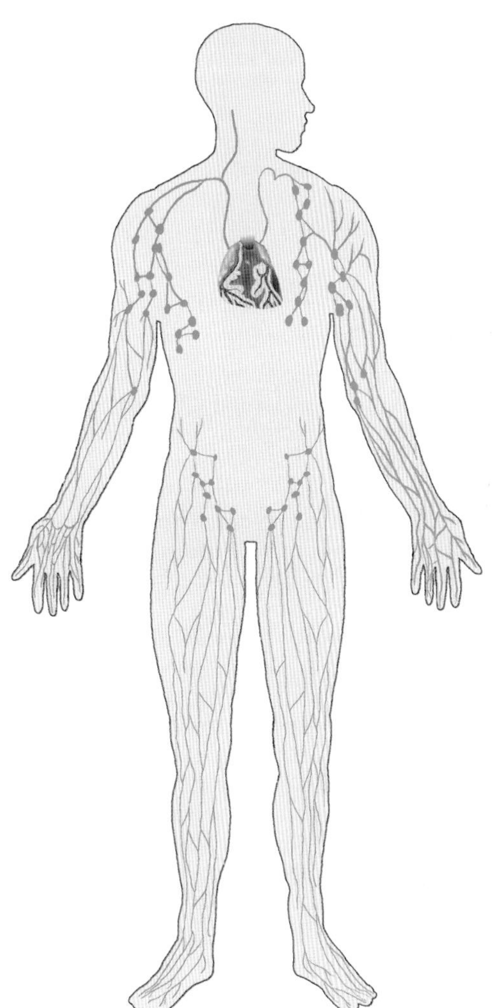

Figure 9-25 Nodes of upper and lower extremities.

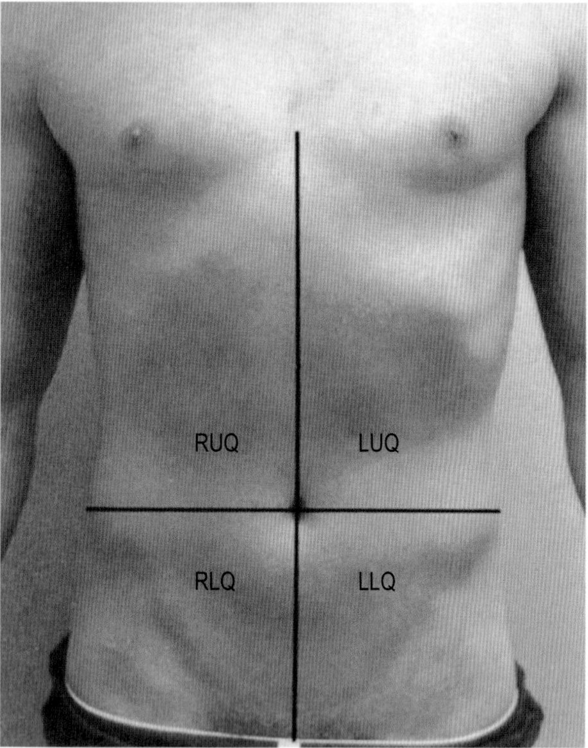

Figure 9-26 Four quadrants of the abdomen. RUQ, right upper quadrant; LUQ, left upper quadrant; RLQ, right lower quadrant; LLQ, left lower quadrant.

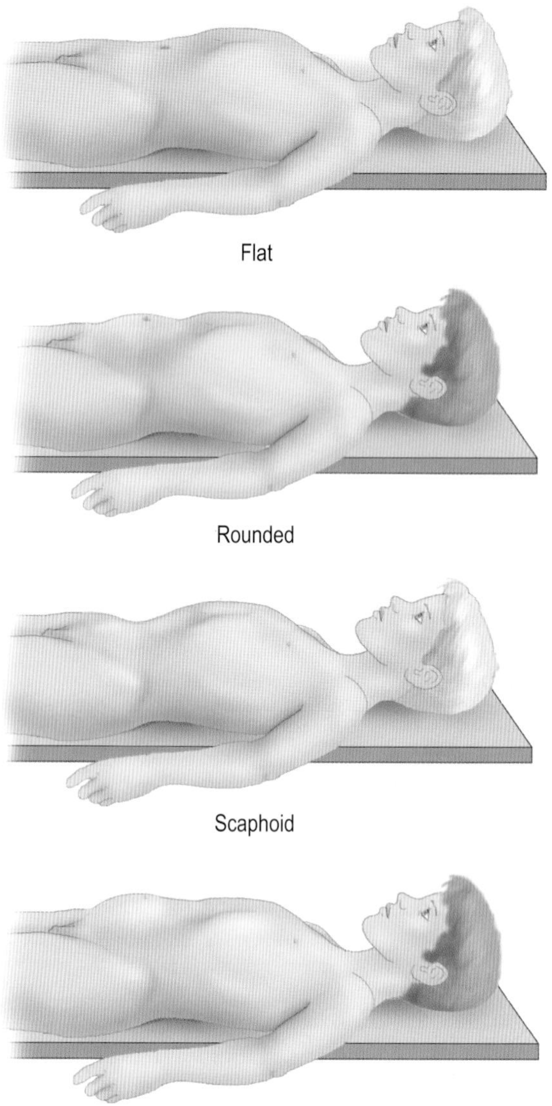

Figure 9-27 Shape of the abdomen.

Auscultation

In general, noting the presence or absence of bowel sounds to assess motility and to discover vascular sounds has limited value in the prehospital setting and to some extent such findings do not affect or determine the approach to patient care. The time needed for complete bowel sound assessment (2 min per quadrant) extends the on-scene time and may be inappropriate. If auscultation is to be performed, though, it should always come before palpation, because palpation may alter the intensity of bowel sounds.

To auscultate bowel sounds, the paramedic holds the diaphragm of the stethoscope on the abdomen with light pressure. If bowel sounds are present, they usually are heard as rumblings or gurgles and should occur irregularly. They may range in frequency from 5 to 35 per minute; auscultation should be performed in all four quadrants. A minimum of 2 min per quadrant is needed to determine that normal bowel sounds are absent. Increased bowel sounds may indicate gastroenteritis or intestinal obstruction, whilst decreased or absent bowel sounds may indicate peritonitis (inflammation of the lining of the abdominal cavity) or ileus (inactive peristaltic activity resulting from one of several causes).

Percussion and palpation

Percussion and palpation of the abdomen may help to detect the presence of fluid, air, and solid masses. The paramedic should use a systematic approach, moving from side to side or clockwise, noting any rigidity, tenderness or abnormal skin temperature or colour. The paramedic should observe the patient's face for signs of pain or discomfort. If the patient is complaining of abdominal pain, the paramedic should examine the painful quadrant last so that the patient will not unnecessarily tighten or 'guard' the abdominal area. The abdominal assessment should begin with a light palpation, using an even pressing motion. As stated before, the paramedic's hands should be warm, and the paramedic should avoid sharp and quick jabs, moving smoothly and carefully; palpation may be done at the same time as percussion. Guarding is the tensing of abdominal muscles by the patient on examination and can indicate inflammation; abdominal rigidity is noticeable and consistent guarding and can be a sign of serious pathology; rebound tenderness, which is pain when pressure is released on the abdomen, can be an indicator of peritonitis.

The paramedic begins percussion by evaluating all four quadrants of the abdomen in turn for tympany and dullness. Tympany is the major sound that should be noted during percussion because of the normal presence of air in the stomach and intestines. Dullness should be heard over organs and solid masses. When percussing the abdomen, proceeding from an area of tympany to an area of dullness

Box 9-5

Abdominal quadrants

Right upper quadrant

- Liver and gallbladder
- Pylorus
- Duodenum
- Head of pancreas
- Right adrenal gland
- Portion of right kidney
- Hepatic flexure of colon
- Portions of ascending and transverse colon

Left upper quadrant

- Left lobe of liver
- Spleen
- Stomach
- Body of pancreas
- Left adrenal gland
- Portion of left kidney
- Splenic flexure of colon
- Portions of transverse and descending colon

Right lower quadrant

- Lower pole of right kidney
- Caecum and appendix
- Portion of ascending colon
- Appendix
- Bladder (if distended)
- Ovary and salpinx
- Uterus (if enlarged)
- Right ureter

Left lower quadrant

- Lower pole of left kidney
- Sigmoid colon
- Portion of descending colon
- Bladder (if distended)
- Ovary and salpinx
- Uterus (if enlarged)
- Left ureter

is best. That way, the change in sound is easier to detect. Individual assessments of the liver and spleen (described in the following paragraphs) may be done if indicated by patient complaint or mechanism of injury. Patients who may require surgery for abdominal illness or injury are best served by assessment that is prompt but detailed enough, stabilization, and transport to an appropriate medical facility.

Percussion and palpation of the liver

The paramedic percusses the liver by starting just above the umbilicus in the right midclavicular line in an area of tympany. Percussion should continue in an upward direction until the change from tympany to dullness occurs; this change usually occurs slightly below the costal margin and indicates the lower border of the liver. To determine the upper border of the liver, the percussion should begin in the same midclavicular line at the midsternal level, proceeding downward until the tympany from the lung area changes to dullness (usually between the fifth and seventh intercostal spaces). Liver size is related to age and sex; the liver usually is proportionately larger in adults than in children and is larger in males than in females.

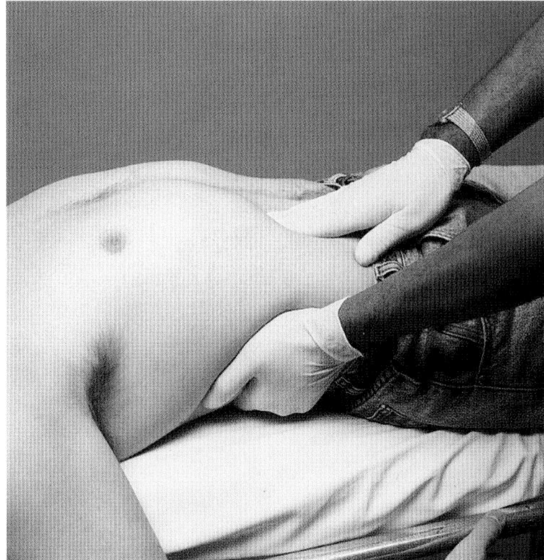

Figure 9-28 Palpation of the liver.

For palpation of the liver, the patient should be supine and comfortable and should have a relaxed abdomen. The paramedic should perform the examination from the patient's right side and should begin by placing the left hand under the patient in the area of the eleventh and twelfth ribs (Figure 9-28). The right hand should be placed on the abdomen, with the fingers pointing toward the patient's head and extended, resting just below the edge of the costal margin. The conscious patient should be instructed to breathe deeply through the mouth. During exhalation, the paramedic presses upward with the hand under the patient and gently pushes in and up with the right hand. If the paramedic feels the liver, it should be firm and non-tender; a healthy liver usually cannot be palpated unless the patient is thin.

Percussion and palpation of the spleen

For percussion of the spleen, the patient must be lying supine or in a right lateral recumbent position. Percussion should begin at the area of lung tympany, just posterior to the midaxillary line on the left side. When percussing downward, a change from tympany to dullness should be audible between the sixth and tenth ribs; large areas of dullness suggest an enlarged spleen. Stomach contents and air-filled or faeces-filled intestines make splenic assessment by percussion difficult. These and other factors may affect percussion tones of dullness and tympany.

Palpation is a more useful assessment technique for evaluating the spleen; the patient should be lying supine with the paramedic positioned at the patient's left side. The paramedic places the left hand under the patient, supporting the lower left rib cage, and places the right hand just below the patient's lower left costal margin (Figure 9-29). The paramedic should palpate the area gently by lifting up the left hand and pressing down with the right hand. A normal spleen usually cannot be palpated in an adult. A palpable spleen is probably enlarged three times its normal size.

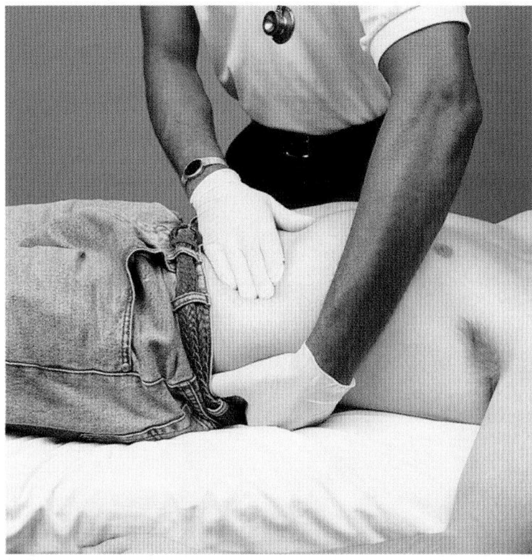

Figure 9-29 Palpation of the spleen.

Careless palpation of the spleen may risk rupture of the organ, thus palpation must be performed with caution.

Genitourinary system

Examination of the genitalia of either sex of patient can be awkward; the patient and the paramedic may feel uncomfortable. When possible, paramedics of the same sex as the patient should perform these assessments; if that is not possible, a second person should act as a chaperone and be present during the examination.

The external genitalia should be inspected visually to note any swelling, redness, discharge, bleeding, or evidence of trauma. Discoloration or tenderness of the genital tissue may be the result of traumatic bruising. Ulcers, vesicles and discharges (with or without pain) indicate sexually transmitted disease. If touching the anal area is necessary, the paramedic should change the gloves afterward; changing gloves helps to prevent bacteria from being introduced into the vaginal area.

> **Critical Thinking**
>
> Examination of a patient's genitalia in the presence of another care provider is advisable. Why might this be important?

Male genitalia

When examining the male genitalia, the paramedic should inspect the area visually; the paramedic should look for bleeding and signs of trauma. The shaft of the penis should be non-tender and flaccid. Rarely, patients with leukaemia, sickle cell disease or spinal injury may have a persistent painful erection (priapism). The urethral opening should be free of blood (a possible result of pelvic trauma) and should also be free of discharge (a sign of sexually transmitted disease). The scrotum should be non-tender and slightly asymmetrical. A swollen or painful scrotum may result from infection, herniation, testicular torsion or trauma; discoloration of the genitals is called Coopernail's sign and may indicate peritoneal bleeding.

Anus

Examination of the anus is indicated in the presence of rectal bleeding or trauma to the area. Examination can be done with the patient in one of several positions but most patients will find the side-lying position to be most comfortable. The paramedic should protect the patient's privacy and use proper drapes. Inspection of the sacrococcygeal and perineal areas may reveal abnormal findings such as lumps, ulcers, inflammation, rashes and excoriations. Excoriations are surface injuries caused by scratching or abrasions. Inflamed external haemorrhoids are common in adults and pregnant women.

Musculoskeletal system

When examining the upper and lower extremities, a paramedic should pay attention to function and structure. The patient's general appearance, body proportions, and ease of movement are important factors; in particular, the paramedic should note any limitation in the range of motion or any unusual increase in the mobility of a joint. Abnormal findings include the following:

- signs of inflammation
  - swelling
  - tenderness
  - increased heat
  - redness
- decreased function
- asymmetry
- crepitus
- deformities
- decreased muscular strength
- atrophy.

Examining upper and lower extremities

A full assessment of the upper and lower extremities includes an evaluation of the skin and tissue overlying the muscles, cartilage, and bones, and of the joints for soft tissue injury, discoloration, swelling and masses. The upper and lower extremities should be symmetrical in structure and muscularity. The paramedic should assess the circulatory status of each extremity by determining skin colour, temperature, sensation and the presence of distal pulses. The paramedic should assess bones, joints and surrounding tissues of the extremities for structural integrity and continuity; muscle tone should be firm and non-tender. The paramedic assesses joints for function by moving each joint through its full range of motion; a normal range of motion occurs without pain, deformity, limitation or instability.

Hands and wrists

The paramedic should inspect both hands and wrists for contour and positional alignment (Figure 9-30) and should palpate the wrists, hands, and joints of each finger for tenderness, swelling, or deformity. To determine range of motion, ask the patient to flex and extend the wrists, make a fist, and touch the thumb to each fingertip; all movements should be performed without pain or discomfort.

Elbows

The paramedic should inspect and palpate the elbows in the flexed and extended positions (Figure 9-31a, b). To determine the range of motion of the elbow, the paramedic should ask the patient to rotate the hands from palm up to palm down. The paramedic should inspect the grooves between the epicondyle and olecranon by palpation; pain and tenderness should not be present when pressing on the lateral and medial epicondyle.

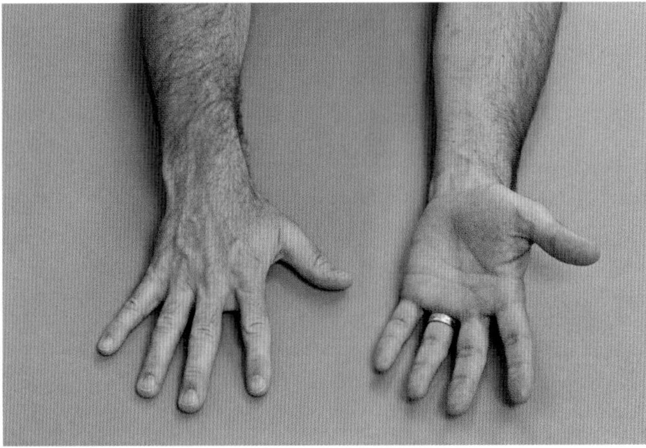

Figure 9-30 Hands and wrists.

Shoulders and related structures

The paramedic should inspect and palpate the shoulders for symmetry and integrity of the clavicles, scapulae, and humeri; pain, tenderness, or asymmetrical contour may indicate a fracture or dislocation. The patient should be able to shrug the shoulders and also be able to raise and extend both arms without pain or discomfort. The paramedic should palpate the following regions, noting any tenderness or swelling (Figure 9-32):

- sternoclavicular joint
- acromioclavicular joint
- subacromial area
- bicipital groove.

Ankles and feet

The paramedic should inspect the patient's feet and ankles for contour, position, and size; tenderness, swelling, and deformity are abnormal findings on palpation and the toes should be straight and aligned with each other. The paramedic can determine range of motion by requesting the patient to bend the toes, point the toes, and rotate the feet inward and outward from the ankle (Figure 9-33a–c). These movements should be possible without pain or discomfort. The paramedic should inspect all surfaces of the ankles

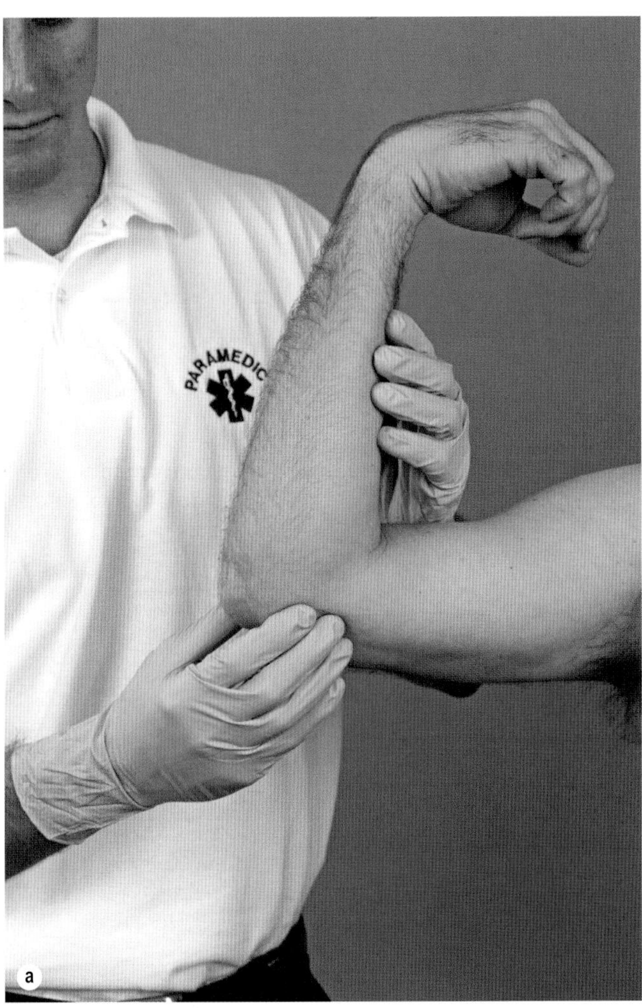

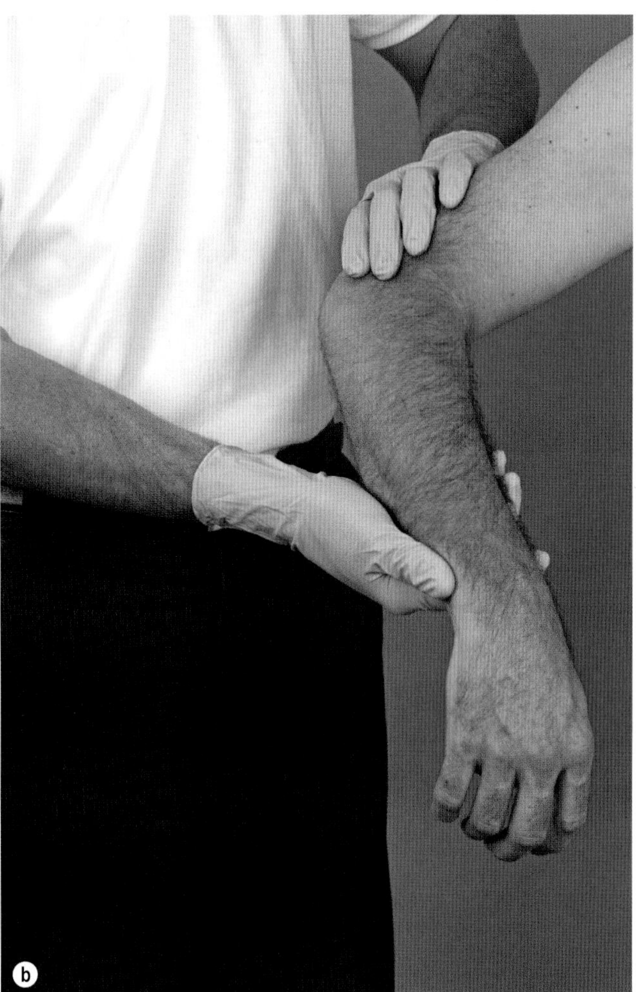

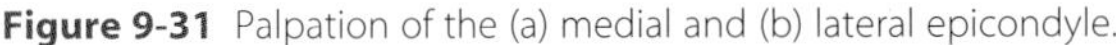

Figure 9-31 Palpation of the (a) medial and (b) lateral epicondyle.

and feet for deformities, nodules, swelling, calluses, corns and skin integrity.

Pelvis, hips and knees

The paramedic may check the structural integrity of the pelvis, although caution must be exercised to avoid worsening injury in situations where pelvic injury is obvious (for example by visualization); there is a risk of increasing instability in any pelvic fracture and worsening any internal haemorrhage, and palpation may not provide any further useful information (Figure 9-34). Deformity and point tenderness of the pelvis may be signs of fracture and these signs may mask major structural and vascular injury.

The paramedic should inspect and palpate the hips for instability, tenderness, and crepitus. A mobile patient should be able to walk without discomfort; a supine patient should be able to raise the legs and knees and rotate the legs inward and outward.

The paramedic should inspect and palpate the knees for swelling and tenderness. The patella should be smooth, firm, non-tender, and midline in position; the patient should be able to bend and straighten each knee without pain.

Spine

A full physical examination includes an assessment of the spine. This begins with a visual assessment of the cervical, thoracic, and lumbar curves; from the patient's side, the paramedic should note any curvature of the spine, including curvature associated with abnormal lordosis, kyphosis, and scoliosis (Figure 9-35). In addition, the paramedic should look for any differences in the height of the shoulders or iliac crests (hips) that may result from abnormal spinal curvature.

Critical Thinking

Consider a case in which no deformity of the spine is found during an examination. Can spine fracture or dislocation be ruled out?

Cervical spine

The patient's neck should be in a midline position. If the patient is alert and denies neck pain, the paramedic should palpate the posterior aspect for point tenderness and swelling; the only palpable landmark should be the spinous process of the seventh cervical vertebra at the base of the neck (Figure 9-36). In the absence of suspected injury, the paramedic tests range of motion by directing the patient to bend the head forward, backward, and from side to side. These movements should not cause pain or discomfort. Use of an appropriate C-spine immobilization algorithm (such as JRCALC clinical practice guidelines) should be considered; for immobilization need to be excluded, the patient should be a fully alert and cooperative adult, who is not under drug or alcohol influences, is free of distracting inju-

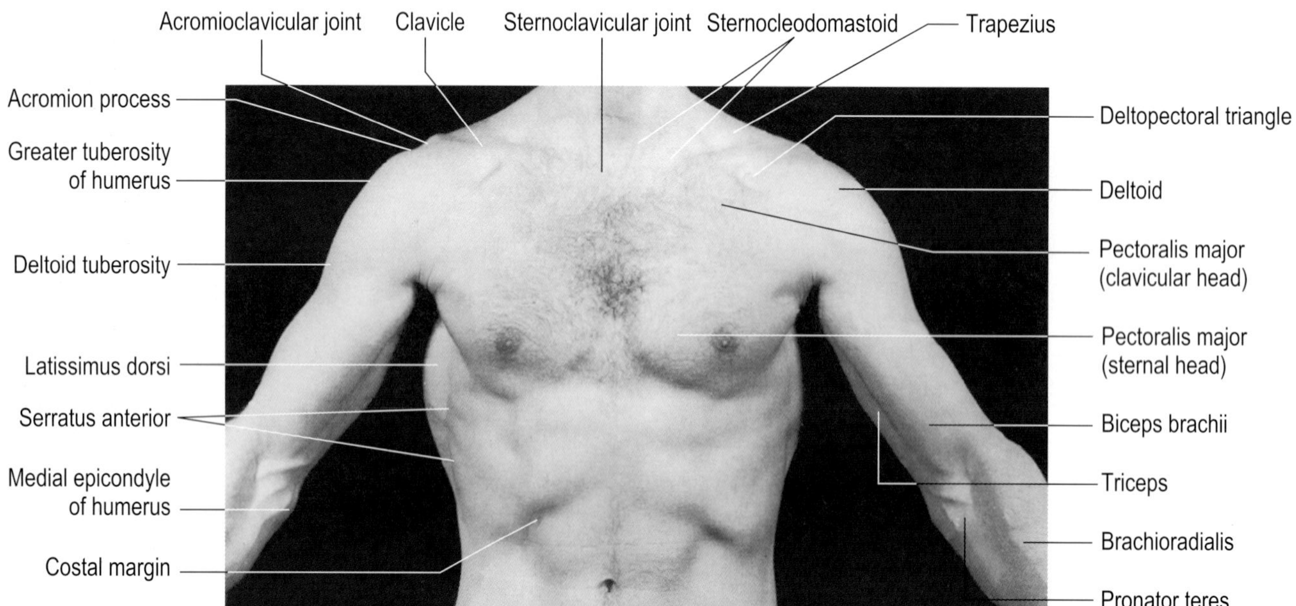

Figure 9-32 Evaluation of shoulder and related structures.

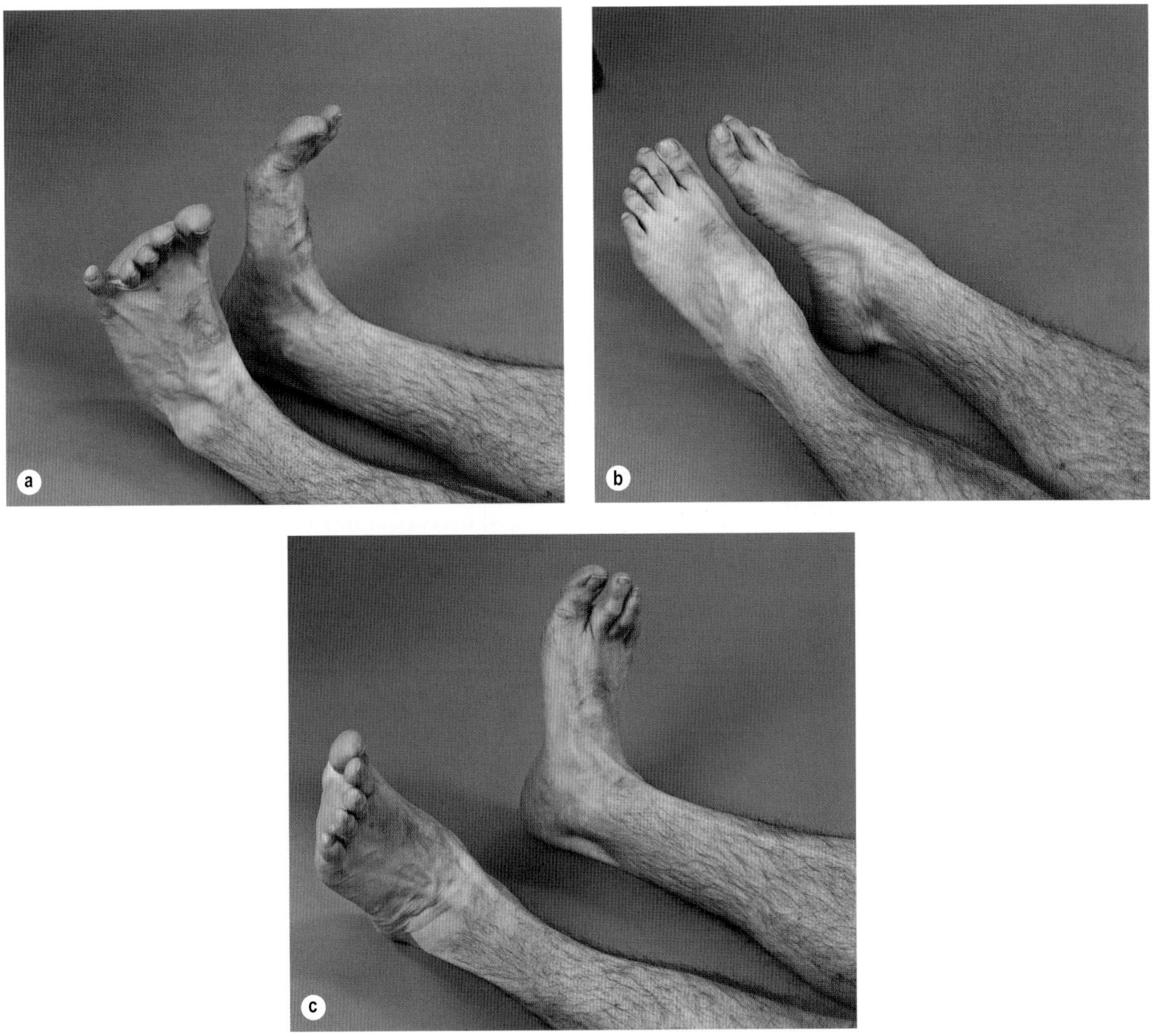

Figure 9-33 Motor function of the foot and ankle. (a) Bend toes. (b) Point toes. (c) Rotate feet in and out.

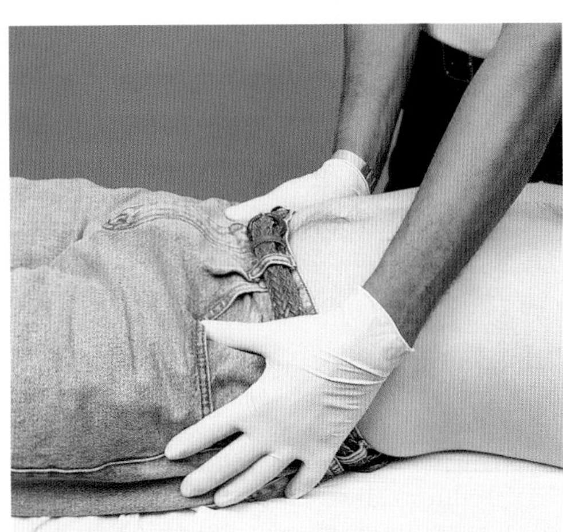

Figure 9-34 Palpating the pelvis.

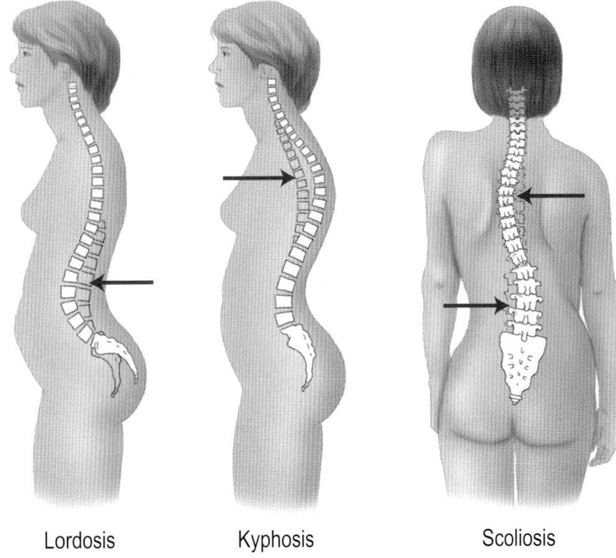

Figure 9-35 Lordosis, kyphosis and scoliosis.

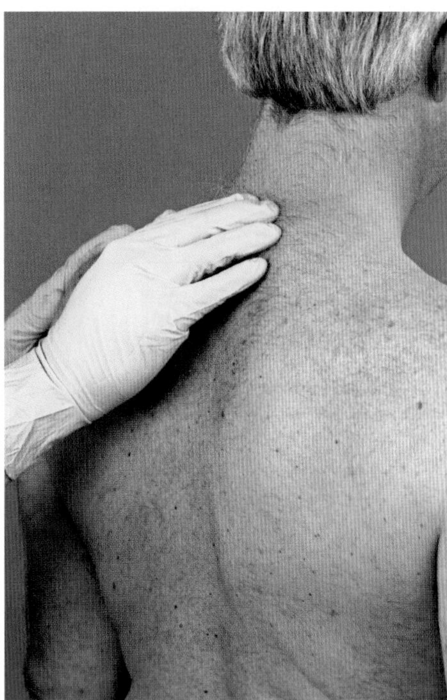

Figure 9-36 Palpation of the seventh cervical spinous process.

ries and has no midline cervical or spinal pain or tenderness on examination and no neurological deficit.

Note

The paramedic will need to test range of motion; however, the paramedic should never attempt to move the neck of a person who is unconscious. The paramedic also should never attempt this with a person who is unable or unwilling to do so on his or her own. Spontaneous cervical muscle spasm frequently is associated with significant cervical spine injury in the trauma victim.

Thoracic and lumbar spine

The paramedic should inspect the thoracic and lumbar areas for signs of injury, swelling, and discoloration. Palpation should begin at the first thoracic vertebra and move downward to the sacrum. Under normal conditions, the spine is non-tender to palpation. The paramedic can evaluate range of motion by requesting the patient to bend at the waist forward and backward and to each side and also to rotate the upper trunk from side to side in a circular motion. Again, assessment for any neurological deficit such as sensory alteration or loss should be undertaken.

Nervous system

The details of an appropriate neurological examination vary greatly and usually depend on the origin of the patient's complaint. For example, the assessment may depend on whether the complaint refers to the peripheral nervous system or the central nervous system. The assessment and examination of the nervous system may be performed separately; however, neurological assessment often is completed during other assessments. A neurological examination may be organized into five categories:

- mental status and speech
- cranial nerves
- motor system
- sensory system
- reflexes.

Mental status and speech

As discussed before, a healthy patient should be oriented to person, time, and place, and able to organize their thoughts and speak freely (provided they have no hearing or speech impediments). Abnormal findings include unconsciousness, confusion, slurred speech, aphasia, dysphonia and dysarthria.

Cranial nerves

The 12 cranial nerves can be categorized as sensory, somatomotor and proprioceptive, and parasympathetic. The following methods can be used to assess each of the cranial nerves:

Nerve	Nerve function and test
Cranial nerve I	Olfactory: Test sense of smell.
Cranial nerve II	Optic: Test for visual acuity (previously described).
Cranial nerves II and III	Optic and oculomotor: Inspect the size and shape of the pupils; test the pupil response to light.
Cranial nerves III IV, and VI	Oculomotor, trochlear, abducens: Test extraocular movements by asking the patient to look up and down, to the left and right, and diagonally up and down to the left and right (the six cardinal directions of gaze).
Cranial nerve V	Trigeminal: Test motor movement by asking the patient to clench the teeth while you palpate the temporal and masseter muscles. Test sensation by touching the forehead, cheeks, and jaw on each side.
Cranial nerve VII	Facial: Inspect the face at rest and during conversation, noting symmetry, involuntary muscle movements (tics) or abnormal movements. Ask the patient to raise the eyebrows, frown, show upper and lower teeth, smile, and puff out both cheeks. The paramedic can assess strength of the facial muscles by asking the patient to close their eyes tightly so they cannot be opened and gently attempting to raise the eyelids. Observe for weakness or asymmetry.
Cranial nerve VIII	Acoustic: Assess hearing acuity (previously described).
Cranial nerves IX and X	Glossopharyngeal and vagus: Assess the patient's ability to swallow with ease; to produce saliva; and to produce normal voice sounds. Instruct the patient to hold the breath, and assess for normal slowing of the heart rate. Testing for the gag reflex also will test the cranial nerves.

Cranial nerve XI	Spinal accessory: Ask the patient to raise and lower the shoulders and to turn the head.
Cranial nerve XII	Hypoglossal: Ask the patient to stick out the tongue and to move it in several directions.

Critical Thinking

Why should abnormal findings in examination of one or more of the cranial nerves concern you?

Motor system

An evaluation of a patient's motor system includes observing the patient during movement as well as observing the patient at rest. The paramedic should evaluate abnormal involuntary movements for quality, rate, rhythm, and fullness of range and other body movement assessments include posture, level of activity, fatigue and emotion.

Muscle strength

Muscle strength should be bilaterally symmetrical and the patient should be able to provide reasonable resistance to opposition. One way to evaluate muscle strength in the upper extremities is to ask the patient to extend the elbow and ask the patient to pull the arm toward the chest against opposing resistance (Figure 9-37a). Assess muscle strength in the lower extremities by asking the patient to push the soles of the feet against the paramedic's palms, then ask the patient to pull the toes toward the head. The paramedic provides opposing resistance (Figure 9-37b). The patient should be able to perform both of these actions easily without evident fatigue. Other methods to evaluate muscle strength and agility include testing for flexion, extension, and abduction of the upper and lower extremities.

Coordination

To evaluate a patient's coordination, the paramedic should assess the patient's ability to perform rapid alternating movements; these include point-to-point movements, gait, and stance.

One point-to-point movement that the patient can perform easily is to touch the finger to the nose, alternating hands. Another test is to ask the patient to touch each heel to the opposite shin. Both movements should be done numerous times and quickly to assess coordination, which should be smooth, rapid, and accurate.

Gait can be evaluated in many ways. A healthy patient should be able to perform each of the following tasks without discomfort or losing balance:

- walk heel to toe
- walk on the toes
- walk on the heels
- hop in place
- do a shallow knee bend
- rise from a sitting position without assistance.

Stance and balance can be evaluated by using Romberg's test and the pronator drift test. To perform Romberg's test, the paramedic asks the patient to stand erect with the feet together and arms at the sides (Figure 9-38). The patient's eyes initially should be open and then closed. Although slight swaying is normal, a loss of balance is abnormal (a positive Romberg's sign). A patient should be able to stand in this position with one foot raised for 5 s without losing balance.

Note

The paramedic should stay close to the patient being tested for gait, stance and balance. That way, the paramedic can help to prevent injury from a fall or loss of balance. The paramedic also should consider the patient's age and physical condition in deciding the appropriateness of these examinations.

The pronator drift test (also known as an arm drift test) is performed by asking the patient to close their eyes and hold both arms out from the body (Figure 9-39). A normal test will reveal that both arms move the same or both arms do not move at all; abnormal findings include one arm that does not move in concert with the other or one arm that drifts down compared with the other.

Sensory system

The sensory pathways of the nervous system conduct sensations of pain, temperature, position, vibration, and touch; a healthy patient is expected to be responsive to each of these stimuli. Common assessments of the sensory system include evaluating the patient's response to pain and light touch. Each of the responses should be considered in relation to dermatomes.

In conscious patients the paramedic should perform a sensory examination with light touch on each hand and each foot. If the patient cannot feel light touch or is unconscious, the paramedic may evaluate sensation by gently pricking the hands and soles of the feet with a sharp object. The paramedic should make sure the object will not penetrate the skin (e.g. a paper clip or cotton swab). The sensory examination should proceed from head to toe; the examination should compare symmetrical areas on each side of the body and the distal and proximal areas of the body. A lack of sensory response may indicate spinal cord or nervous system damage.

Reflexes

Although some reflex testing is not commonly undertaken in paramedic practice, testing a patient's reflexes can evaluate the function of certain areas of the nervous system as they relate to sensory impulses and motor neurons. Reflexes may be categorized as superficial reflexes and deep tendon reflexes (Table 9-3); both types of reflexes should be tested as part of a thorough neurological examination.

Superficial reflexes

Superficial reflexes are elicited by sensory afferents from skin and include the upper abdominal, lower abdominal, cremasteric (for males) and plantar reflexes. All superficial reflexes are tested using the edge of a tongue blade (or similar object) or the end of a reflex hammer; an absent

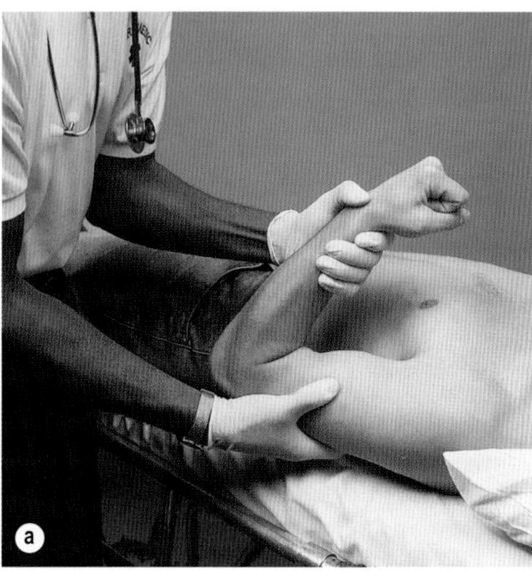

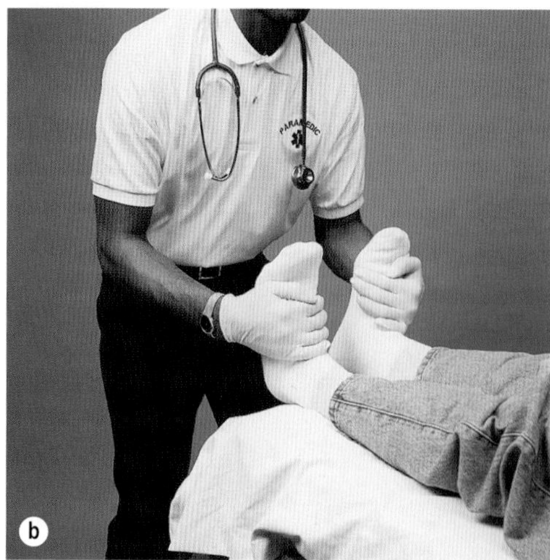

Figure 9-37 Evaluating muscle strength of the upper (a) and lower (b) extremities.

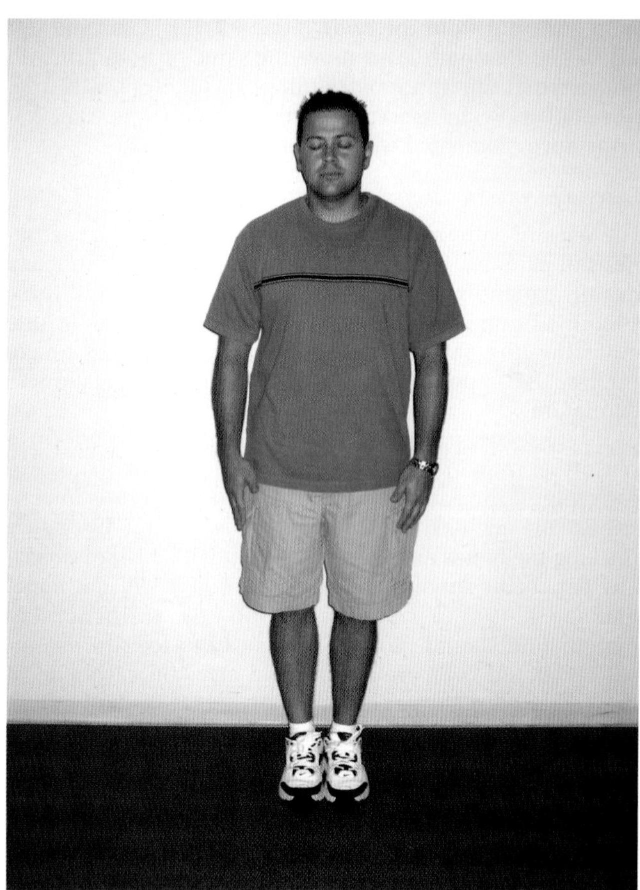

Figure 9-38 Romberg's test.

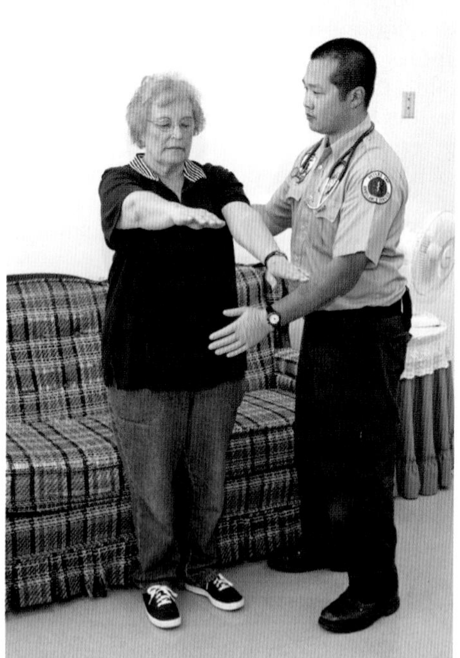

Figure 9-39 Pronator drift test.

reflex may indicate an upper or lower motor neuron disorder.

- *Upper and lower abdominal reflex:* Place the patient supine. Gently stroke each quadrant of the abdomen with the tongue blade. A normal reflex is a slight movement of the umbilicus toward each area that is stroked.
- *Cremasteric reflex:* Place the patient supine. Gently stroke the inner thigh (proximal to distal). The testicle and scrotum should rise on the side that is stroked.
- *Plantar reflex:* Place the patient with legs extended. Gently stroke the lateral side of the foot from heel to the ball and then across the foot to the medial side. Fanning of all the toes should occur with the direction

Table 9-3 Superficial and deep tendon reflexes

Reflex	Spinal level evaluated
SUPERFICIAL	
Upper abdominal	T7, T8 and T9
Lower abdominal	T10 and T11
Cremasteric	T12, L1 and L2
Plantar	L4, L5, S1 and S2
DEEP TENDON	
Biceps	C5 and C6
Brachioradial	C5 and C6
Triceps	C6, C7 and C8
Patellar	L2, L3 and L4
Achilles	S1 and S2

Modified from Rudy EB 1984 Advanced neurological and neurosurgical nursing. Mosby, St Louis.

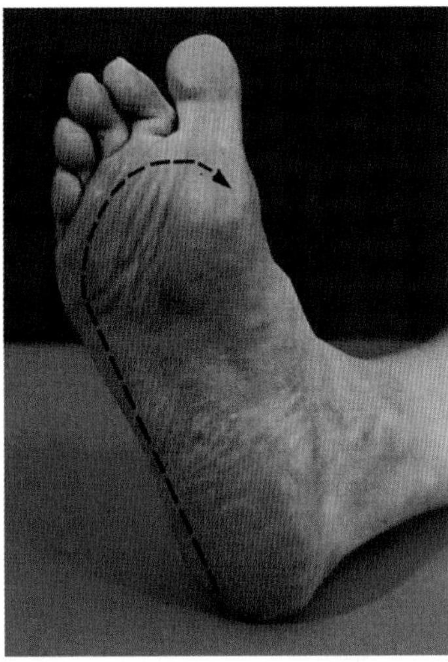

Figure 9-40 Plantar reflex indicating the direction of the stroke and the Babinski sign – dorsiflexion of the great toe with or without fanning of the toes.

of the stroke (Figure 9-40). The Babinski sign is present when there is dorsiflexion of the great toe with or without fanning of the other toes. (An abnormal finding in older children and adults, but a normal response in children less than 2 years of age.)

Deep tendon reflexes

Deep tendon reflexes are elicited by sensory afferents from muscle rather than bone. They include the biceps reflex, brachioradial reflex, triceps reflex, patellar reflex and the Achilles reflex. These reflexes should be tested on each extremity with a reflex hammer and a comparison made for visible and palpable responses. Deep tendon reflexes are graded using the scoring system in Table 9-4 and are recorded on a stick figure. Diminished or absent reflexes may indicate damage to lower motor neurons or the spinal cord, whilst hyperactive reflexes may suggest a motor neuron disorder.

Table 9-4 Scoring deep tendon reflexes

Grade	Deep tendon reflex response
0	No response
1+	Sluggish or diminished
2+	Active or expected response
3+	More brisk than expected, slightly hyperactive
4+	Brisk, hyperactive, with intermittent or transient clonus

All reflexes are tested with the patient in a sitting position in the following manner (Figure 9-41a–f).

- *Biceps reflex:* Flex the patient's arm to 45 degrees at the elbow. Palpate the biceps tendon in the antecubital fossa. Place your thumb over the tendon and your fingers under the elbow. Strike your thumb with the reflex hammer. Contraction of the biceps muscle should cause visible or palpable flexion of the elbow.
- *Brachioradial reflex:* Flex the patient's arm up to 45 degrees. Rest the patient's forearm on your arm with the hand slightly pronated. Strike the brachioradial tendon (about 4–5 cm above the wrist) with the reflex hammer. Pronation of the forearm and flexion of the elbow should occur.
- *Triceps reflex:* Flex the patient's arm at the elbow up to 90 degrees and rest the patient's hand against the side of the body. Palpate the triceps tendon and strike it with the reflex hammer, just above the elbow. Contraction of the triceps muscle should cause visible or palpable extension of the elbow.
- *Patellar reflex:* Flex the patient's knee to 90 degrees, allowing the lower leg to hang loosely. Support the leg with your hand. Strike the patellar tendon just below the patella. Contraction of the quadriceps muscle should cause extension of the lower leg.
- *Achilles reflex:* Flex the patient's knee to 90 degrees. Keep the ankle in a neutral position and hold the heel of the patient's foot in your hand. Strike the Achilles tendon at the level of the ankle malleoli. Contraction of the gastrocnemius muscle should cause plantar flexion of the foot.

Differential and working impression

The differential impression is an adaptation of the differential diagnosis. On completion of the initial assessment, taking of a history and performing a physical examination, it will be possible to develop a working impression. In EMS it is generally accepted that patient assessment has limitations and, without some additional diagnostic techniques, formulating a firm diagnosis is not possible. However, the notion of a working impression is that the history and examination will lead the paramedic to have a strong sense of what is wrong. It is important of course that

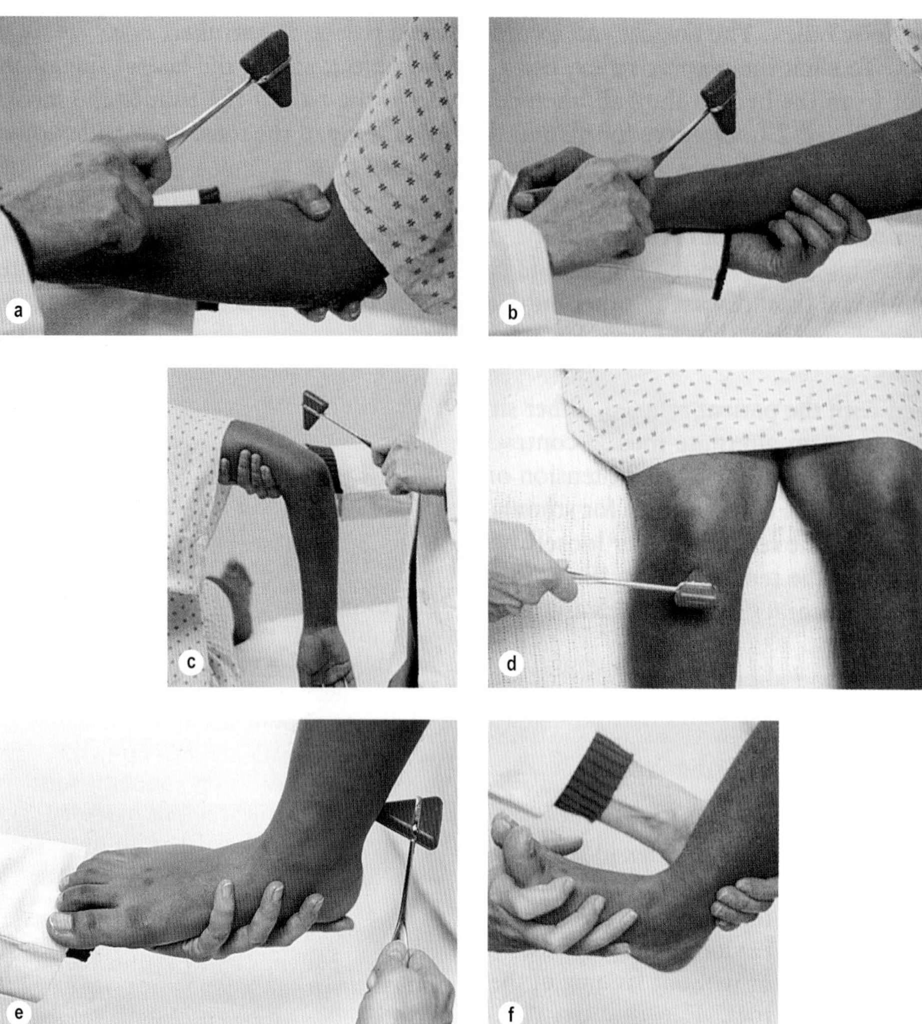

Figure 9-41 Location of the tendons for evaluation of deep tendon reflexes.

this working impression is just that and it is open to adjustment in the light of revised findings. Differential impressions are other possible reasons for the patient's presentation but which have been ruled out or deemed less likely causes.

Effective assessment

Assessment-based management 'puts it all together'. The paramedic gathers, weighs, and synthesizes the information, makes decisions based on this information and then takes appropriate actions required for the patient's care.

As described throughout this text, effective assessment depends on two things: the patient's history and the physical examination. Often as much as 80% of a medical diagnosis is based on the patient's history.[4] The paramedic's knowledge of disease helps him or her to hold a high degree of suspicion for possible illness and helps the paramedic to focus the history towards the complaint and associated problems. The paramedic must focus the examination toward body systems associated with the complaint as well. Some field situations may impair the thoroughness of the examination; for example, unsafe scenes or entrapment may hinder this process. Still, the paramedic must not overlook the value of the careful physical examination and be cautious in not performing the examination too quickly.

Pattern recognition

Paramedics first need to obtain the patient's history and perform the physical examination, then compare the details gathered with their knowledge base of illness and disease. They must ask whether the history and physical examination match a pattern of illness. For example, consider a 55-year-old man with chest pain and shortness of breath. This person matches a possible pattern for acute coronary syndrome. However, a 20-year-old woman with similar complaints would be unlikely to match this pattern. Another example is a 4-year-old who is in respiratory distress and drooling; this patient matches a pattern for epiglottitis. Consider an older woman with distended neck veins and respiratory congestion who produces a pink, frothy sputum when she coughs; this person matches a pattern for congestive heart failure. Pattern recognition makes it possible for the paramedic to form a field impression and to begin a treatment plan. Consequently, the greater the paramedic's knowledge, the better. Likewise, the greater the quality of the assessment details, the greater the chance for a correct assessment and good decision making.

Critical Thinking

How can pattern recognition lead you down the wrong path?

Field impression and action plan

The paramedic forms a field impression of the patient's condition from pattern recognition and gut instinct that comes from experience. Once the paramedic forms a field impression, the paramedic can form an action plan; this plan is based on the patient's condition and the environment. Using the previous example of the two patients with chest pain, the field impression of the 55-year-old patient most likely leads to an action plan that includes the administration of oxygen, electrocardiograph monitoring, intravenous therapy, administration of aspirin, pain relief, and perhaps drug therapy for cardiac rhythm disturbances or administration of fibrinolytics. The 20-year-old patient's action plan most likely includes administration of oxygen, electrocardiograph monitoring to evaluate cardiac rhythm, and a more thorough assessment to detect a recent respiratory illness to rule out the possibility of pleurisy or pneumonia.

Note

The paramedic should not ignore a so-called 'gut' instinct; if something seems wrong, the paramedic should keep looking. Gut instincts (intuition) often help the paramedic to identify subtle physical findings. These findings are hard to quantify (e.g. patient affect or dull and lack-lustre eyes).

Following the field impression and the action plan, the paramedic provides appropriate clinical interventions. The paramedic bases this treatment on knowledge of the clinical practice guidelines and on judgement, that is, knowing when and how to apply the guidelines; judgement also involves knowing when it is appropriate to deviate from the protocols. For example, consider the administration of IV glucose to an unconscious diabetic patient; this patient is over 50 years of age, may have had a stroke and glucose administration can exacerbate cerebral damage. The cause of altered mental status indicates the need for the paramedic to deviate from a common protocol used to manage patients with suspected hypoglycaemia.

Critical Thinking

How can you continue to improve your patient care judgement?

Physical examination of infants and children

Examining the ill or injured child calls for special assessment skills. Children differ physiologically, psychologically, and anatomically from adults, and paediatric patient assessment must take age and development into account.

Approaching the paediatric patient

The assessment and management objectives in caring for critically ill or injured children are similar to those for any other patient but the approach must differ. The initial encounter with the sick or injured child sets the tone for the entire patient care episode so the paramedic must consider the patient's age. The paramedic must also be sensitive to how the child perceives the emergency environment. The paramedic should consider the following six guidelines when approaching the paediatric patient:[2]

1. Remain calm and confident. The parent's anxiety is infectious. Stay under control and take charge of the situation in a gentle but firm manner.
2. Do not separate the child from the parent unless absolutely necessary. In fact, once parents are reassured, encourage them to touch, hold or cuddle the child when such actions are practical. This comforts the parents and the child.
3. Establish rapport with the parents and the child. Much of a child's fear and anxiety reflects the parent's behaviour. When the family is calm, the child is reassured and is less fearful.
4. Be honest with the child and parent. In simple, direct, non-medical language, explain to the parent and the child what is happening as it occurs. When a procedure is going to hurt, inform the child. Never lie. Do not give the impression that there are options when none exist. For example, do not say, 'Would you like to go for a ride in the ambulance?' The child may answer 'No'.
5. Whenever possible, assign one emergency caregiver to stay with the child; this person should obtain the history and be the primary person to initiate therapy. Even in a few moments, one person who remains on the child's level can establish a trusting relationship.
6. Observe the patient before the physical examination. If possible, the paramedic should at first assess the alert child with no touching. After the physical examination begins, the child's behaviour may change radically; this may make it difficult to assess whether the behaviour is a reaction to a physical state or to the perceived intrusion. The paramedic usually can assess the patient's general appearance, skin signs, level of consciousness, respiratory rate and behaviour easily before approaching the patient. During this observation, the paramedic should also note any area of the body that looks painful but avoid manipulating this area until the end of the examination. The paramedic should inform the child that he will give warning before he touches the area.

Critical Thinking

The next time you are in a room with an infant or small child, try this 'across the room' assessment technique. What can you tell about the level of distress and cardiopulmonary function by doing this?

General appearance

A child's general appearance is assessed best at a distance. While the patient is in safe, familiar surroundings (e.g. a parent's arms), the paramedic visually should assess the child's level of consciousness, spontaneous movement, respiratory effort and skin colour. The child's body position can also offer helpful information. For example, the child may be lying limp or sitting upright to aid breathing. Other clues may help determine the child's willingness to cooperate during the examination. These clues may include crying, eye contact, concentration and distractibility.

A visual inspection of the child's general appearance can be helpful. Appearance is a fairly reliable indicator of the patient's need for emergency care; children who are seriously ill or injured usually do not attempt to hide their state and their actions generally reflect the severity of the situation. Therefore the patient's appearance is a valuable tool for the paramedic. Table 9-5 provides the key aspects of general appearance in initial assessment of the paediatric patient.

Table 9-5 Components of general appearance for assessment

Assessment finding	Evaluation considerations
Alertness	How perceptive is the child, and how responsive is the child to the presence of a stranger or to other aspects of the environment?
Distractibility	How readily does a person, sound or object draw the child's attention? For example, drawing a child's attention to a toy when the child initially appeared disinterested in the surroundings is a positive sign.
Consolability	Can a distressed child be comforted? For example, stopping a child from crying by speaking softly or offering a pacifier or a toy is an encouraging sign.
Speech or cry	Is the speech or cry strong or spontaneous? Weak or muffled? Hoarse? Absent unless stimulated? Absent altogether?
Spontaneous activity	Does the child appear flaccid? Do the extremities move only in response to stimuli, or are movements spontaneous?
Colour	Is there pallor, a flushed appearance, cyanosis, or mottling? Does the skin colouring of the trunk differ from that of the extremities?
Respiratory efforts	Are there intercostal, supraclavicular, or suprasternal retractions in the resting state? Nasal flaring also indicates respiratory difficulty.
Eye contact	Does the child appear to gaze aimlessly, or does the child maintain eye contact with objects or persons? Even small infants, when well, preferentially fix their gaze on a face rather than other objects.

Physical examination

A physical examination is best conducted with a knowledge of the development of children and changes that occur within age groups. The guidelines that follow vary according to the child's development. However, these guidelines may be used as a reference during the examination. Parents and family members also may be a source of information. The paramedic may direct questions regarding 'normal' behavior and activity levels to the parents.

Birth to 6 months

Children under 6 months of age are, typically, not frightened by the approach of a stranger, therefore physical examination is fairly easy. During the examination, the paramedic should maintain the child's body temperature.

Healthy and alert infants are usually in constant motion. They may have a lusty cry. If the patient is under 3 months of age, poor head control is normal. Infants are 'abdominal breathers'; this causes the stomach to protrude and the infant's chest wall to retract during inspiration. This diaphragmatic involvement may give the impression of laboured breathing. Skin colour, nasal flaring and intercostal muscle retraction are the best indicators of respiratory insufficiency.

In the infant, assessing the fontanelles is particularly important (Figure 9-42). These sutures between the flat bones of the skull are fairly wide to allow a 'give' in the skull during the birth process; the anterior fontanelle, known as the soft spot, is usually present up to the age of 18 months and should be level with the skull or slightly depressed and

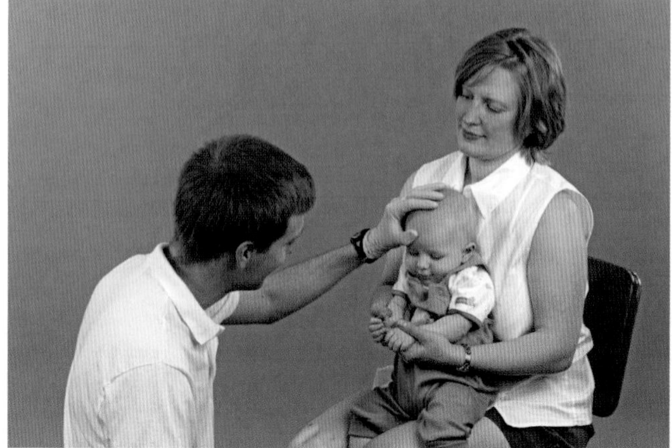

Figure 9-42 Palpation of the anterior fontanelle.

soft. The fontanelle usually bulges during crying and may feel firm if the child is lying down. In the absence of injury, the fontanelle is best examined with the child in an upright position. A sunken fontanelle may indicate dehydration, and a bulging fontanelle in the non-crying upright infant may indicate an increase in intracranial pressure.

7 months to 3 years

Patients from 7 months to 3 years of age often are difficult to evaluate; they have little capacity to understand the emergency event. In addition, they are likely to experience emotional problems as a result of illness, injury or hospitalization. Children of this age fear strangers and may show separation anxiety. If possible, parents should be present and should be allowed to hold the child during the examination (Figure 9-43). The paramedic should approach the child with a quiet, reassuring voice. If time permits, the paramedic should allow the patient to become accustomed to the examination environment.

During the physical assessment, the paramedic should explain each activity in short, simple sentences. The paramedic should give this explanation even though it may not improve cooperation. The best approach is to be gentle and firm. Another good idea is to complete the examination as quickly as possible. If physical restraint is necessary and if patient care activities will not be hindered, the paramedic should restrain the child with hands rather than mechanical devices (e.g. backboards).

4 to 10 years

Children in the 4–10-year age group are developing a capacity for rational thought; they may be cooperative during the physical examination. Depending on the child's age and the emergency scenario, the child may be able to provide a limited history of the event. These children also may experience separation anxiety; moreover, they may view their illness or injury as punishment and the paramedic should approach the child slowly and speak in quiet and reassuring tones. Questions should be simple and direct.

During the examination, the paramedic should allow the child to take part by holding the stethoscope, penlight, or other pieces of equipment; this 'helping' activity may lessen the child's fear. Helping also may improve the paramedic–patient relationship. Children of this age group have a limited understanding of their bodies. They also are reluctant to allow the paramedic to see or touch their 'private parts' (seldom necessary in the prehospital setting). The paramedic should explain all examination procedures simply and completely and advise the child of any expected pain or discomfort.

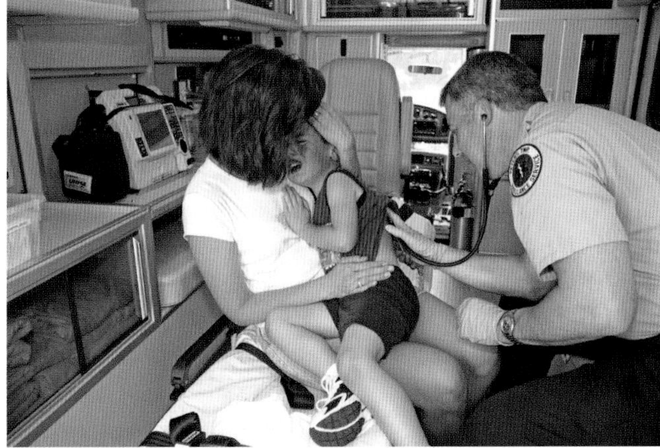

Figure 9-43 Examining a child.

Adolescents (11 to 18 years of age)

Adolescents generally understand what is happening; they usually are calm, mature and helpful. These patients are more adult than child, therefore the paramedic should treat them as such. Adolescents are preoccupied with their bodies and may be concerned about modesty, disfigurement, pain, disability and death. If appropriate, the paramedic should give reassurance about these concerns during the examination.

During the patient interview, the paramedic should respect the patient's need for privacy. Some adolescents may hesitate to reveal relevant history; this hesitancy may be even more obvious in the presence of family and friends. If the adolescent gives vague answers or seems uncomfortable, the paramedic should interview the parents and patient privately. The paramedic should consider the possibility of alcohol or other drug use, as well as the possibility of pregnancy.

Physical examination of older adults

As with paediatric patients, age-related physiological and psychological variations may create special challenges in patient assessment of older adults. The paramedic should not assume that all older adults are victims of age-related disorders. Individual differences in knowledge, mental reasoning, experience, and personality influence how these patients respond to examination.

Communicating with the older adult

Some older adults have sensory losses. This may make communications more difficult. Hearing and visual impairments, for example, are not uncommon. In addition, some older adults experience some memory loss and may become easily confused. Extra time may be needed to communicate effectively with these patients.

The paramedic should remain close to the patient during the interview. The older adult generally perceives a reassuring voice and gentle touch as comforting. Short and simple questions are best. The paramedic may need to speak louder than usual and may need to repeat questions. The paramedic must be patient and careful not to patronize or offend patients by assuming that they have a hearing impairment or cannot understand a particular line of questioning.

Patient history

Older patients often have multiple health problems present at the same time. Patients may be vague and non-specific when describing their presenting complaint. This makes it hard to isolate a non-apparent injury or illness and normal signs and symptoms of illness or injury may be absent because of decreased sensory function in some older adult patients.

Older patients with many health problems often take several medications, which increase the risk of illness from use and misuse. The paramedic should try to gather a full medication history and be alert to the relationship among drug interactions, disease and the ageing process.

As part of the history, the paramedic should assess the patient's functional abilities and any recent changes in daily activities. Many older adults attribute these changes to age; they may not mention them unless asked. These details may help indicate patient conditions that are not readily observable. Moreover, they may reveal the need for other pertinent lines of questioning. Examples of functional activities to be discussed with the patient include the following:

- walking
- getting out of bed
- dressing
- driving a car
- using public transportation
- preparing meals
- taking medications
- sleeping habits
- bathroom habits.

Physical examination

During examination, the paramedic should ensure the older adult patient's comfort. The paramedic should explain procedures clearly and answer all questions sensitively. Many older patients with chronic illness may have lived with pain or discomfort for a long time and their perception of what is painful may be different from that of other patients. The paramedic should observe for signs such as grimacing or wincing during the examination; these signs may indicate pain or a possible injury site. If the situation permits, the paramedic should perform the examination slowly and gently with consideration to the patient's feelings and needs.

Many older adults believe they will die in a hospital. If transportation is needed, patients may become fearful and anxious. The paramedic should be sensitive to these concerns. If appropriate, the paramedic can reassure patients that their condition is not serious. The paramedic should attempt to calm these patients and advise them that they will be well cared for in the hospital. The paramedic should record all examination findings carefully.

Note

The paramedic must have a wide range of knowledge and skills to perform a comprehensive physical examination. This knowledge and skill also will aid the paramedic in making good clinical care decisions. This chapter presents the techniques of the basic physical examination. In addition, this chapter reviews the relevant pathophysiological significance of the physical findings. Some of the techniques presented are not used routinely with patients in the prehospital setting. Some apply to the examinations performed in the field. However, other techniques more likely will be performed in the expanded scope of practice activities. A list of text and further reading specific to physical examination and assessment is provided at the end of the chapter.

Summary

- The examination techniques commonly used in the physical examination are inspection, palpation, percussion, and auscultation.
- Equipment used during the comprehensive physical examination includes the stethoscope, blood pressure cuff, pen-torch and occasionally the ophthalmoscope and otoscope.
- The physical examination is performed in a systematic manner. The examination is a step-by-step process. Emphasis is placed on the patient's present illness and presenting complaint.
- The physical examination is a systematic assessment of the body that includes the relevant systems related to the presenting complaint and is done in either a systems-based or integrated assessment format.
- The first step in any patient care encounter is to note the patient's appearance and behaviour. This includes assessing for level of consciousness and assessment of posture, gait and motor activity; dress, grooming, hygiene and breath or body odours; facial expression; mood, affect and relation to person and things; speech and language; thought and perceptions; and memory and attention.
- During the general survey, the paramedic should evaluate the patient for signs of distress, apparent state of health, skin colour and obvious lesions, height and build, sexual development and weight. The paramedic also should assess vital signs.
- The comprehensive physical examination should include an evaluation of the texture and turgor of the skin, hair and fingernails and toenails.
- Examination of the structures of the head and neck involves inspection, palpation and auscultation.
- A full knowledge of the structure of the thoracic cage is needed and assists in performing a good respiratory and cardiac assessment. Air movement creates turbulence as it passes through the respiratory tree and produces breath

Summary—cont'd

sounds during inhalation and exhalation. In the prehospital setting the paramedic must examine the heart indirectly; however, the paramedic can obtain details about the size and effectiveness of pumping action through a skilled assessment that includes palpation and auscultation.

- The four quadrants of the abdomen and their contents provide the basis for inspection, auscultation, percussion and palpation of this body region. In some cases the abdomen is divided into nine regions.
- An examination of the genitalia of either sex can be awkward for the patient and the paramedic, although it may on occasions be necessary for the paramedic to inspect the genitalia for bleeding and signs of trauma.
- Examination of the anus is indicated in the presence of rectal bleeding or trauma to the area.
- When examining the upper and lower extremities, the paramedic should direct his or her attention to function and structure.
- Assessment of the spine begins with a visual assessment of the cervical, thoracic and lumbar curves and continues with a region-by-region examination for pain, swelling and range of motion.
- A neurological examination may be organized into five categories: mental status and speech, cranial nerves, motor system, sensory system and reflexes.
- When approaching the paediatric patient, the paramedic should remain calm and confident and should observe the child before beginning the physical examination. The paramedic should ensure the child and parent are kept together if possible and establish a honest rapport with parents and child. One caregiver should be assigned to the child.
- The paramedic should not assume that all older adults are victims of disorders related to ageing. Individual differences in knowledge, mental reasoning, experience, and personality influence how these patients respond to examination.

References

1. Epstein O, Perkin GD, Cookson J, de Bono DP 2003 Clinical examination, 3rd edition. Mosby, Edinburgh
2. Seidel J, Henderson D, eds 1987 Prehospital care of pediatric patients, California EMSC project. American Academy of Pediatrics, Los Angeles
3. Seidel H, Ball J, Dains J, Benedict GW 2006 Mosby's guide to physical examination, 6th edition. Mosby/Elsevier, St Louis
4. Douglas G, Nicol F, Robertson C 2005 Macleod's clinical examination, 11th edition. Mosby Churchill Livingstone, Edinburgh

Further reading

Jarvis C 2004 Physical examination and health assessment, 4th edition. Saunders/Elsevier, St Louis

Skinner S 2005 Understanding clinical investigation, 2nd edition. Elsevier/Baillière Tindall, Edinburgh

CHAPTER 10

Differential Impressions and Clinical Decision Making

Chapter contents

Objectives

Upon completion of this chapter, the paramedic student will be able to:

1. List the key elements of paramedic practice.
2. Discuss the limitations of protocols, standing orders, and patient care algorithms.
3. Outline the key components of the critical thinking process for paramedics.
4. Identify elements necessary for an effective critical thinking process.
5. Describe situations that may necessitate the use of the critical thinking process while delivering prehospital patient care.
6. Describe the six elements required for effective clinical decision making in the prehospital setting.

Key terms

application of principle A component of critical thinking in which the examiner makes patient care decisions based on conceptual understanding of the situation and interpretation of data gathered from the patient.

concept formation A component of critical thinking that refers to all elements that are gathered to form a general impression of the patient.

data interpretation A component of critical thinking in which the examiner gathers the necessary data to form a field impression and working diagnosis.

evaluation A component of critical thinking in which the examiner assesses the patient's response to care.

reflection in action A component of critical thinking (usually performed during the event) in which the examiner evaluates patient care during the actual episode of patient contact and changes practice in a dynamic 'on the spot' way.

reflection on action A component of critical thinking (usually performed after the event) in which the examiner evaluates a patient care episode for possible improvement in similar future responses.

The spectrum of prehospital care

As described in Chapters 7 and 9, the paramedic must have a wide base of knowledge and skills to make good patient care decisions in the prehospital setting. On any given workday, the paramedic may be exposed to obvious critical life threats, potential life threats, and non-life-threatening situations (Box 10-1); in all of these situations, the paramedic is expected to provide proper care and treatment.

Protocols, standing orders and patient care algorithms (such as resuscitation algorithms) help to promote a standardized approach to patient care for classic presentations which clearly define and outline performance parameters. In a number of circumstances these protocols or algorithms are appropriate as they provide a formal approach to a very set problem. The use of patient group directives (PGDs) for drug administration is another good example. However, widespread use of these more didactic approaches has, in some circumstances, limitations. First, they may not apply to non-specific patient complaints; the calls that do not 'fit' the model. Second, these standards may not take into account multiple disease aetiologies or multiple treatment modalities, and, thirdly, they may promote linear thinking ('cookbook medicine'). In many circumstances healthcare, including paramedic practice, is moving away from rigid protocols or algorithms towards a more guidelines-based

Box 10-1

Spectrum of prehospital care

Obvious critical life threats

- Major multisystem trauma
- Devastating single-system trauma
- End-stage disease presentations
- Acute presentations of chronic conditions

Potential life threats

- Serious multisystem trauma
- Multiple disease aetiologies

Non-life-threatening presentations

- Minor illness or injury
- Emergency medical services system misuse

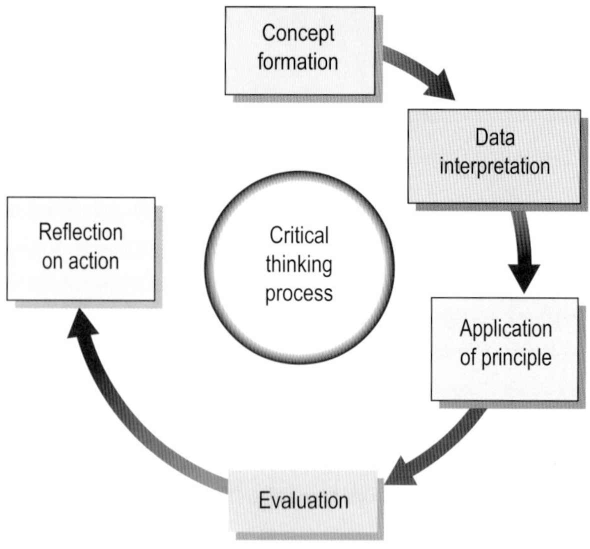

Figure 10-1 Critical thinking process.

approach. Guidelines provide a strong direction or 'framework' of care but recognize that in some circumstances deviation or adaptation of the procedure or practice may be required. Resuscitation algorithms are a good example: they provide a very clear framework for responding to a patient in, for example, a ventricular fibrillation cardiac arrest but also recognize that some of the scenarios may occur in an unusual context and modification of the normal procedure is required: for instance, a hypothermic patient will require different management approaches in cardiac arrest compared with one who is normothermic. Therefore, it is essential paramedics develop critical thinking skills, which will assist in unique patient care situations.

In order to develop critical thinking skills the paramedic must have a good base of knowledge and understanding: this is obtained by theoretical acquisition of areas such as anatomy, physiology, pathophysiology, clinical assessment and so on. In order to relate why a patient may have dysrhythmias on an ECG requires an understanding, for instance, of the cardiac conduction system. Secondly, previous experience contributes to the thinking processes involved; having seen many patients with a breathing problem will allow you to become familiar with common (and, in time, less common) presentations and how they are managed. The risk, of course, is that over-familiarity may make a paramedic complacent, so caution must always be exercised. However, the combination of theoretical knowledge and understanding and the practical 'street' experience is essential to allow effective clinical decision making to take place. The paramedics' approach to a particular call or patient is also important. In many situations, the paramedic will be dealing with a non-time-critical patient and the considered (perhaps reflective) approach to assessment and management can be adopted, with time taken to consider a range of factors in determining what is wrong with the patient and what the best options of care and management might be. On occasions, however, in a critical patient a more instinctive approach may be required as time is of the essence and key interventions must be delivered quickly; in this case care is more reactive as the situation requires prompt attention and the focus is on the most important/specific and key aspects of the call.

Critical thinking process for paramedics

Specific aspects, stages, and sequences are linked with the critical thinking process.[1] These include concept formation, data interpretation, application of principle, evaluation, and reflection on action (Figure 10-1).

Concept formation

Concept formation refers to all elements gathered to form a general impression of the patient: it is the 'what' of the patient story. These elements are described in Chapters 7 and 9 and include the following:

- scene assessment (mechanism of injury, social setting, etc.)
- presenting complaint
- patient history
- patient affect
- initial assessment and physical examination
- diagnostic tests.

Scenario: part one

Your crew has been dispatched to a local park for a person with 'difficulty breathing'. On your arrival at the scene, you find an 18-year-old female sitting on a park bench surrounded by her friends; the scene is safe. She is crying and tells you that she cannot catch her breath. You attempt to calm the patient and provide her with supplemental oxygen. You obtain a history from the patient and her friends that she and her boyfriend have argued recently and that she became emotional during the argument. Her lung sounds are clear. She has no allergies and no significant medical history other than a recent sinus infection and denies any injury or pain. Aside from her increased respiratory rate, her vital signs are within normal range. Consider your concept formation for this patient.

Critical Thinking

What effect would wrong or incomplete concept formation have on your critical thinking process during patient care? How can you enhance your concept formation skills while in your paramedic programme?

Data interpretation

Following concept formation, the paramedic must gather the needed data to form a working impression, which is the 'working phase' of patient care. These data comprise a range of findings, including vital signs, the patient history or results of the physical examination. The data should then be applied to the relevant anatomy, physiology, and pathophysiology, and the paramedic's previous experience in providing patient care will also influence this application. The application in some circumstances is simple: for example, in a patient with leg pain localized to the ankle. However, in some scenarios the data can be very general (signs of fever or collapse in a patient) which means that multiple systems and areas of the body might be involved. During the interpretation of data, the paramedic tries to get a full picture of the patient's situation; the paramedic's attitude can affect the success of this phase as the interaction between the paramedic and patient can affect data acquisition and interpretation (see Chapter 6). In some cases, the paramedic may need to condense these data and discuss the patient with the GP or the out of hours service.

The next step in data interpretation is to make sense of it and apply it to likely processes: the use of 'diagnostic sieves' may assist in this: for instance, if there is structural abnormality, a so-called surgical sieve[2] may be useful which is made up of components such as congenital, traumatic, infective, vascular, metabolic/nutritional, toxic, neoplastic or degenerative causes. Once these aspects have been considered, then it is necessary to come to a working impression about what is wrong, against which other possible differential impressions are considered and tested/explored to rule them in or out. Once the data interpretation is complete, the principles of clinical care and management can be considered and applied.

Scenario: part two

While assessing this patient, you recall a similar emergency call, where you provided care to a young male with difficulty breathing. He had just lost a big tennis match and at first you assumed that the patient was having breathing difficulty because of emotions that resulted from his loss. Like the female patient you are caring for now, this male patient had no allergies and no significant medical history and denied any recent injury. His vital signs were within normal range. However, lung sounds were diminished slightly on the patient's left side and the patient also complained of mild pain on inspiration. You administered supplemental oxygen and conveyed the patient to the emergency department. After obtaining a chest X-ray film, the emergency department doctor confirmed your suspicion of a spontaneous pneumothorax (which resolved during the patient's hospitalization). Compare this interpretation of data to that of the female patient you are caring for now.

Application of principle

The next step in the critical thinking process is the application of principles of proper patient care; these principles are based on the paramedic's conceptual understanding of the situation and are also based on the interpretation of the data gathered from the patient. Once the paramedic establishes the field impression and working diagnosis, the paramedic initiates treatment and intervention through protocols and standing orders or direct/online medical direction.

Scenario: part three

Based on your experience, your knowledge of patient care, and your interpretation of the data gathered from your patient, you decide that she is hyperventilating. You initiate proper treatment with calming measures and encourage her to slow her respiratory rate. Although the female patient you are caring for presented much like the male patient you recall, your working impression is different. You reach this conclusion because the female patient had clear, bilateral lung sounds and denied any pain on respiration.

Evaluation

The paramedic must evaluate the patient's response to the care on an ongoing basis. Evaluation includes the following:

- Reassessment of the patient (ongoing assessment).
- Reflection on action (effectiveness of the intervention).
- Revision of differential impressions (leading to a change in the working impression).
- Review of the appropriateness of any protocol or guideline applicable to the patient.
- Revision of the treatment or intervention as needed.

Scenario: part four

After you have provided calming measures and oxygen to your patient, she has slowed her breathing and appears to be more relaxed. You reassess the patient and find that her vital signs remain normal and her lung sounds remain clear. Based on these findings, you know that your working impression of hyperventilation was correct and that there is no need to change your treatment. After discussing it on scene with your colleague the decision is made that the patient's condition does not warrant transportation to hospital and you provide verbal and written advice regarding warning signs and what to do if the problem reoccurs ('red flags' and 'safety netting').

Reflection on action

Reflection on action occurs after the event and usually occurs through a critique of the call. In this the paramedic evaluates the care episode for improvement in similar future responses. Reflection on action provides paramedics with an avenue to add to or alter their experience base.

Scenario: part five

On the way back to station, you discuss the call with a paramedic student; this student has just begun her practice placement. Like you, she instantly thought that the patient was hyperventilating because of the argument that she had had with her boyfriend. The paramedic student admitted that she had read about a spontaneous pneumothorax in her studies. However, she had never seen a patient who had one and moreover conceded she might not have considered this possibility when caring for this patient. You discuss the pathology of a pneumothorax (including the development of tension pneumothorax) with her and the importance of assessing bilateral lung sounds in a patient who is having trouble breathing. This reflection on action reinforces your data interpretation skills and adds to the student's experience base.

Fundamental elements of critical thinking for paramedics

For an effective critical thinking process, some basic elements must be present. These elements include adequate knowledge and the ability to do the following:

- Focus on specific and multiple elements of data at the same time.
- Gather and organize data and form concepts.
- Identify and deal with medical ambiguity. This may include patients who do not fit the model.
- Differentiate between relevant and irrelevant data.
- Analyse and compare similar situations from past experience.
- Recall cases in which the working diagnosis was wrong.
- Articulate decision-making reasoning and construct arguments to support or discount the decision.

All of these elements were present in the previous scenario. At the scene the paramedic dealt with the patient's symptoms and dealt with the input of friends as well. In addition, he focused on assessment and history finding and he offered initial emergency care; the paramedic did this all within moments of arriving at the patient's side. He gathered and organized the data and then concluded that the patient fitted the model for hyperventilation syndrome. The paramedic also decided that the patient's sinus infection was not likely related to her present respiratory troubles. He recalled a certain case in which his initial working diagnosis of hyperventilation syndrome was wrong. The paramedic used clinical decision making to support his diagnosis of hyperventilation syndrome, which was based on his experience and on his assessment findings.

Field application of assessment-based patient management

Assessment-based patient management places huge responsibility on the paramedic. The paramedic must have a systematic means of analysing a patient's problems, determining how to solve them, carrying out a plan of action, and evaluating effectiveness of the treatment. The success of assessment-based patient management in the prehospital setting depends on an integration of interpersonal skills, scientific knowledge, and physical activities (skills).

The patient crisis severity spectrum

Emergency medical services are set into daily action for many reasons, yet few prehospital calls present true threats to life. Minor medical and trauma events often call for less critical thinking and result in fairly easy decision making for the paramedic. Likewise, patients with clear life threats pose limited critical thinking challenges because they often fit the model for standardized treatment (e.g. cardiac arrest). However, some patients fall in the spectrum between minor and life-threatening events and these patients pose the most critical thinking challenges for the paramedic. Examples include patients with mild to moderate respiratory distress or diffuse abdominal pain; either of these situations could be minor or could have life-threatening elements.

Thinking under pressure

Hormonal influences from the fight-or-flight response can have both positive and negative effects on critical decision making. The response may offer greater visual acuity and auditory keenness and also allow for improved reflexes and strength. These can be helpful when one must make decisions and act on them. The negative aspects of the response may include reduced critical thinking skills as a result of a decrease in the ability to concentrate and assess. The key to strong performance under pressure is mental conditioning; this results in instinctive performance and automatic responses for technical procedures.

Mental checklist for thinking under pressure

Mental conditioning takes a good deal of practice. A checklist for thinking under pressure may help the paramedic to concentrate during stressful events. The mental checklist the paramedic should use is as follows:

- Stop and think.
- Scan the situation.
- Decide and act.
- Maintain clear and effective control.
- Regularly and continually re-evaluate the patient.

Critical Thinking

Do you think you can improve your performance under pressure by practising imaginary critical situations in your head? Why or why not?

Practising this checklist when under pressure will result in behaviours that refine clinical decision making. One of these positive behaviours is staying calm (not panicking). Another is assuming a plan for the worst case (erring on the side of the patient). A third is maintaining a systematic assessment pattern. In addition, the paramedic can learn to balance the various styles of situation analysis, data processing, and decision making. Applying the styles of situational analysis (reflective versus impulsive), data processing (divergent versus convergent), and decision making (anticipatory versus reactive) allows the paramedic to provide the best possible care in most situations. In time, paramedics are able to apply all of these approaches with skill.

Situational analysis: reflective versus impulsive

In most patient care situations, paramedics should avoid closing off the pursuit of data too quickly; one may do this to try to reach a correct working diagnosis. For example, consider a patient who has abdominal pain in his lower right quadrant; this patient should not be automatically considered to have a working impression of appendicitis; this is an impulsive decision because the patient fits the model. Instead the paramedic should take time to reflect on other conditions; for example a condition such as food poisoning could be the cause of the patient's pain. In other situations (e.g. a patient with foreign body airway obstruction), the impulsive decision to clear the patient's airway with chest thrusts and back blows would be the most prudent course of action to follow.

Data processing: divergent versus convergent

Paramedics should avoid the trap of gathering only partial data, which may lead them down the wrong diagnostic or therapeutic path (a result of impulsive situational analysis); this is known as convergent data processing. The convergent approach may be best in some cases (e.g. giving a standard drug dose to a patient in cardiac arrest) but may hinder care in complex cases (e.g. an older adult patient with multiple presenting complaints). A divergent approach in data processing looks at all sides of a case. The paramedic does this before arriving at a solution (e.g. multiple illnesses and polypharmacy in the older patient).

Decision making: anticipatory versus reactive

A paramedic's decision making can be seen as anticipatory or reactive. With reactive decision making, one waits until a problem occurs before starting treatment; this can affect patient care negatively and an example of this is waiting to address respiratory compromise in a patient with an allergic reaction until the patient has trouble breathing. The process that healthcare workers should use is anticipatory decision making, which is based on ongoing data collection and evaluation of the patient's condition. Using the same example, the paramedic applying this kind of decision making would treat early signs and symptoms of an allergic reaction by administering oxygen and medications and would have intubation equipment ready to manage the patient's airway; this would be in anticipation of respiratory compromise.

Putting it all together: the six Rs

To put all components required for effective clinical decision making into action, the paramedic can think in terms of the six Rs listed next (Figure 10-2):

1. *Read* the patient. The paramedic should observe the patient's level of consciousness and skin colour and note the patient's position along with any obvious deformity or asymmetry. The paramedic can determine

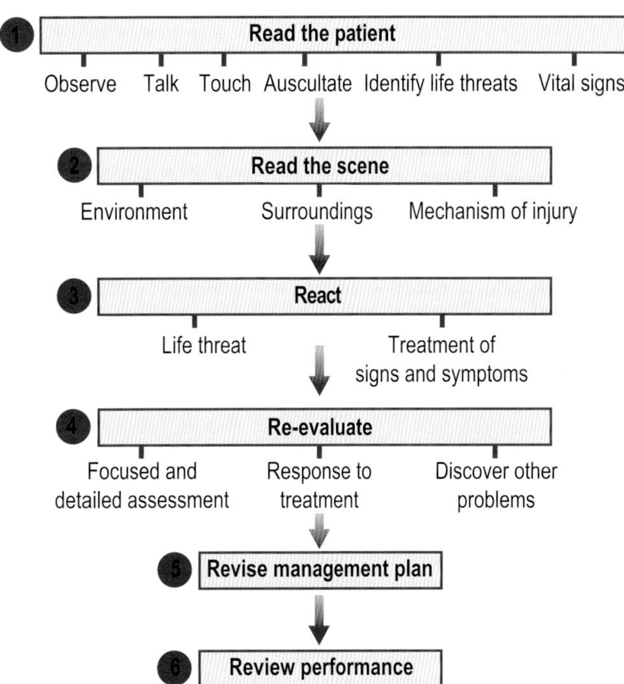

Figure 10-2 The six Rs.

the presenting complaint by talking to the patient and identify the presence of a worsening or pre-existing condition. The paramedic should evaluate skin temperature and moisture and assess the pulse for rate, strength, and regularity. Auscultation of the lungs will reveal upper or lower airway problems. The paramedic should identify all life threats and obtain an accurate set of vital signs.

Note

Vital signs can be used as a triage tool. The paramedic can use vital signs to estimate severity. Vital signs also can help the paramedic identify the majority of life-threatening conditions. The paramedic should remember that the patient's age and physical and medical conditions can affect vital signs. Currently used medication also can affect vital signs.

2. *Read* the scene. As a part of the scene size-up, the paramedic should assess general environmental conditions by evaluating the immediate surroundings and attempting to identify any mechanism of injury.
3. *React*. The paramedic should manage all life threats in the order in which they are found. The paramedic should decide on the most common and likely cause of the life threat that fits the patient's initial presentation. The paramedic may not identify a clearly defined and recognizable presentation of medical illness in a priority patient, so treatment should be based on presenting signs and symptoms.
4. *Re-evaluate*. Re-evaluation includes a focused and detailed assessment that analyses the patient's response to management and interventions and may lead the paramedic to find other problems. These problems may not have been evident during the initial assessment.

5. *Revise* management plan. Findings obtained during re-evaluation may require the paramedic to revise the management plan. This revision will address more clearly the needs of the patient. The fact that patient conditions change and that patients do not respond in the same way to identical treatment interventions highlight the importance of ongoing assessment.
6. *Review* performance at call critique. A paramedic can review the details of the call through a critique. This allows for the identification of areas that can be improved on similar calls in the future. The interest and investment of paramedics in the outcome of their personal cases often is the strongest stimulus to change their practice patterns favourably; this process also enhances the paramedic's experience base and in turn leads to improvement of data interpretation skills.

Critical Thinking

Consider a negative or punitive run critique. How do you think this would influence your ability to perform under a similar circumstance in the future?

Unique to the emergency medical services profession is the uncertainty of the prehospital environment. The uncertainty is influenced heavily by factors that do not exist in other medical settings. Paramedics must be able to gather, weigh, and synthesize information. They also must be able to develop and apply proper patient care plans. In addition, they must apply judgement and exercise decision making. They must think and work well under pressure. These are the cornerstones of effective paramedic practice.

Summary

- The paramedic must be able to do several things at the same time and be able to gather, evaluate, and synthesize information. The paramedic also must be able to develop and implement appropriate patient management plans as well as apply judgement and exercise independent decision making. Lastly, the paramedic must be able to think and work effectively under pressure.
- Protocols, standing orders, and patient care algorithms have several limitations; they may not apply to non-specific patient complaints that do not fit the model. They also do not address multiple disease aetiologies or multiple treatment plans. Moreover, they may promote linear thinking.
- The critical thinking process includes concept formation, data interpretation, application of principle, evaluation and reflection on action.
- For effective critical thinking, a paramedic must have a solid knowledge base and be able to deal with a large amount of data all at once as well. The paramedic must be able to organize that data, deal with ambiguity, and relate the situation to similar past experience. The paramedic must also be able to reason and construct arguments to support or discount the decision.
- When using assessment-based patient management, the paramedic must analyse a patient's problems, determine how to solve them, carry out a plan of action and evaluate its effectiveness.
- Effective clinical decision making requires the paramedic to read the patient and the scene. The paramedic must also be able to react, re-evaluate, and revise the management plan and be able to review performance at the end of the call.

References

1. US Department of Transportation, National Highway Traffic Safety Administration 1998 EMT-Paramedic national standard curriculum. Department of Transportation, Washington, DC
2. Burkitt HG, Quick C, Reed J, Raftery A, Deakin P 2007 Essential surgery: problems, diagnosis and management, 4th edition. Churchill Livingstone, Oxford

Further reading

Alfaro-Lefevre R 1999 Critical thinking in nursing: a practical approach. WB Saunders, Philadelphia

Benner P, Hooper-Kyriakidis P, Stannard D 1999 Clinical wisdom and interventions in critical care: a thinking-in-action approach. WB Saunders, Philadelphia

Higgs J, Jones M, Loftus S, Christensen N 2008 Clinical reasoning in the health professions, 3rd edition. Butterworth-Heinnemann, Oxford

Pesut D, Herman J 1999 Clinical reasoning: the art and science of critical and creative thinking. Delmar Learning, Albany, NY

Potter P 2000 Virtual clinical excursions to accompany basic nursing: a critical thinking approach, 5th edition. Mosby, St Louis

CHAPTER **11**

Documentation and Record Keeping

Chapter contents

Objectives

Upon completion of this chapter, the paramedic student will be able to:

1. Identify the purpose of the patient report form.
2. Describe the uses of the patient report form.
3. Outline the components of an accurate, thorough patient report form.
4. Describe the elements of a properly written emergency medical services document.
5. Describe an effective system for documentation of prehospital patient care.
6. Identify differences necessary when documenting special situations.
7. Describe the appropriate method to make revisions or corrections to the patient report form.
8. Recognize consequences that may result from inappropriate documentation.

Key terms

narrative The portion of the patient care report that allows for a chronological description of the call.

pertinent negative findings Findings that warrant no medical care or intervention but that, by seeking them, show evidence of the thoroughness of the examination and history of the event.

pertinent oral statements Statements made by the patient and other on-scene persons.

Note

The requirements for record keeping vary throughout the UK. All patient report forms have to be held for a minimum of 10 years and in the case of children until at least they are aged 25 years. Some authorities may hold records for longer than this. These records are maintained should any litigious activity occur related to that patient; therefore, accurate documentation is essential.

Importance of documentation

There are many reasons for creating thorough written documentation; it provides a tangible and legal record of an incident as well as being used to better understand the patient's initial condition and the type of care given before hospital treatment. The ambulance service and the clinical effectiveness department also may use the report to monitor care in the field, evaluate individual performance, and conduct review conferences and other educational forums. These reports may be used to identify system issues regarding quality improvement and may result in policy changes to improve patient care. For instance, these data may provide information on:

- minimizing time spent on the scene for critical trauma patients
- adding new medications to manage some medical emergencies more effectively
- changing the placement of emergency vehicles during peak response times in certain geographic areas.

The patient report form (PRF) is sometimes also known as a clinical report form or patient care report; differing services and agencies will use differing terms. It offers a means of documenting any unique scene situations which may have affected patient care. For example, traffic may have caused a long response time or entrapped patient may have required prolonged extrication. The PRF also aids in providing evidence of certain patient care skills of the paramedic (e.g. intravenous access, intubation, and defibrillation) which may be useful for continual professional development and re-registration purposes.

General considerations

The PRF (Figure 11-1a, b) should be carefully detailed and legible. The PRF is viewed as a legal document, part of the patient's medical record, and the use of slang terms or

East Midlands Ambulance Service NHS Trust

CONFIDENTIAL PATIENT INFORMATION. Top copy to HQ Bottom copy to hospital or to patient if not transported. 1993588137

1 Incident Number / Call sign / Station
Incident Date / / Call Type ☐ E ☐ U ☐ Dr E ☐ Transfer
Incident location (if different from H/A)
☐ Home ☐ Work ☐ Leisure ☐ Public ☐ AED site ☐ Other
PIN Number:
ID1 P T AES Dr PTS SR Signature
ID2
ID3
AMPDS dispatch AMPDS actual AMPDS code not given ☐

2 Time originated Time Mobile Time at scene/cancelled
Time at patient Time left scene Time at hospital

3 Surname:
First Name:
Home address: GP Name:
Contact details:
Tel no.:
Postcode: L L N N N L L Relatives aware? ☐ Yes ☐ No Relatives following? ☐ Yes ☐ No

4 Patient age: D W M Est Male ☐ Female ☐ Consent to treatment: ☐ Informed ☐ Refused ☐ Presumed
Date of birth: / / Ethnic group

5 **Initial Assessments:** ☐ Calm ☐ Nervous ☐ Uncooperative ☐ Violent ☐ Abusive ☐ Alcohol suspected ☐ Drugs suspected ☐ Hostile situation
Airway & Breathing:
☐ Clear ☐ Obstructed ☐ Noisy ☐ Vomited ☐ Equal air entry
Trachea: ☐ Central ☐ Deviation
☐ Normal ☐ Absent ☐ Shallow ☐ Deep ☐ Regular
☐ Irregular ☐ Paradoxical
Circulation Bleeding: ☐ Internal ☐ External
☐ Radial pulse ☐ Carotid pulse ☐ Strong
☐ Weak ☐ Absent Capillary refill(s): ☐ <2 ☐ >2
☐ Normal ☐ Pale ☐ Clammy ☐ Flushed ☐ Cyanosed
Disability Alert ☐ Pain ☐ Voice ☐ Unconscious ☐
Unconscious / KO'd? ☐ Yes ☐ No ☐ ?? Duration (mins)

6 **Stroke FAST (Face, Arm, Speech Test) Assessment**
Facial weakness ☐ Yes ☐ No ☐ Unable to assess
Affected side ☐ Left ☐ Right
Arm weakness ☐ Yes ☐ No ☐ Unable to assess
Affected side ☐ Left ☐ Right
Speech difficulties ☐ Yes ☐ No ☐ Unable to assess

7 **Chief Complaint**
History of chief complaint, PMH, drugs & allergies
Time of first symptom/incident : ☐ > 24 hours ?
Other relevant information (use to list any patient's property)

8 Time 1st sequence obs : ID | Time 2nd sequence obs : ID
Airway: ☐ Clear ☐ Obstructed ☐ Noisy ☐ Vomited
Breathing: ☐ Normal ☐ Absent ☐ Shallow ☐ Deep ☐ Regular ☐ Irregular ☐ Paradoxical
Resp rate Peak flow UTR ☐
☐ SpO2 On air (%) / SpO2/ETCO2 State O2 % ☐ ETCO2
Circulation: Pulse ☐ Irregular? BP ☐ UTR
Temp °C BM (mmol)
GCS: Eyes, Motor, Verbal E (4) M (6) V (5) Pain score pre-treatment /10 | Pain score post-treatment /10
Pupils: Normal Reactive Size (mm) UTR Left Right Patient unable to score pain ☐

9 **RTA Detail**
☐ Car ☐ Driver ☐ Cyclist ☐ Vehicle roll over ☐ Airbag activated
☐ PSV ☐ Front passenger ☐ Pedestrian ☐ Headrest ☐ SIPS
☐ Van ☐ Rear passenger ☐ Helmet ☐ Trapped > 20 min ☐ Decamped
☐ LGV ☐ M/cyclist ☐ Seatbelt ☐ Extrication Impact speed (mph)
☐ HGV ☐ Pillion ☐ Child restraint ☐ Ejected

10 Show: Deformity Contusion Abrasion Penetration Burns Tenderness Laceration Swelling Burns %
Fracture# Pain Instability Crepitus
Show impact & indicate area of damage and patient position in vehicle FRONT No. of seats

11 **Immobilisation** ☐ C Collar ☐ KED ☐ Longboard ☐ Traction ☐ Box ☐ Vacuum ☐ Scoop If immobilisation refused, please give details:

12 **Airway Management** Suction Postural LMA OPA NPA B/V/M Ventilator Needle Cric. Needle Thorac. ID
Intubation Success Unable Attempts Time Tube size Extubated ID
Cannulation ☐ Pt refused ☐ Pt shut down ☐ IO ☐ Central vein Time Attempts Success Unable Gauge Site ID

13 **Cardiac Monitoring** Refused 3 lead 12 lead Initial Rhythm NSR VF VT ASY PEA ST↑ ST↓ Other (please specify) ECG Rhythm

14 **Cardiac Drugs:** High flow O2 Aspirin GTN IV analgesia PHT
Given / Contra-indicated / Refused / Taken prior to arrival

15 **Cardiac Arrest** Arrest aetiology: ☐ Presumed cardiac ☐ Trauma ☐ Other
☐ Witnessed by crew ☐ Resus attempted by crew
☐ Witnessed by bystander ☐ Resus not attempted by crew
☐ Unwitnessed ☐ Mechanical chest compressions
☐ Bystander CPR ☐ DNAR

16 **Defibrillation** ☐ Manual ☐ AED Total no. of shocks ID

17 Time of collapse / Time bystander CPR started / Time crew CPR started / Time of first shock / Time CPR stopped / Time of ROSC / Time of ROSR

18 **Outcome**
☐ ROSC maintained to arrival at hospital ☐ R.O.L.E. onscene
☐ ROSC during resus not maintained ☐ Resus discontinued by hospital
☐ Return of spontaneous respiration (ROSR) ☐ Resus ongoing at handover

19 **Clinical Impression**
☐ Acute abdo problem ☐ D and or V ☐ Mental health problem
☐ Allergic reaction ☐ Dizziness ☐ Neck injury
☐ Assault ☐ DVT ☐ NOF# (suspected)
☐ Asthma ☐ Dyspnoea ☐ OD (accidental)
☐ Back pain ☐ Emotional/distressed ☐ OD (intentional)
☐ Cardiac arrest ☐ Exacerbation COPD ☐ Obstetric problem
☐ Cardiac problems ☐ Fall < 2m ☐ Off legs/poor mobility
☐ Catheter problem ☐ Fall > 2m ☐ Panic/anxiety attack
☐ Cellulitis ☐ Fracture (suspected) ☐ Rash
☐ Chest infection/pneumonia ☐ GI bleed ☐ Respiratory arrest
☐ Chest pains - cardiac ☐ Haemorrhage ☐ Retention of urine
☐ Chest pains - non cardiac ☐ Gynae problems ☐ STEMI
☐ Collapse ? cause ☐ Head injury ☐ Thermal injury
☐ Confusion ☐ Headache/pain ☐ UTI
☐ Convulsions ☐ ? Intoxicated ☐ Wound
☐ CVA/TIA/ICH ☐ Life extinct ☐ Other
☐ Dehydration ☐ Maternity
☐ Diabetic problem ☐ Meningitis (suspected)

20 **Other information** ☐ CPI ☐ VA ☐ Patient at risk of pressure sore ☐ Patient care pathway in place (e.g. end of life plan, long term care plan)

21 **Prior to Ambulance Arrival** Time of first call for help
First call for help made to: ☐ 999 ambulance ☐ NHSD ☐ GP (requested 999 before attending) ☐ GP (requested 999 not attending) ☐ GP (attended) ☐ Other
First onscene: ☐ EMS (A&E) ☐ EMS (non-A&E) ☐ CFR ☐ Other healthcare professional
Any treatment given prior to ambulance arrival: CPR Shocks Cannulation Intubation — Bystander / Other EMS / CFR / Other Healthcare Professional
NB if any drugs have been given, please record in drugs section using 'given prior to ambulance arrival' column
Comments:

22 **Drugs Administered** Drug name | Refused | Route | Dose | Units / % | Time 1st administered | ID | If drug given prior to ambulance arrival, please indicate by whom: Patient Relative Doctor CFR Other

23 I recognise life extinct in accordance with East Midlands Ambulance Service NHS Trust protocols. ID Signature: Witnessed: Time :

24 **Details for patient conveyed** Destination Department ☐ Pre-alert call made
Handed over to: ☐ Nurse ☐ Doctor ☐ GP ☐ Police ☐ Other
Print name: Handover time
Signature:

25 **Declaration for patient not conveyed**
This section to be completed in respect of the patient who has: 1 *refused treatment and/or transportation to hospital 2 *no need for further treatment 3 *agreed to alternative arrangements.
Referral to other agency: ☐ GP ☐ Social services ☐ Other
I hereby understand and accept: 1*all responsibility for my refusal of treatment and/or transport to hospital 2 *agree no further treatment is necessary 3 * agree with the alternative arrangements above.
Signature of patient:
Signature of witness:
* delete as applicable

(a)

Figure 11-1 (a) Patient care report – front.

Patient Information

On this occasion the Ambulance crew, in consultation with both you and your carers (as appropriate), have decided not to transport you to hospital or other care facility.

The reason for this is:
(please tick)

☐ Your treatment has been completed by the Ambulance crew.

☐ You are being referred to an alternative care provider, best suited to meet your individual needs, who can attend you in your current location.

☐ You have declined consent to either assessment, treatment or transport.

Rarely, an apparently minor problem may reveal itself to be more serious than initially thought or may develop into a more serious condition. This may only become apparent over time so it is important that both the patient and carers remain vigilant.

Some general advice is given below and is applicable to all patients. Specific guidance for certain common conditions is also available and will be highlighted to you by the Ambulance crew.

General Advice

The following conditions are considered potentially life threatening. The patient or carer should dial **999** and ask for an ambulance if the patient:

- Stops breathing
- Loses consciousness
- Develops new or worsening chest pain
- Develops new or worsening difficulty in breathing
- Starts choking
- Develops heavy or uncontrollable blood loss
- Has a fit (unless he or she is a known epileptic and the fit follows the normal pattern for that individual)

If your condition does worsen but does not fall into one of the categories above or if you have **ANY** ongoing concerns then the best source of advice is NHS Direct, a confidential telephone service delivered by trained nursing staff, which is available 24 hours a day, 7 days a week on **08 45 46 47** or online at **www.nhsdirect.nhs.uk**. A self-help guide is also available on the back of your Thompson Local Directory.

For minor illness, your local pharmacist is a valuable source of information and is able to give advice and medication (as appropriate) for most common minor ailments.

Head Injury

Head injury is extremely common, especially in children. Most are minor but in rare cases complications may appear several hours or even days after the initial accident. You should dial **999** and ask for an ambulance if the patient:

- Becomes unconscious, confused, lethargic or unsteady on his/her feet
- Is difficult to wake up
- Has a fit
- Develops a very painful headache which will not go away

You should dial **08 45 46 47** and consult with NHS Direct if the patient:

- Becomes deaf in one or both ears or develops any problems with eyesight
- Develops bleeding from one or both ears
- Vomits

To help your recovery and ensure your safety you should:

- Remain with a responsible adult for the first 48 hours with access to a telephone
- Rest and avoid stressful situations
- Avoid alcohol and drugs except where prescribed by a healthcare professional
- Avoid contact sport for 3 weeks
- Avoid returning to work or operating complex machinery (including driving) until fully recovered

Neck Injury (Whiplash)

Whiplash is the result of a strain on the muscles and ligaments in the neck usually following a sudden deceleration such as a car or motorcycle accident. Given the nature of the incident that has caused your injury, you are advised to undergo a thorough medical assessment. The best treatment is the regular use of analgesia and anti-inflammatory drugs. Your GP or local pharmacist will be able to advise you on the most appropriate drugs for your condition. You should be aware that persistent neck pain can last for several weeks or longer. Professionally prescribed physiotherapy is also of great benefit. The traditional soft collar is of little proven benefit and is now rarely used. If the condition of the patient deteriorates significantly, particularly if there is loss of movement or sensation in a part of the body, then dial **08 45 46 47** and consult with NHS Direct.

Minor Illnesses (cough, cold, fever etc)

Most minor illness is just that and can be effectively treated at home by your GP or local pharmacist. There are, however, a number of pointers you should look out for which indicate a potentially more serious underlying condition. You should dial **999** and ask for an ambulance if the patient:

- Stops breathing
- Develops severe difficulty in breathing and/or the lips turn blue
- Becomes unconscious or, in the case of a child, limp or floppy
- Has a fit (lasting longer than 5 minutes if the patient is a known epileptic or prone to febrile convulsions – see below)
- Develops a rash which does not fade when you press a glass tumbler against it

For other symptoms, you should dial **08 45 46 47** and consult with NHS Direct.

Diabetes (hypoglycaemia)

Hypoglycaemia (a low blood sugar level) may occur in any person. Only known diabetic patients who have previously experienced such an episode are suitable to remain at home post-treatment. Most diabetic hypos can be treated in the home environment with oral carbohydrates or an injection of either glucagon or glucose. It is vitally important that any patient left at home after treatment takes longer acting carbohydrates (such as bread, wholegrain cereals or pasta) as soon as possible or a further episode may occur. Any patient suffering from recurrent hypos should seek medical advice from his/her GP or local diabetic clinic as a matter of urgency.

Fits / convulsions

Only patients with a known history of fitting are suitable to be left at home after treatment. Such patients are usually diagnosed epileptics or children between the ages of around 6 months and 6 years who have a fit secondary to a fever (known as febrile convulsions). You should dial **999** and ask for an ambulance if the patient:

- Has never had a fit before
- The patient is in a dangerous location (usually a public place such as the street etc.)
- Has a fit lasting longer than 5 minutes (in a patient known to suffer fits)
- Has a fit different in nature to that normal for the individual patient
- Is known to suffer prolonged fits requiring medical intervention (status epilepticus)
- Is a known diabetic
- Has developed a rash which does not fade if you push a glass tumbler against it

After a fit patients may be irritable (even aggressive) and often extremely tired. Prolonged periods of sleep are common but a responsible adult should keep an eye on the patient to ensure no further fit occurs and that no evidence of a more serious underlying condition appears over time.

Epileptic patients will usually require no further treatment beyond their prescribed medication, although this may need reviewing if the fits are becoming more frequent. In the case of febrile convulsions, paracetamol suspension may help to reduce fever and the risk of further fitting. This should **ONLY** be given in accordance with the information supplied on the packaging or by the pharmacist. **Paracetamol overdose can be fatal.** If you require any further advice or remain concerned about the condition of the patient, then you should dial **08 45 46 47** and consult with NHS Direct

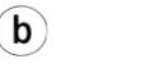

Figure 11-1, cont'd (b) Patient care report – back.

medical abbreviations that are not universally accepted should be avoided (Box 11-1).

There are professional and legal requirements to consider. The Health Professions Council (2008) provides clear requirements on the keeping of accurate records in their Standards of Conduct Performance and Ethics (Box 11-2).[1] Issues around confidentiality are also important and consideration of safe storage and transport must be given; the storage of PRFs on an ambulance between calls on a long shift is an example and care must be taken that PRFs from previous calls are secured in appropriate storage systems as soon as practicable; many emergency medical services (EMS) systems have policies that determine the appropriate methods of storage of PRFs. The Caldicott Report (1997)[2] and the NHS Confidentiality Code of Practice (2003)[3] discussed in Chapter 2 also provide appropriate guidance.

The PRF should include all dates and response times as well as describe any difficulties that were encountered (this should include while en route and during patient treatment, extrication, or transport.) In addition, the report should include observations at the scene, any previous healthcare provided (and by whom), and time of patient extrication, if appropriate (Box 11-3). The times of all significant occurrences and interventions are useful to the receiving healthcare staff. The paramedic should record these as well. In particular, the PRF provides a legal and accurate recording of the following incident times:

- time of call
- time of dispatch
- time of arrival at the scene
- time at patient's side
- time of vital sign assessments
- time(s) of medication administration and procedures
- time of departure from the scene
- time of arrival at the medical facility (when transporting a patient)
- time back in service.

The PRF may be the only way for a paramedic to recall events of an emergency call accurately during testimony that occurs years after the incident so the paramedic must include as much detail as possible in the PRF. This level of detail will be useful for present and future use. (See Chapter 2.)

Critical Thinking

Documentation of specific times on the patient care report is important. How can this information be useful?

The narrative

The narrative portion of the PRF allows for a chronological account of the call and should be written concisely and clearly, using simple words. The paramedic should avoid uncommon abbreviations, unnecessary terms, and duplicate information and use a standard format; this format helps ensure completeness and also assists in quality improvement reviews. Components of the narrative portion of the PRF may include the following:

- presenting complaint
- history of presenting complaint
- pertinent significant medical history (including drug history, allergies and family/social history as necessary)
- pertinent negative findings
- initial assessment and vital signs
- pertinent oral statements
- some patient care activities (including medications and treatments) not noted elsewhere on the form
- patient response to treatment
- vital sign reassessment
- electrocardiogram interpretation
- use of support services
- time and condition of patient on delivery.

Note

Documentation should never be used by the paramedic to construct patient care creatively; if the paramedic did not document the care, it was not done. Conversely, if the care was not done, the paramedic should not document it.

Pertinent negative findings may help to determine the course of treatment; these are findings that warrant no medical care or intervention and by seeking them and recording them the paramedic shows evidence of the thoroughness of the examination and history of the event. Examples of negative findings include the absence of diminished breath sounds, the absence of skin rashes, and the absence of abdominal tenderness. Pertinent oral statements are those made by the patient and other on-scene persons and the paramedic also should record these. Statements that may have an impact on patient care or resolution of the situation include the following:

- mechanism of injury
- patient's behaviour
- initial 'first aid' interventions before EMS arrival
- safety-related information (including disposition of weapons)
- disposal of valuable personal property (e.g. jewellery and wallets).

The paramedic should put into quotation marks on the PRF certain statements; for instance, any statements made directly by patients or others that relate to possible criminal activity, admissions of suicidal intention/ideation or failed skills (examples include unsuccessful attempts to start an intravenous line or to perform endotracheal intubation).

Critical Thinking

Why should you note the previous care given by bystanders in your report?

The narrative also should include the use of support services and mutual aid assistance. Such services might include helicopter services, Fire and Rescue, BASICS and other health and social care practitioners etc. The PRF should list everyone who took part in the patient's care before delivery to the emergency department. Finally, the paramedic should sign

Box 11-1

Common medical abbreviations used in EMS*

°C	degrees centigrade
°F	degrees Fahrenheit
µg	microgram
@	at
AAA	abdominal aortic aneurysm
ABG	arterial blood gas
ACS	acute coronary syndrome
ADL	activities of daily living
AED	automated external defibrillator
AF	atrial fibrillation
AIDS	acquired immune deficiency syndrome
ALS	advanced life support
am	morning
AMI	acute myocardial infarction
ARC	AIDS-related complex
ARDS	acute respiratory distress syndrome; adult respiratory distress syndrome
bid	2 times a day
BLS	basic life support
BM, bm	bowel movement
BP	blood pressure
BSA	body surface area
BVM	bag–valve–mask
c̄w	with
Ca	calcium; cancer; carcinoma
CABG	coronary artery bypass graft
CAD	coronary artery disease
cath.	catheter, catheterize
CC	chief complaint
cc	cubic centimetre
CCP	central chest pain; cardiac chest pain
CCU	coronary care unit; critical care unit
CF	cystic fibrosis
CHF	congestive heart failure
Cl	chlorine
cm	centimetre
cm^3	cubic centimetre
CN	cranial nerves
CNS	central nervous system
CO	carbon monoxide
c/o	complains of
CO_2	carbon dioxide
COPD	chronic obstructive pulmonary disease
CPAP	continuous positive airway pressure
CPR	cardiopulmonary resuscitation
CSF	cerebrospinal fluid
CT	computed tomography
CVA	cerebrovascular accident
CVP	central venous pressure
CVS	cardiovascular system
CXR	chest X-ray
D5W	5% dextrose in water
DIC	disseminated intravascular coagulation
DJD	degenerative joint disease
DH	drug history
DIB	difficulty in breathing
dL	decilitre
DTs	delirium tremens
DOB	date of birth
DNR	do not resuscitate
DVT	deep vein thrombosis
dx, DX	diagnosis
ECF	extracellular fluid
ECG	electrocardiogram
ECT	electroconvulsive therapy
ED	emergency department
EDC	estimated date of confinement
EDD	estimated date of delivery
EEG	electroencephalogram
ENT	ear nose and throat
ESR	erythrocyte sedimentation rate
ESRD	end-stage renal disease
FBC	full blood count
Fe	iron
FEV	forced expiratory volume
FH	family history
FHR	fetal heart rate
FRC	functional residual capacity
g, gm, Gm	gram
GI	gastrointestinal
gr	grain
grav I, II, III, etc.	pregnancy one, two, three, etc.
gt, gtt	drop, drops
GSW	gun shot wound
GU	genitourinary
GYN, Gyn	gynaecological
H_2O	water
H^+	hydrogen ion
Hx	history
h/o	history of
HAV	hepatitis A virus
Hb	haemoglobin
HBV	hepatitis B virus
Hct, HCT	haematocrit
HEENT	head eye ear nose and throat
Hg	mercury
Hgb	haemoglobin
HIV	human immunodeficiency (AIDS) virus
HPC	history of presenting complaint
HSV	herpes simplex virus
ICP	intracranial pressure
ICU	intensive care unit
IDDM	insulin-dependent diabetes mellitus
Ig	immunoglobulin
IgA, etc.	immunoglobulin A, etc.
IM	intramuscular
IPPV	intermittent positive pressure ventilation
IV	intravenous
IVP	intravenous pyelogram
JVD	jugular vein distension
JVP	jugular venous pressure
K	potassium
kg	kilogram
L	litre
LOC	level of consciousness
LBBB	left bundle branch block
LLQ	left lower quadrant
LMP	last menstrual period
LNMP	last normal menstrual period
LUQ	left upper quadrant
LVH	left ventricular hypertrophy
m	metre
MAP	mean arterial pressure
mcg	microgram
MCI	mass casualty incident
mg	milligram

Box 11-1

Common medical abbreviations used in EMS—cont'd

Mg	magnesium
MI	myocardial infarction
MICU	mobile intensive care unit
mL	millilitre
mm	millimetre
mm^3	cubic millimetre
mmHg	millimetres of mercury
MRI	magnetic resonance imaging
MS	multiple sclerosis
N	nitrogen
Na	sodium
NAD	no abnormality detected, no apparent distress
NBM	nil by mouth
NICU	neonatal intensive care unit
NPA	nasopharyngeal airway
NS	normal saline
NSAID	non-steroidal anti-inflammatory drug
NSR	normal sinus rhythm
O_2	oxygen
OD	overdose
OT	occupational therapy
OTC	over-the-counter
oz	ounce
$Paco_2$	partial pressure of carbon dioxide (arterial blood)
Pao_2	partial pressure of oxygen (arterial blood)
para I, II, etc.	unipara, bipara, etc.
PAT	paroxysmal atrial tachycardia
PC	presenting complaint
Pco_2	partial pressure of carbon dioxide
PE	pulmonary embolism; physical examination
PEEP	positive end-expiratory pressure
PERRLA	pupils equal, round, and reactive to light and accommodation
PG	prostaglandin
pH	hydrogen ion concentration (acidity and alkalinity)
PID	pelvic inflammatory disease
pm	evening
PMH	past medical history
PMI	point of maximal impulse
PMS	premenstrual syndrome
PND	paroxysmal nocturnal dyspnoea
PNS	peripheral nervous system
Po_2	partial pressure of oxygen
PO,	po orally
ppm	parts per million
prn	when required; as often as necessary
PT	prothrombin time
PTT	partial thromboplastin time
PUO	pyrexia of unknown origin
PVC	premature ventricular contraction
q	every
q2h	every 2 hours
q3h	every 3 hours
q4h	every 4 hours
qd	every day
qh	every hour
qid	4 times a day
qn	every night
qod	every other day
RA	rheumatoid arthritis
RBBB	right bundle branch block
RDS	respiratory distress syndrome
RHD	rheumatic heart disease
RLQ	right lower quadrant
ROM	range of motion
ROS	review of systems
RS	respiratory system
RTC	road traffic collision
RUQ	right upper quadrant
Rx	take, treatment
SC	subcutaneous
SH	social history
SICU	surgical intensive care unit
SIDS	sudden infant death syndrome
SOB	shortness of breath
STI	sexually transmitted infection
T&A	tonsillectomy and adenoidectomy
TB	tuberculosis
TIA	transient ischaemic attack
tid	3 times a day
TKVO	to keep vein open
URTI	upper respiratory tract infection
UTI	urinary tract infection
VF	ventricular fibrillation
VS	vital signs
VT	ventricular fibrillation, tidal volume
WBC	white blood cell; white blood count
WPW	Wolff–Parkinson–White syndrome

*Note: The abbreviations in common use can vary widely from place to place. Each service provider may have a list of acceptable abbreviations that is the best authority for its records. Caution must be exercised against abbreviations being misinterpreted by other practitioners.

Box 11-2

Importance of documentation

Written documentation provides for the following:

- A tangible record of the incident
- A legal record of the incident
- Professionalism
- Clinical audit, clinical governance, clinical effectiveness
- Quality improvement
- Collection of data

Box 11-3

Prehospital care report data

The prehospital care report data include the following:

- Dates and incident number
- Dispatch code
- Response times
- Difficulties en route
- Communication difficulties
- Scene observations
- Reasons for extended on-scene time
- Previous care provided
- Time of extrication
- Time of patient transport

the PRF. Because a copy of the report is placed in the patient's hospital medical record, leaving a completed copy at the receiving hospital will be necessary. This requires completing the report in a timely fashion at the receiving hospital so that the EMS crew can be available for another call.

> **Note**
>
> The patient report form is valuable; it provides the emergency department staff the advantage of understanding the events and the care rendered in the prehospital setting. The paramedic should leave the report with the patient at the hospital.

Elements of a properly written EMS document

A properly written EMS document is accurate, legible, timely, unaltered, and free of non-professional or extraneous information. A brief description of each of these elements is listed as follows:

1. *Sequential*. The PRF written section (narrative) should normally be completed in a chronological fashion.
2. *Accurate and complete*. All relevant information must be provided in the narrative and check-box sections of the report to ensure accuracy. Completing all areas of the report shows a precise and full document. The paramedic should ensure that medical terms, abbreviations, and acronyms are used properly and are spelled correctly.
3. *Legible*. Legible means that all writing, especially in the narrative part of the report, can be read easily by others. Check-box markings should be clear and consistent from the top page of the report to all underlying pages. In order to ensure this, *never* separate the pages from each other until the PRF is fully completed.
4. *Timely*. The documentation should be completed immediately after the paramedic completes the patient care and before another call is responded to. Delays in recording can result in serious omissions, which may be interpreted as negligent patient care.
5. *Unaltered*. If the paramedic makes errors while writing the report, the paramedic should draw a single line through the error and then the paramedic should date and initial the error (Figure 11-2). Any changes to a completed report should be accompanied by a proper 'revision/correction' supplement with the date and time of revision; procedures will vary but the local policy must be followed.
6. *Free of unprofessional/extraneous information*. The PRF must be free of jargon, slang, personal bias, libellous or slanderous remarks, and irrelevant opinion or impression. It is worth remembering that under UK legislation regarding access to healthcare records (Data Protection Act 1998) patients have a right to review any health records about them; this includes PRFs. The paramedic also should apply these principles of documentation to computer-generated PRFs (Figure 11-3).

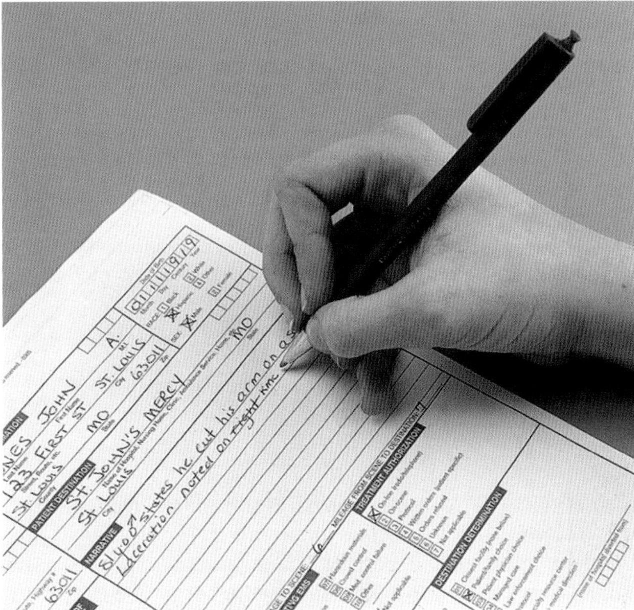

Figure 11-2 Correction of a patient care report.

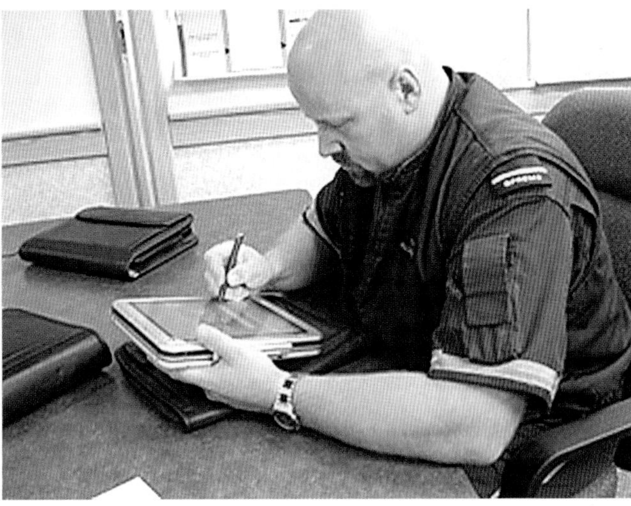

Figure 11-3 Paramedic completing an electronic patient care report.

7. It is recommended that the report is completed in permanent black ink as this is less likely to fade and should copies need to be made will be reproduced more clearly.
8. The person completing the PRF should carefully check it for completeness and accuracy before handing over the copy to the receiving unit/hospital (Box 11-4).

Systems of narrative writing

As with all other aspects of emergency care, the paramedic should develop a systematic approach for writing the narrative portion of the patient care report. Many approaches for writing the narrative can be used; however, the paramedic should adopt only one approach and use it consistently to avoid omissions in report writing. Examples of systems used to write the narrative include the SAMPLE history; SOAP

Box 11-4

Principles of professional record keeping

- Record times accurately.
- Be accurate and record factual information and avoid subjectivity, with direct quotes being placed in speech marks.
- Write clearly and legibly, with data presented chronologically or in an accepted format.
- The record should be completed as soon as is practicable and in any case before leaving the patient in the care of another healthcare professional.
- Mistakes should have a single line drawn through and be signed and dated so that the original can still be seen.
- Avoid jargon, inappropriate abbreviations and statements.
- Write in black ink.

format; CHART format; a physical approach from head to toe; a review of primary body systems; a chronological, call-incident approach; a patient management approach; and others. Regardless of the system used to organize the narrative, the paramedic must ensure that objective (versus subjective) elements of documentation make up the report.

Note

Some information is viewed as objective and can be supported by facts and direct observation; other information is viewed as subjective and cannot be supported by facts. An example of the latter is 'the patient appears depressed'. The paramedic generally should omit such information from the narrative. However, the paramedic should enter the information in the patient's own words using quotes. Some subjective observations should be documented carefully and reported to the receiving unit. An example is a child's behaviour that is suspicious for possible physical or sexual abuse in the home.

The SAMPLE history can be used to organize the narrative part of a written report. To review, the SAMPLE history is comprised of (S) signs and symptoms, (A) allergies, (M) medications, (P) past medical history, (L) last meal or oral intake, and (E) events before the emergency. Sometime the (S) component is not used, leaving AMPLE.

The SOAP format is a method one can use to organize a patient report for most patient care encounters. SOAP is an acronym for the following:

- Subjective data: All patient symptoms, including presenting complaint, associated symptoms, history, current medications and allergies, and information provided by bystanders and family.
- Objective data: Pertinent physical examination information, including vital signs, level of consciousness, physical examination findings, electrocardiogram, pulse oximetry readings, and blood glucose readings.
- Assessment data: The paramedic's clinical impression of the patient based on subjective and objective data.
- Plan of patient management: Treatment that has been provided and any requests for additional treatment.

The CHART format is an alternative to the SAMPLE and SOAP formats. The CHART format includes the following:

- Chief complaint: The patient's primary (presenting) complaint).
- History: History of presenting complaint; significant medical history; current health status; review of systems.
- Assessment: General impression; vital signs; physical examination; diagnostic tests; working impression.
- Rx (treatment): Interventions undertaken/given, effects of interventions.
- Transport: Mode of transportation; ongoing assessment findings, changes during transport.

The physical approach from head-to-toe often is used to organize the narrative after performing a full head-to-toe physical examination. Findings noted in the narrative are in the same order as they were in the exam; for example, the paramedic would begin by noting findings from examining the patient's hand, which, for example, may include looking for clubbing of fingers. The paramedic might end by noting, for example, circulatory findings, in the legs; the paramedic would note the character of a pedal pulse or capillary refill when examining the patient's extremities.

A review of primary body systems also can be used in the narrative; the paramedic may use this review when the examination is performed for a presenting complaint focused on one or two body systems. For example, this may be chest pain with suspected acute coronary syndrome. With this approach, the paramedic limits findings to the cardiac and respiratory systems; findings may include a description of the patient's pain, vital signs, electrocardiogram findings, associated breathing difficulties, significant medical history, allergies and medication use.

The chronological, call-incident approach for writing a narrative begins by noting the time of arrival at the patient's side and initial examination findings, the time of vital sign assessment and reassessment, and a chronological listing of all patient care interventions performed at the scene and en route to the emergency department; this type of report commonly is used to document the events of a patient with major trauma with extended on-scene time. The paramedic also may use this format during a cardiac arrest event when numerous medications and electrical therapy are administered to the patient.

The patient management approach is used to organize and record the complete patient management plan and runs from the start to the finish of an emergency response. This approach might describe in detail how the patient was found, any important assessment findings, and what interventions were performed and why. The patient management approach differs slightly from the others described as it provides a more complete picture of the events at the scene, during care, and during transport of the patient.

Critical Thinking

How many meanings can you think of for the word lethargic? Look it up in the dictionary. Should you use this word to document a patient's mental status? Why?

Special considerations of documentation

Several considerations for documenting patient care deserve special mention. Three of these include a patient's refusal of care or transport, situations and events where transportation is not needed, and situations involving mass casualties. Other situations that require careful documentation (e.g. caring for intoxicated patients and cases of abuse and neglect) are described in Chapters 2 and 40, respectively.

Patient refusal of care or transport

As described in Chapter 2, a patient's refusal of care or transport is a major area of potential liability for paramedics and ambulance services. Thorough documentation of these situations is crucial and should include the following:

- The paramedic's advice to the patient regarding the benefits of treatment and the risks associated with refusing care; the patient must be in receipt of sufficient information about their refusal and be able to comprehend any consequences of this refusal.
- The advice rendered by other healthcare professionals (such as the patient's GP, an 'out of hours' service or other agencies). It is good practice for the paramedic to discuss the patient with their own GP or the out of hours GP service if there is any concern about the patient's condition; this must be fully documented.
- Clinical information (e.g. the patient's level of consciousness) that suggests competency; there are certain circumstances where competence will be in question – for example, drug or alcohol intoxication, hypoglycaemia, and CNS conditions such as head injury.
- The signatures of any witnesses to the event, according to contemporary guidelines; it is good practice to have a witness present to corroborate events, especially if the patient refuses to sign the PRF.
- A complete narrative, including quotations or statements made by others, as well as clear evidence of full assessment and examination.

If the patient refuses care or transport, the paramedic should document the incident carefully. Key signs and symptoms should be identified to the patient and/or others around that would make it important to seek further help; these are often known as 'red flags'. The paramedic should make it clear that the patient may call again for help, despite the initial refusal, and advise about what signs or symptoms to look out for; this is known as 'safety netting'. Where possible, the paramedic should encourage friends or family to stay with the patient.

When care and transportation are not needed

At times, care and transportation of a patient are not warranted; this situation may be the result of the patient's condition or a cancelled request for help. After evaluation of the patient or scene, the paramedic may determine that circumstances do not warrant EMS transport (for example, for a car crash without injuries or a patient who has left the scene). At this point, the paramedic should advise the control room and document the event. If the EMS unit is cancelled en route to the scene, the paramedic should make note of the cancelling authority and time of the cancellation on any particular documentation that the service uses. The cancelling authority, for example, may be the control room or EMS supervisor, and detailed data of the cancellation will be held by the control room in the call notes. Like refusal of care, documentation of these events can protect the paramedic from potential liability.

Situations involving mass casualties

A major incident may involve a large number of patients and consequently comprehensive documentation may have to be postponed; triage tags and major incident cards may be used and it is important that paramedics are aware of the type used in their service. Fuller documentation may need to be delayed until patients are triaged and transported for definitive care (see Chapter 42). These are difficult and unusual situations and in these circumstances, the paramedic should know and follow local documentation procedures.

Document revision/correction

As stated before, revising or correcting a patient report form is sometimes necessary. Some ambulance services may provide separate report forms for this purpose; if a separate report is needed, the paramedic should do the following:

- Note the purpose of the revision or correction and why the information did not appear on the original document.
- Note the date and time the revision or correction was made.
- Ensure that the revision or correction was made by the original author of the document.
- Make the revision or correction as soon as the need for it is realized.

Acceptable methods for making revisions or adding information to a document vary by service. Some include making the change to the original form, including initials, date and time. Other methods include writing the corrections in the narrative or alternatively attaching a new report to the original. Supplemental narratives can be written on a separate form, which should be attached to the original. The paramedic should follow any policies set by their ambulance service for revising or correcting reports.

Consequences of inappropriate documentation

Documentation that is incorrect or incomplete may have serious consequences with medical and legal implications. An inaccurate, incomplete, or illegible PRF may cause caregivers to provide improper care to a patient. For example, consider that a paramedic fails to mention that a patient with a possible infection has an allergy to penicillin; this patient later becomes anaphylactic in the emergency department as a result of a drug given inadvertently. A PRF that is thoroughly completed in a professional manner may influence greatly the decision of a legal professional who is considering the merits of an impending civil action for negligence

Box 11-5

The paramedic's responsibility for documentation

As part of professional responsibility, the paramedic should do the following:

- View the task of documentation as one of utmost importance.
- Assume responsibility for self-assessment of all documentation.
- Appreciate the importance of good documentation among peers.
- Strive to set a good example to others regarding the completion of the documentation task.
- Respect the confidential nature of an emergency medical services report.

or malpractice; the converse also is true if the documentation is not thorough and professional.

Finally, documentation should never become routine to the paramedic (Box 11-5) nor be superficial. Good documentation should be completed in a timely manner and completed with careful attention to detail. This will ensure that the PRF is medically and legally sound.

Note

The patient report form is used effectively to document the essential elements of patient assessment, care, and transport. The report is a legal document. Most importantly, the report helps to ensure that the patient is provided good care and is the paramedic's best protection from liability action.

Presenting the patient (the patient 'handover')

The handover or presenting of the patient in the course of out-of-hospital and hospital care is twofold; it refers to the skills of effective communication as well as the effective transfer of patient information. The paramedic routinely provides patient presentation by face-to-face contact, over the telephone or radio, and in writing. These communication skills are essential and help the paramedic to establish trust and credibility with coworkers and other healthcare team members. Good handovers suggest effective patient assessment and care to the listener, and vice versa, whilst poor handovers can compromise patient care.[2–4] This may occur when the paramedic does not convey patient needs and condition effectively to other healthcare professionals. The following are characteristics of an effective patient presentation:

- The presentation is concise, usually lasting less than 1 minute.
- The presentation is usually free of extensive medical jargon.
- The presentation follows the same basic information pattern.
- The presentation generally follows a standard format.
- The presentation includes pertinent findings and pertinent negatives.

When communicating a patient presentation, the paramedic should begin the report with the end in mind. For instance, the paramedic should anticipate discrete areas of information that others will ask for and the paramedic should be ready to provide those details. For example, details required will usually include:

- patient identification, age, gender
- presenting complaint
- history of presenting complaint (key details)
- medical history (key details)
- vital signs (emphasize the abnormal)
- key pertinent positive and negative findings from clinical assessment
- working impression
- treatment and interventions (key aspects).

Practices will vary but in some emergency departments it may be common practice to give a basic handover to the senior member of staff for purposes of triage and then to provide a more detailed handover to the member of staff who will assess and care for the patient. In all cases ensure that the relevant information is given to the member of staff who needs to have it.

Critical Thinking

Can you think of any areas for improvement for your skills in 'handing over or presenting the patient'?

Electronic patient report forms

Many ambulance services are considering or have implemented some system of electronic patient reporting. The user of the system is provided with a robust and compact laptop or palm computer onto which is loaded patient report form software which allows, at the touch of a screen icon, inputting of patient data. This data can be downloaded via a wireless connection onto the receiving units systems to provide a more streamlined approach to records and patient reports.

Systems can also be adapted to allow the control room data of a call to be transferred directly into the laptop on the ambulance via integration of the mobile data terminal (MDT). It also allows 'live' data transmission from the ambulance to the receiving unit; as the data is inputted, the computer terminals in the emergency department can be updated with the patient details and condition as well as assessment findings and interventions given.

Other benefits are the possible use of clinical decision support systems, more effective clinical audit streams and recording of practitioner's skills and calls attended, as well as a better integration of patient medical notes based in hospitals.

Some aspects are still developmental but the principles of electronic report forms exist already and are being refined constantly.

Summary

- The patient report form (PRF) is used to document the key elements of patient assessment, care and transport.
- The three primary reasons for written documentation are that the healthcare community involved in the patient's care uses it, it is a legal record, and it is essential to data collection.
- The PRF should include dates and response times, difficulties encountered, observations at the scene, previous medical care provided, a chronological description of the call, and significant times.
- A properly written EMS document is accurate, legible, timely, unaltered, and free of non-professional or extraneous information.
- Many approaches for writing the narrative can be used. The paramedic should adopt only one approach. The paramedic should use this approach consistently to avoid omissions in report writing.
- Special documentation is necessary when a patient refuses care or transport. Such documentation is also needed in those cases when care or transportation is not needed. Special documentation is also needed for mass casualty incidents.
- There may be separate forms for revisions or corrections to the PRF.
- Documentation that is inappropriate may have medical and legal implications.

References

1. Health Professions Council 2008 Standards of conduct, performance and ethics. HPC, London
2. Bruce K, Suserud B-O 2005 The handover process and triage of ambulance borne patients: the experience of emergency nurses. Nurs Crit Care 10(4):201–209
3. Scott L, Brice J, Baker C, Shen P 2003 An analysis of paramedic referral reports to physicians in the emergency department trauma room. Prehosp Emerg Care 7:247–251
4. Jenkin A, Abelson-Mitchell N, Cooper S 2007 Patient handover; time for a change? Accid Emerg Nurs 15:141–147

Further reading

Angell L et al 2000 Documentation: the language of nursing. Prentice-Hall, Upper Saddle River, NJ

Department of Health 1997 The Caldicott committee: Report on the Review of Patient-Identifiable Information. Department of Health, London

Department of Health 2003 Confidentiality: NHS code of practice. Department of Health, London

Department of Health 2006 Records management: code of practice. Department of Health, London

Health Professions Council 2007 Standards of proficiency – paramedics. HPC, London

Marelli T, Harper S 2000 Nursing documentation handbook. Mosby, St Louis

Milewski R et al 2000 Documentation: field guide. Jones and Bartlett, Boston

PART THREE

CHAPTER 12

Pharmacology, Venous Access and Drug Administration

Part A: Pharmacology

Chapter contents

Objectives

Upon completion of this part, the paramedic student will be able to:

1. Explain what a drug is.
2. Identify the different types of drug names.
3. Outline drug standards and legislation pertinent to the paramedic profession.
4. Describe the paramedic's responsibilities in drug administration.
5. Distinguish among drug forms.
6. Identify the different routes for drug administration.
7. Discuss factors that influence drug absorption, distribution, and elimination.
8. Describe how drugs react with receptors to produce their desired effects.
9. List variables that can influence drug interactions.
10. Identify special considerations for administering pharmacological agents to pregnant patients, paediatric patients and older patients.
11. Outline drug actions and care considerations for a patient who is given drugs that affect the nervous, cardiovascular, respiratory, gastrointestinal and endocrine systems.
12. Outline drug actions and care considerations for a patient who is taking drugs used in infectious diseases and inflammation.
13. Explain the meaning of drug terms that are necessary to interpret information in drug references safely.

SECTION I

Drug information

Pharmacology

Today's paramedic has access to an increasing array of drugs for administration to patients and clearly has a need to understand how these drugs work, their interactions with other medications that the patient may already be taking, and the effects and side effects of the drugs being administered. In addition, paramedics need to have an understanding of the drugs commonly prescribed to patients as this may provide clues to the patient's condition as well as help to explain some of the findings during patient assessment.

Drug names

In medicine, a drug may be defined as '... any substance with the potential to prevent or cure disease or enhance physical or mental welfare, and in pharmacology to any chemical agent that alters the biochemical physiological processes of tissues or organisms'.[1] Drugs have been identified or derived from five major sources: plants (alkaloids, glycosides, gums, and oils), animals and human beings, minerals or mineral products, microorganisms, and chemical substances made in the laboratory (Box 12-1).

Drugs generally have at least three different names:

1. *Chemical name*: The chemical name is an exact description that describes the chemical composition and molecular structure of the drug, for example 7-chloro-1,3-dihydro-1-methyl-5-phenyl-2H-1,4-benzodiazepin-2-one.
2. *Generic name (non-proprietary name)*: This name is often an abbreviated form of the chemical name, such as diazepam, the generic name of the above-mentioned compound.
3. *Trade name (brand or proprietary name)*: The trade name is a trademark name designated by the drug company that sells the medication. Trade names are proper nouns, and the first letter is capitalized. An example of a trade name is Valium, which is diazepam.

Sources of drug information

Several publications offer information on various drugs, their preparation, and recommended administration. These references include the British National Formulary, the Joint Royal Colleges Ambulance Liaison Committee (JRCALC) guidelines (Box 12-2), medication package inserts, and numerous pharmacology textbooks. In addition, the National Poisons Information Service (NPIS) provides a round-the-clock service for health professionals engaged in the diagnosis, treatment and management of patients who have been poisoned. Paramedics should be familiar with these facilities and with other emergency pharmacology manuals as well. They should also be familiar with the drugs that are administered in prehospital care and the more commonly prescribed medications, e.g. antihypertensives. The internet can be a good source of information about pharmacotherapeutics but caution needs to be applied regarding the source of the information. Although the internet usually

Box 12-1

Examples of drugs and their sources

Plant sources	Animal and human sources
Digoxin	Adrenaline (epinephrine)
Morphine sulphate	Insulin
Atropine sulphate	Adrenocorticotropic hormone
Mineral or mineral product	**Microorganism sources**
Calcium chloride	Penicillin
Iodine	Streptomycin
Iron	
Sodium bicarbonate	
Laboratory-produced chemicals	
Diazepam	
Lidocaine	
Midazolam	

Box 12-2

Drug references

Joint Royal Colleges Ambulance Liaison Committee (JRCALC): Provides information on the drugs available for use by paramedics in the UK. The Committee provide the guidelines that should ordinarily be followed by paramedics in the management of patients.

British National Formulary: The BNF is a manual published by the British Medical Association and Royal Pharmaceutical Society of Great Britain and provides information on all drugs approved for use in the UK. It is updated twice yearly and is also available online. The BNF is considered by many to be the most reliable source of information on medications and drugs.

Medication package inserts: Most medications are packaged with written literature describing product use. These inserts provide valuable information as new drugs are introduced, and the healthcare professional should consult them to become familiar with the product.

National Poisons Information Service: This service comprises six regional centres providing a year-round 24-h service for healthcare staff. They can provide information on the diagnosis, treatment and management of patients who may have been poisoned. Advice can be sought online or via telephone.

Pharmacology textbooks: There is a wide selection of pharmacology textbooks aimed at the healthcare professional. It is recommended that the paramedic selects a book that reflects legislation and nomenclature current in their country of practice.

provides the most up-to-date information, it is imperative that paramedics use only reliable sources.

Drug administration and the law

In Britain, the main pieces of legislation that regulate the use of all medicines include the Medicines Act 1968, the Misuse of Drugs Act 1971, and the Misuse of Drugs Regulations 1985. Amendments have been made to some of these Acts as circumstances and the needs of practitioners and patients have changed, but they remain the foundations of legislation relevant to paramedic practice.

The Medicines Act 1968

This Act controls the manufacture and distribution of all medicines for human and animal use. Responsibility for administration of the Act falls on the incumbent Health and Agricultural Ministers who receive advice from the Commission on Human Medicines. This body was established on 30 October 2005 and combines the functions of the older Medicines Commission and the Committee on Safety of Medicines.

The Act places drugs into three classes:

- General sales list (GSL) – these are medications that can be sold to the public without the supervision of a pharmacist.
- Pharmacy medicines (P) – these may only be sold under supervision of a pharmacist.
- Prescription only medicines (POM) – these may be sold or supplied only in accordance with a prescription from an appropriate practitioner. Nobody may administer a POM except the named patient, an appropriate practitioner, or a person acting in accordance with the directions of a practitioner.
An exemption under part III to schedule 5 of the Prescriptions Only Medicines (Human Use) Order 1997 allows suitably trained paramedics to administer certain drugs in specified circumstances.

The Misuse of Drugs Act 1971

The Act came into operation on 1 July 1973 and serves to regulate the import, export, possession, production and supply of drugs deemed to be dangerous or harmful; it also consolidates and extends earlier legislation. This legislation is largely restrictive and serves to render as unlawful all activities associated with the drugs save for activities provided for under the Act. Drugs that fall within the remit of this Act are termed Controlled Substances and are classified according to the degree of danger they are believed to pose. The use of these drugs in medicine is permitted by the Misuse of Drugs Regulations 1985. The drugs are classified into five schedules in descending order of control; the most stringent controls apply to those in Schedule 1.[2] Morphine is a class A controlled drug under Schedule 2 of the Act; storage, prescription and administration must all be documented in accordance with the Act.[3] It is essential that paramedics are familiar with the procedures required for all drugs but especially for controlled drugs.

Drug regulatory agencies

The main regulating body in the UK is the Medicines and Healthcare products Regulatory Agency (MHRA). The MHRA is a Government agency charged with ensuring that medicines and medical devices work and are acceptably safe.[4] It maintains a watch on medicines and devices and takes action where appropriate. It also aims to make as much information as possible available publicly. The MHRA subjects any new medicines to rigorous scrutiny before they can be used on patients to ensure that they meet standards of quality, safety and efficacy.

National Institute for Health and Clinical Excellence (NICE)

NICE is an independent organization responsible for providing national guidance on the promotion of good health and the prevention and treatment of ill-health.[5] NICE produces guidance in three areas of health: public health, health technology and clinical practice. Once NICE publishes clinical guidance, including the use of drugs, health professionals and their employing organizations are expected to take it fully into account when deciding what treatments to give people.

Critical Thinking

Your patient is acutely ill. She reports taking only a herbal medicine, which is not found in standard drug reference materials. Where can you or the medical staff find information about these alternative therapies?

SECTION II

Mechanisms of drug action

General properties of drugs

Drugs may act in the body in many ways. Some of these actions are desirable (a therapeutic effect) whilst others are considered undesirable or even harmful (a side effect). Drugs may also interact with other drugs and may produce uncommon and sometimes unpredictable effects. In addition, drugs generally exert several effects rather than a single one.

Note

To perform a thorough patient assessment is critical. The paramedic must also obtain a pertinent medical (and drug) history from the patient. Being able to recognize and understand the reasons why certain drugs are prescribed for certain conditions or diseases is important for the paramedic. This knowledge can be important when forming a field impression of what is wrong with a patient based on the assessment and physical findings. With the knowledge of what drugs do, the paramedic should be able to use the right drug to manage the illness, disease, or condition.

One should note that drugs do not confer any new functions on a tissue or organ; they only modify existing functions. The actions of a drug are achieved by a biochemical interaction between the drug and certain tissue components in the body (usually receptors). A drug that interacts with a receptor to stimulate a response is known as an agonist. A drug that attaches to a receptor but does not stimulate a response is called an antagonist. Box 12-3 contains other pharmacological terms and their definitions.

To produce the desired effect, a drug must enter the body and reach appropriate concentrations at its site of action. This process is influenced by three phases of drug activity: the pharmaceutical phase, the pharmacokinetic phase, and the pharmacodynamic phase.

Pharmaceutical phase

Pharmaceutics is the science of preparing and dispensing drugs. One aspect of this field is the study of the ways in which the forms of drugs (solid or liquid) influence pharmacokinetic and pharmacodynamic activities (described in the following sections). All drugs must be in solution to cross the cell membranes to achieve absorption. The term dissolution refers to the rate at which a solid drug goes into solution after ingestion. The faster the rate of dissolution, the more quickly the drug is absorbed.

Pharmacokinetic phase

Pharmacokinetics is the study of how the body handles a drug over a period of time. This includes the processes of absorption, distribution, biotransformation, and excretion. These factors affect a patient's response to drug therapy.

Box 12-3

Pharmacological terminology

Antagonism: the opposition of effects between two or more medications that occurs when the combined (conjoint) effect of two drugs is less than the sum of the drugs acting separately

Contraindications: medical or physiological factors that make it harmful to administer a medication that would otherwise have therapeutic value

Cumulative action: the tendency for repeated doses of a drug to accumulate in the blood and organs, causing increased and sometimes toxic effects; it occurs when several doses are administered or when absorption occurs more quickly than removal by excretion or metabolism

Depressant: a substance that decreases a body function or activity

Drug allergy: a systemic reaction to a drug resulting from previous sensitizing exposure and the development of an immunological mechanism

Drug dependence: a state in which withdrawal of a drug produces intense physical or emotional disturbance; previously known as habituation

Drug interaction: beneficial or detrimental modification of the effects of one drug by the prior or concurrent administration of another drug that increases or decreases the pharmacological or physiological action of one or both drugs

Idiosyncrasy: abnormal or peculiar responses to a drug (accounting for 25–30% of all drug reactions) thought to result from genetic enzymatic deficiencies or other unique physiological variables and leading to abnormal mechanisms of drug metabolism or altered physiological effects of the drug

Potentiation: the enhancement of effect caused by the concurrent administration of two drugs in which one drug increases the effect of the other drug

Side effect: undesirable and often unavoidable effect of using therapeutic doses of a drug; action or effect other than those for which the drug was originally given

Stimulant: a drug that enhances or increases body function or activity

Summation: the combined effect of two drugs such that the total effect equals the sum of the individual effects of each agent:

$$(1+1=2)$$

Synergism: the combined action of two drugs such that the total effect exceeds the sum of the individual effects of each agent:

$$(1+1=3 \text{ or more})$$

Therapeutic action: the desired, intended action of a drug

Tolerance: decreased physiological response to the repeated administration of a drug or chemically related substance, possibly necessitating an increase in dosage to maintain a therapeutic effect (tachyphylaxis)

Untoward effect: a side effect that proves harmful to the patient

Drug absorption

Absorption involves the movement of drug molecules from the entry site to the general circulation. The degree to which drugs attain pharmacological activity depends partly on the rate and extent to which they are absorbed. The rate and extent in turn depend on the ability of the drug to cross the cell membrane through the processes of passive diffusion and active transport. Most drugs enter the cell by passive diffusion although some require a carrier-mediated mechanism to assist them across the membrane.

Absorption begins at the site of administration. The rate and extent of absorption depend on the following factors:[6]

1. *The nature of the absorbing surface (cell membrane) the drug must traverse.* If a drug must pass through a single layer of cells such as the intestinal epithelium, transport is faster than if the drug must pass through several layers of cells (e.g. the skin). In addition, the greater the surface area of the absorbing site, the greater the absorption and the quicker the drug takes effect. For example, the small intestine offers a large absorption area, whereas the stomach has a relatively small absorption surface area.
2. *Blood flow to the site of administration.* A rich blood supply enhances absorption, and a poor blood supply delays it. For example, a patient with diminished blood flow may not respond to intramuscular administration of a drug because diminished circulation reduces absorption. In contrast, intravenous administration of a drug immediately places the drug in the circulatory system, where it is absorbed completely and delivered to its target tissue.
3. *The solubility of the drug.* The more soluble the drug, the more rapidly it is absorbed. For example, drugs that are prepared in oily solutions are absorbed more slowly than drugs dissolved in water or in isotonic sodium chloride.
4. *The pH of the drug environment.* In solution, many drugs exist in an ionized (electrically charged) and non-ionized (uncharged) form. A non-ionized drug is lipid (fat) soluble and readily diffuses across the cell membrane. An ionized drug is lipid insoluble and generally does not cross the cell membrane. Most drugs do not ionize fully following administration, rather they reach equilibrium between their ionized and non-ionized forms, allowing for the non-ionized form to be absorbed. How and to what extent a drug ionizes depends on whether the drug is an acid or a base. An acidic drug such as aspirin is relatively non-ionized and does not dissociate well in an acidic environment (e.g. the stomach) and therefore is absorbed easily there. A drug that is basic in the same acidic environment tends to ionize and is not absorbed easily through the gastric membrane. The reverse occurs when the drug is in an alkaline medium.
5. *The drug concentration.* Drugs administered in high concentrations tend to be absorbed more rapidly than those administered in low concentrations. In some situations, administration of a large dose (loading dose) first that temporarily exceeds the capacity for excretion of the drug is necessary. This rapidly establishes a therapeutic drug level at the receptor site. A smaller dose (maintenance dose) can then be administered to replace the amount of drug excreted. Thus, loading doses are based more on the volume of distribution (of which body size is an important component) and less on capacity for excretion (e.g. renal failure). Maintenance doses are exactly the opposite.

Critical Thinking

Consider a common condition seen in the prehospital setting. This condition requires that drugs be given at higher than usual doses to achieve therapeutic levels. What is the condition?

6. *The form of the drug dosage.* Drug absorption can be manipulated by pharmaceutical processing. An example is a combination of an active drug with another substance that is slowly released or a drug that resists digestive action (enteric coatings).

Routes of drug administration

The mode of drug administration affects the rate at which onset of action occurs and may also affect the resulting therapeutic response. The routes of drug administration are categorized as follows:

- enteral (administration along any portion of the gastrointestinal tract)
- parenteral (administration by any route other than the gastrointestinal tract)
- pulmonary (administration by inhalation or through an endotracheal tube)
- topical (administration by application to the skin and mucous membranes).

The route of administration greatly influences drug absorption (Table 12-1) and is discussed later in this chapter.

Enteral route

Drugs administered along any portion of the gastrointestinal tract are said to use the enteral route (Box 12-4). Administration may be orally, rectally, or through a nasogastric tube.

Table 12-1 Comparison of drug absorption rates by common routes of administration

Route	Rate of absorption
Enteral	Slow
Sublingual	Rapid
Subcutaneous	Slow
Intramuscular	Moderate
Intravenous	Immediate (no absorption required)
Endotracheal	Rapid
Intraosseous	Immediate
Pulmonary	Rapid
Topical	Moderate

Box 12-4

Some emergency drugs administered via the enteral route

Activated charcoal
Aspirin

The enteral method is the safest, most convenient route, yet is also the least reliable and slowest of the common routes because of the frequent changes in the gastrointestinal environment (e.g. with food contents, emotional state, and physical activity). This route allows for four types of absorption: oral absorption, gastric absorption, absorption from the small intestine, and rectal absorption.

Oral absorption

The oral cavity has a rich blood supply; however, little absorption normally occurs in the mouth. Certain drugs, such as glyceryl trinitrate (GTN) tablets and some hormones, are prepared for oral absorption. When administered by sublingual or buccal routes, these drugs rapidly dissolve in the salivary secretions and are absorbed by the oral mucosa. Drugs that are absorbed in the upper gastrointestinal tract enter the systemic circulation and initially bypass gastrointestinal fluids and the liver. Drugs absorbed in the stomach and intestines are absorbed into the portal vein system of the liver and are subject to first-pass metabolism (described later) in the liver. In the sublingual route the medicine is placed under the tongue and the tablet or spray dissolves in the salivary secretions. The effects of sublingual medication are usually clear within a few minutes. With buccal administration the drug is placed between the teeth and mucous membrane of the cheek. As in the sublingual route, absorption by buccal administration usually is rapid.

Critical Thinking

Glyceryl trinitrate spray may be more effective in older patients than the tablet form. Why do you think this is the case?

Gastric absorption

The stomach has a rich blood supply but is not considered an important site of drug absorption. The length of time a medication remains in the stomach varies depending on the pH of the environment and gastric motility. As previously described, weakly acidic drugs tend to remain non-ionized and are readily absorbed into the circulation. In comparison, basic drugs ionize in the stomach and are poorly absorbed. Altering the gastric emptying rate may alter the rate and extent of drug absorption. Many drugs are administered on an empty stomach with sufficient water (225 mL) to ensure rapid passage into the small intestine. Other drugs cause gastric irritation and are usually given with food.

Absorption from the small intestine

The small intestine has a rich blood supply and a larger absorption area than the stomach. Most drug absorption occurs in the upper part of the small intestine. The pH of intestinal fluid is alkaline, which increases the rate of absorption of basic drugs. Prolonged exposure allows more time for drug absorption. An increase in intestinal motility (e.g. diarrhoea) decreases exposure to the intestinal membrane and diminishes absorption.

Box 12-5

Examples of emergency drugs administered via the parenteral route

Amiodarone
Atropine
Dextrose 10%
Diazepam
Adrenaline (epinephrine)
Furosemide
Lidocaine
Morphine
Naloxone
Oxytocin

Rectal absorption

The surface area of the rectum is not large; however, the rectum is vascular and capable of drug absorption. Drugs administered rectally are subject to erratic absorption because of rectal contents, local drug irritation, and the uncertainty of drug retention. Fifty percent of a drug that has been administered rectally is estimated to bypass the liver after absorption. This makes first-pass metabolism by the liver less than that of an orally given dose.

Critical Thinking

The drugs given rectally in emergencies are usually anticonvulsants. Why do you think this route would be chosen over the oral or intravenous route?

Parenteral route

Drugs administered by injection are said to use the parenteral route (Box 12-5). The commonly used parenteral routes for administering medications include the following:

1. *Subcutaneous route*: a subcutaneous injection is given beneath the skin into the connective tissue or fat immediately beneath the dermis. This route is used only for small volumes of drugs (0.5 mL or less) that do not irritate tissue. The rate of absorption is usually slow and can provide a sustained effect.
2. *Intramuscular route*: an intramuscular injection is given into the skeletal muscle. Absorption generally occurs more rapidly than with a subcutaneous injection because of greater tissue blood flow.
3. *Intravenous route*: an intravenous injection is given directly into the bloodstream, bypassing the absorption process. This route produces an almost immediate pharmacological effect. Most intravenous drugs should be administered slowly to help prevent adverse reactions.
4. *Intradermal route*: an intradermal injection is made just below the epidermis. This route is used primarily for allergy testing and to administer local anaesthetics.

5. *Intraosseous route*: an intraosseous injection is given directly into the bone marrow cavity of paediatric (and occasionally adult) patients through an established intraosseous infusion system. Agents infused by this method are thought to circulate via the medullary cavity of the bone. Through the numerous venous channels of long bones, fluids or drugs rapidly enter the central circulation. The length of time from injection to entry into the systemic circulation is thought to equal that of the intravenous route.[7] Emergency medications known to be effective when administered via the intraosseous route include adrenaline (epinephrine) and atropine.
6. *Endotracheal route*: access to the endotracheal route is generally through an endotracheal tube, which allows drug delivery into the alveoli and systemic absorption via the capillaries of the lungs. Because of the large surface area of the alveolar sacs, the rate of absorption by this route is almost as rapid as that of the intravenous route. Administration of drugs via an endotracheal tube is usually reserved for situations in which an intravenous line cannot be established. Medications that can be administered by the endotracheal tube include lidocaine, adrenaline (epinephrine), atropine, and naloxone. This route is erratic and less reliable than intravenous or intraosseous delivery and should therefore be used in adult patients only if first-line routes are unavailable.[8] Drug doses should be doubled when given by this route,[3] although it is suggested that the dose of adrenaline (epinephrine) should be 3 mg diluted to at least 10 mL with sterile water.[8] The paramedic should follow current Trust and JRCALC guidelines.

Note

A mnemonic for the four medications that may be administered via the pulmonary route through an endotracheal tube is LEAN, which stands for lidocaine, epinephrine, atropine and naloxone.

Pulmonary route

Medication can be administered by inhalation. The medication can be in the form of gas or fine mist (aerosol). The most commonly used inhalation medications are bronchodilators (Box 12-6). However, the pulmonary circulation can absorb a number of other medications if necessary, such as drugs for endotracheal administration.

Because of the large surface area and the rich capillary network of the alveoli, drug absorption into the bloodstream is rapid. Bronchodilators and steroids can be given by inhalation devices, such as a nebulizer (described later in this chapter). A nebulizer propels the drug into alveolar sacs. Drugs that are given by a nebulizer device produce mainly local effects but can occasionally produce unwanted systemic effects. An example of these effects is tachycardia, which may be caused by salbutamol.

Box 12-6

Emergency drugs administered via the pulmonary route

Salbutamol
Ipratropium bromide
Entonox
Oxygen

Topical route

In most cases, drugs applied topically to the skin and mucous membranes are absorbed rapidly. They are intended to produce a local effect, such as tetracaine for reducing pain during venepuncture. Only lipid-soluble compounds are absorbed through the skin as the skin acts as a barrier to most water-soluble compounds. To prevent adverse systemic effects, intact skin surfaces should be used as an administration site. Massaging the skin helps to promote drug absorption as the capillaries dilate and local blood flow increases.

Drug distribution

Distribution is the transport of a drug through the bloodstream. The drug is transported to various tissues of the body and ultimately to its site of action. After a drug has entered the circulatory system, it is distributed rapidly throughout the body. The rate at which distribution occurs depends on the permeability of capillaries to the drug molecules.

To review, lipid-soluble drugs readily cross capillary membranes to enter most tissues and fluid compartments. Lipid-insoluble drugs require more time to arrive at their point of action. Cardiac output and regional blood flow also affect the rate and extent of distribution into body tissues. Generally, a drug is distributed first to organs that have a rich blood supply. These organs include the heart, liver, kidneys and brain. Then, depending on its composition, the drug enters tissue with a lesser blood supply, such as muscle and fat.

Drug reservoirs

Drugs may accumulate at certain locations that act as storage sites. At these sites the drugs form reservoirs by binding to specific tissues. As serum levels decline, tissue-bound drug is released from its storage site into the bloodstream. The released drug maintains the desired serum drug levels and may permit sustained release of the drug over time. This allows continued pharmacological effect at the receptor site. The two general processes that create drug reservoirs are plasma protein binding and tissue binding.

As drugs enter the circulatory system, they may attach to plasma proteins (mainly albumin), forming a drug–protein complex.

The extent to which this binding occurs affects the intensity and duration of the effect of the drug. The albumin molecule is too large to diffuse through the membrane of the blood vessel, thus albumin traps the bound drug in the bloodstream. A drug bound to plasma protein is pharmacologically inactive so the protein becomes a circulating drug reservoir. The free drug (unbound drug) exists in proportion to the protein-bound fraction and is the only portion of the drug that is biologically active. As the free drug is eliminated from the body, the drug–protein complex dissociates, and more drug is released to replace the free drug that was metabolized or excreted. This process is summarized in the following equation:

$$\text{Free drug} + \text{protein} \leftrightarrow \text{drug–protein complex}$$

Albumin and other plasma proteins provide a number of binding sites. Yet two drugs can compete for the same site and displace each other. Certain combinations of drugs may be given at the same time. As a result, this competition can have serious consequences. For example, a patient taking the anticoagulant drug warfarin may be given aspirin, which displaces some of the protein-bound warfarin and increases free drug and, thus, activity.

Other factors that influence the binding ability of a drug include the concentration of plasma proteins (especially albumin), the number of binding sites on the protein, the affinity of the drug for the protein, and the acid–base balance of the patient. Various disease states, such as liver disease, alter the ability of the body to handle many medications. These alterations result from a decrease in serum albumin levels (albumin is manufactured by the liver) and a decrease in hepatic metabolism. These and other factors may result in more free drug being available for distribution to tissue sites (increased free drug fraction and enhanced pharmacological response).

A second type of 'drug pooling' occurs in fat tissue and bone. Lipid-soluble drugs have a high affinity for adipose tissue, where these drugs are stored. Because fat tissue has low blood flow, it serves as a stable reservoir for drugs. Some lipid-soluble drugs can remain in body fat for as long as 3 h after administration. Other drugs (e.g. tetracycline) have an unusual affinity for bone and accumulate in bone after being absorbed onto the bone crystal surface.

Critical Thinking

Tetracycline typically is not given to pregnant women because of the harmful effects it has on the development of the baby's teeth. Why would it affect the teeth?

Barriers to drug distribution

The blood–brain barrier and the placental barrier are protective membranes. These membranes prevent the passage of certain drugs into these body sites. The blood–brain barrier consists of a single layer of capillary endothelial cells that line the blood vessels entering the central nervous system. The cells are tightly joined at common borders by continuous intercellular junctions and this special arrangement permits only lipid-soluble drugs to be distributed into the brain and cerebrospinal fluid. Examples of such drugs are general anaesthetics and barbiturates. Drugs that are poorly soluble in fat (e.g. many antibiotics) have trouble passing this barrier so cannot enter the brain.

The placental barrier is made up of membrane layers, which separate the blood vessels of the mother and the fetus. Like the blood–brain barrier, the placental barrier is impermeable to many lipid-insoluble drugs so offers some protection to the fetus. However, the placenta does allow the passage of certain non-lipid-soluble drugs such as steroids, narcotics, anaesthetics, and some antibiotics. If these drugs are given to the pregnant mother, they may affect the developing embryo or fetus or the neonate.

Biotransformation

After absorption and distribution, the body eliminates most drugs, first by biotransformation and then by excretion. Biotransformation (metabolism) is a process in which the drug is chemically converted to a metabolite. The purpose of biotransformation is usually to 'detoxify' a drug and render it less active. The liver is the primary site of drug metabolism; however, other tissues can also be involved, including the plasma, kidneys, lungs and the intestinal mucosa.

Orally administered drugs that are absorbed through the gastrointestinal tract normally travel to the liver before entering the general circulation. When this occurs, a large amount of the drug may be metabolized (first-pass metabolism) before reaching the systemic circulation. This reduces the amount of drug that is available for distribution in the body. Medications affected by this initial biotransformation in the liver may be given in higher dosages or administered parenterally (intravenously or intramuscularly) to bypass the liver.

Individuals metabolize drugs at variable rates. For example, patients with liver, renal, or cardiovascular disease are expected to have prolonged drug metabolism. Infants with immature metabolic capacity and older adults with degenerative metabolic function experience depressed biotransformation. If drug metabolism is delayed, drug accumulation and cumulative drug effects may occur. Therefore the paramedic may need to consider dosage reductions (particularly maintenance doses) for patients in these categories (Figure 12-1).

Excretion

Excretion is the elimination of toxic or inactive metabolites. The kidney is the primary organ for excretion, although the intestine, lungs, and mammary, sweat, and salivary glands may also be involved.

Excretion by the kidneys

A drug can be excreted in the urine unchanged or as a chemical metabolite of its previous form. Renal excretion consists of three mechanisms: passive glomerular filtration, active tubular secretion, and partial reabsorption (Figure 12-2).

Passive glomerular filtration is a simple filtration process and can be measured as the glomerular filtration rate (GFR). The GFR is the total quantity of glomerular filtrate formed each minute in all nephrons of both kidneys (this measure is usually expressed in millilitres). The availability of a drug for glomerular filtration depends on its free concentration in plasma. Unbound drugs and water-soluble metabolites are filtered by the glomeruli; drugs highly bound to protein do not pass through this structure.

After filtration, lipid-soluble compounds are reabsorbed by the renal tubules, thus they re-enter the systemic circulation. Water-soluble compounds are not reabsorbed so are eliminated from the body. Because of the proportional relationship between free and bound drug, as free drug is filtered from the blood, bound drug is released from its binding sites into the plasma. The rate of excretion and the biological half-life of the drug (described later in this chapter) depend on how quickly the bound drug is released.

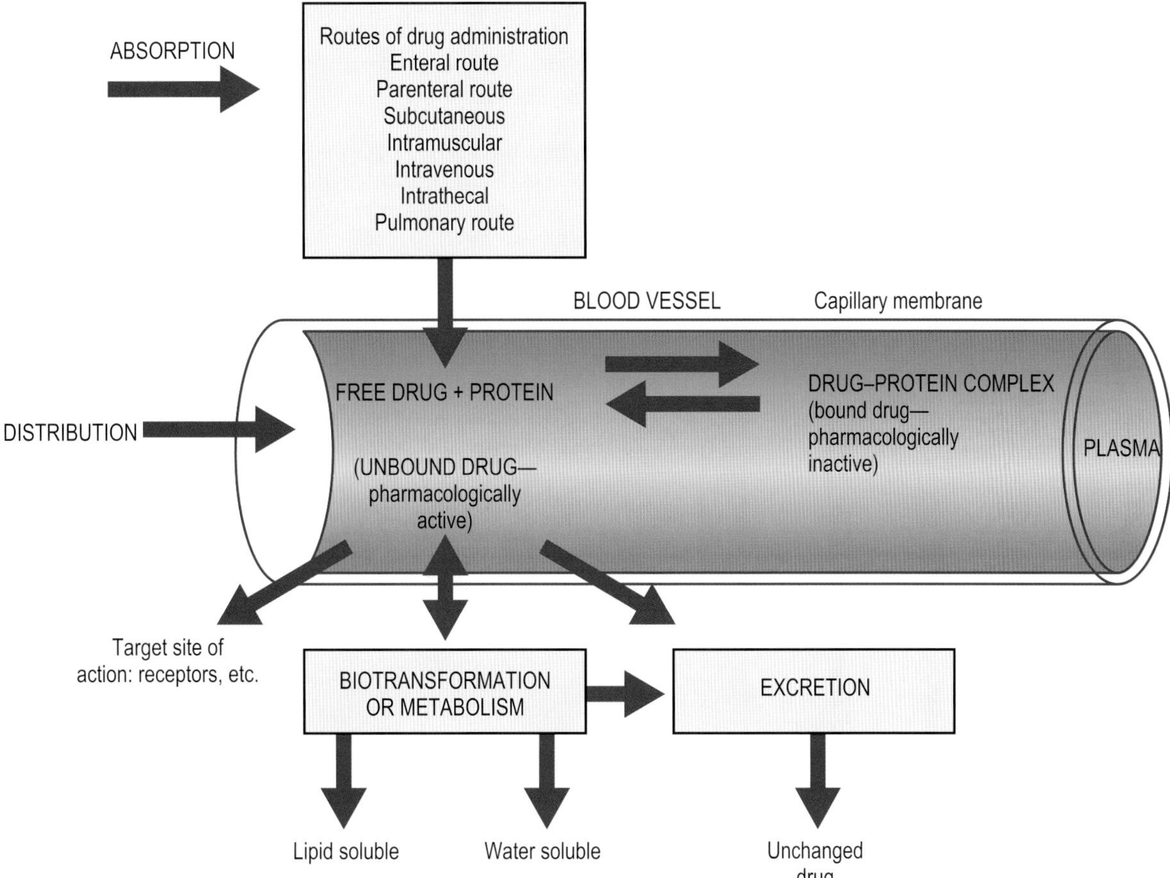

Figure 12-1 Pharmacokinetic phase of drug action, showing absorption, distribution, biotransformation, and excretion of drugs. Only free drug is capable of movement for absorption, distribution to the target site of action, biotransformation, and excretion. The drug–protein complex represents bound drugs; because the molecule is large, it is trapped in the blood vessel and serves as a storage site for the drug.

Critical Thinking

You pick up your patient at the renal dialysis centre. How will you know which medicines you can administer safely?

Active tubular secretion occurs in the renal tubules, where free drug can be transported or secreted from the blood across the structure called the proximal tubule, and from there deposited in the urine. Drugs actively secreted by the renal tubules can compete with other drugs for the same active transport process. An example of competitive drug interaction is that between amiodarone and digoxin. The first drug reduces the removal or clearance of the second drug. (The term clearance refers to the complete removal of a drug by the kidneys.) The result of this competition for removal is an increase in the plasma concentration of the second drug.

Partial reabsorption is the reabsorption from the renal tubule by passive diffusion. Such reabsorption can be influenced greatly by the pH of the tubular urine. Weak acids are excreted more readily in alkaline urine and more slowly in acidic urine. This is because they are ionized in alkaline urine but non-ionized in acidic urine. The reverse is true for weak bases. For example, an increase in urinary pH decreases the reabsorption and increases the clearance of weak acids such as furosemide and aspirin. However, a decrease in urinary pH increases the clearance of weak bases such as amphetamine and tricyclic antidepressants.

As a rule, substances that are completely or almost completely excreted by the normal kidney can be removed by an artificial process that resembles glomerular filtration; this process is haemodialysis. (Chapter 20 describes haemodialysis further.) Haemodialysis can be used to remove a wide variety of substances but is not effective for drugs that are highly tissue or protein bound and is of only limited benefit for the removal of rapidly acting toxins.

Excretion by the intestine

Drugs are eliminated through the intestine by biliary excretion. After liver metabolism the metabolites are carried in bile, passed into the duodenum and eliminated with the faeces. Some drugs are reabsorbed by the bloodstream, returned to the liver and then later excreted by the kidneys.

Excretion by the lungs

Some drugs, such as general anaesthetics, volatile alcohols, and inhaled bronchodilators, can be eliminated by the lungs. Certain factors alter drug elimination via the lungs; these include the rate and depth of respiration and cardiac output. Deep breathing and an increase in cardiac output (which increases pulmonary blood flow) promote excretion. However, respiratory compromise and decreased cardiac

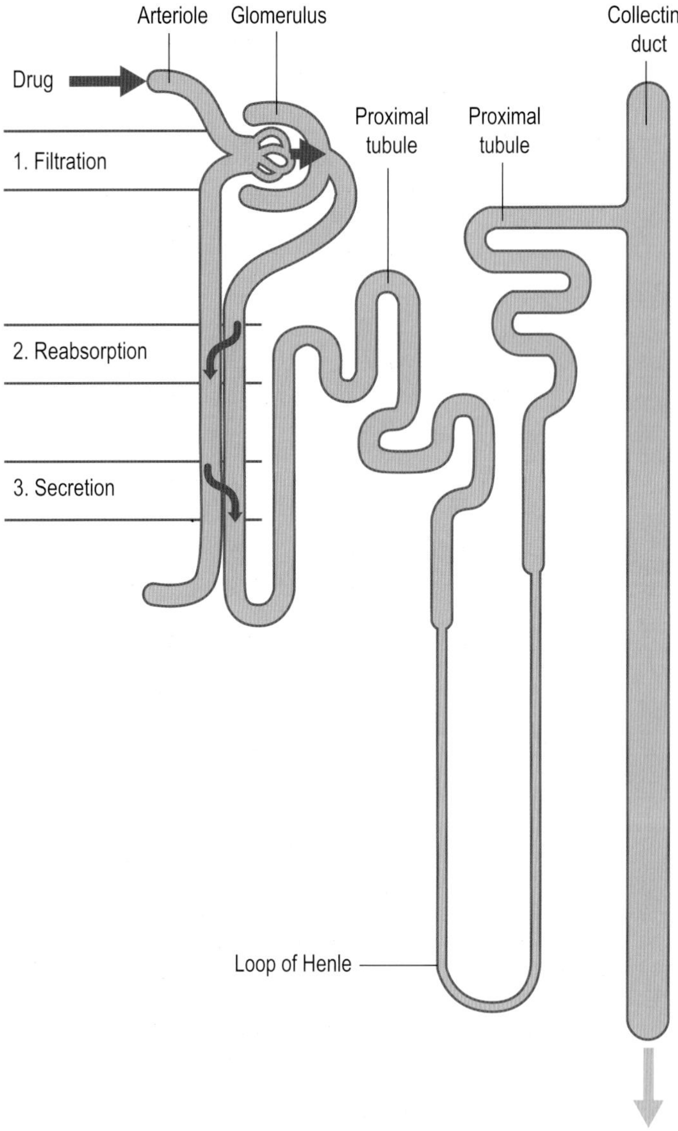

Figure 12-2 Drug excretion process.

output may occur during illness or injury and can prolong the period required to eliminate drugs through the lungs.

Excretion by the sweat and salivary glands
Sweat is an unimportant means of drug excretion. However, this method can cause various skin reactions and can discolour the sweat. Drugs excreted in saliva are usually swallowed and are eliminated in the same manner as other orally administered medicines. Certain substances given intravenously can be excreted into saliva. This may cause the person to complain about the 'taste of the drug', even though it was given intravenously.

Excretion by the mammary glands
Many drugs or their metabolites are excreted through the mammary glands in breast milk. Nursing mothers are advised not to take any medicine except under the supervision of a doctor. Mothers are usually advised to take prescribed medicines right after breast-feeding to diminish any risk to the infant.

Factors that influence the action of drugs

Many factors can alter the response to drug therapy, including age, body mass, gender, pathological state, genetic factors, psychological factors, environment, and time of administration. The paramedic should recognize these factors and should consider individual responses. The paramedic also must consider complications that may result from drug therapy.

Age

For the most part, paediatric and older patients are known to be highly sensitive to drugs. In a child, this sensitivity results in part from the immature hepatic and renal systems. In an older adult, sensitivity results from the natural decline of these systems and possible underlying disease processes. These aspects of body function can reduce the efficiency of excretory and metabolic mechanisms. This can create unexpected responses to drug therapy. Medication doses for children are usually modified based on body weight or surface area (see Chapter 38).

Body mass

Many drugs are given according to body mass (kilograms). An indirect relationship exists between body mass and the final concentration of drug in a patient for any given dosage; for instance, the larger the patient, the lower the concentration for any given dose of drug. The average adult drug dose is determined by a process that determines the amount of a drug that will be needed to produce a particular effect when administered to 50% of the population. This population includes only persons between the ages of 18 and 65 who weigh about 68 kg (110 lb). Therefore the appropriate drug doses for children who weigh less than 68 kg and are less than 18 years old is always based on body mass.

Gender

Drug effects differ in men and women. These differences result partly from size differences and the relative proportions of fat and water in the bodies of men and women. These differences may mean that women have higher concentrations of a drug when the standard dose is administered without consideration of size and also variations in drug distribution.

Environment

Drugs that affect mood and behaviour may be susceptible to the individual's environment and the personality of the user. For example, sensory deprivation and sensory overload may affect a person's response to a drug. The physical environment can also affect the actions of some drugs for some persons. For example, temperature extremes and changes in altitude may increase sensitivity to some drugs.

> **Critical Thinking**
>
> You can alter the environment in the ambulance. How might you do this to promote the action of pain-relieving drugs that you have given your patient?

Time of administration

The presence or absence of food in the gastrointestinal tract affects the manner in which drugs are tolerated and absorbed. Other factors may influence drug activity and reactions to drug therapy. One of these is a person's biological rhythms (e.g. sleep–wake cycles and circadian rhythms).

Pathological state

Illness or injury and the severity of symptoms can play a role in a person's sensitivity to drugs. Illness or injury can affect the type and amount of drug needed to achieve a desired effect. In addition, underlying disease processes such as circulatory, hepatic or renal dysfunction can interfere with the physiological actions of the drug and drug elimination.

Genetic factors

Genetics can alter the response of some persons to a number of drugs. This can occur through inherited diseases, enzyme deficiencies or altered receptor site sensitivities. The results of genetic abnormalities may appear as idiosyncrasies or may be mistaken for drug allergies.

Psychological factors

A patient's belief in the effects of a drug may strongly influence and potentiate drug effects. For example, a placebo can have the same result as a pharmacological agent if the patient thinks it will have the desired effect. In contrast, patient hostility and mistrust can lessen the perceived effects of a drug. The paramedic can enhance the action of a drug by telling the patient that the drug is going to work and when it will take effect.

Pharmacodynamic phase

Pharmacodynamics is the study of how a drug acts on a living organism. This includes the pharmacological response observed relative to the concentration of the drug at an active site in the organism. As stated before, drugs do not confer any new function on a tissue or organ of the body; rather, they modify existing functions. Theories of drug action abound. However, most drug actions are thought to result from a chemical interaction between the drug and various receptors throughout the body. The most common form of drug action is the drug–receptor interaction.

Drug–receptor interaction

For the most part, most drugs are believed to bind to drug receptors to produce their desired effect (Box 12-7). According to this theory, a specific portion of the drug molecule (the active site) selectively combines or interacts with some molecular structure (the reactive site on the cell surface or within the cell). This interaction produces a biological effect. These reactive cellular sites are known as receptors.

The relationship of a drug to its receptor may be thought of as a key fitting into a lock (Figure 12-3). The drug represents the key and the receptor represents the lock. The drug

Box 12-7

Drug–receptor interaction terms

Affinity: the propensity of a drug to bind or attach itself to a given receptor site

Agonist: a drug that combines with receptors and initiates the expected response

Antagonist: an agent that inhibits or counteracts effects produced by other drugs or undesired effects caused by normal or hyperactive physiological mechanisms

Competitive antagonist: an agent with an affinity for the same receptor site as an agonist (The competition with the agonist for the site inhibits the action of the agonist; increasing the concentration of the agonist tends to overcome the inhibition. Competitive inhibition responses are usually reversible.)

Efficacy (intrinsic activity): the ability of a drug to initiate biological activity as a result of binding to a receptor site

Non-competitive antagonist: an agent that combines with different parts of the receptor mechanism and inactivates the receptor so that the agonist cannot be effective regardless of its concentration (Non-competitive antagonist effects are considered to be irreversible or nearly so.)

Partial antagonist: an agent that binds to a receptor and stimulates some of its effects but may antagonize the action of other drugs with greater efficacy (Antagonists frequently share some structural similarities with their agonists.)

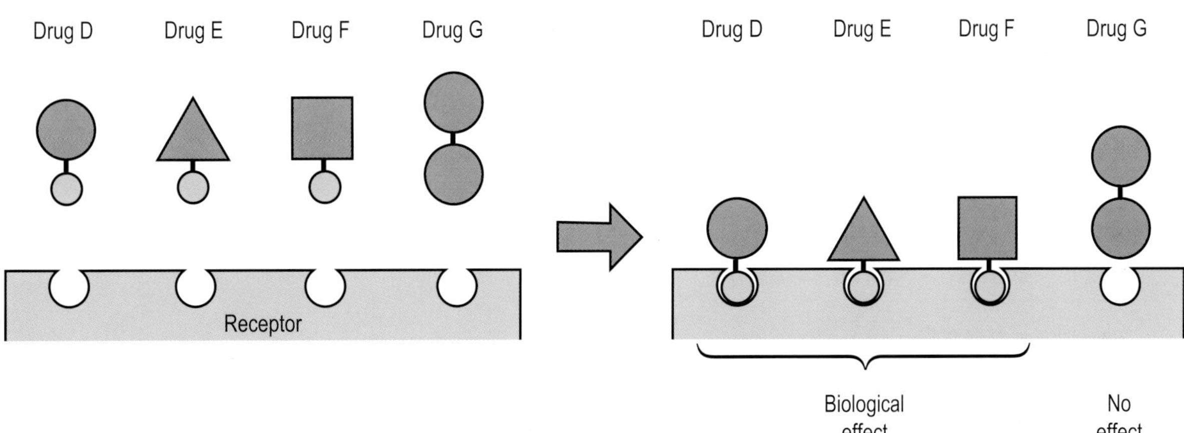

Figure 12-3 Lock-and-key fit between a drug and the receptors through which it acts. The site on the receptor that interacts with a drug has a definite shape. A drug that conforms to that shape can bind and produce a biological response. In this example, only the shape along the lower surface of the drug molecule is important in determining whether the drug binds to the receptor.

molecule with the best fit to a receptor produces the best response. After absorption a drug is believed to gain access to a receptor after it leaves the bloodstream and is distributed to tissues that contain receptor sites. To review, drugs that bind to a receptor and cause an expected physiological response are referred to as agonists. Conversely, drugs that bind to a receptor and the presence of which prevent a physiological response or other drugs from binding are referred to as antagonists.

Drug–response assessment

In the prehospital setting the response to drug therapy can often be assessed by observing the effect of the drug on specific physical findings. Examples include monitoring peak flow after administration of a bronchodilator and pain scoring after administration of an analgesic.

Each drug has its own characteristic rate of absorption, distribution, biotransformation and excretion. Thus the effectiveness of some drugs cannot be monitored solely by the patient's response. For example, medications such as theophylline, digoxin and phenytoin must reach a certain concentration at the target site to achieve the desired effect. Tissue concentrations are often proportional to and can be estimated from drug levels in the blood determined by laboratory analysis. Therapeutic drug levels in the blood, or serum, generally indicate ranges in tissue drug concentration that produce the desired therapeutic response.

Plasma-level profiles (Box 12-8) demonstrate the relationship between the concentration of drug in the plasma and the effectiveness of the drug over time (Figure 12-4). These profiles depend on the rate of absorption, distribution, biotransformation and excretion after drug administration.

The therapeutic range for most drugs is based on the concentration that provides the highest probability of response with the least risk of toxicity.

The dosage (loading and maintenance) required to achieve a therapeutic concentration varies because of the previously described factors that influence the actions of drugs: age, body mass, gender, pathological state, and genetic and psychological factors. In most patients, doses in the therapeutic range have a high probability of producing the desired effect. Moreover, they have a low probability of toxicity. However, some patients fail to respond to doses in the therapeutic range whilst some others may develop drug toxicity.

Biological half-life

The rate of biotransformation and excretion of a drug determines its biological half-life. The biological half-life is defined as the time it takes to metabolize or eliminate 50% of a drug in the body. For example, a 100-mg injection of a

Box 12-8

Plasma-level profile terms

- Duration of action: the period from onset of drug action to the time when a drug effect is no longer seen
- Loading dose: a bolus of a drug given initially to attain a therapeutic plasma concentration rapidly
- Maintenance dose: the amount of drug necessary to maintain a steady therapeutic plasma concentration
- Minimum effective concentration: the lowest plasma concentration that produces the desired drug effect
- Onset of action or latent period: the interval between the time a drug is administered and the first sign of its effect
- Peak plasma level: the highest plasma concentration attained from a dose
- Termination of action: the point at which the effect of a drug is no longer seen
- Therapeutic range: the range of plasma concentrations most likely to produce the desired drug effect with the least likelihood of toxicity (the range between minimum effective concentration and toxic level)
- Toxic level: the plasma concentration at which a drug is likely to produce serious adverse effects

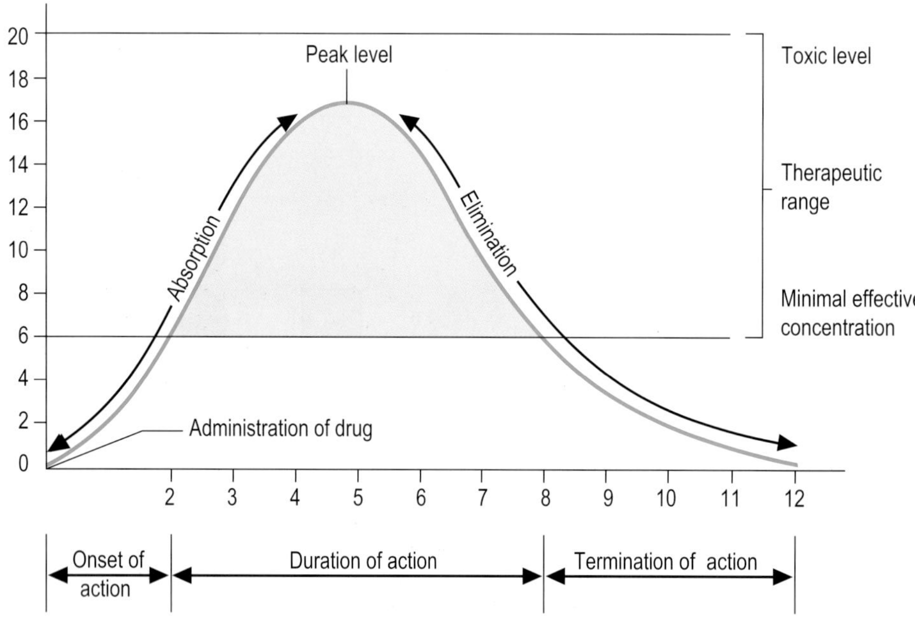

Figure 12-4 Plasma-level profile of a drug.

given drug has a half-life of 4 h, thus 50 mg will be eliminated in the first 4 h, 25 mg (half of the remaining 50 mg) will be eliminated in the second 4 h, and so on. A drug is considered to be eliminated from the body after five half-lives have passed.

Critical Thinking

Adenosine is an intravenous antidysrhythmic medicine that has a half-life of only 1–3 s. How will this brief half-life influence the speed and frequency of administration of this drug?

The half-life of a drug is crucial when determining the rate of administration. A drug that has a short half-life (e.g. 2–3 h) must be administered more often to maintain a therapeutic range than a drug with a long half-life, such as 12 h. The half-life of a drug may be lengthened considerably in persons with liver dysfunction or renal disorders. These and other disease processes may require a reduction in drug dosage, or the interval between doses may have to be lengthened.

Therapeutic index

The therapeutic index (TI) is a measurement of the relative safety of a drug. The index represents the ratio between two factors. The first factor is lethal dose 50 (LD_{50}). This is the dose of a drug that is lethal in 50% of laboratory animals tested. The second factor is effective dose 50 (ED_{50}), which is the dose that produces a therapeutic effect in 50% of a similar population. The TI is calculated as follows:

$$TI = \frac{LD_{50}}{ED_{50}}$$

The closer the ratio is to 1, the greater the danger in administering the drug to human beings. With certain drugs, such as digoxin, the difference between the effective dose and the lethal dose is small. These drugs are said to have a low TI. In contrast, drugs such as naloxone have a wide margin between the effective dose and lethal dose (a high TI).

Drug interactions

Many variables can influence drug interactions, including intestinal absorption, competition for plasma-protein binding, biotransformation, action at the receptor site, renal excretion, and alteration of electrolyte balance. Not all drug interactions are dangerous; some may even be beneficial.

Some drug–drug interactions are clinically important and can even be dangerous. The paramedic should be aware of common drug–drug interactions and the contraindications to drugs contained within the JRCALC guidelines. The following drugs are associated with clinically significant drug–drug interactions:

- anticoagulants
- tricyclic antidepressants
- monoamine oxidase (MAO) inhibitors
- amphetamines
- digitalis glycosides
- diuretics
- antihypertensives.

Other factors that can influence drug interactions include the following:

- drug-induced malabsorption of food and nutrients
- food-induced malabsorption of drugs
- enzyme alterations that affect the metabolism of food or drugs
- alcohol consumption
- cigarette smoking that affects drug metabolism or excretion
- food-initiated alteration of drug excretion.

Note

Grapefruit and its juice can boost blood levels of some drugs as much as 1000%. This occurs through liver enzyme inhibition. Emergency drugs that can be affected include verapamil and midazolam.

Finally, some drugs are incompatible with each other. For example, adrenaline (epinephrine) will precipitate (or crystallize) when mixed with sodium bicarbonate.

Drug forms, preparations and storage

Drugs and drug preparations are available in many forms (Box 12-9). Each one has specific indications, advantages and disadvantages.

Certain rules should guide the manner in which drugs are secured, stored, distributed and accounted for. The paramedic should follow service protocol and also legal requirements. Emergency medical services personnel must be aware that temperature, light, moisture and shelf-life can affect drug potency and effectiveness.

Drug profiles and special considerations in drug therapy

A paramedic should be familiar with the drug profiles of any drug he or she administers. Not all aspects of drug profiles can be committed to memory, thus the paramedic should make regular use of pharmacology references. One should note that paramedics are responsible for safe and effective drug administration and are personally responsible for each drug they give. They are legally, morally, and ethically responsible. As part of the professional practice of patient management, paramedics must do the following:

- Use correct precautions and techniques when administering medications.
- Observe and document the effects of drugs.
- Maintain a current knowledge base regarding changes in trends in pharmacology.
- Establish and maintain professional relationships with other members of the healthcare team.

Box 12-9

Various forms of drug preparations

Preparations for oral use

Liquids

Aqueous solution: substance dissolved in water and syrups
Aqueous suspension: solid particles suspended in liquid
Emulsion: fat or oil suspended in liquid with an emulsifier
Spirits: alcohol solution
Elixir: aromatic, sweetened alcohol and water solution
Tincture: alcohol extract of plant or vegetable substance
Fluid extract: concentrated alcoholic liquid extract of plant or vegetables
Extract: syrup or dried form of pharmacologically active drug, usually prepared by evaporating a solution

Solids

Capsule: soluble case (usually gelatine) that contains liquid, dry, or beaded drug particles
Tablet: compressed, powdered drugs in the form of a small disc
Troche or lozenge: medicated tablets that dissolve slowly in the mouth
Powder or granules: loose or moulded drug substance for administration with or without liquids

Preparations for parenteral use

Ampoule: sealed glass container for liquid injectable medication
Vial: glass container with rubber stopper for liquid or powdered medication
Cartridge or Tubex: single-dose unit of parenteral medication to be used with a specific injecting device

Intravenous infusions (suspended on hanger at bedside)

Flexible collapsible plastic bags (50 to 250 mL): used for continuous infusion of fluid replacement with or without medications
Intermittent intravenous infusions: usually secondary intravenous setup of a small plastic bag (50 to 250 mL) to which medication is added. The infusion runs as a 'piggyback', hung separately from the primary intravenous infusion via a secondary administration tubing set usually for 20–120 min. The primary intravenous solution is run between medication doses.
Heparin lock: a port site for direct administration of intermittent intravenous medications without the need for primary intravenous solution

Preparations for topical use

Liniment: liquid suspension for lubrication that is applied by rubbing
Lotion: liquid suspension that can be protective, emollient, cooling, astringent, antipruritic, or cleansing
Ointment: semisolid medicine in a base for local protective, soothing, astringent or transdermal application for systemic effects (nitroglycerin, scopolamine, oestrogen)
Paste: thick ointment primarily used for skin protection
Plasters: solid preparations that are adhesive, protective or soothing
Cream: emulsion that contains aqueous and oily bases
Aerosol: fine powder or solution in a volatile liquid that contains a propellant

Preparations for use on mucous membranes

Drops for eyes, ears, or nose: aqueous solutions with or without gelling agent to increase retention time in the eye
Topical instillation of aqueous solution of medications: usually for topical action but occasionally for systemic effects (enema, douche, mouthwash, throat spray, gargle)
Aerosol sprays, nebulizers, and inhalers: aqueous solutions of medication delivered in droplet form to the target membrane, such as the bronchial tree (bronchodilators)
Nasal drugs: an alternative route for drugs with poor bioavailability and high molecular weight compounds such as peptides, steroids and vaccines
Foam: powder or solution of medication in volatile liquid with propellant (vaginal foams for contraception)
Suppositories: usually medicinal substances mixed in a firm but malleable base (e.g. cocoa butter) to facilitate insertion into a body cavity (rectum or vagina)

Miscellaneous drug delivery systems

Intradermal implants: pellets that contain a small deposit of medication that are inserted into a dermal pocket; they are designed to allow medication to leach slowly into tissue and usually are used to administer hormones such as testosterone or estradiol
Micropump system: small, external pump attached by belt or implanted that delivers medication via a needle in a continuous steady dose (insulin, anticancer chemotherapy, opioids)
Membrane delivery systems: drug-laden membranes are instilled into the eye to deliver a steady flow of medication (pilocarpine or corticosteroids)

- Understand pharmacodynamics of the drugs they administer.
- Carefully evaluate patients to identify drug indications and contraindications.
- Take a drug history from patients that includes the following information:
  - prescribed medications (name, strength, daily dosage)
  - over-the-counter medications
  - vitamins
  - alternative drug therapies (e.g. homeopathic medicines and herbal medicines)
  - any drug allergies or adverse drug reactions.

The components of a drug profile include the following:

- *Drug names*: usually the generic and trade names; may include chemical names.
- *Classification*: the group to which the drug belongs.
- *Mechanism of action*: the pharmacodynamic properties of a drug; the way in which a drug causes its effects.
- *Indications*: conditions for which the drug is administered.
- *Pharmacokinetics*: how the body handles the drug over time; includes absorption, distribution, biotransformation, excretion, and onset and duration.

- *Side/adverse effects*: untoward or undesired effects that may be caused by the drug.
- *Dosage*: the amount of drug to be administered.
- *Routes of administration*: how the drug is given.
- *Contraindications*: conditions in which it may be harmful to administer the drug.
- *Special considerations*: how the drug may affect paediatric patients, older patients, pregnant patients and other special groups (described next).
- *Storage requirements*: how the drug should be stored.

Special considerations in drug therapy

Special considerations in drug therapy must be taken into account when one is caring for pregnant patients, paediatric patients and older adult patients. These considerations are described next.

Pregnant patients

Before administering any drug to a pregnant patient, the paramedic should consider the expected benefits and the possible risks to the fetus. Drugs given to a pregnant patient may cross the placental barrier and may harm the fetus or may be communicated to a newborn during breast-feeding. The British National Formulary[9] has a complete section dealing with medications during pregnancy, although JRCALC explicitly states which of the drugs authorized for paramedic administration cannot be given to pregnant women.

Paediatric patients

Special considerations for administration of drugs to paediatric patients are presented here and throughout the text. Following is a summary of the pharmacokinetics that influence dosing principles in the neonate, infant and paediatric populations.

Age

The effects of drugs are unpredictable among infants because of the variation in the development and maturation of the organ systems.

> **Critical Thinking**
>
> Drug doses vary for paediatric and neonatal patients. They are almost always related to weight. How can you ensure accuracy of dosing for these patients in critical situations when seconds count, even though you know the wrong dose calculation could be lethal?

Absorption

Drug absorption in infants and children follows the same basic principles as it does in adults. A factor that influences drug absorption is blood flow at the site of intramuscular or subcutaneous administration; this is usually determined by the patient's cardiovascular function. Certain physiological conditions might reduce blood flow to the muscle and subcutaneous tissue. These conditions include shock, vasoconstriction, and heart failure. The smaller muscle mass of the infant further complicates drug absorption because of diminished peripheral perfusion to these areas. For orally administered drugs, underlying gastrointestinal function may influence drug absorption.

Liquids and suspensions disperse quickly in gastrointestinal fluids, thus they are more readily absorbed than tablet or capsule forms. Increases in peristalsis (e.g. diarrhoeal conditions) and lowered gastrointestinal enzyme activities tend to decrease overall absorption of orally or rectally administered medications.

Distribution

Most drugs are distributed in body water. Thus, increases in total body water and extracellular volume can increase the volume of the distribution. Compared with adults, infants have proportionately higher volumes of total body water (70–75% compared with 50–60%). Infants also have a higher ratio of extracellular to intracellular fluid (40% compared with 30%); higher dosages of water-soluble drugs may be needed to have effective blood levels in the newborn.

Another key factor that affects drug distribution is drug binding to plasma proteins. In general, protein binding of drugs is reduced in the infant; therefore the concentration of free drug in plasma is increased. This can result in a greater drug effect or toxicity. Regarding central nervous system effects, the blood–brain barrier in the infant is much less effective than in adults. This allows drugs greater access to this area.

Biotransformation

Various liver enzyme systems for metabolism generally mature unevenly. The infant therefore, has a decreased ability to metabolize drugs, which predisposes the infant to developing toxicity from drugs metabolized by the liver. In addition, many drugs given to infants have slower renal clearance times and longer half-lives. Thus the paramedic must adjust dosages based on age and weight.

Elimination

The GFR is much lower in newborns than in older infants, children and adults. Therefore, drugs eliminated through renal function are cleared from the body slowly in the first few weeks of life. Renal excretory mechanisms progress to maturity after 1 year of age. Before that age, excretion of some substances through the renal system may be delayed because of immaturity. This may result in higher serum levels and a longer duration of action than intended.

Older adult patients

Key changes in drug responses occur with age in most individuals. Factors associated with ageing that significantly affect pharmacokinetics include the likelihood of multiple diseases requiring the use of several drugs (also referred to as polypharmacy). In addition, nutritional problems, decreasing ability to metabolize drugs, and the possibility of decreased drug dosing compliance for a variety of reasons can influence the effects of drugs. This summary is meant to serve as a review of the pharmacokinetics that influence dosing principles in the older adult.

Age

Declines in the functional capacity of most major organ systems begin in young adulthood and continue through life. Older adults do not lose specific function at a quicker rate than young and middle-aged adults; rather, they have less physiological reserves. Decreases in physiological function (GFR, cardiac function, maximal breathing capacity) are generally accepted as beginning no later than age 45. Decreased renal function has the greatest impact on medication administration and drug clearance.

Absorption

Little evidence exists of major changes in drug absorption with age, yet conditions associated with age may alter the rate at which some drugs are absorbed. Examples of these conditions include altered nutritional habits, greater consumption of non-prescription drugs (e.g. antacids and laxatives), and changes in gastric emptying. The reduced production of gastric acid and slowed gastric motility may have an impact and may result in unpredictable rates of dissolution and absorption of weakly acidic drugs.

Distribution

Changes in body composition have been noted in the older adult. Such changes include reduced lean body mass, reduced total body water, and increased fat as a percentage of body mass. Levels of serum albumin – which binds many drugs, especially weak acids – also usually decline. This affects drug distribution as it decreases protein binding of drugs and results in an increase in the amount of free drug in the circulation so that the ratio of bound to free drug may be significantly altered.

Biotransformation

The ability of the liver to metabolize drugs does not appear to decline consistently with age for all drugs, but disorders common with ageing can impair liver function. One such example is congestive heart failure. Hepatic recovery from injury, such as that caused by alcohol or viral hepatitis, declines as well.

Certain drugs are generally believed to be metabolized more slowly in older adults. This is thought to be the case because of decreased liver blood flow, which may lead to drug accumulation and toxicity. The paramedic must use caution when administering medication that is metabolized primarily in the liver to a patient with a history of liver disease. Older patients with severe nutritional deficiencies may also have impaired hepatic function.

Elimination

Renal function is the most critical factor for clearance of most drugs from the body. A natural reduction in renal function occurs with ageing and is usually caused by loss of functioning nephrons and a decrease in blood flow. Both of these result in a decreased GFR. A decrease in renal function caused by decreases in renal blood flow usually occurs because of congestive heart failure. The practical result of renal impairment is a prolongation of the half-life of many drugs and the possibility of accumulation to toxic levels. Other reversible conditions (e.g. dehydration) can cause further reduction in renal clearance of drugs.

Drug administration problems

Older adults commonly do not comply with their drug therapy. Non-compliance may be intentional or unintentional on their part but rarely affects the administration of emergency drugs. Still, the paramedic must be familiar with the most common factors that contribute to drug administration problems in older adults. This is crucial because non-compliance or errors may be a factor in the patient's condition. Following are some common causes of non-compliance and medication errors:

- Non-compliance in taking prescribed medications may result from forgetfulness or confusion, especially if the patient has several prescriptions and different dosing intervals.
- Older patients may forget instructions on the need to complete medication because symptoms have disappeared. Disappearance of symptoms is often regarded as the best reason to stop the therapy.
- Errors in self-administered medications may result from physical disabilities such as arthritis or visual impairment.
- Non-compliance may be deliberate. A patient may be opposed to taking a drug because of past experiences. A careful drug history is especially important when caring for older adults. The paramedic should remember that a patient has the right to refuse medication.

SECTION III

Drugs that affect the nervous system

Review of anatomy and physiology

The effects of many drugs depend upon which branch of the autonomic nervous system they act. The effects also depend on whether the branch is stimulated or inhibited by drug therapy. The following is a discussion of the anatomy and physiology of the nervous system as they pertain to pharmacology (Box 12-10).

The central nervous system (CNS) consists of the brain and spinal cord and serves as the collection point for nerve impulses (Figure 12-5). The peripheral nervous system consists of cranial and spinal nerves and all their branches (those nerves outside the CNS), and connects all parts of the body to the CNS. The somatic nervous system controls functions that are under conscious, voluntary control such as skeletal muscles and sensory neurons of the skin. The autonomic nervous system, mostly motor nerves, controls functions of involuntary smooth muscles, cardiac muscles

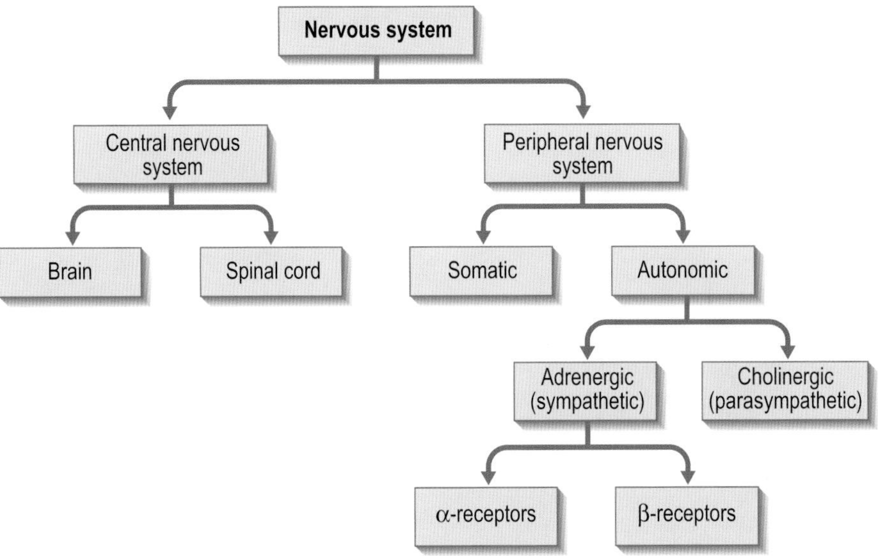

Figure 12-5 Overview of the nervous system.

Box 12-10

Emergency drugs: nervous system

Atropine
Diazepam
Adrenaline (epinephrine)
Morphine
Naloxone
Noradrenaline (norepinephrine)
Pancuronium
Suxamethonium

and glands. Four types of nerve fibres are found in most nerves:

1. Visceral afferent (sensory) fibres, which convey impulses from the internal organs to the CNS.
2. Visceral efferent (motor) fibres, which convey impulses from the CNS to the internal organs, glands, and the smooth and cardiac (involuntary) muscles.
3. Somatic afferent (sensory) fibres, which convey impulses from the head, body wall and extremities to the CNS.
4. Somatic efferent (motor) fibres, which convey impulses from the CNS to the striated (voluntary) muscles.

Simply put, the peripheral (sensory) nervous system receives stimuli from the body; the CNS interprets these stimuli; the peripheral (motor) nervous system initiates responses to the stimuli. Together the visceral afferent and visceral efferent nerve fibres form the autonomic nervous system. In contrast, the somatic afferent and somatic efferent nerve fibres form the somatic nervous system. Thus, the autonomic nervous system and the somatic nervous system can be regarded as subdivisions of the peripheral nervous system (Box 12-11).

Box 12-11

Organization of the nervous system

Central nervous system	Peripheral nervous system
Brain	Cranial nerves
Spinal cord	Visceral afferent nerve fibres
	Visceral efferent nerve fibres
	Somatic afferent nerve fibres
	Somatic efferent nerve fibres
Spinal nerves	Visceral afferent nerve fibres
	Visceral efferent nerve fibres
	Somatic afferent nerve fibres
	Somatic efferent nerve fibres

Autonomic division of the peripheral nervous system

The autonomic division of the peripheral nervous system provides almost every organ with a double set of nerve fibres: sympathetic (also known as adrenergic) and parasympathetic (also known as cholinergic). The cell bodies of the neurons in these two divisions are located in different areas of the CNS; they also exit the spinal cord at different levels. The sympathetic fibres exit from the thoracic and lumbar regions of the spinal cord (thoracolumbar outflow), whilst the parasympathetic fibres exit from the cranial and sacral portions of the spinal cord (craniosacral outflow).

The sympathetic and parasympathetic systems generally work as physiological antagonists on effector organs. That is, one division carries impulses that inhibit a certain function; the other division usually carries impulses that augment that function. There are exceptions to this general rule as certain structures are only innervated by one division or the other. As a rule, the sympathetic system prepares the body for vigorous muscular activity, stress, and emergencies (fight or flight) whilst the parasympathetic system lowers muscular activity, conserves energy, and promotes sedentary activity. The sympathetic and parasympathetic systems generally operate at the same time yet one usually has more dominant effects at any given time.

Autonomic innervation by the sympathetic and parasympathetic nervous system may be viewed as involving a two-

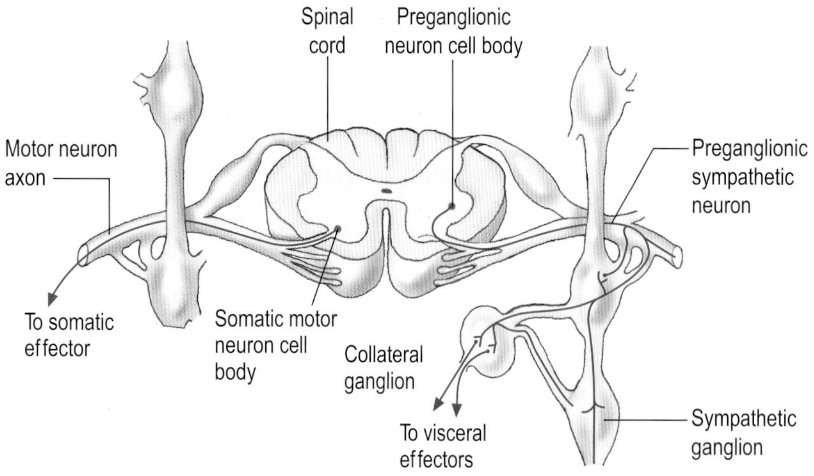

Figure 12-6 Autonomic conduction pathways.

neuron chain. This chain exists in a series between the CNS and the effector organs. This two-neuron chain is composed of a preganglionic neuron, located in the CNS, and a postganglionic neuron, located in the periphery (Figure 12-6). The area that serves as a functional junction between these two neurons is known as a synapse. The preganglionic fibres pass between the CNS and the nerve cell bodies in the peripheral nervous system (ganglia). The postganglionic fibres pass between the ganglia and the effector organ. Many of the sympathetic ganglia lie close to the spinal cord whilst others lie about midway between the spinal cord and the effector organ. The parasympathetic ganglia lie close or within the walls of the effector organ. The difference in location of the ganglia in these two divisions is the anatomical reason for the widespread responses caused by the sympathetic division versus the more localized responses caused by the parasympathetic division.

Neurochemical transmission

Most neurons are insulated electrically from each other and communicate by way of neurotransmitters, which are chemicals that are released from one neuron at the presynaptic nerve fibre. The neurotransmitters cross the synapse, where they may be accepted by the next neuron at a specialized receptor site (neurotransmitters bind only to specific receptors on the postsynaptic membranes). The neurotransmitter is then deactivated or taken up into the presynaptic neuron.

In both the sympathetic and parasympathetic divisions, the neurotransmitter for the preganglionic fibre at the junction between the preganglionic fibre and the synapse is acetylcholine. The neurotransmitter at the junction between the parasympathetic postganglionic fibre and the effector cell is also acetylcholine. Fibres that release acetylcholine are known as cholinergic fibres. All preganglionic neurons of the autonomic division and all postganglionic neurons of the parasympathetic division are cholinergic.

Note

All preganglionic nerves use the same neurotransmitter: acetylcholine.

The neurotransmitter between the sympathetic postganglionic fibre and the effector cell is noradrenaline, which is a member of the catecholamine family. Fibres that release noradrenaline are known as adrenergic fibres (a term derived from noradrenaline). Most postganglionic neurons of the sympathetic division are adrenergic; that is, they release noradrenaline; only a few are cholinergic. The actions of the autonomic nervous system depend on the interaction between the neurotransmitter released by the ganglionic cells and the receptor effector cells; for example, stimulation of the sympathetic nerves causes excitatory effects in some organs and inhibitory effects in others. Likewise, parasympathetic stimulation causes excitation in some organs but inhibition in others.

Note

Two different neurotransmitters exist for postganglionic neurons. All parasympathetic postganglionic neurons release acetylcholine onto their target tissue. Most sympathetic postganglionic neurons release noradrenaline onto their target tissue.

The parasympathetic and sympathetic systems function continuously. They innervate many of the same organs at the same time, thus the opposing actions of the two systems balance one another (most organs, however, are controlled predominantly by one or the other of the two systems). As previously stated, the sympathetic system usually dominates during stressful events; the parasympathetic system is most active during periods of emotional and physical calm.

Transmission of nerve impulses in the autonomic nervous system

Both branches of the autonomic nervous system have multiple receptors. The variety among neurotransmitters and receptors accounts for the differences in response to stimulation of sympathetic and parasympathetic nerves (excitatory or inhibitory).

The parasympathetic nervous system has nicotinic and muscarinic receptors (Figure 12-7). Nicotinic receptors

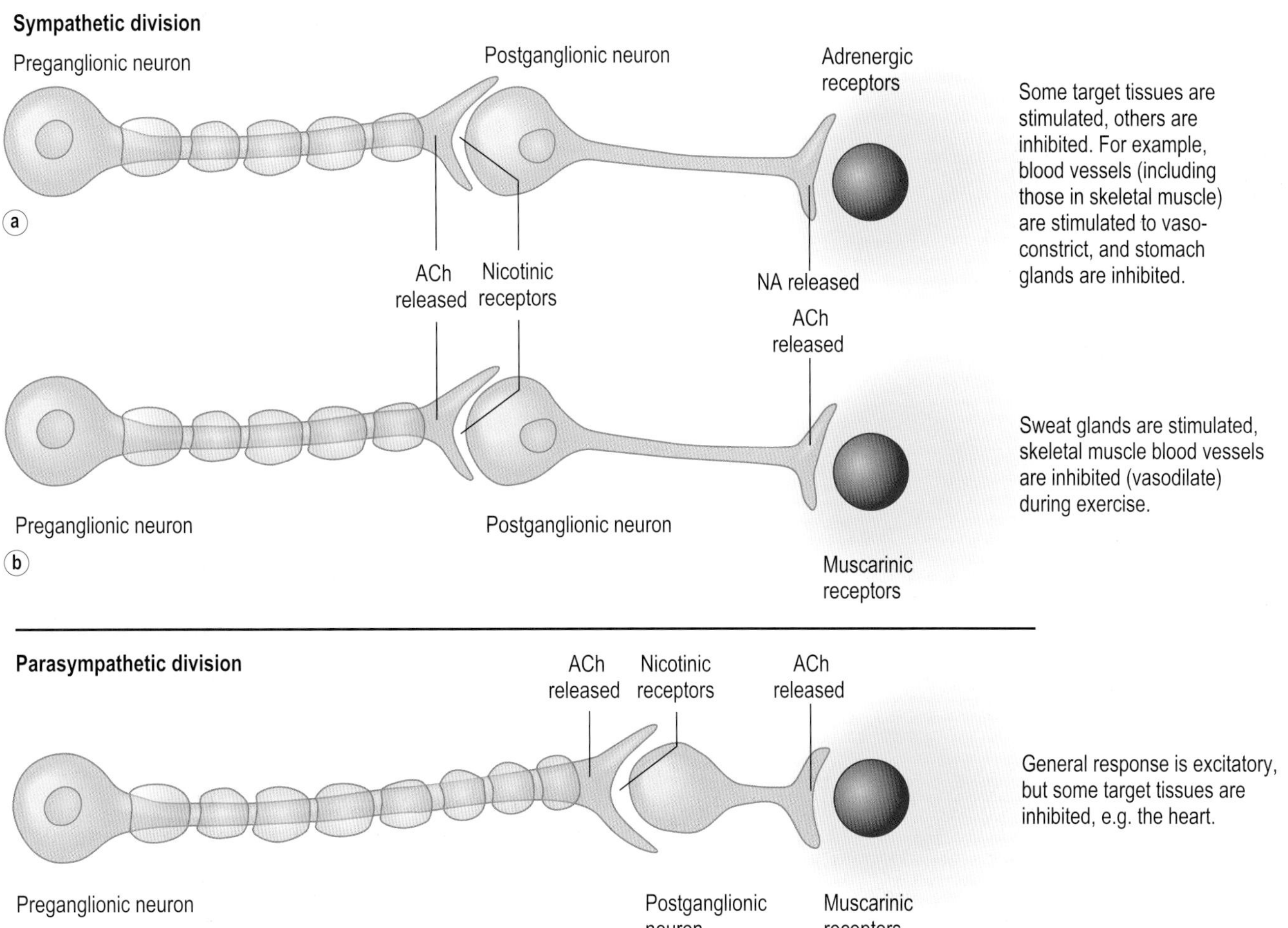

Figure 12-7 Location of the nicotinic, muscarinic, and adrenergic receptors in the autonomic nervous system. Nicotinic receptors are found on the cell bodies of sympathetic and parasympathetic postganglionic cells in the autonomic ganglia. (a) Adrenergic receptors are found in most target tissues innervated by the sympathetic division. (b) Some sympathetic target tissues have muscarinic receptors. (c) All parasympathetic target tissues have muscarinic receptors. NA, noradrenaline; ACh, acetylcholine.

(stimulated by nicotine) are found at the neuromuscular junctions of skeletal muscles and also on the postganglionic neurons of the parasympathetic nervous system. Muscarinic receptors (stimulated by the mushroom poison, muscarine) are found at the neuromuscular junction of cardiac and smooth muscle. They are also found on glands and on the postganglionic neurons of the sympathetic nervous system. Drugs that activate nicotinic receptors typically do not activate muscarinic receptors. The difference between nicotinic and muscarinic receptors is crucial in drug therapy. For example, when acetylcholine binds to nicotinic receptors, an excitatory response occurs; when it binds with muscarinic receptors, it results in excitation or inhibition. This depends on the target tissue in which the receptors are found (Table 12-2). When acetylcholine binds to muscarinic receptors in cardiac muscle, the heart rate slows. When it binds to muscarinic receptors in smooth muscle cells of the gastrointestinal tract, the rate and amplitude of contraction increase. Atropine blocks muscarinic but not nicotinic receptor sites, thus atropine affects the heart rate but does not cause paralysis.

Note

The two types of cholinergic receptors are nicotinic receptors and muscarinic receptors. Nicotinic responses are of fast onset and short duration and are excitatory. Muscarinic receptors are of slow onset and long duration and may be excitatory or inhibitory.

Critical Thinking

Imagine that your patient has eaten some poisonous mushrooms containing muscarine. What signs or symptoms related to pulse rate would you expect? What signs or symptoms related to gastrointestinal tract activity? Lastly, what signs or symptoms related to pupil diameter?

For the sympathetic (adrenergic) nervous system, the major receptor types belong to two structural categories. These are the α-receptors and β-receptors (and their subgroups, described in the following text). Noradrenaline binds to and

Table 12-2 Sites for muscarinic and nicotinic actions of acetylcholine

Site	Muscarinic actions	Nicotinic actions
Cardiovascular		
Blood vessels	Dilation	Constriction
Heart rate	Slowed	Increased
Blood pressure	Decreased	Increased
Gastrointestinal		
Tone	Increased	Increased
Motility	Increased	Increased
Sphincters	Relaxed	–
Glandular secretions	Increased salivary, lacrimal, intestinal and sweat secretion	Initial stimulation and then inhibition of salivary and bronchial secretions
Skeletal muscle	–	Stimulation
Autonomic ganglia	–	Stimulation
Eye	Pupil constriction	–
	Decreased accommodation	–
Blocking agent	Atropine	Tubocurarine
Remarks	Above effects increase as dosage increases	Increased dosage inhibits effects and causes receptor blockade

activates both types of receptor molecules but has greater affinity for α-receptors. The hormone adrenaline is produced by the adrenal medulla and is classified as an adrenergic substance. Adrenaline has nearly equal affinity for both receptors. In tissues containing α- and β-receptor cells, one type is more abundant, so that type has a predominant effect. Both receptors can be excitatory or inhibitory. For example, β-receptors are stimulatory in cardiac muscle, yet they are inhibitory in intestinal smooth muscle (Table 12-3).

Note

The two major types of adrenergic receptors are α and β. Both receptors can be excitatory or inhibitory.

Drugs that affect the autonomic nervous system

The nervous and endocrine systems are responsible for controlling and coordinating body functions. These two systems share three characteristics: a high level of integration in the brain, the ability to influence functions in distant regions of the body, and the extensive use of negative feedback mechanisms. One main difference between the two systems is the mode of transmission of information.

The endocrine system transmission is chiefly chemical and moves via blood-borne hormones. The hormones are not targeted for a specific organ; instead, they diffusely affect many cells and organs at the same time. In contrast, the nervous system mainly relies on rapid electrical transmission of information over nerve fibres. Chemical impulses only carry signals between nerve cells and their effector cells in a localized manner, perhaps affecting only a few cells. Drugs that affect the endocrine system are presented later in this chapter.

Box 12-12

Anatomical and functional terms for the autonomic nervous system

The anatomical names and functional terms for the autonomic nervous system are often used interchangeably: sympathetic or adrenergic, and parasympathetic or cholinergic. The terms parasympathomimetic and sympathomimetic mean to mimic or to produce an effect similar to activation of either system. The words parasympatholytic and sympatholytic mean to block the normal effects seen with activation of either system. The term anticholinergic is synonymous with parasympatholytic.

Anatomical name	Functional term	Primary neurotransmitter
Sympathetic	Adrenergic	Noradrenaline
Parasympathetic	Cholinergic	Acetylcholine

Classifications

The autonomic drugs mimic or block the effects of the sympathetic and parasympathetic divisions of the autonomic nervous system (see Box 12-12). These drugs can be classified into four groups:

1. Cholinergic (parasympathomimetic) drugs, which mimic the actions of the parasympathetic nervous system.
2. Cholinergic blocking (parasympatholytic) drugs, which block the actions of the parasympathetic nervous system.
3. Adrenergic (sympathomimetic) drugs, which mimic the actions of the sympathetic nervous system or the adrenal medulla.

Table 12-3 Autonomic innervation of target tissues

Organ	Effect of sympathetic stimulation	Effect of parasympathetic stimulation
HEART		
Muscle	Increased rate and force (b)	Slowed rate (c)
Coronary arteries	Dilation (b),* constriction (a)*	Dilation (c)
SYSTEMIC BLOOD VESSELS		
Abdomen	Constriction (a)	None
Skin	Constriction (a)	None
Muscle	Dilation (b, c), constriction (a)	None
LUNGS		
Bronchi	Dilation (b)	Constriction (c)
Liver	Release of glucose into blood (b)	None
Skeletal muscles	Breakdown of glycogen to glucose (b)	None
Metabolism	Increase of up to 100% (a, b)	None
GLANDS		
Adrenal glands	Release of adrenaline and noradrenaline (c)	None
Salivary glands	Constriction of blood vessels and slight production of thick, viscous secretion (a)	Dilation of blood vessels and thin, copious secretion (c)
Gastric glands	Inhibition (a)	Stimulation (c)
Pancreas	Inhibition (a)	Stimulation (c)
Lacrimal glands	None	Secretion (c)
Sweat glands		
Merocrine glands	Copious, watery secretion (c)	None
Apocrine glands	Thick, organic secretion (c)	None
GUT		
Wall	Decreased tone (b)	Increased motility (c)
Sphincter	Increased tone (a)	Decreased tone (c)
Gallbladder and bile ducts	Relaxation (b)	Contraction (c)
URINARY BLADDER		
Wall	Relaxation (b)	Contraction (c)
Sphincter	Contraction (a)	Relaxation (c)
EYE		
Ciliary muscle	Relaxation for far vision (b)	Contraction for near vision (c)
Pupil	Dilation	Constriction (c)
Erector pili muscles	Contraction (a)	None
Blood	Increased coagulation (a)	None
Sex organs	Ejaculation (a)	Erection (c)

(a) Mediated by α-receptors; (b) mediated by β-receptors; (c) mediated by cholinergic receptors.
*Normally blood flow through coronary arteries increases as a result of sympathetic stimulation of the heart because of increased demand by cardiac tissue for oxygen. In experiments that isolate the coronary arteries, however, sympathetic nerve stimulation, acting through α-receptors, causes vasoconstriction. The β-receptors are relatively insensitive to sympathetic nerve stimulation but can be activated by drugs.

4. Adrenergic blocking (sympatholytic) drugs, which block the actions of the sympathetic nervous system or adrenal medulla.

Cholinergic drugs

As described earlier, acetylcholine plays a key role in the parasympathetic and sympathetic divisions of the nervous system. Acetylcholine has two major effects in the nervous system: (1) a stimulant effect on the ganglia, adrenal medulla and skeletal muscle (the nicotinic effect) and (2) stimulant effects at postganglionic nerve endings in cardiac muscle, smooth muscle and glands (the muscarinic effect). Drugs that affect nicotinic or cholinergic receptor sites on autonomic ganglia are ganglionic-stimulating drugs (e.g.

nicotine and nicotine gum) and ganglionic-blocking drugs (e.g. mecamylamine).

Cholinergic drugs (choline esters) act directly with cholinergic receptors on postsynaptic membranes, or they act indirectly by inhibiting the enzyme that normally destroys acetylcholine. This inhibition results in an accumulation of acetylcholine, which in turn causes a longer and more intense response at various effector sites. Cholinergic drugs have little therapeutic value and are not for the most part thought of as emergency drugs. Indirect-acting cholinergic drugs are used to treat myasthenia gravis, a condition characterized by weakness of the skeletal muscles. These drugs work to elevate the concentration of acetylcholine at myoneural junctions, which increases muscle strength and function.

Cholinergic blocking (anticholinergic) agents have many uses in emergency medicine. These drugs work by blocking the muscarinic effects of acetylcholine and thus decrease the action of acetylcholine on its effector organ.

The best known cholinergic blocking drug used in emergency care is atropine. Atropine is a belladonna alkaloid that acts as a competitive antagonist. It works by occupying muscarinic receptor sites, which prevents or reduces the muscarinic response to acetylcholine. Large doses dilate the pupils, inhibit accommodation of the eyes, and increase the heart rate by blocking the cholinergic effects of the heart.

Adrenergic drugs

Adrenergic drugs are designed to produce activities like those of neurotransmitters. The three types of adrenergic agents are direct acting, indirect acting and dual acting (direct and indirect).

Direct-acting drugs Three naturally occurring catecholamines are present in the body: adrenaline, noradrenaline and dopamine. Adrenaline is released by the adrenal medulla and acts mainly as an emergency hormone, noradrenaline acts as a critical transmitter of nerve impulses, and dopamine is a precursor of adrenaline and noradrenaline. Dopamine has a transmitter role of its own in certain parts of the CNS. Each of these catecholamines can be produced synthetically to stimulate the same response as the endogenous chemical.

Catecholamines depend on their ability to act directly with α- and β-receptors. Two subgroups of α-receptors have been identified: α_1 and α_2. α_1-receptors are postsynaptic receptors that are located on the effector organs. Their chief role is to stimulate contraction of smooth muscle, which, in the vasculature, results in an increase in blood pressure. α_2-receptors are found on presynaptic and postsynaptic nerve endings. When stimulated, presynaptic receptors inhibit the further release of noradrenaline. Like α_1-receptors, α_2 postsynaptic receptors produce vasoconstriction to increase resistance in blood vessels and thus increase blood pressure.

Beta-receptors are subdivided into β_1- and β_2-receptors based on their response to drugs. However, the division also follows anatomical distinctions. β_1-receptors are located mainly in the heart, β_2-receptors mainly in the bronchiolar and arterial smooth muscle. β-receptors stimulate the heart; dilate bronchioles; dilate blood vessels in the skeletal muscle, brain and heart; and aid in glycogenolysis (Table 12-4).

Note

Use of a memory aid to differentiate the physiological effects of β-receptors may be helpful: A person has one heart (β_1 effects) and two lungs (β_2 effects).

Noradrenaline (norepinephrine) acts mainly on α-receptors and causes almost pure vasoconstriction of the blood vessels. Adrenaline (epinephrine) acts on α- and β-receptors and produces a mixture of vasodilatation and vasoconstriction. The effect depends on the number of α- and β-receptors present in the target tissue. The following are the most important α and β activities in human beings:

1. α activities
   - vasoconstriction of arterioles in the skin and splanchnic area, resulting in a rise in blood pressure and peripheral shunting of blood to the heart and brain from the shifting of blood volume
   - pupil dilatation
   - relaxation of the gut.
2. β activities
   - cardiac acceleration and increased contractility
   - vasodilatation of arterioles supplying the skeletal muscle
   - bronchial relaxation
   - uterine relaxation.

Indirect-acting and dual-acting drugs Indirect-acting adrenergic drugs act indirectly on receptors by triggering the release of the catecholamines adrenaline and noradrenaline. These chemicals then activate the α- and β-receptors. Dual-acting adrenergic drugs have indirect and direct effects. An example of a drug in this group is ephedrine (ephedrine sulphate).

Adrenergic blocking agents may be classified into alpha- and beta-blocking drugs. Alpha-blocking drugs block the vasoconstricting effect of catecholamines and are used in certain cases of hypertension. They are also used to help prevent necrosis when noradrenaline or dopamine has leaked, or extravasated, into the tissues. They have limited clinical application in the prehospital setting.

Note

All drugs with α effects should be administered through a secure intravenous line. This line should be well positioned in a large vein because of the possibility of extravasation and tissue necrosis.

Beta-blocking agents have greater clinical application and are often used in emergency care. These drugs block β-receptors and inhibit the action of β-receptors at the effector site. Beta-blocking agents are grouped into selective beta-blocking agents and non-selective beta-blocking agents. The selective blocking agents block β_1- or β_2-receptors; the non-selective beta-blocking agents block both β_1- and β_2-receptor sites. Selective beta$_1$-blocking agents are also known as cardioselective blockers because they block the β_1-receptors in the heart. Examples of important selective beta$_1$-blocking agents are metoprolol and atenolol. These drugs are

Table 12-4 Actions of autonomic nervous system neuroreceptors

Effector organ or tissue	Receptor	Adrenergic effect	Cholinergic effect
Eye, iris	α_1	Contraction (mydriasis)	–
Radial muscle	β_2	–	Contraction (miosis)
Sphincter muscle	–	Relaxation for far vision	Contraction for near vision
Eye, ciliary muscle	–	–	Secretion
Lacrimal glands	α_1	–	Secretion
Nasopharyngeal glands	β	Secretion of potassium and water	Secretion of potassium and water
Salivary glands		Secretion of amylase	–
Heart			
SA node	β_1	Increased heart rate	Decrease heart rate; vagus arrest
Atrial	β_1	Increased contractility and conduction velocity	Decrease contractility; shorten action potential duration
AV junction	β_1	Increased automaticity and propagation velocity	Decrease automaticity and propagation velocity
Purkinje system	β_1	Increased automaticity and propagation velocity	–
Ventricles	β_1	Increased contractility	–
Arterioles			
Coronary	α_1, β_2	Constriction, dilation	Dilation
Skin and mucosa	α_1, α_2	Constriction	Dilation
Skeletal muscle	α, β_2	Constriction, dilation	Dilation
Cerebral	α_1	Constriction (slight)	–
Pulmonary	α_1, β_2	Constriction, dilation	–
Mesenteric	α_1	Constriction	–
Renal	α_1, β_1, β_2, D	Constriction, dilation	–
Salivary glands	α_1, α_2	Constriction	Dilation
Veins, systemic	α_1, β_2	Constriction, dilation	–
Lung			
Bronchial muscle	β_2	Relaxation	Contraction
Bronchial glands	a_1, β_2	Decreased secretion; increased secretion	Stimulation
Stomach			
Motility	α_1, β_2	Decrease (usually)	Increase
Sphincters	α_1	Contraction (usually)	Relaxation (usually)
Secretion	–	Inhibition (?)	Stimulation
Liver	α, β_2	Glycogenolysis and gluconeogenesis	Glycogen synthesis
Gallbladder and ducts	–	Relaxation	Contraction
Pancreas			
Acini	α	Decreased secretion	Secretion
Islet cells	α_2, β_2	Decreased secretion; increased secretion	–
Intestine			
Motility and tone	α_1, β_1, β_2	Decrease	Increase
Sphincters	α_1	Contraction (usually)	Relaxation (usually)
Secretion	α_2	Inhibition (?)	Stimulation
Adrenal medulla	–	–	Secretion of adrenaline and noradrenaline (nicotinic effect)
Kidney			
Renin secretion	α_1, β_1	Decrease; increase	–
Ureter			
Motility and tone	α_1	Increase	Increase
Urinary bladder			
Detrusor	β_2	Relaxation (usually)	Contraction
Trigone and sphincter	α_1	Contraction	Relaxation
Sex organs, male	α_1	Ejaculation	Erection
Skin			
Pilomotor muscles	α_1	Contraction	–
Sweat glands	α_1	Localized secretion	Generalized secretion
Fat cells	α_2; β_1(β_3)	Inhibition of lipolysis; stimulation of lipolysis	–
Pineal gland	β	Melatonin synthesis	–

AV, atrioventricular; SA, sinoatrial.

antihypertensives and antidysrhythmics that are used in managing hypertension, and may also be used in select patients with suspected myocardial infarction and high-risk unstable angina.

Non-selective beta-blocking agents inhibit both β-receptors in the smooth muscle of the bronchioles and blood vessels. Examples include the anti-anginal anti-hypertensives nadolol and propranolol, and the antihypertensive labetalol. (Labetalol also has some alpha-blocking activity.)

Critical Thinking

Doctors will not usually prescribe a non-selective beta-blocker such as propranolol for patients with a history of asthma. Why is that?

Opiate analgesics and antagonists

Opiate analgesics relieve pain whilst opiate antagonists reverse the effects of some opiate analgesics. Pain has two components: the sensation of pain, which involves the nerve pathways and the brain; and the emotional response to pain. The emotional response may be a result of the individual's anxiety level, previous pain experience, age, gender and culture. Box 12-13 lists and defines classifications of pain.

Opiates are drugs that contain or are extracted from opium. The term opioid refers to synthetic drugs that have pharmacological properties similar to those of opium or morphine. Morphine is the chief alkaloid of opium. Opioids work by binding with opioid receptors in the brain and other body organs, which alters the patient's perception of pain and emotional response to a pain-causing stimulus. Opioid analgesics include morphine, codeine, hydromorphone, meperidine, methadone, pethidine, buprenorphine and tramadol.

Note

Endorphins serve as the body's own supply of opiates. They do this by binding to opiate receptors, thereby blocking pain.

Box 12-13

Classifications of pain

Acute pain: pain sudden in onset that usually subsides with treatment (e.g. pain associated with acute myocardial infarction, acute appendicitis, renal colic, or traumatic injuries)

Chronic pain: persistent or recurrent pain that is difficult to treat (e.g. pain that accompanies cancer and rheumatoid arthritis)

Referred pain: visceral pain felt at a site distant from its origin (e.g. pain from a myocardial infarction felt in the arm)

Somatic pain: pain arising from skeletal muscles, ligaments, vessels, or joints

Superficial pain: pain arising from the skin or mucous membrane

Visceral pain: 'deep' pain arising from smooth musculature or organ systems that may be difficult to localize and is often described as dull or aching

Opioid analgesics may produce undesirable effects such as nausea and vomiting, constipation, urinary retention, cough reflex suppression, orthostatic hypotension, respiratory depression and CNS depression. Most of these effects can be overcome by careful administration and close patient monitoring.

Opioid antagonists block the effects of opioid analgesics, including effects such as opioid-induced respiratory depression and sedation. Opioid antagonists block the effects by displacing the analgesics from their receptor sites. Naloxone (available for use by paramedics), naltrexone, and nalmefene are opioid antagonists.

Opioid agonist–antagonist agents such as buprenorphine have both analgesic and antagonist effects. For example, buprenorphine has a high affinity and exerts an agonist effect at one specific opioid receptor (the mu [μ] receptor), but has an antagonist effect at the kappa (κ) receptor. Buprenorphine will effectively displace a full opioid agonist and limit both the effects and side effects of opioid drugs. These drugs generally have a lower potential for creating dependency than opioid analgesics and the withdrawal symptoms are not as severe as those of the opioid agonist drugs. However, they may bring about withdrawal symptoms in addicts. Their use is limited in emergency care as the effects of the agonist–antagonist opioids adversely affect the level of pain relief that can be achieved by the use of a conventional opiate such as morphine.

Non-opiate analgesics

Non-narcotic analgesics interfere with local mediators released when tissue is damaged in the periphery of the body. These mediators stimulate nerve endings and cause pain. Non-narcotics include paracetamol and non-steroidal anti-inflammatory drugs (NSAID) such as diclofenac and aspirin. NSAID interfere with the production of hyperalgesic and pro-inflammatory prostaglandins by inhibiting cyclo-oxygenase (COX). COX is a key enzyme in the conversion of arachidonic acid to prostaglandins, which themselves are key chemicals that cause hyperalgesia and inflammation. Whereas narcotic agents tend to act at the level of the CNS, many non-narcotic analgesics work peripherally.

Critical Thinking

A non-narcotic analgesic may be selected instead of a narcotic for a paramedic returning to work on the ambulance. Why?

Anaesthetics

Anaesthetic drugs are CNS depressants that have a reversible action on nervous tissue. The three major types of anaesthesia are general, regional, and local. General anaesthesia is achieved by intravenous or inhalation routes and is the most common type of anaesthesia used during surgery to induce unconsciousness. Regional anaesthesia is obtained by injecting a local anaesthetic drug near a nerve trunk or at specific sites in a large region of the body (e.g. spinal block). Local anaesthesia is achieved topically to produce a loss of sensation. It can also be achieved by injection to block an area surrounding an operative field, making it insensitive to pain (e.g. minor wound repair).

Box 12-14

The physiology of sleep

Sleep can be viewed as a series of rhythms. Each has its own brain wave patterns. These rhythms can be divided into two major categories: rapid eye movement (REM) and non-rapid eye movement (non-REM). During sleep, a person moves through REM sleep. Then the person moves through four stages of non-REM sleep. REM, or active, sleep is the time of irregular body activity, vivid dreaming, and rapid eye movements. During REM sleep, the eyes move back and forth under the closed lids as they follow the action of a dream. The heart rate, blood pressure, and respirations may become irregular. During non-REM sleep, the person drifts out of wakeful awareness. The muscles relax, and the blood pressure, heartbeat, and breathing begin to decline. The brain sends signals to the arms, legs, and other large muscles to stop moving. At that point, 'sleep paralysis' occurs. The first REM period lasts nearly 10 min. The whole cycle repeats itself usually four to five times each night. Each cycle lasts an average of 90 min. As the night wears on, REM periods lengthen, and non-REM periods grow shorter. The final REM period of the night may last as long as 1 h.

Anti-anxiety and sedative–hypnotic agents and alcohol

Anti-anxiety and sedative–hypnotic agents and alcohol are presented together because of their similarities in pharmacological action. Anti-anxiety agents are used to reduce feelings of apprehension, nervousness, worry, or fearfulness.

Sedatives and hypnotics are drugs that depress the CNS, produce a calming effect, and help induce sleep (Box 12-14). The major difference between a sedative and a hypnotic is the degree of CNS depression induced by the agent. For example, a small dose of an agent administered to calm a patient is called a sedative; a larger dose of the same agent sufficient to induce sleep is called a hypnotic. Thus, an agent may be a sedative or a hypnotic, depending on the dose used.

As stated before, alcohol has actions that are characteristic of sedative–hypnotic or anti-anxiety drugs. Alcohol is a major source of drug abuse and dependency.

Scattered throughout the brainstem is a group of nuclei, which form the reticular formation. The reticular formation and its neural pathways make up a system known as the reticular activating system. This system is involved with the cycle of sleep and wake. Through these pathways, the reticular activating system collects incoming signals from the senses and viscera and then processes and passes these signals to the higher brain centres. The reticular activating system determines the level of awareness to the environment, thus it also governs actions and responses to the environment. Anti-anxiety and sedative–hypnotic agents and alcohol act by depressing this system.

Classifications

Two prototypical groups of drugs are used to treat anxiety or to induce sleep. These are the benzodiazepines and barbiturates, respectively. Benzodiazepines make up the drug class most often used today to treat anxiety and insomnia. Barbiturates make up an older drug class with many uses, ranging from sedation to anaesthesia.

Benzodiazepines

Benzodiazepines were introduced in the 1960s as anti-anxiety drugs and they are among the most widely prescribed drugs in clinical medicine, partly because of their high therapeutic index. Taken alone, even large doses rarely cause serious effects although there are increasing concerns regarding the use of benzodiazepines in the older population.[10] Benzodiazepines are thought to work by binding to specific receptors in the cerebral cortex and limbic system and, in so doing, enhance the effects of gamma-aminobutyric acid (GABA), an inhibitory neurotransmitter. These drugs are highly lipid soluble and are distributed widely in the body tissues but are also highly bound to plasma protein, usually more than 80%. Benzodiazepines have four actions: anxiety reducing, sedative–hypnotic, muscle relaxing, and anticonvulsant. Most benzodiazepines are Class C drugs under the Misuse of Drugs Act (1971) because of their potential for abuse. Commonly prescribed benzodiazepines are alprazolam, diazepam, oxazepam, midazolam, lorazepam and temazepam.

Critical Thinking

Consider a doctor preparing to reduce a dislocated shoulder. Why would a benzodiazepine be preferred over a narcotic?

Note

Flumazenil is a specific benzodiazepine receptor antagonist. Its use in emergency care is controversial as it fails to show any beneficial effect in adult patients in the clinical practice of an emergency department. Moreover, contraindications are frequently overlooked and this may expose patients to substantial risk of complications.[11]

Barbiturates

Barbiturates were once the most commonly prescribed class of medications for sedative–hypnotic effects; however, they have been virtually replaced by the benzodiazepines. Barbiturates are categorized according to their length of action such that they, may be classed as very short acting, intermediate or long acting. Very short-acting barbiturates, e.g. thiopental, may be used in pre-anaesthesia sedation; intermediate-acting barbiturates such as amobarbital are indicated only for the treatment of severe intractable insomnia. The long-acting barbiturate phenobarbital is still of some value in epilepsy but its use as a sedative is now deemed to be unjustified.[9]

Miscellaneous sedative–hypnotic drugs

The previously discussed drug classes do not include all of the anti-anxiety and sedative–hypnotic drugs. In fact, a number of other anti-anxiety and sedative–hypnotic drugs do not fall into these classes. These agents are more similar to barbiturates than benzodiazepines because they are generally shorter acting. Examples of miscellaneous drugs with anti-anxiety and sedative–hypnotic effects are chloral hydrate, etomidate and zolpidem. In addition to these drugs, antihistamines such as hydroxyzine have pronounced sedative effects.

Alcohol intake and behavioural effects

Alcohol is a general CNS depressant that can produce sedation, sleep and anaesthesia. In addition, alcohol enhances the sedative–hypnotic effects of other drug classes, including all general CNS depressants, antihistamines, phenothiazines, narcotic analgesics and tricyclic antidepressants. If alcohol is taken with other drugs, this enhancement could result in coma or death. Blood alcohol is measured in milligrams per decilitre. Characteristic behavioural effects can be predicted based on the amount of alcohol consumed and blood alcohol levels. Behavioural effects associated with alcohol intake are described further in Chapter 21.

Anticonvulsants

Anticonvulsant drugs are used to treat seizure disorders, the most notable of which is epilepsy. Epilepsy is a neurological disorder characterized by a recurrent pattern of abnormal neuronal discharges within the brain. These discharges result in a sudden loss or disturbance of consciousness, sometimes associated with motor activity, sensory phenomena, or inappropriate behaviour. Epilepsy is the most common serious neurological condition, affecting over 456 000 people in the UK.[12] In 50% of these cases, the cause is unknown (primary or idiopathic epilepsy). Secondary epilepsy is epilepsy that can be traced to trauma, infection, a cerebrovascular disorder, or some other illness. (Epilepsy is discussed further in Chapter 16.)

The exact mode and site of action of anticonvulsant drugs are not understood. In general, these drugs depress the excitability of neurons that fire to initiate the seizure. These drugs also suppress the neurons responsible for generalization of the small focal depolarization, thus preventing the spread of seizure discharge. Anticonvulsants are presumed to modify the ionic movements of sodium, potassium, or calcium across the nerve membrane, thus reducing the response to incoming electrical or chemical stimulation. Benzodiazepines also enhance the effects of major inhibitory neurotransmitters in the CNS. Many patients need drug therapy throughout their lives to control seizure disorders.

Several drugs are available for the control of seizure disorders. The choice of drug depends on the type of seizure disorder (generalized, partial or status). The choice of drug also depends on the patient's tolerance and response to the prescribed medication. Box 12-15 presents classes of anticonvulsant drugs.

Box 12-15

Classes of anticonvulsant drugs

Barbiturates

Phenobarbital

Benzodiazepines

Clonazepam
Diazepam
Lorazepam

Hydantoins

Fosphenytoin
Phenytoin

Succinimides

Ethosuximide

Other

Carbamazepine
Gabapentin
Lamotrigine
Magnesium sulphate
Topiramate
Valproic acid

Central nervous system stimulants

Central nervous system stimulants are classified according to where they exert their major effects in the nervous system: on the cerebrum, the medulla and brainstem, or in the hypothalamic limbic regions. All CNS stimulants work to increase excitability by blocking activity of inhibitory neurons or their respective neurotransmitters, or by enhancing the production of the excitatory neurotransmitters. Some of the more common CNS stimulant drugs are anorectics and amphetamines.

Anorectics

Anorectics are appetite suppressants that are used to treat obesity. They work either by acting on the gastrointestinal tract, or by producing a direct stimulant effect on the CNS. Sibutramine, an example of a CNS anorectic agent, blocks reuptake of serotonin and noradrenaline in the CNS although the mechanism of action is poorly understood. These effects may act to suppress appetite and also to increase metabolic rate.

A newer class of drugs (gastrointestinal lipase inhibitors, or fat blockers) block the absorption of about 30% of dietary fat. These drugs are sometimes used to manage obesity along with a reduced-calorie diet. An example of a gastrointestinal lipase inhibitor is orlistat.

Critical Thinking

Sibutramine is contraindicated in patients with a history of coronary artery disease, congestive heart failure or tachycardia; why do you think these patients are contraindicated?

Amphetamines

Amphetamines stimulate the cerebral cortex and reticular activating system, which increases alertness and responsiveness to environmental surroundings. It is recognized that amphetamines have only a limited field of usefulness and their use has been discouraged due to the risk of dependence and psychotic states.[9] Amphetamines are mainly used to treat attention deficit hyperactivity disorder (ADHD) and narcolepsy. For the most part, ADHD is seen in children and adolescents and is characterized by a short attention span and impulsive behaviour. ADHD is described further in Chapter 25.

Individuals with narcolepsy experience excessive drowsiness, sudden sleep attacks during daytime hours, and sometimes sleep paralysis. Dexamfetamine and modafinil

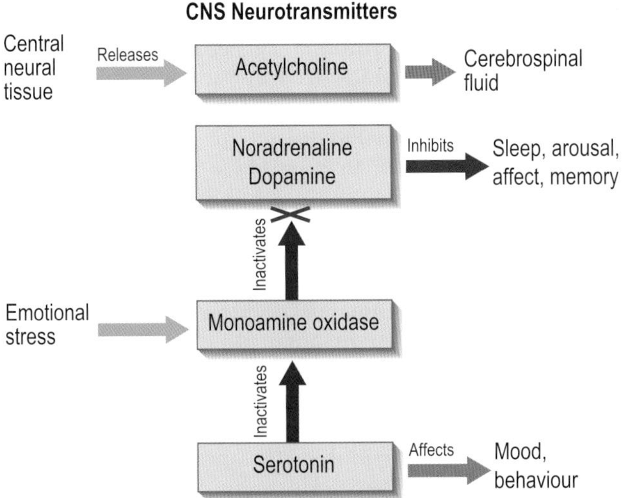

Figure 12-8 Neurotransmitters in the brain and their effects on emotion.

are two amphetamines used to treat narcolepsy in the UK. Methylphenidate (an amphetamine-related drug) is the most commonly used drug in the treatment of ADHD in the UK[13] although there is also an indication for dexamfetamine in the management of children with refractory hyperkinetic states. Paradoxically, amphetamines and other stimulants have a calming effect on children with ADHD, possibly related to an increase in neurotransmitter levels of dopamine. The use of methylphenidate is currently the subject of a review by NICE.

Psychotherapeutic drugs

Psychotherapeutic drugs include antipsychotic agents, antidepressants, and lithium. These drugs are used to treat psychoses and affective disorders, especially schizophrenia, depression, and mania (see Chapter 25).

Central nervous system and emotions

The neurotransmitters acetylcholine, noradrenaline, dopamine and serotonin, and monoamine oxidase (MAO), the enzyme that breaks down certain neurotransmitters, have a major effect on emotion (Figure 12-8). Alterations in the levels of these chemicals are linked to changes in mood and behaviour. Drug therapy alleviates symptoms by temporarily modifying unwanted behaviour.

Note

Acetylcholine is released from central neural tissue into the cerebrospinal fluid during activity. Noradrenaline and dopamine have widespread inhibitory effects. They affect functions such as sleep and arousal, affect, and memory. Serotonin levels affect mood and behaviour. MAO is an enzyme that inactivates dopamine and serotonin, both of which are produced during intense emotional states.

Antipsychotic agents

The main use of antipsychotic drugs is to treat schizophrenia, although they may be used to treat Tourette's syndrome. They may also be used to control disturbing behaviour in patients with senile dementia associated with Alzheimer's disease. Effective antipsychotic (neuroleptic) drugs block dopamine receptors in specific areas of the CNS; they can be classified into the following groups:

- Phenothiazine derivatives
  - Group 1: Chlorpromazine, levomepromazine and promazine
  - Group 2: Pericyazine and pipotiazine
  - Group 3: Fluphenazine, perphenazine, prochlorperazine and trifluoperazine
- Butyrophenones
  - Haloperidol
- Diphenylbutylpiperidines
  - Pimozide
- Thioxanthenes
  - Flupentixol and zuclopenthixol
- Substituted benzamides
  - Sulpiride
- Atypical agents
  - Clozapine
  - Risperidone.

With continued use of antipsychotics, some patients develop supersensitivity of dopamine receptors, which leads to tardive dyskinesia. Tardive dyskinesia is a potentially irreversible neurological disorder characterized by involuntary repetitious movements of the muscles of the face, limbs and trunk. Other identifying features include excessive blinking of the eyelids, lip smacking, tongue protrusion, foot tapping and rocking from side-to-side.

Antidepressants

Antidepressants are used to treat affective disorders (mood disturbances) including depression, mania, and elation. Tricyclic antidepressants, selective serotonin reuptake inhibitors and MAO inhibitors are prescribed for depression; lithium (an antimanic drug) is the preferred treatment for mania.

Note

Depression may be exogenous. That means depression results from a person's response to a loss or disappointment. Exogenous depression is considered normal, is usually temporary, and remits without the use of drug therapy. Endogenous depression, however, lasts 6 months or longer and is characterized by the absence of external causes; it may be the result of genetic or biochemical alterations. Antidepressants are often needed to treat this disorder. Depression is discussed further in Chapter 25.

Tricyclic antidepressants

Tricyclic antidepressants act primarily by blocking the amine reuptake pump on the presynaptic terminal; as a consequence, synaptic levels of noradrenaline and serotonin increase. They are not CNS stimulants as they do not induce stimulatory effects in an individual who is not depressed. Side effects include arrhythmias and heart block, as well the more common side effects of drowsiness, dry mouth, blurred vision (very rarely precipitation of angle-closure glaucoma), constipation, and urinary retention, which are related to anticholinergic effects. Examples include imipramine and amitriptyline.

Critical Thinking

You know that tricyclic antidepressants increase the levels of noradrenaline. Thus, what side effects might you expect in an overdose?

Selective serotonin reuptake inhibitors

Selective serotonin reuptake inhibitors also block the amine reuptake pump but tend to be more selective towards serotonin. Unlike the tricyclics, they do not exert effects on muscarinic (parasympathetic), adrenergic or histaminic receptors, so fewer side effects occur. Most adverse effects are relatively mild, short-lived, and terminate when treatment ends. Examples of selective serotonin reuptake inhibitors are fluoxetine, citalopram, and paroxetine. Suicidal thoughts and behaviour have been linked with the use of antidepressants.

MAO inhibitor antidepressants

Noradrenaline and adrenaline are metabolized by the enzyme monoamine oxidase to prevent accumulation and excessive stimulation of postsynaptic neurons. MAO inhibitors (MAOI) act to increase levels of these neurotransmitters by blocking the degradation normally created by MAO. MAO is also an important enzyme in the metabolism of amines present in food; in particular, tyramine, which is an indirectly acting sympathomimetic agent. When on MAOI the ingestion of food rich in tyramine has the potential to cause the widespread release of noradrenaline, which cannot be broken down because of the inhibition of MAO. Examples of MAOI used to treat depression include isocarboxazid, phenelzine and tranylcypromine. MAOI are used much less frequently than other antidepressants.

Lithium

Lithium is a cation that is closely related to sodium. Both cations are transported actively across cell membranes; however, lithium cannot be pumped out of the cell as effectively as sodium. Lithium therefore accumulates in the cells and results in a decrease in intracellular sodium and perhaps an improvement in the symptoms of a manic state. In addition, lithium appears to enhance some of the actions of serotonin. Lithium may decrease levels of noradrenaline and dopamine, and also appears to block the development of dopamine receptor supersensitivity that may accompany long-term therapy with antipsychotic agents. Lithium carbonate is used to treat manic disorders and comes in capsule, tablet and syrup form (e.g. lithium citrate).

Drugs for specific central nervous system–peripheral dysfunction

Several movement disorders result from an imbalance of dopamine and acetylcholine. Two of the most common are Parkinson's disease (including Parkinsonian syndromes) and Huntington's disease.

Parkinson's disease

Parkinson's disease is a chronic degenerative disease of the basal ganglia that is characterized by varying combinations of rigidity, tremor and bradykinesia (slow movement). The disease most often affects people over the age of 60, although it may occur in younger people. The disease results from abnormally low concentrations of dopamine in specific areas of the brain and may occur after acute encephalitis, as a result of a toxic reaction to chemicals, from the use of some illicit drugs, or as a side effect of treatment with psychotropic drugs that block dopaminergic pathways. It may also be idiopathic in origin. Parkinsonian syndromes mimic the symptoms of Parkinson's disease. They are usually idiopathic but may result from treatment with antipsychotic drugs (drug-induced Parkinsonism) that block dopaminergic receptors (e.g. haloperidol, metoclopramide, and phenothiazines). Symptoms of Parkinson's disease include the following:

- immobile facial expression
- bobbing of the head
- resting tremor
- pill-rolling of the fingers
- shuffling gait
- forward flexion of the trunk
- loss of postural reflexes.

Huntington's disease

Huntington's disease is a dominant gene disorder characterized by progressive dementia and involuntary muscle twitching (chorea). Like Parkinson's disease, Huntington's disease is thought to be related to an imbalance of dopamine, acetylcholine, and perhaps other neurotransmitters.

Drugs with central anticholinergic activity

Drugs that inhibit or block acetylcholine are referred to as anticholinergic. Anticholinergic drugs may be useful in drug-induced Parkinsonism but not in idiopathic Parkinson's disease. They reduce the effects of the central nervous cholinergic excess created by the deficiency of dopamine, thus restoring the normal dopamine–acetylcholine balance in the brain. Common anticholinergic agents include benzatropine (tablets and injections) and trihexyphenidyl hydrochloride.

Drugs that affect dopamine in the brain

Three classifications of drugs affect dopamine in the brain: those that release dopamine, those that increase brain levels of dopamine, and dopaminergic agonists (Box 12-16). Levodopa (L-dopa) is a drug that increases brain levels of

Box 12-16

Drugs that affect dopamine in the brain

Amantadine
Bromocriptine
Carbidopa–levodopa
Levodopa
Pergolide

dopamine and is the current drug of choice in the treatment of movement disorders associated with dopamine–acetylcholine imbalance.

Monoamine oxidase inhibitors

Two types of MAO have been identified. The first is monoamine oxidase A, which metabolizes noradrenaline and serotonin; the second is monoamine oxidase B, which metabolizes dopamine. Selegiline is a selective inhibitor of monoamine oxidase B. It retards the breakdown of dopamine and is often used in conjunction with levodopa because it enhances and prolongs the antiparkinsonism effects of levodopa. (Selegiline allows the dose of levodopa to be reduced.)

Skeletal muscle relaxants

Skeletal muscle contraction is evoked by a nicotinic cholinergic transmission process. Such contractions can be modified by drugs just as the autonomic ganglionic transmission can be. Skeletal muscle relaxants can be classified as central-acting, direct-acting, and neuromuscular blockers.

Central-acting muscle relaxants

Central-acting drugs are used to treat muscle spasms. They are thought to work by producing CNS depression in the brain and spinal cord. Antispasmodic agents include carisoprodol, baclofen and diazepam.

Direct-acting muscle relaxants

Direct-acting muscle relaxants work directly on skeletal muscles to produce muscle relaxation without the central side effects. Dantrolene is an example of a direct-acting muscle relaxant.

Neuromuscular blockers

Neuromuscular blocking drugs produce complete muscle relaxation and paralysis. They do this by binding to the nicotinic receptor for acetylcholine at the neuromuscular junction so that neuromuscular nerve transmission is blocked. Nerve transmission remains blocked for a variable period depending on the type and amount of neuromuscular blocker used.

Neuromuscular blockers are sometimes used to achieve total paralysis before endotracheal intubation (described in Chapter 13), to relieve muscle spasms of the larynx, to suppress tetany, during electroconvulsive therapy for depression, and to allow for breathing control by a respirator. These blocking agents produce complete paralysis, thus a patient's breathing must be supported. The effectiveness of ventilation and oxygenation must be monitored closely. (These muscle relaxants do not inhibit pain or seizure activity.) Examples of neuromuscular blockers include pancuronium, vecuronium and suxamethonium.

SECTION IV

Drugs that affect the cardiovascular system

Review of anatomy and physiology

The heart is made up of many interconnected branching fibres or cells that form the walls of the two atria and two ventricles. Some of these cells are specialized to conduct electrical impulses. Others have contraction as their main role. All of these cells are nourished through a profuse network of blood vessels (coronary vasculature). Cardiac drugs are classified by their effects on these tissues. Boxes 12-17 and 12-18 list cardiac drugs and pharmacological terms that describe their actions.

Cardiac glycosides

Cardiac glycosides are naturally occurring plant substances that have characteristic effects on the heart. These compounds contain a carbohydrate molecule (sugar). When combined with water, the molecule is converted into a sugar plus one or more active substances. Glycosides may work by blocking certain ionic pumps in the cellular membrane, which indirectly increases the calcium concentration to the contractile proteins. A key cardiac glycoside is digoxin. Digoxin is used to treat heart failure and to manage certain tachycardias.

Digitalis glycosides can affect the heart in two distinct ways. First, they increase the strength of contraction (a positive inotropic effect), and second, they have a dual effect on the electrophysiological properties of the heart. They have a modest negative chronotropic effect (slight slowing of the heart rate), and a profound negative dromotropic effect (decreasing conduction velocity of impulses in the heart).

Many patients who take cardiac glycosides develop side effects at one time or another because of the small therapeutic index of the drugs. The symptoms may be neurological, visual, gastrointestinal, cardiac or psychiatric. These symptoms are often vague and can be attributed easily by the patient to a viral illness. It is important to maintain a high index of suspicion in patients who report experiencing flu-like symptoms and are taking cardiac glycosides. The most common side effects of cardiac glycosides are anorexia, nausea or vomiting, visual disturbances (flashing lights, altered colour vision), and cardiac rhythm disturbances (usually slowing with varying degrees of blocked conduction).

Critical Thinking

Proarrhythmias are serious dysrhythmias that are apparently generated by antidysrhythmic agents. All antidysrhythmic drugs have some degree of proarrhythmic effects. The sequential use of two or more antidysrhythmic drugs compounds these effects. As a rule, use of no more than one agent is best to manage dysrhythmias. (That is, of course, unless use of more than one agent is absolutely necessary.)

Box 12-17

Emergency drugs: cardiovascular system

Drugs used to treat dysrhythmias

Adenosine
Amiodarone
Atropine
Beta-adrenergic blockers
Atenolol
Metoprolol
Calcium channel blockers
Diltiazem
Verapamil
Dopamine
Isoproterenol
Lidocaine
Magnesium
Procainamide

Drugs used to optimize cardiac output and blood pressure

Calcium chloride
Digoxin
Dobutamine
Dopamine
Adrenaline (epinephrine)
Furosemide
Nitroglycerin
Noradrenaline (norepinephrine)
Sodium bicarbonate
Vasopressin

Box 12-18

Pharmacological terms to describe actions of cardiovascular drugs

Chronotropic: Chronotropic drugs affect heart rate. If the drug accelerates the heart rate (e.g. isoproterenol), it is said to have a positive chronotropic effect. A drug that decreases the heart rate (e.g. verapamil) is said to have a negative chronotropic effect.

Dromotropic: Dromotropic drugs affect conduction velocity through the conducting tissues of the heart. If a drug speeds conduction, it is said to have a positive dromotropic effect. Examples of drugs with positive dromotropic effects include isoproterenol and phenytoin. Drugs with negative dromotropic effects delay conduction (e.g. verapamil and adenosine).

Inotropic: Inotropic drugs strengthen or increase the force of cardiac contraction (a positive inotropic effect). Some examples include digoxin, dobutamine, adrenaline (epinephrine), and isoproterenol. A drug that weakens or decreases the force of cardiac contraction has a negative inotropic effect. An example of such a drug is propranolol (Inderal).

The toxic effects of cardiac glycosides are dose related and may be increased by the presence of other drugs, such as diuretics. These other drugs may predispose the patient to cardiac rhythm disturbances, which may include bradycardias, tachycardias, and even ventricular fibrillation. For these reasons, patients taking these drugs require close monitoring. Treatment for digitalis toxicity may include correction of electrolyte imbalances, neutralization of the free drug, and use of antidysrhythmics.

Antidysrhythmics

Antidysrhythmic drugs are used to treat and prevent disorders of cardiac rhythm. The pharmacological agents that suppress dysrhythmias may do so by direct action on the cardiac cell membrane (lidocaine), by indirect action that affects the cells (propranolol), or both.

Cardiac rhythm disturbances may be caused by ischaemia, hypoxia, acidosis or alkalosis, electrolyte abnormalities, excessive catecholamine exposure, autonomic influences, drug toxicity, or scarred and diseased tissue. Dysrhythmias result from disturbances in impulse formation, disturbances in impulse conduction, or both.

Classifications

Antidysrhythmic drugs have been classified into categories based on their fundamental mode of action on cardiac muscle.[14] Drugs that belong to the same class do not always produce identical actions. However, all antidysrhythmic drugs have some ability to suppress automaticity.

Class I

Class I drugs are sodium channel blockers that work to stabilize excitable membranes. They are further divided into subclasses (Ia, Ib, and Ic) based on the extent of sodium channel blockade. Class Ia drugs are used for atrial and ventricular dysrhythmias and include quinidine, disopyramide and procainamide. Class Ib drugs have little atrial effect, so use is limited to dysrhythmias of ventricular origin. Examples include lidocaine and phenytoin. Class Ic drugs profoundly slow conduction and are indicated only for control of life-threatening ventricular dysrhythmias. An example of a Class Ic drug is flecainide.

Class II

Class II drugs are beta-blocking agents. These drugs reduce adrenergic stimulation of the heart. Examples include atenolol and propanolol.

Critical Thinking

How might the signs of shock in a patient taking digoxin or propranolol vary from what might be expected normally?

Class III

Class III drugs prolong the duration of the action potential and the refractory period. Unlike other antidysrhythmic agents, drugs in this class do not suppress automaticity and also have no effect on conduction velocity. These drugs are thought to arrest dysrhythmias that result from the re-entry of blocked impulses. An example of such a drug is amiodarone.

Class IV

Class IV drugs are also known as calcium channel blockers. These drugs are thought to work by blocking the inflow of calcium through the cell membranes of the cardiac and smooth muscle cells. This action depresses the myocardial and smooth muscle contraction, decreases automaticity, and in some cases decreases conduction velocity. Examples of calcium channel blockers include verapamil and diltiazem.

Antihypertensives

In England, 34% of men and 30% of women have hypertension; the figures are slightly lower in Scotland, whilst it is difficult to provide comparative figures for Wales and Northern Ireland due to variations in the reporting methods.[15] Hypertension has been related directly to an increased incidence of stroke, cerebral haemorrhage, heart and renal failure, and coronary heart disease. The exact mechanism of action of many antihypertensive drugs is unknown. The ideal antihypertensive drug should accomplish the following:

- maintain blood pressure within normal limits for various body positions
- maintain or improve blood flow without compromising tissue perfusion or blood supply to the brain
- reduce the workload of the heart
- have no undesirable side effects
- permit long-term administration without intolerance.

Classifications

Certain drugs are used to reduce blood pressure in patients with chronic hypertension. These drugs are usually given in low-dose combinations and are titrated to effect. These drugs include diuretics, sympathetic blocking agents (sympatholytic drugs), vasodilators, angiotensin-converting enzyme (ACE) inhibitors, calcium channel blockers, and the newer class, angiotensin II receptor antagonists.[16] The National Institute for Clinical Excellence make evidence-based recommendations for pharmacological management of hypertension in the UK (Figure 12-9).

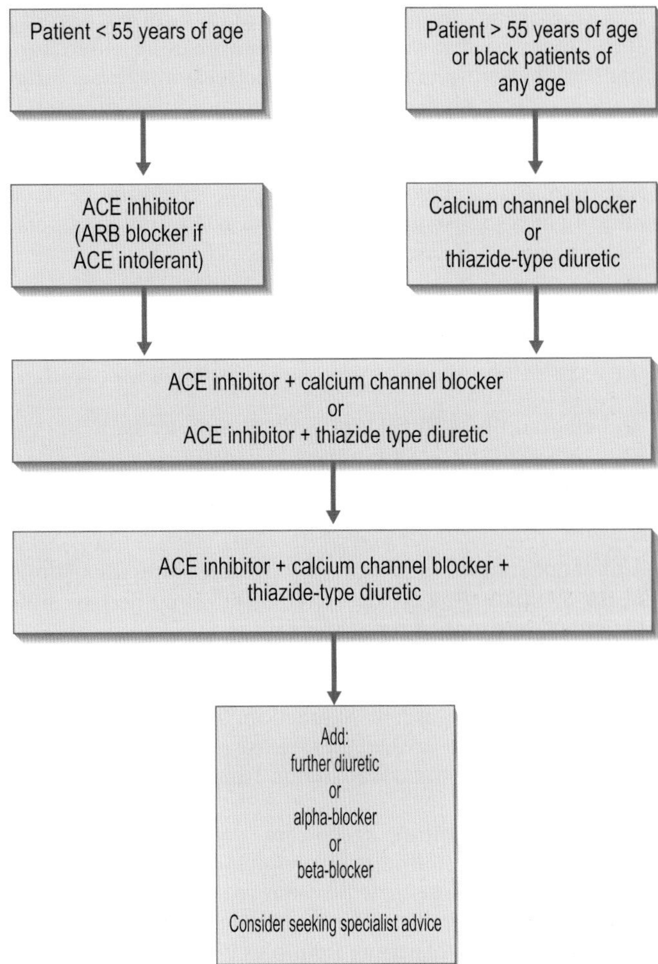

Figure 12-9 NICE guidelines on management of hypertension.

Diuretics

Diuretics promote water loss from the body into the urine. They generally act upon the nephron and cause a decrease in plasma and extracellular fluid volume, which is reflected in a decrease in preload and stroke volume. These responses result in a lowering of the blood pressure.

Thiazides are diuretics that decrease sodium reabsorption by the kidneys, which results in a more concentrated fluid entering the collecting ducts and slows down water reabsorption. Thiazide and thiazide-like diuretics also have an effect on the peripheral arterioles, which leads to vasodilatation and a further reduction in blood pressure. Many antihypertensive agents cause retention of sodium and water, yet thiazides may be given concomitantly to help prevent this side effect. An example of a thiazide diuretic is bendrofluazide.

Loop diuretics are strong, short-acting agents that inhibit sodium and chloride reabsorption in the loop of Henle. These drugs cause excessive loss of potassium and also cause an increase in the excretion of sodium and water. Loop diuretics have fewer side effects than most other antihypertensives; however, hypokalaemia and profound dehydration can be a result of their use. These agents are prescribed to patients who have renal insufficiency and may also be given to patients who cannot take other diuretics. An example of a loop diuretic is furosemide.

Note

Many drugs are excreted by the kidneys. Thus, patients with renal system dysfunction (acute or chronic renal failure) may accumulate drugs in their systems. These patients often require modifications in drug doses and dosing intervals. These changes are in addition to diet modification and fluid restriction.

Potassium-sparing agents can be effective as an antihypertensive when they are used in combination with other diuretics. They promote sodium and water loss without a loss of potassium. These agents are used to treat hypertensive patients who become hypokalaemic from other diuretics and also for patients who are apparently resistant to the antihypertensive effects of other diuretics. Potassium-sparing agents are also used to treat some oedematous states. (An example of such is cirrhosis of the liver with ascites.) An example of a potassium-sparing agent is spironolactone.

Sympathetic blocking agents

Sympathetic blocking agents may be classified as beta-blocking agents and adrenergic-inhibiting agents. Beta-blocking agents are used to treat cardiovascular disorders, including patients with suspected myocardial infarction, high-risk unstable angina, and hypertension. These drugs work by decreasing cardiac output and inhibiting renin secretion from the kidneys. Both actions result in lower blood pressure. Beta-blocking drugs compete with adrenaline for available β-receptor sites as well. This inhibits tissue and organ response to beta stimulation. Examples of beta-blocking agents include the following:

- $beta_1$-blocking agents (cardioselective)
  - acebutolol
  - atenolol
  - metoprolol
- $beta_1$- and $beta_2$-blocking agents (non-selective)
  - labetalol (also has $alpha_1$-blocking properties)
  - nadolol
  - propranolol.

Adrenergic-inhibiting agents work by modifying the actions of the sympathetic nervous system. They are effective antihypertensive drugs. Arterial pressure is influenced through various mechanisms of the heart, blood vessels and kidneys. Sympathetic stimulation increases the heart rate and force of myocardial contraction, constricts arterioles and venules, and causes the release of renin from the kidneys. Blocking this sympathetic stimulation can reduce blood pressure.

Adrenergic-inhibiting agents are classified as centrally acting adrenergic inhibitors or peripheral adrenergic inhibitors. The mechanism by which many of these agents work is unknown. Generally, most of these agents are believed to have multiple sites of action. Examples include the following drugs:

- methyldopa
- prazosin hydrochloride
- doxazosin.

Vasodilator drugs

Vasodilator drugs act directly on the smooth muscle walls of the arterioles, veins, or both. They lower peripheral resistance, causing a reduction in blood pressure. This lower blood pressure stimulates the sympathetic nervous system and activates the baroreceptor reflexes, which, in turn, leads to an increase in heart rate, cardiac output and renin release. Medications that inhibit the sympathetic response are usually given with vasodilator drugs.

In addition to their use as antihypertensives, some vasodilator drugs work to treat angina pectoris (ischaemic chest pain). For example, nitrates dilate veins and arteries, which leads to venous pooling of blood and reduces the blood returned to the heart. Thus these effects reduce left ventricular end-diastolic volume and pressure. The subsequent decrease in wall tension helps to reduce myocardial oxygen demand and also relieves the chest pain of myocardial ischaemia. Vasodilator drugs are classified as arteriolar dilators and arteriolar and venous dilators. Examples of each include the following:

- Arteriolar dilator drugs
  - diazoxide
  - hydralazine
  - minoxidil
- Arteriolar and venous dilator drugs
  - sodium nitroprusside
  - nitrates and nitrites
  - amyl nitrite inhalant
  - isosorbide dinitrate
  - nitroglycerin sublingual tablet
  - intravenous nitroglycerin.

Angiotensin-converting enzyme (ACE) inhibitor drugs

The renin–angiotensin–aldosterone system plays a key role in maintaining blood pressure as well as helping to regulate sodium and fluid balance. A disturbance in this system can result in hypertension. In addition, kidney damage can result in an inability to regulate the release of renin through normal feedback mechanisms. This causes elevated blood pressure in some patients.

Angiotensin II is a strong vasoconstrictor that raises blood pressure and also causes the release of aldosterone. Aldosterone contributes to sodium and water retention. By inhibiting conversion of the precursor angiotensin I to the active molecule angiotensin II (which is brought about through ACE), the renin–angiotensin–aldosterone system is suppressed and blood pressure is lowered. Examples of ACE inhibitors include captopril, enalapril, benazepril and lisinopril.

Calcium channel blockers

Calcium channel blocking agents such as verapamil, amlodipine,˙ felodipine and diltiazem reduce peripheral vascular resistance by inhibiting the contractility of vascular smooth muscle. They dilate coronary vessels through the same mechanism. The effects of these drugs are important in treating hypertension, decreasing the oxygen requirements of the heart (through decreased afterload), and increasing oxygen supply (by abolishing coronary artery spasm), thus relieving the causes of angina pectoris. The various drugs in this class differ in degree of selectivity for coronary (and peripheral) vasodilation or decreased cardiac contractility.

Angiotensin II receptor antagonists

Angiotensin II receptor antagonists are a new class of antihypertensive agent. They block the renin–angiotensin–aldosterone system more completely than ACE inhibitors. They lower blood pressure by selectively inhibiting the actions of angiotensin II receptors that include vasoconstriction, renal tubular sodium reabsorption, aldosterone release, and stimulation of central and peripheral sympathetic activity. These drugs are used to manage hypertension in those who cannot deal with the adverse effects of ACE inhibitors. (Some of these effects include cough and angioedema.) The drugs appear to be equally effective in lowering systolic and diastolic pressure and are now being studied for their effectiveness in treating congestive heart failure, diabetic nephropathy, and vascular diseases such as atherosclerosis. Drugs in this classification include candesartan, irbesartan and losartan.

SECTION V

Drugs that affect the blood

Anticoagulants, fibrinolytics and blood components

Bleeding and thrombosis are altered states of haemostasis. An understanding of the drugs that affect blood coagulation and of the use of fibrinolytic agents and blood components is crucial. In the prehospital arena, these concepts will assist in the management of patients.

Agents that affect blood coagulation

Drugs that affect blood coagulation may be classified as antiplatelet, anticoagulant and fibrinolytic agents.

Platelets are small cell fragments in the blood that provide the initial step in normal repair of blood vessels. Blood coagulation is a process that results in the formation of a stable fibrin clot that entraps platelets, blood cells, and plasma. The end result of this process is called a blood clot or thrombus. Abnormal thrombus formation is the major cause of myocardial infarction (from coronary thrombosis) and stroke (from cerebral vascular thrombosis).

The coagulation process also occurs in the venous system, although the underlying mechanisms responsible for the thrombosis differ. Arterial thrombi are commonly associated with atherosclerotic plaques, hypertension, and turbulent blood flow that damages the endothelial lining of blood vessels. Damage to the endothelium causes platelets to stick and aggregate in the arterial system. Arterial thrombi are made up mostly of platelets, but they also involve the chemical substances that contribute to the coagulation process (in particular, fibrinogen and fibrin). Myocardial infarctions and strokes are often the result of arterial thrombi.

The three major risk factors for various thromboses are stasis, localized trauma and hypercoagulable states. Stasis is reduced blood flow and results from immobilization or venous insufficiency. Stasis is responsible for the increased incidence of deep vein thrombosis in most bedridden patients. Localized trauma may initiate the clotting cascade and may cause arterial and venous thrombosis. Hypercoagulability of the blood is the cause of the increased incidence of deep vein thrombosis in women who take birth control pills. Hypercoagulability is also responsible for many of the familial thrombotic disorders (see Chapter 15).

Antiplatelet agents

Drugs that interfere with platelet aggregation are known as antiplatelet or antithrombic drugs. These drugs are sometimes prescribed as a prophylactic and may be prescribed for patients at risk of developing arterial clots. They are also prescribed for those who have suffered myocardial infarction or stroke, and those with certain valvular heart diseases, valvular prostheses and various intracardiac shunts. Among the most common antiplatelet drugs are aspirin, dipyridamole and clopidogrel.

Anticoagulant agents

Anticoagulant drug therapy is used to prevent intravascular thrombosis. The therapy works by decreasing blood coagulability and is commonly used to prevent postoperative thromboembolism. Anticoagulant agents are also used during haemodialysis and in reperfusion therapy for some patients with acute coronary syndromes. Anticoagulant therapy is a preventive measure against future clot formation. The therapy has no direct effect on a blood clot that has formed already or on ischaemic tissue injured by inadequate blood supply as a result of a thrombus. The major side effect of anticoagulant therapy is haemorrhage and bleeding complications. Examples of anticoagulant agents include warfarin and heparin.

Note

Platelet adhesion, activation, and aggregation that result in the formation of an arterial thrombus are pivotal in the pathogenesis of acute coronary syndromes (acute myocardial infarctions). Recent studies indicate that the administration of a glycoprotein IIb/IIIa receptor antagonist may reduce ischaemic complications after plaque fissure or rupture. (These drugs inhibit glycoprotein receptors in the membrane of platelets and help prevent platelet aggregation.) These drugs may be included along with aspirin, heparin and beta-blockers during in-hospital reperfusion therapy for select patients. Examples of glycoprotein IIb/IIIa inhibitors include abciximab, eptifibatide and tirofiban.

Fibrinolytic agents

Fibrinolytic drugs dissolve clots after their formation. They do so by promoting the digestion of fibrin. Fibrinolytic therapy has become the treatment of choice for treating acute myocardial infarction in certain groups of patients and has recently become the treatment of choice in managing some stroke patients. The goal is to re-establish blood flow and prevent ischaemia and tissue death. Fibrinolytic therapy has been used in acute pulmonary embolism, deep vein thrombosis, and peripheral arterial occlusion. Fibrinolytics are used in the prehospital setting in the UK for management of acute ST elevation myocardial infarction (STEMI). These drugs include reteplase and tenecteplase (see Chapter 15).

Critical Thinking

Fibrinolytics have the potential to dissolve clots, which in turn may reverse the serious effects of myocardial infarction and stroke. So why are fibrinolytics not given to everyone who is suspected of having these conditions?

Antihaemophilic agents

Haemophilia (further described in Chapter 22) is a group of hereditary bleeding disorders. With these, a person lacks one of the factors needed for the coagulation of blood. These disorders are characterized by persistent and uncontrollable bleeding that can occur after even a minor injury. Bleeding may occur into joints, the urinary tract, and at times the

CNS. Haemophilia A is the classic form of haemophilia and is caused by a deficiency of factor VIII. Haemophilia B is also known as Christmas disease and results from a deficiency in factor IX complex. Replacement therapy of the missing clotting factor can be effective in managing haemophilia.

Note

Coagulation factors refer to the 13 proteins contained in blood plasma. These proteins interact to produce a blood clot.

Box 12-19

Examples of antihyperlipidaemic drugs

Atorvastatin
Fenofibrate
Fluvastatin
Gemfibrozil
Pravastatin
Simvastatin

Haemostatic agents

Haemostatic agents hasten clot formation which in turn reduces bleeding. Systemic haemostatic agents (e.g. tranexamic acid) are generally used to control rapid blood loss after surgery by inhibiting fibrinolysis. Topical haemostatic agents (e.g. hemocollagene sponges) are used to control capillary bleeding during surgical and dental procedures.

Blood and blood components

The healthy body maintains a normal balance of blood and its components. However, illness and injury such as haemorrhage, burns, and dehydration may affect this balance. These conditions may impair this balance and require replacement therapy. The usual treatment of choice is to replace the sole blood component that is deficient. Replacement therapy may include transfusing the following:

- whole blood (rarely used)
- packed red blood cells
- fresh-frozen plasma
- plasma expanders
- platelets
- coagulation factors
- fibrinogen
- albumin
- gamma globulins.

Antihyperlipidaemic drugs

Hyperlipidaemia refers to an excess of lipids in the plasma. Several types of hyperlipidaemia occur; all are associated with elevated levels of cholesterol and triglycerides. This condition is thought to play a role in the development of atherosclerosis, thus antihyperlipidaemic drugs are sometimes used along with diet and exercise to control serum lipid levels (Box 12-19). Antihyperlipidaemic drugs do not reverse existing atherosclerosis.

SECTION VI

Drugs that affect the respiratory system

Review of anatomy and physiology

The respiratory system includes all structures that are involved in the exchange of oxygen and carbon dioxide. Serious narrowing of any portion of the respiratory tract may be an indication for drug therapy (Box 12-20). Emergencies involving the respiratory system are usually caused by reversible conditions such as asthma, emphysema with infection, and foreign body airway obstruction (see Chapter 13).

Smooth muscle fibres line the tracheobronchial tree and directly influence the diameter of the airways. The bronchial smooth muscle tone is maintained by impulses from the autonomic nervous system. Parasympathetic fibres from the vagus nerve stimulate bronchial smooth muscle through the release of acetylcholine. This neurotransmitter interacts with the muscarinic receptors on the membranes of the cell, producing bronchoconstriction.

Sympathetic fibres mainly affect β_2-receptors in the lungs through the release of adrenaline from the adrenal medulla and the release of noradrenaline from the peripheral sympathetic nerves. The adrenaline reaches the lungs by way of the circulatory system. Adrenaline interacts with β_2-receptors to produce smooth muscle relaxation and bronchodilatation, thus the β_2-receptor plays the dominant role in bronchial muscle tone. (Although β_1-receptors are also found on bronchial smooth muscle, their ratio to β_2-receptors is 1 : 3.)

Bronchodilators

Bronchodilator drugs are the primary treatment for obstructive pulmonary disease such as asthma, chronic bronchitis, and emphysema. These drugs are classified as sympathomimetic drugs or xanthine derivatives. Many of these drugs are administered by inhalation via a nebulizer or pressure cartridge (see Chapter 14).

Sympathomimetic drugs

Sympathomimetic drugs are grouped according to their effects on receptors. Non-selective adrenergic drugs have α, β_1 (cardiac), and β_2 (respiratory) activity. Non-selective β-adrenergic drugs have β_1 and β_2 effects. Selective β_2-receptor drugs act primarily on β_2-receptors in the lungs (bronchial

Box 12-20

Emergency drugs: respiratory system

Ipratropium bromide
Chlorphenamine
Adrenaline (epinephrine) 1:1000
Salbutamol

Box 12-21

α, β_1, and β_2 activities of adrenergic drugs used as bronchodilators

α effects

Systemic effects
Vasoconstriction
Increased blood pressure

Inhalation
Decreased bronchial congestion
Increased duration of action for co-administered β_2 drugs

β_1 effects

Systemic effects
Cardiac stimulation
Increased heart rate
Increased force of contraction
Possible palpitations and dysrhythmmias
Relaxation of gastrointestinal tract

Inhalation
Some bronchodilatation and increased heart rate
Fewer effects than with subcutaneous administration

β_2 effects

Systemic effects
Bronchodilatation
Stimulation of skeletal muscles (tremors)
Vasodilatation (mainly in blood vessels supplying muscle)
Glycogenolysis

Central nervous system effects
Anxiety
Dizziness
Inhalation
Insomnia
Irritability
Nervousness
Sweating
Lower incidence of systemic effects than with subcutaneous administration

smooth muscle). Box 12-21 summarizes the α, β_1, and β_2 activities of the adrenergic drugs used as bronchodilators.

The β_2-selective drugs are most commonly used as bronchodilators because they lessen the incidence of unwanted cardiac effects caused by β_1-adrenergic agents. Patients with hypertension, cardiac disease, or diabetes can better tolerate this group of bronchodilators. Examples of selective β_2-receptor drugs include salbutamol, fenoterol, terbutaline, salmeterol and formoterol.

Xanthine derivatives

The xanthine group of drugs includes caffeine, theophylline and theobromine. These drugs relax smooth muscle (particularly bronchial smooth muscle), stimulate cardiac muscle and the CNS, increase diaphragmatic contractility, and promote diuresis through increased renal perfusion. The action of various theophylline compounds depends on the concentration of theophylline, which is the active ingredient. Theophylline products vary in their rate of absorption and therapeutic effects. Aminophylline and theophylline are some of the many theophylline-containing preparations. Theophylline preparations are not generally considered a first-line drug in the treatment of acute reactive airway disease such as asthma.

Other respiratory drugs

A number of other drugs can be used to treat asthma and other obstructive pulmonary diseases. These drugs include prophylactic asthmatic agents such as cromolyn sodium; aerosol corticosteroid agents such as beclometasone dipropionate; dexamethasone; antileukotrienes such as montelukast; and muscarinic antagonists (anticholinergics) such as ipratropium. These drugs reduce the allergic or inflammatory response to a variety of stimuli and also have an effect on bronchial smooth muscle. In the acute care setting, intravenously administered steroids (e.g. methylprednisolone) may be given in an attempt to decrease the inflammatory response and improve airflow.

Mucokinetic drugs

Mucokinetic drugs are used to move respiratory secretions, excessive mucus and sputum along the tracheobronchial tree. These agents work by altering the consistency of these secretions so that they can be removed from the body more easily. Persons with chronic pulmonary disease often use mucokinetic drugs. These drugs help to clear their respiratory passages and improve ciliary activity in the airways.

Mucokinetic drugs include diluents (water, saline solution), aerosols, and mucolytic drugs or expectorants.

Note

Mucus is a normal secretion produced by the surface cells in the mucous membranes. Sputum is an abnormal viscous secretion that consists mainly of mucus and originates in the lower respiratory tract.

Oxygen and miscellaneous respiratory agents

Oxygen is mainly used to treat hypoxia and hypoxaemia. Oxygen is a colourless, odourless and tasteless gas that is essential for sustaining life. (Oxygen and oxygen delivery are described in detail in Chapter 13.)

Direct respiratory stimulants

Direct respiratory stimulants are known as analeptics. These act directly on the medullary centre of the brain to increase the rate and depth of respirations. These drugs are considered inferior to mechanical ventilatory measures to treat respiratory depression and to counteract drug-induced respiratory depression caused by anaesthetics. An example of a direct respiratory stimulant is doxapram.

Reflex respiratory stimulants

Spirits of ammonia is given by inhalation and acts as a reflex respiratory stimulant. The noxious vapour is used sometimes in cases of fainting and works by irritating sensory nerve receptors in the throat and stomach. These nerve receptors send afferent messages to the control centres of the brain to stimulate respiration.

Respiratory depressants

Respiratory depressants include opiates and barbiturate drugs previously described. Respiratory depression is a common side effect of these drugs; however, they are seldom given to inhibit rate and depth of respiration intentionally.

Cough suppressants

The cough is a protective reflex to expel harmful irritants and may be productive when removing irritants or secretions from the airway. The cough may also be non-productive (dry and irritating) and prolonged. The cough can result from an underlying disorder, thus treatment with antitussive drugs may be indicated. Box 12-22 presents a few narcotic and non-narcotic antitussive agents.

Box 12-22

Examples of narcotic and non-narcotic antitussive agents

Narcotic agent

Codeine

Non-narcotic agents

Benzonatate (Tessalon)

Dextromethorphan (Sucrets, Robitussin DM)

Antihistamines

Histamine is a chemical mediator found in almost all body tissues. The concentration is highest in the skin, lungs, and gastrointestinal tract. The body releases histamine when exposed to an antigen, such as pollen or insect stings, which results in increased localized blood flow, increased capillary permeability, and swelling of the tissues. In addition, histamine produces contractile action on bronchial smooth muscle.

Allergic responses involving histamine and other chemical mediators include local effects such as angioedema, eczema, rhinitis, urticaria, and asthma. Systemic effects from the release of histamine and certain other mediators may result in anaphylaxis (see Chapter 18).

Antihistamines compete with histamine for receptor sites to prevent the physiological action of histamine. Two types of histamine receptors are H_1 receptors (these act mainly on the blood vessels and the bronchioles) and H_2 receptors (these act mainly on the gastrointestinal tract). In addition to blocking some actions of histamine, antihistamines also have anticholinergic or atropine-like action. This may result in tachycardia, constipation, drowsiness, sedation and inhibition of secretions. Most antihistamines have a local anaesthetic effect as well, which may soothe the skin irritation caused by an allergic reaction. The chief clinical use of antihistamines is for allergic reactions; however, they are also sometimes prescribed to control motion sickness or as a sedative or antiemetic. Examples of antihistamines are chlorphenamine, promethazine, and the newer H_1 receptor antagonists loratadine, cetirizine and fexofenadine.

SECTION VII

Drugs that affect the gastrointestinal system

Review of anatomy and physiology

The gastrointestinal system is composed of the digestive tract, the biliary system, and the pancreas. The primary function of the gastrointestinal system is to provide the body with water, electrolytes, and other nutrients used by cells. Drug therapy for the gastrointestinal system can be divided into two groups: drugs that affect the stomach and drugs that affect the lower gastrointestinal tract. In emergency care, conditions of the stomach or gastrointestinal tract that may require drug therapy are usually limited to nausea and vomiting.

Drugs that affect the stomach

Conditions of the stomach that may require drug therapy include hyperacidity, hypoacidity, ulcer disease, nausea, vomiting and hypermotility.

Antacids

Antacids buffer or neutralize hydrochloric acid in the stomach. They are prescribed for the relief of symptoms associated with hyperacidity such as peptic ulcer, gastritis, oesophagitis, heartburn and hiatus hernia. Common over-the-counter antacids include Alka-Seltzer and Gaviscon.

Emetics and antiemetics

Vomiting is an involuntary action coordinated by the emetic centre of the medulla. Vomiting may be initiated through the CNS as a secondary reaction to emotion, pain, or disequilibrium (motion sickness); through irritation of the mucosa of the gastrointestinal tract or bowel; or through stimulation from the chemoreceptor trigger zone of the medulla by circulating drugs and toxins (e.g. opiates or digitalis).

Emetics

Emetics induce vomiting. They are administered infrequently today as part of the treatment for drug overdoses and poisonings. These drugs include apomorphine and syrup of ipecac. The treatment of drug overdoses and poisoning is addressed further in Chapter 21.

Antiemetics

Drugs used to treat nausea and vomiting include antagonists of histamine, acetylcholine and dopamine, and other drugs the actions of which are not understood clearly. These drugs work best when they are given before rather than after nausea and vomiting have begun. For example, drugs used to treat motion sickness or vertigo should be taken 30 min before travelling. Common antiemetics include metoclopramide, ondansetron, chlorpromazine, domperidone and promethazine.

Note

Cannabinoids are drugs that are derived from hemp plants. They have been used experimentally to prevent vomiting in patients who receive cancer chemotherapy. Examples of these drugs include dronabinol and nabilone. These drugs use a synthetic derivative of the active ingredient in marijuana.

H_2 receptor antagonists

As described before, the action of histamine is mediated through H_2 receptors. Histamine has been associated with gastric acid secretion. H_2 receptor antagonists block the H_2 receptors, so reduce the volume of gastric acid secretion and its acid content. Examples of H_2 receptor antagonists include cimetidine, ranitidine and famotidine.

Proton pump inhibitors

Proton pump inhibitors are used to treat symptomatic gastro-oesophageal reflux disease, for short-term treatment of erosive oesophagitis, and for maintenance of erosive oesophagitis healing. The proton pump (potassium adenosine triphosphate enzyme system) is the final pathway for secretion of hydrochloric acid by the parietal cells of the stomach. Proton pump inhibitors decrease hydrochloric acid secretion by inhibiting the actions of the parietal cells. In addition, the gastric pH of the stomach is altered. Examples of proton pump inhibitors include esomeprazole, lansoprazole, omeprazole, pantoprazole and rabeprazole.

Drugs that affect the lower gastrointestinal tract

Constipation and diarrhoea are two common conditions of the lower gastrointestinal tract. Both conditions may require drug therapy. Drugs used to manage these conditions include laxatives and antidiarrhoeals.

Laxatives

Laxatives produce defecation. They are used to evacuate the bowel and to soften hardened stool for easier passage. Situations that may indicate the need for laxative use include the following:

- constipation
- neurological diseases (e.g. multiple sclerosis or Parkinson's disease)
- pregnancy
- rectal disorders
- drug poisoning
- surgery and endoscopic examination.

Numerous types of laxatives are available and many can be bought without a prescription. Regular or excessive use of laxatives is common in older adults and in those with eating disorders. Laxative abuse may result in permanent bowel damage and electrolyte imbalance.

Antidiarrhoeal drugs

Antidiarrhoeal drugs are used to reduce an abnormal frequency of bowel evacuation. Common causes of acute and chronic diarrhoea include bacterial or viral invasion, drugs, diet and numerous disease states (e.g. diabetes insipidus and inflammatory bowel syndromes). Drugs used to treat diarrhoea include the following:

- Adsorbents
  - kaolin
- Anti-motility
  - codeine phosphate
  - co-phenotrope
  - loperamide
  - morphine.

SECTION VIII

Drugs that affect the endocrine system

Review of anatomy and physiology

The endocrine system works to control and integrate body functions. (Box 12-23 presents emergency drugs that affect the endocrine system.) Information from various parts of the body is carried via blood-borne hormones to distant sites. Hormones are natural chemical substances that act after they have been secreted into the bloodstream from endocrine glands (ductless glands that secrete internally). These glands include the anterior and posterior pituitary, thyroid, para-

Box 12-23

Emergency drugs: endocrine system

Dextrose 10%
Glucagon
Insulin
Hydrocortisone
Oxytocin

Box 12-24

Drugs that affect the anterior and posterior pituitary gland

Anterior pituitary gland drugs

Used to treat growth failure in children caused by growth hormone deficiency:
Somatropin

Posterior pituitary gland drugs

Used to treat the symptoms of diabetes insipidus resulting from antidiuretic hormone deficiency:
Vasopressin

Box 12-25

Drugs that affect the thyroid and parathyroid glands

Thyroid drugs

Used to treat hypothyroidism and to prevent goitres:
Thyroid
Iodine products
Levothyroxine

Parathyroid drugs

Used to treat hyperparathyroidism:
Vitamin D
Calcium supplements

Box 12-26

Drugs that affect the adrenal cortex

Glucocorticoids

Betamethasone
Dexamethasone
Methylprednisolone

Mineralocorticoids

Desoxycorticosterone acetate
Fludrocortisone

Adrenal steroid inhibitors

Aminoglutethimide
Metyrapone

thyroid, and adrenal glands and the thymus, pancreas, testes and ovaries. Hormones from the various endocrine glands work together to regulate vital processes, including the following:

- secretory and motor activities of the digestive tract
- energy production
- composition and volume of extracellular fluid
- adaptation (e.g. acclimatization and immunity)
- growth and development
- reproduction and lactation.

Drugs that affect the pituitary gland

The hormones of the anterior and posterior pituitary gland are important for regulating the secretion of other hormones in the body. Box 12-24 lists drugs that affect the anterior and posterior pituitary. (Disorders of the endocrine glands are described further in Chapter 17.)

Drugs that affect the thyroid and parathyroid glands

The thyroid hormone controls the rate of metabolic processes and is required for normal growth and development. Parathyroid hormone regulates the level of ionized calcium in the blood through the release of calcium from bone, the absorption of calcium from the intestine, and controlling the rate of calcium excretion by the kidneys.

Disorders of the thyroid gland include goitre (enlargement of the thyroid gland), hypothyroidism (thyroid hormone deficiency), and hyperthyroidism (thyroid hormone excess). Disorders of the parathyroid include hypoparathyroidism and hyperparathyroidism. Box 12-25 lists the drugs used to treat these disorders.

Drugs that affect the adrenal cortex

The adrenal cortex secretes three major classes of steroid hormones: glucocorticoids (cortisol), mineralocorticoids (primarily aldosterone), and sex hormones. Glucocorticoids raise blood glucose, deplete tissue proteins, and suppress the inflammatory reaction. Mineralocorticoids regulate electrolyte and water balance. Sex hormones are oestrogen, progesterone, and testosterone, and are produced in small amounts by men and women. The sex hormones have little physiological effect under normal circumstances. Box 12-26 lists drugs that affect the adrenal cortex. Two disorders of the adrenal cortex are Addison's disease (adrenal cortical hypofunction) and Cushing's disease (adrenal cortical hyperfunction) (see Chapter 17).

Drugs that affect the pancreas

The pancreas is both an exocrine gland (providing digestive juices to the small intestine) and an endocrine gland. The endocrine portion of the pancreas consists of pancreatic islets (islets of Langerhans), which produce the hormones that enter the circulatory system.

Hormones of the pancreas

The pancreatic hormones play a key role in helping to regulate the concentration of certain nutrients in the circulatory system. The pancreas secretes two major hormones: insulin and glucagon.

Insulin is the primary hormone that regulates glucose metabolism. In general, insulin increases the ability of the liver, adipose tissue, and muscle to take up and use glucose. Glucose not immediately needed for energy is stored in the skeletal muscle, liver, and other tissues. This stored form of glucose is called glycogen.

Glucagon mainly influences the liver although it has some effect on skeletal muscle and adipose tissue. In general, glucagon stimulates the liver to break down glycogen, thus glucose is released into the blood. Glucagon also inhibits the uptake of glucose by muscle and fat cells. The balancing action of these two hormones protects the body from hyperglycaemia and hypoglycaemia.

This balance of hormonal actions is important when one considers the metabolic problems that can occur in diabetes mellitus. The relationship of glucagon and insulin to other hormones and substances such as dextrose 50% (D50) and thiamine (vitamin B_1) is addressed in Chapter 17. Box 12-27 lists drugs that affect the pancreas.

Box 12-27

Drugs that affect the pancreas

Insulin preparations

Short acting
Insulin Aspart
Insulin Glulisine
Insulin Lispro

Intermediate acting
Isophane Insulin
Biphasic Insulin Aspart
Biphasic Insulin Lispro
Biphasic Isophane Insulin

Long acting
Insulin Detemir
Insulin Glargine
Insulin Zinc Suspension

Oral antidiabetic agents

Glibenclamide
Gliclazide
Tolbutamide
Metformin
Acarbose

Hyperglycaemic agents

Dextrose
Glucagon
Hypostop Gel

SECTION IX

Drugs used in infectious disease and inflammation

Antibiotics

Antibiotics are used to treat local or systemic infection. Antibiotics kill or suppress the growth of microorganisms by disrupting the bacterial cell wall, by disturbing the functions of the cell membrane, or by interfering with the metabolic functions of the cell. This group of drugs includes penicillins, cephalosporins and related products; macrolide antibiotics; tetracyclines; fluoroquinolones; and miscellaneous antibiotic agents (e.g. metronidazole and spectinomycin). Antibiotics are much more toxic to bacteria than they are to a patient. Occasionally they may produce hypersensitivity, which can lead to a fatal reaction if the drug is later given to a sensitized patient.

Note

In time, some bacteria that are at first sensitive to antibiotics may become resistant to them. The bacteria develop ways to evade the effect of a drug. Widespread use and misuse of antibiotics leads to the development of resistant strains of bacteria.

Penicillins

Penicillins are active against Gram-positive and some Gram-negative bacteria (Box 12-28). Penicillins are used to treat many infections, including tonsillitis, pharyngitis, bronchitis and pneumonia. Examples of penicillins include amoxicillin, ampicillin, benzylpenicillin, co-amoxiclav and flucloxacillin. Penicillin can produce severe anaphylactic reactions.

Cephalosporins

Cephalosporins (and related products) resemble penicillins but are broad-spectrum antibiotics that are active against Gram-positive and Gram-negative bacteria. Cephalosporins are widely used to treat ear, throat, and respiratory infections and are also useful for treating urinary tract infections. Urinary tract infections are often caused by bacteria that are resistant to penicillin-type antibiotics. Examples of cephalosporins and related products include cefuroxime, ceftazidime, and cefotaxime. About 6–10% of those who are allergic to penicillins are also allergic to cephalosporins.

Macrolide antibiotics

Macrolides (erythromycins) are used to treat infections of the skin, chest, throat, and ears. Macrolides are useful for treating pertussis (whooping cough) and Legionnaires' disease. Examples of macrolides drugs include azithromycin, clarithromycin and erythromycin itself.

Box 12-28

Gram's stain

Gram's stain is an iodine-based stain used to differentiate various types of bacteria. Basically, a specimen is stained with gentian violet, followed by Gram's solution. The specimen is then treated with a decolorizing agent such as acetone, and finally counterstained with a red dye (safranin). Specimens that retain the dark violet stain are known as Gram-positive; those that lose the violet stain after decolorization but take up the counterstain (causing them to appear pink) are Gram-negative. Examples of Gram-positive bacteria are staphylococci, streptococci, and pneumococci. Examples of Gram-negative bacteria are gonococci and meningococci.

Tetracyclines

Tetracyclines are active against many Gram-negative and Gram-positive organisms (broad-spectrum). They are still the treatment of choice for infections caused by *Chlamydia*, and also for conditions such as acne, bronchitis, genital mycoplasma infections, and certain types of pneumonia. Examples of tetracyclines include demeclocycline, doxycycline and tetracycline. Tetracyclines may discolour developing teeth so are not usually prescribed for children under the age of 12 or for pregnant women.

Critical Thinking

Explain how antibiotics and infectious organisms work like a lock and key.

Quinolones

Quinolone antibiotics are the treatment of choice for some human gastrointestinal infections, particularly severe food-borne illness caused by *Campylobacter* or *Salmonella* bacteria. They are also used to treat urinary tract infections, venereal disease, bone and joint infections, some types of pneumonia, and other human illness. Examples of quinolones include ciprofloxacin, moxifloxacin and levofloxacin.

Antifungal and antiviral drugs

As discussed, persons can get an infection from bacterial organisms. In addition, they can be infected by fungi and viral diseases.

Antifungal drugs

Some fungi are harmlessly present at all times in areas of the body such as the mouth, skin, intestines, and vagina. These fungi are prevented from multiplying through competition from bacteria and the actions of the immune system. Fungal infections are more common and serious in persons taking antibiotics long term (antibiotics destroy the bacterial competition), in those who are immunosuppressed as a complication of illness (e.g. infection with the human immunodeficiency virus), and in those who are taking corticosteroids or immunosuppressant drugs (described later in this chapter). Fungal infections can be classified broadly into superficial infections, subcutaneous infections, and deep infections (Box 12-29). Examples of antifungal drugs include fluconazole, terbinafine and nystatin. About 50 species of fungi can cause illness and sometimes fatal disease in human beings.

Box 12-29

Categories of fungal infections

Examples of superficial infections

Candidiasis (thrush): Affects the genitals or inside of the mouth and vaginal and intertriginous areas

Tinea (including ring worm, athlete's foot, jock itch): Affects external areas of the body

Examples of subcutaneous infections (rare)

Mycetoma (Madura foot): Occurs in tropical countries

Sporotrichosis: May follow inoculation of spores through a puncture or scratch

Examples of deep infections

Aspergillosis

Blastomycosis

Candidiasis (that spreads from its usual site to the oesophagus, urinary tract, or other internal sites)

Cryptococcosis

Histoplasmosis

Antiviral drugs

To date, few effective drugs exist to treat minor viral infections such as colds. In fact, few drugs exist for use in any viral infections. This is due partly to the relative delay in the onset of symptoms that occurs in viral diseases which makes drug therapy difficult once the disease is established. Some viral infections are trivial and harmless (e.g. warts) but others are serious diseases such as influenza, rabies, acquired immune deficiency syndrome (AIDS) and probably some types of cancers (Table 12-5).

Examples of specific antiviral drugs include aciclovir, which is effective against herpes infection. Others are zidovudine, lamivudine, which are used to treat human immunodeficiency virus (HIV) infection, and entecavir, which is used against viral hepatitis.

Protease inhibitors

The manner in which protease inhibitors work is not understood clearly. Yet they appear to inhibit the replication of retroviruses (e.g. HIV) in acute and chronically infected cells. Side effects and adverse reactions of these drugs include nausea and vomiting, headache, malaise, fever and flu-like symptoms. Examples of protease inhibitors include indinavir, ritonavir and saquinavir.

Note

The administration of antiviral drugs and protease inhibitors for a healthcare worker who has had significant occupational exposure to body fluids that may contain HIV or another virus known or suspected to be resistant to antiviral drugs is important and is a post-exposure prophylaxis recommendation by the Department of Health.[17]

Table 12-5 Common viruses and viral diseases or conditions

Viral family	Diseases or conditions
Papovavirus	Warts
Adenovirus	Cold sores, genital herpes, chickenpox, herpes zoster (shingles), congenital abnormalities (cytomegalovirus)
Picornavirus	Poliomyelitis, viral hepatitis A and B, respiratory infections, myocarditis, rhinovirus (common cold)
Togavirus	Yellow fever, encephalitis
Orthomyxovirus	Influenza
Paramyxovirus	Mumps, measles, rubella
Coronavirus	Common cold
Rhabdovirus	Rabies
Retrovirus	Acquired immune deficiency syndrome, degenerative brain disease, possibly cancer

Other antimicrobial drugs and antiparasitic drugs

Various drugs are used to treat atypical microbial infection (e.g. *Mycobacterium tuberculosis* and *M. leprae*) and infection and disease caused by parasite and insect vector (e.g. trichomoniasis and malaria). Box 12-30 lists examples of these drugs and their classifications.

Note

Malaria is still a prevalent disease in tropical areas and may be carried into the UK by refugees and immigrants. Tuberculosis is on the rise in individuals with AIDS and also in the homeless, those who are drug dependent, and those taking immunosuppressant drugs.

Box 12-30

Examples of antimicrobial and antiparasitic drugs

Antimalarial agents
Hydroxychloroquine
Chloroquine

Antituberculous agents
Capreomycin
Cycloserine
Isoniazid
Rifampicin
Streptomycin

Amoebicidal agents
Diloxanide
Metronidazole
Tinidazole

Anthelmintic agents
Mebendazole
Piperazine

Antiprotozoal agents
Metronidazole (Flagyl)

Leprostatic agents
Clofazimine (Lamprene)
Dapsone (DDS)

Cephalosporins
Cefaclor
Cefalezin
Cefotaxime
Cefradine
Cefuroxime
Cefalexin

Quinolones
Ciprofloxacin
Levofloxacin

Penicillins
Amoxicillin
Ampicillin
Benzylpenicillin
Co-amoxiclav
Phenoxymethylpenicillin

Anti-inflammatory drugs

Inflammation

Inflammation is a defence mechanism of body tissues in response to physical trauma, foreign biological and chemical substances, surgery, radiation, and electricity. Regardless of the event producing inflammation, the response is similar. For example, if bacterial infection or an injury to the tissues occurs, chemical mediators are released or activated. These mediators cause vasodilatation and increased blood flow (localized warmth and redness at the site). This process brings phagocytes and other leukocytes to the area to prevent the spread of infection by limiting the infected site. Finally, phagocytes clean the area and the damaged tissues are repaired.

Inflammation can be localized or systemic. Local inflammation is confined to a specific area of the body and produces symptoms such as redness, heat, swelling, pain, and loss of function. Systemic inflammation occurs in many parts of the body. In addition to local symptoms at the inflammation site, red bone marrow produces and releases large numbers of neutrophils that promote phagocytosis, pyrogens stimulate fever production, and increased vascular permeability may, in severe cases, result in decreased blood volume. Drugs used to treat inflammation or its symptoms may be classified as analgesic–antipyretic drugs and NSAID. A number of medications have both properties.

Analgesic–antipyretic drugs

An antipyretic drug is one that reduces fever. The temperature-regulating mechanism of the body is located in the anterior hypothalamus. Normally, the set point of this hypothalamic centre is about 37.0°C (98.4°F). When an inflammatory response occurs in the body, endogenous pyrogens are released by the phagocytic leukocytes, and fever is produced. Analgesic–antipyretic drugs work by reversing the effect of the pyrogen on the hypothalamus so that the set point of the hypothalamus is returned to normal. The analgesic effects of these drugs act on peripheral pain receptors to block activation. Examples of these drugs include paracetamol and aspirin/acetylsalicylic acid.

NSAID

Aspirin is the oldest model of the NSAID. New drugs have been developed and, like aspirin, these drugs are analgesic, antipyretic and anti-inflammatory. These drugs are often prescribed for patients with various inflammatory conditions such as rheumatoid arthritis. The newer drugs may also be prescribed for those who cannot tolerate aspirin. In addition, these drugs may be used to treat painful joint disorders (with or without inflammation) such as osteoarthritis, low back pain, and gout. One should note that, like aspirin, the other NSAID may decrease platelet activity, which could result in gastrointestinal bleeding. Long-term use of some NSAID has been linked to an increased risk for heart attack and stroke.

Note

Gout is a metabolic disease associated with high levels of uric acid in the blood (hyperuricaemia). Gout is characterized by attacks of acute pain, swelling, and tenderness of joints. The condition is treated with uricosuric drugs, colchicine and NSAID.

NSAID are thought to act by inhibiting specific enzymes so that prostaglandins (substances that promote inflammation and pain) are not formed. Examples of these drugs include the following:

- aspirin
- diclofenac
- ibuprofen
- indometacin
- naproxen
- sulindac
- ketorolac
- cyclooxygenase-2 inhibitors
- celecoxib.

Summary

- A drug may be defined as any substance taken by mouth; injected into a muscle, blood vessel or cavity of the body; or applied topically to treat or prevent a disease or condition.
- Drugs can be identified by three types of names. These include the chemical name; generic or non-proprietary name; and trade, brand, or proprietary name.
- In Britain, the main pieces of legislation that regulate the use of all medicines include the Medicines Act 1968, the Misuse of Drugs Act 1971, and the Misuse of Drugs Regulations 1985.
- The main regulating body in the UK is the Medicines and Healthcare products Regulatory agency (MHRA). The MHRA is a Government agency charged with ensuring that medicines and medical devices work and are acceptably safe.
- NICE is an independent organization responsible for providing national guidance on the promotion of good health and the prevention and treatment of ill-health. NICE produces guidance in three areas of health: public health, health technology, and clinical practice. Once NICE publishes clinical guidance, including the use of drugs, health professionals and their employing organizations are expected to take it fully into account when deciding what treatments to give people.
- Paramedics are held responsible for the safe and effective administration of drugs. In fact, they are responsible for each drug they provide to a patient. They are legally, morally, and ethically responsible.
- Drug allergies can be divided into four classifications based on the mechanism of the immune reaction. They are type I (anaphylactic), type II (cytotoxic), type III (serum sickness) and type IV (contact dermatitis) reactions.
- The parasympathetic and sympathetic nervous systems function continuously. They innervate many of the same organs at the same time. The opposing actions of the two systems balance each other. In general, the sympathetic system dominates during stressful events. The parasympathetic system is most active during times of emotional and physical calm.
- The degree to which drugs attain pharmacological activity depends partly on the rate and extent to which they are absorbed. Absorption in turn depends on the ability of the drug to cross the cell membrane. The rate and extent of absorption depend on the nature of the cell membrane the drug must cross, blood flow to the site of administration, solubility of the drug, pH of the drug environment, drug concentration, and drug dosage form.
- The route of drug administration influences drug absorption. These routes can be classified as enteral, parenteral, pulmonary, and topical.
- Distribution is the transport of a drug through the bloodstream to various tissues of the body and ultimately to its site of action. After absorption and distribution, the body eliminates most drugs. The body first biotransforms the drug and then excretes the drug. The kidney is the primary organ for excretion; however, the intestine, lungs, and mammary, sweat and salivary glands also may be involved.

Summary—cont'd

- Many factors can alter the response to drug therapy, including age, body mass, gender, pathological state, genetic factors and psychological factors.
- Most drug actions are thought to result from a chemical interaction. This interaction is between the drug and various receptors throughout the body. The most common form of drug action is the drug–receptor interaction.
- Many variables can influence drug interactions, including intestinal absorption, competition for plasma-protein binding, biotransformation, action at the receptor site, renal excretion and alteration of electrolyte balance.
- Narcotic analgesics relieve pain. Narcotic antagonists reverse the narcotic effects of some analgesics. Non-narcotic analgesics interfere with local mediators released when tissue is damaged in the periphery of the body. These mediators stimulate nerve endings and cause pain.
- Anaesthetic drugs are CNS depressants that have a reversible effect on nervous tissue. Anti-anxiety agents are used to reduce feelings of apprehension, nervousness, worry or fearfulness. Sedatives and hypnotics are drugs that depress the CNS. They produce a calming effect. They also help induce sleep. Alcohol is a general CNS depressant that can produce sedation, sleep and anaesthesia.
- Anticonvulsant drugs are used to treat seizure disorders. Most notably they treat epilepsy.
- All CNS stimulants work to increase excitability. They do this by blocking activity of inhibitory neurons or their respective neurotransmitters or by enhancing the production of the excitatory neurotransmitters.
- Psychotherapeutic drugs include antipsychotic agents, antidepressants and lithium. These drugs are used to treat psychoses and affective disorders, especially schizophrenia, depression and mania.
- Several movement disorders can result from an imbalance of dopamine and acetylcholine. Drugs that inhibit or block acetylcholine are referred to as anticholinergic. Three classes of drugs affect brain dopamine: those that release dopamine, those that increase brain levels of dopamine, and dopaminergic agonists.
- The autonomic drugs mimic or block the effects of the sympathetic and parasympathetic divisions of the autonomic nervous system. These drugs are classified into four groups: cholinergic (parasympathomimetic) drugs, cholinergic blocking (parasympatholytic) drugs, adrenergic (sympathomimetic) drugs, and adrenergic blocking (sympatholytic) drugs.
- Skeletal muscle relaxants can be classified as central acting, direct acting, and neuromuscular blockers.
- Cardiac drugs are classified by their effects on specialized cardiac tissues. Cardiac glycosides are used to treat congestive heart failure and certain tachycardias. Antidysrhythmic drugs are used to treat and prevent disorders of cardiac rhythm. The pharmacological agents that suppress dysrhythmias may do so by direct action on the cardiac cell membrane (lidocaine), by indirect action that affects the cell (propranolol), or both.
- Antihypertensive drugs used to reduce blood pressure are classified into four major categories: diuretics, sympathetic blocking agents (sympatholytic drugs), vasodilators and ACE inhibitors. Calcium channel blockers are also used to treat persons with hypertension who do not respond to other drug therapies.
- Drugs that affect blood coagulation may be classified as antiplatelet, anticoagulant, or fibrinolytic agents. Drugs that interfere with platelet aggregation are known as antiplatelet or antithrombic drugs. Anticoagulant drug therapy is designed to prevent intravascular thrombosis. The therapy decreases blood coagulability. Fibrinolytic drugs dissolve clots after their formation. These drugs work by promoting the digestion of fibrin.
- Haemophilia is a group of hereditary bleeding disorders. These disorders involve a deficiency of one of the factors needed for the coagulation of blood. Replacing the missing clotting factor can help manage haemophilia.
- Haemostatic agents speed up clot formation, thus reducing bleeding. Systemic haemostatic agents are used to control blood loss after surgery. They work by inhibiting the breakdown of fibrin. Topical haemostatic agents are used to control capillary bleeding. They are used during surgical and dental procedures.
- The treatment of choice in managing a loss of blood or blood components is to replace the sole blood component that is deficient. Replacement therapy may include transfusing whole blood (rare), packed red blood cells, fresh-frozen plasma, plasma expanders, platelets, coagulation factors, fibrinogen, albumin or gamma globulins.
- Hyperlipidaemia refers to an excess of lipids in the plasma. Antihyperlipidaemic drugs are sometimes used along with diet and exercise to control serum lipid levels.
- Bronchodilator drugs are the primary form of treatment for obstructive pulmonary disease such as asthma, chronic bronchitis and emphysema. These drugs may be classified as sympathomimetic drugs and xanthine derivatives.
- Mucokinetic drugs are used to move respiratory secretions, excessive mucus and sputum along the tracheobronchial tree.
- Oxygen is used chiefly to treat hypoxia and hypoxaemia.
- Direct respiratory stimulant drugs act directly on the medullary centre of the brain. These drugs are analeptics. They increase the rate and depth of respiration.
- Spirits of ammonia is a reflex respiratory stimulant. The drug is administered by inhalation.
- A cough may be prolonged or result from an underlying disorder. In such a case, treatment with antitussive drugs may be indicated.
- The main clinical use of antihistamines is for allergic reactions. They are also used to control motion sickness or as a sedative or antiemetic.

Summary—cont'd

- Drug therapy for the gastrointestinal system can be divided into drugs that affect the stomach and drugs that affect the lower gastrointestinal tract. Antacids buffer or neutralize hydrochloric acid in the stomach. Digestant drugs promote digestion in the gastrointestinal tract. They do this by releasing small amounts of hydrochloric acid in the stomach. Drugs used to induce vomiting may be administered as part of the treatment of certain drug overdoses and poisonings. Drugs used to treat nausea and vomiting include antagonists of histamine, acetylcholine and dopamine, and other drugs the actions of which are not understood clearly.
- H_2 receptor antagonists are used to treat peptic ulcer disease by protecting the gastric mucosa. H_2 receptor antagonists block the H_2 receptors and also reduce the volume of gastric acid secretion and its acid content.
- Two common conditions of the lower gastrointestinal tract may require drug therapy: constipation and diarrhoea. Drugs used to manage these conditions include laxatives and antidiarrhoeals.
- The endocrine system works to control and integrate body functions. A number of drugs are used to treat disorders of the anterior and posterior pituitary, the thyroid and parathyroid glands, and the adrenal cortex.
- The pancreatic hormones play a key role in regulating the amount of certain nutrients in the circulatory system. The two main hormones secreted by the pancreas are insulin and glucagon. Imbalances in either of these may call for drug therapy. This therapy is meant to correct metabolic derangements.
- Antibiotics are used to treat local or systemic infection. This group includes penicillin, cephalosporins, and related products; macrolide antibiotics; tetracyclines; and miscellaneous antibiotic agents.
- Persons can be infected by bacterial organisms, fungi, and viruses. Examples of antifungal drugs include fluconazole, terbinafine, and nystatin.
- Few drugs exist for use in any viral infections. One antiviral drug is aciclovir, which is effective against herpes infection. Others include zidovudine and lamivudine, which are used to treat HIV infection; and entecavir, which is used against viral hepatitis.
- Drugs used to treat inflammation or its symptoms may be classified as analgesic–antipyretic drugs and NSAID. A number of medications have both properties.

References

1. World Health Organization Lexicon of alcohol and drug terms. Online. Available http://www.who.int/substance_abuse/terminology/who_lexicon/en/ 23 January 2009
2. Galbraith A, Bullock S, Manias E, Hunt B, Richards A 1999 Fundamentals of pharmacology; a text for nurses and health professionals. Pearson Education, London
3. Joint Royal Colleges Ambulance Liaison Committee 2006 UK Ambulance Service Clinical Practice Guidelines 2006. JRCALC. Online. Available http://jrcalc.org.uk/guidelines.html
4. Medicines and Healthcare Product Agency, http://www.mhra.gov.uk/
5. National Institute for Health and Clinical Excellence, About NICE. Online. Available http://www.nice.org.uk/aboutNICE 23 January 2009
6. McKenry L, Salerno E 1989 Mosby's pharmacology in nursing, 18th edition. Mosby, St Louis
7. Pratt J 1989 Intraosseous infusion. Int Pediatr 4(1):19
8. Nolan JP, Deakin CD, Soar J, Böttiger BW, Smith G 2005 European Resuscitation Council guidelines for resuscitation 2005 Section 4. Adult advanced life support. Resuscitation 67(S1):S39–S86
9. British Medical Association and Royal Pharmaceutical Society of Great Britain. British National Formulary 53. March 2007. Online. Available http://www.bnf.org.uk/bnf/ 23 January 2009
10. Terrell KM, Heard K, Miller DK 2006 Prescribing to older ED patients. Am J Emerg Med 24(4):468–478
11. Mathieu-Nolf M, Babé MA, Coquelle-Couplet V, Billaut C, Nisse P, Mathieu D 2001 Flumazenil use in an emergency department: a survey. J Toxicol Clin Toxicol 39(1):15–20
12. Joint Epilepsy Council 2005 Epilepsy prevalence, incidence and other statistics. Joint Epilepsy Council, Leeds
13. Lord J, Paisley S 2000 The clinical effectiveness and cost effectiveness of methylphenidate for hyperactivity in childhood. National Institute for Clinical Excellence, London
14. Gonzalez E, Kannewurf BS, Ornato JF 1998 Intravenous amiodarone for ventricular arrhythmias: overview and clinical use. Resuscitation 39:33
15. British Heart Foundation. Coronary Heart Disease Statistics 2005, Section 9 Blood Pressure. Online. Available http://www.heartstats.org/datapage.asp?id=5340 23 January 2009
16. National Institute for Clinical Excellence. Hypertension: management of hypertension. NICE, London
17. Department of Health 2004 HIV post-exposure prophylaxis, Guidance from the UK Chief Medical Officers' Expert Advisory Group on AIDS. Online. Available http://www.dh.gov.uk/publications 23 January 2009

Part B: Venous Access and Medication Administration

Chapter contents

Objectives

Upon completion of this part, the paramedic student will be able to:

1. Become familiar with SI units and prefixes, and equivalences of weight, volume and amount of substance.
2. Identify the steps in the calculation of drug dosages.
3. Calculate the correct volume of drug to be administered in a given situation.
4. Compute the correct rate for an infusion of drugs or intravenous fluids.
5. List measures for ensuring the safe administration of medications.
6. Describe actions paramedics should take if a medication error occurs.
7. List measures for preserving asepsis during parenteral administration of a drug.
8. Explain drug administration techniques for the enteral and parenteral routes.
9. Describe the steps for safely initiating an intravenous infusion.
10. Identify complications and adverse effects associated with intravenous access.
11. Describe the steps for safely initiating intravenous access.
12. Describe the steps for safely initiating an intraosseous infusion.
13. Explain drug administration techniques for percutaneous routes.
14. Identify special considerations in the administration of pharmacological agents to paediatric patients.
15. Explain the technique for obtaining a venous blood sample.
16. Describe the safe disposal of contaminated items and sharps.

Key terms

gram A metric unit of mass equal to 1/1000 of a kilogram.

kilogram A metric unit of mass equal to 1000 grams, or 2.2046 pounds.

litre A metric unit of capacity equal to 1 cubic decimetre or 1.759 pints.

medical asepsis The removal or destruction of disease-causing organisms or infected material.

metre A metric unit of length equal to 1000 millimetres.

microgram A metric unit of mass equal to 1/1 000 000 of a gram.

milligram A metric unit of mass equal to 1/1000 of a gram.

millilitre A metric unit of capacity equal to 1/1000 of a litre.

Système Internationale The metric system of measurement.

Certain key skills are required of all paramedics. The ability to insert a needle or an intravenous catheter into a vein safely (i.e. gain venous access) is a crucial skill. A paramedic also must be able to administer prescribed medications. These skills, and the patient care they require, are critical to medication therapy.

Critical Thinking

Mathematical skills are important in the administration of drugs. These skills include multiplication and division, figuring percentages, and working with Roman numerals, fractions, decimal fractions, and proportions. Paramedics must have a good working knowledge of these principles. They also must be adept at calculations.

Mathematical equivalents used in pharmacology

Système Internationale

Système International (SI) is generally accepted as the unit of measurement in UK pharmacy and medical practice; it is also known as the metric system and makes calculations easier than the traditional imperial system (stones, pounds, ounces etc.) The use of the SI system was introduced into the NHS in 1975[18] and should be used by paramedics. About 92% of the countries of the world use the metric system.

Definitions of units

The basic metric units of measurement are the metre, the litre and the gram. The metre is the unit for linear measurement; the litre is the unit for capacity or volume; and the gram is the unit for weight.

The basic units of the metric system can be divided or multiplied by 10, 100 or 1000 parts to form secondary units. These secondary units differ from each other by 10 or some multiple of 10. Subdivisions of these basic units are made when the decimal is moved to the left. Multiples of the basic unit are made when the decimal is moved to the right. The names of the secondary units are formed by putting a Greek or Latin prefix on the primary unit (Table 12-6).

The metre (m) is the unit of length from which the other metric units of length are derived (Figure 12-10). Centimetres (cm) and millimetres (mm) are the primary linear measurements used in medicine. For example, they are used to measure the size of body organs and to measure blood pressure.

The litre (L) is the unit of capacity or volume (Figure 12-11). A fractional part of a litre is expressed in millilitres (mL) or cubic centimetres (cc). The litre is equal to 1000 mL, so one millilitre is 1/1000 of a litre. The unit of measure ml or mL should be used to express fractional parts of a litre.

The gram (g) is the metric unit used in weighing drugs and various pharmaceutical preparations (Figure 12-12). The gram equals the weight of 1 mL of distilled water at 4 °C. A kilogram (kg) is equal to 1000 g, or 2.2 pounds. A milligram (mg) is equal to 1/1000 of a gram. A microgram (μg) is equal to 1/1 000 000 of a gram.

Table 12-6 Common metric prefixes

Prefix	Meaning
kilo-	1000 times greater
deci-	10 times less
centi-	100 times less
milli-	1000 times less
micro-	1 million times less

Metric style of notation

The British National Formulary makes the following recommendations regarding documentation of metric units:[19]

- The unnecessary use of decimal points should be avoided, e.g. 3 mg, not 3.0 mg.
- Quantities of 1 gram or more should be written as 1 g, etc.

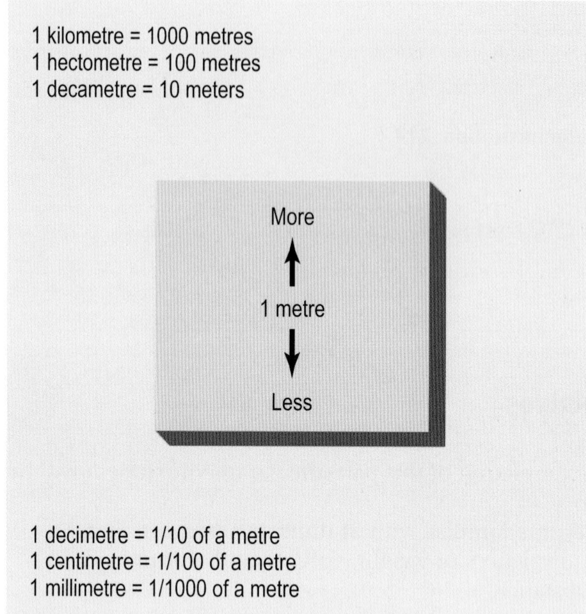

Figure 12-10 The metre measures length.

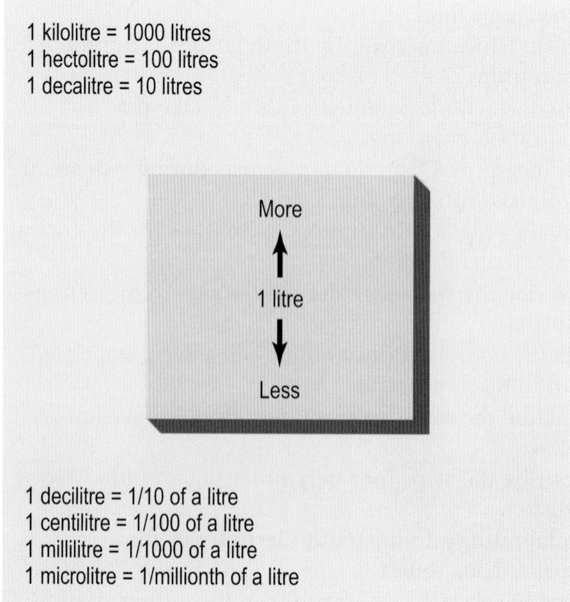

Figure 12-11 The litre measures capacity.

- Quantities less than 1 g should be written in milligrams, e.g. 500 mg, not 0.5 g.
- Quantities less than 1 mg should be written in micrograms, e.g. 100 μg, not 0.1 mg.
- When decimals are unavoidable a zero should be written in front of the decimal point where there is no other figure, e.g. 0.5 mL, not .5 mL.
- Use of the decimal point is acceptable to express a range, e.g. 0.5 to 1 g.

The paramedic should also remember that:

- Units are not capitalized (gram, not Gram).
- Unit abbreviations are not followed by a full stop (mL, not m.L. or mL.).
- A single space is left between the quantity and the symbol (24 kg, not 24kg).
- Unit abbreviations are not pluralized (kg, not kgs).
- As a rule, fractions are not used, only decimal notation (0.25 kg, not ¼ kg).

Critical Thinking

Placing a 0 to the left of the decimal point reduces the likelihood of a drug dosing error. Why?

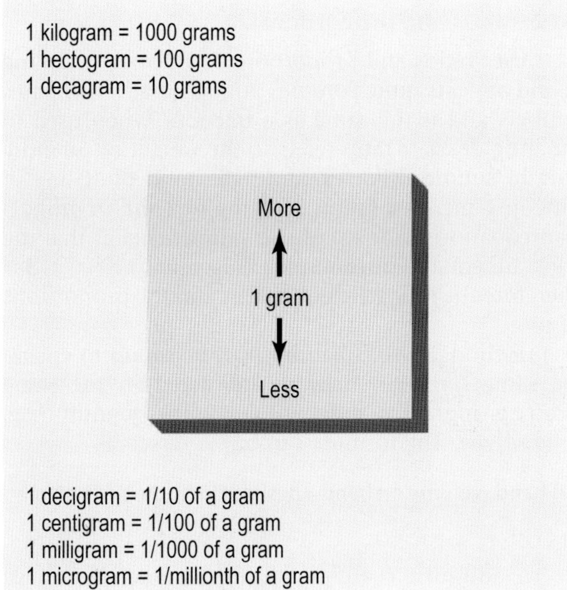

Figure 12-12 The gram measures weight.

Temperature conversions

Normal body temperature is 37°Celsius (centigrade), or 98.6°Fahrenheit. A simple formula can be used to convert temperatures. To convert a Celsius reading to Fahrenheit, multiply the Celsius reading by 9/5. Then add 32. To convert a Fahrenheit reading to Celsius, subtract 32 from the Fahrenheit reading. Then multiply by 5/9 (Figure 12-13).

Note

Remember these temperature conversion formulas:

Celsius to Fahrenheit: (°C × 9/5) + 32

Fahrenheit to Celsius: (°F – 32) × (5/9)

Drug calculations

While providing emergency care, the paramedic may need to calculate adult and paediatric drug dosages and infusion rates, as well as the strength of drug solutions and diluted solutions. These tasks involve the use of basic maths skills in a logical order and require a working knowledge of decimals, fractions, ratios, and proportions.

Calculation methods

Paramedics should choose a method of calculation that is precise and reliable. To perform drug calculations, paramedics should:

- Convert all units of measure to the same unit and system.
- Check the computed dosage to determine whether it is reasonable.
- Use one dosage calculation method consistently.

Conversion of units of measure

Most emergency drug preparations do not require conversion. Most drugs are packaged in milligrams and administered in milligrams. However, some drugs, such as atropine, are packaged in milligrams but administered in micrograms (μg). These drugs must be converted to like units. When conversion to like units is required, the conversion must be done before the drug dose is calculated.

Example

You are to administer a dose of 500 μg atropine as a bolus. You have 1 mg of the drug in 5 mL of solution. The choice is to convert the dosage to milligrams or convert the presentation to micrograms. BNF recommends that dosages

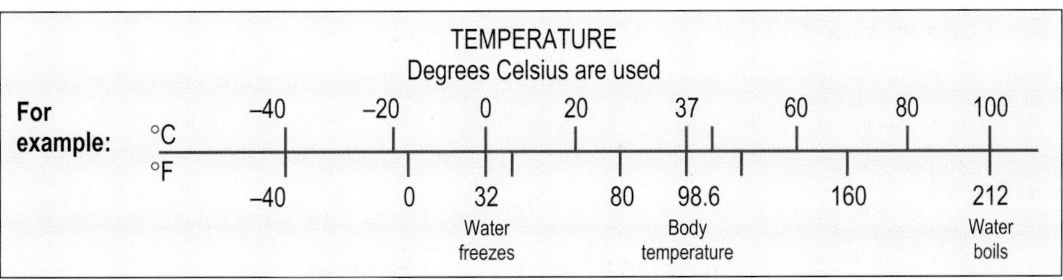

Figure 12-13 Temperature conversions.

below 1 mg should be stated as micrograms, so it would be logical to convert the presentation to micrograms:

$$1\,\text{mg in } 5\,\text{mL} = 1000\,\mu\text{g in } 5\,\text{mL}$$

Thus, for a dose of 500 µg, you would need

$$500/1000 \times 5\,\text{mL} = 2.5\,\text{mL}$$

Critical Thinking

Imagine that you failed to convert the 500 µg of atropine to 0.5 mg in this example. Would you overdose or underdose your patient?

Note

Maths tip: Move the decimal point to the right when multiplying (converting the measurement to smaller units). Move it to the left when dividing (converting the measurement to larger units).

When the dose is given per unit of weight (kg), the patient's weight needs to be calculated in kilograms. This may necessitate a conversion from pounds to kilograms and should be done before the total dose to be given is calculated.

Example

You are to give 1 mg/kg of lidocaine to a patient who weighs 132 lb. Divide 132 by 2.2 to convert pounds to kilograms (132 lb /2.2 = 60 kg). The total dose equals 1 mg/kg multiplied by 60 kg. This equals 60 mg.

$$132\,\text{lb}/2.2 = 60\,\text{kg}$$

$$1\,\text{mg/kg} \times 60\,\text{kg} = 60\,\text{mg}$$

Assessment of computed doses

Many emergency drugs are packaged in units that contain enough drug for a normal adult dose. After doing the maths, the paramedic should decide whether the answer is reasonable – that is to say that the paramedic should be able to recognize a gross error.

Example

You are to administer 8 mg of diazepam. It is supplied in a 2 mL ampoule that contains 10 mg of the drug; therefore, a reasonable calculation of volume would be less than 2 mL.

Methods of calculation

Many drug calculations can be performed almost intuitively because many drugs are packaged to supply one adult dose. However, a paramedic should never rely on intuitive calculations, no matter how simple the drug dose may seem. The three methods of calculation discussed below are in common use.

Method 1: basic formula ('desire over have')

For method 1, information must be substituted in the following formula:

$$\frac{D}{H} \times Q = X$$

In this formula, D is the desired dose to be given and H is the known dose on hand. Q is the unit of measure or volume on hand and X is the unit of measure to be given. Many consider 'desire over have' to be the easiest formula to use. It works for nearly all emergency drug calculations.

Example

You are to administer 40 mg of furosemide. You have an 8 mL pre-filled syringe that contains 80 mg of the drug. How many millilitres will you give? Using the desire over have formula, calculate the dose.

$$\frac{40\,\text{mg}}{80\,\text{mg}} \times 8\,\text{mL} = X$$

$$\frac{40}{10} \times 1\,\text{mL} = X$$

$$4 \times 1\,\text{mL} = X$$

$$X = 4\,\text{mL}$$

Note

Maths tip: When using the basic formula, always divide the bottom number into the top number.

Method 2: ratios and proportions

Method 2 uses ratios and proportions to calculate the drug dosage, and appears quite complex at first. A ratio compares two numbers and is the same as a fraction. When used to calculate drug doses, a ratio refers to the weight or quantity of a drug in solution. For example, the ratio of 10 mg of morphine in 1 mL of solution is 10 mg to 1 mL. A proportion is an equation made up of two ratios; it states that the two ratios are equal. For example, ⅔ is equal to 4/6 (2 : 3 = 4 : 6); therefore the ratios are equivalent and the proportions are true.

To use method 2, the equation must be set up to ensure that the same units of measure are stated in the same sequence (e.g. mg : mL = mg : x mL). x is the quantity (e.g. mL) to be solved. The formula can be expressed as

Dose on hand : volume on hand = desired dose : desired volume

Example

You are to administer 40 mg of furosemide. You have 100 mg of the drug in 10 mL of solution. How many millilitres will you give? Calculate the dose using ratios and proportions:

$$100\,\text{mg} : 10\,\text{mL} = 40\,\text{mg} : x\,\text{mL}$$

Multiply inside numbers (means) and outside numbers (extremes). Drop the unit of measurement terms:

Means

100 mg : 10 mL :: 40 mg : *x* mL

Extremes

Note

Maths tip: Remember the phrases middle for means and end for extremes. In a proportion, the product of the means is always equal to the product of the extremes.

Solve the proportion by dividing both sides of the equation by the number before *x* (100).

$$\frac{100x}{100} \times \frac{400}{100} = 4\ \text{mL}$$

To check your answer, multiply the means and then multiply the extremes. The sum product will be equal if the proportion is true.

$$\left.\begin{array}{r} 100 \times 4 = 400 \\ 10 \times 40 = 400 \end{array}\right\} \text{Sum parts are equal}$$

Method 3: dimensional analysis

Dimensional analysis works well for complex drug calculations. These may call for several conversions of a similar basic dimensional unit so that all units of measure are changed to like units (e.g. milligrams). Dimensional analysis is based on the same tenet as the basic formula; however, it does not require memorization of the 'desire over have' equation. All conversion factors are set up in one equation. They are separated by multiplication signs.

Note

Maths tip: When using dimensional analysis, convert all units to the easiest maths operation. This reduces the chance of error.

Example

You are to administer 0.8 mg of naloxone. The drug is packaged in 1 mL of solution containing 0.4 mg of the drug.

Step 1: Set up the equation, placing the desired unit of measure in the answer to the left of the equal sign. Place the first factor to the right of the equal sign. Make sure it is the same unit as the answer.

$$\text{mL} = \frac{1\,\text{mL}}{0.4\,\text{mg}} \times \frac{0.8\,\text{mg}}{1}$$

Step 2: Cancel like units of measure in the numerator and denominator, and reduce the fraction, if needed:

$$\text{mL} = \frac{1\,\text{mL}}{0.4\,\cancel{\text{mg}}} \times \frac{0.8\,\cancel{\text{mg}}}{1}$$

Note

Maths tip: The only unit remaining after cancelling the like units should be the unit of the answer. If this is not the case, the equation is set up incorrectly.

Step 3: Multiply the numerators and then the denominators.

$$\text{mL} = \frac{1\,\text{mL}}{0.4} \times \frac{0.8}{1} = \frac{0.8\,\text{mL}}{0.4}$$

Step 4: Divide the numerator by the denominator to solve the equation.

$$\text{mL} = \frac{0.8\,\text{mL}}{0.4} = 2\,\text{mL}$$

Calculating intravenous flow rates

To calculate intravenous (IV) flow rates, paramedics must know three factors. First, they must know the volume to be infused; second, they must know the period of time, in minutes, over which the fluid is to be infused; and third, they must know the number of drops (gtt) per millilitre the infusion set delivers (drop factor). The flow rate can then be calculated using the following equation:

$$\text{gtt/min} = \frac{\text{Volume to be infused} \times \text{drop factor}}{\text{Duration of infusion (min)}}$$

Example

You are to give 250 mL of normal saline over 90 min. Your infusion set delivers 10 gtt/mL. Calculate the drops per minute using the above formula.

$$\text{gtt/min} = \frac{250\,\text{mL} \times 10\,\text{gtt/mL}}{90\,\text{min}} = \frac{2500\,\text{gtt}}{90\,\text{min}}$$

$$= 27.7 \text{ or } 28\,\text{gtt/min}$$

Note

The two intravenous (IV) infusion sets most often used in emergency care are microdrip tubing and macrodrip tubing. Microdrip tubing delivers 60 gtt/mL. Macrodrip tubing delivers 10, 15, or 20 gtt/mL. Maths tip: When a drop factor of 60 is used, the gtt/min always equals the mL/h infusion.

Critical Thinking

When would it be best to use microdrip tubing? When would it be better to use macrodrip tubing?

Calculating infusion rates

Although not current practice for most UK paramedics, there may be occasions when the paramedic needs to administer medications via a continuous IV infusion. Calculating the correct drip rate is crucial to avoid overdosing or underdosing the patient. To properly calculate and give a prescribed drug by continuous infusion, paramedics must know three things. First, they must know the prescribed dose. Second, they must know the concentration of the drug in 1 mL of solution. Third, they must know the drop factor of the IV infusion set. The example below is not of a currently licensed UK paramedic drug but illustrates the steps required to calculate the drip rate:

$$\text{gtt/min} = \frac{\text{Volume to be infused} \times \text{drop factor}}{\text{Concentration of drug in 1 mL}}$$

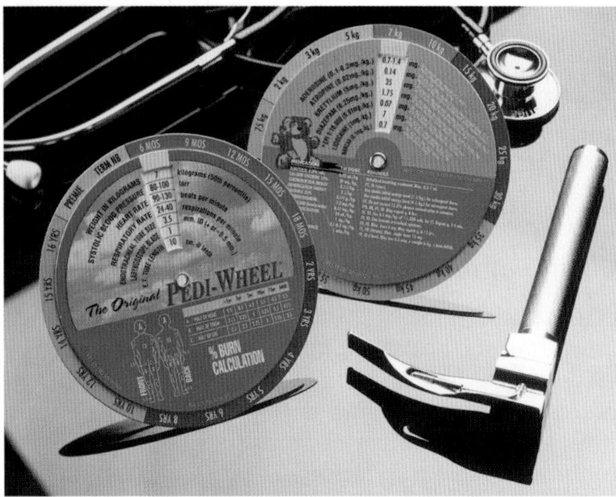

Figure 12-14 PediWheel.

Example

You are to administer a procainamide infusion at 3 mg/min. You have 1 g of the drug in 250 mL of 5% dextrose in water (D5W). The infusion set delivers 60 gtt/mL. How many drops per minute will you deliver?

Convert all units to like measurements and calculate the concentration of the drug in 1 mL.

$$1\,\text{g} = 1000\,\text{mg}$$
$$1000\,\text{mg} \div 250\,\text{mL} = 4\,\text{mg/mL}$$

Calculate the drops per minute using the IV drip formula:

$$\text{gtt/min} = \frac{3\,\text{mg/min} \times 60\,\text{gtt/mL}}{4\,\text{mg in 1mL}} = \frac{180}{4} = 45\,\text{gtt/min}$$

Calculating drug dosages for infants and children

The doses of some medications for infants and children are administered in the same proportion to body weight as the doses for adults. Others are given in much reduced doses due to differences in the child's ability to metabolize the drug. Paediatric drug doses are most often calculated in the prehospital setting by using the 'age-per-page' facility in the JRCALC.[3] Other memory aids include charts, tapes, dosage books, and dosage wheels (Figure 12-14). The most precise way to calculate a paediatric drug dose is based on the child's body surface area. Body surface area as a function of weight is described in Chapter 38.

Drug administration

During the administration of any drug, safety should always be a high priority.

Safety considerations and procedures

Paramedics should follow these guidelines when administering drugs to patients:

- Focus on the procedure and avoid distractions (including when preparing the medicines).
- Verify that the patient is not allergic to the medication. Strictly follow these five patient rights of drug administration: Make sure the right patient receives the right dose of the right drug via the right route at the right time. Also make sure to document the drug administration accurately and thoroughly. This is the sixth patient right of drug administration.
- Make a habit of reading the label of the medicine and comparing it to the guidelines at least three times before administration:

  First – when removing the drug from the drug kit or supply area

  Second – when preparing the medication for administration

  Third – just before administering the drug to the patient (before the container is discarded).
- Always check the correct route of administration. Some medications can be prepared for administration by several routes. For instance, the route could be intramuscular or intravenous.
- Never give a medicine from an unlabelled container. Also, never give a medicine from a container on which the label is not legible.
- It is best practice to have a colleague check the drug and any calculations prior to administration.
- Handle multidose vials carefully. Use aseptic technique. This way, medicines are not wasted or contaminated.
- When preparing more than one injection, always label the syringe immediately. Keep the medication container with the syringe. Do not rely on your memory to recall which solution is in which syringe.
- Never administer a medicine that is unlabelled and that was prepared by someone else. In doing so, you accept the blame. You will be responsible for accuracy, dose, and correct medication.
- Never administer a medication that is out-of-date. Likewise, never give one that looks discoloured, cloudy, or in any other way unusual, or as if someone has tampered with it.
- If the patient or your colleagues express doubt or concern about a medication or dose, recheck it. Do not administer it until you are sure no error has been made. Remember that the patient has the right to refuse a medication.
- Carefully monitor the patient for any adverse effects. Monitor for at least 5 min after you give the medication. (Intramuscular and oral medicines may require longer monitoring.)
- Document all medications given. This includes the name of the drug, the dosage, and the time and route of administration. When documenting parenteral medications, note the site of injection. The patient's response, adverse as well as intended, is also recorded.
- It is critical to return and dispose of any unused medication. Follow all guidelines set by your local Trust.

Critical Thinking

Your clinical preceptor hands you an unlabelled syringe of medication and tells you to give it by means of intramuscular injection. What do you do?

Medication errors

The exact incidence of medication errors in the NHS is unknown; however, errors are consistently reported to account for between 10% and 20% of all adverse events. It follows that the direct cost of medication errors in NHS hospitals may be £200–400 million per year.[20] Common causes of medication errors include the following:

- The prescriber ordered the wrong dose of medication.
- Drug calculations were incorrect.
- Drugs were administered via the wrong route.
- The drug was given to the wrong patient.

If a medication error occurs, paramedics should do the following:

- Accept responsibility for the error.
- Advise receiving medical staff.
- Assess and monitor the patient. Monitor for effects of the drug.
- Document the error. Make sure to follow Trust procedures for the reporting of drug errors.
- Make changes in their personal practice technique to help prevent such an error in the future.

Medical asepsis

Medical asepsis is the removal or destruction of disease-causing organisms or infected material. Medical asepsis is performed by using clean technique (rather than sterile technique). Clean technique requires hygienic measures, cleaning agents, antiseptics, disinfectants and barrier fields.

Note

Sterile technique means using sterile equipment and sterile fields that are free of all forms and types of life. This is also known as surgical asepsis. Clean technique focuses on destroying or inhibiting only pathogens (not all forms and types of life).

Antiseptics and disinfectants

Antiseptics and disinfectants are chemical agents that are used to kill specific groups of microorganisms. They generally do not work very well against spores of bacteria and fungi, many viruses, and some resistant bacterial strains. Disinfectants are used only on non-living objects as they are toxic to living tissue. Antiseptics are applied to living tissue as they are more dilute, to prevent cell damage. Some chemical agents have both antiseptic and disinfectant properties. Examples of these are alcohol and some chlorine compounds (Box 12-31).

Universal precautions in medication administration

Universal precautions should be a crucial part of an encounter with a patient. When administering drugs, paramedics should follow handwashing and gloving procedures. Face shields should be used during administration of endotracheal drugs.

Box 12-31

Examples of antiseptics and disinfectants

Antiseptics

- Hexachlorophene
- Silver nitrate
- Benzoyl peroxide

Disinfectants

- Cresol
- Carbolic acid
- Lysol

Note

Many consider handwashing the most crucial step in reducing the risk of transmission of organisms from one person to another or from one site to another on a patient.[6] Handwashing protects both the paramedic and the patient. If soap and water are not available, a sanitizing gel or wipe should be used.

Enteral administration of medications

Enteral medications are drugs that are administered and absorbed through the gastrointestinal tract and were discussed earlier in this chapter. Enteral drugs are given by means of oral, gastric or rectal administration.

Oral route

The oral route is the most frequently used method of drug administration. The patient should be in an upright or sitting position and the pill, tablet or capsule should be placed in the patient's mouth and swallowed with enough fluid (120–250 mL) to make sure the drug reaches the stomach.

Critical Thinking

Think of some clinical situations in which oral administration of a drug would not be the best technique. Why is this so?

Many oral drugs come in solid and liquid forms (Box 12-32). If the medication is in a suspension, the stock bottle or unit dose should be shaken thoroughly before the drug is poured for administration. A drug not packaged as a unit dose should be measured in a medicine cup or a medicine dropper or by syringe.

Rectal administration of medications

Some drugs, such as suppositories, are made for rectal administration (Box 12-33). Other drugs can be given by the rectal route when vascular access cannot be established; for example, diazepam.

Parenteral administration of medications

Parenteral drugs are administered outside the gastrointestinal tract. This term usually refers to injections. Drugs

Box 12-32

Forms of solid and liquid oral medications

- Caplets
- Capsules
- Time-released capsules
- Lozenges
- Pills
- Tablets
- Elixirs
- Emulsions
- Suspensions
- Syrups

Box 12-33

Procedure for administering rectal drugs via rectal tube*

1. Carefully restrain the child. If possible, place the child in a knee-chest or lateral recumbent position with the legs flexed at the hips and the knees. Remove as little of the patient's underwear as possible.
2. Hold the tube in between your thumb and index finger. DO NOT SQUEEZE. Lubricate the distal end of the rectal tube.
3. Insert the lubricated tube just beyond the external sphincter (aiming just above the junction of the skin and mucous membranes and toward the rectal wall).
4. Empty the contents of the tube into the rectum. Do not release the tube until it has been removed from the rectum.
5. Aid drug retention by squeezing the buttocks together with manual pressure.

*Although the procedure is described for a child, it is also appropriate for adults.

are administered parenterally by the intradermal, subcutaneous, intramuscular, intravenous and intraosseous routes. (Percutaneous medications are also discussed in this section.)

Note

Parenteral administration of drugs can be very hazardous. This is because drugs given by injection are usually thought to be irretrievable. Also, a slight risk of infection exists because the skin is broken. Other possible hazards associated with parenteral administration include cellulitis or abscess formation, necrosis, skin sloughing, nerve injury, prolonged pain and periostitis (inflammation of connective tissue covering bones). The use of aseptic technique, ensuring an accurate drug dosage, finding the proper site for the injection, and administering the injection at the proper rate are essential to minimize the risk of harm.

Equipment used for injections

Syringes and needles

The choice of syringe and needle depends on three factors: (1) the route of administration, (2) the characteristics of the fluid (e.g. aqueous or oil based), and (3) the volume of medication. Syringes in common use today are made of disposable plastic. Sizes range from 1 mL tuberculin and insulin syringes to 60 mL irrigation syringes.

Tuberculin syringes are marked in 0.01 mL gradients. They should be used when the volume to be given is small. Insulin syringes are available in 0.5 and 1 mL volumes and are marked in 1-unit increments. When used with the specified strength of insulin, this syringe allows the patient to draw up the correct dose easily without doing any calculations. Tuberculin and insulin syringes should not be substituted for each other. Figure 12-15 shows syringes used to accurately measure varying amounts of liquids and liquid medications.

Needles vary in length and gauge. Lengths range from 15 mm to 75 mm or longer. Gauges range from 12 gauge (large lumen) to 30 gauge (small lumen). Smaller lumen (larger gauge) needles are usually used for intradermal injections. Subcutaneous injections are usually given with a 23- or 25-gauge needle. Intramuscular injections are usually given with a 19- or 21-gauge needle; occasionally a 16- or 18-gauge needle is used.

In 2004, the Ambulance Service Association in partnership with the Health Protection Agency and Health and Safety Executive published 'National guidance and procedures for infection control'; this document also contained a section on the safe management of sharps[22] (Box 12-34) (see also Chapter 24). In the US, the Occupational Safety and Health Administration recommended needleless systems or

Box 12-34

Prevention of needle and sharps injuries

Needlestick Injuries are common and grossly under-reported in the NHS, yet infection rates are relatively low.[21] However, the risk of transmission of disease is real and should be avoided as much as possible. These diseases include human immunodeficiency virus (HIV) infection, hepatitis B and C, syphilis, herpes simplex, herpes zoster, and tuberculosis. The following precautions can help prevent exposure to these pathogens:[22]

- Sharps must not be passed directly from hand to hand and handling should be kept to a minimum.
- Needles and cannulae should not be resheathed.
- Discard sharps directly into a sharps container immediately after use and at the point of use. NEVER leave clinical sharps lying around.
- Sharps should be discarded using a single-handed technique. Do not hold the sharps container in the other hand. Do not ask someone else to hold it.
- Needles must not be bent or broken prior to use or disposal.
- Needle and syringes must not be disassembled.
- Sharps containers should be placed on a level, stable surface. They should not be placed on the floor or above shoulder height. Wall-mounted boxes should be used in vehicles.

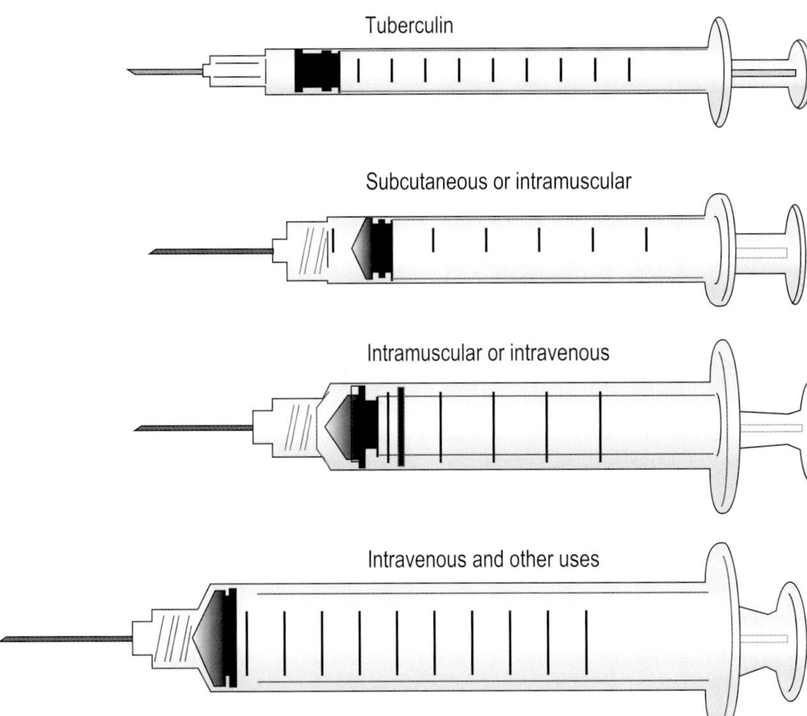

Figure 12-15 Syringes.

'needle safe' devices (sharps with engineered sharps protection). These devices collect body fluids or deliver medications without the use of a needle, thus they help to prevent blood exposure and needlestick injury. Examples of these devices include self-sheathing hypodermic syringes, self-blunting phlebotomy needles, retracting lancets, and disposable retracting scalpels.

Containers used for parenteral medications

Medications given by injection are usually supplied in three forms. They come in single-dose ampoules, multidose vials, or prefilled syringes. Single-dose ampoules are glass containers that hold one dose of a medication for injection. After use, the ampoule is thrown away. Multidose vials are glass containers that come with rubber stoppers. These permit several medication doses to be withdrawn for injection.

Paramedics must prepare a medication for injection. To do this, they must pick the right needle and syringe. The size of the syringe must be in proportion to the volume of solution to be given. To withdraw medication from an ampoule or vial, the paramedic should follow these steps:

1. Assemble the equipment (alcohol swab or gauze, syringe, 18-gauge needle to withdraw medication if using an ampoule, and appropriate-gauge needle for injection).
2. Compute the volume of medication to be given.
3. If using a vial (Figure 12-16a–c):
   - **(a)** Clean the rubber stopper with alcohol.
   - **(b)** Using the needle chosen for the injection, inject a volume of air into the vial equivalent to the amount of solution to be withdrawn. (This prevents the formation of a vacuum in the vial. A vacuum can make the solution hard to withdraw.) Withdraw the volume required and remove the syringe from the vial.
   - **(c)** Gently push in the plunger of the syringe to expel air from the solution.
4. If using an ampoule (Figure 12-17a–d):
   - **(a)** Lightly tap or shake the ampoule to dislodge any solution from the neck of the container.
   - **(b)** Use an ampoule breaker or wrap the neck of the glass ampoule with an alcohol swab or gauze dressing to protect the fingers.
   - **(c)** Grasp the ampoule, snap off the top, and discard the top in an appropriate medication disposal container. (The ampoule is designed to break easily when pressure is exerted at the neck.)
   - **(d)** Carefully insert an 18-gauge needle (a filter needle, if recommended by the drug manufacturer to retain particles in the solution) into the solution without allowing it to touch the edges of the ampoule and draw the solution into the syringe.
   - **(e)** Carefully remove the 18-gauge needle and discard it in the appropriate container. Attach the needle to be used for injection.
   - **(f)** Gently push in the plunger of the syringe to expel air.

Some hospitals and ambulance services require the use of a filter needle. This is a precaution against the inclusion of

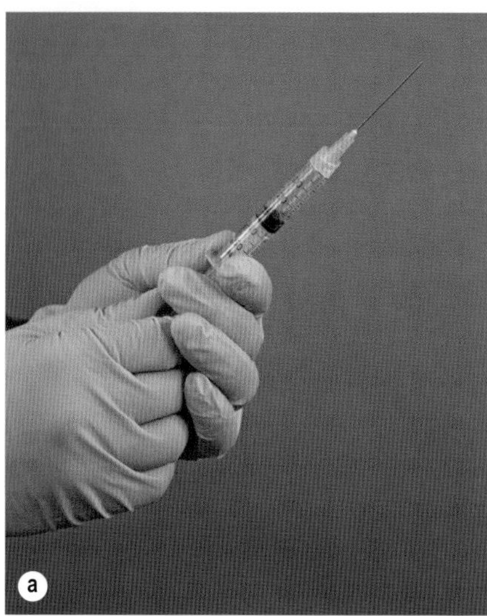

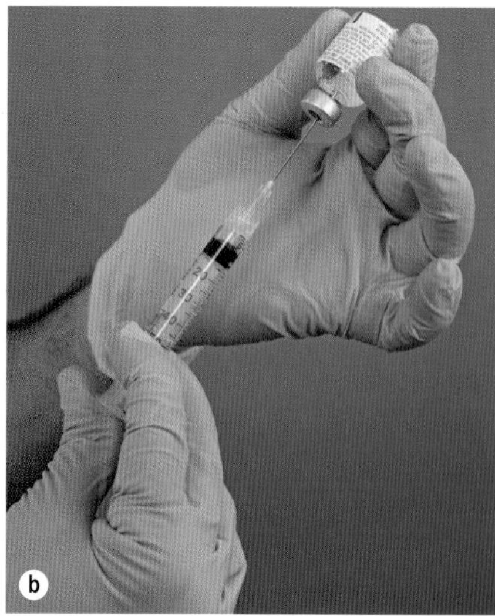

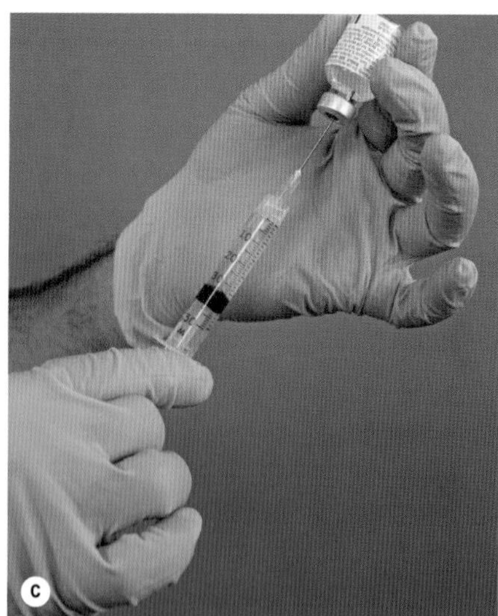

Figure 12-16 Withdrawing medication from a vial. (a) An amount of air equal to the volume to be given is drawn into the syringe. (b) The air is injected into the drug vial. (c) The drug is drawn into the syringe.

glass particles when medications are withdrawn from an ampoule. A further precaution is the use of in-line tubing filters for intravenous injections.

Note

Some medications are dry powders that must be reconstituted before administration. An example is glucagon. Carefully read the manufacturer's information. Use the correct amount of the diluent prescribed for this purpose. Always mix the diluent and powder in the closed vial before withdrawing the dose. Some drugs are packaged in a vial that contains the diluent and powder in two compartments (Mix-o-Vial).

Prefilled syringes

Several manufacturers make prefilled syringes (Figure 12-18a–c). The techniques for activating and using the products vary. Paramedics should be familiar with the devices used by their own Trust. The technique for activating a common type of prefilled syringe is as follows:

1. Calculate the volume of medication to be administered.
2. Remove the protective caps from the syringe barrel and medication cartridge.
3. Hold the cartridge and syringe barrel upside down and screw the cartridge into the syringe barrel.
4. Gently push in the plunger of the syringe to expel air.

Preparing the injection site

The injection site is prepared by cleansing the area using aseptic technique. Controversy still exists regarding the appropriate solution and technique to use, but current practice recommends the use of alcohol-based solution, such as 70% chlorhexidine in spirit.

The steps in preparing the injection site are as follows:

1. Thoroughly scrub the site with the appropriate cleanser to remove dirt, dead skin and other surface contaminants.
2. Clean the site, using overlapping, concentric circles and moving outward from the site.
3. Allow the site to dry.

Intradermal injections

An intradermal injection is made just below the epidermis or outer layer of skin (Figures 12-19 and 12-20a, b). This site is commonly used for allergy testing and for administration of local anaesthetics. A tuberculin syringe is usually used for intradermal injections as the volume injected is usually less than 0.5 mL. Common sites for intradermal injections are the medial surface of the forearm and the back. The steps for administering an intradermal injection are as follows:

1. Choose the injection site and cleanse the skin surface.
2. Hold the skin taut with one hand.
3. With the other hand, hold the syringe (with the needle bevel up) at a 10- to 15-degree angle to the injection site.
4. Gently puncture the skin. Insert the needle until the bevel is completely under the skin surface. Inject the medication. (Intradermal injections usually produce a raised wheal that resembles a mosquito bite.)
5. Withdraw the needle and dispose of the equipment appropriately.

Subcutaneous injections

Subcutaneous injections are given to place medication below the skin into the subcutaneous layer (Figure 12-21). The volume of such an injection is usually less than 0.5 mL. It is administered through a 23- or 25-gauge needle. In the pre-hospital setting, the drug most often given by this route is

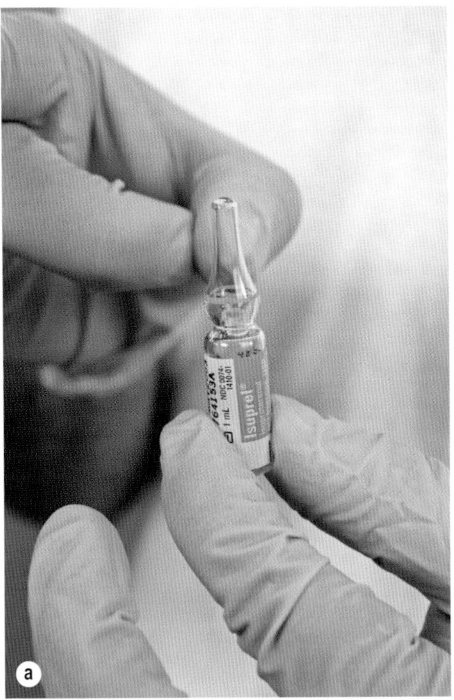

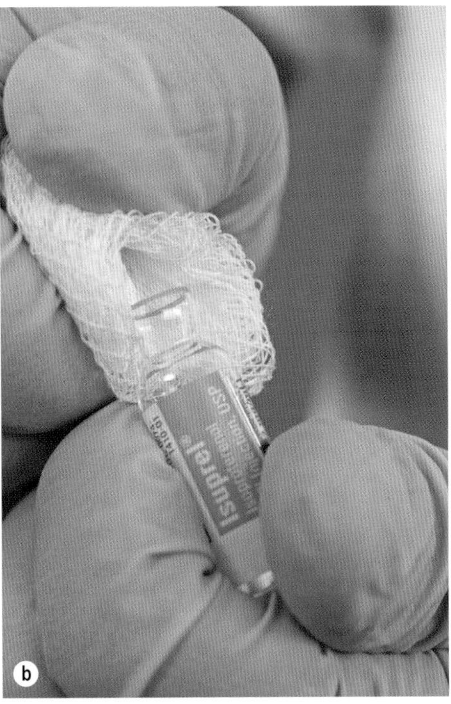

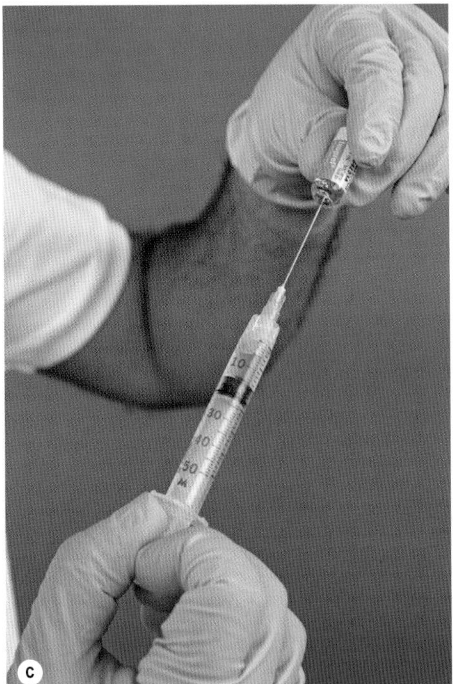

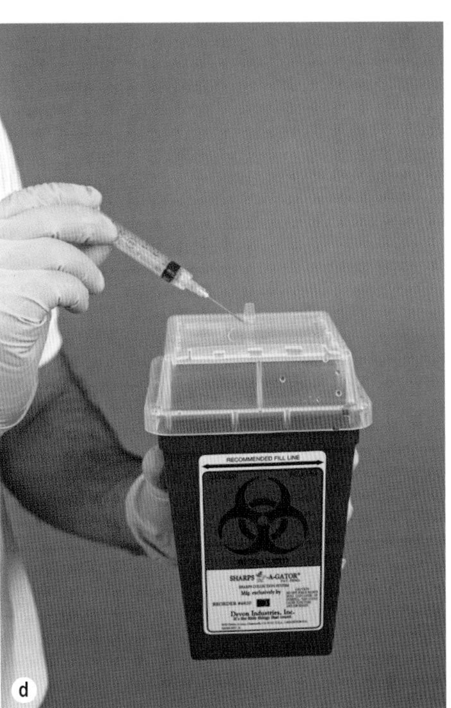

Figure 12-17 Withdrawing medication from an ampoule. (a) The ampoule is tapped to remove drug from the neck. (b) The top of the ampoule is broken off with a gauze pad. (c) The drug is withdrawn from ampoule. Care must be taken to make sure the needle does not touch the sides of the ampoule. (d) Sharps are discarded in an appropriate container.

adrenaline (epinephrine). The steps for subcutaneous injections are as follows (Figure 12-22a–d):

1. Choose the injection site and cleanse the area.
2. Elevate the subcutaneous tissue by gently pinching the injection site.
3. With the needle bevel up, insert the needle at a 45-degree angle in one quick motion.
4. Pull back slightly on the plunger (aspirate) to ensure needle placement. If no blood is aspirated, gently but smoothly inject the medication. If blood is present on aspiration, withdraw the needle, discard the medication and equipment, and begin again.
5. After the injection, withdraw the needle at the same angle at which it was inserted. Use an alcohol swab to massage the site. This helps distribute medication and promote absorption by dilating blood vessels in the area and increasing blood flow.

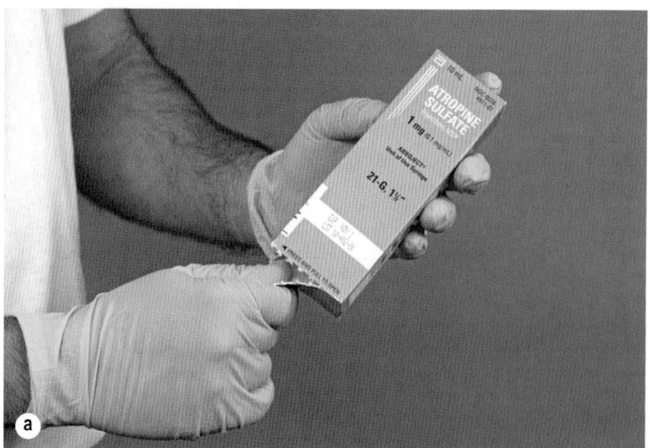

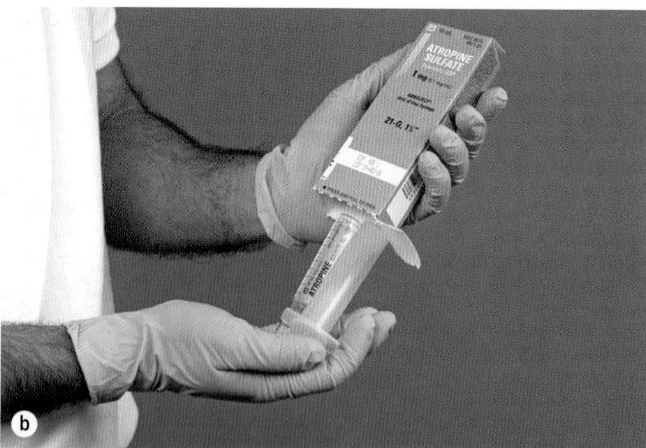

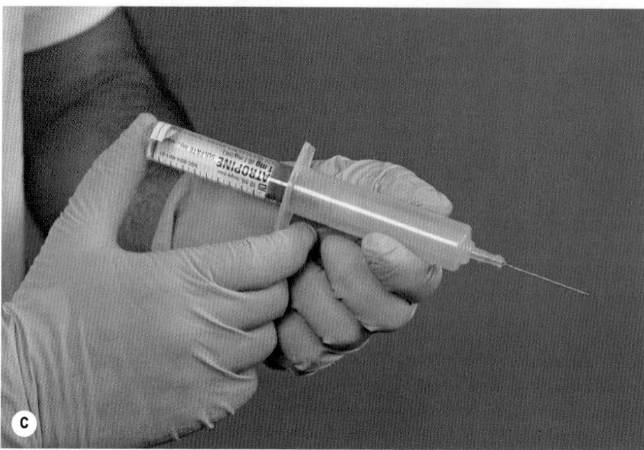

Figure 12-18 Prefilled medication syringe. (a) Drug in packaging. (b) Components in box. (c) Assembled syringe with needle.

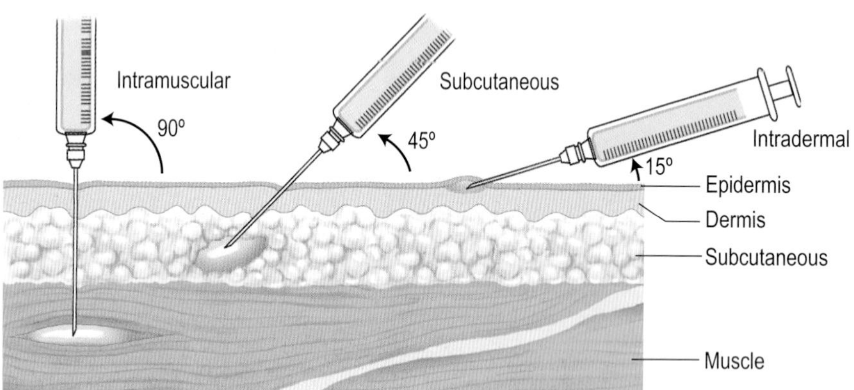

Figure 12-19 Comparison of angle of injection and deposition of medication for intramuscular, subcutaneous, and intradermal injections.

Intramuscular injections

Deeper injections are made into muscle tissue. These pass through the skin and subcutaneous tissue. They are given when a drug is too irritating to be injected subcutaneously or when a greater volume or faster absorption is desired. (Irritation may still occur via this route.) A maximum volume of 5 mL may be given by intramuscular injection in a large muscle mass (e.g. gluteal muscle).

The type of needle used depends on four factors: (1) the site of the injection; (2) the condition of the tissue; (3) the size of the patient; and (4) the type of drug to be injected (i.e. small-lumen needles are used for thin solutions, and larger-lumen needles are used for suspensions and oils). Because the muscle layer is below the subcutaneous layer, a longer-needle generally is used (usually 25 mm and 19- or 21-gauge). The procedures for intramuscular injections are mostly the same as those described before

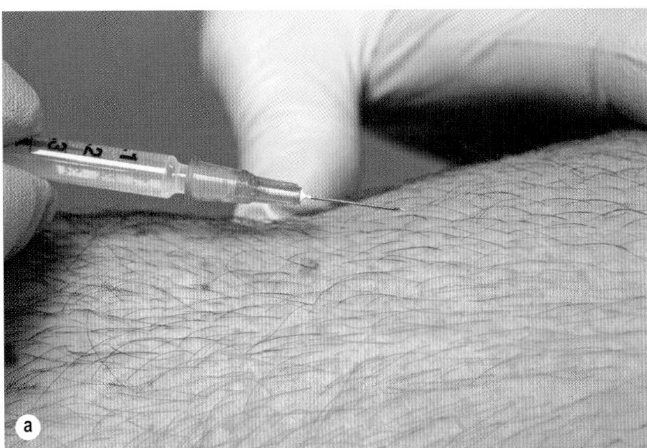

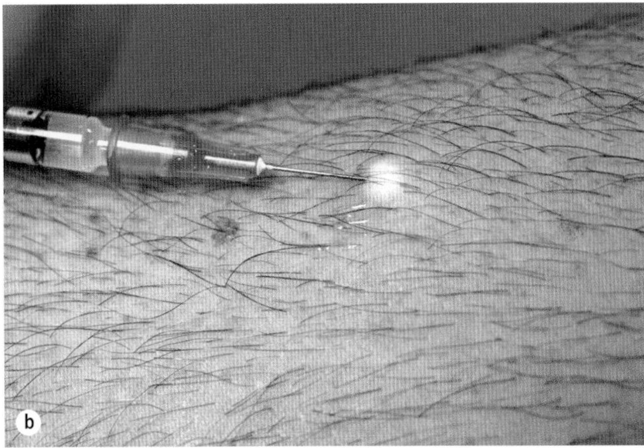

Figure 12-20 Intradermal injection. (a) Choose the site and cleanse the skin. Then, with the bevel up, insert the needle at a 15-degree angle. (b) Wheal produced by the injection.

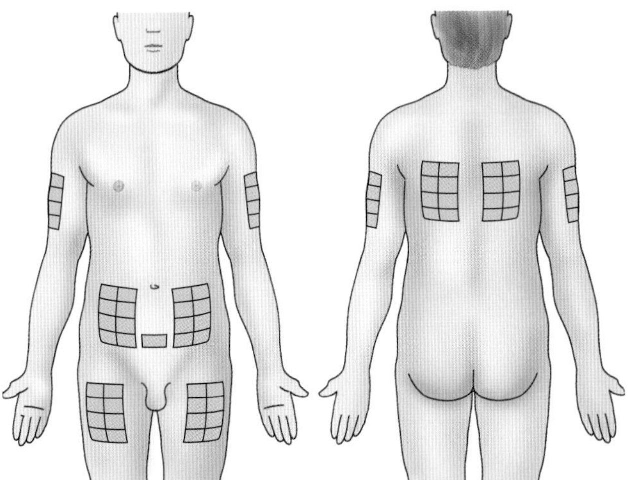

Figure 12-21 Sites commonly used for subcutaneous injections.

(Figure 12-23a–e). However, the needle is inserted at a 90-degree angle. Also, the skin is held taut, not pinched.

Several muscles are commonly used for intramuscular injections. These are the deltoid muscle, several gluteal muscles (dorsogluteal site), the vastus lateralis muscle, the rectus femoris muscle, and the ventrogluteal muscle. The deltoid muscle is located in the upper arm. It forms a triangular shape, with the base of the triangle along the acromion process and the peak of the triangle ending approximately one-third of the way down the lateral aspect of the upper arm (Figure 12-24). This muscle is small and can accommodate only small doses of injection (1 mL or less). When injections are made in this location, care must be taken to avoid hitting the radial nerve. The patient should be sitting upright or lying flat and they should be told to relax the arm muscles.

The dorsogluteal site consists of several gluteal muscles and can be identified in two ways. The first method is to divide the buttocks on one side into imaginary quadrants; the medication is administered into the upper outer quadrant. The second method is to locate the posterior-superior iliac spine and the greater trochanter of the femur. An imaginary line is drawn between the two landmarks; the injection is given up and out from this line (Figure 12-25). This site should not be used for children under 3 years of age as the muscles are not yet well developed and the proximity of the sciatic nerve (the largest nerve in the body) poses a risk. Large, well-developed muscles can accommodate an injection of up to 5 mL; however, volumes over 3 mL may be uncomfortable for the patient. When an injection is administered at the dorsogluteal site, the patient should be lying prone with the toes pointing inward to promote muscle relaxation. Another complication of gluteal injections is inadvertent injection into the hip joint. The paramedic can minimize this risk by paying attention to anatomical landmarks.

The vastus lateralis and the rectus femoris muscles lie side by side in the thigh. They are not generally used by paramedics as sites for injection but the technique is described for completeness. To identify the necessary landmarks, the paramedic should place one hand on the patient's upper thigh and one hand on the lower thigh. The area between the hands is the middle third of the thigh and the middle third of the underlying muscle (Figure 12-26). The vastus lateralis lies lateral to the midline and is the preferred injection site for children. It is well developed in all patients and has few major blood vessels and nerves that can be injured. The rectus femoris is most often used for self-injection because of its accessibility. Acceptable volumes for injection vary with the age of the patient and the size of the muscle. Up to 5 mL may be injected into a well-developed adult. The patient should be sitting upright or lying supine and should be advised to relax the muscles.

The ventrogluteal muscle is accessible when the patient lies in a supine or lateral recumbent position. The paramedic should palpate the greater trochanter using the palm, with the index finger pointing to the anterior-superior iliac spine. The paramedic's remaining three fingers should extend toward the iliac crest. The injection is made into the centre of the V formed by the fingers (Figure 12-27). This injection site may be used for all patients. It is a desirable site because it has no large nerves or fat tissue and may accommodate up to 5 mL of drug in adults.

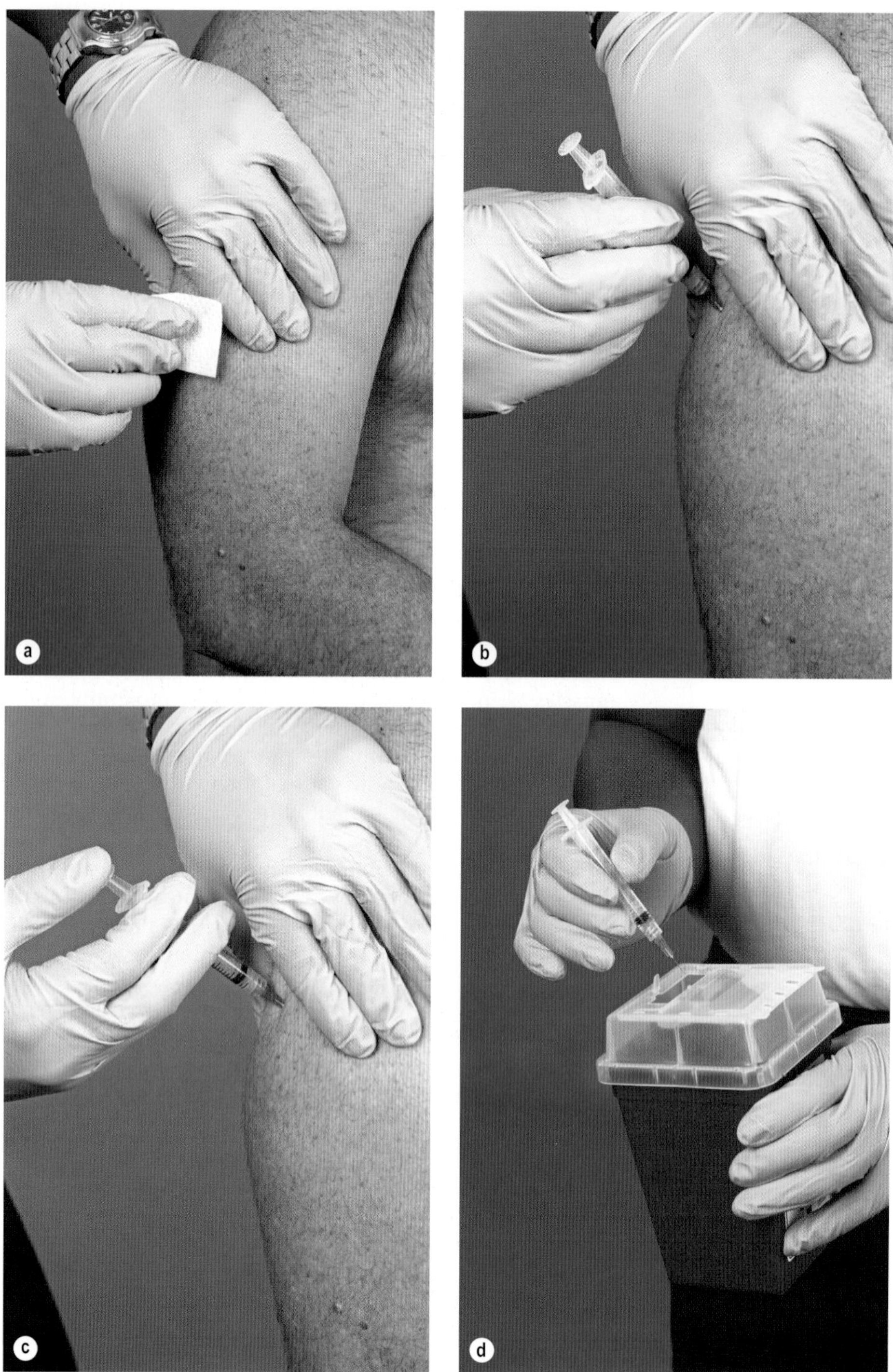

Figure 12-22 Subcutaneous injection. (a) Cleanse the skin. Then, grasp it to maximize the amount of subcutaneous tissue available. (b) Insert the needle. Pull back on the plunger to aspirate (to check needle placement). (c) Slowly push in the plunger to deliver the medication. (d) Remove the needle. Discard it in an appropriate container.

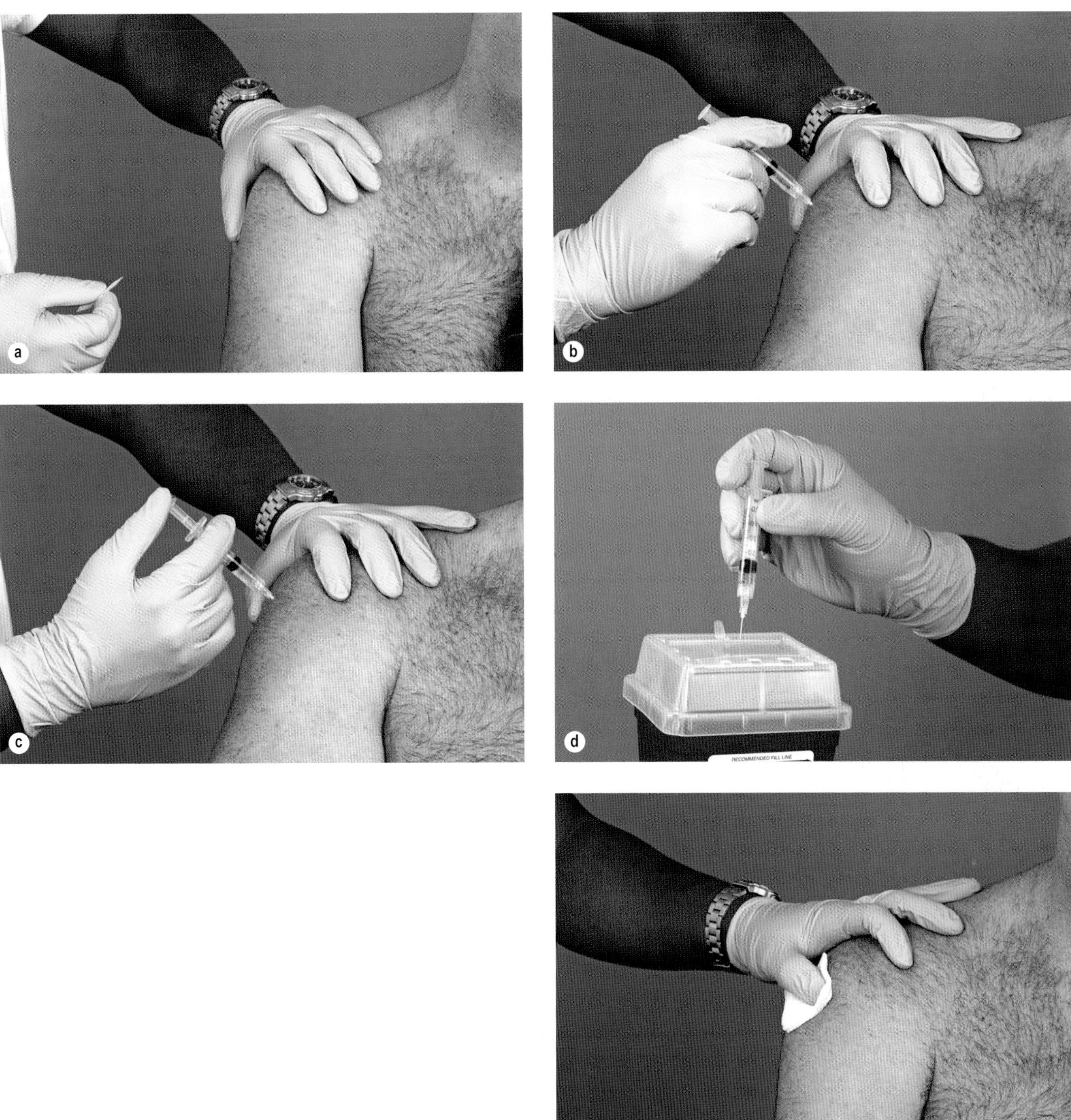

Figure 12-23 Intramuscular injection. (a) Choose the site. Cleanse the skin and pull it tight. (b) Insert the needle. Pull back on the plunger to aspirate (to check needle placement). (c) Slowly push in the plunger to deliver the medication. (d) Remove the needle. Discard it in an appropriate container. (e) Massage the skin over the injection site.

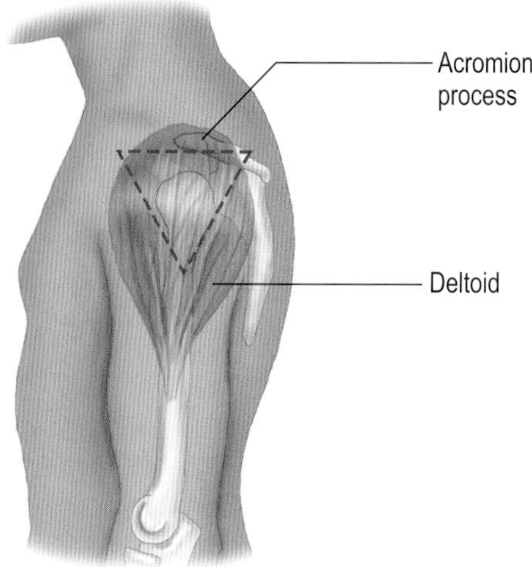

Figure 12-24 The injection site for the deltoid muscle roughly forms an inverted triangle, with the acromion process as the base. The muscle may be visible in well-developed patients.

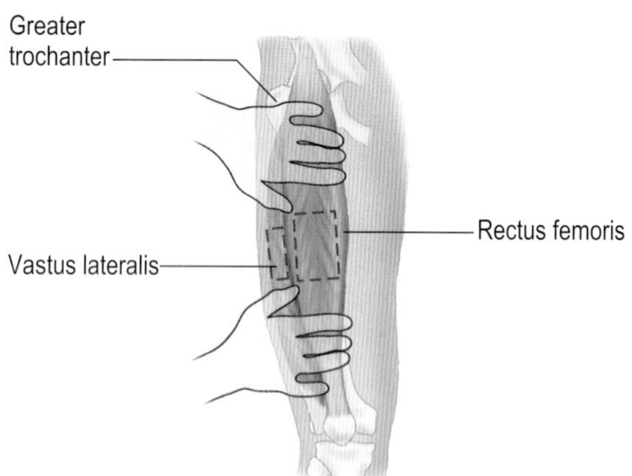

Figure 12-26 The injection sites for the vastus lateralis muscle and the rectus femoris muscle can be defined through landmarks. One hand is placed below the greater trochanter. The other hand is placed above the knee. The space between the two hands defines the middle third of the underlying muscle. The rectus femoris is on the anterior thigh. The vastus lateralis is on the lateral side.

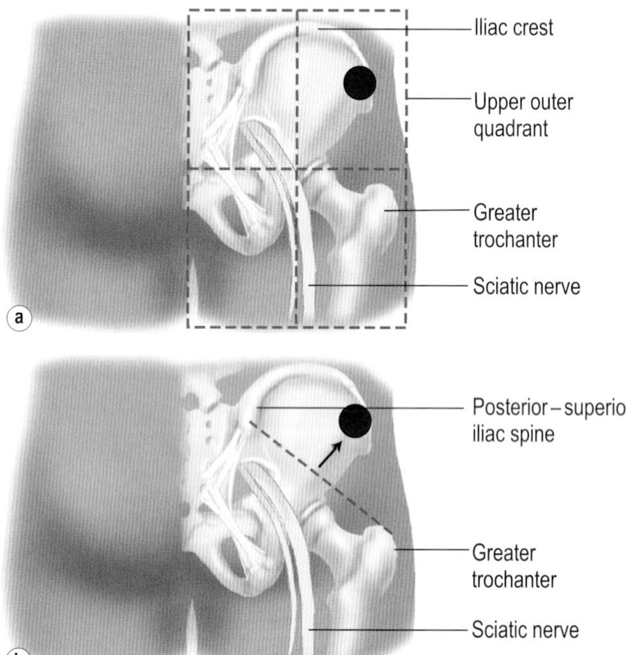

Figure 12-25 The injection area for the dorsogluteal site can be defined in two ways. (a) The buttocks can be divided on one side into imaginary quadrants. The centre of the upper outer quadrant should be used as the injection site. (b) The posterior-superior iliac spine and the greater trochanter are located by palpation. An imaginary line is drawn between the two. The injection site should be above and out from that line.

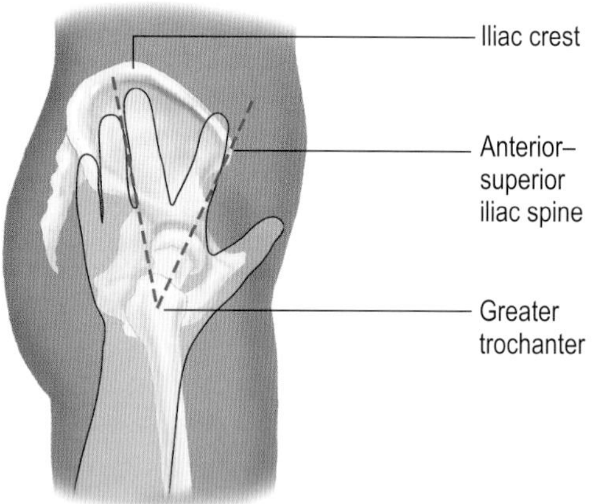

Figure 12-27 The injection site for the ventrogluteal muscle is defined by placing the palm of one hand on the trochanter of the femur. A V is then made with the fingers of that hand. One side runs from the greater trochanter to the anterior-superior iliac spine. The other side runs from the greater trochanter to the iliac crest. The injection is made into the centre of the V.

Intravenous therapy

Intravenous cannulation is used to gain access to the body's circulation. It is indicated for three reasons: the first is to administer fluids; the second is to administer drugs; and the third is to obtain specimens for laboratory determinations. The intravenous route puts the drug directly into the bloodstream, so bypasses all barriers to drug absorption. Intravenous cannulation may also be considered as a prophylactic measure in certain circumstances.

> **Critical Thinking**
>
> There are benefits to choosing the upper extremity for intravenous access in an adult. What are they?

Intravenous fluid administration

In the prehospital setting, the route of choice for fluid therapy is through a peripheral vein in an extremity. If the arms have no major injury, upper extremity veins should

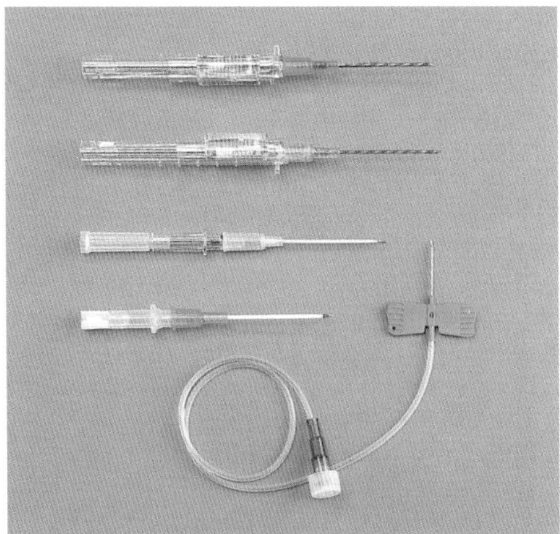

Figure 12-28 Various types of intravenous (IV) catheters.

be used. If upper extremity sites are not available, lower extremity sites may be used. IV fluids often used in the prehospital setting include normal saline, sodium lactate solution, and mixtures of glucose and water. For the most part, normal saline and lactated Ringer solution are used for fluid replacement. They also are used as a means of administering a drug.

Types of intravenous catheters

The three main types of intravenous catheters are (1) the hollow needle (butterfly) type; (2) the indwelling plastic catheter over a hollow needle (e.g. Venflon); and (3) the indwelling plastic catheter inserted through a hollow needle (e.g., Intracath; this type is seldom used in the prehospital setting) (Figure 12-28).

Hollow needles are not advised for IV fluid replacement in the prehospital setting as it is very difficult to stabilize the needle. In some cases a butterfly catheter may be used for a paediatric patient if it can be stabilized adequately. This can sometimes be achieved by using arm boards or other immobilization devices. In the prehospital setting, use of the over-the-needle catheter is preferred as it is easily secured and more comfortable for the patient.

Peripheral intravenous insertion

The areas most commonly used for peripheral intravenous therapy are the hands and the arms (including the antecubital fossae [ACF]). Other sites include the long saphenous veins and the external jugular veins; however, the incidences of embolism and infection are higher at the latter two sites. Figures 12-29 to 12-31 show sites and techniques for peripheral cannulation.

Another factor in the selection of a puncture site for intravenous therapy is the patient's clinical status. Injuries or diseases involving an extremity interfere with the use of veins in that extremity for venepuncture or venous cannulation. Examples of such conditions include trauma, dialysis fistula, and a history of mastectomy.

Steps

1. If the patient is conscious, explain the procedure and gain consent. Give the reason why intravenous therapy is necessary and describe the procedure.

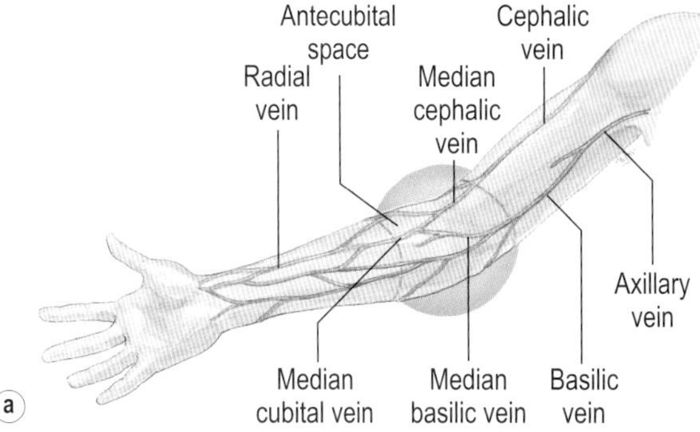

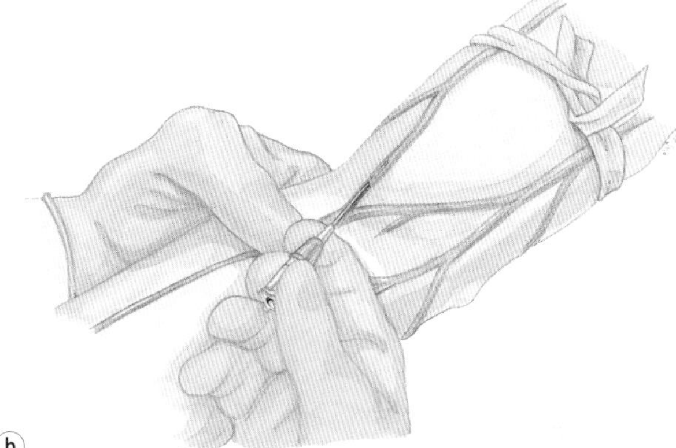

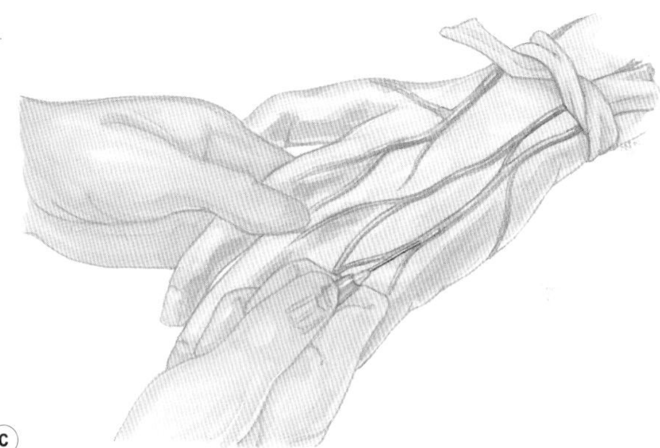

Figure 12-29 (a) Veins of the upper extremity. (b) Antecubital venepuncture. (c) Dorsal hand venepuncture.

2. Assemble the equipment (Figure 12-32a, b)
   - **(a)** Inspect the prescribed fluid for contamination, appearance, and expiration date. Never use fluids that are cloudy, outdated, or in any way suspect for contamination.
   - **(b)** Prepare the microdrip or macrodrip infusion set. Attach the infusion set to the bag of solution.
3. Clamp the tubing and squeeze the reservoir on the infusion set until it fills halfway. Then open the clamp and flush the air from the tubing. Close the clamp.
4. Select the catheter. A large-bore catheter (14- to 16-gauge) should be used for fluid replacement; a smaller-bore catheter (18- to 20-gauge) should be used for 'keep open' lines. 'Keep open' lines are used to maintain hydration and to establish a channel for IV medication if needed.

5. Prepare other equipment:
   - Alcohol, chlorhexidine/alcohol, or iodine wipes to cleanse the skin
   - Sterile dressings or 4×4 gauze pads
   - Adhesive tape, torn or cut into several strips or proprietary cannula dressing
   - Venous tourniquet (a blood pressure cuff may be used).
6. Put on gloves for personal and patient protection.
7. Select the puncture site. If using an upper extremity, allow the patient's arm to hang dependent, and apply the tourniquet several inches above the antecubital space. (The tourniquet should be just tight enough to tamponade venous vessels but not occlude arterial flow.) When selecting a suitable vein, begin by looking at the dorsum of the hand and forearm. Choose a vein that is fairly straight and easily accessible. The forearm is better than the hand because it allows hand movement and is more easily secured after cannulation. If a second puncture attempt is necessary, the second puncture should always be proximal to the first puncture. Therefore the vein selected for initial cannulation should be the most distal suitable vein. Avoid veins near joints, where immobilization is difficult, and veins near injured areas. If the long saphenous vein is chosen, begin site selection near the medial malleolus of the foot. To locate the external jugular vein, place the patient in a supine head-down position and turn the patient's head toward the opposite side.
8. Prepare the puncture site and cleanse the area:
   - **(a)** Thoroughly clean the site with alcohol to remove dirt, dead skin, blood, and other surface contaminants. Allow the area to dry.
   - **(b)** Clean the site using overlapping, concentric circles and moving outward.
9. Stabilize the vein by applying distal pressure and tension to the point of entry (Figure 12-33a). With the bevel up, pass the needle through the skin and into the vein from the side or directly on top (Figure 12-33b). (Using a 'bevel down' technique in infants and children may facilitate entry into constricted peripheral veins.[22]) Advance the needle and catheter about 2 mm beyond the point where blood return in the hub of the needle was first encountered. Slide the catheter over the needle and into the vein. While stabilizing the catheter, withdraw the needle (Figure 12-33c). Apply pressure on the proximal end of the catheter to stop escaping blood. Obtain blood samples, if authorized and needed, with a syringe or Vacutainer.
10. Release the tourniquet and attach the IV tubing (Figure 12-33d). Open the tubing clamp and allow fluid infusion to begin at the prescribed flow rate (Figure 12-33e).

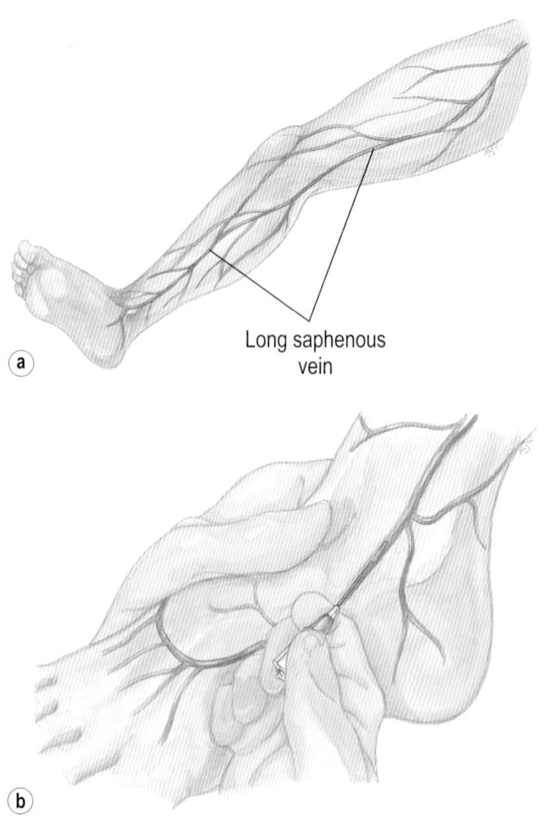

Figure 12-30 (a) Long saphenous vein. (b) Venepuncture of the long saphenous vein.

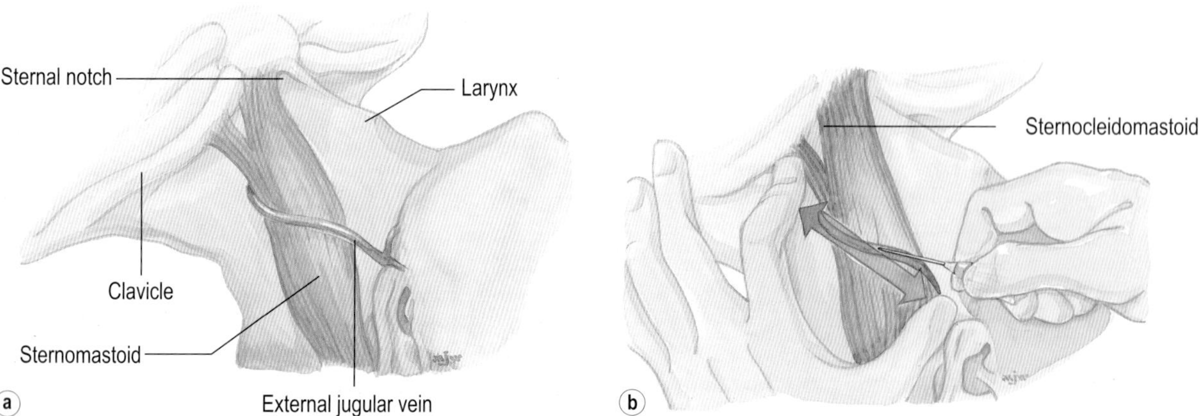

Figure 12-31 (a) Anatomy of the external jugular vein. (b) External jugular venepuncture.

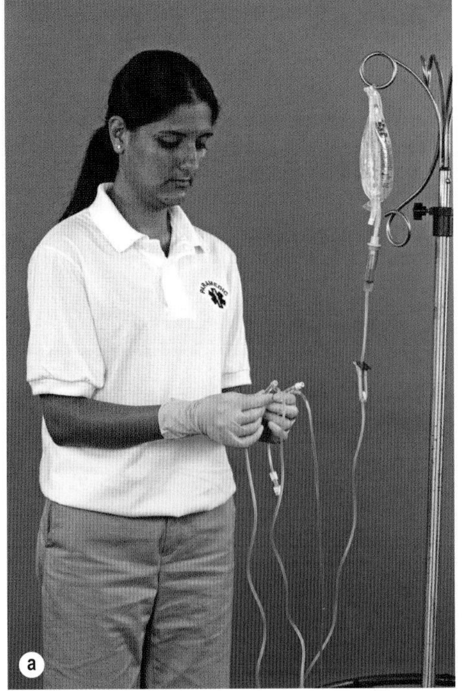

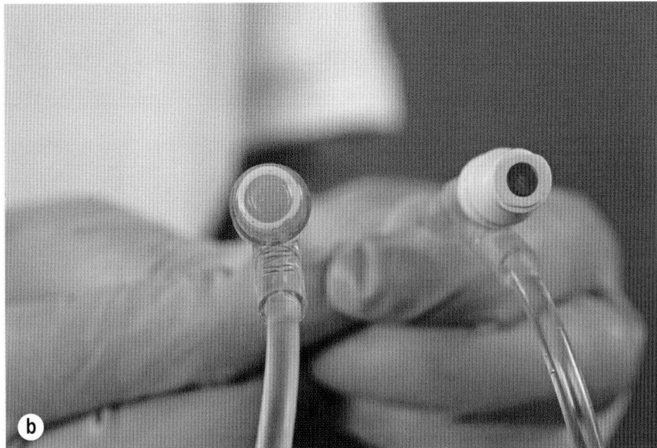

Figure 12-32 (a) Intravenous infusion setup. (b) Needle and needleless ports.

11. Cover the puncture site with a dressing to ensure asepsis and to secure the line. Anchor the tubing and secure the catheter. Catheter movement can increase the risk of phlebitis and cause migration of pathogens along the cannula into the vein.
12. Document the infusion procedure.

External jugular cannulation

The paramedic should only consider accessing the external jugular vein after all other avenues of peripheral venous cannulation have been exhausted. As a result this procedure is to be carried out in adults only, and only to aid drug or fluid delivery in a cardiac or respiratory arrest when peripheral access is unobtainable. It is absolutely contraindicated in any patient with an unidentifiable external jugular vein.

Steps

1. Prepare equipment and puncture site as above.
2. Position the patient supine with the patient's head turned to opposite side from procedure.
3. Aim to have the patient in the Trendelenburg position where possible to minimize the risk of air entrainment during the procedure.
4. Align the cannula in the direction of the vein with the point aimed toward the ipsilateral shoulder.
5. Stabilize the vein between your fingers.
6. Make a puncture midway between the angle of the jaw and the midclavicular line, 'tourniqueting' the vein lightly with one finger above the clavicle.
7. Flash back should be seen as with cannulation of any vein. A 2 ml syringe attached to the cannula to aspirate blood will aid in confirmation of placement and minimize the risk of air embolus.
8. Do not allow air to be drawn into the cannula.
9. Secure the line as normal.

Complications of intravenous techniques

Several possible complications are associated with all intravenous techniques. These include local complications, systemic complications, infiltration, and air embolism.

Local and systemic complications

Local complications may involve haematoma formation, thrombosis, cellulitis and phlebitis. Systemic complications include the following:

- sepsis
- pulmonary embolism
- catheter fragment embolism
- fibre embolism originating from cotton or paper fibres in the catheter irrigation solution, leading to foreign body reactions
- arterial puncture.

Infiltration

Infiltration may occur when the needle or catheter has been displaced or when blood or fluid leaks from around the catheter and escapes into the tissues (extravasation). It can also occur if a vein is punctured more than once during initiation of IV access. Signs and symptoms include the following:

- coolness of the skin at the puncture site
- swelling at the puncture site, with or without pain
- sluggish or absent flow rate.

If infiltration is suspected, the paramedic should lower the fluid reservoir to a dependent position to check for backflow of blood into the tubing. (The absence of backflow

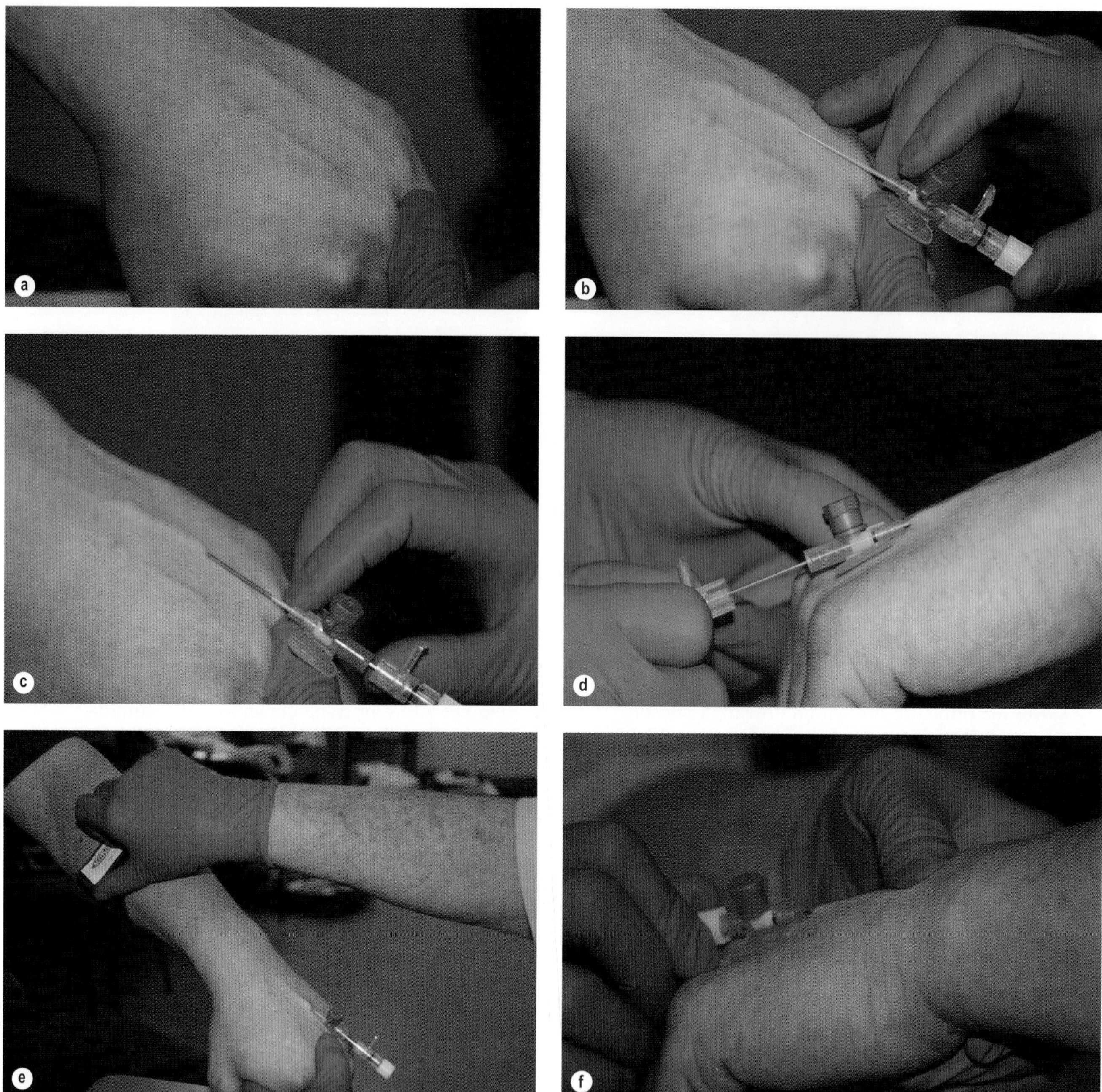

Figure 12-33 Technique for intravenous catheterization. (a) Stabilize the vein by applying distal pressure and tension to the point of entry. (b) With the bevel up, pass the needle into the vein from the side or directly on top. (c) When you see a 'flashback', slide the catheter over the needle and into the vein. (d) While stabilizing the catheter, withdraw the needle. (e) Release the tourniquet, apply distal pressure to minimize leakage, and then attach the bung or infusion. (f) Open the tubing clamp. Adjust the infusion to begin at the prescribed flow rate.

suggests infiltration.) If any of the signs and symptoms are present, the intravenous flow should be discontinued (Box 12-35). The needle or catheter should be removed immediately and a pressure dressing should be applied to the site. An alternative puncture site should be chosen and the infusion restarted with new equipment. The incident must be documented.

Air embolism

Air embolism is uncommon but it can be fatal. The volume of air that the human bloodstream can tolerate has not been firmly established; however, fatalities have been reported after 100 mL of air entering the cardiovascular system.[23] A total of 10 mL of air can be fatal in a critically ill patient.

Box 12-35

Discontinuation of an intravenous infusion

To discontinue an intravenous (IV) infusion and remove the intravenous catheter, follow these steps:

1. Put on gloves.
2. Carefully remove any securing tapes and dressings.
3. Close the drip chamber to stop the flow of fluid.
4. Place sterile gauze over the insertion site and apply gentle pressure with one hand. With the other hand, quickly withdraw the catheter, pulling straight back from the angle of insertion.
5. Apply firm pressure to the insertion site for 2–5 min to prevent bleeding or bruising.
6. Cover the insertion site with a bandage.
7. Appropriately dispose of all equipment.

The embolism is caused by air entering the bloodstream via the catheter tubing. The risk of air embolism is greatest when a catheter is passed into the central circulation, where negative pressure may actually pull in air. Air can enter the circulation either on insertion of the catheter or when the tubing is disconnected to replace solutions or add new extension tubing. With subsequent pumping, blood foaming occurs in the heart. If enough air enters the heart chamber, it can impede the flow of blood, which, in turn, can lead to shock.

Signs and symptoms of air embolism include hypotension, cyanosis, weak rapid pulse, and loss of consciousness. If air embolism is suspected, the following steps should be taken:

1. Close the tubing.
2. Turn the patient on the left side with the head down. (If air has entered the heart chambers, this position may keep the air in the right side of the heart and away from the cardiac valves. The pulmonary artery may absorb small air bubbles.)
3. Check tubing for leaks.
4. Administer high-concentration oxygen.
5. Notify receiving hospital.

Accidental disconnection of the IV tubing may occur during patient movement and can cause an air embolism. The chance of an air embolism can be minimized by making sure that all tubing connections are secure and changing fluid containers before they are empty.

Intravenous medications

Medications can be administered via the intravenous route directly into the circulating blood. Intravenous medications can be given by injection or infusion. An intravenous injection can be given through a previously established intravenous cannula or infusion line, or directly into the vein with a sterile needle or butterfly device. An intravenous infusion is given by adding a drug to an infusing intravenous solution such as normal saline. Another method is to dilute the drug in a larger volume of fluid and administer the medication through a volume-control, in-line device (e.g. burette, Volutrol, infusion pump). Sometimes the medication is given by intermittent infusion through an existing infusion site (intravenous piggyback or secondary set) [not discussed in this text].

Intravenous injections normally involve a small amount of medication (usually less than 5 mL). These are called intravenous push or intravenous bolus medications. To give such an injection (Figure 12-34a–d), the paramedic should clean the injection port of the IV line with alcohol or remove the cap from the needleless port. The prescribed medication is then injected at the appropriate rate depending upon the type of medication and the patient's response. Most intravenous tubing has one-way valves to prevent backflow of medication. If such a valve is not present or cannot be identified, the tubing above the injection site should be clamped during drug administration. After the injection, the infusion of fluids is continued.

Intravenous infusions for drug administration can take several forms. To add a medication to the fluid reservoir of an established intravenous line, the paramedic should follow these steps (Figure 12-35):

1. Compute the volume of the drug to be added to the fluid reservoir.
2. Draw up the prescribed dose into a syringe. If prefilled syringes are used, note the volume of medication in the syringe and the dose to be used.
3. Cleanse the rubber sleeve of the fluid reservoir with an alcohol swab.
4. Puncture the rubber sleeve (if a needle is used) and inject the prescribed medication into the fluid reservoir.
5. Withdraw the needle (if a needleless system is not used) and discard the needle and syringe. Gently mix the medication with the fluid by agitating the reservoir.
6. Label the fluid reservoir with (1) the name of the medication added, (2) the amount of the medication added, (3) the resultant concentration of the medication in the reservoir, (4) the date and time the infusion was prepared, and (5) the name of the paramedic who prepared the infusion.
7. Calculate the rate of administration in drops per minute as prescribed.

A number of in-line, volume-control devices allow more accurate delivery of medication diluted in precise amounts of fluids than is possible by simply setting the drip rate manually. These devices are often used to give intravenous medications to children and adults who need precise doses. Medications that can readily cause toxicity when given too rapidly (e.g. antidysrhythmics, vasopressors) are well suited to this delivery method. In-line devices include electronic flow rate regulators that regulate fluid passage by means of a magnetically activated metal ball valve. They also include infusion pumps that exert pressure on tubing or fluid by pumping against pressure gradients. It is likely that only critical care paramedics will be using these devices; they should follow the instructions of the equipment's manufacturer and also familiarize themselves with these devices before using them (Figure 12-36).

Another device used to administer a drug intravenously is a drug pump. Drug pumps are used by patients who need a slow injection of medication in the home; for example,

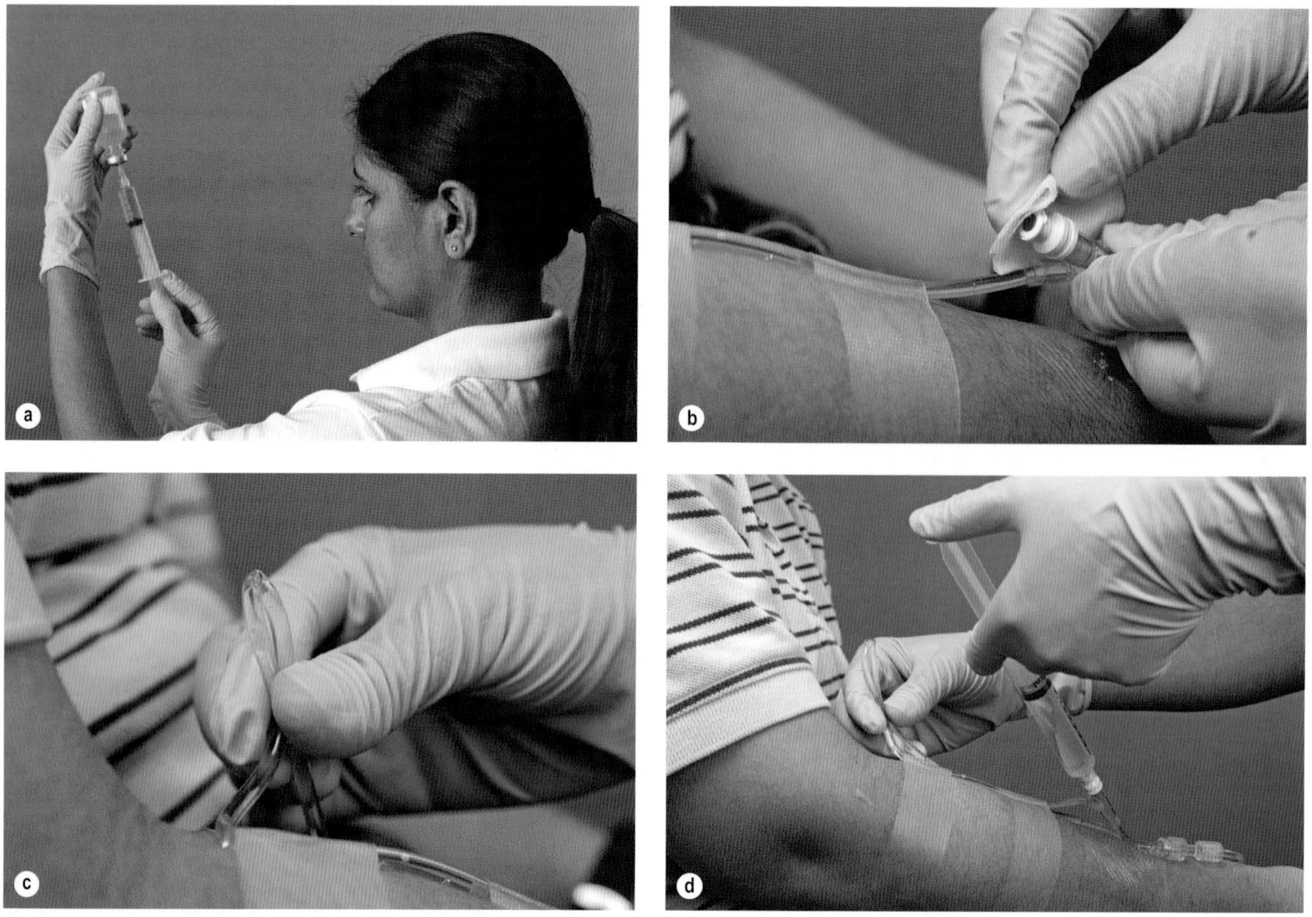

Figure 12-34 Administration of a drug by intravenous (IV) route. (a) Prepare the correct volume of the drug. Cleanse the injection port. (b) If the tubing does not have a one-way valve, pinch the line to clamp it. (c) Inject the drug at the recommended rate. (d) Resume IV flow (with a small flush if indicated) and monitor the patient.

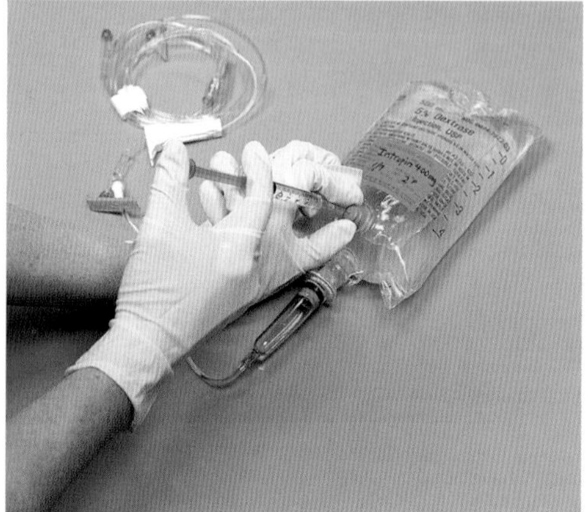

Figure 12-35 Adding medication to an intravenous reservoir.

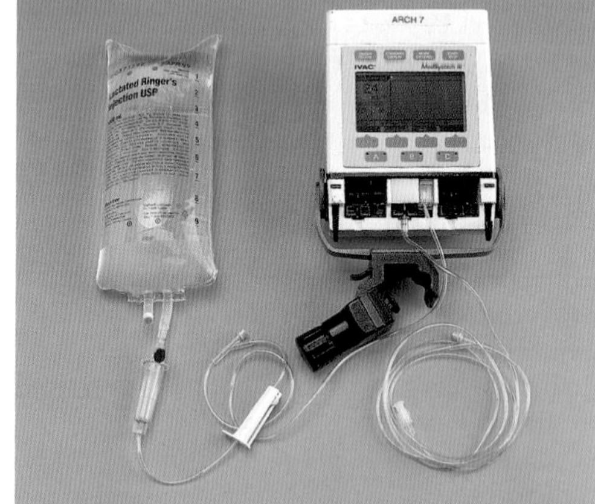

Figure 12-36 Intravenous infusion pump.

patients who are undergoing cancer chemotherapy. These devices usually consist of a syringe with a battery attachment that regulates the injection of medication. Drug pumps are used to give medication subcutaneously but can also be attached to indwelling vascular devices. Such devices include the Port-A-Cath or Hickman catheter.

Intraosseous medications

Studies have shown that intraosseous (IO) infusion is relatively safe and effective in children. The procedure should be used where two attempts at peripheral venous access have failed, or where no suitable vein is apparent within a reasonable timeframe in children requiring urgent venous access.[3]

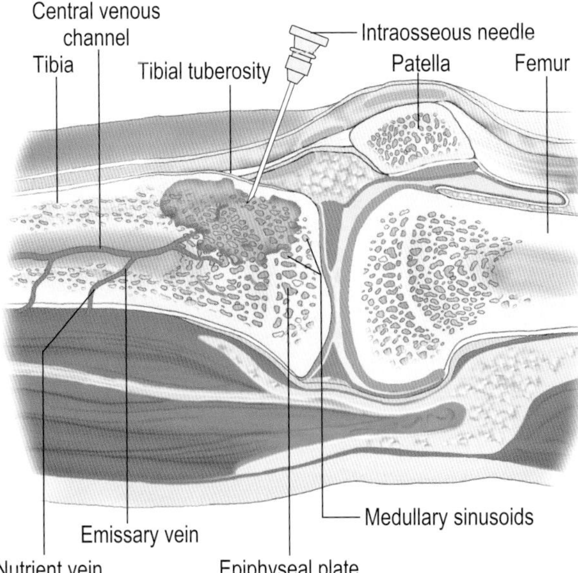

Figure 12-37 Obtaining intraosseous access.

IO is the first choice in cardiorespiratory arrest and decompensated failure states in young children. JRCALC no longer provide guidance on the maximum age for use of this technique so the paramedic should follow the guidelines of their employing Trust. Normally the IO route will only be used on unconscious children; if IO access is attempted on a conscious child, the paramedic should remember to use a local anaesthetic.[3]

Fluids and drugs infused through IO access pass quickly from the marrow cavities of long bones into the sinusoids. They then pass to large venous channels and emissary veins and into the systemic circulation. Normal saline, sodium lactate solution, G10W, plasma, blood and most advanced life-saving (ALS) medications may be infused quickly by this route (Figure 12-37). Drugs administered by the IO route should be followed by a saline flush of at least 5 mL. This ensures that the drug is delivered into the central circulation.

IO infusion should generally only be considered for unconscious children and only when peripheral cannulation is unobtainable. Example scenarios include cardiopulmonary arrest and peripheral vascular collapse (as in shock, major trauma or burns). The procedure may also be indicated in children in whom vascular access is impaired by obesity or oedema, and in children with life-threatening status asthmaticus. Paramedics should follow service guidelines regarding indications for IO infusion.

Note

The intraosseous space can be thought of as a 'non-collapsable vein'. This space is surrounded by bone and is directly connected to the central circulation. In the absence of trauma to the bone, the IO space remains patent, even when peripheral veins collapse.

The site of choice for initiation of this procedure in children is the tibia, one to two fingerbreadths below the tubercle on the anteromedial surface. An alternative choice is the femur, two to three fingerbreadths above the lateral condyles in the midline. The procedures for initiating IO infusion in the tibia of a child and in the sternum of an adult are shown in Figure 12-38a–e.

Necessary equipment

- Alcohol wipes.
- Tape.
- Bone marrow needle or commercial intraosseous needle.
- IV tubing (paediatric infusion set).
- IV fluids.

Insertion technique

1. Put on gloves for personal and patient protection.
2. Cleanse the site as previously described for peripheral cannulation.
3. Prepare the needle for insertion. Insert the needle pointing away from the epiphyseal plate. Advance it to the periosteum.
4. Using a boring or screwing motion, advance the needle until it penetrates the bone marrow (usually noted by decreased resistance and a slight popping sound).
5. Remove the stylet.
6. Aspirate bone marrow into a saline-filled syringe. (Bone marrow may not always be aspirated.)
7. Infuse saline by syringe to ensure placement of the needle and to clear clots.
8. Secure the needle with tape and a securing screw if so equipped (although the needle is usually well stabilized by the bone).
9. Attach a three-way tap extension, and infuse fluid boluses using a 20 or 50 mL syringe. Fluids will not usually run freely from an infusion set.
10. Apply a dressing to the site and immobilize the limb.
11. Document the procedure.

Contraindications

- Fracture of the site or proximal to the site.
- Traumatized extremity.
- Cellulitis.
- Burns that may be infected by the technique.
- Congenital bone disease.

Potential complications

Technical

- Subperiosteal infusion from improper placement.
- Penetration of posterior wall of medullary cavity, resulting in soft tissue infusion.
- Slow infusion from clotting of marrow.

Systemic

- Osteomyelitis (occurs in fewer than 0.6% of cases, usually with prolonged infusion).
- Fat embolism (rare).

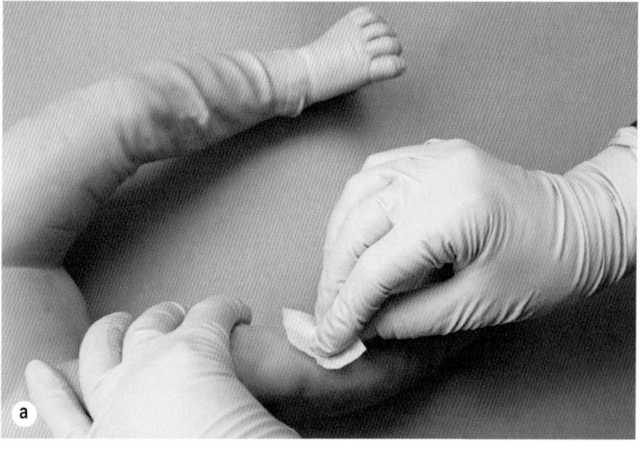

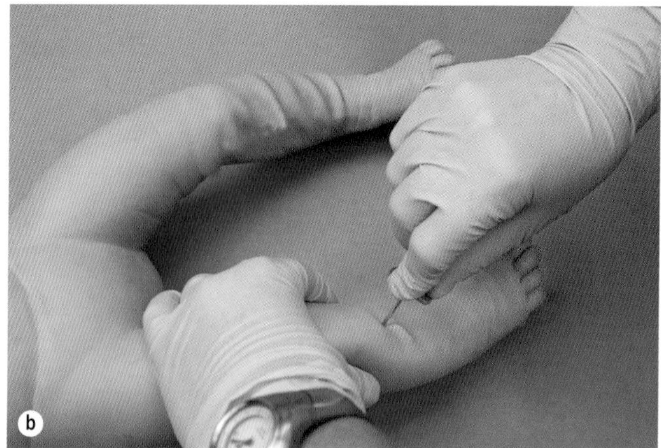

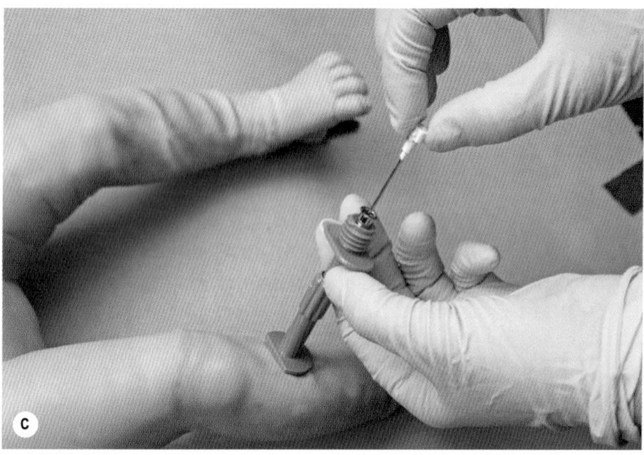

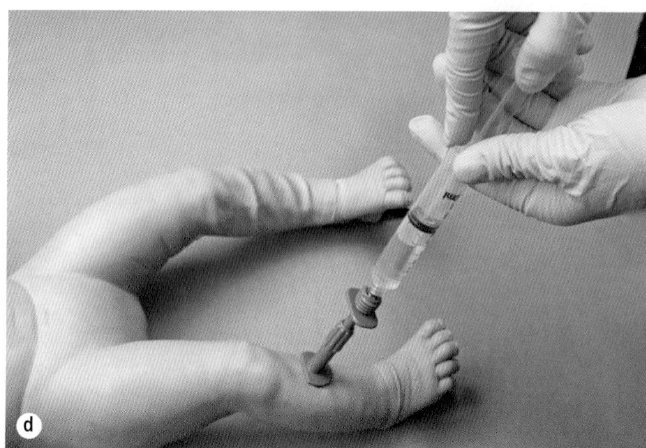

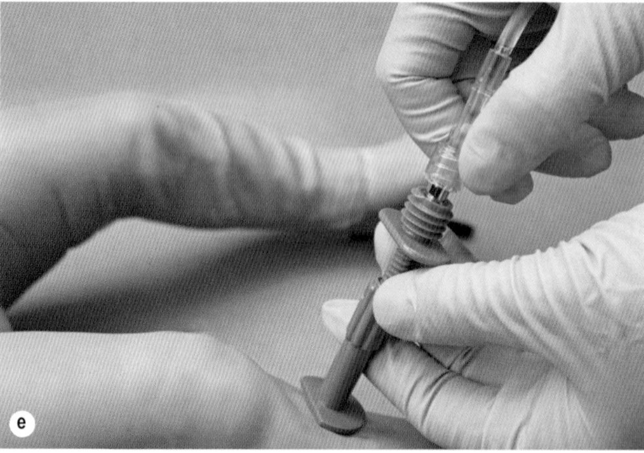

Figure 12-38 Intraosseous infusion. (a) Cleanse the site. (b) Using a screwing motion, insert the bone marrow needle away from the epiphyseal plate. Advance the needle until a pop is felt (this occurs when the needle penetrates the marrow). (c) Remove the stylet. (d) Aspirate for marrow and then flush with saline. (e) Attach the intravenous tubing, and adjust the infusion to the prescribed flow rate. Check for signs of infiltration.

- Slight periostitis at the injection site (usually clears within 2 to 3 weeks).
- Infection (acceptably low rate, comparable to that with other infusion techniques).
- Fracture.

Administration of percutaneous medications

Percutaneous drug administration is the administration of drugs that are absorbed through the mucous membranes or skin. These include topical drugs, sublingual drugs, buccal drugs, inhaled drugs, endotracheal drugs, and drugs for the eye, nose and ear.

Topical drugs

UK paramedics do not routinely apply topical drugs but it is important to recognize drugs that are commonly used in patch form as they may affect the patient unfavourably during illness. Drugs that may be administered topically in the form of a patch include: opioid analgesics such as buprenorphine and fentanyl; vasodilator drugs such as glyceryl trinitrate; dopamine receptor agonists used in

Parkinson's disease, such as Rotigotene; estrogen and hormone replacement therapy patches; and nicotine patches.

Paramedics should be able to recognize the different types of patches and should remove them if indicated. Usual sites for the patches are behind the ear and on the chest, back, hip and upper arms.

Sublingual drugs

The most frequently prescribed sublingual drugs are nitrates (e.g. glyceryl trinitrate), which are used to treat angina pectoris. The tablet should be placed under the tongue, where it dissolves. The patient should not drink fluids while the drug is being absorbed. If the patient inadvertently swallows the tablet, the effects are severely impaired by the 'first-pass' effect.

Buccal drugs

Buccal drugs are held between the patient's cheek and gum and dissolve to achieve their desired effects. As with sublingual drugs, the patient should not drink fluids whilst the drug is being absorbed. Glucose gel preparations are an example of an emergency medication administered via the buccal route.

Inhaled drugs

In addition to oxygen and nitrous oxide, several other drugs may be administered by means of inhalation. These include bronchodilators, corticosteroids, antibiotics, and mucokinetic agents delivered through aerosolization.

Aerosols are liquid or solid particles of a substance dispersed in gas or solution. The effectiveness of aerosolization therapy depends on the number of droplets that can be suspended in the gas or solution, the particle size (diameter in microns), output (mL/min), and the rate and depth of the patient's breathing. Rapid, shallow breathing reduces the number and retention of droplets that reach the deep bronchioles of the lungs. The delivery of drugs by this method has certain advantages over other routes. Specifically, these are rapid onset of the drug's effect and fewer or less intense systemic side effects.

Aerosols are made by devices called nebulizers. Intermittent positive-pressure breathing (IPPB) devices are designed for in-hospital use. Out-of-hospital devices include metered-dose inhalers (pressure cartridges) and handheld nebulizers. Handheld nebulizers operate by means of a compressed air or oxygen source regulated by a flowmeter.

Metered-dose inhaler

The metered-dose inhaler (MDI) is now the most commonly used device in aerosol therapy (Figure 12-39). It is convenient and delivers a measured dose with each push of the cartridge. MDIs are usually prescribed for self-treatment of asthma. Medications prepared in MDIs include salbutamol, beclometasone and ipratropium bromide. Paramedics do not generally administer medications using these devices but may be called upon to prepare and supervise self-administration; the following procedure should be used to maximize effectiveness of the drug:

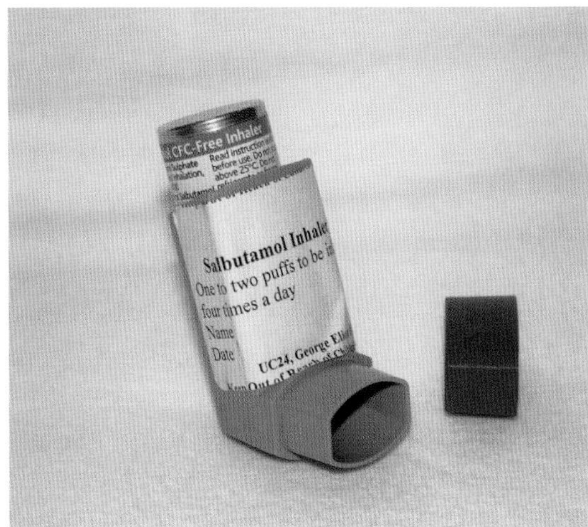

Figure 12-39 Metered-dose inhaler (MDI).

1. Remove the mouthpiece and protective cap from the canister (the drug container).
2. Carefully snap off the cap and turn the mouthpiece sideways.
3. Insert the canister stem into the hole inside the mouthpiece.
4. Shake the canister and mouthpiece well.
5. Invert the MDI and ask the patient to hold it close to their mouth. Instruct the patient to exhale, pushing as much air from the lungs as possible.
6. The patient should place the mouthpiece in their mouth. Instruct the patient to close the lips loosely around it, with the tongue underneath the mouthpiece. As the patient inhales deeply over 5 s, guide them to press down on the canister quickly and then release it.
7. Instruct the patient to hold his or her breath 5 to 10 s before exhaling.
8. Repeat the procedure in 5 to 10 min to take advantage of possibly deeper penetration by a second round of therapy (if required). Most MDI medications are administered using aero chambers (spacers). These are beneficial devices for children and for patients with problematic conditions. For example, some patients might need additional time to inhale the medication. Others may lack coordination. Still others may be hampered by a high level of anxiety or by a diminished ability to inhale for 5 s. Aero chambers allow the patient to receive the maximum benefit of the drug and do not require exact synchronization.

> **Critical Thinking**
>
> What happens to the medication if the patient does not use the metered-dose inhaler (MDI) properly?

Nebulizers

Nebulizers are another means of administering some medications via inhalation in the prehospital setting. Various manufacturers make disposable nebulizer kits. The kits may include a mouthpiece or, more commonly in UK paramedic practice, an aerosol mask, oxygen tubing, and reservoir

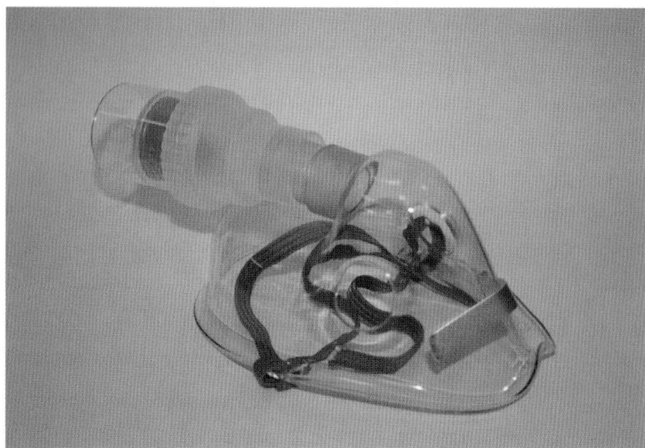

Figure 12-40 A nebulizer mask.

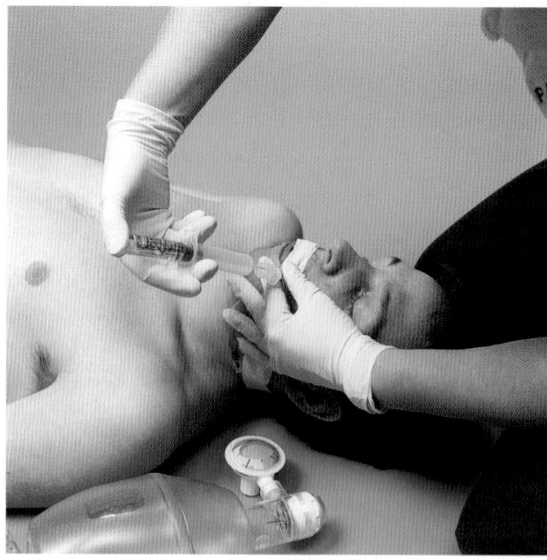

Figure 12-41 Administration of a drug through an endotracheal (ET) tube.

tubing (Figure 12-40). These devices are attached to a non-humidified portable or on-board oxygen source and use the Bernoulli principle to create an aerosol mist (sometimes referred to as a jet or pneumatic nebulizer). Some patients may have home nebulizer units that are powered by battery or electricity. Medications appropriate for nebulization therapy include salbutamol and ipratropium bromide.

The specific procedure may vary and depends on the patient's ability to tolerate the treatment by mask. Paramedics should follow these steps:

1. Using aseptic technique, mix the prescribed drug as recommended in JRCALC guidelines; then instill it into the nebulizer. Some medications come in a packaged unit dose and have a fixed amount of diluent (usually 0.9% normal saline).
2. Connect the nebulizer to the oxygen supply via the tubing or compressed gas (depending on local arrangements). The paramedic should closely monitor the COPD patient if powering the nebulizer with oxygen, as CO_2 retention may occur (Chapter 14).
3. Adjust the oxygen flowmeter to a rate of 6 to 8 L/min to create a steady, visible mist, and to prevent the build-up of exhaled carbon dioxide in the mask.
4. When the mist is visible, begin treatment. Instruct the patient to inhale slowly and deeply by mouth and encourage them to hold a breath for 3–5 s before exhaling. This results in topical deposition of the aerosol particles deep within the tracheobronchial tree. Inhalation and exhalation should be continued until the aerosol canister is depleted of the medication. Repeat treatments are not usually given more often than every 15–20 min (usually to a maximum of three). Treatment of severe asthma, however, may include continuous administration of nebulized beta-agonists, tailored to the patient's response.

The patient must be cooperative to undergo nebulization therapy and the individual must be able to follow instructions to breathe deeply so that the drug can be absorbed. This therapy would be ineffective if the patient is unable to inhale the drug sufficiently or if bronchospasm is too severe. In such cases, administration via another route may be necessary, warranting rapid transportation to an appropriate facility.

Notable changes in the heart rate or dysrhythmias may occur during nebulization therapy. If these occur, treatment should be stopped and the patient conveyed to hospital with ongoing supportive treatment. Paramedics and ambulance crews should avoid the medication vapour stream during nebulization therapy.

Endotracheal drugs

The endotracheal (ET) route of drug administration is an alternative. It may be used when intravenous or intraosseous access cannot be established. Emergency drugs that may be administered by this route are lidocaine, adrenaline (epinephrine), and atropine. When giving medication by this route, paramedics should follow these steps (Figure 12-41):

1. Make sure the ET tube is in the correct position. This can be checked by direct visualization and by auscultation (see Chapter 13).
2. Make sure oxygenation and ventilation of the patient's lungs are adequate.
3. Prepare the medication (per JRCALC guidelines). In adults the ET dose is two or three times that of the IV dose. In adults this equates to 3 mg of adrenaline (epinephrine), 6 mg of atropine, and 200 mg of lidocaine. The normal presentation for these drugs in paramedic practice is either the IMS system or prefilled syringes; these presentations require no further dilution. If using an alternative format, the paramedic should dilute the dose to 10 mL with normal saline (or prepare a 10 mL normal saline flush, per protocol).
4. Remove the air source from the ET tube. Inject the medication through a catheter deep into the tube, or inject it directly into the tube and follow with one or two full ventilations. This helps to ensure that the medication penetrates as deeply as possible into the pulmonary tree (which enhances absorption).
5. Monitor the patient for the desired therapeutic effect and for any side effects.

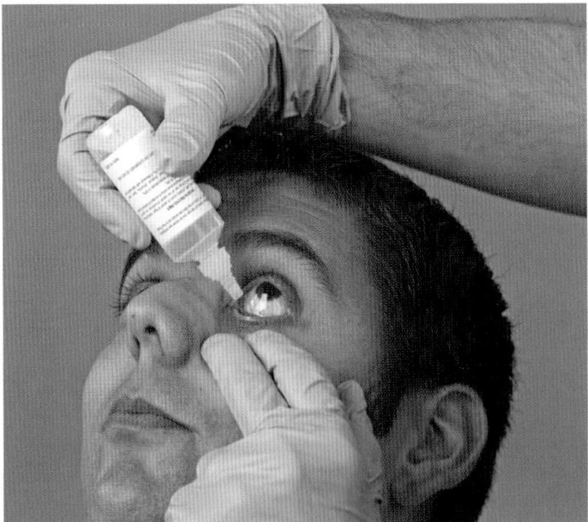

Figure 12-42 Administration of eye medication.

Drugs for the eye, nose and ear

Eye medications are usually in the form of drops or ointments. To administer these drugs, the paramedic should have the patient lie down or sit with the head tilted back. Stabilizing the patient's head with one hand, the paramedic uses the thumb or fingers of the other hand to pull down the lower lid gently. The medication should be applied into the conjunctival sac of the lower lid, never onto the eyeball (Figure 12-42).

Nose drops are best administered with the patient lying down with the head over the edge of a bed in a midline position. The drops are instilled into each nostril. The patient should be instructed not to blow the nose for several minutes to allow absorption of the drug. To administer a nasal spray, the paramedic should have the patient inhale through one nostril whilst blocking the other and squeezing the spray applicator. The patient's head should be upright or tilted back during administration of the drug (Figure 12-43). The paramedic should not use this route unless authorized to do so.

Ear medications are usually in the form of drops. The patient should lie down with the affected ear up. With adults or children over age 3, the paramedic should gently pull the top of the ear up and back to straighten the ear canal. The prescribed number of drops is then instilled. In children under age 3, the ear is pulled down and straight back. The patient should remain in the ear-up position for about 10 min to allow the medicine to disperse. To prevent contamination of the drops, the paramedic should not allow the tip of the dropper to come into contact with the ear canal. Placing a cotton ball in the ear canal after administration of the drug may reduce seepage of the drops onto the face.

Special considerations for paediatric patients

Administering drugs to infants and children can be quite difficult, especially in emergency situations. The following guidelines may be helpful for this process:

- Try to establish a positive relationship with the child. Accept fearful or anxious behaviour as a natural response.

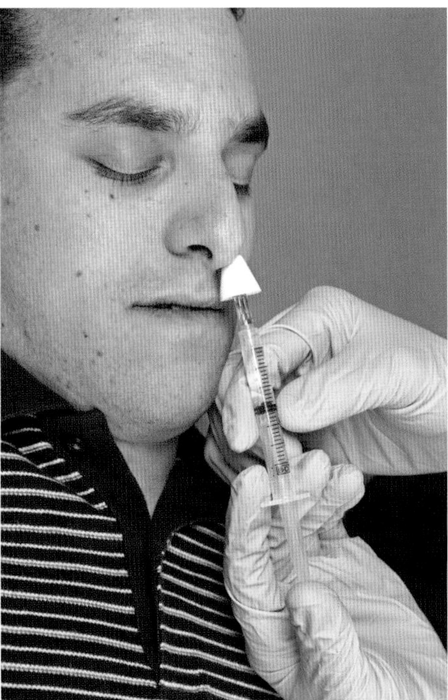

Figure 12-43 Nasal administration of naloxone.

- Be honest with the child when explaining a medication or procedure that will be unpleasant or painful.
- If appropriate, allow the child to help administer the medication (e.g. by holding the medicine cup or by placing a pill in the mouth).
- Use mild physical restraint only if it is required. Explain to the child why it is needed.
- Enlist the assistance of parents or other caregivers when possible.
- When parenteral medications are required, make sure to stabilize the injection site well and to give the injection quickly. Two or more individuals should be available to hold a child over 4 years of age, even if the child promises to 'be still'.
- Remember when administering medications that the younger and smaller the child, the smaller the margin for error.

Obtaining a blood sample

Venous blood samples are often obtained in the prehospital setting for glucose testing but are rarely taken for laboratory determinations performed in the hospital in the UK. If possible, these samples should be obtained when an IV line is established. If they are to be obtained from the IV site, this should be done before any fluids are infused. When authorized to take a blood sample from an IV site, the paramedic should follow these steps:

1. Prepare all equipment in advance.
2. After removing the needle from the IV catheter, exert manual pressure above the IV site to prevent the free flow of blood from the catheter.

Table 12-7 Types of blood sample tubes

Stopper colour	Additive/preservative	Tests done on blood sample	Comments
Green	Heparin	Electrolytes, glucose; not enzymes	Invert tube several times. Heparin prevents blood from clotting without killing cells
Lavender	EDTA anticoagulant	Blood cell count, Hb, Hct, ESR	Invert tube several times to prevent clotting. EDTA tubes are used to collect samples for whole-blood haematology testing
Light blue	Sodium citrate	PT, aPTT, fibrinogen levels	Tube must be filled completely. Invert tube several times to prevent clotting. Sodium citrate tubes are used to collect samples primarily for coagulation studies. Such tests are often needed for patients with bleeding problems (e.g. in the abdomen, brain, or elsewhere)
Red	None	Serum electrolytes, liver and other enzymes, therapeutic drug levels, blood bank procedures	The tube need not be inverted, because the objective is to produce a clot. Some companies make tubes with clot activators, which hasten clotting to speed testing. Paramedics should make sure they know which kind of tube they have

Modified from Miller CD 1996 EMS Pocket Guide. JEMS, Hong Kong.
aPTT, activated partial thromboplastin time; EDTA, ethylenediamine tetraacetic acid; ESR, erythrocyte sedimentation rate; Hb, haemoglobin; Hct, haematocrit; PT, prothrombin time.

3. While stabilizing the site, insert the Vacutainer into the hub of the IV catheter.
4. Push blood collection vacuum tubes (Table 12-7) into the barrel of the Vacutainer to draw blood from the IV catheter.
5. After obtaining the required specimens, attach the IV tubing and begin infusion.
6. Label the sample with the patient's name and the time and date it was obtained.

Critical Thinking

Why should a venous blood sample never be drawn above an IV infusion site?

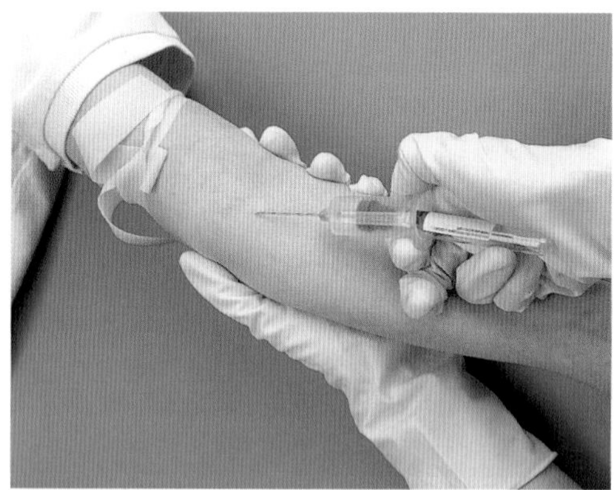

Figure 12-44 Obtaining a blood sample with a Vacutainer.

If no IV line is to be used, the paramedic must obtain the blood sample using a Vacutainer (Figure 12-44) or a needle and syringe and then transfer the sample to an evacuation tube. The steps for obtaining a blood sample using a needle and syringe are as follows:

1. Apply a tourniquet above the selected site.
2. Cleanse the site as previously described for venepuncture.
3. Using an 18- or 20-gauge needle attached to a 10- or 12-mL syringe, enter the vein.
4. With an even, steady motion, draw back on the plunger to obtain the sample.
5. After the sample has been obtained, release the tourniquet, withdraw the needle, and apply manual pressure to the site.
6. Immediately transfer the sample to the appropriate evacuation tube. Do not force additional blood into the tube; each tube has the correct amount of vacuum for the amount of blood required in the vial. Forcing blood into a vacuum tube can cause expulsion of contents and can lead to unnecessary injury or exposure to contents.
7. Label the sample with the patient's name and the time and date it was obtained.

Disposal of contaminated items and sharps

Needles and other sharp objects can injure the patient, the paramedic, coworkers, and others. They can also be a source of infection with hepatitis or the human immunodeficiency virus (HIV). Needles should not be capped, bent, or broken before disposal; rather, they should be discarded with the syringe intact in a special container (i.e. sharps container) that is clearly marked. These containers should be puncture-proof and leak-proof. When full (as indicated by the 'full line', which is usually no more than three-quarters of the space), the container should be discarded according to established policies for disposition of contaminated items and sharps.

Summary

- Système International (SI) is generally accepted as the unit of measurement in UK pharmacy and medical practice; it is also known as the metric system and makes calculations easier than the traditional imperial system.
- Paramedics should choose a drug calculation method that is precise and reliable. Paramedics should
  (1) Convert all units of measure to the same size and system.
  (2) Assess the computed dosage to determine whether it is reasonable.
  (3) Use one method of dose calculation consistently.
- Many drug calculations can be performed almost intuitively. Nevertheless, paramedics should never rely on intuitive calculations. Methods of calculation include the basic formula (desire over have), ratios and proportions, and dimensional analysis.
- Intravenous flow rates can be calculated using the following formula:

$$\text{Drops/min} = \frac{(\text{volume to be infused} \times \text{drops/mL of infusion set})}{\text{total time of infusion (min)}}$$

- Safety procedures should be a high priority during the administration of any medication. The paramedic must make sure the right patient receives the right dose of the right drug via the right route at the right time.
- An incident involving a medication error may occur. In such a case, paramedics should take responsibility for their actions. They should quickly advise ambulance control and assess and monitor the patient for effects of the drug. They must document the error as required by Trust policies. In addition, they must change their personal practice to prevent a similar error in the future.
- Medical asepsis is accomplished by using clean technique, which involves hygienic measures, cleaning agents, antiseptics, disinfectants, and barrier fields.
- Enteral drugs are administered and absorbed through the gastrointestinal tract. They are given by the oral, gastric, and rectal routes. Parenteral drugs are administered outside the intestine and are usually injected. Parenteral drugs are given by the intradermal, subcutaneous, intramuscular, intravenous, and intraosseous routes.
- In the prehospital setting, the route of choice for fluid replacement is through a peripheral vein in an extremity. The over-the-needle catheter is generally preferred in this setting.
- Several possible complications are associated with all intravenous techniques. These include local complications, systemic complications, infiltration, and air embolism.
- Cannulation of the central veins presents specific dangers. These are in addition to the complications common to all intravenous methods.
- Fluids and drugs that are infused by the intraosseous route pass from the marrow cavities into the sinusoids. Next, they pass into large venous channels and emissary veins, and then they pass into the systemic circulation. The site of choice for IO infusions in children is the tibia, one to two fingerbreadths below the tubercle on the anteromedial surface.
- Percutaneous drugs are absorbed through the mucous membranes or skin. These include topical drugs, sublingual drugs, buccal drugs, inhaled drugs, endotracheal drugs, and drugs for the eye, nose, and ear.
- Administering drugs to infants and children can be quite difficult. This is especially true in emergency situations. Paramedics frequently calculate paediatric drug doses by using memory aids. Some of these aids include charts, tapes, and dosage books.
- Venous blood samples may be obtained when intravenous access is established and Trust guidelines allow. They should be obtained before any fluids are infused. If no IV line is to be used and a blood sample is still needed, it must be obtained with a needle and syringe (or a special vacuum needle and sleeve).
- Needles should not be capped, bent, or broken before disposal. Rather, they should be left on the syringe and discarded in an appropriate, clearly marked container that is puncture-proof and leak-proof.

References

18. Lapham R, Agar H 2003 Drug calculations for nurse, a step-by-step approach. Oxford University Press. Oxford
19. British Medical Association and Royal Pharmaceutical Society of Great Britain 2007 British National Formulary 53. March 2007. Online. Available http://www.bnf.org.uk/bnf/ 8 August 2007
20. Department of Health 2004 Building a safer NHS for patients; improving medication safety. Department of Health, London
21. Elder A, Paterson C 2006 Sharps injuries in UK health care: a review of injury rates, viral transmission and potential efficacy of safety devices. Occupational Medicine 56(8):566–574
22. Ambulance Service Association and Health Protection Agency 2004 National Guidance and Procedures for Infection Prevention and Control. Ambulance Service Association, London
23. Needle and cannula technique 1977 Abbott Laboratories, Chicago

PART FOUR

CHAPTER 13

Airway Management and Ventilation

Chapter contents

Objectives

Upon completion of this chapter, the paramedic student will be able to:

1. Discuss the assessment and management of medical or traumatic obstruction of the airway.
2. Outline the causes and effects of and preventive measures for pulmonary aspiration.
3. Outline the essential parameters for evaluating the effectiveness of the airway and breathing.
4. Describe the indications, contraindications, and techniques for delivery of supplemental oxygen.
5. Discuss methods of patient ventilation based on the indications, contraindications, potential complications, and use of each method.
6. Describe the use of manual airway manoeuvres and mechanical airway adjuncts based on the indications, contraindications, potential complications, and techniques for each.
7. Describe assessment techniques and devices used to ensure adequate oxygenation, correct placement of the tracheal tube, and elimination of carbon dioxide.
8. Explain variations in assessment and management of airway and ventilation problems in paediatric patients.
9. Given a patient scenario, identify possible alterations in oxygenation and ventilation based on a knowledge of gas exchange and the mechanics of breathing.

Key terms

anatomical dead space The volume of the conducting airways from the external environment down to the terminal bronchioles.

atelectasis An abnormal condition characterized by the collapse of lung tissue; it prevents the respiratory exchange of oxygen and carbon dioxide.

compliance The ease with which the lungs and thorax expand during pressure changes. The greater the compliance, the easier the expansion.

Fick principle The principle used to determine cardiac output. It assumes that the amount of oxygen delivered to an organ is equal to the amount of oxygen consumed by that organ plus the amount of oxygen carried away from that organ.

gag reflex A normal neural response triggered by touching the soft palate or posterior pharynx.

hypocarbia A state of diminished carbon dioxide in the blood; also known as hypocapnia.

hypoxaemia A state of decreased oxygen content of arterial blood.

hypoxia A state of decreased oxygen content at the tissue level.

intrapulmonic pressure The pressure of the gas in the alveoli.

intrathoracic pressure The pressure in the pleural space; also known as intrapleural pressure.

minute volume The amount of gas inhaled or exhaled in 1 minute. It is found by multiplying the tidal volume by the respiratory rate.

physiological dead space The sum of the anatomical dead space plus the volume of any non-functional alveoli.

pulmonary ventilation The movement of air into and out of the lungs. This process brings oxygen into the lungs and removes carbon dioxide.

respiration The exchange of oxygen and carbon dioxide between an organism and the environment.

tidal volume The volume of air inspired or expired in a single, resting breath.

The absence of an adequate airway and ineffective ventilation are major causes of preventable death and cardiopulmonary complications in all patients. A thorough understanding of the respiratory system and mastery of airway management and ventilation are important aspects of prehospital emergency care.

SECTION I

Respiratory pathophysiology

A common cause of poor ventilation is upper airway obstruction. This type of obstruction is typically caused by inhalation of food, a foreign body, or fluid (vomitus, saliva, blood, neutral liquids). Establishing and maintaining a clear airway in any patient who has poor ventilation from any cause is the most critical lifesaving manoeuvre a paramedic can perform. It should always be a first-order priority of patient care. Early detection, early intervention, and education of the general public in basic life support measures are major factors in preventing unnecessary deaths from airway compromise.

Note

Brain damage may occur 4 to 6 minutes after interruption of breathing and circulation. After 6 minutes of circulatory arrest, brain damage almost always occurs. After 10 minutes of circulatory arrest, some portions of the brain have been irreversibly damaged to the point of death.[1]

Foreign body airway obstruction (FBAO)

Death caused by FBAO is an uncommon but potentially treatable condition. Immediate removal of the obstruction might have prevented the resulting hypoxaemia, unconsciousness or cardiopulmonary arrest that caused these deaths. The management of foreign body airway obstruction by healthcare providers is summarized in Figure 13-1 and Table 13-1.[1]

Note

Methods to relieve foreign body airway obstruction (FBAO) in an unconscious victim of any age have been simplified for lay rescuers. Lay rescuers are to begin standard cardiopulmonary resuscitation (CPR) when an unrelieved, responsive choking victim becomes unresponsive, or when an unresponsive person suspected of having a foreign body airway obstruction is encountered, evaluated, and treated. The only difference from regular CPR is that the lay rescuer should open the airway widely whenever ventilations are attempted. This is to look for a foreign object and remove it if seen. Blind finger sweeps are not to be used by lay rescuers for victims of any age.

Airway obstruction in a conscious patient

Meat is the most common cause of foreign body airway obstruction in conscious adults although a variety of other foods and foreign objects are responsible for obstruction in children and in some adults. Factors associated with choking include large, poorly chewed pieces of food, an elevated blood alcohol level, and poorly fitting dentures. The patient is often middle-aged or older.

Critical Thinking

How can you relieve a foreign body airway obstruction using only your hands?

Foreign bodies may cause partial or complete airway obstruction. A patient with a partly obstructed airway can usually speak and cough forcefully in an effort to expel the object.

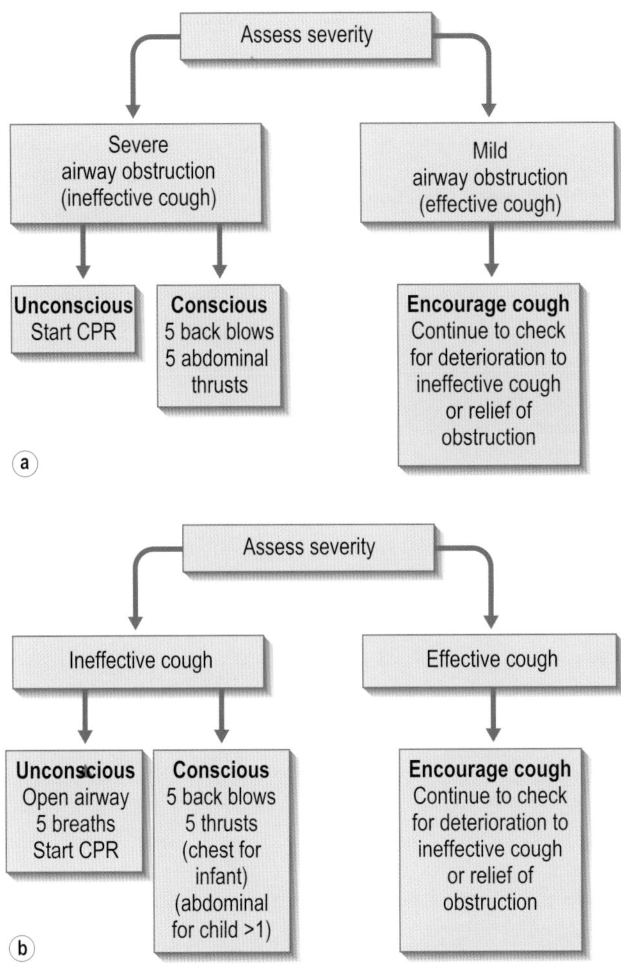

Figure 13-1 (a) Foreign body airway obstruction (adult). (b) Foreign body airway obstruction (child). With permission of Resuscitation Council (UK) www.resus.org.uk

If air exchange is adequate, the rescuer should not intervene but should encourage the patient to continue coughing and observe for changes.[1] If the obstruction persists or air exchange becomes inadequate (evidenced by a silent cough, wheezing, increased respiratory difficulty, decreased air movement, and cyanosis), the patient should be managed as though a complete airway obstruction existed.

Patients with complete airway obstruction cannot speak (aphonia), exchange air or cough. They often grasp the neck between the thumb and fingers; this is a universal sign of choking. These patients need immediate rescuer intervention because complete airway obstruction causes hypoxaemia and can lead to an acute myocardial infarction in patients with atherosclerotic cardiovascular disease. Airway obstruction inevitably leads to cardiac arrest if not corrected within minutes.

Airway obstruction in an unconscious patient

Although upper airway obstruction may lead to loss of consciousness and cardiopulmonary arrest, more often the obstruction results from unconsciousness and cardiopulmonary arrest.[2] The primary source of upper airway obstruction in an unconscious patient is the tongue.

The tongue is attached to the mandible by the muscles that form the floor of the mouth. The normal tone of these muscles allows for air exchange by keeping the posterior pharynx open. If a patient is unconscious or has neuromuscular dysfunction, relaxation of these muscles may cause the airway to be blocked by the tongue. Airway obstruction by the tongue is common in the following situations:

- cardiac arrest
- trauma
- stroke
- intoxication with alcohol, barbiturates or psychotropic drugs
- paralysis caused by muscle relaxants
- myasthenia gravis
- fractured facial and nasal bones.

Laryngeal spasm and oedema

Spasmodic closure of the vocal cords may be caused by an aggressive intubation technique (tracheal intubation is discussed later in this chapter). It may also occur during extubation (removal of the tracheal tube), especially if the patient is semiconscious. There is a suggestion that laryngeal spasm is best managed with aggressive ventilation and a forceful upward pull on the jaw; however, the success with this technique is variable. At times it may require the use of muscle relaxants which are not currently licensed for use by UK paramedics. Maintaining steady pressure against the cords with the tracheal tube sometimes overcomes the spasmodic closure.

Swelling of the glottic and subglottic tissues of the airway can also close off the larynx. The formation of oedema may result from inflammatory or mechanical causes such as epiglottitis, croup, allergic reaction, thermal injuries, strangulation, blunt trauma or drowning. Associated swelling may partly or completely obstruct the airway. Aggressive airway management is required for the patient's survival when this occurs.

Fractured larynx

The most common cause of external trauma to the larynx is a motor vehicle crash. If a trauma patient has localized laryngeal pain on palpation or swallowing, stridor, hoarseness, difficulty with speech (dysphonia) or haemoptysis (coughing up blood), a fracture of the larynx should be suspected. Laryngeal injury can result in a lack of support for the vocal cords, which may cause them to collapse into the tracheal–laryngeal opening leading to airway obstruction. Subcutaneous emphysema, dysphagia (difficult swallowing), and throat discomfort that increases with coughing or swallowing indicate the possibility of an impending airway obstruction as a result of a fracture. The paramedic should remain alert to the possibility of laryngeal fracture; this is important because laryngeal oedema can rapidly close off the airway.

Examples of injury that may cause laryngeal fracture include a clothesline injury and blunt trauma to the neck. A laryngeal fracture requires rapid intervention before laryngeal oedema and haemorrhage cause complete closure.

Table 13-1 Management of foreign body airway obstruction

GENERAL SIGNS OF CHOKING	
Attack occurs whilst eating	
Victim may clutch his/her neck	
Signs of mild airway obstruction	**Signs of severe airway obstruction**
Response to question 'are you choking?'	*Response to question 'are you choking?'*
Victim speaks and answers yes	Victim unable to speak Victim may respond by nodding
Other signs	*Other signs*
Victim is able to speak, cough, and breathe	Victim unable to breathe Breathing sounds wheezy Attempts at coughing are silent Victim may be unconscious
ADULT FBAO (MAY ALSO BE SUITABLE FOR CHILDREN OVER 1 YEAR OF AGE)	
1. If the victim shows signs of mild airway obstruction:	
Encourage him/her to continue coughing but do nothing else	
2. If the victim shows signs of severe airway obstruction and is conscious:	
Give up to five back blows	
• Stand to the side and slightly behind the victim • Support the chest with one hand and lean the victim well forwards so that when the obstructing object is dislodged it comes out of the mouth rather than goes further down the airway • Give **up to** five sharp blows between the shoulder blades with the heel of your hand	
Check to see if each back blow has relieved the airway obstruction. The aim is to relieve the obstruction with each blow rather than necessarily to give all five	
If five back blows fail to relieve the airway obstruction give **up to** five abdominal thrusts	
• Stand behind the victim and put both arms around the upper part of his/her abdomen • Lean the victim forwards • Clench your fist and place it between the umbilicus and the xiphoid process • Grasp this hand with your other hand and pull sharply inwards and upwards • Repeat **up to** five times	
3. If the victim becomes unconscious:	
• Support the victim to the ground • Begin CPR from point 5B of the Adult BLS sequence.	
NB – in the unconscious choking patient, chest compressions should be initiated even if a pulse is present	
CHILD FBAO	
General signs of FBAO	
Witnessed episode Coughing or choking Sudden onset Recent history of playing with or eating small objects	
Ineffective coughing	**Effective cough**
Unable to vocalize Quiet or silent cough Unable to breathe Cyanosis Decreasing level of consciousness	Crying or verbal response to questions Loud cough Able to take a full breath before coughing Fully responsive
CONSCIOUS CHILD WITH FBAO	
• If the child is still conscious but has absent or ineffective coughing, give back blows • If back blows do not relieve the FBAO, give chest thrusts to infants or abdominal thrusts to children	

Table 13-1 Management of foreign body airway obstruction—cont'd

BACK BLOWS

In an infant

- Support the infant in a head-downwards, prone position, to enable gravity to assist removal of foreign body
- A seated or kneeling rescuer should be able to support the infant safely across her/his lap
- Support the infant's head by placing the thumb of one hand at the angle of the lower jaw, and one or two fingers from the same hand at the same point on the other side of the jaw
- Do not compress the soft tissues under the infant's jaw as this will exacerbate the airway obstruction
- Deliver **up to** five sharp back blows with the heel of one hand in the middle of the back between the shoulder blades
- The aim is to relieve the obstruction with each blow rather than to give all five

In a child over 1 year

- Back blows are more effective if the child is positioned head down
- A small child may be placed across the rescuer's lap as with an infant
- If this is not possible, support the child in a forward-leaning position and deliver the back blows from behind

IF the blows fail to dislodge the object, and the child is still conscious, use chest thrusts for infants or abdominal thrusts for children. **DO NOT USE ABDOMINAL THRUSTS ON INFANTS**

Chest thrusts for infants

- Turn the infant into a head-downwards supine position. This is achieved safely by placing your free arm along the infant's back and encircling the occiput with your hand
- Support the infant down your arm, which is placed down (or across) your thigh
- Identify the landmark for chest compression (lower sternum approximately a finger's breadth above the xiphisternum)
- Deliver **up to** five chest thrusts. These are similar to chest compressions but sharper in nature and delivered at a slower rate

Abdominal thrusts for children over 1 year

- Stand or kneel behind the child. Place your arms under the child's arms and encircle his/her torso
- Clench your fist and place it between the umbilicus and xiphisternum
- Grasp this hand with your other and pull sharply inwards and upwards
- Repeat this **up to** five times
- Ensure that pressure is not applied to the xiphoid process or the lower rib cage as this may cause abdominal trauma

Following chest or abdominal thrusts, reassess the child:

- If the object has not been expelled and the victim is still conscious, continue the sequence of back blows and chest (for infant) or abdominal (for children) thrusts

UNCONSCIOUS CHILD WITH FBAO

- If the child with a FBAO is, or becomes, unconscious, place him/her on a firm, flat surface

Airway opening

- Open the mouth and look for any obvious object
- If one is seen, make an attempt to remove it with a single finger sweep

Do not attempt blind or repeated finger sweeps – these can impact the object more deeply into the pharynx and cause injury

Rescue breaths

- Open the airway and attempt five rescue breaths
- Assess the effectiveness of each breath; if a breath does not make the chest rise, reposition the head before making the next attempt

Chest compressions and CPR

- Attempt five rescue breaths and, if there is no response, proceed immediately to chest compression regardless of whether the breaths were successful
- Follow the sequence for single rescuer
- When the airway is opened for attempted delivery of rescue breaths, look to see if the foreign body can be seen in the mouth
- If an object is seen, attempt to remove it with a single finger sweep
- If it appears that the obstruction has been relieved, open and check the airway as above. Deliver rescue breaths if the victim is not breathing
- If the child regains consciousness and is breathing effectively, place in the side-lying position and monitor vital signs

DO NOT DELAY UNNECESSARILY ON SCENE

Further information can be found at the Resuscitation Council website: www.resus.org.uk

Tracheal trauma

Trauma to the trachea is rare but serious. The most common site of tracheal injury is the area bordered by the cricoid cartilage and the third tracheal ring. This injury seldom occurs as an isolated event but is more often associated with injuries to the surrounding oesophagus and cervical spine. Central nervous system (CNS) injuries and abdominal and thoracic trauma also usually accompany tracheal injury. (Tracheal trauma is described in more detail in Chapter 31.)

Aspiration by inhalation

Aspiration is the active inhalation of food, a foreign body or fluid (e.g. vomitus, saliva, blood, neutral liquids) into the airway. Depending on the type and degree of aspiration, the syndrome may cause spasm, mucus production, atelectasis, a change in pH (if the substance is acidic), or coughing. Prevention of aspiration is far superior to any known treatment. Aspiration is prevented mainly by controlling and maintaining the airway. Paramedics should be prepared for the risk of aspiration in patients with a diminished level of consciousness.

The majority of deaths from foreign body aspiration occur in younger children.[3] Running with food or other objects in the mouth, seizures and forced feeding are among the risk factors in this age group. Hot dogs and peanuts are foods children commonly aspirate. In adults, obstruction may be caused by dental or nasal surgery, loss of consciousness, swallowing of poorly chewed food, and alcohol intoxication.

Large food particles and other foreign bodies can block the airway, causing hypoventilation of lower lung segments. The size of the particle determines which airway is obstructed and to what extent. Approximately 74% of foreign bodies are found in the right mainstem bronchus and 21% in the left main bronchus.[4] (The left mainstem bronchus branches from the trachea at a 45–60-degree angle, thus foreign body occlusion of this bronchus is less likely than of the right mainstem bronchus, which is shorter, wider, and more vertical.) When the larynx or trachea is completely obstructed, the victim can die from asphyxiation within minutes.

The average adult stomach has a capacity of 1.4 L and it manufactures an additional 1.4 L of gastric juices in each 24-h period. Hydrochloric acid is manufactured by special cells in the gastric mucosa and with the assistance of a protein-dissolving enzyme (pepsin); this acid helps break down large pieces of food into smaller ones.

Vomitus contains not only partly digested food particles but also acidic gastric fluid. Saliva is a watery, slightly acidic fluid secreted in the mouth by the major salivary glands and the smaller salivary glands in the mucous membranes that line the mouth. Saliva contains the digestive enzyme amylase, which helps break down carbohydrates. Saliva also contains a number of other substances, including minerals (e.g. sodium, calcium and chloride); proteins; mucin (the principal constituent of mucus); urea; white blood cells; debris from the lining of the mouth; and bacteria.

The consequences of aspiration of neutral liquids (liquids that are neither acidic nor basic) are easier to reverse with supportive therapy than are the consequences of aspiration of acids or bases. Nonetheless, aspiration of a large volume of neutral liquids is also associated with a high mortality rate.

Pathophysiology of aspiration

Two conditions are associated with a high risk of aspiration: (1) a diminished level of consciousness and (2) mechanical disturbances of the airway and gastrointestinal (GI) tract.

A diminished level of consciousness may be caused by trauma, alcohol or other drug intoxication, a seizure disorder, cardiopulmonary arrest, a stroke or a CNS dysfunction. The common element of these conditions is depression or loss of the gag reflex, with or without a full stomach. The gag reflex is a normal neural reflex triggered by touching the soft palate or posterior pharynx.

Iatrogenic obstructions (i.e. those caused by medical procedures) are a common type of mechanical obstruction. This type of obstruction results from the use of various devices to control upper airway problems. Examples include removal of certain airway devices (risk of vomiting on removal), placement of a nasogastric tube (the artificial opening through the oesophageal sphincter increases the risk of regurgitation and aspiration), and intubation, which requires an adequate seal at the tracheal orifice to prevent aspiration. These mechanical airway devices are discussed later in this chapter.

Other mechanical or structural problems that may lead to a high risk of aspiration include tracheostomy and oesophageal motility disorders such as hiatus hernia and oesophageal reflux. Other individuals at risk include those with intestinal obstructions.

The chance of aspiration increases whenever vomiting occurs. Vomiting follows stimulation of the vomiting centre of the medulla. This can result from irritation anywhere along the GI tract, from information passed to the medulla from the frontal lobes of the brain, or from disturbances in the balance mechanism of the inner ear. Once this centre is stimulated, the following seven events occur:

1. A deep breath is taken.
2. The hyoid bone and larynx are elevated, thereby opening the pre-oesophageal sphincter.
3. The opening of the larynx closes.
4. The soft palate is elevated, closing the posterior nares.
5. The diaphragm and the abdominal muscles contract forcefully. This compresses the stomach and increases the intragastric pressure.
6. The lower oesophageal sphincter relaxes. The stomach contents are propelled into the lower oesophagus.
7. If the patient is unconscious or unable to protect the airway, pulmonary aspiration may occur.

Effects of pulmonary aspiration

The severity of pulmonary aspiration depends on the pH of the aspirated material, the volume of the aspirate, and whether particulate matter (e.g. food) and bacterial contamination are present in the aspirate. It is generally accepted that when the pH level of an aspirated material is 2.5 or lower, severe pulmonary damage occurs. When the pH is below 1.5, the patient usually dies. The mortality rate among patients who aspirate material that is grossly contaminated (as occurs in bowel obstruction) approaches 100%.

The toxic effects on the lungs from gastric acid (which has a pH of less than 2.5) can be equated with those of chemical burns. These are severe injuries that produce pulmonary changes such as destruction of surfactant-producing alveolar cells, alveolar collapse and destruction, and destruction of pulmonary capillaries. The permeability of the capillaries increases, with massive flooding of the alveoli and bronchi with fluid. The resulting pulmonary oedema creates areas of hypoventilation, shunting, and severe hypoxaemia. The massive fluid shift from the intravascular area to the lungs may also produce hypovolaemia severe enough to require volume replacement.

Note

The risk of pulmonary aspiration can be minimized by continuously monitoring the patient's mental status, properly positioning the patient to allow for drainage of secretions, limiting ventilation pressures to avoid gastric distension, and using suction devices and oesophageal or endotracheal (ET) intubation. Airway protection should be provided if the risk of aspiration exists. It also should be provided promptly after an occurrence of aspiration.

SECTION II

Airway evaluation

Essential parameters of airway and respiratory evaluation

This discussion is limited to essentials of airway evaluation that are used to identify immediate signs of life-threatening airway compromise. The airway may be partially or completely obstructed at the upper or lower levels of the respiratory tract; evaluation of the airway and respiration seeks to identify the level of any airway problem so that optimum management techniques can be applied. The essentials of airway evaluation involve a physical assessment of the airway and ventilation (look, listen, feel) and a focused history.

Recognition of airway problems

Airway management begins with an assessment of the patency of the airway. Those who have a fully patent airway are normally easy to recognize whilst those with a partial or complete airway obstruction will require a greater assessment. Respiratory distress may be caused by upper or lower airway obstruction, inadequate ventilation, impairment of the respiratory muscles, ventilation–perfusion mismatching (ventilated alveoli that are not perfused, or perfused alveoli that are not ventilated), diffusion abnormalities, or impairment of the nervous system. Dyspnoea is often associated with hypoxia.

Note

Recognition and management of respiratory failure are crucial to the patient's survival. The brain can survive only a few minutes of anoxia. All therapies will fail if the airway is not adequate.

Respiratory rate, regularity and effort

The normal respiratory rate in a resting adult is 12 to 20 breaths per minute. Regularity is defined as a steady inspiratory and expiratory pattern. Breathing at rest should be effortless and should be marked by only subtle changes in rate or regularity.

Patients in respiratory distress often compensate for their inability to breathe easily by sitting upright with the head tilted back (upright sniffing position), by leaning forward on the arms (tripod position), or by lying down with the head and thorax slightly elevated (semi-Fowler's position). These patients frequently avoid lying flat, or supine.

Critical Thinking

Why would lying flat on the back (i.e. in the supine position) most likely worsen respiratory distress?

Observation techniques

Visual clues can aid the recognition of airway problems. Paramedics should note the patient's preferred position to facilitate breathing and assess the rise and fall of the patient's chest. Other visual clues to respiratory distress include the following:

- gasping for air
- cyanosis
- nasal flaring
- pursed-lip breathing
- retraction of the intercostal or subcostal muscles, suprasternal notch, and supraclavicular fossa during respirations (Figure 13-2).

Auscultation and palpation techniques

Air movement can be evaluated by listening to respirations without using a stethoscope (Figure 13-3). A stethoscope is used to assess air movement in both lung fields. Palpation of the chest wall helps determine the presence or absence of paradoxical (contrary) motion of the chest wall, inspiration, expiration, and any retraction of accessory muscles.

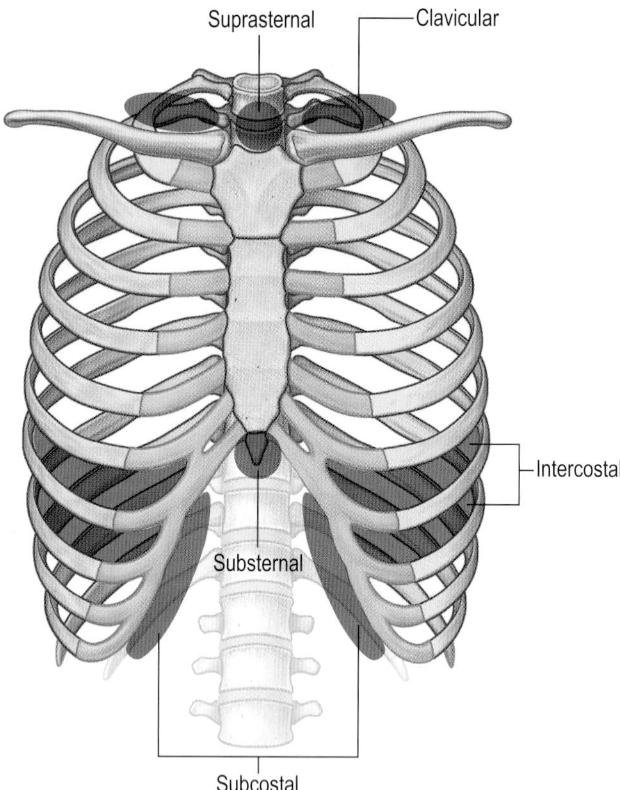

Figure 13-2 Areas of chest muscle retractions.

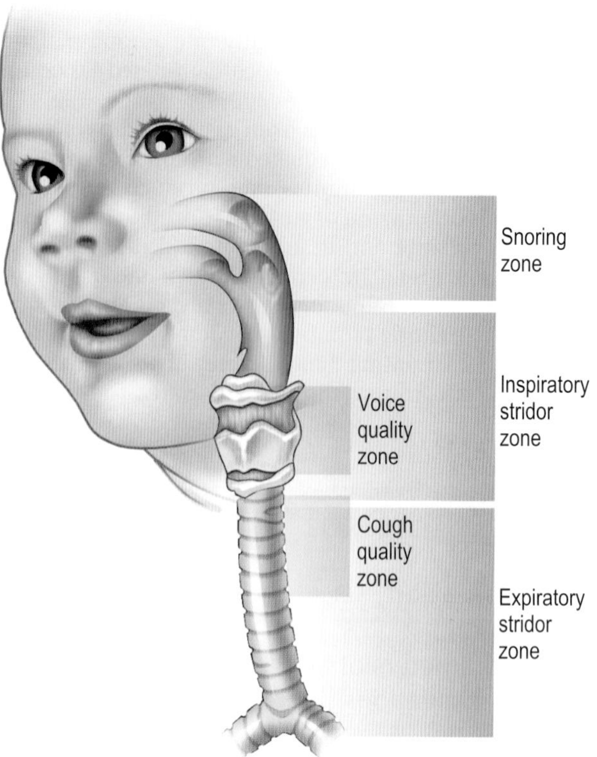

Figure 13-3 A loud, gasping snore suggests enlarged tonsils or adenoids. With inspiratory stridor, the airway is compromised at the level of the supraglottic larynx, vocal cords, subglottic region, or upper trachea. Expiratory stridor, or central wheeze, results from narrowing or collapse of the lower trachea or bronchi. Airway noise during both inspiration and expiration often represents a fixed obstruction of the vocal cords or subglottic space. Hoarseness or a weak cry is a by-product of obstruction of the vocal cords. If a cough is croupy or low pitched, a tracheal disorder should be suspected.

Note

Pulsus paradoxus is an exaggeration of the normal blood pressure variation that occurs with breathing. It is defined as a fall in systolic pressure of 10 mmHg or more on spontaneous inspiration. At times it is associated with a change in the quality of the pulse. The condition is occasionally observed in patients with asthma or chronic obstructive pulmonary disease (COPD) and in victims of blunt or penetrating chest trauma (see Chapter 27). Pulsus paradoxus is difficult to measure. The paramedic should rely on more obvious signs and symptoms of respiratory distress.

Other signs of respiratory distress

Other signs that indicate possible causes of respiratory distress include resistance or changing compliance when assisting or delivering respirations with a bag-valve-mask (seen in asthma, COPD and tension pneumothorax), and the presence of pulsus paradoxus.

History

Obtaining a history to determine the progression and duration of the dyspnoeic event also helps guide the direction of patient care. For example, the paramedic should ask whether the event was sudden in onset or occurred over time. If it occurred over time, the length of that period should be determined. The paramedic should ask whether any known causes or triggers initiated the difficulty breathing and should establish if the respiratory distress is continuous or recurring. Other questions that should be asked in obtaining a patient's history include the following:

- What makes it better?
- What makes it worse?
- Do any other symptoms occur at the same time (e.g. cough, chest pain, fever)?
- Has any treatment with drugs been attempted?
- Has the patient taken all medications and treatments as prescribed?

It is also crucial to determine whether the patient has been previously evaluated or hospitalized for this condition and whether the person has ever been intubated because of respiratory problems.

Changes in the respiratory pattern

As previously stated, the breathing process should be comfortable, regular and performed without distress. Abnormal respiratory patterns are commonly seen in ill or injured patients (Figure 13-4 and Box 13-1). Recognizing these patterns may help paramedics to determine the proper patient care.

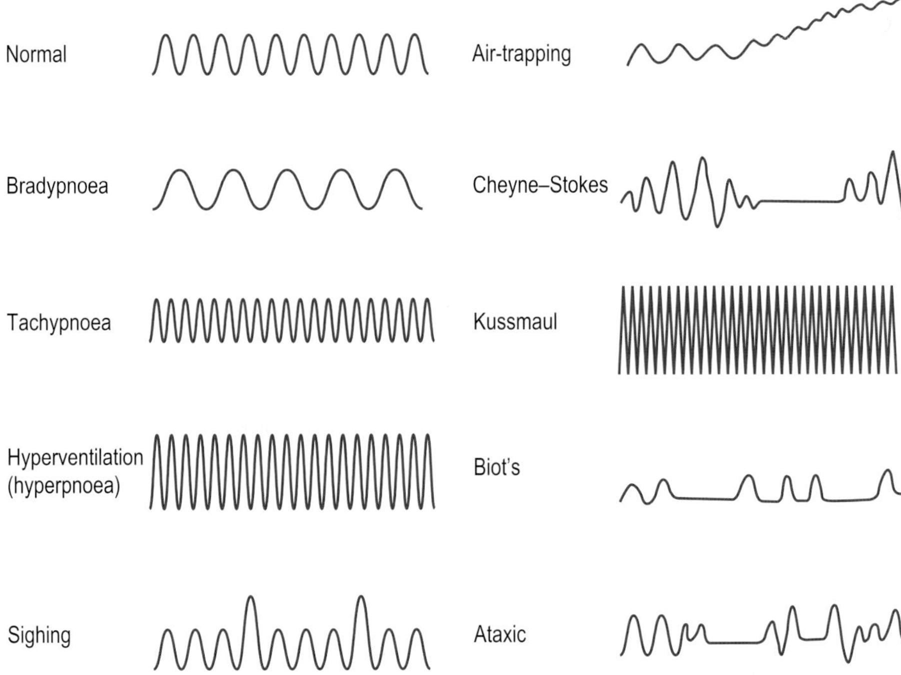

Figure 13-4 Patterns of respiration. The horizontal axis indicates the relative rate; the vertical swings indicate the relative depth.

Some influences on the rate and depth of breathing

The rate and depth of breathing will

Increase with	*Decrease with*
Acidosis (metabolic)	Alkalosis (metabolic)
Anxiety	Central nervous system lesions (cerebrum)
Aspirin poisoning	Myasthenia gravis
Oxygen need (hypoxaemia)	Narcotic overdoses
Pain	Obesity (extreme)
Central nervous system lesions (pons)	

Inadequate ventilation

Inadequate ventilation is said to occur when the body cannot compensate for increased oxygen demand or cannot maintain a normal range of oxygen/carbon dioxide balance. Numerous factors can cause inadequate ventilation, including infection, trauma, brainstem injury, and a noxious or hypoxic atmosphere. A patient who has inadequate ventilation may have a number of symptoms, and may display various respiratory rates and breathing patterns. Some medical experts distinguish between inadequate ventilation caused by a problem in the mechanics of breathing (usually defined by the PCO_2) and inadequate oxygenation but normal ventilation, as seen in pulmonary embolus and often pneumonia.

Supplemental oxygen therapy

Supplemental oxygen therapy may be provided for two reasons: (1) enriched oxygen in the atmosphere increases the oxygen content in pulmonary capillary blood; and (2) increasing the available oxygen allows the patient to compensate without increasing the work of breathing.

Oxygen sources

The most common form of oxygen used in the prehospital setting is pure oxygen gas, delivered in litres per minute (LPM). This gas is stored under pressure in stainless steel or lightweight alloy cylinders (Figure 13-5). These cylinders have been colour-coded in the UK to distinguish various compressed gases. Steel oxygen cylinders are black bodied with a white neck whilst the more modern lightweight cylinders tend to have a white body. Common sizes of oxygen cylinders that are used in emergency care include the following:

- D cylinder (340 L of oxygen)
- CD cylinder (460 L of oxygen)
- F cylinder (1360 L of oxygen)
- HX cylinder (2300 L of oxygen).

Box 13-1

Abnormal respiratory patterns

Agonal respiration: A type of breathing that usually follows a pattern of gasping succeeded by apnoea. It generally indicates the onset of respiratory arrest or the breathing pattern of a dying person.

Ataxic pattern: A type of cluster or irregular breathing pattern characterized by a series of inspirations and expirations. Ataxic respiration is usually associated with a structural or compressive lesion in the medullary respiratory centres.

Biot pattern: A respiratory pattern involving irregular respirations varying in depth and interrupted by intervals of apnoea (absence of breathing). Although similar to Cheyne–Stokes respiration, this pattern lacks the repetitiveness of that type and is often irregular. Biot respiration is usually seen in patients with head injuries who have increased intracranial pressure. Unlike Cheyne–Stokes respiration, the Biot ataxic pattern frequently produces ventilatory failure and may lead to apnoea.

Bradypnoea: A persistent respiratory rate slower than 12 breaths per minute. This abnormal rate may be a result of the patient guarding against respiratory discomfort caused by chest wall injury, respiratory failure, cerebral vascular accident (CVA), pulmonary infection, or narcotic poisoning. However, bradypnoea is more commonly caused by respiratory drive depression that occurs secondary to neurological disturbances.

Central neurogenic hyperventilation: A pattern of breathing marked by rapid and regular ventilations at a rate of about 25 per minute. Increasing regularity, rather than rate, is an important diagnostic sign because it indicates an increasing depth of coma.

Cheyne–Stokes respiration: A regular, periodic pattern of breathing with equal intervals of apnoea followed by a crescendo–decrescendo sequence of respirations. Cheyne–Stokes respirations are thought to represent a level of cortical dysfunction of the brain. Although some children and older adults breathe in this pattern during sleep, it is usually seen in patients who are seriously ill or injured.

Eupnoea: Normal breathing.

Hyperventilation: A persistent, rapid, deep respiration that often results in hyperpnoea. Compared with tachypnoea, hyperpnoea is usually slower and much deeper. Its causes include exercise, anxiety, metabolic disturbances (e.g. diabetic ketoacidosis), and central nervous system (CNS) illness.

Kussmaul respiration: An abnormally deep, very rapid sighing respiratory pattern characteristic of diabetic ketoacidosis or other metabolic acidosis.

Tachypnoea: A persistent respiratory rate that exceeds 20 breaths per minute. It may be common in patients who are in pain, frightened, or anxious. The many other causes of tachypnoea include fractured ribs, pneumonia, pneumothorax, pulmonary embolus, and pleurisy.

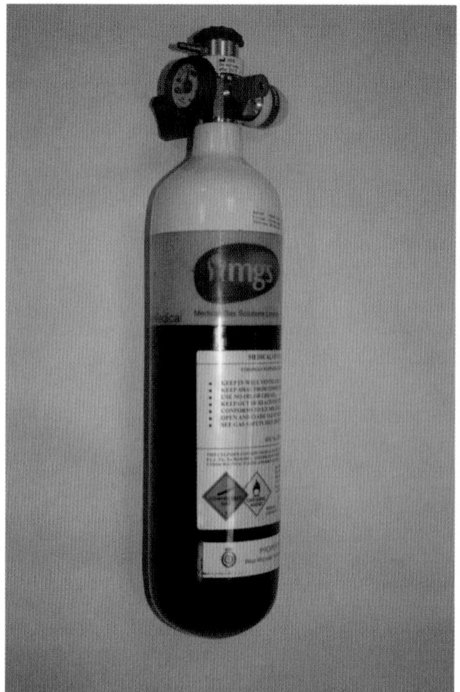

Figure 13-5 CD lightweight oxygen cylinder. The cylinder holds 690 L.

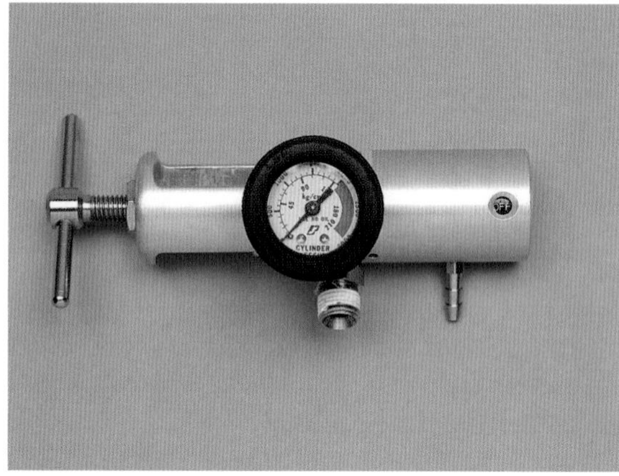

Figure 13-6 Therapy regulator.

CD and HX cylinders are filled to a maximum pressure of 23000 kPa (3300 psi), thus safety is critical when this equipment is handled. Where the cylinder does not have an integrated regulator, the paramedic should ensure that the correct regulator is firmly attached before moving an oxygen cylinder. A cylinder should never be handled by the neck assembly alone. Most oxygen cylinders are considered 'empty' at 1400 kPa (200 psi) (this is the safe residual pressure). As a rule, cylinders with less than 3500 kPa (500 psi) are too low to keep in service.

Regulators

High-pressure regulators are used to transfer cylinder gas from tank to tank. They are attached to cylinder stems and allow cylinder gas to be delivered under high pressure. Therapy regulators are used to deliver a safe pressure of oxygen to patients (Figure 13-6). They are attached to the cylinder stem. Therapy regulators work through a regulator mechanism whereby 350 kPa (50 psi) escape pressure is reduced ('stepped down') to 206 kPa (30 psi) for safe delivery to the patient. On the new lightweight cylinders, these are integrated into the cylinder.

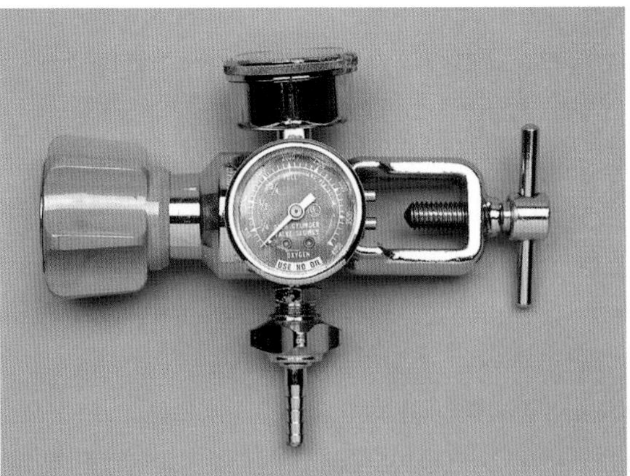

Figure 13-7 Flowmeter.

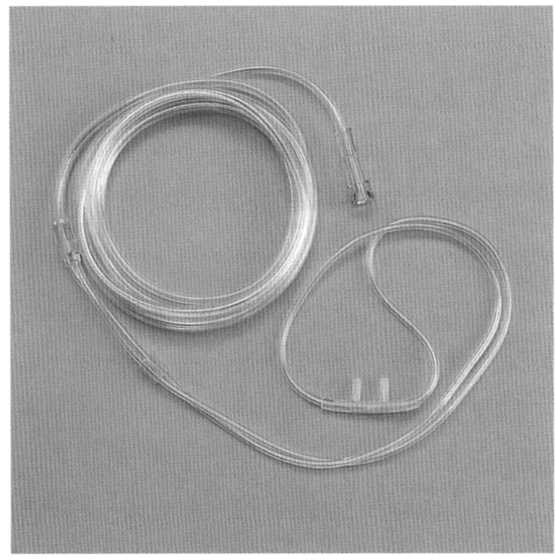

Figure 13-8 Nasal cannula.

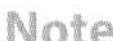

Note

Therapy regulators (used for delivery of oxygen to patients) are attached to smaller oxygen cylinders by a yoke assembly with a pin index safety system. This system prevents the paramedic from using a regulator with the wrong type of gas. It requires that the yoke pins match the corresponding holes in the valve assembly for oxygen to be delivered. Larger oxygen cylinders have valve assemblies with a threaded outlet specific to medical oxygen.

Table 13-2 Oxygen delivery devices

Device	Flow rate (L/min)	Oxygen (O_2) % delivered
Nasal cannula	1–6	24–44
Simple facemask	6–10	35–60
Partial rebreather mask	6–10	35–60
Non-rebreather mask	10–15	80–95
Venturi mask	4–8	24–50

Flowmeters

Flowmeters control the amount of oxygen that is delivered to the patient (Figure 13-7). These devices are connected to the pressure regulator and adjusted to deliver oxygen at a set number of litres per minute. Disposable humidifiers may be attached to the flowmeter although this is not common practice in the UK. Humidifiers provide moisture to the dry oxygen coming from the supply cylinder. Humidified oxygen is desirable for long-term oxygen administration and for patients with croup, epiglottitis or bronchiolitis (see Chapter 14).

Oxygen delivery devices

Patients who have spontaneous respirations can receive supplemental oxygen through several different oxygen delivery devices. Oxygen masks are divided into two groups: low-flow masks such as a nasal cannula, simple facemask, partial rebreather mask and non-rebreather mask; and high-flow masks, sometimes called the Venturi mask (Table 13-2). Low-flow masks deliver oxygen at less than the peak inspiratory flow rate so therefore deliver a variable concentration of oxygen, depending on how the patient is breathing. High-flow masks deliver oxygen at a rate above the peak inspiratory flow rate, hence they are noisier, but deliver fixed concentrations of oxygen irrespective of the patient's breathing.

A person breathing normally inspires approximately 15 L/min of air (this is the inspiratory flow rate and varies through respiration). Assuming a constant flow rate, if the paramedic administers 3 L/min to a person who is breathing normally via a nasal cannula, the patient would be breathing 3 L/min of 100% oxygen and 12 L/min of air (21% oxygen). The concentration of oxygen delivered to the patient is therefore $[(1 \times 3) + (0.21 \times 12)] \times 100/15 = 37\%$. In someone with respiratory distress, the inspiratory flow rate can reach 30 L/min, in which case the patient would be breathing 3 L/min of 100% oxygen plus 28 L/min of air (21% oxygen). Perform the calculation as above and see how the inspired oxygen concentration has changed. Venturi masks avoid this problem by delivering a constant mixture of oxygen and air at above the maximum inspiratory flow rate.

Nasal cannula

The nasal cannula (Figure 13-8) delivers low-concentration oxygen by way of two small plastic prongs placed into the nostrils. Nasal cannulae should not be used in patients with poor respiratory effort, severe hypoxia or apnoea, nor should they be used in patients who breathe primarily through the mouth. As a rule, the nasal cannula is well tolerated but it does not deliver high-volume/high-concentration oxygen. The relationship of approximate oxygen concentration to litres per minute flow is listed in Table 13-3.

It is difficult to obtain oxygen concentrations greater than 30–35% with a nasal cannula because the patient continues to mouth breathe during oxygen administration. The mouth breathing reduces the concentration of oxygen inspired through the nose. The device is also ineffective if the patient's nose is blocked by blood or mucus. For these reasons, use of the nasal cannula is limited to patients who would benefit from low-concentration oxygen delivery. This may include

Table 13-3 Approximate oxygen concentration for litres per minute flow

Litres per minute	Oxygen concentration
1	24%
2	28%
3	32%
4	36%
5	40%
6	44%

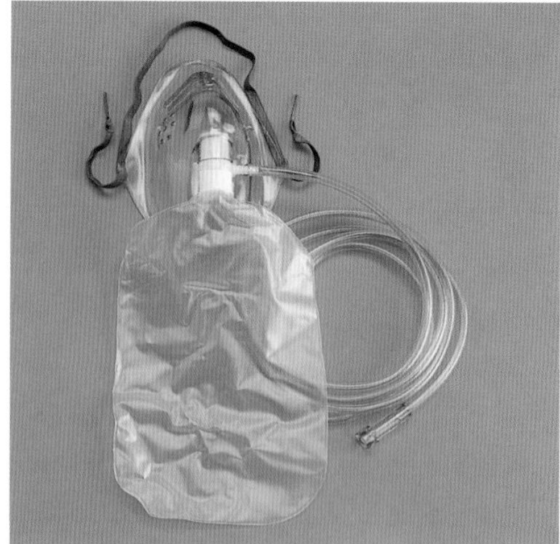

Figure 13-10 Partial rebreather mask.

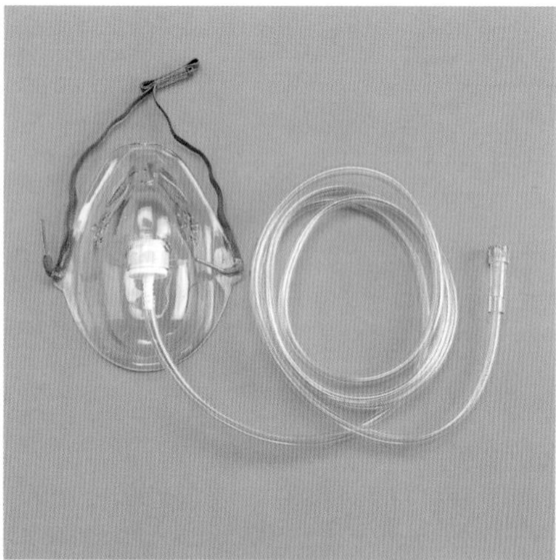

Figure 13-9 Simple facemask.

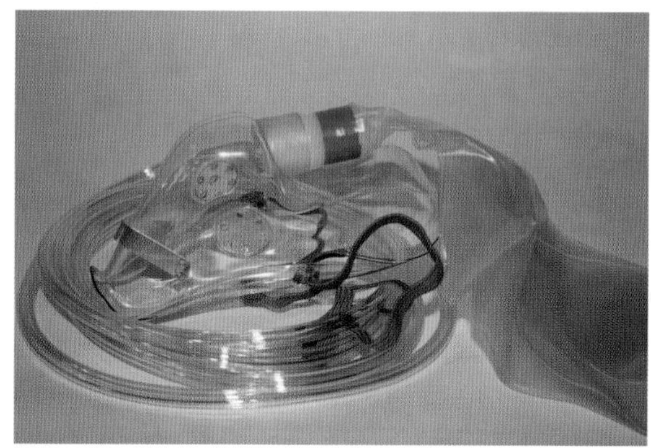

Figure 13-11 Non-rebreather mask.

some patients with chest pain and patients who have chronic pulmonary disease. The maximum oxygen flow rate for a nasal cannula is 6 L/min.

Simple facemask

The simple facemask (Figure 13-9) is a soft, clear plastic mask that conforms to the patient's face. Small perforations in the mask allow atmospheric gas to be mixed with oxygen during inhalation and also permit the patient's exhaled air to escape. Oxygen concentrations of 35–60% can be delivered through this device with a flow rate of 6 to 10 L/min. A flow rate of less than 6 L/min can produce an accumulation of carbon dioxide in the mask; therefore oxygen delivery through any facemask should always exceed this minimum. Flow rates above 10 L/min do not enhance oxygen concentration. All masks must be well fitted to the patient's face for optimal benefit; leaks reduce the oxygen concentration.

Partial rebreather mask

The partial rebreather mask (Figure 13-10) has an attached oxygen reservoir bag, which should be filled before the patient uses the mask. This device has vent ports covered by one-way disks to allow a portion of the patient's exhaled gas to enter the reservoir bag and be reused. The remainder of the carbon dioxide-loaded gas escapes into the atmosphere. Oxygen concentrations of 35–60% can be delivered with a flow rate that prevents the reservoir bag from collapsing completely on inspiration. Partial rebreather masks should not be used in patients with apnoea or poor respiratory effort. As with the simple facemask, delivery of volumes above 10 L/min with this device does not enhance oxygen concentration.

Non-rebreather mask

The non-rebreather mask (Figure 13-11) is similar in design to the partial rebreather. However, a flutter valve assembly in the mask piece stops the patient's exhaled air from returning to the reservoir bag. This device delivers oxygen concentrations up to and above 95%. The flow rate must be adequate to keep the reservoir bag partly inflated during inspiration (patients with severe respiratory distress may need up to 20 L/min to maintain inflation of the reservoir bag). Paramedics should ensure that the mask is seated firmly over the patient's mouth and nose and that the reservoir bag is never less than two-thirds full. This device is most often used in patients who need high-concentration oxygen delivery (10–15 L/min). Like other masks, it should not be used in patients with apnoea or poor respiratory effort.

Critical Thinking

What could happen if the oxygen source is disconnected from a non-rebreather mask?

Venturi mask

The Venturi mask (Figure 13-12) is a high-airflow oxygen entrainment delivery device. It delivers a precise fraction of inspired oxygen (FiO_2) at typically low concentrations. The device was originally designed to deliver 30–40% concentrations; however, it has since been adapted to deliver higher oxygen percentages. The Venturi mask uses 'jet mixing' of atmospheric gas and oxygen to achieve the desired mixture.

Colour-coded adapters in various sizes are attached to the mask to control the oxygen flow rate (standard size adapters are 3, 4 and 6 L/min). The colour codes and adapters state the exact litre flow to use to obtain the precise FiO_2. Choosing a different litre flow greatly alters the FiO_2 delivered. The various Venturi masks deliver 24–50% oxygen and are advised for patients who are at risk of CO_2 retention when higher concentrations of supplementary oxygen are delivered; this includes, for example, patients with chronic obstructive pulmonary disease. The main benefit of the Venturi mask is that it allows precise regulation of the FiO_2. It also permits the paramedic to titrate oxygen for the patient with COPD so as not to induce CO_2 retention, whilst allowing enrichment of supplemental oxygen. Care must be taken to match the proper FiO_2 to the correct flow rate, otherwise the Venturi mask does not deliver the indicated FiO_2.

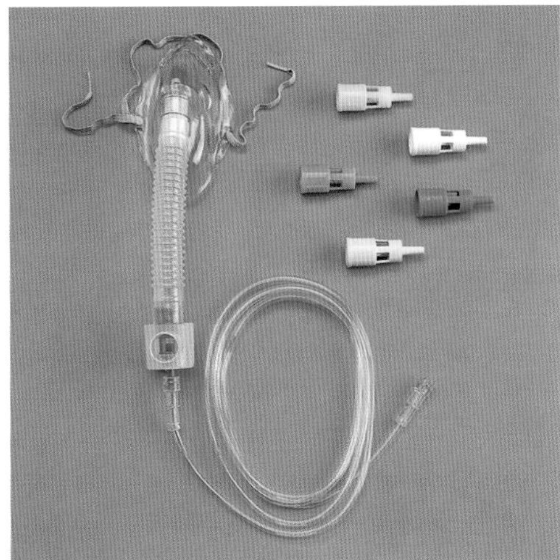

Figure 13-12 Venturi mask.

Ventilation

Patient ventilation can be provided by several methods in the prehospital setting. These include rescue breathing (mouth to mouth, mouth to nose, mouth to stoma), mouth-to-mask breathing, bag–valve–mask devices, and automatic transport ventilators. The use of bag–valve–mask devices with supplementary oxygen should be used in preference to exhaled air ventilation.

Rescue breathing

As discussed before, inspired air has an oxygen concentration of about 21%, of which about 4% is used by the body. The remaining 17% is exhaled. Ventilation by rescue breathing can provide adequate oxygenation to a patient with respiratory insufficiency where no other equipment is available.

Rescue breathing has some advantages. First, no equipment is needed, and second, it is immediately available. However, it also has disadvantages such as the limitation of the vital capacity of the rescuer (about 500 to 600 mL is needed to ventilate an adult). Another drawback is the low amount of oxygen delivered in expired air compared with other methods of ventilation with supplemental oxygen. Also, a rescuer may find it difficult to force air past any obstructions in the airway. The risk exists that a disease will be transmitted through direct body fluid contact. Complications common to all rescue breathing techniques include the following:

- hyperinflation of the patient's lungs
- gastric distension
- blood/body fluid contact concerns
- rescuer hyperventilation.

Critical Thinking

What are two harmful effects of gastric distension during artificial ventilation?

Mouth-to-mouth method[1] (should not be used where resuscitation equipment is available)

Paramedics should use the following guidelines in delivering ventilations mouth to mouth:

1. If no spinal injury is suspected, position the patient with optimal head-tilt and chin-lift. (If spinal injury is suspected, maintain in-line stabilization and maintain an open airway through the jaw-thrust without head-tilt technique, described later in this chapter.) If this technique does not open the airway, use the head-tilt chin-lift manoeuvre. If necessary, clear the airway of vomitus, body fluids, and foreign objects.
2. Pinch the soft part of the victim's nose closed, using the index finger and thumb of your hand on their forehead.
3. Allow the victim's mouth to open, but maintain chin-lift.
4. Take a normal breath and place your lips around the victim's mouth, making sure that you have a good seal.

5. Blow steadily into their mouth whilst watching for the chest to rise; take about one second to make the chest rise as in normal breathing; this is an effective rescue breath.
6. Maintaining head-tilt and chin-lift, take your mouth away from the victim and watch for the chest to fall as air comes out.
7. Repeat the process for as long as is necessary.

Mouth-to-mouth breathing usually results in the exchange of saliva between the victim and the rescuer. Transmission of the hepatitis B virus (HBV) and the human immunodeficiency virus (HIV) during rescue breathing has not been documented. However, rare instances of herpes transmission during cardiopulmonary resuscitation (CPR) have been reported.[2] When possible, personal barrier protection devices should be used.

Mouth-to-nose method

Mouth-to-nose ventilation is very similar to the technique described for mouth-to-mouth rescue breathing. The differences in the mouth-to-nose method are as follows:

- If no spinal injury is suspected, the rescuer must keep one hand on the patient's forehead to maintain an open airway while using the other hand to close the patient's mouth. If a spinal injury is suspected, the jaw-thrust without head-tilt technique should be used. The rescuer's cheek is used to seal the patient's mouth.
- The patient's nose is left open.
- The rescuer's mouth is placed over the patient's nose with as tight a seal as possible.
- During passive exhalation by the patient, the rescuer's mouth is removed from the patient's nose and the patient's mouth is opened for exhalation. The head-tilt or jaw-thrust position must be maintained to ensure an open airway.
- Mouth-to-nose ventilation may be appropriate for patients who have injuries to the mouth and lower jaw and for patients with missing teeth or dentures (which makes a tight seal around the mouth difficult). It also may overcome psychological barriers in having mouth-to-mouth contact with a patient.

Ventilation of infants and children

To provide ventilation to infants and children, the paramedic should use the mouth-to-mouth-and-nose technique as described below:

Child above 1 year[1]

1. Position the patient with a slight head-tilt and chin-lift sufficient to open the airway. Hyperextension of a paediatric patient's neck may block the airway. (Use spinal precautions as needed [see Chapter 32].)
2. Pinch the soft part of the nose closed with the index finger and thumb of your hand on the forehead.
3. Open the child's mouth a little, but maintain the chin upwards.
4. Take a breath and place your lips around the child's mouth, making sure that you have a good seal.
5. Blow steadily into the mouth over about 1–1.5 s watching for chest rise.
6. Maintaining head-tilt and chin-lift, take your mouth away from the victim and watch for their chest to fall as air comes out.
7. Take another breath and repeat this sequence five times. Identify effectiveness by seeing that the child's chest has risen and fallen in a similar fashion to the movement produced by a normal breath.

Infant[1]

1. Ensure a neutral position of the head and apply chin-lift.
2. Take a breath and cover the mouth and nasal apertures of the infant with your mouth, making sure you have a good seal. If the nose and mouth cannot both be covered in the older infant, the rescuer may attempt to seal only the infant's nose or mouth with her/his mouth (if the nose is used, close the lips to prevent air escape).
3. Blow steadily into the infant's mouth and nose over 1–1.5 s sufficient to make the chest visibly rise.
4. Maintaining head-tilt and chin-lift, take your mouth away from the victim and watch for their chest to fall as air comes out.
5. Take another breath and repeat this sequence five times.

Mouth-to-stoma method

A stoma is a temporary or permanent surgical opening in the neck of a patient who has had a laryngectomy or tracheostomy (Figure 13-13). The airway of such a patient has been surgically interrupted and the larynx is no longer connected to the trachea (Box 13-2).

The stoma created by a laryngectomy is large and round; the edge of the tracheal lining can be seen attached to the skin. The stoma in patients is usually no more than several millimetres in diameter. It usually contains one or two concentric tubes (one fitting inside the other) made of plastic

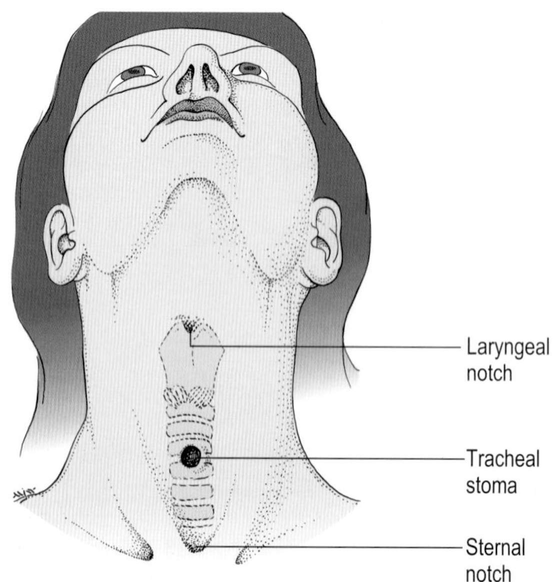

Figure 13-13 Stoma.

Box 13-2

Special considerations for patients who have had a laryngectomy

When providing care for a patient who has had a laryngectomy, paramedics sometimes may need to suction the tracheostomy tube or remove, clean, and replace a tube that has become obstructed by mucus. (Patients who have had a laryngectomy have a less effective cough. As a result, mucus plugs often obstruct breathing tubes.)

The steps for suctioning a breathing tube are as follows:

1. Pre-oxygenate the patient.
2. Inject 3 mL of sterile saline down the trachea.
3. Step 2 usually results in coughing. If it does not, instruct the patient to exhale.
4. Insert the suction catheter into the trachea until resistance is met (without negative pressure).
5. Step 4 usually results in coughing. If it does not, instruct the patient to cough or exhale.
6. Suction while withdrawing the catheter.

If the breathing tube cannot be cleared and requires replacement, follow these steps:

1. Lubricate a same-size tracheostomy tube or tracheal tube (5 mm or larger).
2. Instruct the patient to exhale.
3. Gently insert the tube 1 to 2 cm (about ½ to ¾ inch) beyond the balloon cuff.
4. Inflate the cuff.
5. Confirm the patient's comfort and verify the patency and proper placement of the tube.

Stenosis (spontaneous narrowing of a stoma) may be life threatening. It also makes replacing a tracheostomy tube difficult or impossible. When stenosis is a factor, an tracheal tube must be placed before total obstruction occurs.

or metal. The method of ventilating these patients is the same, regardless of the type of stoma.

Stomas and breathing tubes may become clogged with secretions, encrusted mucus and foreign matter, leading to inadequate ventilation. If cleaning is needed, wipe the neck opening with gauze. If the breathing tubes are clogged, they can be removed or suctioned. The tracheostomy tube or stoma is suctioned by passing a sterile suction catheter through the external opening into the trachea. Do not insert the catheter more than 7–12 cm (3–5 inches) into the trachea. Once the airway is partly open, begin ventilations by the mouth-to-stoma method (mouth-to-stoma ventilation is bacteriologically cleaner than the mouth-to-mouth method) by using a paediatric-size pocket mask over the top of the stoma or by securing the airway with an endotracheal (ET) tube placed through the stoma.

The technique for stoma ventilation is basically the same as that for other methods of artificial ventilation. However, the patient's head should be kept straight (rather than tilted back), with the patient's shoulders slightly elevated; this position allows more effective ventilation. If the patient's chest does not rise or if air is heard to escape through the patient's upper airway, the patient may be a 'partial neck breather'. These patients are able to inhale and exhale some air through their nose and mouth. If this occurs, the patient's nostrils must be pinched closed and the mouth sealed with the palm of one hand during ventilation.

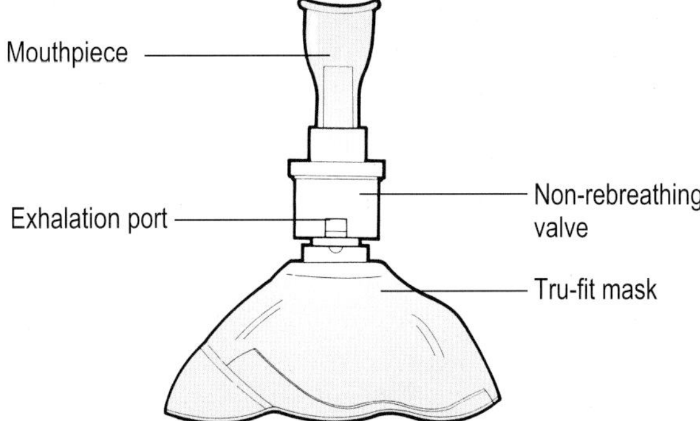

Figure 13-14 Mouth-to-mask device.

Mouth-to-mask devices

Mouth-to-mask devices are used as an alternative to mouth-to-mouth methods of ventilation. These masks are constructed of a clear, flexible material and are available with one-way valves, bacterial filters and ports for supplemental oxygen delivery (Figure 13-14). They are made by a number of manufacturers and are available in a variety of sizes. The mouth-to-mask technique confer several advantages:

- it eliminates direct contact with the patient's mouth and nose
- it provides more effective ventilation than the mouth-to-mouth method
- it is aesthetically more acceptable than mouth-to-mouth ventilation
- supplemental oxygen delivery is possible
- the one-way valve eliminates exposure to exhaled gases and sputum
- the mask is easy to apply.

Technique

The mask device can be used in patients with or without spontaneous respirations. If the device is immediately available, it is the preferred method of initial ventilation for the patient (Figure 13-15). To apply the mask, the paramedic should follow these steps:

1. If no spinal injury is suspected, position the patient with optimal head-tilt and chin-lift. The use of an oropharyngeal or nasopharyngeal airway is indicated in an unconscious patient. (If a spinal injury is suspected, spinal precautions should be used.)
2. Connect the one-way valve to the mask. Oxygen tubing should be connected to the inlet port with an oxygen flow rate of 10 to 12 L/min. Using supplemental oxygen provides a higher concentration of oxygen in the inspired air. An oxygen flow rate of 10 L/min, combined with rescuer ventilations, can supply an oxygen concentration of 50%.
3. Position yourself at the patient's head (cephalic technique) or side (lateral technique). Clear the airway of secretions, vomitus, and foreign objects. Place the mask on the patient's face and create an airtight seal.

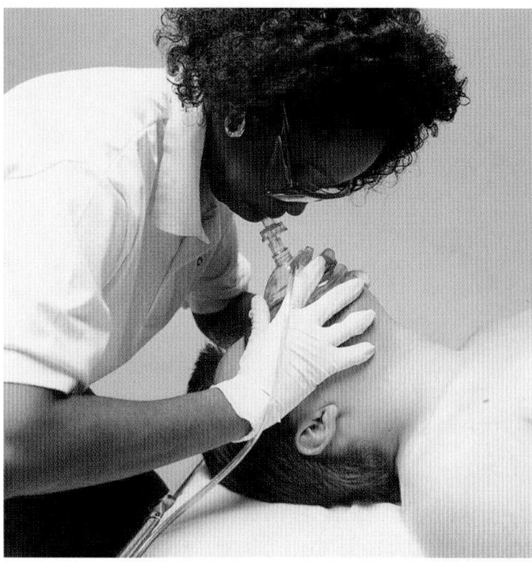

Figure 13-15 Mouth-to-mask ventilation technique (cephalic technique).

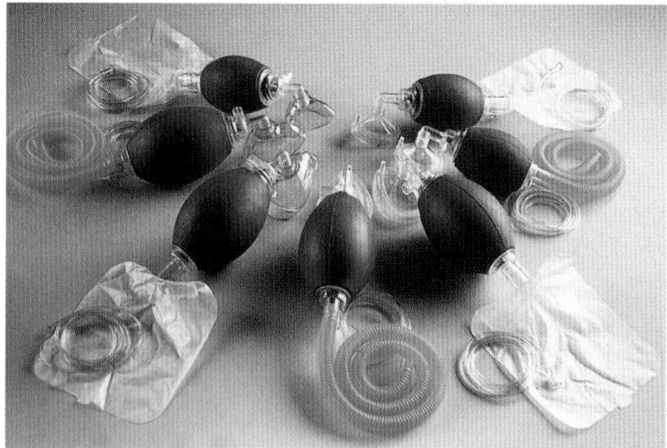

Figure 13-16 Disposable and reusable adult and paediatric bag–valve devices.

Box 13-3

Application of cricoid pressure

Applying pressure to the solid ring of the cricoid cartilage can occlude the oesophagus. This reduces the risk of regurgitation and aspiration. This type of pressure can also help to minimize gastric distension during bag–mask ventilation. Cricoid pressure should not be applied if vomiting occurs due to the risk of oesophageal rupture. It may be indicated if the patient is unconscious while intubation or artificial ventilation is performed.

Cricoid pressure should be used with caution if cervical spine injury is suspected, because it may cause additional damage to the spine. Complications include laryngeal trauma with excessive force and oesophageal rupture from unrelieved high gastric pressures.

Using the thumb side of the palm with both hands, apply pressure to the sides of the mask. If using the cephalic technique, apply upward pressure to the mandible just in front of the ear lobes, using the index, middle, and ring fingers of both hands, while maintaining head-tilt. If using the lateral technique, seal the mask by placing the index finger and thumb of the hand closer to the top of the patient's head along the border of the mask and place the thumb of the other hand along the lower margin of the mask. Place the remaining fingers of the hand closer to the patient's feet and lift the jaw while performing a head-tilt chin-lift.

4. Blow into the opening of the mask, observing chest rise and fall. If available, a second rescuer should apply cricoid pressure (Box 13-3). This helps prevent gastric inflation during positive-pressure ventilation and reduces the chance of regurgitation and aspiration.
5. Remove the mask from the patient's face to allow for passive exhalation.

If oxygen is not available, the tidal volumes and inspiratory times for mouth-to-mask ventilation should be the same as for mouth-to-mouth breathing (500–600 mL delivered over 1 s). If supplemental oxygen is used with the facemask, provide a minimum flow rate of 10–12 L/min.

Bag–valve devices

Bag–mask devices consist of a self-inflating bag and a non-rebreathing valve (Figure 13-16). They can be used with a mask, an tracheal tube, or another invasive airway device. An adequate bag–valve unit should have: (1) a self-refilling bag that is disposable or easily cleaned or sterilized; (2) a non-jam valve system that allows a minimum oxygen inlet flow of 15 L/min; (3) a non-pop-off valve; (4) standard 15 and 22 mm fittings; (5) a system for delivering high-concentration oxygen through an inlet port at the back of the bag or by an oxygen reservoir; and (6) a non-rebreathing valve.[6]

The device should also perform in all common environmental conditions and under extremes of temperature. It should be available in both adult and paediatric sizes.

Note

All paramedics should be proficient in delivering effective oxygenation and ventilation with a bag-valve device to adults, children, and infants. It is the preferred method of ventilatory support.[7]

When the bag–valve device is compressed, air is delivered to the patient through a one-way valve. The air inlet to the bag is closed during delivery. When the bag is released, the patient's expired gas passes through an exhalation valve into the atmosphere, which prevents the patient's exhaled air from re-entering the bag–valve device. As the patient exhales, atmospheric air and supplemental oxygen from the reservoir refill the bag.

Use of the bag–valve device with a mask may be difficult due to the problem of creating an effective seal between the mask and the patient's face whilst maintaining an open airway. For this reason it has been recommended that two rescuers use the device. One should hold the mask and maintain the airway while the second compresses the bag with two hands. If three rescuers are available, one rescuer can be solely responsible for maintaining the mask seal while providing spinal precautions as indicated.

When properly used, the bag–valve device has many benefits. The rescuer can provide a wide range of inspiratory pressures and volumes to adequately ventilate patients of varying sizes and underlying pathological conditions. It can be used to assist patients with shallow respirations and it performs adequately in extremes of environmental temperatures. Oxygen concentrations ranging from 21% (room air concentration) to nearly 100% (using supplemental oxygen and a reservoir) can be achieved. In addition, manual compression of the bag can give the rescuer a sense of the patient's lung compliance, which is an advantage over mechanical methods of ventilation.

Technique

Ventilation with the bag–valve device is best accomplished when the patient has been intubated. If the patient has not been intubated, the bag–valve device may be used with a mask. The following technique is recommended for use with the bag–valve device:

1. The rescuer is positioned at the top of the patient's head.
2. If no spinal injury is suspected, place the patient in the optimal head-tilt chin-lift position, with the patient's head elevated in extension. (If a spinal injury is suspected, spinal precautions should be used.) If the jaw-thrust manoeuvre does not produce an open airway, use the head-tilt-chin lift manoeuvre.
3. Clear the airway of secretions, vomitus, and foreign objects. If the patient is unconscious, insert an oropharyngeal or nasopharyngeal airway. The patient's mouth should remain open under the mask.
4. Connect an oxygen source, and then flush the reservoir with high-concentration oxygen.
5. Place the mask on the patient's face, making a tight seal. This can be accomplished by placing the thumb on the nose area and an index finger on the chin, and then spreading the remaining fingers along the mandible. The anterior displacement of the mandible must be maintained. To compress the bag, the rescuer's other hand presses the bag against his or her body (e.g. the thigh), or another rescuer compresses the bag with two hands. The two-person operator technique is the preferred method for bag–mask ventilation.[7] The bag should be compressed smoothly, delivering approximately 500 to 600 mL for the average adult over 1 s to produce visible chest rise.
6. Avoid hyperventilating the patient as this has been shown to cause increased thoracic pressure, decreased cerebral and coronary perfusion, and poorer survival rates in animals and adults.[7]

Paediatric considerations

Smaller bag–valve devices are needed for infants and children; this helps to reduce the chances of over-inflation and barotrauma. Bag–valve devices are used mainly for paediatric patients who are in respiratory arrest. Bag–valve devices equipped with a fish-mouth- or leaf-flap-operated outlet valve should not be used to provide supplemental oxygen to a spontaneously breathing infant or child. If the valve fails to open during inspiration, the child receives only the exhaled gases from within the mask itself. For this reason, bag devices for ventilation of full-term neonates, infants, and children should have a minimum volume of 450 to 500 mL.[8] At least 10 to 15 L/min of oxygen flow is needed to maintain an adequate oxygen volume in the reservoir of a paediatric bag (Figure 13-17).

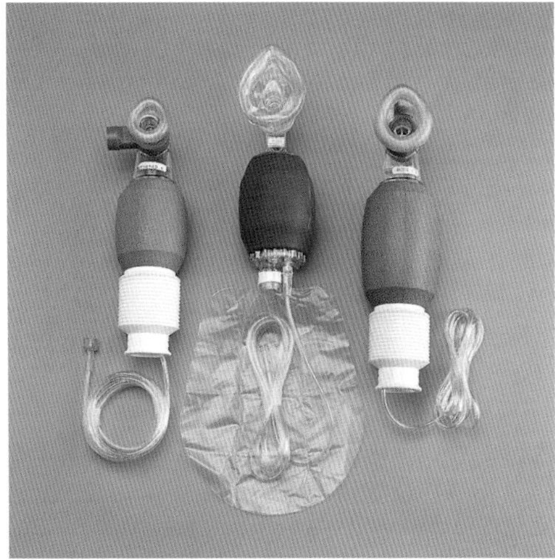

Figure 13-17 Paediatric bag–valve devices.

> **Note**
>
> A child's flat nasal bridge makes achieving a mask seal difficult. In addition, compressing the mask against the face may result in obstruction. The mask seal is best achieved with jaw displacement using two rescuers to provide bag–mask ventilation.

Technique

The following procedure is used to artificially ventilate a paediatric patient with a bag–valve device:

1. Ensure a proper mask fit by using a length-based resuscitation tape or by measuring from the bridge of the nose to the cleft of the chin.
2. Ensure a proper mask position and seal. Place the mask over the mouth and nose (avoid compressing the eyes). With one hand, place a thumb on the mask at the apex and place the index finger on the mouth at the chin (like a C clamp). With gentle pressure, push down on the mask to establish an adequate seal. Maintain the airway by lifting the bony prominence on the chin, with the remaining fingers placed on the mandible, forming an E. Avoid putting pressure on the soft area under the chin.
3. Provide ventilations at a rate of 12–20 breaths/min.
4. Deliver each breath in 1 s; both rescuers should make sure it produces visible chest rise.
5. Assess bag–mask ventilation by observing adequate rise and fall of the chest, by listening for lung sounds at the third intercostal space and midaxillary line, and by checking for improvement in skin colour or heart rate, or both.

6. Avoid hyperventilating the patient as this has been shown to cause increased thoracic pressure, decreased cerebral and coronary perfusion, and poorer survival rates in animals and adults.[9]

Critical Thinking

What should you do if you find that it is suddenly harder to ventilate a patient who is not intubated?

Automatic transport ventilators

Several time-cycled, gas-powered ventilators are available for field use or intrahospital transport of patients who require ventilatory support (Figure 13-18). Most of these ventilators consist of a plastic control module connected by tubing to any 350 kPa (50 psi) gas source (e.g. air or different concentrations of oxygen, including 100% oxygen). The exit valve of the control module is connected by one or two tubes (based on the model) to the patient valve assembly to deliver selected tidal volumes (400–1200 mL for adults, 200–600 mL for children). Another control selects respiratory rates from 8 to 22 breaths per minute for adults and rates from 8 to 30 breaths per minute for children. Most ambulance-use ventilators are not to be used in children under 5 years of age. Most units provide a 40 L/min flow of oxygen, which remains constant despite changes in the patient's airway or lung compliance.

Note

In the cardiac arrest situation, portable mechanical ventilators should be set at 10 breaths a minute for intubated patients (adults and children) and compressions should be uninterrupted.[9,10]

The volume of gas delivered by the automatic ventilator is determined by the length of time the manual trigger is depressed or by the inspiratory effort of the spontaneously breathing patient. Most units are designed to limit the inspiratory pressure to 60–80 cmH_2O. When this pressure is reached, an alarm sounds and excess gas flow is vented off, preventing possible lung damage. Mechanical ventilators allow the paramedic to use both hands to obtain a tight face-to-mask seal on a patient who has not been intubated. Cricoid pressure can also be applied with one hand while the other hand seals the mask on the face. They also allow the paramedic to perform other tasks when the ventilator is used on a patient who has been intubated. Most ventilators should not be used in patients who are awake, who have an obstructed airway, and/or who have increased airway resistance (e.g. pneumothorax, asthma, pulmonary oedema).

Airway management

Science and technology have produced many devices for supporting airway management; however, the paramedic must not neglect basic airway management procedures. A basic procedure that secures a safe and functional airway is better than a more technically difficult procedure. Airway management should progress rapidly from the least to the most invasive procedures and devices (see algorithm on next page). Paramedics should also make sure they are always equipped with the appropriate personal protective equipment for these procedures (Box 13-4).

Note

Unconscious patients lack the muscular tone and control to maintain a patent airway. For this reason, an airway must be established and maintained in the initial assessment of all unconscious patients. Any injury severe enough to cause loss of consciousness is severe enough to cause spinal injury. Spinal precautions should be considered in all trauma patients who need airway management or ventilatory support until an X-ray film of the spine has been made.

Box 13-4

Personal protective equipment

The Ambulance Service Association and Health Protection Agency recommend that healthcare workers, in addition to taking the normal precautions for personal protection from communicable diseases, use masks, gloves, plastic apron and eye/mouth/nose protection when splashing of blood or other body fluids is likely. During airway management, certain patient reactions may occur. These may include vomiting and coughing. Exposure to blood and other body fluids also is possible. Because of these possibilities, the paramedic should observe barrier precautions.

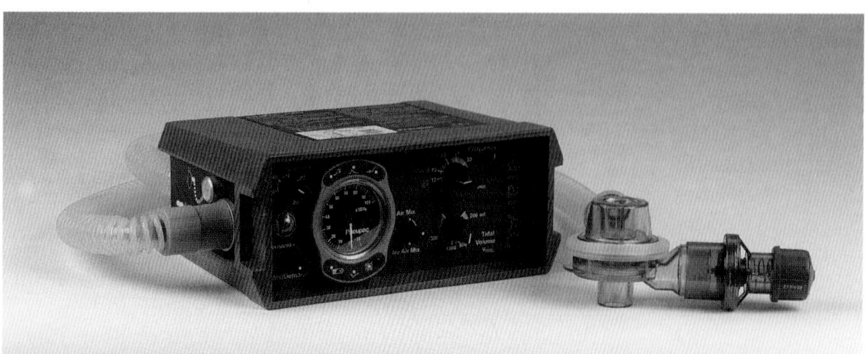

Figure 13-18 Pneupac® paraPAC with alarms.

Manual techniques for airway management

Manual techniques for airway management include the head-tilt chin-lift method, the jaw-thrust, and the jaw-thrust without head-tilt. The paramedic should not use manual manoeuvres to open the airway in patients who are responsive or when attempts to open the patient's mouth are met with resistance. All such manoeuvres are hazardous if spinal injury is a factor. In addition, none of these manoeuvres protects against aspiration.

The head-tilt chin-lift manoeuvre (Figure 13-19) is preferred for opening the airway when a spinal injury is not suspected. The head-tilt is performed by placing one hand on the victim's forehead and applying firm backward pressure with the palm to tilt the head back. The fingers of the other hand then are placed under the bony part of the lower jaw (near the chin) and lifted to bring the chin forward. These fingers support the jaw and help to maintain the head-tilt position.

The jaw-thrust manoeuvre (Figure 13-20) may be used to gain additional forward displacement of the mandible if no spinal injury is suspected. This is achieved by grasping the angles of the patient's lower jaw and lifting with both hands, one on each side. This displaces the mandible forward while tilting the head back. However, if the paramedic is unable to open the airway with the jaw-thrust manoeuvre, the head-tilt chin-lift manoeuvre should be performed. An open airway remains the highest priority, even for the unresponsive trauma victim.

If a spinal injury is suspected, the jaw-thrust without head-tilt manoeuvre (Figure 13-21) should be used to open the airway. During this manoeuvre, the patient's head should be stabilized and the cervical spine should be immobilized with neutral, in-line stabilization. The jaw-thrust manoeuvre should then proceed without extension of the neck.

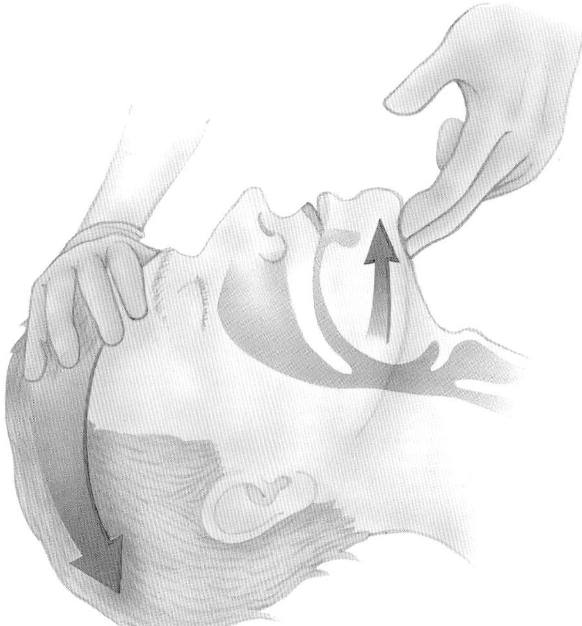

Figure 13-19 Head-tilt chin-lift manoeuvre.

Suction

Suction can be used to remove vomitus, saliva, blood, food and other foreign objects that might block the airway or increase the likelihood of pulmonary aspiration by inhalation. Many factors can predispose a person to aspiration. For this reason, every patient should be considered a possible aspiration victim.

Suction devices

Fixed and portable mechanical suction devices are available through a number of manufacturers. Fixed suction devices are mounted in patient care areas of hospitals and nursing homes, and they are used in many emergency vehicles. These systems are electrically operated by vacuum pumps or powered by the vacuum produced by a vehicle engine manifold. Fixed suction devices furnish an air intake of at least 40 L/min. They provide a vacuum of more than 300 mmHg when the tube is clamped.

Portable suction devices may be oxygen or air powered, electrically powered, or manually powered (Figures 13-22 and 13-23). To operate effectively, these devices should furnish an air intake of no less than 20 L/min.

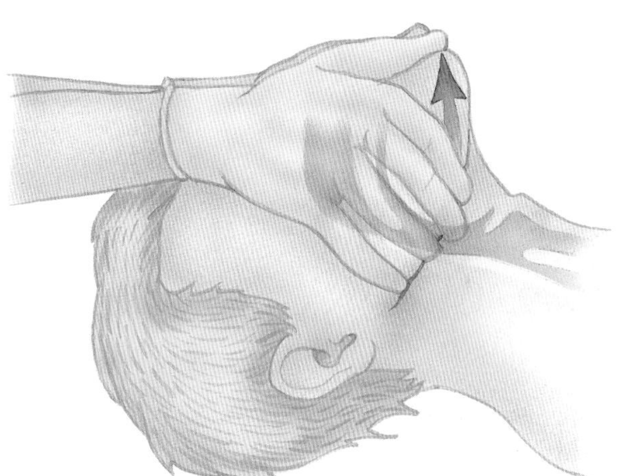

Figure 13-20 Jaw-thrust manoeuvre.

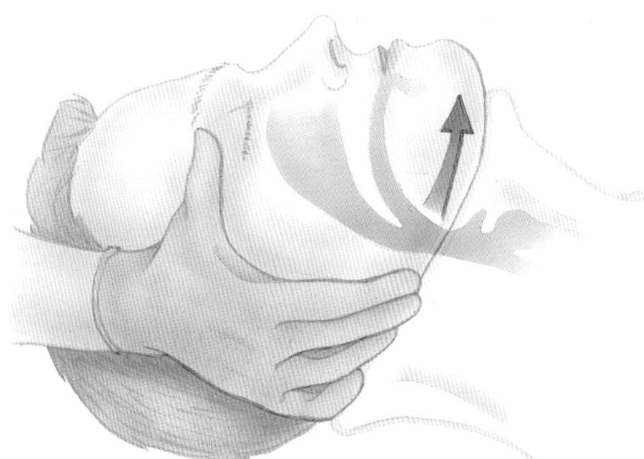

Figure 13-21 Jaw-thrust without head-tilt manoeuvre.

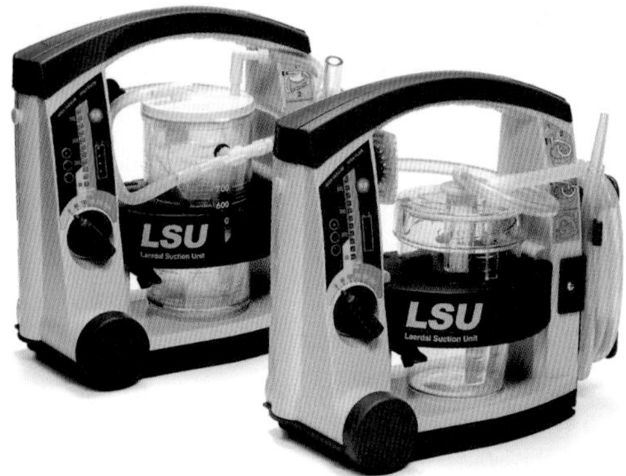

Figure 13-22 Portable suction unit. With Kind permission of Laerdal Ltd.

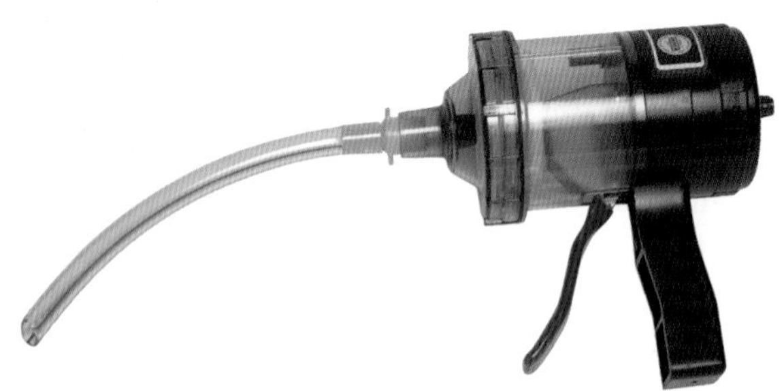

Figure 13-23 Manual suction unit. With Kind permission of Vitalograph Ltd.

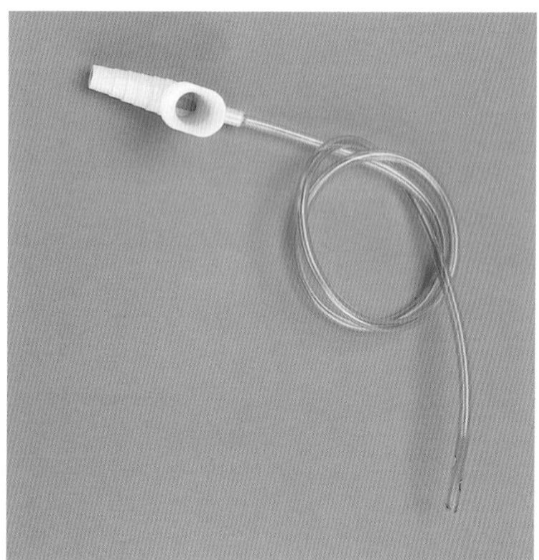

Figure 13-24 Soft (whistle-tip) suction catheter.

Suction catheters

Suction catheters are used to clear secretions and debris from the oral cavity and airway passages. The two broad classifications of catheters are soft-tip suction catheters and Yankauer suction catheters.

The soft-tip catheter is a narrow, flexible tube that is used primarily for tracheobronchial suctioning to clear secretions through either an tracheal tube or the nasopharynx (Figure 13-24). This catheter is designed with moulded ends and side holes to cause minimal trauma to the mucosa and should be lubricated before insertion. A side opening in the proximal end is covered with the thumb to produce suction. Using sterile technique, the paramedic advances the catheter to the desired location and then applies suction intermittently as the catheter is withdrawn.

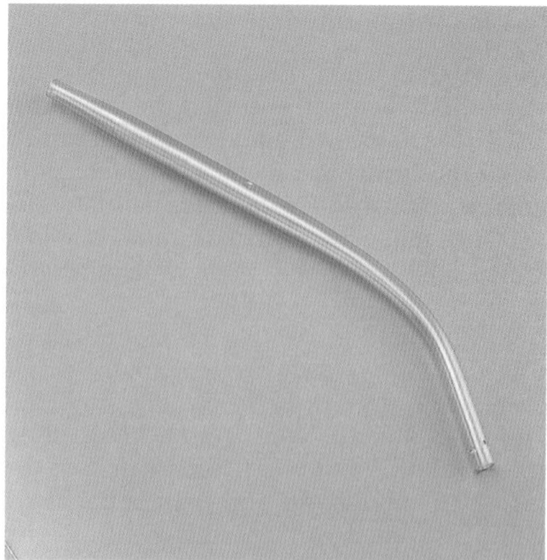

Figure 13-25 Rigid (tonsil-tip [Yankauer]) suction catheter.

The Yankauer suction catheter is a rigid pharyngeal catheter that is used to clear secretions, blood clots, and other foreign material from the mouth and pharynx (Figure 13-25). The device is carefully inserted into the oral cavity under direct visualization and then slowly withdrawn while suction is activated.

Before any suctioning is begun, all equipment should be checked. The suction should be set between 80 and 120 mmHg. (Higher suction is needed for tracheobronchial suctioning.) If possible, the patient's lungs should be oxygenated with 100% oxygen for at least 2 min before suction is initiated. Suction should be applied for no longer than 10–15 s in adult patients and for no longer than 5 s in paediatric patients. If more suctioning is needed, the patient's lungs should be reoxygenated first. Possible complications from suctioning include the following:

- sudden hypoxaemia that occurs secondary to decreased lung volume during the application of suction
- severe hypoxaemia that may lead to cardiac rhythm disturbances and cardiac arrest
- airway stimulation that may increase arterial pressure and cardiac rhythm disturbances
- coughing that may result in increased intracranial pressure with reduced blood flow to the brain and increased risk of herniation in patients with head injury
- soft tissue damage to the respiratory tract.

The following section is not currently within the remit of the UK paramedic but has been included for completeness and in anticipation of future developments.

Tracheobronchial suctioning (not currently a UK paramedic skill)

Before tracheobronchial suctioning is performed through an tracheal tube (Figure 13-26a–d), the patient must be oxygen-

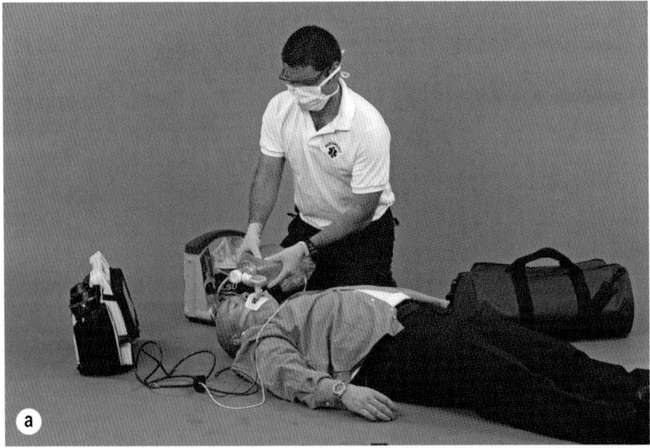

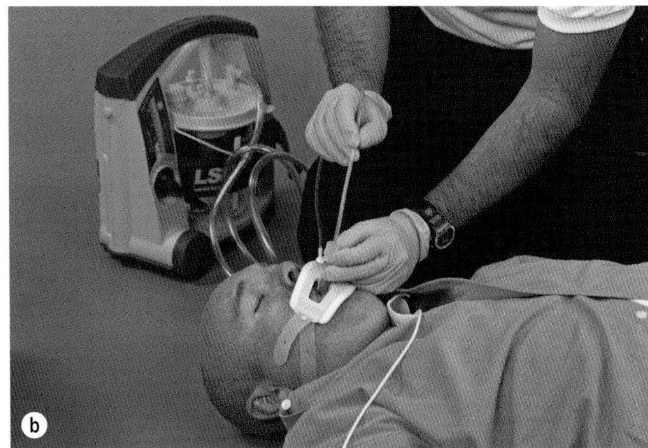

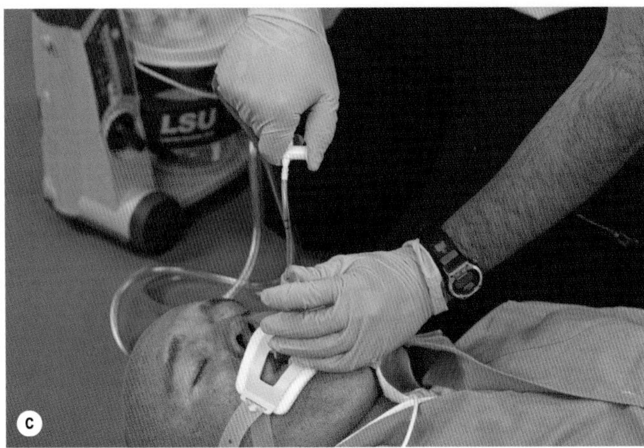

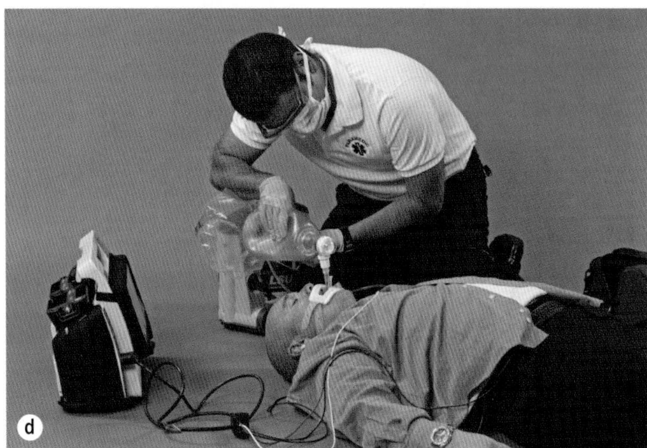

Figure 13-26 Tracheobronchial suctioning. (a) Bag the intubated patient with a bag–valve device. (b) Introduce the suction catheter through the tracheal tube without suction. (c) Withdraw the catheter with suction intermittently applied while observing the electrocardiographic (ECG) rhythm. (d) Ventilate the patient and re-evaluate the respiratory status.

ated with 100% oxygen for 5 min.[8] For tracheal suctioning, a Y- or T-piece or a lateral opening should lie between the suction tube and the source of the on–off suction control. Using sterile technique, the paramedic advances the catheter to the desired location (about the level of the carina). Suction is applied intermittently by closing the side opening as the catheter is withdrawn in a rotating motion. The patient's cardiac rhythm should be monitored throughout the procedure. If dysrhythmias or bradycardia develop, suctioning should stop. The patient then should be manually ventilated and oxygenated. Before suctioning is resumed, the patient should be ventilated with 100% oxygen for about 30 s.

Note

It may be necessary to inject 3–5 mL of sterile saline down the endotracheal (ET) tube to loosen secretions before suctioning.

Gastric distension

Gastric distension results from the trapping of air in the stomach. As the stomach enlarges, it pushes against the diaphragm and interferes with lung expansion. The abdomen becomes more and more distended (especially in small children). Resistance may be felt to bag–mask ventilation.

Management of gastric distension begins by slightly increasing the bag–mask ventilation inspiratory time. (Large-volume suction should be readily available.) If possible, the patient should be placed in a left lateral recumbent position. Manual pressure should be slowly applied to the upper stomach or epigastric region. Gastric distension that cannot be managed with these techniques may require insertion of a gastric tube (Figure 13-27).

Gastric tubes

Gastric distension is very common in patients who are ventilated but have not been intubated. Gastric decompression for gastric distension or vomiting control can be achieved through nasogastric (NG) or orogastric emptying or decompression of the stomach. Gastric decompression is done with extreme caution in patients who have oesophageal trauma or oesophageal disease, and should not be performed if an oesophageal obstruction is present. NG decompression should not be attempted in a patient with facial trauma or oesophageal varices (large, swollen veins in the oesophagus that are susceptible to haemorrhage).

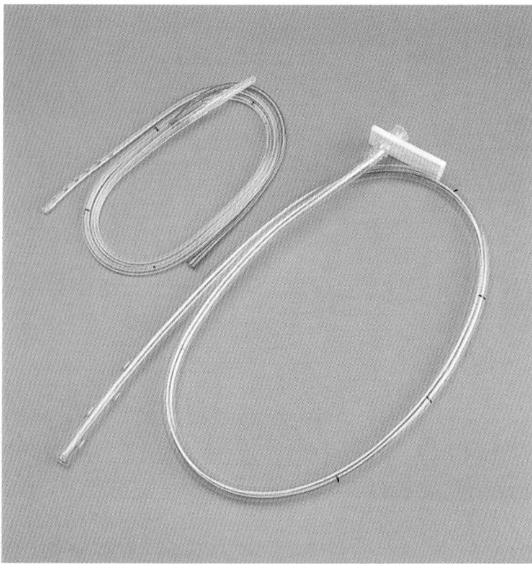

Figure 13-27 Top, nasogastric/orogastric tube. Bottom, oral gastric lavage tube.

Nasogastric decompression (Figure 13-28a–d)

1. Prepare the patient.
   (a) Place the head in a neutral position.
   (b) Pre-oxygenate.
   (c) Instil a topical anaesthetic or intravenous (IV) lidocaine (per standing order).
   (d) Locate the larger nostril.
2. Measure the NG tube to the correct insertion length and lubricate it with viscous lidocaine or water-soluble lubricant per protocol.
3. Advance the tube gently along the nasal floor and into the stomach. (Having the patient swallow during insertion may help advance the tube into the oesophagus and prevent tracheal insertion.)
4. Confirm placement.
   (a) Auscultate the epigastric region while injecting 30–50 mL of air.
   (b) Note gastric contents in the NG tube.
   (c) Ensure that no reflux appears around the NG tube.
5. Secure the NG tube in place and attach to suction if indicated.

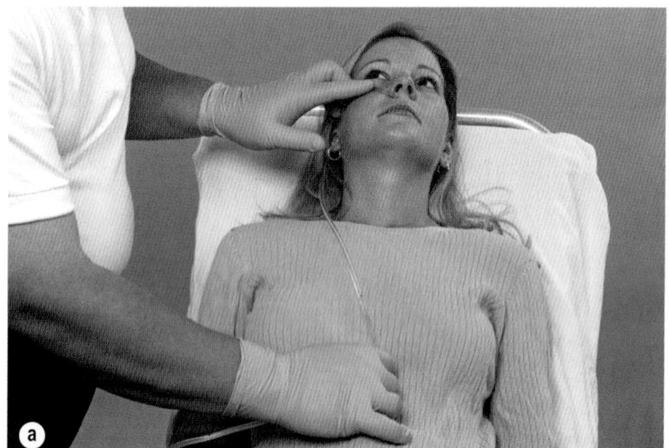

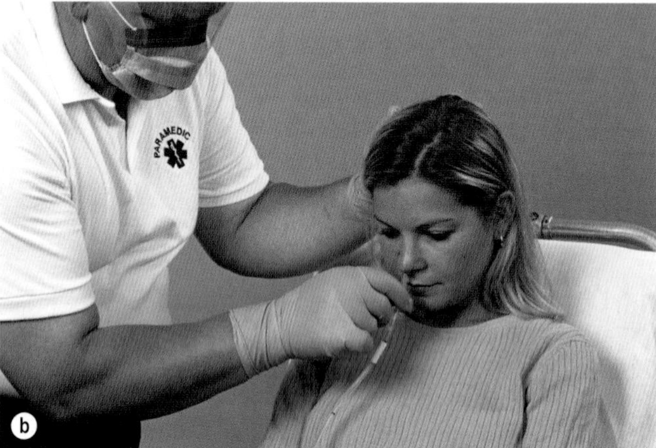

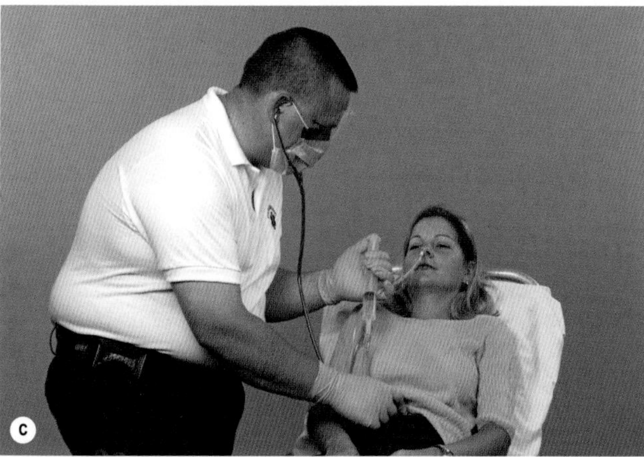

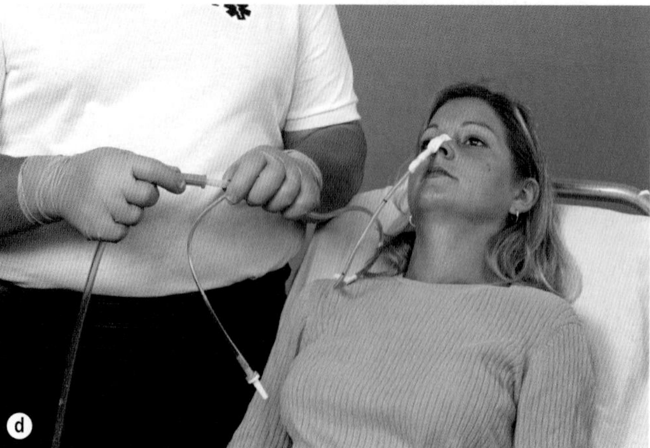

Figure 13-28 (a) Position the patient. Measure the tube from the nose to the ear, and from the ear to the xiphoid process. (b) Lubricate the tube and insert it into the largest nostril. Advance the tube to the proper length. (c) Verify correct placement of the tube by injecting 30 to 50 mL of air while auscultating over the epigastric area. (d) Secure the tube and attach the suction unit.

Orogastric decompression

1. Prepare the patient and tube as described above for NG insertion.
2. Introduce the orogastric tube down the midline of the oropharynx and into the stomach.
3. Confirm placement. Secure the orogastric tube as described above for NG insertion.

Complications of gastric decompression

Whatever the method chosen, gastric decompression is uncomfortable for the patient. It may induce nausea and vomiting even when the gag reflex is suppressed. In addition, gastric tubes interfere with mask seals and with visualization of airway structures during intubation. Complications of the procedures include nasal, oesophageal or gastric trauma, tracheal placement, and gastric tube obstruction.

Mechanical adjuncts in airway management

The use of mechanical devices for airway management should never delay manual opening of the airway. These devices should be used only after efforts have been made to open the airway manually.

Nasopharyngeal airway (nasal airway)

Nasal airways (Figure 13-29) are used to maintain an open airway passage in unconscious patients or in patients who are responsive but not alert enough to control their own airway. Insertion of a nasal airway may be useful as a temporary airway maintenance manoeuvre or may be used to control the airway in patients with seizures or possible cervical spine injury. It may also be used before nasotracheal intubation (described later in this chapter). In addition, it can serve as a guide for insertion of a nasogastric tube.

> **Critical Thinking**
>
> Think about two or three specific patient conditions that would warrant the use of a nasal airway.

Description

Nasal airways are soft and pliable. They have a gentle curve, and the outer end is flared. Nasal airways are available in a variety of sizes to accommodate infants and adults, and range in length from 17 to 20 cm (about 7 to 8 inches), and in size from 12 to 36 French. (As with most other catheters, the French scale system is used to indicate internal diameter. Each unit of the scale equals about ⅓ mm. A 21 French catheter, for example, is 7 mm [about ⅓ inch] in diameter.)

It has widely been taught that the correct size of a nasopharyngeal airway is related to the patient's little finger or nostril (anterior nares). It has now been shown that these measurements do not correlate with the anatomy.[12] The length of the airway is more important in determining appropriate size than diameter. If too short, the airway would fail to separate the soft palate from the posterior wall of the pharynx, and if too long, could enter either the larynx and aggravate laryngeal reflexes or the space between the epiglottis and the tongue (vallecula) where the airway could become obstructed. The ideal length of a nasopharyngeal airway is one which lies within 1 cm of the epiglottis. This corresponded to a nares–epiglottis length of 150 mm in men and 130 mm in women (corresponding to a size 7 and 6 Portex nasopharyngeal airway, respectively).[12]

Insertion

The nasal airway should be lubricated with a water-soluble lubricant. This helps to ease the airway through the nasal cavity. The device is placed in the nostril with the bevelled tip (designed to protect nasal structures) directed toward the nasal septum. The airway is gently passed close to the midline, along the floor of the nostril, following the natural curve of the nasal passage. The airway should not be forced. If resistance is encountered, rotating the tube slightly may help, or insertion can be attempted through the other nostril (Figure 13-30).

After insertion, the nasal airway rests in the posterior pharynx behind the tongue. If the patient begins to gag, the tube may be stimulating the posterior pharynx. It may be necessary to remove the airway or withdraw it 0.5 to 1 cm (¼ to ½ inch) and reinsert it. The paramedic should maintain displacement of the mandible with the head-tilt chin-lift

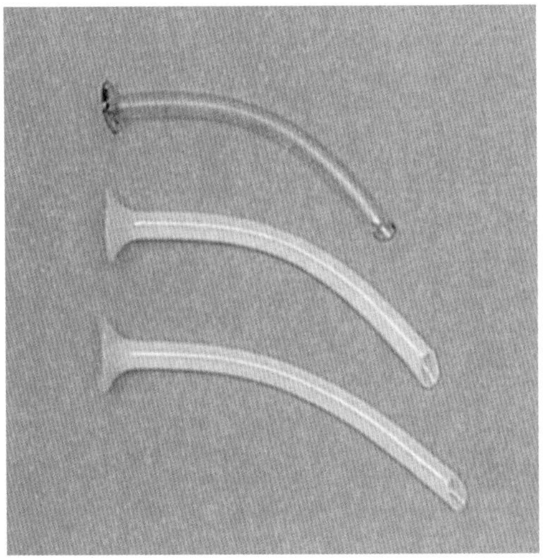

Figure 13-29 Nasal airways.

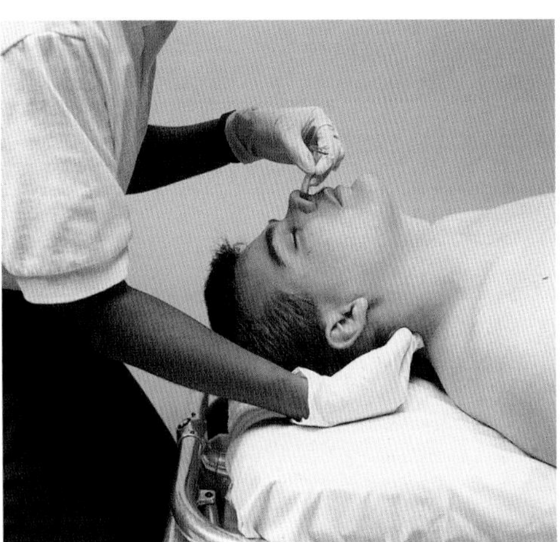

Figure 13-30 Insertion of a nasal airway.

or jaw-thrust without head-tilt manoeuvre when using this airway.

Note

The ATLS course and manual taught that basal skull fracture constitutes a contraindication to the use of nasal airways but, in the absence of any other method of opening the airway, nasopharyngeal airway insertion is a safe procedure, where the benefits of the procedure far outweigh the small risk of intracranial penetration.[12]

Advantages

- A nasal airway is well tolerated by conscious and semiconscious patients with an intact gag reflex.
- Insertion is a quick procedure.
- A nasal airway may be used when insertion of an oropharyngeal airway is contraindicated or difficult because of oral trauma or soft tissue injury.

Possible complications

- Long nasal airways may enter the oesophagus.
- The airway may precipitate laryngospasm and vomiting in patients with a gag reflex.
- The airway may injure the nasal mucosa, causing bleeding and possibly airway obstruction.
- Small-diameter airways may become obstructed by mucus, blood, vomitus and the soft tissues of the pharynx.
- A nasal airway does not protect the lower airway from aspiration.
- Suctioning through a nasal airway is difficult.

Oropharyngeal airway (oral airway)

Oral airways are designed to prevent the tongue from obstructing the glottis. They are indicated in unconscious or semiconscious patients who have no gag reflex and who are not intubated.

Description

The oral airway is a semicircular device designed to hold the tongue away from the posterior wall of the pharynx. Most oropharyngeal airways are made of disposable plastic. The two types of airways most often used are the Guedel airway and the Berman airway. The Guedel airway is distinguished by its tubular design. The Berman airway is distinguished by the airway channels along each side of the device (Figure 13-31).

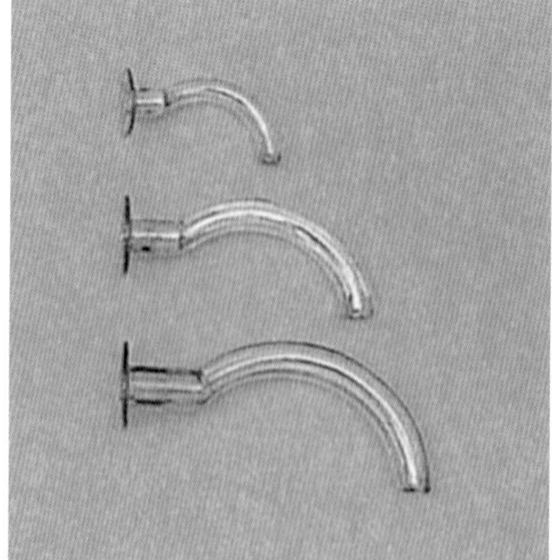

Figure 13-31 Oral airways.

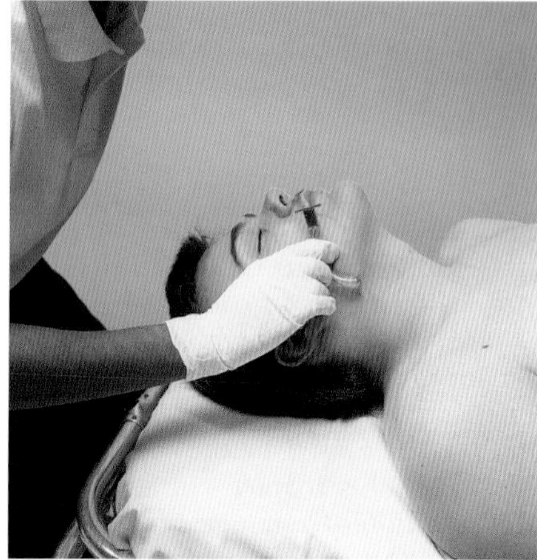

Figure 13-32 Measuring an oral airway.

Note

The cuffed oropharyngeal airway (COPA) is a modified oral airway. It has a distal inflatable cuff and proximal standard 15 mm connector that allows attachment of a bag–mask device to the airway. The COPA may be a useful adjunct in airway management during resuscitation.

Like nasopharyngeal airways, oral airways are available in a variety of sizes, ranging from infant to adult. The size is based on the distance in millimetres from the flange to the distal tip. The proper size for the patient may be determined by placing the airway next to the face so that the flange is at the level of the patient's central incisors and the bite block segment is parallel to the patient's hard palate. The airway should extend from the corner of the mouth to the tip of the ear lobe or the angle of the jaw (Figure 13-32).

The most common sizes are 2, 3 and 4 for small, medium and large adults, respectively.[10]

Insertion

Before an oral airway is inserted, the mouth and pharynx should be cleared of all secretions, blood, or vomitus. In an adult or older child, the oral airway may be inserted upside down or at a 90-degree angle (Figure 13-33a). This helps the paramedic to avoid catching the tongue during insertion. As the oral airway passes the crest of the tongue, it is rotated into the proper position. It should be situated against the posterior wall of the oropharynx. Another method of insertion is recommended for paediatric patients (Figure 13-33b). (It can also be used in adults.) A tongue blade is used to displace the tongue inferiorly and anteriorly. The airway is then inserted and moved posteriorly toward the back of the oropharynx, following the normal curve of the oral cavity. Regardless of the method of insertion, trauma to the face

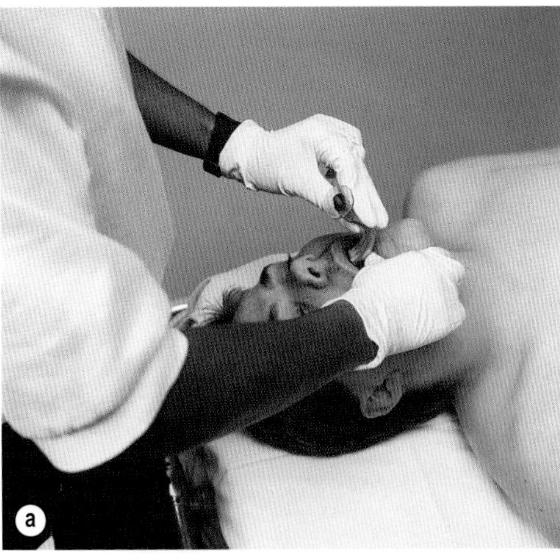

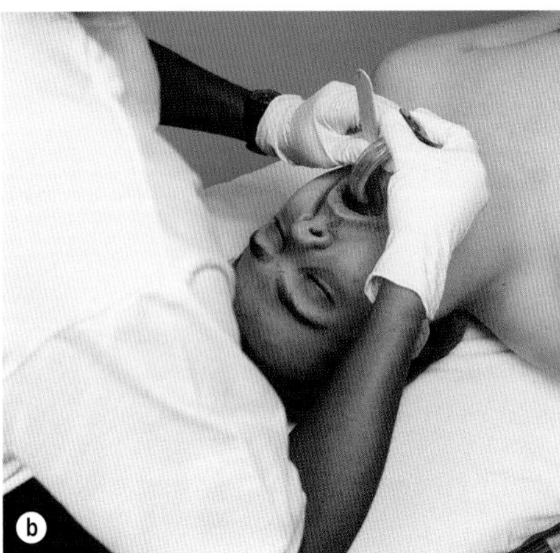

Figure 13-33 (a) Inserting an airway upside down. (b) Alternative method of inserting an oral airway.

and oral cavity should be avoided. In addition, the paramedic should be sure the patient's lips and tongue are not caught between the teeth and the airway.

> **Critical Thinking**
>
> Why is this method of oral airway insertion used for infants and young children?

Proper placement of the airway is confirmed by observable chest wall expansion accompanied by good breath sounds on auscultation of the lungs during ventilation. The paramedic must remember that even with an oral airway in place, the patient's head must be kept in proper position to help ensure a patent airway.

Advantages

- An oral airway secures the tongue forward and down, away from the posterior pharynx.
- It provides easy access for airway suction.
- It serves as a bite block to protect an tracheal tube and the airway in the event of convulsions.

Possible complications

- Oral airways that are too small do not provide a passageway between the tongue and posterior oropharynx.
- Long airways may press the epiglottis against the entrance of the trachea, producing a complete airway obstruction.
- The airway may stimulate vomiting and laryngospasm in a patient with a gag reflex.
- The airway does not protect the lower airway from aspiration.
- Improper insertion may push the tongue back, causing it to obstruct the airway.

Advanced airway procedures

Advanced airway procedures described in this text include the laryngeal mask airway (LMA) and tracheal intubation. Both these procedures require special training and should only be used by practitioners authorized and competent in their use. The paramedic should be aware that long-term complications may result from these procedures even when the procedures are properly performed. Such complications include aspiration, tracheal stenosis, transient dysphagia and voice changes.

Laryngeal mask airway

The LMA is an advanced airway control device. It should be used in the prehospital setting as part of a stepwise approach to airway management. Ventilation using the LMA is more efficient and easier than with a bag–mask[13] so, when an LMA can be inserted without delay it is preferable to avoid bag–mask ventilation altogether.[10] The LMA may also be considered when access to the patient is limited, when an unstable neck injury may be present, as a rescue device when ET intubation is unsuccessful, or when appropriate positioning of the patient for tracheal intubation is impossible.

> **Note**
>
> The LMA does not offer full protection against aspiration. However, aspiration is uncommon with this device. A small number of patients cannot be ventilated adequately with the LMA. Also, it is contraindicated in conscious patients and in those with an intact gag reflex.

Description

The LMA is available in several sizes (ranging from size 1 for neonates to size 5 for adults.) It consists of a proximal tube with standard adapters for connecting ventilatory devices. The tube is connected to a distal mask that is inflated by means of a pilot tube and balloon (Figure 13-34).

Insertion

The LMA is inserted through the mouth into the pharynx. It is advanced until resistance is felt as the distal portion of the tube locates in the hypopharynx. When the device has been properly inserted, the black line marked on the LMA rests midline against the patient's upper lip. Inflating the cuff seals the larynx and leaves distal opening of the tube just

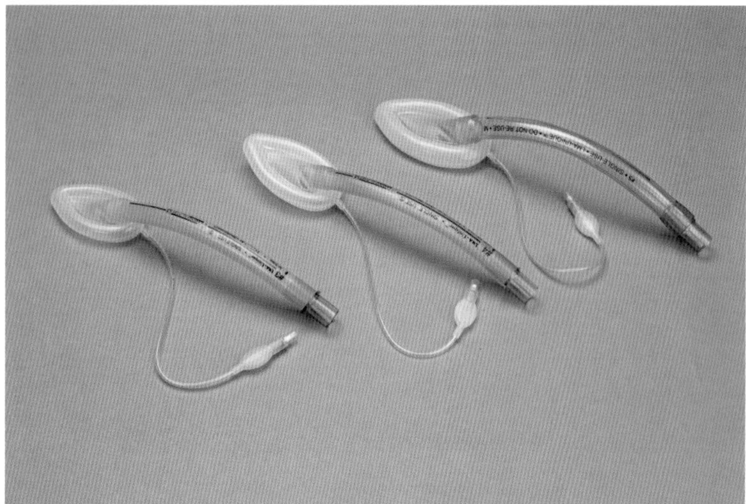

Figure 13-34 Laryngeal mask airways.

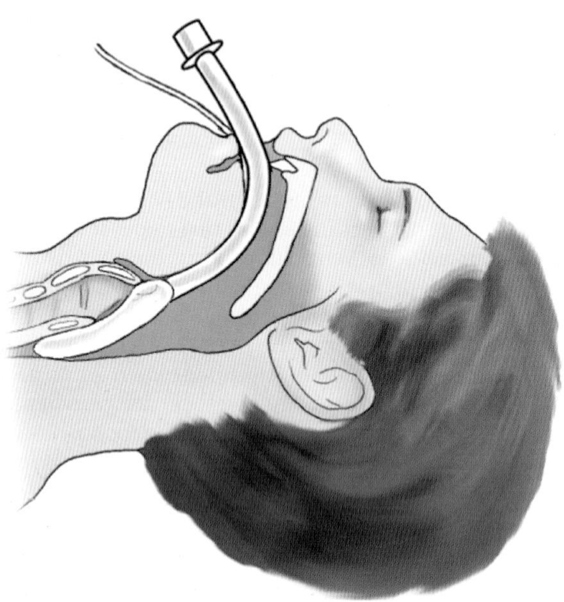

Figure 13-35 A patient with a laryngeal mask airway (LMA).

above the glottis, providing a clear and secure airway. After the pilot cuff has been inflated, proper placement is confirmed by observing equal rise and fall of the chest, by ensuring bilateral breath sounds, and with end-tidal CO_2 detectors, and pulse oximetry monitoring (in a patient who has a perfusing rhythm) (Figure 13-35). The LMA may be hard to maintain during patient movement, which can make it difficult to use during patient transport. The paramedic should consider using a cervical collar to minimize movement of the LMA during patient handling and transportation.

Necessary equipment

- Water-soluble lubricant
- Syringes
- Bag–valve device
- Oxygen source and connecting tubing
- Suction equipment
- Stethoscope.

Common advantages

- Less skilled training or maintenance is required than for ET intubation.
- Laryngoscopy and visualization of the vocal cords are not required.
- Minimal spinal movement is required for insertion.

Common disadvantages

- The patient must be unresponsive and have no gag reflex.
- Not all patients can be adequately ventilated with the LMA.
- The airway must be removed when the patient becomes responsive or agitated.
- Risk of gastric distension.

Common contraindications

- Presence of a gag reflex
- Caustic ingestion
- Oesophageal trauma or disease.

Tracheal intubation

Tracheal intubation is seen as the 'gold standard' for controlling the airway in patients who are unable to maintain an open airway. In the context of cardiac arrest (the most likely indication for non-pharmacologically assisted intubation in the UK) there is insufficient evidence to support or refute the use of any specific technique to maintain an airway and provide ventilation in adults.[30] Tracheal intubation should be considered in the following situations:

- The rescuer is unable to ventilate an unconscious patient with conventional methods (mouth-to-mask method, bag–mask device).
- The patient cannot protect his or her own airway (coma, respiratory and cardiac arrest).
- Prolonged artificial ventilation is needed.

Tracheal intubation has the following advantages:

- The airway is isolated, which prevents aspiration of material into the lower airway.
- Ventilation and oxygenation are easier.
- Suctioning of the trachea and bronchi is easier.
- Wasted ventilation and gastric insufflation are prevented during positive-pressure ventilation.
- A route is provided for administration of some medications (e.g. lidocaine, adrenaline [epinephrine], atropine, naloxone and vasopressin).

Tracheal intubation has the following disadvantages:

- Time delay in placing the tube during which the patient is not being ventilated.
- Risk of misplacement of the tracheal tube (unrecognized misplacement of an tracheal tube by paramedics occurs in 5.8–25% of prehospital intubations).[14,15]
- Requires significant skill to achieve.
- Risk of hyperventilation of the patient, particularly when ventilating manually, which is linked with adverse haemodynamic effects and decreased cerebral perfusion.[16–18]
- Interferes with other important skills – e.g. defibrillation, chest compressions.
- Risk of damage to teeth, mouth and upper airway.

Description

The common tracheal tube is a flexible tube that is open at both ends (Figure 13-36). The proximal end has a standard 15 mm adapter which connects to various oxygen delivery devices for positive-pressure ventilation. The end of the tube that is inserted into the trachea is bevelled to aid placement between the vocal cords. The adult tube size (5 or larger) has a balloon cuff that closes off the remainder of the tracheal opening. This cuff prevents aspiration of fluids around the tube and minimizes air leakage during ventilation. The cuff is attached to a small pilot tube which has a one-way inflating valve with a port designed to fit a standard syringe. A properly positioned tracheal tube with the cuff inflated allows administration of high concentrations of oxygen at controlled pressures.

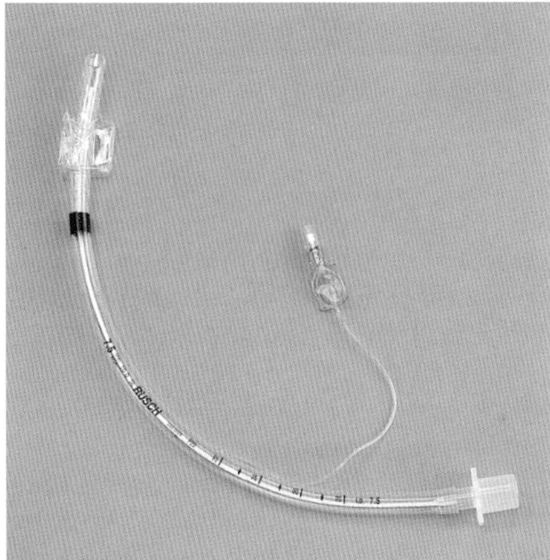

Figure 13-36 Endotracheal (ET) tube.

Tracheal tube sizes

The markings on the tracheal tube indicate the internal diameter of the tube in millimetres. (The tubes are available in graduated sizes from 2.5–10 mm.) The length of the tube from the distal end is indicated in centimetres at several levels. Recommended tracheal tube sizes are 9 mm internal diameter for men, 8 mm internal diameter for women and 7 mm internal diameter for adolescents.[19] Tube sizes are expressed simply as 'size 7' or 'size 8', without the millimetre designation.

Infant and paediatric tracheal tubes are available with and without balloon cuffs. Cuffed tracheal tubes are indicated only for children over the age of 8 to 10 years. The traditional view that young children have a cylindrical narrowing at the cricoid ring is being challenged. Recent research shows that the anterior–posterior view is cylindrical but that the lateral view is funnel shaped. It is now believed that the narrowest part of the child's airway is at the glottis level. Uncuffed tracheal tubes are still recommended for this age group due to the risk of barotrauma. Cuffed tracheal tubes for young children may be appropriate when high ventilatory pressures are indicated. This may occur with status asthmaticus and acute respiratory distress syndrome (ARDS) (see Chapter 14).

Various methods can be used to determine the correct tracheal tube size for infants and children but the most reliable method is to use the 'age per page' guidelines in JRCALC, or to use length-based resuscitation tapes (for children up to 35 kg) (see Chapter 38). Suggested sizes for tracheal tubes for adult and paediatric patients are listed in Table 13-4.[20]

Necessary equipment

A laryngoscope is required for visualization of the glottis during tracheal intubation. Although various makes are available, all have a number of features in common. The standard laryngoscope includes a handle made of plastic or stainless steel. The handle contains the batteries for the light source and attaches to a plastic or stainless steel blade with a bulb placed in the distal third. The electrical contact between the blade and the handle is made at a connection point called the fitting. The indentation of the blade is attached to the bar of the handle. When the blade is elevated to a right angle with the laryngoscope handle, the blade snaps into place and the bulb lights (Figure 13-37). (Failure of the bulb to light may be the result of a loose connection between the bulb and the bulb socket, a damaged bulb, or faulty batteries.) Other necessary equipment includes a 10 mL syringe for cuff inflation, water-soluble lubricant, and suction equipment.

Two types of blades (available in various sizes) are used with the laryngoscope: a straight blade, such as the Miller, Wisconsin or Flagg blade (Figure 13-38), and a curved blade, such as a MacIntosh blade (Figure 13-39). The tip of a straight blade is applied directly to the epiglottis to expose the vocal cords. A straight blade is usually recommended for infant intubation because it provides greater displacement of the tongue into the floor of the mouth and better visualization of the glottic structures.

Critical Thinking

Ask several paramedics and anaesthesiologists which laryngoscope blade they prefer and why.

Table 13-4 Paediatric weight, OPA, LMA and tracheal tube*

Age	Approximate weight (kg)	Oropharyngeal airway	Laryngeal mask airway	ETT internal diameter (mm)	ETT length (cm)
Birth	3.5	00	1	3.0	10
1 month	4.4	00	1	3.0	10
3 months	6.0	00	1.5	3.5	11
6 months	7.8	00	1.5	4.0	12
9 months	8.9	00	1.5	4.0	12
12 months	9.8	00 or 0	1.5	4.5	13
18 months	11.1	00 or 0	2.0	4.5	13
2 years	12.2	0 or 1	2.0	5.0	14
3 years	14.4	1	2.0	5.0	14
4 years	16.4	1	2.0	5.0	15
5 years	18.5	1	2.0	5.5	15
6 years	20.6	1	2.5	6.0	16
7 years	23.0	1 or 2	2.5	6.0	16
8 years	25.8	1 or 2	2.5	6.5	17
9 years	28.6	1 or 2	2.5	6.5	17
10 years	31.8	2 or 3	3.0	7.0	18
11 years	35.3	2 or 3	3.0	7.0	18

*These are approximate sizes and should be adjusted on the basis of clinical experience. Tracheal tube selection should be based on the child's age or size. One size larger and one size smaller ETT should be selected to allow for individual variations.

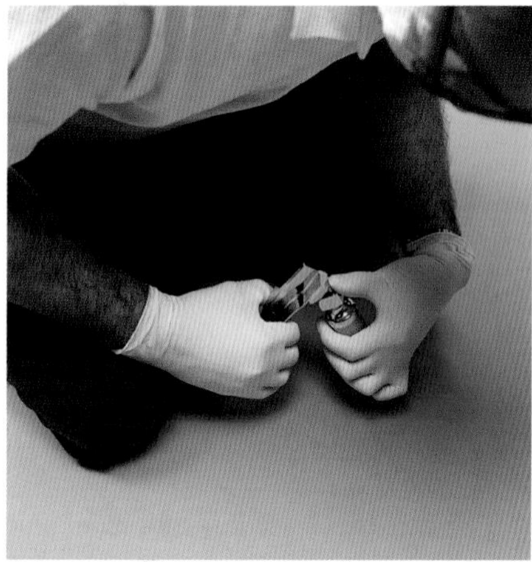

Figure 13-37 Attaching a blade to the handle of a laryngoscope.

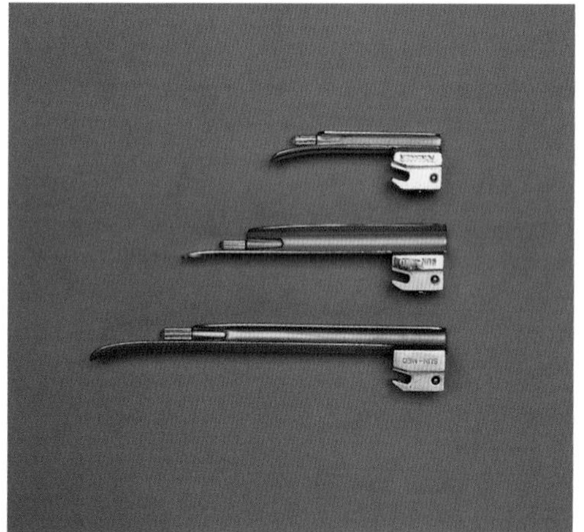

Figure 13-38 Types of straight laryngoscopic blades.

The curved blade design is intended to displace the tongue to the left and to elevate the epiglottis without touching it. It is suggested that this blade provides more room for passage of the tracheal tube and it is generally selected for older children and adults. The choice of blade is a matter of personal preference and the patient's anatomy. Paramedics should acquire expertise in using both curved and straight blades; some patients can be intubated more easily with one type than the other. Occasions may also arise when only one type of blade is available. Versatility with both curved and straight blades may improve the patient's chances of survival.

A malleable stylet (preferably plastic coated) may be inserted through the tracheal tube before intubation (Figure 13-40) although this is not common practice in the UK. The stylet conforms to any desired configuration and may facilitate proper placement of the tracheal tube. If used, the stylet must be recessed at least 1 to 2 cm (½ to ¾ inch) from the distal end of the tracheal tube to prevent injury to the patient. Recession of the stylet tip is maintained by bending the proximal end of the stylet over the proximal rim of the adapter so that it does not advance through the lumen with manipulation of the tracheal tube. If the stylet is allowed to

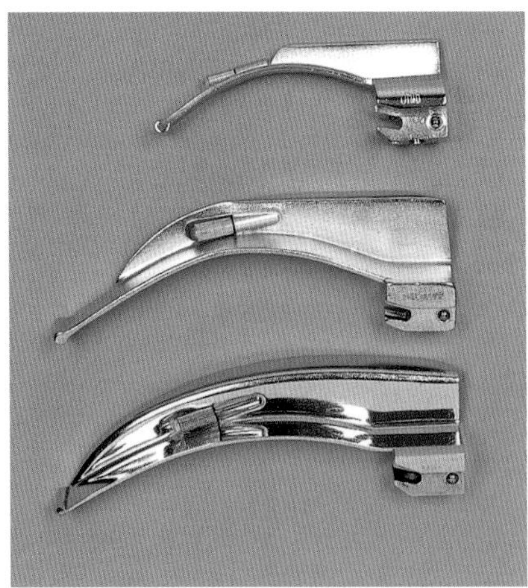

Figure 13-39 Types of curved laryngoscopic blades.

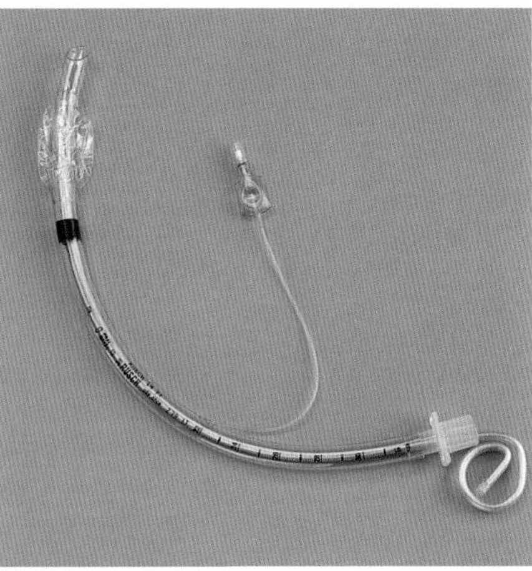

Figure 13-40 Tracheal (ET) tube with malleable stylet.

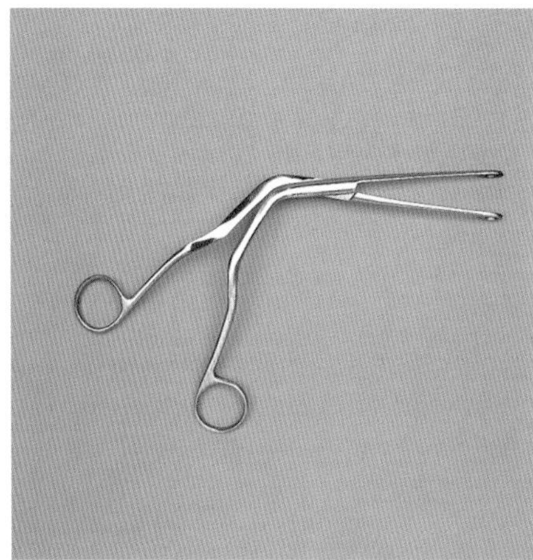

Figure 13-41 Magill forceps.

extend beyond the distal end of the tube, the mucosal surface of the larynx or trachea or the vocal cords may be damaged. A gum elastic bougie can be used to assist with tracheal tube placement. This large flexible device is placed in the trachea, after which the tracheal tube is passed over the bougie and into position in the trachea. Several studies suggest that the gum elastic bougie with coudé tip is more effective than a stylet for intubation when a good view of the glottis is not available.[21,22]

The paramedic also has the use of Magill forceps (Figure 13-41). This is a scissors-style clamp with circular tips that may be used to help direct the tip of the tracheal tube into the larynx during intubation and to remove some foreign bodies.

Preparing for intubation

The patient should be ventilated by other standard procedures before intubation (e.g. bag–valve device). The paramedic should assess the adequacy of ventilation by observing the chest rise and fall during ventilation, by auscultating for breath sounds, and by noting the patient's skin colour. Before intubation, the patient should be ventilated with 100% oxygen. In the pulseless patient, the goal should be to not interrupt chest compressions for more than 10 s. Interruptions for intubation should be minimized by preparing equipment beforehand. Chest compressions should be interrupted only for the placement of the tube and should resume immediately the tube is distal to the vocal cords. When more than one attempt is required, the patient should receive adequate ventilation, oxygenation, and chest compressions before each attempt. The patient's lungs should then be well ventilated and oxygenated for 15–30 s by other means before intubation is attempted again. Pulse oximetry and the electrocardiogram (ECG) should be monitored continuously during intubation attempts. It is reasonable to suggest that no more than three intubation attempts should be made.[23]

Before intubation, all equipment should be examined and tested for defects. The paramedic should check the integrity of the cuff of the tracheal tube by inflating the balloon with 5–8 mL of air and checking for leaks in the cuff or inlet port. The blade of the laryngoscope should be snapped into place to examine the light bulb. The bulb should be secured in its socket and checked for brightness ('light, bright, and tight').

Anatomical considerations

The orotracheal method is the only route currently taught to and authorized for use by paramedics in the UK. It is performed under direct visualization of the glottic opening.

- The trachea is in the midline of the neck and has its superior entry at the level of the glottic opening. With orotracheal intubation the vocal cords should be visualized while the tube is passed to ensure entry into the trachea.
- The uvula is suspended from the midline of the soft palate. It is used as a guide for correct placement of the laryngoscope.
- The epiglottis is attached to the base of the tongue. It should be visualized and elevated to expose the glottis and vocal cords. Pressure on the solid ring of the cricoid can block the oesophagus, reducing the risk of regurgitation during the intubation attempt. It also may help to better visualize the entrance of the trachea by pushing it slightly posteriorly.

The trachea extends to the level of the second intercostal space anteriorly, at which point it divides into the left and right mainstem bronchi. The right main bronchus branches off at a very slight angle to the trachea, whereas the left branches at a 45–60-degree angle.

Note

An tracheal tube that has been advanced too far most often enters the right main bronchus, bypassing and occluding the origin of the left main bronchus. If this occurs, atelectasis and pulmonary insufficiency of the left lung may result. Therefore it is crucial that the paramedic evaluate tracheal tube placement by auscultating both lungs. With proper tracheal tube placement, breath sounds should be of almost equal intensity over both lung fields. Certain pathological conditions (e.g. haemopneumothorax, surgical removal of a lung) may result in unequal breath sounds even when an tracheal tube is in the proper position (Box 13-5).

Orotracheal intubation

In preparation for orotracheal intubation, a patient who is not a trauma victim should be placed in the sniffing position (Figure 13-42). In this position, the neck is flexed at the fifth and sixth cervical vertebrae. The head is extended at the first and second cervical vertebrae. This allows the three axes of the mouth, pharynx, and trachea (oropharyngeolaryngeal axis) to be aligned for direct visualization of the larynx. (When trauma is not a factor, it may help to place a few layers of towels or a pillow under the patient's head to elevate it.)

Box 13-5

Removal of foreign bodies by direct laryngoscopy

Direct laryngoscopy and use of Magill forceps to remove foreign bodies should be attempted only after manual techniques for clearing the airway have proved unsuccessful. The steps for removing a foreign body from the airway by direct laryngoscopy are as follows:

1. Assemble the necessary laryngoscopic equipment. (Have suction ready for immediate use in case of vomiting.)
2. Place the supine patient in the sniffing position (see Figure 13-42) with the head extended.
3. Ventilate the patient with supplemental oxygen if possible.
4. Insert the laryngoscope, visualizing the glottic opening and surrounding structures.
5. If foreign matter is seen, grasp it with Magill forceps and remove it from the airway.
   Note: Forceps removal of foreign matter should be attempted only with direct visualization of the obstruction. Even then, caution must be exercised to avoid soft tissue damage from the teeth of the forceps.
6. If spontaneous respirations resume within 5 s, remove the blade of the laryngoscope and monitor the patient.
7. If spontaneous respirations do not resume, insert an tracheal tube, administer 100% oxygen, and assess the patient's circulatory status.

If complete foreign body obstruction of the upper airway cannot be relieved, needle cricothyroidotomy or transtracheal jet insufflation may be warranted. These advanced airway procedures provide oxygenation until tracheal intubation or tracheostomy can be performed in a controlled setting.

The orotracheal tube should be lubricated. Also, a stethoscope, bougie and/or stylet, and suction equipment (with large-bore catheters) should be readily available. As in all advanced airway procedures, the patient's lungs should be ventilated with 100% oxygen before intubation. The orotracheal intubation procedure is as follows (Figure 13-43a–f):

1. Position yourself at the patient's head.
2. Inspect the oral cavity for secretions and foreign material. Suction the mouth and pharynx if needed.
3. Open the patient's mouth with the fingers of the right hand. Retract the patient's lips on the teeth or gums to avoid pinching them in the blade. The 'crossed-finger technique' may be useful in opening the patient's mouth. To perform this procedure, cross the right thumb and index finger to form an X. Place the thumb on the patient's lower incisors and the index finger on the patient's upper incisors; apply crossed-finger pressure to open the patient's mouth.
4. Grasp the lower jaw with the right hand and draw it forward and upward. Remove any dentures.
5. Holding the laryngoscope in the left hand, insert the blade into the right side of the mouth, displacing the tongue to the left. Move the blade toward the midline and the base of the tongue and identify the uvula. Working gently and avoiding pressure on the lips and teeth are essential.
6. When using a curved blade, advance the tip of the blade into the vallecula, the space between the base of the tongue and the pharyngeal surface of the epiglottis (Figure 13-44a, b). When using a straight blade, insert the tip under the epiglottis (Figure 13-45). The glottic opening is exposed by exerting upward traction on the handle. Never use a prying motion with the handle and do not use the teeth as a fulcrum.
7. Advance the tracheal tube through the right corner of the mouth and, under direct vision, through the vocal cords (Figure 13-46). If a stylet has been used, it should be removed from the tube after the tube passes through the cords into the trachea.
8. After viewing the vocal cords, ensure that the proximal end of the cuffed tube has advanced past the cords about 1 to 2.5 cm (½ to 1 inch) (Figure 13-47). The

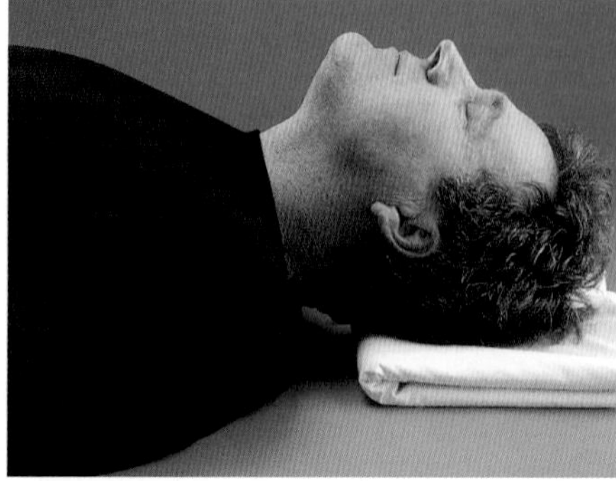

Figure 13-42 Sniffing position.

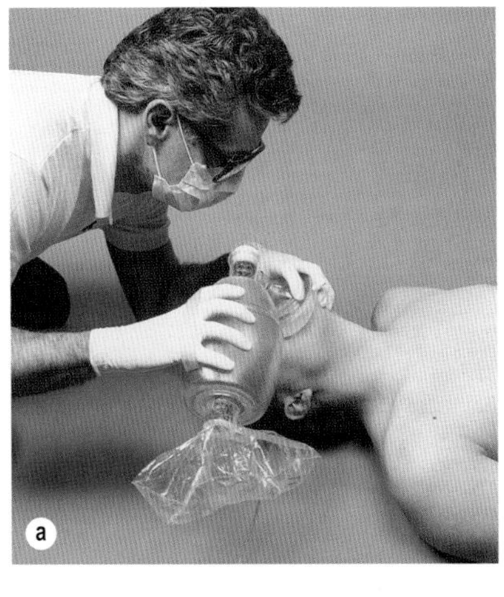

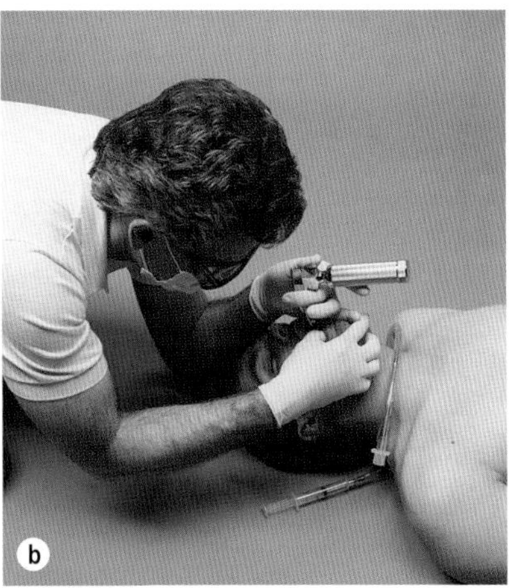

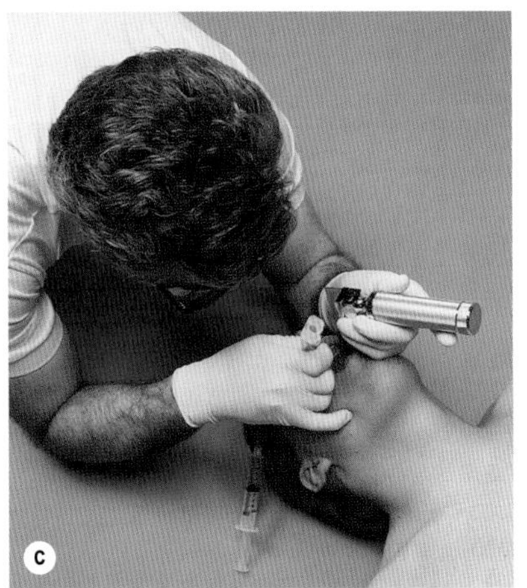

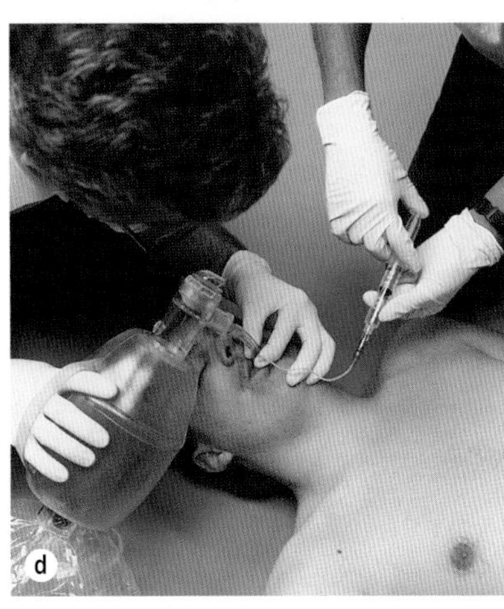

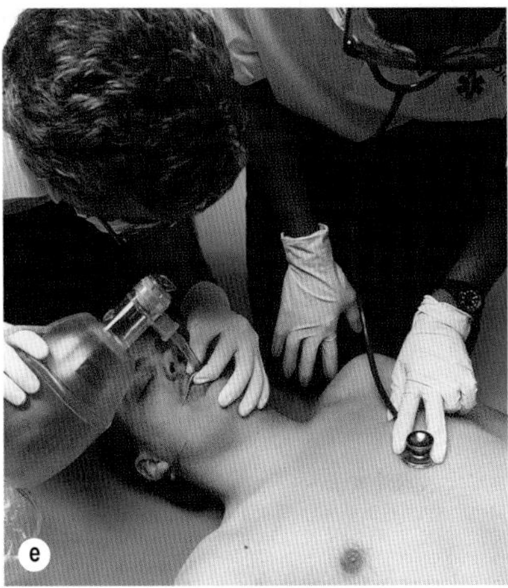

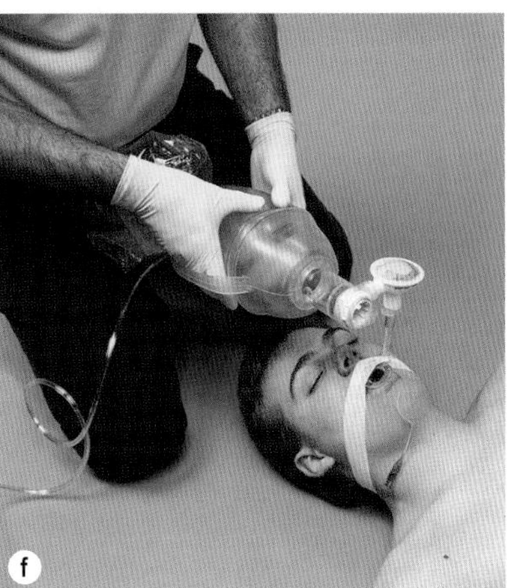

Figure 13-43 Orotracheal intubation. (a) Before intubation, ventilate the patient's lungs with 100% oxygen. (b) Holding the laryngoscope in the left hand, insert the blade into the right side of the patient's mouth, displacing the tongue to the left. (c) Advance the endotracheal (ET) tube through the right corner of the mouth and, under direct vision, through the vocal cords. (d) Inflate the cuff with about 10 mL of air. Ventilate the patient's lungs with a mechanical airway device. (e) Confirm correct placement of the tracheal tube by primary and secondary confirmation methods. (f) Secure the tracheal tube in place and provide ventilatory support with supplemental oxygen.

tip of the tube should then be halfway between the vocal cords and the carina. This position allows some displacement of the tube tip during flexion or extension of the patient's neck without extubation or movement of the tip into the mainstem bronchus. (In the average adult, the distance from teeth to carina is 27 cm (about 11 inches.) The paramedic should observe the depth markings on the tracheal tube during intubation. In the average adult, the tube is properly positioned when the patient's teeth are between the 19 and 23 cm marks on the tube. This places the tip of the tube 2 to 3 cm [¾ to 1½ inches] above the carina.) The average tube depth in men is 22 cm (about 9 inches) ('teeth and tube at 22'). The average tube depth in women is 21 cm (about 8½ inches).

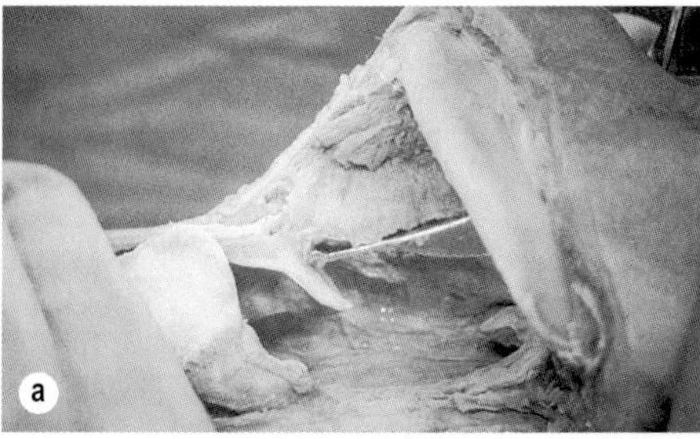

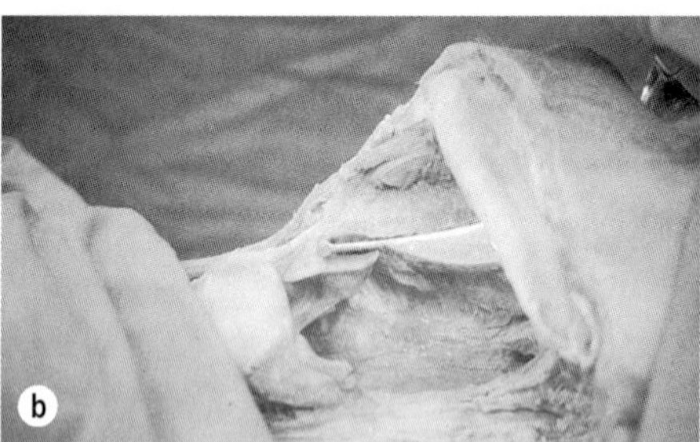

Figure 13-44 (a) When a curved laryngoscopic blade is used, the tip of the blade is inserted into the vallecula. (b) Direct pressure is exerted on the blade upward and toward the feet, using a lifting motion to expose the vocal cords.

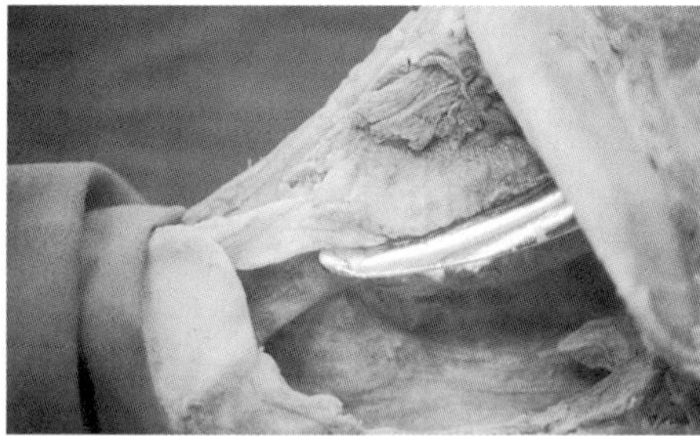

Figure 13-45 A straight laryngoscopic blade is used to lift the epiglottis, directly exposing the vocal cords.

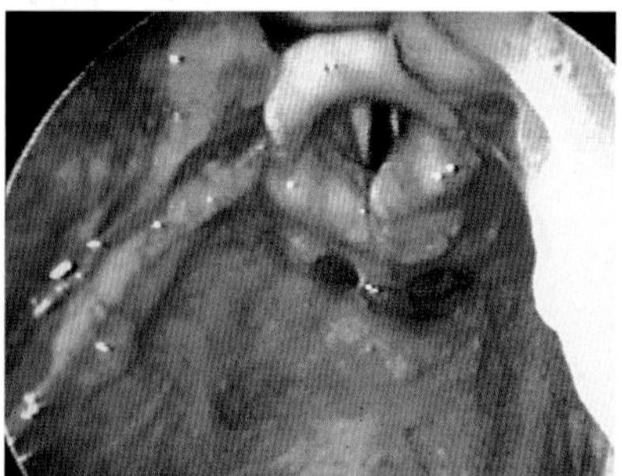

Figure 13-46 View of the vocal cords.

9. Inflate the cuff to prevent any air leaks around the tracheal cuff seal. Avoid high cuff pressures as these have been shown to cause mucosal damage.[24]
10. Attach the tube to a mechanical airway device and ventilate the patient's lungs.
11. During ventilation, confirm accurate tube placement using primary and secondary confirmation methods.[10]

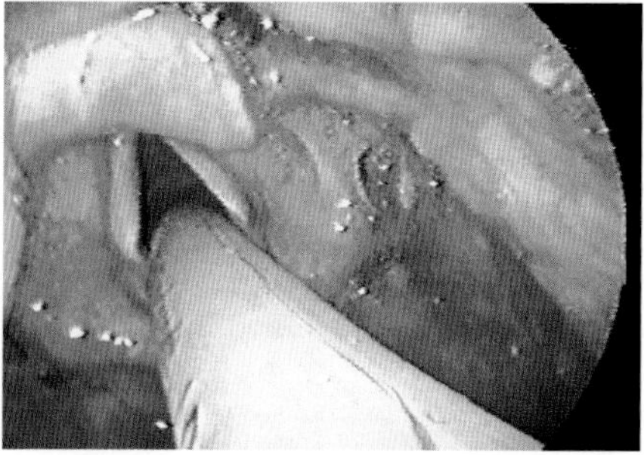

Figure 13-47 Endotracheal (ET) tube passing through the vocal cords.

Primary confirmation methods

Primary assessment includes observation of chest expansion bilaterally, auscultation over the lung fields bilaterally in the axillae (breath sounds should be equal and adequate) and over the epigastrium (breath sounds should not be heard).[10] If chest expansion and lung sounds are absent or there are gurgling sounds across the epigastrium, the tube should be removed. Reattempt intubation after oxygenating the patient's lungs with 100% oxygen for 15–30 s or choose an alternative airway management strategy. When appropriate tube placement has been confirmed, reconfirm and note the tube mark at the front of the patient's teeth. Secure the tube to the patient's head and face with tape or a commercially available device and then re-evaluate lung sounds to ensure that the tube was not inadvertently repositioned. Finally, insert an oral airway or bite block. This prevents the patient from biting down and blocking the airway.

Note

If breath sounds are decreased or absent in the left lung, the orotracheal tube may have passed into the right mainstem bronchus, effectively bypassing the origin of the left main bronchus. If this is the case, the cuff should be deflated and the tube withdrawn 1–2 cm (about ½ to ¾ inch). The cuff then should be re-inflated and tube placement should be verified as above.

Secondary confirmation methods

A second method of determining correct tube placement requires the use of mechanical devices. These include end-tidal carbon dioxide detectors, oesophageal detectors and pulse oximetry for patients who have a perfusing rhythm. Tube confirmation should include both clinical and mechanical methods. Do not rely on a single method. Confirm correct placement immediately after intubation and each time a patient is moved.

End-tidal carbon dioxide detectors Capnography is the measurement of carbon dioxide concentrations in exhaled air and is made possible by end-tidal carbon dioxide detectors. End-tidal carbon dioxide detectors are designed to help verify tracheal tube placement and to reveal inadvertent oesophageal intubation. These devices provide a non-invasive estimate of alveolar ventilation, carbon dioxide production, and arterial carbon dioxide content. Their use as an adjunct to assessment of tracheal tube placement is strongly encouraged.[10]

Note

The colour indicators of colorimetric carbon dioxide (CO_2) detectors can be affected by vomitus. They also can be affected if the patient recently drank a carbonated beverage (if the tracheal tube is placed in the oesophagus).

The two types of carbon dioxide detectors are disposable colorimetric devices and electronic monitors. Colorimetric devices are made of plastic and contain a chemical indicator in the upper part that is sensitive to carbon dioxide gas. When the detector is attached to an tracheal tube, the colour of the indicator changes with elevated carbon dioxide concentrations such as would be expected in the trachea but not in the oesophagus (Figure 13.48). A memory aid for colorimetric devices is as follows: yellow (yes, the tracheal tube is correctly placed in the trachea); tan (think about it; the tracheal tube may not be in the trachea); and purple (problem; the tracheal tube is not in the trachea). Colorimetric devices provide limited information and can only be used for short periods. Exposure to secretions may render them ineffective.

Note

Cardiac output is very low during cardiopulmonary resuscitation. Consequently, the carbon dioxide detector may show no colour change even when the endotracheal (ET) tube is in the trachea. In such cases, a second method of confirming tube placement should be used, such as an oesophageal detector.

Electronic devices can confirm successful tracheal tube placement within seconds of an intubation attempt, as well as subsequent tracheal dislodgement.[10] An infrared analyser measures the percentage of carbon dioxide gas at each phase of respiration (Figure 13-49). Capnometers provide a numerical reading of exhaled CO_2 levels. The information may also be displayed in a digital waveform using a capnograph with printout capability (similar to an ECG tracing) (Box 13-6). Both colorimetric and electronic devices may be useful as indicators of circulation during some cardiac arrest situations because an increase in end-tidal carbon dioxide concentrations seems to be related to effective perfusion during external chest compression.[25] Some capnometers can be used in patients who have not been intubated (i.e. using a device that resembles a nasal cannula). They are helpful in determining the effectiveness of EMS treatments.

Critical Thinking

Your patient is in full arrest; therefore the measurements from your end-tidal carbon dioxide ($EtCO_2$) detector are inconclusive. Also, you can't get the oxygen saturation monitor to work. You are not sure whether you hear breath sounds clearly. What should you do?

Bulb- and syringe-type oesophageal detectors Oesophageal detection devices (e.g. the Toomey syringe) are attached to the end of the tracheal tube (Figure 13-50a, b). They operate on the principle that the oesophagus is a collapsible tube and will create a vacuum when air is removed from the oesophagus. This occurs with the bulb device after it is compressed or when air is withdrawn by the syringe device if the tracheal tube is in the oesophagus. If the tracheal tube has been correctly placed in the trachea, the bulb device easily refills with air or the syringe device is easily aspirated when the plunger is pulled back. Several studies have shown limitations of the oesophageal detector device[26–28] so the ODD should be used to supplement the other techniques previously discussed.

Pulse oximetry

Pulse oximeters (Figure 13-51) help determine how well the patient is being oxygenated by measuring the transmission of red and near-infrared light through arterial beds. Haemoglobin absorbs red and infrared light waves differently when it is bound with oxygen (oxyhaemoglobin) and when it is not (reduced haemoglobin). Oxyhaemoglobin absorbs more infrared than red light whilst reduced haemoglobin

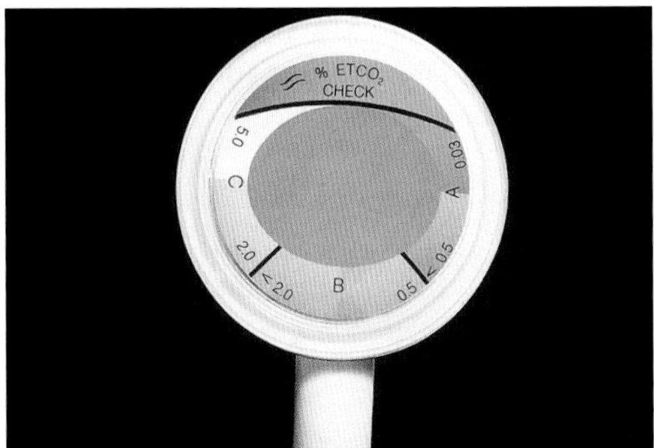

Figure 13-48 Colorimetric end-tidal carbon dioxide (CO_2) detector.

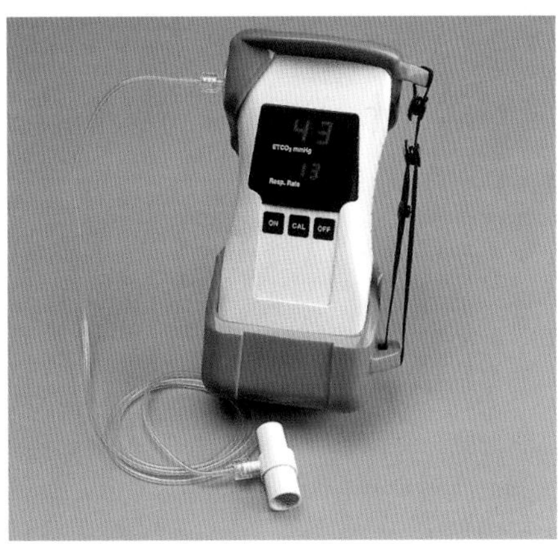

Figure 13-49 Digital (or electronic) end-tidal carbon dioxide (CO_2) detector.

Box 13-6

Capnography waveforms

Capnography waveforms on the monitor screen are condensed to provide assessment information in a 4-second view. Printouts of waveforms provide the same information in 'real time' and may differ in duration from that of the monitor screen. The following are example waveforms for both intubated and non-intubated patients.*

Normal ranges:

Arterial $PaCO_2$	35–45 mmHg
Capnography $EtCO_2$	35–45 mmHg (4–6 vol%)

Capnography – intubated patients

May be used to:
Verify tracheal tube placement
Monitor or detect tracheal tube dislodgement
Monitor loss of circulatory function
Assess adequacy of CPR compressions
Confirm return of spontaneous circulation

Capnography – non-intubated patients

May be used to:
Assess asthma and COPD
Document and monitor procedural sedation
Detect apnoea or inadequate breathing
Measure hypoventilation
Evaluate hyperventilation

End-tidal CO_2

Causes of elevated end-tidal CO_2

Decreased ventilation secondary to:
- Head trauma
- Overdose
- Respiratory failure (severe asthma, COPD)
- Sedation
- Stroke

Increased CO_2 production
- Fever
- Shivering

Causes of low end-tidal CO_2

Ventilation problem
- Oesophageal intubation
- Airway obstruction

Inadequate blood flow
- Cardiac arrest
  - Lower if poor compressions
  - Lower values predict poor outcome
- Tension pneumothorax
- Pericardial tamponade
- Reduced cardiac output

Ventilation–perfusion (VQ) mismatch
- Pulmonary embolism

Decreased production of CO_2
- Hypothermia

Sampling error
- Inadequate tidal volume delivery
- CO_2 sampling tubing blocked 1*473

*Level of sedation and severity of conditions may affect respiratory rate and $EtCO_2$ level in patients.

Box 13-7

Oxygen saturation and partial pressure (Po_2)

With 90% saturation, Po_2 drops to 60 mmHg
With 75% saturation, Po_2 drops to 40 mmHg
With 50% saturation, Po_2 drops to 27 mmHg

absorbs more red than infrared light. Pulse oximetry reveals arterial saturation by measuring this difference.

The oximeter probe is placed on an area of thin tissue, such as a finger, toe, or ear lobe. One side of the probe sends wavelengths of light through the arterial bed; the other side detects the presence of red or infrared light. Using this balance of red and infrared colours, the oximeter calculates the oxygen saturation of the blood and displays it on the monitor screen.

The percentage of haemoglobin saturated with oxygen is denoted as the Sao_2. It depends on a number of factors, including the Pco_2, pH, temperature, and whether the haemoglobin is normal or altered. The lower range of normal for the Sao_2 is 93–95%, the upper range is 99–100%. Once the Sao_2 falls below 90% (corresponding to a Po_2 of 60 mmHg), further decreases are associated with a marked decline in oxygen content (Box 13-7).

Difficulties and inaccuracies may result from the use of pulse oximeters. Therefore, paramedics should consider them only as another tool to assist the monitoring of a patient's oxygenation levels. Circumstances that may produce false readings include the following:[29]

- dyshaemoglobinaemia (haemoglobin saturation with compounds other than oxygen [e.g. carbon monoxide, methaemoglobinaemia])
- excessive ambient light (sunlight, fluorescent lights) on the oximeter's sensor probe
- patient movement
- hypotension
- hypothermia/vasoconstriction
- patient use of vasoconstrictive drugs
- patient use of nail polish
- jaundice.

Potential complications from intubation procedures

- Lacerated lips or tongue (oral)
- Dental trauma from the laryngoscope (oral)
- Lacerated pharyngeal or tracheal mucosa
- Tracheal rupture
- Avulsion of an arytenoid cartilage
- Vocal cord injury
- Vomiting and aspiration of stomach contents
- Significant release of adrenaline and noradrenaline, leading to hypertension, tachycardia, or cardiac rhythm disturbances
- Vagal stimulation (particularly in infants and children), resulting in bradycardia and hypotension

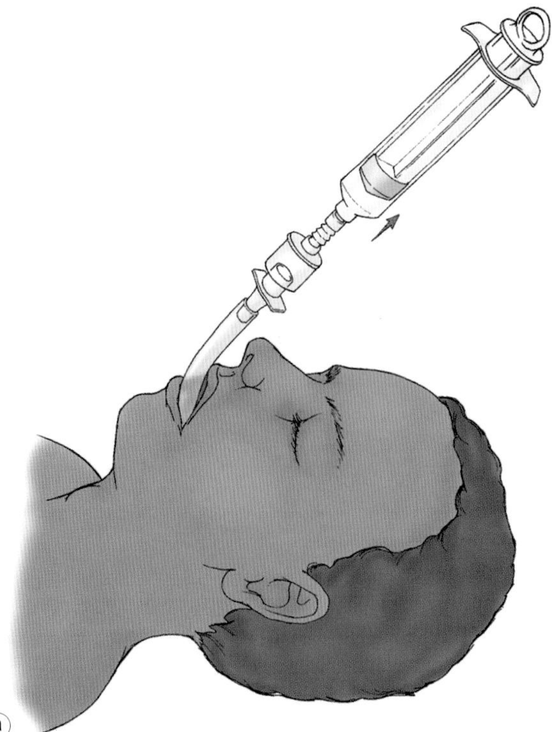

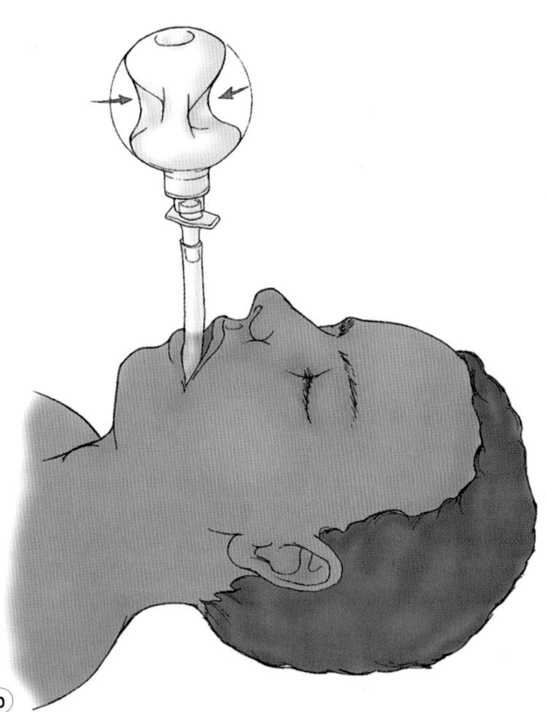

Figure 13-50 Oesophageal intubation detector. (a) Syringe. (b) Bulb.

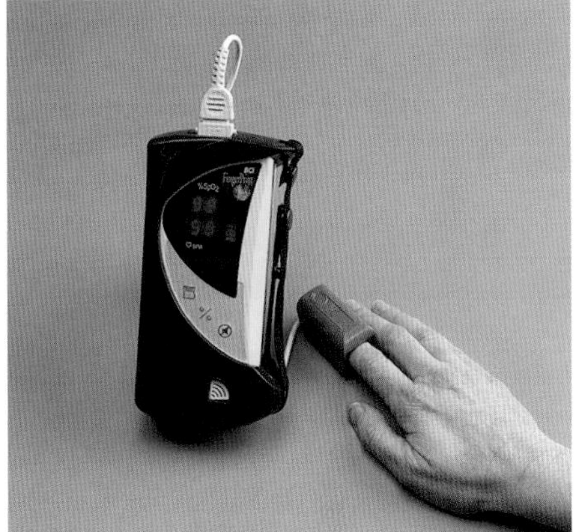

Figure 13-51 Pulse oximeter.

- Increased intracranial pressure in patients with a head injury
- Accidental intubation of the oesophagus
- Accidental intubation of a bronchus
- In addition, rupture of the cuff, inflation port malfunction, or severance or kinking of the inflation tube may cause cuff malfunction and air leakage.

Intubation with spinal precautions

Nasal or oral intubation may be performed in patients suspected of having a spinal injury. The procedure is as follows:

1. Auscultate for bilateral breath sounds while manual or mechanical ventilations are in progress. This provides a baseline.
2. One rescuer should apply manual in-line stabilization from the patient's side. The rescuer places the hands over the patient's ears. The little fingers should be under the occipital skull. The thumbs should be on the face over the maxillary sinuses. Stabilization (without distraction) should be maintained in a neutral position throughout the procedure. Thin padding under the patient's head may be necessary to maintain neutral, in-line positioning.
3. In one method of intubation, the primary paramedic is positioned at the patient's head. The legs straddle the patient's shoulders and arms, and the patient's head is secured between the paramedic's thighs. The grip of the primary rescuer in this position and of the other rescuer (from the side) prevents the head from moving during the intubation. In this position, the primary paramedic may need to lean back to visualize the vocal cords (Figure 13-52). With another method, the primary paramedic lies prone at the patient's head, and the other rescuer (at the patient's side) maintains the in-line position alone (Figure 13-53).

Face-to-face orotracheal intubation

Face-to-face orotracheal intubation (Figure 13-54) may be used when the paramedic cannot take a position above the patient's head (e.g. the patient is in a sitting position). In this method of intubation, a second rescuer maintains in-line immobilization of the patient's neck and head from behind the patient. The primary rescuer takes a position

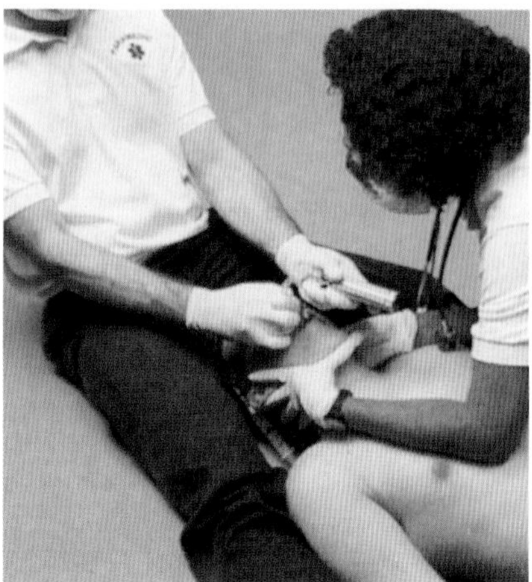

Figure 13-52 Intubation in a sitting position.

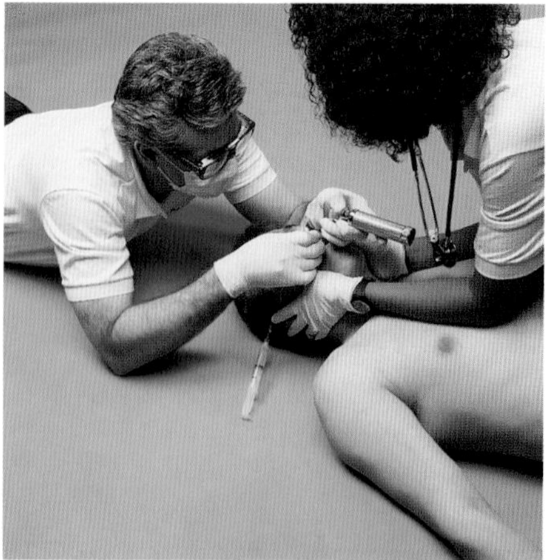

Figure 13-53 Intubation in a prone position.

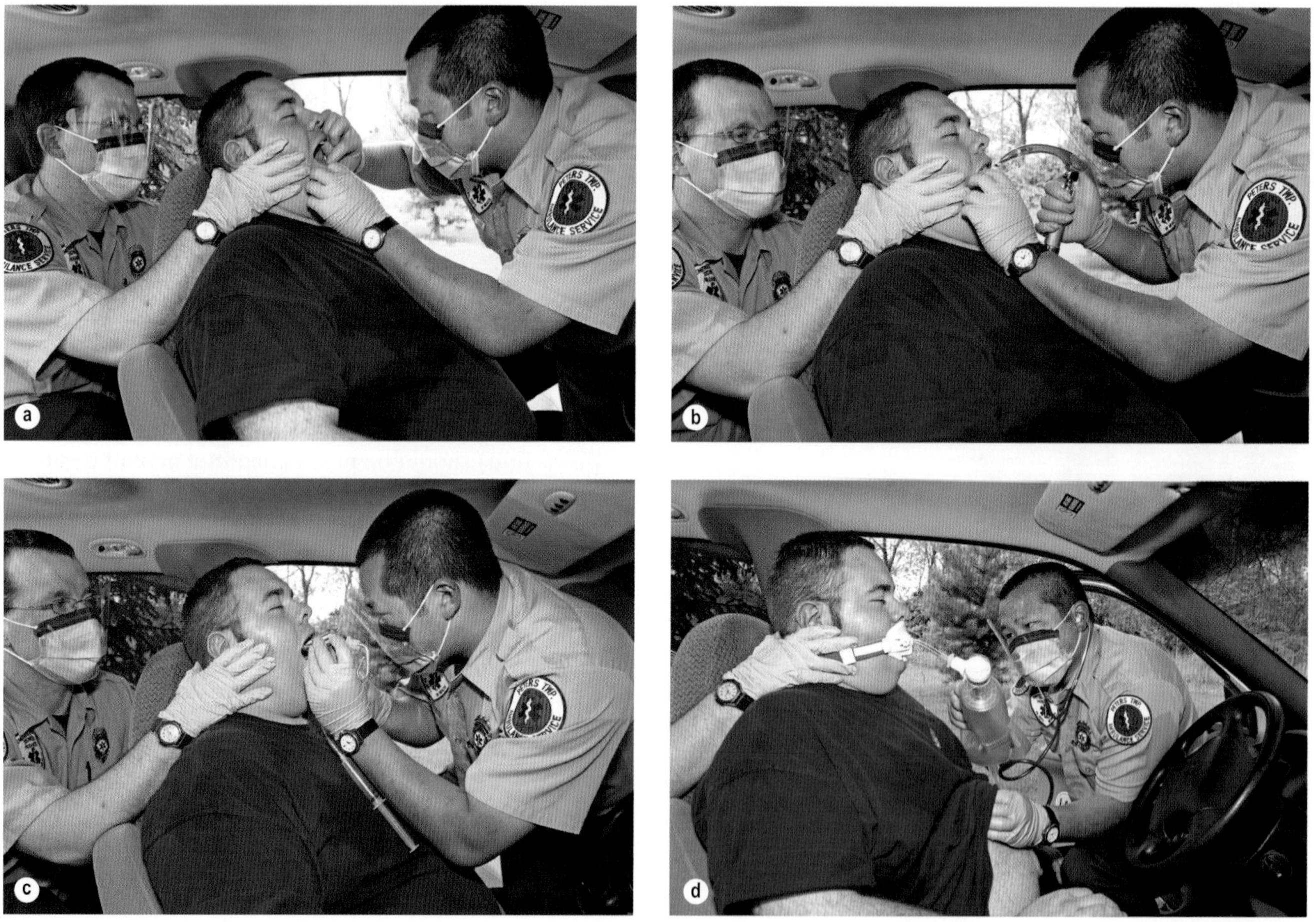

Figure 13-54 Face-to-face orotracheal intubation. (a) One rescuer maintains in-line immobilization. The primary rescuer takes a position facing the patient and opens the person's mouth. The primary rescuer then should follow these steps: (b) Holding the laryngoscope in the right hand, insert it into the patient's mouth. (c) With the left hand, pass the endotracheal (ET) tube into the mouth and through the vocal cords. (d) Inflate the cuff. Ventilate the patient and confirm correct placement of the tube. Secure the tube in place.

facing the patient and opens the patient's mouth with the left hand. The laryngoscope is held in the right hand, and the blade is inserted into the patient's mouth, following the normal curve of the tongue. After visualizing the vocal cords from a position above the patient's mouth, the primary rescuer passes an tracheal tube between the cords with the left hand. The cuff is inflated, and the syringe removed. The patient then is ventilated with a bag–mask device. After proper placement has been confirmed as previously described, the tracheal tube is secured in place.

Extubation

The tracheal tube is not usually removed in the prehospital setting; however, the patient may develop intolerance to the tube. If time allows, the patient's lungs should first be ventilated with 100% oxygen. To remove the tracheal tube, the paramedic should tilt the patient or backboard to one side and proceed as follows:

1. Have suction available. (The oral cavity and the area above the cuff should be suctioned before the tracheal tube is removed.)
2. Deflate the cuff completely.
3. Swiftly withdraw the tube on cough or expiration.
4. Assess the patient's respiratory status.
5. Provide high-concentration oxygen; assist ventilations as needed.

Note

Patients who are awake are at high risk of laryngospasm immediately after extubation. Also, they may be difficult to re-intubate should respiratory distress or failure occur again.

Advantages of tracheal intubation

- It provides complete airway control.
- It helps prevent aspiration.
- It prevents gastric distension.
- It may provide a route for administration of some drugs.
- Positive-pressure ventilation can be delivered.
- Tracheal suctioning is possible.
- High concentrations of oxygen and large volumes of ventilation can be delivered.

Special considerations for paediatric intubations

In addition to the differences in airway and ventilation procedures for paediatric patients, the anatomical differences of the paediatric airway must be considered.[30] These anatomical differences include the following:

1. The infant's upper airway is relatively small; the tongue is disproportionately large. Therefore, posterior displacement of the tongue easily obstructs the airway. In addition, the larger tongue of the paediatric patient tends to make laryngoscopy more difficult.
2. The epiglottis is shaped like the Greek letter omega (ω). It is narrower and longer in children than in the adult. Because of this, the epiglottis is more difficult to control with a laryngoscopic blade. The larynx lies more anteriorly in relation to the base of the tongue than in the adult and is elevated under the base of the tongue, making visualization more difficult. The glottic opening is at the third cervical vertebra in premature neonates, the third to fourth cervical vertebra in term neonates, and the fourth to fifth cervical vertebra in adults.
3. During the first few months of life, the infant's vocal cords slope from back to front. As a result, the tracheal tube frequently gets hung up in the angle formed by the cords. This problem can be minimized by rotating the tracheal tube or by having a second rescuer perform the Sellick manoeuvre during intubation.
4. The cricoid cartilage is arguably the narrowest part of the airway in the infant and young child although new evidence suggests it may still be the glottis. As the child reaches 8 to 10 years of age, the vocal cords become the narrowest part. This remains the case into adulthood.
5. The distance from the vocal cords to the carina varies and can be correlated with the patient's height. This distance is about 4 to 5 cm (2 to 2½ inches) at birth and 6 to 7 cm (3 to 3½ inches) by 6 years of age. During placement of the tracheal tube, the tube should be advanced until breath sounds are lost unilaterally (usually on the left side). It should then be withdrawn slowly until breath sounds return, indicating that the tube tip is at the carina. After the return of breath sounds, the tube should be withdrawn 2 to 3 cm (¾ to 1½ inches) farther, placing it at a safe distance above the carina and below the cords. The tube should then be secured with tape or a commercial device.
6. Children use the diaphragm as the major muscle for ventilation so require full diaphragmatic excursion to breathe. Gastric distension caused by swallowing air or artificial ventilation can inhibit the child's respiratory efforts. Infants are nose breathers until 3 to 5 months of age.
7. Deciduous teeth begin to develop at about 6 months and are lost between 6 and 8 years. They may become dislodged during airway procedures such as intubation and oral airway insertion and by the child biting on the airway.

Note

The correct depth of insertion of an endotracheal (ET) tube in children over age 2 can be approximated by adding one half the patient's age to 12.

$$\text{Depth of insertion (cm)} = \text{age}/2 + 12$$

As an alternative, the depth of insertion can be estimated by multiplying the internal diameter of the tube by 3.[7]

$$\text{Depth of insertion (cm)} = \text{tracheal tube internal diameter} \times 3$$

During any airway procedure, the paramedic should remember that the airway structures of children are very fragile and easily damaged. Therefore, great care must be taken not to injure these patients.

Pharmacological adjuncts to airway management and ventilation

The use of pharmacological adjuncts to airway management is being taught to paramedics on critical care courses; the techniques described below MUST NOT be used unless the paramedic is authorized to do so.

Sedation is sometimes used in airway management and ventilation to reduce anxiety, induce amnesia, and decrease the gag reflex. Possible indications for sedation include combative patients, patients who require aggressive airway management but who are too alert to tolerate intubation, and agitated trauma patients. The classes of drugs commonly used for sedation in these situations are tranquillizers, barbiturates, benzodiazepines and narcotics.

Note

Sedating a patient with a poor airway is risky. The patient may suffer respiratory arrest.

Paralytic agents in emergency intubation

Paralysis involves the use of neuromuscular blocking drugs and may be used for emergency intubation. These drugs are indicated for combative patients who need to be intubated; for instance, a patient suffering a head injury may be agitated and combative. These drugs should not be used in the following situations:

- patients who will be difficult to ventilate (e.g. patients with facial hair)
- patients who will be difficult to intubate (e.g. patients with short necks, obstructions).

Pharmacology

As described in Chapter 12, neuromuscular blockers produce skeletal muscle paralysis. They do this by binding to the nicotinic receptor for acetylcholine (ACh) at the neuromuscular junction. To review, this junction is the point of contact between the nerve ending and the muscle fibre. When nerve impulses pass through this junction, ACh and other chemicals are released, which causes the muscle to contract. The two types of neuromuscular blocking drugs are depolarizing agents and non-depolarizing agents.

Depolarizing agents invade the neuromuscular junction and bind to the receptors for ACh. These drugs produce depolarization of the muscular membrane and often lead to fasciculations (uncontrollable muscle twitching). These drugs may also lead to some muscular contractions. An example of a depolarizing agent is succinylcholine. Suxamethonium has a rapid onset of action yet it has the briefest duration of action of all the neuromuscular blocking drugs. This makes it the drug of choice for emergency tracheal intubation.

Non-depolarizing agents also bind to the receptors for ACh; however, they block the uptake of ACh at the neuromuscular junction without initiating depolarization of the muscle membrane. Examples of non-depolarizing drugs include vecuronium and pancuronium. These drugs have a longer onset and duration than depolarizing agents.

Neuromuscular blocking agents produce complete paralysis, so ventilatory support must be provided. Ventilation and oxygenation must be closely monitored to ensure that they are adequate. If the patient is conscious, the paramedic should explain the effects of the medication before administering it. Administration of atropine should be strongly considered, particularly in children, before a blocking agent is administered. Lidocaine given prior to administration of a blocking agent may blunt any increase in intracranial pressure associated with intubation. Finally, diazepam, etomidate, midazolam, or another sedative approved by the Trust should be used in any conscious patient to whom a blocking agent is administered; neuromuscular blocking agents do not inhibit pain or seizure activity.

Rapid sequence intubation

Rapid sequence intubation (RSI) involves the administration of a potent sedative and a neuromuscular blocking agent at the same time for the purpose of ET intubation. The blocking agent most often used is suxamethonium. RSI provides optimal intubation conditions. It also minimizes the risk of aspiration of gastric contents. RSI is indicated in the following situations:[31]

- emergency intubation is warranted
- the patient has a 'full' stomach
- intubation is predicted to be successful (Box 13-8)
- if intubation fails, ventilation is predicted to be successful.

Box 13-8

Signs for assessing the difficulty of intubation

The potential difficulty of an intubation can be judged by the accessibility of the oropharynx. Visibility of the oropharynx ranges from complete visualization, including the tonsillar pillars (indicating an easy intubation), to no visualization at all, with the uvula pressed against the tongue (indicating a difficult intubation).

Other situations that indicate a potentially difficult intubation include the following:

- an immobilized trauma patient
- children
- a short neck that makes visualization of the cords more difficult
- prominent upper incisors that limit working space
- receding mandible that may limit the line of vision
- limited jaw opening
- limited cervical mobility
- upper airway conditions (e.g. burns, neck injury, epiglottitis)
- facial trauma
- laryngeal trauma.

RSI is not indicated for patients in cardiac arrest or deeply comatose patients when immediate intubation is required. Relative contraindications include concern that intubation or mask ventilation would be unsuccessful; significant facial or laryngeal oedema, trauma or distortion; or a spontaneously breathing patient who requires upper airway muscle tone and positioning (e.g. upper airway obstruction, epiglottitis).[32]

RSI is an organized approach to tracheal intubation. It involves specific steps and actions that lead to rapid sedation and paralysis without positive-pressure ventilation once the procedure begins. The purpose of RSI is to achieve optimal and rapid tracheal intubation in patients who are at risk for aspiration. RSI requires special training and authorization and should not be carried out by non-authorized paramedics. The effectiveness of RSI performed in the field should be monitored through a quality improvement process. RSI is intended to take the patient from a conscious, breathing state to a state of unconsciousness and is accomplished with complete neuromuscular paralysis. Intubation is performed without interposed mechanical ventilation. The six steps of RSI (the six 'Ps') are preparation, pre-oxygenation, pre-treatment, paralysis (with sedation), placement of the tube, and post-intubation management (Box 13-9). Each step is described below.

Technique

1. *Preparation*

- Assess the patient for difficulty of intubation (e.g. using the Mallampati score in Box 13-8).
- Prepare all drugs and equipment.
- Ensure one or more patent IV lines.
- Explain the procedure to the patient.

2. *Pre-oxygenation (to be done simultaneously with preparation)*

- Pre-oxygenate the patient with 100% oxygen for 5 min (an essential step of the 'no-bagging' approach of RSI).
- Consider the use of a pulse oximeter.

3. *Pre-treatment (to be done 3 min before intubation)*

- Consider lidocaine to protect against a rise in intracranial pressure and to prevent laryngospasm.
- Consider beta-blockers or opioids to reduce sympathoadrenal response (e.g. a drop in blood pressure) to intubation.

4. *Paralysis (with sedation)*

- Administer a sedative (per protocol) to produce unconsciousness. This should be immediately followed by a rapid push of the neuromuscular blocker (see the EDI).

Box 13-9

The six 'Ps' of rapid sequence intubation

1. Preparation
2. Pre-oxygenation
3. Pre-treatment
4. Paralysis (with sedation)
5. Placement of the tube
6. Post-intubation management

Critical Thinking

How would you decide whether a patient needs more sedation after a paralytic has been given?

- Apply cricoid pressure as the patient loses consciousness to prevent vomiting. (Once neuromuscular blockade has been established, active vomiting cannot occur.)
- Do not initiate ventilations unless the patient's oxygen saturation falls below 90%.
- Within 45 s of administration of suxamethonium, the patient will be relaxed enough for intubation.

5. *Placement*

- Perform orotracheal intubation and confirm placement.

6. *Post-intubation management*

- Secure the tube in place.
- Begin mechanical ventilation.
- Monitor the patient continuously.

If RSI is unsuccessful and the patient cannot be intubated, the patient's airway should be managed by other means (e.g. cricothyroidotomy).

Translaryngeal cannula ventilation

Translaryngeal cannula ventilation is also known as percutaneous transtracheal ventilation and needle cricothyroidotomy. It may be valuable in the initial stabilization of a patient whose airway cannot be managed by the usual manual measures. It may also be valuable in patients who cannot be intubated by oral or nasal means. It is a temporary procedure. It provides oxygenation when the airway is obstructed as a result of oedema of the glottis, fracture of the larynx or severe oropharyngeal haemorrhage. Translaryngeal cannula ventilation requires special training and should not be carried out by those not authorized to do so.

Description

Translaryngeal cannula ventilation provides high-volume, high-pressure oxygenation of the lungs. This occurs through cannulation of the trachea below the glottis. The procedure delivers a large volume of oxygen through a small port at high pressure to the lungs. This oxygen delivery (350 kPa (50 psi)) is much greater than can be achieved with other methods (e.g. 7 kPa (1 psi) with a therapy regulator).

Necessary equipment

- A 12- or 14-gauge over-the-needle catheter with a 5 or 10 mL syringe.
- Alcohol swabs.
- Adhesive tape or appropriate ties.
- Pressure-regulating valve and pressure gauge attached to a high-pressure (206–412 kPa (30–60 psi)) oxygen supply. (Most oxygen cylinders and regulators can provide 350 kPa (50 psi) at 15 L/min or when opened to flush.)
- High-pressure tubing connecting the high-pressure regulating valve to a hand-operated release valve (1.5 m tubing is recommended).

- A release valve connected by tubing to the catheter (this may be provided via a Y- or T-connector, through a three-way stopcock directly attached to the high-pressure tubing, or by cutting a hole in the oxygen line to provide a 'whistle-stop' effect).

Technique

The steps in translaryngeal cannula ventilation are as follows (Figure 13-55a–d):

1. Make sure the patient is supine. Also make sure the cricothyroid membrane has been identified. (If a spinal injury is suspected, in-line stabilization may be provided as for nasal and tracheal intubation.)
2. Stabilize the larynx using the thumb and middle finger of one hand. With the other hand, palpate the small depression below the thyroid cartilage (the 'Adam's apple'). Slide the index finger down to locate the cricothyroid membrane.
3. Insert the needle of the syringe downward through the midline of the membrane at a 45–60-degree angle toward the patient's carina. Apply negative pressure to the syringe during insertion. The entrance of air into the syringe indicates that the needle is in the trachea (Figure 13-56a).
4. Advance the catheter over the needle toward the carina and remove the needle and syringe (Figure 13-56b). Care must be taken not to kink the catheter when removing the needle and syringe.
5. Hold the hub of the catheter to prevent accidental dislodgement while providing ventilation. Remove the end of the oxygen tubing from the hub of the cannula and connect it to the oxygen regulator. Provide for a release valve as described before.

Critical Thinking

What conditions could make it difficult to locate the anatomical landmarks for translaryngeal cannulation or cricothyroidotomy?

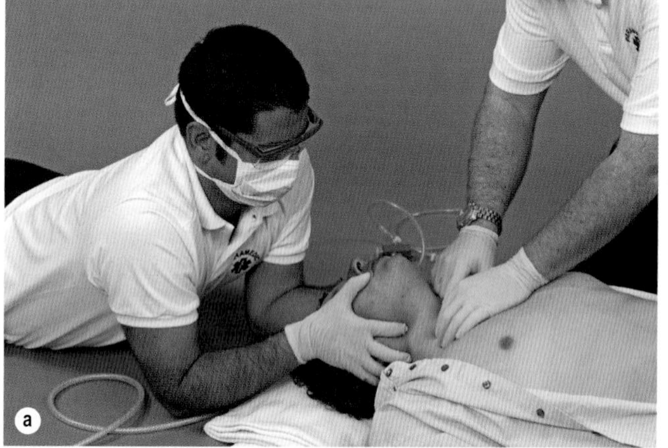

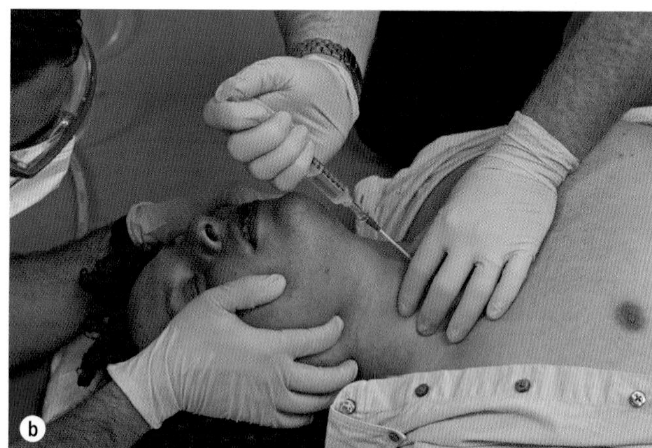

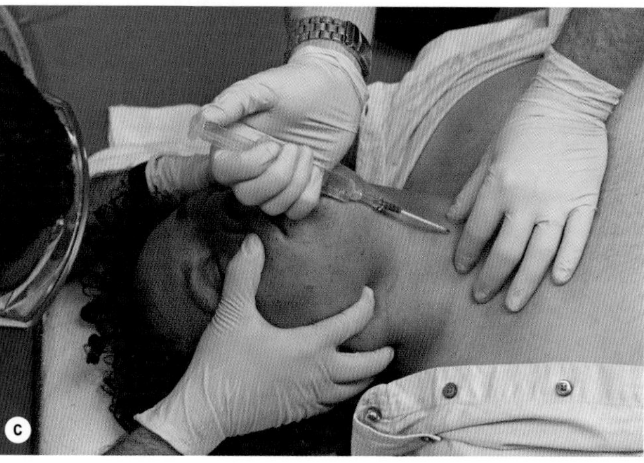

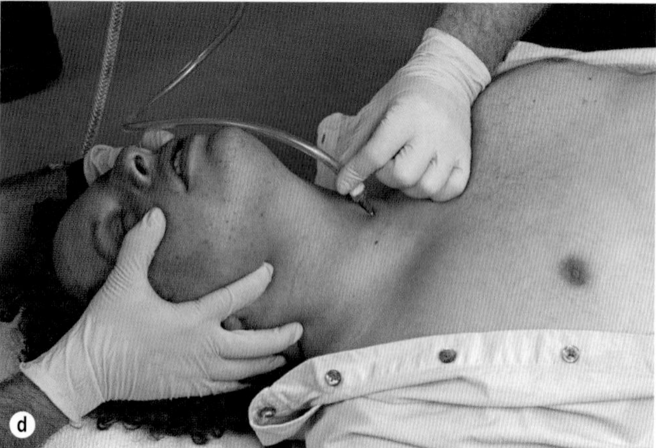

Figure 13-55 Translaryngeal cannula ventilation. (a) Stabilize the larynx and identify the cricothyroid membrane. (b) Insert the needle of the syringe downward through the midline of the membrane toward the carina. (c) While inserting the needle, draw back on the plunger of the syringe. If air enters the syringe, the needle is in the trachea. (d) After removing the needle and syringe, stabilize the catheter and connect the end of the oxygen tubing from the hub of the cannula to the oxygen regulator. Provide for a release valve.

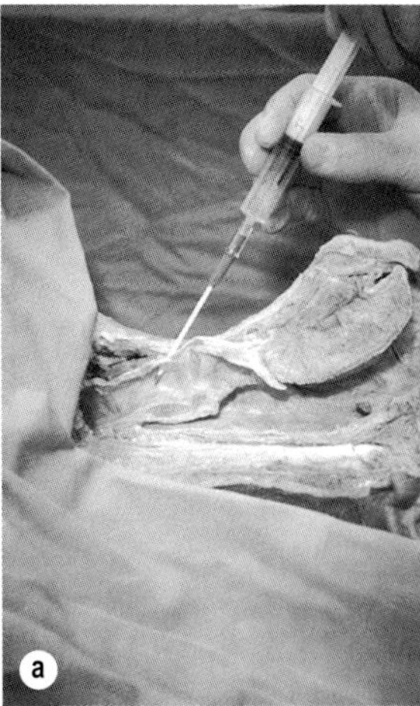

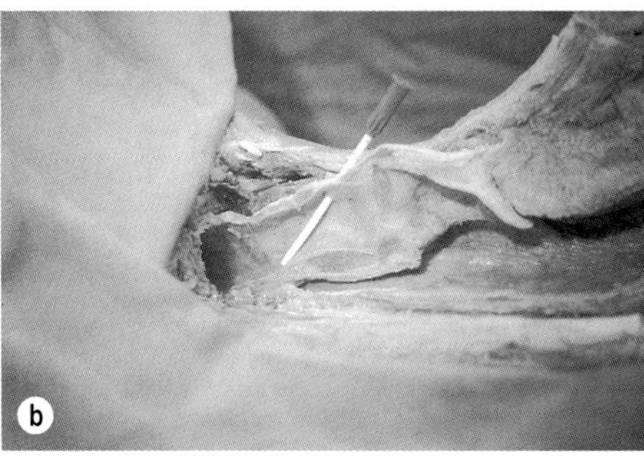

Figure 13-56 (a) Insert a large-bore catheter through the cricothyroid membrane, directing it toward the feet. While inserting the catheter, draw back on the plunger of the syringe; when air enters the syringe, the needle is in the airway. (b) Slide the catheter off the stylet into the larynx.

When the release valve is closed, oxygen under pressure is introduced into the trachea. The pressure is adjusted to a level that allows adequate lung expansion. The patient's chest must be observed closely. The release valve must be opened to allow for exhalation. The correct ratio of inflation to deflation varies. It depends on whether upper airway obstruction is present. For an open upper airway, an inspiratory to expiratory ratio of 1:4 s is adequate. Ratios may need to be extended to prevent barotrauma (injuries caused by excessive pressures, such as pneumothorax, when the upper airway is obstructed.[33]

Note

If the chest remains inflated during exhalation, a complete upper airway obstruction may be present. In such cases a longer expiratory time should be allowed. If this does not produce adequate deflation, a second large-bore catheter may be inserted through the cricothyroid membrane next to the first one. If the chest remains distended, a cricothyroidotomy is needed.

Advantages

- It is the least invasive of surgical procedures.
- It can be initiated quickly.
- When performed by a trained paramedic, it is simple, inexpensive, and effective.
- Minimal spinal movement is needed for insertion.

Disadvantages

- The technique is an invasive procedure.
- Constant monitoring is required.
- Jet ventilation is required
- The airway is not protected.
- The procedure does not allow for efficient elimination of carbon dioxide.
- The patient's lungs may be adequately ventilated for only 30–45 min.

Possible complications

- High pressure during ventilation and air entrapment may cause pneumothorax.
- Haemorrhage may occur at the insertion site. The thyroid and oesophagus also may be perforated if the needle is advanced too far.
- Direct suctioning of secretions is impossible.
- Subcutaneous emphysema may occur.

Removal

Translaryngeal cannula ventilation is a temporary emergency procedure. It provides time for the use of other airway management techniques. Removal should follow only after successful orotracheal or nasotracheal intubation or after a cricothyroidotomy or a tracheostomy has been performed. Removal involves withdrawing the catheter and dressing the wound.

Summary

- A key aspect of emergency care is a full understanding of the respiratory system. Another is mastery of airway management and ventilation techniques.
- Causes of inadequate ventilation include upper airway obstruction and aspiration by inhalation. The most crucial lifesaving action for any patient who has respiratory problems from any cause is establishing and maintaining an open airway. This should always be the first priority of patient care.
- Essential parameters of airway evaluation include rate, regularity, effort, and recognition of airway problems that might indicate respiratory distress.
- The most common form of oxygen used in the prehospital setting is pure oxygen gas. This is delivered in litres per minute (LPM). Therapy regulators are used to deliver a safe pressure of oxygen to patients. Flowmeters control the amount of oxygen delivered to the patient. Several oxygen delivery devices provide supplemental

Summary—cont'd

oxygen to patients who have spontaneous respirations. They are the nasal cannula, simple facemask, partial rebreather mask, non-rebreather mask and Venturi mask.

- In the prehospital setting, ventilation can be provided in several ways. These methods include rescue breathing (mouth-to-mouth, mouth-to-nose, mouth-to-stoma), mouth-to-mask breathing, use of bag–valve devices and automatic transport ventilators.
- Emergency airway management should progress rapidly from the least to the most invasive techniques. Manual techniques for airway management include the head-tilt chin-lift method, the jaw-thrust and the jaw-thrust without head-tilt.
- Suction catheters are used to clear the air passages of secretions and debris.
- Mechanical devices for airway management include the nasal airway, oral airway, tracheal intubation, laryngeal mask airway and translaryngeal cannula ventilation.
- End-tidal carbon dioxide detectors, pulse oximeters, and oesophageal detectors can help the paramedic determine whether an tracheal tube has been placed correctly.
- In the management of a child's airway, the differences in the paediatric airway must be considered. Compared to the adult airway, the child's upper airway structures have very different proportions. Their orientation to each other also differs. Smaller bag–valve devices are needed for infants and children. These reduce the chance of over-inflation and barotrauma.
- Rapid sequence intubation (RSI) involves administration of a potent sedative and a neuromuscular blocking drug at the same time. These are administered for the purpose of ET intubation.

References

1. Resuscitation Council UK. Resuscitation Guidelines 2005. Online. Available www.resus.org.uk 3 February 2009
2. American Heart Association 1997 Basic life support for healthcare providers. American Heart Association, Dallas TX
3. Rovin JD, Rodgers BM 2000 Pediatric foreign body aspiration. Pediatr Rev 21:86–90
4. Asif M, Shah SA, Khan F, Ghani R. Foreign body inhalation: site of impaction and efficacy of rigid bronchoscopy. *J Ayub Med Coll Abbottabad* 2007; 19(2): 46–48
5. American Heart Association 2001 ACLS provider manual. American Heart Association, Dallas TX
6. Handley AJ, Koster R, Monsieurs K, Perkins GD, Davies S, Bossaert L 2005 European Resuscitation Council Guidelines for Resuscitation 2005: Section 2. Adult basic life support and use of automated external defibrillators. Resuscitation 67(S1):S7–S23
7. American Heart Association 1997 Paediatric advanced life support. American Heart Association, Dallas TX
8. Biarent D, Bingham R, Richmond S, et al 2005 European Resuscitation Council Guidelines for Resuscitation 2005: Section 6. Paediatric life support. Resuscitation 6(S1):S97–S133
9. Nolan JP, Deakin CD, Soar J, Böttiger BW, Smith G 2005 European Resuscitation Council Guidelines for Resuscitation 2005: Section 4. Adult advanced life support. Resuscitation 67(S1):S39–S86
10. American Heart Association 1997 Paediatric advanced life support. American Heart Association, Dallas TX
11. Roberts K, Porter K 2003 How do you size a nasopharyngeal airway? Resuscitation 56:19–23
12. Alexander R, Hodgson P, Lomax D, Bullen C 1993 A comparison of the laryngeal mask airway and Guedel airway, bag and facemask for manual ventilation following formal training. Anaesthesia 48:231–234
13. Jones JH, Murphy MP, Dickson RL, Somerville GG, Brizendine EJ 2004 Emergency physician-verified out-of-hospital intubation: miss rates by paramedics. Acad Emerg Med 11:707–709
14. Katz SH, Falk JL 2001 Misplaced tracheal tubes by paramedics in an urban emergency medical services system. Ann Emerg Med 37:62–64
15. Aufderheide TP, Lurie KG 2004 Death by hyperventilation a common and life-threatening problem during cardiopulmonary resuscitation. Crit Care Med 32:S345–S351
16. Aufderheide TP, Sigurdsson G, Pirrallo RG, et al 2004 Hyperventilation-induced hypotension during cardiopulmonary resuscitation. Circulation 109:1960–1965
17. O'Neill JF, Deakin CD 2007 Do we hyperventilate cardiac arrest patients? Resuscitation 73:82–85
18. Dolenska S, Dahal P, Taylor A 2004 Essentials of airway management. Greenwich Medical, London
19. Joint Royal Colleges Ambulance Liaison Committee. UK Ambulance Service Clinical Guidelines v4. 2006. http://www2.warwick.ac.uk/fac/med/research/hsri/emergencycare/prehospitalcare/jrcalcstakeholderwebsite/guidelines/
20. Gataure PS, Vaughan RS, Latto IP 1996 Simulated difficult intubation. Comparison of the gum elastic bougie and the stylet. Anaesthesia 51(10):935–938
21. Noguchi T, Koga K, Shiga Y, Shigematsu A 2003 The gum elastic bougie eases tracheal intubation while applying cricoid pressure compared to a stylet. Can J Anaesth 50(7):712–717
22. Wang HE, Yealy DM 2006 How many attempts are required to accomplish out-of-hospital tracheal intubation? Acad Emerg Med 13:372–377
23. Galinski M, Tréoux V, Garrigue B, et al 2006 Intracuff pressures of tracheal tubes in the management of airway emergencies: the need for pressure monitoring. Ann Emerg Med 47(6):545–547
24. Garnet R, Ornato JP, Gonzalez ER, et al 1987 End-tidal carbon dioxide monitoring during cardiopulmonary resuscitation. JAMA 257(4):1379
25. Pelucio M, Halligan L, Dhindsa H 1997 Out-of-hospital experience with the syringe esophageal detector device. Acad Emerg Med 4:563–568
26. Takeda T, Tanigawa K, Tanaka H, et al 2003 The assessment of three methods to verify tracheal tube placement in the emergency setting. Resuscitation 56(2):153–157
27. Tanigawa K, Takeda T, Goto E, Tanaka K 2000 Accuracy and reliability of the

self-inflating bulb to verify tracheal intubation in out-of-hospital cardiac arrest patients. Anesthesiology 93:1432–1436

28. Mackreth B 1990 Assessing pulse oximetry in the field. JEMS 15(6):56
29. Advanced Life Support Group 2005 Prehospital paediatric life support, 2nd edition. BMJ Books, London
30. Marx JA, Hockberger RS, Walls RM, et al 2002 Rosen's Emergency medicine: concepts and clinical practice, 5th edition. Mosby, St Louis
31. American Heart Association 2000 Guidelines 2000 for cardiopulmonary resuscitation and emergency cardiovascular care. International Consensus on Science. Circulation 102(8):302
32. Stothert JC, Stout MJ, Lewis LM, et al 1990 High pressure transtracheal ventilation: the use of large-gauge intravenous-type catheters in the totally obstructed airway. Am J Emerg Med 8:184

PART FIVE

CHAPTER **14**

Respiratory Emergencies

Chapter contents

Objectives

Upon completion of this chapter, the paramedic will be able to:

1. Distinguish the pathophysiology of respiratory emergencies related to ventilation, diffusion, and perfusion.
2. Describe the causes, complications, signs and symptoms, and prehospital management of patients diagnosed with obstructive airway disease, pneumonia, adult respiratory distress syndrome, pulmonary thromboembolism, upper respiratory infection, spontaneous pneumothorax, hyperventilation syndrome and lung cancer.

Key terms

bronchiectasis An abnormal dilatation of the bronchi caused by a pus-producing infection of the bronchial wall.

hyperventilation syndrome Abnormally deep or rapid breathing that leads to excessive loss of carbon dioxide, resulting in respiratory alkalosis.

spontaneous pneumothorax A condition that results when a subpleural bleb ruptures, allowing air to enter the pleural space from within the lung.

status asthmaticus A severe, prolonged asthma exacerbation that has not been broken with repeated doses of bronchodilators.

Each year, respiratory disease is responsible for one in five deaths in the UK (around 110 000 deaths) and accounts for 845 000 hospital admissions.[1] Respiratory disease is one of the most common causes of emergency admission to hospital.[2] In 2004, the cost of respiratory disease to the NHS was £6.6 billion.[1] Patients with respiratory emergencies require the highest priority of care, therefore the paramedic must be able to assess a patient with respiratory distress quickly, identify the cause, initiate management, and provide appropriate care en route to the hospital.

Pathophysiology

A variety of problems can affect the respiratory system's ability to achieve gas exchange. Specific disorders responsible for respiratory emergencies include those related to ventilation, diffusion, and perfusion. Risk factors associated

Box 14-1

Risk factors associated with the development of respiratory disease

Intrinsic factors

Genetic predisposition may influence the development of these conditions:

- Asthma
- Obstructive lung disease
- Cancer.

Cardiac or circulatory disorders may influence the development of these conditions:

- Pulmonary oedema
- Pulmonary emboli.

Stress may increase the following:

- Severity of respiratory complaints
- Frequency of exacerbations of asthma and chronic obstructive pulmonary disease (COPD).

Extrinsic factors

Smoking increases the following:

- Prevalence of COPD and cancer
- Severity of virtually all respiratory disorders.

Environmental pollutants increase the following:

- Prevalence of COPD
- Severity of all obstructive airway disorders.

Table 14-1 Ventilation, diffusion and perfusion problems

Problem	Example
VENTILATION	
Upper airway obstruction	Foreign body, epiglottitis
Lower airway obstruction	Asthma, airway oedema
Chest wall impairment	Trauma, muscular dystrophy
Neurogenic dysfunction	Central nervous system (CNS)-depressant drugs, stroke
DIFFUSION	
Inadequate oxygen in ambient air	Fire environment, carbon monoxide (CO) poisoning
Alveolar disorder	Lung disease, inhalation injury
Interstitial space disorder	Pulmonary oedema, near-drowning
Capillary bed disorder	Severe atherosclerosis
PERFUSION	
Inadequate blood volume or haemoglobin levels	Shock, anaemia
Impaired circulatory blood flow	Pulmonary embolus
Capillary wall disorder	Trauma

with the development of respiratory disease are listed in Box 14-1. Key public health strategies for avoiding respiratory illness include: smoking prevention and cessation programmes, controlling air pollution, and law surrounding smoke-free workplaces and public locations. The following brief discussion of physiology serves as a review.

There are many pulmonary diseases, each of which acts in different ways on a number of body systems. However, all respiratory problems (acute or chronic) can be categorized as affecting ventilation, diffusion, or perfusion. Treatment can be started rapidly and effectively once the problem has been identified as a ventilation, diffusion or perfusion problem (or a combination of defects) (Table 14-1).

Ventilation

Ventilation is the process of air movement into and out of the lungs. For ventilation to occur, the following must be intact:

- neurological control (to initiate ventilation)
- nerves between the brainstem and the muscles of respiration
- functional diaphragm and intercostal muscles
- patent upper airway
- functional lower airway
- alveoli that are functional and have not collapsed.

Specific pathophysiologies associated with ventilation include upper and lower airway obstruction, chest wall impairment, and problems in neurological control. Emergency treatments for ventilation problems include making sure the upper and lower airways are open and clear and providing assisted ventilations.

Diffusion

Diffusion is the process of gas exchange. This gas exchange occurs between the air-filled alveoli and the pulmonary capillary bed. Gas exchange is driven by simple diffusion. In simple diffusion, gases move from areas of higher concentration to areas of lower concentration. (This occurs until the concentrations are equal.) For diffusion to occur, the following must be intact:

- alveolar and capillary walls that are not thickened
- interstitial space between the alveoli and capillary wall that is neither enlarged nor filled with fluid.

Specific pathophysiologies associated with diffusion include inadequate oxygen concentration in ambient air, alveolar disorders, interstitial space disorders, and capillary bed disorders. Emergency treatment for diffusion problems includes providing high-concentration oxygen. Treatment is also directed at reducing inflammation in the interstitial space.

Perfusion

Perfusion is the process of circulation of the blood through the lung tissues (capillary bed). For perfusion to occur, the following must be intact:

- adequate blood volume
- adequate haemoglobin in the blood
- pulmonary capillaries that are not blocked
- efficient pumping by the heart that provides a smooth flow of blood through the pulmonary capillary bed.

Specific pathophysiologies associated with perfusion include inadequate blood volume, impaired circulatory blood flow, and capillary wall disorders. Emergency treatment for perfusion problems includes providing an adequate circulating blood volume. In addition, the blood must have enough haemoglobin to carry adequate oxygen supplies. Treatment may also be needed to increase the heart's ability to pump effectively.

Scene size-up and rescuer safety

Sometimes the air a patient is breathing may not have enough oxygen or may have poisonous or toxic gases. This can lead to breathing difficulties. During the scene size-up, it is critical to ensure a safe environment for all emergency medical services (EMS) workers. This should be done before treatment efforts are started. Rescue personnel with special training and equipment should be used as needed to ensure scene safety.

Patient care

Initial assessment

A primary focus of the initial assessment is to detect any life-threatening conditions. This and starting resuscitation take priority over detailed assessment. Signs of life-threatening respiratory distress in adults include the following:

- alterations in mental status
- severe cyanosis
- absent breath sounds
- audible stridor
- inability to speak one or two words without dyspnoea
- tachycardia
- pallor and diaphoresis
- recession and/or the use of accessory muscles to assist breathing.

Focused history and physical examination

The paramedic should find out the patient's chief complaints. These may include dyspnoea, chest pain, productive or non-productive cough, haemoptysis (coughing up blood from the respiratory tract), wheezing, and signs of respiratory infection (e.g. fever, increased sputum production). The history should focus on the patient's previous experiences with similar or the same symptoms. The patient's objective description of severity is often an accurate indicator of the severity of the current episode if the condition is chronic.

Asking the patient, 'What happened the last time you had an attack this bad?' is very useful for predicting what will happen with this episode. The following is a sample of questions that might be asked in order to obtain a focused history for a patient with respiratory distress. This format uses the acronym OPQRST (onset, provocation, quality, region/radiation, severity and time). Sample questions include the following:

- *Onset:* What were you doing when the breathing difficulty began? Do you think anything might have triggered it? Did your breathing difficulty begin gradually or was it sudden in onset? Did you experience any pain when the breathing difficulty began?
- *Provocation:* Does lying down or sitting up make your breathing better or worse? Do you have any pain when you breathe? If so, does the pain increase when you take a deep breath or does it stay the same?
- *Quality:* Is it more difficult to breathe when you inhale or exhale? If you have pain when you breathe, would you describe it as sharp or dull?
- *Region/Radiation:* If you have pain where is the pain, does it radiate anywhere else?
- *Severity:* On a scale of 1 to 10 (with 10 being the worst), how would you rate the difficulty of your breathing?
- *Time:* What time did the breathing difficulty start? Has it been constant since it began? If you've had this type of difficulty before, how long did it last?

Unknown pulmonary diagnosis

If paramedics do not know a patient's diagnosed condition, they should try to determine whether it is related mainly to ventilation, diffusion or perfusion or to a combination of defects. They may be able to determine this from the patient's medication history. After obtaining a history of the current illness, paramedics should obtain a medication history that includes current medications, medication allergies, cardiac medications, and pulmonary medications (e.g. oxygen therapy; inhaled, oral, or parenteral sympathomimetics; inhaled or oral corticosteroids; antibiotics).

Note

It is important to ask patients whether they have been intubated before because of breathing difficulty. A history of previous intubation indicates severe pulmonary disease and suggests that intubation may be required again.

Physical examination

The physical examination begins with a general impression of the patient. The paramedic should note the patient's position, mental status, ability to speak, respiratory effort and skin colour (see Chapter 7). Vital signs should be assessed, with the following considerations kept in mind:

- Pulse rate: Tachycardia is a sign of hypoxaemia but may result from the use of sympathomimetic medications. Bradycardia caused by respiratory problems is a pre-terminal sign.
- Blood pressure: Hypertension may result from the use of sympathomimetic medications.
- Respiratory rate: The respiratory rate is not an accurate sign of respiratory status unless it is very slow. Trends are essential in evaluating a patient with chronic respiratory disease. A slowing rate in a patient who is not improving suggests exhaustion and impending respiratory insufficiency. Abnormal patterns (see Chapter 13) that may be seen in patients with respiratory disease include tachypnoea, Cheyne–Stokes respirations, central neurogenic hyperventilation, Kussmaul respirations, ataxic respirations, apneustic respirations and apnoea.

The patient's face and neck should be assessed for pursed-lip breathing and use of accessory muscles. Pursed-lip breathing helps maintain pressure in the airways (even during exhalation), which helps to support bronchial walls that have lost their support as a result of disease. The use of accessory muscles can quickly result in respiratory fatigue. The patient should be questioned about sputum production. An increasing amount of sputum suggests infection. Thick, green or brown sputum may indicate pneumonia; yellow or pale grey sputum may be related to allergic or inflammatory causes; pink, frothy sputum is associated with severe and late stages of pulmonary oedema. The patient should be evaluated for jugular vein distension as it may be a sign of right-sided heart failure resulting from severe pulmonary congestion.

The patient's chest should be inspected for injury and for any indicators of chronic disease (e.g. barrel chest from long-standing chronic obstructive pulmonary disease). Other components of the chest examination include noting accessory muscle use or recession to facilitate breathing, evaluating chest wall symmetry, and auscultating the patient's lungs for normal and abnormal breath sounds.

The patient's extremities should be assessed for peripheral cyanosis, clubbing of the fingers, and carpopedal spasm. Peripheral cyanosis is caused when a large amount of the haemoglobin in the blood is not carrying oxygen. Clubbing is an abnormal enlargement of the ends of the fingers that indicates long-standing chronic hypoxaemia. Carpopedal spasms are spasms of the hands, thumbs, feet, or toes that are often associated with hypocapnia and result from long periods of rapid, deep respiration. All of these are crucial findings in a patient with respiratory disease and should be documented on the patient report form.

Diagnostic testing

Diagnostic testing that may be appropriate for some patients with respiratory disease includes pulse oximetry, the use of peak flow meters, and capnometry. Pulse oximeters measure oxygen saturation; peak flow meters (described later in this chapter) provide a baseline assessment of airflow for patients with obstructive lung disease; and capnometry can help determine proper placement of an endotracheal tube in intubated patients. Pulse oximetry and capnometry are described in Chapter 13.

Obstructive airway disease

Obstructive airway disease is a major health problem in the UK. There are an estimated 3 million people with COPD in the UK,[3] although only an estimated 900 000 are correctly diagnosed.[4] Predisposing factors that contribute to obstructive pulmonary disease include smoking, environmental pollution, industrial exposures, and various pulmonary infectious processes. Obstructive airway disease is a triad of distinct diseases that often coexist; they are chronic bronchitis and emphysema (together referred to as chronic obstructive pulmonary disease [COPD]) and asthma. These diseases are presented separately in this chapter; however, the paramedic must remember that patients often have all three in different degrees.

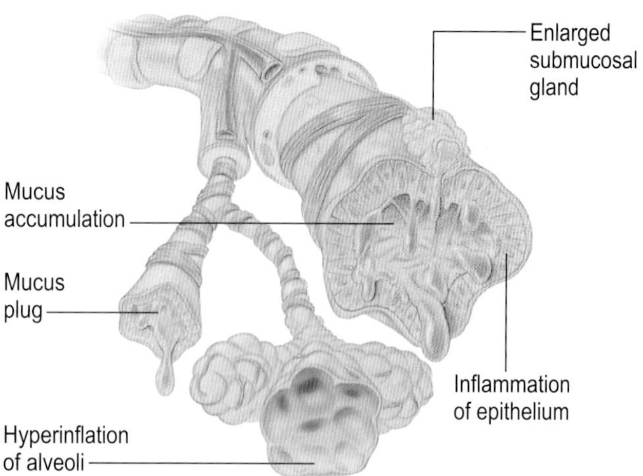

Figure 14-1 Chronic bronchitis. Bronchi are filled with excess mucus.

Critical Thinking

Will patients with chronic obstructive pulmonary disease (COPD) always be able to 'name' their disease when you ask about their history?

Chronic bronchitis

Chronic bronchitis is a condition involving inflammatory changes and excessive mucus production in the bronchial tree (Figure 14-1). Its prevalence is estimated at 45 per 10 000 of the general population, with a peak of 204 per 10 000 in the 75–84 age group.[5] The disease is characterized by an increase in the number and size of mucus-producing glands, which results from prolonged exposure to irritants (most often the irritant is cigarette smoke). The condition is diagnosed clinically by the presence of cough with sputum production on most days for at least 3 months of the year and for at least 2 consecutive years.[6] The alveoli are not seriously affected and diffusion remains relatively normal.

Patients with severe chronic bronchitis have a low oxygen pressure (Po_2) and often appear cyanotic. They have a low Po_2 because of changes in the ventilation–perfusion relationships in the lung, and hypoventilation. The hypoventilation leads to hypercapnia (high levels of carbon dioxide [CO_2]), hypoxaemia (low levels of oxygen [O_2]), and increases in arterial carbon dioxide pressure (Pco_2). Patients with chronic bronchitis have frequent respiratory infections, which eventually cause scarring of lung tissue. In time, irreversible changes occur in the lung, which may lead to emphysema or bronchiectasis. Bronchiectasis is an abnormal dilatation of the bronchi and is caused by a pus-producing infection of the bronchial wall.

Emphysema

Emphysema results from pathological changes in the lung and is the end stage of a process that progresses slowly for many years. The disease is characterized by permanent abnormal enlargement of the air spaces beyond the terminal bronchioles, destruction of the alveoli, and collapse of the alveoli (Figure 14-2). The disease reduces both the number

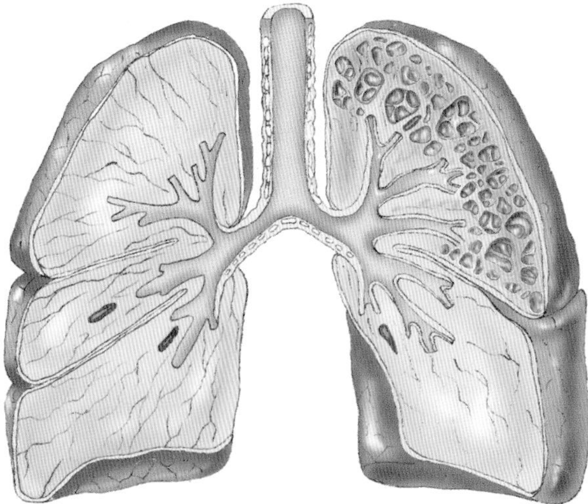

Figure 14-2 Cystic changes of lobar emphysema resulting from destruction of alveoli.

of alveoli available for gas exchange and the elasticity of the remaining alveoli. This loss of elasticity leads to trapping of air in the alveoli, thus increasing residual volume, whereas vital capacity remains somewhat normal.

The reduction in arterial Po_2 leads to increased production of red blood cells (called polycythaemia, i.e. an elevated haematocrit value). This elevation in haematocrit is much more common in the chronic bronchitic than in the mainly emphysemic patient because the chronic bronchitic is more often chronically hypoxaemic. Decreases in alveolar membrane surface area and in the number of pulmonary capillaries in the lung reduce the area for gas exchange and increase resistance to pulmonary blood flow.

Patients with emphysema have some resistance to airflow into and out of the lungs, yet most of the hyperexpansion is caused by air trapped in the alveoli as a result of the loss of elasticity (Figure 14-3a, b). Patients with chronic bronchitis have increased airway resistance during inspiration and expiration whilst patients with emphysema have increased airway resistance only on expiration. Expiration is normally a passive, involuntary act, but it becomes a muscular act in patients with COPD. Over time, the chest becomes rigid (barrel shaped) and the patient has to use accessory muscles of the neck, chest, and abdomen to move air into and out of the lungs. Full deflation of the lungs becomes more and more difficult. Often the patient with emphysema is thin due to poor dietary intake and an increased calorific consumption required by the work of breathing (Table 14-2). Patients with emphysema often develop bullae (thin-walled cystic lesions in the lung) from the destruction of alveolar walls. When bullae collapse, they increase the problems with air exchange seen in these patients and can lead to pneumothorax.

Critical Thinking

What effect might application of a cervical collar, use of a short spine board or vest, and immobilization supine on a long backboard have on a patient with chronic obstructive pulmonary disease (COPD) who has sustained trauma?

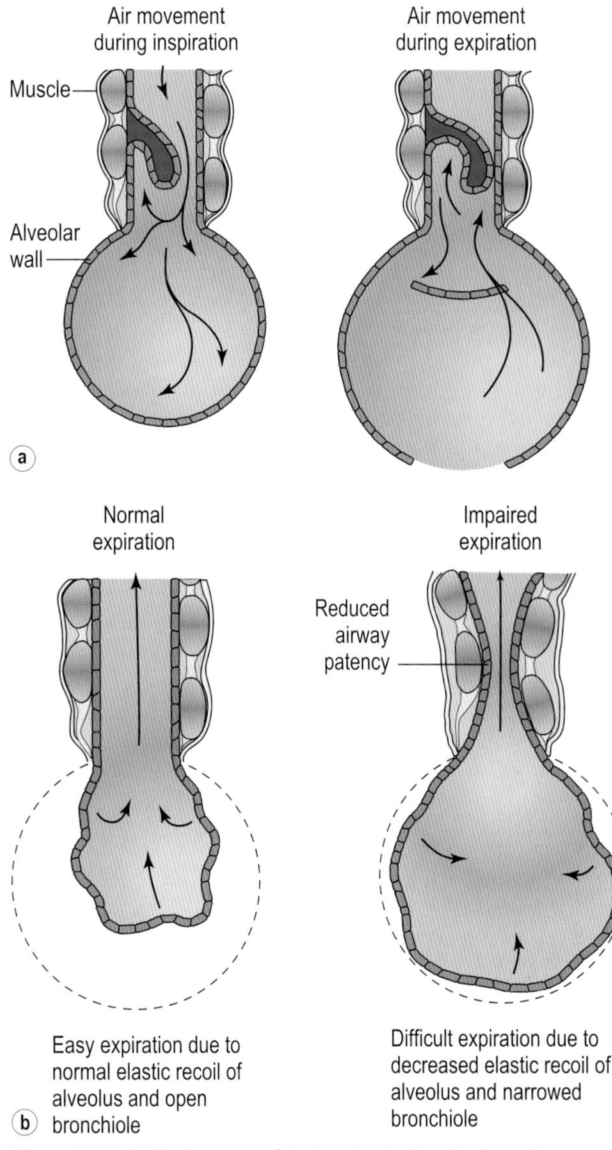

Figure 14-3 (a) Mechanisms of air trapping in chronic obstructive pulmonary disease (COPD): mucus plugs and narrowed airways cause air trapping and hyperinflation on expiration. During inspiration, the airways enlarge, allowing gas to flow past the obstruction. This mechanism of air trapping occurs in asthma and chronic bronchitis. (b) Mechanism of air trapping in emphysema: Damaged or destroyed alveolar walls no longer support and hold open the airways, and alveoli lose their property of elastic recoil. Both these factors contribute to airway collapse during expiration.

Table 14-2 Comparison of signs and symptoms of emphysema and chronic bronchitis

Emphysema	Chronic bronchitis
Thin, barrel-chest appearance	Typically overweight
Non-productive cough	Productive cough with sputum
Wheezing and rhonchi	Coarse rhonchi
Pink complexion	Chronic cyanosis
Extreme dyspnoea on exertion	Mild, chronic dyspnoea
Prolonged inspiration (pursed-lip breathing)	Resistance on inspiration and expiration

Assessment of COPD

Patients with COPD usually are aware of and have adapted to their illness. A request for emergency care indicates that a significant change has occurred in the patient's condition. The patient with COPD usually has an acute episode of worsening dyspnoea that is manifested even at rest, an increase or change in sputum production, or an increase in the malaise that accompanies the disease. Other common complaints include inability to sleep and recurrent headaches.

Paramedics responding to the call are likely to find the patient with COPD in respiratory distress. Often the patient is sitting upright. The person may be leaning forward to aid breathing. The individual frequently is using pursed-lip breathing to maintain positive airway pressures, in addition to using accessory muscles. Increased hypoxaemia and hypercarbia may be indicated by tachypnoea, diaphoresis, cyanosis, confusion, irritability and drowsiness.

Other physical findings include wheezes, rhonchi and crackles. Breath sounds and heart sounds may also be diminished, which is due to reduced air exchange and the increased diameter of the thoracic cavity. In late stages of decompensation, the patient may have peripheral cyanosis, clubbing of the fingers, and signs of right-sided heart failure. The patient's electrocardiogram (ECG) may reveal cardiac dysrhythmias or signs of right atrial enlargement; these include tall, peaked P waves in leads II, III, and aV_F (see Chapter 15).

Management of COPD

The main goal of prehospital care for COPD patients is to manage time-critical features if they are present. If the paramedic is confident that the diagnosis is an exacerbation of COPD then they should seek to establish if the patient has a personalized treatment plan available and work to implement the plan. Paramedics should ensure the patency of the airway and work to improve airflow through the use of bronchodilators.[7] It should be remembered that drug therapy can cause serious side effects and complications, particularly if the patient has self-medicated before the paramedics arrive. It is crucial for paramedics to obtain a thorough medical history regarding medication use, home oxygen use, and drug allergies.

An intravenous (IV) line should be considered in all patients in respiratory distress, and a cardiac monitor should be applied. If the patient has a productive cough, coughing should be encouraged and any sputum should be collected for laboratory analysis.

A small proportion of COPD patients are chronically hypoxic and may develop loss of respiratory drive when administered high concentrations of oxygen. This leads to hypoventilation with subsequent hypercapnia and deranged blood gases. Pulse oximetry (SpO_2) is a useful guide to oxygen concentration in COPD patients but it should be remembered that it does not indicate carbon dioxide levels. Current guidelines suggest that where there are no features of life-threatening or severe COPD, then oxygen should be administered in a controlled manner to maintain SpO_2 levels at between 90% and 92%.[7] Oxygen should not be withheld from those whose primary diagnosis indicates a requirement for high-concentration O_2 such as serious trauma and myocardial infarction.

The medications used in the prehospital setting to relieve bronchospasm and reduce constricted airways are the beta agonist salbutamol and the anticholinergic ipratropium bromide (see JRCALC guidelines for dosages).[7] The use of systemic corticosteroids is of no proven benefit in acute exacerbation of COPD so should not be used.[7]

Asthma

Approximately 5.2 million people are living with asthma in the UK; it is responsible for 1400 deaths per annum (1 death every 7 hours).[8] In 2002 there were nearly 70 000 hospital admissions due to asthma, and a further 4.1 million GP consultations. In addition, confidential inquiries into asthma deaths have often concluded that the fatality could have been avoided through better routine and emergency care, avoiding delay in getting help during the final attack, or by taking the prescribed medication.[9,10] Asthma is most common in children and young adults although it can occur in any decade of life. Aggravating factors tend to be extrinsic (external) in children and intrinsic (internal) in adults (Figure 14-4). Childhood asthma often improves or resolves with age. Adult asthma usually persists.

Pathophysiology of an asthma exacerbation

Asthma generally occurs in acute episodes of variable duration. Between these episodes, the patient is somewhat free of symptoms. The exacerbation is characterized by reversible airflow obstruction caused by bronchial smooth muscle contraction; hypersecretion of mucus, resulting in bronchial plugging; and inflammatory changes in the bronchial walls. The increased resistance to airflow leads to alveolar hypoventilation, marked ventilation–perfusion mismatching (leading to hypoxaemia), and carbon dioxide retention (stimulating hyperventilation) (Figure 14-5). The obstruction of inspiration and marked obstruction of expiration causes pressure to remain high in the airways, as a result of air trapping in the lungs.

During an acute asthma exacerbation, the combination of increased airway resistance, increased respiratory drive, and air trapping creates excessive demand on the muscles of respiration. This leads to greater use of accessory muscles and increases the chance of respiratory fatigue. If laboured breathing continues, high pressures in the thorax can reduce the amount of blood returning to the left ventricle (left ventricular preload), resulting in a drop in cardiac output and systolic blood pressure (near-fatal asthma). Pulsus paradoxus may also be seen. If the episode continues, hypoxaemia and changes in blood flow and blood pressure may lead to death. Most asthma-related deaths occur outside the hospital. In the prehospital setting, cardiac arrest in patients with severe asthma has been linked to the following factors:[11]

- severe bronchospasm and mucus plugging, which leads to asphyxia (the most common cause of asthma-related deaths)
- cardiac dysrhythmias caused by hypoxia
- tension pneumothorax (often bilateral).

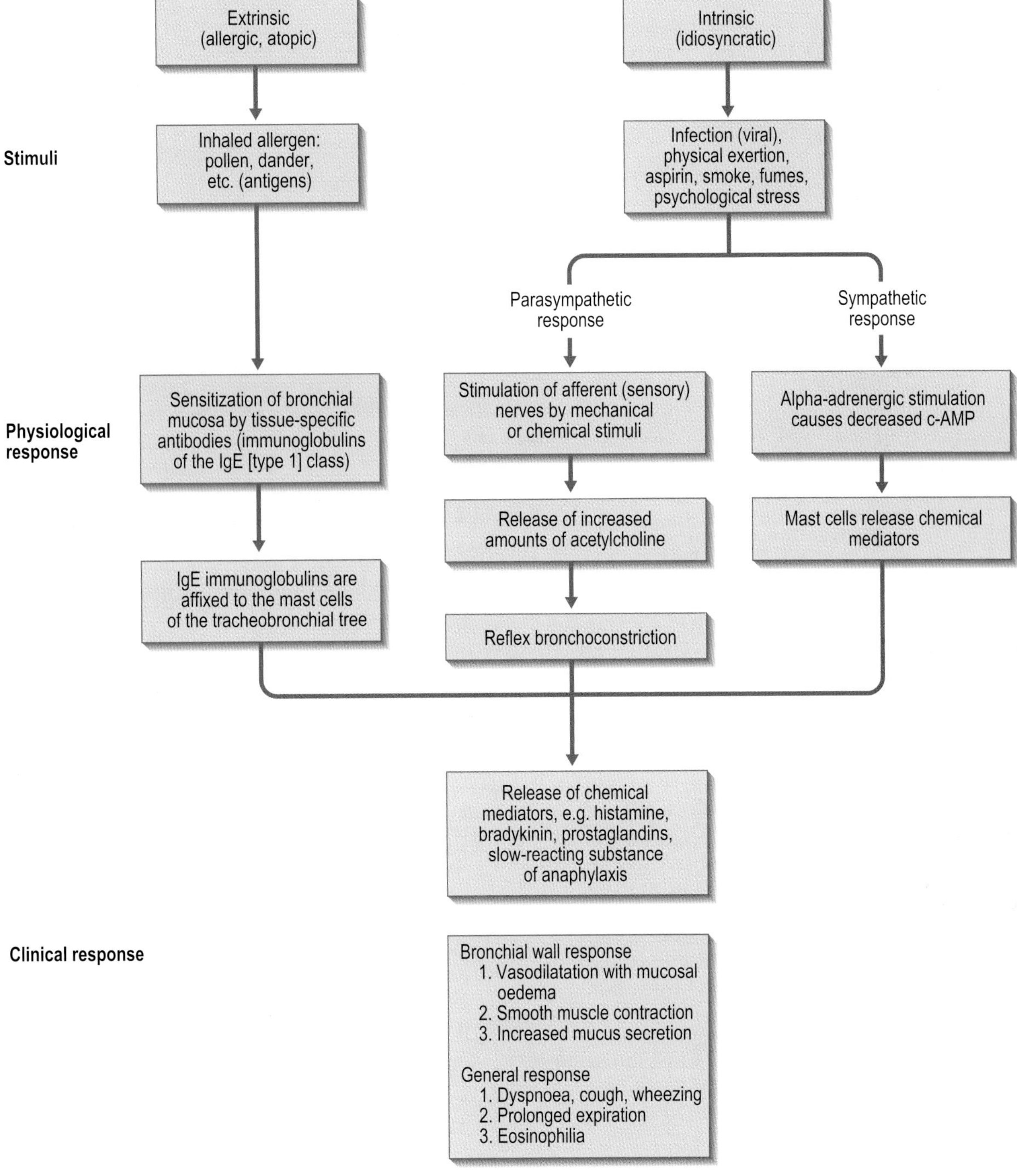

Figure 14-4 Extrinsic and intrinsic bronchial asthma.

Note

Caution: Thoracic decompression in a patient with severe refractory asthma without a pneumothorax might result in puncture of the visceral pleura of the hyperinflated lung, producing a pneumothorax (most likely under tension).[12]

Other conditions that may be present in patients with near-fatal asthma include cardiac disease, pulmonary disease, acute allergic bronchospasm or anaphylaxis, drug use or misuse (beta-blockers, cocaine and opiates), and recent discontinuation of long-term corticosteroid therapy (associated with adrenal insufficiency).

Assessment

When paramedics arrive, the asthmatic patient is usually sitting upright, and may be leaning forward with hands on knees (tripod position). The typical asthmatic patient is in obvious respiratory distress and often uses accessory muscles to aid breathing. Respirations are rapid and loud, and audible wheezing may be present.

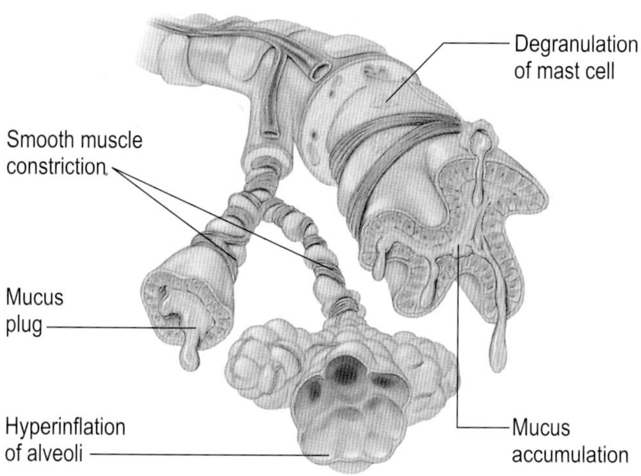

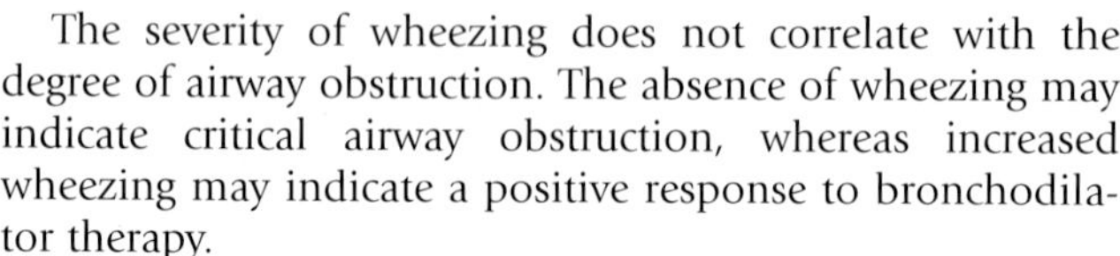

Figure 14-5 With bronchial asthma, thick mucus, mucosal oedema, and smooth muscle spasm obstruct the small airways. Breathing becomes laboured, and expiration is difficult.

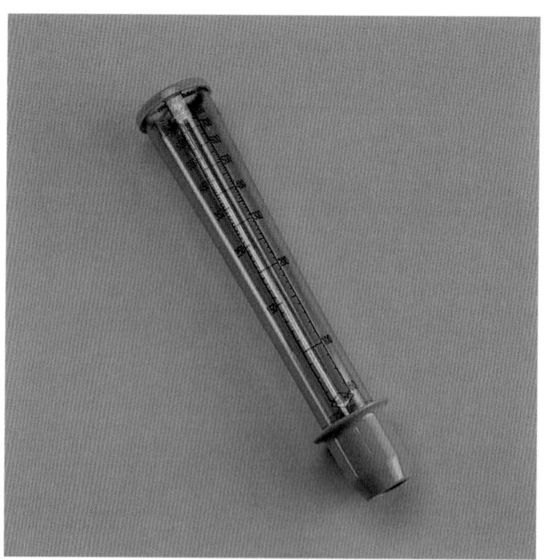

Figure 14-6 Peak flow meter.

The severity of wheezing does not correlate with the degree of airway obstruction. The absence of wheezing may indicate critical airway obstruction, whereas increased wheezing may indicate a positive response to bronchodilator therapy.

The patient's mental status should be noted and monitored carefully. Lethargy, exhaustion, agitation and confusion are serious signs of impending respiratory failure. An initial history must be obtained quickly. Questions about the onset of the current problem, its relative severity, the precipitating cause, medication use, and allergies should be specific and to the point. It is crucial to find out whether the patient has needed intubation to manage previous asthma attacks.

On auscultation, a prolonged expiratory phase may be noted. Usually wheezing is heard from the movement of air through the narrowed airways. Inspiratory wheezing (unlike inspiratory stridor) does not indicate upper airway occlusion; rather it suggests that the large and midsize muscular airways are obstructed. This indicates greater obstruction than if expiratory wheezes alone are heard. Inspiratory wheezes may also suggest that the large airways are filled with secretions. A silent chest (i.e. no audible wheezing or air movement) may indicate such severe obstruction that the flow of air is too low to generate breath sounds. Other signs of severe asthma include the following:

- reduced level of consciousness
- diaphoresis and pallor
- recession
- inability to complete a sentence
- poor, floppy muscle tone
- pulse rate greater than 130 beats per minute
- respirations greater than 30 breaths per minute
- pulsus paradoxus greater than 20 mmHg
- altered mental status or severe agitation.

Pulmonary function tests

Pulmonary function tests measure the peak expiratory flow rate (PEFR). They can help to determine the severity of an asthma attack (Box 14-2) and also help the paramedic assess the effectiveness of treatment of the airway obstruction. Peak flow meters (Figure 14-6) should be used in the prehospital setting for this purpose. Their use requires a cooperative patient and may also require coaching by the paramedic.

Box 14-2

Severity of asthma

Moderate exacerbation	Acute severe	Life-threatening
Increasing symptoms PEFR >50–75% best or predicted No features of severe asthma	Any one of: PEFR 33–50% best or predicted Respiratory rate ≥25/min Pulse rate ≥110/min Inability to complete sentences in one breath	In a patient with severe asthma any one of: PEFR <33% best or predicted Sp_{O_2} <92% Silent chest Cyanosis Feeble respiratory effort Bradycardia, dysrhythmia, hypotension Exhaustion, confusion, coma

Adapted from Scottish Intercollegiate Guidelines Network and British Thoracic Society. British Guidelines on the Management of Asthma. 2003. SIGN and BTS.

To determine a baseline airflow (before drug administration), the paramedic should instruct the patient to inflate the lungs fully and forcefully exhale as quickly as possible into the flow meter. (Children should be reminded to breathe out as if they were blowing out candles or blowing up a balloon.) The reading is recorded in litres per minute. This measurement should be taken two more times and the highest of the three readings recorded as the peak value flow. The recorded value is then compared with standard tables based on height, gender, and race (Table 14-3 and Figure 14-7). A PEFR measurement between 33% and 50% of predicted norm is considered acute severe asthma, a peak flow of <33% of expected

Table 14-3 Predicted average peak expiratory flow for normal children and adolescents. For use with EU/EN13826 scale PEF meters only.

Height (m)	Height (ft)	Predicted EU PEFR (L/min)	Height (m)	Height (ft)	Predicted EU PEFR (L/min)
0.85	2′9″	**87**	**1.30**	4′3″	**212**
0.90	2′11″	**95**	**1.35**	4′5″	**233**
0.95	3′1″	**104**	**1.40**	4′7″	**254**
1.00	3′3″	**115**	**1.45**	4′9″	**276**
1.05	3′5″	**127**	**1.50**	4′11″	**299**
1.10	3′7″	**141**	**1.55**	5′1″	**323**
1.15	3′9″	**157**	**1.60**	5′3″	**346**
1.20	3′11″	**174**	**1.65**	5′5″	**370**
1.25	4′1″	**192**	**1.70**	5′7″	**393**

Normal PEF values in children correlate best with height; with increasing age, larger differences occur between the sexes. These predicted values are based on the formulae given in Coates JE, Lung Function, 4th edition, adapted for EU scale Mini-Wright peak flow meters by Clement Clarke International.

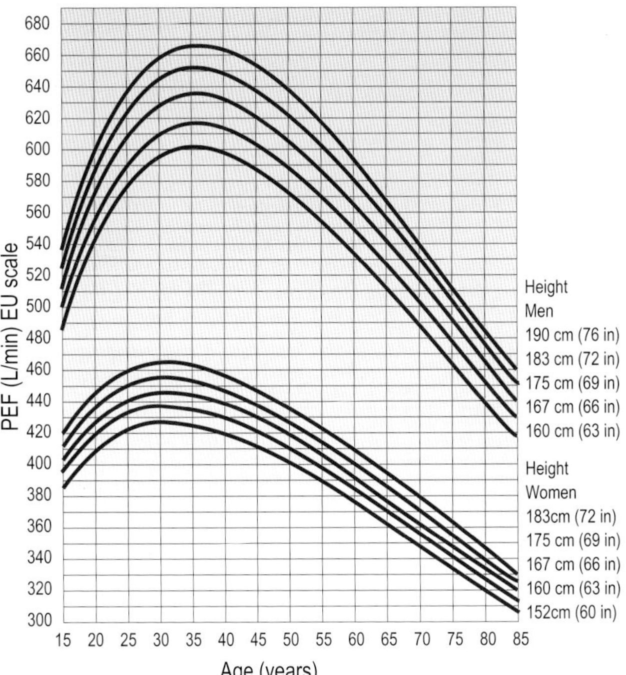

Figure 14-7 Predicted average peak expiratory flow rate for normal adults. For use with EU/EN13826 scale PEF meters only. Adapted by Clement Clarke International from Nunn AJ, Gregg I 1989 BMJ 298:1068–1070.

is life-threatening. Peak flow measurements should be repeated throughout the course of management to evaluate the patient's response to drug therapy. It is not always practicable to obtain a PEFR but it is best practice wherever possible.

Note

Most children under 5 years of age cannot adequately perform peak expiratory flow rate (PEFR) tests. Also, this test should not be used with a patient in severe respiratory distress. Drug therapy to reverse the bronchospasm is the priority.

Management

After administration of high-concentration oxygen, drug therapy is provided. Drug therapy is based on the patient's age and the patient's use of medications before the arrival of paramedics. Salbutamol should be administered via an oxygen-driven nebulizer at 6–8 L/min. If the asthma is severe or life-threatening, ipratropium bromide should be added to the salbutamol. Hydrocortisone should be considered if there is a delay in getting the patient to hospital, although it should be borne in mind that the sooner steroids are administered the better (where indicated). In rare cases, the patient may not respond to oxygen or bronchodilator therapy. If any of the following features are present, then the paramedic should administer adrenaline (epinephrine) as per guidelines:[7]

- life-threatening asthma
- failing ventilation
- continued deterioration despite O_2 and nebulizer therapy.

Note

Adrenaline (epinephrine) is not indicated in the management of life-threatening asthma in children.

Note

Asthma attacks are true medical emergencies. Deterioration of the patient's condition can be rapid and can also be fatal. The paramedic must monitor the patient carefully and continuously. Initial patient management should be directed at ensuring an adequate airway, providing supplemental oxygen, and reversing the bronchospasm.

Critical Thinking

Consider that the patient is unable to hold the nebulizer mouthpiece or needs to be ventilated using a bag–mask device. What can you do to promote bronchodilatation?

Status asthmaticus

Status asthmaticus is a severe, prolonged asthma attack that has not been broken with repeated doses of bronchodilators. It may be of sudden onset (for example, it may result from spasm of the airways), or it can be subtle in onset, resulting from a viral respiratory infection or prolonged exposure to one or more allergens. Status asthmaticus is a true emergency that calls for early recognition and immediate transport of the patient. These patients are in danger of respiratory failure.

The treatment of patients for status asthmaticus is the same as that for acute asthma attacks, yet the urgency of rapid transport is more important. In addition, these patients are usually dehydrated and may benefit from IV fluid administration. The patient's respiratory status should be monitored closely and high-concentration oxygen should be administered. The need for intubation and aggressive ventilatory support should be anticipated and transportation to an appropriate receiving facility expedited.

Critical Thinking

When a patient treated for status asthmaticus is reassessed, would decreasing respiratory and heart rates indicate a good outcome or a bad one? Why?

Differential considerations

Wheezing is commonly associated with asthma but it may be present in all types of obstructive lung disease as well as other conditions that cause dyspnoea (Table 14-4). For example, tachypnoea, wheezing and respiratory distress may indicate heart failure, pneumonia, pulmonary oedema, pulmonary embolism, pneumothorax, toxic inhalation, foreign body aspiration, and various other pathological states. Appropriate emergency care is based on the patient assessment and an accurate history.

Table 14-4 Disease and symptoms associated with wheezing

Disease	Symptoms
Asthma	Productive cough, tightness in chest
Bacterial pneumonia	Productive cough, pleuritic pain
Chronic bronchitis	Chronic, productive cough
Emphysema	Cough
Foreign body aspiration	Cough
Heart failure	Cough, orthopnoea, nocturnal dyspnoea
Pneumothorax	Sudden, sharp pleuritic pain
Pulmonary disease	Tachypnoea, cough, congestion
Pulmonary embolism	Sudden, sharp pleuritic pain
Toxic inhalation	Cough, pain

Pneumonia

Pneumonia is a group of specific infections (not a single disease) that cause an acute inflammatory process of the respiratory bronchioles and the alveoli. (Figure 14-8) It is very common in the UK, with around 1 in 100 people suffering each year.[13] The risk of dying has fallen dramatically since doctors have been prescribing antibiotics for the condition but pneumonia remains the fifth most common cause of death.[14] Pneumonia can be caused by bacterial, viral or fungal infection; associated risk factors include cigarette smoking, alcoholism, exposure to cold, and extremes of age (the very young and very old). These diseases may be spread by respiratory droplets or by contact with infected individuals. They may also be spread by breathing in bacteria from one's own nose and mouth.

Pneumonia is typically classified as viral, bacterial or aspiration. Pneumonia generally manifests with classic signs and symptoms (typical pneumonia), including a productive cough, pleuritic chest pain, and fever that produces 'shaking chills'. It may also cause non-specific complaints, particularly in older adults and debilitated patients. Non-specific complaints may include a non-productive cough, headache, fatigue and sore throat (atypical pneumonia) (Box 14-3).

Note

Community-acquired pneumonia is an infection that is acquired from the environment. This category includes infections acquired indirectly as a result of the use of medications that change the body's ability to fight off disease. The occurrence of these infections has risen in recent years. This is due to the increased percentage of the population over age 65 and to the increasing number of patients taking immunosuppressive drugs for malignancy, transplantation or autoimmune disease.

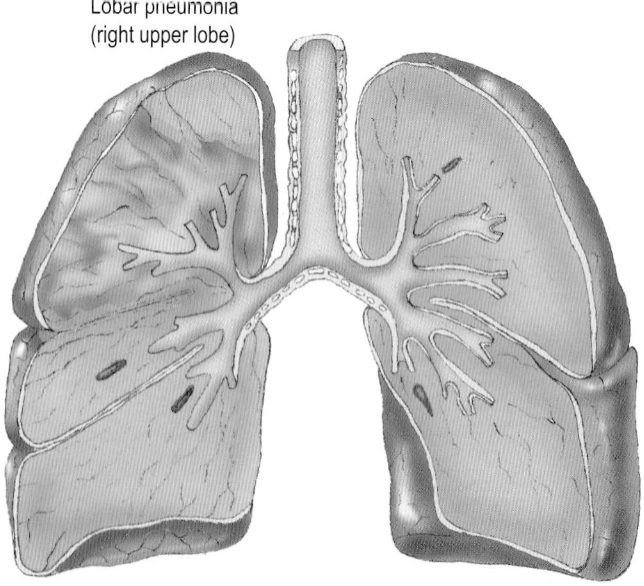

Figure 14-8 Pneumonia is an inflammatory process of the respiratory bronchioles and alveoli. It is caused by infection.

Box 14-3

Influenza

Influenza is an acute, febrile disease that affects the entire body. It is associated with viral infection of the upper and lower respiratory tracts. It is usually characterized by the abrupt onset of a severe, protracted cough, fever, headache, muscle ache and mild sore throat. Of all the viruses, the influenza and parainfluenza viruses are the most common causes of serious respiratory infections. Moreover, they have high morbidity and mortality rates.

Influenza viruses A, B and C (and their many strains) are known for their potential to quickly cause respiratory infections after exposure. (It usually occurs within 24–48 h.) The virus is inhaled in respiratory droplets from infected individuals (such as when an infected person sneezes). The droplets penetrate the surface of upper respiratory tract mucosal cells and eventually spread to the lower respiratory tract. There the virus causes cell inflammation and destruction of the cilia. Without the cilia, clearing the airways of infected mucus is more difficult; consequently, a secondary bacterial infection often develops. This may result in pneumonia or acute respiratory failure and is particularly the case in patients with chronic lung disease.

Influenza has the potential for widespread epidemics in high-risk populations (these include adults and children with chronic cardiorespiratory or metabolic disorders, residents of nursing homes and other institutions, and healthcare workers). Current vaccines are effective against some strains of the virus and have minimal side effects. If uncomplicated, influenza is self-limiting with acute symptoms lasting 2–7 days. These are followed by a convalescent period of about 1 week.

Aspiration pneumonia

Aspiration pneumonia is an inflammation of the lung tissue (parenchyma) that results when foreign material enters the tracheobronchial tree. The syndrome is common in patients who have an altered level of consciousness (e.g. from head injury, seizure activity, use of alcohol or other drugs, anaesthesia, infection, shock) and in intubated patients and those who have aspirated foreign bodies. Factors common to victims of aspiration include depression of the cough or gag reflex, inability of the patient to handle secretions or gastric contents, and inability to protect the airway.

Aspiration pneumonia may be non-bacterial (for example, it may develop after aspiration of stomach contents, toxic materials or inert substances); this is typically called pneumonitis to distinguish it from infectious pneumonia or bacterial pneumonia (as a secondary complication). Bacterial aspiration pneumonia has a poor prognosis, even with antibiotic therapy.

The physiological effects of aspiration pneumonia are based on the volume and pH of the aspirated substances. If the pH is below 2.5 (as may occur in the aspiration of stomach contents), atelectasis, pulmonary oedema, haemorrhage and cell necrosis may occur. The alveolar–capillary membrane may be damaged as well. This, in turn, may lead to fluid build-up in the alveoli and, in severe cases, it may lead to adult respiratory distress syndrome (described in the next section). The patient's signs and symptoms vary with the scenario and the severity of the insult (e.g. near-drowning, foreign body aspiration, aspiration of gastric contents). Clinical features may include dyspnoea, cough, bronchospasm, wheezes, rhonchi, crackles, cyanosis, and pulmonary and cardiac insufficiency. Of these patients, 25–45% develop pulmonary infection.

Critical Thinking

What measures can the paramedic take to reduce a patient's risk of aspiration?

Management

Prehospital care for patients with pneumonia includes airway support, oxygen administration, ventilatory assistance as needed, cardiac monitoring, and transport for evaluation by a physician. Bronchodilator drugs may also be indicated for some patients. In cases of aspiration, suctioning of the airway may be required.

General patient management usually includes bed rest, analgesics, decongestants, expectorants, antipyretics, and antibiotic therapy. In severe cases, bronchoscopy, intubation, and mechanical ventilation may be required for some patients.

Adult respiratory distress syndrome

Adult respiratory distress syndrome (ARDS) is a fulminant form of respiratory failure characterized by acute lung inflammation and diffuse alveolar–capillary injury.[15] All disorders that result in ARDS cause severe pulmonary oedema. The syndrome develops as a complication of injury or illness such as trauma, gastric aspiration, cardiopulmonary bypass surgery, Gram-negative sepsis, multiple blood transfusions, oxygen toxicity, toxic inhalation, drug overdose, pneumonia and infections. Regardless of the specific cause, increased capillary permeability (high-permeability non-cardiogenic pulmonary oedema) results in a clinical condition in which the lungs are wet and heavy, congested, haemorrhagic and stiff, with decreased perfusion capacity across alveolar membranes. The lungs become non-compliant, which requires the patient to increase the pressure in the airways to breathe.

The pulmonary oedema associated with ARDS leads to severe hypoxaemia, intrapulmonary shunting, reduced lung compliance and, in some cases, irreversible parenchymal lung damage. Unique to this syndrome is the fact that most patients who develop this condition have healthy lungs before the event that caused the disease. ARDS is more common in men than in women. The mortality rate is over 65%. Complications include respiratory failure, cardiac dysrhythmias, disseminated intravascular coagulation, barotrauma, congestive heart failure and renal failure (Box 14-4).

Management

All patients with ARDS should be given high-concentration oxygen and ventilatory support. Depending on the underlying cause of ARDS, prehospital management may include fluid replacement to maintain cardiac output and peripheral perfusion; drug therapy to support mechanical ventilation;

Box 14-4

Severe acute respiratory syndrome (SARS)

SARS, a viral disease, emerged in China in November 2003. To date, SARS has affected about 8000 people in 29 countries, including the UK. More than 770 SARS-related deaths have been reported worldwide. SARS is thought to be caused by a new member of the coronavirus family. It is spread by direct contact with the respiratory secretions or body fluids of an infected person. Signs and symptoms of the disease include cough, shortness of breath, difficulty breathing, hypoxia, chills, and body ache (clinical findings of respiratory illness), as well as fever over 38 °C.

The exact aetiology of the illness has not yet been determined and no specific treatment recommendations have been made. The Health Protection Agency recommends that healthcare workers should use respirators, correctly fitted, for contact with possible or probable cases of SARS. A mask should be used only if a respirator is not available, on the grounds that, although not recommended, it is better to wear a mask than no protection at all. It is unlikely that respirators will be routinely available to EMS personnel in the UK.

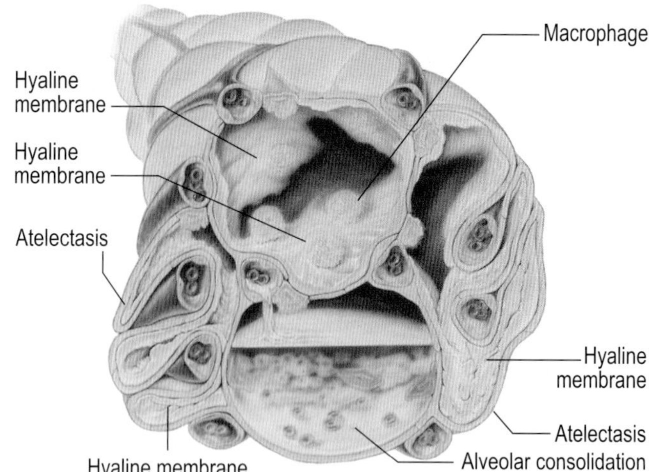

Figure 14-9 Cross-sectional view of alveoli in adult respiratory distress syndrome.

the use of pharmacological agents (e.g. corticosteroids) to stabilize pulmonary, capillary, and alveolar walls; and diuretics (all of these treatments are controversial).

Patients with ARDS usually have tachypnoea, laboured breathing, and impaired gas exchange 12–72 h after the initial injury or medical crisis. The syndrome often results from another illness or injury; therefore, paramedics should consider the cause of the underlying problem. They should also provide supplemental oxygen and ventilatory support to improve arterial oxygenation (assessed by pulse oximetry). Most patients with moderate to severe respiratory distress require mechanical ventilation. This ventilation includes the use of positive end-expiratory pressure (PEEP) or continuous positive airway pressure (CPAP). Both of these provide positive-pressure ventilation and increase Po_2 by reducing pressure in the lungs. Although not commonly available for paramedic use in the UK, PEEP and CPAP are discussed due to the potential for their use in the future.

Note

Positive end-expiratory pressure (PEEP) and continuous positive airway pressure (CPAP) may have unfavourable effects on the circulation. Such effects include decreased venous return, decreased cardiac output, and pulmonary barotrauma.

Positive end-expiratory pressure

PEEP maintains a degree of positive pressure at the end of exhalation. This keeps the alveoli open and pushes fluid from the alveoli back into the interstitium or capillaries (Figure 14-9). In the prehospital setting, ventilatory support with PEEP can be provided through intubation and the use of a Boehringer valve or other special PEEP delivery devices. The Boehringer valve is a cylinder in which a metal ball is suspended. It is connected to the expiratory port of a bag-valve device. The valve (available in pressures of 5, 10 and 15 cmH_2O) creates PEEP by forcing the patient to exhale against the weight of the metal ball.

Continuous positive airway pressure

CPAP transmits positive pressure into the airways of a spontaneously breathing patient throughout the respiratory cycle. The increase in airway pressure allows for better diffusion of gases and re-expansion of collapsed alveoli. This results in improvement of gas exchange and a reduction in the work of breathing. CPAP can be applied invasively in a patient with spontaneous breathing (through an ET tube) or through a face or nose mask. Mask CPAP is provided through a tight-fitting facemask, which is connected to a battery-operated or oxygen-driven breathing circuit. This breathing circuit may have a fixed or adjustable fraction of inspired oxygen (Fio_2) and a fixed or adjustable pressure valve that delivers pressures of 5–10 cmH_2O. CPAP reduces the inspiratory work of breathing and lowers mean airway pressures. In addition to its use in patients with pulmonary oedema, CPAP may benefit patients with acute blunt and penetrating pulmonary injury and those with obstructive airway disease.[16] Trials of CPAP are taking place in the UK; implementation of CPAP will be largely dependent upon the results of these trials.

Biphasic positive airway pressure

Biphasic positive airway pressure (BiPAP) combines partial ventilatory support and CPAP. This allows the pressure to vary during each breath cycle. When the patient inhales, the pressure is similar to CPAP. When the patient exhales, the pressure drops, making it easier to breathe. BiPAP is applied by facemask or nosemask through a non-invasive ventilator device with two settings. The device provides a 5 cmH_2O pressure difference between inspiratory positive airway pressure (IPAP) and expiratory positive airway pressure (EPAP). BiPAP is a leak-tolerant system (CPAP is not). It allows IPAP and EPAP settings to be titrated (adjusted) to reach a desired PEEP range. In selected patients with respiratory distress caused by COPD, pulmonary oedema, pneumonia, and asthma, BiPAP may eliminate the need for ET intubation.

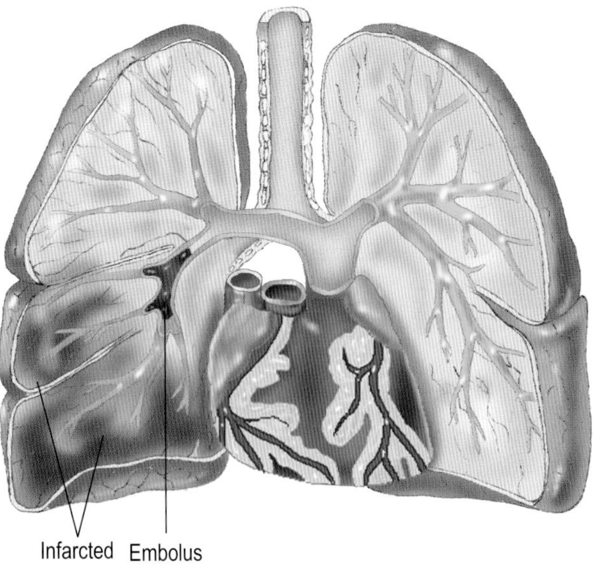

Figure 14-10 Pulmonary embolism (PE) is the blockage of a pulmonary artery by foreign matter, such as a thrombus. The blockage usually arises from a peripheral vein, fat, air, or tumour tissue. The result is obstruction of the blood supply to the lung tissue.

Pulmonary thromboembolism

Pulmonary thromboembolism (pulmonary embolism [PE]) is a blockage of a pulmonary artery. The artery is blocked by a clot or other foreign material that has travelled there from another part of the body (Figure 14-10). Usually, pulmonary emboli originate in the lower extremities. PE is a somewhat common disorder, especially after surgery, although there are no reliable studies indicating the incidence/prevalence in the UK.[17] In 2002, PE was recorded as the cause of death in 3016 patients in England and Wales.[18]

PE usually begins as a venous disease. It is most often caused by migration of a thrombus from the large veins of the lower extremities, but it can also occur as a result of fat, air, sheared venous catheters, amniotic fluid or tumour tissue. The clot or embolus dislodges and travels through the venous system to the right side of the heart. From there it migrates to the pulmonary arteries, obstructing the blood supply to a section of lung. The most common sites of thrombus formation are the deep veins of the legs and pelvis. Six factors that contribute to the development of venous thrombosis are listed in Box 14-5.

When one or more pulmonary arteries are blocked, an area does not receive blood flow; however, it continues to be ventilated. In response to the lack of blood flow, vasoconstriction occurs. If the vascular obstruction is severe (blockage of 60% or more of the pulmonary vascular supply), hypoxaemia, acute pulmonary hypertension, systemic hypotension, and shock may rapidly occur, with subsequent death.

Signs and symptoms

An embolus may be small, moderate or massive; thus, patients with PE may have very different presentations. A patient may have a wide variety of signs and symptoms depending upon the location and size of the clot. They may include dyspnoea, cough, haemoptysis (rare), pain, anxiety, syncope, hypotension, diaphoresis, tachypnoea, tachycardia, fever, and distended neck veins. In addition, chest splinting, pleuritic pain, pleural friction rub, crackles, and localized wheezing may be present. The paramedic should consider a pulmonary embolism in any patient who has cardiorespiratory problems that cannot otherwise be explained, particularly when risk factors are present.

Box 14-5

Contributing factors in the development of venous thrombosis

Venostasis
- Extended travel
- Prolonged bed rest
- Obesity
- Advanced age
- Burns
- Varicose veins

Venous injury
- Surgery of the thorax, abdomen, pelvis, or legs
- Fractures of the pelvis or legs

Increased blood coagulability
- Malignancy
- Use of oral contraceptives
- Congenital or acquired coagulation disorders

Pregnancy

Disease
- Chronic lung disease
- Congestive heart failure
- Sickle cell anaemia
- Cancer
- Atrial fibrillation
- Myocardial infarction
- Previous pulmonary embolism
- Previous deep vein thrombosis
- Infection
- Diabetes mellitus

Multiple trauma
- Long bone fracture
- Pelvic fracture

Critical Thinking

Consider that you need to distinguish a PE from other conditions with similar signs and symptoms. What information in the patient assessment may help?

Management

Prehospital care is mainly supportive. Supplemental high-concentration oxygen should be administered, a cardiac monitor applied, pulse oximetry used, and an IV line considered. The patient should be transported in a position of comfort. Definitive care requires hospitalization and in-hospital treatment with fibrinolytic or heparin therapy.

Upper respiratory infection

Upper respiratory infections (URIs) affect the nose, throat, sinuses and larynx. They are among the most common of all illnesses and include the common cold, pharyngitis, tonsillitis, sinusitis, laryngitis and croup. They are rarely life-threatening but they may exacerbate underlying pulmonary conditions. They may also lead to significant infections in patients with suppressed immune function. A key action for preventing the spread of respiratory infections is hand washing.

A variety of bacteria and viruses can cause URIs; signs and symptoms include the following:

- sore throat
- fever
- chills
- headache
- facial pain (sinusitis)
- purulent nasal drainage
- halitosis (bad breath)
- cervical adenopathy (enlarged cervical lymph nodes)
- erythematous pharynx (pharyngeal inflammation/irritation).

Critical Thinking

When might an upper respiratory infection (URI) become life-threatening? Think of two or three examples.

Management

Most URIs are self-limiting and require little or no prehospital treatment. Prehospital care is aimed at relieving the symptoms, especially for patients who have underlying lung conditions. With such conditions, oxygen administration may be indicated, as may the administration of bronchodilators or corticosteroids. The paramedic should follow local guidelines regarding management and hospitalization of patients with URI.

Spontaneous pneumothorax

A primary spontaneous pneumothorax usually results when a bleb ruptures (a bleb is a cystic lesion on a lobe of the lung). This allows air to enter the pleural space from within the lung. This type of pneumothorax may occur in seemingly healthy individuals who are usually between 20 and 40 years of age. Often these patients are tall, thin men with long, narrow chests.

Most primary spontaneous pneumothoraces that are well tolerated by the patient occupy less than 20% of a lung (partial pneumothorax). Signs and symptoms include shortness of breath and chest pain that often is sudden in onset, pallor, diaphoresis and tachypnoea. In severe cases in which the pneumothorax occupies more than 20% of the hemithorax, the following signs and symptoms may be present:

- altered mental status
- cyanosis
- tachycardia
- decreased breath sounds on the affected side
- local hyperresonance to percussion
- subcutaneous emphysema.

In severe cases, a spontaneous pneumothorax may generate a tension pneumothorax. When this occurs, venous return to the heart is impaired. This can lead to total cardiovascular collapse.

Management

Prehospital care is based on the patient's symptoms, particularly the degree of respiratory distress. For most cases, the administration of oxygen is all that is required. Airway, ventilatory and circulatory support may be required in severe cases but this is rare. Patients with a spontaneous pneumothorax who require ventilation should be managed very carefully; they are at high risk of developing a tension pneumothorax. Patients should be transported in a position of comfort and monitored en route to hospital. ECG monitoring should be undertaken alongside standard respiratory assessments. If signs and symptoms of tension pneumothorax develop, needle chest decompression should be performed.

Hyperventilation syndrome

Hyperventilation syndrome is defined 'as a rate of ventilation exceeding metabolic needs and higher than that required to maintain a normal level of plasma CO_2.'[7] It is most often seen in anxious patients but physiological hyperventilation is also a natural response to a number of more serious conditions (see below). The paramedic should consider hyperventilation to be indicative of a more serious condition until proven otherwise; this will minimize the risk of inappropriate treatment being applied. In the purely anxious patient, the hypocarbia increases the amount of bound calcium, which leads to relative hypocalcaemia. This electrolyte imbalance in turn leads to tetany, paraesthesia, and carpopedal spasm (cramping of the muscles of the hands and feet). The following conditions can cause hyperventilation syndrome:

- anxiety
- hypoxia
- pulmonary disease
- cardiovascular disorders
- metabolic disorders
- neurological disorders
- fever
- infection
- pain
- pregnancy
- drug use.

Critical Thinking

How can you distinguish between hyperventilation caused by anxiety and hyperventilation caused by a serious medical illness or toxic ingestion?

Signs and symptoms of hyperventilation syndrome include dyspnoea with rapid breathing and a high minute volume, chest pain, facial tingling, paraesthesia, dizziness, feelings of euphoria and carpopedal spasm. Other assessment findings vary, based on the cause of the syndrome.

Management

If airway, breathing or circulation need correction, then the cause is unlikely to be hyperventilation syndrome; in this case the normal medical approach should be adopted and the underlying condition managed. If the syndrome clearly is caused by anxiety, prehospital care is mainly supportive and consists of calming measures and reassurance. The paramedic should aim to restore $P\text{CO}_2$ over a period of time and should aim to achieve this by coaching the patient's respirations. Treatment with a paper bag to encourage the rebreathing of CO_2 is no longer considered appropriate due to the potential for harm should the hyperventilation be secondary to increased oxygen demand from a medical cause.[19] If the hyperventilation is severe or complicated by illness or drug ingestion, transport for evaluation by a physician is indicated.

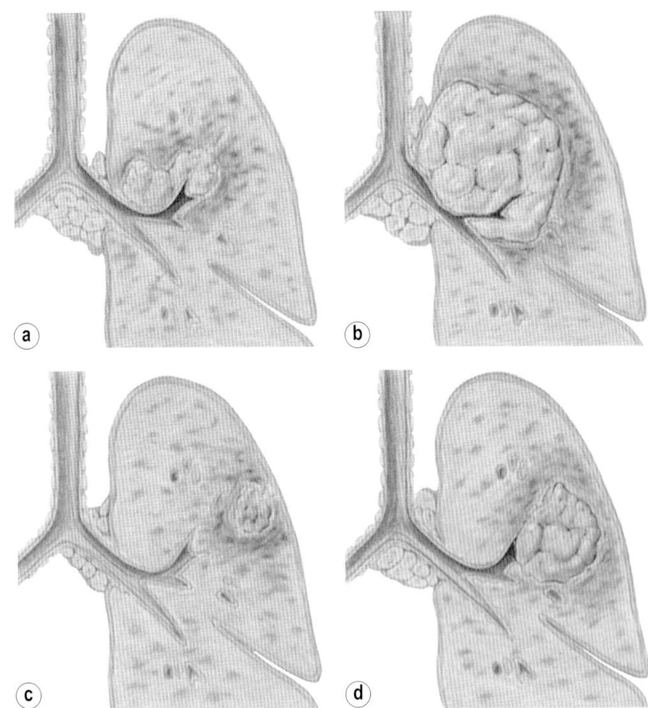

Figure 14-11 Cancer of the lung. (a) Squamous cell carcinoma. (b) Small cell (oat cell) carcinoma. (c) Adenocarcinoma. (d) Large cell carcinoma.

Lung cancer

Lung cancer is epidemic in the UK. An estimated 32 000 new cases are reported each year.[20] Most cases of lung cancer develop in individuals between 55 and 79 years of age. Of the new cases reported, most patients die of the disease within 1 year; 20% have local lung involvement; 25% have spread to the lymph system, and 55% have distant metastatic cancer.[16] The most common cause of lung cancer is cigarette smoking. Heavy smokers (more than 20 cigarettes a day) have a 25 times greater chance of developing lung cancer than non-smokers.[21] Other risk factors include passive smoking (exposure to someone else's cigarette smoke) and exposure to asbestos, radon gas, dust, coal products, ionizing radiation and other toxins.

Pathophysiology

Like other cancers, lung cancer is the uncontrolled growth of abnormal cells. At least a dozen different cell types of tumours are associated with primary lung cancer (Figure 14-11). The two major cell types of lung cancer are small cell lung cancer and non-small cell lung cancer (which is subcategorized as squamous cell carcinoma, adenocarcinoma, and large cell carcinoma). Each cell type has a different growth pattern and has also a different response to treatment. Most abnormal cell growth begins in the bronchi or bronchioles. The lung is also a fairly common site of metastasis for cancers from other primary sites (e.g. breast cancer).

Signs and symptoms

The signs and symptoms of early-stage disease are often nonspecific and include coughing, sputum production, lower airway obstruction (noted by wheezing) and respiratory illness (e.g. bronchitis). Smokers often attribute them to the effects of smoking. As the disease progresses, signs and symptoms may include the following:

- cough
- haemoptysis (which may be severe)
- dyspnoea
- hoarseness or voice change
- dysphagia
- weight loss/anorexia
- weakness.

Patients with cancer may call paramedics because of complications resulting from chemotherapy or radiation therapy. Such therapy is toxic to both normal body cells and malignant cells. Associated complaints often include nausea and vomiting, fatigue and dehydration. These patients should be offered emotional and psychological support.

Critical Thinking

Should you assume that patients who have been diagnosed with lung cancer want 'do not resuscitate' (DNR) status?

Management

Most patients with lung cancer are aware of their disease. Prehospital management includes airway, ventilatory, and circulatory support; oxygen administration (based on symptoms and pulse oximetry); and transport for evaluation by a physician. Depending on the severity of the patient's condition, drug therapy such as bronchodilators and corticosteroids may be indicated to improve breathing. Analgesia may also be required if the patient is in pain, although the paramedic should ascertain what medication the patient has already taken, to avoid unintentional overdose. End-stage patients may have advance directives or 'do not resuscitate' (DNR) orders. In these cases emotional support should also be offered to the family and loved ones.

Summary

- Diseases responsible for respiratory emergencies include those related to ventilation, diffusion and perfusion.
- Obstructive airway disease is a triad of distinct diseases that often coexist. These are chronic bronchitis, emphysema and asthma. The patient with chronic obstructive pulmonary disease usually has an acute episode of worsening dyspnoea that is manifested even at rest, an increase or change in sputum production, or an increase in the malaise that accompanies the disease. The main goal of prehospital care for these patients is the correction of hypoxaemia through improved airflow.
- Asthma, or reactive airway disease, is characterized by reversible airflow obstruction caused by bronchial smooth muscle contraction; hypersecretion of mucus, resulting in bronchial plugging; and inflammatory changes in the bronchial walls. The typical patient with asthma is in obvious distress. Respirations are rapid and loud. Initial medications in the prehospital setting probably will have a short onset of action.
- Pneumonia is a group of specific infections (bacterial, viral or fungal). These infections cause an acute inflammatory process of the respiratory bronchioles and the alveoli. Pneumonia usually manifests with classic signs and symptoms that include a productive cough and associated fever that produces 'shaking chills'. Prehospital care of patients with pneumonia includes airway support, oxygen administration, ventilatory assistance as needed, IV fluids, cardiac monitoring, and transport.
- Adult respiratory distress syndrome is a fulminant form of respiratory failure. It is characterized by acute lung inflammation and diffuse alveolar-capillary injury. It develops as a complication of illness or injury. In ARDS, the lungs are wet and heavy, congested, haemorrhagic and stiff, with decreased perfusion capacity across alveolar membranes. Management includes airway and ventilatory support.
- Pulmonary thromboembolism is a blockage of a pulmonary artery by a clot or other foreign material. When one or more pulmonary arteries is blocked by an embolism, a section of lung is ventilated but hypoperfused. Prehospital care is mainly supportive and includes oxygen administration, IV access, and transport for definitive care.
- Upper respiratory infections affect the nose, throat, sinuses and larynx. Signs and symptoms of a URI include sore throat, fever, chills, headache, cervical adenopathy and an erythematous pharynx. Prehospital care is based on the patient's symptoms.
- A primary spontaneous pneumothorax usually results when a subpleural bleb ruptures. This allows air to enter the pleural space from within the lung. Signs and symptoms include shortness of breath and chest pain that are often sudden in onset, pallor, diaphoresis and tachypnoea. Prehospital care is based on the patient's symptoms and degree of distress.
- Hyperventilation syndrome is abnormally deep or rapid breathing that results in an excessive loss of carbon dioxide. If the syndrome clearly is caused by anxiety, prehospital care is mainly supportive (i.e. calming measures and reassurance). The paramedic may suspect that the syndrome is a result of illness or drug ingestion. If this is the case, care may include oxygen administration and airway and ventilatory support.
- Lung cancer is an expression of the uncontrolled growth of abnormal cells. As the disease progresses, signs and symptoms may include cough, haemoptysis, dyspnoea, hoarseness and dysphagia. Prehospital management includes airway, ventilatory, and circulatory support.

References

1. British Thoracic Society 2006 The burden of lung disease: a statistical report from the British Thoracic Society, 2nd edition. British Thoracic Society, London
2. Parshall MB 1999 Adult emergency visits for chronic cardiorespiratory disease: does dyspnoea matter? Nurs Res 48(2):62–70
3. Stang P, Lydick E, Silberman C, et al 2000 The prevalence of COPD: using smoking rates to estimate disease frequency in the general population. Chest 117:354S–359S
4. British Lung Foundation 2003 Lung Report III (2003). British Lung Foundation, London
5. McGuire A, Irwin DE, Fenn P, et al 2001 The excess cost of acute exacerbations of chronic bronchitis in patients aged 45 and older in England and Wales. Value Health 4(5):370–375
6. Medical Research Council 1965 Definition and classification of chronic bronchitis for clinical and epidemiological purposes. Lancet i:775–779
7. Joint Royal Colleges Ambulance Liaison Committee 2006 UK Ambulance Service Clinical Guidelines v4. 2006. Online. Available http://jrcalc.org.uk/guidelines.html
8. Asthma UK. Where do we stand? Asthma in the UK today. 2004. Online. Available http://www.asthma.org.uk/how_we_help/publishing_reports/index.html 4 February 2009
9. Burr ML, Davies BH, Hoare A, et al 1999 A confidential inquiry into asthma deaths in Wales. Thorax 54:985–989
10. Bucknall CE, Slack R, Godley CC, et al 1999 Scottish Confidential Inquiry into Asthma Deaths (SCIAD), 1994–1996. Thorax 54:978–984
11. American Heart Association 2000 Guidelines 2000 for cardiopulmonary resuscitation and emergency cardiovascular care, International Consensus on Science. Circulation 102(8):237
12. American Heart Association 2000 Guidelines 2000 for cardiopulmonary resuscitation and emergency cardiovascular care, International Consensus on Science. Circulation 102(8):240
13. British Thoracic Society Standards of Care Committee 2001 BTS guidelines for the management of community acquired pneumonia in adults. Thorax 56(Suppl 4):IV1–64

14. Guest JF, Morris A 1997 Community-acquired pneumonia: the annual cost to the National Health Service in the UK. Eur Resp J 10:1530–1534
15. McCance L, Huether S 1988 Pathophysiology: the biologic basis for disease in adults and children, 3rd edition. Mosby, St Louis
16. Rosen P, Barkin R 1998 Emergency medicine: concepts and clinical practice, 4th edition. Mosby, St Louis
17. McManus R, Fitzmaurice D 2007 Thromboembolism. BMJ Clinical Evidence. Online. Available http://www.clinicalevidence.com/ceweb/conditions/cvd/0208/0208_background.jsp 4 February 2009
18. Hogg K, Dawson D, Mackway-Jones K 2006 Investigating pulmonary embolism in the emergency department with lower limb plethysmography: Manchester Investigation of Pulmonary Embolism Diagnosis (MIOPED) study. Emerg Med J 23:94–98
19. Callaham M 1989 Hypoxic hazards of traditional paper bag rebreathing in hyperventilating patients. Ann Emerg Med 18(6):622–628
20. Forman D, Stockton D, Møller H et al 2003 Cancer prevalence in the UK: results from the EUROPREVAL study. Ann Oncol 14(4):648–654
21. American Lung Association, data and statistics. Online. Available http://www.lungusa.org/site/c.dvLUK90DE/b.33347/k.AC09/Data_Statistics.html

CHAPTER 15

Cardiology

Chapter contents

Chapter contents

Objectives

Upon completion of this chapter, the paramedic student will be able to:

1. Identify risk factors and prevention strategies associated with cardiovascular disease.
2. Describe the normal physiology of the heart.
3. Discuss electrophysiology as it relates to the normal electrical and mechanical events in the cardiac cycle.
4. Outline the activity of each component of the electrical conduction system of the heart.
5. Outline the appropriate assessment of a patient who may be experiencing a cardiovascular disorder.
6. Describe basic monitoring techniques that permit electrocardiogram interpretation.
7. Explain the relationship of the electrocardiogram tracing to the electrical activity of the heart.
8. Describe in sequence the steps in electrocardiogram interpretation.
9. Identify the characteristics of normal sinus rhythm.
10. When shown an electrocardiogram tracing, identify the rhythm, site of origin, possible causes, clinical significance, and prehospital management that is indicated.
11. Describe prehospital assessment and management of patients with selected cardiovascular disorders based on knowledge of the pathophysiology of the illness.
12. List indications, contraindications, and prehospital considerations when using selected cardiac interventions, including basic life support, monitor–defibrillators, defibrillation, implantable cardioverter defibrillators, synchronized cardioversion, and transcutaneous cardiac pacing.
13. List indications, contraindications, dose, and mechanism of action for pharmacological agents used to manage cardiovascular disorders.
14. Identify appropriate actions to take in the prehospital setting to terminate resuscitation.

Key terms

atrioventricular dissociation A conduction disturbance in which atrial and ventricular contractions occur rhythmically but are unrelated to each other.

automaticity A property of specialized excitable tissue that allows self-activation through spontaneous development of an action potential.

bundle of Kent An accessory pathway between the atria and ventricles outside of the conduction system; a congenital anomaly that causes Wolff–Parkinson–White syndrome.

cardiac ejection fraction The percentage of ventricular blood volume released during a contraction.

hypertensive encephalopathy A set of symptoms – including headache, convulsions, and coma – that results solely from elevated blood pressure.

P wave The first complex of the electrocardiogram, representing depolarization of the atria.

paroxysmal nocturnal dyspnoea An abnormal condition of the respiratory system characterized by sudden attacks of shortness of breath, profuse sweating, tachycardia, and wheezing that awaken a person from sleep; often associated with left ventricular failure and pulmonary oedema.

paroxysmal supraventricular tachycardia An ectopic rhythm in excess of 100 beats per minute and usually faster than 170 beats per minute that begins abruptly with a premature atrial or junctional beat and is supported by an atrioventricular nodal re-entry mechanism or by an atrioventricular re-entry involving an accessory pathway.

P-R interval The time elapsing between the beginning of the P wave and the beginning of the QRS complex in the electrocardiogram.

premature atrial complex A cardiac dysrhythmia characterized by an atrial beat occurring before the expected excitation and indicated on the electrocardiogram as an early P wave.

premature junctional contraction A cardiac dysrhythmia that occurs during sinus rhythm earlier than the next expected sinus beat and is caused by premature discharge of an ectopic focus in the atrioventricular junctional tissue.

premature ventricular complex A cardiac dysrhythmia characterized by a ventricular beat preceding the expected electrical impulse and indicated on the electrocardiogram as an early, wide QRS complex without a preceding related P wave.

proarrhythmia A new or worsened rhythm disturbance seemingly generated by antidysrhythmic therapy.

QRS complex The principal deflection in the electrocardiogram, representing ventricular depolarization.

Q-T interval The time elapsing from the beginning of the QRS complex to the end of the T wave, representing the total duration of electrical activity of the ventricles.

R-on-T phenomenon The occurrence of a ventricular depolarization during a vulnerable period of relative refractoriness.

refractory period The period after effective stimulation during which excitable tissue fails to respond to a stimulus of threshold intensity.

resting membrane potential The electrical charge difference inside a cell membrane measured relative to just outside the cell membrane.

ST segment The early part of repolarization in the electrocardiogram of the right and left ventricles.

Starling's law of the heart A rule that the force of the heartbeat is determined by the length of the fibres making up the myocardial walls.

T wave A deflection in the electrocardiogram after the QRS complex, representing ventricular repolarization.

threshold potential The value of the membrane potential at which an action potential is produced as a result of depolarization in response to a stimulus.

torsades de pointes An unusual bidirectional ventricular tachycardia.

U wave The gradual deviation from the T wave in the electrocardiogram, thought to represent the final stage of repolarization of the ventricles.

ventricular bigeminy A cardiac rhythm disturbance characterized by two ventricular beats in rapid succession followed by a longer interval.

ventricular tachycardia A tachycardia that usually originates in the Purkinje fibres.

ventricular trigeminy A cardiac dysrhythmia characterized by three ventricular beats in rapid succession followed by a longer interval.

It is estimated that over 250 000 people suffer from acute coronary syndrome (ACS) each year in the UK, with up to a third dying prior to reaching hospital and with a further 8–13% dying after admission. A large number of these deaths can be prevented by rapid entry into the emergency medical services system, prompt provision of cardiopulmonary resuscitation, and early defibrillation as well as the administration of pharmacological agents and where necessary definitive interventions such as percutaneous cardiac intervention (PCI).

Critical Thinking

How many of your friends or family have had a heart attack or stroke? How has that illness affected their lives?

Risk factors and prevention strategies

Although death rates from myocardial infarction have declined over the past several decades, coronary heart disease (CHD) and its associated complications such as acute coronary syndrome (ACS) are still a major cause of morbidity and mortality and are still a prominent medical emergency in the UK. The decline in death rates is due in large part to heightened public awareness, increased availability of automated external defibrillators and Department of Health strategies (e.g. National Service Framework (NSF) for CHD) as well as improved cardiovascular diagnosis and therapy, use of cardiovascular drugs by persons at high risk, improved revascularization techniques, and improved and more aggressive risk factor modification.

Risk factors and risk factor modifications

Persons at high risk for cardiovascular disease include those with diabetes, hypertension, hypercholesterolaemia, hyperlipidaemia, a family history of premature cardiovascular disease, and known coronary artery disease. Their risk can be increased considerably if they have additional risk factors such as obesity, cigarette smoking, and a sedentary lifestyle (Box 15-1). Clearly, some risk factors cannot be changed.

Box 15-1

Risk factors for cardiovascular disease

Risk factors

- Age
- Carbohydrate intolerance
- Cigarette smoking
- Cocaine use
- Diabetes
- Family history
- Hypercholesterolaemia
- Hyperlipidaemia
- Hypertension
- Prior myocardial infarction

Possible contributing risk factors

- Obesity
- Oral contraceptive use
- Personality type
- Poor diet
- Psychosocial tensions
- Sedentary lifestyle
- Stress

Other risk factors, however, can be changed or modified through the following health promotion strategies:

- cessation of smoking
- management and control of blood pressure, diabetes, cholesterol, and lipid disorders by healthcare providers
- exercise
- weight loss
- diet
- stress reduction.

Modifying cardiovascular risk factors can slow the rate of development of arterial disease and reduce the incidence of acute myocardial infarction, sudden death, renal failure and stroke.

Prevention strategies

Paramedics and other healthcare professionals can support and practise prevention activities against the development of cardiovascular disease, which include educational programmes about nutrition in their communities, cessation of smoking (and smoking prevention for children), early recognition and management of hypertension and cardiac symptoms, and prompt intervention (including cardiopulmonary resuscitation and early use of an automated external defibrillator). These and other prevention strategies may help reduce risk factors at a young age and they also may have the greatest impact on risk factor modification.

SECTION I

Anatomy and physiology of the heart

Anatomy

The coronary arteries are the sole suppliers of arterial blood to the heart, delivering 200–250 mL of blood to the myocardium each minute during rest (Figure 15-1). The left coronary artery carries about 85% of the blood supply to the myocardium and the right coronary artery carries the rest. The coronary arteries begin just above the aortic valve where the aorta exits the heart, run along the epicardial (outer) surface and then divide into smaller vessels as they penetrate the myocardium and the endocardial (inner) surface.

The left main coronary artery supplies the left ventricle, interventricular septum, and part of the right ventricle and has two main branches; the left anterior descending and the circumflex arteries. The right coronary artery supplies the right atrium and ventricle, part of the left ventricle, and the conduction system; its two major branches are the right anterior descending and the marginal branch. In addition to the blood supply provided by these arteries, many connections (anastomoses) exist between arterioles to provide backup (collateral) circulation. These anastomoses play a key role in providing alternative routes of blood flow in the event of blockage in one or more of the coronary vessels.

> **Critical Thinking**
>
> Why is collateral circulation important?

Coronary capillaries allow for the exchange of nutrients and metabolic wastes and they merge to form coronary veins; these veins deliver most of the blood to the coronary sinus. The coronary sinus empties directly into the right atrium and is the major vein draining the myocardium.

Physiology

The heart can be thought of as two pumps in one. One is a low-pressure pump (right atrium and right ventricle) and supplies blood to the lungs. The second is a high-pressure pump (left atrium and left ventricle) and supplies blood to the body. The right atrium receives venous blood from the systemic circulation and from the coronary veins; most of this deoxygenated blood in the right atrium then passes to the right ventricle as the ventricle relaxes from the previous contraction. Once the right ventricle receives about 70% of its volume, the right atrium contracts and the blood remaining in the atrium is pushed into the ventricle. Contraction of the right ventricle pushes blood against the tricuspid valve (forcing it closed) and through the pulmonic valve (forcing it open); this allows the blood to enter the lungs via the pulmonary arteries. From the pulmonary arteries, the deoxygenated blood enters the capillaries in the lungs where gas exchange takes place.

From the lungs the blood travels through four pulmonary veins back to the left atrium. The mitral (bicuspid) valve opens, and blood flows to the left ventricle. Once the left ventricle receives about 70% of its volume, the left atrium contracts; the remaining blood is pushed into the ventricle. The blood passing from the left atrium to the left ventricle opens the bicuspid valve when the ventricle relaxes to complete left ventricular filling. As the left ventricle contracts, blood is pushed against the bicuspid valve (closing it) and against the aortic valve (opening it), which allows blood to enter the aorta. From the aorta, blood is distributed first to the heart itself and then throughout the systemic arterial circulation.

> **Note**
>
> The atria work mainly as 'primer pumps'. Under most conditions, the ventricles can pump enough blood to maintain adequate blood flow to the body without the help of the atria; however, under stress, the heart may pump 300–400% more blood than during rest; in such conditions, the priming action of the atria becomes key in maintaining pumping efficiency.

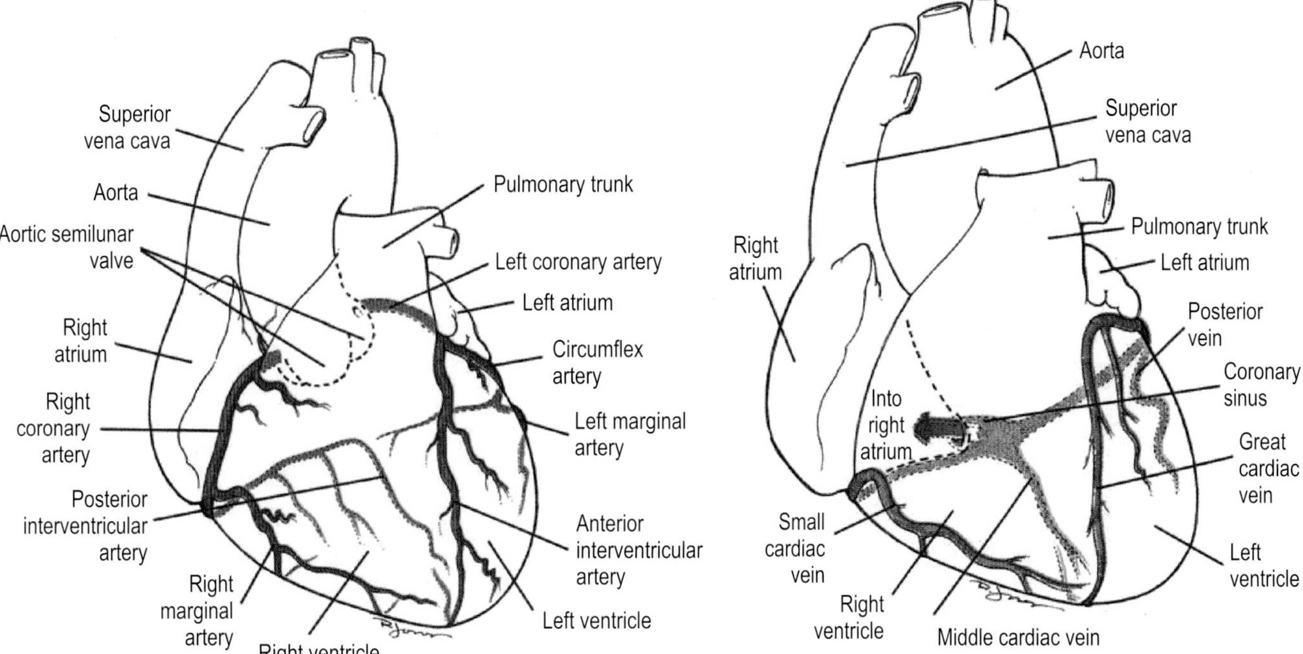

Figure 15-1 Blood vessels providing circulation of the heart. (a) Arteries. (b) Veins. The anterior surface of the heart is represented. The vessels of the anterior surface are seen directly and have a darker colour, whereas the vessels of the posterior surface are seen through the heart and have a lighter colour.

Cardiac cycle

The pumping action of the heart is a product of rhythmic, alternate contraction (systole) and relaxation (diastole) of the atria and ventricles. (When systole and diastole are used without reference to specific chambers, they mean ventricular systole or diastole.) These heartbeats occur about 70 times per minute in resting adults and these rhythmic contractions of the heart chambers are responsible for blood movement (Figure 15-2a–c).

Ventricular systole and diastole

As the ventricles begin to contract, ventricular pressure exceeds atrial pressure, causing the atrioventricular valves to close. As the contraction proceeds, ventricular pressure continues to rise, until it exceeds that in the pulmonary artery on the right side of the heart and in the aorta on the left side. At that time, the pulmonary and aortic valves open and blood flows from the ventricles into those arteries (ejection).

After ventricular contraction, ventricular relaxation begins and ventricular pressure falls rapidly. When the pressure falls below the pressure in the aorta or the pulmonary trunk, blood is forced back toward the ventricles; this closes the pulmonic and aortic valves. As ventricular pressure drops below atrial pressure, the tricuspid and bicuspid valves open and blood flows from the atria into the ventricles. Atrial systole occurs during ventricular diastole.

> **Critical Thinking**
>
> What would happen if the valves were scarred and became stiff?

Stroke volume

The stroke volume is the amount of blood ejected from the heart with each ventricular contraction and depends on three factors: preload (the volume of blood returning to the heart), afterload (the resistance against which the heart muscle must pump) and myocardial contractility.

Preload

During diastole, blood flows from the atria into the ventricles; known as the end-diastolic volume, it normally reaches 120–130 mL. As the ventricles empty during systole, their volume decreases to 50–60 mL (end-systolic volume) and therefore the amount of blood ejected during each cardiac cycle (stroke volume) is about 70 mL.

In a patient with a healthy heart the capacity to increase stroke volume is great; the strong contraction of a heart during exercise, for example, can reduce the volume returning to each ventricle to as little as 10–30 mL. If large amounts of blood flow into the ventricles during diastole, their end-diastolic volume can be as much as 200–250 mL and in this way, stroke volume can increase to more than double that of normal. The ability of the heart to pump more strongly when it has a larger preload is explained by Starling's law of the heart.

> **Critical Thinking**
>
> When you blow up a balloon, why does the balloon act like the heart muscle?

According to Starling's law (Figure 15-3), myocardial fibres contract more forcefully when they are stretched (this ability of stretched muscle to contract with increased force is a

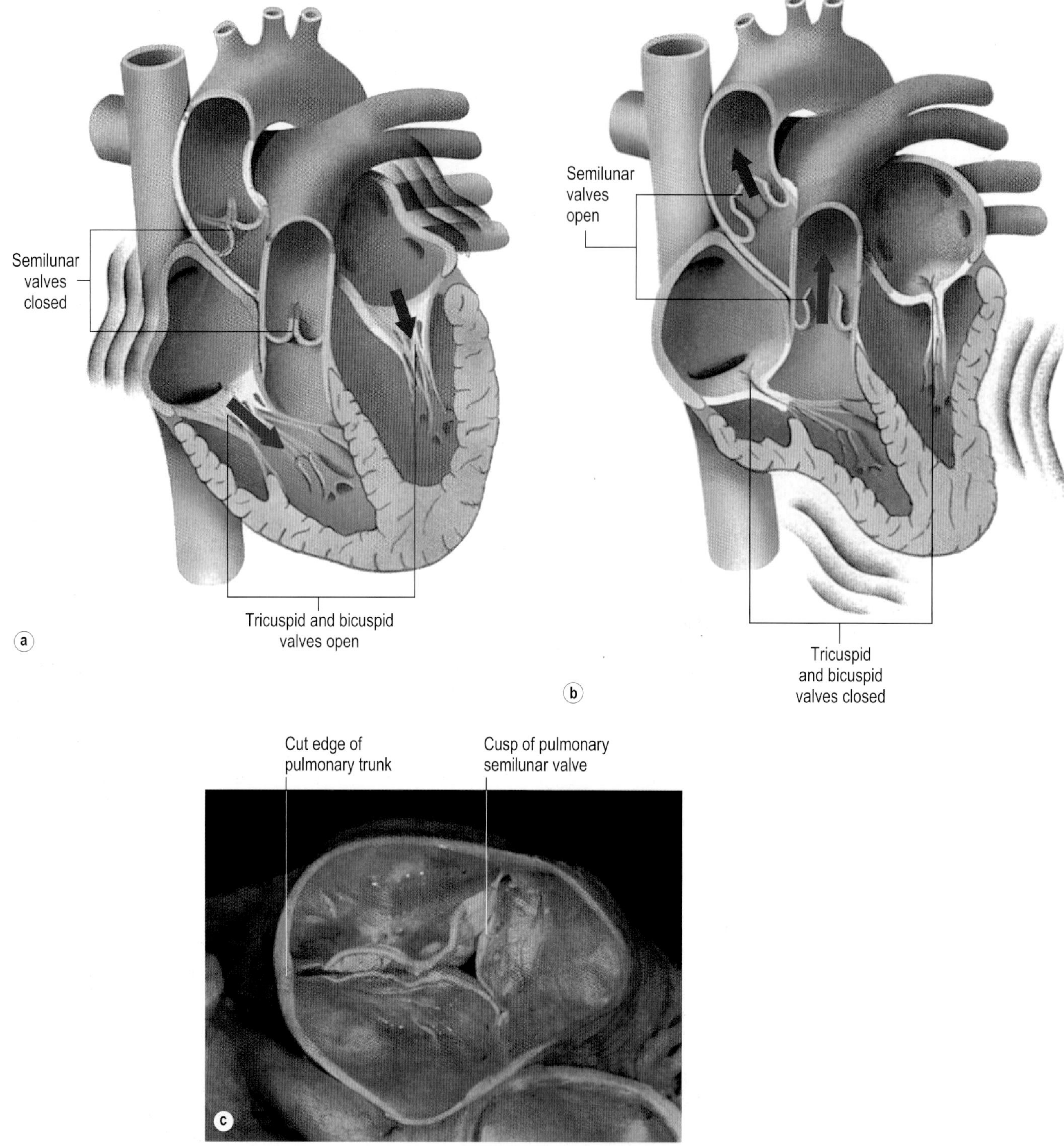

Figure 15-2 Heart action. (a) During atrial systole (contraction), cardiac muscle in the atrial wall contracts, forcing blood through the AV valves and into the ventricles. (b) During the ventricular systole that follows, the AV valves close, and blood is forced out of the ventricles through the semilunar valves into the arteries. (c) The pulmonary semilunar valves as seen from above (superior).

quality of all striated muscle; it is not just a quality of cardiac muscle.) When the ventricles are filled with larger-than-normal volumes of blood (increased preload), they contract with greater-than-normal force to deliver all of the blood to the systemic circulation.

The most important feature of the ability of the heart to handle changes in venous blood return is that changes in arterial pressure have minimal effect on cardiac output. In other words, the heart can pump a small amount of blood or a large amount; the amount depends on the amount of

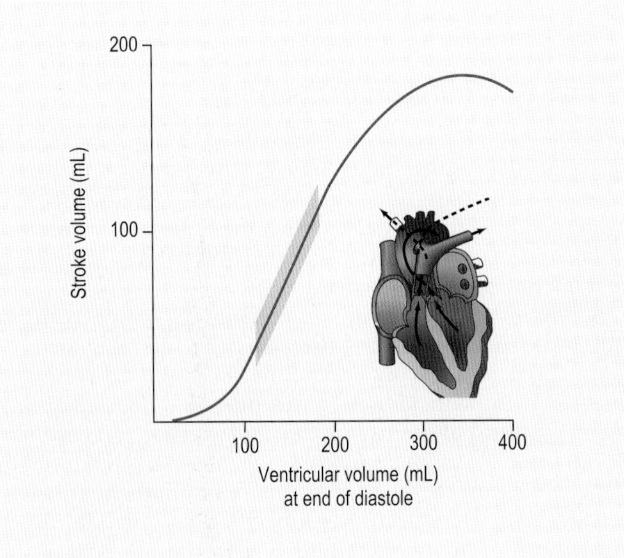

Figure 15-3 Starling's law of the heart.

venous return. The heart just adapts as long as the total quantity of blood does not exceed the limit that the heart can pump. Venous return is the most important factor in stroke volume, with arterial pressure causing a lesser effect in the form of afterload. Starling's law and its effect on stroke volume can be applied only up to a certain limit of muscle fibre stretching. Beyond that limit, muscle fibre stretch actually diminishes the strength of contraction and at that point the heart begins to fail.

Note

Preload is more important in determining cardiac output than is afterload.

Afterload

Afterload is a result of peripheral vascular resistance. An increase in peripheral vascular resistance decreases stroke volume which is due to the increased pressure in the aorta that the ventricular muscle must overcome to open the aortic valve and push blood through. However, a decrease in peripheral vascular resistance increases stroke volume if there is enough volume of fluid in the system.

Critical Thinking

What condition will increase the afterload?

Myocardial contractility

The unique function of the myocardial muscle fibres and the influence of the autonomic nervous system play a major role in the function of the heart. Ischaemia or various drugs can decrease myocardial contractility; ischaemia can decrease the total number of working myocardial cells. (This occurs in myocardial infarction.) Hypoxia or the administration of beta-blockers can decrease the ability of the separate myocardial cells to contract.

Cardiac output

Cardiac output is the amount of blood pumped by the ventricles per minute. Cardiac output can increase by increasing the heart rate, stroke volume, or both and is calculated as follows:

$$\text{Cardiac output} = \text{Stroke volume} \times \text{Heart rate}$$

Peripheral vascular resistance changes cardiac output by affecting the stroke volume. Vasodilation of the arteries, for example, decreases afterload and this produces an increase in cardiac output. In contrast, vasoconstriction increases afterload and tends to decrease cardiac output. However, the body responds to the decrease by constricting the venous circulation, which increases the amount of blood returning to the heart and causes the heart to contract more forcefully (Starling's law); these actions help to maintain or increase cardiac output.

Nervous system control of the heart

In addition to the heart regulating its behaviour, the autonomic nervous system also controls the behaviour of the heart, greatly influencing the heart rate, conductivity, and contractility. The autonomic nervous system innervates the atria and ventricles; the atria are well supplied with large numbers of sympathetic and parasympathetic nerve fibres but the ventricles are mainly supplied by sympathetic nerves.

The parasympathetic nervous system mainly is concerned with vegetative functions. In contrast, the sympathetic nervous system helps prepare the body to respond to stress. These sympathetic and parasympathetic control systems work in a check-and-balance manner and stimulate the heart to increase or decrease cardiac output according to the metabolic demands of the body.

Critical Thinking

Consider how you regulate the hot and cold taps in a shower. How is the behaviour of the autonomic nervous system similar?

Parasympathetic control

Parasympathetic control of the heart is through the vagus nerve; control by these nerve fibres has a continuous restraining influence on the heart, primarily by decreasing the heart rate and, to a lesser extent, contractility. The vagus nerve may be stimulated in several ways such as the Valsalva manoeuvre, carotid sinus massage (described later in this chapter), pain, and distension of the urinary bladder. Airway adjunct insertion and airway suctioning can also stimulate a vagal response. Acetylcholine is the chemical mediator of the parasympathetic nervous system.

Strong parasympathetic stimulation can decrease the heart rate to 20 or 30 beats per minute, yet such stimulation generally has little effect on stroke volume. In fact, stroke volume may increase with a decreased heart rate because the longer time interval between heartbeats allows the heart to fill with a larger amount of blood and thus contract more forcefully (Starling's law).

Sympathetic control

Sympathetic nerve fibres originate in the thoracic region of the spinal cord and form groups of nerve fibres called ganglia. Their postganglionic fibres release the chemical noradrenaline, which stimulates an increase in the heart rate (positive chronotropic effect). Noradrenaline also stimulates an increase in the force of muscle contraction (positive inotropic effect); sympathetic stimulation of the heart causes coronary arteries to dilate and causes constriction of peripheral vessels. These two effects, dilation and constriction, help to increase blood and oxygen supply to the heart. The cardiac effects of noradrenaline result from stimulation of alpha- and beta-adrenergic receptors.

Note

As described in Chapter 12, inotropic refers to the force of energy of muscular contractions; chronotropic refers to the regularity and rate of the heartbeat; and dromotropic refers to conduction velocity. The effects are classified as positive or negative. For example, a positive inotropic effect would increase the strength of contraction but a negative dromotropic effect would decrease the speed of conduction.

Strong sympathetic stimulation of the heart may significantly increase the heart rate; when rates are very high (greater than 150 beats per minute), the time available for the heart to fill is decreased, resulting in a decreased stroke volume.

Hormonal regulation of the heart

Impulses from the sympathetic nerves are sent to the adrenal medulla at the same time that they are sent to all blood vessels. In response, the adrenal medulla secretes the hormones adrenaline and noradrenaline into the circulating blood in response to increased physical activity, emotional excitement or stress.

Adrenaline has basically the same effect on cardiac muscles as noradrenaline, increasing the rate and force of contraction. In addition, adrenaline causes blood vessels to constrict in the skin, kidneys, gastrointestinal tract, and other organs (viscera) and causes dilation of skeletal and coronary blood vessels. Adrenaline from the adrenal glands takes longer to act on the heart than direct sympathetic innervation does, yet the effect lasts longer. Noradrenaline causes constriction of peripheral blood vessels in most areas of the body and stimulates cardiac muscle as well.

Role of electrolytes

Myocardial cells, like all other cells of the human body, are bathed in an electrolyte solution. The major electrolytes that affect cardiac function (described in the next section) are calcium, potassium, and sodium. Magnesium is a major intracellular cation and plays an important role as well.

Critical Thinking

What drugs can alter the normal balance of electrolytes in the body?

SECTION II

Electrophysiology of the heart

Caring for patients with cardiac disease is based on understanding how the heart works, including the mechanical and electrical functions; understanding why and how the electrical conduction system can malfunction is crucial for the paramedic. The paramedic also must understand the effect that lack of oxygen to the cells (myocardial ischaemia) has on cardiac rhythms. Two basic groups of cells within the myocardium are vital for cardiac function; one group is the specialized cells of the electrical conduction system, which are responsible for the formation and conduction of electrical current. The second group is the working myocardial cells, which possess the property of contractility and do the actual pumping of the blood.

Electrical activity of cardiac cells and membrane potentials

Ions are either positively or negatively charged particles; the charge depends on the ability of the ion to accept or to donate electrons. In solutions containing electrolytes, particles with unlike (opposite) charges attract each other, and the particles with like charges push away from each other; this results in a tendency to produce ion pairs, which help keep the solution neutral.

Electrically charged particles may be thought of as small magnets; they require energy to pull them apart if they have opposite charges. They also require energy to push them together if they have like electrical charges; therefore separated particles with opposite charges have an electrical magnetic-like force of attraction that gives them potential energy (Figure 15-4). The electrical charge creates a membrane potential between the inside and the outside of the cell; this electrical charge (potential difference) between the inside and outside of cells is expressed in millivolts (1 mV equals 0.001 volt) and this potential energy is released when the cell membrane separating the ions becomes permeable.

Resting membrane potential

When the cell is in its resting state, the electrical charge difference is the resting membrane potential; the term potential

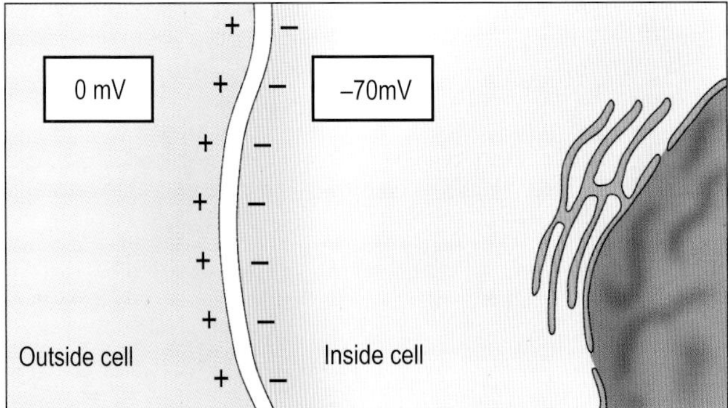

Figure 15-4 Electrical activity of cardiac cells and membrane potentials.

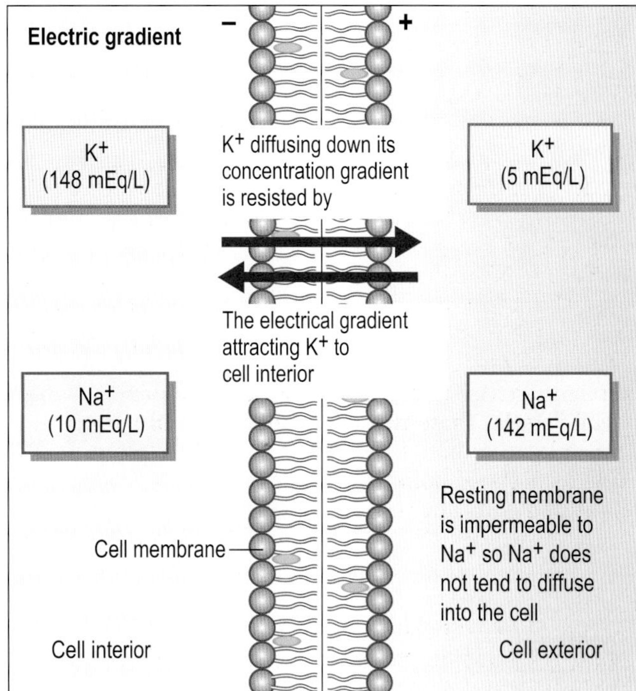

Figure 15-5 At equilibrium (resting conditions), the tendency for potassium ions to diffuse out of the cell is opposed by the potential difference (electrical gradient) across the cell membrane. Because the resting membrane is not permeable to sodium ions, sodium ions do not tend to diffuse into the cell. Sims/illustrator Rusty Jones.

is used in the electrical sense as a synonym for voltage. The inside of the cell is negative compared with the outside of the cell membrane. The resting membrane potential is recorded from the inside of the cell; therefore the resting membrane potential is reported as a negative number (about –70 to –90 mV).

The resting membrane potential is a result of the balance between two opposing forces. One of these forces is the concentration gradient of ions (mainly potassium) across a permeable cell membrane; the other is the electrical forces produced by the separation of positively charged ions from their negative ion pair. The resting membrane potential mainly is established by the difference between the intracellular potassium ion level and the extracellular potassium ion level. The ratio of 148:5 produces a large chemical gradient for potassium ions to leave the cell, yet the negative intracellular charge relative to the extracellular charge tends to keep potassium ions in the cell (Figure 15-5).

Sodium ions are positively charged ions on the outside of the cell and have a chemical and electrical gradient. This gradient tends to cause them to move intracellularly. Depolarization (electrical conduction) takes place when sodium ions rush into the cell, making the cell more positive on the inside compared with the outside.

Diffusion through ion channels

The cell membrane is relatively permeable to potassium, less permeable to calcium and chloride and minimally permeable to sodium. The cell membrane appears to have individual protein-lined channels which allow passage of a specific ion or group of ions. Permeability is influenced by electrical charge, size, and the proteins that open and close the channels (gating proteins).

The potassium ion channels are smaller than the sodium ion channels and prevent sodium from passing into the cell. Potassium ions are small enough to pass through sodium ion channels, but the cell favours sodium entering the cell during rapid depolarization (the rapid entry of sodium ions into cells). Rapid depolarization creates a local area of current known as the action potential. After one patch of membrane is depolarized, the electrical charge spreads along the cell surface, which opens more channels (Figure 15-6a, b).

Note

Depolarization occurs when the resting membrane potential changes from being more negatively charged on the inside of the cell to being more positively charged on the inside of the cell and is followed by muscle contraction. Repolarization occurs when charges inside the cell return to normal (become more negatively charged on the inside), allowing the cell to return to its normal resting state.

The contribution of unpaired ions to the resting membrane potential depends on two factors. The first factor is the diffusion of ions through the membrane by way of the ion channels; this creates an imbalance of charges. The second factor is the active transport of ions through the membrane by way of the sodium–potassium exchange pump, also creating an imbalance of charges.

Critical Thinking

Which of these processes of electrolyte transfer requires energy for it to occur?

Sodium–potassium exchange pump

The specialized sodium–potassium exchange pump actively pumps sodium ions out of the cell and potassium ions into the cell and separates the ions across the membrane against

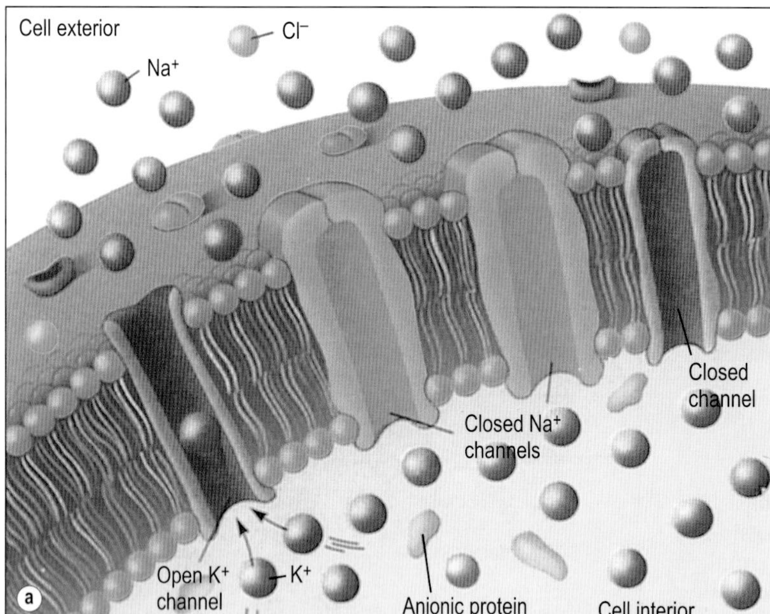

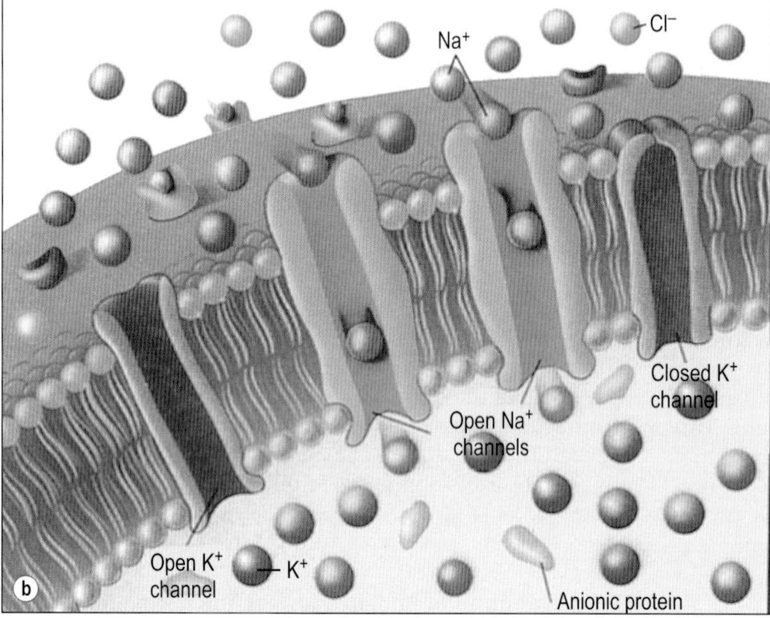

Figure 15-6 Effect of a stimulus that causes a voltage change across the cell membrane on the permeability of the cell membrane. (a) Sodium channels remain closed in a resting or unstimulated cell membrane. (b) Depolarization of the cell membrane causes sodium channels to open. Sodium ions then diffuse down their concentration gradient into the cell, causing depolarization of the cell membrane.

their concentration gradients. Potassium ions are transported into the cell, increasing their intracellular concentration, sodium ions are transported out of the cell, increasing their extracellular concentration (Figure 15-7).

The sodium–potassium exchange pump normally transports three sodium ions out for every two potassium ions taken in so more positively charged ions are transferred outward than inward; this returns the cell to its resting state. In the resting state of the cell, the number of negative charges inside the cell is equal to the number of positive charges outside the cell.

Pharmacological actions

In cardiac muscle, sodium and calcium ions can enter the cell through two separate channel systems in the cell membrane known as fast channels and slow channels. Fast channels are sensitive to small changes in membrane potential; as the cell drifts toward threshold level (the point at which a cell depolarizes), fast sodium channels open, resulting in a rush of sodium ions into the cell and rapid depolarization. The slow channel has selective permeability to calcium and to a lesser extent to sodium. Calcium plays an electrical role and contributes to the number of positive charges in the cell as well as playing a contractile role and is the ion required for cardiac muscle contraction to occur.

An understanding of ion channels helps the paramedic understand how the heart rate and contractility responds to drugs. For example, calcium channel blockers selectively block the slow channel. Examples of such drugs are verapamil and diltiazem. These drugs limit the movement of calcium ions into the cell without altering its voltage. Other examples,

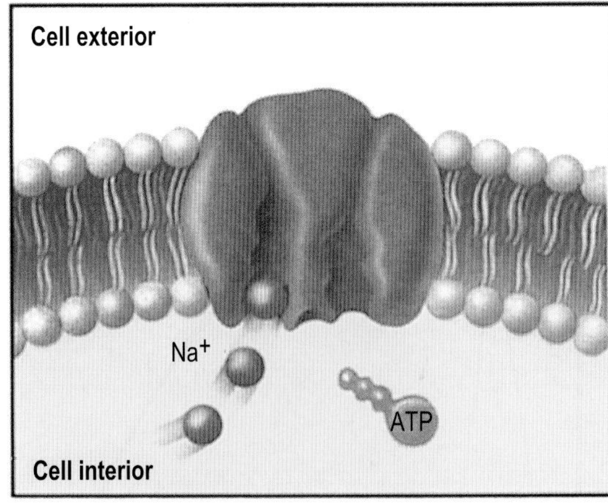

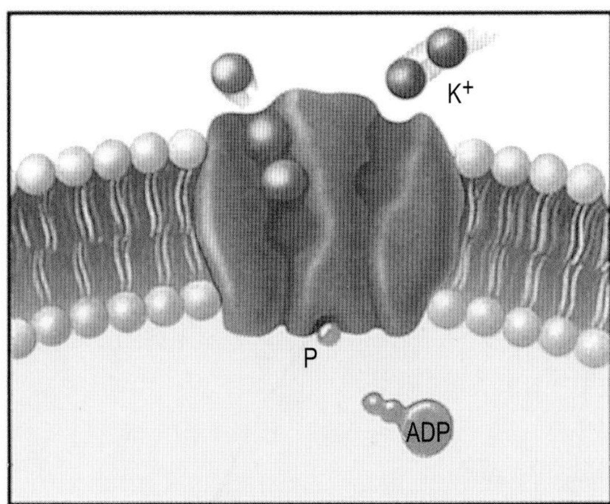

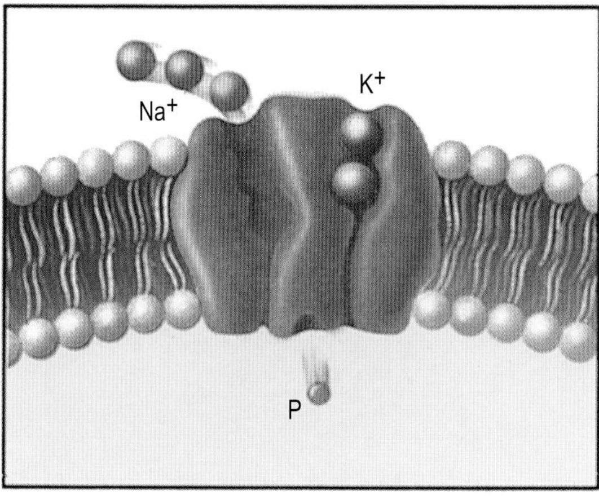

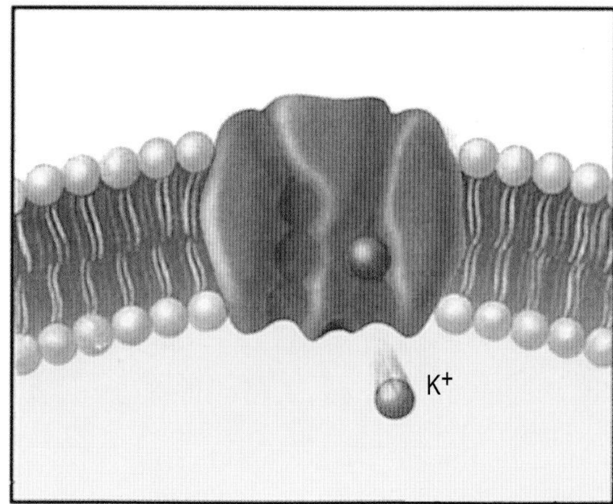

Figure 15-7 The sodium–potassium exchange pump actively transports sodium ions out of the cell across the cell membrane and potassium ions into the cell across the cell membrane. Adenosine triphosphate is used as the energy source, and the pump can transport up to three sodium ions for every two potassium ions transported.

such as procainamide and flecainide (both type I antidysrhythmics), owe much of their antidysrhythmic effects to their ability to block the fast inward sodium channel.

Cell excitability

Nerve and muscle cells are capable of producing action potentials known as excitability. When these cells are stimulated, a series of changes in the resting membrane potential normally causes depolarization of a small region of the cell membrane. The stimulus may be strong enough to depolarize a cell membrane to a level called the threshold potential. If this is the case, an explosive series of permeability changes takes place, causing an action potential to spread over the entire cell membrane.

Propagation of action potential

An action potential at any point on the cell membrane acts as a stimulus to adjacent regions of the cell membrane and the excitation process, once started, is spread along the length of the cell and onto the next cell and so on. A stimulus that is strong enough to cause a cell to reach threshold and depolarize (action potential) spreads quickly from one cell to another – the 'all-or-none' principle. The cardiac action potential can be divided into five phases (phases 0 to 4) (Figure 15-8).

Phase 0

Phase 0 is the rapid depolarization phase and represents the rapid upstroke of the action potential occurring when the cell membrane reaches threshold potential. During this phase, the fast sodium channels open momentarily and the sodium channels permit rapid entry of sodium into the cell. As the positively charged ions flow into the cell, the inside of the cell becomes positively charged compared with the outside, leading to muscular contraction.

Phase 1

Phase 1 is the early rapid repolarization phase; the fast sodium channels close, the flow of sodium into the cell stops, and potassium continues to be lost from the cell. This results in a decrease in the number of positive electrical charges inside the cell and a drop in the membrane potential, which returns the cell membrane to its resting permeability state.

Phase 2

Phase 2 is the plateau phase, a prolonged phase of repolarization of the action potential. During this phase, calcium enters the myocardial cells, triggering a large secondary release of calcium from intracellular storage sites and initiating contraction. Calcium slowly enters the cell through the slow calcium channels and simultaneously potassium con-

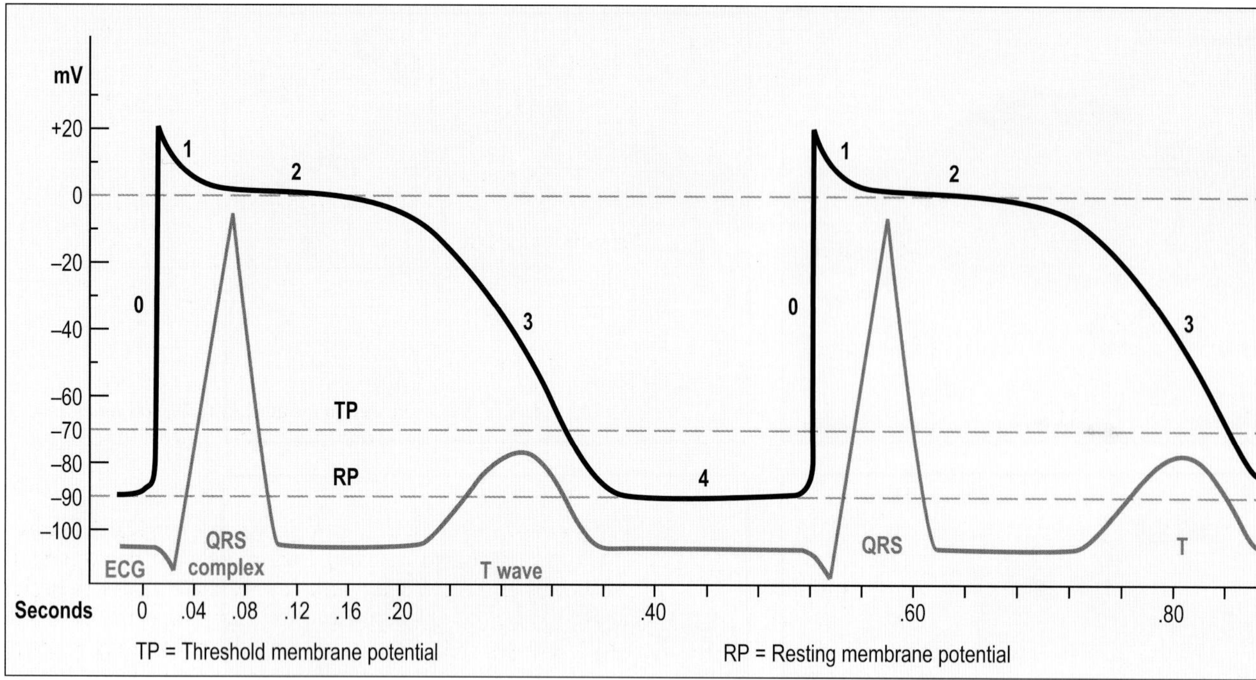

Figure 15-8 Cardiac action potential of myocardial cells.

tinues to leave the cell. The inward calcium current maintains the cell in a prolonged depolarization state, allowing time for completion of one muscle contraction before another depolarization begins; this phase also stimulates the release of intracellular stores of calcium and aids in the contraction process.

Phase 3

Phase 3 is the terminal phase of rapid repolarization, resulting in the inside of the cell becoming negative and the membrane potential returning to its resting state. This phase is initiated by closing of the slow calcium channels and by an increase in permeability with an outflow of potassium. Repolarization is completed by the end of this phase.

Phase 4

Phase 4 represents the period between action potentials, when the membrane has returned to its resting membrane potential. During this phase, the inside of the cell is negatively charged compared with the outside; however, the cell still has an excess of sodium inside and potassium outside which activates the sodium–potassium exchange pump. The excess sodium is transported out of the cell and the potassium is transported back into the cell. During phase 4, pacemaker cells have a slow depolarization from their most negative membrane potential to a level at which threshold is reached, and phase 0 begins all over again.

Refractory period of cardiac muscle

Cardiac muscle, like all excitable tissue, has a refractory period or resting period. During the absolute refractory period, the cardiac muscle cell cannot respond to any stimulation. If the depolarization phase of cardiac muscle is prolonged, the refractory period also is prolonged (Figure 15-9).

The refractory period ensures that the cardiac muscle is fully relaxed before another contraction begins. The refractory period of the ventricles is of about the same duration as that of the action potential but the refractory period of the atrial muscle is much shorter than that of the ventricles. This allows the rate of atrial contraction to be much faster than that of the ventricles. There also is a relative refractory period; during this time, the muscle cell is harder than normal to excite but can still be stimulated.

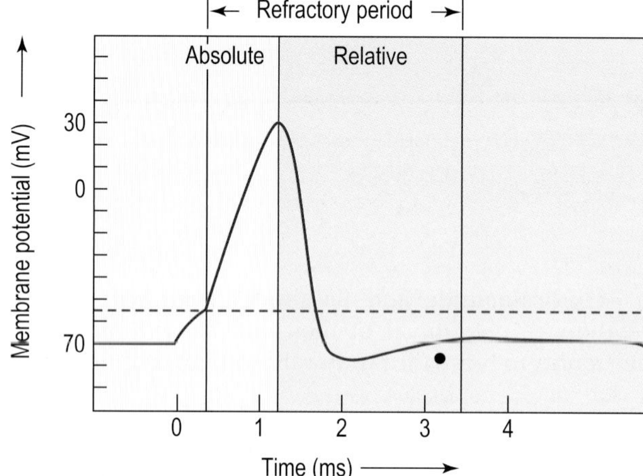

Figure 15-9 Refractory period.

Critical Thinking

How are the relative and absolute refractory periods of the heart similar to the flushing mechanism of your toilet?

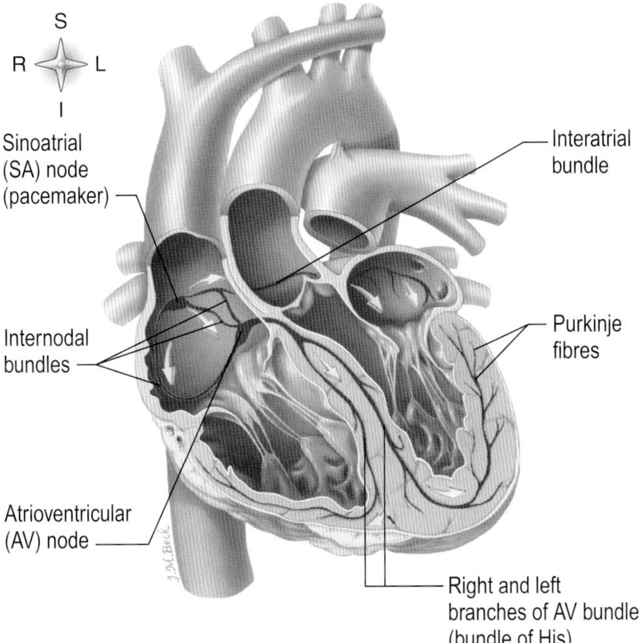

Figure 15-10 Conduction system of the heart. Impulses (arrows) travel across the wall of the right atrium from the SA node to the AV node. The AV bundle extends from the AV node through the fibrous skeleton and into the interventricular septum, where it divides into right and left bundle branches. The bundle branches descend to the apex of the ventricle and then branch repeatedly for distribution throughout the ventricular walls.

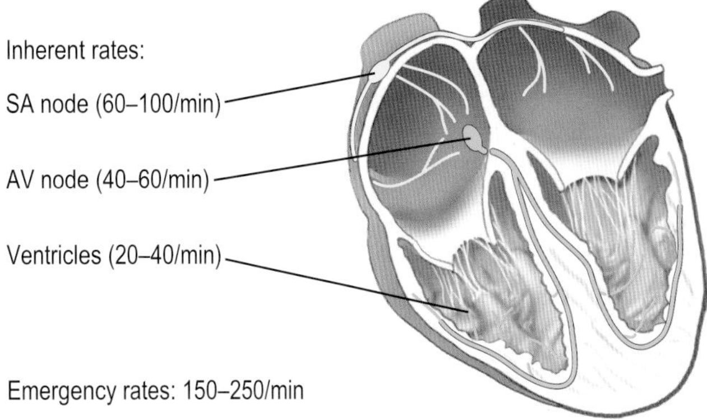

Figure 15-11 Intrinsic pacemakers in the atria, AV node, and ventricles can discharge at their own inherent rate when normal pacemaking fails.

Electrical conduction system of the heart

The conduction system of the heart has two nodes in the right atrium and a bundle branch (Figure 15-10), named according to their location. The sinoatrial (SA) node is located by the opening of the superior vena cava and the atrioventricular (AV) node is located by the right atrioventricular valve. The atrioventricular node and the bundle of His form the atrioventricular junction which serves as the only electrical link between the atria and ventricles in a normal heart. The bundle of His reaches into the interventricular septum, where the bundle of His divides into right and left bundle branches. The left bundle branch then subdivides into the anterior and posterior branches, which provide pathways for impulse conduction; a third branch of the left bundle branch also innervates the interventricular septum and the base of the heart.

The right and left bundle branches are on either side of the septum, reach to the apical portions of the right and left ventricles and then subdivide into smaller branches. The smallest branches are called Purkinje fibres which spread electrical impulses through the myocardial fibres resulting in contraction of the heart muscle. The rapid conduction along these fibres causes all ventricular cells to contract at more or less the same time.

Pacemaker activity

In skeletal and most smooth muscle, the individual cells contract only in response to hormones or nerve impulses from the central nervous system; unlike most other muscle cells, cardiac fibres have specialized cells that are known as pacemaker cells, which can generate electrical impulses spontaneously (automaticity). Pacemaker cells depolarize in a rhythmic and repetitive manner; pacemaker cells can depolarize without an outside stimulus. Sometimes the SA node may fail to generate an electrical impulse; if this occurs, other pacemaker cells take over and are capable of spontaneous depolarization and subsequent spread of an action potential; however, their rate is slower.

Sequence of excitation in cardiac muscle

Under normal conditions the chief pacemaker of the heart is the SA node because it reaches its threshold for depolarization at a faster rate than other pacemakers do. The rapid rate of the SA node normally prevents the slower pacemakers from taking over. If impulses from the SA node do not develop normally, however, the next pacemaker to reach its threshold level would take over the pacemaker duties. The SA node receives blood supply from the right coronary artery (RCA) and occlusion is likely cause the node to become ischaemic with resultant dysrhythmias (usually bradycardia).

Because of automaticity, cardiac cells can act as a fail-safe means for initiating electrical impulses. The backup cells (intrinsic pacemakers) are arranged in cascade fashion: the further from the sinoatrial node, the slower the intrinsic firing rate. In order, the location of cells with pacemaker capabilities and rates of spontaneous discharge are the sinoatrial node (60–100 discharges per minute); atrioventricular junctional tissue (40–60 discharges per minute); and the ventricles, including the bundle branches and Purkinje fibres (20–40 discharges per minute) (Figure 15-11).

From the SA node the excitation spreads throughout the right atrium; through internodal tracts (which includes the Bachman bundle), impulses travel directly from the right to the left atrium and to the base of the right atrium, resulting in virtually simultaneous contraction of both atria. About 0.04 s is required for the impulse of the sinoatrial node to spread to the atrioventricular node. From there, propagation of the action potentials within the atrioventricular node is slow compared with the rate in the rest of the conducting system. As a result, a delay of 0.11 s occurs from the time the action potentials reach the atrioventricular node until they pass to the atrioventricular bundle. The total delay of 0.15 s allows atrial contraction to be completed before ventricular contraction begins. Again the RCA supplies the AV node (in the majority of subjects) and occlusion may result in bradydysrhythmias.

After leaving the AV node, the impulse picks up speed travelling rapidly through the bundle of His and the left and right bundle branches, passes quickly through the individual Purkinje fibres and then ends in near simultaneous stimulation and contraction of the left and right ventricles. Ventricular contraction begins at the apex. Once stimulated, the special arrangement of muscle layers in the wall of the heart produce a 'wringing' action that proceeds toward the base of the heart.

Autonomic nervous system – effects on pacemaker cells

The effects of autonomic nervous system stimulation on the heart rate are mediated by acetylcholine (causes the cell membrane of the sinoatrial node to take more time to reach its threshold, therefore decreasing heart rate) and noradrenaline. Parasympathetic effects also may result from stimulation of the vagus nerve (e.g. vigorous carotid sinus massage). Excessive vagal stimulation may result in asystole (an absence of electrical and mechanical activity in the heart) and is why asystole at times is referred to as the ultimate bradycardia.

Critical Thinking

What else can cause vagal stimulation?

Noradrenaline increases the heart rate by increasing the rate of depolarization, causing an increase in pacemaker discharge rate in the SA node. As a result, sympathetic stimulation leads to an increase in the heart rate and increase in cardiac contractility.

Mechanisms of ectopic electrical impulse formation

An ectopic beat results when cells other than those in the SA node cause the heart to contract and are called premature beats because they occur early in the cycle before the SA node would normally discharge. The new pacemaker is called an ectopic focus. Depending on the location of the ectopic focus, the premature beats may be of atrial origin (premature atrial complexes), junctional origin (premature junctional contractions), or ventricular origin (premature ventricular complexes). The ectopic focus may be intermittent or sustained and may assume the pacemaker duties of the heart (i.e. the pacemaker site that fires the fastest controls the heart).

The two basic ways ectopic impulses are generated are by enhanced automaticity and re-entry.

Enhanced automaticity

Enhanced automaticity is caused by an acceleration in depolarization, with cells reaching threshold prematurely, causing an increase in the rate of electrical impulse formation in potential pacemakers.

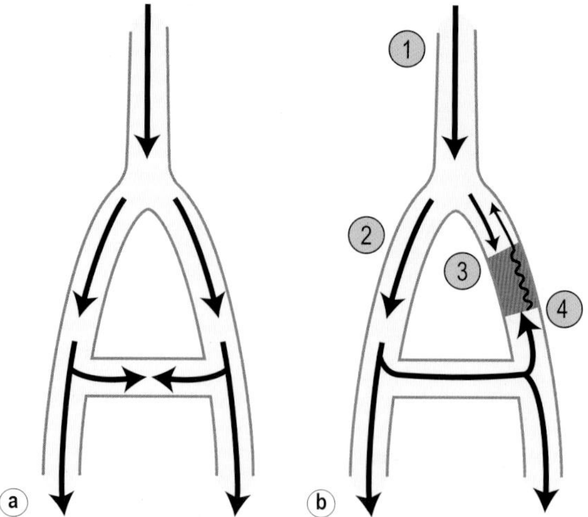

Figure 15-12 Re-entry within terminal Purkinje fibres. (a) Conduction through normal Purkinje fibres. The conduction velocity is uniform. (b) Conduction through a severely depressed segment of terminal Purkinje fibres. The impulse (1) travels normally through normal tissue (2) and is blocked at the severely depressed tissue (3) but returns, with delay, through this tissue from the opposite direction (4).

Enhanced automaticity is responsible for dysrhythmias in Purkinje fibres and other myocardial cells and may occur following release of excess catecholamine (i.e. noradrenaline and adrenaline), digitalis toxicity, hypoxia, hypercapnia, myocardial ischaemia or infarction, increased venous return (preload), hypokalaemia or other electrolyte abnormalities, or atropine administration.

Re-entry

Re-entry is the reactivation of myocardial tissue for the second or subsequent time by the same impulse (Figure 15-12) and occurs when the progression of an electrical impulse is delayed and/or blocked in one or more segments of the electrical conduction system of the heart. A delayed or blocked impulse can enter cardiac cells that have just become repolarized and may produce single or repetitive ectopic beats. Re-entry dysrhythmias can occur in the SA node, atria, AV junction, bundle branches, or Purkinje fibres. Re-entry is the most common mechanism in producing ectopic beats, including cases of premature ventricular complexes, ventricular tachycardia, ventricular fibrillation, atrial fibrillation, atrial flutter, and paroxysmal supraventricular tachycardia.

The re-entry mechanism requires that at some point conduction impulses (which have different conduction speeds and refractory characteristics through the heart) take parallel pathways. A premature impulse, for example, may find one branch of a conducting pathway still refractory from the passage of the last normal impulse. If the impulse passes (somewhat slowly) along a parallel conducting pathway, by the time the impulse reaches the previously blocked pathway, the blocked pathway may have had time to recover its ability to conduct. If the two parallel paths connect at an area of excitable myocardial tissue, the depolarization process from the slower path may enter the now repolarized tissue and give rise to a new impulse spawned from the original impulse. Common causes of delayed or blocked electrical impulses include myocardial ischaemia, certain drugs and hyperkalaemia.

SECTION III

Assessment of the patient with cardiac disease

Assessment

Any initial assessment must involve a global overview of the patient's general condition; a so-called 'first impression'. This will include a primary survey for patients who are not alert and orientated. The first impression may reveal clues about the patient by, for example, their posture, facial expression and general appearance as well as clues related to perfusion.

After this, a focused evaluation of any patient should include three things: a presenting complaint, a patient history and a physical examination. These elements are crucial in determining the cause of the emergency, assist in directing initial patient care, and help in anticipating issues during transport to a healthcare facility. The following discussion of patient assessment explains the approach to the patient with a cardiovascular problem.

Critical Thinking

What emotions might the patient who has called you for a cardiovascular complaint be feeling?

Presenting complaint

As cardiovascular disease may cause a variety of symptoms, the paramedic should obtain an appropriate history of each symptom and consider this to form a working impression of any patient with a possible cardiac event. Common presenting complaints include chest pain or discomfort, including shoulder, arm, neck, or jaw pain or discomfort; dyspnoea; syncope; and abnormal heartbeat or palpitations.

In some patients (e.g. some women, older adults and patients with diabetes), cardiovascular problems commonly have atypical symptoms, including mental status changes, abdominal or gastrointestinal symptoms (including persistent heartburn) and vague complaints of being ill.

Chest pain or discomfort

Whilst chest pain or discomfort is the most common presenting complaint of patients with ACS, many causes of chest pain are not related to cardiac disease (e.g. pulmonary embolus, pleurisy and reflux oesophagitis). The OPQRST-ASPN method is one method used to evaluate the presenting complaint (and can be easily adapted to other presenting complaints such as breathlessness, dizziness, etc.); it should be used to obtain the following information when possible:

Onset/origin: Was the onset sudden (seconds or a few minutes) or more gradual (over many minutes or longer)? What were you doing when the pain began? Have you ever had this type of pain before? Is it the same or different from last time?

Provoke/palliate: Try to determine the events surrounding the patient's symptoms. What do you think might have caused this pain? What were you doing at the time of onset? Does anything you do make the pain better or worse? Does the pain go away when you rest? Have you taken a nitrate (GTN – glyceryl trinitrate) for the pain, and if so, did it help? Does the pain get worse when you exercise, walk or when you eat certain foods?

Quality: Ask the patient to describe the character of the pain or discomfort using his or her own words. Common descriptions for the quality of chest pain associated with a cardiac event include sharp, tearing, burning, heavy, and squeezing.

Region/radiation: Ask the patient to localize the pain. With one finger, point to where the pain hurts most. Does the pain move (radiate) to another area of the body or does it stay in one place? If the pain moves, where does it move to? (Cardiac chest pain often radiates to the arms, neck, jaw, and back.)

Severity: Asking the patient to rate the pain or discomfort, whilst subjective, helps to establish a baseline. On a scale of 1 to 10, with 10 being the worst pain you have ever had/imagine and 1 being no pain, what number would you use to describe this pain? If you have had pain like this before, is it worse than the last time, or not as bad as the last time?

Time: Try to determine the length of the pain episode and document it. How long have you had this pain? Is the pain better or worse than it was when you called emergency medical services? Is the pain constant, or does it come and go?

Associated symptoms: Other than the main presenting complaint, are there any other symptoms?

Pertinent negatives: Symptoms that might reasonably be expected to be present but are not.

Critical Thinking

What factors may influence a person's perception and description of pain?

Note

Chest pain is one of the most common complaints of cocaine users. The use of cocaine can cause serious cardiac toxicity because of the effect of the drug on the heart. Cocaine also stimulates the central nervous system and that also stimulates the cardiovascular system. Although rare, acute myocardial infarction can occur in these patients, even in the absence of risk factors for coronary heart disease.

Dyspnoea

Dyspnoea often is associated with myocardial infarction and is also a main symptom of pulmonary congestion that is caused by heart failure (usually left sided). It can be more common at night, waking the patient from their sleep with a feeling of gasping for air. Other common causes of dyspnoea that may be unrelated to heart disease include chronic obstructive pulmonary disease, respiratory infection, pulmonary embolus, and asthma. Historical factors important in differentiating breathing difficulties include the following:

- duration and circumstances of onset of dyspnoea (paying particular attention to reported dyspnoea at night)
- anything that aggravates or relieves the dyspnoea, including medications or exercise
- previous episodes
- associated symptoms such as cough (productive/non-productive)
- orthopnoea (does the patient need several pillows to prop themselves up with at night?)
- previous cardiac problems.

Syncope (fainting)

Syncope is caused by a sudden decrease in oxygenated blood to the brain. Cardiac causes of syncope result from events that decrease cardiac output. The most common cardiac disorders associated with syncope are dysrhythmias. Other causes of syncope in the patient include stroke, drug or alcohol intoxication, aortic stenosis, pulmonary embolism and hypoglycaemia. In the older patient, syncope may be the only symptom of a cardiac problem, whilst young people who are healthy may have a syncopal episode. This episode may result from stimulation of the vagus nerve (vasovagal syncope), producing hypotension and bradycardia. The history of a syncopal event should include the following:

- pre-syncope aura (nausea, weakness, light-headedness)
- circumstances of occurrence (e.g. patient's position before the event, severe pain or emotional stress)
- duration of syncopal episode
- symptoms before syncopal episode (palpitation, seizure, incontinence)
- other associated symptoms
- previous episodes of syncope.

Critical Thinking

Syncopal events often occur in public places, such as a church. How can you decrease the feelings of embarrassment that the patient may have during this situation?

Abnormal heartbeat and palpitations

Many patients are aware of their own heartbeat and may be even more aware if it is irregular (skipping beats) or rapid (fluttering). Palpitations are sometimes a normal occurrence but may indicate a serious dysrhythmia. Important information to obtain from these patients includes the following:

- pulse rate
- regular versus irregular rhythm
- circumstances of occurrence
- duration
- associated symptoms (chest pain, diaphoresis, syncope, confusion, dyspnoea)
- previous episodes and frequency
- medication (drug stimulant) or alcohol use.

Significant medical history

Medical history is a vital part of any patient assessment. If possible, the paramedic should determine the following:

1. Is the patient taking prescription medications, particularly cardiac medications? Common medications that should alert the paramedic to a possible acute coronary event include nitrates, atenolol and other beta-blockers, digoxin, furosemide and other diuretics, antihypertensives, and drugs such as statins. The paramedic should ask the patient about his or her concordance with medications as well. The paramedic should also ask about the use of any non-prescription drugs such as over-the-counter medications, aspirin, and herbal supplements. Alcohol use or recreational drug use may be a contributing factor in the patient's presenting complaint. (This may include, for example, the use of cocaine or methamphetamines.)
2. Is the patient being treated for any other illness? A medical history that includes angina, previous myocardial infarction, coronary artery bypass (Box 15-2) or angioplasty procedures increases the likelihood of a significant coronary event. Chronic illness such as heart failure, hypertension, diabetes, and lung disease are also indicators that heart disease may be present. A history of transient ischaemic attack (TIA) and stroke, for example, also indicates probable circulatory disease.
3. Does the patient have any allergies? Few emergency drugs given in the prehospital setting have the potential to cause an allergic reaction but medication allergies (e.g. an allergy to radiographic dye) may be important in the course of the patient's care. The paramedic should document these allergies and report them to medical direction.
4. Does the patient have risk factors for ACS? Examples of risk factors include older age, tobacco use, diabetes, family history of heart disease, obesity, an increased serum cholesterol level (hypercholesterolaemia) and recreational drug use.
5. Does the patient have an implanted pacemaker or implantable cardioverter defibrillator? The presence of these devices (described later in this chapter) indicates a significant coronary history.

Physical examination

The classic presentation of myocardial infarction is pain or discomfort beneath the sternum which often lasts more than 30 min and is described as crushing, pressure, squeezing or burning. Associated signs and symptoms may include apprehension, diaphoresis, dyspnoea, nausea and vomiting, and a sense of impending doom (e.g. patients feel that they are going to die). Yet at times the presentation is atypical. The paramedic's skill in gathering a relevant medical history and performing a focused physical examination

Box 15-2

Coronary bypass surgery

Coronary bypass surgery is a commonly performed heart surgery whereby blood vessels from another part of the body are used to 'bypass' diseased coronary arteries. This improves blood flow in the heart. The goal of improved blood flow is to reduce chest pain and to lessen the risk of myocardial infarction. This surgical procedure is sometimes referred to as CABG (coronary artery bypass grafting) or cabbage. A patient may undergo one, two, three or more bypass grafts, depending on how many coronary arteries are blocked. Three-way and four-way coronary bypass surgery is common.

Coronary bypass surgery may be performed with or without a heart-lung machine ('on-pump' 'off-pump' surgery). During surgery, an artery is removed from the patient's chest wall or arm (internal mammary artery or radial artery) and is sewn to the coronary artery below the site of blockage. If a vein (usually the saphenous vein taken from the patient's leg) is used, it is attached to the aorta and then grafted to the coronary artery below the blocked area. In either case, the surgery allows blood to flow more freely through the grafts to nourish the heart muscle. Grafts normally remain open and function well for 10 to 15 years, after which bypass surgery may be needed again.

There are several alternatives to CABG that may be appropriate for some patients. Two alternatives are specific drug therapy (e.g. thrombolytics) and atherectomy (plaque removal). Another is balloon angioplasty. In this procedure a balloon catheter is placed over a guidewire. The catheter is used to insert a mesh-like stent into a narrowed section of a coronary artery. Once positioned, the balloon is inflated. This opens the stent and pushes it against the arterial wall. The balloon is then deflated and removed, leaving the stent permanently in place to keep the artery open. Newer stents are coated with medication (drug-eluting stents) that prevents the growth of cells around the stent. This lessens the chance of the artery closing again (restenosis). Stents also may be placed without angioplasty.

will direct the patient care; for example, patients with myocardial ischaemia may deny that they have chest pain and need to be asked specifically about a tightness or squeezing in the chest.

Critical Thinking

Think of a way to ask a patient a question about chest pain that cannot be answered with a simple yes or no.

When caring for a patient who has chest pain caused by cardiac problems, the paramedic should understand that the patient is frightened; chest pain is associated with life-threatening consequences and these patients should be calmed and reassured to decrease their anxiety.

Initial assessment

In most medical emergencies involving conscious patients, the main elements of the initial assessment (airway, breathing and circulation) can be evaluated during the initial paramedic–patient encounter. For example, an appropriate verbal exchange between the paramedic and the conscious patient will establish that the patient is alert, orientated, and has adequate cardiorespiratory function. However, the initial assessment for a patient with a possible coronary event should include a more in-depth evaluation of the patient's level of consciousness, respirations, pulse and blood pressure.

A change in the patient's level of consciousness (e.g. light-headedness or confusion) may indicate decreased cerebral perfusion caused by poor cardiac output. If possible, the paramedic should determine the normal level of functioning for the patient. The paramedic can do this by interviewing the patient, family members, or others who are familiar with the patient (e.g. neighbours and nursing staff). In addition, the paramedic should evaluate the patient's vital signs and include a respiratory assessment, an assessment of the patient's pulse for rate and regularity, and an initial measurement of the patient's blood pressure. These findings will give the paramedic a baseline from which to guide patient care.

Physical examination

The physical examination of the patient with cardiac disease should be organized and complete. The paramedic should use a look–listen–feel approach (see Chapter 9) and consider the main systems, as a minimum, to be assessed (cardiovascular and respiratory).

Look

- *Skin*: Pale and diaphoretic skin may indicate peripheral vasoconstriction and sympathetic stimulation. Cyanosis is an indicator of poor oxygenation and pulse oximetry should be used to measure haemoglobin oxygenation.
- *Jugular veins*: An increase in central venous pressure from heart failure and cardiac tamponade can produce distension of internal jugular veins, and jugular veins are best evaluated with the patient's head elevated at 45 degrees and rotated away; distension may be hard to assess in obese patients.
- *Peripheral and presacral oedema*: Oedema can result from chronic back pressure in the systemic venous circulation and is most obvious in dependent areas; for example, these areas may include the ankles and the sacral region of patients who are bedridden. Oedema can be classified as non-pitting, with minimal or no depression of tissue occurring after removal of finger pressure, or can be pitting, with depression of tissue remaining after removal of finger pressure (press for 1 min with one finger in one place).
- *Additional indicators of cardiac disease*: More subtle signs of cardiac disease that may be found on a visual inspection include a midsternal scar from coronary surgery, a GTN patch on the skin, an implanted pacemaker or implantable cardioverter defibrillator in the left upper chest (Figure 15-13) or abdominal wall, and medical alert identification necklaces or bracelets. Chest shape can indicate the existence of COPD.

Listen

- *Lung sounds*: The paramedic should assess the patient's chest visually for accessory muscle use in breathing

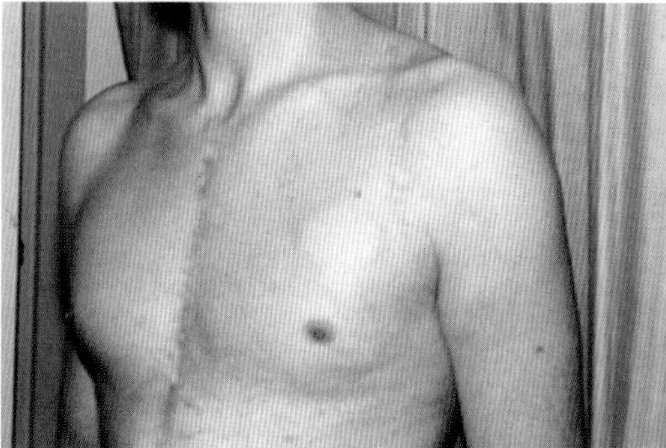

Figure 15-13 Midsternal scar and implanted cardiac device.

before listening to lung sounds. Lung sounds should be clear and equal bilaterally. Adventitious breath sounds may indicate pulmonary congestion or oedema.

Critical Thinking

What breath sounds might you hear if the patient has congestive heart failure or pulmonary oedema?

- *Heart sounds*: Abnormal heart sounds may indicate congestive heart failure in adult patients (Box 15-3). Heart sounds are best heard at the point of maximum impulse which is where the apical impulse is most readily visible or palpable and is often in the fifth intercostal space, just medial to the left midclavicular line. Heart sounds are difficult to distinguish in the prehospital setting but abnormalities may be detected at times. A third heart sound (S3 gallop) might be heard which suggests heart failure.
- *Carotid artery bruit*: Bruits are murmurs that indicate turbulent blood flow through a vessel, commonly from atherosclerosis. The presence of a bruit in a patient with cardiac disease is evaluated at the carotid artery with a stethoscope and should always be assessed before performing carotid sinus massage (described later in this chapter). If a carotid artery bruit is present, carotid sinus massage is contraindicated as the procedure may dislodge plaque in the artery and cause a stroke.

Feel

- *Skin*: The paramedic should assess the patient's skin with the back of the hand for diaphoresis or fever.

Box 15-3

Heart sounds

Heart sounds typically can be auscultated with a stethoscope during ventricular systole and diastole. When the ventricles contract, both AV valves close at nearly the same time. This closure causes a vibration of the valves and surrounding fluid. Vibration results in a low-pitched sound (often described as a 'lubb'). Closing of the aortic and pulmonary semilunar valves at the end of ventricular systole produces a higher-pitched sound (described as 'dubb'). These normal heart sounds are referred to as S_1 and S_2, respectively.

Rarely, a third heart sound can be heard near the end of the first third of diastole (S_3). The third heart sound (caused by turbulent flow of blood into the ventricles) may be normal but may be an indicator of congestive heart failure. A fourth heart sound (S_4) may be heard during the end of diastole. This sound is thought to result from turbulence and chamber stretching from the atrial contraction during this part of the cardiac cycle and is often a sign of congestive heart failure in adults. The S_3 and S_4 contribute to 'gallop' rhythms, which are useful clinical indicators of congestive heart failure. Heart sounds are difficult to distinguish in the field. The evaluation of heart sounds should never delay emergency care or transport; they do not alter prehospital patient management.

S_1: First heart sound occurs with closure of AV valves during ventricular systole.

S_2: Second heart sound occurs with closure of aortic and pulmonic valves and signifies the beginning of ventricular diastole.

S_3: Extra heart sound is heard after S_2 and is compatible with heart failure but not always present. It also may be a normal finding in some patients.

S_4: Extra heart sound is heard in late diastole (just before S_1); it is associated with atrial contractions and often is heard in patients with congestive heart failure.

- *Pulse*: The paramedic should assess the pulse for rate, regularity, and equality. A pulse deficit between peripheral and apical pulse sites may indicate a rhythm disturbance or vascular disease; this should be noted and reported when handing over the patient.
- *Thorax and abdomen*: The paramedic should check the thorax and abdomen of a patient with cardiac disease for chest wall tenderness and pulsating masses, as chest wall tenderness is not uncommon in patients with acute myocardial infarction. A pulsating mass or distension in the abdomen or epigastric area may indicate an abdominal aneurysm.

SECTION IV

Electrocardiogram monitoring

The electrocardiogram is a graphic representation of the electrical activity of the heart and is produced by the electrical events in the atria and ventricles; it is an important diagnostic tool, which helps to identify a number of cardiac abnormalities. These include abnormal heart rates and rhythms, abnormal conduction pathways, hypertrophy or atrophy of portions of the heart, and the approximate location of ischaemic or infarcted cardiac muscle.

An evaluation of the electrocardiogram requires a systematic approach. The paramedic analyses the electrocardiogram and then relates it to the clinical assessment of the patient,

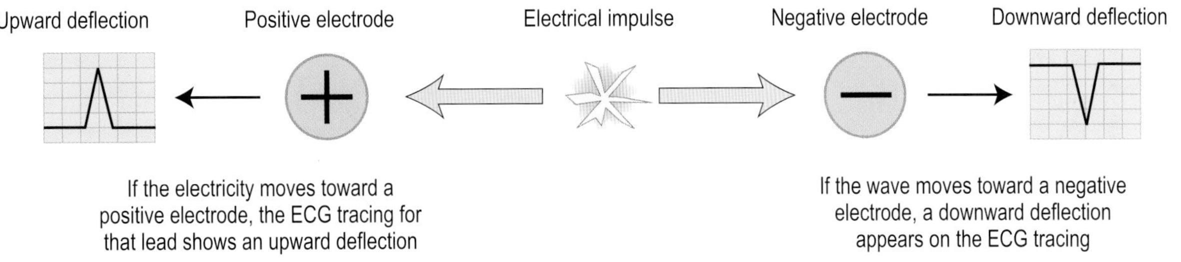

Figure 15-14 Rule of electrical flow.

but remember it is a 'picture' of the electrical activity of the heart and does not offer details on mechanical events such as force of contraction or blood pressure.

Critical Thinking

Aside from blood pressure, how will you evaluate the mechanical activity of the heart?

Basic concepts of electrocardiogram monitoring

The summation of all the action potentials transmitted through the heart during the cardiac cycle can be measured on the surface of the body; this measurement is obtained by applying electrodes on the surface of the body. These electrodes are connected to an electrocardiogram machine and voltage changes are fed to the machine, amplified, and displayed visually on the oscilloscope, graphically on electrocardiogram paper, or both. Voltage may be positive (seen as an upward deflection on the electrocardiogram tracing); negative (seen as a downward deflection on the electrocardiogram tracing); or isoelectric, when no electrical current is detected (seen as a straight baseline on the electrocardiogram tracing).

Electrocardiogram leads

Electrocardiogram machines can offer many views of the electrical activity of the heart by monitoring voltage changes using electrodes applied to the body. Each pair of electrodes is referred to as a lead. A standard electrocardiogram views the electrical activity of the heart from 12 leads.

An electrocardiogram lead can consist of either two surface electrodes, one positive and the other negative (bipolar), or the lead consists of one positive surface electrode and one reference point (unipolar). Bipolar leads constitute the standard limb leads (I to III). Unipolar leads make up the augmented voltage limb leads (aV_R, aV_L, and aV_F) and the precordial leads (V_1 to V_6) (Table 15-1).

Each lead assesses the electrical activity of the heart from a slightly different view and produce different electrocardiogram tracings. If the electricity moves toward a positive electrode, the electrocardiogram tracing for that lead shows an upward deflection, but if the wave moves away from a positive electrode, a negative deflection appears on the electrocardiogram tracing (Figure 15-14).

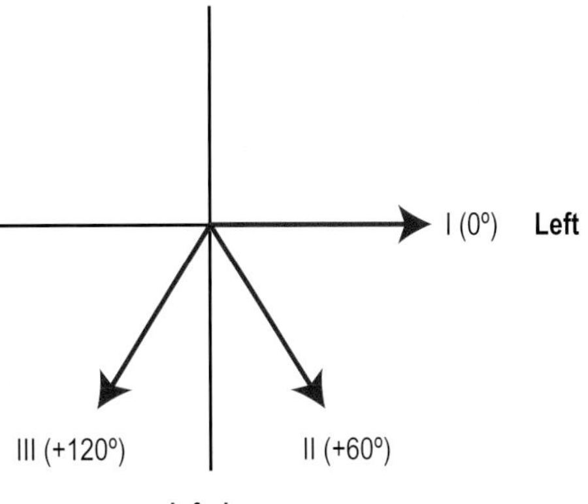

Figure 15-15 Electrical vantage points of the three standard limb leads.

Table 15-1 Comparison of various leads

Leads	Type of lead	Polarity
I, II, III	Limb lead	Bipolar
aV_R, aV_L, aV_F	Limb lead	Unipolar
V_1–V_6	Chest lead	Unipolar

From Phalen T 1996 The 12-lead ECG in acute myocardial infarction. Mosby, St Louis.

Standard limb leads

Standard limb leads record the difference in electrical potential between the left arm, the right arm, and the left leg electrodes, which represent the axes (the average direction of the electrical activity of the heart) of the standard limb leads (forming Einthoven's triangle). If these axes are moved so that they cross a common midpoint without altering their orientation, they form a triaxial reference system (this is three intersecting lines of reference). Lead I is a lateral (leftward) lead. It assesses the electrical activity of the heart from a vantage point that is defined as 0 degrees on a circle. This circle is divided into an upper negative 180 degrees and a lower positive 180 degrees. Leads II and III are inferior leads. They assess the electrical activity of the heart from vantage points of +60 degrees and +120 degrees, respectively (Figure 15-15). The electrodes of the three bipolar leads are placed on the following areas of the body:

Lead	Positive electrode	Negative electrode
I	Left arm	Right arm
II	Left leg	Right arm
III	Left leg	Left arm

Augmented limb leads

Augmented limb leads record the difference in electrical potential between the respective extremity lead sites and a reference point with zero electrical potential at the centre of the electrical field of the heart. As a result, the axis of each lead is formed by the line from the electrode site (on the right arm, left arm, or left leg) to the centre of the heart. The aV_R, aV_L, and aV_F leads intersect at different angles than the standard limb leads and produce three other intersecting lines of reference, which together with the standard limb leads make up the hexaxial reference system. Augmented limb leads use the same set of electrodes as the standard limb leads and measure an axis between the two bipolar leads by electronically combining the negative electrodes. Augmented limb leads augment the voltage of the positive lead to increase the size of the electrocardiogram complexes.

Lead aV_L acts as a lateral (leftward) lead. It records the electrical activity of the heart from a vantage point that looks down from the left shoulder (−30 degrees). Lead aV_F acts as an inferior lead. It records the electrical activity of the heart from a vantage point that looks up from the left lower extremity (+90 degrees). Lead aV_R is a distant recording electrode. It looks down at the heart from the right shoulder. Based on these lead descriptions, the lateral, or left-sided, leads are I and aV_L. The inferior leads are II, III, and aV_F (Figure 15-16).

In some cases ECG monitoring may be varied by use of modified chest leads MCL_1 and MCL_6. These approximate to V_1 and V_6, respectively.

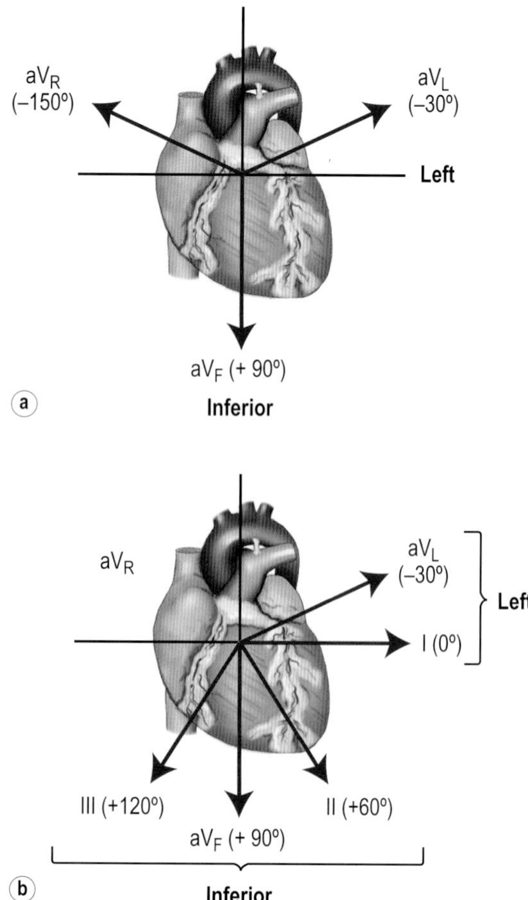

Figure 15-16 (a) Electrical vantage points of the three augmented limb leads. (b) Combined electrical vantage points. Leads II, III, and aV_F are considered inferior leads; leads I and aV_L are considered lateral leads.

Critical Thinking

Why is aV_R seldom used in electrocardiogram analysis? What 'view' of the heart does it provide?

Routine electrocardiogram monitoring

Routine monitoring of cardiac rhythm in the prehospital setting, emergency department, or coronary care unit usually is obtained in lead II and is the best lead to monitor for dysrhythmias because of its ability to display waves on the ECG that represent atrial depolarization (P waves). A good deal of information can be gathered from a single monitoring lead and, in most cases, cardiac monitoring by a single lead is sufficient as the paramedic can determine the rate and regularity as well as conduction duration in various parts of the heart.

However, single-lead monitoring has its limitations; it may fail to reveal various abnormalities (particularly ST segment changes that signal myocardial injury or infarction) in the electrocardiogram tracing.

12-lead electrocardiogram monitoring

A 12-lead electrocardiogram is obtained through 10 electrodes: four limb leads (right arm, right leg, left arm, left leg) and six chest leads (V_1 to V_6) (Figure 15-17). The four limb leads provide readings of leads I, II, and III and aV_F, aV_L, and aV_R. Each lead of the 12-lead electrocardiogram views the left ventricle from the position of its positive electrode. Monitoring 12 leads is performed with a 12-lead monitor which obtains the leads at the same time and provides a readout in conventional three- or four-column format. As described later in this chapter, 12-lead electrocardiogram monitoring can be used to do the following:

- Identify ST segment and T wave changes relative to myocardial ischaemia, injury, and infarction.
- Identify ventricular tachycardia in wide-complex tachycardia.
- Determine the electrical axis and the presence of fascicular blocks.
- Determine the presence and location of bundle branch blocks.

Precordial leads

The six precordial leads used in 12-lead electrocardiogram monitoring are projected through the anterior chest wall toward the patient's back (the negative end of each chest

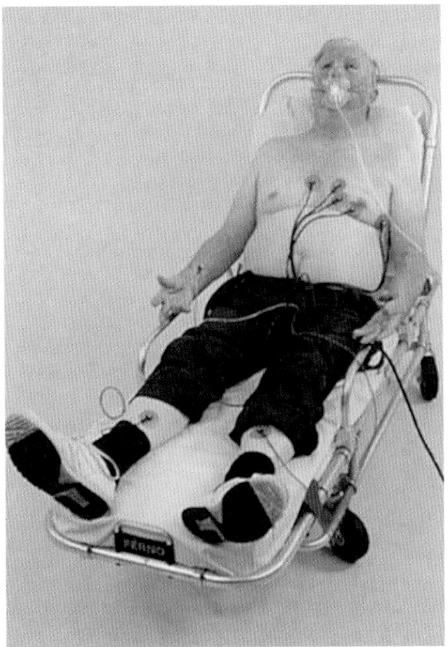

Figure 15-17 To obtain a 12-lead electrocardiogram when using a 12-lead monitor or machine, simply attach the cables to the electrodes, ask the patient to be still, and push the record button. Acquisition requires only 10 seconds.

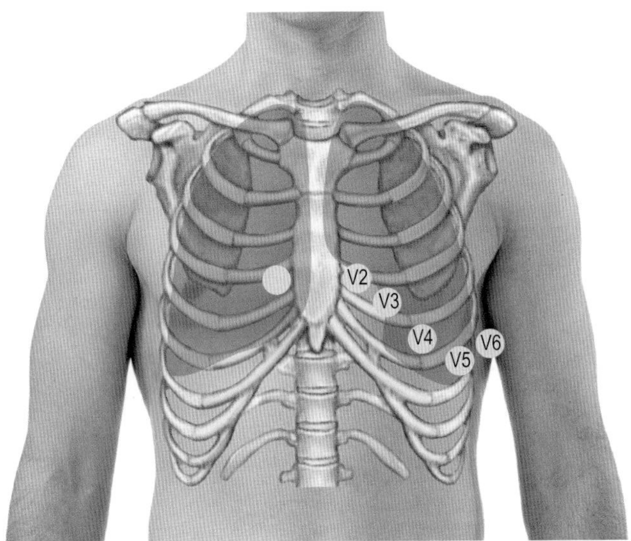

Figure 15-18 Proper chest lead placement.

lead) (Figure 15-18). These positive leads are placed on the chest in reference to specific thoracic landmarks and record the electrical activity of the heart in the transverse or horizontal plane. Leads V_1 and V_2 are septal leads, V_2 to V_4 are anterior leads and V_4 to V_6 are lateral precordial leads (Box 15-4).

Proper placement of the chest leads at specific intercostal spaces is essential for an accurate reading. One method to locate the appropriate intercostal spaces is as follows[2] (Figure 15-19a–m):

1. Locate the jugular notch and move downward until the sternal angle (Angle of Louis) is found.
2. Follow the articulation to the right sternal border to locate the second rib; just below the second rib is the second intercostal space.
3. Move down two intercostal spaces and position the V_1 electrode in the fourth intercostal space, just to the right of the patient's sternum.
4. Move across the sternum to the corresponding intercostal space and position V_2 to the left of the patient's sternum.
5. From V_2, palpate down one intercostal space and follow the fifth intercostal space to the midclavicular line to place the V_4 electrode.
6. Place lead V_3 midway between V_2 and V_4.
7. Place V_5 in the anterior axillary line in a straight line with V_4 (where the arm joins the chest).
8. Place V_6 in the midaxillary line, level with V_4 and V_5. (It may be more convenient to place V_6 first, and then V_5.) In women, try to place the V_4 to V_6 electrodes under the left breast to avoid any errors in the electrocardiogram tracing that may occur from breast tissue although in certain circumstances over the breast tissue may be the only option.

Box 15-4

Posterior and right-sided electrocardiogram

The wall of the right ventricle and the posterior ventricular walls are areas of the heart that are hard to evaluate with the six precordial leads. Electrocardiogram monitoring that includes 12 leads either right sided (V_4R, V_5R and V_6R leads) or posterior (V_7–V_9) increases sensitivity for myocardial infarctions that occur in these areas (e.g. isolated posterior myocardial infarction). V_4R is placed in the right midclavicular line, 5th intercostal space, with V_5R and V_6R continuing around the right side at the same level, in the anterior and mid axillary lines respectively. The posterior leads are placed at the same level as V_4–V_6 but continue round the back of the patient, with V_7 being in the posterior axillary line, V_9 being subscapularis to the left of the spinal column and V_8 being between V_7 and V_9 (see also Fig. 15-93).

Note: Right-sided and posterior electrocardiograms are being performed more often in prehospital settings.

Critical Thinking

Consider that your patient is female. You are performing 12-lead electrocardiogram tracing. What measures can you take to decrease her potential discomfort or embarrassment?

Some manufacturers now produce chest ECG electrodes for 12-lead use that are interconnected and prespaced to help overcome placement error, although they are not commonly used in UK paramedic practice.

Critical Thinking

What effect will improper lead placement have on the 'view' of the heart and the analysis of the electrocardiogram tracing?

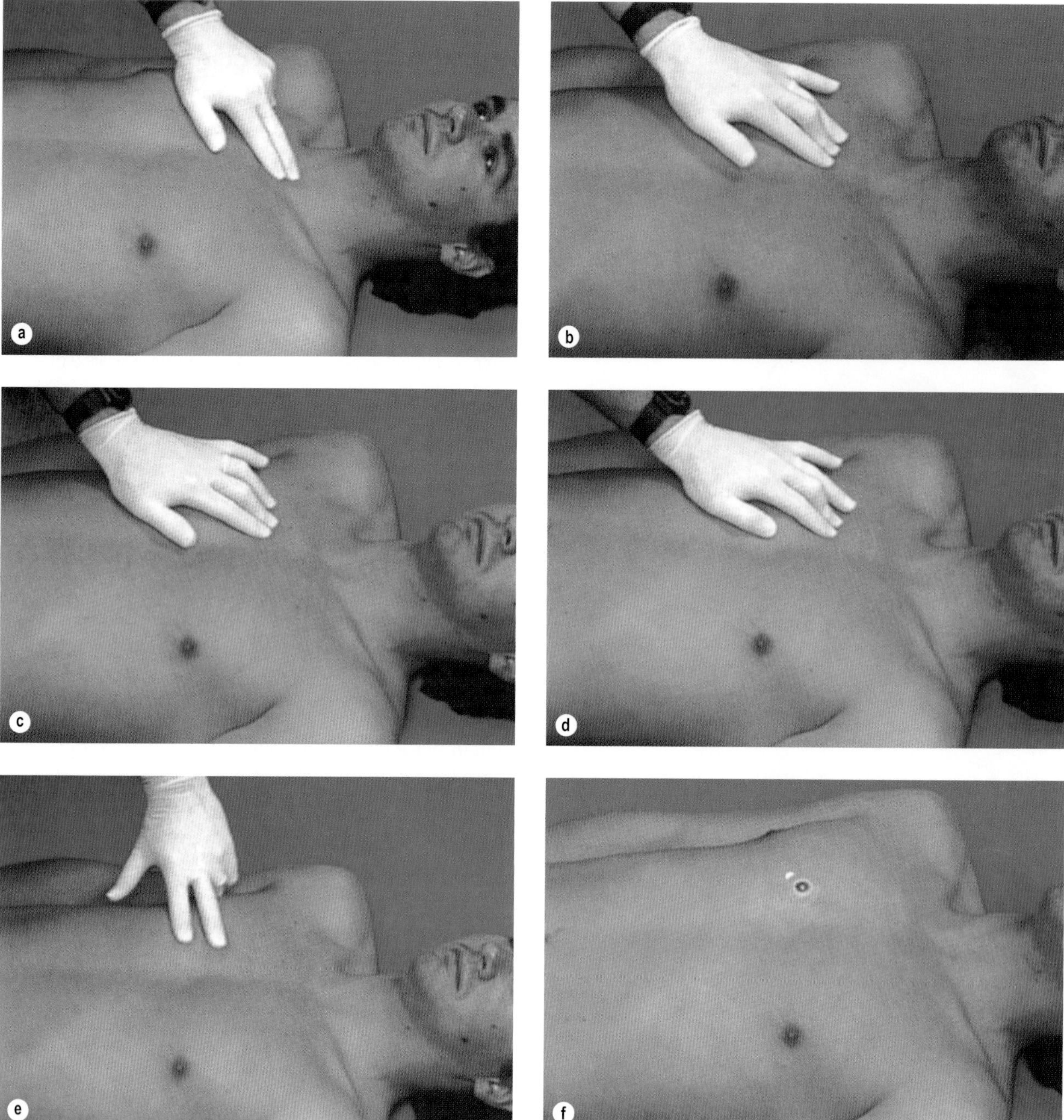

Figure 15-19 Step-by-step skill.
a Locate the jugular notch.
b Palpate for the angle of Louis.
c Follow the angle of Louis to the patient's right until it articulates with the second rib.
d Locate the second intercostal space (immediately below the second rib).
e From the second intercostal space the third and fourth intercostal spaces can be found.
f Lead V_1 is positioned in the fourth intercostal space just to the right of the sternum.

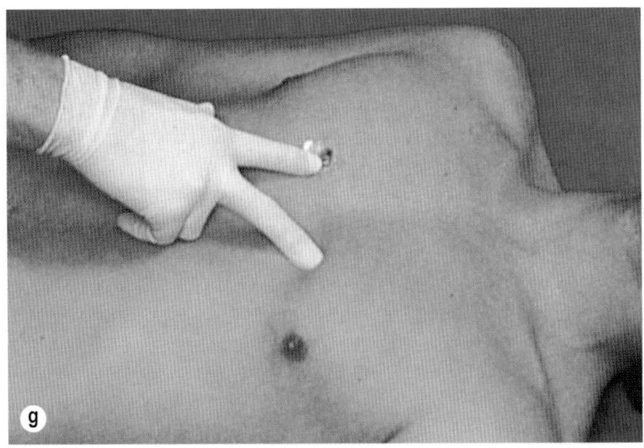

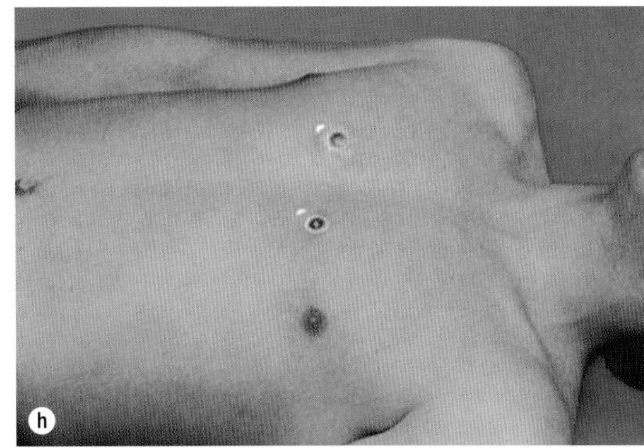

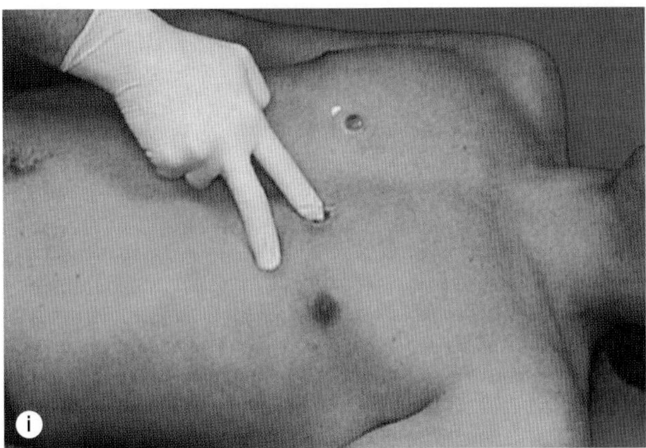

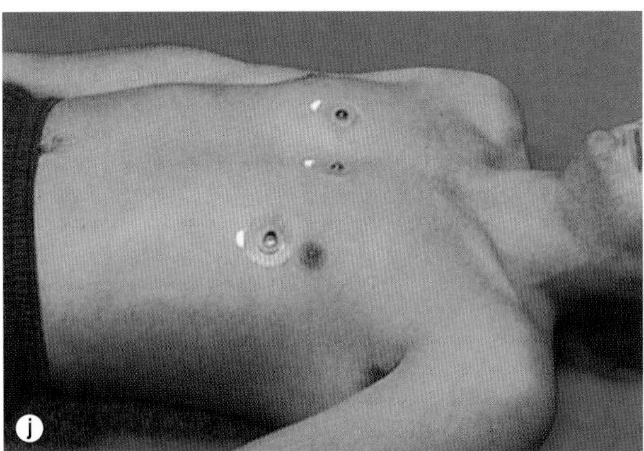

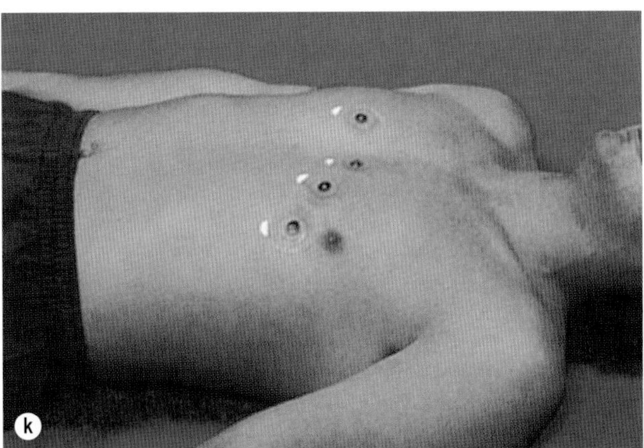

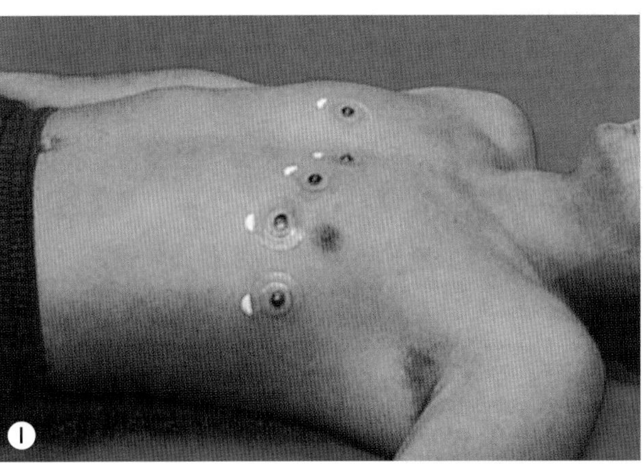

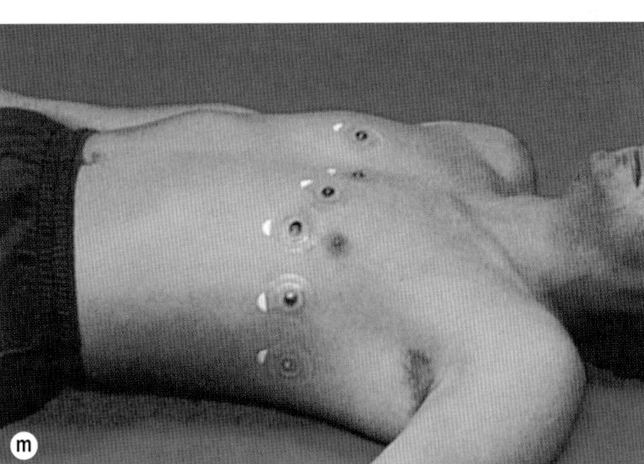

Figure 15-19, cont'd

g From the V_1 position, find the corresponding intercostal space on the left side of the sternum.

h Place the V_2 electrode in the fourth intercostal space just to the left of the sternum.

i From the V_2 position, locate the fifth intercostal space and follow it to the midclavicular line.

j Position the V_4 electrode in the fifth intercostal space in the midclavicular line.

k Lead V_3 is positioned halfway between V_2 and V_4.

l Lead V_5 is positioned in the anterior axillary line, level with V_4.

m Lead V_6 is positioned in the midaxillary line, level with V_4.

Application of monitoring electrodes

The most commonly used electrodes for continuous electrocardiogram monitoring are pregelled, stick-on discs, which can be applied easily to the chest wall. The paramedic should observe the following guidelines to minimize artefacts in the signal and to make effective contact between the electrode and the skin:

> **Critical Thinking**
>
> Why should alcohol or benzoin not be used under defibrillator pads?

1. Choose an appropriate area of skin, avoiding large muscle masses and large quantities of hair, which may prevent the electrode from lying flat against the skin.
2. Cleanse the area with alcohol to remove dirt and body oil. Consider lightly abrading the area by vigorous rubbing with gauze. If necessary, trim excess body hair before placing the electrodes. When attaching electrodes to the extremities, use locations that will minimize artefact (deltoid aspect of arms and the thighs).
3. Attach the electrodes to the prepared site (do this as soon as practicable, as maximizing 'time on skin' will allow better impulse conduction). Place the precordial electrodes so that the cables can be directed down the abdomen to avoid lead wire strain.
4. Attach the electrocardiogram cables to electrodes. Most electrocardiogram cables are marked for right arm, left arm, and left leg application.
5. Turn on the electrocardiogram monitor and obtain a baseline tracing.

If the signal is poor, the paramedic should recheck the cable connections. The paramedic also should check the effectiveness of the patient's skin contact with the electrodes; common causes of a poor signal include body hair, dried conductive gel, poor electrode placement, and diaphoresis.

Problems with ECG acquisition

- Ensure the electrodes are fresh and in date. Damaged or dried out electrodes will not provide a good quality signal. When connecting electrodes, be cautious that pressure is not placed on the centre disc as this may damage the metal sensor inside.
- Monitoring cables should be intact and free from any damage or wear; interference and a poor quality recording may result if this occurs. Cables should be replaced if damaged.
- Patient movement: if the baseline wanders or moves, then any analysis of the ECG (especially ST segments) is unreliable and difficult to undertake. Patient movement due to thoracic movement when breathing is a possible cause, as is vehicle movement; ECG analysis in a moving vehicle is best avoided if at all possible. Cable movement, poor chest/skin preparation and electrical interference are all other reasons likely to cause a poor recording.

Electrocardiogram graph paper

The paper used in recording electrocardiograms is standardized to allow comparative analysis of an electrocardiogram wave. The graph paper is divided into squares 1 mm in height and width and further divided by darker lines every fifth square vertically and horizontally. Each large square is 5 mm high and 5 mm wide (Figure 15-20).

As the graph paper moves past the stylus of the electrocardiogram machine, it measures time and amplitude. Time is measured on the horizontal plane (side to side). When the electrocardiogram is recorded at the standard paper speed of 25 mm/s, each small square is equal to 1 mm (0.04 s) and each large square (the dark vertical lines) is equal to 5 mm (0.20 s); these squares measure the length of time it takes an electrical impulse to pass through a specific part of the heart.

Amplitude is measured on the vertical axis (top to bottom) of the graph paper. Each small square of the graph paper is equal to 0.1 mV and each large square (five small squares) is equal to 0.5 mV. The sensitivity of the 12-lead electrocardiogram machine is standardized; when properly calibrated, a 1-mV electrical signal produces a 10-mm deflection (two large squares) on the electrocardiogram tracing. Most modern ECG machines calibrate automatically but those equipped with calibration buttons should have a calibration curve placed at the beginning of the first electrocardiogram tracing (generally a 1-mV burst, represented by a 10-mm 'block' wave).

Time-interval markings are denoted by short vertical lines and usually are located on the top of the electrocardiogram graph paper. When the electrocardiogram is recorded at the standard paper speed, the distance between each short vertical line is 75 mm (3 s); each 3-s interval contains 15 large squares (0.2 s multiplied by 15 squares equals 3 s). These markings are used as a method of heart rate calculation (i.e. counting the number of QRS complexes in 6 s and multiplying by 10).

Relationship of the electrocardiogram to electrical activity

Each waveform seen on the oscilloscope or recorded on the electrocardiogram graph paper represents the conduction of an electrical impulse through a certain part of the heart. All waveforms begin and end at the isoelectric line, which represents the absence of electrical activity in cardiac tissue. A deflection above the baseline is positive, indicating an electrical flow toward the positive electrode. A deflection below the baseline is negative, indicating an electrical flow away from the positive electrode.

The normal electrocardiogram consists of a P wave, QRS complex, and T wave. At times, a U wave also can be seen after the T wave. If present, the U wave usually is a positive deflection and may be associated with electrolyte abnormalities. Other key parts of the electrocardiogram that should

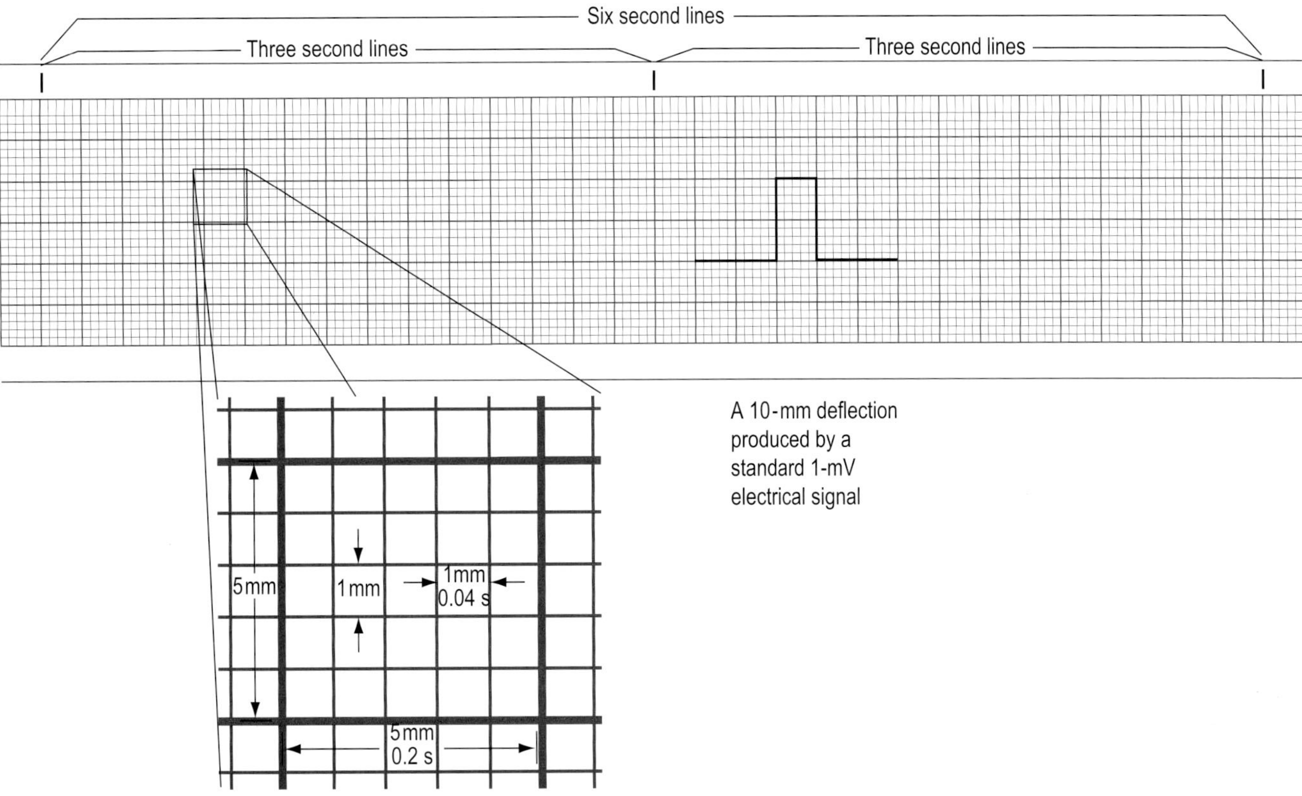

Figure 15-20 Electrocardiogram graph paper.

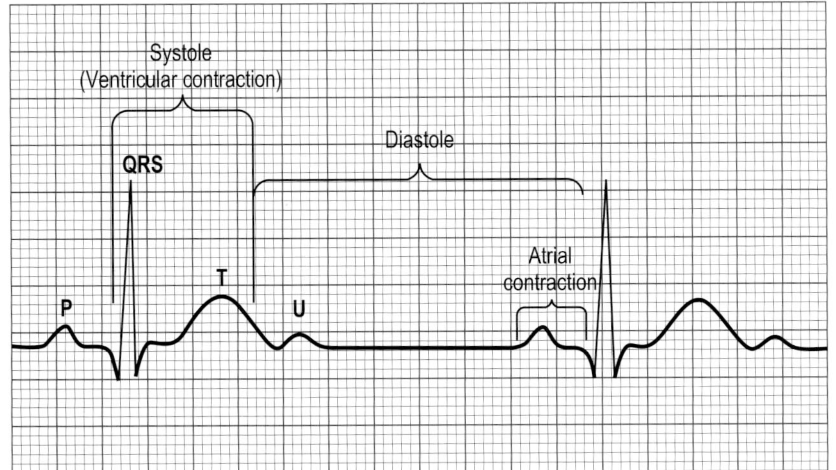

Figure 15-21 Summary of the electrical basis of the electrocardiogram.

be evaluated include the P-R interval, ST segment, and Q-T interval. The combination of these waves represents a single heartbeat, or one complete cardiac cycle (Figure 15-21). The electrical events of the cardiac cycle are followed by their mechanical counterparts. The descriptions of electrocardiogram waveform components refer to those that would be seen in lead II monitoring.

P wave

The P wave is the first positive (upward) deflection on the electrocardiogram, representing atrial depolarization, is usually rounded and precedes the QRS complex. The P wave begins with the first positive deflection from the baseline and ends at the point where the wave returns to the baseline. The duration of the P wave normally is 0.10 s or less, and its amplitude is 0.5–2.5 mm. The P wave usually is followed by a QRS complex; however, if conduction disturbances are present, a QRS complex does not always follow each P wave.

P-R interval

The P-R interval is the time it takes for an electrical impulse to be conducted through the atria and the AV node up to the instant of ventricular depolarization. The P-R interval is measured from the beginning of the P wave to the beginning of the next deflection on the baseline (the onset of the QRS complex). The normal P-R interval is 0.12 to 0.20 s (three to five small squares on the graph paper) and depends on the heart rate and the conduction characteristics of the AV node. When the heart rate is fast, the P-R interval normally is of shorter duration than when the heart rate is slow. A normal P-R interval indicates that the electrical impulse has been conducted through the atria, AV node, and bundle of His normally and without delay.

QRS complex

The QRS complex generally is composed of three individual waves: the Q, R and S waves. The QRS complex begins at the point where the first wave of the complex deviates from the baseline. It ends where the last wave of the complex begins to flatten at, above, or below the baseline. The direction of the QRS complex may be predominantly positive (upright), predominantly negative (inverted), or biphasic (partly positive, partly negative). The shape of the normal QRS complex is narrow and sharply pointed (when conduction is normal). Its duration generally is 0.08 to 0.12 s (two to three small squares on the graph paper) or less, and its amplitude normally varies from less than 5 mm to more than 15 mm.

The Q wave is the first negative (downward) deflection of the QRS complex on the electrocardiogram but it may not be present in all leads and represents depolarization of the interventricular septum or a pathological change. The R wave is the first positive deflection after the P wave. Subsequent positive deflections in the QRS complex that extend above the baseline and that are taller than the first R wave are called R prime (R′), R double prime (R″), and so on. The S wave is the negative deflection that follows the R wave. Subsequent negative deflections are called S prime (S′), S double prime (S″), and so on. Although there may be only one Q wave, there can be more than one R wave and one S wave in the QRS complex. The R and S waves represent the sum of electrical forces resulting from depolarization of the right and left ventricles (Figure 15-22).

Critical Thinking

What is the importance of a QRS complex duration of 0.12 s?

The QRS complex follows the P wave and marks the approximate beginning of mechanical systole of the ventricles, which continues through the onset of the T wave. The QRS complex represents ventricular depolarization and includes the conduction of an electrical impulse from the AV node through the bundle of His, Purkinje fibres and the right and left bundle branches; this impulse results in ventricular depolarization.

ST segment

The ST segment represents the early phase of repolarization of the right and left ventricles. It immediately follows the QRS complex and ends with the onset of the T wave. The point at which it takes off from the QRS complex is called the J point. In a normal electrocardiogram, the ST segment begins at baseline and has a slight upward slope.

The position of the ST segment commonly is judged as normal or abnormal using the baseline of the P-R or T-P interval as a reference. Deviations above this baseline are referred to as ST segment elevation. Deviations below baseline are referred to as ST segment depression (Figure 15-23a–d). Certain conditions can cause depression or elevation of the P-R interval, thus affecting the reference for ST segment abnormalities. Usually the baseline from the end of the T wave to the beginning of the P wave maintains its isoelectric position and can be used as a reference. Abnormal ST segments may be seen in infarction, ischaemia, and pericarditis; after digitalis administration; and in other disease states.

T wave

The T wave represents repolarization of the ventricular myocardial cells, occurring during the last part of ventricular contraction. The T wave is identified as the first deviation from the ST segment and ends where the T wave returns to the baseline and may be above or below the isoelectric line. The T wave usually is slightly rounded and slightly asymmetrical. Deep and symmetrically inverted T waves may indicate cardiac ischaemia and a T wave elevated more than half the height of the QRS complex (peaked T wave) may indicate new onset of ischaemia of the myocardium or hyperkalaemia.

Q-T interval

The Q-T interval is measured from the beginning of the QRS complex to the end of the T wave (Figure 15-24), represent-

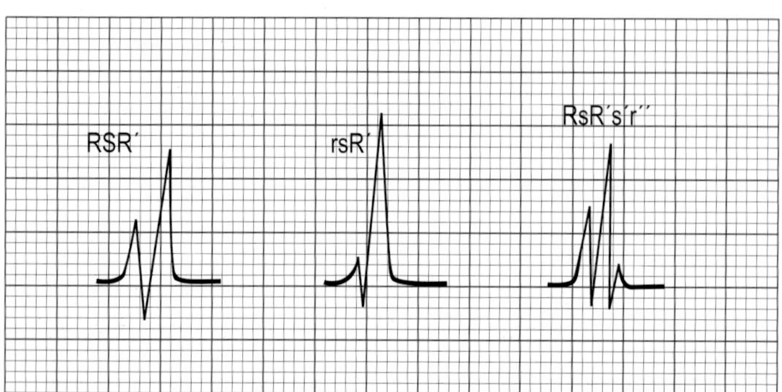

Figure 15-22 QRS complexes with more than one positive or negative deflection.

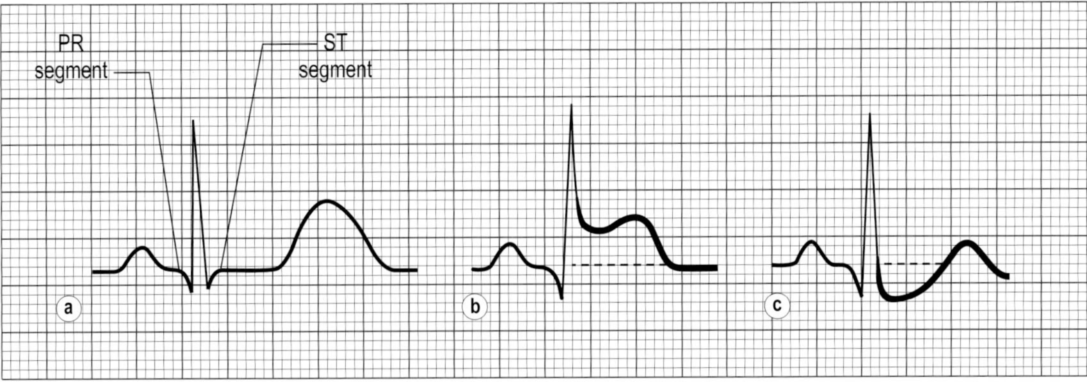

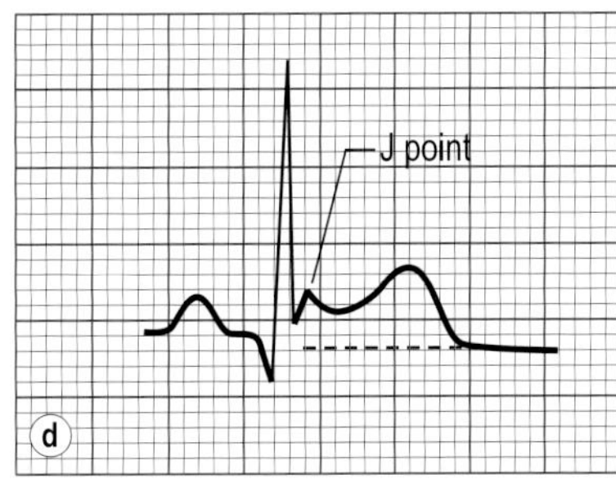

Figure 15-23 ST segment deviations. (a) Use of the PR segment as a baseline. (b) The ST segment is elevated with respect to the PR-segment baseline. (c) The ST segment is depressed with respect to the PR-segment baseline. (d) J point (ST segment elevation). A prominent notch marks the takeoff of the ST segment.

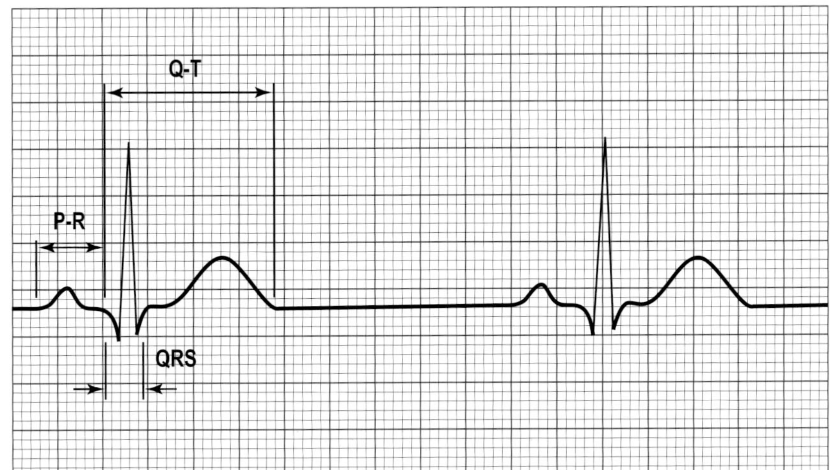

Figure 15-24 P-R, Q-T and QRS intervals.

ing the time from the beginning of ventricular depolarization until the end of ventricular repolarization. During the start of the Q-T interval, the heart is completely unable to respond to electrical stimuli. (This is the absolute refractory period.) During the latter portion of this interval (from the peak of the T wave onward), the heart may be able to respond to premature stimuli. This is called the relative refractory period. During this period, premature impulses may depolarize the heart. Commonly prescribed medications may prolong the Q-T interval, especially class I and class III antidysrhythmics. These antidysrhythmics, by virtue of their effect on the Q-T interval, may lead to potentially lethal dysrhythmias, including ventricular tachycardia, ventricular fibrillation, and an unusual bidirectional ventricular dysrhythmia called torsades de pointes (described later in this chapter). Genetic abnormalities (e.g. Brugada syndrome), hypokalaemia, hypomagnesaemia, hypocalcaemia and hypothermia may also prolong the Q-T interval, while hypercalcaemia and digoxin shorten it.

Note

If the heart rate is fewer than 100 beats per minute, the Q-T interval probably is prolonged if it is greater than half of the R-R interval.

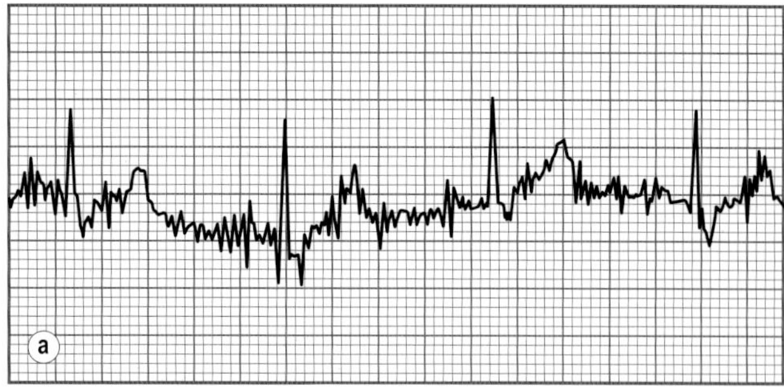

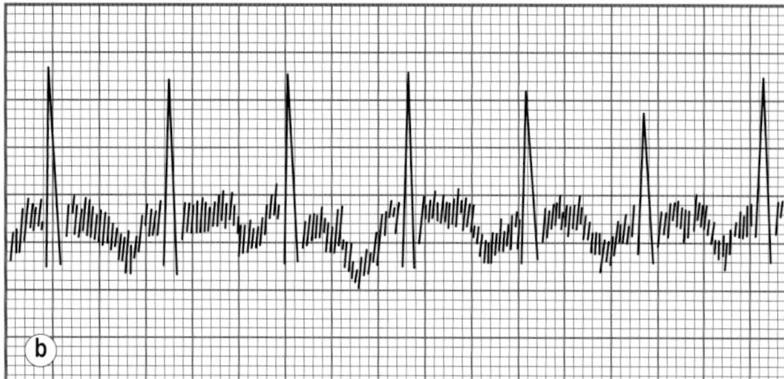

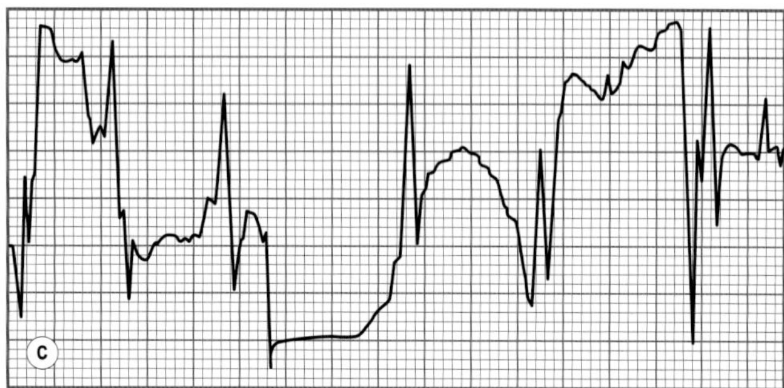

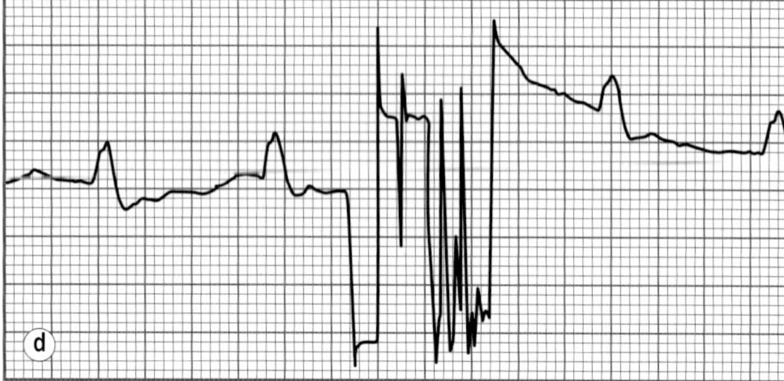

Figure 15-25 Artefacts. (a) Muscle tremors. (b) Alternating current (electrical) interference. (c) Loose electrodes. (d) Biotelemetry.

Artefacts

Artefacts are marks on the electrocardiogram display or tracing caused by activities other than the electrical activity of the heart (Figure 15-25). Common causes of artefacts are improper grounding of the electrocardiogram machine, patient movement, loss of electrode contact with the patient's skin, patient shivering or tremors, and external chest compression. Two types of artefacts deserve special mention. One is alternating current interference (electrical interference), the other biotelemetry-related interference.

Alternating current interference may occur in a poorly grounded electrocardiogram machine or when an electrocardiogram is obtained near high-tension wires, transformers and some household appliances. This results in a thick baseline made up of electrical interference waves. The P waves may not be discernible because of the interference but the QRS complex usually is visible. Alternating current interference may also be caused by the patient or the lead cable touching a metal object such as a bed rail; placing a blanket between the metal object and the patient may correct the interference.

Biotelemetry-related interference may occur when biotelemetry electrocardiogram signals are received poorly, as a result of weak batteries or from electrocardiogram transmission in areas with poor signalling conditions. Interference also may result if the transmitter is located a distance away from a base station receiver. Biotelemetry-related interference may produce sharp spikes and waves that have a jagged appearance.

SECTION V

Electrocardiogram interpretation – steps in rhythm analysis

Evaluation of an electrocardiogram requires a systematic approach to analysing a given rhythm. Numerous methods can be used for rhythm interpretation; this text uses a method that first looks at the QRS complex (the most important observation in life-threatening dysrhythmias); followed by P waves and the relationship between the P waves and the QRS; rate; rhythm; and finally the P-R interval. Regardless of the method chosen to analyse a given rhythm, the paramedic should use a consistent format. This section of the text discusses rhythm interpretation as it pertains to standard 3-lead electrocardiogram monitoring. Evaluation of 12-lead electrocardiogram monitoring is presented later in this chapter.

Five questions the paramedic must ask in any rhythm analysis to determine the presence or potential for life-threatening rhythm disturbances are as follows:

1. Is the patient sick?
2. What is the heart rate?
3. Are there normal-looking QRS complexes?
4. Are there normal-looking P waves?
5. What is the relationship between the P waves and the QRS complexes?

Critical Thinking

What does the electrocardiogram tell you about perfusion?

Step 1: Analyse the QRS complex

The paramedic should analyse the QRS complex for regularity and width. QRS complexes should be less than 0.12 s wide (less than three small squares), are supraventricular in origin and are normal. Complexes that are equal to or greater than 0.12 s wide may indicate a conduction abnormality in the ventricles or may indicate that the focus originates in the ventricles and is abnormal (Figure 15-26a–e). When evaluating an abnormal QRS width, the paramedic should identify the lead with the widest QRS complex because a portion of the QRS complex may be hidden or hard to see in some leads.

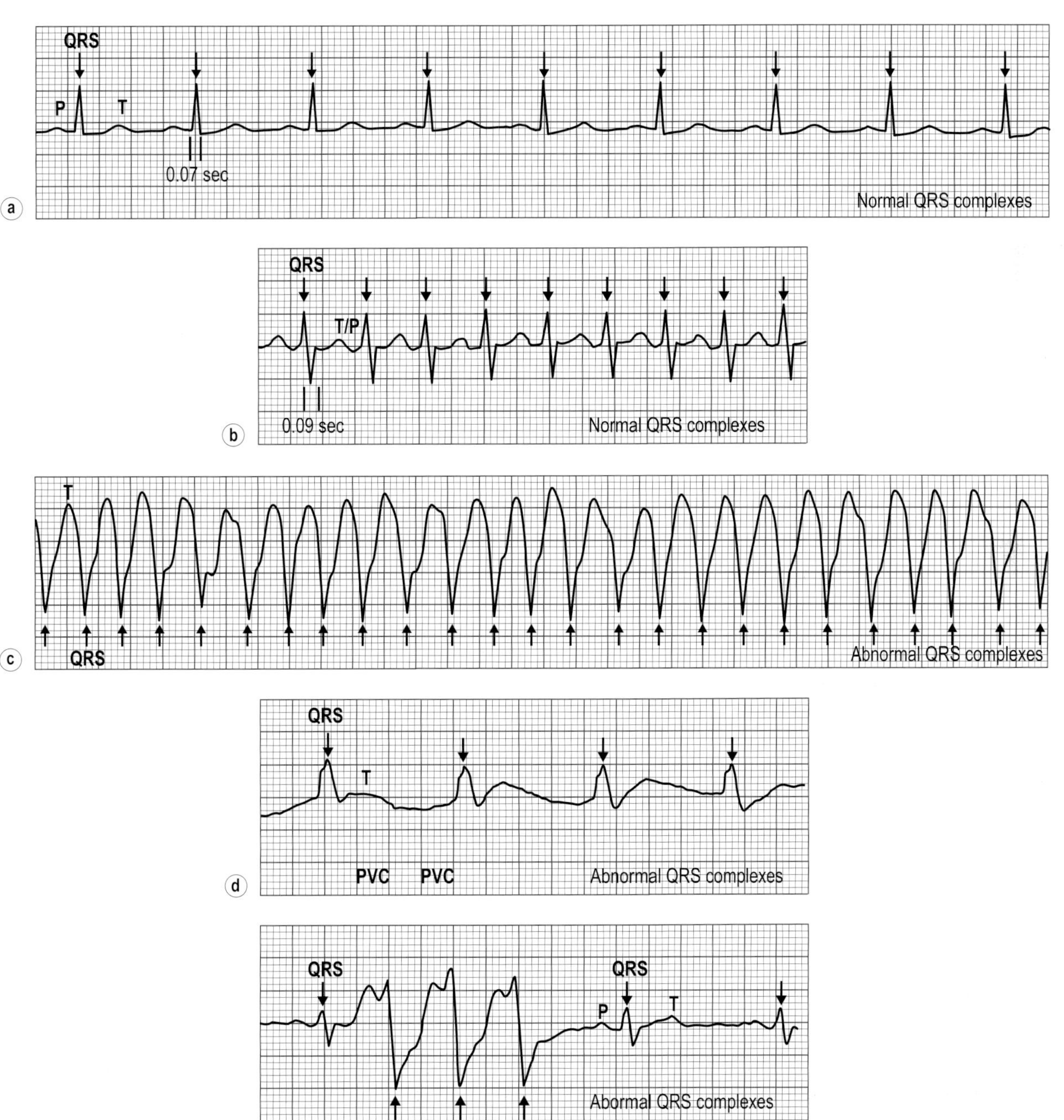

Figure 15-26 (a) and (b) Normal QRS complexes. (c–e) Abnormal QRS complexes.

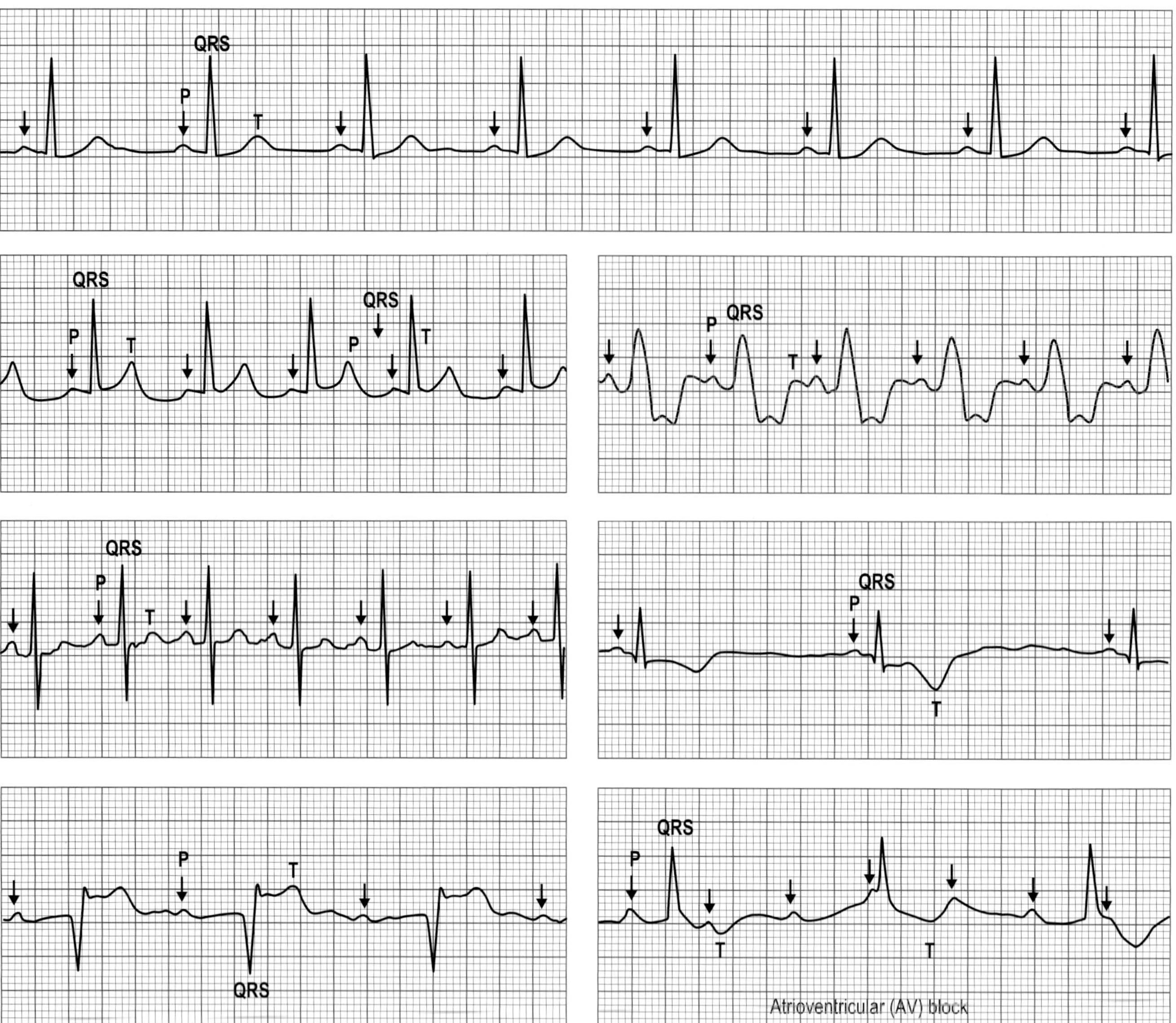

Figure 15-27 Normal P waves.

Step 2: Analyse the P waves

The normal P wave in lead II is positive and smoothly rounded and usually precedes each QRS complex, indicating that the pacemaker originates in the SA node (Figure 15-27). Therefore the paramedic should observe the following five components when evaluating P waves:

1. Are P waves present?
2. Are the P waves regular (can they be mapped out similar to R-R intervals [described later])?
3. Is there one P wave for each QRS complex, and is there a QRS complex following each P wave?
4. Are the P waves upright or inverted?
5. Do they all look alike? (P waves that look alike and are regular are likely from the same pacemaker.)

Step 3: Analyse the rate

Analysis of the heart rate may be done in a number of ways. The methods for calculating the heart rate presented in this text are heart rate calculator rulers, the triplicate method, the R-R method and the 6-s count method.

The heart rate is determined by analysing the ventricular rate (QRS complex). An adequate rate of ventricular contraction is responsible for cardiac output; however, if the atrial and ventricular rates differ (as may occur in certain dysrhythmias), they should be calculated separately. The normal adult heart rate is between 60 and 99 beats per minute. If the ventricular rate is less than 60 beats per minute, it is considered a bradycardia; if the rate is equal to or greater than 100 beats per minute, it is considered a tachycardia.

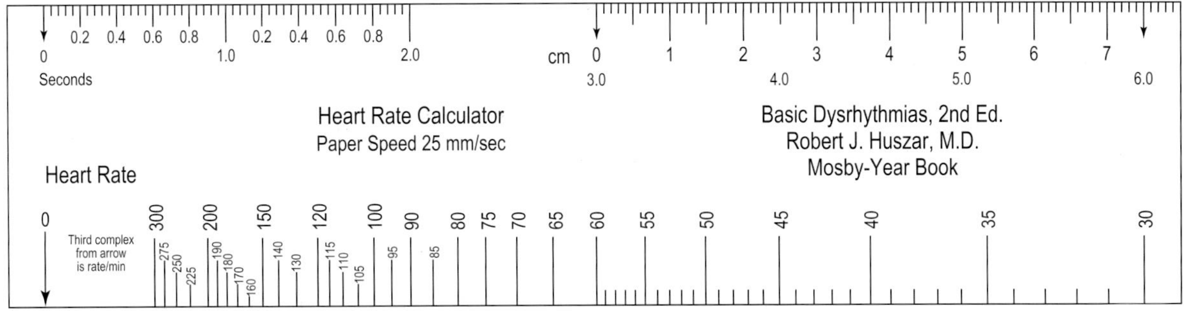

Figure 15-28 Heart rate calculator ruler.

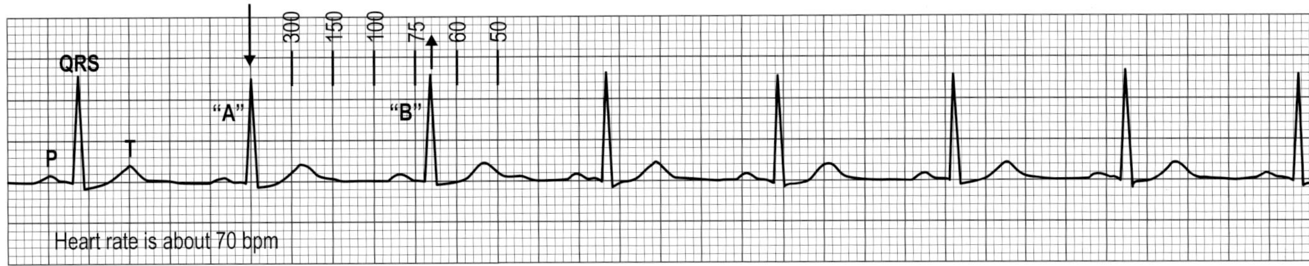

Figure 15-29 Triplicate method.

Heart rate calculator rulers

Heart rate calculator rulers (Figure 15-28) are available from a number of manufacturers. The paramedic should follow the directions that come with the rulers. Heart rate calculator rulers are reasonably accurate if the rhythm is regular although a mechanical device or tool should not be relied on solely to determine the heart rate because one may not be readily available.

Triplicate method

The triplicate method of determining the heart rate (Figure 15-29) is accurate only when the rhythm is regular and the heart rate is greater than 50 beats per minute. The method requires memorizing two sets of numbers. These are 300-150-100 and 75-60-50. These numbers are derived from the distance between the heavy black lines (each representing $\frac{1}{300}$ minute). Thus two $\frac{1}{300}$-minute units are equal to $\frac{2}{300}$ minute, which is equal to $\frac{1}{150}$ minute, or a heart rate of 150 beats per minute; three $\frac{1}{300}$-minute units are equal to $\frac{3}{300}$ minute, which is equal to $\frac{1}{100}$ minute, or a heart rate of 100 beats per minute. Using these triplicates, the paramedic can calculate heart rate as follows:

1. Select an R wave that lines up with a dark vertical line.
2. Number the next six dark vertical lines consecutively from left to right as 300-150-100 and 75-60-50.
3. Identify where the next R wave falls with reference to the six dark vertical lines. If the R wave falls on 75, the heart rate is 75 beats per minute. If the R wave falls halfway between 100 and 150, the heart rate is about 125 beats per minute.

R-R method

The R-R method may be used several different ways to calculate the heart rate. Like the triplicate method, the rhythm must be regular to obtain an accurate reading. However, the R-R method works equally well for slow rates. The three methods are as follows:

Method 1. Measure the distance in seconds between the peaks of two consecutive R waves. Then divide this number into 60 to obtain the heart rate (Figure 15-30).

Method 2. Count the large squares between the peaks of two consecutive R waves. Divide this number into 300 to obtain the heart rate (Figure 15-31).

Method 3. Count the small squares between the peaks of two consecutive R waves. Divide this number into 1500 to obtain the heart rate (Figure 15-32).

6-s count method

The 6-s count method (Figure 15-33) is the least accurate method of determining the heart rate but is useful, however, for quickly obtaining an approximate rate in regular and irregular rhythms.

As previously stated, the short vertical lines at the top of most electrocardiogram graph papers are divided into 3-s intervals when run at a standard speed of 25 mm/s. Two of these intervals are equal to 6 s. The heart rate is calculated by counting the number of QRS complexes in a 6-second interval and then multiplying by 10.

Critical Thinking

Which of these rate calculation methods is fastest? Which is most accurate?

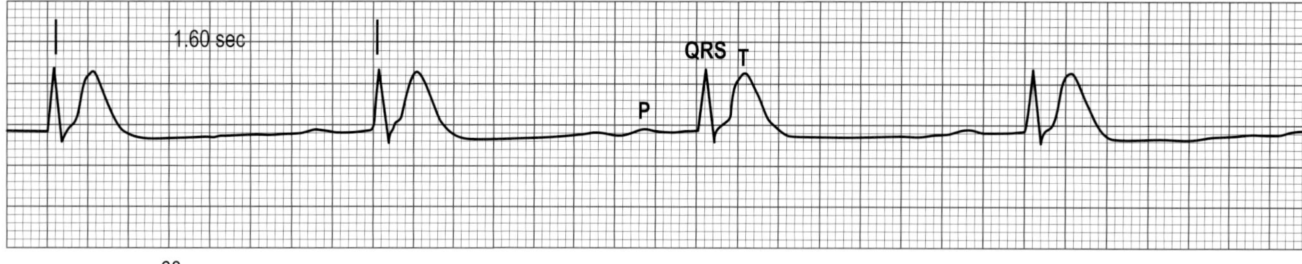

Heart rate = $\frac{60}{1.6 \text{ sec}}$ = 37.5 or, rounded off, 38

Figure 15-30 R-R interval method 1.

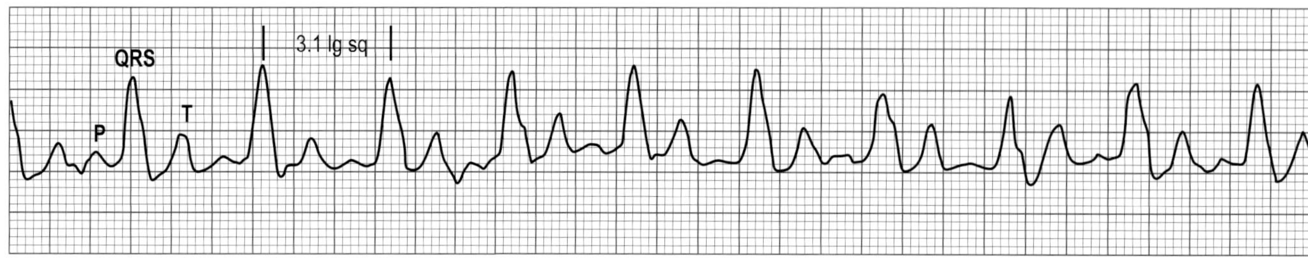

Heart rate = $\frac{300}{3.1 \text{ lg sq}}$ = 97

Figure 15-31 R-R interval method 2.

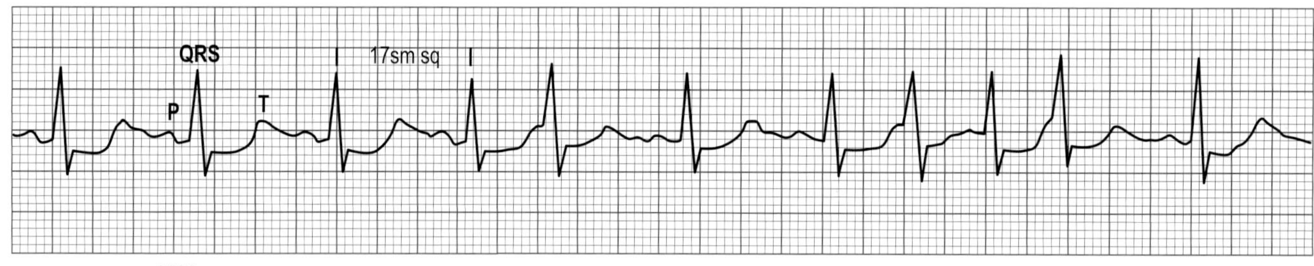

Heart rate = $\frac{1500}{17 \text{sm sq}}$ = 88

Figure 15-32 R-R interval method 3.

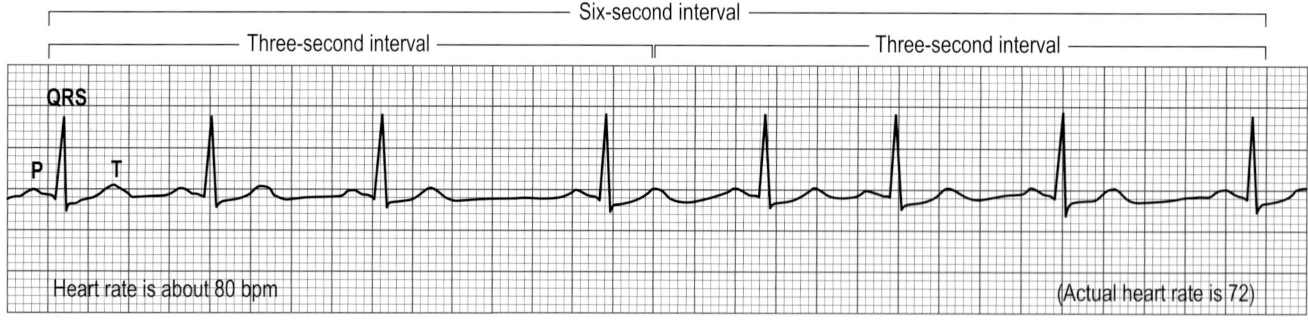

Figure 15-33 Six-second count method.

Step 4: Analyse the rhythm

To analyse the ventricular rhythm, the paramedic should compare the R-R intervals on the electrocardiogram tracing in a systematic way from left to right. This measurement may be taken using electrocardiogram calipers or pen and paper. Using calipers, the paramedic should place one tip of the caliper on the peak of one R wave and adjust the other tip so that it rests on the peak of the adjacent R wave; the paramedic then uses the caliper to map the distance of the R-R interval to evaluate evenness and regularity.

In the absence of calipers, the paramedic may use a similar method of evaluating the R-R interval using pen and paper. The paramedic places the straight edge of the paper near the

The distances between the R waves are determined:

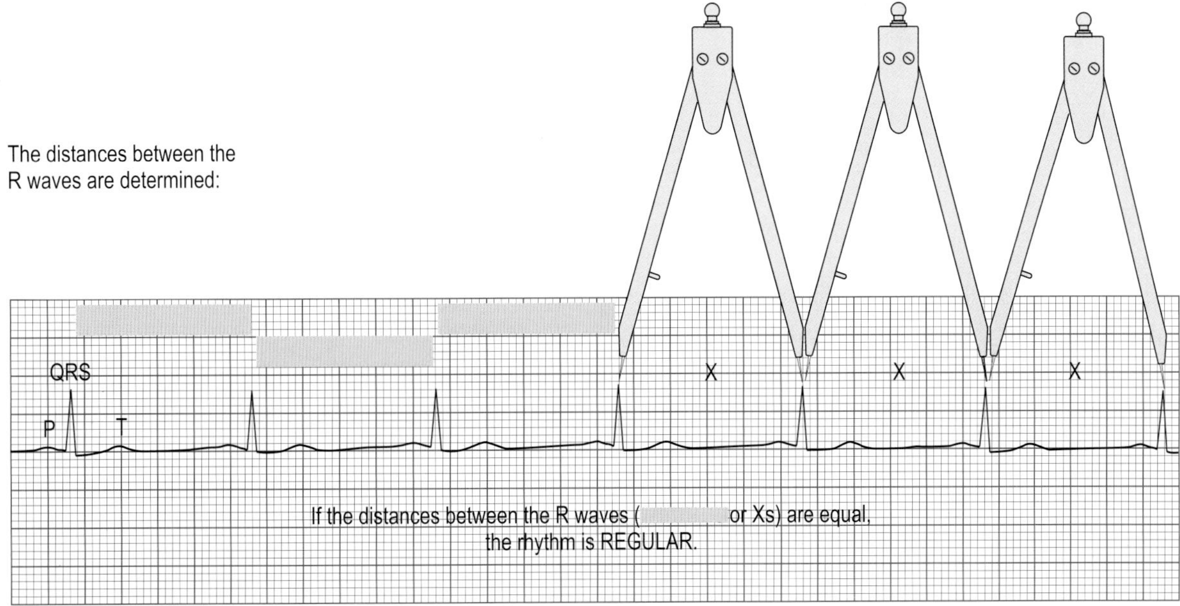

1. by estimating the R-R intervals,

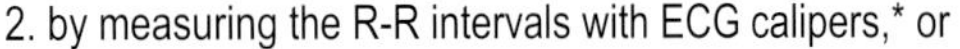

2. by measuring the R-R intervals with ECG calipers,* or

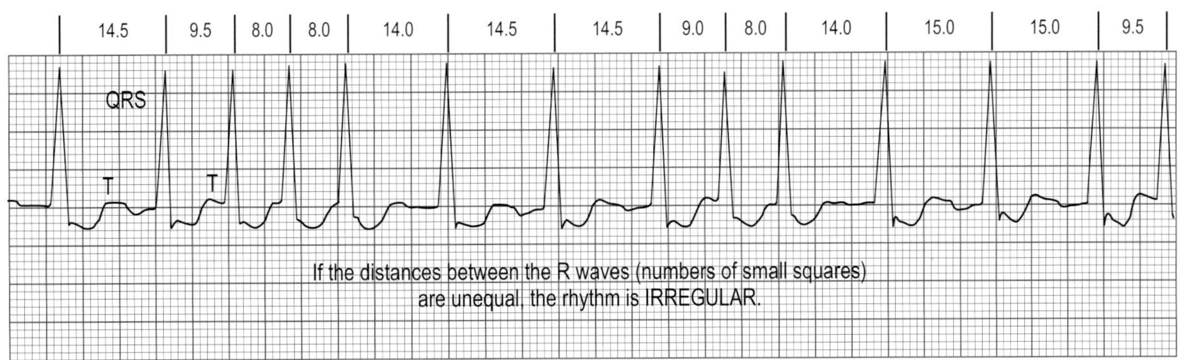

3. by counting the small squares between the R waves.

* If calipers are not available, mark off the distance between two R waves on a piece of paper and compare this distance with the other R-R intervals.

Figure 15-34 Determining the rhythm.

peaks of the R waves and marks off the distance between the two other consecutive R waves. The paramedic then compares this R-R interval with the other R-R intervals in the electrocardiogram tracing (Figure 15-34).

If the distances between the R waves are equal or vary by less than 0.16 s (four small squares), the rhythm is regular. If the shortest and longest R-R intervals vary by more than 0.16 s, the rhythm is irregular. Irregular rhythms may be classified further. They may be classified as regularly irregular. In this case, the irregularity has a pattern; it is also called 'group beating'. Irregular rhythms also may be occasionally irregular. In this case, only one or two R-R intervals are unequal. Finally, irregular rhythms may be irregularly irregular. In this case, the rhythm is totally irregular. No relationship is seen between the R-R intervals (Figure 15-35a–d).

Step 5: Analyse the P-R interval

The P-R interval indicates the time it takes for an electrical impulse to be conducted through the atria and AV node and should be constant across the electrocardiogram tracing. A prolonged P-R interval (greater than 0.20 s) indicates a delay in the conduction of the impulse through the AV node or bundle of His and is called an AV block. A short P-R interval (less than 0.12 s) indicates that the impulse progressed from the atria to the ventricles through pathways other than the AV node (Figure 15-36); this is known as an accessory pathway syndrome, the most common of which is Wolff–Parkinson–White syndrome (described later in this chapter).

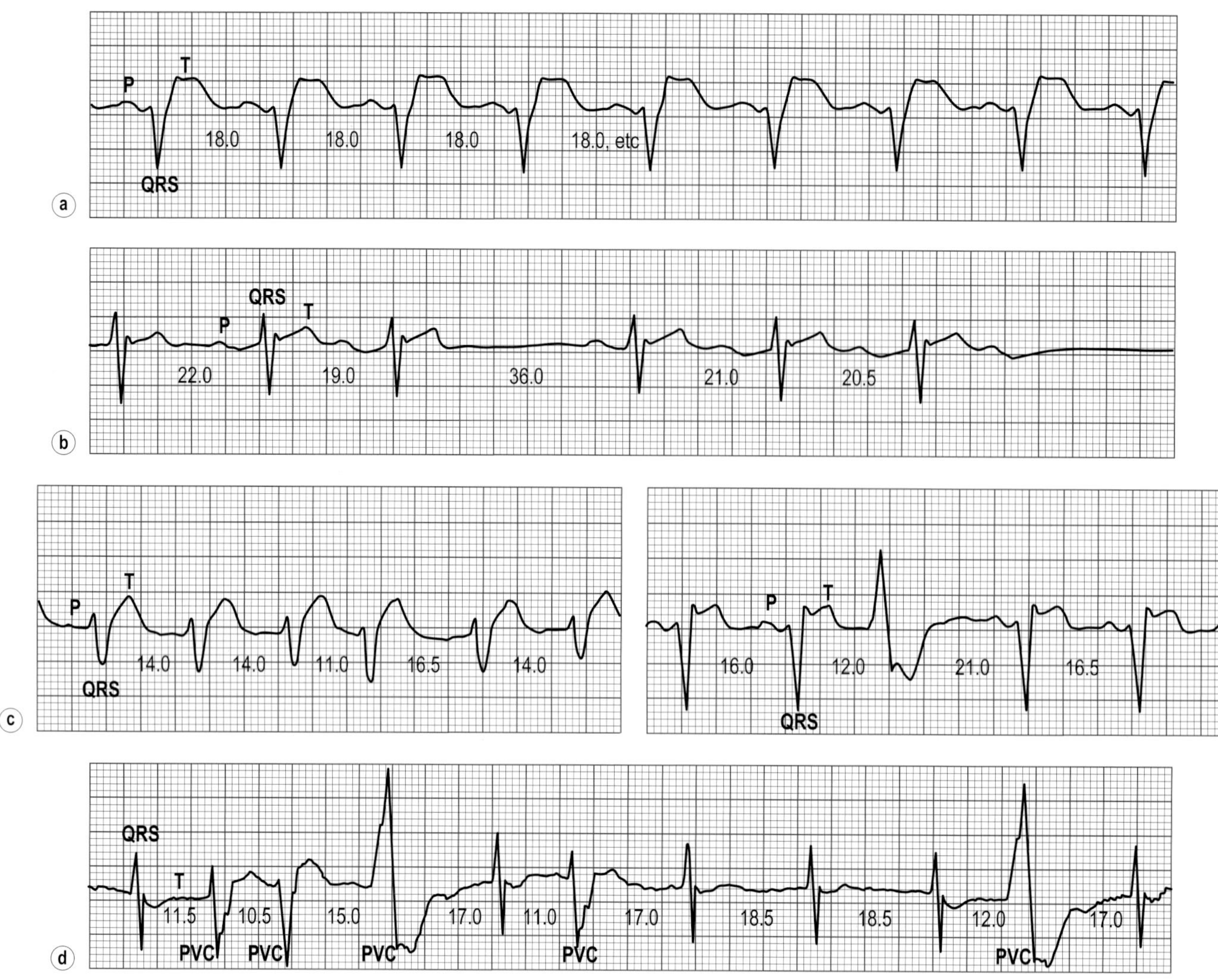

Figure 15-35 (a) Regular rhythm. (b) Regularly irregular rhythm. (c) Occasionally irregular rhythm. (d) Irregularly irregular rhythm.

Analysing a rhythm using the five steps

To review, the normal sequence of atrial and ventricular activation as it relates to the electrocardiogram tracing is as follows: each P wave (atrial depolarization) is followed by a normal QRS complex (ventricular depolarization) and T wave (ventricular repolarization). All QRS complexes are preceded by P waves; the P-R interval is within normal limits, and the R-R interval is regular. The five steps in electrocardiogram rhythm interpretation can be applied to the rhythm in Figure 15-37.

SECTION VI

Introduction to dysrhythmias

Cardiac dysrhythmias can result from a number of physiological, pharmacological and disease processes, including the following:

- myocardial ischaemia or necrosis
- autonomic nervous system imbalance
- distension of heart chambers
- acid–base abnormalities
- hypoxaemia
- electrolyte imbalance
- drug effects or toxicity
- electrical injury
- hypothermia
- central nervous system injury.

In addition to these potential causes of dysrhythmias, some cardiac rhythm disturbances are normal and may be seen even in patients who have healthy hearts (e.g. a patient may have sinus tachycardia from stress or anxiety). Regard-

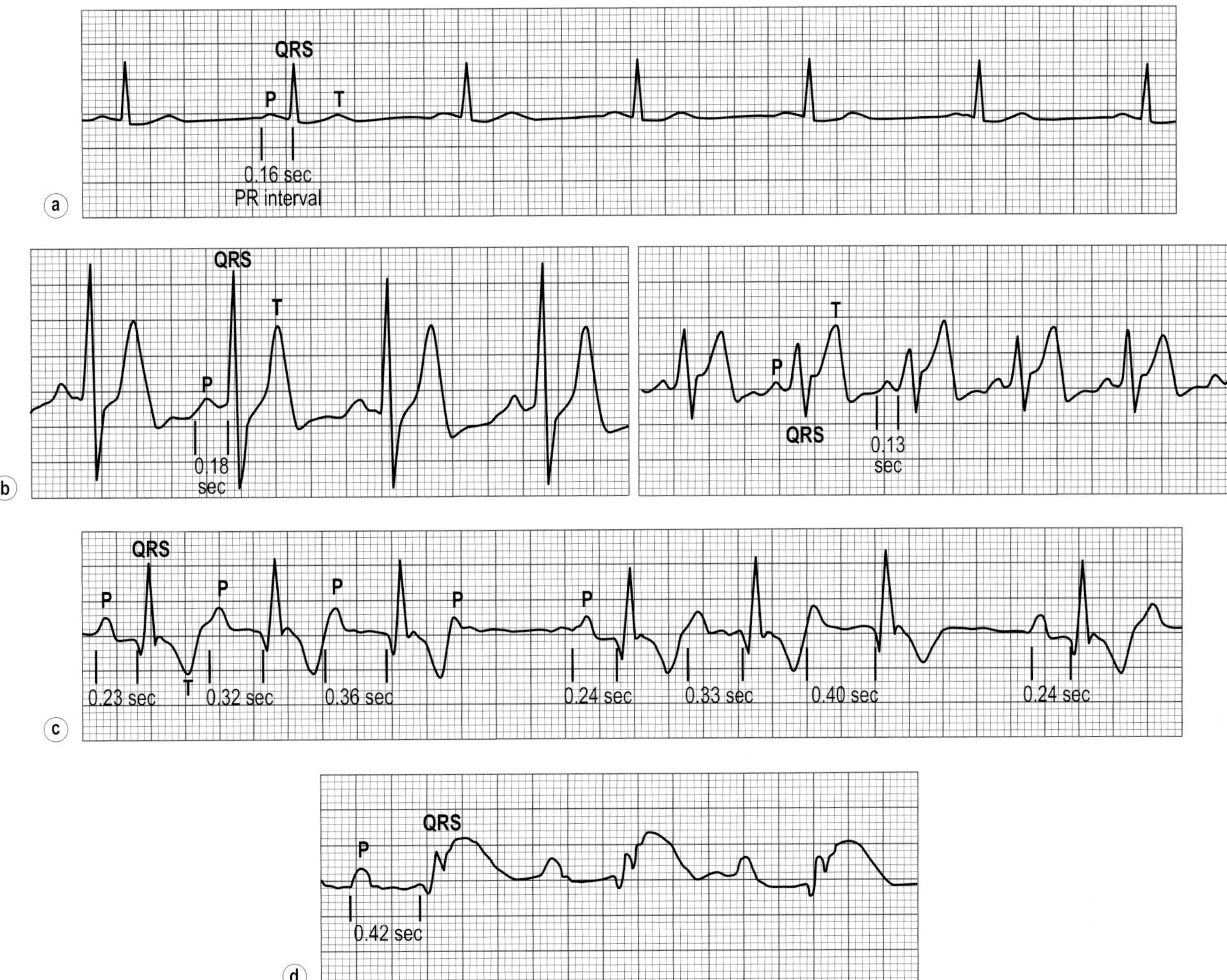

Figure 15-36 (a) and (b) Normal P-R intervals. (c) and (d) Abnormal P-R intervals.

less of the cause or type of dysrhythmia, management should focus on the patient and the underlying cause and not just on the dysrhythmias alone.

Note

Special considerations regarding cardiac rhythm disturbances and resuscitation for infant and paediatric patients are addressed in Chapters 37 and 38.

Classification of dysrhythmias

Classification by rate and pacemaker site

The classification of dysrhythmias can be based on a number of factors, including changes in automaticity versus disturbances in conduction, cardiac arrest (lethal) rhythms and non-cardiac arrest (non-lethal) rhythms, and site of origin. For learning purposes, this text classifies rhythms by rate and pacemaker site (e.g. ventricular tachycardia and sinus bradycardia) and includes the following five groups:

1. Dysrhythmias originating in the SA node
   a. Sinus bradycardia
   b. Sinus tachycardia
   c. Sinus dysrhythmia
   d. Sinus arrest
2. Dysrhythmias originating in the atria
   a. Wandering pacemaker
   b. Premature atrial complex
   c. Paroxysmal supraventricular tachycardia
   d. Atrial flutter
   e. Atrial fibrillation
3. Dysrhythmias originating in the AV node and surrounding tissues
   a. Premature junctional contraction
   b. Junctional escape complexes or rhythms
   c. Accelerated junctional rhythm

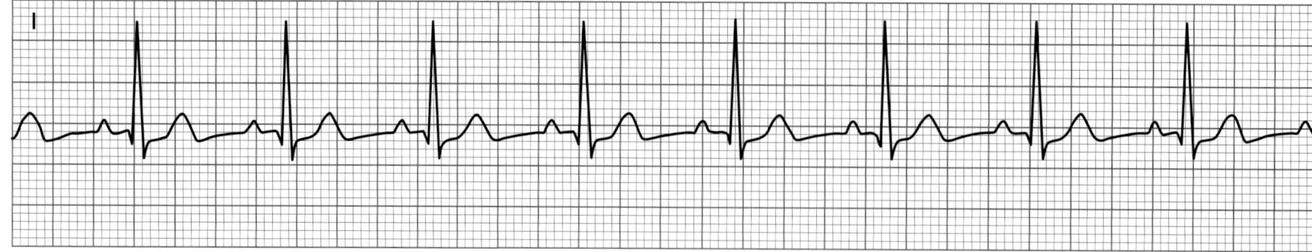

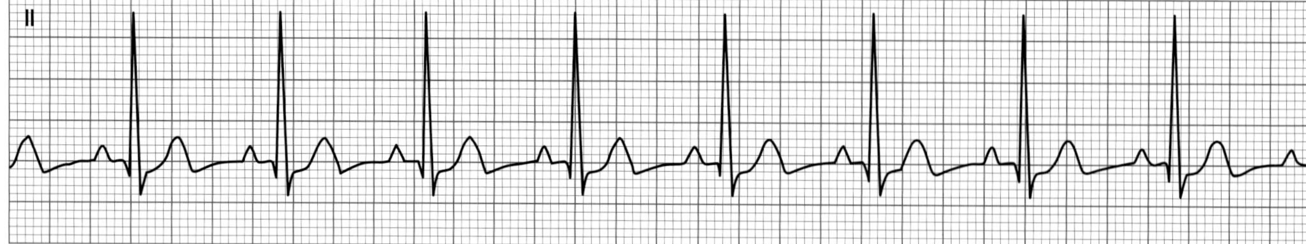

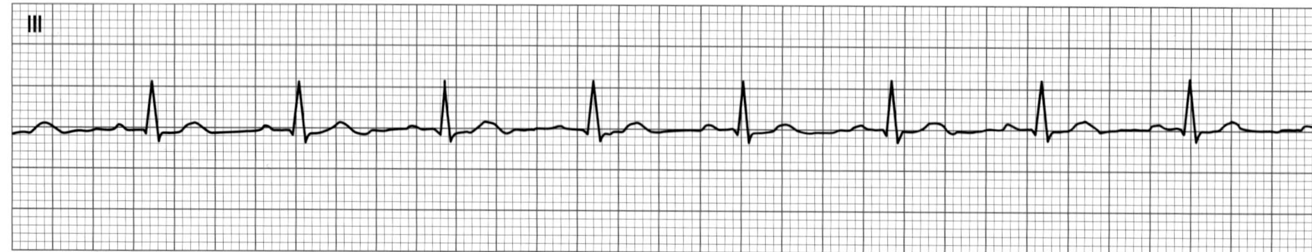

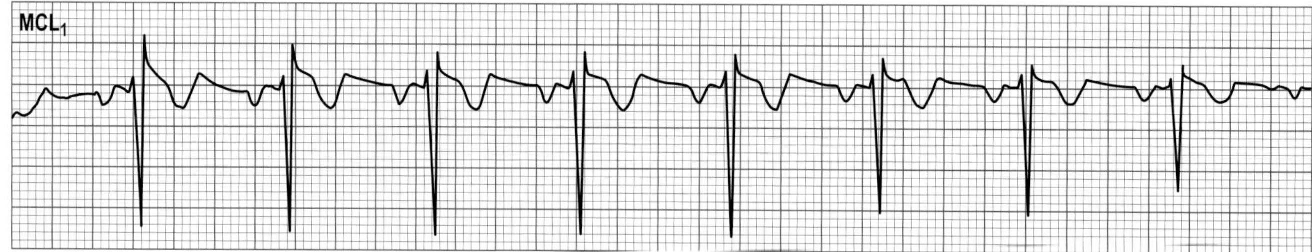

Figure 15-37 Normal sinus rhythm.

4. Dysrhythmias originating in the ventricles
   a. Ventricular escape complexes or rhythms
   b. Premature ventricular complex
   c. Ventricular tachycardia
   d. Ventricular fibrillation
   e. Asystole
   f. Artificial pacemaker rhythms
5. Dysrhythmias that are disorders of conduction
   a. Atrioventricular blocks
      (1) First-degree AV block
      (2) Second-degree AV block type I (or Wenckebach)
      (3) Second-degree AV block type II
      (4) Third-degree AV block
   b. Disturbances of ventricular conduction
   c. Pulseless electrical activity
   d. Pre-excitation syndrome: Wolff–Parkinson–White syndrome

Note

Broadly speaking, there are only four cardiac arrest rhythms. These are ventricular fibrillation, pulseless ventricular tachycardia, asystole, and various pulseless electrical activity rhythms. The two non-cardiac arrest rhythms (known as periarrest rhythms) that are important to consider in prehospital care are those that are too slow (fewer than 60 beats per minute) and those that are too fast (more than 120 beats per minute).

The text presents each dysrhythmia in lead II. For comparison, the same dysrhythmia also is shown as it would appear in leads I and III. The text discusses how to recognize the dysrhythmia and the emergency treatment for patients with each dysrhythmia. All treatments in this chapter follow the recommendations of the European Resuscitation Council and/or Resuscitation Council UK as well as the JRCALC Clinical Practice Guidelines.

Use of algorithms for classification

Algorithms are lists used to summarize information; some algorithms contain prehospital and in-hospital management recommendations. The following eight guidelines apply to the use of all algorithms:

1. First, manage (treat) the patient, not the monitor. THIS IS MOST IMPORTANT.
2. Algorithms for cardiac arrest presume that the condition under discussion continually persists, that the patient remains in cardiac arrest, and that cardiopulmonary resuscitation is always performed.
3. Apply different interventions when appropriate indications exist.
4. The algorithms are designed to outline the most common assessments and actions performed for the majority of patients, but they are not designed to be all-inclusive or restrictive. The flow diagrams present treatments mostly in sequential order of priority. A treatment or pharmacological agent may have a class recommendation (Box 15-5). The footnotes to the algorithm contain additional important information related to assessment, treatment and evaluation.
5. Adequate airway, ventilation, oxygenation, chest compression and defibrillation are more important than administration of medications. These measures take precedence over initiating an intravenous line or injecting pharmacological agents.
6. If IV or IO access is not available, some medications (adrenaline [epinephrine], lidocaine, atropine and naloxone) may be administered via an endotracheal tube. The endotracheal dose is 2 to 2½ times the intravenous dose for adults. Plasma concentrations are unreliable though and the optimal dose of these drugs given via this route unknown. Note, do not give drugs via a laryngeal mask as most of the drug is likely to be deposited on the larynx and therefore dosing will be very unreliable.
7. With a few exceptions, intravenous medications should always be administered rapidly in bolus method.
8. After each intravenous medication, give a 20–30-mL bolus of intravenous fluid. This may enhance delivery of drugs to the central circulation. This delivery may take 1–2 min.

Box 15-5

Classes of recommendations 2005

Class I

Benefit significantly outweighs any possible harm
High-level prospective studies supports the treatment
Treatment should be performed/ administered

Class IIa

Benefit outweighs risk
Weight of evidence support the treatment
Treatment is considered acceptable and useful

Class IIb

Benefit equals or is greater than the risk
Evidence documented only short-term benefit or lower-level evidence supported its use
Therapy may be considered

Class III

Risk is greater than benefit
Therapy is not indicated
Not proven to be helpful
May harm the patient
Research is continuing
No consensus recommendation for or against use

Adapted from American Heart Association 2005 American Heart Association Guidelines for Cardiopulmonary Resuscitation and Emergency Cardiovascular Care. Circulation 112(24)(Suppl.).

Dysrhythmias originating in the SA node

Most sinus dysrhythmias result from increases or decreases in vagal tone (parasympathetic nervous system). The SA node generally receives sufficient inhibitory parasympathetic impulses from the vagus nerve to keep the SA node within the normal rate of 60 to 100. However, if vagal nerve activity increases, the heart rate becomes bradycardic. If the vagus nerve is slowed or blocked, the heart rate increases and results in sinus tachycardia. Dysrhythmias that originate in the SA node include sinus bradycardia, sinus tachycardia, sinus dysrhythmia and sinus arrest. Electrocardiogram features common to all SA node dysrhythmias include the following:

- normal duration of QRS complex (in the absence of bundle branch block)
- upright P waves in lead II
- similar appearance of all P waves
- normal duration of P-R interval (in the absence of AV block).

Sinus bradycardia

Description

Sinus bradycardia results from slowing of the pacemaker rate of the SA node (Figure 15-38).

Aetiology

The following are possible causes of sinus bradycardia:

- intrinsic sinus node disease
- increased parasympathetic vagal tone
- hypothermia
- hypoxia
- raised intracranial pressure
- drug effects (e.g. digitalis, beta-blockers and calcium channel blockers)
- myocardial infarction.

Rules for interpretation (lead II monitoring)

Sinus bradycardia has the following characteristics on the electrocardiogram:

QRS complex: Less than 0.12 s, provided there is no ventricular conduction disturbance.

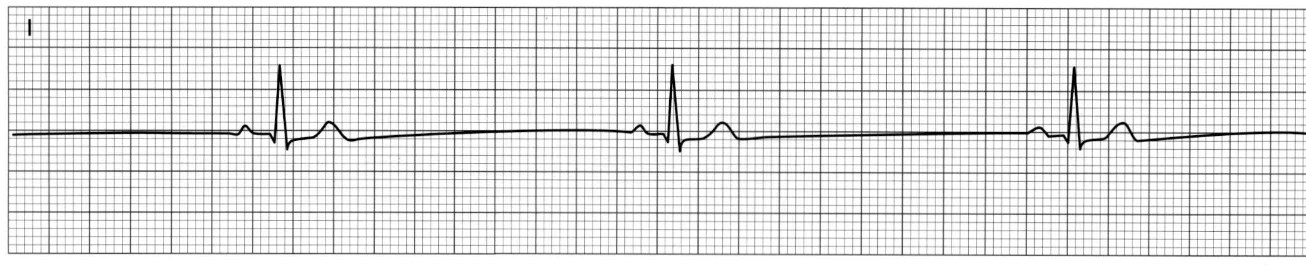

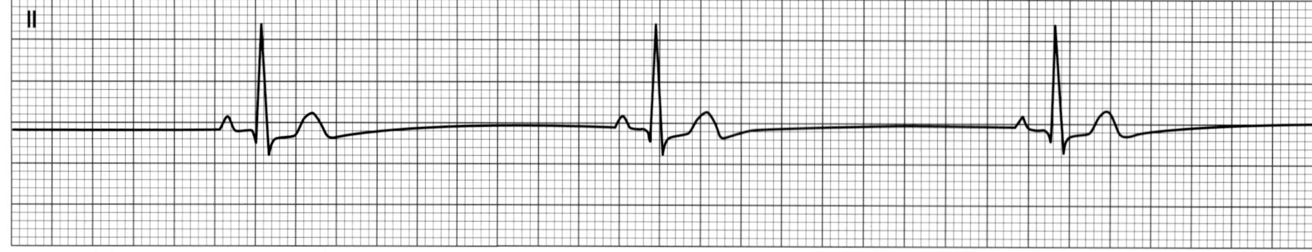

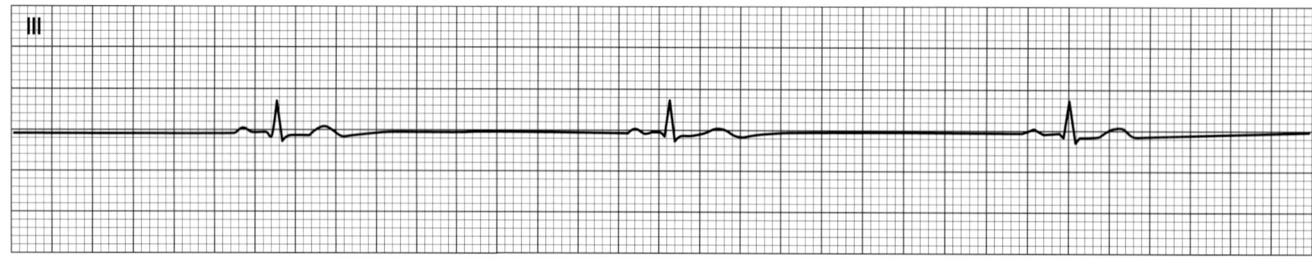

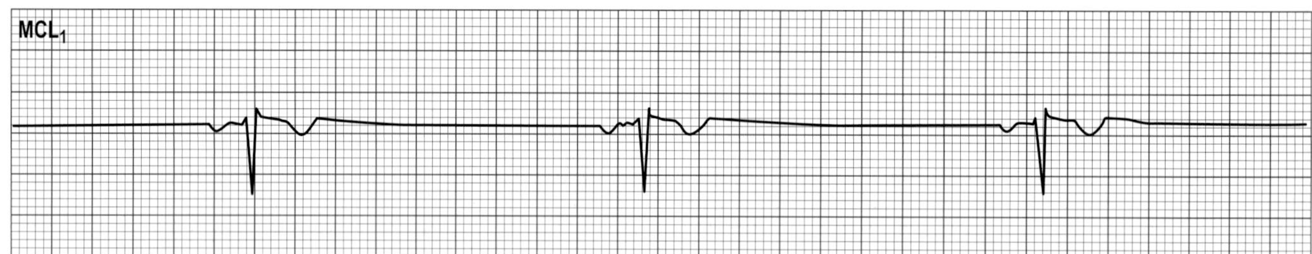

Figure 15-38 Sinus bradycardia.

P waves: Normal and upright; one P wave before each QRS complex.

Rate: Less than 60 beats per minute.

Rhythm: Regular.

P-R interval: 0.12 to 0.20 s and constant (normal), provided no AV block is present.

Clinical significance

Decreased rate may compromise cardiac output, resulting in hypotension or other signs of shock, angina pectoris, or central nervous system symptoms (e.g. light-headedness, vertigo, and syncope). Sinus bradycardia can result from nausea and vomiting, as well as overstimulation of the vagus nerve that can result in fainting (vasovagal syncope). However, sinus bradycardia may be beneficial. It may reduce myocardial oxygen consumption when the patient is having a heart attack. Sinus bradycardia also may follow the use of carotid sinus pressure (carotid sinus massage). This dysrhythmia is common during sleep and in well-conditioned athletes.

> **Critical Thinking**
>
> Take a poll of your classmates. How many have a resting heart rate 60 beats per minute?

Management (Figure 15-39)

Provide basic care of oxygen, IV access and record a 12-lead ECG. Assess the patient for any adverse sign(s) which might include systolic BP less than 90 mmHg, heart rate less than 40, ventricular dysrhythmias or evidence of heart failure; adverse signs/symptoms are usually rate dependent (at less than 50 beats per minute). Consider the potential risk of asystole; recent asystole, Mobitz II AV block, 3rd degree AV block, particularly with a rate under 40, and ventricular standstill for more than 3 s all increase the risk, and complications should be anticipated. Management for symptomatic bradycardia is aimed at increasing the heart rate to improve cardiac output and includes oxygen, atropine, and, where permitted, transcutaneous pacing (described later in

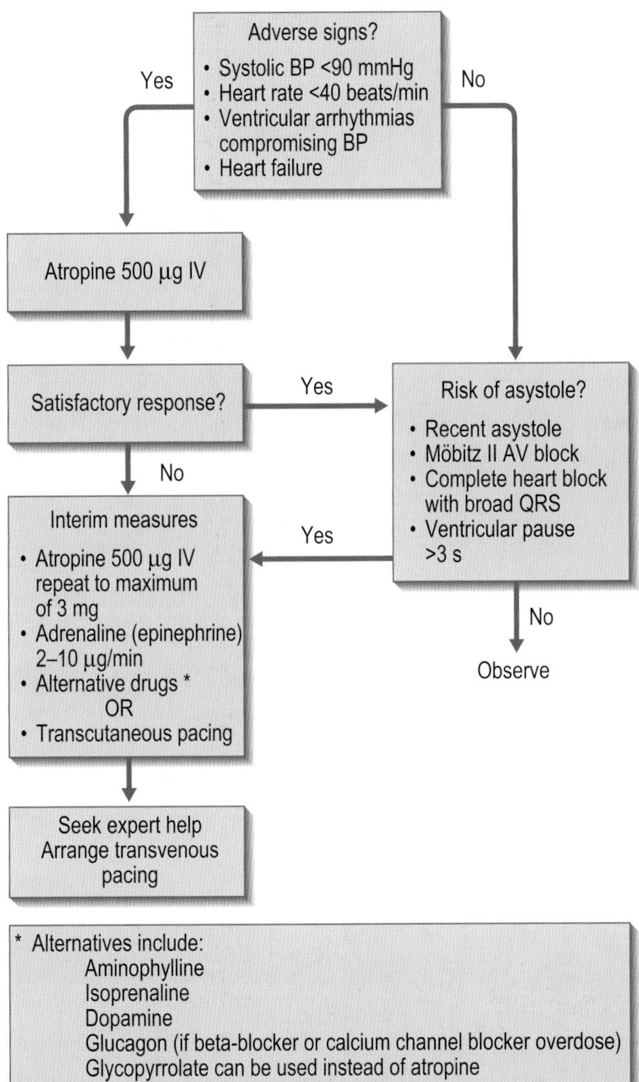

Figure 15-39 Bradycardia algorithm.

this chapter). Transcutaneous pacing is considered a class I intervention for all symptomatic bradycardias; if the patient fails to respond to atropine or is critically unstable, the paramedic, if permitted, should begin pacing immediately. Pacing is indicated for symptomatic bradycardias that are related to a conduction delay or block at or below the His–Purkinje level (infranodal). The paramedic should consider sedation for the patient to decrease discomfort caused by the electrical pacer stimuli. 'Fist' pacing may be effective in very extreme bradycardia, given by repeated blows or thumps with a closed fist (similar in manner to a pre-cordial thump) to the left lower sternum at a rate of 50–70/min; this may buy time if external pacing, described above, is not available.

For mild symptoms related to the bradycardia, atropine may be administered intravenously. Administration may be repeated every 3–5 min as needed. The frequency of atropine administration is based on the patient's condition. Atropine should be administered at shorter intervals, every 3 min, for severely unstable patients.

Atropine should be used with caution in the patient with an acute myocardial infarction. Atropine can increase the heart rate, increasing myocardial oxygen demand and in turn can worsen ischaemia or increase the size of the infarction.

Additional interventions, currently beyond the normal scope of UK paramedics, might include administration of isoprenaline and dopamine as intravenous infusions depending on the patient presentation.

Sinus tachycardia

Description

Sinus tachycardia results from an increase in the rate of sinus node discharge (Figure 15-40).

> **Critical Thinking**
>
> What effect will the excitement and commotion of the arrival of your ambulance likely have on the heart rate and blood pressure of a conscious, alert patient?

Aetiology

Sinus tachycardia is common and may result from multiple factors, including the following:

- exercise
- fever
- anxiety
- pain
- ingestion of caffeine or alcohol
- smoking
- hypovolaemia
- hyperthyroidism
- anaemia
- congestive heart failure
- administration of atropine or any vagolytic or sympathomimetic drug (e.g. cocaine, phencyclidine, adrenaline [epinephrine] and isoprenaline).

Rules for interpretation (lead II monitoring)

Sinus tachycardia has the following characteristics on the electrocardiogram:

QRS complex: Less than 0.12 s, provided there is no ventricular conduction disturbance.

P waves: Normal and upright; one before each QRS complex.

Rate: Equal to or greater than 100 beats per minute.

Rhythm: Regular.

P-R interval: 0.12 to 0.20 s (normal), provided no AV conduction block is present.

Clinical significance

Sinus tachycardia in healthy individuals generally is not significant. If tachycardia is associated with myocardial infarction, however, it may increase the oxygen requirements of the heart, increase myocardial ischaemia, and predispose the patient to more serious rhythm disturbances. Cardiac output may be compromised at rates above 120 as ventricular refilling is reduced.

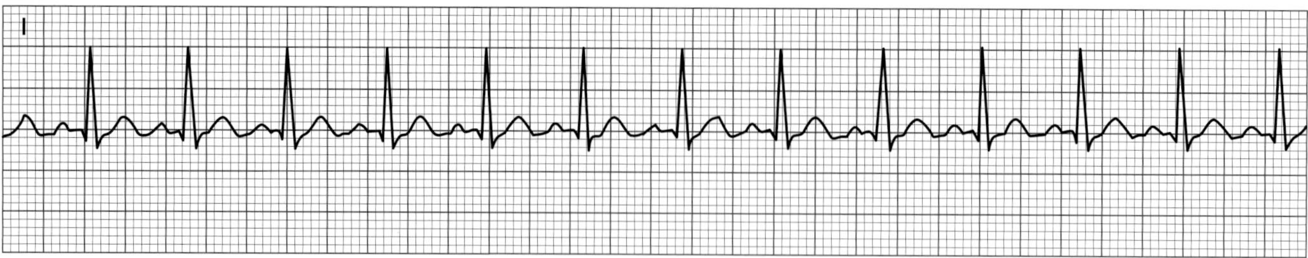

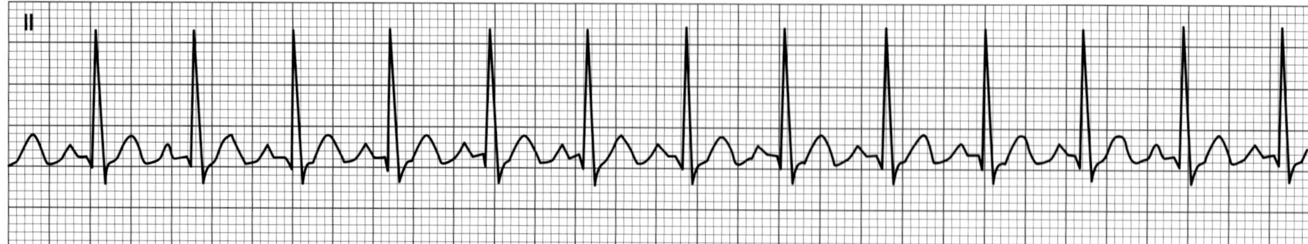

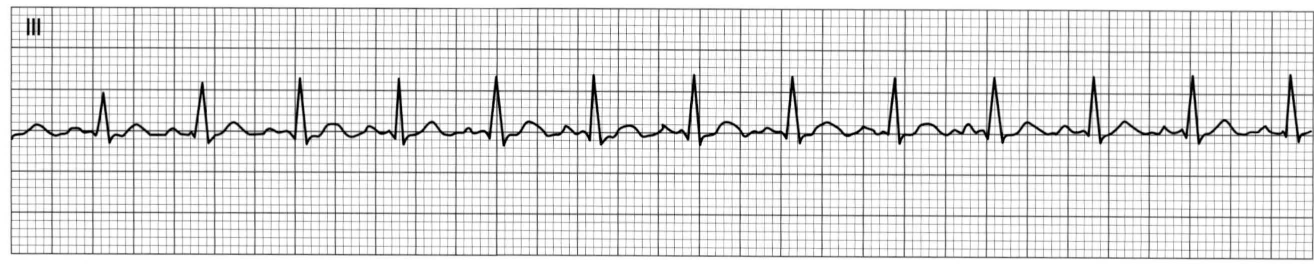

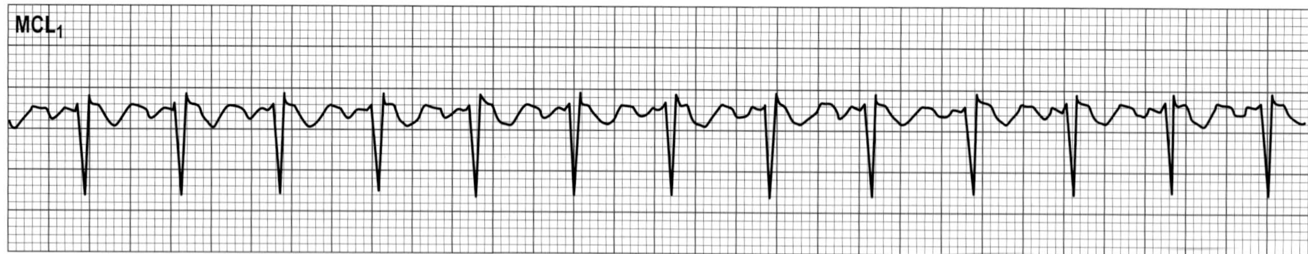

Figure 15-40 Sinus tachycardia.

Management

Sinus tachycardia usually does not require treatment. When the underlying cause is removed, the tachycardia usually resolves gradually and spontaneously.

Sinus dysrhythmia

Description

Sinus dysrhythmia is present when the difference between the longest and shortest R-R intervals is greater than 0.16 s (Figure 15-41).

Aetiology

Sinus dysrhythmia usually is normal. It often is related to the respiratory cycle and to changes in intrathoracic pressure causing the heart rate to increase during inspiration and to decrease during expiration. Although sinus dysrhythmia sometimes occurs normally in younger and healthy persons, it is more common in patients with heart disease or myocardial infarction. It also is more common in patients receiving certain drugs such as digoxin and morphine.

Rules for interpretation (lead II monitoring)

Sinus dysrhythmia has the following characteristics on the electrocardiogram:

QRS complex: Less than 0.12 s, provided no ventricular conduction disturbance is present.

P waves: Normal and upright; one P wave before each QRS complex.

Rate: Usually 60 to 99 beats per minute (varies with respiration).

Rhythm: Irregular (changes occur in cycles and usually follow the patient's respiratory pattern).

P-R interval: 0.12 to 0.20 s and constant (normal).

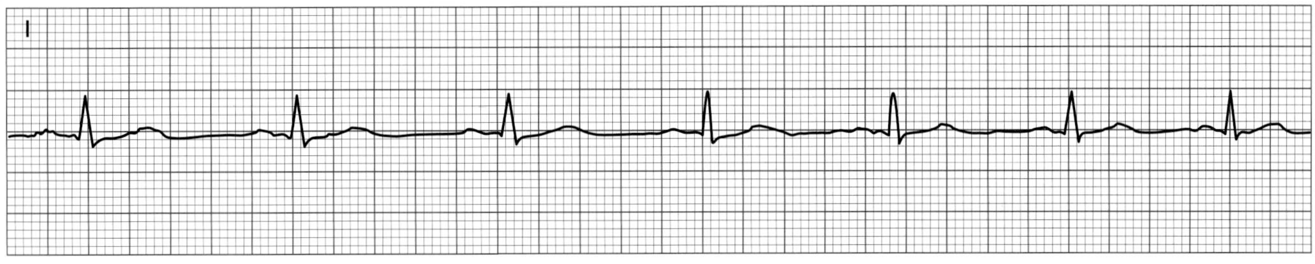

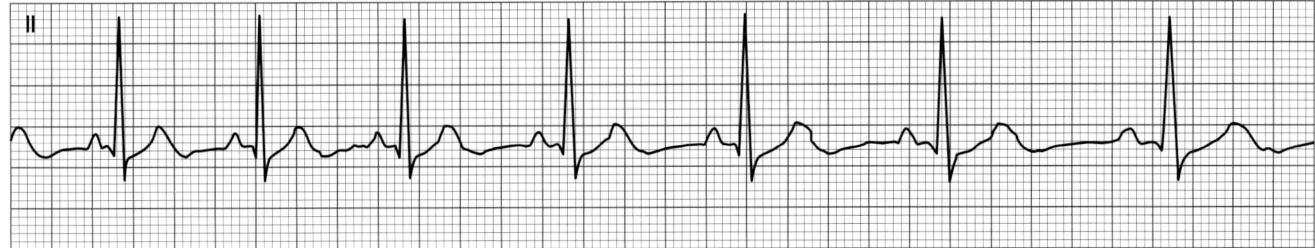

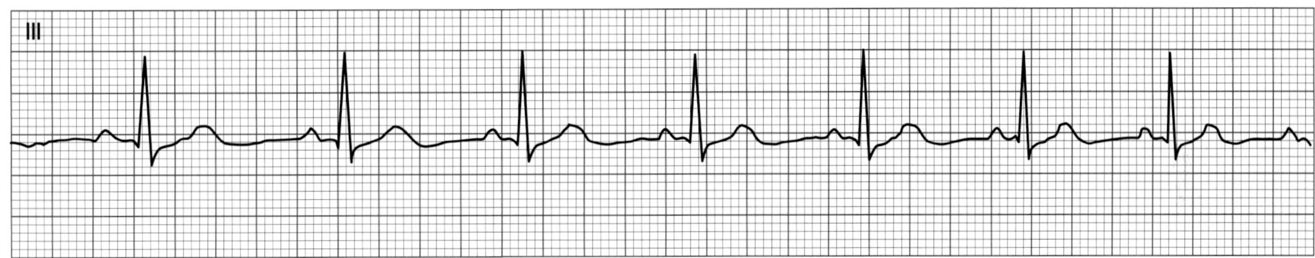

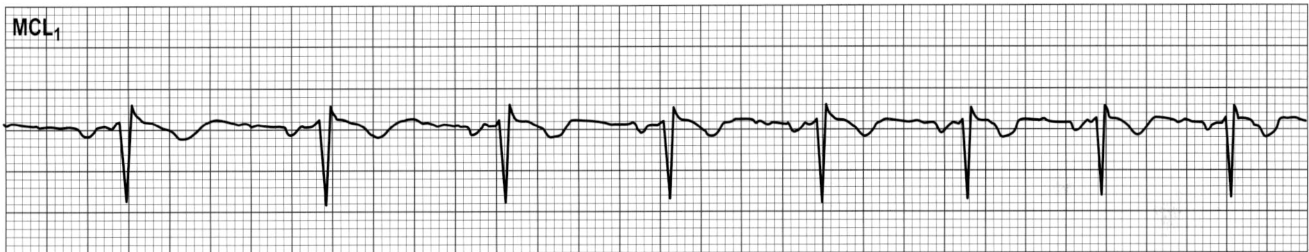

Figure 15-41 Sinus dysrhythmia.

Clinical significance

Sinus dysrhythmia is common in children, young adults and older adults. It may be associated with palpitations, dizziness and syncope (rare).

Management

Sinus dysrhythmia usually is not significant. It seldom requires treatment.

Sinus arrest

Description

Sinus arrest results from a problem with the ability of the SA node to fire automatically (Figure 15-42), causing short periods of cardiac standstill. This occurs until lower-level pacemakers discharge (escape beats) or the sinus node resumes its normal function.

Aetiology

Sinus arrest may be precipitated by an increase in parasympathetic tone on the SA node, hypoxia or ischaemia, excessive administration of digitalis or propranolol, hyperkalaemia or damage to the SA node (acute myocardial infarction, degenerative fibrotic disease).

Rules for interpretation (lead II monitoring)

Sinus arrest has the following characteristics on the electrocardiogram:

QRS complex: Less than 0.12 s, provided there is no bundle branch conduction disturbance.

P waves: Normal and upright. If the electrical impulse is not generated by the SA node or blocked from entering the atria, atrial depolarization does not occur and the P wave is dropped.

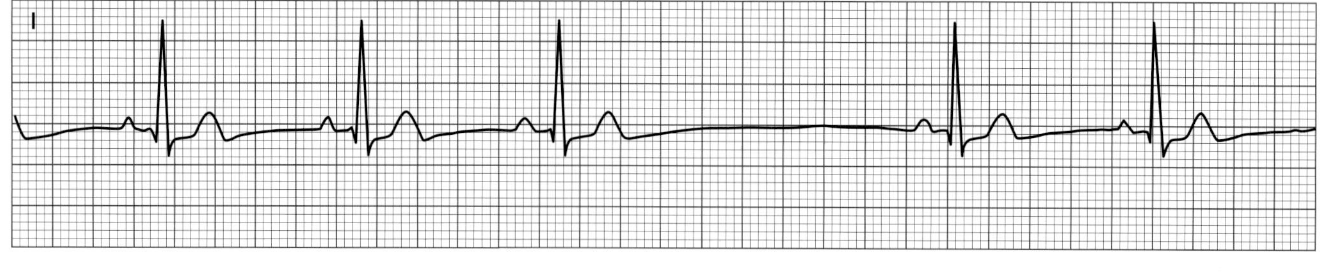

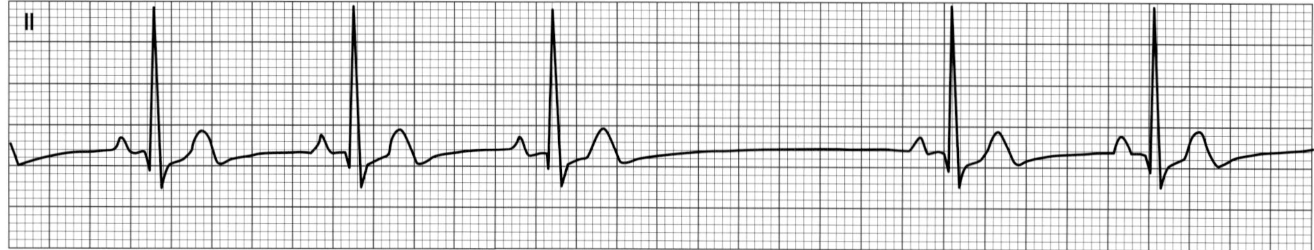

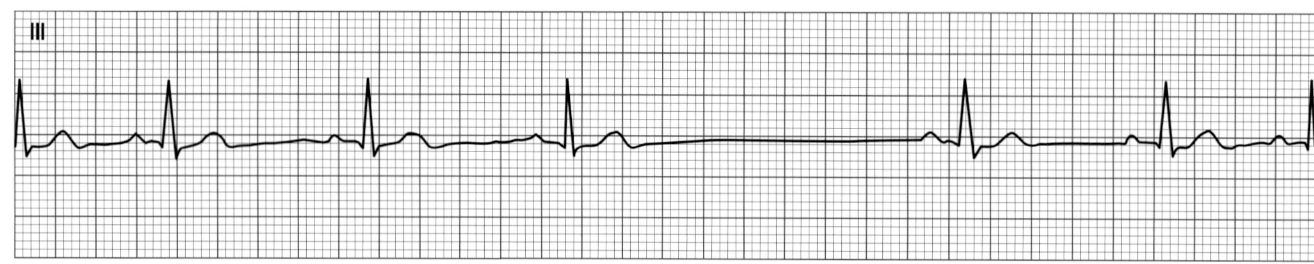

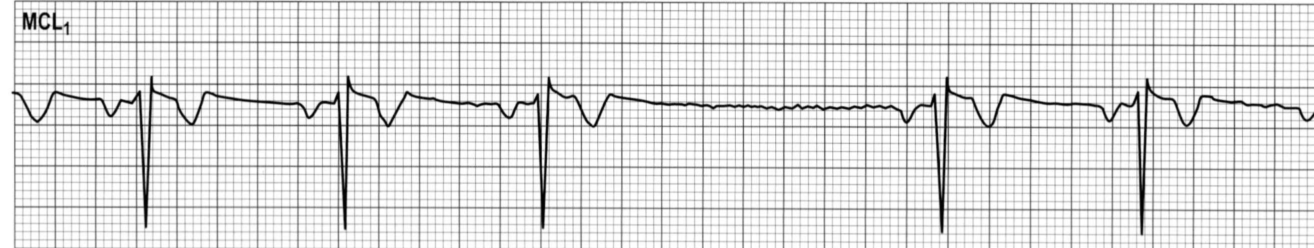

Figure 15-42 Sinus arrest.

Rate: Normal to slow, depending on the frequency and duration of sinus arrest.

Rhythm: Irregular when sinus arrest is present.

P-R interval: P-R intervals (when the P wave is present) of the underlying rhythm are normal (0.12 to 0.20 s) in the absence of AV block. Junctional escape beats may occur with no P waves.

Clinical significance

Frequent or prolonged episodes of sinus arrest may decrease cardiac output; the overall heart rate slows and the atria do not contract, so ventricular filling is reduced. If an escape pacemaker does not take over, ventricular asystole may result. This would cause light-headedness followed by syncope. With this dysrhythmia, there is danger that sinus node activity will cease completely or that an escape pacemaker may not take over pacing, which would result in asystole.

Management

If the patient is asymptomatic, close observation is all that is required. In patients with bradycardia that produces symptoms, management may include the administration of atropine or transcutaneous cardiac pacing (Figure 15-39).

Dysrhythmias originating in the atria

Atrial dysrhythmias may begin in the tissues of the atria or in the AV junction. Common causes of atrial dysrhythmias are ischaemia, hypoxia and atrial dilation caused by congestive heart failure, mitral valve abnormalities or increased pulmonary artery pressures. Atrial dysrhythmias include wandering pacemaker, premature atrial complexes, paroxysmal supraventricular tachycardia, atrial flutter and atrial fibrillation. Electrocardiogram features common to all atrial dysrhythmias (provided there is no ventricular conduction disturbance) include the following:

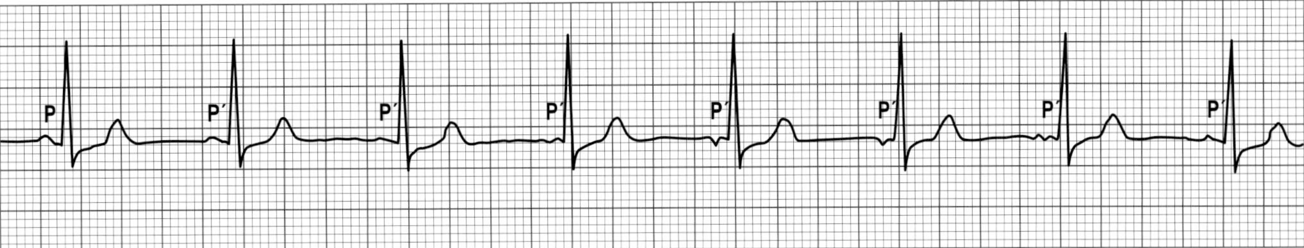

Figure 15-43 Wandering atrial pacemaker.

- normal QRS complexes
- P waves (if present) that differ in appearance from sinus P waves
- abnormal, shortened, or prolonged P-R intervals.

Wandering pacemaker

Description

Wandering pacemaker (or wandering atrial pacemaker) occurs when the pacemaker shifts from the sinus node to another pacemaker site in the atria or the AV junction (Figure 15-43). The shift in the site usually is transient, back and forth along the SA node, atria, and AV junction.

Aetiology

Wandering pacemaker is a type of sinus dysrhythmia that may be normal in the very young, older adults and well-conditioned athletes. The dysrhythmia is generally caused by pressure on the vagus nerve related to respiration; this stimulation or pressure on the vagus nerve causes the SA node and AV junction pacemaker rates to slow and may be seen in those with lung diseases. Other causes include associated underlying heart disease and the administration of digitalis. Another type of wandering atrial pacemaker is multifocal atrial tachycardia, which looks like a wandering pacemaker. However, multifocal atrial tachycardia is associated with rates often in the 120–150/min range and is always considered pathological. Multifocal atrial tachycardia is most often found in patients with severe chronic obstructive pulmonary disease and treatment of the lung disease may help to stop this rhythm. Multifocal atrial tachycardia often is mistaken for atrial fibrillation with rapid ventricular response.

Rules for interpretation (lead II monitoring)

Wandering pacemaker has the following characteristics on the electrocardiogram:

QRS complex: Usually less than 0.12 s provided no conduction block occurs in the bundle branches.

P waves: Change in P wave morphology from beat to beat. In lead II the P waves may be upright, rounded, notched, inverted, biphasic, or buried in the QRS complex.

Rate: Usually 60 to 99 beats per minute. The rate may slow gradually when the pacemaker site shifts from the SA node to the atria or AV junction and may increase when the pacemaker site shifts back to the SA node.

Rhythm: Irregular.

P-R interval: Varies.

Clinical significance

A wandering pacemaker usually does not produce serious signs and symptoms but other atrial dysrhythmias (such as atrial fibrillation) sometimes result from this dysrhythmia.

Management

Sometimes a wandering pacemaker is a benign rhythm and no management is required. Multifocal atrial tachycardia, however, may be precipitated by acute exacerbation of emphysema, congestive heart failure or acute mitral valve regurgitation. Management is aimed at the underlying cause and oxygen administration is usually the initial treatment of choice for multifocal atrial tachycardia.

Premature atrial complex

Description

A premature atrial complex is a single electrical impulse originating in the atria, outside the sinus node (Figure 15-44) creating a premature atrial complex (P wave). If conducted through the AV node, the impulse also causes a QRS complex before the next expected sinus beat. Because the premature atrial complex usually depolarizes the SA node prematurely, the timing of the SA node is reset; the next expected P wave of the underlying rhythm appears earlier than it would have if the SA node had not been disturbed (non-compensatory pause). Premature atrial complexes may originate from a single ectopic pacemaker site or they may originate from multiple sites in the atria. Premature atrial complexes probably result from enhanced automaticity or a re-entry mechanism.

> **Critical Thinking**
>
> What will you feel when you palpate the pulse of a patient with premature atrial complexes?

Aetiology

Premature atrial complexes may result from the following:

- increase in catecholamines and sympathetic tone
- use of caffeine, tobacco, or alcohol
- use of sympathomimetic drugs (adrenaline [epinephrine], salbutamol, noradrenaline [norepinephrine])
- electrolyte imbalance

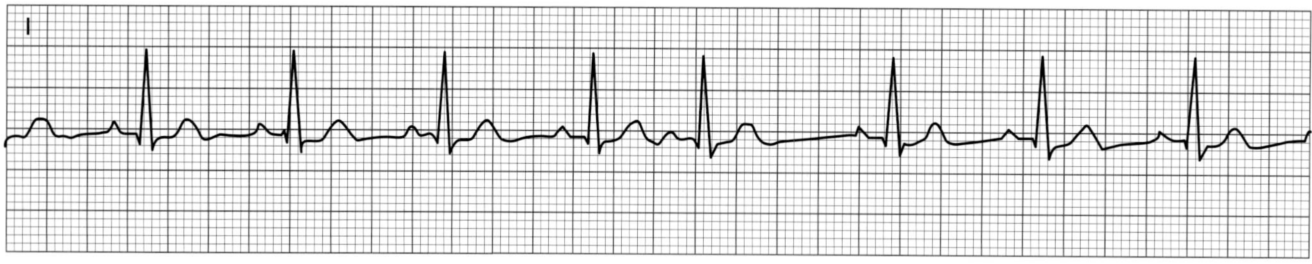

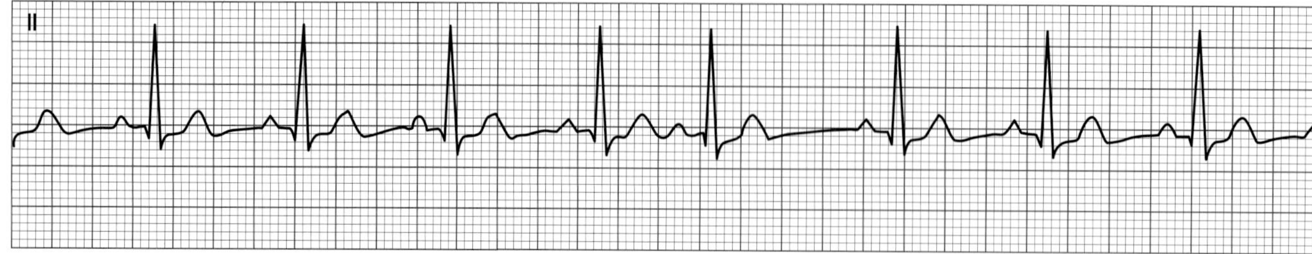

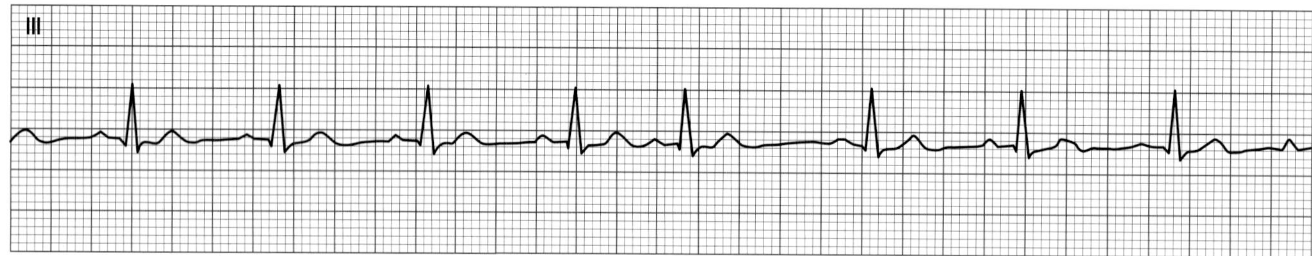

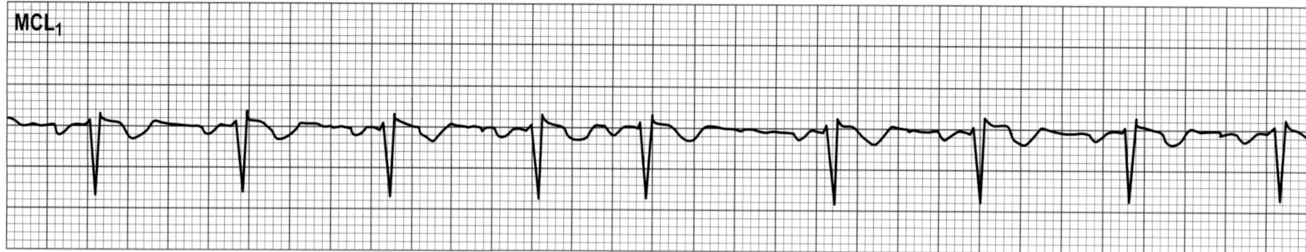

Figure 15-44 Premature atrial complex.

- hypoxia
- digitalis toxicity
- cardiovascular disease
- in some cases, no apparent cause.

Rules for interpretation (lead II monitoring)

Premature atrial complexes have the following characteristics on the electrocardiogram:

QRS complex: Usually less than 0.12 s. The QRS complex may be greater than 0.12 s and appear bizarre if the premature atrial complex is conducted abnormally. The QRS complex may be absent as a result of a temporary complete AV block (non-conducted premature atrial complex) that occurs during the refractory period of the AV node or ventricles.

P waves: The P wave of a premature atrial complex differs in shape from a sinus P wave. It occurs earlier than the next expected sinus P wave and may be so early that it is superimposed or hidden in the preceding T wave. The paramedic should evaluate the preceding T wave to see whether its morphology is altered by the presence of a P wave.

Rate: Depends on the underlying rhythm.

Rhythm: Usually the underlying rhythm is sinus and regular with irregular premature beats when the premature atrial complexes occur.

P-R interval: Usually in the normal range but differs from those of the underlying rhythm. The P-R interval of a premature atrial complex varies from 0.20 s when the pacemaker site is near the SA node to 0.12 s when the pacemaker site is near the AV junction.

Note

Premature atrial complexes with aberrancy may resemble premature ventricular complexes. Distinguishing between these two types of dysrhythmias is important so as to manage the patient properly.

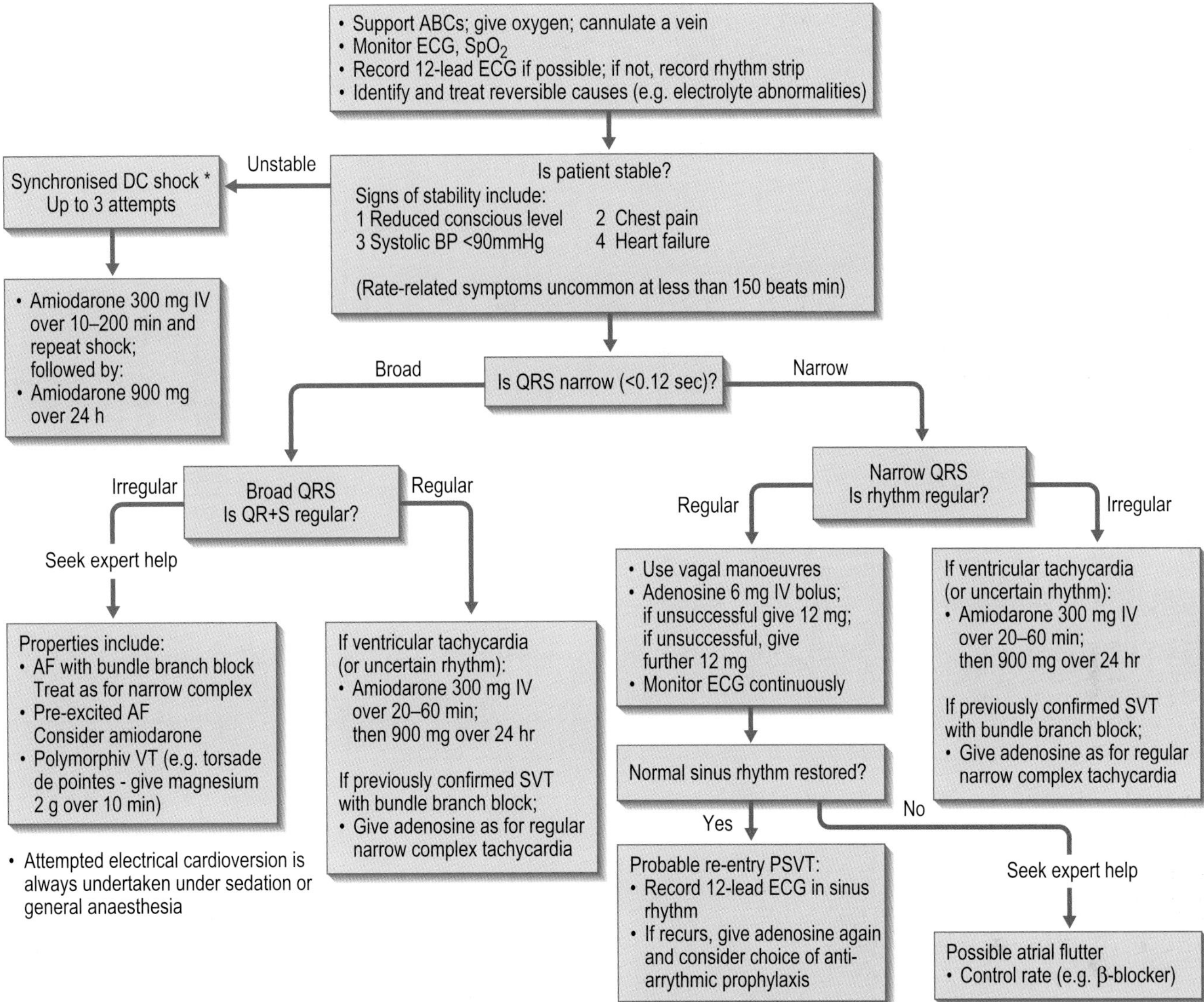

Figure 15-45 Tachycardia algorithm. From the Resuscitation Council (UK).

Clinical significance

Isolated premature atrial complexes in healthy patients are not significant but frequent premature atrial complexes that occur in patients with heart disease may lead to serious supraventricular dysrhythmias such as multifocal atrial tachycardia, atrial tachycardia, atrial flutter, atrial fibrillation or paroxysmal supraventricular tachycardia.

Management

Prehospital care usually only requires observation. If non-conducted premature atrial complexes are frequent and the patient becomes symptomatic from bradycardia, transcutaneous cardiac pacing or atropine may be indicated (Figure 15-39).

Supraventricular tachycardia and paroxysmal supraventricular tachycardia (re-entry SVT)

Description

Supraventricular tachycardias include paroxysmal re-entry SVT, non-paroxysmal atrial tachycardia, multifocal atrial tachycardia, junctional tachycardia, atrial flutter, and atrial fibrillation (Figure 15-45) and are collectively termed 'narrow complex tachycardias'. This section considers paroxysmal SVT, a SVT that begins abruptly, which is now more often termed re-entry SVT.

Note

Junctional tachycardia, ectopic atrial tachycardia, and multifocal atrial tachycardia are known as automatic supraventricular tachycardia.

Paroxysmal supraventricular tachycardia can originate in the atria or AV junction (Figure 15-46). Paroxysmal atrial tachycardia starts in the atria, whereas paroxysmal junctional tachycardia starts in the junction. The dysrhythmia results from rapid atrial or junctional impulse firing that overrides the rate of the SA node; the impulse re-enters the AV node at the same time that it is conducted to the ventricles (to produce the QRS complex). The cycle and the tachycardia

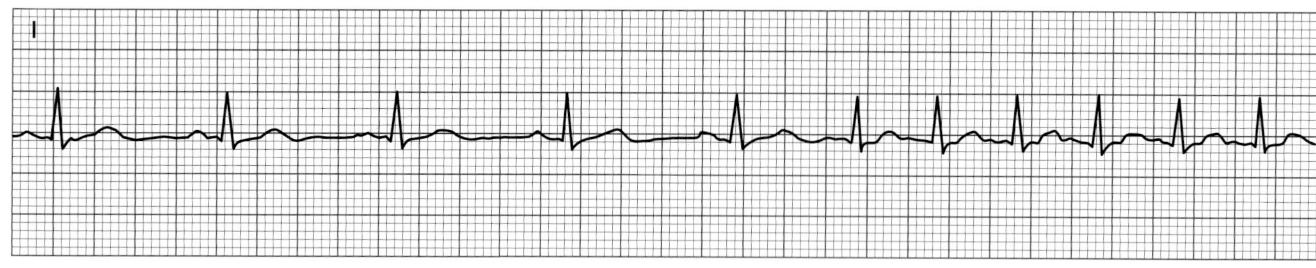

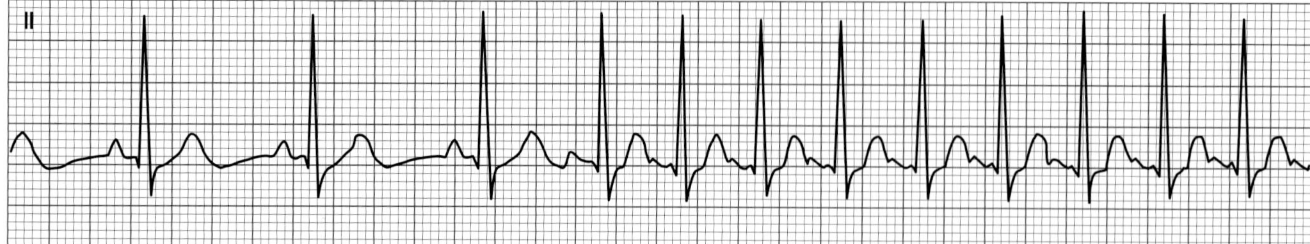

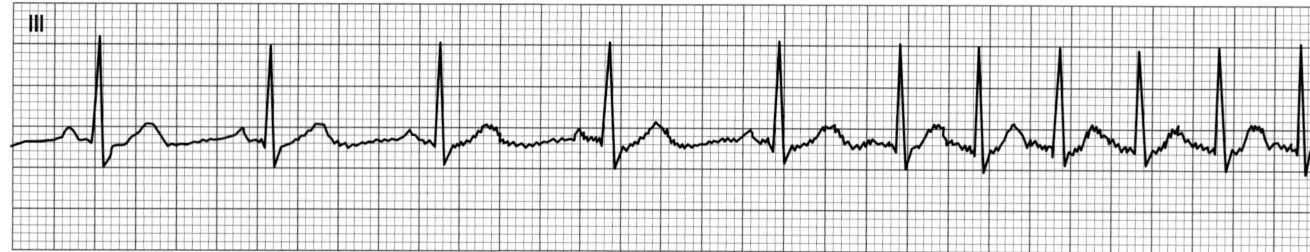

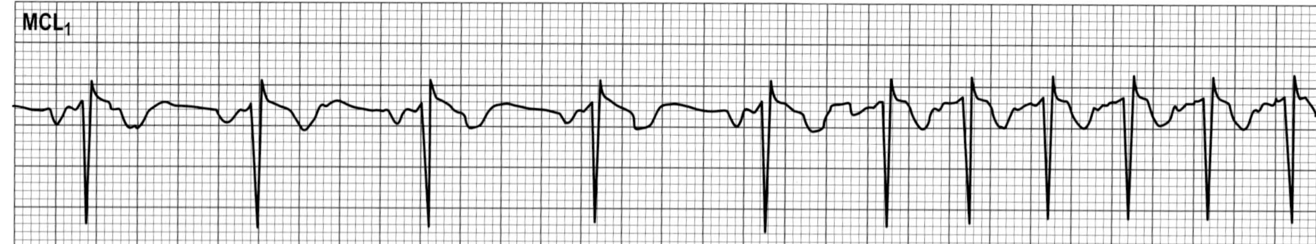

Figure 15-46 Paroxysmal supraventricular tachycardia.

continue until the re-entry pathway is interrupted. Paroxysmal SVT is characterized by repeated episodes (paroxysms) of atrial tachycardias; these episodes often have a sudden onset (lasting minutes to hours) as well as an abrupt termination as well.

Aetiology

In most cases, paroxysmal SVT is a re-entry tachycardia; the electrical impulses are caught in a cycle that continuously circulates around the AV node. Paroxysmal SVT may occur at any age, is not commonly associated with underlying heart disease and is rare in patients with myocardial infarction. Precipitating factors include stress, overexertion, tobacco use and caffeine consumption and common in patients who have Wolff–Parkinson–White syndrome.

Rules for interpretation (lead II monitoring)

Paroxysmal SVT has the following characteristics on the electrocardiogram:

QRS complex: Less than 0.12 s, provided no ventricular conduction disturbance is present.

P waves: The ectopic P waves differ from the normal sinus P waves. In lead II the P waves may be normal and upright if the pacemaker site is near the SA node but inverted if they originate near the AV junction. The P waves frequently are buried in preceding T or U waves or QRS complexes and therefore cannot be identified.

Rate: 150 to 250 beats per minute.

Rhythm: Regular except at onset and termination.

P-R interval: If P waves are discernible, the P-R interval often is shortened but may be normal or, rarely, prolonged.

Clinical significance

Paroxysmal SVT may occur in patients who have healthy hearts. Patients may tolerate it well for short periods although quite often the dysrhythmia is accompanied by palpitations, nervousness and anxiety. A rapid ventricular rate may prevent the ventricles from filling fully and can compromise cardiac output in patients with existing heart disease. Decreased perfusion may cause confusion, vertigo, light-headedness and syncope and may precipitate angina pectoris, hypotension or congestive heart failure. In addition, paroxysmal SVT increases the oxygen requirement of the heart; this may increase myocardial ischaemia and may increase the frequency and severity of the patient's chest pain.

Note

The distinctions among ventricular tachycardia, non-paroxysmal SVT, and paroxysmal SVT may be difficult to make. However, they are crucial. Two critical points to remember are these. First, if the patient displays serious signs and symptoms, particularly if the ventricular rate is greater than 150 beats per minute, the paramedic should prepare for immediate cardioversion, if permitted. Second, if the tachycardia complex appears wide, the paramedic should manage the rhythm as ventricular tachycardia; these two clinical rules should help manage the most difficult tachydysrhythmias.

Management

The paramedic should manage symptomatic paroxysmal SVT promptly, which will help to reverse the consequences of the reduced cardiac output and increased workload on the heart. If the patient is stable (conscious with normal blood pressure and without chest pain, congestive heart failure, or pulmonary oedema), the paramedic should attempt the following techniques to terminate paroxysmal SVT.

Vagal manoeuvres

Vagal manoeuvres slow the heart and decrease the force of atrial contraction by stimulating the vagus nerve and may be used to interrupt and end paroxysmal supraventricular tachycardia. The patient should be stable. Continuous electrocardiogram monitoring and an intravenous line must be in place before beginning these procedures. In addition, atropine and airway equipment should be readily available. Vagal manoeuvres carry some degree of risk (in the context of carotid sinus massage) and great care must be exercised if undertaking the technique.

Valsalva manoeuvre The paramedic should place the patient in a sitting or semisitting position with the head tilted down. The paramedic then instructs the patient to take in a deep breath and to bear down as if to have a bowel movement. The forced expiration against a closed glottis stimulates the vagus nerve and may terminate the tachycardia; the procedure may be repeated if unsuccessful. An adaptation is to take a 50 mL syringe with a bladder tip and encourage the patient to blow into it, to 'try to push the plunger out' (which they will not manage!); this will have the same effect.

Ice pack manoeuvre Placing an ice pack on the patient's anterior neck may stimulate the vagus nerve because of the mammalian diving reflex (see Chapter 23). In the paediatric patient, this technique is performed with a facecloth soaked in ice water. The facecloth is placed across the patient's face, about to nostril level. The paramedic should not attempt the ice pack manoeuvre if ischaemic heart disease is present or suspected; the procedure may be repeated if unsuccessful.

Unilateral carotid sinus pressure Whilst this procedure is described in JRCALC guidelines and contemporary texts it must be used with great caution. Carotid sinus pressure stimulates the carotid bodies located in the carotid arteries. The body interprets this localized pressure as an increase in blood pressure, which activates the autonomic nervous system and stimulates the vagus nerve. The heart rate slows in an attempt to lower blood pressure. The paramedic should auscultate the carotid arteries for the presence of a bruit (described in Chapter 9) before applying carotid sinus pressure. The paramedic should not apply carotid sinus pressure if bruits are present, if the patient is an older adult, or if the patient is known to have carotid artery disease or cerebral vascular disease. Possible complications from the procedure include cerebral emboli, stroke, syncope, sinus arrest, asystole and increased degree of AV block. The procedure for carotid sinus massage is as follows:

1. Position yourself behind the patient, who is lying supine with the neck extended and the head turned away from the side of the applied pressure.
2. Gently palpate each carotid artery to confirm the presence of equal pulses. If pulses are unequal, or if one is absent, do not apply carotid sinus pressure.
3. Auscultate (while the patient holds his or her breath for 4–5 s) for the presence of bruits.
4. To apply carotid sinus pressure, place the index and middle fingers over the artery on the neck just below the angle of the jaw. Compress the artery firmly against the vertebral column while massaging the area; inform the patient that he or she may experience some pain or discomfort. Maintain pressure no longer than 5–10 s and discontinue the massage immediately if bradycardia or signs of heart block develop or if the tachycardia breaks. Apply pressure to only one carotid sinus at a time; applying bilateral carotid sinus pressure may interfere with cerebral circulation.
5. Observe the electrocardiogram monitor and run a strip during the procedure and obtain a tracing. Repeat the procedure in 2–3 min if it is ineffective.

Critical Thinking

You perform carotid sinus massage on a patient with bruits or known carotid artery disease. What might occur?

Pharmacological therapy

If vagal manoeuvres fail or are contraindicated and the patient remains unstable, drugs that might be given for narrow complex tachycardias might include adenosine, verapamil, beta-blockers or digoxin, although these are not currently licensed for use by paramedics in the UK. Amiodarone is also indicated in symptomatic narrow complex tachycardia (RCUK, 2005) although it is not within the remit of JRCALC (2006) guidelines.

Whilst several drug treatments are available for narrow complex tachycardias (ventricular rate 150), serious signs and symptoms point to poor perfusion and instability from tachycardias, and synchronized electrical cardioversion is the treatment of choice. Cardioversion should commence with a synchronized shock of 120–150 J biphasic energy (200 J monophasic). If this fails, give two further shocks, increasing the energy up to the maximum the machine will permit (RCUK, 2005). Sedation should be considered before the cardioversion (if time permits).

Cardioversion encompasses vagal, pharmacological, and electrical therapy but in this context, the term is used to describe electrical cardioversion.

Critical Thinking

Why is the drug midazolam an ideal sedative before cardioversion?

Atrial flutter

Description

Atrial flutter is almost always a result of a rapid atrial re-entry focus (Figure 15-47). Atrial flutter not slowed by pre-existing AV block usually manifests a 2 : 1 AV conduction ratio; 50% of the atrial impulses are conducted through the ventricles and may look like supraventricular tachycardia. However, conduction ratios, which may be constant or variable, of 3 : 1, 4 : 1 and greater are not uncommon which produce a discrepancy between atrial and ventricular rates. Atrial flutter may be seen with atrial fibrillation (atrial fib-flutter). Rarely, atrial flutter may conduct 1 : 1 resulting in rapid ventricular rates that cause the patient to become unstable quickly.

Aetiology

Atrial flutter usually is seen in middle-aged and older patients who have heart disease. At times, atrial flutter also occurs in

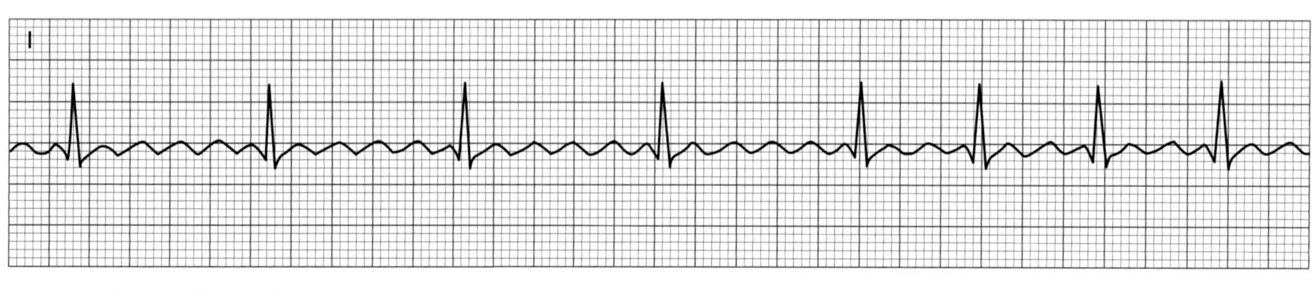

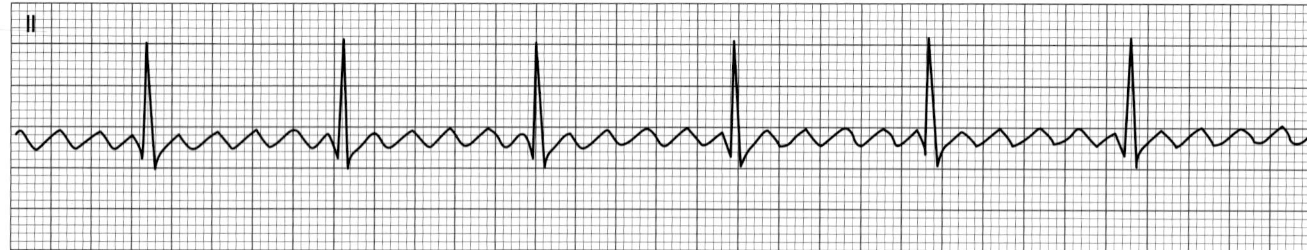

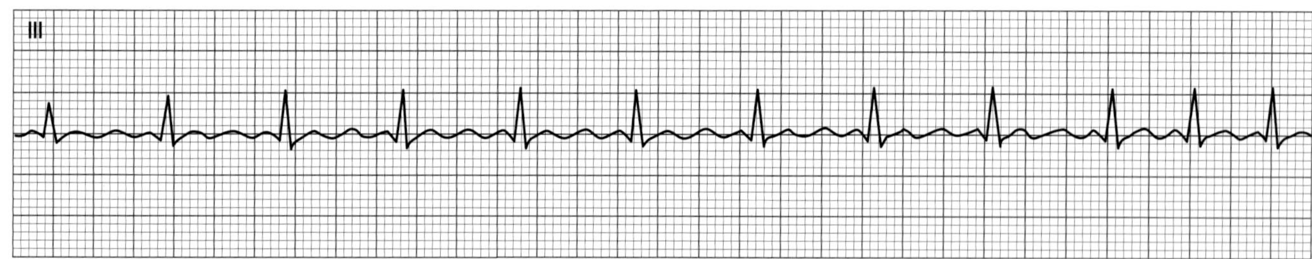

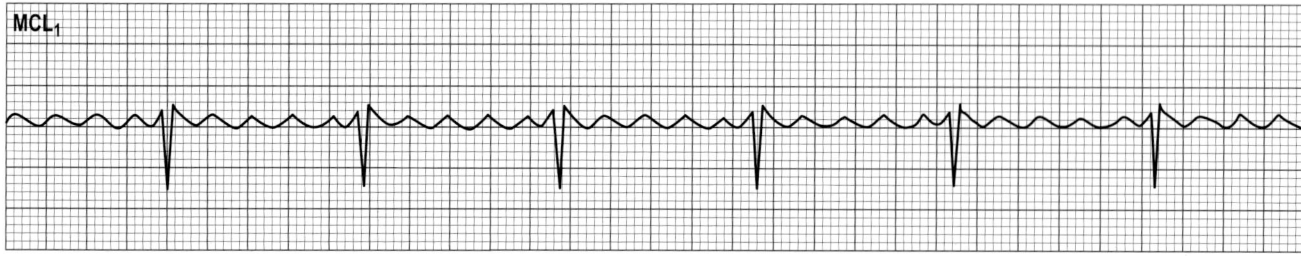

Figure 15-47 Atrial flutter.

patients who have healthy hearts. The dysrhythmia commonly is associated with the following:

- cardiomyopathy
- cardiac hypertrophy
- digitalis toxicity (rare)
- hypoxia
- congestive heart failure
- pericarditis
- myocarditis.

Rules for interpretation (lead II monitoring)

Atrial flutter has the following characteristics on the electrocardiogram:

QRS complex: Less than 0.12 s, unless ventricular conduction disturbance (aberrancy) is present.

P waves: Normal P waves are absent. The flutter waves (F waves) usually resemble a saw-tooth or picket fence pattern. The flutter waves represent atrial depolarization in an abnormal direction that is followed by atrial repolarization.

Flutter waves may be hard to identify when there is a 2 : 1 ratio of atrial to ventricular complexes. The paramedic should suspect 2 : 1 flutter when the rhythm is regular and the ventricular rate is 150 beats per minute.

Rate: The atrial rate is 250–300 beats per minute; the ventricular rate is regular but often is less than the atrial rate.

Rhythm: The atrial rhythm is regular; the ventricular rate is usually regular. However, the ventricular rate may be irregular if the AV conduction ratio varies.

P-R interval: Usually is constant but may vary.

Clinical significance

With a normal ventricular rate, atrial flutter usually is well tolerated by the patient. A rapid ventricular rate produces the same signs and symptoms of decreased cardiac output as seen in patients with atrial tachycardia. In addition, in some flutter rhythms (particularly a 2 : 1 atrial flutter), the atria do not contract regularly and empty before each ventricular contraction, leading to loss of the 'atrial kick' resulting in incomplete filling of the ventricles and possibly decreasing cardiac output further.

Note

The pulse rate of a patient with this dysrhythmia (and other tachycardias) might not be the same as the heart rate. This is because not all heart contractions produce enough output of blood to create a palpable pulse.

Atrial fibrillation

Description

Atrial fibrillation results from multiple areas of re-entry within the atria (Figure 15-48) or from ectopic atrial pacemakers; the activity of the SA node is suppressed completely by atrial fibrillation. Atrial fibrillation produces chaotic impulses too numerous for all to be conducted by the AV node through the ventricles. AV conduction is random, resulting in an irregular ventricular response, which is usually rapid unless the patient is taking medication (e.g. digoxin) to slow the ventricular rate.

Aetiology

Sudden onset (paroxysmal) atrial fibrillation may occur in young adults after heavy alcohol ingestion as well as a result of acute stress. It usually does not require treatment. Chronic atrial fibrillation may be intermittent and is often associated with rheumatic heart disease, congestive heart failure, and atherosclerotic heart disease. Chronic atrial fibrillation (found quite commonly in the older population) usually requires drug therapy with digitalis (or calcium channel blocker or beta-blocker) therapy, which slows the ventricular rate to 80–100 beats per minute. Atrial fibrillation may be a stable rhythm that does not require management. Less commonly, atrial fibrillation may occur in cardiomyopathy, acute myocarditis and pericarditis, and chest trauma and rarely is caused by digitalis toxicity. However, a slow, regular ventricular response with atrial fibrillation could be the result of digitalis toxicity. It is worth noting that due to the increased risk of atrial clot development and resultant emboli in the circulation, many patients with atrial fibrillation may be on anticoagulants such as warfarin.

Rules for interpretation (lead II monitoring)

Atrial fibrillation has the following characteristics on the electrocardiogram:

QRS complex: Less than 0.12 s, provided there is no ventricular conduction disturbance.

P waves: P waves and organized atrial contractions are absent. Fibrillation waves (f waves) may be fine (less than 1 mm) or coarse (greater than 1 mm). Fine f waves may be so small that they appear as a wavy or flat (isoelectric) line or absent. The f waves are irregularly shaped, rounded (or pointed), and dissimilar.

Rate: The atrial rate is 350–700 beats per minute (cannot be counted); the ventricular rate varies greatly, depending on conduction through the AV node (average 150–180 beats per minute, if uncontrolled).

Rhythm: Irregularly irregular.

P-R interval: None.

Note

Irregularly irregular rhythms are most likely to be atrial fibrillation.

Clinical significance

The atrial kick is lost in atrial fibrillation, reducing cardiac output by as much as 15%. This loss, coupled with a rapid ventricular response, may cause cardiovascular decompensation (angina pectoris, myocardial infarction, congestive heart failure, or cardiogenic shock).

Management of atrial fibrillation/atrial flutter

A risk of emboli formation exists when atrial fibrillation or atrial flutter has been present for more than 48 hours,

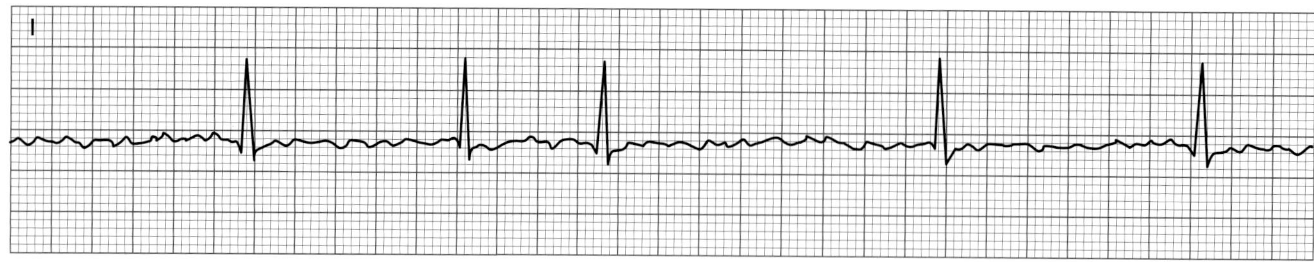

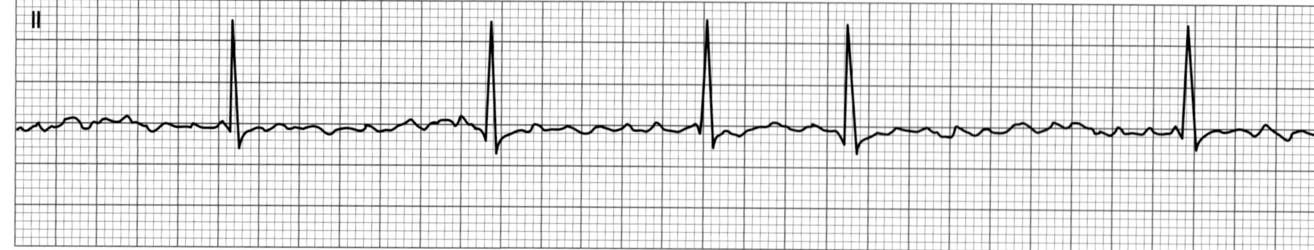

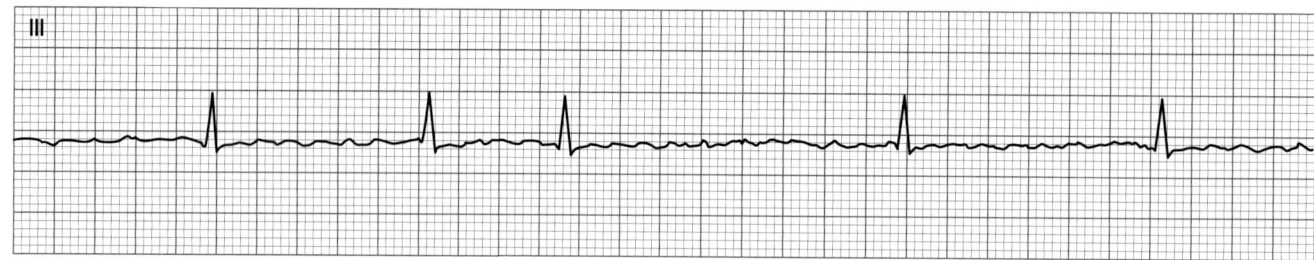

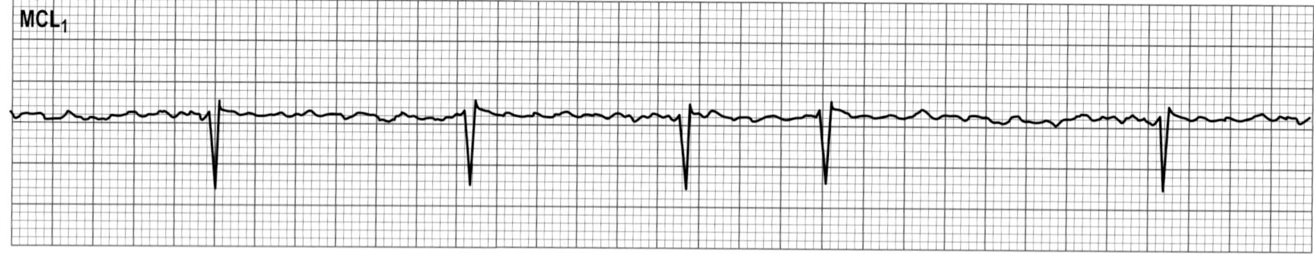

Figure 15-48 Atrial fibrillation.

increasing the risk of 'throwing a clot' or systemic embolization. This most often occurs when the atrial fibrillation is converted suddenly to a sinus rhythm. Electrical cardioversion and the use of antidysrhythmic agents that may convert the rhythm should be avoided unless the patient is unstable or haemodynamically compromised and converting atrial fibrillation or atrial flutter without first giving the patient drugs that prevent blood from clotting is not recommended.

Prehospital management of atrial fibrillation is usually supportive but more specialist in-hospital management may include the use of beta-blockers or digoxin (or amiodarone if a new onset less than 48 hours old).

The use of calcium channel blocking agents and beta-blocking agents warrants caution in the presence of congestive heart failure because of their negative inotropic properties. Beta-blocking agents also should be used with caution in patients with asthma and chronic obstructive pulmonary disease. Other drugs that may be effective to convert the rhythm are ibutilide or flecainide, which should only be used if the patient developed atrial fibrillation within the previous 48 hours or less.

Critical Thinking

What signs or symptoms would make you think these patients are unstable?

Dysrhythmias sustained or originating in the AV junction

When the SA node and the atria cannot generate the electrical impulses needed to begin depolarization because of factors such as hypoxia, ischaemia, myocardial infarction and drug toxicity, the AV node or the area surrounding the AV node may assume the role of the secondary pacemaker.

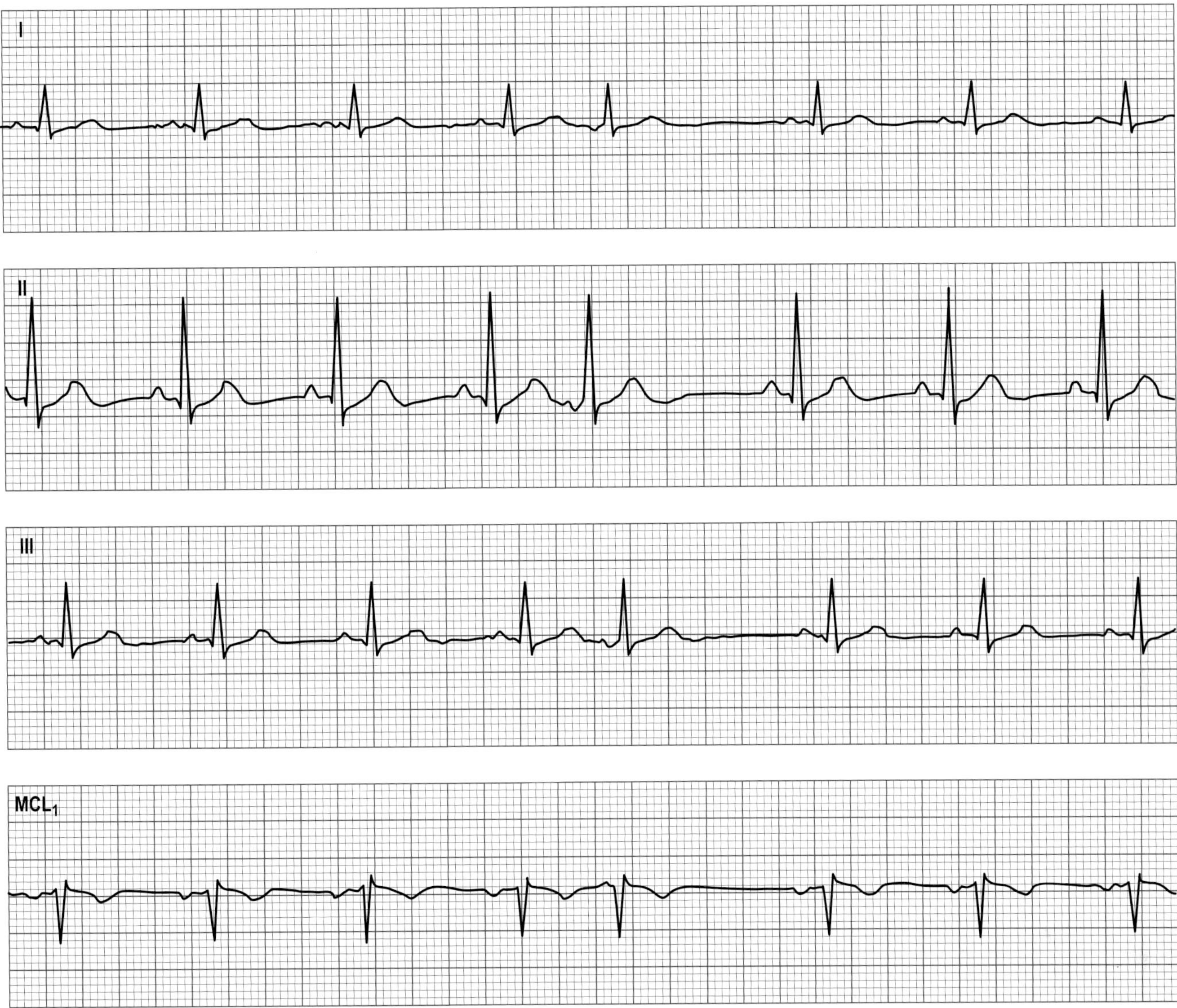

Figure 15-49 Premature junctional contractions.

Rhythms that start in the AV node or AV junctional area are junctional rhythms. This type of rhythm usually is a benign dysrhythmia yet the paramedic must assess the rhythm to determine the patient's tolerance of the rhythm disturbance. Dysrhythmias that originate in the AV junction include premature junctional contractions, junctional escape complexes or junctional escape rhythms, and accelerated junctional rhythm.

In junctional rhythms, electrical impulses travel in a normal pathway from the AV junction through the bundle of His and bundle branches to the Purkinje fibres. The pathway ends in the ventricular muscle. Conduction through the ventricles proceeds normally and the QRS complex is usually within normal limits of 0.04–0.12 s. However, the impulse that depolarizes the atria travels in a backward or retrograde motion which results in one of the following three P wave characteristics: (1) inverted P waves in lead II with a short P-R interval, (2) absent P waves, or (3) retrograde P waves.

Premature junctional contraction

Description

A premature junctional contraction results from a single electrical impulse from the AV junction (Figure 15-49); the impulse occurs before the next expected sinus impulse.

Aetiology

Isolated premature junctional contractions may occur in a healthy person without apparent cause but more often are a result of heart disease or drug toxicity and usually result from enhanced automaticity or a re-entry mechanism. Premature junctional contractions have several causes:

- digitalis toxicity
- other cardiac medications (quinidine, procainamide)
- increased vagal tone on the SA node
- sympathomimetic drugs (e.g. cocaine and methamphetamines)

- hypoxia
- congestive heart failure
- damage to the AV junction.

Critical Thinking

Will the P wave be visible if it occurs during the QRS wave? Why?

Rules for interpretation (lead II monitoring)

Premature junctional contractions have the following characteristics on the electrocardiogram:

QRS complex: Usually less than 0.12 s, provided there is no ventricular conduction disturbance.

P waves: May be associated with premature junctional contractions. P waves can occur before, during, or after the QRS complex or can be absent. If present, P waves are abnormal, differing in size, shape, and direction from normal P waves.

Rate: The heart rate is that of the underlying rhythm.

Rhythm: Usually regular, except when premature junctional contractions are present.

P-R interval: Usually less than 0.12 s if the P wave precedes the QRS complex.

Clinical significance

Occasional premature junctional contractions usually are not significant.

Management

No management is required.

Junctional escape complexes or rhythms

Description

A junctional escape beat or rhythm (series of beats) occurs when the rate of the SA node falls below that of the AV junction (Figure 15-50) and may also occur when the electrical impulses from the SA node or atria fail to reach the

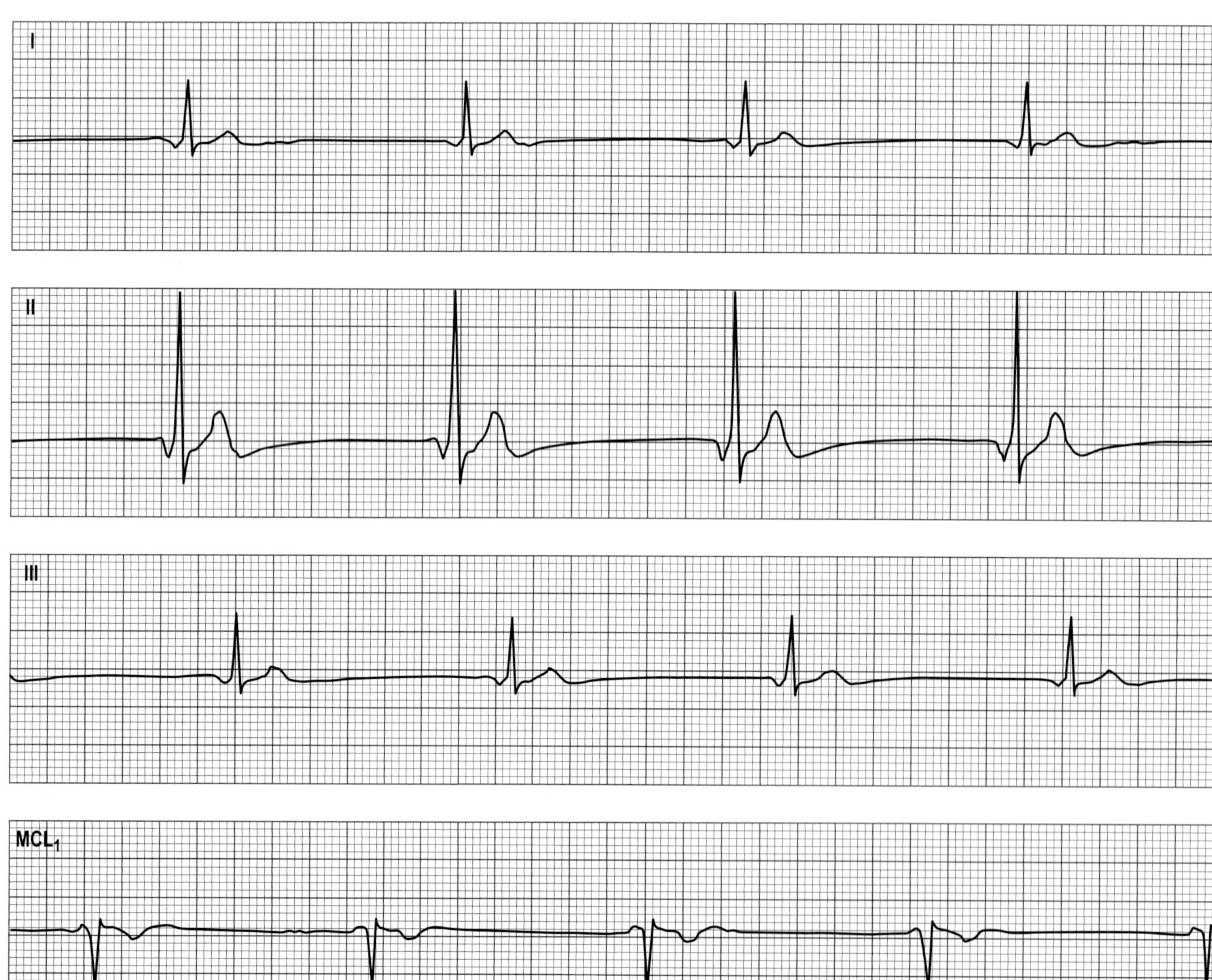

Figure 15-50 Junctional escape complex or rhythm.

AV junction because of SA or AV block. The escape complex or rhythm provided by the AV junction serves as a safety mechanism, which prevents cardiac standstill. The AV junction begins firing at an inherent rate of 40–60 beats per minute within about 1.0–1.5 s of not receiving an impulse from the SA node.

Aetiology

A junctional escape complex or a junctional escape rhythm is a normal response and may result from an increased vagal tone on the SA node, a pathological slowing of the SA discharge, or a complete AV block.

Rules for interpretation (lead II monitoring)

Junctional escape complexes or rhythms have the following characteristics on the electrocardiogram:

QRS complex: Usually less than 0.12 s, provided no pre-existing bundle branch block is present.

P waves: May be present (with or without relationship to QRS complex) or absent. If P waves are present, they may occur before, after, or during the QRS complex. Depending on the pacemaker site, P waves may differ from normal P waves in size, shape and direction and may be upright or inverted.

Rate: Usually 40–60 beats per minute but may be less.

Rhythm: The ventricular rhythm usually is regular in junctional rhythm; it may be irregular if an isolated junctional escape complex is present.

P-R interval: If P waves precede the QRS complex, the P-R interval commonly is shortened (less than 0.12 s) and constant.

Clinical significance

Junctional escape rhythms can cause decreased cardiac output causing signs and symptoms that are similar to those of other bradycardias, such as light-headedness, hypotension, and syncope. As a rule, patients tolerate junctional rhythms of 50 beats per minute or greater.

Management

Patients who are stable do not need to be treated. If the patient is symptomatic or if ventricular irritability is present, drug therapy (beginning with atropine) may be indicated. In severe cases and in patients unresponsive to atropine, external pacing may be necessary. If the SA node is diseased or damaged, the patient may need a permanent pacemaker once admitted to hospital (see Figure 15-39).

Accelerated junctional rhythm

Description

Accelerated junctional rhythm results from increased automaticity of the AV junction (Figure 15-51) causing it to discharge faster than its intrinsic rate of 40–60 beats per minute which in turn overrides the main (SA node) pacemaker. The rate of this dysrhythmia (usually 60–99 beats per minute) does not truly constitute a tachycardia and the dysrhythmia is termed accelerated junctional rhythm. In this text, rapid junctional rhythms equal to or greater than 100 beats per minute (junctional tachycardia) and caused by a re-entry mechanism are discussed with other supraventricular tachycardias.

Aetiology

An accelerated junctional rhythm is commonly a result of digitalis toxicity, with other possible causes including excessive catecholamine administration, damage to the AV junction, inferior wall myocardial infarction (described later in this chapter), and rheumatic fever.

Rules for interpretation (lead II monitoring)

Accelerated junctional rhythm has the following characteristics on the electrocardiogram:

QRS complex: Usually is less than 0.12 s, provided there is no pre-existing bundle branch block.

P waves: May be present (with or without relationship to the QRS complex), absent (retrograde AV block), or buried in the QRS complex. If present, P waves usually are inverted and appear before or after the QRS complex.

Rate: Usually 60–99 beats per minute.

Rhythm: Regular.

P-R interval: If the P wave occurs before the QRS complex, the P-R interval will be less than 0.12 s. If the P wave follows the QRS complex, it technically is an R-P interval and usually is less than 0.20 s.

Clinical significance

Accelerated junctional rhythm usually is well tolerated by the patient but the presence of heart disease and lack of oxygen to the heart muscle may cause more serious dysrhythmias.

Management

Accelerated junctional rhythm generally requires no immediate treatment.

Critical Thinking

Do you need to start an intravenous line on these patients, since no drug therapy is indicated?

Dysrhythmias originating in the ventricles

Ventricular dysrhythmias usually are considered a threat to life. Ventricular rhythm disturbances generally result from failure of the atria and/or AV junction to initiate an electrical impulse as well as resulting from enhanced automaticity or re-entry pathways in the ventricles. Enhanced automaticity and re-entry can lead to premature ventricular complexes, ventricular tachycardia, and even ventricular fibrillation which are often are associated with myocardial ischaemia or infarction. The ventricle is the least efficient pacemaker of the heart, normally generating only 20 to 40 impulses per minute but may discharge at rates up to 99 impulses per minute (accelerated idioventricular rhythm) or even faster (ventricular tachycardia) because of increased automaticity. Dysrhythmias originating in the ventricles include ventricu-

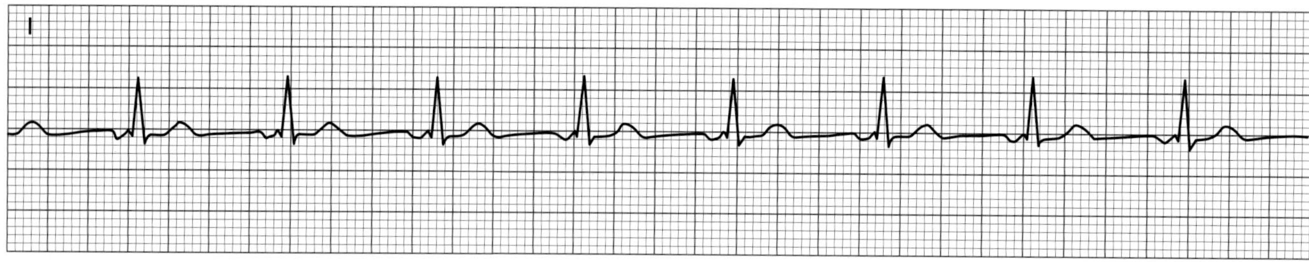

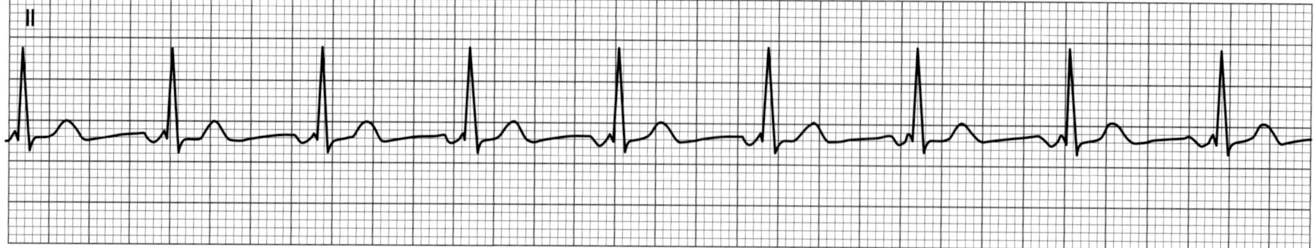

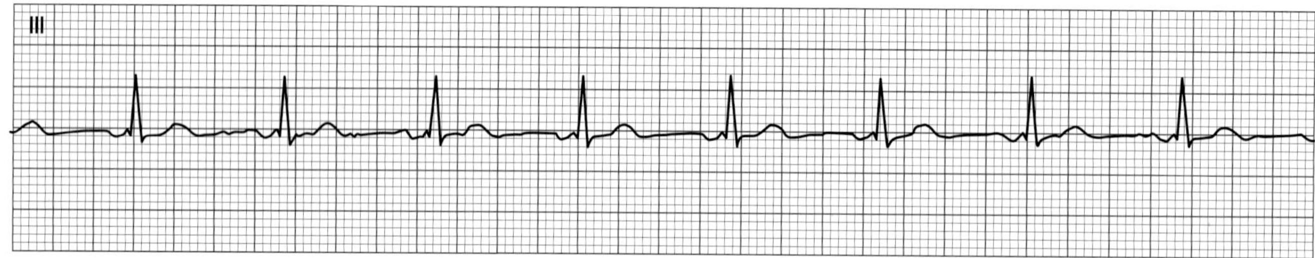

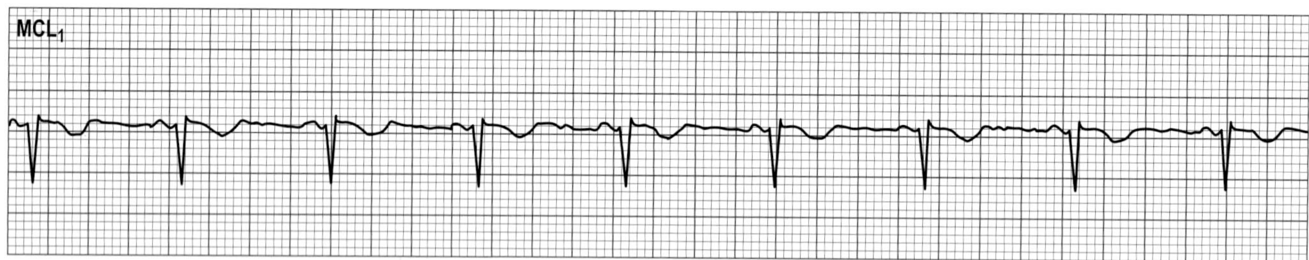

Figure 15-51 Accelerated junctional rhythm.

lar escape complexes or rhythms, premature ventricular complexes, ventricular tachycardia, ventricular fibrillation, asystole, and artificial pacemaker rhythm.

Because electrical impulses of ventricular origin start in the lower portion of the heart (the ventricular muscle, bundle branches or Purkinje fibres), the electrical impulse must travel in a retrograde conduction pathway to depolarize the atria, but, depending on site of initiation, may travel in an antegrade direction to depolarize the ventricles. Regardless of the direction of depolarization, the normal, rapid conducting pathways are bypassed, producing the following three electrocardiogram features:

1. QRS complexes are wide and bizarre in appearance. They are 0.12 s or greater in duration.
2. P waves may be hidden in the QRS complex (due to the atria being depolarized at about the same time as the ventricles) or they may be superimposed on every second or third QRS complex when ventricular tachycardia with AV dissociation (P waves that have no set relation to the QRS complexes) is present.
3. ST segments usually deviate from baseline. T waves frequently are sloped off in the opposite direction of the QRS complex.

Ventricular escape complexes or rhythms

Description

A ventricular escape complex (isolated impulse) or rhythm (series of complexes) is also known as idioventricular rhythm (Figures 15-52 and 15-53). The dysrhythmia results when impulses from higher pacemakers fail to fire or to reach the ventricles or when the rate of discharge of higher pacemaker sites falls to less than that of the ventricles. Like the junctional escape complex or rhythm, this dysrhythmia serves as a compensatory mechanism to prevent cardiac standstill.

Aetiology

Ventricular escape rhythms occur in two ways. First, the rate of impulse formation of the dominant pacemaker

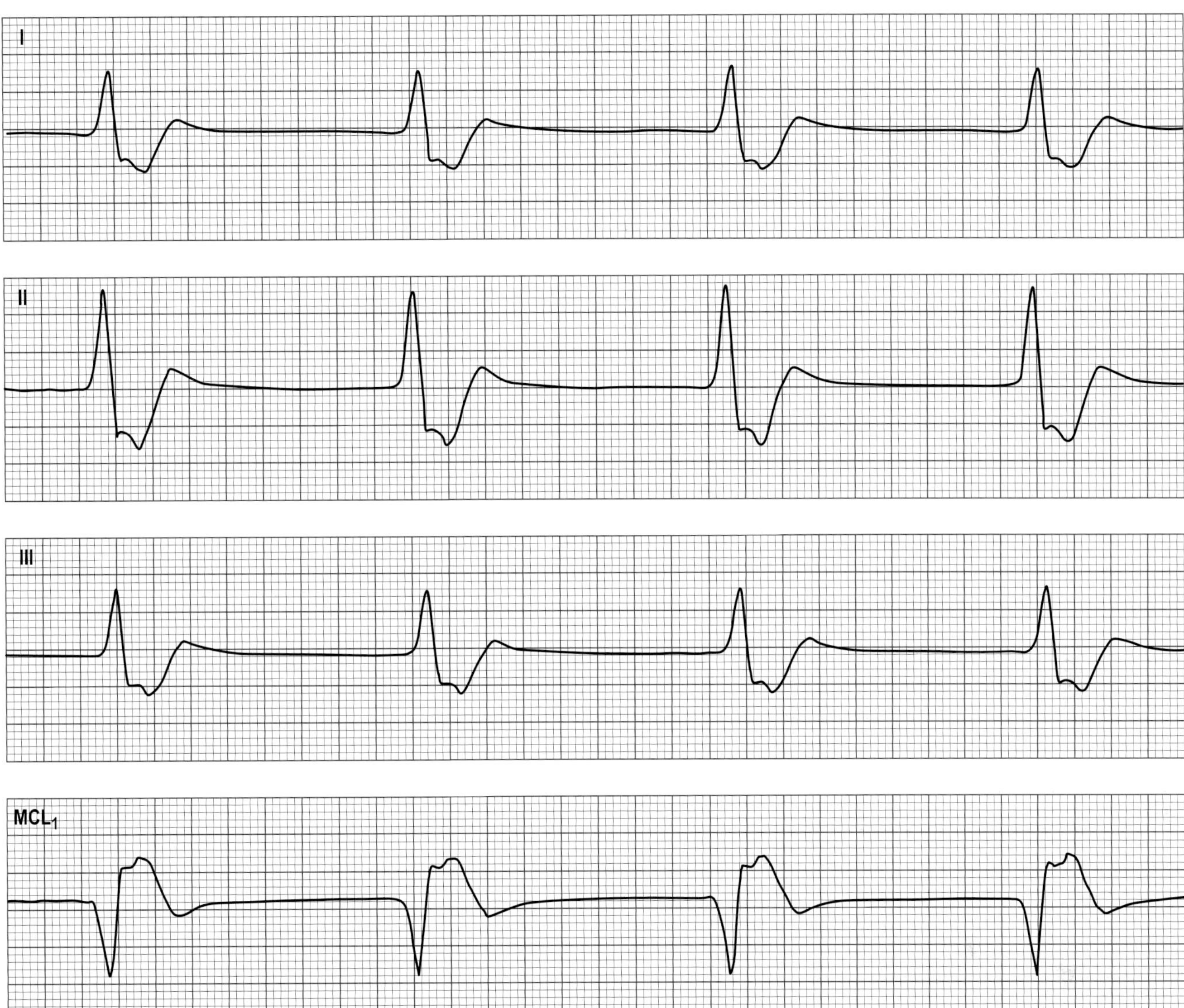

Figure 15-52 Ventricular escape rhythm.

(usually the SA node) can fall below that of the ventricles. Second, the escape pacemaker in the AV junction can fail or fall below that of the pacemaker in the ventricles. This dysrhythmia often is seen as the first rhythm after defibrillation.

Rules for interpretation (lead II monitoring)

Ventricular escape complexes or rhythms have the following characteristics on the electrocardiogram:

QRS complex: Generally exceed 0.12 s and are bizarre in appearance. The shape of the QRS complex may vary in any given lead.

P waves: May be absent. If they are present and have no set relationship to the QRS complex, then a third-degree AV block should be suspected.

Rate: Usually 20–40 beats per minute; may be lower.

Rhythm: The ventricular rhythm usually is regular but may be irregular.

P-R interval: If P waves are present, the P-R interval is variable and irregular.

Clinical significance

A ventricular escape rhythm generally produces symptoms such as hypotension, decreased cardiac output, and decreased perfusion of the brain and other vital organs, often resulting in syncope and shock. Patient assessment is essential because the escape rhythm may be perfusing or non-perfusing (pulseless electrical activity).

Management

If the rhythm is perfusing, management must be directed at increasing the heart rate by administering oxygen, with transcutaneous cardiac pacing and drug therapy being other options in a hospital setting. Managing the escape rhythm with lidocaine is contraindicated. If the rhythm is non-perfusing, the paramedic should initiate basic life support measures and follow advanced life support guidelines for cardiac arrest (Figure 15-54).

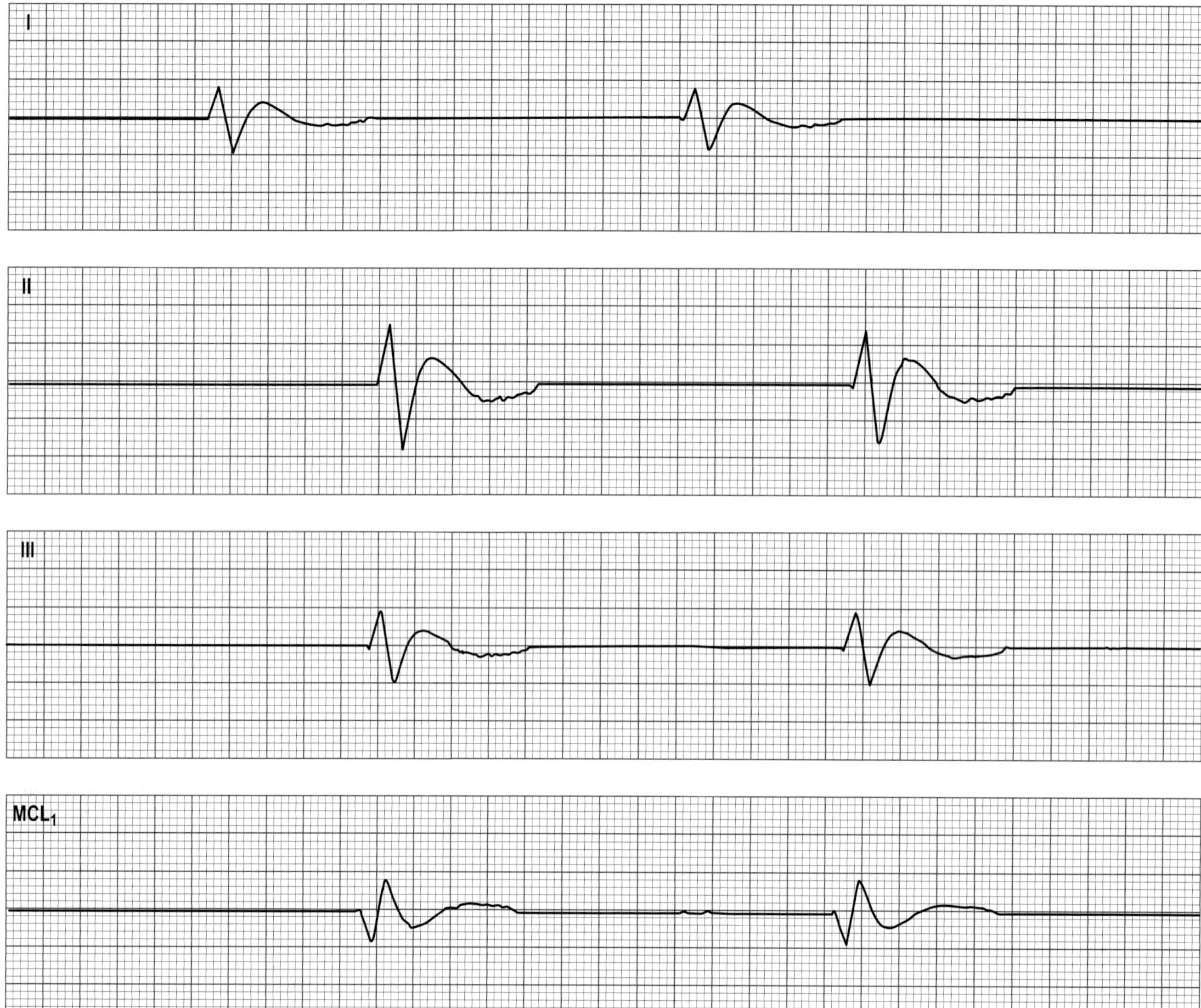

Figure 15-53 'Dying heart' or agonal rhythm.

> **Critical Thinking**
>
> Why might lidocaine be harmful in this situation?

Premature ventricular complex

Description

A premature ventricular complex is a single ectopic impulse arising from an irritable focus in either ventricle (bundle branches, Purkinje fibres or ventricular muscle) that occurs earlier than the next expected sinus beat (Figure 15-55). This dysrhythmia is common and can occur with any underlying cardiac rhythm as a result of enhanced automaticity or a re-entry mechanism.

When the ventricles initiate a premature ventricular complex, the atria may or may not respond and depolarize. If atrial depolarization does not occur, a P wave is seen on the electrocardiogram. If atrial depolarization does occur, the P wave occurs but often is hidden in the QRS complex. The reason for this is the timing and large electrical force of ventricular depolarization blocking out the electrical activity from the atrial depolarization. The altered sequence of ventricular depolarization results in a wide, bizarre QRS complex. Depolarization may be deflected in the opposite direction from the QRS complex in the underlying rhythm or it may be deflected in the same direction, depending on the location of the focus and the lead selected. The T wave that immediately follows the premature ventricular complex usually is deflected in the opposite direction from the QRS complex of the premature ventricular complex because of the altered sequence of repolarization.

Why is the QRS deflection opposite the underlying rhythm?

A premature ventricular complex does not usually depolarize the SA node or interrupt its rhythm; the P wave of the underlying rhythm that follows the premature ventricular

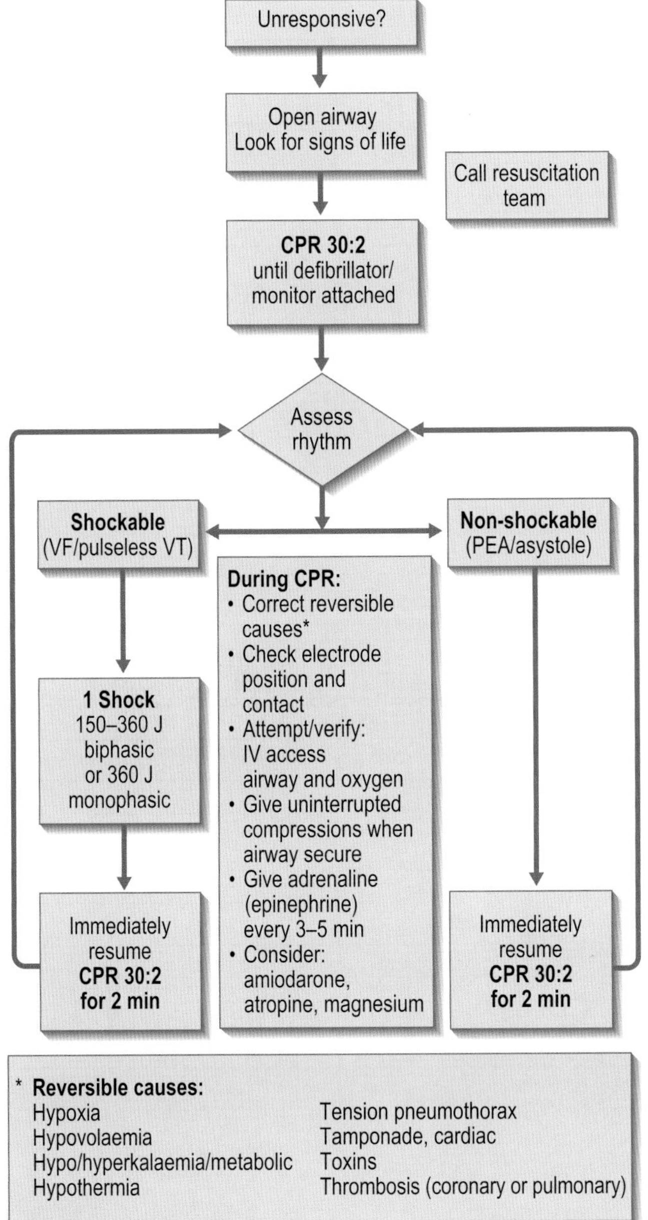

Figure 15-54 ACLS pulseless arrest algorithm. From The Resuscitation Council UK.

complex occurs at its expected time but is obstructed by the premature ventricular complex and finds the ventricles refractory. Therefore, the ectopic impulse usually is followed by a full compensatory pause. Compensatory pauses are confirmed by measuring the interval between the R wave before the premature ventricular complex and the R wave after it. If the pause is compensatory, the distance is at least twice the R-R interval of the underlying rhythm. At times, a premature ventricular complex falls between two sinus beats without interrupting the rhythm and is called an interpolated premature ventricular complex (Figure 15-56).

Premature ventricular complexes may originate from a single ectopic pacemaker site (unifocal premature ventricular complexes) or from multiple sites in the ventricles (multifocal premature ventricular complexes) (Figure 15-57). Unifocal premature ventricular complexes look alike, whilst multifocal premature ventricular complexes have varying shapes and sizes.

Multifocal premature ventricular complexes are thought of as more dangerous than unifocal premature ventricular complexes, as they usually result from increased myocardial irritability. A premature ventricular complex that occurs at about the same time as ventricular activation by a normal impulse can cause ventricular depolarization to occur at the same time; this fusion beat results in a QRS complex that has the characteristics of a premature ventricular complex and the QRS complex of the underlying rhythm (Figure 15-58). Fusion beats confirm that the ectopic impulse is located in the ventricle rather than the atria.

Frequently, premature ventricular complexes occur in patterns of grouped beating. Ventricular bigeminy occurs when every other complex is a premature ventricular complex, ventricular trigeminy occurs when every third complex is a premature ventricular complex, and quadrigeminy occurs when every fourth complex is a premature ventricular complex (Figure 15-59). Consecutive premature ventricular complexes that are not separated by a complex of the underlying rhythm also can occur on the electrocardiogram: couplets, or salvos, are two premature ventricular complexes in a row, and triplets are three premature ventricular complexes in a row (a definition for ventricular tachycardia). These terms may also be used to describe patterns of premature atrial complexes and premature junctional contractions.

Like multifocal premature ventricular complexes, frequently occurring premature ventricular complexes usually indicate that the ventricles are highly irritable which can trigger life-threatening dysrhythmias such as ventricular tachycardia and ventricular fibrillation. This is especially the case if they occur during the T wave (relative refractory phase) of the cardiac cycle, as during this period the heart muscle is at its greatest electrical instability.

During this period, some of the ventricular muscle fibres may be repolarized partially, with others repolarized completely and still others being completely refractory. Stimulation of the ventricles in the vulnerable period by an electrical impulse such as a premature ventricular complex, cardiac pacemaker, or cardioversion may cause ventricular fibrillation or ventricular tachycardia. The occurrence of a ventricular depolarization during the relative refractory period is known as the R-on-T phenomenon (Figure 15-60).

Aetiology

Isolated premature ventricular complexes do occur in healthy persons without apparent cause and usually are of no significance. Pathological premature ventricular complexes usually are a result of one or more of the following:

- myocardial ischaemia
- hypoxia
- acid–base and electrolyte imbalance
- hypokalaemia
- congestive heart failure
- increased catecholamine and sympathetic tone (as in emotional stress)
- ingestion of stimulants (alcohol, caffeine, tobacco)
- drug toxicity

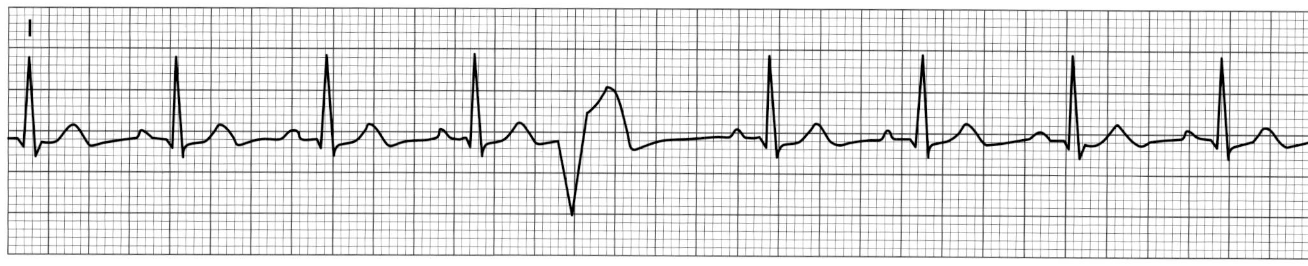

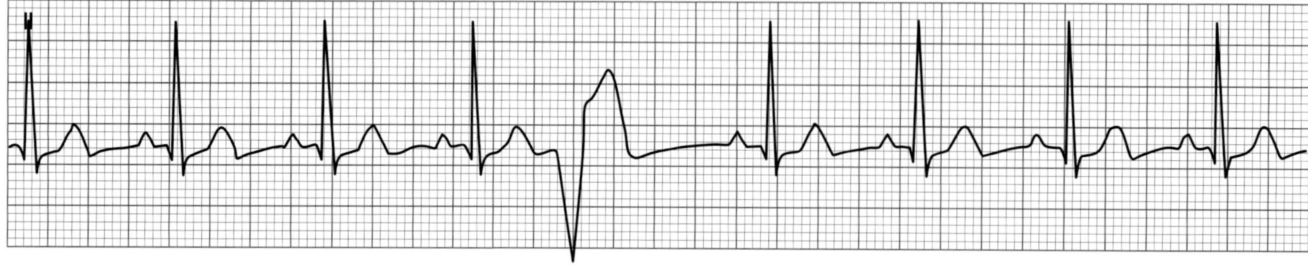

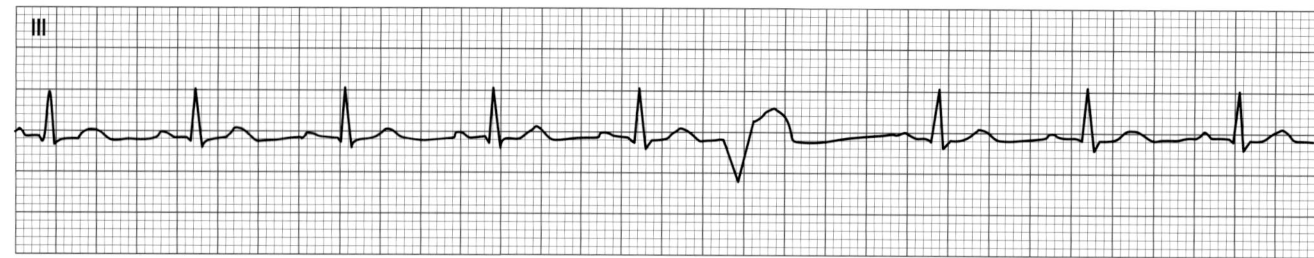

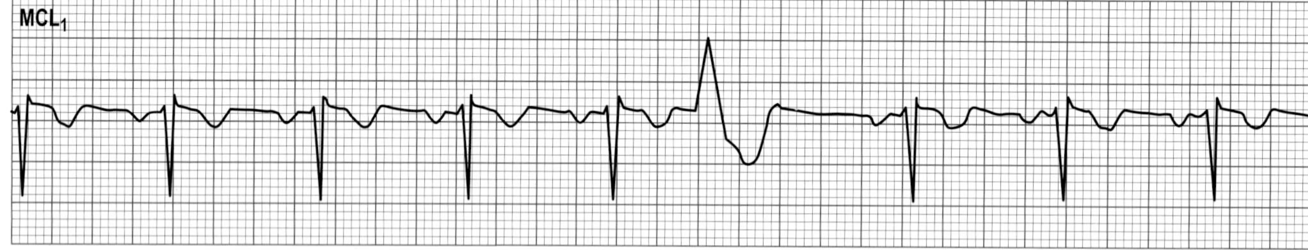

Figure 15-55 Premature ventricular complexes.

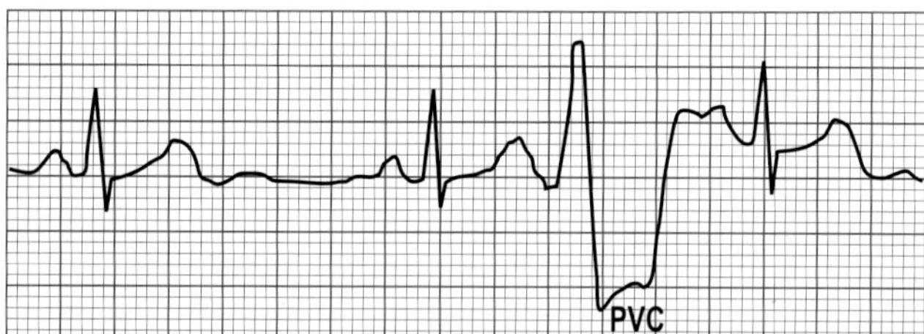

Figure 15-56 Interpolated premature ventricular complex.

- sympathomimetic drugs (cocaine; stimulants such as phencyclidine and adrenaline [epinephrine]).

Rules for interpretation (lead II monitoring)

Premature ventricular complexes have the following characteristics on the electrocardiogram:

QRS complex: Equal to or greater than 0.12 s; frequently distorted and bizarre.

P waves: May be present or absent. If they are present, they usually are of the underlying rhythm and have no relationship to the premature ventricular complex.

Rate: Depends on the underlying rhythm and the number of premature ventricular complexes.

Rhythm: Premature ventricular complexes interrupt the regularity of the underlying rhythm.

P-R interval: None.

Clinical significance

Premature ventricular complexes that occur in patients without heart disease do not usually produce serious signs and symptoms, although these patients may complain of skipped beats. Premature ventricular complexes that occur with heart disease (myocardial ischaemia) may result from enhanced automaticity, a re-entry mechanism, or both and may trigger lethal ventricular dysrhythmias. Premature ventricular complexes do not permit complete ventricular filling and may produce a diminished or non-palpable pulse (non-perfusing premature ventricular complex). If the pre-

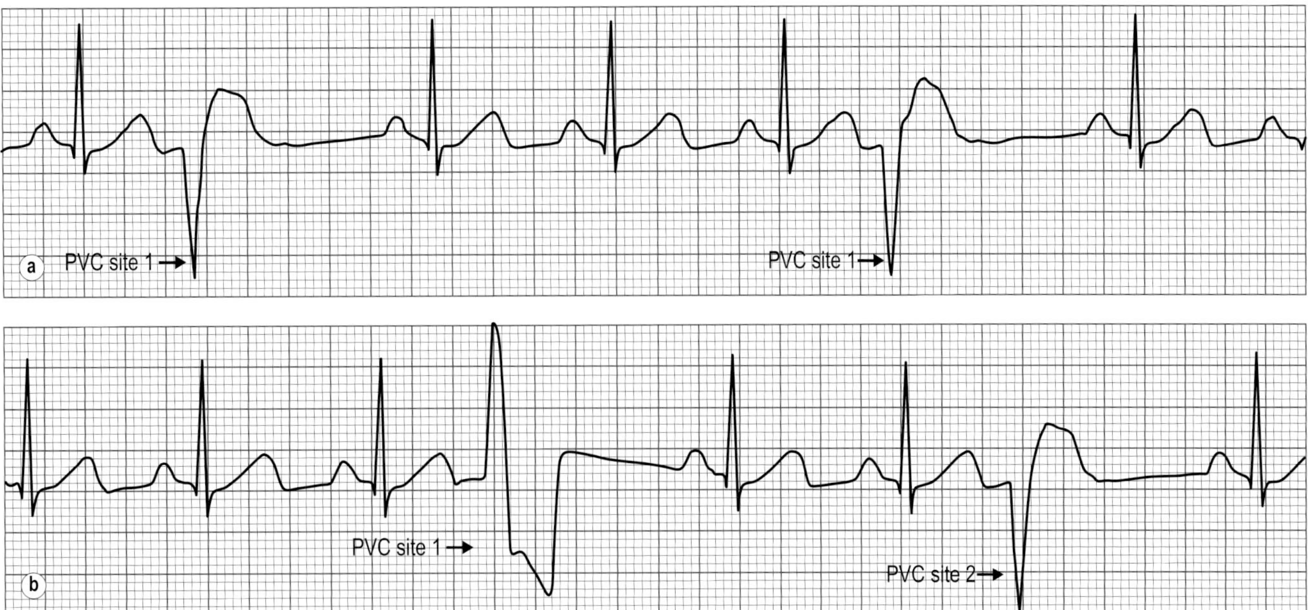

Figure 15-57 (a) Unifocal premature ventricular complexes. (b) Multifocal premature ventricular complexes.

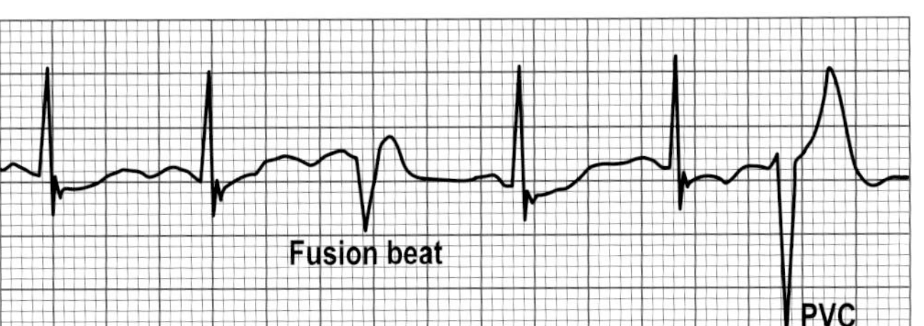

Figure 15-58 Fusion beat with premature ventricular complex.

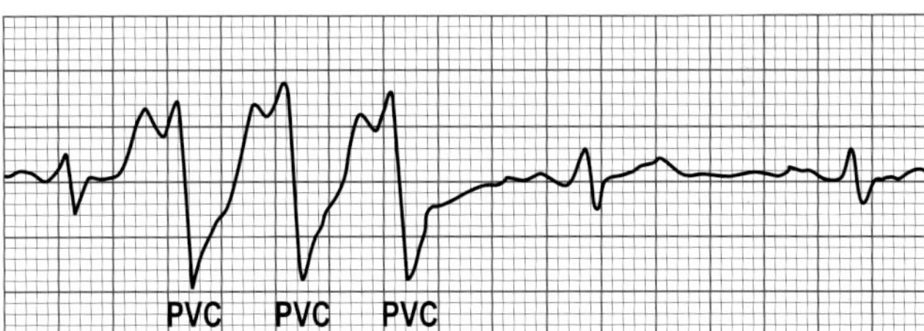

Figure 15-60 R-on-T phenomenon (unifocal premature ventricular complexes).

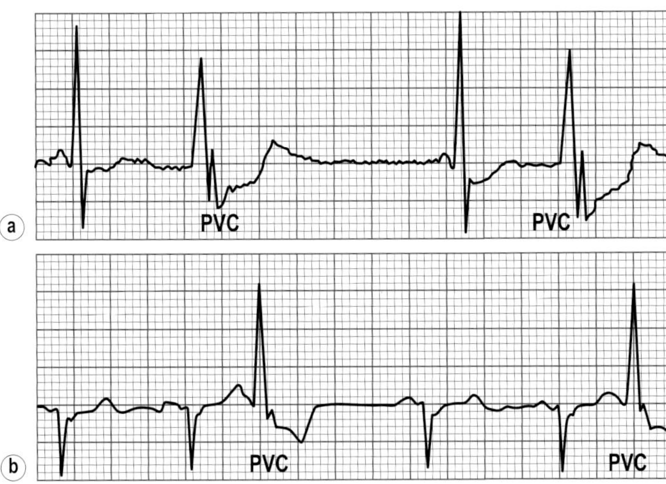

Figure 15-59 (a) Bigeminy (unifocal premature ventricular complexes). (b) Trigeminy (unifocal premature ventricular complexes).

mature ventricular complexes occur often and early enough in the cardiac cycle, cardiac output drops.

Warning signs of serious ventricular dysrhythmias in patients with myocardial ischaemia include frequent premature ventricular complexes, the presence of multifocal premature ventricular complexes, early premature ventricular complexes (R-on-T phenomenon), and patterns of grouped beating.

Management

Premature ventricular complexes that occur in patients without symptoms and without known heart disease seldom require treatment, but in patients with myocardial ischaemia, frequent premature ventricular complexes must be treated promptly with oxygen. In hospital, antidysrhythmic drugs (e.g. beta-blockers) may be given and serum potassium will be checked with any hypokalaemia being treated promptly.

> **Critical Thinking**
>
> Consider this situation. A lidocaine drip is not regulated properly and infuses too rapidly. What signs and symptoms might the patient develop?

Ventricular tachycardia

Description

Ventricular tachycardia is a dysrhythmia defined by three or more consecutive ventricular complexes occurring at a rate of more than 100 beats per minute (Figure 15-61). The origin of ventricular tachycardia is enhanced automaticity or re-entry; this dysrhythmia starts suddenly, is triggered by a premature ventricular complex and overrides the primary

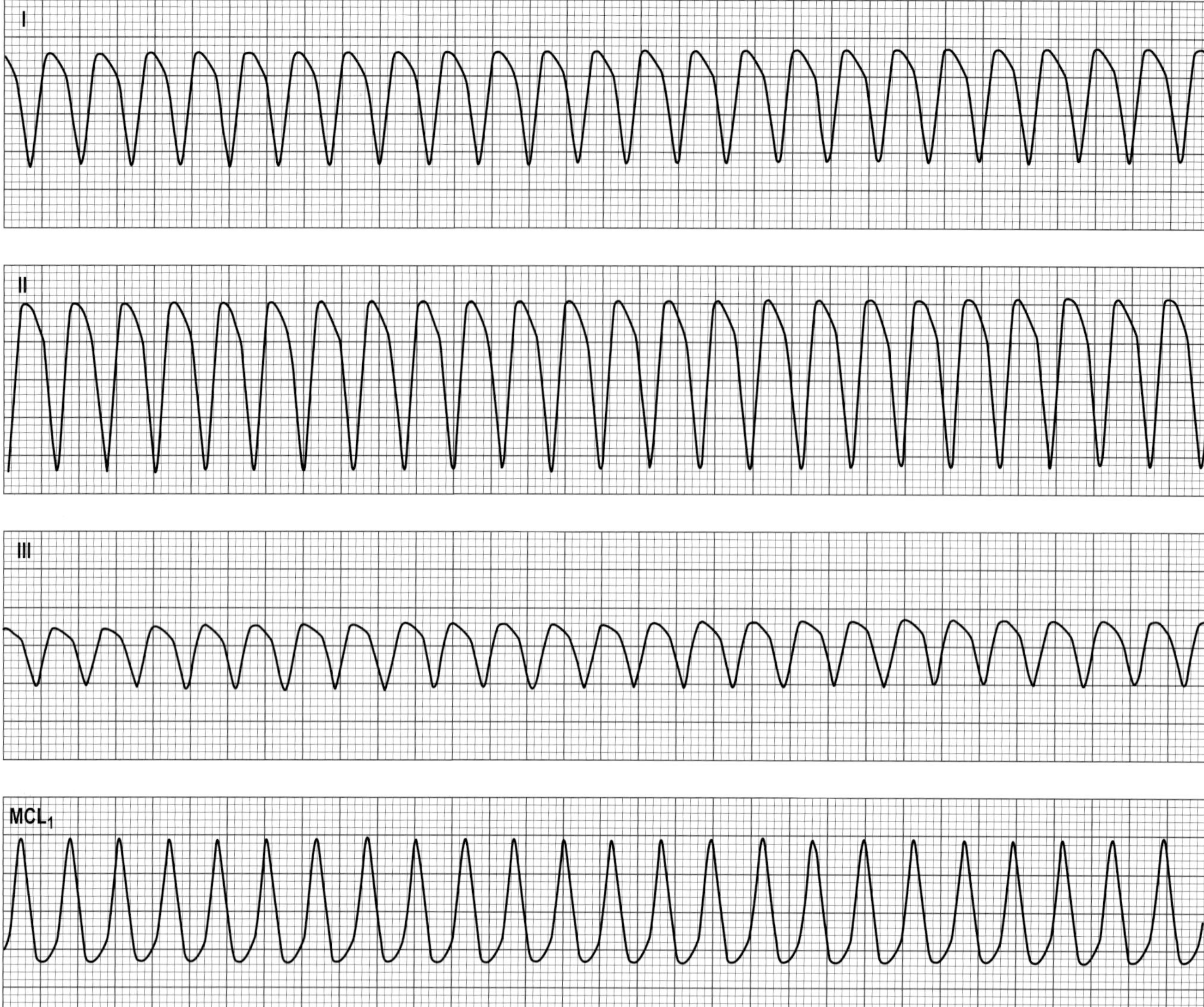

Figure 15-61 Ventricular tachycardia.

pacemaker. During ventricular tachycardia, the atria and ventricles do not beat in step with each other. If ventricular tachycardia continues, the patient's condition may become compromised, causing altered levels of consciousness and loss of perfusing pulses. However, some patients in ventricular tachycardia may be uncompromised and the misconception that ventricular tachycardia cannot be associated with adequate blood pressure may result in a patient being inappropriately managed.

Aetiology

Like premature ventricular complexes, ventricular tachycardia usually occurs in the presence of myocardial ischaemia or significant cardiac disease. Other causes of ventricular tachycardia include the following:

- acid–base and electrolyte imbalance
- hypokalaemia
- congestive heart failure
- increased catecholamine and sympathetic tone (as in emotional stress)
- ingestion of stimulants (alcohol, caffeine, tobacco)
- drug toxicity (digitalis, tricyclic antidepressants)
- sympathomimetic drugs (cocaine, methamphetamines)
- prolonged Q-T interval (may be caused by drugs, metabolic problems, or be congenital).

Note

Patients with a history of previous acute coronary syndrome, who are now experiencing a wide-complex tachycardia, have a high risk of being in ventricular tachycardia.

Rules for interpretation (lead II monitoring)

Ventricular tachycardia has the following characteristics on the electrocardiogram:

QRS complex: Equal to or greater than 0.12 s and usually distorted and bizarre. The QRS complexes generally are identical (monomorphic), but if fusion beats are present, one or more QRS complexes may differ in size, shape, and direction (polymorphic); polymorphic VT is depicted by differing shaped QRS complexes, of which torsades de pointes is an example.

P waves: May be absent. If present, P waves have no set relation to the QRS complex (AV dissociation). P waves occur at a slower rate than the ventricular focus and are superimposed on the QRS complexes.

Rate: Usually between 100 and 250 beats per minute

Rhythm: Usually regular (unless drug induced) but may be slightly irregular.

P-R interval: If P waves are present, the P-R interval varies widely.

Note

AV dissociation may precipitate cannon A waves which are waves of pulse pressure that are visible in the jugular veins of a patient in ventricular tachycardia. The cannon A waves result from the right atrium pumping against a closed tricuspid valve that in turn directs the waves of pressure into the jugular veins. AV dissociation is diagnostic of ventricular tachycardia.

Clinical significance

Ventricular tachycardia usually indicates significant heart disease. The rapid rate and the loss of atrial kick cause a drop in cardiac output and decreased coronary artery and cerebral perfusion. The severity of symptoms varies with the rate of the ventricular tachycardia and how much heart disease is present but monomorphic ventricular tachycardia is considered to be less sinister than polymorphic ventricular tachycardia. Ventricular tachycardia may be perfusing or non-perfusing; that is, it may produce a pulse or it may not. Importantly, ventricular tachycardia also may lead to ventricular fibrillation and the paramedic must be alert to sudden patient deterioration.

Management

Treatment of patients with ventricular tachycardia is based on their signs and symptoms and the presence or absence of torsades de pointes (Figure 15-62). As with other supraventricular tachycardias, the paramedic should obtain a history and identify the rhythm (see Figure 15-45) and if the patient is stable, a 12-lead ECG should be promptly obtained.

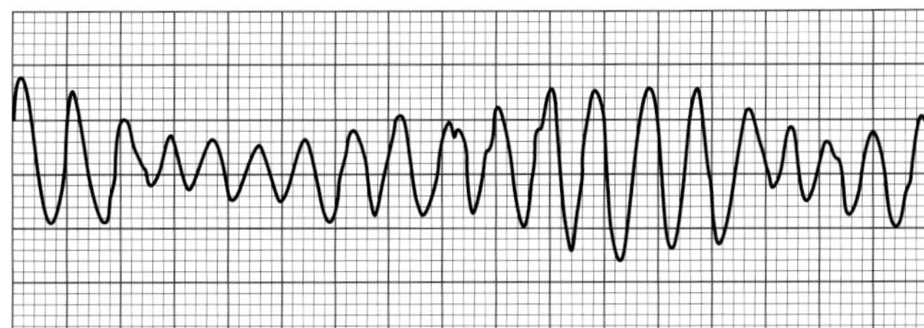

Figure 15-62 Torsades de pointes.

Ventricular tachycardia treatment depends on whether the QRS complex is monomorphic (having the same morphology or fixed shape) or polymorphic (having varying morphology). The paramedic should remember, however, that any wide-complex tachycardia that occurs with signs and symptoms of compromise – such as chest pain, dyspnoea, decreased level of consciousness, or hypotension or other signs of shock – requires immediate management. Patients who have ventricular tachycardia without a pulse should be treated as if it were ventricular fibrillation.

Monomorphic ventricular tachycardia treatment guidelines follow current resuscitation guidelines for ALS and take into account degree of compromise; signs and symptoms of compromise include systolic blood pressure less than 90 mmHg, heart failure, chest pain and decreased level of consciousness. Monomorphic ventricular tachycardia in a stable patient can be managed with amiodarone. Unstable patients with monomorphic ventricular tachycardia should receive immediate synchronized cardioversion; however, the patient will require sedation and this skill is currently not common UK paramedic practice. This should begin with an initial shock of 120–150 J biphasic or 200 J monophasic; if there is no response to the first shock, the energy should be gradually increased (in stepwise fashion). Polymorphic ventricular tachycardia can degenerate into ventricular fibrillation quickly, and similarly therefore requires immediate intervention. If the patient's rhythm is torsades de pointes (a particular form of polymorphic ventricular tachycardia), the rhythm may be the result of a prolonged Q-T interval. Medications that prolong the Q-T interval should be discontinued, electrolyte imbalances should be corrected, and IV magnesium sulphate will be given in hospital.

Note

Drugs given to treat dysrhythmias also can cause dysrhythmias; this is called proarrhythmic. Sequential use of two or more antidysrhythmic drugs increases the incidence of bradycardias, hypotension, and torsades de pointes. Avoiding use of more than one antidysrhythmic agent in treating narrow or wide QRS complex tachydysrhythmias is strongly recommended. In most cases, after an adequate dose of a single drug is unsuccessful in ending the dysrhythmia, synchronized cardioversion is the next treatment.

12-lead strategies for wide-complex tachycardias

If an unstable patient's QRS complex is wide (greater than 0.12 s) and fast (greater than 150 beats), immediate management as per current guidelines is indicated. If the patient is stable, however, the following steps in multi-lead assessments may help distinguish between ventricular tachycardia and other wide-complex tachycardias:[5]

1. Assess leads I, II, III, V_1 and V_6. If the QRS complex is negative in leads I, II and III and positive in V_1, the rhythm indicates ventricular tachycardia (Figure 15-63). If these criteria are not met, proceed to step 2.
2. Assess the QRS deflection in $V_1$and V_6. Regardless of the QRS deflection in leads I, II, and III, positive QRS deflections with a single peak, a taller left 'rabbit ear',

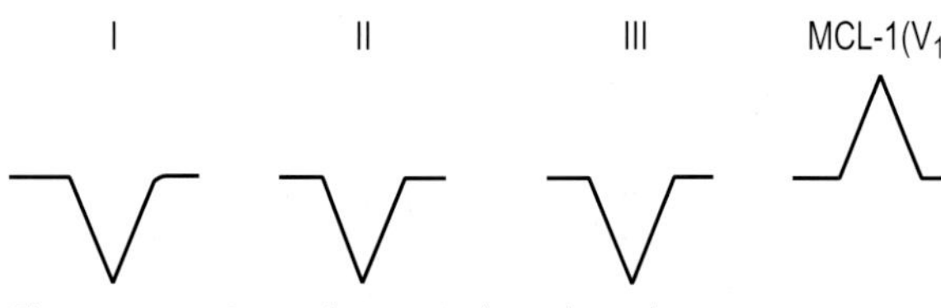

Figure 15-63 Criteria for ventricular tachycardia. .

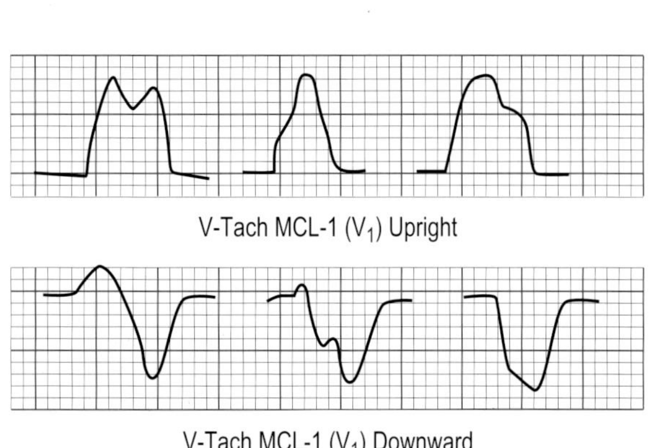

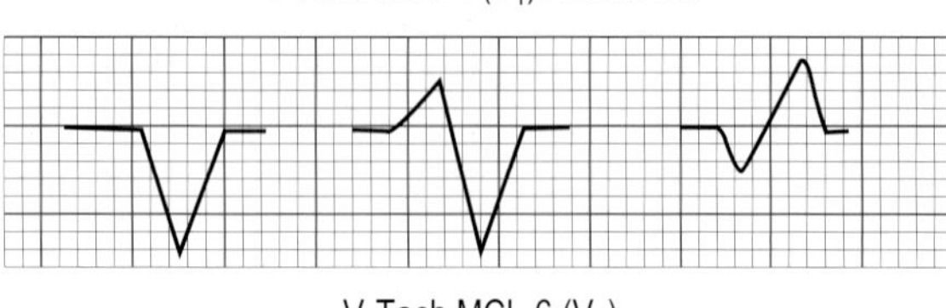

Figure 15-64 Step 1: A QRS complex that is negative in leads I, II, III, and positive in MCL1 (V_1) indicates ventricular tachycardia. Step 2: Assess the QRS complex in MCL1 (V_1) and MCL6 (V_6). Step 3: Assess the QRS complex in leads I, II, III and MCL1 (V_1).

or an RS complex with a fat R wave or slurred S wave in V_1 indicates ventricular tachycardia. A negative QS complex, a negative RS complex, or any wide Q wave in V_6 also indicates ventricular tachycardia (Figure 15-64).

3. A negative QRS complex in lead I, positive QRS complex in leads II and III, and a negative QRS complex in V_1 indicates ventricular tachycardia.
4. If all precordial leads (V leads) are positive or negative (precordial concordance), the rhythm indicates ventricular tachycardia (Figure 15-65).
5. If the RS interval is greater than 0.12 s in any V lead (increased ventricular activation time), the rhythm indicates ventricular tachycardia (Figure 15-66).

Note

These steps involve identifying the predominant direction of flow of impulses in the heart (axis), further described later in this chapter.

Note

Non-ventricular tachycardia precordial concordance may occur in patients who have Wolff–Parkinson–White syndrome and associated left bundle branch block.

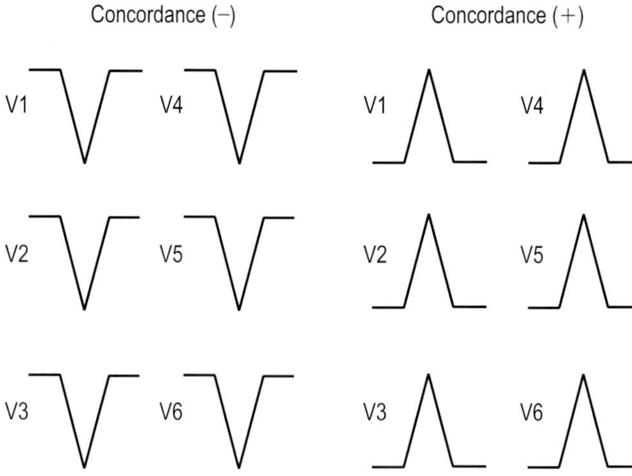

Figure 15-65 Ventricular tachycardia–concordance.

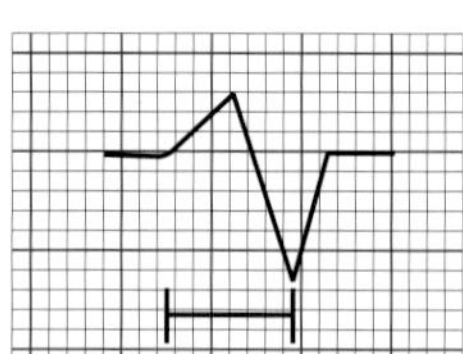

VT (RS interval is 0.16 s)

Figure 15-66 RS interval.

Critical Thinking

Why is it crucial to distinguish between ventricular tachycardia and wide-complex tachycardias in stable patients?

Critical Thinking

How will you manage a patient with ventricular tachycardia, chest pain or difficulty breathing if you cannot establish an intravenous line?

Ventricular fibrillation

Description

Ventricular fibrillation is a quivering of the ventricles, organized ventricular contraction does not occur and results in pulselessness (Figure 15-67). Ventricular fibrillation is the most common initial rhythm disturbance in sudden cardiac arrest and results from multifocal re-entry foci in the ventricles.

Aetiology

Ventricular fibrillation most commonly is associated with significant heart disease. The dysrhythmias also may be precipitated by premature ventricular complexes, the R-on-T phenomenon (rarely), or a sustained ventricular tachycardia. Other causes include the following:

- myocardial ischaemia
- acute myocardial infarction

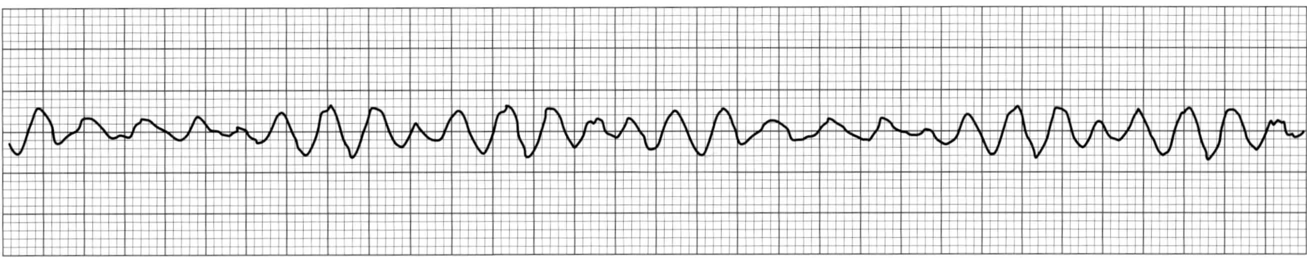

Figure 15-67 Ventricular fibrillation.

- third-degree AV block with a slow ventricular escape rhythm
- cardiomyopathy
- digitalis toxicity
- hypoxia
- acidosis
- electrolyte imbalance (hypokalaemia, hyperkalaemia, submersion)
- electrical injury
- drug overdose or toxicity (cocaine, tricyclic antidepressants).

Rules for interpretation (all leads)

Ventricular fibrillation has the following characteristics on the electrocardiogram:

QRS complex: Absent.

P waves: Absent.

Rate: No coordinated ventricular contractions are present. The unsynchronized ventricular impulses occur at rates from 300 to 500 beats per minute.

Rhythm: Irregularly irregular.

P-R interval: Absent.

Because organized depolarizations of the atria and ventricles are absent, P waves, QRS complexes, ST segments and T waves are absent. Ventricular fibrillatory waves are seen on the ECG screen as bizarre, rounded or pointed and considerably different in shape. They vary at random from positive to negative as well. These waves represent twitching of small individual groups of muscle fibres. Fibrillatory waves less than 3 mm in amplitude are called fine ventricular fibrillation whilst those greater than 3 mm are called coarse ventricular fibrillation (Figure 15-68). The fibrillatory waves may be fine and resemble ventricular asystole.

> **Note**
>
> Coarse ventricular fibrillation usually indicates the recent onset of ventricular fibrillation and is more readily converted by prompt defibrillation. The presence of fine ventricular fibrillation that approaches asystole often means that a considerable delay has occurred since collapse and that successful defibrillation is more difficult.[2]

Clinical significance

Ventricular fibrillation causes all life functions to cease because of the lack of circulating blood flow. The dysrhythmia initially may result in light-headedness, followed within seconds by loss of consciousness, apnoea, and if untreated, death.

Management

For adult resuscitation, management of ventricular fibrillation and pulseless ventricular tachycardia is the most important sequence because most adult cardiac arrests result from these two rhythm disturbances and the vast majority of successful resuscitations result from the appropriate management of these two dysrhythmias (see Figure 15-54).[1] Ventricular fibrillation and pulseless ventricular tachycardia are managed alike: basic life support (if a defibrillator is not immediately available), defibrillation, endotracheal intubation and pharmacological therapy, as per current resuscitation guidelines.

When cardiac arrest is present, there is no blood flow. Chest compressions create a small amount of blood flow to the vital organs, such as the brain and heart. The importance of chest compressions is now greater than ever before, and in unwitnessed arrests, 2 min of basic life support is given before defibrillation. Other key aspects to emphasize are that chest compressions should not be delayed and reducing the 'time off chest' is important; interruptions MUST be minimized. The rate of compressions is 100 per minute, ensuring appropriate compression depth and allowing the chest to fully recoil after each compression; there is equal time allowed for compression as relaxation.

This same train of thought applies to defibrillation: 'CPR first', and minimize interruptions in chest compressions. If an EMS provider does not witness the arrest in the out-of-hospital setting, the EMS crew may give 2 min of basic life support before attempting defibrillation. If the arrest is witnessed and the rhythm is shockable, one shock should be delivered, and then CPR should be resumed immediately, beginning with chest compressions. CPR should be continued for another 2 min, before checking the rhythm again. Theory holds that even when a shock eliminates ventricular fibrillation, several minutes are required for a normal rhythm to return and for the heart to create more blood flow. A brief period of chest compressions can deliver oxygen and sources of energy to the heart, increasing the likelihood that the heart will be able to effectively pump blood after the defibrillatory shock. Therefore, even if the rhythm changes after a shock, a 2-min cycle of basic life support is continued unless there are obvious signs of life. In addition, chest compressions should not be interrupted until the defibrillation process is undertaken; analysis in an automated mode may require compressions to be stopped to avoid a 'motion detected' error and care should be taken to analyse the ECG screen to confirm the rhythm only when compressions have

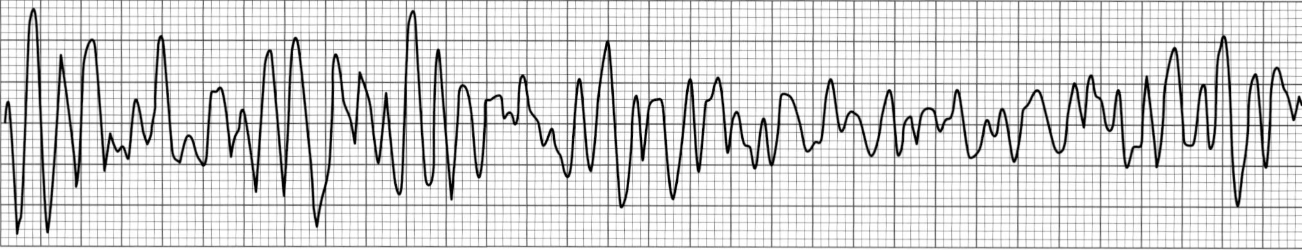
Coarse VF

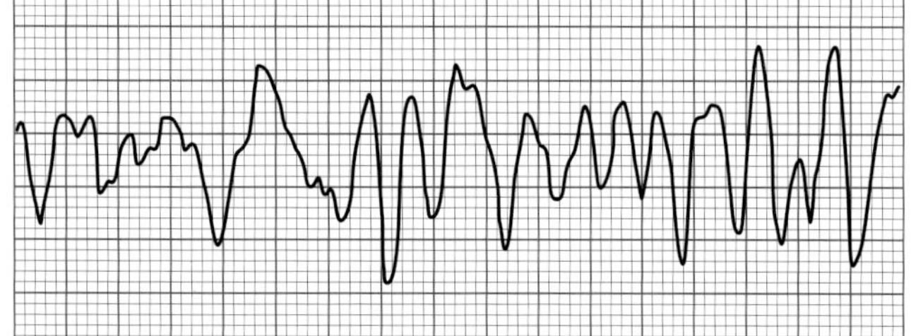
Coarse VF

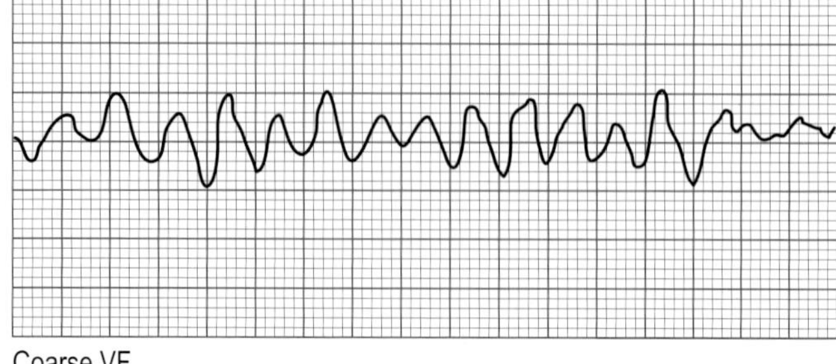
Coarse VF

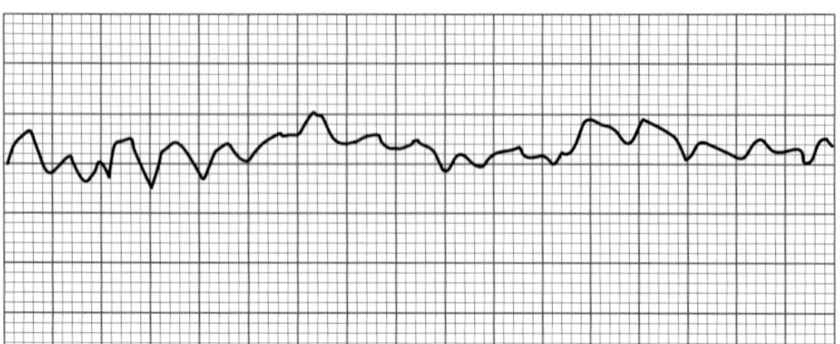
Coarse VF

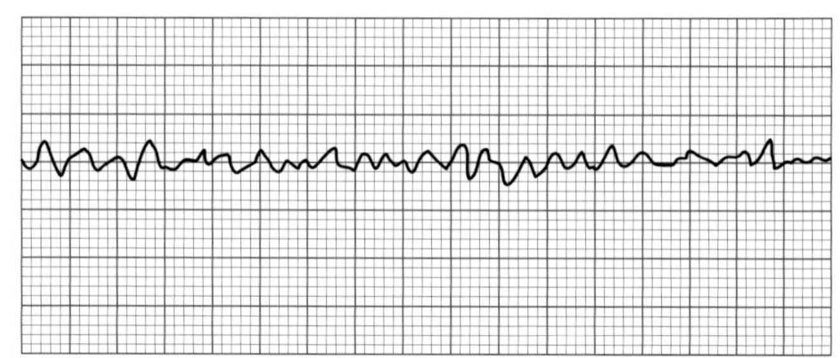
Coarse VF

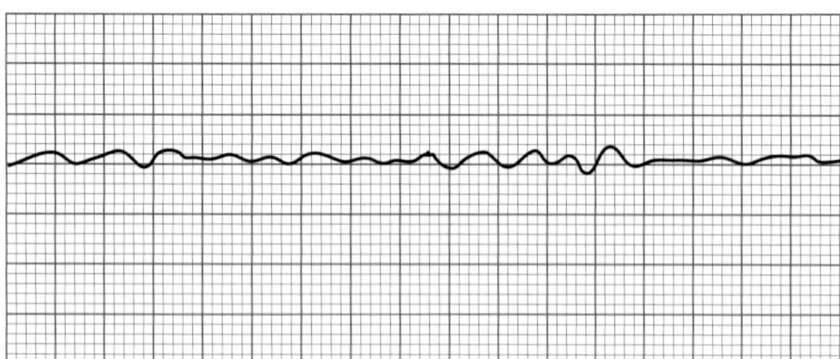
Fine VF

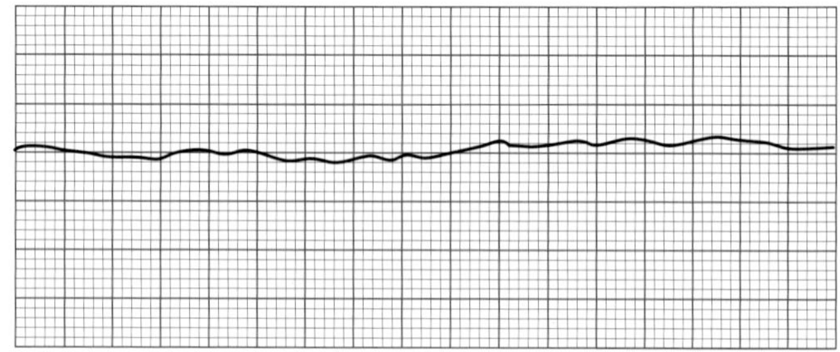
Fine VF

Figure 15-68 Coarse and fine ventricular fibrillation.

been paused, otherwise 'compression complexes' may be seen.

Rhythm checks should be brief, and pulse checks should be performed only if an organized rhythm is observed (see Figure 15-54).

Ventricular asystole

Description

Ventricular asystole (cardiac standstill) refers to the absence of all ventricular activity (Figure 15-69).

Aetiology

Ventricular asystole may be the cause of cardiac arrest and may also occur in complete heart block when there is no escape pacemaker. The dysrhythmia usually is associated with extensive heart disease and often follows ventricular tachycardia, ventricular fibrillation, pulseless electrical activity, or an agonal escape rhythm in the dying heart.

Rules for interpretation (all leads)

Ventricular asystole has the following characteristics on the electrocardiogram:

QRS complexes: Absent.
P waves: Absent or present.
Rate: Absent.
Rhythm: Absent.
P-R interval: Absent.

Clinical significance

Ventricular asystole produces no cardiac output and is an ominous dysrhythmia. Asystole often confirms death. The chance for resuscitation is small.

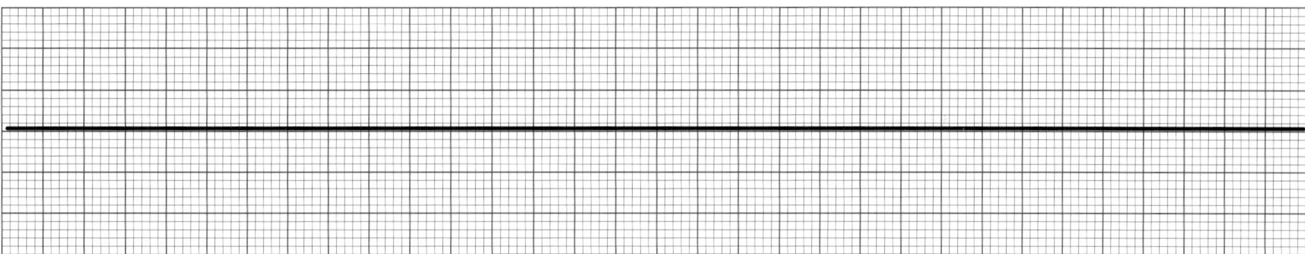

Figure 15-69 Ventricular asystole.

Management

The management of ventricular asystole is as per current guidelines and includes basic life support with effective CPR, advanced airway, and pharmacological therapy of adrenaline (epinephrine) and atropine (Figure 15-54). If fine ventricular fibrillation is suspected, defibrillation is indicated; however, defibrillating asystole 'just in case' is not recommended. The stopping of resuscitation efforts in the prehospital setting after meeting 'recognition of life extinct' (ROLE) is indicated for this patient situation. However, potential reversible causes of asystole should be considered before cessation of resuscitative efforts and these include hypoxia, hyperkalaemia, hypothermia, drug overdose and acidosis.

> **Critical Thinking**
>
> What benefit is there to the community and to the patient's family when resuscitation is halted in the field after following all appropriate guidelines?

Artificial pacemaker rhythms

Description

Artificial pacemakers generate a rhythm (Figure 15-70) by regular electrical stimulation of the heart through an electrode implanted in the heart. The electrode is connected to a power source (a battery cell implanted subcutaneously, typically the right or left side of the chest). The tip of the pacemaker wire is at the apex of the right ventricle (ventricular pacemaker), in the right atrium (atrial pacemaker), or in both locations (dual-chamber pacemaker). These devices are placed in patients with complete heart block or in patients who have episodes of severe symptomatic bradycardia.

Some pacemakers, known as fixed-rate or asynchronous pacemakers, fire continuously at a preset rate regardless of the patient's own electrical activity. They rarely are used today. Other pacemakers fire only if the patient's own rate drops below the preset rate of the pacemaker; they act as an escape rhythm and are known as demand pacemakers. Atrial and ventricular demand pacemakers pace the atria and ventricles when the intrinsic rate of the paced chamber drops dangerously low. Atrial synchronous ventricular pacemakers are in step with the patient's atrial rhythm; this type paces the ventricle after the patient's atria contract. This pacemaker is useful in patients with normal sinus node activity but various degrees of AV block. AV sequential pacemakers pace the atria first and then the ventricles when normal impulses are absent or slowed in either or both chambers. If regular atrial activity is too slow, for example, then both chambers are paced sequentially to maintain the atrial kick. If the atrial rate is adequate, the atrial pacer does not fire. The ventricular pacemaker still fires if the ventricular rate is below a preset rate. This pacemaker is ideal for sick sinus syndrome and sinus arrest.

A class of newer pacemakers are rate-responsive pacemakers. These pacemakers can adjust their pacing rates to a patient's needs, by sensing when cardiac output should be increased. Several methods of sensing metabolic activity are used. However, the most popular rate-responsive pacers detect patient movement to determine the best firing rate. These devices are popular and they can increase cardiac output and increase tolerance of physical activity. At times these pacemakers may increase the patient's pacing rate inappropriately; for example if they sense muscle movement that is not caused by increased patient activity.

Rules for interpretation (lead II monitoring)

Artificial pacemaker rhythms have the following characteristics on the electrocardiogram:

QRS complex: If pacemaker induced, QRS complexes are 0.12 s or greater. Their appearance usually is bizarre, resembling a premature ventricular complex. The pacemaker is said to be 'capturing' if each pacemaker spike elicits a QRS complex. If only the atria are being paced, the QRS complexes usually are normal, provided no bundle branch block is present. With demand pacemakers, some of the patient's own QRS complexes may be present. These normal QRS complexes occur without pacemaker spikes.

P waves: May be present or absent, normal or abnormal. The relationship of the P waves to the pacemaker (QRS) complex varies by type of artificial pacemaker. Pacemaker spikes precede QRS complexes induced by ventricular pacemakers, whereas dual-chambered pacemakers also produce an atrial spike followed by a P wave. The pacemaker spike is a narrow deflection on the oscilloscope and represents the electrical discharge of the pacemaker. Pacemaker spikes indicate only that a pacemaker is discharging. They provide no information about ventricular contraction or perfusion.

Rate: Varies according to the preset rate of the pacemaker. Typically the rate is 60 to 80 beats per minute.

Rhythm: Regular if pacing is constant; irregular if pacing occurs only on demand.

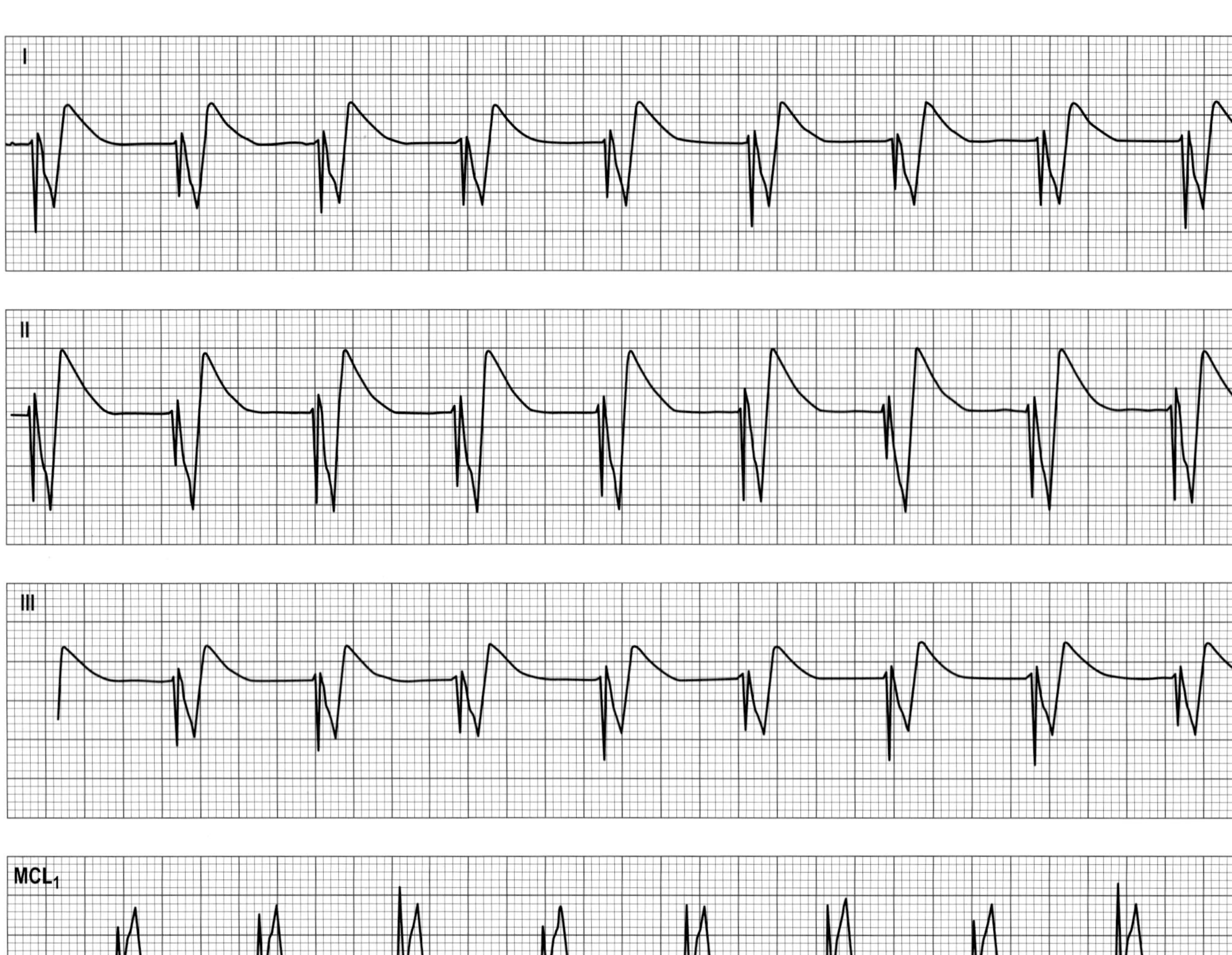

Figure 15-70 Artificial pacemaker rhythms.

P-R interval: The presence and duration of P-R intervals depend on the underlying rhythm and vary by the type of artificial pacemaker.

Critical Thinking

If the pacemaker fails, what rhythms might you see on the monitor?

Clinical significance

Pacemaker spikes indicate that the patient's heart rate is being regulated by an artificial pacemaker. Pacemaker spikes followed by QRS complexes indicate electrical capture; if spikes do not elicit a QRS complex, the pacemaker is not capturing the ventricle electrically and there will be no ventricular contraction. A large percentage of pacemaker failures occur within the first month after implantation (Box 15-6).

Management

Pacemaker failure is a true emergency, requiring immediate recognition and rapid transport for definitive care, which may include battery replacement or temporary pacemaker insertion. The paramedic should not delay transport while attempting to stabilize these patients. The following five principles apply to treating patients with pacemakers:

1. When examining an unconscious patient, be alert for battery packs implanted under the skin. Also be alert for any medical alert information.
2. Manage all dysrhythmias per the appropriate algorithm.
3. Manage ventricular irritability with appropriate drug therapy without fear of suppressing ventricular response to a pacemaker rhythm.
4. Defibrillate patients with artificial pacemakers in the usual manner. However, do not discharge paddles directly over the implanted battery pack.
5. Transcutaneous cardiac pacing, if indicated, may be used in the usual manner.

Box 15-6

Four potential causes of pacemaker malfunction

1. Battery failure: Most implanted pacemakers today use a lithium-iodine cell power source. This source provides stable voltage output for about 80–90% of the life of the battery. (The battery life is 5–10 years or more.) Battery failure usually slows the pacemaker rate. It also usually decreases the spike amplitude. If the battery fails, the patient may have bradycardia or asystole.
2. Runaway pacemakers: Runaway pacemakers are ones that develop rapid discharge rates that may reach 300 beats per minute. This occurs as the batteries decrease their voltage output. This type of failure rarely is seen in pacemakers used today because the newer power sources provide a gradual increase in rate as their batteries run low.
3. Failure of the sensing device in demand pacemakers: Demand pacemakers may fail to shut off when patients have an adequate rate of their own. When this occurs, there is a competition between the natural and artificial pacemakers of the heart. The pacemaker may discharge during the vulnerable period of the cardiac cycle. This may result in dysrhythmias.
4. Failure to capture: A failure of the pacemaker to capture may result from a variety of causes. These may include battery failure, loose or broken catheter electrode wires, inoperable electrodes, and a shift in the location of the catheter tip. In such cases, pacemaker spikes usually are present. However, they are not followed by P waves or QRS complexes.

Besides pacemakers, implantable cardioverter defibrillators also are common; the battery packs of these devices are located in the subcutaneous tissues of the abdominal wall. Emergency cardiac care can be given as usual. These devices present no danger to rescuers but paramedics should wear gloves to help avoid unpleasant sensations when the device discharges. Implantable cardioverter defibrillators are described further later in this chapter.

Dysrhythmias that are disorders of conduction

Delay or blockage of the electrical impulse conduction in the heart is called a heart block and can occur anywhere in the atria between the SA node and the AV node or in the ventricles between the AV node and the Purkinje fibres. These conduction problems can be caused by diseased tissue in the conduction system or by a physiological block, as in atrial fibrillation or atrial flutter. Causes of heart blocks include AV junctional ischaemia, AV junctional necrosis, degenerative disease of the conduction system, electrolyte imbalances (e.g. hyperkalaemia) and drug toxicity, especially with digitalis.

Classifications

Conduction blocks may be classified based on several characteristics: site of block (e.g. left bundle branch block), degree of block (e.g. second-degree AV block), or category of AV conduction disturbances (e.g. type I). This text presents the dysrhythmias by degree and location. One should note, however, that the term degree does not reflect directly the gradients of severity when applied to the classification of heart blocks; any evaluation of heart block must consider the specific rates of the atria and ventricles, the patient's clinical presentation, and the findings of a complete history and physical examination before one determines the clinical severity of AV conduction disturbances. The dysrhythmias discussed in this section include first-degree AV block; second-degree AV block type I (or Wenckebach); second-degree AV block type II; third-degree AV block (complete heart block); and ventricular conduction disturbances, including bundle branch blocks and hemiblocks.

Atrioventricular blocks

The discussion of conduction disturbances of the heart begins with the AV blocks.

First-degree AV block

Description

First-degree AV block is not a true block (Figure 15-71) but is a delay in conduction, usually at the level of the AV node. First-degree AV block is not considered a rhythm in itself because it usually is superimposed on another rhythm. The paramedic must also identify the underlying rhythm (e.g. sinus bradycardia with first-degree AV block).

Aetiology

First-degree AV block may occur for no apparent reason. The dysrhythmia sometimes is associated with myocardial ischaemia, acute myocardial infarction, increased vagal (parasympathetic) tone, or digitalis toxicity.

Rules for interpretation (lead II monitoring)

First-degree AV block has the following characteristics on the electrocardiogram:

QRS complex: Typically normal (less than 0.12 s), with an AV conduction ratio of 1 : 1 (a QRS complex follows each P wave).

P waves: Present, identical waves that precede each QRS complex.

Rate: The rate is that of the underlying sinus or atrial rhythm.

Rhythm: The rhythm is that of the underlying rhythm.

P-R interval: A prolonged (greater than 0.20 s), constant P-R interval is the hallmark of first-degree AV block and often is the only alteration in the electrocardiogram.

Clinical significance

As a general rule, first-degree AV block has little or no clinical significance because all of the impulses are conducted to the ventricles. Rarely, though, a newly developed first-degree AV block may progress to a more serious AV block.

Management

This dysrhythmia usually does not require treatment.

Second-degree AV block type I (Wenckebach)

Description

Type I second-degree AV block is an intermittent block (Figure 15-72) occurring at the level of the AV node. The conduction delay progressively increases from beat to beat until conduction to the ventricle is blocked. This dysrhythmia produces a characteristic cyclical pattern in which the P-R intervals get progressively longer until a P wave occurs that is not followed by a QRS complex. By the time the SA node fires again, AV conduction has had time to recover, then the sequence repeats.

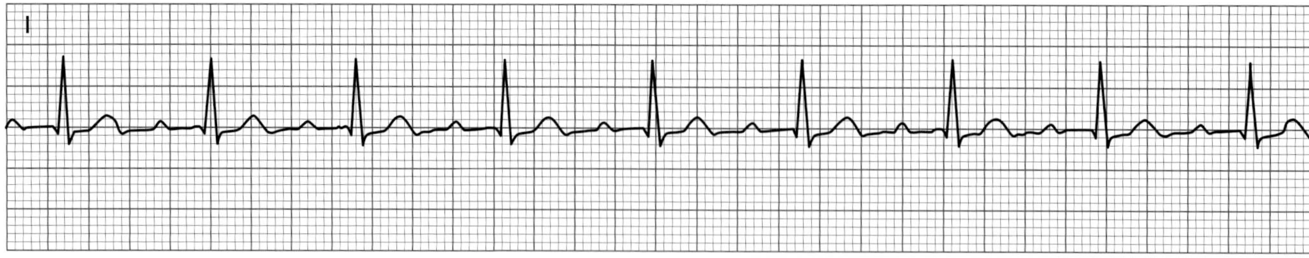

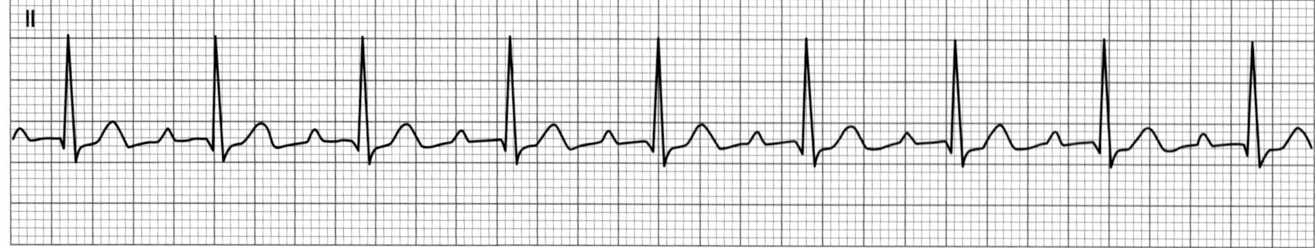

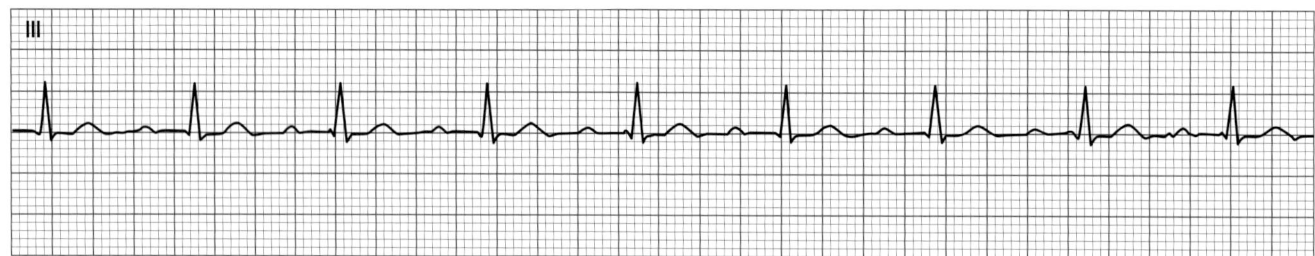

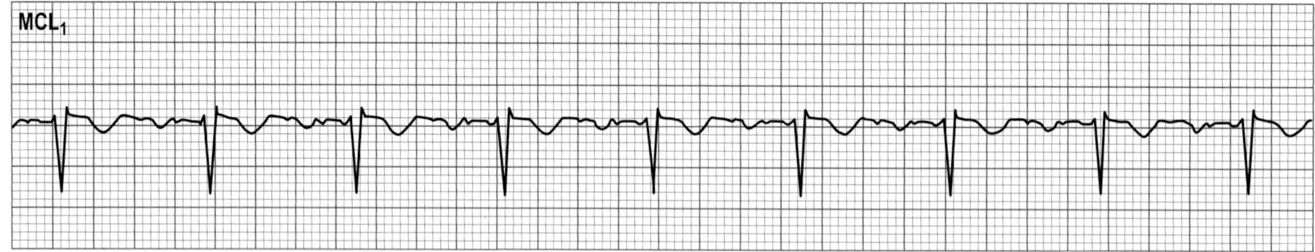

Figure 15-71 First-degree AV block.

Aetiology

Type I second-degree AV block often occurs in acute myocardial infarction or acute myocarditis; other causes include increased vagal tone, ischaemia, drug toxicity (digitalis, beta-blockers, verapamil), head injury and electrolyte imbalance.

Rules for interpretation (lead II monitoring)

Second-degree AV block type I has the following characteristics on the electrocardiogram:

QRS complex: Usually less than 0.12 s. Commonly, the AV conduction ratio (P waves to QRS complexes) is 5:4, 4:3, 3:2, or 2:1; the pattern may be constant or variable. A constant 2:1 block makes it difficult to distinguish between type I and type II blocks.

P waves: Upright and uniform and preceding the QRS complex when the QRS complex occurs.

Rate: The atrial rate is that of the underlying sinus or atrial rhythm. The ventricular rate may be normal or slow but always is slightly less than the atrial rate.

Rhythm: The atrial rhythm is regular; the ventricular rhythm is irregular (characteristic group beating).

P-R interval: Progressively lengthens before the non-conducted P wave. The P-P interval is constant, but the R-R interval decreases until the dropped beat (producing grouping of QRS complexes).

Clinical significance

Type I second-degree AV block usually is a transient and reversible phenomenon but it can progress to a more serious AV block. If dropped beats occur often, the patient may show signs and symptoms of decreased cardiac output.

Note

AV block, in which the P-R interval before a dropped beat is prolonged and the P-R interval after the dropped beat is shortened by comparison, is the most common form of second-degree block.

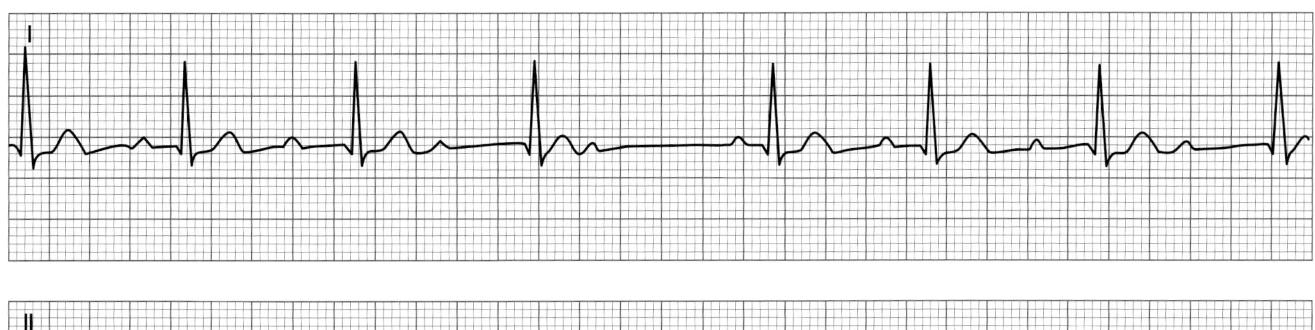

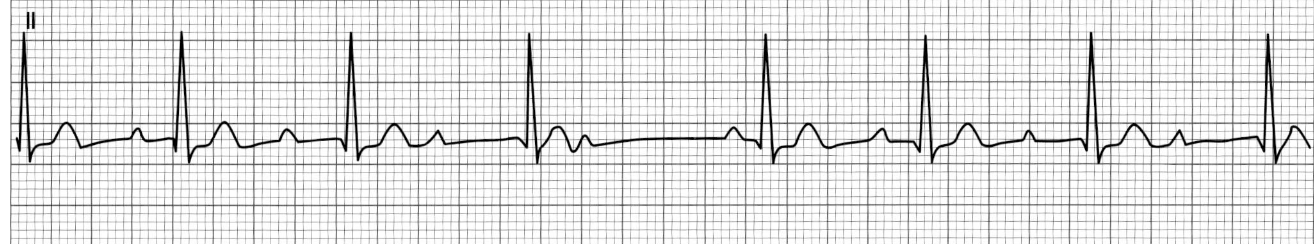

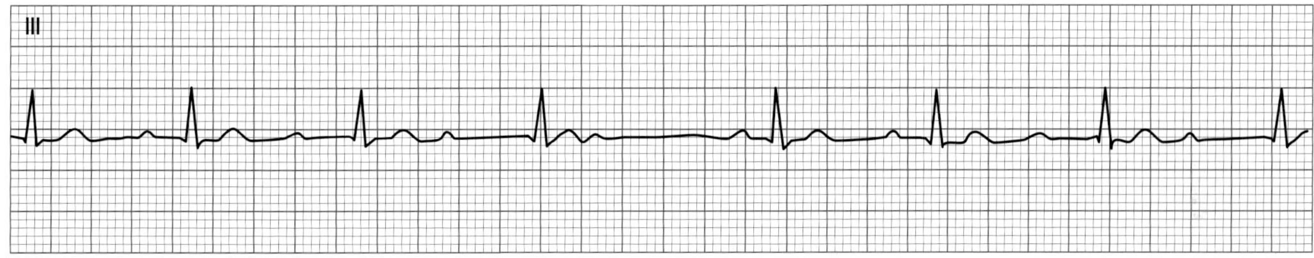

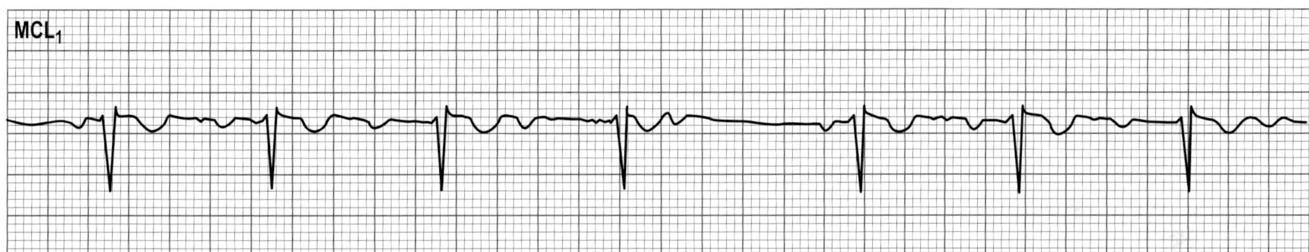

Figure 15-72 Second-degree AV block, type I.

Management

No management is required if the patient is asymptomatic. If the dropped beats compromise the heart rate and cardiac output, administration of atropine, transcutaneous cardiac pacing, or both, may be indicated (see Figure 15-39).

Second-degree AV block type II

Description

Type II second-degree AV block is an intermittent block (Figure 15-73). This dysrhythmia occurs when atrial impulses are not conducted to the ventricles. Unlike type I, this block is characterized by consecutive P waves being conducted with a constant P-R interval before a dropped beat. This variation of AV block usually occurs in a regular sequence with the conduction ratios (P waves to QRS complexes), such as 2:1, 3:2, and 4:3 (Figure 15-74). Type II second-degree AV block usually occurs below the bundle of His.

When at least two consecutive P waves fail to be conducted to the ventricles, the AV block is referred to as a high-grade AV block (Figure 15-75). Clinically, serious high-grade AV blocks and those that are less serious are distinguished by the atrial and ventricular rates. A 2:1 block might be considered high grade (and certainly is clinically significant) when the patient's underlying atrial rate is 60 beats per minute. However, such a block is of much less concern if the patient's atrial rate is 120 beats per minute.

A type II 2:1 AV block sometimes may be difficult to distinguish from a type I 2:1 AV block. When assessing a patient who has two atrial complexes for each QRS complex, the paramedic should evaluate the normal cycle. If the normally conducted cycle has a prolonged P-R interval (greater than 0.20 s), a narrow QRS complex (less than 0.12 s, indicating the absence of bundle branch block), and an adequate escape rate, the patient probably has a type I 2:1 AV block. If the conducted QRS complex has a normal P-R interval, a wide QRS complex (greater than 0.12 s, which indicates the presence of a bundle branch block), and an adequate escape rate, a type II 2:1 AV block is most likely (Figure 15-76).

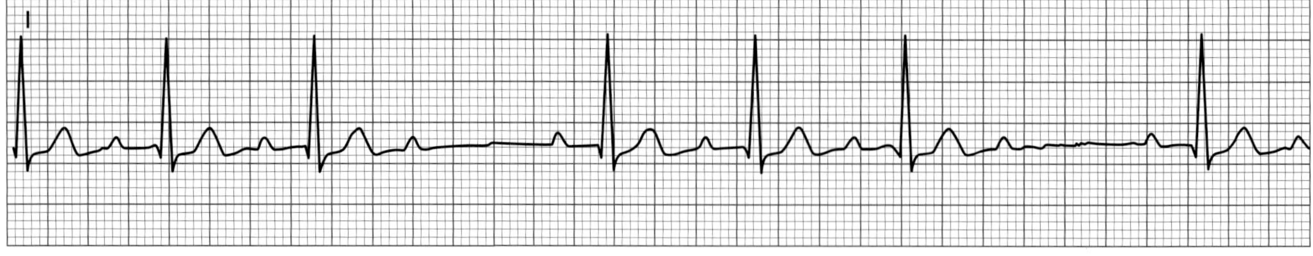

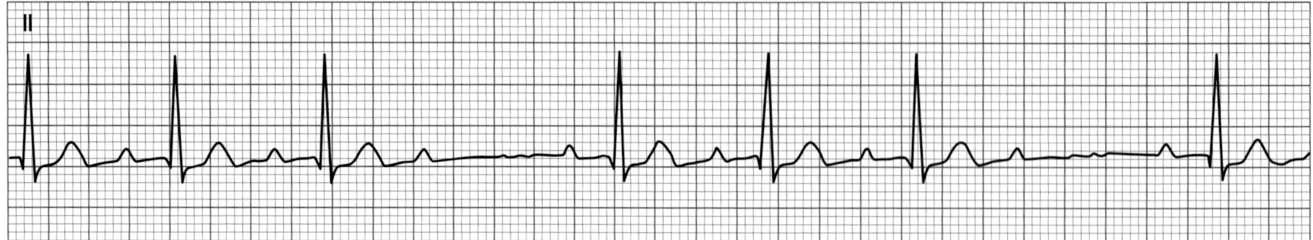

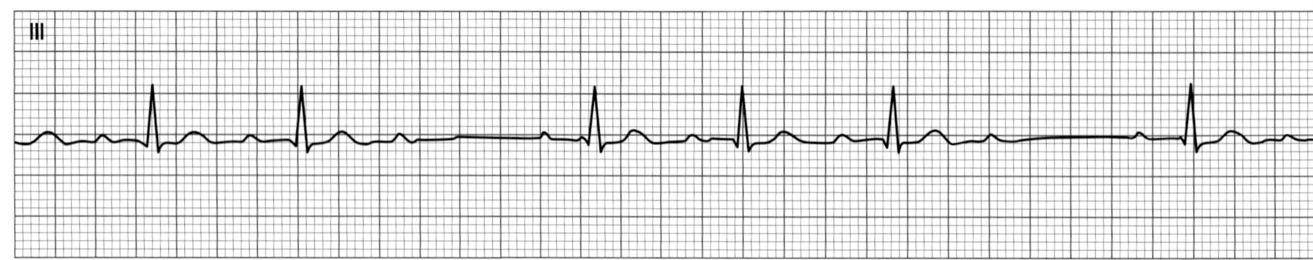

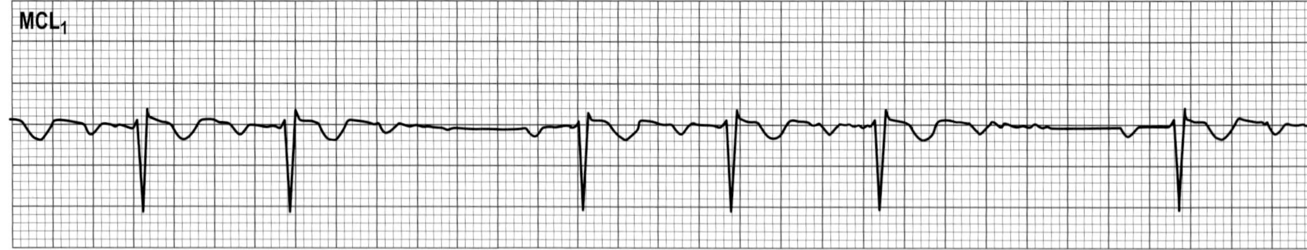

Figure 15-73 Second-degree AV block, type II.

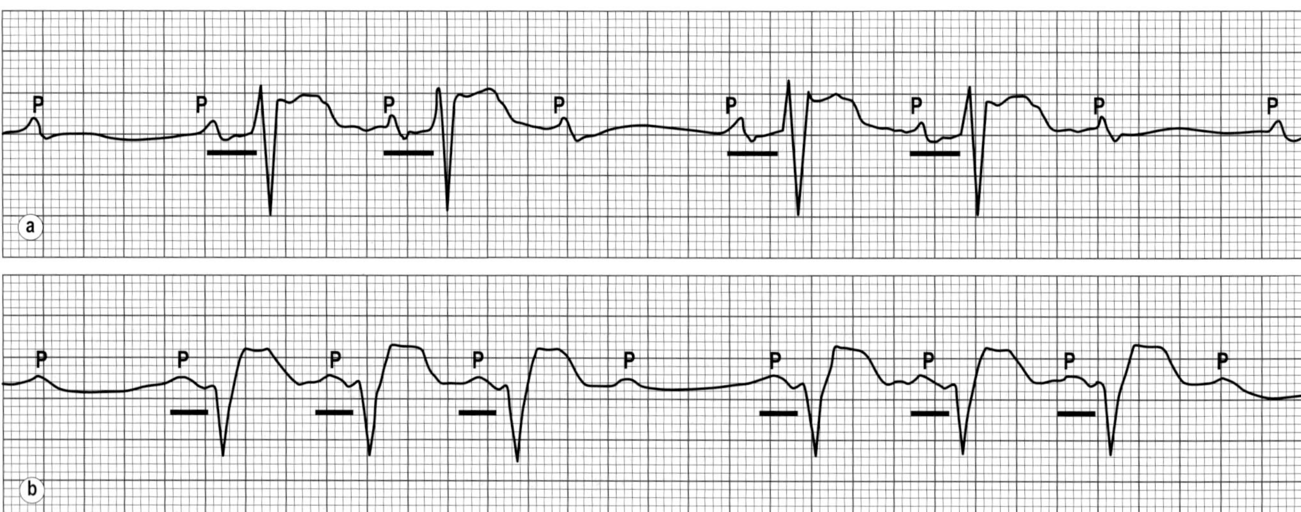

Figure 15-74 (a) A 3 : 2 AV block. (b) A 4 : 3 AV block.

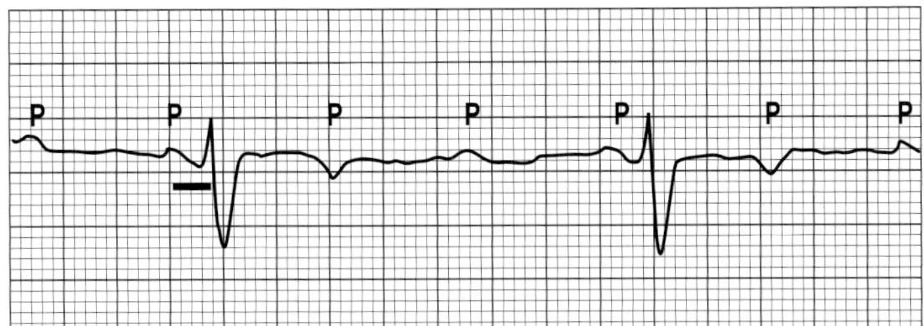

Figure 15-75 A 3:1 high-grade AV block.

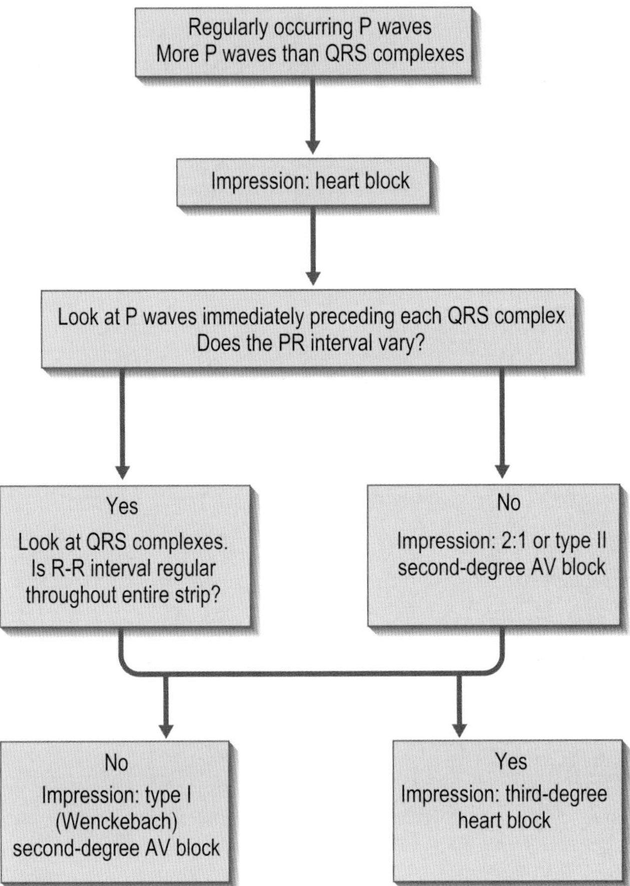

Figure 15-76 Identifying heart blocks.

Aetiology

Type II second-degree AV block usually is associated with acute myocardial infarction that occurs in the septum. Unlike type I second-degree AV block, type II normally does not result solely from increased parasympathetic tone or drug toxicity.

Rules for interpretation (lead II monitoring)

Second-degree AV block type II has the following characteristics on the electrocardiogram:

QRS complex: May be abnormal (equal to or greater than 0.12 s) because of bundle branch block.

P waves: Upright and uniform. Some P waves will not be followed by QRS complexes.

Rate: The atrial rate is unaffected and is that of the underlying sinus, atrial, or junctional rhythm. The ventricular rate is less than that of the atrial rate and is often bradycardic.

Rhythm: Regular or irregular, depending on whether the conduction ratio is constant or variable.

P-R interval: Usually is constant for conducted beats and may be greater than 0.20 s.

Clinical significance

Type II second-degree AV block is a serious dysrhythmia and considered malignant in the emergency setting (unlike type I AV blocks, which usually are considered benign). Slow ventricular rates may result in signs and symptoms of hypoperfusion. This dysrhythmia may progress to a more severe heart block and may even progress to ventricular asystole.

Management

Regardless of the patient's initial condition, pacemaker insertion is the treatment for the patient. Prehospital care for symptomatic patients may consist of transcutaneous cardiac pacing and possibly the administration of atropine (see Figure 15-39).

Third-degree heart block

Description

Third-degree AV block results from complete electrical block at or below the AV node (infranodal) (Figure 15-77). The dysrhythmia is said to be present when the opportunity for conduction between the atria and the ventricles is present but conduction does not occur. In this condition the SA node serves as the pacemaker for the atria with an ectopic focus serving as a pacemaker in the ventricles. The result is that P waves and QRS complexes occur rhythmically, yet the rhythms are unrelated to each other (AV dissociation). The only electrical link between the atria and the ventricles is the AV node and bundle of His.

Note

Atropine should be used with caution in patients with complete heart block and wide-complex ventricular escape beats and also for patients with type II second-degree heart block; atropine may increase the degree of block or cause third-degree AV block. Many patients with heart block cannot be managed effectively in the prehospital setting solely with medication and immediate transport to an emergency department is indicated.

Aetiology

Common causes of third-degree AV block include increased vagal tone (which may produce a transient AV dissociation),

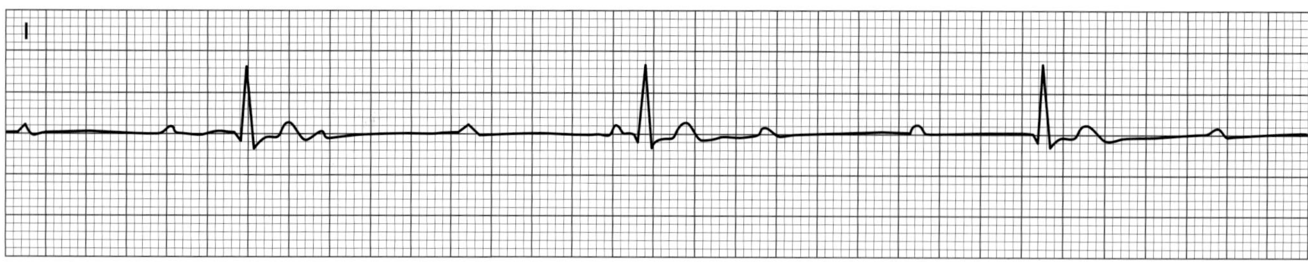

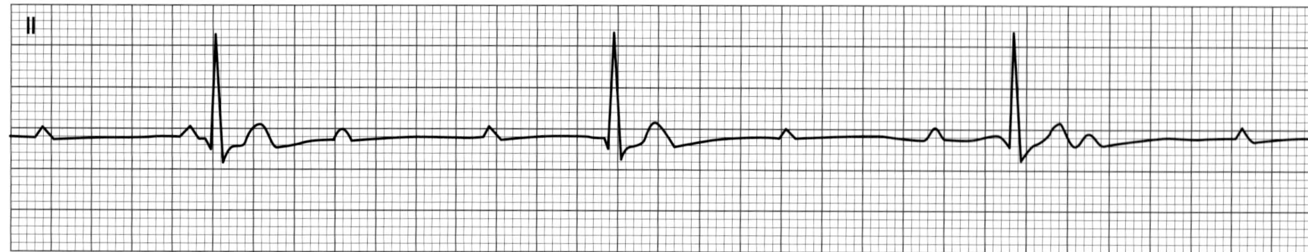

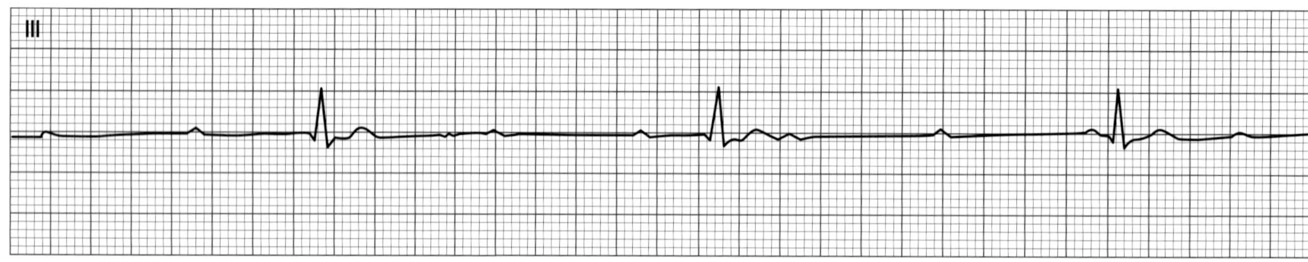

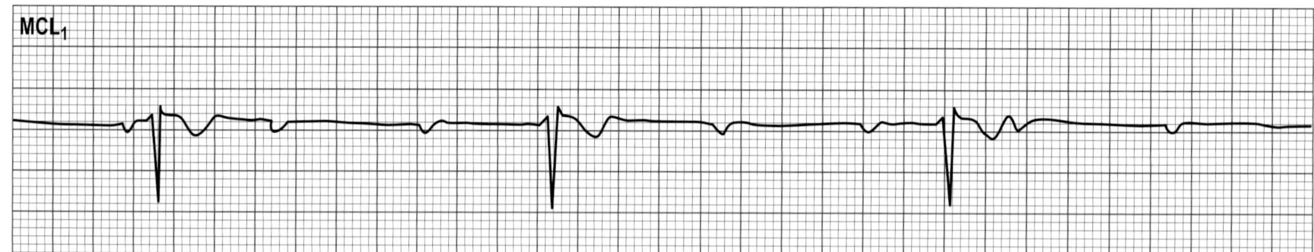

Figure 15-77 Third-degree AV block.

septal necrosis, acute myocarditis, digitalis, beta-blocker or calcium channel blocker toxicity, and electrolyte imbalance. The dysrhythmia also may occur in older adults from chronic degenerative changes in the conduction system.

Critical Thinking

When P waves and QRS complexes do not appear to be related to each other on the electrocardiogram, the paramedic should look at the shape of QRS-T waves. QRS-T waves altered by superimposed P waves suggests AV dissociation; AV dissociation suggests third-degree AV block.

Rules for interpretation (lead II monitoring)

Third-degree heart block has the following characteristics on the electrocardiogram:

QRS complex: May be less than 0.12 s if the escape focus is below the AV node and above the bifurcation of the bundle branches or 0.12 s or greater if the escape focus is ventricular. A narrow QRS complex in third-degree heart block is less common than a wide QRS complex.

P waves: Present but with no relationship to the QRS complexes. In cases of atrial flutter or fibrillation, complete heart block is manifested by a slow, regular ventricular response.

Rate: The atrial rate is that of the underlying sinus or atrial rhythm. The ventricular rate typically is 40–60 beats per minute if the escape focus is junctional and less than 40 beats per minute if the escape focus is in the ventricles.

Rhythm: The atrial and ventricular rhythms usually are regular. The rhythms are independent of each other.

P-R interval: No relation exists between atrial and ventricular activity (Figure 15-78).

Clinical significance

The patient may have signs and symptoms of severe bradycardia and decreased cardiac output; these are the result of

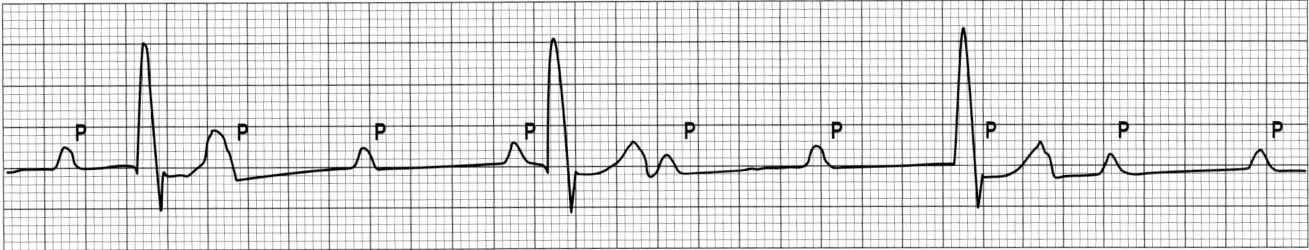

Figure 15-78 Third-degree block demonstrating P waves superimposed on the QRS complex and T waves.

slow ventricular rate and asynchronous action of the atria and ventricles. Third-degree AV block associated with wide QRS complexes is an ominous sign; the dysrhythmia is potentially lethal and patients with this rhythm often present as unstable.

Note

Complete AV block in the presence of atrial fibrillation often is caused by drug toxicity (usually digitalis). Almost always some AV block occurs with atrial fibrillation or flutter, yet complete AV block is recognized by a slow, regular ventricular response (response is usually less than 60 beats per minute). The QRS complex may be normal if the escape focus is from above the bifurcation of the bundle branches.

Management

Pacemaker insertion is the definitive treatment for symptomatic third-degree AV block and is also the treatment for asymptomatic third-degree heart block with bundle branch block. Initial prehospital care includes consideration of atropine (but with consideration of its limitations discussed elsewhere in this chapter) or transcutaneous cardiac pacing if possible. Other indicated drugs (outside current UK paramedic practice) might include adrenaline (epinephrine), isoprenaline, dopamine or aminophylline; if the bradycardia is due to calcium channel or beta-blocker overdose, glucagon might be considered.

Transcutaneous cardiac pacing is a key intervention for all symptomatic bradycardias and should be applied as soon as possible if the patient's condition is unstable (see Figure 15-39). Atropine (a parasympatholytic) is unlikely to help patients with complete heart block. The vagus nerve innervates the atria, and the focus controlling the heart in a third-degree block is most often in the ventricles; atropine will likely have no effect on the ventricular rate.

Critical Thinking

What should you tell the patient before initiating transcutaneous cardiac pacing?

Ventricular conduction disturbances

Ventricular conduction disturbances (bundle branch blocks and hemiblocks) are delays or interruptions in the transmission of electrical impulses. These disturbances occur below the level of bifurcation of the bundle of His. Identifying these blocks is important as it helps to identify the patient who is at an increased risk of severe bradycardia and third-degree heart block and is especially true when the patient has other forms of AV block. Common causes of bundle branch block include the following:

- acute heart failure
- acute myocardial infarction
- aortic stenosis
- cardiomyopathy
- hyperkalaemia
- infection (e.g. carditis)
- ischaemic heart disease
- trauma.

Bundle branch anatomy

To review, the bundle of His begins at the AV node and divides to form the left and right bundle branches (Figure 15-79). The right bundle branch continues toward the apex and spreads throughout the right ventricle. The left bundle branch subdivides into the anterior and posterior fascicles and spreads throughout the left ventricle. Conduction of electrical impulses through the Purkinje fibres stimulates the ventricles to contract.

With normal conduction, the first part of the ventricle to be stimulated is the left side of the septum, and then the electrical impulse traverses the septum to stimulate the other side. Shortly thereafter, the left and right ventricles at the same time are stimulated. The left ventricle is normally much larger and thicker than the right ventricle so the electrical activity predominates over that of the right ventricle.

Common electrocardiogram findings

When an electrical impulse is blocked from passing through the right or left bundle branch, one ventricle depolarizes and contracts before the other; ventricular activation no longer occurs at the same time and the QRS complex widens (often with a slurred or notched appearance known as 'rabbit ears'). The hallmark of bundle branch block is a QRS complex that is equal to or greater than 0.12 s. The two criteria for bundle branch block recognition are as follows:

- a QRS complex equal to or greater than 0.12 s
- QRS complexes produced by supraventricular activity.

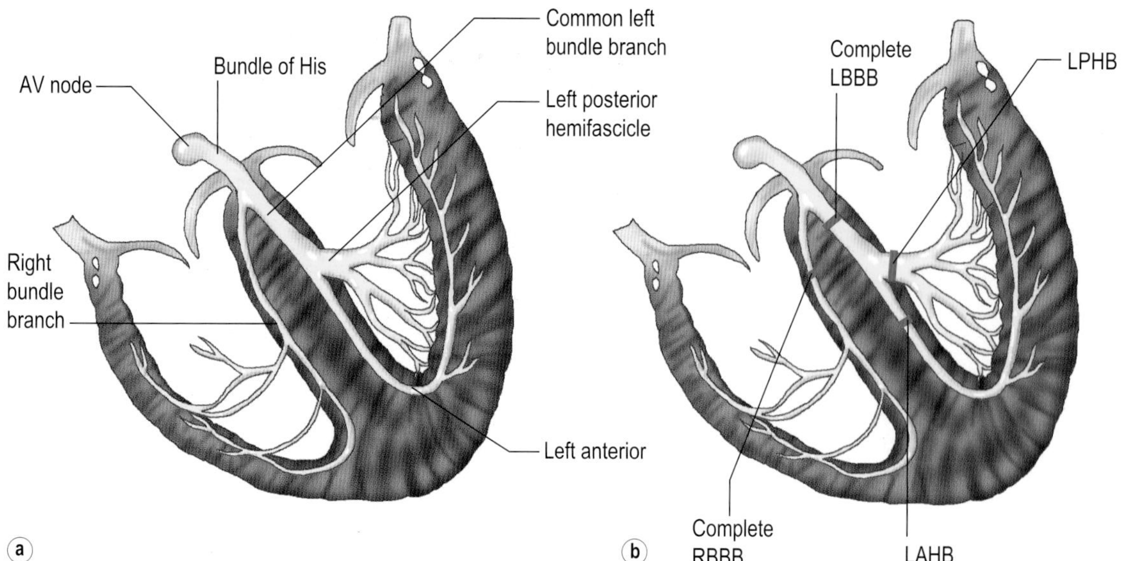

Figure 15-79 (a) Simplified illustration showing the major divisions of the ventricular conduction system. After passing through the AV node and the bundle of His, the electrical impulse is carried to the right and common left bundle branches. The latter structure divides into the left anterior and posterior hemifascicles. (b) Possible sites of block and the conduction deficits that may be produced.

> **Note**
>
> Bundle branch block and hemiblock (fascicular block) are terms used to describe abnormal conduction of impulses from above the bundle branches to the ventricles. These patterns of abnormal or aberrant conduction must be recognized as different from beats of ventricular origin. Beats of ventricular origin can have similar QRS complex shapes.

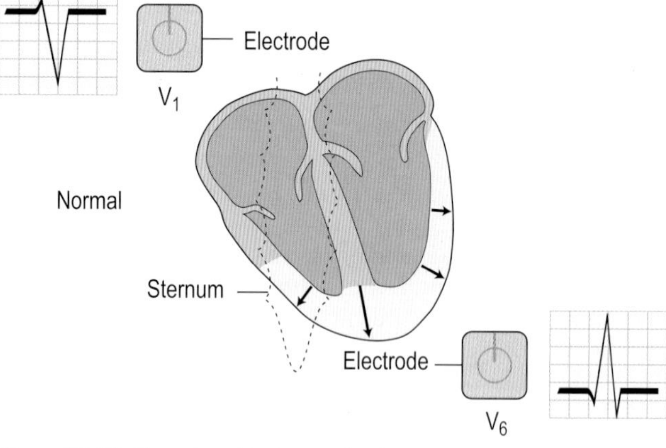

Figure 15-80 Normal ventricular conduction.

Ventricular conduction disturbances are identified best by monitoring leads V_1 and V_6. These leads permit the easiest differentiation of the right and left bundle branch blocks. For electrocardiogram evaluation the paramedic should ensure that the electrodes are placed properly for leads I, II, and III. Lead V_1 looks at right and left bundle branches and should be monitored during transport of these patients.

Normal conduction

In normal ventricular stimulation the electrical impulse reaches the septum first, then travels from the left endocardium to the right endocardium of the septum (Figure 15-80). This impulse generates a small R wave in V_1. The rest of the impulses are conducted mainly away from the V_1 electrode. This yields a negative deflection; during normal conduction, V_1 mainly is negative. The QRS complex usually is 0.08–0.12 s wide (the same as any other narrow QRS complex).

Right bundle branch block

In right bundle branch block the left bundle branch performs normally and activates the left side of the heart before the right (Figure 15-81). When the left ventricle is initially

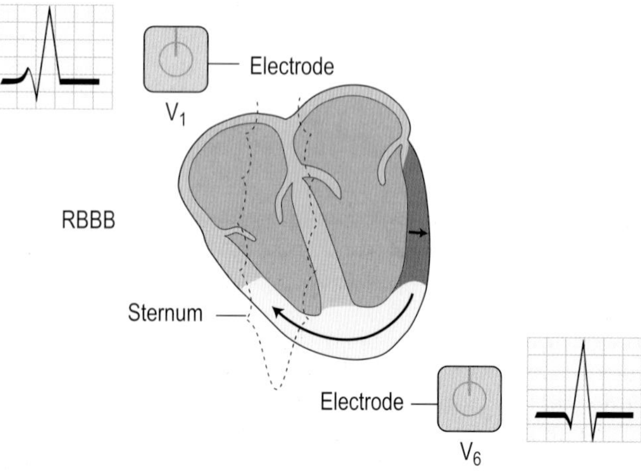

Figure 15-81 Right bundle branch block.

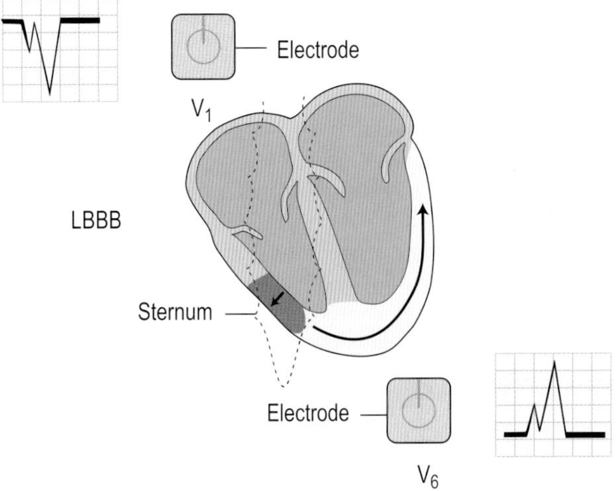

Figure 15-82 Left bundle branch block.

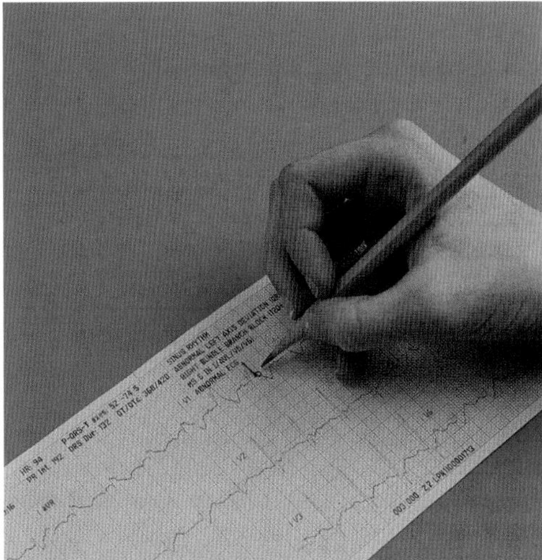

Figure 15-83 To distinguish left from right bundle branch blocks, find the J point of the QRS complex, draw a line backward into the QRS complex, and fill in the triangle created by this line and the last portion of the QRS complex. The direction the triangle points distinguishes the two types of blocks.

activated, the impulse travels away from the V_1 electrode, yielding a negative deflection (S wave). The electrical impulse then travels across the interventricular septum and activates the right ventricle. Because the impulse is coming back toward the V_1 electrode, a large positive deflection (R wave) occurs. This results in the RSR′ pattern seen in V_1 in patients with right bundle branch block. The QRS (or in this case, RSR) complex is at least 0.12 s. Whenever the two criteria for bundle branch block are met and V_1 displays an RSR′ pattern, right bundle branch block should be suspected.

Left bundle branch block

In the more serious left bundle branch block, the fibres that usually stimulate the interventricular septum are blocked, which alters normal septal activation and sends it in the opposite direction (Figure 15-82). This yields an initial Q wave in V_1 instead of the normal small R wave. The right ventricle then is activated, producing a positive deflection R wave in V_1; this impulse travels across the interventricular septum to the left ventricle. Because the impulse is leading away from V_1, the lead shows a deep, wide S wave (QS pattern) (Figure 15-83). As with right bundle branch block, the activation takes at least 0.12 s. Whenever the two criteria for bundle branch block are met and a QS pattern is seen in V_1, a left bundle branch block should be suspected (Box 15-7). Patients with new left bundle branch block have lost a lot of myocardium; left ventricular failure may develop and may lead to death.

Anterior hemiblock

Anterior hemiblocks (anterior hemifascicular blocks) occur more often than posterior hemiblocks (posterior hemifascicular blocks). The anterior fascicle of the left bundle branch is a longer and thinner structure and its blood supply comes mainly from the left anterior descending coronary artery. Anterior hemiblock is characterized by left axis deviation in a patient who has a supraventricular rhythm (Figure 15-84). Other electrocardiogram findings associated with an anterior hemiblock include a normal QRS complex (less than 0.12 s) or a right bundle branch block, a small Q wave followed by a tall R wave in lead I, and a small R wave followed by a deep S wave in lead III. In a patient who has an anterior hemiblock with a right bundle branch block, impulses can be conducted only through the ventricles by way of the posterior fascicle of the left bundle branch. These patients are at high risk of developing complete heart block.

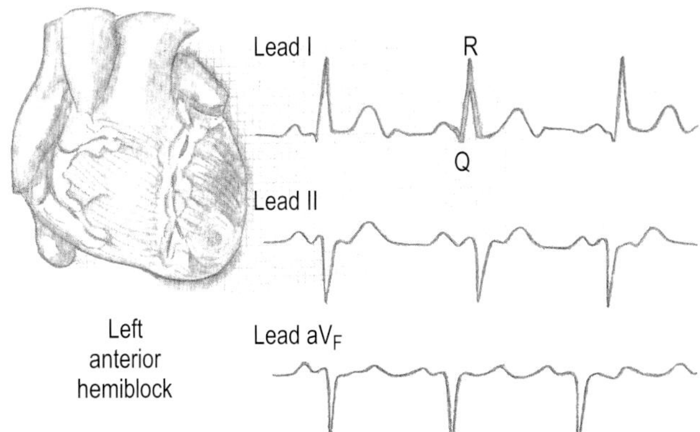

Figure 15-84 Anterior hemiblock.

Box 15-7

Determining right or left bundle branch block

When lead MCL_1 is monitored, the bundle branch block may be determined by the following procedure (see also Figure 15-83).

1. Find a QRS complex that is at least 0.12 s wide.
2. Count backward three small boxes from the beginning of the QRS and move straight up to see the J point.
3. Draw a line backward from the J point into the QRS complex.
4. Fill in the triangle that is created by this line and the last portion of the QRS complex.
5. If the triangle points up, it is a right bundle branch block.
6. If the triangle points down, it is a left bundle branch block.

Critical Thinking

What rhythms are produced by supraventricular activity?

Posterior hemiblock

The posterior fascicle of the left bundle branch is not blocked as easily as the anterior fascicle. As a result, posterior hemiblock occurs less often. Posterior hemiblock is identified by right axis deviation with a normal QRS complex or a right bundle branch block (Figure 15-85). A diagnosis of posterior hemiblock requires excluding right ventricular hypertrophy. This is difficult to do in the prehospital setting, if not impossible. For practical purposes, posterior hemiblock can be assumed in patients with right axis deviation and a QRS complex of normal width or with a right bundle branch block. (Other electrocardiogram findings that indicate the presence of a posterior hemiblock include a small R wave followed by a deep S wave in lead I and a small Q wave followed by a tall R wave in lead III.)

Bifascicular block

Bifascicular block refers to the blockage of two of three pathways for ventricular conduction; this condition occurs with right bundle branch block with anterior or posterior hemiblock and in left bundle branch block. Bifascicular block decreases myocardial contractility and cardiac output. Patients with this condition may develop complete heart block suddenly and without warning. As a rule, the more branches that have impaired conduction, the greater the chance a patient will develop complete AV block (especially in patients with acute myocardial infarction).

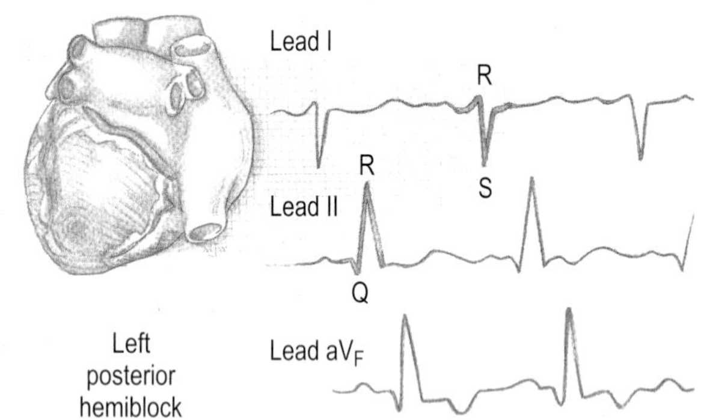

Figure 15-85 Posterior hemiblock.

Multilead determination of the axis and hemiblocks

The axis is the direction of impulse flow in the heart that stimulates contraction. Identifying the axis can be useful in determining the presence of hemiblocks. They are evaluated best by looking at the QRS complexes in leads I, II, and III. The axis is considered normal when the QRS deflection is positive (upright) in all bipolar leads; physiological left (which may be normal in some patients) when the QRS deflection is positive in leads I and II but negative (inverted) in lead III; pathological left when the QRS deflection is positive in lead I and negative in leads II and III (indicating an anterior hemiblock); right axis when the QRS deflection is negative in lead I, negative or positive in lead II, and positive in lead III (pathological in any adult and indicative of a posterior hemiblock); and extreme right ('no man's land') when the QRS deflection is negative in all three leads (indicating that the rhythm is ventricular in origin) (Table 15-2).

Management of bundle branch blocks and hemiblocks

No specific treatment is necessary for bundle branch blocks or hemiblocks. However, if other conditions (e.g. hypoxia, ischaemia, electrolyte imbalance or drug toxicity) are causing a block, these conditions should be treated. Some emergency medications administered to patients with cardiac disease (e.g. procainamide, digoxin, and verapamil or diltiazem) can slow electrical impulse conduction through the AV node. Those at such risk include the following:

- any patient with type II AV block
- any patient with evidence of disease in both bundle branches
- any patient with two or more blocks of any kind (e.g. prolonged P-R interval and anterior hemiblock, right bundle branch block and anterior hemiblock, type I AV block, and left bundle branch block).

Prehospital care for these patients should include management of any accompanying signs and symptoms, transport, constant electrocardiogram monitoring, and anticipation of the possible need for external pacing. Emergency pacing has been recommended for the following four indications:

1. Hemodynamically compromising bradycardias.
2. Bradycardias with malignant escape rhythms unresponsive to pharmacological therapy.

Table 15-2 Identifying axis by QRS complex

	QRS Complex			
Axis	**Lead I**	**Lead II**	**Lead III**	**Indications**
Normal	Upright	Upright	Upright	May be normal
Physiological left	Upright	Upright	Inverted	May be normal
Pathological left	Upright	Inverted	Inverted	Anterior hemiblock
Right axis	Inverted	Inverted or upright	Upright	Posterior hemiblock
Extreme right	Inverted	Inverted	Inverted	Ventricular in origin

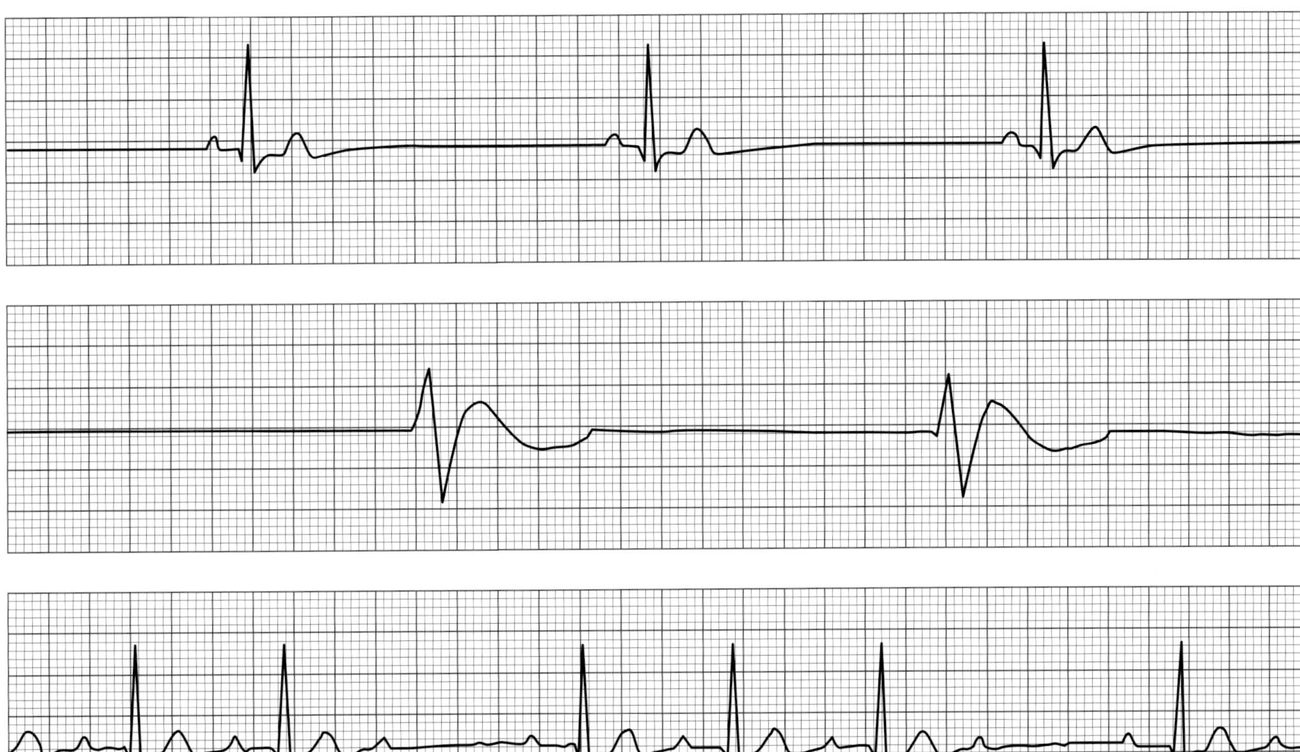

Figure 15-86 Various pulseless electrical activity rhythms as seen in lead II.

3. Overdrive pacing of refractory supraventricular or ventricular tachycardia unresponsive to pharmacological therapy or cardioversion.
4. Bradyasystolic cardiac arrest (in rare situations).

Considerations should be given to pacing readiness in the setting of acute myocardial infarction for patients with symptomatic sinus node dysfunction; type II second-degree AV block; third-degree heart block; or newly acquired left, right, or alternating bundle branch block or bifascicular block.[1]

Pulseless electrical activity

The term pulseless electrical activity (Figure 15-86) is defined as the absence of a detectable pulse and the presence of some type of electrical activity other than ventricular tachycardia or ventricular fibrillation. The outcome of pulseless electrical activity almost always is poor; that is, unless an underlying cause can be identified and corrected. The paramedic must maintain circulation for the patient with basic and advanced life support techniques while searching for a correctable cause.

Critical Thinking

What rhythms might you see on the monitor when a patient is in pulseless electrical activity?

Correctable causes of pulseless electrical activity are cardiac tamponade, tension pneumothorax, hypoxaemia, acidosis, hyperkalaemia, hypothermia and overdoses of, for example, tricyclic antidepressants, beta-blockers and digitalis. Other less correctable causes include massive myocardial damage from infarction, prolonged ischaemia during resuscitation, profound hypovolaemia, and massive pulmonary embolism. Patients in profound shock of any type (including anaphylactic, septic, neurogenic and hypovolaemic) may have pulseless electrical activity. The paramedic should manage tension pneumothorax with needle decompression. If the patient is hypoxic, the paramedic should manage the patient by good airway management, improving oxygenation and ventilation. If acute hypovolaemia is present (because of haemorrhage), the paramedic should begin fluid resuscitation. The paramedic should manage acidosis by ensuring adequate cardiopulmonary resuscitation and hyperventilation. Calcium is a specific therapy (not in current UK paramedic practice) for hyperkalaemia and calcium channel blocker toxicity. Both of these conditions can produce pulseless electrical activity. Besides calcium channel blockers, other drugs when taken in toxic amounts can produce wide-complex pulseless electrical activity. These overdoses can be managed with specific therapy, which may be effective in re-establishing a perfusing rhythm (see Figure 15-54).

Critical Thinking

What patient care measures should you take in this case?

Pre-excitation syndromes

Pre-excitation syndrome (anomalous or accelerated AV conduction) is associated with an abnormal conduction pathway between the atria and ventricles. This pathway bypasses the AV node, bundle of His, or both, allowing the electrical impulses to initiate depolarization of the ventricles earlier than usual. The most common pre-excitation syndrome is Wolff–Parkinson–White syndrome.

Wolff–Parkinson–White syndrome

Description

In some hearts, an accessory muscle bundle (known as the bundle of Kent or the Kent fibres) connects the lateral wall of the atrium and the ventricle, bypassing the AV node. This produces an early activation of the ventricle (Wolff–Parkinson–White syndrome). Wolff–Parkinson–White syndrome is thought to be of minor clinical significance; that is, unless a tachycardia is present, in which case the syndrome can become life threatening.

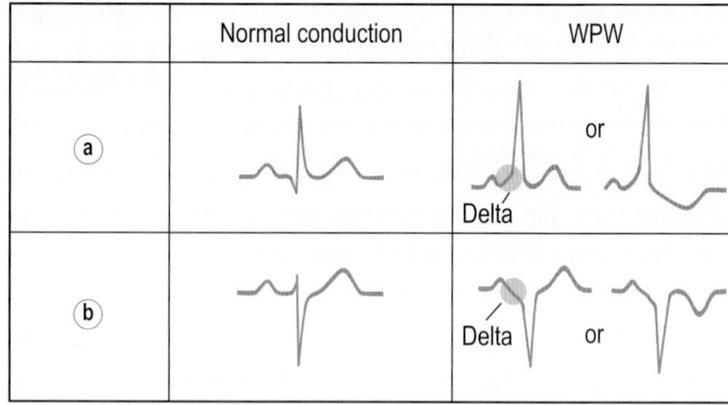

Figure 15-87 Characteristic findings in Wolff–Parkinson–White syndrome (short P-R interval, QRS widening, and delta wave) compared with normal conduction. (a) Usual appearance of Wolff–Parkinson–White syndrome in leads where the QRS complex is predominantly upright. (b) Appearance of Wolff–Parkinson–White syndrome; the QRS complex is predominantly negative.

Aetiology

Wolff–Parkinson–White syndrome may occur in young, healthy persons (mainly men) without apparent cause. The syndrome also may occur in multiple members of a family and it may be present in successive generations.

Rules for interpretation (lead II monitoring)

Wolff–Parkinson–White syndrome has the following characteristics on the electrocardiogram:

QRS complex: May be normal or wide (depending on whether conduction is retrograde or anterograde along the bundle of Kent). Conduction that occurs normally down the AV node and simultaneously in an anterograde fashion along the accessory pathway results in a meeting of the two waves or depolarization that forms a fusion (delta wave). A delta wave is evidenced by slurring or notching of the onset of the QRS complex and is a diagnostic finding in Wolff–Parkinson–White syndrome. Not all leads show the delta wave. One should note that QRS widening may simulate right or left bundle branch block.

P waves: Normal.

Rate: Normal unless associated with rapid supraventricular tachycardia.

Rhythm: Regular.

P-R interval: Usually less than 0.12 s because the normal delay at the AV node does not occur.

The three characteristic electrocardiogram findings in Wolff–Parkinson–White syndrome are a short P-R interval, a delta wave and QRS widening (Figure 15-87).

Clinical significance

Patients with Wolff–Parkinson–White syndrome are highly susceptible to bouts of paroxysmal supraventricular tachycardia, due to the accessory pathway providing a ready-made re-entry circuit, allowing continued transmission of the impulse from the atria to the ventricles. The majority of tachydysrhythmias seen in Wolff–Parkinson–White syndrome occur with the wave of depolarization progressing from the AV node to the bundle of His to the accessory pathway. In the accessory pathway the impulse is conducted in a retrograde direction to the atria; therefore the majority of tachydysrhythmias seen in Wolff–Parkinson–White syndrome are narrow complexes. Patients with Wolff–Parkinson–White syndrome may have attacks of paroxysmal tachydysrhythmias for many years. However, these attacks are not always benign. The AV node may be bypassed. Conduction rates also can greatly exceed those in patients whose AV node is part of the re-entry circuit, leading to rapid tachycardias and may precipitate congestive heart failure and even death from ventricular fibrillation.

Management

Recognition of Wolff–Parkinson–White syndrome is crucial. Differentiating the syndrome from ventricular tachycardia and uncomplicated supraventricular tachycardia is key; many emergency drugs used to manage other re-entry tachycardias are contraindicated in Wolff–Parkinson–White syndrome. AV nodal blocking agents such as adenosine, calcium channel blockers, digoxin, and possibly beta-blockers, should not be administered. These drugs can cause a paradoxical increase in the ventricular response to the rapid atrial impulses of atrial fibrillation. Management must be based on the patient's signs and symptoms; if the patient's heart rate is normal, no emergency care is required. If the patient has a rapid tachycardia, emergency treatment to restore normal rhythm is needed and is aimed at blocking conduction through the accessory pathways from the atria to the ventricle.

Prehospital care may include pharmacological therapy for specific dysrhythmias, vagal manoeuvres, and cardioversion (if authorized) for severe clinical deterioration. Verapamil and diltiazem are contraindicated in wide-QRS complex tachycardia because these drugs can speed conduction down the accessory pathway (greater than 280 beats per minute), which may lead to ventricular fibrillation and sudden death. Therefore, in patients with wide-QRS complex tachycardia, the drug treatment depends on signs and symptoms and their severity.

Drug therapy such as amiodarone and the use of cardioversion in unstable patients is likely to be considered.

SECTION VII

Specific cardiovascular diseases

Pathophysiology and management of cardiovascular disease

Many true medical emergencies are cardiovascular in nature. Cardiovascular emergencies often result from atherosclerosis of the coronary arteries or peripheral arteries. The following specific medical conditions are discussed in this section:

- acute coronary syndromes
- atherosclerosis
- angina pectoris
- myocardial infarction
- left ventricular failure and pulmonary oedema
- right ventricular failure
- cardiogenic shock
- cardiac tamponade
- thoracic and abdominal aneurysm
- acute arterial occlusion
- non-critical peripheral vascular disorders
- hypertension.

Acute coronary syndromes

Acute myocardial infarction and unstable angina are part of a spectrum of clinical disease, collectively known as acute coronary syndromes (ACS) which is the most common cause of sudden cardiac death. The pathophysiology of both conditions is a ruptured or eroded atheromatous plaque. ECG findings that are common to ACS include ST segment elevation, ST segment depression, and T wave abnormalities (described later in this chapter). As with other life-threatening conditions, time is of the essence in managing these patients. Primary goals of therapy for patients with ACS include the following:

- Reduce the amount of myocardial necrosis that occurs in patients with myocardial infarction, preserving left ventricular function, and preventing heart failure.
- Prevent major adverse cardiac events: death, non-fatal myocardial infarction, and the need for urgent revascularization.
- Treat acute, life-threatening complications of ACS, such as ventricular fibrillation, pulseless ventricular tachycardia, symptomatic bradycardias and unstable tachycardias.

Pathophysiology of atherosclerosis

Atherosclerosis is a disease process characterized by progressive narrowing of the lumen of medium and large arteries (e.g. the aorta and its branches, cerebral arteries, and coronary arteries). The process results in the development of thick, hard atherosclerotic plaque, referred to as atheromata or atheromatous lesions. These lesions are found most often in areas of turbulent blood flow including vessel bifurcations or in vessels with decreased lumen diameter.

Atherosclerosis is thought to result from damage to the endothelial cell from mechanical or chemical injury and perhaps excess inflammation (Box 15-8). This response includes platelet adhesion and clotting. Smooth muscle cells may move from the middle muscle layer into the lining of the artery, and in the lining the muscle cells form an atheroma. Over time, the atheromata become fibrous and hardened and then eventually partially or fully obstruct the opening of the arteries. In most cases, some collateral circulation develops to make up for the narrowed vessels.

Major risk factors

Atherosclerosis occurs to some extent in all middle-aged and older persons but the disease occurs in some young persons as well. Atherosclerosis is thought to have a hereditary tendency and is usually seen at a younger age in men than in women. Associated risk factors include age, family history of heart disease, and diabetes. Some other risk factors (modifiable risk factors) can be reduced or eliminated and include cigarette smoking, lack of physical exercise, obesity, hypertension and hypercholesterolaemia; in fact, evidence suggests that plaque formation is not only preventable but also reversible.

Effects

Atherosclerosis has two major effects on blood vessels and it is worth remembering that these effects can be found in other arteries not just the coronary arteries. First, the disease disrupts the innermost lining of the vessels, causing a loss of vessel elasticity and an increase in the formation of clots. Second, the atheroma reduces the diameter of the vessel lumen, decreasing the blood supply to tissues. Both effects result in an insufficient supply of nutrients to the tissue, which is especially true under conditions of increased tissue demand for nutrients and oxygen.

The severity of this insufficiency is related to the extent of narrowing (stenosis) of the blocked artery as well as how long the atheroma took to develop, and the patient's ability to develop collateral circulation around the obstruction. For example, a patient who gradually develops an atherosclerotic occlusion in an artery of a lower extremity may compensate well through collateral circulation and experience only mild, intermittent pain during periods of exercise. In contrast, sudden-onset occlusion in a coronary artery

Box 15-8

Role of inflammation in heart attacks

Studies have suggested that painless inflammation deep within the body plays an important role in the trigger of heart attacks. The inflammation may arise from sources such as chronic gum disease, lingering urinary tract infections, and others. Inflammation may weaken the walls of the blood vessels, allowing fatty build-ups to burst. Inflammation can be measured in those at risk for heart disease by testing the blood for elevated white blood cell count and for C-reactive protein. This is a chemical in the blood that is necessary for fighting injury and infection. C-reactive protein can be lowered with cholesterol-lowering drugs, aspirin, and other medications and through diet and exercise.

(following an acute thrombus) almost always results in ischaemia, injury, and necrosis to the area of the myocardium supplied by the affected artery.

Angina pectoris

Angina pectoris is a symptom of myocardial ischaemia; the term literally means 'choking pain in the chest'. Angina is caused by an imbalance between myocardial oxygen supply and demand. The result is a build-up of lactic acid and carbon dioxide in ischaemic tissues of the myocardium; these metabolites irritate nerve endings that produce anginal pain. The most common cause of angina pectoris is atherosclerotic disease of the coronary arteries. A temporary occlusion caused by spasm of a coronary artery with or without atherosclerosis (Prinzmetal's angina) also can cause angina pectoris. Emotional stress and any activity that increases myocardial oxygen demand may cause anginal pain, particularly in patients with atherosclerosis. Myocardial ischaemia in turn may put the patient at risk for cardiac dysrhythmias.

Note

Several conditions can mimic signs and symptoms of heart disease and angina pectoris. These include cholecystitis, peptic ulcer disease, aneurysm, hiatal hernia, pulmonary embolism, pancreatitis, pleural irritation and respiratory infection (Box 15-9).

Stable angina

Angina pectoris generally is classified as stable or unstable. Stable angina usually is precipitated by physical exertion, cold weather, a large meal or emotional stress, with pain lasting 1–5 min but in some circumstances up to 15 min. Angina is relieved by rest, GTN or oxygen. Stable angina attacks usually are similar and are always relieved by the same mode of therapy.

Box 15-9

Other conditions that may mimic angina pectoris

- Acromioclavicular disease
- Chest wall syndrome
- Chest wall trauma
- Chest wall tumours
- Cholecystitis
- Costochondritis
- Dyspepsia
- Oesophageal disease
- Gastric reflux
- Herpes zoster
- Hiatal hernia
- Pancreatitis
- Peptic ulcer disease
- Pleural irritation
- Pneumothorax
- Pulmonary embolism
- Respiratory infection
- Thoracic aortic dissection

Unstable angina

Unstable angina (preinfarction angina) denotes an anginal pattern that has changed in its ease of onset, frequency, intensity, duration or quality. (This includes any new-onset anginal chest pain.) Unstable angina may occur during periods of light exercise or at rest. The pain usually lasts 10 min or more and is relieved less promptly with cessation of activity or GTN than is stable angina. Unstable angina mimics acute myocardial infarction and these are sometimes difficult to differentiate in the prehospital setting. Patients with unstable angina are at increased risk of acute myocardial infarction and sudden death.

The pain of angina usually is described by the patient as a pressure, squeezing, heaviness or tightness in the chest. Although 30% of patients with angina feel pain only in the chest, others describe the pain as radiating to the shoulders, arms, neck and jaw and through the chest to the back. Associated signs and symptoms include anxiety, shortness of breath, nausea or vomiting and diaphoresis. The patient history often reveals previous attacks of angina and often the patient will have taken GTN before arrival of emergency medical services. If so, the paramedic should determine the age of the GTN prescription (GTN is unstable and quickly loses its strength), the amount of GTN taken, and its effect. If the pain is not relieved by rest and medication, the paramedic should suspect a myocardial infarction.

Management

All patients with chest pain and signs and symptoms of myocardial ischaemia should be managed as though an acute myocardial infarction were evolving (Table 15-3). The goal of management is to increase the coronary blood supply, decrease the myocardial oxygen demand, or both. Management guidelines include the following:

1. Place the patient at rest physically and emotionally.
2. Administer oxygen.
3. Administer aspirin.
4. Initiate intravenous therapy for any drugs that may be needed.
5. If pain is present on arrival of emergency medical services, use pharmacological therapy. This may include sublingual or topical GTN followed by morphine.
6. Monitor the electrocardiogram for dysrhythmias. Whenever possible (and if scene time is not delayed), record a 3-lead or 12-lead electrocardiogram, or both, during pain. (The electrocardiogram may be normal during a pain-free period.) Also measure, record, and communicate any ST segment changes.
7. Transport the patient for further evaluation.

Myocardial infarction

Acute myocardial infarction occurs with a sudden and total blockage or near blockage of blood flowing through an affected coronary artery to an area of heart muscle, resulting in ischaemia, injury, and necrosis to the area of the myocardium distal to the occlusion. Acute myocardial infarction most often is associated with atherosclerotic heart disease.

Table 15-3 Likelihood of ischaemic aetiology and short-term risk

Part I: Chest pain patients without ST-segment elevation: likelihood of ischaemic aetiology

	A. High likelihood: High likelihood that chest pain is of ischaemic aetiology if patient has *any* of the findings in the column below:	**B. Intermediate likelihood: Intermediate likelihood that chest pain is of ischaemic aetiology if patient has NO findings in column A and *any* of the findings in the column below:**	**C. Low likelihood: Low likelihood that chest pain is of ischaemic aetiology if patient has NO findings in column A or B. Patients may have any of the findings in the column below:**
History	• Chief symptom is chest or left arm pain or discomfort *plus* Current pain reproduces pain of prior documented angina *and* Known CAD including MI	• Chief symptom is chest or left arm pain or discomfort • Diabetes mellitus	• Probably ischaemic symptoms • Recent cocaine use • Age 70 years • Male sex
Physical exam	• Transient mitral regurgitation • Hypotension • Diaphoresis • Pulmonary oedema or rales	• Extracardiac vascular disease	• Chest discomfort reproduced by palpation
ECG	• New (or presumed new) transient ST deviation (≥0.5 mm) *or* T wave inversion (≥2 mm) with symptoms	• Fixed Q waves • T-wave flattening or T-wave inversion in leads with dominant R waves	• Normal ECG *or* Abnormal ST segments or T waves that are not new
Cardiac markers	• Elevated troponin I or T	Any finding in column B above *plus* • Elevated CK-MB	• Normal • Normal

Part II: Risk of death or non-fatal MI over the short term in patients with chest pain with high or intermediate likelihood of ischaemia (columns A and B in Part I)

	High risk: Risk is high if patient has *any* of the following findings:	**Intermediate risk: Risk is intermediate if patient has *any* of the following findings:**	**Low risk: Risk is low if patient has NO high- or intermediate-risk features; may have any of the following:**
History	• Accelerating tempo of ischaemic symptoms over prior 48 h	• Prior MI *or* • Cerebrovascular disease *or* • CABG, prior aspirin use	• Peripheral-artery disease *or* • New-onset functional angina (Class III or IV) in past 2 weeks without prolonged rest pain (but with moderate or high likelihood of CAD)
Character of pain	• Prolonged, continuing (>20 min) rest pain	• Prolonged (>20 min) rest angina is now resolved (moderate to high likelihood of CAD) • Rest angina (<20 min) or relieved by rest or sublingual nitrates	
Physical exam	• Pulmonary oedema secondary to ischaemia • New or worse mitral regurgitation murmur • Hypotension, bradycardia, tachycardia • S_3 gallop or new or worsening rales • Age >75 years	• Age >70 years	

Table 15-3 Likelihood of ischaemic aetiology and short-term risk—cont'd

Part II: Risk of death or non-fatal MI over the short term in patients with chest pain with high or intermediate likelihood of ischaemia (columns A and B in Part I)

	High risk: Risk is high if patient has *any* of the following findings:	**Intermediate risk: Risk is intermediate if patient has *any* of the following findings:**	**Low risk: Risk is low if patient has NO high- or intermediate-risk features; may have any of the following:**
ECG	• Transient ST-segment deviation (≥0.5 mm) with rest angina • New or presumably new bundle branch block • Sustained VT	• T-wave inversion ≥2 mm • Pathologic Q waves or T waves that are not new	• Normal or unchanged ECG during an episode of chest discomfort
Cardiac markers	• Elevated cardiac troponin I or T	Any of the above findings *plus* • Elevated CK-MB	• Normal • Normal

Modified from Braunwald et al 2002 Circulation 106:1893–1900.

Table 15-4 Localization of a myocardial infarction

Location of MI	**Indicative changes (leads facing affected area)**	**Reciprocal changes (leads opposite affected area)**	**Affected coronary artery**
Anterior	V_3, V_4	V_7, V_8, V_9	Left coronary artery
			• LAD: diagonal branch
Anteroseptal	V_1, V_2, V_3, V_4	V_7, V_8, V_9	Left coronary artery
			• LAD: diagonal branch
			• LAD: septal branch
Anterolateral	I, aV_L, V_3, V_4, V_5,	II, III, aV_F, V_7, V_8,	Left coronary artery
	V_6	V_9	• LAD: diagonal branch and/or
			• Circumflex branch
Inferior	II, III, aV_F	I, aV_L	Right coronary artery (most common): posterior descending branch or
			Left coronary artery: circumflex branch
Lateral	I, aV_L, V_5, V_6	II, III, aV_F	Left coronary artery
			• LAD: diagonal branch and/or
			• Circumflex branch
			Right coronary artery
Septum	V_1, V_2	V_7, V_8, V_9	Left coronary artery
			• LAD: septal branch
Posterior	V_7, V_8, V_9	V_1, V_2, V_3	Right coronary or left circumflex artery
Right ventricle	V_1R–V_6R	I, aV_L	Right coronary artery
			• Proximal branches

LAD, Left anterior descending.

Precipitating events

The process of myocardial infarction is complex. It generally begins with the formation of an atherosclerotic plaque involving the intimal layer of a coronary artery that disrupts the smooth arterial lining and results in an uneven surface. This creates turbulent blood flow. The plaque may rupture causing injured tissue to be exposed to circulating platelets. This results in the formation of a thrombus that occludes the artery, and as the thrombus enlarges, it further reduces blood flow in the coronary vessel.

Acute thrombotic occlusion is generally accepted as the cause of most myocardial infarctions. Other factors that may lead to acute myocardial infarction include coronary spasm, coronary embolism, severe hypoxia, haemorrhage into a diseased arterial wall, and reduced blood flow after any form of shock, all of which may result in an inadequate amount of blood reaching the myocardium.

Types and locations of infarcts

The myocardial cells beyond the occluded artery die (infarct) from lack of oxygen. The size of the infarct is determined by the needs of the tissue supplied by the occluded vessel, by the presence of collateral circulation, and by the time it takes to re-establish blood flow. Therefore emergency care is directed at the following:

- increasing oxygen supply by administering supplemental oxygen
- decreasing the metabolic needs and providing collateral circulation
- re-establishing perfusion to the ischaemic myocardium as quickly as possible after the onset of symptoms.

The majority of acute myocardial infarctions involve the left ventricle or interventricular septum, which are supplied by either of the two major coronary arteries, although some patients sustain damage to the right ventricle. If the occlusion is in the left coronary artery, the result is an anterior, lateral, or septal wall infarction. Inferior wall infarction (of the inferior-posterior wall of the left ventricle) is usually a result of right coronary artery occlusion (Table 15-4).

Infarction also can be classified into one of three ischaemic syndromes based on the rupture of an unstable plaque in an epicardial artery: unstable angina, non-Q wave myocardial infarction, and Q wave myocardial infarction. All three of these ACS share common risk factors and the management of each overlaps a good deal. Sudden cardiac death may occur with any of these syndromes. It is worth emphasizing that the current terminology of non-ST segment elevation myocardial infarction (NSTEMI) and ST segment elevation myocardial infarction (described later) do not correlate directly to non-Q wave and Q wave infarction as some non-Q wave infarctions present initially as STEMI. The key point is that STEMI and NSTEMI refer to the 12-lead ECG findings in the earlier stages of ischaemia and injury, whereas Q wave development reflects the end point of infarction when the use of fibrinolytics/thrombolytics may be much less effective

1. Unstable angina. In unstable angina the early thrombus has not obstructed coronary blood flow completely. This partial occlusion produces symptoms of ischaemia. The blockage eventually may result in complete occlusion and produce a non-Q wave myocardial infarction. Fibrinolytic therapy (described later in this chapter) is not effective in unstable angina. In fact, such therapy may accelerate the occlusion. Therapy with antiplatelet agents, however, is most effective at this time because the thrombus is rich in platelets.
2. Non-Q wave myocardial infarction. Non-Q wave myocardial infarction occurs as microemboli from the thrombus become lodged in the coronary arteries, producing minimal damage to the myocardium although these patients are at increased risk of progression to myocardial infarction. Non-Q wave infarcts are evident only with ST segment depression or T wave abnormalities.
3. Q wave myocardial infarction. A Q wave myocardial infarction occurs when the thrombus occludes the coronary vessel for a prolonged period and is diagnosed by the development of abnormal Q waves in two or more contiguous (adjacent) leads. (Abnormal Q waves are greater than 5 mm in depth or greater than 0.04 s in duration) (Figure 15-88). The clot is rich in thrombin and early management with fibrinolytics may help to limit the size of the infarct.

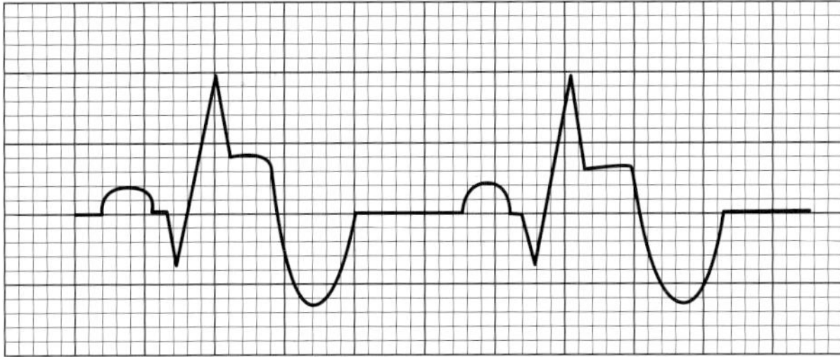

Figure 15-88 Pathological Q waves.

Death of myocardium

When blood flow to the myocardium ceases, a series of events begins. Cells switch from aerobic to anaerobic metabolism, resulting in the release of lactic acid and an increase in tissue carbon dioxide levels. These changes contribute to ischaemic pain (angina). As cells lose their ability to maintain their electrochemical gradients, they begin to swell and depolarize, and are considered to be injured. These initial changes are reversible, but within a few hours, if collateral flow and reperfusion are inadequate, much of the muscle distal to the occlusion dies (infarcted). The area surrounding the necrotic tissue may survive because of collateral circulation but this may become the origin of dysrhythmias (Figure 15-89).

Scar tissue replaces the infarcted area in a process that takes about 8 weeks. The process starts with deposits of connective tissue on about the twelfth day. Scar tissue is durable, but lacks elasticity, does not contract, and conducts electrical impulses poorly in the damaged area of the myocardium. The left ventricle, however, can lose as much as 25% of its muscle and still function as an effective pump. Areas with poor perfusion after a large myocardial infarction may not develop strong scar tissue and may result in an aneurysm. Such an aneurysm can greatly decrease the effective ventricular contractility or may lead to the development of serious dysrhythmias.

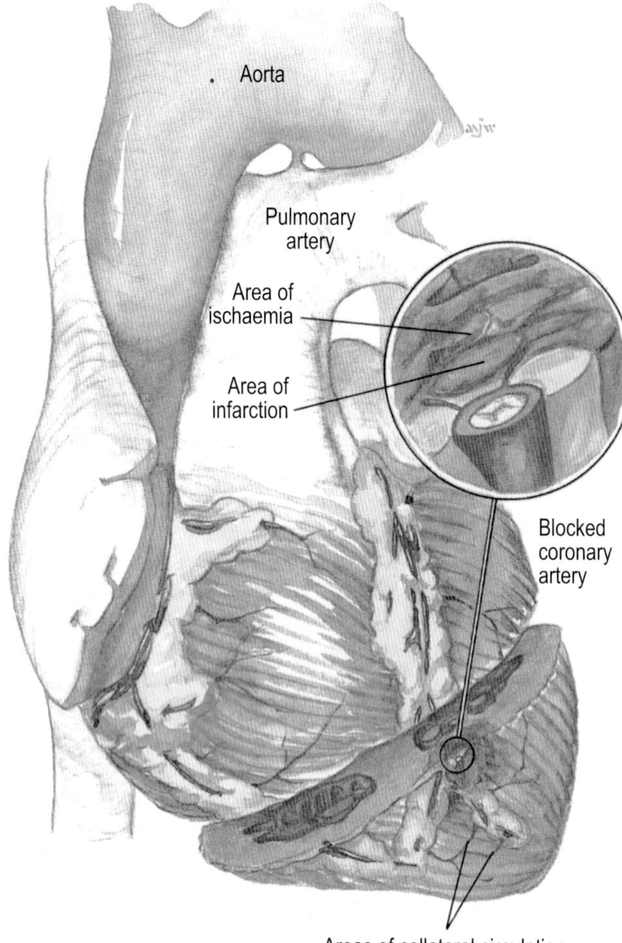

Figure 15-89 Area of infarct.

The damaged myocardium is most susceptible to rupture during the first 1 to 2 weeks after a myocardial infarction because the scar tissue has not reached adequate strength. For this reason, patient activity is limited and prevention of hypertension and excitement during this period also is usually necessary. Even so, the length of hospitalization of patients with uncomplicated myocardial infarctions has decreased; most patients resume activity within 2 to 3 days and leave the hospital within 7 to 10 days. Many patients get an exercise test before they are discharged which determines the patient's exercise tolerance level and whether ischaemia or dysrhythmias are present during exercise. The result of this test helps determine what activities the patient may resume after discharge.

Deaths following myocardial infarction

Deaths following myocardial infarction usually result from lethal dysrhythmias (ventricular tachycardia, ventricular fibrillation and cardiac standstill), pump failure (cardiogenic shock and congestive heart failure), or myocardial tissue rupture (rupture of the ventricle, septum or papillary muscle). Fatal dysrhythmias are the most common cause of death from myocardial infarction. Deaths that occur within the first 2 h after the onset of illness or injury are sudden deaths. The majority of patients who suffer sudden death have no immediate warning symptoms.

Note

Sudden death is defined as a sudden dysrhythmic death that occurs within the first 4 hours of cardiac ischaemic symptoms. More than 50% of cardiac deaths occur with no evidence of infarction on post mortem when resuscitation attempts fail. Sudden death without infarction is a main reason for the widespread availability of automated external defibrillators. (Another reason is the fact that the most common death-producing dysrhythmia is ventricular fibrillation.)

Signs and symptoms

Some patients with acute myocardial infarction – particularly diabetic patients, some women, and those in the older age groups – may have only symptoms of dyspnoea, syncope or confusion. However, substernal chest pain is present in 70–90% of patients with acute myocardial infarction. The pain generally has the same characteristics and locations as anginal pain and may radiate to the arms, neck, jaw or back. The following signs and symptoms may accompany the pain and occasionally are present even in the absence of pain (silent myocardial infarction):

- agitation
- anxiety
- cyanosis
- diaphoresis
- dyspnoea
- nausea and vomiting
- palpitations
- sense of impending doom.

Critical Thinking

How can the prehospital recognition of acute myocardial infarction affect the care of the patient at the hospital?

The chest pain associated with acute myocardial infarction is often constant and not altered or alleviated by GTN or other cardiac medications, rest, changes in body position or breathing patterns. With angina pectoris, the onset often occurs during periods of activity but by contrast, the onset of pain in more than half of all patients with acute myocardial infarction occurs during rest. Most patients have had warning anginal pains (pre-infarction angina) hours or days before the attack. Many patients deny the possibility of an evolving myocardial infarction and may blame the chest pain or discomfort on unrelated causes such as fatigue or indigestion. Denial delays the request for emergency medical services assistance during the most critical phase of the illness. Death from myocardial infarction occurs outside of hospital in up to a half of all cases, in the first few hours of symptom onset; these deaths are due mostly to dysrhythmias, predominantly ventricular fibrillation.

Critical Thinking

Why do you think patients deny that their signs and symptoms may be due to a heart attack?

Vital signs vary. They depend on the extent of damage to the heart muscle and conduction system and the degree and type of autonomic nervous system response. Inferior myocardial infarctions often show a mainly parasympathetic response. In contrast, anterior myocardial infarctions commonly show a mainly sympathetic response. For example, the patient's blood pressure may be normal, elevated (sympathetic discharge), or low (parasympathetic discharge or pump failure). The pulse rate depends on the presence or absence of dysrhythmias and may be normal, tachycardic, bradycardic, regular, or irregular. Respirations may be normal or increased.

Common electrocardiogram findings

When the heart muscle is damaged, the damaged area is unable to contract effectively. The area remains in a constant depolarized state. The flow of current between the pathologically depolarized and normally repolarized areas can produce ST segment elevation (Figure 15-90), ischaemic ST segment depression, or normal or non-diagnostic changes in the ST segment or T waves. Using these ECG findings can classify the patient into one of three groups:

1. ST segment elevation MI (STEMI): ST segment elevation or presumed new left bundle branch block is characterized by ST segment elevation greater than 1 mm (0.1 mV) in two or more contiguous precordial leads or two or more adjacent limb leads (some criteria require a minimum of 2 mm elevation in the precordial leads).
2. High-risk unstable angina/non-ST elevation myocardial infarction (NSTEMI): Ischaemic ST segment depression equal to or greater than 0.5 mm (0.05 mV) or dynamic T wave inversion with pain or discomfort. Non-persistent or transient ST segment elevation equal to or greater than 0.5 mm (0.05 mV) for more than 20 min is also included in this category.
3. Normal or non-diagnostic changes in ST segment or T wave: These findings are inconclusive. This classification includes patients with normal ECGs and those with ST segment deviation of less than 0.5 mm (0.05 mV) or T wave inversion less than or equal to 0.2 mV. Special cardiac studies and testing are needed for these patients.

ST segment elevation is best measured by drawing a baseline from the end of the T wave to the start of the P wave. ST segment elevation, however, is not always present on an initial ECG tracing; this is true even when a patient is experiencing a myocardial infarction. Therefore, it is important to repeat ECGs in symptomatic patients as ST segment changes may become apparent soon after. Whether ST segment elevation is present or not in a symptomatic patient presenting with signs of ACS, the paramedic should pre-alert the receiving unit and record (and if able transmit) an ECG for evaluation. Even if infarction is present, ST segment elevation is a poor indicator of whether the infarction will be Q wave or non-Q wave infarction. In addition, ST segment elevation can be caused by conditions other than acute myocardial infarction. These conditions include the following:

- left bundle branch block
- some ventricular rhythms
- left ventricular hypertrophy
- pericarditis
- ventricular aneurysm
- early repolarization.

Use of a 12-lead electrocardiogram to assess infarcts

Early recognition and management of acute myocardial infarction sometimes can salvage a damaged myocardium ('time is muscle'). Paramedics can play an important role in identifying these patients by using the five-step analysis for infarct recognition:[2]

Step 1: Identify the rate and rhythm. The recognition and management of life-threatening rhythms is more important than obtaining a 12-lead electrocardiogram monitoring for infarct location.

Step 2: Identify the area of infarct. ST segment elevation is the most reliable indicator during the first hours of infarction and can be present before serious tissue damage has occurred. If ST segment elevation is present in a patient with chest pain, the paramedic should identify the degree of elevation and visualize cardiac anatomy to predict which coronary artery is occluded. The paramedic should use a systematic approach for multilead assessment. One method is to begin by monitoring the inferior leads (II, III, aV_F), followed by septal leads (V_1, V_2), anterior leads (V_3, V_4), and lateral leads (V_5, V_6, I, aV_L). The paramedic then evaluates each lead for ST segment elevation (the most important sign of injury), deep symmetrically inverted T waves (a sign of ischaemia), ST segment depression (a reciprocal change to ST elevation), and pathological Q waves (Figure 15-91).

> **Note**
>
> Sulphonylurea drugs (diabetes drugs), such as glibenclamide or glipizide, may lessen the magnitude of ST segment elevation in the presence of an infarct.* Therefore a careful check of all patients with a cardiac event for a diabetic history is crucial.
>
> *Diabetes drugs can mask severity of heart attack, Reuters Health Sep 29, 2003.

At times, the extent of the infarction can be gauged by the number of leads showing ST segment elevation; the degree of ST segment elevation is also important. For example, large infarcts often show an ST elevation of 7 mm or more in inferior leads and an ST elevation of 12 mm or more in anterior leads. ST segment elevation or new or presumably new left bundle branch block is suspicious for injury. Also, consider the use of the 12 lead ECG to assess for right sided or posterior changes (Figure 15-92).

Step 3: When evaluating the electrocardiogram, the paramedic must consider other conditions that could be responsible for ST segment changes (as described before). These 'infarct impostors' also may be present in a patient who is experiencing acute myocardial infarction. With the exception of left bundle branch block (which makes the interpretation of myocardial infarction difficult), left ventricular hypertrophy looks

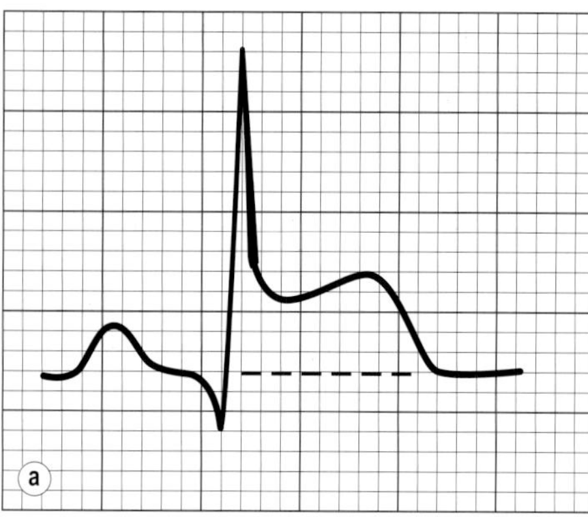

Tracking the evolution of a myocardial infarction

You can use your patient's electrocardiogram to track the progression of his myocardial infarction through five phases: the hyperacute phase, early acute phase, later acute phase, fully evolved phase, and healed phase.

Hyperacute phase

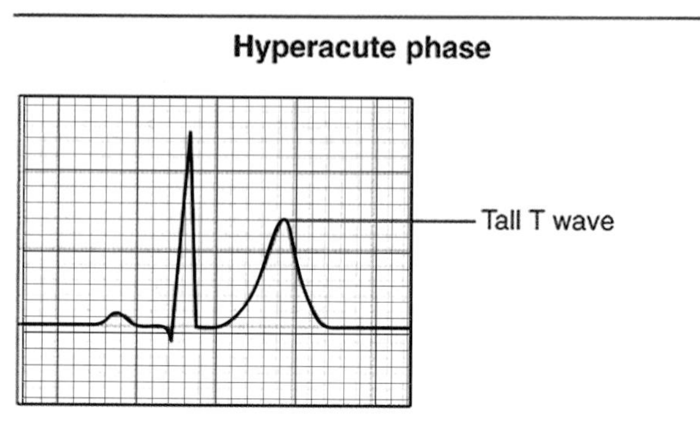

Early acute phase

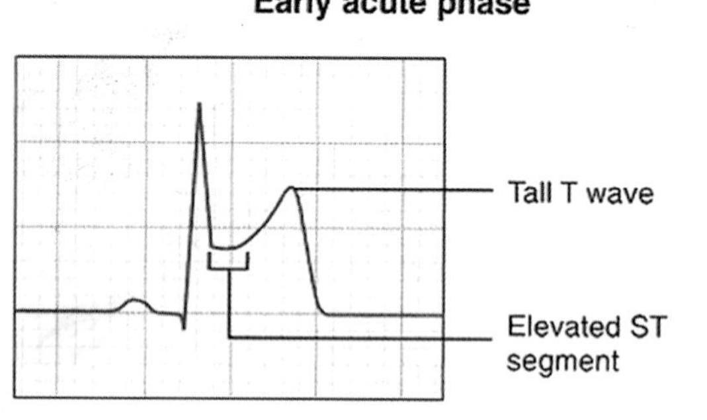

Later acute phase

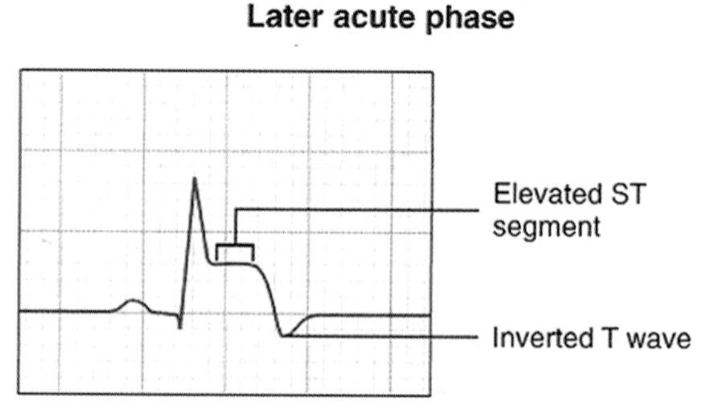

Fully evolved phase

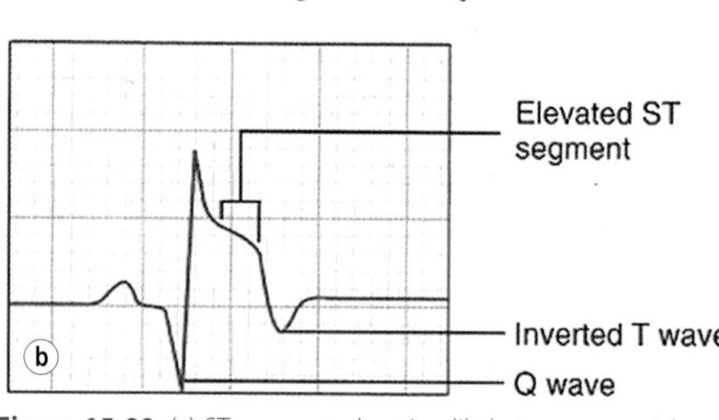

Healed phase

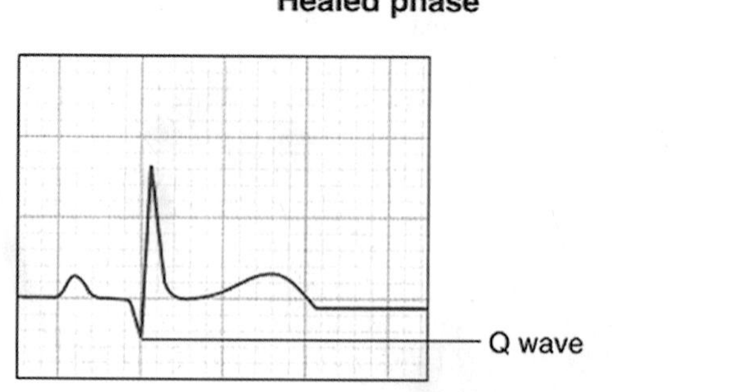

Figure 15-90 (a) ST segment elevation likely to present with acute injury. (b) From Phalen and Aehelert 2006 The 12 lead ECG in acute coronary syndromes, 2nd edition. Elsevier, Edinburgh.

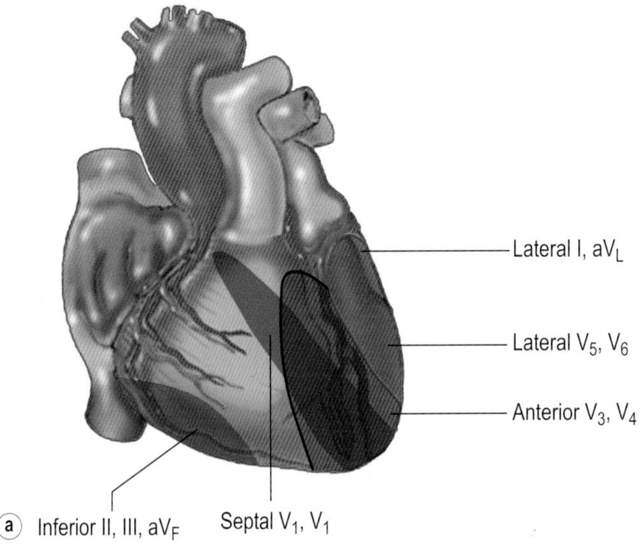

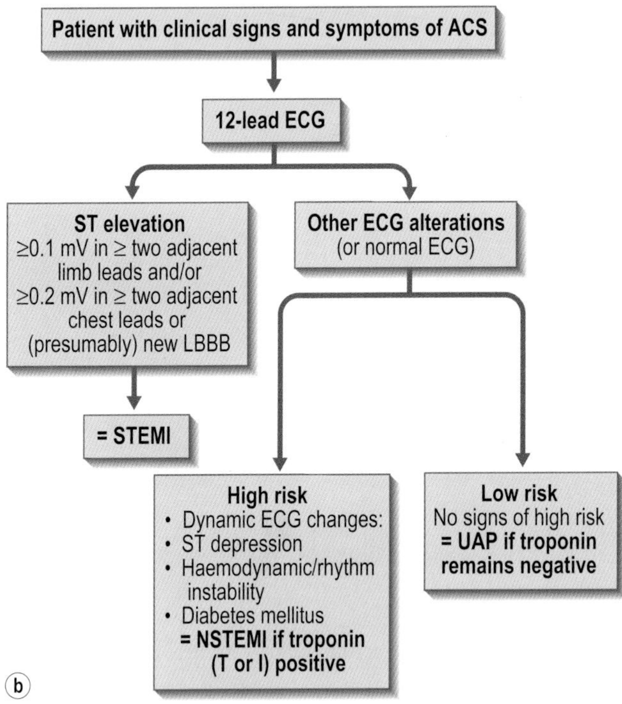

Figure 15-91 (a) Multilead assessment of the heart. (b) Classification of ACS. From Baskett and Nolan 2005 A pocket book of European Resuscitation Council Guidelines for Resuscitation 2005. Elsevier, Edinburgh, p 88.

less like an infarction. Ventricular rhythms often produce Q waves and ST segment elevation and will not have reciprocal ST depression. Electrocardiogram changes with pericarditis are subtle. In addition, early repolarization produces no clinical symptoms.

Step 4: Assess the patient's clinical presentation. An assessment of the clinical condition is just as crucial as the electrocardiogram findings and obtaining a thorough patient history and performing a physical examination should be incorporated into the electrocardiogram interpretation. Not all patients with acute myocardial infarction have classic signs and symptoms, so the paramedic should maintain a high degree of suspicion in the absence of pain; this should be the case especially with diabetic patients, older adults and postmenopausal women. A significant number of patients with acute myocardial infarction have no early electrocardiogram changes. The clinical picture is therefore important.

Step 5: Recognize the infarction and initiate care. When all indications point to acute myocardial infarction, the paramedic will need to take steps to speed the process of data collection, clinical evaluation, and thrombolysis (when appropriate) or percutaneous coronary intervention (PCI). This will help to reduce the time from infarct to treatment. Clinical presentation and electrocardiogram findings that suggest an acute myocardial infarction must be confirmed by medical direction to determine whether fibrinolytic therapy is appropriate.

Management of an uncomplicated acute myocardial infarction

All patients with anginal chest pain are assumed to have an acute myocardial infarction until proven otherwise (Figure 15-93). Any patient with chest pain should be transported to a medical facility for further evaluation; this is regardless of the apparent severity on emergency medical services arrival, the patient's age, or associated complaints. The primary goals of prehospital care are to relieve pain and apprehension, to prevent the development of serious dysrhythmias, and to limit the size of the infarct.

The paramedic should obtain a full patient history while conducting the physical examination and during initial patient care. Time is of the essence. Thus the following aspects of patient care are a high priority:

1. Place the patient at rest or in a comfortable position. This will help to decrease anxiety and the heart rate. Thus it will decrease oxygen demand.
2. Administer oxygen via a facemask. Concentrations vary; higher concentrations may not be necessary in uncomplicated presentations but patients with respiratory compromise need a higher oxygen concentration. Caution should be exercised in those with COPD.
3. Initiate transport quickly; the need to minimize on-scene times is vital. Not transporting under visual and audible warnings will need to be considered in order to decrease patient anxiety, but prompt transport and early arrival at the receiving unit must never be compromised.
4. Administer aspirin.
5. Measure pulse oximetry.
6. Establish an intravenous line.
7. Obtain baseline vital signs and repeat the assessment often. Vital sign assessment should include auscultation of the lungs for heart failure indicators.
8. Attach electrocardiogram electrodes, obtain 12-lead ECG, document initial rhythm, and monitor for dysrhythmias. Repeat the 12-lead ECG as necessary.

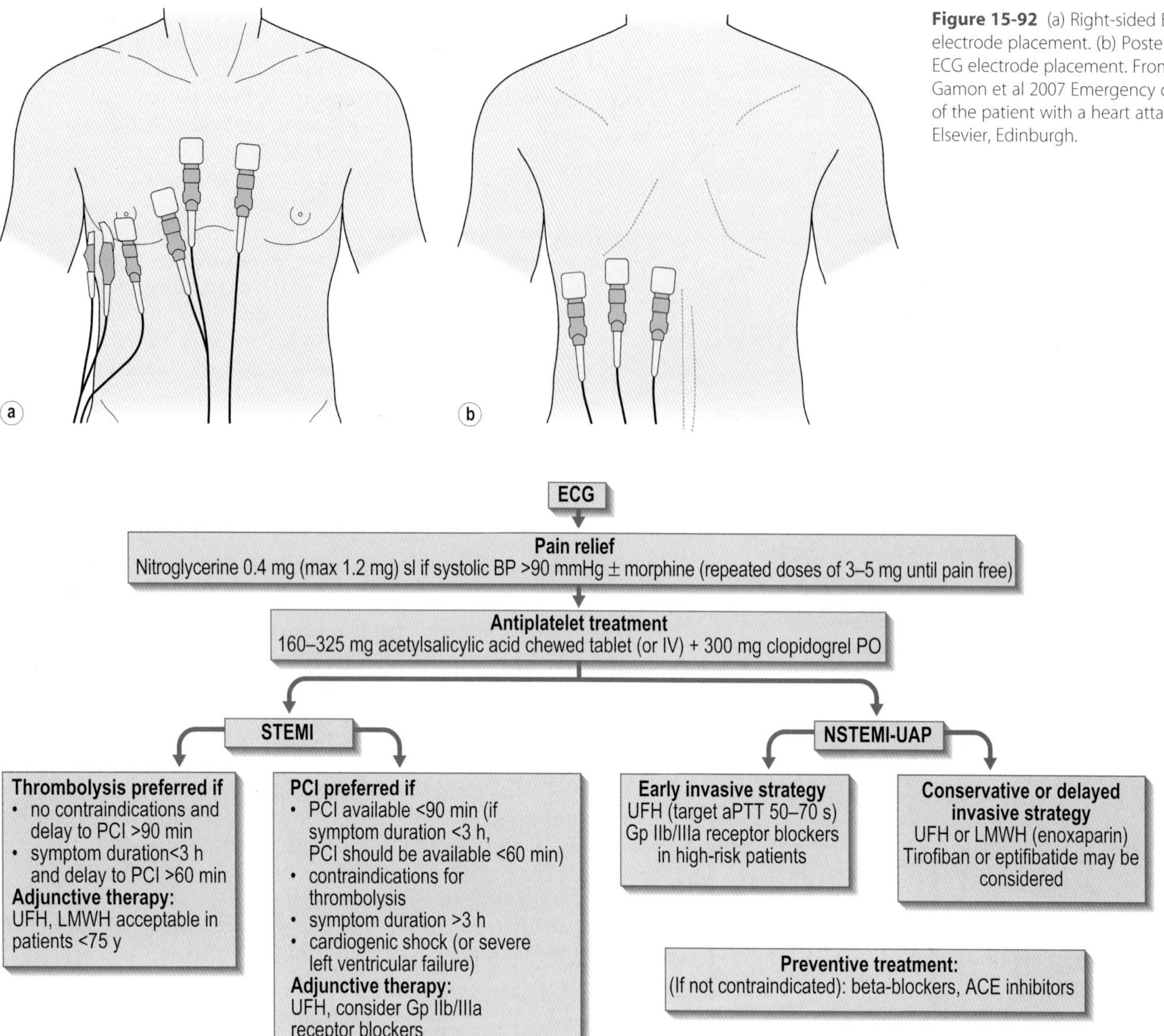

Figure 15-92 (a) Right-sided ECG electrode placement. (b) Posterior ECG electrode placement. From Gamon et al 2007 Emergency care of the patient with a heart attack. Elsevier, Edinburgh.

Figure 15-93 Acute coronary syndrome algorithm. From Baskett and Nolan 2005 A pocket book of European Resuscitation Council Guidelines for Resuscitation 2005. Elsevier, Edinburgh, p 88.

9. Pain score and administer medications for the relief of pain and the management of dysrhythmias:
   a. Medications that may be used for analgesia and to decrease preload and afterload include GTN and morphine.
   b. Medications that may be used to manage the various dysrhythmias in UK paramedic practice are limited to lidocaine (not in common use), atropine, and amiodarone.

   GTN is an effective analgesic for ischaemic chest pain. It also has beneficial haemodynamic effects, including dilation of arterioles and veins in the periphery, and the dilation of the coronary arteries, thereby decreasing preload. This decreases the workload of the heart and lowers myocardial oxygen demand. Because of these haemodynamic effects, GTN should not be used in patients with:
   - hypotension (systolic blood pressure less than 90 mmHg or more than 30 mmHg above baseline)
   - extreme bradycardia (heart rate less than 50 bpm)
   - tachycardia (heart rate more than 100 bpm).

   GTN also should be given with extreme caution (if at all) to patients with suspected inferior wall myocardial infarction with possible right ventricular involvement as right ventricular infarction is commonly associated with hypotension. GTN is also contraindicated in patients who have taken medication for erectile dysfunction within the last 24 h (longer for some preparations).
10. Where indicated, against the appropriate check sheet, thrombolysis (fibrinolytic) therapy may be administered. Even if the patient does not meet all the criteria within the guidelines for prehospital thrombolysis (PHT), completion will allow the receiving unit to quickly assess whether PHT can be given on arrival at hospital, as on occasions the criteria may differ in that environment.

Prehospital thrombolysis (PHT) and fibrinolytic therapy

Studies have shown that an acute intracoronary thrombus can be dissolved (thereby restoring blood flow to the ischaemic area) with salvage of ischaemic myocardium if PHT is administered within 6 h after the onset of symptoms. However, time literally is muscle, and mortality is significantly reduced by much earlier administration; evidence suggests that in the first 3 h of onset of pain, in a STEMI, each minute of delay contributes to several days of life lost. Consequently the National Service Framework for Coronary Heart Disease (NSF for CHD) has much stricter criteria, calling for PHT within the first hour from making the initial call for help. Ideally, PHT can often be initiated within 30–60 min of the call for help.

Common agents in the UK include streptokinase, alteplase, tenecteplase and reteplase; the last two are given in the prehospital environment as they are in a bolus form. These agents work by affecting the clotting cascade to dissolve the coronary thrombus. Plasminogen is converted to plasmin (the active form), the plasmin degrades fibrin, the basic component of a clot (thrombus), hence the coexisting term 'fibrinolytic'; aspirin and heparin are part of the 'fibrinolytic package'.

Aspirin has been long demonstrated to have a key role as an adjunct in PHT and even on its own can reduce mortality rates to some extent. Absolute contraindication is uncommon and if it is not tolerated, in-hospital use of clopidogrel is occurring more often.

Heparin is given concurrently with PHT with low molecular weight heparin (LMWH) being favoured. A fibrinolytic agent can dissolve beneficial and pathological thrombi and the drug is administered selectively. Most emergency medical services systems using PHT establish inclusion–exclusion criteria such as the JRCALC model checklist for PHT. However, common absolute contraindications are history of stroke, neoplasms, recent trauma, surgery or head injury in the past 4 weeks, gastric haemorrhage in the past 3 months, pregnancy, a known bleeding disorder or clinical evidence of aneurysm or aortic dissection.

During PHT, specific care needs to be given. It is vital that the appropriate checklist is completed and consent has been obtained. Heparin should be given prior to the thrombolytic agent. Reperfusion dysrhythmias can appear dramatic but are usually self-limiting. Frequent assessment of the ECG should be made, with repeat vital signs being recorded every 5–10 min, including level of consciousness and oxygen saturation levels. The patient should be monitored for any signs of bleeding at any external sites as well as signs of internal bleeding with signs of shock or altered levels of consciousness.

There are some complications of PHT that need to be mentioned; bleeding is the most common occurrence with intracranial bleed being the most concerning and the risk is greater in advanced age and those with lower body weight. Allergic reactions and low blood pressure are complications associated with the early generation drugs but current PHT agents such as tenecteplase and reteplase have much lower incidences of these complications. Finally, failure to reopen (recanalize) an occluded artery or reoccurrence of an occlusion after initial PHT are also potential complications.

The development of PCI should be mentioned. Whilst PHT has undoubtedly saved many lives, in some centres in the UK ambulance crews are able to identify suitable patients and transport directly for interventions such as insertion of stents and angioplasty. Some groups of patient have improved outcomes with PCI (for example where there is heart failure or where there is doubt about the STEMI diagnosis, as well as those in cardiogenic shock). Equally, where PHT is contraindicated or where it is several hours after onset of symptoms, PCI provides an opportunity for myocardium to be salvaged and in some circumstances will allow a second chance where the initial PHT has failed to recanalize an occluded artery. It is argued that PCI is superior to thrombolysis (although the evidence is based on hospital-based thrombolysis) in returning blood flow to the affected artery as well as reducing the incidence of reocclusion and consequent infarction. It also has the benefit of avoiding the risk of cerebral haemorrhage.

Congestive heart failure

Congestive heart failure is a condition in which the heart is unable to pump blood at a rate to meet the metabolic needs of the tissues. According to the British Heart Foundation, it affects close to 1 million people over 45 years old in the UK. Congestive heart failure most often is caused by volume overload, pressure overload, loss of myocardial tissue and impaired contractility, which can impair left ventricular function. Congestive heart failure in terms of left ventricular failure and pulmonary oedema and of right ventricular failure is considered below.

Left ventricular failure and pulmonary oedema

Left ventricular failure occurs when the left ventricle fails to work as an effective forward pump, causing a back-pressure of blood into the pulmonary circulation. This condition may be caused by a number of forms of heart disease, including ischaemic, valvular and hypertensive heart disease. If left unmanaged, significant left ventricular failure results in pulmonary oedema.

In left ventricular failure, blood is delivered to the left ventricle, but not fully ejected from the ventricle. The increase in end-diastolic blood volume increases left ventricular end-diastolic pressure which in turn is transmitted to the left atrium; pressure is then transmitted to the pulmonary veins and capillaries. As pulmonary capillary hydrostatic pressure increases, the plasma portion of blood is forced into the alveoli, where it mixes with air, resulting in the typical finding in pulmonary oedema: foamy, blood-tinged sputum. If left unmanaged, the progressive fluid build-up can result in death from hypoxia. Myocardial infarction is a common cause of left ventricular failure; all patients with pulmonary oedema (particularly those with an abrupt onset) also should be suspected of having an acute myocardial infarction.

Note

Paroxysmal nocturnal dyspnoea is an abnormal condition of the respiratory system, characterized by sudden attacks of shortness of breath, profuse sweating, tachycardia, and wheezing that awaken a person from sleep. This dyspnoea is often associated with left ventricular failure and pulmonary oedema.

Box 15-10

Signs and symptoms of left ventricular failure

- Severe respiratory distress
  - Orthopnoea
  - Spasmodic cough that may produce foamy, blood-tinged sputum
  - History of paroxysmal nocturnal dyspnoea (a sudden episode of dyspnoea that occurs after lying down)
- Severe apprehension, agitation, confusion
- Cyanosis (if severe)
- Diaphoresis
- Adventitious lung sounds
  - Bilateral crackles that do not clear with coughing (usually present at the base of the lungs and up to the level of the scapulae)
  - Rhonchi (fluid in upper airways)
  - Wheezes (reflex airway spasm, sometimes referred to as cardiac asthma)
- Jugular vein distension (indicative of back-pressure through the right heart and into the venous system)
- Abnormal vital signs
  - Blood pressure: possibly elevated
  - Pulse rate: rapid to compensate for low stroke volume; possibly irregular if dysrhythmias are present
  - Regular alterations of weak and strong beats without changes in the length of cycle (pulsus alternans)
  - Respirations: rapid, laboured
- Level of consciousness (Patient may be anxious, agitated, uncooperative, or obtunded because of poor cerebral perfusion or hypoxia)
- Chest pain
  - Presence or absence of pain
  - Possible masking by respiratory distress

Left ventricular failure results in a reduction of stroke volume that in turn initiates several compensatory mechanisms that restore cardiac output and organ perfusion (tachycardia, vasoconstriction, and activation of the renin–angiotensin–aldosterone system). However, these mechanisms often increase myocardial oxygen demand and further decrease the ability of the myocardium to contract. Box 15-10 lists the signs and symptoms of left ventricular failure and pulmonary oedema.

Management

Pulmonary oedema is an acute and critical emergency and may lead to death unless treated rapidly. Emergency management is directed at decreasing the venous return to the heart, improving myocardial contractility, decreasing myocardial oxygen demand, improving ventilation and oxygenation, and rapidly transporting the patient to a medical facility.

Emergency care entails patient positioning, oxygenation, ventilatory support as needed, and pharmacological therapy. As in any other true emergency, the paramedic should perform a full but focused patient history and examination while initiating treatment. No characteristic electrocardiogram changes are associated with pulmonary oedema but the paramedic should obtain an initial tracing and monitor the patient's rhythm continuously for evidence of myocardial irritability and dysrhythmias.

The paramedic should place the patient in a sitting position with the legs dependent, which increases lung volume and vital capacity, diminishes the work of respiration and decreases venous return to the heart.

The paramedic should administer high-concentration oxygen using a well-fitted facemask, preferably a high-concentration mask to optimize the amount of inspired oxygen. Some patients may require (and will tolerate) positive-pressure assistance including continuous positive airway pressure (CPAP) or biphasic positive airway pressure (BiPAP). Positive pressure assistance helps reduce pulmonary oedema and also reduces the need for high levels of inspired oxygen. If possible, the paramedic should use a pulse oximeter to ensure arterial oxygen saturation of at least 90%. If this cannot be achieved with 100% oxygen or if there are signs of cerebral hypoxia or progressive hypercapnia, endotracheal intubation and assisted ventilations may be indicated.

The following three medications may be used to decrease venous return, enhance contractile function of the myocardium and reduce dyspnoea:

1. GTN
   a. Induction of peripheral vasodilation.
   b. Possible reduction of preload and afterload, thereby reducing the myocardial workload and improving cardiac function.
2. Furosemide
   a. Direct relaxant (dilating) effect on the venous system within 5 min.
   b. Diuretic effect that reduces intravascular volume.
   c. May lead to electrolyte imbalance.
3. Morphine
   a. Decrease of venous return by dilation of the capacitance vessels of the peripheral venous bed (reduces preload).
   b. Reduction of myocardial work.
   c. Reduction of anxiety.

All of these medications can lower blood pressure and care must be taken in patients with pulmonary oedema and hypotension (blood pressure less than 100 mmHg systolic).

If the patient has signs of bronchoconstriction, salbutamol may be a useful adjunct, although care must be exercised to avoid significant increases in heart rate and therefore workload of the heart.

Critical Thinking

What happens to the diffusion of oxygen and carbon dioxide in the lungs during this process?

Right ventricular failure

Right ventricular failure most often results from left ventricular failure that produces elevated pressure in the pulmonary vascular system. This pressure causes resistance to pulmonary blood flow and increases the workload of the right side of the heart to overcome the resistance. Over time, the right ventricle fails as an effective forward pump, causing back-pressure of blood into the systemic venous circulation. When the pressure in the systemic venous circulation becomes too high, the plasma portion of the blood is forced out into the interstitial tissues of the body. This results in oedema, particularly in the dependent areas of the body such as the lower extremities and the sacrum of patients who are bedridden. Right ventricular failure can result from several diseases, including chronic hypertension (in which left ventricular failure usually precedes right ventricular failure), chronic obstructive pulmonary disease, pulmonary embolism, valvular heart disease, and infarction of the right ventricle.

Box 15-11 lists the signs and symptoms of right ventricular failure. When left and right ventricular failure occur at the same time, signs and symptoms of each may be present. Table 15-5 can help the paramedic differentiate between the two.

Box 15-11

Signs and symptoms of right ventricular failure

- Tachycardia
- Venous congestion
  - Engorged liver, spleen or both
  - Venous distension: distension and pulsation of the neck veins
- Peripheral oedema
  - Lower extremities or entire body (anasarca)
  - Sacral region in bedridden patients
  - Pitting oedema
- Fluid accumulation in serous cavities
  - Abdominal cavity (ascites)
  - Pericardium (pericardial effusion)*
- History
  - Often previous myocardial infarction in patients with chronic congestive failure
  - Frequent medication history of digitalis and diuretics to control heart failure

*Note: Patients often can tolerate large quantities of effusion without compromise when the effusion develops over an extended period.

Management

Right ventricular failure is often a chronic condition and not a medical emergency in itself. If right ventricular failure is associated with pulmonary oedema or hypotension, it may be a medical emergency. The paramedic should be prepared to manage the patient for either of these situations, which includes the following:

1. Placing the patient at rest in a sitting or semi-Fowler position (head elevated).
2. Administering high-concentration oxygen.
3. Obtaining baseline vital signs and an electrocardiogram tracing.
4. Initiating an intravenous line to keep the vein open or to manage hypotension.
5. Monitoring the electrocardiogram.
6. Managing symptoms of left ventricular failure, if present.

Note

Hypotension caused by right ventricular failure (often seen in right ventricular infarction) can mimic cardiogenic shock. In this case, fluid administration helps normalize left ventricular filling. Administration of fluids is crucial and helps the hypotensive patient regain a normal blood pressure as opposed to the hypotension associated with cardiogenic shock, where administration of fluids worsens the condition. Management may include 250-mL intravenous boluses of normal saline over 5–10 min, helping increase myocardial strength (Starling's law) and contractility. Close observation of the patient and vital signs is crucial.

Cardiogenic shock

Cardiogenic shock is the most extreme form of pump failure, occurring when left ventricular function is so compromised that the heart cannot meet the metabolic needs of the body. The result is a significant decrease in stroke volume (resulting from ineffective myocardial contraction), cardiac output and blood pressure, all of which result in an inadequate supply of blood to the organs. Cardiogenic shock occurs in

Table 15-5 Symptoms and signs of chronic heart failure

Right ventricular dysfunction		Left ventricular dysfunction		Non-specific findings	
Symptoms	**Signs**	**Symptoms**	**Signs**	**Symptoms**	**Signs**
Abdominal pain	Peripheral oedema	Dyspnoea on exertion	Bibasilar crackles	Exercise intolerance	Tachycardia
Anorexia	Jugular venous distension	Paroxysmal nocturnal dyspnoea	Pulmonary oedema	Fatigue	Pallor
Nausea	Engorged liver	Orthopnoea	S_3 gallop	Weakness	Cyanosis of digits
Bloating	Engorged spleen	Tachypnoea	Pleural effusion	Nocturia	Cardiomegaly
Constipation	–	Cough	Chest pain	Central nervous system symptoms	Agitation
Ascites	–	Haemoptysis	Diaphoresis		

5–10% of patients with acute myocardial infarction or may be the result of acute left- or right-sided heart failure or can be present for a short time in the post-resuscitation phase of cardiac arrest and defibrillation.

By definition, cardiogenic shock is present when shock persists after correction of existing dysrhythmias, volume deficit, or decreased vascular tone. Cardiogenic shock is usually caused by extensive myocardial infarction (often involving more than 40% of the left ventricle) or by diffuse ischaemia. Even with aggressive therapy, cardiogenic shock has a mortality rate of 70% or higher.

In addition to the signs and symptoms of myocardial infarction, patients in cardiogenic shock show clinical evidence of hypoperfusion to vital organs and significant systemic hypotension similar to that found in other forms of shock and this makes it difficult to differentiate the exact cause of shock. This evidence includes the following:

- acidosis
- altered level of consciousness
- cool, clammy, cyanotic, or ashen skin
- hypoxaemia
- profound hypotension (systolic blood pressure usually less than 80 mmHg)
- pulmonary congestion (crackles)
- sinus tachycardia or other dysrhythmias
- tachypnoea.

In the early stages of cardiogenic shock, the patient's heart tries to compensate; the heart rate increases and where able also increases contractility and cardiac output. If the condition is managed inadequately, the heart progresses toward hypodynamic failure with depressed contractility, reduced stroke volume, and subsequent hypoperfusion (see Chapter 28).

Management

Patients in cardiogenic shock are ill and require rapid transport to a medical facility. Transport should not be delayed on scene; prehospital care should include airway management and ventilatory support with high-concentration oxygen, placement of the patient in a supine position (or semi-Fowler position, if the patient is dyspnoeic), insertion of an intravenous line, electrocardiogram monitoring, correction of dysrhythmias, and frequent evaluation of vital signs (including auscultation of the lungs and observation for jugular venous distension). A patient in respiratory failure may require intubation and ventilatory support.

Critical Thinking

Consider unstable patients with signs and symptoms indicating cardiogenic shock. How should you respond when they ask you, 'Am I going to die?'

Drug therapy may include drugs that strengthen the force of contraction (inotropic agents) to improve cardiac output such as dopamine or dobutamine and the use of vasodilator drugs to reduce afterload which are generally reserved for in-hospital care settings. In such settings, blood pressure can be evaluated more accurately. If left-sided heart failure and pulmonary oedema also are present, they should be treated at the same time.

Critical Thinking

What dose of each of these drugs should be given for this condition?

Cardiac tamponade

Cardiac tamponade (described in Chapter 27) is defined as impaired diastolic filling of the heart caused by increased intrapericardial pressure and volume. As the pressure of the build-up in pericardial fluid compresses the atria and ventricles, they are unable to fill adequately, resulting in a decrease in ventricular filling and stroke volume. The condition may have a gradual onset, resulting from, for example, a cancerous growth or infection, or the condition may be acute, resulting from trauma to the chest, including cardiopulmonary resuscitation. Cardiac tamponade also may result from renal disease or hypothyroidism. Signs and symptoms of cardiac tamponade include the following:

- chest pain
- decreased systolic pressure (a late sign)
- ectopy
- electrocardiogram changes (usually inconclusive)
- elevated venous pressure (an early sign) with associated jugular vein distension
- faint or muffled heart sounds
- low-voltage QRS complexes and T waves
- pulsus paradoxus
- ST segment elevation or non-specific T wave changes
- tachycardia.

As described in Chapter 27, the most important reliable signs of cardiac tamponade are elevated venous pressure associated with hypotension and tachycardia (Beck's triad).

Critical Thinking

Why would fluid resuscitation with large amounts of fluid not be indicated in this situation?

Management

First, the paramedic must obtain a thorough history to attempt to identify the cause of cardiac tamponade and then perform a physical examination. Prehospital care is directed at ensuring an adequate airway and ventilatory support and providing rapid transport for further evaluation and possible drainage of the pericardial sac (pericardiocentesis). A fluid bolus may help support the circulatory system temporarily if the patient becomes hypotensive but definitive management requires drainage of the pericardial sac; cardiac tamponade may result in death if the condition is not relieved.

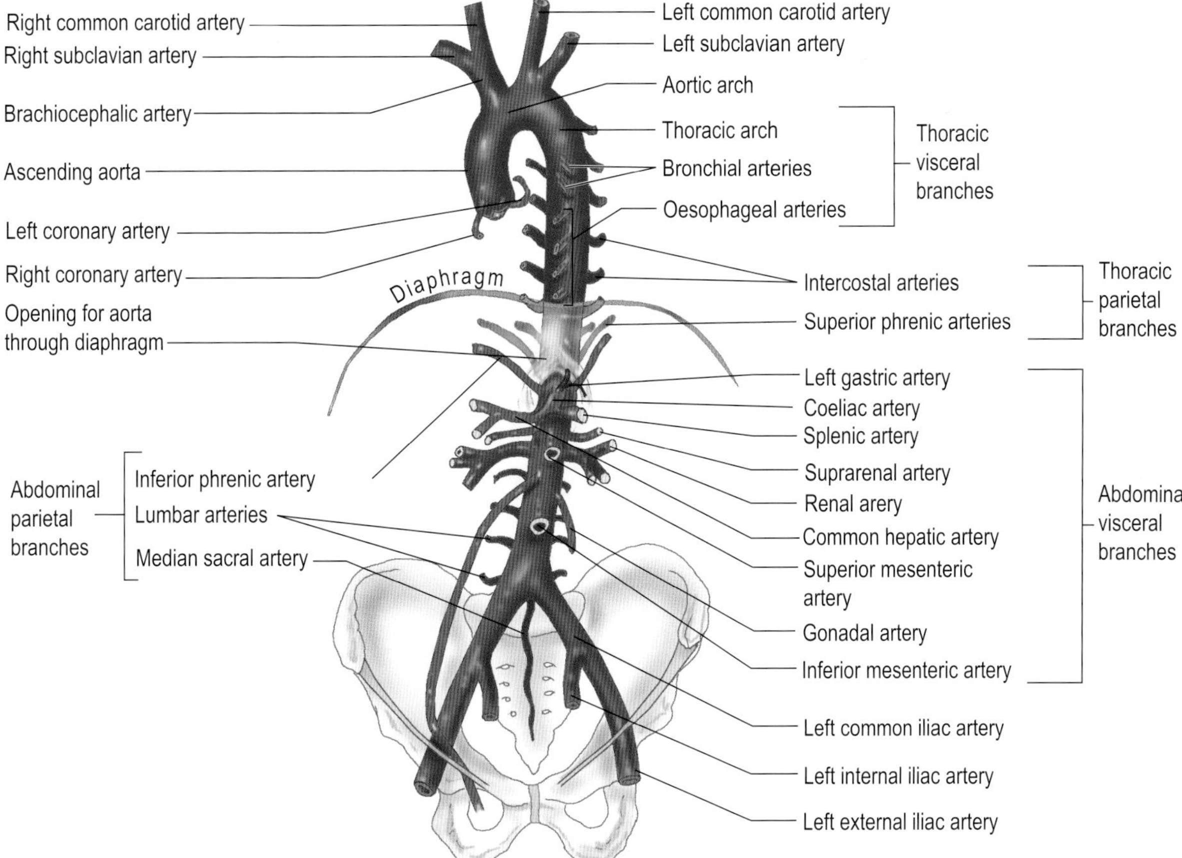

Figure 15-94 Branches of the aorta: aortic arch, thoracic aorta, abdominal aorta, and their branches.

Critical Thinking

Why is drainage of the pericardial sac not done routinely in the prehospital setting?

Thoracic and abdominal aortic aneurysms

Aneurysm is a non-specific term that means 'dilation of a vessel'. Aneurysm may result from atherosclerotic disease (most common), infectious disease (primarily syphilis), traumatic injury or certain genetic disorders (e.g. Marfan syndrome). Figure 15-94 illustrates the branches of the aorta. Abdominal aortic aneurysm and dissecting aneurysm of the aorta are considered here.

Most aneurysms develop at a weak point in the wall of an artery, which results from degenerative changes in the medial layer. Weakening of the supportive elements of the vessel wall allows dilation, creating turbulence and increasing lateral pressure. The aneurysm tends to enlarge over time as the lateral pressure increases in the dilated segment and may eventually rupture, producing a risk of life-threatening haemorrhage.

Abdominal aortic aneurysm

Abdominal aortic aneurysms affect about 2% of the population. The most common site for an abdominal aortic aneurysm is below the renal arteries and above the branching of the common iliac arteries. Abdominal aortic aneurysm is 10 times more common in men and is most prevalent between the ages of 60 and 70. An abdominal aneurysm is usually asymptomatic as long as it is stable, but if the aneurysm begins to expand or leak, symptoms will indicate impending rupture (Box 15-12).

Rupture of an abdominal aortic aneurysm may begin with a small tear in the intima that allows blood to leak into the wall of the aorta. As the process continues with increasing pressure, the tear may extend through the outer layer of the vessel, which may cause bleeding into the retroperitoneal space. If bleeding is tamponaded by the retroperitoneal tissues, the patient may be normotensive on the arrival of emergency medical services. If the rupture opens into the peritoneal cavity, however, massive fatal haemorrhage may follow; in either case, major blood loss results, and hypovolaemic shock ensues. The patient will typically complain of back or abdominal pain, and due to the peritoneal irritation may feel the need to have a bowel movement. There may be a palpable abdominal mass that is pulsating.

Often a patient with a rupturing aneurysm will have syncope followed by hypotension with bradycardia despite a large amount of blood loss. The reason for bradycardia is stimulation of the vagus nerve as the aorta has fibres of the vagus nerve wrapped around it. When the aorta tears, the

Box 15-12

Signs and symptoms of a leaking or ruptured abdominal aortic aneurysm

- Unexplained hypotension (that results from haemorrhage or a compensatory vasovagal response mechanism)
- Unexplained syncope (as the aneurysm ruptures, blood pressure drops transiently to zero, producing sudden cerebral hypoperfusion and syncope)
- Sudden onset of abdominal or back pain (described as tearing or ripping) from the physical trauma itself or from inflammation
- Low back or flank pain (radiating to the thigh, groin, testicle or perineum) that is unrelieved by rest or changes in position
- Signs of peritoneal irritation
- Urge to defecate (caused by retroperitoneal leakage of blood)
- Pulsatile, tender mass that may be palpated when greater than 5 cm and that usually is located above the umbilicus, left of the midline
- Distal pulses (femoral artery and below) that may be present or absent, depending on the patient's blood pressure, the occurrence of a dissection, and the degree of peripheral vascular disease
- Possible presentation as bleeding in the gastrointestinal tract if the aneurysm erodes into it

tear stretches these fibres, which in turn produces bradycardia. The bradycardia is present despite the hemorrhagic shock condition, which usually produces hypotension and tachycardia in the patient.

Management

Patients with a leaking or a ruptured abdominal aneurysm appear ill and often need immediate surgery to repair the vessel. Twenty percent of patients with an abdominal aortic aneurysm rupture their aneurysm before reaching the hospital, and 80% of these patients die; early recognition and rapid transport can prevent the death of these patients.

In most cases, prehospital care should be limited to gentle handling, oxygen administration, cardiac monitoring (myocardial infarctions may be associated with advanced aneurysms), initiation of intravenous fluids (cautiously) while en route to the receiving hospital, and alerting the receiving facility to prepare for imminent surgery. Pulsatile masses (if present) are fragile and in most cases are membrane thin; the paramedic should avoid aggressive examination or deep palpation of the mass as this may cause the mass to rupture. Examination, if needed, can be made by auscultation, possibly revealing a sound similar to that of a systolic murmur or bruit.

The management of hypotension varies and depends on whether the aneurysm is leaking or ruptured. A patient with a suspected leaking aneurysm can be maintained with mildly hypotensive blood pressure to try to prevent rupture during the transport; the hypotension associated with small leaks is thought to result from a compensatory vasovagal mechanism. In these patients, fluid resuscitation should be minimal and less aggressive than in patients who have a ruptured aneurysm.

If rupture has occurred, hypotension, tachycardia and loss of the pulsating mass may develop suddenly, the patient may become unresponsive and subsequently often suffer full cardiac and respiratory arrest. These patients require rapid and aggressive resuscitation (intubation, ventilation, fluid replacement, and rapid transport for surgery).

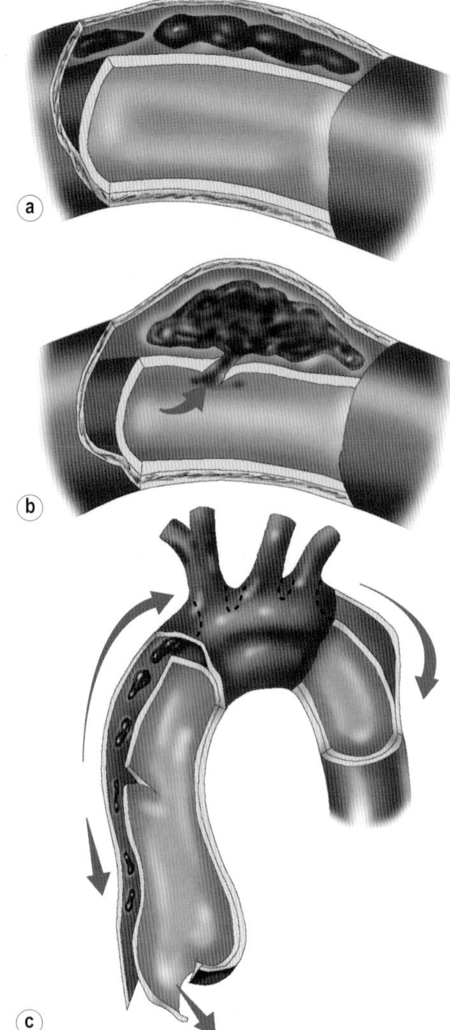

Figure 15-95 Pathogenesis of dissecting aneurysms. (a) Medial and intimal degeneration in aortic wall set stage. (b) Haemodynamic forces acting on aortic wall produce intimal tear, directing bloodstream into diseased media. (c) Resulting dissecting haematoma is propagated in both directions by pulse wave produced with each myocardial contraction.

Acute dissecting aortic aneurysm

Acute dissection (separation of the arterial wall) is the most common aortic catastrophe, affecting 5 to 10 persons per million population each year (three times as many as ruptured abdominal aortic aneurysm). Factors that can lead to the development of dissecting aneurysm are systemic hypertension, atherosclerosis, congenital abnormalities, degenerative changes in the connective tissue of the aortic media (cystic medial necrosis), trauma and pregnancy. The syndrome affects men twice as often as women and is more common in those of African descent.

A dissecting aneurysm of the aorta results from a small tear in the intimal layer of the vessel wall (Figure 15-95). After the tear, the process of dissection begins and allows blood to move between the inner and outer layers. This creates a false passage between the layers of the vessel wall. Blood that enters the false passage results in the formation of a haematoma. As a result, this can rupture through the outer wall (adventitia) at any time, usually into the pericardial or pleural cavity.

Any area of the aorta may be involved but in the majority of cases the site of a dissecting aneurysm is in the ascending aorta. Once begun, the aneurysm may extend distally or proximally to involve all of the thoracic and abdominal aorta and tributaries, the coronary arteries, the aortic valve, and the carotid and subclavian vessels. Any vessels (including the carotid and other aortic arch vessels) bypassed by the dissection have their blood flow decreased. As a result, aortic dissection may cause the following:

- syncope
- stroke
- absent or reduced pulses
- heart failure resulting from sudden aortic valve regurgitation
- pericardial tamponade
- acute myocardial infarction.

Signs and symptoms

The signs and symptoms of a dissecting aortic aneurysm depend on the site of the intimal tear (ascending or descending aorta) and the extent of dissection. More than 70% of patients with acute dissecting aneurysm of the aorta complain of severe pain in the back, epigastrium, abdomen or extremities. They often describe this pain as the most intense pain they have ever experienced, characterized by the patient as 'ripping', 'tearing', or 'sharp and cutting, like a knife'; it is usually sudden in onset. Pain often originates in the back (between the scapulae) and possibly extends down into the legs. The patient with acute dissection may appear shocked, with pallor, sweating, and peripheral cyanosis (from impaired perfusion), even when blood pressure is normal or elevated. If the patient is hypotensive, the paramedic should suspect cardiac tamponade or aortic rupture.

Critical Thinking

What other condition has signs and symptoms similar to abdominal aortic aneurysm?

It may be difficult to distinguish the pain of aortic dissection from that of myocardial infarction or pulmonary embolism in the prehospital setting. The following distinctive features may help:

1. Severity of pain is maximal from the onset (compared with crescendo pain characteristic of acute myocardial infarction).
2. Pain may migrate from the anterior portion of the chest or interscapular area downward as dissection progresses.
3. Significant differences in blood pressure occur between the left and right arm or between the arms and the legs.
4. Peripheral pulses are unequal.
5. Neurological deficits result from occlusion of a cerebral vessel.

Note

Blood pressure may differ significantly in the two arms if the dissection occludes either subclavian artery, leading to loss of blood pressure in the affected upper extremity.

Management

The goals of managing suspected aortic dissection in the prehospital setting are the relief of pain and rapid transport to a medical facility. The transport should not be delayed; analgesics should be administered en route to the hospital. The emergency medical services crew should be ready to initiate advanced life support measures. Other prehospital care measures include the following:

- gently handling the patient
- decreasing anxiety
- administering high-concentration oxygen
- beginning a large-bore intravenous line of crystalloid solution (fluids should be kept to a minimum unless severe hypotension is present)
- giving analgesia (e.g. morphine) in small incremental doses titrated against response if the diagnosis is strongly suspected.

Definitive in-hospital care generally includes reducing the myocardial contractile force to stop progressive dissection (with antihypertensives and beta-blockers), monitoring of intra-arterial pressure, and possibly surgical repair.

Acute arterial occlusion

Sudden occlusion of an artery can occur and most commonly is caused by trauma, embolus or thrombosis. The severity of the ischaemic episode depends on the site of occlusion and also on how much collateral circulation is around the blockage. Vascular occlusion caused by thrombosis is a complication of atherosclerosis, whereas occlusions caused by emboli may indicate an abnormal cardiac rhythm, particularly atrial fibrillation.

Critical Thinking

Why does atrial fibrillation put the patient at increased risk for emboli?

Arterial occlusion may follow blunt or penetrating trauma; it often is associated with long bone fractures. These injuries vary from injuries to the lining of a vessel to a vessel being severed completely; the occlusion usually is evident because there are no signs of circulation in the tissue or limb.

An embolism occurs when a blood clot breaks away and enters the arterial system. The clot travels until it reaches a narrow point in a vessel, often at a branching site of an artery. Ninety percent of peripheral emboli originate in the heart, therefore a history of cardiac disease (e.g. dysrhythmia, myocardial infarction, or valvular heart disease) favours a diagnosis of embolic occlusion, particularly when the patient has an asymptomatic opposite extremity with normal pulses. The most common sites of embolic occlusion are the abdominal aorta, common femoral artery, popliteal artery, carotid artery, brachial artery and mesenteric artery (Figure 15-96).

Thrombosis usually results from atherosclerotic disease and usually occurs at a site of severe narrowing of a vessel. Unlike an embolus, thrombosis usually develops over time. As the thrombosis gets larger, collateral blood supply also can become occluded, causing progressive ischaemia. The location of the ischaemic pain often is related to the site of occlusion:

- terminal portion of the abdominal aorta: pain in both hips or lower limbs
- iliac artery: pain in the buttocks or hip on the involved side
- femoral artery: claudication (cramp-like pain) in the calf of the involved leg
- mesenteric artery: severe abdominal pain.

If severe ischaemia persists, muscle necrosis occurs. Thrombotic occlusion is seen most often in men, smokers, and those over 60 years of age. Common sites of atherosclerotic (thrombotic) occlusions are depicted in Figure 15-97.

Signs and symptoms

Regardless of the origin of the occlusion, the signs and symptoms of ischaemia are the same and include the following:

- pain in the extremity that may be severe and sudden in onset or absent as a result of paraesthesia
- pallor (skin also may be mottled or cyanotic)
- lowered skin temperature distal to the occlusion
- changes in sensory and motor function
- diminished or absent pulse distal to the injury
- bruit over the affected vessel
- slow capillary filling
- sometimes shock (particularly in mesenteric occlusion).

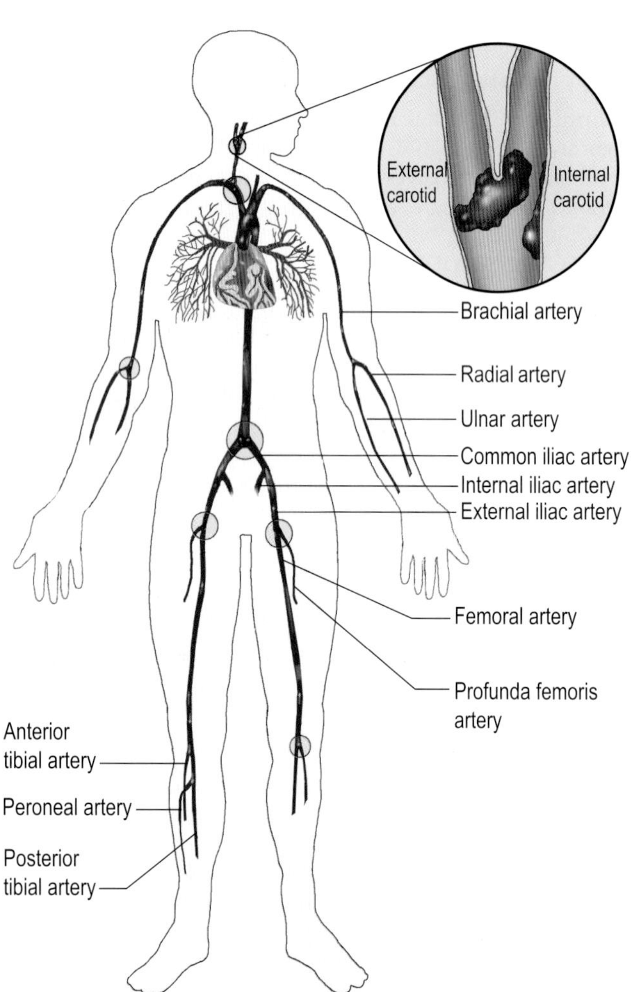

Figure 15-96 Common sites of embolic arterial occlusion.

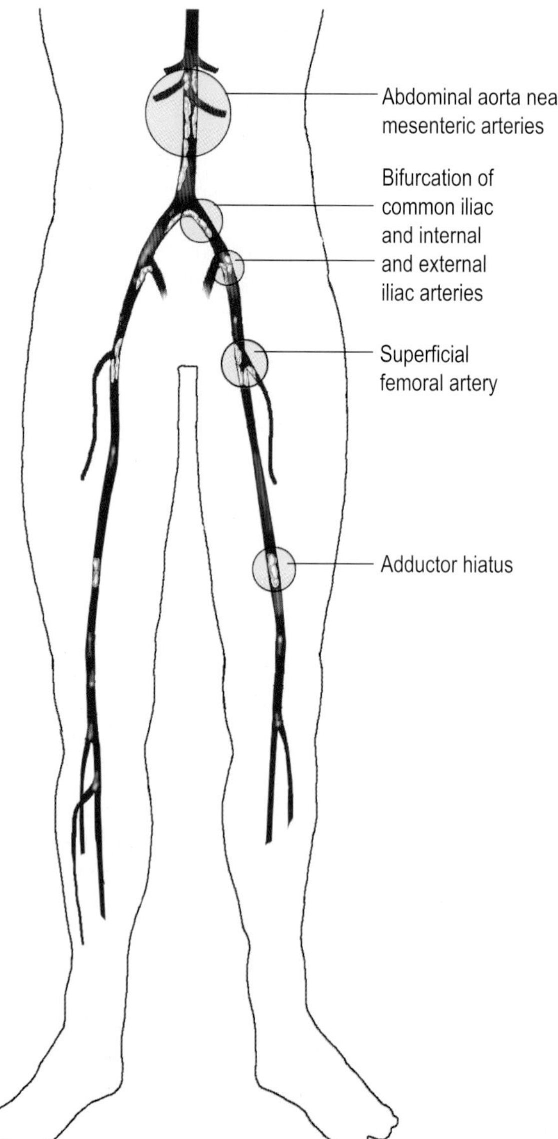

Figure 15-97 Common sites of atherosclerotic occlusive disease.

Note

Some patients with vascular occlusion will have unequal blood pressure readings in the arms. Systolic readings in the arms that differ by 15 mmHg or more suggest vascular disease; a normal difference of 5–10 mmHg exists between arms.

Management

Acute arterial occlusion in an extremity is serious and painful; occlusion may be limb-threatening if blood flow is not re-established within 4 to 8 h. The affected limb should be immobilized and protected and the patient must be transported for further evaluation. Patients with mesenteric occlusion should be managed for shock with oxygen and intravenous fluids. Analgesics may also be indicated for pain relief. In-hospital, definitive care may include anti-coagulant or fibrinolytic therapy, transluminal arterial dilation using a balloon catheter, embolectomy, or vascular reconstruction.

Non-critical peripheral vascular conditions

Non-critical peripheral vascular conditions include varicose veins, superficial thrombophlebitis and acute deep vein thrombosis. Of these conditions, deep vein thrombosis is the only one that can cause life-threatening pulmonary embolus. Predisposing factors to venous thrombosis include the following:

- oral contraceptives
- coagulopathies
- history of trauma
- malignancy
- pregnancy
- recent immobilization (e.g. leg fracture)
- sepsis
- smoking
- stasis or inactivity (e.g. bedridden patients or long air flights)
- varicose veins (usually a benign condition).

Acute deep vein thrombosis

Occlusion of the deep veins is a serious, common problem. Occlusion may involve any portion of the deep venous system but is much more common in the lower extremities. Risk factors for deep vein thrombosis include recent lower extremity trauma, recent surgery, advanced age, recent myocardial infarction, inactivity, confinement to bed, congestive heart failure, cancer, previous thrombosis, oral contraceptive therapy and obesity. Signs and symptoms of acute deep vein thrombosis include the following:

- pain
- oedema
- warmth
- erythema or bluish discoloration
- tenderness.

Management

Patients with acute deep vein thrombosis require hospitalization. Prehospital care usually is limited to immobilization and elevation of the extremity and transport for further evaluation. Deep vein thrombosis in the calf of the leg usually is much less serious than deep vein thrombosis of the thigh, as the latter has a higher incidence of associated pulmonary embolus. Definitive care includes bed rest, administration of anticoagulants or occasionally fibrinolytic agents, and on occasion thrombectomy.

Hypertension

Hypertension is a common disorder, afflicting over 20% of the UK population, and is directly responsible for several thousand deaths per year. Hypertension often is defined by a resting blood pressure consistently greater than 140/90 mmHg. The several categories of hypertension are based on the level of blood pressure, symptomatology, and urgency of need for intervention (Table 15-6 and Box 15-13). For the purpose of this textbook, two general categories are presented: chronic hypertension and hypertensive emergencies, including hypertensive encephalopathy. A common cause of hypertension is the patient who has stopped taking the medication or other therapy prescribed by their doctor.

Table 15-6 Classification of blood pressure levels (in mmHg) in people without diabetes

Category*	Systolic blood pressure	Diastolic blood pressure
Optimal	<120	<80
Normal	<130	<85
High normal	130–139	85–89
Mild hypertension	140–159	90–99
Moderate hypertension	160–179	100–109
Severe hypertension	≥180	≥110
Isolated systolic hypertension	≥140	<90

*When systolic and diastolic readings fall into different categories, the higher blood pressure category should apply.

Box 15-13

Signs and symptoms of hypertensive emergencies

- Altered mental status
- Changes in visual acuity
- Electrocardiogram changes
- Epistaxis
- Headache
- Nausea and vomiting
- Paroxysmal nocturnal dyspnoea
- Seizures
- Shortness of breath
- Tinnitus
- Vertigo

Chronic hypertension

Chronic hypertension has an adverse effect on the function of the heart and blood vessels, requiring the heart to perform more work than normal. This leads to hypertrophy of the cardiac muscle and left ventricular failure. Chronic hypertension increases the rate at which atherosclerosis develops, which in turn increases the probability of cardiovascular, cerebrovascular, and peripheral vascular disease and the risk of aneurysm formation. Conditions commonly associated with chronic, uncontrolled hypertension are cerebral haemorrhage and stroke, myocardial infarction, renal failure (caused by vascular changes in the kidney), and development of thoracic or abdominal aortic aneurysm.

Many persons with established hypertension have elevated peripheral resistance and elevated cardiac output (a function of Starling's law) that results from an increase in the heart rate and stroke volume. The heart responds to the increased workload that results from high peripheral resistance by becoming enlarged, and whilst the enlarged heart may work well for many years, in time the heart will no longer be able to maintain adequate blood flow and the patient may develop symptoms of failure.

Any hypertension-related problem – such as pulmonary oedema, dissecting aortic aneurysm, toxaemia of pregnancy, or stroke – requires stabilization and prompt, appropriate management. The hypertension associated with these situations often is a result of a primary problem. Managing the primary problem (e.g. toxaemia) often makes it easier to control the patient's blood pressure, but the primary problem may not easily be correctable. In situations such as dissecting aortic aneurysm, controlling the blood pressure is also key to managing the primary problem. A life-threatening problem that develops from unmanaged or partially managed hypertension may lead to a hypertensive emergency.

Hypertensive emergencies

Hypertensive emergencies are conditions in which an increase in blood pressure leads to significant, irreversible damage to organs that can occur within hours if the hypertension is not treated. The organs most likely to be at risk are the brain, heart and kidneys. This now uncommon condition is experienced by 1% of all hypertensive patients whose illness is poorly controlled or unmanaged. As a rule, the diagnosis is based on loss of organ function but is also based on the rate of the rise in blood pressure, not the level of blood pressure (although diastolic blood pressure usually is greater than 100 mmHg). All hypertensive emergencies (except hypertension in ischaemic stroke) require a 5–20% reduction in blood pressure within a few hours of discovery to avoid permanent organ damage. For blood pressure readings to range from 220/120 mmHg to 240/140 mmHg in hypertensive emergencies is not uncommon.

Hypertensive emergencies include the following clinical conditions: (1) myocardial ischaemia with hypertension, (2) aortic dissection with hypertension, (3) pulmonary oedema with hypertension, (4) hypertensive intracranial haemorrhage, (5) toxaemia, and (6) hypertensive encephalopathy. Hypertension per se may not be the cause of the first five conditions but they all can be made worse by untreated hypertension. The sixth condition, hypertensive encephalopathy, results solely from elevated blood pressure and concurrently raised intracranial pressure.

Persistent hypertension produces brain damage (hypertensive encephalopathy), results in a decrease in blood and oxygen to the brain (cerebral hypoperfusion) and also damages the tissues that make up the blood–brain barrier; this results in fluid exudation into the brain tissue. Hypertensive encephalopathy may progress over several hours from initial symptoms of severe headache, nausea, vomiting, aphasia, hemiparesis and transient blindness to seizures, stupor, coma and death. The condition is a true emergency. It requires immediate transport to a medical facility for definitive care. The goal of therapy is controlled but rapid lowering of blood pressure to normalize cerebral blood flow; if blood pressure is lowered too fast, infarction of end organs (heart, kidney, brain) may occur.

Critical Thinking

Why do patients fail to take medicines that are prescribed for hypertension?

Prehospital management of these patients includes the following:

- supportive care
- calming the patient
- oxygen therapy
- intravenous line to keep the vein open
- electrocardiogram monitoring
- rapid transport.

In most cases, drug therapy for hypertensive emergencies is not initiated in the prehospital setting; normal supportive measure of managing ABCs, oxygen therapy, ECG monitoring, and IV access are the main interventions, although diazepam may be given if convulsions occur.

Critical Thinking

How will fluid leak into the brain affect intracranial pressure and cerebral perfusion pressure?

SECTION VIII

Techniques of managing cardiac emergencies

This section addresses various procedures, techniques and equipment used in managing cardiac emergencies. These include basic life support, mechanical cardiopulmonary resuscitation devices, monitor–defibrillators (manual, fully automated and semiautomated), defibrillation, automatic implantable cardioverter defibrillators, synchronized cardioversion and transcutaneous cardiac pacing. This section also offers an overview of managing a cardiac arrest as it applies to working within an advanced life support system. The reader is encouraged to review the dysrhythmias and drug therapy presented previously in this text. In the UK, information about best practice is that found within the guidance from the Resuscitation Council UK; the most up-to-date algorithms are found via their website.

Basic cardiac life support

Basic cardiac life support provides circulation and respiration of a victim of cardiac arrest until advanced life support (ALS) is available. The best hospital discharge rate – a measure of resuscitation success – is achieved in patients for whom CPR (cardiopulmonary resuscitation) is initiated within the first minutes of the arrest and who, in addition, are provided with additional interventions and ALS management within 8 min of their arrest. The victim whose heart and breathing have stopped for less than 4 min has an excellent chance for recovery if CPR is administered immediately. After 4–6 min without circulation, brain damage may occur; after 6 min, brain damage will almost always occur. Cardiac arrest most often is associated with cardiovascular disease and is precipitated by ventricular fibrillation or ventricular asystole and may also result from non-cardiac causes such as poisonings, drug overdose, toxic inhalation, trauma, and foreign body airway obstruction.

Physiology of circulation via external chest compression

Two mechanisms are thought to be responsible for blood flow during cardiopulmonary resuscitation. The first is direct compression of the heart between the sternum and the spine, increasing pressure within the ventricles enough to provide blood flow to the lungs and body organs. The second mechanism to provide blood flow is the increased pressure in the chest cavity that gets transmitted to the vessels in the chest. This causes forward blood flow through the heart. Which mechanism contributes more to blood flow is unknown and other mechanisms not currently known may be involved as well but chest compressions generate only about 20–30% of the normal output of the heart. However, the most recent evidence emphasizes the importance of good chest compressions and minimizing 'time off chest' as it will take several chest compressions to restore the coronary blood flow return to its previous state if compressions are interrupted.

Research has been conducted for many years on ways to improve cardiopulmonary resuscitation; these methods include simultaneous chest compressions and ventilation, abdominal compression with synchronized ventilation, cardiopulmonary resuscitation augmented by pneumatic antishock garments, interposed abdominal compression, continuous abdominal binding, and plunger mechanisms for chest compression that cause active compression and active expansion. However, no alternative method has been shown to improve survival or circulation unequivocally (Figure 15-98).

Mechanical cardiopulmonary resuscitation devices

A number of mechanical devices have been designed to produce external chest compressions; most operate to decrease intrathoracic pressure during decompression of the chest, thereby improving venous return to the heart. Some devices provide chest compression and synchronized ventilation in the patient with cardiac arrest (Figure 15-99). These devices help to standardize cardiopulmonary resuscitation technique, eliminate rescuer fatigue, free other rescuers to participate in advanced life support procedures, and ensure adequate compression during patient transport. In addition, these devices permit acceptable electrocardiogram recordings during compressions and defibrillation without interruption of cardiopulmonary resuscitation. The use of these devices is usually limited to adult patients, requires special training and is not widely used in out-of-hospital settings.

Monitor–defibrillators

Cardiac monitor–defibrillators are classified as manual or automated external defibrillators. The latter may be semi-automated or fully automated. The paramedic should be familiar with the monitor–defibrillators used in their particular clinical area.

Manual monitor–defibrillators

Monitor–defibrillators are available from a number of equipment manufacturers in a variety of designs and capabilities. All consist of the following:

- pad electrodes (with 'quick look' capability) (it is uncommon to have paddles on newer machines)
- defibrillator controls
- synchronizer switch
- oscilloscope
- patient cable and lead wires
- controls for monitoring.

In addition, some manual monitor–defibrillators contain special features such as data recorders, transcutaneous cardiac pacing capabilities, oxygen saturations and capnography, 12-lead monitoring and non-invasive blood pressure monitoring.

Automated external defibrillators

Automated external defibrillators (Figure 15-100) analyse the electrocardiogram signal, by evaluating the frequency, amplitude and shape of the electrocardiogram waves. They are designed to be used by persons with minimal training, increasing the number of persons who are able to use a

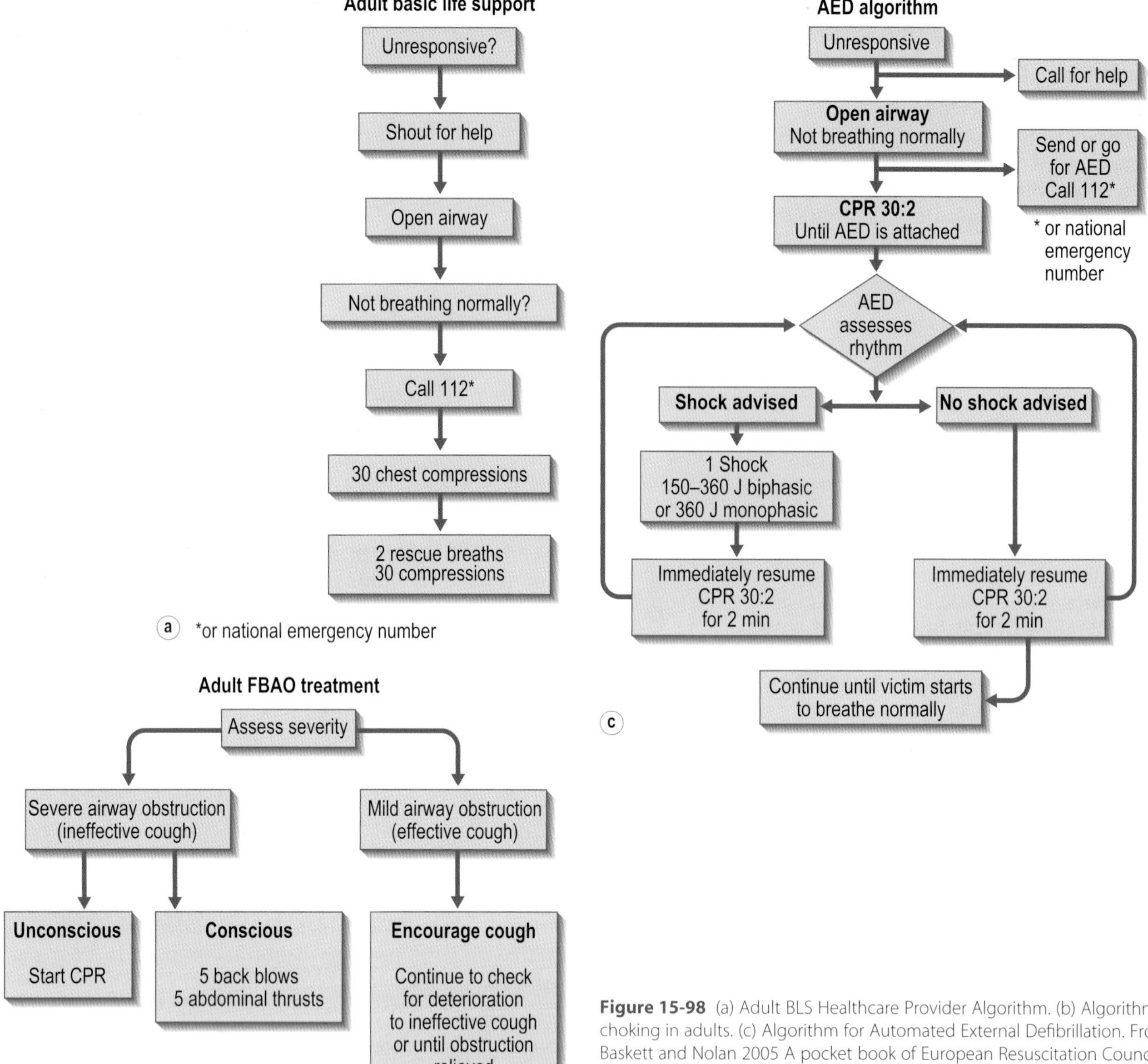

Figure 15-98 (a) Adult BLS Healthcare Provider Algorithm. (b) Algorithm for choking in adults. (c) Algorithm for Automated External Defibrillation. From Baskett and Nolan 2005 A pocket book of European Resuscitation Council Guidelines for Resuscitation 2005. Elsevier, Edinburgh, p 14, 29 & 32. Copyright European Resuscitation Council, www.erc.edu, 2009.

defibrillator in a cardiac arrest emergency. Automated external defibrillators are available for adult and paediatric patients.

All automated external defibrillators are attached to the patient by two adhesive monitor–defibrillator pads (electrodes) and connecting cables. Automated external defibrillators are available from a number of manufacturers, have a variety of features and controls as well and most units provide programmable modules, data recorders, and voice messages to the operator. All users should become familiar with the automated external defibrillator device used in their system and must follow the recommendations of the manufacturer.

A fully automated defibrillator requires only that the operator attach the defibrillation pads and turn on the device. The rhythm is analysed in the internal circuitry of the automated external defibrillator; if a shockable rhythm is detected, the automated external defibrillator charges capacitors and delivers a shock.

A semiautomated defibrillator requires the operator to press an 'analyse' button to interpret the rhythm and a 'shock' button to deliver the shock. The operator presses the shock control only when the automated external defibrillator identifies a shockable rhythm and 'advises' the operator to press the shock button.

Critical Thinking

What safety measure is still the duty of the automated external defibrillator operator?

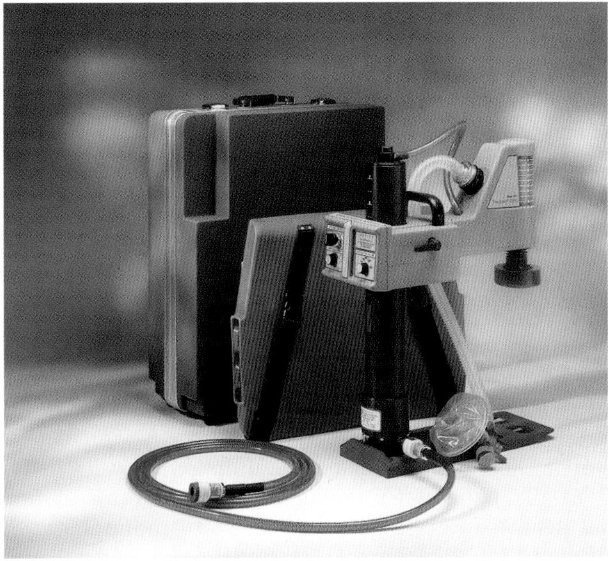

Figure 15-99 Mechanical cardiopulmonary resuscitation device.

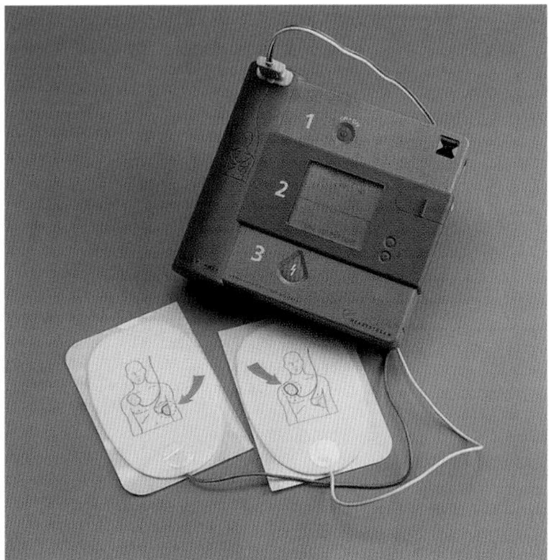

Figure 15-100 R2 automated defibrillator.

Automated external defibrillators have four safety features:

1. They can analyse electrocardiogram waves.
2. They have built-in filters that check for QRS-like signals, radio transmission waves, electrical interference, and loose or poor electrode contact.
3. Most are programmed to detect spontaneous patient movements, continued heartbeat and blood flow, and movement of the patient by others.
4. They make multiple evaluations of the rhythm before making a shock advisory or delivering a shock.

Biphasic technology

In the past, defibrillation has used mostly monophasic waveforms, in which the current travels in only one direction from positive pad to negative pad; these defibrillators require high energy to defibrillate a patient effectively and may deliver more energy than is needed for some patients. These machines also require large batteries, energy storage capacitors, inductors, and large, high-voltage mechanical devices.

The majority of defibrillators developed and sold over the past few years use biphasic waveform technology. This technology predicts a patient's energy requirements and chest wall impedance; the shock then is delivered by a current that travels in one direction, is stopped, and then is reversed to travel in the opposite direction, allowing for effective defibrillation to occur with lower energy for most patients. Therefore the energy settings for biphasic are typically around 150–200 J, whereas monophasic energy settings for all shock delivery is now recommended at 360 J. Biphasic waveforms are more effective at lower energy than are monophasic waveforms, and automated external defibrillators (using smaller batteries) have become smaller, lighter, more durable and less expensive to manufacture.

Defibrillation

Defibrillation is the delivery of electrical current through the chest wall, to terminate ventricular fibrillation and pulseless ventricular tachycardia. The shock depolarizes a large mass of myocardial cells at once. If about 75% of these cells are in the resting state (depolarized) after the shock is delivered, a normal pacemaker may resume discharging. Early defibrillation is supported by the following rationale:

- The most frequent initial rhythm in sudden cardiac arrest is ventricular fibrillation.
- The most effective management for ventricular fibrillation is electrical defibrillation.
- The probability of successful defibrillation decreases rapidly over time.
- Ventricular fibrillation tends to convert to asystole within a few minutes.

The modern defibrillator is designed to deliver an electrical shock via pads (or on occasion paddles) to the patient's chest. The defibrillator accepts the electrical charge from the battery source, stores the charge in the capacitor, then releases the current into the patient in a short, controlled burst (within 5–30 ms).

Paddle electrodes

Paddle electrodes are designated by location of use as 'apex' or 'sternum'. This allows the operator to view an approximation of lead II though the 'quick look' function. If the paddles are reversed in polarity or location, a negative QRS complex is noted; in defibrillation the position of the paddles is unimportant.

> **Note**
>
> Most services use defibrillators with adhesive pad electrodes instead of paddles. Care should be taken to ensure pad electrodes are applied in accordance with manufacturer's instructions.

The position of the defibrillation electrodes (pads or paddles) on the chest wall is important during shock delivery (Figure 15-101) and they should be placed so that the

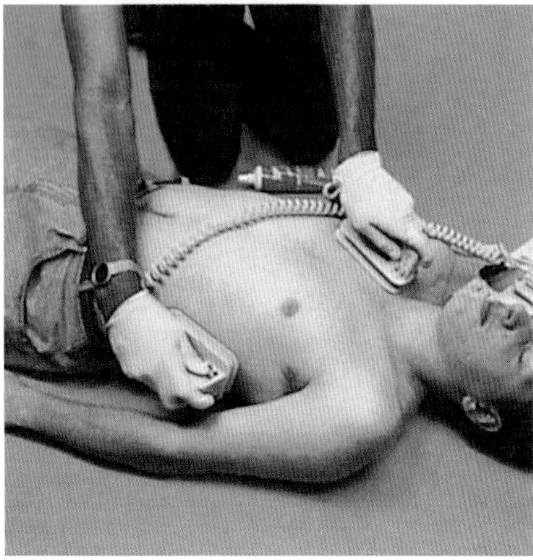

Figure 15-101 Correct paddle placement for defibrillation.

heart (mainly the ventricles) is in the path of the current and the distance between the electrodes and the heart is minimized, which helps ensure adequate delivery of current through the heart. Bone is not a good conductor, so the paddles should not be placed over the sternum. One paddle should be placed to the right of the upper sternum below the right clavicle, and the other to the left of the nipple in the midaxillary line. The anterior–posterior position also is acceptable and can be considered in the case of refractory episodes where initial shocks are unsuccessful. Most manufacturers have adult and paediatric paddles available. Adult paddles are usually 10–13 cm in diameter; paediatric paddles are used for children and the recommended size of the padde/pad is 8–12 cm for children over 1 year of age/more than 10 kg or 4.5 cm in diameter for children less than 1 year of age/under 10 kg.

The resistance to current by the chest wall is called impedance, which is determined by body size, bone structure, skin properties, underlying health conditions and other variables. The greater the resistance, the less current delivered. Dry, unprepared skin has high impedance. To reduce resistance (if using paddles) the paramedic should place gel pads between the paddles and the skin; paste or gel is not now recommended as it often smears and may contribute to arcing. The paramedic should hold the paddles firmly in place with about 8 kg of pressure in adults and 5 kg in children 1–8 years. Prepackaged self-adhesive monitor–defibrillator pads are mostly used now. Whichever method is chosen to decrease impedance, the paramedic should take care to prevent contact (bridging) between the two conductive areas on the chest wall; if contact between the two areas is made, superficial burns of the skin may result. The effective current also may bypass the heart (arcing) and even when gel pads or adhesive pads and proper techniques are used, minor skin damage may occur.

Stored and delivered energy

Electrical energy is commonly measured in joules (watt seconds). One joule of electrical energy is the product of 1 V (potential) multiplied by 1 A (current) multiplied by 1 s. Delivered energy is about 80% of stored energy because of losses within the circuitry of the defibrillator and resistance to the flow of current across the chest wall. As a rule, 80% of stored energy approximates the number of joules delivered to the patient. Current guidelines recommend one initial defibrillation be attempted at 360 J monophasic or equivalent biphasic energy (150–200 J) followed by 2 min of CPR (Box 15-14). The paediatric defibrillation is 4 J/kg repeated after each 2-min cycle of CPR as required. If the defibrillator (when using automated or semiautomated) is not configured to deliver paediatric defibrillation energy levels, then adult energy setting may be used in those children over 25 kg (around 8 years of age). It is worth remembering though that ventricular fibrillation is quite uncommon in children, compared with adults.

> **Box 15-14**
>
> **Current-based defibrillation**
>
> Current-based defibrillation has been studied as an alternative to traditional defibrillation. With current-based defibrillation, the defibrillator operator selects electrical current (A) versus energy (J). This method avoids the problem of low-energy selection in the presence of high impedance (resulting in current flow that is too low and failure to defibrillate). It also avoids the problem of high-energy selection in the presence of low impedance (resulting in excessive current flow, myocardial damage, and failure to defibrillate). The optimal current for ventricular defibrillation[2] appears to be 30–40 A.

Procedure

The following is the recommended procedure for defibrillation:

1. Turn on defibrillator.
2. Select energy level at 360 J for monophasic defibrillators or 150–200 J for biphasic.
3. Set 'lead select', switch on 'pads/paddles' (or lead I, II, or III if monitor leads are used).
4. Apply gel pads on patient's chest if using paddles.
5. Position paddles or remote defibrillation pads on patient (sternum-apex).
6. Visually check the monitor display and assess the rhythm. Remember the rhythm cannot be accurately assessed during CPR as compression complexes/ interference will be seen. (Subsequent steps assume a shockable rhythm is present.)
7. Announce to team: 'Stand clear, analysing.'
8. Press the analyse button if using semiautomatic mode
9. Announce to team: 'Stand clear, charging the defibrillator!'
10. Select the appropriate energy and press the 'charge' button.
11. When defibrillator is fully charged, state quickly in a forceful voice the following (or some suitable equivalent) before each shock: – 'Stand clear, shocking.' As you do this but BEFORE delivering the shock, check to make sure you are clear of contact with the patient, the stretcher, and the equipment, make a visual check to ensure that no one continues to touch the patient or stretcher and, in particular, do not forget about the person providing ventilations. That person's hands should not be touching the ventilatory adjuncts,

including the tracheal tube. Turn oxygen off or direct flow away from the patient's chest.
12. If using paddles, apply correct pressure on both paddles.
13. Press the shock button.
14. Give 2 min of CPR (approximately five cycles of CPR).
15. After 2 min, check the monitor. If a shockable rhythm remains, repeat the sequence above.
16. Increase energy levels for biphasic machines as required; monophasic will always be given at 360 J.

Operator and personnel safety

The following guidelines are designed to ensure safe defibrillator use:

1. Make certain that all personnel are clear of the patient, bed, and defibrillator before making a defibrillation attempt.
2. Do not make contact with the patient (except through the defibrillator paddle handles if using these).
3. Avoid if possible the use of gel or coupling material, which can become a contact between the patient's chest and the paddle handles; use gel pads instead or better still adhesive pad electrodes for 'hands free' defibrillation. Do not discharge pads or paddles over a pacemaker or implantable cardioverter defibrillator generator or GTN paste. Remove GTN patches before defibrillation.
4. To prevent gel from the patient's chest from being transferred to the paddle handles, do not have one person perform cardiopulmonary resuscitation and defibrillation alternately.
5. Apply gel or paste before turning on the defibrillator.
6. Do not 'open air' discharge the defibrillator to get rid of an unwanted charge; reduce the energy setting on the dial or turn the defibrillator off to 'dump' the charge (depending on machine type).
7. Do not fire the defibrillator with the paddles placed together; this can cause pits on the paddles that can increase the risk of burns to the patient.
8. Treat equipment with respect. It is safe when used properly. Do not touch the metal electrodes or hold the paddles to your body when the defibrillator is on.
9. Clean the paddles after use; even dry gel presents a conductive pathway that could endanger the operator during a subsequent defibrillation attempt or equipment checkout procedure.
10. Routinely check the defibrillator (including batteries) to make sure the equipment is functioning properly. Follow the recommendations of the manufacturer.
11. Reduce the risk of oxygen combustion by keeping any free flow oxygen well away from the patient during defibrillation (such as bag–valve–mask devices with oxygen attached) unless the patient is intubated and the connections are secure, in which case the risk of oxygen seepage from the circuit is minimal and poses little or no risk. Where there is not closed circuit, such as using other airway devices, best practice suggests removing the oxygen source to at least 1 m away from the patient's chest.

Defibrillator use in special environments

On occasion a patient requires defibrillation in a special environment (e.g. in inclement weather); the guidelines in operator and personnel safety always apply. However, additional precautions are taken in special situations.

A patient can be defibrillated in wet conditions, such as near water, in rain or in snowy weather; the patient's chest should be kept dry between the defibrillator electrode sites. The operator's hands and the paddle handles should be kept as dry as possible and it is best to use adhesive defibrillation electrodes. In heavy rain, it would be safest to find shelter in, for example, the ambulance.

Depending on the defibrillator and its equipment specifications, the device may not be guaranteed to work properly in non-pressurized aircraft. In addition, some electrical interference may occur between the radio equipment in the aircraft and the monitor–defibrillator or vice versa; this is affected by the distance and angle between the defibrillator and the radio equipment. Studies have demonstrated that defibrillation with current equipment would be expected to be safe in all types of rotary aircraft used for emergency medical transport; however, the medical crew should always inform the pilot(s) when electrical therapy is being used. In addition, the paramedic should consult with the pilot(s) to make sure the flight instruments are well shielded from electromagnetic interference.

Implantable cardioverter defibrillators

Implantable cardioverter defibrillators commonly are implanted through an incision in the sternum, which is similar to that used for coronary artery bypass surgery. However, left lateral thoracotomy, subcostal, and subxiphoid approaches also are used (Figure 15-102). During

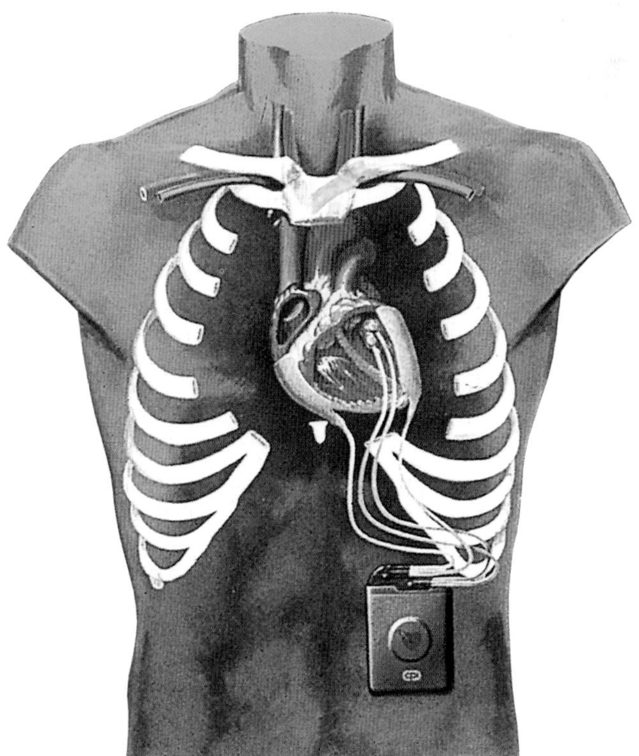

Figure 15-102 Automatic implantable cardioverter defibrillator.

implantation, the two defibrillation patches of the implantable cardioverter defibrillator are placed on the epicardium; the patches are usually opposite each ventricle to increase the effectiveness of the device. The device is tested in the operating theatre; a pair of sensors is attached to the surface of the left ventricle to monitor cardiac rhythm and the leads are connected to the biphasic defibrillator device. The device is placed surgically in the left upper quadrant of the abdomen; an outline of the generator usually can be felt or seen under the patient's skin.

Critical Thinking

What type of patients will have these devices?

The implantable cardioverter defibrillator works by monitoring the patient's cardiac rhythm, rate, and QRS complex morphology. When a monitored ventricular rate exceeds the pre-programmed rate, the implantable cardioverter defibrillator delivers a shock of about 6 to 30 J through the patches to restore a normal sinus rhythm. The device requires 10–30 s to sense ventricular tachycardia or ventricular fibrillation and to charge the capacitor before delivering the shock. If defibrillation does not restore a normal sinus rhythm, the implantable cardioverter defibrillator will charge again and then it will deliver up to four shocks. A complete sequence of five shocks, if required, may take up to 2 min. If the tachycardia or fibrillation persists after five shocks, no further shocks are delivered. Once a slower rhythm is restored (i.e. sinus or idioventricular) for at least 35 s, the device can deliver another series of up to five shocks if ventricular tachycardia or ventricular fibrillation recurs.

Critical Thinking

Consider a conscious patient whose device is firing repeatedly in response to the presence of a ventricular rhythm. How can you lessen the patient's discomfort and anxiety?

The paramedic must manage patients with implantable cardioverter defibrillators as if they did not have a device, following standard advanced life support protocols if the patient is in cardiac arrest or in any other way medically unstable. It is recommended that the following guidelines are followed when caring for a patient with an implantable cardioverter defibrillator:

1. If the implantable cardioverter defibrillator discharges while the rescuer is touching the victim, the rescuer may feel the shock but the shock will not be dangerous. Personnel shocked by implantable cardioverter defibrillators report sensations similar to contact with an electrical current.
2. Implantable cardioverter defibrillators are protected against damage from traditional external defibrillation shocks. However, they require an implantable cardioverter defibrillator readiness check after external defibrillation occurs.
3. If ventricular fibrillation or ventricular tachycardia is present despite an implantable cardioverter defibrillator, an external shock should be given immediately, because the implantable cardioverter defibrillator is likely to have failed to defibrillate the heart. After an initial series of shocks, the implantable cardioverter defibrillator will become operative again only if a period of non-fibrillatory rhythm occurs to reset the unit.
4. Implantable cardioverter defibrillator units generally use patch electrodes, which cover a portion of the epicardial surface. They may reduce the amount of current delivered to the heart from external defibrillation shocks, and if external shocks of up to 360 J fail to defibrillate a patient with an implantable cardioverter defibrillator, the chest electrode positions should be changed immediately (e.g. anterior-apex to anteroposterior) and the external shocks be repeated. Different electrode positions may increase transthoracic current flow, which may facilitate defibrillation.

Because the implantable cardioverter defibrillator can be deactivated and activated with a magnet, patients with implantable cardioverter defibrillators should be kept away from strong magnets. This will prevent accidental deactivation or reactivation of the device. The ability to use a magnet to deactivate and reactivate many of these devices can be useful when the unit is not working properly; however, use of a handheld magnet to turn the unit off or back on should be considered only with the advice and under the direction of expert clinicians.

Synchronized cardioversion

Synchronized cardioversion is used to terminate dysrhythmias other than ventricular fibrillation and pulseless ventricular tachycardia. Defibrillation (unsynchronized cardioversion) delivers the shock on the operator's command and with no regard as to where the shock occurs in the cardiac cycle. In contrast, synchronized cardioversion is designed to deliver the shock about 10 ms after the peak of the R wave of the cardiac cycle, avoiding the vulnerable relative refractory period of the ventricles. Synchronization may reduce the energy required to end the dysrhythmia and may decrease the chance of causing another dysrhythmia.

When the defibrillator is placed in the synchronized mode, the electrocardiogram displayed on the oscilloscope shows a marker denoting where in the cardiac cycle the energy will be discharged. This marker should appear on the R wave; if it does not, the paramedic should select another lead. Adjustment of the electrocardiogram size may be needed if the marker does not appear. The procedure for synchronized cardioversion is as for defibrillation but with the addition of the following key points:

1. Consider sedation.
2. Turn on defibrillator (monophasic or biphasic).
3. Attach the monitoring cable to the patient and ensure proper display of the patient's rhythm.
4. Enlarge the synchronization mode by pressing the 'sync' control button.
5. Look for markers on R waves indicating sync mode.

6. If necessary, adjust monitor gain until sync markers occur with each R wave.
7. Apply gel pads to skin on patient's chest if using paddles.
8. Position paddles or remote defibrillation pads on patient (sternum-apex).
9. Visually check the monitor display and assess the rhythm.
10. Announce to the team members, 'Stand clear, charging the defibrillator!'
11. Select the appropriate energy and press 'charge' button.
12. When defibrillator is fully charged, state quickly in a forceful voice the following (or some suitable equivalent) before each shock: – 'Stand clear, shocking.' As you do this but BEFORE delivering the shock, check to make sure you are clear of contact with the patient, the stretcher, and the equipment, make a visual check to ensure that no one continues to touch the patient or stretcher and, in particular, do not forget about the person providing airway interventions or ventilation. That person's hands should not be touching the ventilatory adjuncts, including the tracheal tube. Turn oxygen off or direct flow away from the patient's chest.
13. If using paddles, apply correct pressure on both paddles.
14. Press the shock button.
15. Remember to hold the paddles on chest until the shock is delivered as there may be a momentary delay.
16. Check the monitor and check for continued presence of a pulse. If tachycardia persists, increase the joules according to the electrical cardioversion algorithm.
17. Reset the sync mode after each synchronized cardioversion because most defibrillators default back to the unsynchronized mode. This default allows an immediate shock if the cardioversion produces ventricular fibrillation.

Transcutaneous cardiac pacing

Transcutaneous cardiac pacing (also known as external cardiac pacing) is an effective emergency therapy for bradycardia, complete heart block, asystole and suppression of some malignant ventricular tachydysrhythmias. They are used to treat bradycardia and asystole.

Artificial pacemakers

Artificial pacemakers (Figure 15-103) deliver repetitive electrical currents to the heart and can act as a substitute for a natural pacemaker. The natural pacemaker may have become blocked or dysfunctional. The patient with severe sinus bradycardia, heart block, or idioventricular rhythm who is capable of generating a pulse with cardiac contractions may respond to an external pacing device and produce a perfusing pulse. Sinus bradycardia may also be paced, but generally responds well to atropine. Most patients in cardiac arrest do not respond to pacing because the heart does not receive adequate perfusion and the heart cannot achieve effective contractions.

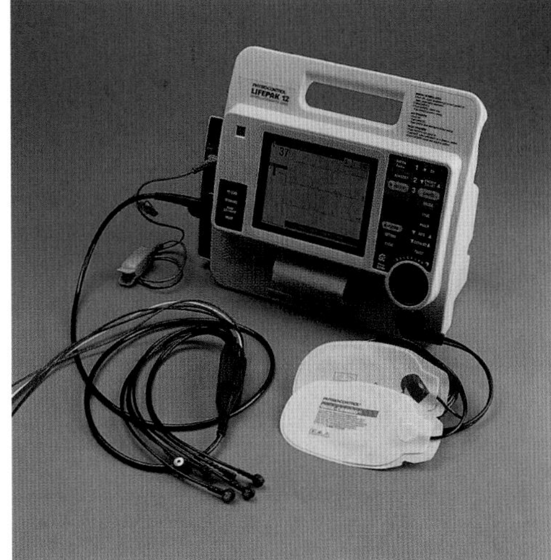

Figure 15-103 Lifepak 12 3D Biphasic defibrillator.

The two modes of transcutaneous cardiac pacing are non-demand (asynchronous) pacing and demand pacing. Most devices provide both modes. An asynchronous pacemaker delivers timed electrical stimuli at a selected rate, which occurs regardless of the patient's own cardiac activity. These pacing devices are used less often than demand pacers. That is because they may discharge during the vulnerable period of the cardiac cycle (producing the R-on-T phenomenon). The asynchronous mode generally is used only as a last resort, usually in asystole. This mode also can be used when an artefact on the electrocardiogram interferes with the ability of the machine to sense the patient's own heart beat. Another use for asynchronous pacing is in overriding the high heart rates in tachydysrhythmias (e.g. torsades de pointes); this should be attempted only if other means of controlling the dysrhythmia have failed.

Demand pacing senses the patient's QRS complex; the pacemaker delivers electrical stimuli only when needed. Demand pacing is much safer to apply than the non-demand mode. When the pacemaker senses an intrinsic beat, the pacemaker is inhibited. If no beats are sensed, the pacemaker delivers pacing stimuli at a selected rate. The device usually is set to discharge at a rate between 70 and 80 beats per minute beginning with 50 mA; the charge then is increased in increments of 5 to 10 mA of electricity, and mechanical capture is achieved. Generally, the patient's clinical condition (blood pressure, level of consciousness, skin colour and temperature) improves at this point.

The paramedic should ensure that each pacemaker spike on the oscilloscope is followed by a QRS complex. If not, the current should be increased gradually until there is consistent capture. Unfortunately, motion artefact often makes electrocardiogram confirmation of electrical capture difficult; the only accurate method of monitoring mechanical function of the heart produced by the pacing device is the presence of a pulse with each QRS complex and so the patient's pulse must be constantly monitored. The paramedic should assess the patient's pulse rate and blood pressure on the patient's right side. This will help to minimize interference from muscle artefact.

Procedure

The procedure for transcutaneous pacing is as follows:

1. Gather the required equipment.
2. Explain the procedure to the patient and prepare the patient's chest: dry, remove excess hair, etc.
3. Connect the patient to a cardiac monitor and obtain a rhythm strip.
4. Obtain baseline vital signs.
5. Apply pacing electrodes (avoid large muscle masses) and attach the pacing cable and pacing device; the electrodes should be placed in the anterior–posterior position, avoiding the diaphragm, ensuring any diagrams or instructions are followed.
6. Select the pacing mode (usually demand mode).
7. Select the pacing rate (usually between 60 and 90 beats per minute); set the current (begin with a low setting of no more than 50 mA and then increase the current until ventricular capture is obtained).
8. Activate the pacemaker, observing the patient and the electrocardiogram.
9. Obtain rhythm strips as appropriate.
10. Continue monitoring the patient and anticipate further therapy. Remember that pacing will cause discomfort and the patient is likely to require analgesia and/or sedation.

Note

As with synchronized cardioversion, selecting the 'pacing mode' should result in the appearance of light markers on intrinsic beats. Paramedics should ensure that this occurs as they will know the demand mode is activated and working properly.

Indications and contraindications

The primary indications for transcutaneous cardiac pacing in the prehospital setting are symptomatic bradycardia, heart block associated with reduced cardiac output that is unresponsive to atropine, or pacemaker failure. As stated before, cardiac pacing is rarely effective in cardiac arrest and is ineffective in pulseless electrical activity unless the underlying cause of pulseless electrical activity is corrected. Use of cardiac pacing is not advised in patients with open wounds or burns to the chest or for patients in a wet environment.

Critical Thinking

Why should patient movement be minimized during transcutaneous cardiac pacing?

Electrode placement

Proper electrode placement is key in providing effective external pacing (Figure 15-104a–c). The paramedic should apply the negative (anterior) electrode to the left of the sternum. The electrode should be centred as close as possible to the point of maximal cardiac impulse. The paramedic should place the positive (posterior) electrode directly behind the anterior electrode, to the left of the thoracic spinal column. In rare cases the posterior placement cannot be used; then the positive electrode can be placed in line with the patient's left nipple at the midaxillary line. (Anterior–anterior placement may produce pronounced chest muscle twitching.) The electrodes should be applied to clean, dry skin without localized trauma or infection.

The conscious patient most likely will experience some pain and discomfort during transcutaneous cardiac pacing. This is related directly to the intensity of muscle contractions and the amount of applied current. Ideally, analgesia or sedation of the patient should be provided.

Box 15-15

Related terminology

Resuscitation: To provide efforts to return spontaneous pulse and breathing to the patient in full cardiac arrest

Survival: Resuscitation of a patient who survives to hospital discharge

Return of spontaneous circulation: Resuscitation of a patient to the point of having a pulse without cardiopulmonary resuscitation; may or may not have return of spontaneous respirations; the patient may or may not survive

Cardiac arrest and sudden death

It is becoming increasingly evident that patients who cannot be resuscitated in the prehospital setting rarely survive; this is the case even if they are resuscitated temporarily in the emergency department (Box 15-15). The patient's best chance for survival is to have rapid and appropriate treatment in the field. However, endotracheal intubation and intravenous access take time to complete and maintaining ventilation and compressions and rapidly transporting the patient to the nearest medical facility should be considered. Initial defibrillation should always be attempted as soon as possible. However, prolonged field resuscitation in the face of difficulties in implementing the full range of ALS interventions may make the attempt futile.

Much research is under way in the area of emergency cardiac care; some of the research deals with various drugs to improve cardiac and neurological outcomes after resuscitation. A fairly large number of patients regain cardiac function but never regain consciousness and a great deal of interest has arisen in how to improve cerebral perfusion after cardiac arrest. This research may lead to a variety of new drugs to be used by paramedics during resuscitation in the future.

Termination of resuscitation

According to JRCALC Clinical Practice Guidelines, UK paramedics are expected to provide basic life support and advanced life support as part of their professional duty to respond. However, in some circumstances, resuscitation attempts will be futile and specific criteria have been devised to guide the paramedic into appropriate decision making.

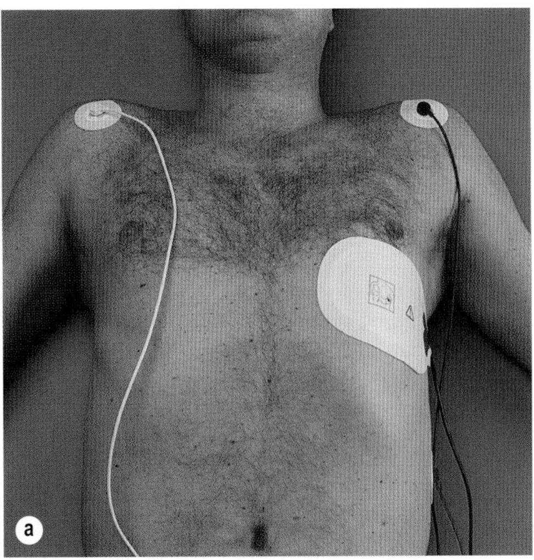

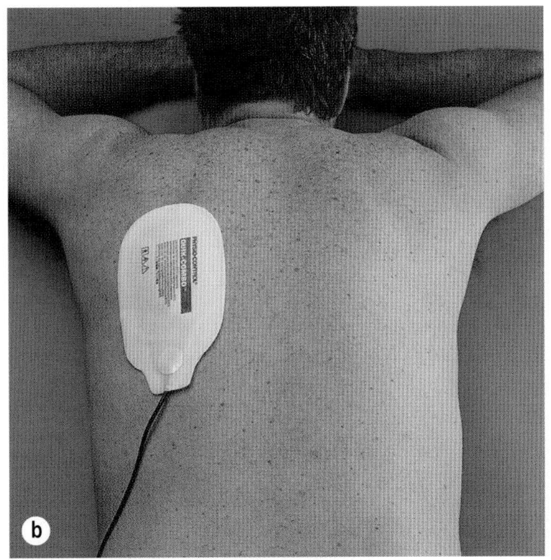

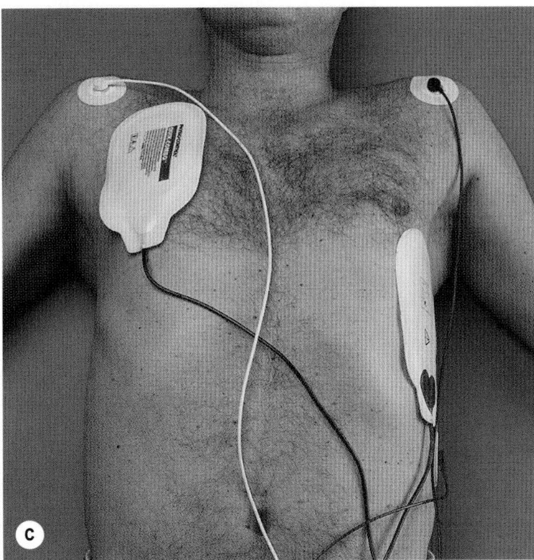

Figure 15-104 Proper electrode attachment for external pacing. (a) and (b) Preferred anterior–posterior placement. (c) Alternative anterior–anterior placement.

These criteria are to be found in the Recognition of Life Extinct section of the JRCALC Clinical Practice Guidelines.

Consideration must also be taken of the existence of any advance directives (e.g. lasting power of attorney) that indicates a patient should not be resuscitated. Appropriate policy must be followed in this case.

Paramedics must also consider specific circumstances where successful resuscitation might be possible: for instance, have reversible causes been ruled out and has there been consideration of unusual clinical features such as drowning or profound hypothermia, young age, toxins or electrolyte abnormalities, and drug overdose, which may be indicators that continued resuscitation is appropriate?

Critical Thinking

Consider that you have just terminated resuscitation in the home. What resources can you contact to help the family?

Special considerations

In addition to the needs of the patient, grief support for the family must be considered. Support services vary by agency but often a paramedic (or other emergency medical services personnel) will need to stay with the family for a period of time. At times, a community agency referral will be arranged.

Police officers (including HM Coroner's Officer) may have more duties at the scene as part of their professional role. These duties may include an on-scene determination that the patient be assigned to a forensic medical examiner, who may determine whether the death or event is suspicious.

Summary

- Persons at high risk for cardiovascular disease include those with diabetes, a family history of premature cardiovascular disease, and prior myocardial infarction. Prevention strategies include community educational programmes in nutrition, cessation of smoking (smoking prevention for children), and screening for hypertension and high cholesterol.
- The left coronary artery carries about 85% of the blood supply to the myocardium. The right coronary artery carries the rest. The pumping action of the heart is a product of rhythmic, alternate contraction and relaxation of the atria and ventricles. The stoke volume is the amount of blood ejected from each ventricle with one contraction. Stroke volume depends on preload, afterload, and myocardial contractility. Cardiac output is the amount of blood pumped by each ventricle per minute.
- In addition to the intrinsic control of the body in regulating the heart, extrinsic control by the parasympathetic and sympathetic nerves of the autonomic nervous system is a major factor influencing the heart rate, conductivity, and contractility. Sympathetic impulses cause the adrenal medulla to secrete adrenaline and noradrenaline into the blood.
- The major electrolytes that influence cardiac function are calcium, potassium, sodium, and magnesium. The electrical charge (potential difference) between the inside and outside of cells is expressed in millivolts. When the cell is in a resting state, the electrical charge difference is referred to as a resting membrane potential. The specialized sodium–potassium exchange pump actively pumps sodium ions out of the cell. It also pumps potassium ions into the cell. The cell membrane appears to have individual protein-lined channels. These channels allow for passage of a specific ion or group of ions.
- Nerve and muscle cells are capable of producing action potentials. This property is known as excitability. An action potential at any point on the cell membrane stimulates an excitation process. This process is spread down the length of the cell and is conducted across synapses from cell to cell.
- The contraction of cardiac and skeletal muscle is believed to be activated by calcium ions. This results in a binding between myosin and actin myofilaments.
- The conduction system of the heart is composed of two nodes and a conducting bundle. One of the nodes is the SA node. The other is the AV node.
- Common chief complaints of the patient with cardiovascular disease include chest pain or discomfort, including shoulder, arm, neck, or jaw pain or discomfort; dyspnoea; syncope; and abnormal heartbeat or palpitations. Paramedics should ask patients suspected of having a cardiovascular disorder whether they take prescription medications, especially cardiac drugs. Paramedics should ask whether patients are being treated for any serious illness as well. They also should ask whether patients have a history of myocardial infarction, angina, heart failure, hypertension, diabetes, or chronic lung disease. In addition, paramedics should ask whether patients have any allergies or have other risk factors for heart disease.
- After performing the initial assessment of the patient with cardiovascular disease, the paramedic should look for skin colour, jugular venous distension, and the presence of oedema or other signs of heart disease. The paramedic should listen for lung sounds, heart sounds, and carotid artery bruit. The paramedic should feel for oedema, pulses, skin temperature, and moisture.
- The electrocardiogram represents the electrical activity of the heart. The electrocardiogram is generated by depolarization and repolarization of the atria and ventricles.
- Routine monitoring of cardiac rhythm in the prehospital setting usually is obtained in lead II. This is the best lead to monitor for dysrhythmias because it allows visualization of P waves. A 12-lead electrocardiogram can be used to help identify changes relative to myocardial ischaemia, injury, and infarction; distinguish ventricular tachycardia from supraventricular tachycardia; determine the electrical axis and the presence of fascicular blocks; and determine the presence of bundle branch blocks.
- The paper used to record electrocardiograms is standardized. This allows comparative analysis of an electrocardiogram wave.
- The normal electrocardiogram consists of a P wave, QRS complex, and T wave. The P wave is the first positive deflection on the electrocardiogram. The P wave represents atrial depolarization. The P-R interval is the time it takes for an electrical impulse to be conducted through the atria and the AV node up to the instant of ventricular depolarization. The QRS complex represents ventricular depolarization. The ST segment represents the early part of repolarization of the right and left ventricles. The T wave represents repolarization of the ventricular myocardial cells. Repolarization occurs during the last part of ventricular systole. The Q-T interval is the period from the beginning of ventricular depolarization (onset of the QRS complex) until the end of ventricular repolarization or the end of the T wave.
- The steps in electrocardiogram analysis include analysing the QRS complex, P waves, rate, rhythm and P-R interval.
- Dysrhythmias originating in the SA node include sinus bradycardia, sinus tachycardia, sinus dysrhythmia, and sinus arrest. Most sinus dysrhythmias are the result of increases or decreases in vagal tone.
- Dysrhythmias originating in the atria include wandering pacemaker, premature atrial complexes, paroxysmal supraventricular tachycardia, atrial flutter and atrial fibrillation. Common causes of atrial dysrhythmias are

Summary—cont'd

ischaemia, hypoxia and atrial dilation caused by congestive heart failure or mitral valve abnormalities.

- When the SA node and the atria cannot generate the electrical impulses needed to begin depolarization because of factors such as hypoxia, ischaemia, myocardial infarction, and drug toxicity, the AV node or the area surrounding the AV node may assume the role of the secondary pacemaker. Dysrhythmias originating in the AV junction include premature junctional contractions, junctional escape complexes or rhythms, and accelerated junctional rhythm.
- Ventricular dysrhythmias pose a threat to life. Ventricular rhythm disturbances generally result from failure of the atria, AV junction, or both to initiate an electrical impulse. They also may result from enhanced automaticity or re-entry phenomena in the ventricles. Dysrhythmias originating in the ventricles include ventricular escape complexes or rhythms, premature ventricular complexes, ventricular tachycardia, ventricular fibrillation, asystole and artificial pacemaker rhythm.
- Partial delays or full interruptions in cardiac electrical conduction are called heart blocks. Causes of heart blocks include AV junctional ischaemia, AV junctional necrosis, degenerative disease of the conduction system and drug toxicity. Dysrhythmias that are disorders of conduction are first-degree AV block, type I second-degree AV block (Wenckebach), type II second-degree AV block, third-degree AV block, disturbances of ventricular conduction, pulseless electrical activity and pre-excitation (Wolff–Parkinson–White) syndrome.
- Atherosclerosis is a disease process characterized by progressive narrowing of the lumen of medium and large arteries. Atherosclerosis has two major effects on blood vessels. First, the disease disrupts the intimal surface. This causes a loss of vessel elasticity and an increase in thrombogenesis. Second, the atheroma reduces the diameter of the vessel lumen. Thus, this decreases the blood supply to tissues.
- Angina pectoris is a symptom of myocardial ischaemia. Angina is caused by an imbalance between myocardial oxygen supply and demand. Prehospital management includes placing the patient at rest, administering oxygen, initiating intravenous therapy, administering GTN and possibly morphine, monitoring the patient for dysrhythmias, and transporting the patient for physician evaluation.
- Acute myocardial infarction occurs when a coronary artery is blocked and blood does not reach an area of heart muscle. This results in ischaemia, injury, and necrosis to the area of myocardium supplied by the affected artery. Death caused by myocardial infarction usually results from lethal dysrhythmias (ventricular tachycardia, ventricular fibrillation, and cardiac standstill), pump failure (cardiogenic shock and congestive heart failure), or myocardial tissue rupture (rupture of the ventricle, septum, or papillary muscle). Some patients with acute myocardial infarction, particularly those in the older age groups, have only symptoms of dyspnoea, syncope or confusion. However, substernal chest pain is usually present in patients with acute myocardial infarction (70–90% of patients). ST segment elevation greater than or equal to 0.5 mV in at least two contiguous electrocardiogram leads indicates an acute myocardial infarction. However, some patients infarct without ST segment elevation changes. Other conditions also can produce ST segment elevation. Prehospital management of the patient with a suspected myocardial infarction should include placing the patient at rest; administering oxygen; frequently assessing vital signs and breath sounds; initiating intravenous access; monitoring for dysrhythmias; administering medications such as GTN, morphine, and aspirin; and screening for risk factors for fibrinolytic therapy.
- Left ventricular failure occurs when the left ventricle fails to function as an effective forward pump. This causes a back-pressure of blood into the pulmonary circulation. This in turn may lead to pulmonary oedema. Emergency management is directed at decreasing the venous return to the heart, improving myocardial contractility, decreasing myocardial oxygen demand, improving ventilation and oxygenation, and rapidly transporting the patient to a medical facility.
- Right ventricular failure occurs when the right ventricle fails as a pump. This causes back-pressure of blood into the systemic venous circulation. Right ventricular failure is not usually a medical emergency in itself; that is, unless it is associated with pulmonary oedema or hypotension.
- Cardiogenic shock is the most extreme form of pump failure. It usually is caused by extensive myocardial infarction. Even with aggressive therapy, cardiogenic shock has a mortality rate of 70% or higher. Patients in cardiogenic shock need rapid transport to a medical facility.
- Cardiac tamponade is defined as impaired filling of the heart caused by increased pressure in the pericardial sac.
- Abdominal aortic aneurysms are usually asymptomatic. However, signs and symptoms will signal impending or active rupture. If the vessel tears, bleeding initially may be stopped by the retroperitoneal tissues. The patient may be normotensive on the arrival of emergency medical services. If the rupture opens into the peritoneal cavity, however, massive fatal haemorrhage may follow.
- Acute dissection is the most common aortic catastrophe. Any area of the aorta may be involved. However, in 60–70% of cases the site of a dissecting aneurysm is in the ascending aorta, just beyond the takeoff of the left subclavian artery. The signs and symptoms depend on the site of the intimal tear. They also depend on the extent of dissection. The goals of managing suspected aortic dissection in the prehospital setting are relief of pain and immediate transport to a medical facility.

Summary—cont'd

- Acute arterial occlusion is a sudden blockage of arterial flow. Occlusion most commonly is caused by trauma, an embolus, or thrombosis. The most common sites of embolic occlusion are the abdominal aorta, common femoral artery, popliteal artery, carotid artery, brachial artery and mesenteric artery. The location of ischaemic pain is related to the site of occlusion.
- Non-critical peripheral vascular conditions include varicose veins, superficial thrombophlebitis and acute deep vein thrombosis. Of these conditions, deep vein thrombosis is the only one that can cause a life-threatening problem. This problem is pulmonary embolus.
- Hypertension often is defined by a resting blood pressure that is consistently greater than 140/90 mmHg. Chronic hypertension has an adverse effect on the heart and blood vessels. It requires the heart to perform more work than normal. This leads to hypertrophy of the cardiac muscle and left ventricular failure. Conditions associated with chronic, uncontrolled hypertension are cerebral haemorrhage and stroke, myocardial infarction, and renal failure.
- Hypertensive emergencies are conditions in which a blood pressure increase leads to significant, irreversible end-organ damage within hours if not treated. The organs most likely to be at risk are the brain, heart, and kidneys. As a rule, the diagnosis is based on altered end-organ function and the rate of the rise in blood pressure, not on the level of blood pressure.
- Effective basic cardiac life support is critical to maintain the circulation and respiration of a victim of cardiac arrest. Basic life support is continued until advanced cardiac life support is available. Two mechanisms are thought to be responsible for blood flow during cardiopulmonary resuscitation. One is direct compression of the heart between the sternum and the spine. This increases pressure within the ventricles to provide blood flow to the lungs and body organs. The second one is increased intrathoracic pressure transmitted to all intrathoracic vascular structures. This creates an intrathoracic-to-extrathoracic pressure gradient. This gradient causes blood to flow out of the thorax. A number of mechanical devices provide external chest compression. Others provide chest compression with ventilation in the cardiac arrest patient.
- Cardiac monitor–defibrillators are classified as manual or automated external defibrillators. Defibrillation is the delivery of electrical current through the chest wall. Its purpose is to terminate ventricular fibrillation and certain other non-perfusing rhythms.
- Implantable cardioverter defibrillators work by monitoring the patient's cardiac rhythm. When a monitored ventricular rate exceeds the pre-programmed rate, the implantable cardioverter defibrillator delivers a shock of about 6 to 30 J through the patches. This is an attempt to restore a normal sinus rhythm.
- Synchronized cardioversion is designed to deliver a shock about 10 ms after the peak of the R wave of the cardiac cycle. (Thus the device avoids the relative refractory period.) Synchronization may reduce the amount of energy needed to end the dysrhythmia. It also may decrease the chances of causing another dysrhythmia.
- Transcutaneous cardiac pacing is an effective emergency therapy for bradycardia, complete heart block, asystole, and suppression of some malignant ventricular dysrhythmias. Proper electrode placement is important for effective external pacing.
- What is becoming more and more evident is that patients who cannot be resuscitated in the prehospital setting rarely survive. This is the case even if they are resuscitated temporarily in the emergency department. Cessation of resuscitative efforts in the prehospital setting should follow system-specific criteria established by medical direction.

Further reading

ACC/AHA 2001 guidelines for the evaluation and management of chronic heart failure in the adult: executive summary. Circulation 104:2926–3007

American Heart Association 2005 AHA 2005 Guidelines for Cardiopulmonary Resuscitation and Emergency Cardiovascular Care. Circulation 112(24):Suppl Resuscitation Council UK website www.resus.org.uk

American Heart Association/Centers for Disease Control and Prevention Scientific Statement 2003 Markers of inflammation and cardiovascular disease: application to clinical and public health practice. Circulation 107:499–511

Baskett P, Nolan J 2005 A pocket book of European Resuscitation Council guidelines for resuscitation 2005. Elsevier, Edinburgh

British Heart Foundation Statistics website http://www.heartstats.org/homepage.asp?id=6

Department of Health 2000 National Service Framework for Coronary Heart Disease.

Gamon R, Quinn T, Parr B, et al 2007 Emergency care of the patient with a heart attack. Elsevier, Edinburgh

JRCALC Clinical Practice Guidelines website http://www2.warwick.ac.uk/fac/med/research/hsri/emergencycare/prehospitalcare/jrcalcstakeholderwebsite/

Marriott H, Conover M 1989 Advanced concepts in

arrhythmias, 2nd edition. Mosby, St Louis

Page B 1998 12-lead ECG interpretation workshop. Multi-lead Medics, St Louis

Phalen T, Aehelert B 2006 The 12 lead ECG in acute coronary syndromes, 2nd edition. Elsevier, Edinburgh

Scottish Intercollegiate Guidelines Network/ NICE 2007 Management of chronic heart failure: national clinical guidelines available at http://www.sign.ac.uk/pdf/sign95.pdf

Taigman M, Cannon S 1990 Reading bundle branch blocks. J Emerg Med Serv JEMS 15(5):41

CHAPTER **16**

Neurology

Chapter contents

Objectives

Upon completion of this chapter, the paramedic student will be able to:

1. Describe the anatomy and physiology of the nervous system.
2. Outline pathophysiological changes in the nervous system that may alter the cerebral perfusion pressure.
3. Describe the assessment of a patient with a nervous system disorder.
4. Describe the pathophysiology, signs and symptoms, and specific management techniques for each of the following neurological disorders: coma, stroke and intracranial haemorrhage, convulsion disorders, headaches, brain neoplasm and brain abscess, and degenerative neurological diseases.

Key terms

amyotrophic lateral sclerosis One of a group of rare disorders in which the nerves that control muscular activity degenerate in the brain and spinal cord; also called Lou Gehrig disease.

Bell's palsy A condition in which paralysis of the facial muscles is caused by inflammation of the seventh cranial nerve; the condition usually is one sided and temporary and often develops suddenly.

central pain syndrome Infection or disease of the trigeminal nerve (cranial nerve V).

cluster headache A type of headache that occurs in bursts (clusters); also known as a histamine headache.

convulsion A temporary change in behaviour or consciousness caused by abnormal electrical activity in one or more groups of neurons in the brain.

dystonia A condition characterized by local or diffuse changes in muscle tone, resulting in painful muscle spasms, unusually fixed postures, and strange movement patterns.

epilepsy A condition characterized by a tendency of the individual to have recurrent convulsions (excluding those that arise from correctable or avoidable circumstances).

migraine A severe, incapacitating headache that often is preceded by visual and/or gastrointestinal (GI) disturbances.

multiple sclerosis A progressive disease of the central nervous system in which scattered patches of myelin in the brain and spinal cord are destroyed.

muscular dystrophy An inherited muscle disorder of unknown cause marked by a slow but progressive degeneration of muscle fibres.

myoclonus A condition characterized by rapid, uncontrollable contractions or spasms of muscles that occur at rest or during movement.

Parkinson's disease A disease caused by degeneration or damage (of unknown origin) to nerve cells in the basal ganglia in the brain.

peripheral neuropathy Diseases and disorders that affect the peripheral nervous system, including the spinal nerve roots, cranial nerves, and peripheral nerves.

sinus headache A headache characterized by pain in the forehead, nasal area, and eyes.

spina bifida A congenital defect in which part of one or more vertebrae fails to develop completely, leaving a portion of the spinal cord exposed.

status epilepticus Continuous convulsion activity lasting 30 min or longer, or a recurrent convulsion without an intervening period of consciousness.

tension headache A headache caused by muscle contraction in the face, neck, and scalp.

Acute disorders of the nervous system require rapid assessment and management. Paramedics must combine knowledge and skills with appropriate and aggressive intervention. These actions can help reduce mortality and morbidity. Proper recognition and treatment are the foundation for the greatest potential for rehabilitation and recovery.

Anatomy and physiology of the nervous system

The nervous system is divided into two parts (Figure 16-1). These two parts are the central nervous system (CNS) and the peripheral nervous system (PNS). The ability of the human body to maintain a state of balance (homeostasis) is chiefly the result of the nervous system's ability to coordinate and regulate the body's activities. The CNS consists of the brain and spinal cord, both of which are encased in and protected by bone. A total of 43 pairs of nerves originate from the CNS to form the PNS: 12 pairs of cranial nerves originate from the brain and 31 pairs of spinal nerves originate from the spinal cord.

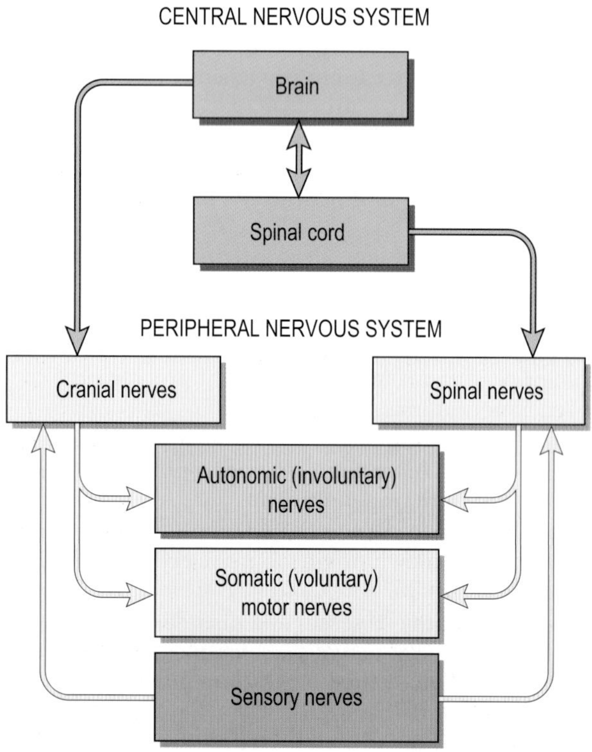

Figure 16-1 Divisions of the nervous system.

Cells of the nervous system

The cells of the nervous system include neurons (the basic units of the nervous system) and connective tissue cells known as neuroglia (specialized cells that protect and hold functioning neurons together). Each neuron has three main parts (Figure 16-2): (1) the cell body, which has a single, relatively large nucleus with a prominent nucleolus; (2) one or more branching projections, called dendrites; and (3) a single, elongated projection, known as an axon. Dendrites transmit impulses to the cell bodies whilst axons transmit impulses away from the cell bodies. Axons are surrounded by supportive and protective sheaths. In the CNS (unmyelinated axons), these sheaths are formed by the cytoplasmic extensions of neuroglial cells. In the PNS (myelinated axons), the sheaths are formed by Schwann cells.

Bundles of parallel axons with their associated sheaths are white and are called white matter. The action potential, which is initiated in the neuron body, is propagated through the axons via conduction pathways or nerve tracts from one area of the CNS to another. In the PNS, bundles of axons and their sheaths are called nerves. Collections of nerve cells are greyer in colour and are called grey matter, which is the site of integration in the nervous system. The outer surface of the cerebrum and the cerebellum consists of grey matter, which forms the cerebral cortex and the cerebellar cortex.

Types of neurons

Neurons are classified as sensory neurons, motor neurons or interneurons, based on the direction in which they transmit impulses. Sensory neurons transmit impulses to the spinal cord and brain from all parts of the body. Motor neurons transmit impulses in the opposite direction, away from the brain and spinal cord, as well as transmitting impulses only to muscle and glandular epithelial tissue. Interneurons (called central or connecting neurons) conduct impulses from sensory neurons to motor neurons; sensory neurons also are called afferent neurons and motor neurons are called efferent neurons.

Impulse transmission

The transmission of nerve impulses in the nervous system is similar to the conduction of electrical impulses through the heart. In its resting state, the neuron is positively charged on the outside and negatively charged on the inside. When stimulated by pressure, temperature, or chemical changes, the permeability of the neuron's membrane to sodium ions increases. As a result, positively charged sodium ions rush into the interior of the neuron. This inward movement begins a wave of depolarization which travels down the axon, resulting in the propagation of an action potential (Figure 16-3).

> **Critical Thinking**
>
> Think of examples of a pressure, a temperature and a chemical stimulus to a nerve.

In unmyelinated axons, action potentials are spread along the entire axon membrane. Myelinated axons, however, have interruptions in the myelin sheaths, known as nodes of

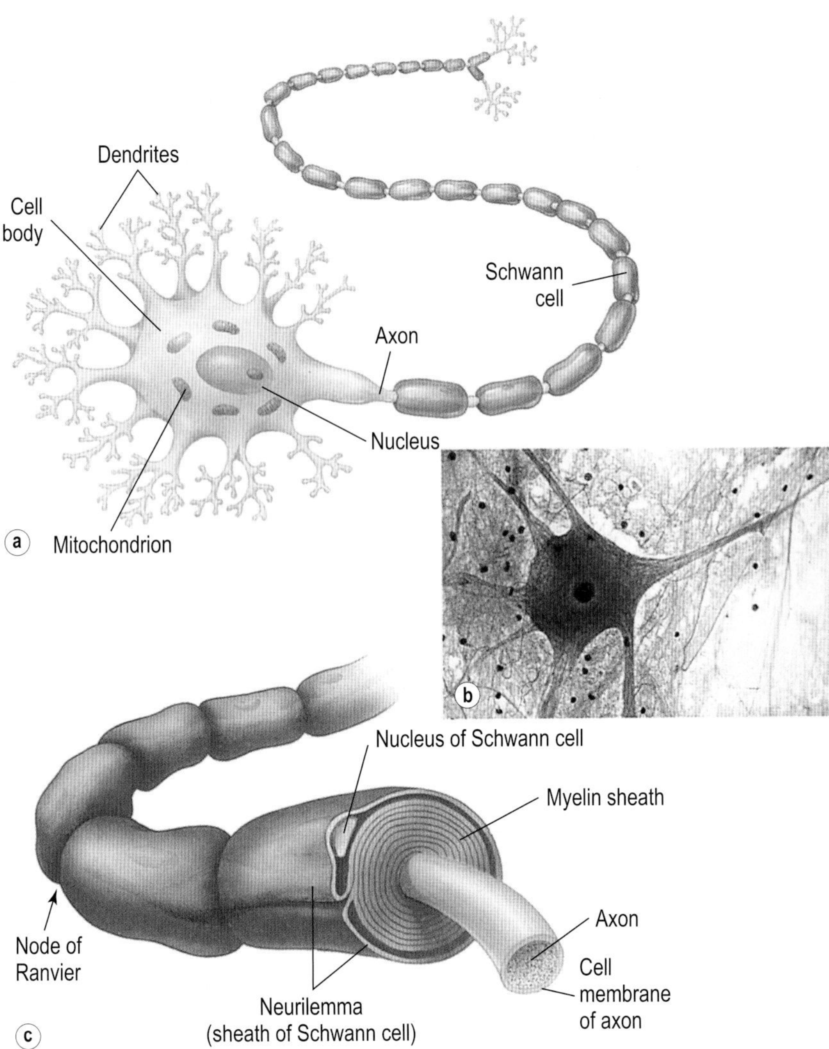

Figure 16-2 (a) Typical neuron showing dendrites, a cell body, and an axon. (b) Photomicrograph of a neuron. (c) Segment of a myelinated axon cut to show detail of the concentric layers of the Schwann cell filled with myelin.

Ranvier. These nodes allow nerve impulses to 'jump' from one node to the next without spreading along the entire length of the cell (saltatory conduction), therefore myelinated axons conduct action potentials faster than unmyelinated axons.

Synapse

The membrane-to-membrane contact that separates the axon endings of one neuron (presynaptic neuron) from the dendrites of another neuron (postsynaptic neuron) is known as a synapse. The structures that compose a synapse are the presynaptic terminal, the synaptic cleft, and the plasma membrane of the postsynaptic neuron. Within each presynaptic terminal are synaptic vesicles, containing neurotransmitter chemicals (Figure 16-4).

Each action potential arriving at the presynaptic terminal initiates a series of specific events that result in the release of the neurotransmitter substance. The neurotransmitter chemical rapidly diffuses the short distance across the synaptic cleft, then binds to specific receptor molecules on the postsynaptic membrane. After an impulse is generated and is conducted by the postsynaptic neurons, neurotransmitter activity ends rapidly. Several substances have been identified as neurotransmitters; others are thought to be neurotransmitters. Well-known neurotransmitters include acetylcholine, noradrenaline, adrenaline and dopamine.

Reflexes

One type of route travelled by nerve impulses is a reflex or reflex arc. A reflex is the basic unit of the nervous system that is capable of receiving a stimulus and generating a response. Reflexes allow conduction of impulses in one direction and have several basic components: a sensory receptor, a sensory neuron, interneurons, a motor neuron, and an effector organ. Individual reflexes vary in complexity; some function to remove the body from painful stimuli, some prevent the body from suddenly falling or moving as a result of external forces, and others are responsible for maintaining a relatively constant blood pressure, body fluid pH, blood carbon dioxide level and water intake. All reflexes are homeostatic; that is, they function to maintain healthy survival.

Action potentials initiated in sensory receptors spread along sensory axons in the PNS to the CNS, where they synapse with interneurons. Interneurons synapse with motor

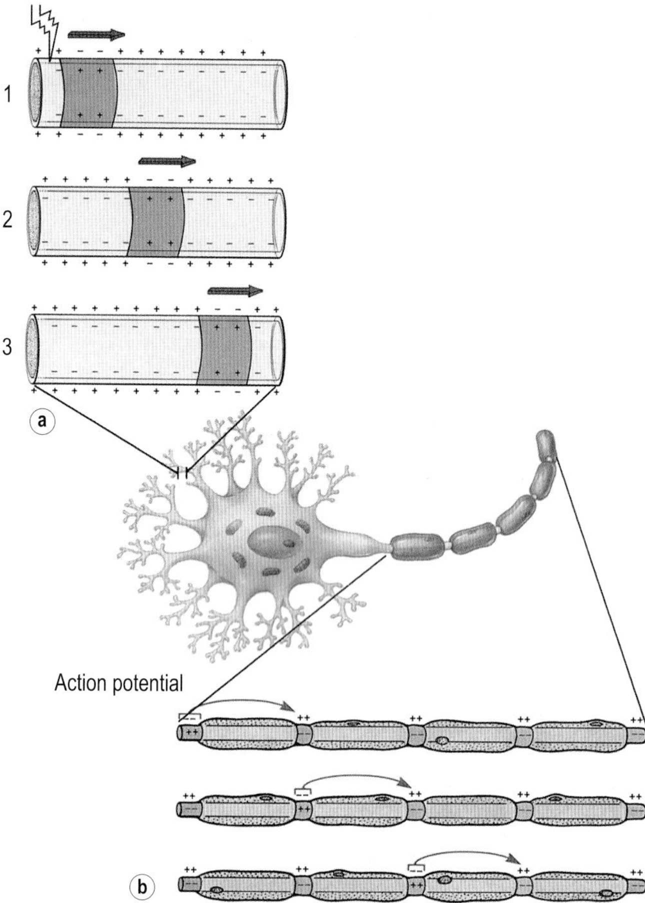

Figure 16-3 Conduction of nerve impulses. (a) In unmyelinated fibre, a nerve impulse (action potential) is a self-propagating wave of electrical disturbance. (b) In myelinated fibre, the action potential 'jumps' around the insulating myelin in a rapid type of conduction called saltatory conduction.

neurons in the spinal cord, which send their axons out of the spinal cord and through the PNS to muscles or glands. This causes the effector organ to respond. Figure 16-5 shows the transmission of nerve impulses that result in the patellar (knee-jerk) reflex.

Blood supply

The arterial blood supply to the brain comes from the vertebral arteries and the internal carotid arteries (Figure 16-6). The right and left vertebral arteries (supplying the cerebellum) enter the cranial vault through the foramen magnum and unite to form the midline basilar artery. The basilar artery branches to supply the pons and the cerebellum; it divides again to form the posterior cerebral arteries which supply the posterior portion of the cerebrum.

The internal carotid arteries enter the cranial vault through the carotid canals; these vessels give rise to the anterior cerebral arteries. The anterior cerebral arteries supply blood to the frontal lobes of the brain and end by forming the middle cerebral arteries; these supply a large portion of the lateral cerebral cortex. A posterior communicating artery branches off each internal carotid artery and connects with the ipsilateral posterior cerebral artery. The two posterior cerebral arteries are connected at their common origin from the basilar artery. The anterior cerebral arteries are connected by an anterior communicating artery and they complete a circle around the pituitary gland and the brain. This is the circle of Willis. The circle of Willis provides an important safeguard, helping to ensure the supply of blood to all parts of the brain in the event of a blockage in one of the vertebral or internal carotid arteries.

The veins that drain blood from the head form the venous sinuses (these are the spaces in the dura mater surrounding the brain); eventually they drain into the internal jugular

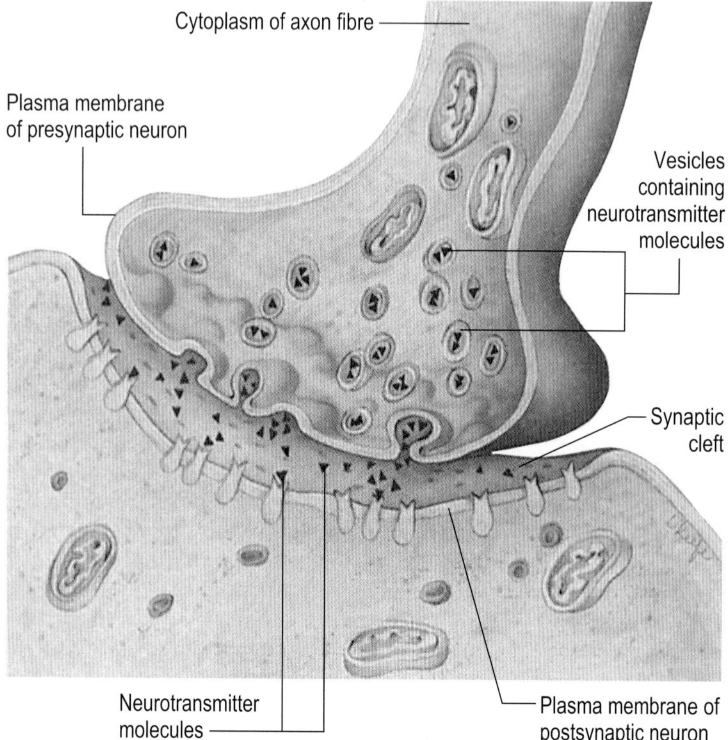

Figure 16-4 Components of a synapse. The diagram shows an axon terminal of a presynaptic neuron and a synaptic cleft. When an action potential arrives at the axon terminal of a presynaptic neuron, neurotransmitter molecules are released from vesicles in the axon terminal into the synaptic cleft. The combining of neurotransmitter and receptor molecules in the plasma membrane of the postsynaptic neuron initiates impulse conduction in the postsynaptic neuron.

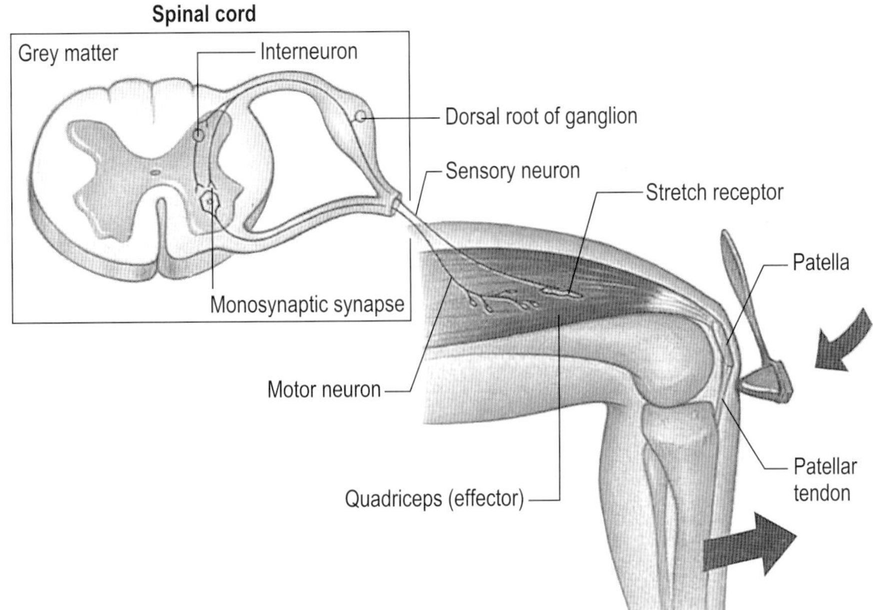

Figure 16-5 Neural pathway involved in the patella (knee-jerk) reflex.

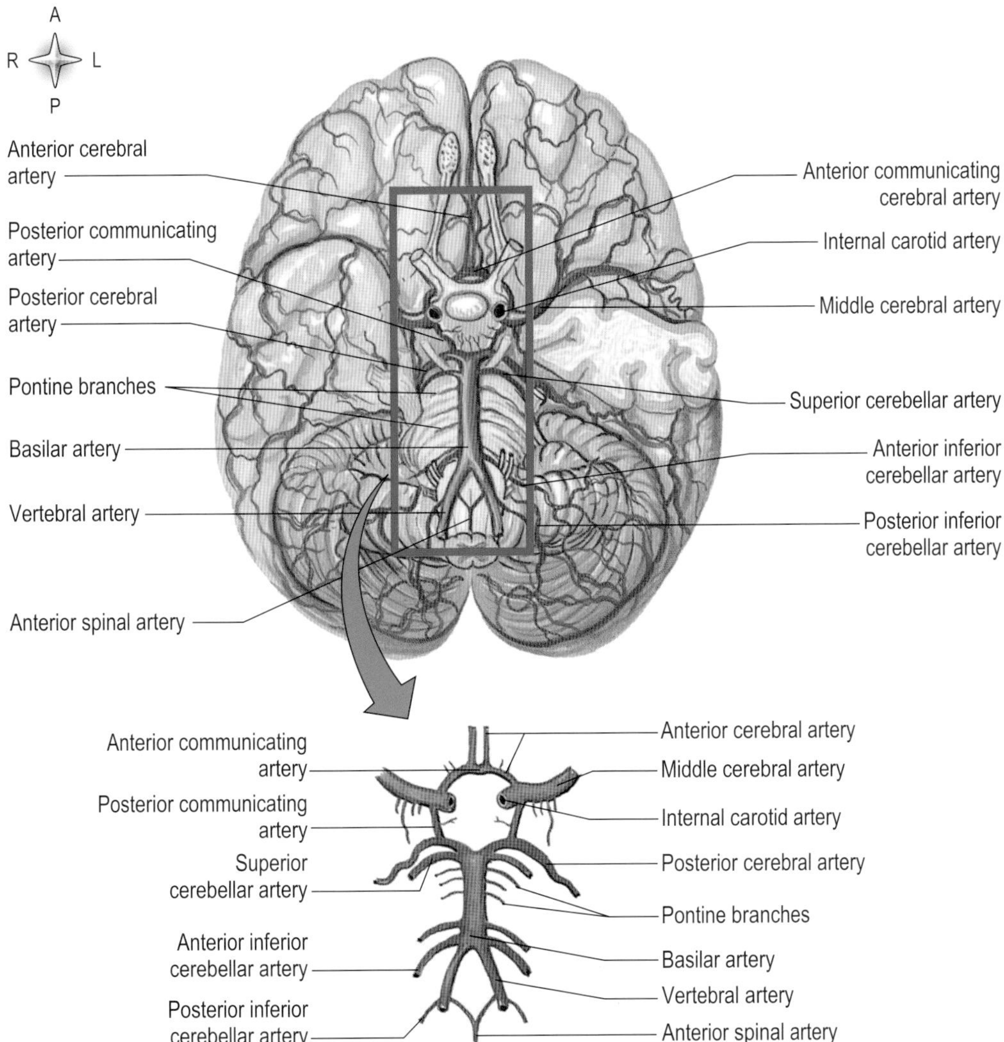

Figure 16-6 Inferior view of the brain showing vertebral, basilar, and internal carotid arteries and their branches.

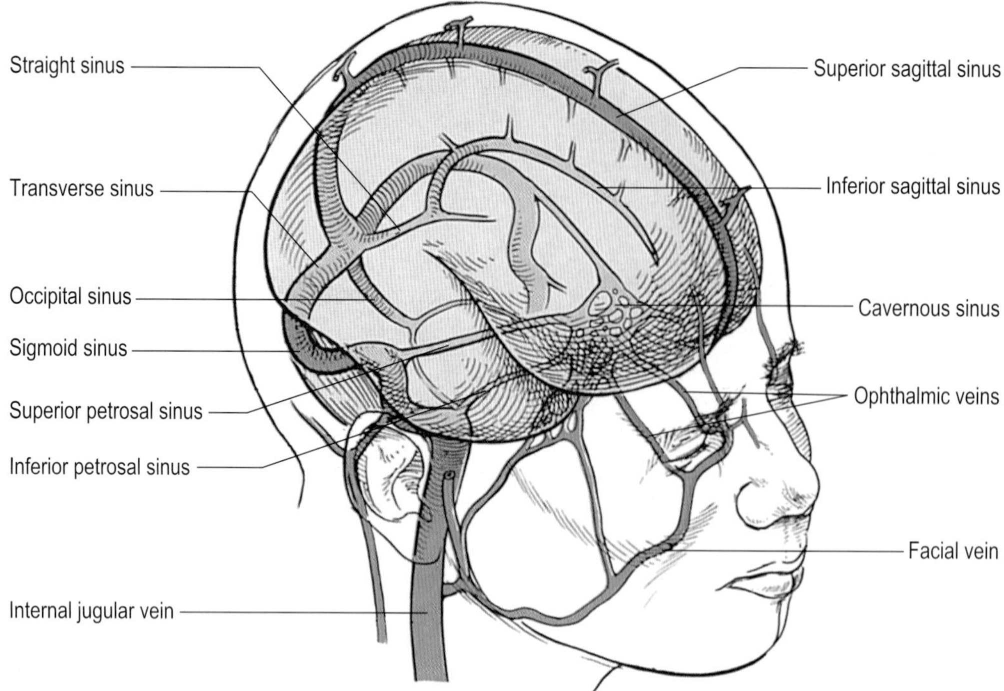

Figure 16-7 Venous sinuses associated with the brain.

veins (Figure 16-7). These veins exit the cranial vault and join with several other veins that drain the external head and face. The internal jugular veins join the subclavian veins on each side of the body.

Ventricles

Each cerebral hemisphere contains a large space (known as a lateral ventricle) that is filled with cerebrospinal fluid (CSF). The lateral ventricles are connected posteriorly whilst a third ventricle is located in the centre of the diencephalon between the two halves of the thalamus. The two lateral ventricles communicate with the third ventricle through two interventricular foramina and the third ventricle communicates with the fourth ventricle (located in the superior region of the medulla) by way of a narrow canal, known as the cerebral aqueduct. The fourth ventricle is continuous with the central canal of the spinal cord.

Critical Thinking

What happens if the flow in one of these canals becomes obstructed?

Divisions of the brain

The major divisions of the adult brain are the brainstem (medulla, pons, midbrain and site of the reticular formation), cerebellum, diencephalon (hypothalamus and thalamus) and cerebrum (Figure 16-8).

Neurological pathophysiology

Some neurological emergencies are a consequence of structural changes or damage, circulatory changes, or alterations in intracranial pressure (ICP) that affect cerebral blood flow (CBF). Three structures occupy the intracranial space; brain tissue, blood, and water. Brain tissue contains mostly water, both intracellular and extracellular. Blood is contained within the major arteries in the base of the brain; in arterial branches, arterioles, capillaries, venules, and veins in the substance of the brain; and in the cortical veins and dural sinuses. Water is located in the ventricles of the brain, in the CSF, and in extracellular and intracellular fluid. Normally the volumes of brain tissue, blood, and water are such that the pressure inside the skull is maintained within a millimetre of mercury above atmospheric pressure.

Cerebral perfusion pressure

Cerebral blood flow depends on the cerebral perfusion pressure (CPP), which is the pressure gradient across the brain. CBF remains constant when the CPP is 50 to 160 mmHg. If the CPP falls below 40 mmHg, cerebral blood flow declines; this critically affects cerebral metabolism. As explained in Chapter 31, the CPP is estimated as the mean arterial pressure (MAP) minus the ICP. With mild to moderate elevation of the ICP, the MAP usually rises; the rise in the MAP causes cerebral blood vessels to constrict and prevents the increase in blood volume and CBF that normally would occur.

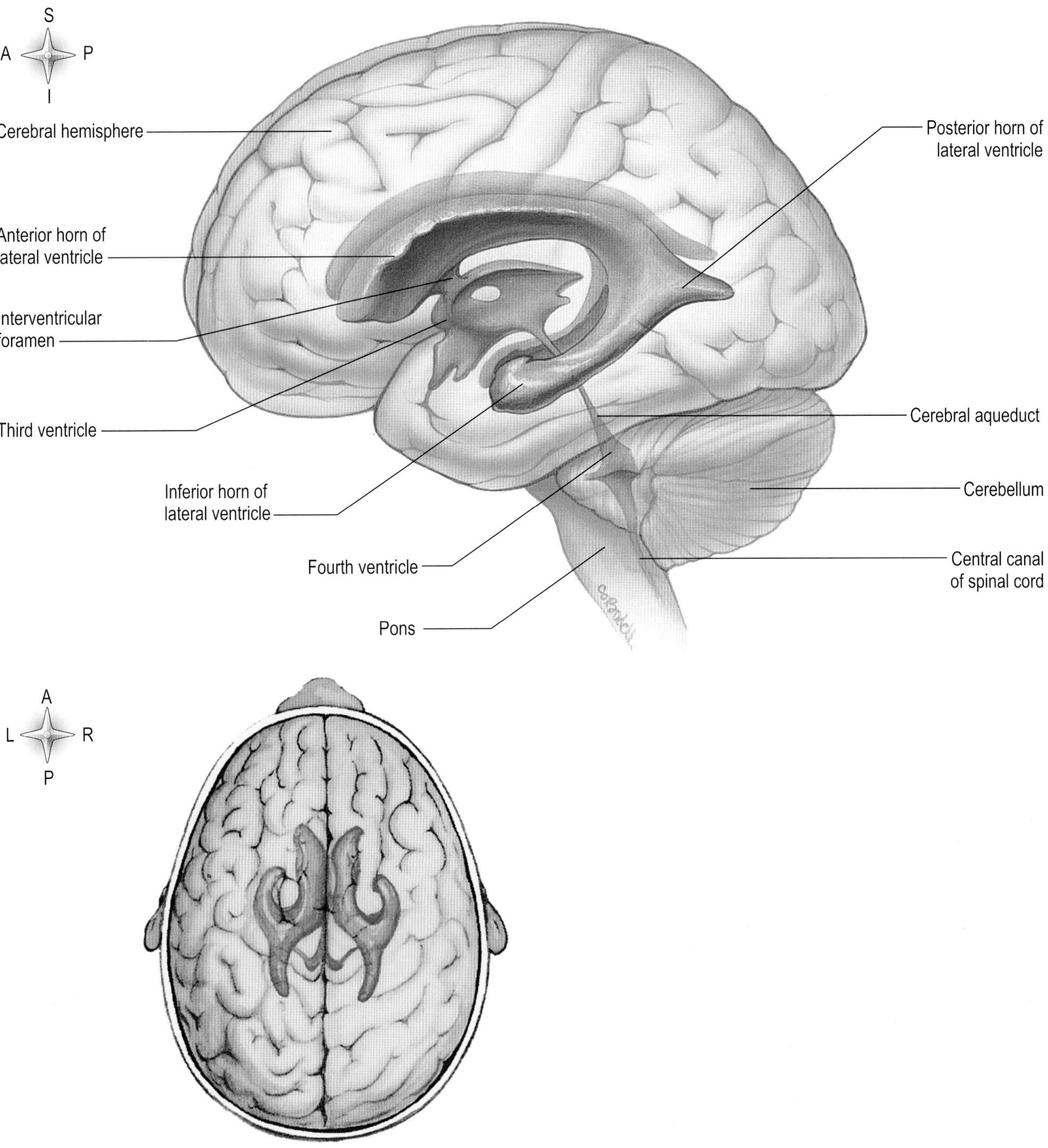

Figure 16-8 Divisions of the brain.

Critical Thinking

Relate the difficulty created for cerebral blood flow by increased intracranial pressure to having a person push on a door from the outside while you try to open it from the inside. How much harder is it for you to open the door?

On the other hand, if the MAP falls, the cerebral arteries dilate, increasing cerebral blood flow; therefore with an MAP of about 60 to 150 mmHg, cerebral blood flow may be maintained in a constant state. However, when ICP elevations are marked (greater than 22 mmHg), perfusion of brain tissue often decreases despite a rise in the systemic arterial pressure. If a mass or cerebral oedema develops, an immediate reduction in the volume of one or more of these components (brain tissue, blood, or water) must occur to prevent the ICP from rising and compressing brain tissue.

Assessment of the nervous system

The assessment approaches used in non-traumatic neurological emergencies are very similar to those used for neurological trauma. The following discussion of patient assessment focuses on non-traumatic neurological emergencies; assessment of neurological trauma is addressed in Chapter 31.

As with all patient encounters, care of a patient with a non-traumatic neurological emergency begins with the initial assessment. Paramedics should have a systematic approach for examining these patients, which helps to ensure that they do not miss signs and symptoms that may indicate an urgent condition. The goals of emergency care are (1) management of the airway, (2) stabilization and support of the cardiovascular system, (3) intervention to interrupt ongoing cerebral injury, and (4) protection of the patient from further harm while at the scene and during transport to an appropriate medical facility.

Initial assessment

The paramedic should begin the initial assessment by determining the patient's level of consciousness; an open and patent airway also must be ensured. If the patient is unconscious when paramedics arrive and there is reason to suspect a cervical spine injury, the patient's airway should be opened with spinal precautions and the cervical spine immobilized. It is important to remember that an unconscious patient is unable to maintain the airway and so airway adjuncts may be indicated. The patient's airway and breathing also should be closely monitored for respiratory deterioration or respiratory arrest which may result from an increased ICP. The patient should be closely watched for vomiting or aspiration of stomach contents; suction should be readily available.

Note

The mantra of the cardiologist is 'time is muscle'. Many neurologists agree that in a similar way rapid assessment and management of the patient suffering stroke or other neurological emergency and transport to definitive care is the most prudent course of action.

Support of breathing and administration of supplemental oxygen should be provided for any patient experiencing a neurological emergency whose oxygen saturation is less than 95%. Increased carbon dioxide pressure (PCO_2) or decreased oxygen pressure (PO_2) results in dilation of the blood vessels. As the PCO_2 drops, blood volume and blood flow to the brain are reduced.

Physical examination

A patient with neurological illness may be difficult to assess, particularly if the patient's mental function is impaired. Key elements of the physical examination may offer clues to the cause of the neurological emergency and include the patient history, the history of the event, vital signs, and respiratory patterns.

History

After any life-threatening problems have been identified and managed, the paramedic should attempt to compile a thorough history with information from the patient (when possible) or from family members or bystanders. The following are the six important elements of the patient history:

1. The patient's presenting complaint
2. Details of the presenting illness
3. Pertinent underlying medical problems with particular consideration of:
   a. Cardiac disease
   b. Lung disease
   c. Neurological disease (e.g. multiple sclerosis)
   d. Previous stroke
   e. History of convulsions or epilepsy
   f. Diabetes
   g. Hypertension
4. Alcohol or other drug use
5. Previous history of similar symptoms
6. Recent injury (particularly head trauma).

If a loss of consciousness was involved, the paramedic should ascertain the events that led up to the unconscious state. This information may include the patient's position (sitting, standing, lying down), whether the person complained of a headache, and whether convulsive activity or a fall occurred. At times no history is available or is very uncertain and in such cases paramedics should assume that the onset of unconsciousness was acute which might be from causes such as an intracranial haemorrhage. In addition, they should be alert for any environmental clues such as evidence of current prescribed medications, medical alert identification, recreational drugs, or alcohol or drug paraphernalia.

Critical Thinking

How could having one of the conditions listed in the six important elements of the patient's history result in a change in the patient's neurological status?

Vital signs

The patient's vital signs should be checked and frequently recorded. This is important because the vital signs may change rapidly in patients with a neurological emergency. The patient's electrocardiogram (ECG) also should be monitored for dysrhythmias; these commonly occur with neurological problems (for example there is a link between atrial fibrillation and the risk of stroke).

The early stages of increased ICP are marked by an increase in systolic pressure, a widened pulse pressure, and a decrease in the pulse and respiratory rate (Cushing triad) (Figure 16-9). In the terminal stages, the ICP continues to rise and brain tissue is compressed. As this occurs, body temperature

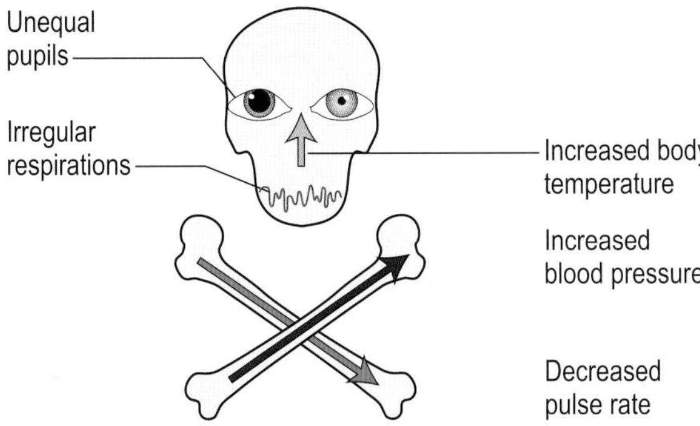

Figure 16-9 Cushing triad.

usually remains elevated and the pulse rate generally drops. Also, the blood pressure falls, particularly after herniation occurs; thus hypotension is a late and very serious sign.

Respiratory patterns

The respiratory pattern of a patient with a neurological emergency may be normal or abnormal. Sometimes respiratory arrest is caused by damage to the lower respiratory centres in the medulla and respiratory abnormalities of rate and rhythm may occur. These abnormalities may provide clues to which area of the brain is involved and possibly indicate the severity of the neurological problem. Apnoea can occur with loss of consciousness even with relatively minor head trauma. However, acute respiratory arrest usually results from involvement of the medullary respiratory centre (brainstem compression or infarct). Damage to neural pathways (anywhere from the cortex down to the medulla) more often produces changes with the respiratory rhythm/pattern, rather than respiratory arrest. Abnormal respiratory patterns (see Chapter 14) include the following:

- Cheyne–Stokes respiration
- central neurogenic hyperventilation
- ataxic respiration
- apneustic respiration
- diaphragmatic breathing.

Critical Thinking

Consider a patient who has ataxic or apneustic respirations. Which respiratory control centre is likely affected?

Neurological evaluation

Some neurological problems are obvious (e.g. paralysis); others may be subtle (e.g. a decreasing level of awareness). A sudden or rapidly worsening level of consciousness is the single most suggestive sign of a serious neurological condition.

Use of the mnemonic device AVPU (alert, verbal, painful, unresponsive) and the Glasgow Coma Scale (see Chapter 31) are quick, easy ways to determine the patient's baseline neurological status that allow comparisons for future management. Evaluation should be repeated and recorded often, so changes in the patient's mental state can be detected as soon as possible.

When evaluating a patient's neurological status, the paramedic should report and record patient information with descriptive terms. These terms should be specific to responses to certain stimuli; for example, 'The patient has no recall of the event'; 'The patient moves on command'; and 'The patient does not open his eyes to painful stimuli'. Using clear descriptions of the patient's response allows others involved in the patient's care to follow the progression of the condition.

Posturing, muscle tone and paralysis

Significant neurological emergencies may be associated with abnormal or unusual posturing, paralysis of a limb or several limbs, or both. Generally, disturbances of posture result from flexor spasms, extensor spasms, or flaccidity. Abnormal flexor response of one or both arms with extension of the legs is called decorticate rigidity; this abnormal posturing is thought to result from damage to the cortex of the brain. Abnormal extensor response of the arms with extension of the legs is called decerebrate rigidity; decerebrate rigidity has a worse prognosis than decorticate rigidity. It is thought to result from damage to the subcortical areas of the brain. Flaccidity usually is caused by brainstem or cord dysfunction and has a dismal prognosis.

Abnormal reflexes are not uncommon with decorticate or decerebrate rigidity. Associated with this may be a positive Babinski sign (see Chapter 9). The patient with this type of brain damage may be incontinent of urine or faeces, or both.

Pupillary reflexes

Examination of the pupils is very important in the unconscious patient; often drug use can at least be suspected based on the appearance and reaction of the pupils (Figure 16-10). If deviations from normal (in relative symmetry, size, and prompt reaction to light) are observed, it is crucial to note whether these deviations are unilateral or bilateral. If both pupils are dilated and do not react to light, the brainstem has probably been damaged; it may also occur when the brain has not received enough oxygen.

Note

The response of the pupils must be considered in conjunction with the patient's mental status. If the patient is awake, alert, and orientated, yet the pupils are unresponsive and dilated, this condition is most likely the result of, for example, topical medications used to induce pupillary dilation rather than a neurological problem.

Pupillary constriction is controlled by parasympathetic fibres, which originate in the midbrain and accompany the oculomotor nerve (cranial nerve III). Pupillary dilation involves fibres that travel the entire brainstem and return in the cervical sympathetic nerves. Midbrain injury interrupts both pathways. Generally it results in fixed, midsize pupils. Compression of the third cranial nerve interrupts parasympathetic nerve actions and is manifested by a unilateral,

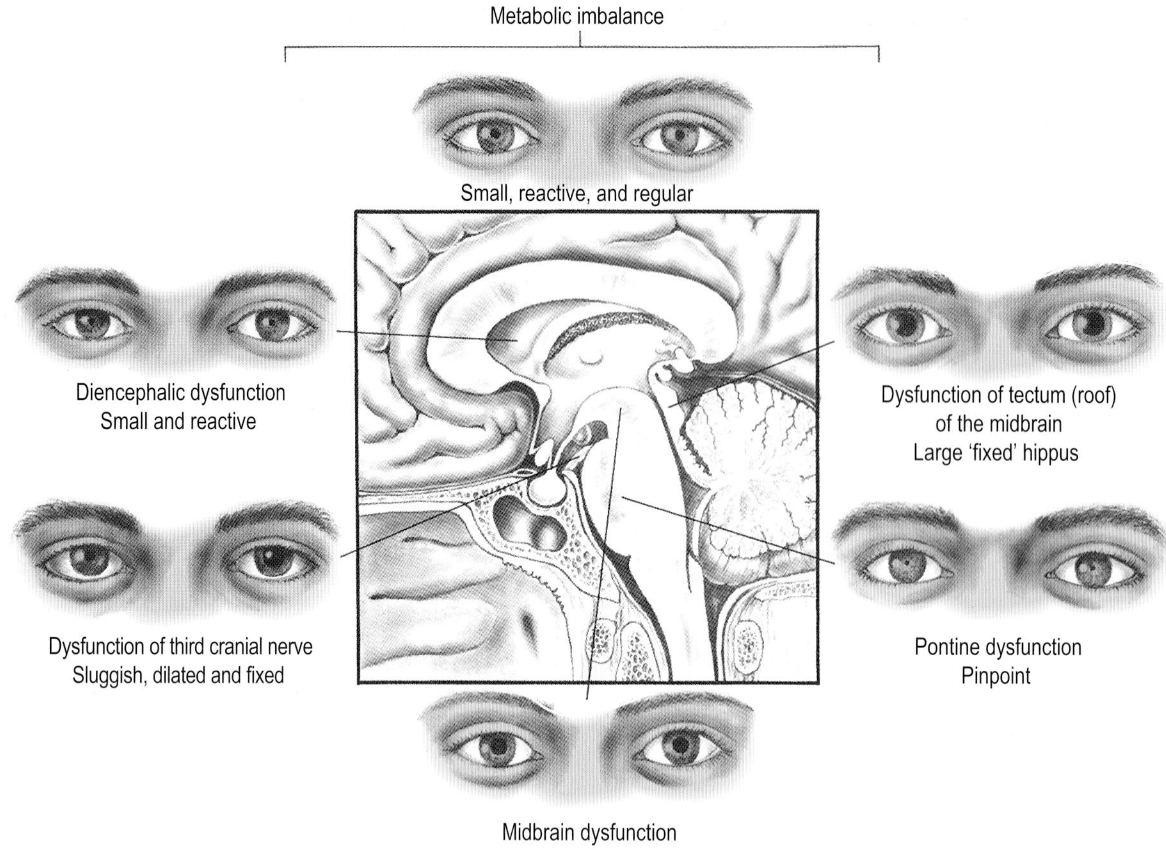

Figure 16-10 Pupils at different levels of consciousness.

fixed, dilated pupil. Any unconscious patient who suddenly develops a fixed, dilated pupil probably has suffered a significant brain injury that requires immediate transport to the proper medical facility.

Extraocular movements

Conscious patients should be able to move their eyes in full directional ranges. Paramedics can evaluate extraocular movements by asking the patient to follow their finger movements; for this test, the paramedic moves a finger to the extreme left and then up and down and to the extreme right and then up and down. Any deviations from normal should be recorded.

> **Critical Thinking**
>
> Which cranial nerves control eye movements?

A deviation of both eyes to either side (conjugate gaze) at rest implies damage to brain tissue (a lesion). The lesion may have an irritative focus; in this focus, the eyes look away from the lesion. Alternatively, they may have a destructive focus; in this focus, the eyes look toward the lesion. A deviation of the eyes to opposite sides (dysconjugate gaze) at rest implies damage to the brainstem (Figure 16-11).

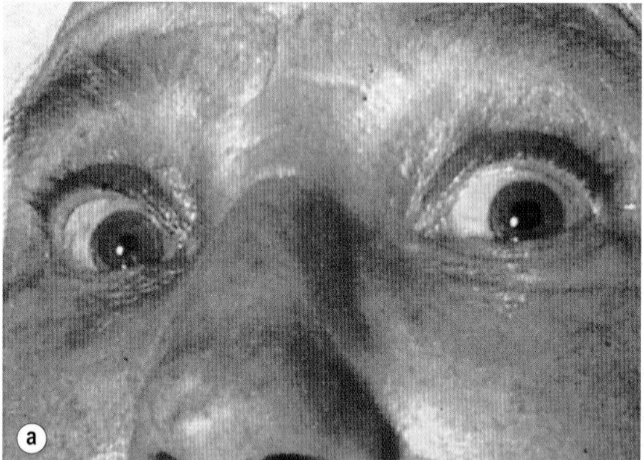

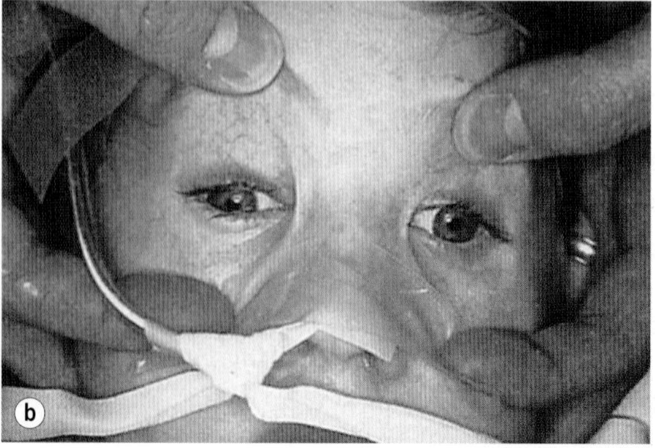

Figure 16-11 (a) Conjugate gaze. (b) Dysconjugate gaze.

Pathophysiology and management of specific central nervous system disorders

Disorders of the nervous system have many causes. Specific causes discussed in this chapter include structural and metabolic coma, stroke and intracranial haemorrhage (including transient ischaemic attack), convulsion disorders, headaches, and brain neoplasm and brain abscess. Several degenerative neurological diseases also are discussed.

Coma

Coma is an abnormally deep state of unconsciousness where the patient cannot be aroused by external stimuli. In general terms, only two mechanisms produce coma; structural lesions (e.g. a tumour or abscess) are one mechanism and depress consciousness by destroying or pressing on the reticular activating system in the brainstem. The other mechanism is toxic–metabolic conditions. These involve the presence of toxins or the lack of oxygen or glucose. Either type of toxic–metabolic condition may result in depression of the cerebrum, with or without depression of the reticular activating system.

Within these two primary mechanisms there are six general causes of coma (Box 16-1). A mnemonic aid that may be useful for remembering the common causes of coma is AEIOU-TIPS (Box 16-2).

Box 16-1

Six general causes of coma

Structural origin

- Intracranial bleeding
- Head trauma
- Brain tumour or other space-occupying lesions

Metabolic system

- Anoxia
- Hypoglycaemia
- Diabetic ketoacidosis
- Thiamine deficiency
- Kidney and liver failure
- Postictal phase of convulsion

Drugs

- Barbiturates
- Narcotics
- Hallucinogenics
- Depressants
- Alcohol

Cardiovascular system

- Hypertensive encephalopathy
- Shock
- Dysrhythmias
- Stroke

Respiratory system

- Chronic obstructive pulmonary disease
- Toxic inhalation (e.g. carbon monoxide poisoning)

Infection

- Meningitis
- Sepsis

Structural versus toxic–metabolic coma

Structural and toxic–metabolic causes of coma differ in two major ways. In patients with coma of structural origin, the neurological signs often are one-sided or asymmetrical. In toxic–metabolic coma, the neurological findings often are the same on both sides of the body. In addition, coma of toxic–metabolic origin often is slow to develop, whereas structural damage often occurs rapidly. Changes in pupil responses are the most important physical sign in distinguishing between structural and toxic–metabolic causes of coma. Normal pupil responses suggest that the coma has a toxic–metabolic cause, whereas unresponsive or asymmetrical pupils suggest structural damage.

Note

Coma-like states can be mimicked by some psychiatric conditions; a hysterical coma is one example. In these conditions, the unconscious state has no physical cause. Patients who appear unconscious as a result of a psychiatric condition often vigorously blink and move the eyes and usually also respond to annoying physical or verbal stimuli. In contrast, patients with organic sources of coma are unresponsive.

Unlike metabolic coma, structural coma follows a progressive pattern of deterioration, caused by local pressure or compression in the brain. The syndrome is often sudden in onset. The patient's signs and symptoms are often one-sided, or asymmetrical (e.g. hemiparesis). As a rule, structural lesions damage the reticular activating system as a result of increased ICP and herniation of the brain; this type of injury requires rapid surgical correction.

A knowledge of the difference between toxic–metabolic coma and structural coma can help the paramedic to understand what is likely to occur next in the patient's condition.

Assessment and management

Regardless of the cause of coma, prehospital care is directed at support of vital functions, prevention of further deterioration of the patient's condition, and possible administration

Box 16-2

Common causes of coma: AEIOU-TIPS

A – Acidosis or alcohol
E – Epilepsy
I – Infection
O – Overdose
U – Uraemia
T – Trauma
I – Insulin
P – Psychosis
S – Stroke

of medications, intravenous (IV) fluids, or both, to manage potentially reversible causes of coma. As always, airway maintenance and ventilatory support with supplemental oxygen are the first priorities in patient care; rapid transport for definitive care may be indicated.

If respirations are abnormally slow or shallow, ventilations should be supported. If the patient is unconscious and has no gag reflex, the trachea should be managed with advanced airway adjuncts. After securing the airway, the paramedic should take the following steps to treat a patient in a coma of unknown origin:

1. Cannulate the patient to achieve IV access.
2. Monitor the patient's ECG.
3. If hypoglycaemia is suspected, use a glucometer or other device to measure blood glucose levels and treat if low.
4. Where there is suspicion that opiates may be the cause of the unconsciousness, administer naloxone.
5. If the patient remains in a comatose state, transport the person in a lateral recumbent position (if not contraindicated). This aids drainage of secretions and also minimizes the chance of aspiration of stomach contents. Closely monitor the patient's airway and have suction readily available. On prolonged journeys, consider protecting the patient's eyes from corneal drying; this can be done by gently closing them and covering the lids with moist gauze pads.

Note

Thiamine is a B vitamin (B_1). It usually is found in adequate amounts in the normal diet. However, chronic alcoholism interferes with the intake, absorption, and utilization of thiamine. Serious neurological syndromes may occur where there is a thiamine deficiency.

Note

Patients who are dependent on opiates may have frank withdrawal symptoms. The paramedic should be prepared for a patient to become violent as the naloxone reverses the opiate adverse effects. Repeated doses of naloxone may be needed as the duration of some opiates may be longer than that of naloxone. Doses should be titrated to prevent any respiratory depression reoccurring.

Stroke and intracranial haemorrhage

Stroke is also known as cerebrovascular accident (CVA) or 'brain attack'. It is a sudden interruption in blood flow to the brain affecting a patient's normal neurological functioning. Stroke is a serious disease in England and Wales, with over 130 000 people having a stroke and 20 000 suffering a TIA each year. Stroke accounts for over 56 000 deaths per year, with a million or more living with the effects of stroke.[1] Around half of these people will require some form of health and social care support for their day-to-day activities. Individuals who are more likely to suffer a stroke have prior risk factors that can be classified as modifiable and non-modifiable. Modifiable risk factors include the following:

- high blood pressure
- cigarette smoking
- transient ischaemic attacks
- heart disease
- diabetes mellitus
- hypercoagulopathy
- high red blood cell count and sickle cell anaemia
- carotid bruit.

Non-modifiable risk factors include the following:

- age
- gender (men are at greater risk than women)
- race (African-Americans are at greater risk than Caucasians)
- prior stroke
- heredity.

The best way to prevent strokes is to identify individuals who are at risk and as many risk factors as possible must be controlled, by, for example, modification of poor health habits and drug therapy.

Pathophysiology

As described before, blood reaches the brain through four major vessels; two carotid arteries which provide about 80% of cerebral blood flow and the two vertebral arteries which combine to form the single basilar artery (supplying the remaining 20% of CBF). These two systems are interconnected at various levels, the principal level being the circle of Willis. In addition, collateral blood flow can be supplied to the brain through connections from blood vessels in the face to the dura and arachnoid coverings of the brain. The amount of collateral circulation varies from individual to individual. Beyond this, however, there is no collateral circulation in the depths of the brain and occlusion of any one of the more distal vessels may result in ischaemia and infarction.

Normally, the CBF is maintained through autoregulation of cerebral vessels which constrict or dilate to preserve perfusion pressure even when the patient is hypotensive. Arterial cerebral perfusion is regulated by the level of oxygen and glucose supplied (ischaemia and acidosis are profound vasodilators). Vessel occlusion or haemorrhage causes a sudden cessation of circulation to a portion of the brain. Autoregulatory mechanisms cannot readily correct this problem and uncorrected ischaemia that results within a short period of time leads to neuronal dysfunction and death. The onset and symptoms of the stroke depend on the area of the brain involved.

Critical Thinking

How much oxygen and glucose can the brain store for emergency situations?

Types of stroke

Stroke is a general term that refers to the neurological manifestations of a critical decrease in blood flow to a portion of the brain, regardless of the cause. There are two primary categories of stroke: ischaemic stroke (those caused by clots)

Box 16-3

Classification of strokes

Ischaemic strokes

Ischaemic strokes are caused by blood clots. This type of stroke accounts for 85% of all strokes. This is the only type of stroke for which fibrinolytics are administered. Ischaemic strokes are divided into two classes, depending on the cause:

1. Cerebral thrombosis
2. Cerebral embolism

Haemorrhagic strokes

Haemorrhagic strokes are caused by ruptured blood vessels. The two classes of haemorrhagic stroke are:

1. Intracerebral haemorrhage
2. Subarachnoid haemorrhage

Table 16-1 Differentiation of ischaemic and haemorrhagic strokes

Ischaemic strokes	Haemorrhagic strokes
Most common	Least common
Usually the result of atherosclerosis or tumour in the brain	Usually the result of cerebral aneurysms, AV malformations, hypertension
Develop slowly	Develop abruptly
Long history of vessel disease	Commonly occur during stress or exertion
May be associated with valvular heart disease and atrial fibrillation	May be associated with use of cocaine and other sympathomimetic amines
History of angina, previous strokes	May be asymptomatic before rupture

and haemorrhagic stroke (those caused by bleeding). Each of these is subdivided into two classes; for ischaemic stroke, these are cerebral thrombosis and cerebral embolism, and for haemorrhagic stroke, they are intracerebral haemorrhage and subarachnoid haemorrhage (Box 16-3).

Determining the origin of a stroke frequently is difficult in the prehospital setting and is often unnecessary. However, a paramedic who understands the various signs and symptoms of each type of stroke is better equipped to anticipate the course of patient care (Table 16-1). Documenting a thorough history and physical examination also helps others involved in the patient's care.

Ischaemic stroke

About 85% of strokes are the ischaemic type. They are caused by a cerebral thrombosis that occurs as a result of atherosclerotic plaques or pressure from a mass in the brain itself. Stroke caused by cerebral thrombosis is usually associated with a long history of blood vessel disease; most of these patients are older and also have evidence of atherosclerotic disease in other areas of the body (angina pectoris, claudication, previous strokes). The signs and symptoms of thrombotic stroke are usually slower to develop than those of cerebral haemorrhage; signs and symptoms include the following:

- hemiparesis or hemiplegia on the side of the body opposite the lesion
- numbness (decreased sensation) on the side of the body opposite the lesion
- aphasia
- confusion or coma
- convulsions
- incontinence
- diplopia (double vision)
- monocular blindness (painless visual loss in one eye)
- numbness of the face
- dysarthria (slurred speech)
- headache
- dizziness or vertigo
- ataxia.

Cerebral embolus

A stroke caused by an embolus results when an intracranial vessel is blocked by a foreign substance; the vessel is occluded by a fragment of a foreign substance originating outside the CNS. Common sources of cerebral emboli include atherosclerotic plaques (originating from large vessels of the head, neck, or heart). Thrombi that develop on the valves or in the chambers of the heart are very common in patients with heart valve disease and atrial fibrillation. Other, rare causes include air embolism from a chest injury and fat embolism after long bone injury, and bacterial and fungal infections of the heart can also produce emboli. Women taking oral contraceptives and patients with sickle cell disease have an increased risk of developing a stroke (by both thrombotic and embolic origin). Signs and symptoms of cerebral embolus are similar to those of thrombotic stroke but embolic signs and symptoms develop more quickly and often are associated with an identifiable cause (e.g. atrial fibrillation).

Haemorrhagic stroke

Cerebral haemorrhage accounts for about 15% of all strokes. A haemorrhage may occur anywhere in the brain and its structures, including the epidural, subdural, subarachnoid, intraparenchymal, and intraventricular spaces. The most common causes are cerebral aneurysms, arteriovenous (AV) malformations, and hypertension. Cerebral aneurysms and AV malformations are congenital anomalies and can run in families. They often are asymptomatic until they rupture. Unlike thrombotic and embolic strokes, which have relatively high survival rates, cerebral haemorrhages are fatal in 50–80% of cases.

Haemorrhagic strokes often occur during stress or exertion. Cocaine and other sympathetic-type drugs also may contribute to intracranial haemorrhage, through rapid elevation of blood pressure. The onset of the stroke is sudden, beginning with a headache, often described as the worst headache of the patient's life. The headache is accompanied by nausea, vomiting, and loss of consciousness; often the patient loses consciousness or experiences a convulsion at the time of the haemorrhage. As the haemorrhage expands, intracranial pressure (ICP) increases, causing the patient to become comatose, with increasing hypertension and bradycardia (Cushing reflex).

Critical Thinking

Why do you think mortality is higher for haemorrhagic stroke than for embolic stroke?

Transient ischaemic attacks

Transient ischaemic attacks (TIAs) are often referred to as little or ministrokes. They are episodes of cerebral dysfunction that affect a specific portion of the brain lasting minutes to several hours; the patient returns to normal within 24 h without permanent neurological deficit. A TIA is thought to be the most important indication of impending stroke; about 5% of patients who have a TIA go on to have a complete stroke within 1 month if untreated.

The signs and symptoms of a TIA are the same as those that characterize stroke, including weakness, paralysis, numbness of the face, and speech disturbances. All these correspond to vascular occlusion of a specific cerebral artery. Most patients who experience a TIA are hospitalized for close observation, evaluation, and treatment of vascular disease (e.g. endarterectomy, anticoagulant therapy).

Role of paramedics in stroke care

The role of a paramedic in stroke care is currently evolving. The paramedic's role is to quickly identify a stroke event, manage appropriately, and quickly transport to a facility for rapid, hospital-based evaluation and treatment. Key points in the management of stroke include the seven Ds: detection, dispatch, delivery, door, data, decision and drug (Box 16-4). (The first three Ds are the responsibility of the public and emergency medical services [EMS] providers.) The Royal College of Physicians, in their 'National Clinical Guideline for Diagnosis and Initial Management of Acute Stroke and Transient Ischaemic Attack (TIA)'[2] refer explicitly to prompt recognition and decision making in the prehospital setting.

Note

About 85% of strokes occur at home and therefore health promotion has focused on early recognition and care of individuals who suffer stroke as well as preventative measures to reduce the risk of occurrence. Similar to the ALS chain of survival a stroke chain of survival would be:

1. Rapid recognition and reaction to stroke warning signs.
2. Rapid EMS dispatch.
3. Rapid EMS transport and hospital prenotification.
4. Rapid diagnosis and treatment in the hospital.

Box 16-4

Seven Ds of stroke management*

Detection: A patient, family member, or bystander recognizes the signs and symptoms of a stroke or transient ischaemic attack (TIA) and calls EMS for help.

Dispatch: EMS dispatchers prioritize the call regarding a suspected stroke and dispatch the appropriate EMS team with high transport priority.

Delivery: EMS providers respond rapidly, confirm the signs and symptoms of stroke, and transport the patient (delivery) to an appropriate medical facility.

Door: An appropriate medical facility is a hospital that can provide fibrinolytic therapy within 1 h of arrival at the emergency department (ED) door.

Data: A computed tomography (CT) scan is obtained.

Decision: Candidates for fibrinolytic therapy are identified.

Drug: Eligible patients are treated with fibrinolytic therapy.

*The first three Ds are the responsibility of the public and emergency medical services (EMS) providers. The fourth D is the responsibility of EMS, and the last three Ds are performed in the hospital.

Assessment

The initial examination of a patient who may have suffered a stroke (or TIA) follows the same sequence as for any other ill or injured patient in the emergency setting. The priorities are to maintain a patent airway and to provide adequate ventilatory support with supplemental oxygen if required. If the patient is conscious and able to talk, a thorough history should be obtained. The following are important components of the patient history:

- time of symptom onset
- previous neurological symptoms (TIAs)
- previous neurological deficits
- initial symptoms and their progression
- alterations in level of consciousness
- precipitating factors
- dizziness
- palpitations
- significant past medical history
  - hypertension
  - diabetes mellitus
  - cigarette smoking
  - oral contraceptive use
  - cardiac disease
  - sickle cell disease
  - previous stroke.

In addition to the abnormal neurological signs and symptoms described previously, other methods such as assessment tools can be used to determine existence of stroke. These include Face Arm Speech Test (FAST), Cincinnati Prehospital Stroke Scale (CPSS), Los Angeles Prehospital Stroke Screen (LAPSS) and Melbourne Ambulance Stroke Screen (MASS). The FAST assess for facial weakness, arm weakness and speech disturbance and is adapted from the CPSS,[3] which evaluates three major physical findings: facial droop, arm drift, and speech (Box 16-5).

Los Angeles Prehospital Stroke Screen

The LAPSS is another way to diagnose stroke. This screening tool requires the examiner to rule out other causes of altered level of consciousness (e.g. hypoglycaemia or convulsion). The examiner then must identify asymmetry (right versus left) in facial smile/grimace, grip, and arm strength (Box 16-6). Asymmetry in any category indicates a possible stroke. Like the CPSS, the LAPSS can be used quickly in the prehospital setting and has a specificity of 97% and a sensitivity of 93%.

Management (Figure 16-12)

Once the diagnosis of a stroke is suspected, time in the field must be reduced, as treatment must begin as soon as possible; less than 3 h from onset is required for the use of fibrinolytics. Whenever possible, the paramedic should

Box 16-5

Cincinnati Prehospital Stroke Scale (CPSS)

Facial droop (have patient show teeth or smile)

- Normal—Both sides of face move equally well.
- Abnormal—One side of face does not move as well as the other side.

Arm drift (patient closes eyes and holds both arms out)

- Normal—Both arms move the same or both arms do not move at all (other findings, such as pronator grip, may be helpful).
- Abnormal—One arm does not move or one arm drifts down compared with the other.

Speech (have the patient say, 'You can't teach an old dog new tricks')

- Normal—Patient uses correct words with no slurring.
- Abnormal—Patient slurs words, uses inappropriate words, or is unable to speak.

Note: The presence of a single abnormality on the CPSS has a sensitivity of 59% and a specificity of 89% when scored by prehospital providers.

Box 16-6

Los Angeles Prehospital Stroke Screen (LAPSS)

For evaluation of acute, non-comatose, non-traumatic neurological complaint: If items 1 through 6 are all checked 'Yes' (or 'Unknown'), notify the receiving hospital before arrival of the potential stroke patient. If any are checked 'No,' follow the appropriate treatment protocol.

Interpretation: Ninety-three percent of patients with stroke have positive findings (all items checked 'Yes' or 'Unknown') (sensitivity = 93%). Of those with positive findings, 97% will have a stroke (specificity = 97%). The patient may still be having a stroke even if LAPSS criteria are not met.

Criteria	Yes	Unknown	No
1. Age >45	[]	[]	[]
2. History of convulsions or epilepsy absent	[]	[]	[]
3. Symptom duration <24 hours	[]	[]	[]
4. At baseline, patient is not wheelchair bound or bedridden	[]	[]	[]
5. Blood glucose between 4 and 10 mmol/L?	[]	[]	[]
6. Obvious asymmetry (right vs. left) in any of the following three categories (must be unilateral):	[]	[]	[]

	Equal	R Weak	L Weak
Facial smile/grimace	[]	[] Droop	[] Droop
Grip	[]	[] Weak grip	[] Weak grip
	[]	[] No grip	[] No grip
Arm strength	[]	[] Drifts down	[] Drifts down
	[]	[] Falls rapidly	[] Falls rapidly

establish the time of onset of stroke signs and symptoms. If the patient awoke with the symptoms, the time of onset should be recorded as the last time they were known to be normal; this is important for determining whether fibrinolytics can be administered. Prehospital care is directed at managing the patient's airway, breathing, and circulation, and monitoring vital signs. Besides life support, the most important care a paramedic can provide a stroke victim is quick identification of the possible stroke and rapid transport of the patient for definitive care.

Note

Many hospitals now have dedicated stroke units staffed with a multidisciplinary team experienced in managing stroke.

Airway

Paralysis of the muscles of the throat, tongue and mouth can lead to partial or complete airway obstruction and can be a major problem in acute stroke. Frequent suctioning of the oropharynx and nasopharynx may be required to prevent aspiration of saliva. If possible, the patient should be positioned to aid drainage of oral secretions.

Critical Thinking

How can you detect paralysis of the muscles of the throat, tongue and mouth on your physical examination?

Breathing

Inadequate ventilation should be managed with oxygen and positive-pressure ventilation, and hypoxia (<95% saturation on oximetry) managed by supplemental oxygen. Hypoxia and hypercarbia can occur as a result of inadequate ventilation, contributing to cardiac and respiratory instability.

Circulation

Cardiac arrest is uncommon but may result from a respiratory arrest. Cardiac dysrhythmias occur frequently and the patient's ECG and blood pressure require constant monitoring. A difference in blood pressure readings in the upper extremities of 10 mmHg or more may indicate aortic dissection and compromise of the brain's blood supply.

Note

Many patients develop hypertension after a stroke. However, this usually does not require emergency treatment. Elevated blood pressure after a stroke is not a hypertensive emergency unless the patient has other medical complications, such as an acute myocardial infarction (AMI) or left ventricular failure. Management of hypertension in the prehospital setting is not recommended in cases of suspected stroke.

Other supportive measures

If the airway is patent and the patient's condition permits, the individual should be kept supine but the head should

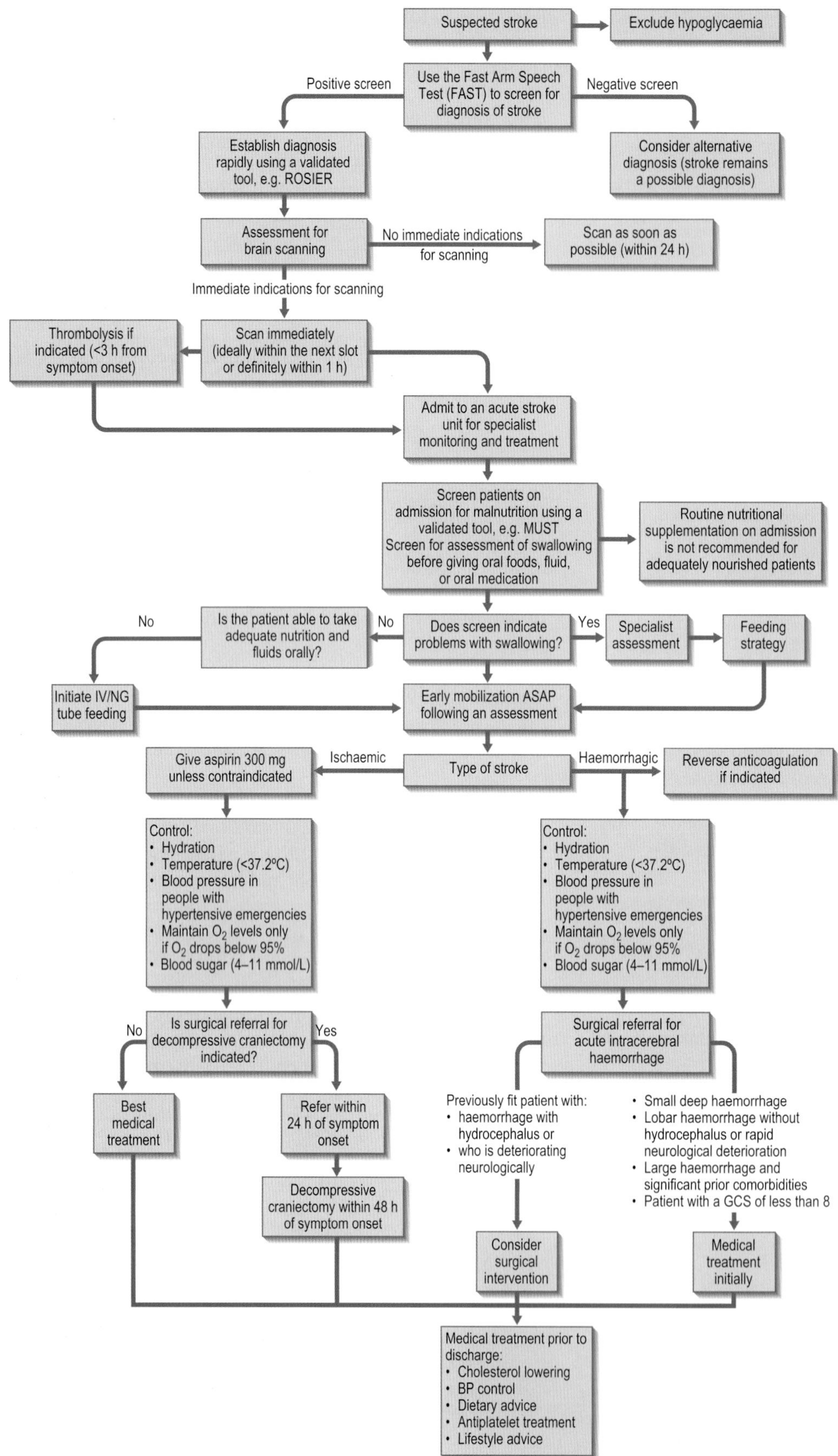

Figure 16-12 Algorithm for suspected cases of stroke. Reproduced with permission from National Institute for Health and Clinical Excellence (2008). CG 68 Stroke: diagnosis and initial management of acute stroke and transient ischaemic attack (TIA). London: NICE. Available from www.nice.org.uk/CG068.

be elevated 15 degrees. The patient should be nil by mouth and it is useful for a family member or other person (such as close friend) to travel with the patient, in case more history is needed. Other patient care measures the paramedic can provide while en route to the receiving hospital include the following:

1. IV access should be obtained (give IV fluids carefully to manage hypotension if necessary).
2. Blood glucose analysis can be performed (dextrose should be administered only if indicated to prevent the blood sugar level dropping below 4 mmol/L).
3. A 12-lead ECG should be recorded to supplement the 3-lead ECG monitoring already in place.
4. Paralysed extremities should be protected.
5. Normal body temperature should be maintained.
6. Any convulsions should be controlled with benzodiazepines.
7. Comfort measures and reassurance should be provided.
8. Care should be taken to ensure gentle but prompt transport to the receiving hospital with a relevant pre-alert: consider transfer to a specialist unit if local policy/practice allows.

Paramedics must keep in mind that stroke patients have experienced a catastrophic event, one that may seriously affect their quality of life. They often are frightened, embarrassed, confused and frustrated with their inability to move or communicate, have special physical and emotional needs and deserve a compassionate, caring approach.

In-hospital treatment

On arrival at the emergency department, the non-haemorrhagic stroke patient is evaluated as a possible candidate for fibrinolytic therapy. This evaluation includes an emergency neurological stroke assessment, which identifies the patient's level of consciousness and also identifies the type, location, and severity of the stroke. This assessment is aided by use of the Glasgow Coma Scale and other standardized scales. These scales and other in-hospital diagnostic studies help to measure neurological function, which correlates with the severity of the stroke and the long-term outcome. These studies also help to identify stroke patients who would benefit from fibrinolytic therapy. Rapid evaluation of the computed tomography (CT) scan is critical to rule out an intracranial haemorrhage, which is a contraindication for fibrinolytic therapy. Fibrinolytics have potential adverse effects and evaluation by a physician with inclusion–exclusion criteria to ensure the patient is a candidate for fibrinolytic therapy is necessary.

Convulsive disorders

A convulsion is a brief alteration in behaviour or consciousness, caused by abnormal electrical activity of one or more groups of neurons in the brain. The annual incidence of convulsion is estimated to be about 0.5% of the population, with the highest incidence among feverish children under 5 years of age. (Febrile convulsions are further addressed in Chapter 38.)

> **Critical Thinking**
>
> What feelings may parents experience after seeing their child have a febrile convulsion? How should you respond to those feelings?

The underlying cause of convulsions is not well understood. However, a convulsion is generally believed to result from a structural lesion or problems with brain metabolism which results in changes in the brain cell's permeability to sodium and potassium ions. When such changes occur, the neurons' ability to depolarize and emit an electrical impulse sometimes results in convulsion activity. Convulsions may be caused by several factors, including the following:

- stroke
- head trauma
- toxins (including alcohol or other drug withdrawal)
- hypoxia
- hypoperfusion
- hypoglycaemia
- infection
- metabolic abnormalities
- brain tumour or abscess
- vascular disorders
- eclampsia
- drug overdose.

In the prehospital setting, determining the cause of a convulsion is not as important as other measures such as managing the complications and recognizing whether the convulsion is reversible with therapy (e.g. whether it is caused by hypoglycaemia). A tendency to have recurrent convulsions is called epilepsy. (This does not include convulsions that arise from correctable or avoidable causes, such as alcohol withdrawal.)

Types of convulsions

All convulsions are pathological, may arise from almost any region of the brain and therefore have many clinical manifestations. The two most common types are generalized convulsions and partial (focal) convulsions.

Generalized convulsions

As the name implies, generalized convulsions do not have a definable origin (focus) in the brain, although focal convulsions may progress to generalized convulsions. This class includes petit mal (absence convulsions) and grand mal (tonic–clonic) convulsions. Petit mal convulsions occur most often in children between the ages of 4 and 12 and are characterized by brief lapses of consciousness without loss of posture; often no motor activity is seen. However, some children have eye blinking, lip smacking, or isolated contraction of muscles. These convulsions usually last less than 15 s. During this time, the patient is unaware of the surroundings. These convulsions are followed by the patient's immediate return to normal. Most patients have remission by age 20 but later may develop grand mal convulsions.

Grand mal convulsions are common and are associated with significant morbidity and mortality. Grand mal convulsions may be preceded by an aura such as an olfactory or auditory sensation. Often the patient recognizes the aura as a warning of the imminent convulsion; the convulsion is characterized by a sudden loss of consciousness associated with loss of organized muscle tone.

Critical Thinking

What could cause death after a grand mal convulsion?

The tonic phase is marked by a sequence of extensor muscle tone activity (sometimes flexion) and apnoea; tongue biting and bladder or bowel incontinence may occur. The tonic phase lasts only seconds and is followed by a bilateral clonic phase (rigidity alternating with relaxation). This usually lasts 1–3 min. During the clonic phase, a massive autonomic discharge occurs, resulting in hyperventilation, salivation, and tachycardia.

After the convulsion, the patient usually experiences a period of drowsiness or unconsciousness; this resolves over minutes to hours. On regaining consciousness, the patient often is confused and fatigued and may show signs of a transient neurological deficit; this part of the convulsion is known as the postictal phase. Grand mal convulsions may be prolonged or may recur before the patient regains consciousness. When this occurs, the patient is said to be in status epilepticus (see discussion later in the chapter).

Partial convulsions

In generalized convulsions, a specific convulsion focus is unknown. In contrast, partial convulsions arise from identifiable cortical lesions. Partial convulsions may be classified as simple or complex. Simple partial convulsions result mainly from convulsion activity in the motor or sensory cortex. Simple motor convulsions usually manifest as clonic activity that is limited to one body part. (For instance, this might be one hand, one arm or leg, or one side of the face.) Simple sensory convulsions result in symptoms such as tingling or numbness of a body part or abnormal visual, auditory, olfactory, or taste symptoms. Patients with partial convulsions generally do not lose consciousness. They usually maintain a somewhat normal mental status. However, the convulsion focus may spread and lead to a generalized tonic–clonic convulsion. Partial convulsion activity that spreads in an orderly way to surrounding areas is known as a jacksonian convulsion.

Complex partial convulsions arise from focal convulsions in the temporal lobe (psychomotor convulsions) and manifest mainly as changes in behaviour. The classic complex partial convulsion is preceded by an aura and followed by abnormal repetitive motor behaviour (automatisms) such as lip smacking, chewing, or swallowing. During this time the patient will have no memory of the event. These convulsions usually are brief, lasting less than 1 min, and the patient usually regains normal mental status quickly. Like simple partial convulsions, complex partial convulsions also may progress to a generalized tonic–clonic convulsion.

Note

A hysterical convulsion can mimic a true convulsion. However, it stems from psychological causes. These convulsions are not considered true convulsions because they have no physical cause. Also, they do not respond to the usual treatments. Hysterical convulsions, or pseudoconvulsions, usually can be ended by sharp commands or painful stimuli (e.g. a sternal rub). These manoeuvres may help to distinguish between pathological and psychogenic convulsion activity.

Assessment

The assessment process is determined by the patient's convulsion state; in most cases the patient's convulsion has ended before paramedics arrive. If possible, the assessment should include a thorough history and physical examination, including a neurological evaluation.

History

If the patient is in the postictal phase of the convulsion, information can be gathered from family members or bystanders who saw the event. Important components of the patient history include the following:

1. History of convulsions
   a. Frequency
   b. Compliance in taking prescribed medications (e.g. phenytoin, sodium valproate, carbamazepine and lamotrigine)
2. Description of convulsion activity
   a. Duration of convulsion
   b. Typical or atypical pattern of convulsion for the patient
   c. Presence of aura
   d. Generalized or focal
   e. Incontinence
   f. Tongue biting
3. Recent or past history of head trauma
4. Recent history of fever, headache, nuchal rigidity (suggesting meningeal irritation)
5. Past significant medical history
   a. Diabetes
   b. Heart disease
   c. Stroke.

Physical examination

During the physical examination, maintaining a patent airway is always of prime importance. The paramedic also should be alert for signs of trauma (head and neck trauma, tongue injury, oral lacerations). These injuries may have occurred before or during the convulsion. The patient's mouth should be inspected for gingival hypertrophy (swelling of the gums) as this is a sign of chronic phenytoin therapy. Other components of the physical examination include the following:

- level of sensorium, including presence or absence of amnesia
- cranial nerve evaluation, particularly pupillary findings

- motor and sensory evaluation, including coordination (abnormalities may be caused by metabolic disturbances, meningitis, intracranial haemorrhage and drug use)
- evaluation for hypotension, hypoxia and hypoglycaemia
- presence of urine or faeces (suggesting bladder or bowel incontinence)
- automatisms
- cardiac dysrhythmias.

Critical Thinking

What are signs and symptoms of phenytoin toxicity?

Syncope versus convulsion

It may be difficult to determine whether the patient has experienced a syncopal episode or a convulsion. The main difference is in the symptoms the patient experiences before and after the event. The factors listed in Table 16-2 may aid differentiation of these two events.

Management

The first step in managing a patient with convulsion activity is to protect the patient from injury. This is best achieved by removing obstacles in the patient's immediate area and, if necessary, the patient can be moved to a safe environment such as a carpeted or soft, grassy area. At no time should a patient with convulsion activity be restrained, nor should objects be forced between the patient's teeth to maintain an airway. Restraining activity may harm the patient or paramedic crew. Forcing objects into the oral cavity in an effort to secure an airway or prevent the patient from biting the tongue may evoke vomiting, aspiration, or spasm of the larynx.

Most patients with an isolated convulsion can be properly managed in the postictal phase by being placed in a lateral recumbent position. This allows drainage of oral secretions and aids suctioning (if needed). Supplemental oxygen should be administered. The patient should be moved to a quiet place (away from onlookers); patients often are embarrassed or self-conscious after a convulsion, especially if incontinence has occurred. Paramedics should be sensitive to the physical and emotional needs of the patient.

Some patients should always be transported to the emergency department for further evaluation; these include patients who have a history of convulsions but who experienced a convulsion that is different from the usual one, and patients with a convulsion that is complicated by an unusual event (e.g. trauma). All patients who have experienced a convulsion for the first time should be transported to the emergency department for evaluation by a physician. Depending on the patient's status and convulsion history, an IV line may be necessary to administer drug therapy such as benzodiazepines. However, few patients who experience an isolated convulsion require drug therapy in the prehospital setting.

Status epilepticus

Status epilepticus is ongoing convulsion activity that lasts for a prolonged period of time (5–20 min) or recurrent convulsions without a period of consciousness between them. Status epilepticus is a true emergency; without immediate management, it can result in permanent neurological damage, respiratory failure, and death. Associated complications of status epilepticus include aspiration, brain damage, and fracture of long bones and the spine. The most common cause in adults is failure to take prescribed anticonvulsant medications.

Management

As in all patients with convulsions, management priorities include managing the airway and providing ventilatory support, protecting the patient from injury, and transporting the patient to a medical facility for evaluation by a physician. In addition, management includes stopping the convulsion activity with anticonvulsant medications (e.g. diazepam or lorazepam).

After the airway has been secured with oral or nasal adjuncts (or with intubation of the trachea during the flaccid period between convulsions), high-concentration oxygen should be administered. If required, ventilation should be supported with a bag-valve device. IV access should be established. It should be secured well with an IV dressing and/or

Table 16-2 Differentiation of syncope and convulsion

Characteristic	Syncope	Convulsion
Position	Syncope usually starts when patient is in standing position	Convulsion may start with patient in any position
Warning	Patient usually has a warning period of lightheadedness	Patient has little or no warning
Level of consciousness	Patient usually regains consciousness immediately on becoming supine; fatigue, confusion, and headache last less than 15 min	Patient may remain unconscious for minutes to hours; fatigue, confusion, and headache last longer than 15 min
Tonic–clonic activity	Clonic movements (if present) are of short duration	Tonic–clonic movements occur during unconscious state
Electrocardiographic (ECG) analysis	Bradycardia is caused by increased vagal tone associated with syncope	Tachycardia is caused by muscular exertion associated with convulsion activity

tape and roller bandage. Administration of the following medications may be considered:

- dextrose if hypoglycaemia is confirmed to correct hypoglycaemia that caused the convulsion or replace blood glucose lost during convulsion activity
- lorazepam or diazepam to stop the spread of the convulsion focus.

While administering these drugs, paramedics should closely monitor the patient's blood pressure and respiratory status and be prepared for respiratory arrest. If the patient's blood pressure begins to fall or if the respiratory rate or effort decreases, paramedics should stop the drug therapy and manage any resulting effects.

Headache

Headaches are painful and bothersome, although most are minor health concerns and are easily managed with analgesics. Headaches are categorized according to their underlying cause. The types of headaches are the tension headache, migraine, cluster headache, and sinus headache. Therapies that may be useful in managing these headaches include prescription and over-the-counter medications, herbal remedies, meditation, acupressure, aromatherapy, and others. Headache is an extremely common medical complaint; 40% of the population will have what they consider to be a serious headache at some time during their lives. The pain associated with headaches arises from the meninges and from the scalp and its blood vessels and muscles.

Tension headaches are caused by muscle contractions of the face, neck and scalp. They have a variety of causes, including stress, persistent noise, eyestrain and poor posture. The pain of tension headaches (usually described as dull, persistent, and non-throbbing) may last for days or weeks, causing variable degrees of discomfort. These headaches can be short-lived and infrequent, or chronic in nature. Most tension headaches can be managed effectively with analgesics such as aspirin, paracetamol or ibuprofen.

Migraines are severe, incapacitating headaches which often are preceded by visual and/or GI disturbances. These headaches usually begin with an intense, throbbing pain on one side of the head that may spread and are often accompanied by nausea and vomiting. The symptoms of migraines are associated with constriction and dilation of blood vessels that may be brought on by an imbalance of serotonin or hormone fluctuations. Migraines also can be triggered by excessive caffeine use, various foods, changes in altitude, and extremes of emotions. A wide range of medications are prescribed for migraines, including beta-blockers, calcium channel blockers, antidepressants, and serotonin-inhibiting drugs.

Cluster headaches are headaches that occur in bursts (clusters), often beginning several hours after a person falls asleep. The pain may be severe and is located in and around one eye, with possible nasal congestion and tearing. The painful episode often lasts 30 min to 2 h, then diminishes or disappears, recurring a day or so later. The headaches may occur every day for weeks or months before going into long periods of remission. Cluster headaches also are known as histamine headaches, as they are associated with the release of histamine from the body tissues. They are marked by symptoms of dilated carotid arteries, fluid accumulation under the eyes, tearing or lacrimation, and rhinorrhea. Cluster headaches generally are managed with antihistamines, corticosteroids, and calcium channel blockers. Cluster headaches seem to be more common in heavy smokers than in non-smokers and alcohol consumption and certain foods also may be implicated. The vast majority of sufferers are men.

Sinus headaches are characterized by pain in the forehead, nasal area and eye and often produce a feeling of pressure behind the face. Allergies or inflammation or infection of the membranes lining the sinus cavities usually are responsible for the discomfort. Sinus headaches are managed with medications such as analgesics, antihistamines, and antibiotics to treat infection.

Management

Many causes of headaches can be avoided. For example, 'triggers' can be identified, such as irregular meals, prolonged travel, noisy environments and food additives (in susceptible individuals). Headaches such as those described in the preceding paragraphs seldom require prehospital emergency care. However, a full history of the headache should be obtained; this helps to identify a more serious cause of the headache, should one be present. For example, the headache may be a sign of an aneurysm, infection, bleed or a stroke and care must be taken not to assume the headache is one of the more benign conditions identified above: if in doubt, refer on for more detailed evaluation. Important assessment findings include the following:

- the patient's general health
- previous medical conditions
- medications used
- previous experience with headaches
- the time of onset.

After a patient history has been obtained and a neurological examination performed, prehospital care for patients with tension headaches, migraines, cluster headaches and sinus headaches is mainly supportive. It may be appropriate to refer the patient on to their own general practitioner or the out of hour's service.

Brain neoplasm and brain abscess

A brain tumour, or neoplasm, is a mass in the cranial cavity which may be either malignant or benign. Heredity may play a role in the development of brain tumours and they are associated with several risk factors, including exposure to radiation, tobacco use, dietary habits, some viruses and the use of some medications. The effects of the tumour depend on its size, location, and growth rate, and whether any evidence of haemorrhage or oedema exists. Brain tumours may cause local and generalized manifestations; local effects are caused by the destructive action of the tumour on a particular site in the brain and by compression, which reduces cerebral blood flow (Figure 16-13). These effects are varied and may include the following:[5]

- convulsions
- visual disturbances
- unstable gait
- cranial nerve dysfunction.

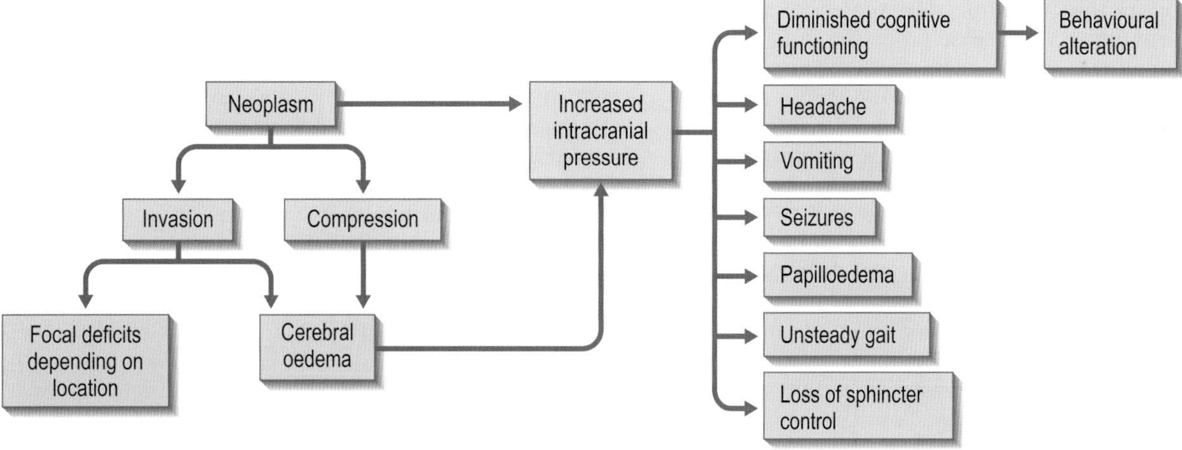

Figure 16-13 Origin of signs and symptoms associated with an intracranial neoplasm.

> **Note**
>
> CNS tumours include both brain tumours and spinal cord tumours. The incidence of these tumours tends to increase up to age 70 and then decreases. CNS tumours are the second most common group of tumours in children.[5]

Lesions inside the cranial vault cause pain, by distending or stretching the arteries and other pain-sensitive structures of the head and neck. Headache may be present but often is a late finding in the absence of haemorrhage, which may cause a sudden onset of pain. The main treatment for a cerebral tumour is surgical or radiosurgical excision; surgical decompression may be used if total excision is not possible. Chemotherapy and radiation also may be used.

A brain abscess is a build-up of purulent material (pus) surrounded by a capsule within the brain and develops from a bacterial infection. The infection often begins in the nasal cavity, middle ear, or mastoid cells and may also develop after surgery or penetrating cranial trauma, especially when bone fragments are retained in cranial tissue. Clinical manifestations of a brain abscess are associated with intracranial infection (e.g. fever) and an expanding intracranial mass (e.g. nausea, vomiting, convulsions, and changes in mental status). Headache is the most common early symptom. The removal of fluid from the abscess or excision accompanied by antibiotic therapy generally is recommended to manage this disorder (controversial). The incidence of brain abscess is about 1 per 100 000 hospital admissions and is twice as common in men as in women. The median age for abscess formation is 30 to 40 years of age.

Management

Prehospital care of a patient with a brain neoplasm or abscess may range from providing comfort and emotional support during patient transport to managing convulsion activity and providing airway, ventilatory, and circulatory resuscitation. If the patient's condition permits, a focused history should be obtained and a neurological evaluation should be performed. Elements of the focused history for these patients should include the following:

- past significant medical history (e.g. surgical removal of a tumour, radiation therapy)
- history and description of any headache
- dizziness or loss of consciousness
- convulsion activity
- GI disturbances (vomiting, diarrhoea)
- new onset of poor coordination, difficulty walking, or maintaining balance
- behavioural or cognitive changes
- weakness or paralysis
- vision disturbances.

Degenerative neurological diseases

There are many degenerative neurological diseases, the pathophysiology of which is not fully understood. Some diseases may involve Schwann cells, the CSF, or axons of the CNS, while others may result from circulatory and immunological disorders and exposure to bacterial toxins and chemicals. The following specific neurological diseases are discussed in this chapter:

- muscular dystrophy
- multiple sclerosis
- dystonia
- Parkinson's disease
- central pain syndrome
- Bell's palsy
- amyotrophic lateral sclerosis
- peripheral neuropathy
- myoclonus
- spina bifida
- polio.

Muscular dystrophy

Muscular dystrophy is an inherited muscle disorder caused by a genetic defect affecting the muscle and marked by a slow but progressive degeneration of muscle fibres. Different forms of the disease are classified by the age at which the symptoms appear (but commonly in preschool-age children), the rate at which the disease progresses, and the way in which it is inherited. Duchenne muscular dystrophy is the most common type, affecting 1 or 2 in 10 000 male children. It is inherited through a recessive sex-linked gene, therefore only males are affected and only females can pass on the disease.

Muscular dystrophy often is first diagnosed by the child's GP, who notices that the child is slow in learning to sit up and walk. The disease is confirmed through blood tests that reveal high levels of enzymes released from damaged muscle cells, through nerve conduction studies, and sometimes with muscle biopsy. Muscular dystrophy rarely is diagnosed before age 3. As the disease progresses, the child tends to walk with a waddle and has difficulty climbing stairs. Muscles (especially those in the calves) become bulky as wasted muscle is replaced by fat. By about age 12, affected children are no longer able to walk, and few survive their teenage years. Death usually results from pulmonary infections and heart failure.

Critical Thinking

How can you determine a child's baseline level of functioning?

No effective treatment exists for muscular dystrophy. Parents or siblings of an affected child should receive genetic counselling. Some types of muscular dystrophy can be diagnosed before birth; this can be done through blood analysis and amniocentesis.

Multiple sclerosis

Multiple sclerosis (MS) is a progressive disease of the CNS where scattered patches of myelin in the brain and spinal cord are destroyed. It is believed to be an autoimmune disease in which the body's defence system begins to treat the myelin in the CNS as foreign, gradually destroying it (demyelination), with subsequent scarring and nerve fibre damage.

MS is the most common acquired disease of the nervous system in young adults. It affects about 1 in every 1000 individuals and the ratio of women to men with the disease is 3 to 2. The symptoms, which may be active briefly in early adult life and resume years later, vary according to the parts of the brain and spinal cord affected and range from numbness and tingling to paralysis and incontinence and may last several weeks to several months. Damage to the white matter in the brain may lead to fatigue, vertigo, clumsiness, unsteady gait, slurred speech, blurred or double vision, and facial numbness or pain. Some patients may have mild relapses and long symptom-free periods throughout life whilst others may gradually become disabled from the first attack and are bedridden and incontinent in early middle life.

Critical Thinking

Consider the patient who has been receiving long-term steroid therapy. This person is at risk for what conditions?

The disease is usually diagnosed by ruling out other diseases. Diagnostic tests that may help to identify MS include lumbar puncture, CT scanning, and magnetic resonance imaging (MRI) studies. Affected patients are managed with medications (e.g. corticosteroids, antidepressants, immune system medications) that help to control symptoms of an acute episode and to prevent it from getting worse. The disease also is managed with physical therapy to help maintain mobility and independence. Currently no cure exists for the disease.

Dystonia

The term dystonia refers to local or diffuse changes in muscle tone (usually abnormal muscle rigidity). These changes cause painful muscle spasms, unusually fixed postures, and strange movement patterns. Localized dystonia may result from torticollis (a painful neck spasm) as well as from scoliosis (an abnormal curvature of the spine). More generalized dystonia results from various neurological disorders such as Parkinson disease and stroke and may also be a feature of schizophrenia or a side effect of some antipsychotic drugs. Dystonia sometimes is managed with medications such as benzatropine (an antimuscarinic drug), which may help to reverse the symptoms and to prevent their recurrence.

Parkinson's disease

Parkinson's disease is caused by degeneration of and damage to the part of the brain producing dopamine (substantia nigra) which causes dopamine shortage direct effects on smooth muscle contraction. This causes tremor, joint rigidity, and slow movement. Parkinson's disease affects about 130 in 100 000 persons, usually when reaching their 60s, and more men than women. Left untreated, the disease progresses over 10 to 15 years to severe weakness and incapacity and is a leading cause of neurological disability in people over 60 years of age.

Parkinson's disease usually begins as a slight tremor in one hand, arm or leg. In the early stages, the tremor is worse while the limb is at rest. In the later stages, the disease affects both sides of the body and causes stiffness, weakness and trembling of the muscles. Other symptoms include an unusual walking pattern (shuffling) that may break into uncontrollable, tiny running steps; constant trembling of the hands, sometimes accompanied by shaking of the head; a permanent rigid stoop; and an unblinking, fixed facial expression. Late in the disease, intellect may be affected. Speech becomes slow and hesitant as well. Depression is common.

At first, Parkinson's disease is managed with counselling, exercise and special aids in the home. As the disease progresses, management may include various combinations of drugs to provide relief from specific symptoms, such as dopamine receptor agonist drugs, levodopa (levodopa is converted by the body into dopamine) and monoamine-oxidase-B inhibitors such as selegiline. Other management measures may include brain surgery to reduce tremor and rigidity and transplantation of dopamine-secreting adrenal tissue (experimental).

Central pain syndrome

Central pain syndrome refers to infection or disease of the trigeminal nerve (cranial nerve V). A common form of the syndrome is tic douloureux (trigeminal neuralgia) where patients complain of paroxysmal episodes of excruciating pain (often described as recurrent bursts of an electric shock) that affect the cheek, lips, gums or chin on one side of the face. The episode usually is very brief, lasting only a few seconds to minutes, but may be so intense that the person is unable to function during the attack. The pain often causes wincing; hence the name tic douloureux (literally, 'painful twitch'). Central pain syndrome is unusual in individuals under age 50 but may be associated with MS in younger people. Attacks occur in bouts that may last weeks at a time.

The pain of trigeminal neuralgia usually begins from a trigger point on the face. It can be brought on by touching, washing, shaving, eating, drinking or talking. The cause of the syndrome is unclear, therefore management is difficult. Treatment includes the use of drugs to inhibit nerve impulses (commonly carbamazepine or phenytoin) and sometimes surgery if the cause is a tumour or lesion.

Bell's palsy

Bell's palsy (facial palsy) is a paralysis of the facial muscles caused by inflammation of the seventh cranial nerve (Figure 16-14). It usually is one-sided and temporary and often develops suddenly. Bell's palsy is the most common cause of facial paralysis, affecting 1 in 60–70 people in a lifetime. The cause of the inflammation is unclear but it has been associated with many past or present infectious processes, including Lyme disease, herpes viruses, mumps, and infection with the human immunodeficiency (HIV) virus.

Critical Thinking

In the field, should you diagnose and release a patient who has Bell's palsy?

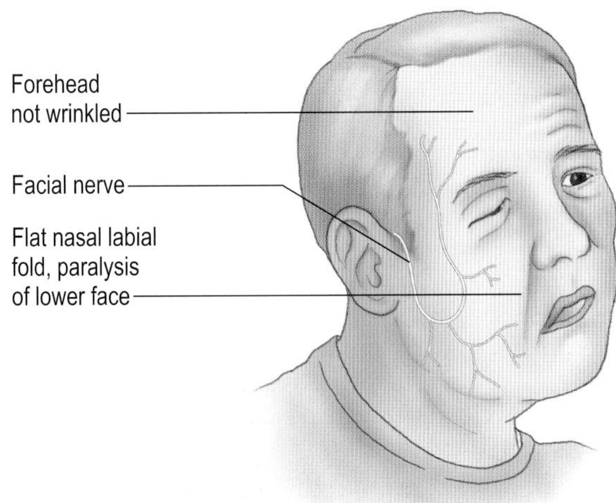

Figure 16-14 Bell's palsy.

Bell's palsy usually causes the eyelid and corner of the mouth to droop on one side of the face and is sometimes associated with numbness and pain. Depending on which branches of the nerve are affected, taste may be impaired, or sounds may seem oddly loud. Management involves the use of corticosteroids (controversial) to reduce inflammation of the nerve, or aciclovir if thought to be caused by herpes viral infection, as well as analgesics. Recovery usually is complete within 2 weeks to 2 months. A key component of therapy is to protect the affected eye from corneal drying and injury as the paralysis may prevent the eyelid from closing. Prevention of these conditions is best accomplished through the use of lubricating ointments and eye patches. Caution must be taken that the facial weakness is not indicative of stroke; if there is any doubt, the patient must be further evaluated in hospital.

Amyotrophic lateral sclerosis

Amyotrophic lateral sclerosis (ALS), also called Lou Gehrig disease, is one of a group of rare disorders (motor neuron diseases) where the nerves that control muscular activity degenerate in the brain and spinal cord. ALS usually affects people over the age of 50 and is more common in men than in women. The incidence is about 1–2 per 100 000 people and about 10% of ALS cases are familial.[5]

Motor neuron diseases may involve deterioration of both upper and lower neuron tracts. When only muscles of the tongue, jaw, face, and larynx are involved, the term progressive bulbar palsy is used. When only corticospinal processes are affected, the term primary lateral sclerosis is used. When only lower motor neurons are affected, the term progressive spinal muscular atrophy is used. ALS is used to describe neuron signs that predominate in the extremities and trunk.

Patients with ALS often first notice weakness in the hands and arms and it is often accompanied by involuntary quivering (fasciculations). The disease progresses to involve the muscles of all four extremities and those involved in respiration and swallowing. In the final stages of the disease, patients often are unable to speak, swallow, or move; however, awareness and intellect are maintained. Death usually occurs 2 to 4 years after the diagnosis due to involvement of the respiratory muscles, aspiration pneumonia, and general inanition (starvation, failure to thrive). In some cases, life can be prolonged through the use of feeding tubes and ventilators. Care generally is aimed at providing emotional support and easing discomfort.

Critical Thinking

Why is there a tendency to treat patients with ALS as if they have impaired intelligence?

Peripheral neuropathy

As the name implies, peripheral neuropathy refers to diseases and disorders that affect the peripheral nervous system, including the spinal nerve roots, cranial nerves, and peripheral nerves. Most neuropathies arise from damage to or irritation of either the axons or their myelin sheaths which slows or fully blocks the passage of electrical signals. The various types of peripheral neuropathy are classified according to the site and distribution of damage. For example, damage to sensory nerve fibres may cause numbness and tingling, sensations of cold, or pain that often starts in the hands and feet and spreads toward the central body. Damage to motor nerve fibres may cause muscle weakness and muscle wasting. Damage that occurs to the nerves of the autonomic nervous system may result in blurred vision, impaired or absent sweating, fluctuations in blood pressure (and associated syncope), GI disorders, incontinence and impotence.

Some peripheral neuropathies have no identifiable cause but others may be related to specific causes, including the following:

- diabetes
- dietary deficiencies (especially of vitamin B)
- alcoholism
- uraemia
- leprosy
- lead poisoning
- drug intoxication
- viral infection (e.g. Guillain–Barré syndrome)
- rheumatoid arthritis
- systemic lupus erythematosus
- malignant tumours (e.g. lung cancer)
- lymphomas
- leukaemia
- inherited neuropathies (e.g. peroneal muscular atrophy).

When possible, management is aimed at the underlying cause, such as blood glucose control in a diabetic patient, and better nutrition. If management is successful and the cell bodies of the damaged nerves have not been destroyed, full recovery from the neuropathy is possible.

Myoclonus

Myoclonus refers to rapid and uncontrollable muscular contractions (jerking) or spasms of one or more muscles which occur at rest or during movement. The syndrome may be associated with disease of nerves and muscles or may be a symptom of a brain disorder (e.g. encephalitis) or convulsion disorder. Myoclonus can occur in healthy individuals. An example is a limb 'jump' that sometimes happens just before a person falls asleep. The condition is treated with medications to reduce the patient's symptoms and may include barbiturates, benzodiazepines, and phenytoin.

Spina bifida

Spina bifida is a congenital (neural tube) defect in which part of one or more vertebrae fails to develop completely, leaving a portion of the spinal cord exposed. The condition can occur anywhere on the spine but is most common in the lower back. Although the cause is unknown, spina bifida occurs in about 1 in every 1000 births and is more likely to occur with extremes of maternal age. A woman who has given birth to one child with spina bifida is 10 times more likely than the average woman to give birth to another affected child (indicating the need for genetic counselling).

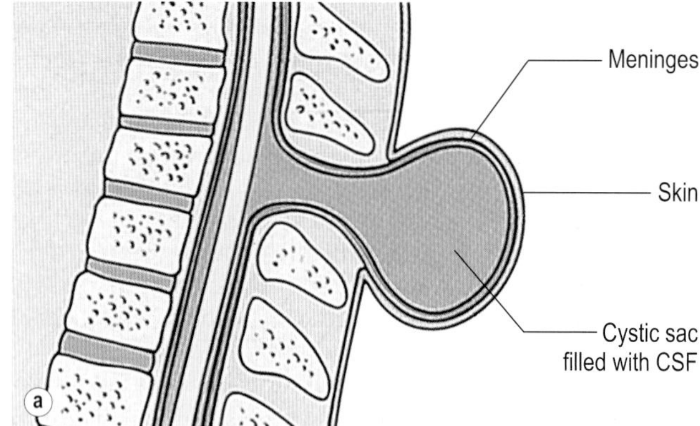

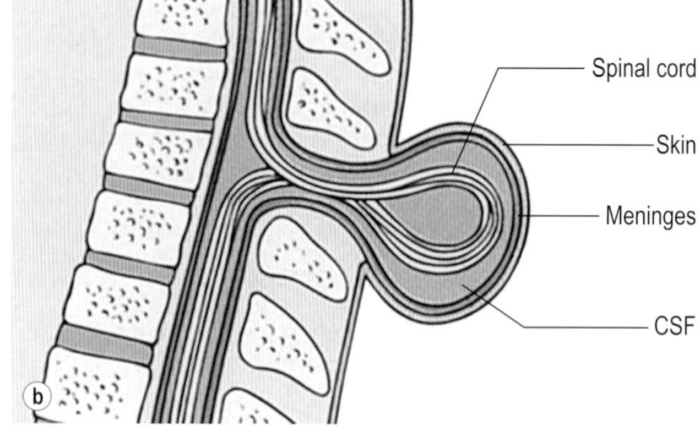

Figure 16-15 (a) Meningocele. (b) Myelomeningocele.

Types of spina bifida

The severity of spina bifida depends on how much nerve tissue is exposed after the neural tube has closed. The four types of spina bifida are spina bifida occulta, meningocele, myelomeningocele and encephalocele. Currently the condition has no cure. Treatment includes surgery, medications, and physical therapy. Most patients with spina bifida live into adulthood.

Spina bifida occulta is the most common and least serious form. There is little external evidence of the defect. Meningocele (Figure 16-15a) is a type of spina bifida in which the nerve tissue of the spinal cord usually is intact and covered with a membranous sac of skin and does not usually cause functional problems. However, it requires surgical repair early in life. Myelomeningocele (Figure 16-15b) is the severest form of spina bifida. The child often is severely handicapped and this type of spina bifida is marked by a raw swelling over the spine and a malformed spinal cord that may or may not be contained in a membranous sac. The legs of these children often are deformed. The condition causes partial or complete paralysis and loss of sensation in all areas below the level of the defect. Associated abnormalities of myelomeningocele include hydrocephalus (excess CSF in the skull) with brain damage, cerebral palsy, epilepsy, and developmental delay. In the fourth and very rare type of spina bifida, encephalocele, the protrusion occurs through the skull. Severe brain damage is common with this condition.

Polio

Polio (poliomyelitis) is caused by the poliovirus, which attacks with variable severity. It may range from a not very apparent infection, to a febrile illness without neurological after-effects, to aseptic meningitis, and finally to paralytic disease (including respiratory paralysis) and possibly death. The incidence of polio has declined in many parts of the world since the development of the Salk and Sabin vaccines in the 1950s. However, the disease may affect non-immune adults and indigent (particularly immigrant) children and remains a risk for anyone not vaccinated and travelling in some parts of Africa or Asia. Polio vaccinations are given during infancy and preschool ages.

Critical Thinking

Ask your older friends or relatives about their memories of the polio epidemic. How did it affect their lives?

People infected with the poliovirus can pass large amounts of the virus in their faeces which then may be spread directly or indirectly to others by fingers-to-food transmission and by airborne transmission. Signs and symptoms of polio differ in the non-paralytic and paralytic forms. Fever, headache, sore throat, and malaise are common to both forms. However, the paralytic form of polio also is associated with generalized pain, weakness, muscle spasms, and paralysis of limbs and other muscles. If the infection spreads to the brainstem, the person may find it difficult or may be unable to swallow or breathe. A full recovery can be made from non-paralytic polio. Of those who become paralysed, more than half eventually make a full recovery but some patients may develop 'post-polio deterioration' and may have new weakness and pain from recovered muscles. The disease is confirmed though CSF analysis, throat culture, or testing of faecal samples.

Summary

- The human body's ability to maintain a state of balance, or homeostasis, results from the nervous system's regulatory and coordinating activities. The blood supply to the brain comes from the vertebral arteries and the internal carotid arteries.
- Some neurological emergencies are a consequence of structural changes or damage, circulatory changes, or alterations in intracranial pressure that affect cerebral blood flow.
- The initial survey should begin by determining the patient's level of consciousness and by ensuring an open and patent airway. Key elements of the physical examination that may provide clues to the nature of the neurological emergency include the patient history and the history of the event, vital signs, and respiratory patterns.
- Coma is an abnormally deep state of unconsciousness. The patient cannot be aroused from this state by external stimuli. In general, two mechanisms produce coma: structural lesions and toxic–metabolic states.
- Stroke is a sudden interruption in blood flow to the brain that results in a neurological deficit. Strokes can be classified as ischaemic strokes or haemorrhagic strokes.
- A convulsion is a brief alteration in behaviour or consciousness. It is caused by abnormal electrical activity of one or more groups of neurons in the brain. In the prehospital setting, determining the cause of a convulsion is not as important as other measures. These include managing the complications and recognizing whether the convulsion is reversible with therapy (e.g. it is caused by hypoglycaemia).
- The four fairly common types of headaches are tension headaches, migraines, cluster headaches and sinus headaches.
- A brain tumour, or neoplasm, is a mass in the cranial cavity. This mass can be either malignant or benign. Heredity may play a role in the development of brain tumours. They also are associated with several risk factors. These include exposure to radiation, tobacco use, dietary habits, some viruses and the use of some medications.
- A brain abscess is a build-up of purulent material (pus) surrounded by a capsule within the brain. It develops from a bacterial infection. The infection often starts in the nasal cavity, middle ear or mastoid bone.
- Muscular dystrophy is an inherited muscle disorder. The cause is unknown. The disease is marked by a slow but progressive degeneration of muscle fibres.
- Damage to the white matter of the brain in multiple sclerosis may lead to fatigue, vertigo, clumsiness, unsteady gait, slurred speech, blurred or double vision, and facial numbness or pain.
- The term dystonia refers to local or diffuse changes in muscle tone. These may cause painful muscle spasms, unusually fixed postures, and strange movement patterns.
- Parkinson's disease usually begins as a slight tremor in one hand, arm or leg. In the later stages, the disease affects both sides of the body, causing stiffness, weakness, and trembling of the muscles.
- The term central pain syndrome refers to infection or disease of the trigeminal nerve.
- Bell's palsy is paralysis of the facial muscles. It is caused by inflammation of the seventh cranial nerve. The condition is usually one-sided and temporary. It often develops suddenly.
- Amyotrophic lateral sclerosis is also called Lou Gehrig disease. It is one of a group of rare nervous system disorders. In these disorders, the nerves that control

Summary—cont'd

muscular activity degenerate in the brain and spinal cord.

- Peripheral neuropathies usually arise from damage to or irritation of either the axons or their myelin sheaths. This slows or fully blocks the passage of electrical signals.
- The term myoclonus refers to rapid and uncontrollable muscle contractions or spasms. These occur at rest or during movement.
- Spina bifida is a congenital defect in which part of one or more vertebrae fails to develop completely. This leaves a portion of the spinal cord exposed.
- Polio is caused by a virus. The severity of the disease can range from unapparent infection, to a febrile illness without neurological after-effects, to aseptic meningitis, and finally to paralytic disease and possibly death.

References

1. Department of Health 2006 Mending hearts and brains; clinical case for change: Report by Professor Roger Boyle, National Director for heart disease and stroke. Department of Health, London
2. Royal College of Physicians (England) 2008 Stroke: National clinical guideline for diagnosis and initial management of acute stroke and transient ischaemic attack (TIA). Royal College of Physicians, London
3. Kothari R, Hall K, Brott T, Broderick J 1997 Early stroke recognition: developing an out-of-hospital stroke scale. Acad Emerg Med 4(10):986–990
4. National Institute for Health and Clinical Excellence 2008 CG68: clinical guideline for stroke/stoke algorithm. Online. Available http://www.nice.org.uk/guidance/index.jsp?action=download&o=41318 6 February 2009
5. McCance K, Huether S 2006 Pathophysiology: the biologic basis for disease in adults and children, 5th edition. Mosby, St Louis

CHAPTER 17

Endocrinology

Chapter contents

Objectives

Upon completion of this chapter, the paramedic student will be able to:

1. Describe how hormones secreted from endocrine glands help the body to maintain homeostasis.
2. Describe the anatomy and physiology of the pancreas and how its hormones work to maintain normal glucose metabolism.
3. Discuss pathophysiology as a basis for key signs and symptoms, patient assessment, and patient management for diabetes and diabetic emergencies of hypoglycaemia, diabetic ketoacidosis, and hyperosmolar hyperglycaemic non-ketotic coma.
4. Discuss pathophysiology as a basis for key signs and symptoms, patient assessment, and patient management for disorders of the thyroid gland.
5. Discuss pathophysiology as a basis for key signs and symptoms, patient assessment, and patient management of Cushing syndrome and Addison's disease.

Key terms

Addison's disease A rare and potentially life-threatening disorder caused by a deficiency of the corticosteroid hormones normally produced by the adrenal cortex.

Cushing syndrome A condition caused by an abnormally high circulating level of corticosteroid hormones produced naturally by the adrenal glands.

gluconeogenesis The formation of glucose from fatty acids and proteins rather than carbohydrates.

glycogenolysis The breakdown of glycogen to glucose.

hyperosmolar hyperglycaemic non-ketotic (HHNK) coma A diabetic coma in which the level of ketone bodies is normal. It is caused by hyperosmolarity of extracellular fluid and results in dehydration of intracellular fluid.

ketogenesis The formation or production of ketone bodies.

myxoedema A condition that results from a deficiency in thyroid hormone.

thyrotoxicosis A term that refers to any toxic condition that results from thyroid hyper-function.

The endocrine system and the nervous system allow the body to regulate many functions. Some patients that paramedics treat will have endocrine system disorders. These disorders can range from minor changes in functioning to life-threatening conditions.

Anatomy and physiology of the endocrine system

The endocrine system is composed of ductless glands and tissues that produce and secrete hormones. The major endocrine glands are the pituitary, thyroid, and parathyroid glands; the adrenal cortex and medulla; the pancreatic islets; and the ovaries and testes (Figure 17-1). Other specialized groups of cells that secrete hormones are found in the kidneys and the mucosa of the gastrointestinal (GI) tract.

Endocrine gland functions

Endocrine glands secrete hormones directly into the bloodstream and serve to regulate various metabolic functions. The products of endocrine glands travel via the blood (or tissue fluids) so are able to exert their effects on the entire body. The endocrine hormones are released either in response to a change in the cellular environment or to maintain a normal level of certain hormones or substances. This integrated chemical and coordination system enables reproduction, growth and development, and the regulation of energy. Target organs and body tissues have hormone receptors and are able to respond to a certain hormone.

Critical Thinking

How are hormones and their target organs like a lock and key?

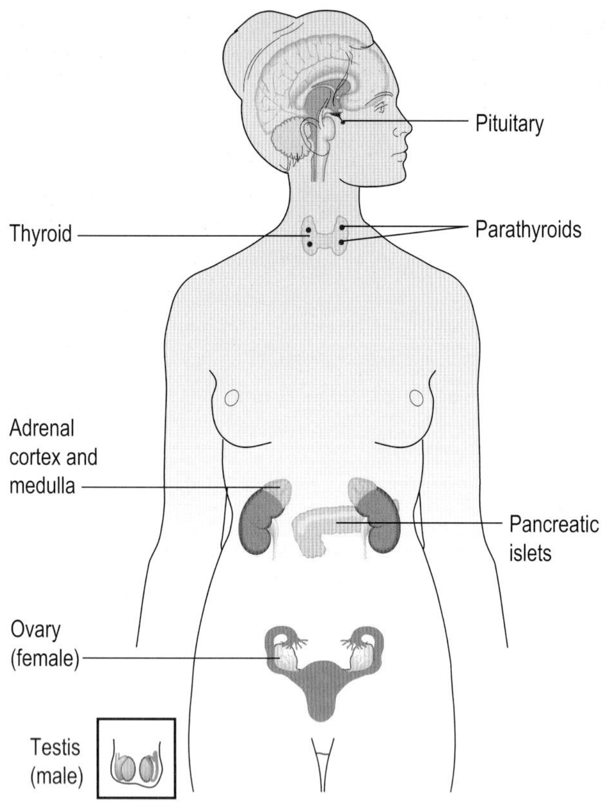

Figure 17-1 Major endocrine glands.

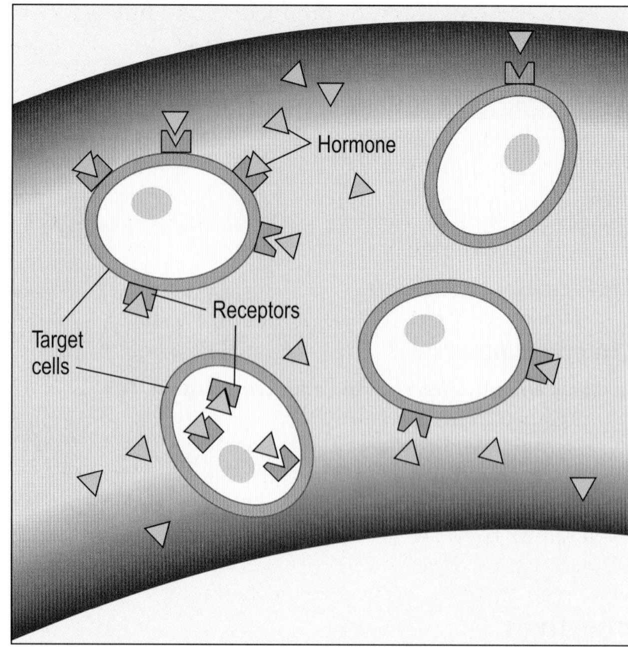

Figure 17-2 Target cell concept. Cells with fewer receptor sites bind with less hormone than cells with many receptor sites.

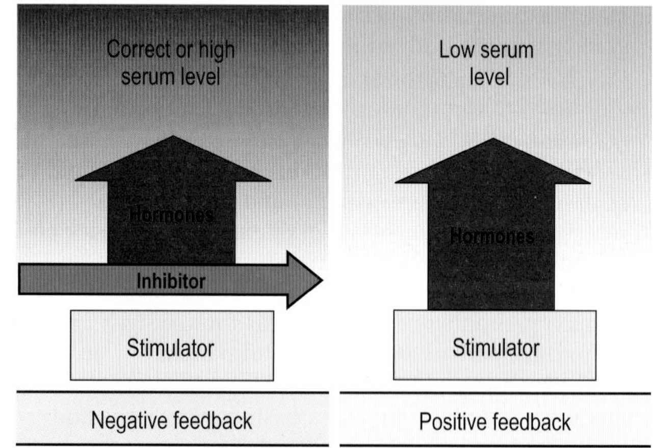

Figure 17-3 Negative feedback.

Hormone receptors

Most hormones can be categorized as proteins, polypeptides, derivatives of amino acids, or lipids. Each hormone may affect a specific organ or tissue, or it may have a general effect on the entire body. Hormones may also be classified as steroid or non-steroid. Steroid hormones are manufactured by endocrine cells from cholesterol, and include cortisol, aldosterone, oestrogen, progesterone and testosterone. Nonsteroid hormones are synthesized chiefly from amino acids and include insulin and parathyroid hormone, amongst others.

Hormones affect only cells with appropriate receptors and act to initiate specific cell functions or activities. Hormone receptor sites may be on the cell membrane or in the interior of the cell. Cells with fewer receptor sites bind with less hormone than cells with many receptor sites (Figure 17-2). Abnormalities in, or the presence of specific hormone receptors can result in endocrine disorders. This happens because the target cells completely reject the hormone for that receptor.

Regulation of hormone secretion

All hormones operate with feedback systems that help to maintain an optimal internal environment (Figure 17-3). These feedback systems are either positive or negative. An example of positive feedback can be found in childbirth. The hormone oxytocin stimulates and enhances labour contractions. As the baby moves towards the birth canal, pressure receptors in the cervix send messages to the brain to produce oxytocin. Oxytocin travels to the uterus through the bloodstream, where it stimulates the muscles in the uterine wall to contract more strongly. The contractions intensify and increase until the baby is outside the birth canal. When the stimulus to the pressure receptors ends, oxytocin production stops. Labour contractions also stop.

Negative feedback is the mechanism most commonly used to maintain homeostasis and works by reversing a change in a controlled condition such as blood glucose levels. For example, after a person eats a chocolate bar, the following occurs:

1. Glucose from the ingested lactose or sucrose is absorbed in the intestine, causing a rise in the level of glucose in the blood.
2. The increase in the blood glucose concentration stimulates the pancreas to release insulin. Insulin facilitates the entry of glucose into the cells, causing a fall in blood glucose level.
3. When the blood glucose level has dropped sufficiently, the endocrine cells in the pancreas stop producing and releasing insulin.

On the other hand, hormone production is stimulated when serum levels of the hormone fall. For example, the hypothalamus receptors monitor blood levels of thyroid hormones. Low blood levels of thyroid-stimulating hormone (TSH) cause the release of TSH-releasing hormone from the hypothalamus. This, in turn, causes the release of TSH from the anterior pituitary. TSH travels to the thyroid, where it promotes the production of thyroid hormones. These, in turn, regulate the metabolic rate and body temperature.

Specific disorders of the endocrine system

Disorders of the endocrine system arise from the effects of an imbalance in the production of one or more hormones. They also arise from the effects of a change in the body's ability to use the hormones produced. The clinical effects of endocrine gland disorders are determined by the degree of dysfunction. They are also determined by the individual's age and gender. Specific disorders of the endocrine system in this chapter include those found in Table 17-1.

Table 17-1 Specific disorders of the endocrine system

Gland	Disorder
Pancreas	Diabetes mellitus (types 1 and 2)
	Hyperosmolar hyperglycaemic non-ketotic (HHNK) coma
Thyroid	Hyperthyroidism
	Hypothyroidism
	Myxoedema
	Thyrotoxic crisis (thyroid storm)
	Thyrotoxicosis
Adrenal	Addison's disease
	Cushing syndrome

Disorders of the pancreas: diabetes mellitus

Diabetes mellitus is a systemic disease of the endocrine system that usually results from a dysfunction of the pancreas. It is a complex disorder of fat, carbohydrate, and protein metabolism that affects more than 1.8 million people in the UK, both children and adults.[1] Diabetes mellitus is potentially lethal and can put the patient at risk for several kinds of true medical emergencies. A recent report suggests that more than 1 in 10 (11.6%) deaths among 20–79-year-olds in England can be attributed to diabetes.[2]

Anatomy and physiology of the pancreas

The pancreas is important in the absorption and use of carbohydrates, fat, and protein, and is the chief regulator of glucose levels in the blood. The pancreas is a retroperitoneal organ adjacent to the duodenum on the right and extending to the spleen on the left. The healthy pancreas has exocrine and endocrine functions. To review, exocrine glands secrete substances through a duct onto the inner surface of an organ or the outer surface of the body; endocrine glands are those that secrete chemicals directly (not through a duct) into the bloodstream. The exocrine portion consists of acini (glands that produce pancreatic juice) and a duct system that carries the pancreatic juice to the small intestine. The endocrine portion consists of pancreatic islets (islets of Langerhans) that produce hormones (Figure 17-4).

Islets of Langerhans and pancreatic hormones

About 500 000 to 1 million pancreatic islets are dispersed among the ducts and the acini of the pancreas. Each islet is composed of beta cells, alpha cells, and other cells. The beta cells secrete insulin at a daily average of 0.6 units per kilogram of body weight. The alpha cells secrete glucagon. Nerves from both divisions of the autonomic nervous system innervate the pancreatic islets, and each islet is surrounded by a well-developed capillary network.

Critical Thinking

Consider that part of a patient's pancreas must be removed as a result of traumatic injury. Will the patient still be able to produce insulin and glucagon?

Insulin

Insulin is a small protein that is released by the beta cells when blood glucose levels rise. The main functions of insulin are to increase glucose transport into cells, increase glucose metabolism by cells, increase liver glycogen levels, and decrease the blood glucose concentration toward normal (Box 17-1). Many of the functions of insulin antagonize the effects of glucagon.

Glucagon

Glucagon is a protein released by the alpha cells when blood glucose levels fall. Glucagon has two major effects. One effect is to increase blood glucose levels, which it does by stimulating the liver to release glucose stores from glycogen and other glucose storage sites (this is called glycogenolysis). The other effect is to stimulate gluconeogenesis (glucose formation) through the breakdown of fats and fatty acids, thereby maintaining normal blood glucose levels (Figure 17-5).

Growth hormone

Growth hormone (GH) is a polypeptide hormone. It is produced and secreted by the anterior pituitary gland. GH secretion is triggered by many physiological stimuli such as exercise, stress, sleep, and hypoglycaemia. GH acts as an insulin antagonist, thereby decreasing insulin actions on cell membranes. This reduces the capacity of muscles and adipose and liver cells to absorb glucose.

Box 17-1

Primary functions of insulin

- To increase glucose transport into cells
- To increase glucose metabolism by cells
- To increase liver glycogen levels
- To decrease blood glucose concentration toward normal levels

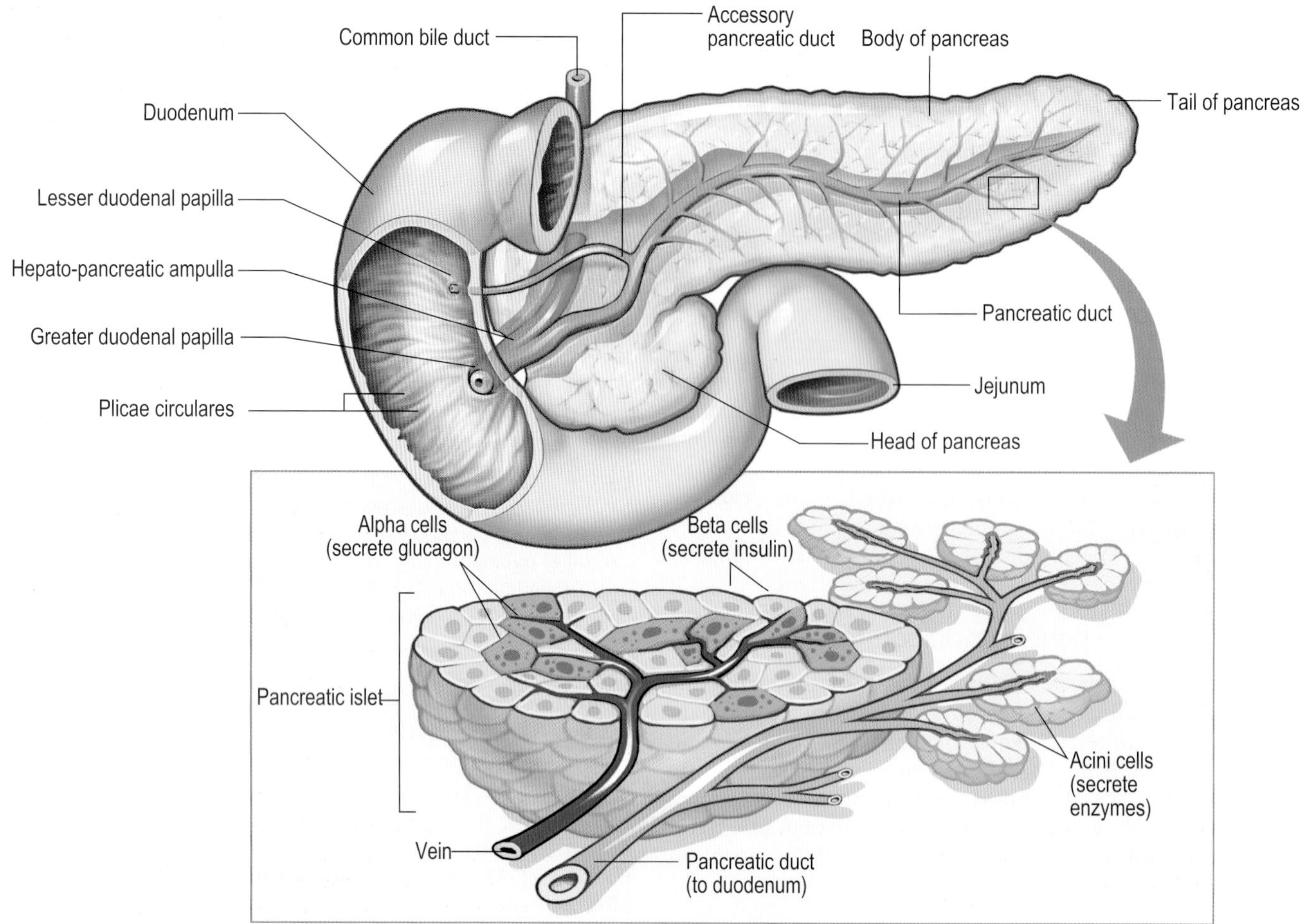

Figure 17-4 Two pancreatic islets (islets of Langerhans), or hormone-producing areas, are evident among the pancreatic cells that produce the pancreatic digestive juice.

Regulation of glucose metabolism

Under normal conditions, the body maintains the serum glucose level in the blood at 3.9–6.1 mmol/L. An understanding of food intake and digestion is required to understand glucose metabolism.

Dietary intake

The three main organic components of food are carbohydrates, fats and proteins (food also contains minerals and vitamins). Carbohydrates are found in all sugary, starchy foods and provide a ready source of near-instant energy. They are the first food substances to enter the bloodstream after a meal is ingested. Carbohydrates yield the simple sugar glucose. If not 'burned' for immediate energy, glucose is stored in the liver and muscles as glycogen for short-term energy needs or converted into fat by adipose tissue and stored for intermediate and long-term needs.

Process of digestion

Before food compounds can be used by body cells, they must be digested and absorbed into the bloodstream. Digestion begins in the mouth and is accomplished by physical forces (chewing) and chemical (enzymatic) forces. This begins the process that reduces the food to soluble molecules and particles small enough to be absorbed. After food is swallowed, it enters the stomach. There, various nutrients are absorbed into the circulatory system. These nutrients include glucose, salts, water, and some other substances (alcohol and certain other drugs). The remaining material (chyme) is shunted from the stomach into the intestine for further digestion.

The duodenum signals the release of hormones that mobilize the pancreas to contribute its molecule-splitting enzymes and the gallbladder to release bile salts. These enzymes and salts neutralize acids and help emulsify fats. Carbohydrates are absorbed as simple sugars, fats are absorbed as fatty acids and glycerol, and proteins are absorbed as amino acids. These nutrients are then carried from the intestine to the liver by way of the portal vein. Water and remaining salts are absorbed from food residues reaching the colon. The liver synthesizes glycogen from the absorbed glucose, lipoproteins from the absorbed fatty acids, and many proteins required for health from absorbed amino acids.

Carbohydrate metabolism The secretion of insulin is controlled by chemical, neural and hormonal means. An increased concentration of blood glucose, parasympathetic stimulation, and gastrointestinal hormones involved with regulation of digestion cause beta cells of the pancreas to release insulin after dietary intake of carbohydrates. Insulin travels through the blood to target tissues, where it combines with specific chemical receptors on the surface of the cell membrane to permit glucose to enter the cell (Table 17-2). This allows the cells to use glucose for energy and also pre-

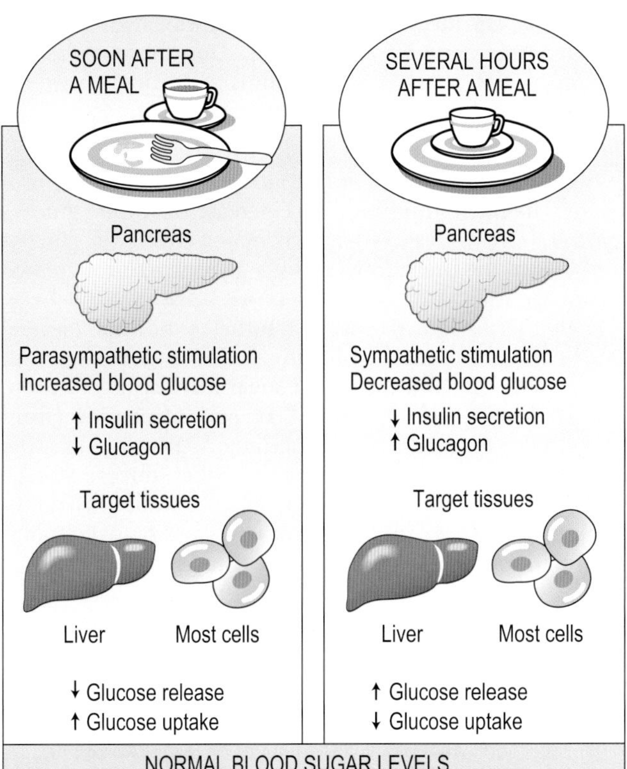

Figure 17-5 Regulation of insulin and glucagon secretion. Sympathetic stimulation and decreasing concentrations of glucose increase the secretion of glucagon, which acts primarily on liver cells to increase the rate of glycogen breakdown and the secretion of glucose from the liver. The release of glucose from the liver helps maintain blood glucose levels. Increasing blood glucose levels has an inhibitory effect on glucagon secretion. Increasing concentrations of glucose and amino acids stimulate the beta cells of the islets to secrete insulin. In addition, parasympathetic stimulation causes insulin secretion. Insulin acts on most tissues to increase the uptake of glucose and amino acids. As the blood levels of glucose and amino acids decrease, the rate of insulin secretion also decreases.

vents the breakdown of alternative energy sources (proteins and fat cells). In addition, it promotes the uptake of glucose into the liver, where it is converted to glycogen for storage. This rapid uptake and storage of glucose normally prevents a large increase in blood glucose levels, even just after a normal meal.

Critical Thinking

Why do diabetics eat carbohydrates instead of protein or fat when they sense that their glucose level is too low?

When the blood glucose level begins to fall, the liver releases glucose back into the circulating blood. Thus, the liver removes glucose from the blood when it is in excess after dietary intake and returns it to the blood when it is needed between meals. Under normal circumstances, about 60% of the glucose in a meal is stored in the liver as glycogen and released later.

If the muscles are not exercised after a meal, much of the glucose transported into the muscle cells by insulin is stored as muscle glycogen. Muscle glycogen differs from liver glycogen in that it cannot be reconverted into glucose and released into the circulation. The stored glycogen must be used by the muscle for energy.

The brain is quite different from other body tissues with regard to glucose uptake. Insulin has little or no effect on the uptake or use of glucose by the brain; the cells of the brain do not have adequate storage capacity. Also, because the brain normally uses only glucose for energy, it cannot depend on stored supplies of glycogen. Thus it is essential that serum glucose be maintained at a level that provides adequate energy to these tissues. When the serum glucose level falls too low, signs and symptoms of hypoglycaemia can develop quickly. These include progressive irritability, altered mental states, fainting, convulsions, and even coma.

Fat metabolism Only a limited amount of glycogen can be stored in the liver and skeletal muscles. Therefore one-third of any glucose passing through the liver is converted to fatty

Table 17-2 Effects of insulin and glucagon on target tissues

Target tissue	Response to insulin	Response to glucagon
Skeletal muscle, cardiac muscle, cartilage, bone, fibroblasts, leukocytes, and mammary glands	Increased glucose uptake and glycogen synthesis; increased uptake of certain amino acids	Little effect
Liver	Increased glycogen synthesis; increased use of glucose for energy (glycolysis)	Rapid increase in the breakdown of glycogen to glucose (glycogenolysis) and release of glucose into the blood
	Increased formation of glucose (gluconeogenesis) from amino acids and, to some degree, from fats	
	Increased metabolism of fatty acids, resulting in increased ketones in the blood	
Adipose cells	Increased glucose uptake, glycogen synthesis, fat synthesis, and fatty acid uptake; increased glycolysis	High concentrations cause breakdown of fats (lipolysis); probably unimportant under most conditions
Nervous system	Little effect except to increase glucose uptake in the satiety centre	No effect

From Seeley R 1992 Anatomy and physiology, 2nd edition. Mosby, St Louis.

acids. Under the influence of insulin, fatty acids are converted to triglycerides (storable fats) and stored in adipose tissue. In the absence of insulin, the stored fat is broken down so that the plasma concentration of free fatty acids rapidly increases. An inadequate level of insulin in the blood can result in high levels of triglycerides and cholesterol (in the form of lipoproteins) in the plasma. This is thought to contribute to the development of atherosclerosis in patients with serious diabetes.

If needed (as in the absence of insulin), fatty acids in the liver can be metabolized and used for energy. A by-product of the breakdown of fatty acids in the liver is acetate. Acetate is converted to acetoacetic acid and beta hydroxybutyric acid. These products are released into the circulating blood as ketone bodies. Ketone bodies may cause acidosis and coma (diabetic ketoacidosis) in the diabetic patient.

Protein metabolism Insulin causes proteins, as well as carbohydrates and fats, to be stored. Amino acids (through the actions of GH and insulin) are actively transported into the various cells of the human body. Most amino acids are used as building blocks to form new proteins (protein synthesis.) However, some enter the metabolic cycle by being converted to glucose after initial breakdown in the liver.

In the absence of insulin, protein storage stops whilst protein breakdown (particularly in muscle) begins. This releases large amounts of amino acids into the circulation, which are used directly for energy or as substrates for gluconeogenesis. The degradation of the amino acids leads to increased urea excretion in the urine. This 'protein wasting' has serious effects in diabetes mellitus and leads to extreme weakness and dysfunction of many organs.

Glucagon and its functions

Glucagon has several functions that oppose the functions of insulin. The most important is to increase the blood glucose concentration. Glucagon has two major effects on glucose metabolism: the breakdown of liver glycogen and increased gluconeogenesis.

As the serum glucose level returns to normal (several hours after dietary intake), insulin secretion decreases with continued fasting and the blood sugar level begins to drop. As a result, glucagon, cortisol, GH, and adrenaline (from sympathetic stimulation) are secreted. This initiates the release of glucose from glycogen and other glucose storage sites. Glycogen is converted back to glucose and released into the blood. Uptake of glucose by most tissues helps to maintain the blood glucose at levels necessary for normal function (Figure 17-6).

> **Critical Thinking**
>
> What signs and symptoms will the patient have in response to the release of adrenaline when blood glucose falls?

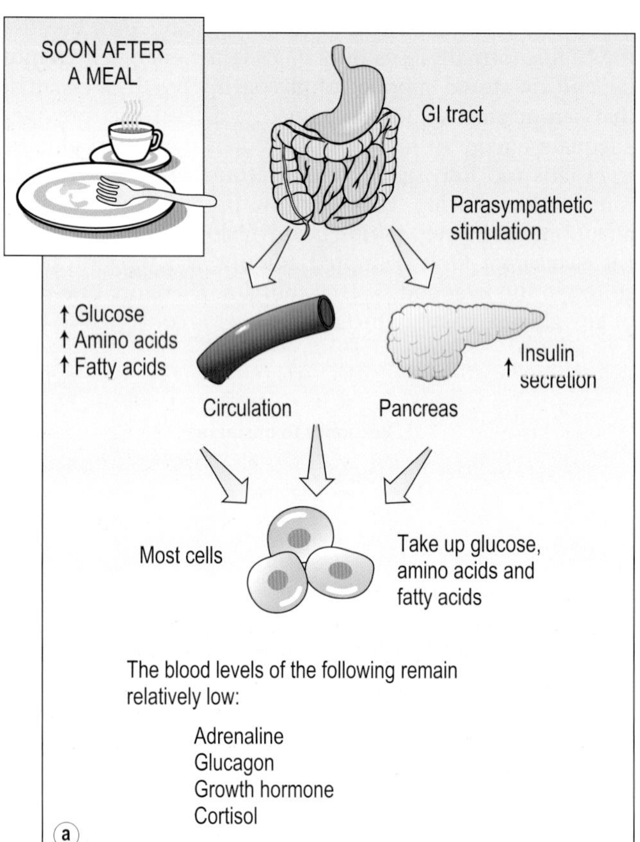

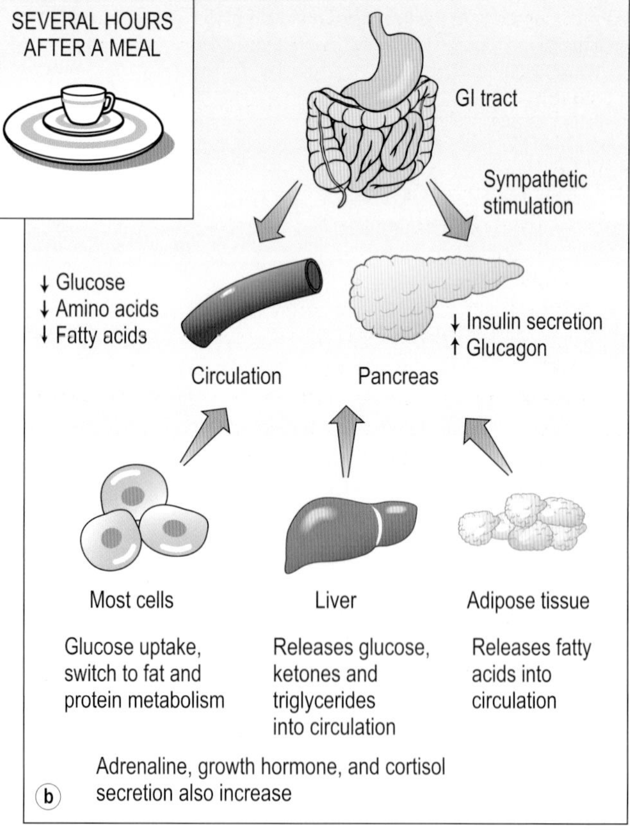

Figure 17-6 (a) Soon after a meal, glucose, amino acids, and fatty acids enter the bloodstream from the intestinal tract. Glucose and amino acids stimulate insulin secretion. Cells take up the glucose and amino acids and use them in their metabolism. (b) Several hours after a meal, absorption from the intestinal tract decreases, and the blood levels of glucose, amino acids, and fatty acids decrease. As a result, insulin secretion decreases, and glucagon, adrenaline, and growth hormone (GH) secretion increases. Cell uptake of glucose decreases, and usage of fats and proteins increases.

In summary, the four mechanisms for achieving adequate blood glucose regulation are as follows:

1. The liver functions as a blood glucose buffer system. It removes glucose from the blood when it is in excess (and stores it as glycogen), and returns glucose to the blood when the glucose concentration and insulin secretion decline.
2. Insulin and glucagon function as a feedback control system. They work to maintain normal serum glucose concentrations. When serum glucose levels rise, insulin is secreted to lower them towards normal. On the other hand, when serum glucose levels fall, glucagon is secreted to raise the serum glucose level towards normal.
3. Low serum glucose levels stimulate the sympathetic nervous system to secrete adrenaline. Adrenaline and, to a lesser degree, noradrenaline have a glucagon-like effect that promotes liver glycogenolysis.
4. GH and cortisol play a role in less immediate regulation of serum glucose levels. They are secreted in response to more prolonged hypoglycaemic episodes. (For example, this might be a late overnight fast.) They tend to increase the rate of glucose production (gluconeogenesis). They tend to decrease the rate of glucose use.

Pathophysiology of diabetes mellitus

Diabetes UK estimates that 1.8 million people have diagnosed diabetes with up to a further 1 million people living with undiagnosed type 2 diabetes in the UK. They suggest that life expectancy for those with type 1 diabetes is reduced by an average of 20 years and by up to 10 years in type 2.[1] The NHS spends close to £10 million per day treating diabetes and its effects.[1] The disease is characterized by a deficiency of insulin or the inability of the body to respond to insulin. The disease is often associated with an increased intake of fluid (polydipsia), excretion of large quantities of urine containing glucose (polyuria, glucosuria), and weight loss. Diabetes mellitus is generally classified as type 1 or type 2. Type 1 is insulin-dependent diabetes mellitus (IDDM) and type 2 is non-insulin-dependent diabetes mellitus (NIDDM). A new classification system endorsed by the World Health Organization classifies four types of diabetes: type 1, type 2, 'other specific types', and gestational diabetes, to address the continuum of hyperglycaemia and insulin requirements.[3]

Type 1 diabetes mellitus

Type 1 diabetes is characterized by inadequate production of insulin by the pancreas. This form of diabetes affects 1 in every 10 diabetics. It may occur any time after birth but it usually occurs in teenagers and young adults. Heredity is a factor in type 1 diabetes. The disease appears to be an autoimmune phenomenon that results from a genetic abnormality or susceptibility that causes the body to destroy its own insulin-producing cells. The genetic aspects of type 1 diabetes are complex but on average:[1]

- if a mother has the condition, the risk of developing it is 2–3%
- if a father has the condition, the risk of developing it is 8–9%
- if both parents have the condition, the risk of developing it is 30%.

Type 1 diabetes requires lifelong treatment with insulin injections, exercise, and diet regulation. The symptoms of type 1 diabetes include polyuria, polydipsia, dizziness, blurred vision, and rapid, unexplained weight loss.

Type 2 diabetes mellitus

Type 2 diabetes is usually characterized by a decrease in the production of insulin by the pancreatic beta cells and diminished tissue sensitivity to insulin. The disease most often occurs in adults over 40 years of age and in those who are overweight; obesity predisposes a person to this form of diabetes because larger amounts of insulin are needed for metabolic control in obese individuals than in those with normal weight. Others at increased risk for type 2 diabetes are people from African Caribbean and Asian backgrounds.[4] Type 2 diabetes tends to develop around 5 years sooner in these groups,[5] and prevalence of the condition is at least five times higher amongst these communities.[6]

Critical Thinking

Would patients with type 1 or type 2 diabetes have an increased risk of complications related to this disease?

Most patients with type 2 diabetes require oral hypoglycaemic medications, exercise, and dietary regulation to control their illness. A small number of patients require insulin injection. Warning signs (if present) are gradual and include all of those associated with type 1 diabetes. Fatigue, changes in appetite, and tingling, numbness, and pain in the extremities are also indicators.

Effects of diabetes mellitus

Most effects of diabetes mellitus can be attributed to one of the following three effects of decreased insulin levels:

1. Decreased use of glucose by the body cells, with a resultant increase in the serum glucose level.
2. Markedly increased mobilization of fats from the fat storage areas, causing abnormal fat metabolism, which may result in the short term in ketoacidosis and in the long term in severe atherosclerosis.
3. Depletion of protein in body tissues and muscle wasting.

Loss of glucose in the urine

When the amount of glucose entering the kidneys rises above the kidneys' ability to reabsorb it, a significant portion of the glucose 'spills' into the urine. The loss of glucose in the urine causes diuresis due to the osmotic effect of glucose, which prevents the kidneys from reabsorbing fluid (osmotic diuresis). The effect is dehydration.

Acidosis in diabetes

The shift from carbohydrate to fat metabolism results in the formation of strongly acidic ketone bodies (called ketoacids). Continuous production of ketoacids leads to a metabolic acidosis. The respiratory system at least partly compensates for this acidosis (indicated by Kussmaul respirations) but the kidneys' ability to clear the acid is overwhelmed by the continuous production of ketone bodies. Profound acidosis eventually occurs. This acidosis, along with the usually severe dehydration that occurs as a result of the osmotic diuresis, can lead to death. Treatment of this condition can be lifesaving.

Diabetes mellitus is a systemic disease with many long-term complications, including the following:

- blindness (the leading cause of blindness in people of working age in the UK)[7]
- kidney disease (diabetic nephropathy [diabetic kidney disease] develops in about one-third of people with diabetes)[8]
- peripheral neuropathy, which results in nerve damage to the hands and feet and an increased incidence of foot infections
- autonomic neuropathy, which damages the nerves controlling voluntary and involuntary functions and may affect sexual function, bladder and bowel control, and blood pressure
- heart disease and stroke
- high blood glucose and blood fat levels contribute to atherosclerosis
- people with diabetes have an up to fivefold increased risk of developing cardiovascular disease and are at least two to three times as likely to have a stroke compared to those without the condition[9]
- peripheral vascular disease (also secondary to atherosclerosis), which results in the need for amputations.

Management

The treatment of diabetes mellitus consists of drug therapy (insulin or oral hypoglycaemic agents), diet regulation, and exercise. These therapies allow patients to control their serum glucose levels and help restore normal metabolism. Pancreatic transplants remain an experimental treatment for diabetes mellitus.

Insulin

Genetically engineered human insulin is available in rapid-, intermediate- and long-acting preparations. (Insulin is administered by injection; it is a protein that would be digested if it were consumed orally.) An insulin-dependent diabetic usually takes one or two doses of a long-acting insulin preparation each day. The person also takes additional amounts of a rapid-acting insulin (lasting only a few hours) at meal times.

Another way for the patient to self-administer insulin is with an insulin infusion pump. These devices allow for a continuous dose of insulin and are adjusted so that the blood glucose level is constantly controlled. The patient must regularly monitor the glucose level to ensure adequate medication control. Medication balance is delicate; the same dosage of insulin that appears correct at one time may be too much or too little at another time. This depends on various factors such as exercise and infection.

Oral hypoglycemic agents

- Sulphonylureas: act mainly by augmenting insulin secretion and consequently are effective only when some residual pancreatic beta-cell activity is present. Commonly prescribed sulphonylureas include chlorpropamide, glibenclamide, gliclazide, glimepiride, glipizide and tolbutamide.[10]
- Biguanides: Metformin is the only available biguanide and exerts its effect mainly by decreasing gluconeogenesis and by increasing peripheral utilization of glucose; since it acts only in the presence of endogenous insulin it is effective only if there are some residual functioning pancreatic islet cells.[10]
- Thiazolidinediones, pioglitazone and rosiglitazone, reduce peripheral insulin resistance, leading to a reduction of blood glucose concentration.[10]

Diabetic emergencies

Three life-threatening conditions may result from diabetes mellitus: hypoglycaemia (insulin shock), hyperglycaemia (diabetic ketoacidosis) and hyperosmolar hyperglycaemic non-ketotic (HHNK) coma.

Hypoglycemia

Hypoglycaemia is a syndrome related to blood glucose levels below about 4 mmol/L. Symptoms usually occur at levels less than 3.3 mmol/L or at slightly higher blood glucose levels if the fall has been rapid. The condition may also occur in patients who are not diabetic and is usually the result of excessive response to glucose absorption, physical exertion, alcohol or drug effects, pregnancy and lactation, or decreased dietary intake. In diabetics, hypoglycaemic reactions are usually caused by the following:

- too much insulin (or oral hypoglycaemic medication)
- decreased dietary intake (a delayed or missed meal)
- unusual or vigorous physical activity
- administration of certain antibiotics (with oral hypoglycaemic agents).

Less common causes and predisposing factors include the following:

- chronic alcoholism (alcohol depletes liver glycogen stores)
- adrenal gland dysfunction
- liver disease (i.e. hepatic insufficiency or failure)
- malnutrition
- pancreatic tumour
- cancer
- hypothermia
- sepsis
- administration of beta-blockers (e.g. propranolol)
- administration of salicylates in ill infants or children
- intentional overdose with insulin, oral hypoglycaemic agents or salicylates.

Signs and symptoms The signs and symptoms of hypoglycaemia usually appear quickly (often within minutes). They are related to the release of adrenaline as the body tries to compensate for a drop in blood sugar. In the early stages, the patient may complain of extreme hunger. He or she may demonstrate one or more of the following signs and symptoms because of decreased glucose availability to the brain:

- nervousness, trembling
- irritability

- psychotic (combative) behaviour
- weakness and poor coordination
- confusion
- appearance of intoxication
- weak, rapid pulse
- cold, clammy skin
- drowsiness
- seizures
- coma (in severe cases).

Hypoglycaemia should be suspected in any diabetic patient with behavioural changes, confusion, abnormal neurological signs, or unconsciousness. This condition is a true emergency that requires immediate administration of glucose to prevent permanent brain damage or death.

Critical Thinking

Why might a call for a patient with diabetic ketoacidosis (DKA) be dispatched as a behavioural emergency?

Diabetic ketoacidosis

Diabetic ketoacidosis (DKA) results from an absence of or resistance to insulin (Box 17-2). The low insulin level prevents glucose from entering the cells, causing an accumulation of glucose in the blood. Consequently, the cells become starved of glucose and begin to use other sources of energy (principally fat). The metabolism of fat generates fatty acids and glycerol. The glycerol provides some energy to the cells, but the fatty acids are further metabolized to form ketoacids, resulting in acidosis.

Any acidosis increases the loss of potassium from the cells into the blood. This results in a high potassium concentration in the urine and a loss of total body potassium. In addition, the sodium concentration outside the cells usually decreases and is replaced by increased amounts of hydrogen ions, which adds greatly to the acidosis. As blood sugar rises, the patient undergoes massive osmotic diuresis. This, combined with vomiting, causes dehydration and shock. The associated electrolyte imbalances may cause cardiac dysrhythmias and altered neuromuscular activity, including seizures.

Signs and symptoms The signs and symptoms of DKA are usually related to diuresis and acidosis. They are normally slow in onset (over 12–48 h) and include the following:

Box 17-2

Common causes of diabetic ketoacidosis

- Inadequate insulin dose
- Failure to take insulin
- Infection
- Increased stress (trauma, surgery)
- Increased dietary intake
- Decreased metabolic rate
- Other, less common predisposing factors, including significant emotional stress, alcohol consumption (often associated with hypoglycaemia), and pregnancy

- diuresis
- warm, dry skin
- dry mucous membranes
- tachycardia, thready pulse
- postural hypotension
- weight loss
- polyuria
- polydipsia
- acidosis
- abdominal pain (usually generalized)
- anorexia, nausea, vomiting
- acetone breath odour (fruity odour)
- Kussmaul respirations in an attempt to reduce carbon dioxide levels
- decreased level of consciousness.

DKA patients are seldom deeply comatose. Patients who are unresponsive should be assessed for another cause, such as head injury, stroke or drug overdose.

Critical Thinking

How can you distinguish Kussmaul respirations from hyperventilation?

HHNK coma

HHNK is a life-threatening emergency that most often occurs in older patients with type 2 diabetes or in patients with undiagnosed diabetes. The syndrome is easily mistaken for DKA but differs from DKA in that enough insulin may be present to prevent metabolism of fats (ketogenesis) and the development of ketoacidosis. However, the amount of insulin may not be enough to prevent glucose use by peripheral tissues or to reduce gluconeogenesis by the liver. HHNK develops from sustained hyperglycaemia that produces a hyperosmolar state. This is followed by an osmotic diuresis that results in marked dehydration and electrolyte losses. These patients usually have greater hyperglycaemia (blood glucose levels of up to 50 mmol/L) than those with DKA because they tend to be more dehydrated. They also have less ketone formation because the presence of insulin in the liver directs free fatty acids into non-ketogenic pathways, which results in less acidaemia than in patients with DKA (Figure 17-7).

HHNK tends to develop slowly, often over several days, and it has a high mortality rate. Early signs and symptoms are mostly related to volume depletion and include polyuria and polydipsia. Associated signs and symptoms may include orthostatic hypotension, dry mucous membranes, and tachycardia. CNS dysfunction may result in lethargy, confusion and coma. Precipitating factors of HHNK coma include the following:

- advanced age
- pre-existing cardiac or renal disease
- inadequate insulin secretion or action (type 2 diabetes)
- increased insulin requirements (stress, infection, trauma, burns, myocardial infarction)
- medication use (thiazide and thiazide diuretics, glucocorticoids, phenytoin, sympathomimetics, propranolol, immunosuppressants)
- supplemental parenteral and enteral feedings.

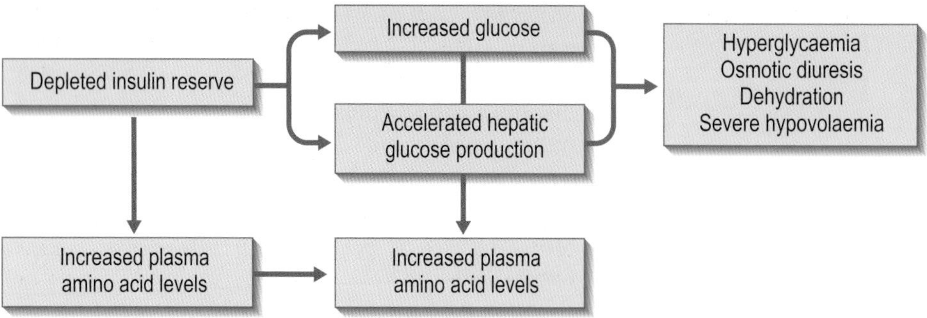

Figure 17-7 Pathophysiology of hyperosmolar hyperglycaemic non-ketotic (HHNK) coma.

Assessment of the diabetic patient

A patient with a diabetic emergency may have a range of signs and symptoms. Many of these may mimic other, more commonly encountered conditions. Thus, the paramedic must have a high degree of suspicion for illness related to diabetes.

In addition to the patient assessment measures appropriate for any emergency patient encounter (initial assessment, physical examination, and treatment of life-threatening illness or injury), the paramedic should search for medical alert information, insulin syringes and diabetic medications (insulin is usually kept in the refrigerator). Important components of the patient history in the assessment of diabetic patients include onset of symptoms, food intake, insulin or oral hypoglycaemic use, alcohol or other drug consumption, predisposing factors (exercise, infection, illness, stress), and any associated symptoms.

Management of the conscious diabetic patient

If the diabetic patient is conscious and able to talk, a pertinent history should be obtained. The paramedic should do this while assessing the patient's airway, breathing, and circulation. A blood glucose measurement should be taken (Figure 17-8) and, if appropriate, the patient should be given oral glucose (sugary drink, chocolate bar/biscuit or glucose gel) until the blood glucose levels have improved to at least 5 mmol/L.[11]

Where the level of consciousness has reduced, the patient is uncooperative or there is a risk of aspiration, and the blood glucose reading indicates hypoglycaemia, JRCALC are recommending the administration of 10% glucose.[11] Paramedics also have the option to administer glucagon and the decision as to which is the most appropriate intervention remains a clinical decision. JRCALC advocate that glucagon should be administered where intravenous access cannot be gained.[11] IV glucose is the most reliable treatment for accidental hypoglycaemia, and once venous access is established it also has the fastest effect.[12] However, the time to gain venous access and the problems associated with the procedure need to be considered when making a clinical decision. Some patients who have experienced a diabetic reaction may be treated at the scene and released, whilst others may need to be transported for evaluation by a physician. The paramedic should follow the established service guidelines or seek medical advice if unsure.

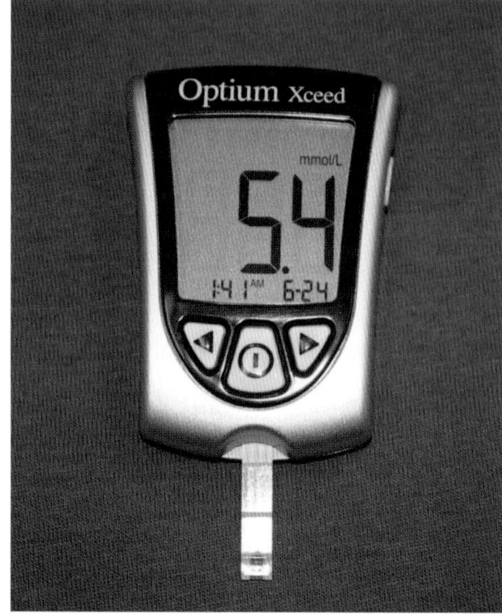

Figure 17-8 Glucometer for measuring serum glucose levels.

Critical Thinking

What steps should you take before leaving the scene if the patient refuses transport after treatment with dextrose?

Management of the unconscious diabetic patient

Prehospital management of any unconscious patient should be directed at airway management, administration of high-concentration oxygen, and ventilatory and circulatory support. An intravenous cannula should be inserted and 10–20 mL of fluid should be flushed to ensure patency of the cannula. If the patient is hypoglycaemic, 10% glucose should be administered in doses of 10 g (100 mL) and repeated every 5 min as required to a maximum dose of 30 g (300 mL).[11]

Note

A patient's age (over 50) and clinical history may suggest a transient ischemic attack (TIA) or stroke. In such a case, administration of a concentrated glucose solution may worsen cerebral damage. Otherwise, a patient in a coma of unknown origin should be given glucose (if indicated by testing). (This is especially true if hypoglycaemia cannot be ruled out.)

If an IV line cannot be established, intramuscular administration of glucagon may help to raise serum glucose levels. It does this by stimulating the breakdown of liver glycogen but it is not effective in chronic alcoholics and those with liver disease. Definitive treatment for patients with DKA or HHNK requires administration of insulin, fluid replacement, electrolyte monitoring and in-hospital observation.

Differential diagnosis

Determining the cause of a diabetic emergency may be difficult in the prehospital setting. When the paramedic is not sure of the cause, all diabetic patients should receive glucose if indicated by testing. The difference in signs and symptoms in diabetic emergencies should help to identify the cause (Table 17-3).

Disorders of the thyroid gland

Common disorders of the thyroid gland include hyperthyroidism and hypothyroidism. Hyperthyroidism is an excess of thyroid hormones in the blood, which may result in thyrotoxicosis. Hypothyroidism is an insufficiency of thyroid hormones in the blood, which may result in myxoedema.

Thyrotoxicosis

The term thyrotoxicosis refers to any toxic condition that results from overproduction of thyroid hormone by the thyroid gland. Hyperthyroidism and thyrotoxicosis are used interchangeably, although this is inaccurate as thyrotoxicosis may occur without associated hyperthyroidism.[13] Thyrotoxic crisis (thyroid storm) is a rare and life-threatening condition resulting from overactivity of the thyroid gland. The crisis may occur spontaneously, or it may be brought on by stress in individuals who have undiagnosed or partially treated hyperthyroidism.[13] Precipitating factors include infection, respiratory or cardiovascular disorders, emotional distress, dialysis, or inadequate preparation for thyroid surgery. The most common cause of thyrotoxicosis is Graves' disease; this is an autoimmune disease characterized by generalized

Table 17-3 Differential considerations in diabetic emergencies

Findings	Hypoglycaemia	Hyperglycaemia	HHNK coma
HISTORY			
Food intake	Insufficient	Excessive	Excessive
Insulin dosage	Excessive	Insufficient	Insufficient
Onset	Rapid	Gradual	Gradual
Infection	Uncommon	Common	Common
GASTROINTESTINAL TRACT			
Thirst	Absent	Intense	Intense
Hunger	Intense	Absent	Intense
Vomiting	Uncommon	Common	Uncommon
RESPIRATORY SYSTEM			
Breathing	Normal or rapid	Deep or rapid	Shallow/rapid
Breath odour	Normal	Acetone smell	Normal
CARDIOVASCULAR SYSTEM			
Blood pressure	Normal	Low	Low
Pulse	Normal, rapid, or full	Rapid or weak	Rapid or weak
Skin	Pale or moist	Warm or dry	Warm or dry
NERVOUS SYSTEM			
Headache	Present	Absent	
Consciousness	Irritability	Restless	Irritable
	Seizure or coma	Coma (rare)	Seizure or coma
URINE			
Sugar	Absent	Present	Present
Acetone	Usually absent	Usually present	Absent
Serum glucose levels	<4 mmol/L	>16.5 mmol/L	>33 mmol/L
Treatment response	Immediate (after glucose)	Gradual (within 6–12 h)	Gradual (within 6–12 h after medication and fluid replacement)

(Note: if the hypoglycaemic episode and fluid retention after medication is prolonged or severe, response may be delayed and may require more than one dose)
From Clark F et al 1993 Pharmacological basis of nursing, 4th edition. Mosby, St Louis.
HHNK, hyperosmolar hyperglycaemic non-ketotic.

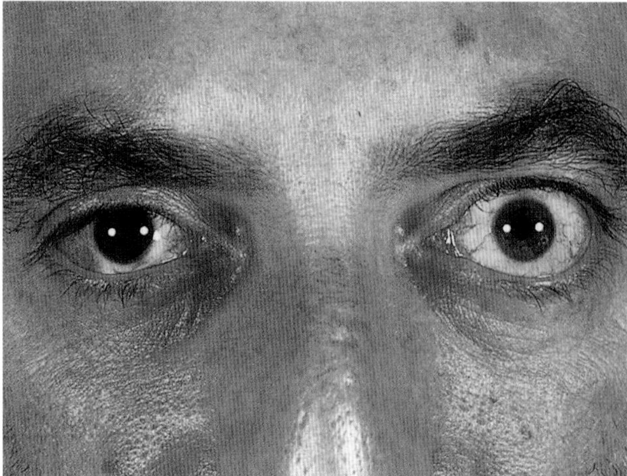

Figure 17-9 Protrusion of the eyes in a patient with Graves' disease. From Epstein O et al 2003 Clinical examination, 3rd edition. Mosby, St Louis.

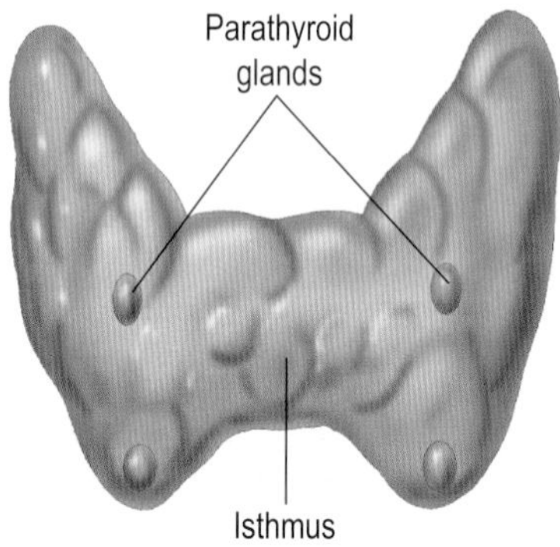

Figure 17-10 Thyroid gland.

enlargement of the gland (goitre), which leads to a swollen neck and, often, protruding eyes (exophthalmos) (Figure 17-9). Graves' disease occurs more commonly in women and may arise from an autoimmune process in which an antibody stimulates the thyroid cells.

Anatomy and physiology of the thyroid gland

The thyroid gland is situated in the front of the neck just below the larynx. It consists of two lobes, one on each side of the trachea, joined by a narrower portion of tissue called the isthmus (Figure 17-10).

Thyroid tissue is composed of two types of secretory cells; follicular cells and parafollicular cells (or C cells). Follicular cells make up most of the gland and are arranged in the form of hollow, spherical follicles. They secrete the iodine-containing hormones thyroxine (T4) and triiodothyronine (T3). Parafollicular cells occur singly or in small groups in the spaces between the follicles and secrete the hormone calcitonin, which helps regulate the level of calcium in the body.

Thyroid hormones play a key role in controlling body metabolism. They are essential in children for normal physical growth and mental development. The secretion of T3 and T4 is controlled by a feedback system that involves the pituitary gland and the hypothalamus. (The secretion of calcitonin is regulated directly by the level of calcium in the blood, independent of the pituitary gland or hypothalamus.)

> **Box 17-3**
>
> **Causes of thyroid gland disorders**
>
> - Congenital defects
> - Genetic disorders
> - Infection (thyroiditis)
> - Tumours (benign or malignant)
> - Autoimmune disorders
> - Hormonal disorders during puberty or pregnancy
> - Nutritional disorders

Disorders of the thyroid gland may result from defects in the gland itself or from disruption of the hypothalamic–pituitary hormonal control system (Box 17-3). The disease advances in a slow fashion and may have non-specific signs and symptoms over months to years before culminating in an acute episode. Non-specific signs and symptoms of thyroid hyperfunction include fatigue, anxiety, palpitations, sweating, weight loss, diarrhoea and heat intolerance.

In acute episodes of thyrotoxic crisis, signs and symptoms are those related to adrenergic hyperactivity. They may include the following:

- severe tachycardia
- heart failure
- cardiac dysrhythmias
- shock
- hyperthermia
- restlessness
- agitation and paranoia
- abdominal pain
- delirium
- coma.

The paramedic should consider other causes of symptoms related to adrenergic hyperactivity – most notably the use of cocaine and amphetamines, hypoglycaemia, and withdrawal from alcohol and other drugs.

> **Critical Thinking**
>
> What medical emergencies could produce signs and symptoms similar to those of thyroid storm?

Management

Mild hyperthyroidism requires no emergency therapy so is best managed with physician follow-up. By comparison, thyrotoxic crisis is a true emergency requiring immediate treatment. Emergency care efforts are directed at providing airway, ventilatory, and circulatory support and rapid transport to an appropriate medical facility. In-hospital care focuses on inhibiting hormone synthesis, blocking hormone release and the peripheral effects of thyroid hormone with antithyroid drugs, and providing general support of the patient's vital functions.

Table 17-4 lists the signs and symptoms caused by hyperthyroidism and hypothyroidism.

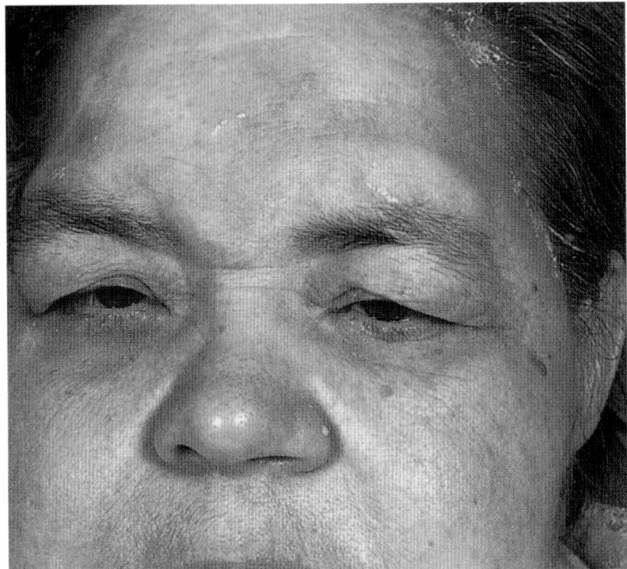

Figure 17-11 Myxoedema. From Epstein O et al 2003 Clinical examination, 3rd edition. Mosby, St Louis.

Table 17-4 Features of hyperthyroidism and hypothyroidism

Hyperthyroidism	Hypothyroidism
Signs and symptoms	
Exophthalmos	Facial oedema
Goitre	Jugular venous distention (sometimes goitre)
Warm, flushed skin	Cool skin
Fever	Cold intolerance
Agitation/psychosis	Coma
Hyperactivity	Weakness
Weight loss	Weight gain
Common medications	
Iodine	Levothyroxine
Carbimazole	Liothyronine
Propylthiouracil	

Myxoedema

Myxoedema is a condition that results from a deficiency in thyroid hormone. It may be associated with inflammation of the thyroid gland (e.g. Hashimoto thyroiditis) or atrophy of the thyroid gland and may also be a consequence of treatment for hyperthyroidism. Myxoedema causes the build-up of mucinous material in the skin, which results in thickening and coarsening of the skin and other body tissues (most notably the lips and nose) (Figure 17-11). The condition is most common in adults (especially women) over age 40.

Myxoedema coma is a rare condition that is characterized by hypothermia and mental obtundation in addition to myxoedema. Myxoedema coma is a medical emergency that may be precipitated by the following factors:

- exposure to cold
- infection (usually pulmonary)
- congestive heart failure
- trauma
- drugs (sedatives, hypnotics, anaesthetics)
- stroke
- internal haemorrhage
- hypoxia
- hypercapnia
- hyponatraemia
- hypoglycaemia.

Management

Prehospital care is directed at managing life-threatening conditions (airway, ventilatory and circulatory compromise) and providing rapid transport to an appropriate medical facility for evaluation by a physician. Once other causes of the coma have been ruled out and the patient's condition has been stabilized, treatment of myxoedema can begin. Treatment involves oral administration of thyroxine, which must be continued for life.

Disorders of the adrenal glands

Cushing syndrome and Addison's disease are two disorders of the adrenal glands. Cushing syndrome is a rare disease caused by an excessive level of cortisol irrespective of the cause. Addison's disease is caused by inactivity of the adrenal cortex.

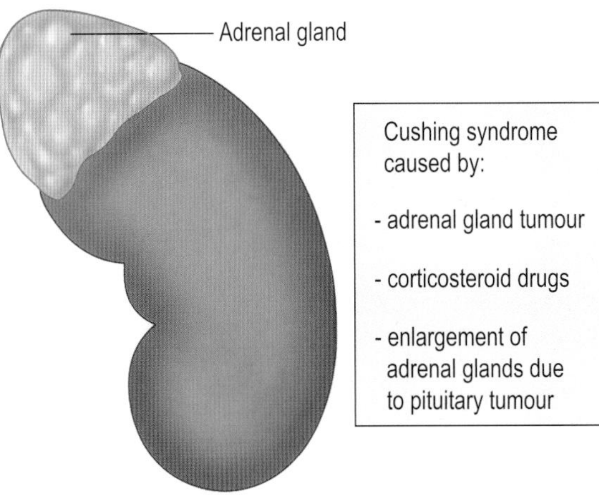

Figure 17-12 Adrenal gland.

Cushing syndrome

Cushing syndrome is caused by an abnormally high circulating level of corticosteroid hormones that are produced naturally by the adrenal glands (Figure 17-12). This condition may be produced directly by an adrenal gland tumour, which causes excessive secretion of corticosteroids, or it may be produced by administration of corticosteroid drugs (these are used to treat conditions such as rheumatoid arthritis, inflammatory bowel disease, and asthma). It may also be produced by enlargement of both adrenal glands as a result of a pituitary tumour. The pituitary gland controls the activity of the adrenal gland by producing adrenocorticotropic hormone (ACTH). ACTH stimulates the cortex of the adrenal gland to grow. Cushing syndrome is rare and mainly affects women of 30 to 50 years of age.

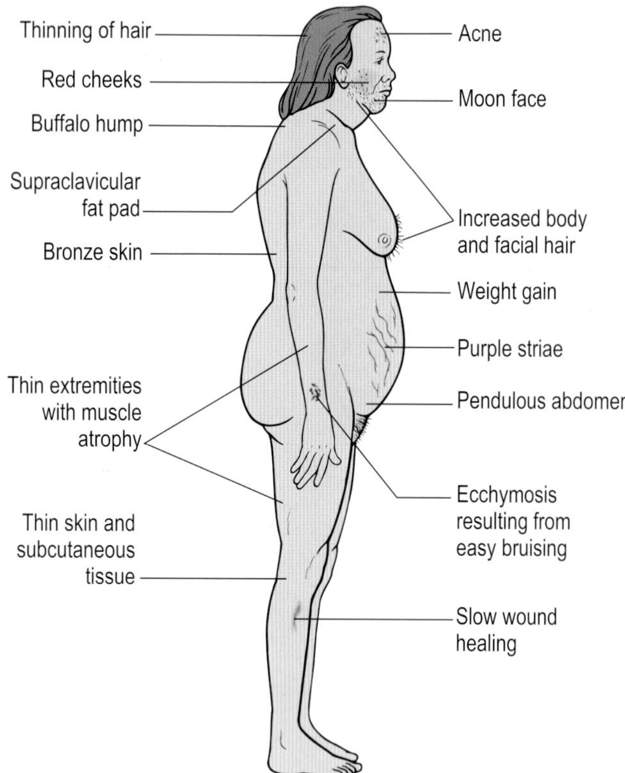

Figure 17-13 Cushing syndrome. From Lewis SM, Collier IC, Heitkemper MM 1996 Medical-surgical nursing: assessment and management of clinical problems, 4th edition. Mosby, St Louis.

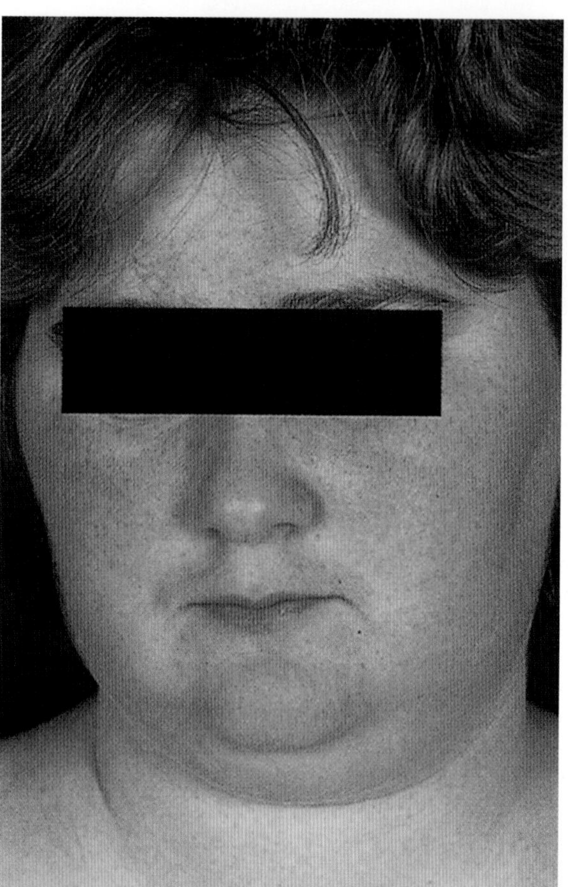

Figure 17-14 Moon-faced appearance in a patient with Cushing syndrome. From Epstein O et al 2003 Clinical examination, 3rd edition. Mosby, St Louis.

People with Cushing syndrome have a characteristic appearance (Figure 17-13). The face appears round ('moon face') and red (Figure 17-14), and the trunk tends to become obese from disturbances in fat metabolism. The limbs become wasted from muscle atrophy; acne develops, and purple stretch marks may appear on the abdomen, thighs and breasts. The skin often thins and bruises easily whilst weakened bones are at increased risk of fracture. Other features of the disease include the following:

- increased body and facial hair
- hump on the back of neck ('buffalo hump')
- supraclavicular fat pads
- weight gain
- hypertension
- psychiatric disturbances (depression, paranoia)
- insomnia
- diabetes mellitus.

Critical Thinking

How do you think patients who suffer from Cushing syndrome feel about their body image?

Management

Prehospital care for patients with Cushing syndrome is mainly supportive. The disease is diagnosed through measurement of hormone levels in the blood and urine, and by radiological imaging (e.g. computed tomography [CT] scan). If the cause of the syndrome is overtreatment with corticosteroid drugs, the condition is usually reversible when the drug dosages are adjusted. If the cause is a tumour or overgrowth of the adrenal gland, the gland may require surgical removal. If the tumour is in the pituitary gland, the usual treatment involves surgery, radiation, and medication. Treatment is usually successful although lifelong hormone replacement therapy is required.

Addison's disease

Addison's disease is a rare but potentially life-threatening disorder. The disease is caused by a deficiency of the corticosteroid hormones cortisol and aldosterone, which are normally produced by the adrenal cortex. The disorder can be caused by any disease process that destroys the adrenal cortices. (Such disease processes may include adrenal haemorrhage or infarction, infections [tuberculosis, fungi, viruses], and autoimmune diseases.) However, the most common cause of Addison's disease is shrinking of the adrenal tissue. When this occurs, production of corticosteroid hormones is inadequate to meet the body's metabolic requirements. Signs and symptoms associated with this disease include the following:

- progressive weakness
- progressive weight loss
- progressive anorexia

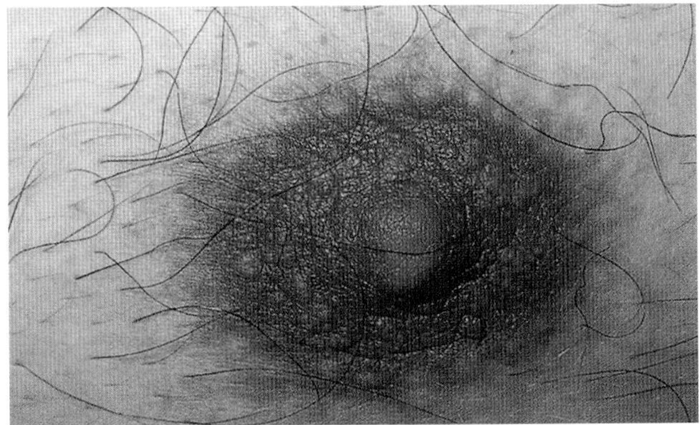

Figure 17-15 Hyperpigmentation of the areola in a patient with Addison's disease. From Epstein O et al 2003 Clinical examination, 3rd edition. Mosby, St Louis.

- skin hyperpigmentation (caused by increased hormone production by the pituitary gland, which stimulates melanin) (Figure 17-15)
- hypotension
- hyponatraemia
- hyperkalaemia
- GI disturbances (nausea, vomiting, diarrhoea).

Addison's disease usually has a slow onset and a chronic course with symptoms developing gradually over months to years. However, acute episodes (Addisonian crisis) may be brought on by emotional and physiological stress. Examples of such stressors include surgery, alcohol intoxication, hypothermia, myocardial infarction, severe illness, trauma, hypoglycaemia and infection. During these events, the adrenal glands cannot increase the production of the corticosteroid hormones to help the body cope with stress. As a result, blood glucose levels drop; the body loses the ability to regulate the content of sodium, potassium and water in body fluids (causing dehydration and extreme muscle weakness); blood volume and blood pressure fall; and the body may not be able to maintain circulation efficiently. In these situations, airway, ventilatory and circulatory support are required in the prehospital setting.

Table 17-5 Features of adrenal gland disorders

Corticosteroid excess (Cushing syndrome)	Adrenal insufficiency (Addison's disease)
Signs and symptoms	
Weight gain	Weight loss
Weakness	Weakness
Hump on back of neck	Hypotension
Slow healing	Gastrointestinal disorders
Increased body and facial hair	Skin hyperpigmentation
Common medications	
Metyrapone	Dexamethasone
	Fludrocortisone

Management

Prehospital management of any Addisonian patient should follow the normal stepwise approach to identify and manage any problems associated with airway, breathing and circulation. 100 mg of hydrocortisone should then be administered slowly via the IV route in adults (or as per JRCALC guidelines for children from 1–11 years).[11] Where intravenous access cannot be achieved, the IM route can be used. In-hospital treatment involves maintaining the patient's vital functions and correcting any sodium deficiency and dehydration. After the life-threatening episode has been managed, treatment consists of administration of corticosteroids. The patient may be advised to increase the dosage of these drugs during times of emotional and physiological stress. Table 17-5 presents a comparison of the signs and symptoms of Cushing syndrome and Addison's disease.

Summary

- The endocrine system consists of ductless glands and tissues, which produce and secrete hormones. Endocrine glands secrete their hormones directly into the bloodstream and exert a regulatory effect on various metabolic functions. All hormones operate within feedback systems (either positive or negative). These systems work to maintain an optimal internal environment.
- The pancreatic islets are composed of beta cells, alpha cells and other cells. The beta cells secrete insulin; the alpha cells secrete glucagon; the other cells are of questionable function. The chief functions of insulin are to increase glucose transport into cells, increase glucose metabolism by cells, increase the liver glycogen level, and decrease the blood glucose concentration toward normal. Glucagon has two major effects: (1) to increase blood glucose levels by stimulating the liver to release glucose stores from glycogen and other glucose storage sites (glycogenolysis) and (2) to stimulate gluconeogenesis through the breakdown of fats and fatty acids, thereby maintaining a normal blood glucose level.
- Diabetes mellitus is characterized by a deficiency of insulin or an inability of the body to respond to insulin. Diabetes generally is classified as type 1 or type 2. Type 1 is insulin dependent, type 2 is non-insulin dependent. Type 1 diabetes requires lifelong treatment consisting of insulin injections, exercise, and diet regulation. Most patients with type 2 diabetes require oral hypoglycaemic medications, exercise, and dietary regulation to control the illness.
- Hypoglycaemia is a syndrome related to blood glucose levels below 4 mmol/L. Any diabetic patient with behavioural changes or unconsciousness should be treated for hypoglycaemia. This condition is a true emergency that requires immediate administration of glucose to prevent permanent brain damage or death.

- Diabetic ketoacidosis results from an absence of or a resistance to insulin. The signs and symptoms of DKA are related to diuresis and acidosis and are usually slow in onset.
- Hyperosmolar hyperglycaemic non-ketotic coma is a life-threatening emergency. It often occurs in older patients with type 2 diabetes or in undiagnosed diabetics. The hyperglycaemia produces a hyperosmolar state, which is followed by an osmotic diuresis, dehydration and electrolyte losses.
- Important components of the patient history in the assessment of diabetic patients include the onset of symptoms, food intake, insulin or oral hypoglycaemic use, alcohol or other drug consumption, predisposing factors, and any associated symptoms.
- Any patient with a glucose reading below 4 mmol/L and signs and symptoms consistent with hypoglycaemia should be given dextrose.
- Thyroid hormones play a key role in controlling body metabolism. They are essential in children for normal physical growth and development.
- Thyrotoxicosis is any toxic condition that results from over activity of the thyroid gland.
- Thyrotoxic crisis (thyroid storm) is a life-threatening condition resulting from an overactive thyroid gland.
- Myxoedema is a condition that results from a thyroid hormone deficiency. Myxoedema coma is a rare illness that is characterized by hypothermia and mental obtundation. It is a medical emergency.
- Cushing syndrome is caused by an abnormally high circulating level of corticosteroid hormones. These are produced naturally by the adrenal glands.
- Addison's disease is a rare but life-threatening disorder. It is caused by a deficiency of the corticosteroid hormones cortisol and aldosterone. These are normally produced by the adrenal cortex.

References

1. Diabetes UK: Diabetes in the UK 2004. Online. Available http://www.library.nhs.uk/diabetes/ August 15 2008
2. Diabetes UK: Shocking new statistics, 2008. Online. Available http://www.diabetes.org.uk August 15 2008
3. Expert Committee on the Diagnosis and Classification of Diabetes Mellitus 1997 Report of the Expert Committee on the Diagnosis and Classification of Diabetes Mellitus. Diabetes Care 20:1183–1197
4. Mather HM, Chaturverdi N, Fuller JH 1998 Mortality and morbidity from diabetes in South Asians and Europeans: 11 year follow-up of the Southall Diabetes Survey, London, UK. Diabet Med 15:53–59
5. Greenhalgh PM 1997 Diabetes in British South Asians: nature, nurture and culture. Diabet Med 14:10–18
6. Coronary Heart Disease Statistics. British Heart Foundation Statistics Database. 2003. Online. Available http://www.heartstats.org/homepage.asp
7. Kohner E, Allwinkle J, Andrews J, et al 1996 Report of the Visual Handicap Group. Diabet Med 13(Suppl. 4):S13–S26
8. Diabetes and kidney disease: time to act. International Diabetes Federation, 2003. Online. Available http://www.idf.org/webdata/docs/your%20guide_EN.pdf
9. Yudkin JS, Blauth C, Drury P, et al 1996 Prevention and management of cardiovascular disease in patients with diabetes mellitus: an evidence base. Diabet Med 13(Suppl. 4):S101–S121
10. Royal Pharmaceutical Society of Great Britain and British Medical Association. British National Formulary 55. March 2008. Online. Available www.bnf.org
11. Joint Royal Colleges Ambulance Liaison Committee. UK Ambulance Service Clinical Guidelines 2006. Online. Available http://jrcalc.org.uk/guidelines.html 9 February 2009
12. Boyd R. IV glucose is the most reliable treatment for accidental hypoglycaemia. Once venous access is established it is also has the fastest effect. BestBets 2004. Online. Available http://www.bestbets.org/bets/bet.php?id=85 August 15 2008
13. McCance KL, Heuther SE 2006 Pathophysiology; the biological basis for disease in adults and children, 5th edition. Elsevier Mosby, St. Louis

Further reading

Becker K, et al 2001 Principles and practice of endocrinology and metabolism, 3rd edition. Lippincott Williams & Wilkins, Philadelphia

Kacsoh B 2000 Endocrine physiology. McGraw-Hill/Appleton Lange, New York

William R, et al 2002 Williams textbook of endocrinology, 10th edition. WB Saunders, Philadelphia

CHAPTER 18

Allergies and Anaphylaxis

Chapter contents

Objectives

Upon completion of this chapter, the paramedic student will be able to:

1. Describe the antigen–antibody response.
2. Differentiate between an allergic reaction and a normal immune response.
3. Describe signs and symptoms and management of local allergic reactions based on an understanding of the pathophysiology associated with this condition.
4. Identify allergens associated with anaphylaxis.
5. Describe the pathophysiology, signs and symptoms, and management of anaphylaxis.

Key terms

eosinophil chemotactic factor of anaphylaxis A group of active substances, including histamine and leukotrienes, that are released during an anaphylactic reaction.

leukotrienes A class of biologically active compounds that occur naturally in leukocytes and that produce allergic and inflammatory reactions.

sensitization An acquired reaction in which specific antibodies develop in response to an antigen.

thromboxanes Antagonistic prostaglandin derivatives that are synthesized and released by degranulating platelets, causing vasoconstriction and promoting the degranulation of other platelets.

Anaphylaxis is an allergic reaction which is an immediate, systemic, life-threatening reaction. It is associated with major changes in the cardiovascular, respiratory, and cutaneous systems. The prompt recognition and the proper drug therapy are vital to patient survival.

Antigen–antibody reaction

An antigen is a substance that induces the formation of antibodies. Antigens can enter the body by injection, ingestion, inhalation or absorption. The antibodies bind to the antigen that produced them; antibodies then aid in neutralizing the antigens and removing them from the body. This normal antigen–antibody reaction protects the body from disease by activating the immune response (Figure 18-1).

The immune responses normally are protective; however, they can become oversensitive. They can become directed toward harmless antigens to which human beings often are exposed; when this occurs, the response is termed allergic. The antigen or substance causing the allergic response is called an allergen. Common allergens include drugs, insects, foods, latex, animals, pollens and moulds (Box 18-1). The healthy body responds to an antigen challenge through a collective defence system, known as immunity. Immunity may be natural (present at birth), acquired (resulting from exposure to a specific antigenic agent or pathogen) or induced artificially through immunization.

Allergic reaction

An allergic reaction is marked by an increased physiological response to an antigen after a previous exposure (sensitization) to the same antigen. The allergic reaction starts when a circulating antibody (immunoglobulin G [IgG] or M [IgM]) combines with a specific foreign antigen, resulting in hypersensitivity reactions, or with antibodies bound to mast cells or basophils (IgE). Hypersensitivity reactions are divided into four distinct types; type I (IgE-mediated allergic reactions), type II (tissue-specific reactions), type III (immune-complex–mediated reactions), and type IV (cell-

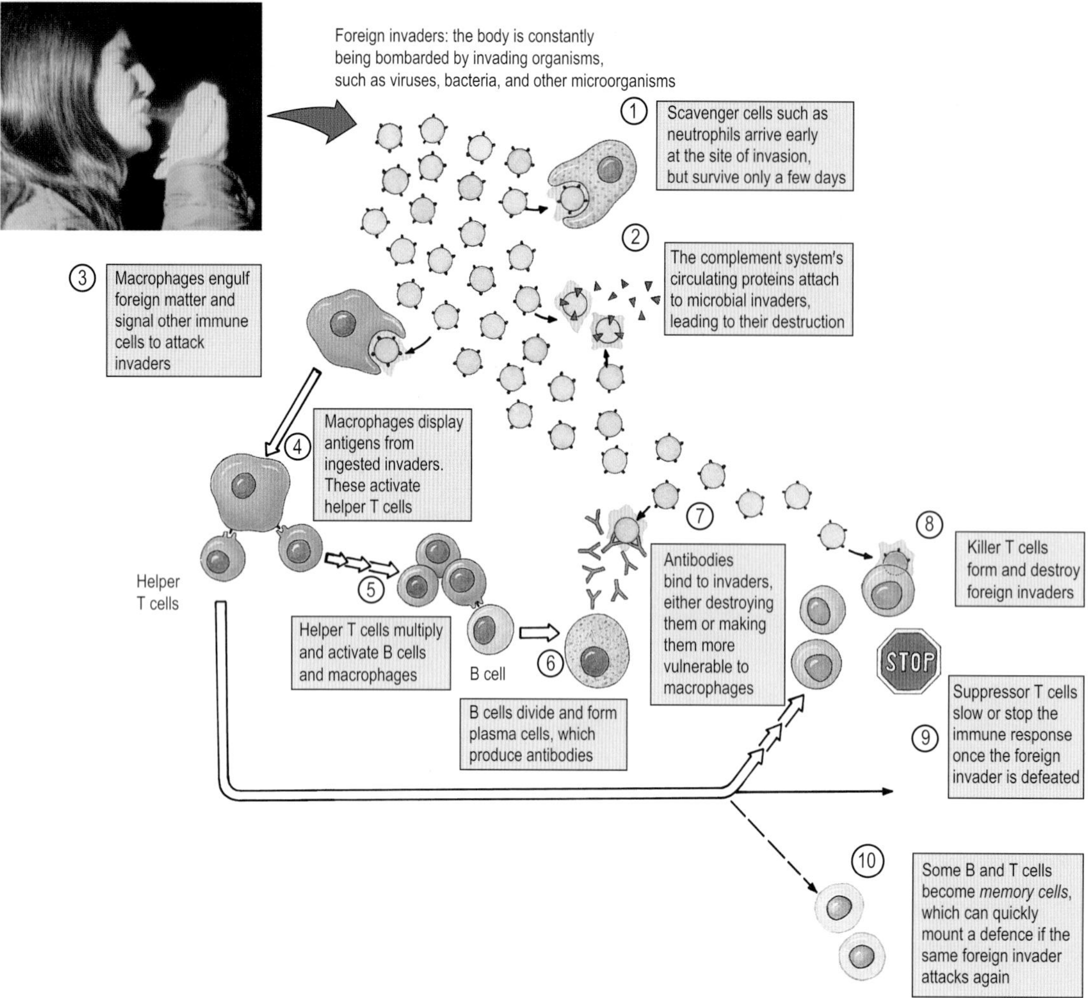

Figure 18-1 A brief summary of the immune response.

mediated reactions). A type I or immediate hypersensitivity reaction is the most dramatic. It may lead to life-threatening anaphylaxis. Box 18-2 gives examples of antigens that may cause hypersensitivity reactions (including anaphylaxis). Patients who have a known sensitivity to these or other agents should avoid exposure.

Note

Anaphylactoid reactions are allergic reactions that are not mediated by an antigen–antibody reaction. These reactions present exactly like anaphylaxis. The distinction is not crucial in relation to treatment of an acute attack.[1]

Localized allergic reaction

Localized allergic reactions (type IV) do not involve the entire body. In these cases, the sites of mast cell and basophil mediator release are limited. Common signs and symptoms of localized allergic reaction include the following:

- conjunctivitis
- rhinitis
- angioedema
- urticaria
- contact dermatitis (Figure 18-2).

Localized allergic reactions are best managed with drugs that compete for receptor sites with histamine, which prevent histamine from performing its physiological actions. Common antihistamines include over-the-counter oral and nasal decongestants and prescription and non-prescription drugs such as chlorphenamine. Other medications that may be helpful for some local reactions include steroids and topical creams.

Anaphylaxis

The term anaphylaxis comes from Greek, meaning 'against or opposite of protection'. Anaphylaxis is the most extreme form of an allergic reaction, with a lifetime incidence of 75 per 100 000 of the UK population. There is evidence that the prevalence may be increasing, with admission rates to English hospitals increasing in the period 1990 to 2004 by around 700%. Once experienced, the risk of recurrence is around 1 in 12 per annum. Anaphylaxis accounts for at least 20 deaths per annum in the UK;[2] evidence suggests that cardiac arrest occurs around 30–35 min after food ingestion reactions and in insect stings within 15 min. All of these factors mean that rapid recognition and aggressive therapy are essential.

Box 18-1

Latex allergies

Today there is significant concern about latex allergy, especially among healthcare workers. The first published account of contact urticaria related to glove use was published in 1979; however, latex allergy was relatively unknown until after the acquired immunodeficiency syndrome epidemic in the mid-1980s and the resulting tremendous increase in glove usage. The prevalence of sensitization to latex has been reported to range from 2.9% to 4.7% among healthcare workers and from 7% to 10% among operating room staff. (In addition to latex gloves, healthcare workers and latex-sensitive patients can be exposed to latex on medical instruments, surgical equipment, and other appliances.) Those persons considered at high risk for latex allergy include the following:

- Individuals who have had significant and early exposure to latex (e.g. patients with spina bifida or genitourinary anomalies, and others who have had multiple surgeries and catheterizations).
- Persons with a genetic propensity to develop allergies.
- Asthmatics.
- Healthcare workers, police officers and fire service personnel who regularly use latex gloves.
- Workers in some occupations (e.g. rubber manufacturing employees, hairdressers, food handlers, car mechanics, etc.).

Symptoms of latex allergy can range from mild discomfort to life-threatening anaphylaxis. Most often the first manifestation of a latex allergy is urticaria that typically is localized to the hands but may be widespread. A type I latex allergy can manifest itself in symptoms that include rash, lacrimation, rhinitis, wheezing, bronchospasm, laryngeal oedema, hypotension, dysrhythmia, and, rarely, respiratory or cardiac arrest.

Many healthcare facilities and hospitals, emergency medical services, and other public service agencies have addressed this issue by developing 'latex safe' environments and by using latex-free equipment for patients with latex allergy. For the healthcare provider the need for education, early recognition, prevention strategies, and the implementation of safe and effective practice is essential. It is recommended that healthcare workers wear low-protein, powder-free gloves when latex gloves are necessary and synthetic gloves when the risk of exposure to blood-borne pathogens is low. Nitrile gloves give protection for paramedics but remove the risk of latex allergy. Individuals not exposed to blood or body fluids (e.g. food handlers and maintenance workers) should avoid latex gloves altogether. All patients should be questioned about latex allergy; persons with latex allergy should wear appropriate medical-alert identification. Sensitivity to latex should be documented on the patient report form, and this information should be conveyed to the A&E department or receiving unit.

Source: Korniewicz D 1999 Latex allergy: a current challenge. Asepsis on the Web 20(3). Online. Available http://web.archive.org/web/20000618085817/www.jnjmedical.com/asepsis/latex_allg.asp.

Critical Thinking

Consider the list of allergens in Box 18-2. Based on this list, what are some likely locations to which you may be dispatched to care for a patient who is experiencing an anaphylactic reaction?

Box 18-2

Agents that may cause allergies and anaphylaxis

Drugs and biological agents

Antibiotics
Anticancer agents
Aspirin
Cephalosporins
Chemotherapeutics
Insulin
Local anaesthetics
Muscle relaxants
Non-steroidal anti-inflammatory agents
Opiates
Vaccines
Incorrectly matched blood products

Insect bites and stings

Bees
Ants
Wasps

Foods

Fish (especially shellfish)
Egg
Soya
Food additives
Milk
Nuts
Sesame and sunflower seeds
Strawberries/mango
Wheat

Other

IV contrast agents
Animal fur

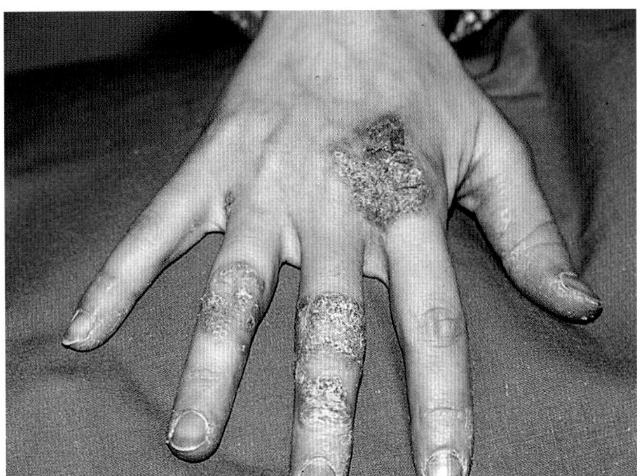

Figure 18-2 Contact dermatitis caused by a delayed hypersensitivity leading to vesicles and scaling at the sites of contact.

Causative agents

Almost any substance can cause anaphylaxis; the antigenic agents most frequently associated with anaphylaxis are drugs, particularly antibiotics (by ingestion or injection) and anaesthetics, envenomation by stinging insects, and food (especially nuts and shellfish). Regardless of the offending antigen, the risk of anaphylaxis in sensitive persons increases with each exposure; to a lesser extent, the risk increases with the length of exposure or site of inoculation.

Pathophysiology

As described before, a person first must be exposed to a specific antigen to develop type I hypersensitivity. In the first exposure the antigen enters the body by injection, ingestion, inhalation or absorption, then the antigen activates the immune system. In susceptible persons, large amounts of IgE antibody are produced. Immunoglobulin E antibodies leave the lymphatic system and bind to the cell membranes of basophils that are circulating in the blood and to mast cells that are in tissues surrounding the blood vessels. These antibodies remain on the cells and are inactive until the same antigen is introduced into the body a second time (Figure 18-3). With the next exposure to the specific antigen, the allergen cross-links at least two of the cell-bound IgE molecules, which results in degranulation (release of internal substances) of the mast cells and basophils and the onset of an anaphylactic reaction (Box 18-3).

The degranulation of the target cell is associated with the release of pharmacologically active chemical mediators from inside the affected basophils and mast cells. These chemicals include histamine, leukotrienes, eosinophil chemotactic factor of anaphylaxis, heparin, kinins, prostaglandins and thromboxanes; all of these chemicals mediate or trigger an internal systemic response.

Histamine increases the permeability of vessels, causes dilation of capillaries and venules and also causes contraction of smooth muscle in the gastrointestinal tract and bronchial tree. An associated increase in gastric, nasal and lacrimal secretions also occurs, which results in tearing and rhinorrhoea. The increased capillary permeability allows plasma to leak into the interstitial space, decreasing the amount of fluid

Box 18-3

Anaphylaxis

Three conditions must be met to sensitize an individual and generate an anaphylactic response:

1. An antigen-induced stimulation of the immune system with specific immunoglobulin E antibody formation.
2. A latent period after the initial antigenic exposure for sensitization of mast cells and basophils to occur.
3. Subsequent re-exposure to the same specific antigen.

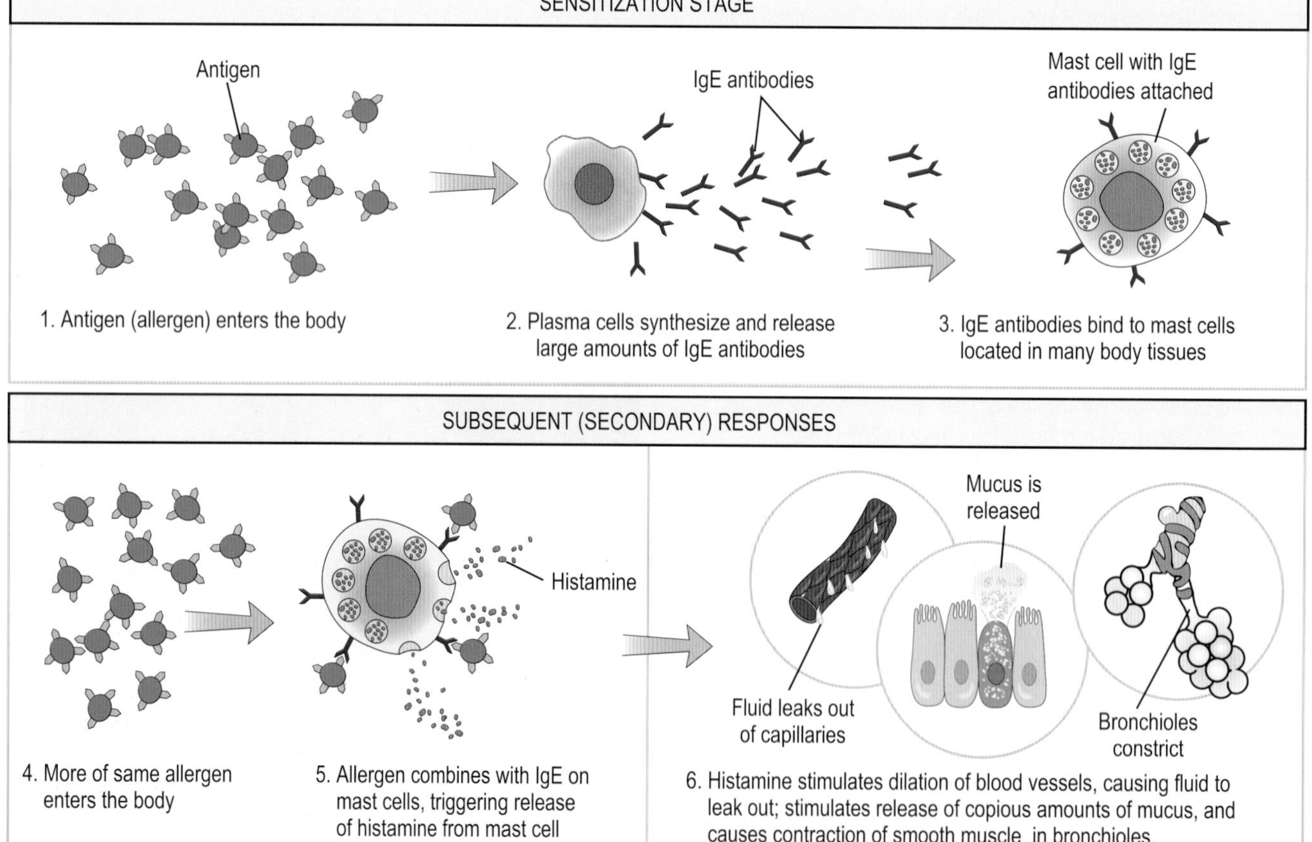

Figure 18-3 Allergic reaction. Antigen stimulates the production of massive amounts of immunoglobulin E, a type of antibody produced by plasma cells. Immunoglobulin E attaches to mast cells. This is the sensitization stage. When the antigen enters again, it binds to the immunoglobulin E antibodies on the mast cells, triggering a massive release of histamine and other chemicals. Histamine, in turn, causes blood vessels to dilate and become leaky. This triggers the production of mucus in the respiratory tract. In some persons the chemicals released by the mast cells also cause the small air-carrying ducts in the lungs to constrict, making breathing difficult.

that is available for the heart to pump; this profound body-wide vasodilation further decreases cardiac preload and this in turn decreases stroke volume and cardiac output. These responses lead to flushing, urticaria, angioedema and hypotension (Figure 18-4). The onset of action of the histamine is rapid, yet the effects of histamine are short lived because it is quickly broken down by enzymes. Figure 18-5 illustrates the pathophysiology of anaphylactic shock.

Leukotrienes are the most potent bronchoconstrictors, which cause wheezing, as well as leading to coronary vasoconstriction and increased vascular permeability. Leukotrienes were formerly known as slow-reacting substances of anaphylaxis (SRS-A) because their effects were delayed relative to histamine; however, the duration of action of these chemicals is much longer than that of histamine.

The process of anaphylaxis attracts eosinophils to the site of allergic inflammation. Eosinophils are thought to contain an enzyme that can deactivate leukotrienes. The remaining chemical mediators (heparin, neutrophil chemotactic factor, and kinins) exert varying effects that may include fever, chills, bronchospasm, and pulmonary vasoconstriction. These complex chemical processes can lead rapidly to upper airway obstruction and bronchospasm, dysrhythmias and cardiac ischaemia, and circulatory collapse and shock.

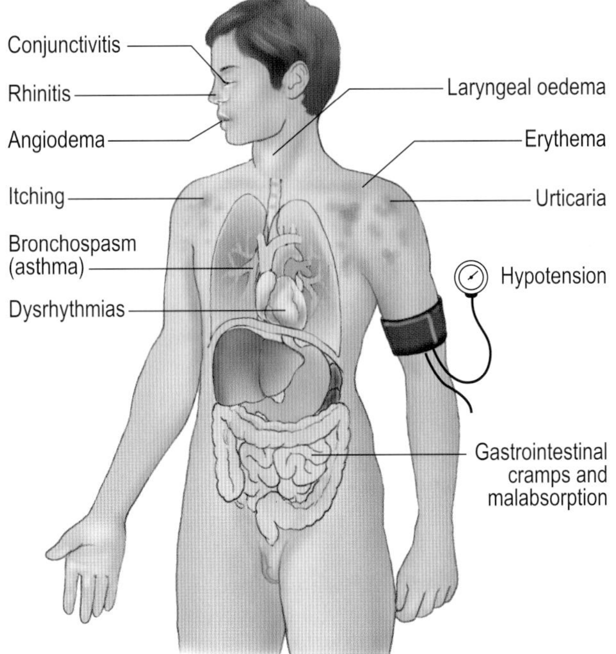

Figure 18-4 Type I hypersensitivity reactions. Manifestations of allergic reactions as a result of type I hypersensitivity include itching, angioedema (swelling caused by exudation), oedema of the larynx, urticaria (hives), bronchospasm (constriction of airways in the lungs), hypotension (low blood pressure), dysrhythmias (irregular heartbeat) because of anaphylactic shock, and gastrointestinal cramping caused by inflammation of the gastrointestinal mucosa.

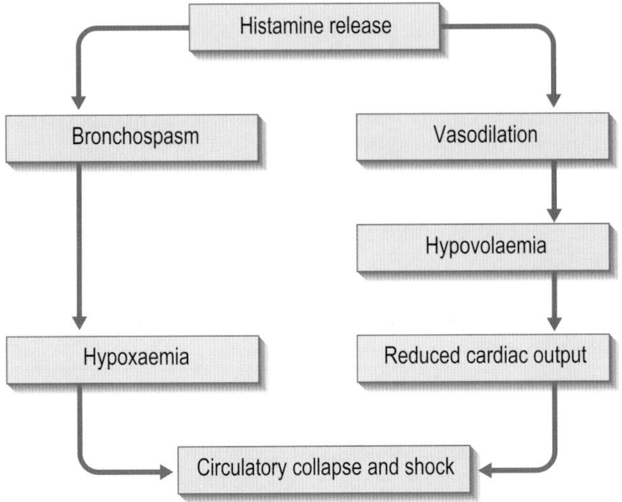

Figure 18-5 Pathophysiology of anaphylactic shock.

Assessment findings

An accurate history and physical assessment are required to tell the difference between severe allergic reactions and other conditions that may mimic anaphylaxis (Table 18-1). Speed of onset is a clue, as the clinical features present within minutes. Consider anaphylaxis when you observe signs or symptoms from two or more body systems. A flawed prehospital assessment in this group can threaten a patient's life. Other conditions that may present similar signs and symptoms to those of anaphylaxis include:

- severe asthma with respiratory failure
- upper airway obstruction
- toxic or septic shock
- pulmonary oedema (with or without myocardial infarction)
- drug overdose
- hypovolaemic shock.

Respiratory effects

The initial signs of a breathing problem associated with anaphylaxis may vary from sneezing and coughing to complete airway obstruction, caused by laryngeal and epiglottic oedema (Box 18-4). The patient may complain of throat tightness and dyspnoea, whilst stridor or voice changes also may be evident. Lower airway bronchospasm and associated hypersecretion of mucus caused by the actions of histamine,

Table 18-1 Conditions that may mimic anaphylaxis

Signs and symptoms	Possible causes
Stridor	Upper airway obstruction
	Foreign body aspiration
	Epiglottitis, angioedema, use of angiotensin-converting enzyme inhibitor, some panic disorders
Bronchospasm	Asthma, chronic obstructive pulmonary disease, bronchitis
Syncope	Vasovagal syncope
	Fitting
	Hypoglycaemia
	Cardiac dysrhythmias

Box 18-4

Signs and symptoms of anaphylaxis

Upper airway

Hoarseness
Laryngeal or epiglottic oedema
Rhinorrhoea
Stridor
Coughing

Lower airway

Dyspnoea
Accessory muscle use
Bronchospasm
Decreased breath sounds
Increased mucus production
Wheezing

Cardiovascular system

Chest tightness
Dysrhythmias
Hypotension
Tachycardia

Gastrointestinal system

Abdominal cramps/distension
Diarrhoea
Nausea
Vomiting

Neurological system

Anxiety/feeling of impending doom
Altered level of consciousness/confusion
Dizziness
Headache
Fitting
Syncope
Weakness

Cutaneous system

Angioedema
Oedema/swelling
Erythema
Pallor
Pruritus
Tearing of the eyes
Urticaria (hives)

leukotrienes, and prostaglandins may produce wheezing and significant respiratory distress, leading to hypoxia (and confusion), cyanosis and an increased respiratory rate. Symptoms can develop with startling rapidity.

Cardiovascular effects

The cardiovascular manifestations of allergic reactions vary, from mild hypotension to collapse and profound shock, with hypotension and decreased level of consciousness. Tachycardia and dysrhythmias are common and may be related to the severe hypoxia and loss of circulating fluid volume that occurs; the patient may complain of chest pain if myocardial ischaemia is present.

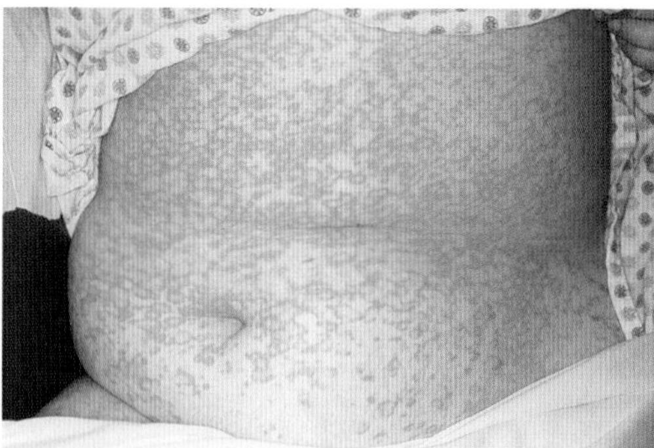

Figure 18-6 Urticaria as a result of an allergic reaction. Courtesy of Gary Quick.

Critical Thinking

Which of these effects has the potential to cause death first?

Gastrointestinal effects

Nausea, vomiting, diarrhoea and severe abdominal cramping may occur in a patient with an anaphylactic reaction. The increased gastrointestinal activity is related to smooth muscle contraction, increased mucus production, and outpouring of fluid from the gut wall into the intestinal lumen initiated by the chemical mediators.

Nervous system effects

The nervous system responses are caused in large part by the impaired gas exchange and shock associated with anaphylaxis. At first the patient may be agitated and speak of a sense of impending doom. As hypoxia and shock worsen, brain functions deteriorate and may result in confusion, weakness, headache, syncope, seizures and coma.

Cutaneous effects

The most visible signs that distinguish anaphylaxis from other medical conditions relate to the skin and are found in over 80% of anaphylactic reactions. These signs are caused by the vasodilation induced by histamine release from the mast cells. Initially the patient may complain of warmth and itching (pruritus); physical examination often reveals diffuse redness and hives (urticaria), which are well-circumscribed wheals of 1–6 cm. Hives may be more reddened or pallid than the surrounding skin and often accompanied by severe itching (Figure 18-6). Significant swelling of the face and tongue and angioedema also may be present. This reflects involvement of deeper capillaries of the skin and mucous membranes. As hypoxia and shock continue, cyanosis appears.

Note

Angioedema is a localized oedematous reaction of the deep dermis or subcutaneous or submucosal tissues, appearing in the form of giant wheals. Patients with angioedema are at high risk for rapid deterioration.

Initial assessment

As in any critical emergency, initial patient care measures are directed at providing adequate airway, ventilatory and circulatory support. Drug therapy is key intervention in anaphylaxis and should be started as quickly as possible. It is important to recognize the condition promptly and watch for deterioration.

Airway assessment is critical because most deaths from anaphylaxis are related directly to upper airway obstruction. The paramedic should evaluate the conscious patient for voice changes, stridor, or a barking cough; complaints of tightness in the neck and dyspnoea should alert the paramedic of impending airway obstruction. The paramedic should evaluate and secure the airway of an unconscious patient, and if air movement is blocked, the paramedic should perform endotracheal intubation. If laryngeal and epiglottic oedema is severe, surgical or needle cricothyrotomy (described in Chapter 13) may be indicated to provide airway access. Early, elective intubation is indicated for patients with hoarseness, lingual oedema, and posterior or oropharyngeal swelling.

Critical Thinking

How significant is stridor as a physical finding?

The paramedic should monitor the patient closely for signs of respiratory distress as indicated by pulse oximetry, skin colour, accessory muscle use, wheezing, diminished breath sounds and abnormal respiratory rates. The patient's circulatory status also may decline quickly and the paramedic should frequently assess pulse quality, rate and location.

History

A history may be hard to obtain yet it can be critical to rule out other medical emergencies that may mimic anaphylaxis. The paramedic should question the patient regarding the presenting complaint and the rapidity of onset of symptoms/signs, which usually appear within 1 to 30 min of introduction of the antigen although the onset of a reaction may be slightly delayed if the exposure is by the oral route.

Important medical history includes previous exposure and response to the suspected antigen as well as identification of the method of exposure to the antigen; injection of an antigen often produces the most rapid and severe response. Other significant history includes chronic or other illness and drugs that are used by the patient; pre-existing cardiac disease or bronchial asthma should cause the paramedic to anticipate severe complications as a result of the allergic reaction. Use of certain drugs, such as beta-blocking agents, may diminish the patient's response to adrenaline (epinephrine), and may necessitate the administration of other medications. The paramedic also should determine whether the patient has an emergency adrenaline (epinephrine) drug kit (e.g. EpiPen) and whether the medication was administered before the arrival of emergency medical services. Some patients with a history of allergic reaction may have taken an oral antihistamine (e.g. chlorphenamine) or they may have used aerosolized adrenaline (epinephrine). The patient's use of these drugs should be ascertained if possible; however, appropriate intervention should not be delayed.

Physical examination

The paramedic should frequently assess vital signs. In severe reactions, most patients are initially tachycardiac, tachypnoeic and hypotensive if deterioration to cardiac arrest has not occurred. The paramedic should inspect the patient's face and neck for angioedema, hives, tearing and rhinorrhoea and should note the presence of erythema or urticaria on other body regions. Along with vital signs, the paramedic should frequently assess airway and breath sounds to evaluate the clinical progress of the patient and commence cardiac monitoring as soon as possible to aid in patient evaluation. Such assessment will also help the paramedic to monitor the effectiveness of interventions.

Key interventions to prevent arrest

Organ involvement in anaphylaxis varies and this makes a standardized approach to patient management difficult. The following key interventions, however, commonly are used to manage anaphylaxis:[1]

1. Place the patient in a position of comfort. Elevate the legs until replacement fluids improve blood pressure. Do not stand the patient up. Protect the airways of unconscious patients by placing them on their side.
2. Administer high-concentration oxygen.
3. Give IM adrenaline (epinephrine), as per current clinical practice guidelines, to all patients with clinical signs of airway swelling, difficulty breathing or shock/hypotension; monitor the ECG as adrenaline (epinephrine) may cause dysrhythmias. Adrenaline (epinephrine) may be repeated every 5 min if required. Additional drugs which should be considered include chlorphenamine, salbutamol (and if transport is unavoidably delayed or prolonged, corticosteroids).
4. Initiate intravenous therapy with normal saline solution if hypotension is present and does not respond rapidly to adrenaline (epinephrine), enough to maintain a distal pulse.
5. Transport the patient for further management. Most patients will be observed carefully in the hospital for up to 24 h. Many patients do not respond promptly to therapy, and symptoms may recur in some patients, a so-called biphasic reaction.

Note

Complications of intravenously administered adrenaline (epinephrine) are significant and include the development of uncontrolled systolic hypertension, vomiting, fits, dysrhythmias and myocardial ischaemia, and therefore the IV route does not fall within normal management of anaphylaxis and is now ONLY advocated in exceptional circumstances by specialist medical staff.

Critical Thinking

How does adrenaline (epinephrine) reverse the signs and symptoms of anaphylaxis?

Other drug therapy

As described above, additional drug therapy may be helpful although adrenaline (epinephrine) is the only drug that can reverse the life-threatening complications of anaphylaxis immediately. Pharmacological agents that may be used with adrenaline (epinephrine) include antihistamine to antagonize the effects of histamine, beta-agonists to improve alveolar ventilation, corticosteroids to prevent a delayed reaction and glucagon or ipratropium (for patients unresponsive to adrenaline [epinephrine], especially those taking antidysrhythmics such as beta-blockers).

Note

Beta-blockers may increase the incidence and severity of anaphylaxis and can produce a paradoxical response to adrenaline (epinephrine).[1] In these cases, glucagon may be effective.

Key interventions during arrest

Cardiac arrest from anaphylaxis may be associated with profound vasodilation, intravascular collapse, tissue hypoxia, and asystole. Special considerations for resuscitation of these patients are described next.[1]

Airway, oxygenation and ventilation

Swelling of the airway can make bag–mask ventilation and endotracheal intubation difficult or ineffective in patients with anaphylaxis. In addition, the landmarks for needle cricothyrotomy may not be visible because of severe swelling in the soft tissues of the neck. Early and effective airway management is crucial for these patients, with recognition of how the patient's airway may be compromised rapidly and mandate rapid transport to hospital.

Support of circulation

Cardiac arrest from anaphylaxis requires rapid and aggressive volume replacement (up to 2 L of crystalloid in 250 mL boluses) to support circulation. In the presence of asystole or slow pulseless electrical activity (the most common arrest rhythms in anaphylaxis), the administration of atropine should be included (see Chapter 15). In addition, cardiac arrest from anaphylaxis may respond to prolonged periods of cardiopulmonary resuscitation. This may be the case especially when the patient is young and has a healthy heart and cardiovascular system (Figure 18-7).

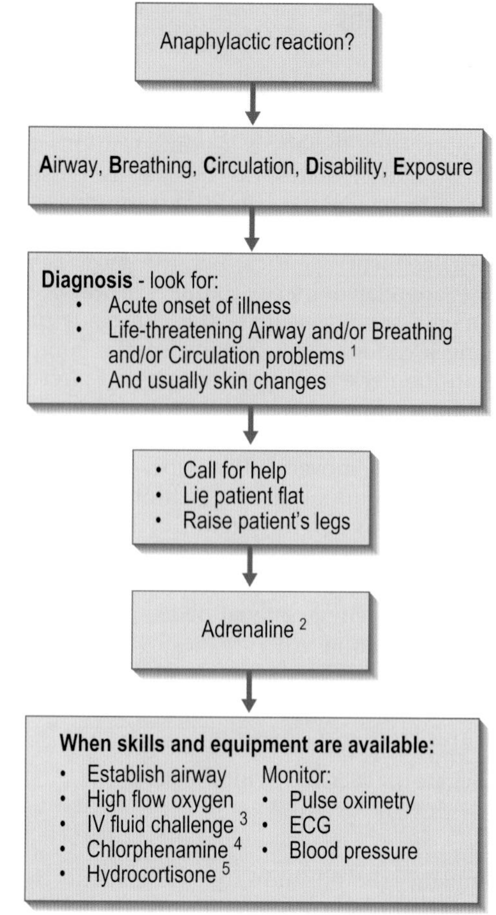

[1] Life-threatening problems:
Airway: swelling, hoarseness, stridor
Breathing: rapid breathing, wheeze, fatigue, cyanosis, SpO_2 <92%, confusion
Circulation: pale, clammy, low blood pressure, faintness, drowsy/coma

[2] Adrenaline (give IM unless experienced with IV adrenaline) IM doses of 1:1000 adrenaline (repeat after 5 min if no better)

• Adult	500 μg IM (0.5 mL)
• Child more than 12 years	500 μg IM (0.5 mL)
• Child 6–12 years	300 μg IM (0.3 mL)
• Child less than 6 years	150 μg IM (0.15 mL)

Adrenaline IV to be given **only by experienced specialists**
Titrate: adults 50 μg; children 1 μg/kg

[3] IV fluid challenge:
Adult: 500–1000 mL
Child: crystalloid 20 mL/kg

Stop IV colloid if this might be the cause of anaphylaxis

	[4] Chlorphenamine (IM or slow IV)	[5] Hydrocortisone (IM or slow IV)
Adult or child more than 12 years	10 mg	200 mg
Child 6–12 years	5 mg	100 mg
Child 6 months to 6 years	2.5 mg	50 mg
Child less than 6 months	250 μg/kg	25 mg

Figure 18-7 Anaphylaxis algorithm. Courtesy of Resuscitation Council UK.

Summary

- Antibodies bind to the antigen that produced them. Antibodies aid in neutralizing the antigen and removing it from the body.
- Allergic reaction is an increased physiological response to an antigen after a previous exposure to the same antigen. Localized allergic reactions do not affect the entire body.
- Anaphylaxis is the most extreme form of allergic reaction. Rapid recognition and aggressive therapy are needed for patient survival.
- Almost any substance can cause anaphylaxis. The risk of anaphylaxis increases with the frequency of exposure.
- Symptoms of anaphylaxis may include sneezing and coughing; airway obstruction; wheezing; hypotension or vascular collapse; chest pain; nausea, vomiting or diarrhoea; and weakness, headache, syncope, seizures or coma.

References

1. Resuscitation Council UK 2008 Emergency treatment for anaphylactic reactions: guidelines for healthcare providers. Resuscitation Council UK, London
2. Pumphrey RS 2004 Fatal anaphylaxis in the UK, 1992–2001. Novartis Found Symp 257:116–128; discussion 128–132, 157–160, 276–285

Further reading

Altman L et al 2000 Allergy in primary care. WB Saunders, Philadelphia

Busse W, Gern J 2003 Contemporary diagnosis and management of allergic diseases and asthma, 3rd edition. Handbooks in Health Care, Newtown, PA

Jevon P 2004 Anaphylaxis: a practical guide. Butterworth-Heinemann, Oxford

Resuscitation Council UK website http://www.resus.org.uk/pages/reaction.pdf

Simmons F, Simons E 1996 Histamine and H-1 receptor antagonists in allergic disease. Marcel Dekker, New York

The Anaphylaxis Campaign website http://www.anaphylaxis.org.uk/

CHAPTER 19

Gastroenterology

Chapter contents

Objectives

Upon completion of this chapter, the paramedic student will be able to:

1. Label a diagram of the abdominal organs.
2. Outline prehospital assessment of a patient who has abdominal pain.
3. Describe general prehospital management techniques for the patient with abdominal pain.
4. Describe signs and symptoms, complications, and prehospital management for the following gastrointestinal disorders: gastroenteritis, gastritis, colitis, diverticulitis, appendicitis, peptic ulcer disease, bowel obstruction, Crohn's disease, pancreatitis, oesophagogastric varices, haemorrhoids, cholecystitis and acute hepatitis.

Key terms

acute gastroenteritis Inflammation of the stomach and intestines with an associated sudden onset of vomiting, diarrhoea, or both.

acute hepatitis An inflammatory condition of the liver associated with the sudden onset of malaise, weakness, anorexia, intermittent nausea and vomiting, and dull right upper quadrant pain, usually followed within 1 week by the onset of jaundice, dark urine, or both.

appendicitis An acute inflammation of the appendix.

bowel obstruction An occlusion of the intestinal lumen that results in blockage of normal flow of intestinal contents.

cholecystitis Inflammation of the gallbladder, most often associated with the presence of gallstones.

chronic gastroenteritis Inflammation of the stomach and intestines that accompanies numerous gastrointestinal disorders.

Crohn's disease A chronic, inflammatory bowel disease of unknown origin, usually affecting the ileum, the colon, or both structures.

diverticulitis Inflammation of one or more diverticula.

diverticulosis The presence of pouch-like herniations through the muscular layer of the colon.

haemorrhoids Swollen, distended veins (internal, external, or both) in the rectoanal area.

involuntary guarding An unconscious rigid contraction of the abdominal muscles; a sign of peritoneal inflammation.

oesophagogastric varices A complex of longitudinal, tortuous veins at the lower end of the oesophagus that become large and swollen as a result of portal hypertension.

pancreatitis Inflammation of the pancreas, which causes severe epigastric pain.

peptic ulcer disease Illness that results from a complex pathological interaction among the acidic gastric juice and proteolytic enzymes and the mucosal barrier.

rebound tenderness A sign of peritoneal inflammation in which pain is caused by the sudden release of fingertip pressure on the abdomen.

referred pain Visceral pain felt at a site distant from its origin.

somatic pain Pain that arises from skeletal muscles, ligaments, vessels or joints.

ulcerative colitis An inflammatory condition of the large intestine characterized by severe diarrhoea and ulceration of the mucosa of the intestine.

visceral pain Deep pain that arises from smooth vasculature or organ systems.

Acute abdominal pain is a common chief complaint in emergency care and may reflect serious illness. The condition accounts for about 5% of all visits to the emergency department each year.[1] This chapter reviews gastrointestinal anatomy and disorders that produce gastrointestinal bleeding and abdominal pain. Appropriate evaluation and management in the prehospital phase of patient care may prevent the development of life-threatening complications.

Gastrointestinal anatomy

The gastrointestinal system provides the body with water, electrolytes, and other nutrients used by the cells. The major organs most often associated with the gastrointestinal system include the oesophagus, stomach, small and large intestines, liver, gallbladder and pancreas (Figure 19-1). The genitourinary system can also produce abdominal pain and bleeding and is dealt with in Chapters 20 and 35.

Assessment of the patient with acute abdominal pain

When caring for a patient with abdominal pain, the paramedic should begin the general assessment by ensuring that the scene is safe. The paramedic should determine whether the nature of the patient's abdominal pain is a result of trauma or a medical condition; this may be evident from the initial scene survey. The nature of the pain may also become evident by obtaining information from the patient, family, or bystanders. The paramedic should inspect the nearby area for medication bottles and signs of alcohol or other drug use as these signs may offer clues about the cause of the patient's condition. Any containers of emesis should be transported with the patient for laboratory analysis.

After the initial survey to ensure adequacy of airway, breathing and circulation, assessment of the patient with acute abdominal pain begins with a thorough history focused on the chief complaint. The paramedic should assess and document the baseline vital signs and perform a systematic physical examination. The examination will help the paramedic to identify abdominal emergencies, which may indicate the development of shock or the need for immediate transport for surgical intervention.

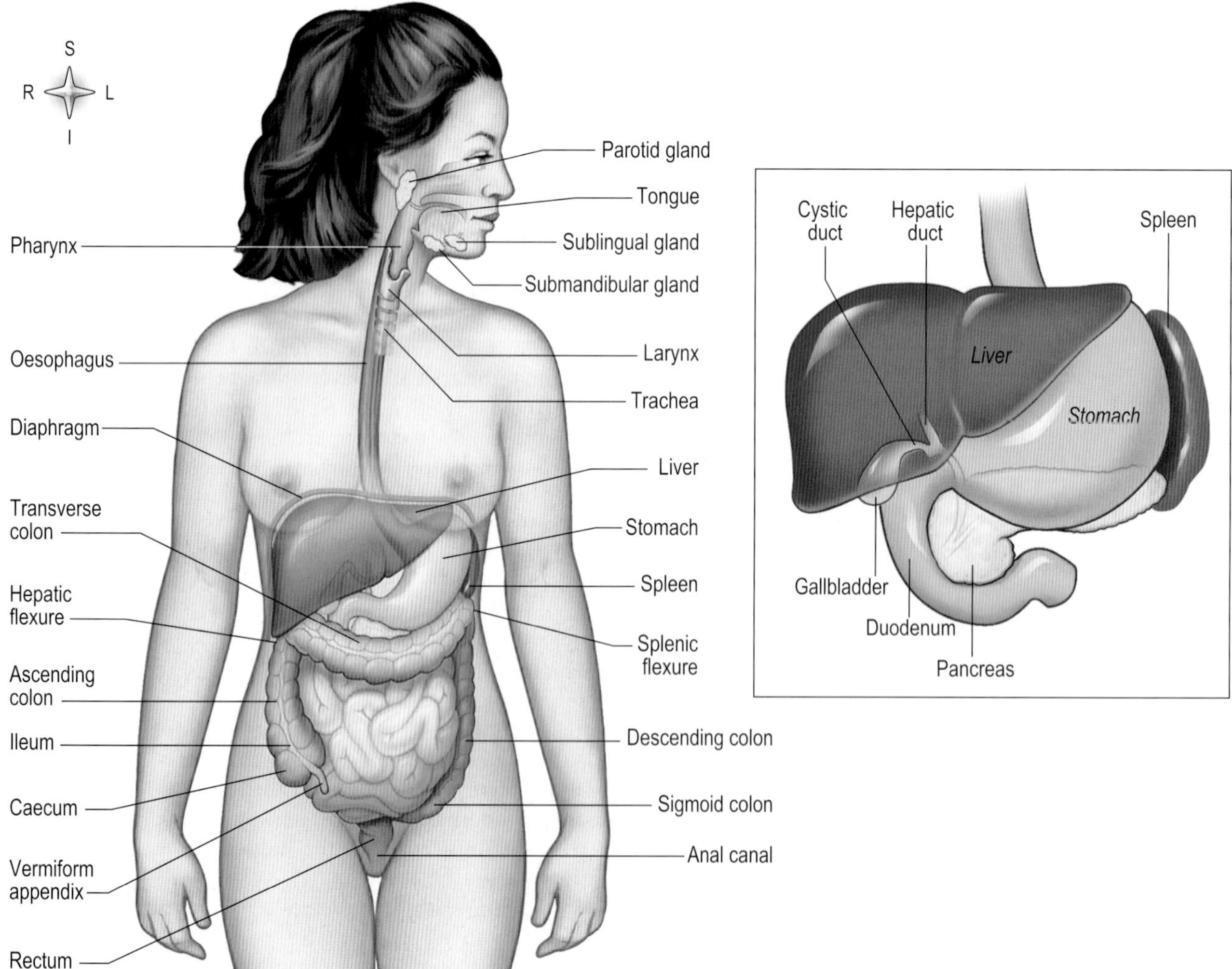

Figure 19-1 Location of digestive organs.

History

When obtaining a history of abdominal pain, the paramedic should attempt to identify the location and type of pain and any associated signs and symptoms. Using the mnemonic OPQRST or a similar method can help the paramedic organize this information. Sample questions that might be included in the OPQRST evaluation include the following:

- O (Onset): Was the onset of pain sudden? What were you doing when it started?
- P (Provocative/palliative): What makes the pain better? What makes the pain worse? Does a sitting or lying position affect your discomfort?
- Q (Quality): What does the pain feel like? Is it sharp, dull, burning, tearing?
- R (Region): Where is the pain located? Does it travel (radiate) to another area of the body or does it stay in the same place?
- S (Severity): Is the pain mild, moderate, or severe? What is the degree of discomfort on a scale of 1 to 10?
- T (Time): When did the pain begin? Is it constant or intermittent? If intermittent, how long does the pain episode last?

Other key elements of a patient history can be obtained through a SAMPLE history (signs and symptoms, allergies, medications, past medical history, last meal or oral intake, and events before the emergency). This will help to identify symptoms, allergies, medical history, last oral intake and important events that preceded the patient's chief complaint. Of particular importance is significant medical history, such as hypertension or cardiac or respiratory disease that may manifest in abdominal pain; medication use; alcohol or other drug use; last bowel movement and any significant changes in the patient's bowel habits; and previous abdominal surgeries. Women of childbearing age should be questioned about menstrual periods (including regularity and the date of the last menstrual period) and the possibility of pregnancy.

Persistent abdominal pain lasting 6 hours or longer warrants patient transport for physician evaluation. Pain management in abdominal pain has been controversial because of the belief that analgesia masks signs and symptoms that are critical for physician evaluation. However, analgesia should not be withheld as there is no conclusive proof that this is the case.[2] Pain has been shown to affect the ability of a patient to concentrate and understand explanations,[3,4] and should be alleviated on humane grounds. Entonox may be considered but may not be effective in abdominal pain. It should be used with caution in patients with marked abdominal distension as the nitrous oxide may increase the volume of gas in the abdomen.[5] In addition, patients should not be permitted to eat or drink anything because surgery may be needed.

Critical Thinking

What factors can influence a patient's perception and description of pain?

Location and type of abdominal pain

To assess a specific disorder, the paramedic can use a method that relates anatomical location of gastrointestinal organs and structures to origin. Box 19-1 lists location of abdominal pain and possible causes of illness. The types of abdominal pain that may result from chronic or acute episodes may be classified as visceral, somatic and referred.

Visceral pain

Visceral pain (or organ pain) is caused by the stimulation of autonomic nerve fibres that surround a hollow organ. Visceral pain can also be caused by the distension or stretching

Box 19-1

Location of abdominal pain and possible origins

Right upper quadrant

Cholecystitis
Hepatitis
Pancreatitis
Perforated ulcer
Renal pain (right)

Left upper quadrant

Gastritis
Pancreatitis
Renal pain (left)

Right lower quadrant

Abdominal aortic dissection or rupture
Appendicitis
Hernia
Ovarian cyst (right)
Ovarian or testicular torsion
Pelvic inflammatory disease
Ruptured ectopic pregnancy
Urinary calculus

Left lower quadrant

Abdominal aortic dissection or rupture
Diverticulitis
Hernia
Ovarian cyst (left)
Ovarian or testicular torsion
Pelvic inflammatory disease
Ruptured ectopic pregnancy
Urinary calculus

Epigastric pain

Abdominal aortic aneurysm
Cholecystitis
Oesophagitis
Gastritis
Myocardial ischaemia
Pancreatitis

Diffuse pain

Generalized peritonitis
Intestinal obstruction
Perforation

of hollow organs or the ligaments. Visceral pain is generally diffuse and may be described as cramping or gas-type pain. Patients usually say that the pain varies in intensity, increasing to a high degree of severity and then subsiding, so is often difficult to localize. Often the pain is centred at the umbilicus or lower in the midline. Visceral pain is often associated with other symptoms of autonomic nerve involvement such as tachycardia, diaphoresis, nausea or vomiting. Common causes of visceral abdominal pain include early appendicitis, pancreatitis, cholecystitis and intestinal obstruction.

Somatic pain

Somatic pain is produced by bacterial or chemical irritation of nerve fibres in the peritoneum (peritonitis). Unlike visceral pain, somatic pain is usually constant and localized to a specific area. The patient often describes the pain as sharp or stabbing. Patients with somatic abdominal pain are generally hesitant to move about and may lie on their back or side with legs flexed to prevent more pain from stimulation of the peritoneal area. These patients often exhibit involuntary guarding of the abdomen during the physical examination and rebound tenderness (signs of peritoneal inflammation). Common causes of somatic pain are appendicitis and an inflamed or perforated viscus (ulcer, gallbladder, or small or large intestine).

Referred pain

Referred pain is pain in a part of the body considerably removed from the tissues that cause the pain. This mechanism results from branches of visceral fibres that synapse in the spinal cord with the same second-order neurons that receive pain fibres from the skin. When these pain fibres are stimulated intensely, pain sensations spread.

A knowledge of referred pain is important because many visceral ailments cause no other symptoms except referred pain. For example, cardiac pain may be referred to the neck and jaw, shoulders, pectoral muscles, and down the arms; biliary pain to the right subscapular area; renal colic to the genitalia and flank area; uterine and rectal pain to the low back; and a leaking aortic aneurysm to the lower back or buttocks. Figure 19-2 illustrates surface areas of referred pain from visceral organs.

Signs and symptoms

Although numerous signs and symptoms may be associated with acute abdominal pain, the following are amongst the most common:[6]

1. Nausea, vomiting, anorexia
   - Appendicitis
   - Biliary tract disease
   - Gastritis
   - High intestinal obstruction
   - Pancreatitis
2. Diarrhoea
   - Inflammatory process (gastroenteritis, ulcerative colitis)
3. Constipation
   - Dehydration, obstruction, medication-induced decreased intestinal motility (codeine, morphine)
4. Change in stool colour
   - Biliary tract obstruction (clay-coloured stools)
   - Lower intestinal bleeding (black, tarry stools)
5. Chills and fever
   - Appendicitis
   - Bacterial infection
   - Cholecystitis
   - Pyelonephritis.

Vital signs

Vital sign assessment should include evaluation and documentation of the patient's blood pressure; pulse rate (includ-

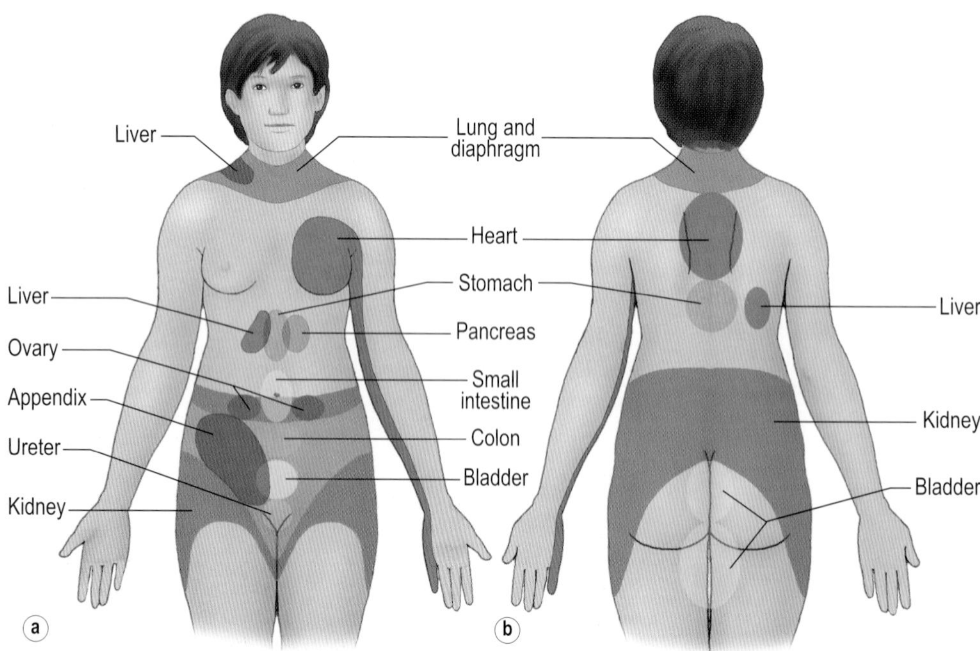

Figure 19-2 Referred pain. (a) Anterior view. (b) Posterior view.

ing electrocardiogram assessment); respiratory rate; and skin colour, moisture, temperature and turgor. If possible, the paramedic should check the patient for orthostatic pulse and blood pressure changes. A rise from a recumbent position to a sitting or standing position associated with a fall in systolic pressure (after 1 min) of 10–15 mmHg and/or a concurrent rise in pulse rate (after 1 min) of 10–15 beats per minute indicates a significant volume depletion and a decrease in perfusion status. The paramedic should also perform an assessment of blood pressure, pulses, and capillary refill in each extremity as a consideration for aortic dissection (described in Chapter 15).

Physical examination

The physical examination of a patient with acute abdominal pain includes the skills of inspection, auscultation, percussion and palpation. If a life-threatening illness is suspected, rapid stabilization and transportation of the patient is the first priority. Further examination can be completed en route to the receiving hospital. Physical examination of the patient's abdomen is described in Chapter 9. However, the following discussion serves as a review. (Male and female physical examinations to evaluate genitourinary complaints are discussed in Chapter 20.)

Inspection

In the initial patient encounter, the paramedic should note the position in which the patient is lying. As stated before, many patients with abdominal peritoneal irritation lie on their sides and often have their knees flexed and pulled in toward their chests. Other visual clues that may indicate abdominal pain are skin colour, facial expressions such as grimacing, and the presence or absence of voluntary movement. The paramedic should remove the patient's clothing and inspect the abdominal wall for the presence of bruises, scars, ascites (Figure 19-3), abdominal distension or abdominal masses.

Auscultation

Determining the presence or absence of bowel sounds by auscultation is usually done in the emergency department.

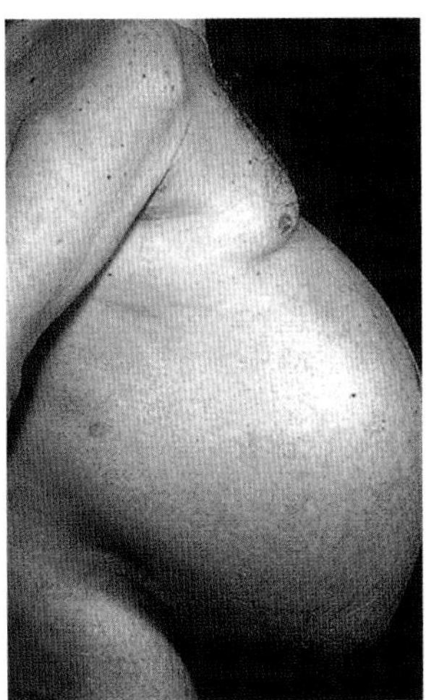
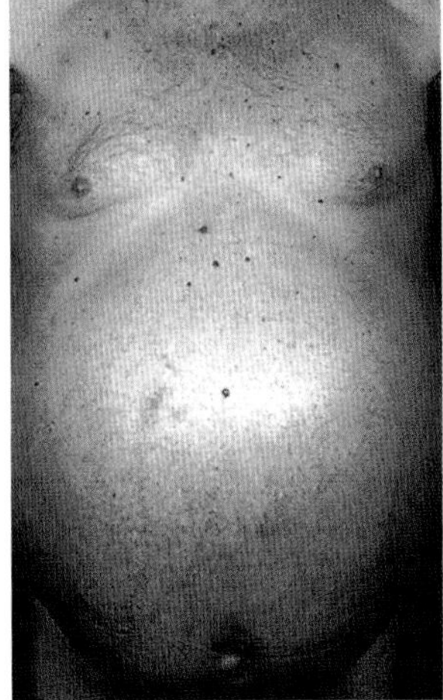

Figure 19-3 Gross ascites in a male patient.

If auscultation is to be performed, it should be done for about 2 min in each quadrant before determining that bowel sounds are absent. (Auscultation should always precede palpation and percussion because these procedures may alter the intensity of bowel sounds.) Bowel sounds that are increased in number, duration or intensity indicate the possibility of gastroenteritis or intestinal obstruction. Bowel sounds that are considerably decreased in number and intensity (or their absence) may indicate peritonitis or ileus (obstruction of the intestine).

Palpation

The paramedic should begin palpation of the abdomen gently and avoid the painful area until after examining the rest of the abdomen. The paramedic should be alert to rigidity or spasm, tenderness or masses, and to the patient's facial expressions. These may provide clues about the severity of the pain. In addition, the paramedic should note whether the abdomen is soft or rigid.

Percussion

If time permits, the paramedic may perform a general assessment of tympany and dullness by percussion to detect the presence of fluid, air or solid masses in the abdomen. The paramedic should use a systematic approach and move from side to side or clockwise. Tenderness and abdominal skin temperature and colour should be noted. To review, tympany is the major sound that should be noted during percussion because of the normal presence of air in the stomach and intestines. Dullness should be heard over organs and solid masses.

Management of the patient with an abdominal emergency

Patients with acute abdominal pain or gastrointestinal bleeding cannot be managed effectively in the prehospital setting. The majority require extensive evaluation in the emergency department, including laboratory analysis, radiological imaging, fluid and medication therapy, and perhaps surgical intervention. The role of the paramedic is to support the patient's airway and ventilatory status, to perform and document an initial patient assessment, including a thorough history, to monitor vital signs and cardiac rhythm, to manage pain, to initiate intravenous therapy for fluid replacement or fluid resuscitation where indicated, and to transport the patient rapidly for physician evaluation.

Specific abdominal emergencies

Abdominal emergencies can result from inflammation, infection, and obstruction. Some disorders may be associated with upper gastrointestinal bleeding; examples of such include lesions, peptic ulceration, and oesophagogastric varices. Some disorders may be associated with lower gastrointestinal bleeding; examples of such include colonic lesions, diverticulosis, and haemorrhoids. Other disorders, such as pancreatitis and cholecystitis, more often are associated with acute abdominal pain in the absence of bleeding. Box 19-2

Box 19-2

Gastrointestinal disorders

- Acute gastroenteritis
- Acute hepatitis
- Appendicitis
- Bowel obstruction
- Cholecystitis
- Chronic gastroenteritis
- Crohn's disease
- Diverticulosis
- Oesophagogastric varices
- Gastrointestinal bleeding
- Haemorrhoids
- Pancreatitis
- Peptic ulcer disease
- Ulcerative colitis

lists the specific gastrointestinal disorders discussed in this chapter.

Gastrointestinal bleeding

Gastrointestinal bleeding is a common clinical problem seen by paramedics. It often requires hospitalization and can vary from a chronic blood loss to a massive, life-threatening haemorrhage. Massive haemorrhage may be hard to stop or control although many bleeding episodes resolve spontaneously. However, it is crucial for a physician to identify the bleeding site to help prevent a recurrence. Bleeding from the gastrointestinal tract can be classified by site of origin as upper or lower gastrointestinal bleeding.

The most common causes of upper gastrointestinal bleeding are peptic ulcer disease and variceal rupture (e.g. oesophageal varices that result from underlying chronic liver disease such as cirrhosis). Other causes include Mallory–Weiss syndrome (an oesophageal laceration that usually results from repeated vomiting or retching), and tumours or cancers of the oesophagus or stomach. Factors that may aggravate upper gastrointestinal bleeding include use of non-steroidal anti-inflammatory drugs such as aspirin and other anti-arthritic drugs, chronic liver disease, blood-thinning medications (e.g. warfarin), and underlying medical conditions such as renal disease, hypertension and cardiorespiratory diseases. The incidence of upper gastrointestinal bleeding is about 100/100 000 adults per year with a mortality rate of 14% in the UK.[7] Risk factors include increasing age, alcohol and tobacco use, and coexisting illness such as hypertension, diabetes, and cardiorespiratory disease.

The most common cause of lower gastrointestinal (colon) bleeding is diverticulosis. Other causes include colon cancers, colon polyps, and inflammatory bowel disorders such as ulcerative colitis and Crohn's disease. These conditions are described later in this chapter. Like upper gastrointestinal bleeding, lower gastrointestinal bleeding may be mild or may be brisk and difficult to control. Common complaints include cramping abdominal pain, diarrhoea (which may be bloody), nausea, vomiting, and changes in the patient's stool and bowel habits.

Gastrointestinal bleeding depends on the acuteness and the source of the blood loss. Mild chronic gastrointestinal blood loss may present without any noticeable bleeding and can result in iron deficiency anaemia. These patients are often unaware that they are bleeding and may or may not notice small amounts of blood with their bowel movements. Patients with severe cases of chronic or acute bleeding can have signs of anaemia such as weakness, pallor, dizziness, shortness of breath or angina (the haematocrit of these patients may be within normal range in the early phase of their haemorrhage).

More serious gastrointestinal bleeding may occur with haematemesis (bloody vomitus). Vomit may be red or have a dark, coffee ground-like appearance. Blood in the stool could present as bright red, dark and clotted, or black and tarry. Presentation depends on the location of the bleeding source. A black, tarry stool (melaena) often indicates an upper gastrointestinal source of bleeding where blood has been partially digested. However, bleeding could also originate from the small intestine or ascending colon. Bright, red blood from the rectum (haematochezia) after a bowel movement usually signifies a bleeding source close to the rectal opening. Such bleeding often results from haemorrhoids; however, conditions such as rectal cancers, polyps, ulcerations or infections can also cause this type of bleeding.

Any source of gastrointestinal bleeding that is active or severe usually requires hospitalization. With hospitalization the hypovolaemia can be managed with intravenously administered fluids or blood transfusions if needed. Attempts to identify and stop the source of haemorrhage may include the use of medications, diagnostic tests (e.g. barium gastrointestinal studies, nuclear scans, angiography, endoscopy and colonoscopy), and other therapeutic measures such as gastric lavage, the placement of a Sengstaken–Blakemore tube (to tamponade bleeding in the oesophagus), and, in some cases, surgery. Prehospital care for patients with active and severe gastrointestinal bleeding includes provision of emotional support, administration of high-concentration oxygen, airway and ventilatory management, and transportation for physician evaluation. Intravenous fluid resuscitation should follow current JRCALC guidelines.

Acute gastroenteritis

Acute gastroenteritis is inflammation of the stomach and intestines with an associated sudden onset of vomiting, diarrhoea, or both. The condition is a common problem worldwide and is responsible for more than 4 million deaths per year in developing countries.[8] The condition may be caused by bacterial or viral infection, parasites (e.g. *Giardia*, responsible for 'traveller's diarrhoea', and *Cyclosporidium*, reported to be contracted in contaminated water), chemical toxins, and other conditions such as allergies, lactose intolerance and immune disorders. The inflammation causes haemorrhage and erosion of the mucosal layers of the gastrointestinal tract. Inflammation can also affect the way in which water and nutrients are absorbed.

Infectious acute gastroenteritis is usually transmitted through the faecal–oral route and by ingestion of infected food or contaminated water. The condition is common in institutional settings (e.g. schools, day care centres and nursing homes) and other group settings (e.g. banquet halls, cruise ships and dormitories) where it can spread quickly. Infectious acute gastroenteritis can also arise among travellers in endemic areas (native populations in endemic areas are generally resistant). Infectious acute gastroenteritis can also arise in populations in disaster areas where water supplies are contaminated. Bacteria that may be responsible for acute gastroenteritis include *Salmonella, Escherichia coli, Campylobacter* and *Staphylococcus*. Contamination generally results from poor sanitation, the lack of safe drinking water, or contaminated food.

As the name implies, acute gastroenteritis is often abrupt and violent. It involves rapid loss of fluids and electrolytes from constant vomiting and diarrhoea. Fluid loss and dehydration may be severe in paediatric patients, the elderly, and in those who are immunosuppressed. Hypokalaemia and hyponatremia, acidosis or alkalosis may develop. Treatment is mainly supportive, requiring intravenous fluid replacement, sedation, bed rest, and medications to control vomiting and diarrhoea. Some forms of gastroenteritis can be treated with antibiotic therapy. Emergency medical services personnel who are working in disaster areas should observe the following guidelines:[6]

- Avoid patient contact if you are ill.
- Know the source of water supplies. Or drink hot beverages that have been boiled or disinfected.
- Avoid habits that aid mucous-oral/mucous membrane transmission.
- Observe body substance isolation precautions. Also observe good hand-washing procedures.

Critical Thinking

What would be your main concern for a patient with a history of severe gastroenteritis?

Chronic gastroenteritis

Chronic gastroenteritis results from inflammation of the stomach and intestines, and can produce long-term changes or damage to the gastric mucosa. The condition is usually due to microbial infection, hyperacidity, or the chronic use of alcohol, aspirin, and other non-steroidal anti-inflammatory medications. Chronic gastroenteritis commonly results from *Helicobacter pylori* infection but may also be caused by other bacteria such as *E. coli, Klebsiella pneumoniae, Enterobacter, Campylobacter jejuni, Vibrio cholerae, Shigella* and *Salmonella*. With the exception of *Shigella* and *Salmonella*, many of the bacteria responsible for chronic gastroenteritis are part of the normal intestinal flora. Thus this precludes effective vaccination against these strains. Other causes of chronic gastroenteritis include the norovirus and rotavirus and parasitic infection from protozoa such as *Giardia* and *Cryptosporidium parvum*. The pathogenic agents responsible for the disease may be contracted via oral–oral transmission or by contaminated food and water. Emergency medical services personnel should follow the same guidelines for personal safety as described previously.

Note

Helicobacter pylori reside between the epithelial surface and the overlying mucosa in the human stomach. The bacteria are more prevalent in lower socioeconomic groups. The bacteria may be spread in adults and children through the oral–oral route. The presence of *H. pylori* is believed to cause mucosal inflammation, which disrupts the normal defence mechanism of the stomach and can lead to ulceration.

Signs and symptoms of chronic gastroenteritis include epigastric pain, nausea and vomiting (which may be severe), fever, anorexia, mucosal bleeding (erosive gastritis) and epigastric tenderness on palpation. In severe cases the patient may have hypovolaemia and shock. The condition is treated with diet regulation, medications (antibiotics, antacids), and fluid replacement or fluid resuscitation if hypovolaemia or dehydration occurs.

Ulcerative colitis

Ulcerative colitis also is known as colitis or proctitis. Ulcerative colitis is an inflammatory condition of the large intestine and is classified as an inflammatory bowel disease. Ulcerative colitis is characterized by ulceration of the mucosa of the intestine; this usually occurs in the rectum and lower part of the colon but may affect the entire colon. The inflammation makes the colon empty often (causing diarrhoea), whilst the ulceration causes bleeding and produces pus. Ulcerative colitis affects men and women equally, and can occur at any age. It most often starts between ages 15 and 30, or less often between ages 50 and 70. Although the cause of ulcerative colitis is unknown, a family history of the disease is present in 10–15% of cases. The cause may be related to the immune system and the way it reacts to a virus or a bacterium that causes chronic inflammation in the intestinal wall. Other possible causes of the disorder include allergies to certain foods (e.g. lactose intolerance) and environmental and psychological factors.

The most common signs and symptoms of ulcerative colitis are fatigue, weight loss, anorexia, rectal bleeding, and the loss of body fluids and nutrients. Some patients have only mild symptoms whilst others experience frequent fever, bloody diarrhoea, nausea and severe abdominal cramping. Some patients with the disease have remissions that last for months or years; most patients' symptoms eventually return. After physician evaluation and stabilization, the condition is usually managed with steroids, electrolytes, antibiotics and diet regulation. Few patients require surgery to manage ulcerative colitis; however, surgical removal of the diseased colon may be indicated in severe cases. Prehospital care is dictated by the severity of the patient's condition. The care may vary from providing only emotional support and transportation to providing airway, ventilatory and circulatory support to manage hypovolaemia and shock.

Note

In patients with acquired immunodeficiency syndrome, the chronic diarrhoea and diffuse colonic involvement of Kaposi's sarcoma (described in Chapter 24) may mimic chronic ulcerative colitis. Undiagnosed signs of human immunodeficiency virus infection also may be the cause. At times, surgical bowel resection may be required in these patients.

Diverticulosis

A diverticulum is a sac or pouch that develops in the wall of the colon (Figure 19-4). A diverticulum is a common development with advancing years and is associated with diets low in fibre. Diverticular outpouchings (a condition known as diverticulosis) tend to develop because of the high pressure within the contracting sigmoid colon that regulates movement of stool into the rectum. The outpouchings are most common at the weakest point in the colon wall, which is on the left side just above the rectum. As a diverticulum expands, it develops a thin wall compared to the rest of the colon. The thin wall may allow bacteria to seep through and cause infection. Often there is a small artery or arteriole in the neck of the diverticulum from which subsequent bleeding may occur.

Most patients with diverticula are completely symptom free; however, up to 30% of these patients experience diverticulitis when one or more diverticula become obstructed with faecal matter. Mild complications of diverticulitis include irregular bowel habits (alternating constipation and diarrhoea), fever, and lower left quadrant pain. Diverticulitis tends to recur within the first 5 years after the onset of symptoms. Definitive care for these patients includes diet regulation, a high-fibre diet to stimulate daily bowel movements, antibiotic therapy, and, sometimes, surgical repair.

Serious complications of diverticular disease are associated with perforation of the bowel. These complications include massive bright red rectal bleeding (or dark stools if bleeding is from a diverticulum in the right colon). Haemorrhage from a diverticulum can occur rapidly, is often painless, and is the most common cause of massive rectal bleeding in older adults. If bacteria escape into the abdomen, peritonitis or an abscess may develop. The haemorrhage often ceases spontaneously but, if bleeding does not stop, emergency surgery may be necessary.

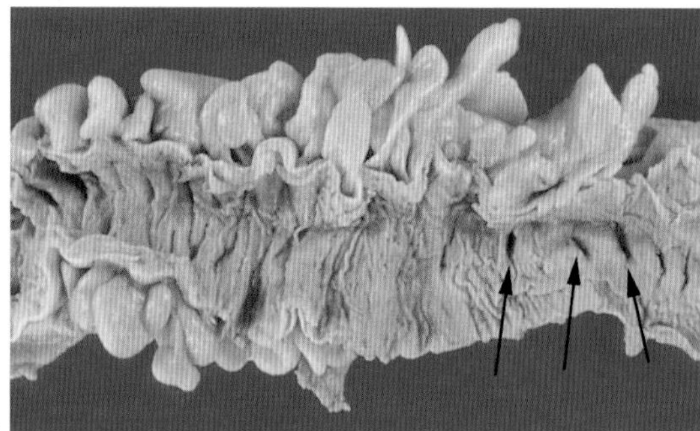

Figure 19-4 Diverticular disease. In diverticular disease the outpouches (arrows) of mucosa seen in the sigmoid colon appear as slit-like openings from the mucosal surface of the opened bowel.

Appendicitis

Appendicitis is a common abdominal emergency. There are approximately 34 000 cases of appendicitis in England each year.[9] The condition may present at any age, but most patients are 8–25 years old; appendicitis is rarely seen in children less than 2 years of age.

Appendicitis occurs when the passageway between the appendix and the caecum is obstructed by faecal matter (a faecalith). It may also be due to an inflammation of the area from viral or bacterial infection. Obstruction of the passageway leads to distension of the appendix. Poor lymphatic and venous drainage allows bacterial infection to develop. If the condition continues, the inflamed organ eventually becomes gangrenous, and then the appendix ruptures into the peritoneal cavity. This results in peritonitis (which may progress to shock) or the development of abscesses.

Because of variations in the position of the appendix, age of the patient and degree of inflammation, the clinical presentation of appendicitis is often inconsistent. (Many other disorders have similar signs and symptoms.) Young children and older adults may also have atypical illness because of reduced inflammatory response associated with extremes of age. This makes appendicitis more difficult to diagnose in these age groups. The classic presentation of appendicitis is abdominal pain or cramping, nausea, vomiting, chills, low-grade fever and anorexia. At first, the pain is periumbilical and diffuse but then becomes intense and localized to the right lower quadrant just medial to the iliac crest (McBurney point). If the appendix ruptures, the patient's pain diminishes before the development of peritoneal signs. The goal of definitive care for appendicitis is surgical appendicectomy before rupture.

Critical Thinking

What other illness presents similar signs or symptoms?

Peptic ulcer disease

Peptic ulcer disease results from a complex pathological interaction among the acidic gastric juice and proteolytic enzymes and the mucosal barrier. Digestion occurs as food passes through the gastrointestinal tract. The stomach produces hydrochloric acid and an enzyme called pepsin to digest the food. From the stomach, food passes into the duodenum. In the duodenum, digestion and nutrient absorption continue. The stomach normally protects itself from the digestive fluids by producing mucus to shield stomach tissues. It also produces bicarbonate to neutralize and break down digestive fluids into substances that are less harmful to stomach tissue. Blood circulation to the stomach lining, cell renewal, and cell repair also help protect the stomach.

Ulcers can form in the lining of the stomach or duodenum where acid and pepsin are present. These sores cause the disintegration and death of tissue as they erode the mucosal layers in the affected areas. If the sores are left untreated, massive haemorrhage or perforation may result. The three most common causes of peptic ulcer disease are *H. pylori* infection, non-steroidal anti-inflammatory drug use, and increased circulatory gastrin from gastrin-secreting tumours (Zollinger–Ellison syndrome),[1] all of which can cause the defence mechanisms of the stomach to fail. Ulcers can develop at any age, yet they are rare among teenagers and even less common in children. Duodenal ulcers usually occur for the first time between the ages of 30 and 50, and are more frequent in men than women.

The patient with a peptic ulcer is usually aware of the condition and often uses over-the-counter antacids. The ulcer pain may be described as a burning or gnawing discomfort in the epigastric region or left upper quadrant (in the case of gastric ulcer). The discomfort develops before meals (classically in the early morning) or during stressful periods, when the production of gastric acids increases. The pain is usually sudden in onset but is often relieved by food intake, antacids, or vomiting. In addition to pain and vomiting of blood, the patient may experience melaena as a result of blood passing through the gastrointestinal tract.

Prehospital care for patients with peptic ulcer disease includes obtaining a pertinent history, evaluating for hypotension, and providing circulatory support as needed. After physician evaluation, definitive care may involve antibiotics, antacids, H_2 receptor antagonists or other medications, and, occasionally, diet regulation (the benefit of which is controversial). Some patients with acute peptic ulcer disease require hospitalization for fluid or blood replacement, or for surgery, if medications are not effective or blood loss is ongoing.

Bowel obstruction

Bowel obstruction is an occlusion of the intestinal lumen that results in blockage of normal flow of intestinal contents. It may be caused by an ileus in which the bowel does not work properly, but more commonly results from mechanical obstruction such as adhesions, hernias (Box 19-3), faecal impaction, polyps and tumours. Other causes of bowel obstruction are intussusception (telescoping of one portion of the intestine into another, which results in decreased blood supply of the involved segment), volvulus (twisting of the intestines), and ingested foreign bodies. Most bowel obstructions occur in the small bowel (accounting for 20% of all hospital admissions for abdominal complaints) and are usually caused by adhesions or hernias.[8] Large bowel obstructions most often result from tumours or faecal impactions.

Box 19-3

Hernia

A hernia is the protrusion of an organ from its normal position through a congenital or acquired opening. Herniation is most often through the musculature of the groin or abdominal wall. Increases in intra-abdominal pressure can cause the peritoneum to push outward through such an opening. (Examples of such increases include those associated with straining, coughing or lifting.) When this occurs, a sac is formed into which various organs within the peritoneal cavity may enter.

Most herniae are uncomplicated. Most herniae also can be placed back into the peritoneal cavity by a physician. If the herniae cannot be placed back, however, the trapped contents of the peritoneal sac (usually a portion of bowel) can become strangulated. These patients often have acute abdominal pain and systemic signs such as fever and tachycardia. Incarcerated or strangulated herniae can lead to serious complications, including intestinal obstruction, perforation and peritonitis. Definitive care for complicated herniae is in-hospital observation, intravenous rehydration, pain medication and surgical repair.

Note

Paralytic ileus, a decrease or absence of intestinal peristalsis, can closely mimic bowel obstructions. This pseudo-obstruction may result from a number of localized or systemic conditions such as medications (especially narcotics), intraperitoneal infection, complications of abdominal surgery, and metabolic disturbances (e.g. decreased potassium levels).

Signs and symptoms of intestinal obstruction include nausea and vomiting, abdominal pain, constipation, and abdominal distension. The speed of onset and degree of symptoms depend on the anatomical site of obstruction (small versus large bowel). The most significant danger is perforation of the bowel with generalized peritonitis and sepsis.

The patient with bowel obstruction often has abdominal pain; dehydration may result from vomiting, decreased intestinal absorption, and fluid loss into the lumen and interstitium (bowel wall oedema). As the affected portion of the bowel distends, its blood supply is decreased and the segment becomes ischaemic. The wall is weakened and perforates, producing peritonitis. If the intestine becomes strangulated, blood or plasma may be lost from the affected intestinal segment. Definitive care involves fluid replacement, antibiotics, placement of a nasogastric tube for decompression, and frequently surgery to correct the obstructing lesion.

Critical Thinking

Have you ever responded to a call for 'constipation'? Did the paramedics consider this diagnosis a possibility? What was the attitude toward the patient?

Crohn's disease

Crohn's disease is a chronic inflammatory bowel disease that usually affects the ileum, the colon, or both structures. The disease may occur in persons of all ages but is primarily a disease of the young adult (most cases are diagnosed before age 30). The disease is thought to be of autoimmune origin and tends to run in families and in certain ethnic groups. Over recent decades the incidence and prevalence of Crohn's disease has been increasing steadily and the incidence is now estimated to be 5–10/100 000 per year with a conservative estimate of prevalence at 50–100/100 000.[10]

The inflammation associated with Crohn's disease may cause blockage of the intestine. This occurs because the disease tends to thicken the intestinal wall with swelling and scar tissue, narrowing the passage. The disease may also cause ulcers that tunnel through the affected area into surrounding tissues such as the bladder, vagina or skin. The areas around the anus and rectum are often involved. The tunnels, called fistulae, are a common complication and often become infected. Other associated complications include arthritis, skin problems, inflammation in the eyes or mouth, kidney stones, gallstones, or other diseases of the liver and biliary system.

Crohn's disease can be difficult to diagnose because its symptoms are similar to those of irritable bowel syndrome and ulcerative colitis. It is characterized by frequent attacks of diarrhoea, severe abdominal pain, nausea, fever, chills, weakness, anorexia and weight loss. Patients with Crohn's and similar diseases often suffer from depression because of the relentless and painful characteristics of these conditions. The paramedic should suspect the disease in any patient with chronic inflammatory colitis and a history of rectal fistulae or abscesses. These patients are frequently hospitalized and may be managed with antibiotics, steroids, antimotility agents to attempt to induce remission, and diet regulation.

Note

The term irritable bowel syndrome or spastic colon is used to describe abnormally increased motility of the small and large intestines. Unlike inflammatory bowel disease, the abdominal pain of irritable bowel syndrome is generally associated with emotional and physical stress. Pain is generally relieved by bowel movement as well.

Pancreatitis

The pancreas secretes digestive juices into the duodenum to help break down food into small molecules that can be absorbed by the body. The gland also secretes insulin and glucagon into the bloodstream, which help to maintain adequate glucose concentration. When the pancreas becomes inflamed (pancreatitis), it releases pancreatic enzymes into the blood, the pancreatic duct and the pancreas itself. This causes further inflammation and autodigestion of the gland. Pancreatitis occurs in two stages: acute and chronic.

Acute pancreatitis occurs suddenly. It occurs soon after the pancreas becomes damaged or irritated by its own enzymes and usually results from obstruction by gallstones in the bile duct or by alcohol abuse. Other less common causes include elevated serum lipids, thromboembolism, drug toxicity, infection, and some surgeries. Around 12 000 patients are hospitalized as a result of acute pancreatitis in the UK each year.[11]

Chronic pancreatitis begins as acute pancreatitis and becomes chronic when the pancreas becomes scarred. This condition usually results from long-term and excessive alcohol consumption although it may also develop from other causes of pancreatitis. Chronic pancreatitis can lead to exocrine and endocrine failure. Rarely pancreatitis leads to pancreatic cancer.

Pancreatitis may cause severe epigastric pain and is often associated with nausea, vomiting, and abdominal tenderness and distension. The abdominal pain is often described as severe, radiating from mid-umbilicus to the patient's back and shoulders. In severe cases the patient has fever, tachycardia and signs of generalized sepsis and shock. These patients are often hospitalized and may be treated with intravenously administered fluids, pain medication, and placement of a nasogastric tube if the patient is vomiting.

Oesophagogastric varices

Oesophagogastric varices are common with liver disease and often result from portal hypertension caused by cirrhosis of the liver. Obstruction to blood flow in the liver, produced by the fibrosis in the liver, increases pressure, and dilates vessels that drain into the liver. This subsequent dilatation of thin-walled veins around the lower oesophagus and upper end of the stomach produces oesophagogastric varices. Varices can rupture and may result in life-threatening haemorrhage. Other causes of oesophageal bleeding include oesophagitis (associated with chronic use of alcohol and non-steroidal anti-inflammatory medications), malignancy, and episodes of prolonged, violent vomiting that produces a tear or laceration in the mucosa of the upper oesophagus (Mallory–Weiss syndrome).

Clinically, a patient with oesophageal bleeding has bright red haematemesis and, if bleeding is profuse, melaena may be evident. The patient may manifest the classic signs of shock as well. Variceal bleeding is usually massive and generally hard to control. Therapeutic intervention includes ensuring a patent airway and fluid resuscitation. Definitive care may include placement of a Sengstaken–Blakemore tube to tamponade bleeding vessels, surgical ligation of the bleeding varices, or transendoscopic injection of a sclerosing agent into the bleeding vessels. The mortality rate for patients with variceal bleeding is about 25%.[1]

Haemorrhoids

Haemorrhoids are swollen, distended veins that are located inside the anus (internal) or under the skin around the anus (external) (Figure 19-5). Haemorrhoids are common during pregnancy and result from fetal pressure in the abdomen and hormonal changes that cause haemorrhoidal vessels to enlarge. Haemorrhoids are present in 50% of all persons by age 50. Irritation of the distended veins is made worse by straining during bowel movements and by rubbing or cleaning around the anus, which may produce itching, bleeding,

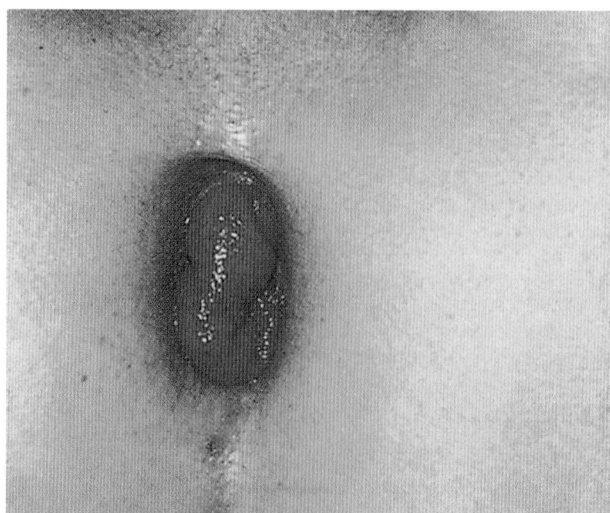

Figure 19-5 Thrombosed external haemorrhoids.

or both. As a rule, haemorrhoidal symptoms subside within a few days.

Pain from haemorrhoids is infrequent unless thrombosis, ulceration or infection is present. Slight bleeding is the most common symptom. (Rarely do haemorrhoids cause significant haemorrhage although recurrent episodes of bleeding may be significant enough to produce anaemia.) The bleeding usually occurs during or after defecation and may be indicated by blood dripping into the toilet after defecation or blood-streaked toilet tissue after wiping. Definitive care includes diet modification, stool softeners, tissue fixation techniques and operative haemorrhoidectomy for severe cases.

Cholecystitis

Cholecystitis is inflammation of the gallbladder. Gallstones are amongst the most common disorders of the gastrointestinal tract, affecting about 10% of people in Western society; more than 80% of people with gallstones are asymptomatic.[11] The disease is more common in women 30 to 50 years of age than men, but becomes more common in both sexes with age. Risk factors for cholecystitis include female sex, oral contraceptive use, increasing age, obesity, diabetes mellitus, chronic alcohol ingestion, and African or Asian ethnicity. The condition may be chronic with recurrent subacute symptoms or acute because of gallstone obstruction.

In 90% of cases, acute cholecystitis is caused by gallstones (composed mainly of cholesterol) in the gallbladder.[12] On occasion the gallstones totally obstruct the neck or cystic duct of the gallbladder. This leads to the common bile duct that empties into the small intestine. The trapped bile becomes concentrated and causes irritation and pressure build-up in the gallbladder, which can lead to bacterial infection and perforation. The increased pressure causes a sudden onset of pain (biliary colic), which radiates to the right upper quadrant or right scapula. Patients with gallbladder disease commonly have their pain episodes at night. Generally, the episodes are associated with recent ingestion of fried or fatty foods. Severe illness, alcohol abuse and, rarely, tumours of the gallbladder can also cause cholecystitis.

Other associated hallmarks of cholecystitis include previous episodes, a family history of gallbladder disease, low-grade fever, nausea, vomiting that may be bile stained and described as bitter (variable), and pain and tenderness on palpation in the right upper quadrant. Passage of stones into the common bile duct with subsequent obstruction may cause shaking chills, high fever, jaundice, and acute pancreatitis. Treatment may include hospitalization, intravenous fluid therapy, antibiotics and placement of a nasogastric tube. Definitive treatment is surgical removal of the gallbladder.

Acute hepatitis

Hepatitis is inflammation of the liver and is the single most important cause of liver disease in the UK and worldwide.

Box 19-4

Risk factors for hepatitis

Hepatitis A

Healthcare practice without body substance isolation precautions
Household or sexual contact with an infected person
Living in an area with hepatitis A virus outbreak
Travelling to developing countries
Engaging in sex with infected partners or multiple partners
Drug use by injection

Hepatitis B

Healthcare practice without body substance isolation precautions
Infant born to mother infected with hepatitis B virus
Engaging in sex with infected partners or multiple partners
Drug use by injection
Receiving haemodialysis

Hepatitis C

Healthcare practice without body substance isolation precautions
Receiving blood transfusion before July 1992
Engaging in sex with infected partners or multiple partners
Drug use by injection
Receiving haemodialysis

Acute hepatitis is associated with the sudden onset of malaise, weakness, anorexia, intermittent nausea and vomiting, and dull right upper quadrant pain. These signs usually are followed within 1 week by the onset of jaundice, dark urine, or both. Although many viruses can infect the liver, the three classes of viruses that are of main concern as causes of acute infectious hepatitis are hepatitis A virus, hepatitis B virus, and hepatitis C virus, formerly known as non-A/non-B hepatitis virus. All types produce similar pathological changes in the liver. These viruses also stimulate an antibody response that is specific to the type of virus causing the disease (Box 19-4). Many hepatitis infections are subclinical; they often present influenza-like symptoms.

The inflammation of hepatitis has many possible causes, including alcohol or other drug use, autoimmune disorders, and toxic bacterial, fungal, parasitic and viral infections. Patients with hepatitis require a physician's evaluation and care. Proper immunization of paramedics is important. Observation of body substance isolation procedures is crucial when paramedics are caring for these patients. Hepatitis is discussed in depth in Chapter 24.

Critical Thinking

Why do you think a person would refuse the chance to be vaccinated against this deadly disease?

Summary

- The major organs most commonly associated with the gastrointestinal system include the oesophagus, stomach, small and large intestines, liver, gallbladder and pancreas.
- After the initial survey, assessment of abdominal pain should begin with a thorough history. The physical examination may help to determine whether the pain is visceral, somatic or referred.
- The most common treatment for abdominal pain occurs at the hospital. The paramedic should provide supportive treatment, manage life threats and transport the patient to an appropriate facility.
- Gastroenteritis is inflammation of the stomach and intestines caused by infectious agents, chemicals or other conditions.
- Gastritis is acute or chronic inflammation of the gastric mucosa. Gastritis commonly results from hyperacidity, alcohol or other drug ingestion, bile reflux, and *H. pylori* infection.
- Colitis is an inflammatory condition of the large intestine. Colitis is characterized by severe diarrhoea and ulceration of the mucosa of the intestine (ulcerative colitis).
- Diverticulosis may result in bright red rectal bleeding if perforation occurs.
- Diverticulitis results when a diverticulum becomes obstructed with faecal matter.
- Appendicitis occurs when the passageway between the appendix and caecum is obstructed by faecal material or by inflammation caused by infection.
- Peptic ulcer disease occurs when open wounds or sores develop in the stomach or duodenum.
- Bowel obstruction is an occlusion of the intestinal lumen. It results in blockage of the normal flow of intestinal contents.
- Crohn's disease is a chronic, inflammatory bowel disease. The disease is of unknown origin.
- Inflammation of the pancreas is called pancreatitis. It causes severe abdominal pain.
- Oesophagogastric varices result from obstruction of blood flow to the liver as a result of liver disease.
- Haemorrhoids are distended veins in the rectoanal area.
- Cholecystitis is inflammation of the gallbladder. It most often is associated with the presence of gallstones.
- Hepatitis is characterized by the sudden onset of malaise, weakness, anorexia, intermittent nausea and vomiting, and dull right upper quadrant pain. These signs usually are followed within 1 week by the onset of jaundice, dark urine, or both.

References

1. Rosen P, Barkin R 1998 Emergency medicine: concepts and clinical practice, 4th edition. Mosby, St Louis
2. Nissman SA, Kaplan LJ, Mann BD 2003 Critically reappraising the literature-driven practice of analgesia administration for acute abdominal pain in the emergency room prior to surgical evaluation. Am J Surg 185(4):291–296
3. Gabbay DS, Dickinson ET 2000 Refusal of base station physicians to authorise narcotic analgesia. Pre Hosp Emerg Care 5(3):293–295
4. Thomas SH, Silen W, Cheema F et al 2003 Effects of morphine analgesia on diagnostic accuracy in emergency department patients with abdominal pain: a prospective, randomized trial. J Am Coll Surg 196(1):18–31
5. Ricard-Hibon A, Chollet C, Saada S, Loridant B, Marty J 1999 A quality control program for acute pain management in out-of-hospital critical care medicine. Ann Emerg Med 34(6):738–744
6. US Department of Transportation, National Highway Traffic Safety Administration 1998 EMT-Paramedic national standard curriculum. US Department of Transportation, Washington, DC
7. Rockall TA, Logan RF, Devlin HB et al 1995 Incidence of and mortality from acute upper gastrointestinal haemorrhage in the United Kingdom. BMJ 311:222–226
8. Frye R et al. Gastroenteritis, bacterial. Online. Available http://www.edmedicine.com/med/topic855.htm 9 February 2009
9. Department of Health. Hospital episode statistics England, Primary diagnosis. Financial year 2007–08. Online. Available http://www.hesonline.nhs.uk/Ease/servlet/ContentServer?siteID=19378categoryID=203
10. Carter MJ, Lobo AJ, Travis SPL, on behalf of the IBD Section of the British Society of Gastroenterology 2004 Guidelines for the management of inflammatory bowel disease in adults. Gut 53(Suppl V):v1–v16
11. Tinto A, Lloyd DAJ, Kang J-Y et al 2002 Acute and chronic pancreatitis – diseases on the rise: a study of hospital admissions in England 1989/90–1999/2000. Aliment Pharmacol Ther 16:2097–2105
12. Indar AA, Beckingham IJ 2002 Acute cholecystitis. BMJ 325:639–643

CHAPTER **20**

Urology

Chapter contents

Objectives

Upon completion of this chapter, the paramedic student will be able to:

1. Label a diagram of the urinary system.
2. Describe pathophysiology, signs and symptoms, assessment, and prehospital management of the patient with urinary retention, urinary tract infection, pyelonephritis, urinary calculus, epididymitis and testicular torsion.
3. Outline the physical examination for patients with genitourinary disorders.
4. Discuss general prehospital management for the patient with a genitourinary disorder.
5. Distinguish between acute and chronic renal failure.
6. Describe the signs and symptoms of renal failure.
7. Describe dialysis and emergent conditions associated with it, including prehospital management.

Key terms

acute renal failure A clinical syndrome that results from a sudden and significant decrease in filtration through the glomeruli, leading to the accumulation of salt, water and nitrogenous wastes within the body.

azotaemia The retention of excessive amounts of nitrogenous compounds in the blood.

chronic renal failure A progressive, irreversible systemic disease caused by kidney dysfunction that leads to abnormalities in blood counts and blood chemistry levels.

dialysis A technique used to normalize blood chemistry in patients with acute or chronic renal failure and to remove blood toxins in some patients who have taken a drug overdose.

disequilibrium syndrome A group of neurological findings that sometimes occur during or immediately after dialysis; thought to result from a disproportionate decrease in osmolality of the extracellular fluid compared with that of the intracellular compartment in the brain or cerebral spinal fluid.

epididymitis An inflammation of the epididymis, a tubular section of the male reproductive system that carries sperm from the testicle to the seminal vesicles.

peritoneal dialysis A dialysis procedure that uses the peritoneum as a diffusible membrane; performed to correct an imbalance of fluid or electrolytes in the blood or to remove toxins, drugs, or other wastes normally excreted by the kidney.

pyelonephritis An inflammation of the kidney parenchyma associated with microbial infection.

testicular torsion A condition in which a testicle twists on its spermatic cord, disrupting its own blood supply.

uraemia The presence of excessive amounts of urea and other nitrogenous wastes produced in the blood.

urinary retention The inability to urinate.

Like gastrointestinal disorders, many genitourinary disorders can produce acute abdominal pain and systemic illness. The treatment for these patients often begins in the prehospital setting. Successful patient recovery often is determined largely by the assessment skills of the paramedic.

Anatomy and physiology review

The urinary system works with other body systems to maintain homeostasis by removing waste products from the

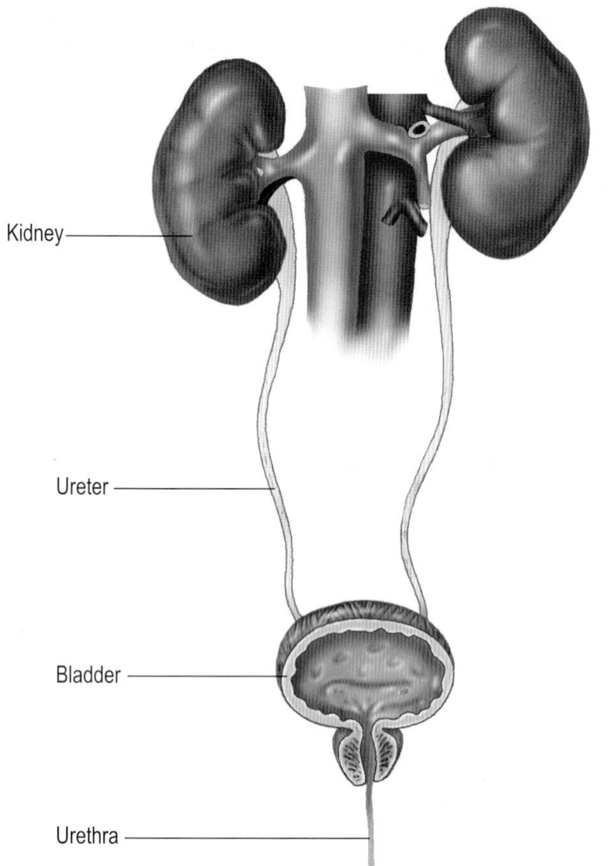

Figure 20-1 Urinary system.

blood. The system also helps to maintain a constant body fluid volume and composition. The urinary system is composed of the kidneys, the ureters, the urinary bladder and the urethra (Figure 20-1).

Many types and causes of renal and urinary tract diseases exist, ranging from mild to acute. Mild urinary tract infections are treatable with antibiotics, whilst acute renal failure requires kidney transplantation or renal dialysis to maintain life. Genitourinary disorders that may cause acute pain include urinary retention, urinary tract infection (UTI), pyelonephritis, urinary calculus, epididymitis and testicular torsion. (Chapter 35 addresses other disorders specific to the female genitourinary system.) Like the pain associated with disorders of the abdomen, genitourinary disorders may produce visceral, somatic and referred pain (see Chapter 19).

Urinary retention

Urinary retention describes the inability to urinate. Possible causes include urethral stricture, an enlarged prostate (benign or malignant prostatic hypertrophy), central nervous system dysfunction, foreign body obstruction, and use of certain drugs such as parasympatholytic or anticholinergic agents. Men are affected with urinary retention more often than are women (most commonly due to an enlarged prostate); however, other common causes can be found in both sexes.

The signs and symptoms of urinary retention include severe abdominal pain (except with central nervous system lesions) that is associated with an urgent need to urinate and a distended bladder. The distended bladder is often palpable. Patients with a progressive obstruction, such as prostatic hypertrophy, often have a history of urinary hesitancy, a poor urinary stream, a sense of incomplete emptying of the bladder, nocturia (excessive urination at night) and overflow incontinence (an overflow of urine from the bladder). In the emergency department, passage of a urethral catheter to empty the bladder is often required. Urinary retention is painful for the patient. The prehospital care is mainly supportive although emergency care practitioners may be able to perform urinary catheterization if appropriate. The cause of the retention should be sought, and if it is not easily correctable following physician examination, the patient may require hospitalization.

Critical Thinking

Have you ever been in a situation when you needed to urinate urgently but could not because of the circumstances? How did you feel?

Urinary tract infection

Over 178 000 patients presented to hospital with urinary tract infections in 2005–2006, and the condition accounted for in excess of 1 million bed days.[1] Urinary tract infections usually develop first in the lower urinary tract (e.g. the urethra or bladder) but may progress to the upper urinary tract (e.g. ureters or kidneys) if not treated. Upper tract infections are often associated with kidney infection (pyelonephritis, described later in this chapter) or abscesses that form within the kidney tissue. These conditions can lead to a reduced kidney function and, in very severe cases, can lead to death if untreated.

The more common lower UTI of the urethra (urethritis) and bladder (cystitis) occurs when enteric flora (particularly *Escherichia coli* normally found in the bowel) enter the opening of the urethra and colonize the urinary tract. These infections are more common in women because the urethra is short and close to the vagina and rectum. The disease also occurs in men (as a result of urethritis, prostatitis, and cystitis) and children. However, urethritis and prostatitis in young men most often results from venereal disease rather than a true UTI. Other factors that may contribute to lower UTI include the use of contraceptive devices (women who use a diaphragm develop infections more often; condoms with spermicidal foam may cause the growth of *E. coli* in the vagina, which may enter the urethra), unsafe sexual practices, the presence of renal stones, bladder catheterization, and a suppressed immune system. In addition, men and women infected with *Chlamydia trachomatis* or *Mycoplasma hominis* can transmit the bacteria to their partner during sexual intercourse. These bacteria could then cause a UTI.

Signs and symptoms of UTI include dysuria, urinary frequency, haematuria and abdominal pain. Often the patient will reveal a history of UTI episodes. In addition, fever, chills, and malaise may be present. Diagnosis is confirmed in the hospital through urinalysis and microscopic examination for blood cells, sediment, and bacteria. Urinary tract infections are generally treated with antibiotic therapy.

Pyelonephritis

Pyelonephritis is inflammation of the kidney parenchyma (upper urinary tract). Inflammation most often occurs as a result of lower UTI. The disease is associated with bacterial infection, particularly in the presence of occasional or persistent backflow (reflux) of infected urine from the bladder into the ureters or kidney pelvis. The bacterial infections may also be carried to one or both kidneys. They may be carried through the bloodstream or lymph glands from the infection that began in the bladder. Pyelonephritis is more common in adult women although the condition can affect persons of any age and either sex. Acute episodes can be severe in the elderly and in persons who are immunosuppressed (e.g. those with cancer or acquired immune deficiency syndrome).

The onset of signs and symptoms of pyelonephritis is usually abrupt and may be mistaken by the patient as resulting from straining the lower back. The condition may be complicated by systemic infection with signs and symptoms that include fever, chills, flank pain, cloudy or bloody urine, nausea and vomiting. Left untreated, pyelonephritis can progress to a chronic condition that can last for months or years and may lead to scarring and possible loss of kidney function. Therapeutic intervention consists primarily of antibiotics, fluid replacement, and sometimes hospitalization.

Critical Thinking

How will you examine the patient for flank pain?

Urinary calculus

Urinary calculi (kidney stones) are pathological concretions that originate in the renal pelvis. They are one of the most painful and most common disorders of the urinary tract, accounting for about 50 000 hospitalizations each year.[1] Between 5% and 15% of the population are affected by kidney stones[2] with recurrence rates close to 50%.[3] Kidney stones result from supersaturation of the urine with insoluble salts. When the level of insoluble salts or uric acid in the urine is high, or the urine lacks citrate (a chemical that normally inhibits the formation of stones), or insufficient water is present in the kidneys to dissolve waste products, kidney stones form. Kidney stones are most common in patients who are between the ages of 20 and 40. The disease is recurrent and is more common in men than in women. Associated risk factors for this condition include dehydration, central nervous system disorders (absent sensory/motor impulses), drug use (anaesthetics, opiates, psychotropic agents, some herbal medicines), and surgery (a postoperative complication).

The chemical composition of the kidney stones depends on the chemical imbalance in the urine. The four most common types of stones are composed of calcium, uric acid, struvite, and cystine. Calcium stones are calcium compounds that are chemically bound to oxalate (most common) or phosphate; they account for about 85% of all kidney stones. Calcium stones typically occur in patients with metabolic (e.g. gout) or hormonal disorders (e.g. hyperparathyroidism). Stones composed of uric acid account for about 10% of kidney stones; their formation is more common in men and there may be a heritable component. Struvite stones (also known as infection stones) are more common in women. These stones are often linked to chronic bacterial UTI or frequent bladder catheterization. Cystine stones are the least common and result from a rare congenital condition in which there are large amounts of cystine (an amino acid in protein) in the urine. Cystine stones are difficult to treat and may require lifelong therapy.

Signs and symptoms of urinary calculus vary according to location. Most stones obstruct the ureter at points of ureteral narrowing in their passage from kidneys to bladder. This produces acute, excruciating pain that originates in the flank area and radiates to the right or left lower abdominal quadrant, groin, and testes (in male patients). Renal or ureteral colic produces severe cyclical pain that occurs as the ureter tries to use forceful contractions to push the stone into the bladder. This pain has been described as having the same intensity as labour pain. The pain may be accompanied by restlessness, nausea and vomiting, urinary urgency or frequency, diaphoresis, low-grade fever, haematuria, dysuria and increased blood pressure (because of the pain). Definitive care includes analgesics (anaesthetics, opiates, psychotropics), fluid replacement, antiemetics, and possible hospital admission. If the calculus does not pass spontaneously, surgical intervention may be required (Box 20-1).

Critical Thinking

Have you cared for or known someone who had a urinary calculus? How did that person describe the pain? What was the level of discomfort?

Epididymitis

Epididymitis is inflammation of the epididymis, a tubular section of the male reproductive system that carries sperm from the testicle to the seminal vesicles. Epididymitis is

Box 20-1

Prevention strategies for recurrent renal calculus

The composition of the stone determines what the patient can do to prevent another stone. Patients may be advised to do the following:

- Increase water consumption.
- Avoid foods containing calcium oxalate (e.g. chocolate, celery, grapes, strawberries, beans and asparagus).
- Take daily supplements of vitamin B_6 and magnesium (to reduce the formation of oxalates).
- Avoid foods that raise uric acid levels (e.g. anchovies and sardines).
- Reduce uric acid by eating a low-protein diet.
- Limit salt intake to reduce the level of calcium oxalate in the urine.

often caused by a bacterial infection that is associated with other structures of the genitourinary tract. Infection tends to occur in sexually active young men. The most common type of epididymitis in young men results from venereal disease.[4]

The signs and symptoms of epididymitis include a gradual onset of unilateral scrotal pain that may radiate to the spermatic cord. At times, tender swelling of the scrotum and testicle occurs, which produces inflammation of one or both testes (orchids). The patient may have a recent history of UTI, fever and malaise as well. After physician evaluation, therapeutic intervention includes antibiotics, bed rest, analgesics and elevation of the scrotum.

Testicular torsion

Testicular torsion is a true urological emergency. In this condition, a testicle twists on its spermatic cord, causing disruption to the blood supply of the testicle. The condition may result from blunt trauma to the scrotal area but is more often spontaneous. The condition occurs in about 1 in 4000 males under the age of 25.[5] It is most common around the age of puberty although it can occur in infancy,[6] and in adult life (approximately 39% of cases occur in adults).[7]

Like epididymitis, testicular torsion results in a tender epididymis and painful swelling of the scrotal sac (Figure 20-2). Unlike epididymitis, though, the patient is usually afebrile. The pain is sudden in onset and is often preceded by vigorous physical activity or an athletic event. The pain is severe and sometimes radiates to the ipsilateral left quadrant. In addition, the pain is unrelieved by rest or scrotal elevation (Prehn's sign) and the scrotum is missing its normal rugae. Pain is often associated with nausea and vomiting. Testicular torsion must be diagnosed and treated within 6 h to prevent loss of the testis from ischaemic infarction.[8] Therapeutic intervention includes the application of ice packs to the scrotum. Intervention also includes manual manipulation by a physician to reduce the torsion and the patient must undergo surgical repair within 4–6 h of onset of the torsion. Thus, rapid transport to the emergency department and early recognition are critical for treatment.

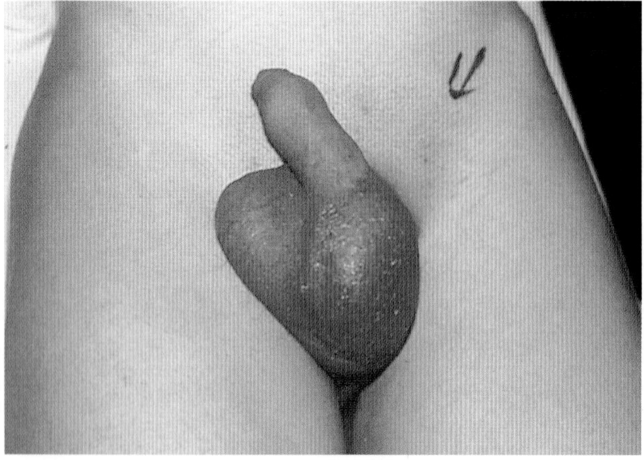

Figure 20-2 Four-day old torsion of the left testis.

Physical examination for patients with genitourinary disorders

As described in Chapter 9, an assessment of the abdomen and genitalia of either sex can be awkward. The assessment can be uncomfortable for the patient and the paramedic. The paramedic should protect the patient's privacy with the proper drapes. When possible, paramedics of the same sex as the patient should perform these examinations. If this is not possible, a chaperone should be present. The examiner should proceed with a calm, caring, and competent attitude, and should keep the patient and significant others informed of all actions. The examination is similar to that performed for abdominal pain (see Chapter 19) and should include the following:

- initial assessment
- focused history
  - OPQRST (Onset/origin, Provokes, Quality, Region, Severity, Time)
  - previous history of similar event
  - nausea or vomiting
  - change in bowel habits or stool (constipation, diarrhoea)
  - change in urinary voiding pattern
  - weight loss
  - last oral intake
  - last bowel movement
- physical examination
  - appearance
  - posture
  - level of consciousness
  - apparent state of health
  - skin colour
  - vital signs
  - abdominal examination (inspection, auscultation, percussion, palpation)
  - genitalia examination (if indicated).

Management and treatment plan

The paramedic should manage patients with genitourinary disorders as any other patient with acute pain, including providing airway, ventilatory and circulatory support; administering high-concentration oxygen (if indicated); electrocardiogram and vital sign monitoring; and rapid, gentle transportation for physician evaluation in the patient's position of comfort. Patients should not be permitted to eat or drink because surgery may be indicated. The administration of analgesics is indicated for these patients and should not be withheld for fear of masking the pain. All patients who have had persistent genitourinary pain or discomfort for more than 6 h should be transported for physician evaluation.

Renal failure

The kidneys play a key role in maintaining homeostasis by controlling extracellular fluid volume, maintenance of proper electrolyte composition and blood pH, and elimination of waste products. If this organ system malfunctions, serious systemic consequences develop, including uraemia (excessive amounts of urea and other nitrogenous waste products in the blood) with subsequent encephalopathy or pericarditis, hyperkalaemia, acidosis, hypertension and volume overload with subsequent congestive heart failure. The disease can be classified as acute or chronic. Classification depends on the duration of renal failure and on the potential for reversibility.

Critical Thinking

Think about why a patient would develop the complications that were just described.

Acute renal failure

Acute renal failure (ARF) is a clinical syndrome that results from a sudden and significant decrease in filtration through the glomeruli that leads to the build-up of high levels of uraemic toxins in the blood. Acute renal failure occurs when the kidneys are unable to excrete the daily load of toxins in the urine. Patients with ARF are separated into two groups based on the amount of urine excreted in 24 h. One group is oliguric (these patients excrete less than 500 mL/day). The other is non-oliguric (these patients excrete more than 500 mL/day). Acute renal failure can threaten the life of a patient, and despite technical improvements in the management of ARF over the last 50 years, mortality rates have remained unchanged at 50%.[9] However, if ARF is recognized early and treated appropriately, it may be readily reversible. Causes of ARF are diverse and include trauma, shock, infection, urinary obstruction, and multisystem diseases.

The onset of ARF can occur within hours. As normal kidney function rapidly deteriorates, urine output frequently decreases (oliguria) or stops completely (anuria). This results in generalized oedema from water and salt retention, acidosis from failure of the kidneys to rid the body of normal acidic products, high concentrations of non-protein nitrogens (especially urea) from failure of the body to secrete metabolic end products, and high concentrations of other products of renal excretion (such as uric acid and potassium). The resulting condition often is termed uraemia. If uraemia is not recognized early and treated appropriately, renal dysfunction leads to the development of heart failure, volume overload, hyperkalaemia, and metabolic acidosis. Acute renal failure may be classified as prerenal, intrarenal, or postrenal in origin (Table 20-1).

Table 20-1 Classification of acute renal failure

Area of dysfunction	Possible causes
Prerenal	Hypovolaemia
	Haemorrhagic blood loss (trauma, gastrointestinal bleeding, complications of childbirth)
	Loss of plasma volume (burns, peritonitis)
	Water and electrolyte losses (severe vomiting or diarrhoea, intestinal obstruction, uncontrolled diabetes mellitus, inappropriate use of diuretics)
	Hypotension or hypoperfusion
	Septic shock
	Cardiac failure or shock
	Massive pulmonary embolism
	Stenosis or clamping of renal artery
Intrarenal	Acute tubular necrosis (post-ischaemic or nephrotoxic)
	Glomerulopathies
	Malignant hypertension
	Coagulation defects
Postrenal	Obstructive uropathies (usually bilateral)
	Ureteral obstruction (oedema, tumours, stones, clots)
	Bladder neck obstruction (enlarged prostate)

From McCance KL, Heuther SE 2002 Pathophysiology: the biologic basis for disease in adults and children, 4th edition. Mosby, St Louis.

Prerenal acute renal failure

Prerenal ARF results from inadequate perfusion of the kidneys. The damaged kidneys are unable to rid the blood of waste products such as urea and creatinine. This condition may be caused by hypovolaemia or impaired cardiac output. Obstruction of renal arteries results in decreased blood flow to the kidneys and an increase in renal vascular resistance that effectively shunts blood away from the kidneys. Many patients with prerenal ARF are critically ill and may have a number of pre-existing medical conditions such as atherosclerosis, chronic liver disease, and heart failure. (Dehydration caused by diuretic use in patients with heart failure is a major cause of prerenal ARF.) In addition, perfusion is often poor within many organs, which may lead to multiple organ failure.

Signs and symptoms of prerenal ARF include dizziness, dry mouth, thirst, hypotension, tachycardia and weight loss. The goal of treatment is to improve kidney perfusion and function by treating the underlying condition (e.g. infection, congestive heart failure and liver failure). Fluids are administered intravenously to most patients to treat dehydration. After this, urine output generally increases and renal function improves.

Intrarenal acute renal failure

Intrarenal ARF is also known as intrinsic ARF and results from conditions that damage or injure both kidneys. Examples include glomerular and other microvascular diseases, tubular diseases, and interstitial diseases that cause direct damage to the kidney parenchyma. Nearly 90% of all cases are caused by ischaemia or toxins. Both of these causes can lead to acute tubular necrosis (death of tubular cells).[10] Ischaemic causes of intrarenal ARF are associated with renal hypoperfusion. These occur most often from haemorrhage, trauma, sepsis and in patients undergoing cardiovascular surgery. Nephrotoxic causes of intrarenal ARF occur most often in the elderly and in patients with chronic renal failure. Drugs and other compounds that can trigger intrarenal ARF include antibiotics, non-steroidal anti-inflammatory drugs, anticancer drugs, radiocontrast dyes, alcohol and other drug use (e.g. cocaine). The condition is also associated with hypertension, autoimmune diseases (e.g. systemic lupus erythematosus) and pyelonephritis.

Signs and symptoms of intrarenal ARF include fever, flank pain, joint pain, headache, hypertension, confusion, seizure and oliguria. The goal of treatment is to restore adequate renal blood flow. This is done by resolving the underlying cause and its complications. In severe cases, renal dialysis (described later in this chapter) may be needed to manage the disease.

Postrenal acute renal failure

Postrenal ARF is caused by obstruction to urine flow to both kidneys. This form of renal failure may be caused by ureteral and urethral obstructions (bilateral calculi, prostatic enlargement, urethral strictures). The blockage of urine causes pressure to build in the renal nephrons and ultimately can cause the nephrons to shut down. The degree of renal failure corresponds directly with the degree of obstruction. Signs and symptoms of postrenal ARF include urine retention; distended bladder; gross haematuria; pain in the lower back, abdomen, groin or genitalia; and peripheral oedema. The condition is reversible by removing the obstruction to urine flow.

Chronic renal failure

Chronic renal failure (CRF) is a progressive, irreversible systemic disease. It develops over months to years as internal structures of the kidney are slowly damaged. Chronic renal failure may be caused by congenital disorders or prolonged pyelonephritis. In the industrialized world, though, CRF more often results from systemic diseases such as diabetes and hypertension and from autoimmune disorders. The kidneys try to make up for renal damage by hyperfiltration within the remaining working nephrons. Over time, hyperfiltration causes further nephron damage and loss of kidney function. Chronic loss of function causes generalized wasting and progressive scarring within all parts of the kidney. This damage results in a reduction in nephron mass and renal mass.

Like ARF, CRF results in the build-up of fluid and waste products in the body. This causes azotaemia (the retention of excessive amounts of nitrogenous compounds in the blood), and uraemia. Most body systems are affected by CRF. Complications of the disease may include hypertension, congestive heart failure, anaemia, electrolyte abnormalities, and others (Table 20-2). There are currently over 37 800 adult patients receiving Renal Replacement Therapy (RRT) in the UK, which gives an indication of the scale of the problem.[11] Once CRF has been diagnosed and the cause has been identified, treatments are started to delay or possibly stop the progressive loss of kidney function. In its final stages, CRF often requires treatment with dialysis (haemodialysis or peritoneal dialysis) or a kidney transplant for the patient to survive. In addition to oliguria, the patient with CRF may exhibit the following six systemic manifestations:

1. Gastrointestinal manifestations
   a. anorexia
   b. nausea
   c. vomiting
2. Cardiopulmonary manifestations
   a. hypertension
   b. pericarditis
   c. pulmonary oedema
   d. peripheral, sacral, and periorbital oedema
   e. myocardial ischaemia
3. Nervous system manifestations
   a. anxiety
   b. delirium
   c. progressive obtundation
   d. hallucinations
   e. muscle twitching
   f. seizures
4. Metabolic or endocrine manifestations
   a. glucose intolerance
   b. electrolyte disturbances
   c. anaemia
5. Personality changes
   a. fatigue
   b. mental dullness
6. Signs of uraemia
   a. pasty, yellow skin discoloration and thin extremities from protein wasting
   b. uraemic frost caused by urea crystals that form on the skin (late finding).

Renal dialysis

Dialysis is a technique used to normalize blood chemistry and is used in patients with acute or chronic renal failure. Dialysis also removes blood toxins in some patients who have taken a drug overdose. The two types of dialysis are haemodialysis and peritoneal dialysis. Both of these bring the patient's blood into contact with a semi-permeable membrane across which water-soluble substances diffuse into a dialysing fluid (dialysate). Eventually, electrolytes are balanced between the patient's blood and the dialysis fluid and waste products are eliminated.

The amount of substance that transfers during dialysis depends on the difference in the concentrations of solutions on the two sides of the semi-permeable membrane, the molecular size of the substance, and the length of time the blood and the dialysate remain in contact with the membrane. In patients with end-stage renal disease, haemodialysis is usually done three times a week with each session lasting 4–5 h.

Haemodialysis

In haemodialysis the patient's heparinized blood is pumped through a surgically constructed arteriovenous fistula. The fistula is a connection between an artery and a vein. An arteriovenous graft, which is a synthetic material grafted between the patient's arteries and vein (Figure 20-3), can also be used. These internal shunts are usually located in the inner aspect of the patient's forearm but may be located in

Table 20-2 Systemic effects of uraemia

System	Manifestations	Mechanisms	Treatment
Skeletal	Osteitis fibrosa (bone inflammation with fibrous degeneration); bone demineralization (principally subperiosteal loss of cortical bone in the fibres, lateral ends of the clavicles, and lamina dura of the teeth); spontaneous fractures, bone pain; osteomalacia (rickets) with end-stage renal failure	Bone resorption associated with hyperparathyroidism, vitamin D deficiency, and demineralization; lowered calcium and raised phosphate levels	Control of hyperphosphataemia to reduce hyperparathyroidism; administration of calcium and aluminium hydroxide antacids, which bind phosphate in the gut, together with a phosphate-restricted diet; vitamin D replacement; avoidance of magnesium antacids because of impaired magnesium excretion
Cardiopulmonary	Hypertension, pericarditis with fever, chest pain, and pericardial friction rub, pulmonary oedema, Kussmaul respirations	Extracellular volume expansion as cause of hypertension; hypersecretion of renin also associated with hypertension; fluid overload associated with pulmonary oedema and acidosis leading to Kussmaul respirations	Volume reduction with diuretics that are not potassium sparing (to avoid hyperkalaemia); angiotensin-converting enzyme (ACE) inhibitors; combination of propranolol, hydralazine, and minoxidil for those with high levels of renin; bilateral nephrectomy with dialysis or transplantation
Neurological	Encephalopathy (fatigue, loss of attention, difficulty problem solving); peripheral neuropathy (pain and burning in the legs and feet, loss of vibration sense and deep tendon reflexes); loss of motor coordination, twitching, fasciculations, stupor, and coma with advanced uraemia	Uraemic toxins associated with end-stage renal disease	Dialysis
Endocrine	Retarded growth in children Osteomalacia Higher incidence of goitre	Decreased growth hormone Elevated parathyroid hormone levels Decreased thyroid hormone	Exogenous recombinant human growth hormone Same as for Skeletal above
Haematological	Anaemia, usually normochromic normocytic; platelet disorders with prolonged bleeding times	Reduced erythropoietin secretion associated with loss of renal mass, leading to reduced red cell production in the bone marrow; uraemic toxins associated with shortened red cell survival	Replacement when indicated Dialysis; recombinant human erythropoietin and iron supplementation; conjugated estrogens; DDAVP (1-desamino-8-D-arginine vasopressin); transfusion
Gastrointestinal	Anorexia, nausea, vomiting; mouth ulcers, stomatitis, ruinous breath (uraemic fetor), hiccups, peptic ulcers, gastrointestinal bleeding, and pancreatitis associated with end-stage renal failure	Retention of urea, metabolic acids, and other metabolic waste products, including methylguanidine	Protein-restricted diet for relief of nausea and vomiting
Integumentary	Abnormal pigmentation and pruritus	Retention of urochromes, contributing to sallow, yellow colour; high plasma calcium levels associated with pruritus	Dialysis with control of serum calcium levels
Immunological	Increased risk of infection that can cause death	Suppression of cell-mediated immunity; reduction in number and function of lymphocytes, diminished phagocytosis	Routine dialysis
Reproductive	Sexual dysfunction: menorrhagia, amenorrhoea, infertility, and decreased libido in women; decreased testosterone levels, infertility, and decreased libido in men	Elevated hormones: luteinizing hormone (LH), follicle-stimulating hormone (FSH), prolactin, and LH-releasing hormone; decreased testosterone, oestrogen, and progesterone	No specific treatment

From McCance KL, Heuther SE 2002 Pathophysiology: the biologic basis for disease in adults and children, 4th edition. Mosby, St Louis.

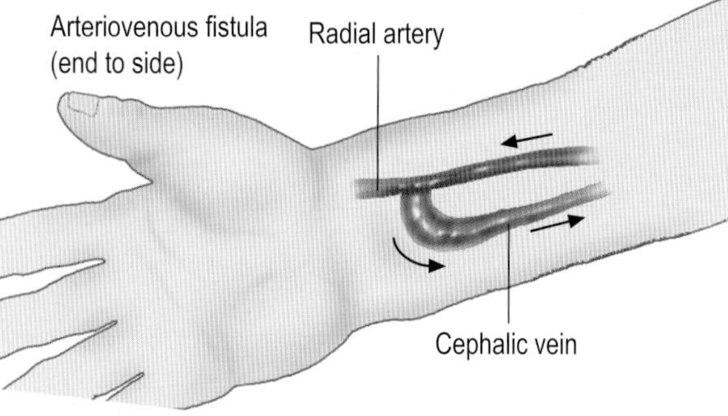

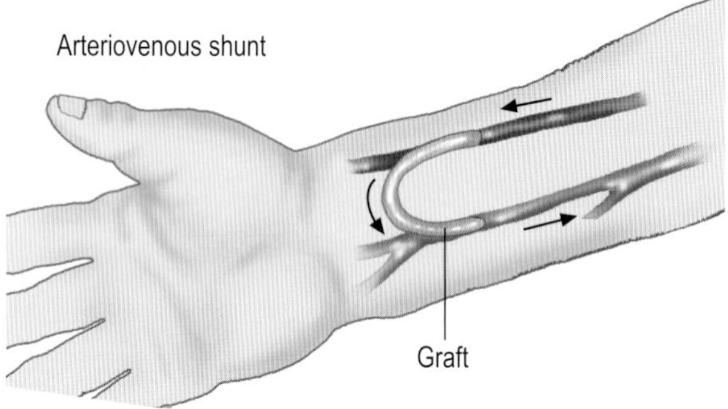

Figure 20-3 Arteriovenous shunts.

the medial aspect of the lower extremity. Some patients may have an external dialysis catheter or a small, button-shaped device (Hemasite). This device is usually located in the upper arm or proximal, anterior thigh. A Hemasite is similar to an arteriovenous graft. However, the Hemasite has an external rubber septum sutured to the skin. A dialysis catheter is inserted into this septum for treatment (see Chapter 41).

Peritoneal dialysis

In peritoneal dialysis the dialysis membrane is the patient's own peritoneum. The dialysate is infused into the peritoneal cavity by a temporary or permanently implanted catheter. Fluid and solutes diffuse from the blood in the peritoneal capillaries into the dialysate. After 1–2 h, equilibration has occurred. At this point, the dialysate is drained and fresh fluid is infused. Peritoneal dialysis works much more slowly than haemodialysis. Over time, though, it is just as effective. In addition, peritoneal dialysis does not require chronic blood access. A major complication of peritoneal dialysis is peritonitis, which usually results when the proper aseptic technique is not used. Peritoneal dialysis may be carried out regularly in the home by the patient or by the family caregiver.

Dialysis emergencies

When caring for a patient with acute or chronic renal failure, the paramedic may encounter emergencies that result from the disease process itself or from complications of dialysis. For example, these patients may experience problems associated with vascular access, haemorrhage, hypotension, chest pain, severe hyperkalaemia, disequilibrium syndrome (described later), and the development of an air embolism. In addition, the paramedic should be aware of problems that may result from concurrent medical illness and its treatment. These problems include decreased ability to tolerate the stress of significant illness or trauma, inadvertent over-administration of intravenous fluid, and altered metabolism and unpredictable action of drugs.

Critical Thinking

Which of these complications could cause an immediate threat to life?

Vascular access problems

Problems associated with vascular access are bleeding at the site of puncture for dialysis, thrombosis, and infection. Bleeding from the fistula or graft is usually minimal and can usually be controlled by direct pressure at the site. (Excessive pressure, though, can cause thrombosis in the graft or fistula.) A potential complication of an internal shunt is the development of a pseudoaneurysm. The aneurysm can rupture, which may cause a large haematoma and possible hypovolaemia. If this occurs, the paramedic should apply direct pressure to the haematoma and assess and treat the patient for significant blood loss. This situation requires rapid transport for physician evaluation.

Fistulae and grafts that become occluded as a result of thrombus formation usually require surgical intervention or the administration of a thrombolytic agent to restore flow. Patients with a surgical anastomosis are instructed to check for the presence of a bruit or 'thrill' periodically. The presence will verify unobstructed circulation. Attempts to clear the graft by irrigation or aspiration are generally not advised. If thrombosis occurs while the patient is undergoing dialysis, the dialysis should be stopped and then intravenous administration of fluids should be initiated in an alternative site. Decreased blood flow is a common trigger of thrombosis and is the main reason that one should not take the blood pressure in the arm with a vascular access.

An infection at the site of vascular access is usually the result of the puncture made during dialysis. Thus, careful sterile technique is the rule when caring for these patients. Routine vascular access using the dialysis route should be discouraged. Vascular access infection should be considered when a dialysis patient has unexplained fever, malaise, or other signs of systemic infection.

Note

When drawing blood or intravenously infusing fluids in a patient with a surgical anastomosis, the paramedic should choose an alternative site. The paramedic should also avoid taking blood pressure measurements and using tourniquets in an extremity with an arteriovenous fistula or graft. Rarely (and perhaps only under direction of a physician), it may be that the internal shunt be used to obtain vascular access. If so, the paramedic must be careful not to puncture the back wall of the vessel. The paramedic must also be sure to use careful aseptic technique during the procedure. Intravenous infusions must be monitored closely to avoid a 'runaway IV'. The intravenous catheter should be taped securely in place as well.

Haemorrhage

Patients who are receiving dialysis have an increased risk of haemorrhage. This risk arises from their regular exposure to anticoagulants during haemodialysis and from the decrease in their platelet function. Thus, a patient who experiences haemorrhage from trauma or a medical condition (e.g. gastrointestinal bleeding) should be monitored closely for signs of hypovolaemia. Most patients on dialysis have anaemia. This lowers their ability to compensate for blood loss when they have acute haemorrhage. Any significant blood loss (whether external or internal) may produce dyspnoea or angina. If haemorrhage from trauma occurs in an extremity with a fistula or graft, the paramedic should control the bleeding and immobilize the extremity. The paramedic should use special care to try to avoid obstructing circulation in the anastomosis.

Hypotension

Hypotension can occur with haemodialysis. This may result from the rapid reduction in intravascular volume, abrupt changes in electrolyte concentrations, or vascular instability that may occur during the procedure. In addition, the patient's mechanisms to cope with these physiological changes may be impaired. This may result in an inability to maintain normal blood pressure. Patients with hypotension caused by dialysis must be managed cautiously with the administration of fluids. The paramedic should be careful not to produce a fluid overload. This may manifest as hypertension and the classic signs of congestive heart failure (Box 20-2). Most patients respond to a small (200–300 mL) fluid challenge. If they do not, other potentially serious causes should be considered.

Chest pain

The episodes of hypotension and mild hypoxaemia that often occur during dialysis may result in myocardial ischaemia and chest pain. The patient may also complain of other symptoms that are associated with decreased oxygen delivery, such as headache and dizziness. These complaints may indicate an evolving myocardial infarction. However, they often are relieved with the administration of oxygen, fluid replacement, and anti-anginal medications. Regardless, all patients with chest pain should be treated as though a myocardial infarction has occurred.

Dysrhythmias that result from myocardial ischaemia may also be associated with dialysis. The most common ischaemic rhythm disturbances are premature ventricular contractions. If dialysis is in progress, the procedure should be stopped. The paramedic may wish to consult with staff at the patient's renal unit for advice.

Box 20-2

Classic signs of congestive heart failure

Crackles
Engorged neck veins
Liver congestion and engorgement
Pitting oedema
Pulmonary oedema
Shortness of breath

Severe hyperkalaemia

Severe hyperkalaemia is an emergency that poses a serious threat to life. It can occur rapidly in patients with acute renal failure. Severe hyperkalaemia often results from poor dietary regulation and missed dialysis treatments. Patients with severe hyperkalaemia may have weakness but are often asymptomatic. Typical electrocardiogram changes initially demonstrate a tall or tented T wave. As the potassium levels rise, conduction slows, resulting in a prolonged P-R interval, depressed ST segments, and sometimes the loss of P waves. This may be followed by a widened QRS complex and delayed conduction in the interventricular conducting system. The electrocardiogram patterns resemble bundle branch blocks. Hyperkalaemic disturbances may not become apparent until dangerous levels of potassium are present. Thus, any patient with renal failure who is in cardiac arrest should be suspected of having severe hyperkalaemia.

Note

Dialysis patients who have chronic renal failure tolerate increased potassium levels better than do those patients with normal kidney function.

Disequilibrium syndrome

Disequilibrium syndrome refers to a group of neurological findings that sometimes occur during or right after dialysis. These symptoms are usually mild (e.g. headache, restlessness, nausea and fatigue) although they may be severe (including confusion, seizures and coma). The syndrome is thought to result from a disproportionate decrease in osmolality of the extracellular fluid compared with that of the intracellular compartment in the brain or cerebrospinal fluid.[12] This results in an osmotic gradient between the blood and the brain, which in turn causes a movement of water into the brain and then cerebral oedema and increased intracranial pressure. If seizures occur, an anticonvulsant may be indicated.

Air embolism

Negative pressure on the venous side of the dialysis tubing or a malfunction in the machine can allow an air embolism to enter the patient's bloodstream. This is a rare occurrence. If air embolism occurs, the embolus may be carried to the right ventricle of the heart. In the heart the embolus may block the passage of blood to the left myocardium. The patient may experience severe dyspnoea, cyanosis, hypotension and respiratory distress. A patient with an air embolus requires high-concentration oxygen and rapid transport to a medical facility. In an effort to trap the embolism where it will be least likely to obstruct blood flow, the paramedic should position the patient on the left side and then transport in the modified Trendelenburg position.

Management

To review, the prehospital management of patients with chronic or acute renal failure includes the following:

- Airway and ventilatory support with supplemental high-concentration oxygen administration.
- Vascular access for fluid replacement, medication therapy (diuretics, antidysrhythmics, vasopressors), or fluid resuscitation if needed.
- Meticulous aseptic technique if intravenous access is ordered by medical direction.
- Electrocardiogram and other vital sign monitoring.
- Rapid transport to an appropriate medical facility.

Summary

- The urinary system removes waste products from the blood. It helps to maintain a constant body fluid volume and composition as well.
- Urinary retention is the inability to urinate.
- Urinary tract infections can involve the upper or lower urinary tract.
- Pyelonephritis is inflammation of the kidney parenchyma.
- Urinary calculi are stones that originate in the kidney.
- Epididymitis is inflammation of the epididymis. The epididymis is the tube that carries sperm from the testicle to the seminal vesicles.
- Testicular torsion is a true emergency. In this condition a testicle twists on its spermatic cord, which disrupts the blood supply to the testicle.
- The physical examination for a patient with a urinary tract problem is similar to that performed for abdominal pain. Patients with genitourinary pain should be managed as any other patient with acute pain.
- Renal failure may result in uraemia, hyperkalaemia, acidosis, hypertension and volume overload with congestive heart failure. Renal failure can be classified as acute or chronic. Classification depends on the duration and on the potential for reversibility.
- Dialysis is a technique used to normalize blood chemistry. Dialysis is used in patients who have acute or chronic renal failure. Dialysis also is used to remove blood toxins. The two dialysis techniques are haemodialysis and peritoneal dialysis. Dialysis emergencies may include problems with vascular access, haemorrhage, hypotension, chest pain, severe hyperkalaemia, disequilibrium syndrome, and air embolism.

References

1. The Information Centre 2007 Hospital episode statistics primary diagnosis: 3 character, 2005–06. Online. Available www.hesonline.nhs.uk 19 August 2008
2. Moe OW 2006 Kidney stones: pathophysiology and medical management. Lancet 367:333–344
3. Sutherland JW, Parks JH, Coe FL 1985 Recurrence after a single renal stone in a community practice. Miner Electrolyte Metab 11:267–269
4. Workowski KA, Berman SM 2006 Sexually transmitted diseases treatment guidelines, 2006. MMWR: Morbid Mortal Weekly Rep 55(RR-11):1–92
5. Sessions AE, Rabinowitz R, Hulbert WC, et al 2003 Testicular torsion: direction, degree, duration and disinformation. J Urol 169:663–665
6. Cuckow PM, Frank JD 2000 Torsion of the testis. Br J Urol Int 86(3):349–353
7. Cummings JM, Boullier JA, Sekhon D, Bose K 2002 Adult testicular torsion. J Urol 167:2109–2110
8. Miller KM 1999 Testicular torsion. Am J Nurs 99(6):33–35
9. Ympa YP, Sakr Y, Reinhart K, Vincent J-L 2005 Has mortality from acute renal failure decreased? A systematic review of the literature. Am J Med 118(8):827–832
10. Prakash J, Sen D, Sarat Kumar N, et al 2003 Acute renal failure due to intrinsic renal diseases: review of 1122 cases. Renal Failure 5(2):225–233
11. UK Renal Registry Report 2005. Online. Available http://www.renalreg.com/Report%202005/Cover_Frame2.htm 2 September 2008
12. Bagshaw SM, Peets AD, Hameed M, et al 2004 Dialysis disequilibrium syndrome: brain death following haemodialysis for metabolic acidosis and acute renal failure – a case report. BMC Nephrol 5:9

CHAPTER 21

Toxicology

Chapter contents

Objectives

Upon completion of this chapter, the paramedic student will be able to:

1. Define poisoning.
2. Describe general principles for assessment and management of the patient who has ingested poison.
3. Describe the causative agents and pathophysiology of selected ingested poisons and management of patients who have taken them.
4. Describe how physical and chemical properties influence the effects of inhaled toxins.
5. Distinguish among the three categories of inhaled toxins: simple asphyxiants, chemical asphyxiants and systemic poisons, and irritants or corrosives.
6. Describe general principles of managing the patient who has inhaled poison.
7. Describe the signs, symptoms, and management of patients who have inhaled cyanide, ammonia, or hydrocarbon.
8. Describe the signs, symptoms, and management of patients injected with poison by insects, reptiles, and hazardous aquatic creatures.
9. Describe the signs, symptoms, and management of patients with organophosphate or carbamate poisoning.
10. Outline the general principles of managing patients with drug overdose.
11. Describe the effects, signs and symptoms, and specific management for selected drug overdose.
12. Describe the short- and long-term physiological effects of ethanol ingestion.
13. Describe signs, symptoms, and management of alcohol-related emergencies.
14. Identify general management principles for the most common toxic syndromes based on knowledge of the characteristic physical findings associated with each syndrome.

Key terms

botulism An often fatal form of food poisoning caused by the bacillus *Clostridium botulinum*.

delirium tremens An acute and sometimes fatal psychotic reaction caused by cessation of excessive intake of alcohol over a long period of time; also known as DTs.

envenomation The injection of snake, arachnid, or insect venom into the body.

gastric lavage Irrigation of the stomach with sterile water or normal saline.

Korsakoff's psychosis A form of amnesia often seen in alcohol-dependent individuals, characterized by a loss of short-term memory and an inability to learn new skills.

Lyme disease An acute, recurrent inflammatory infection transmitted by a tick.

nematocyst A capsule containing thread-like, venomous stinging cells found in some coelenterates.

NPIS National Poisons Information Service.

nystagmus Involuntary rhythmic movements of the eyes.

poison Any substance that produces harmful physiological or psychological effects.

Our environment has a large number of potentially harmful substances (both natural and synthetic.) They can be accidentally or deliberately absorbed, ingested, inhaled, or injected.

SECTION I

Poisonings

A poison can be defined as any substance that produces harmful physiological or psychological effects. Emergencies that involve poisons are a major cause of morbidity and mortality in the United Kingdom. In the UK in 2002, 6612 deaths were attributable to poisonings or exposure to noxious chemicals and approximately 4% of admissions to emergency departments were related to suspected poisoning.[1] The circumstances leading to deaths attributed directly to poisoning were accidental exposure in 30%, deliberate poisoning in 43%, and due to mental or behavioural disorder associated with recreational drug use in 27%.[1]

Critical Thinking

How many substances that fit the definition of a poison are there in or around your home?

National Poisons Information Service

The National Poisons Information Service (NPIS) is a clinical toxicology service for healthcare professionals. The service consists of a network of units across the UK, providing information and advice on the diagnosis, treatment and management of patients who may have been accidentally or deliberately poisoned. Information on management of poisoning is available on its Internet database TOXBASE, or through a consultant-led 24-hour telephone service for more complex cases. The five regional units are located in Edinburgh, Belfast, Newcastle, Birmingham and Cardiff; contact details can be found on the Health Protection Agency (HPA) website.

NPIS units also provide information to government agencies such as the Medicines and Healthcare products Regulatory Agency (MHRA), the Department for Environment, Food and Rural Affairs (DEFRA), and the Pesticide Safety Directorate (PSD); contribute to undergraduate and postgraduate teaching; provide training courses for nurses, doctors, NHS Direct/NHS 24 staff and other medical professionals; and carry out research in the field of clinical toxicology and poisons information.

Use by emergency medical services agencies

NPIS units are a ready source of information for any toxicological emergency. Depending on local communications and protocol, NPIS units may be contacted directly by EMS providers (and other emergency personnel) via telephone or a command and control centre. The immediate determination of potential toxicity is based on the specific agent or agents; the amount ingested; the time of exposure; the weight and medical condition of the patient; and any treatment given before the arrival of EMS.

General guidelines for managing a poisoned patient

Poisons may enter the body through ingestion, inhalation, injection, and absorption. Box 21-1 identifies types of toxicological emergencies that may result in poisoning. Most poisoned patients require only supportive therapy to recover, although a few cases may require the use of lifesaving antidotes. The poisoned patient can often be managed in the prehospital setting using the following guidelines:

1. Ensure adequate airway, ventilation, and circulation. Take action to prevent or reduce the risk of aspiration by carefully watching the patient's airway.
2. Obtain a thorough history, and perform a focused physical examination.
3. Consider hypoglycaemia in a patient who has an altered level of consciousness or is convulsing.
4. Administer naloxone to a patient with respiratory depression where opiate overdose is a possibility.
5. If overdose is suspected, obtain an overdose history from the patient, family, or friends.
6. Consider consulting with NPIS for specific management to prevent further absorption of the toxin (or antidote therapy).

Box 21-1

Types of toxicological emergencies

Unintentional poisoning

Childhood poisoning
Dosage errors
Environmental exposure
Idiosyncratic reactions
Occupational exposure
Drug and alcohol abuse

Intentional poisoning/overdose

Assault/homicide
Chemical warfare
Suicide attempts

7. Frequently reassess the patient; monitor vital signs and electrocardiogram.
8. Safely obtain any substance or substance container of a suspected poison. Transport it along with the patient. The paramedic should collect a sample of the patient's vomitus (if present) for laboratory analysis.
9. Transport the patient for physician examination.

When caring for a patient who has been poisoned, personal safety is the top priority. A toxicological emergency response may involve hazardous materials. It may also involve patient behaviour that is unpredictable or violent. If the scene is not safe, the paramedic crew should retreat to a safe staging area and wait there until the scene has been secured by the appropriate personnel.

Poisoning by ingestion

The majority of all accidental ingestion of poisons occurs in children 1 to 3 years of age. The most common poison exposures in this group result from household products such as petroleum-based agents, cleaning agents and cosmetics; medications; toxic plants; and contaminated foods. Poisoning in adults is often intentional, although unintentional poisoning from exposure to chemicals in the workplace also occurs. Deliberate poisonings may be an attempt at suicide or the result of recreational or experimental drug abuse. They may also result from chemical warfare or acts of terrorism and may even be a factor in assault and murder.

The toxic effects of ingested poisons may be immediate or delayed, depending on the substance that was ingested. For example, corrosive substances such as strong acids and alkalis may produce immediate tissue damage. This is evidenced by burns to the lips, tongue, throat and upper gastrointestinal tract. Other substances, such as medications and toxic plants, usually require absorption and distribution through the bloodstream (and alterations by different organs) to produce toxic effects. Only minimal absorption occurs in the stomach. Thus, poisons may take several hours to enter the bloodstream through the small intestine. Therefore, early management of the ingested poisoning focuses on treating the patient's symptoms and removing the toxin from the stomach or binding it to prevent absorption before the poison enters the intestines.

Assessment and management

The initial assessment and management of a poisoned patient is the same as for any other patient. First, the paramedic should ensure his or her personal safety and then manage immediate threats to the patient's life. During scene size-up, the paramedic crew should be alert for specific clues or details that suggest a toxic emergency. Examples include open medication bottles, scattered pills, vomitus, and open containers of household products. Patient findings that may suggest poisoning include a decreased level of consciousness, airway compromise/injury (e.g. vomitus or pills in the mouth, burns in the oral cavity), abnormal respiratory patterns, and dysrhythmias such as tachycardia and bradycardia.

Note

The paramedic must consider the possibility of poisoning whenever the patient's signs and symptoms cannot be attributed to other explainable conditions (e.g. hypoglycaemia/hyperglycaemia or cardiac dysfunction).

The main goal of physical assessment of poisoned patients is to identify effects on the respiratory system, the cardiovascular system, and the central nervous system. These effects are most likely to produce immediate threats to life. A detailed history of the event and any significant medical or psychiatric history are also important. This information may help to direct treatment in the field or in the emergency department. For example, pre-existing cardiac, liver or renal disease and some psychiatric illnesses may be worsened by a toxic ingestion. These conditions may require care in addition to treating the toxic ingestion.

Respiratory complications

The first priority in managing a poisoned patient after ensuring scene safety is to secure a patent airway. The paramedic should provide adequate ventilatory support and high-concentration oxygen (unless contraindicated). More advanced airway management may be required to protect the airway and prevent aspiration (see Chapter 13). Other respiratory complications that may be associated with poisoning include the early development of non-cardiogenic pulmonary oedema or the later development of adult respiratory distress syndrome (see Chapter 14). Bronchospasm may result from direct or indirect toxic effects.

Cardiovascular complications

The most common cardiovascular complication of poisoning by ingestion is cardiac dysrhythmias. Thus, the paramedic should assess the patient's circulatory status, continually monitor it by electrocardiogram, and frequently check the patient's blood pressure. The presence of tachydysrhythmias or bradydysrhythmias may indicate serious disorders such as hypoxia and acidosis. The development of hypotension is usually associated with decreased vascular tone. Rarely, hypertension develops, which may lead to cerebral vascular haemorrhage.

Neurological complications

The paramedic should perform and record a baseline neurological examination. Deviations from a normal sensorium may range from mild drowsiness and agitation to hallucinations, seizures, coma, and death. Neurological complications may result from the toxin itself (an example of such is lead poisoning in children who have ingested paint chips), or the complications may result from a metabolic or perfusion disorder (for example, this may be poor cardiac output because of cardiac dysrhythmias).

History

The paramedic should obtain a thorough history of the exposure and any significant medical history from the patient, family members, or bystanders. This information may be unreliable (as in cases involving paediatric patients, drug abuse or suicide attempts). However, the paramedic should determine the following if possible:

- What was ingested? (Obtain the poison container and remaining contents unless doing so poses a threat to rescuer safety).
- When was the substance(s) ingested? (This may affect the decision to use activated charcoal or gastric lavage, to induce emesis, or to administer an antidote.)
- How much of the substance was ingested?
- Was an attempt made to induce vomiting? Did the patient vomit?
- Has an antidote or activated charcoal been administered?
- Does the patient have any relevant medical or psychiatric history? Has the patient had episodes of recent depression?

Gastrointestinal decontamination

The goal of managing serious poisonings that occurred by ingestion is to prevent the toxic substance from reaching the small intestine to limit its absorption. This task may be accomplished by gastrointestinal decontamination through the use of activated charcoal, and sometimes gastric lavage or syrup of ipecac. Administration of activated charcoal is not currently within the UK paramedic remit as there is a lack of published data proving efficacy and safety in the prehospital environment. Activated charcoal is discussed here for completeness in the event that future research supports its use by prehospital practitioners.

Activated charcoal

Activated charcoal is administered as a slurry which is ingested orally. It has a highly porous structure and large surface area that makes it effective in adsorbing many poisons within the gastrointestinal tract and therefore preventing systemic absorption. The effectiveness of activated charcoal in reducing drug absorption within the gastrointestinal tract is time dependent; current guidelines do not support its use beyond 1 h of drug ingestion.[2] Paramedics are most likely to reach the patient within this time frame so there is the potential for benefit if activated charcoal were to be administered by paramedics. Unless and until activated charcoal becomes part of the paramedic therapeutic regimen, paramedics should endeavour to transport patients to the emergency department within 1 h of ingestion to maximize the benefits of ED administered activated charcoal.

Activated charcoal is a safe and effective treatment for most toxic ingestions when used in the emergency department. Potential issues associated with its use by paramedics include the risk of vomiting and subsequent charcoal aspiration, potential delays on scene, and the problems associated with cleaning of vomitus in the vehicle. Activated charcoal is not administered when strong acid, strong alkali or ethanol is the toxicant. Other agents not well adsorbed by activated charcoal include cyanide, ferrous sulphate and methanol. If these substances have been ingested, activated charcoal probably should not be given. Activated charcoal comes mixed in an aqueous solution with or without a cathartic (a cathartic is an agent that causes bowel evacuation), which decreases the transit time and expels the charcoal within a short period. Complications of this therapy include poor patient acceptance in consuming the charcoal and the risk of vomiting. In the event that paramedics are permitted to administer activated charcoal they should protect themselves, the patient, and the immediate area from being stained by the activated charcoal. The paramedic should use personal protective measures when administering this agent.

Critical Thinking

Why might a patient be reluctant to take activated charcoal?

Gastric lavage

Gastric lavage is a method of gastrointestinal decontamination that has the advantage of immediate recovery of a portion of gastric contents. This is the case, at least, if gastric lavage is done within 1 h after ingestion while the contents are still in the stomach. As with activated charcoal, paramedics should recognize the benefit of transporting a patient to hospital within 1 h to maximize the benefits of gastric lavage.

Management of specific ingested poisons

Specific ingested poisons discussed in this section include strong acids and alkalis, hydrocarbons, methanol, ethylene glycol, isopropanol, metals (iron, lead and mercury), and poisons from food and plants. Few effective antidotes are available for ingested poisons. Thus, managing the patient's symptoms and preventing absorption are the main goals in caring for the poisoned patient (Table 21-1).

Strong acids and alkalis

Strong acids and alkalis include those found in toilet bowl cleaners, rust remover, ammonia and most liquid drain cleaners (Box 21-2). These acids and alkalis may cause burns to the mouth, pharynx, oesophagus, and sometimes the upper respiratory and gastrointestinal tracts. Perforation of

Table 21-1 Antidotes to common toxins

Toxin	Antidote
Paracetamol	*N*-acetylcysteine
Anticholinergic agents	Physostigmine
Benzodiazepines	Flumazenil
Beta-blockers	Glucagon
Calcium channel blockers	Calcium
Cyanide	Amyl nitrate, sodium nitrate, sodium thiosulphate
Cyclic antidepressants	Bicarbonate
Digoxin	Digoxin immune Fab
Iron	Deferoxamine
Methanol	Ethanol
Opiates	Naloxone
Organophosphates	Atropine, pralidoxime

Box 21-2

Common acid and alkali substances

Acids

Acetic acid
Battery acid
Bleach disinfectants
Hydrochloric acid
Metal cleaners
Phenol
Sulphuric acid
Swimming pool cleaners
Toilet bowl cleaners

Alkalis

Ammonia
Bleach
Disk (button) batteries
Drainpipe and toilet bowl cleaners
Hair dyes and tints
Jewellery cleaners
Metal cleaners or polishes
Paint removers
Sodium or potassium hydroxide (lye)
Washing powders

the oesophagus or stomach may result in vascular collapse, mediastinitis (inflammation of the mediastinum), or pneumoperitoneum (air or gas in the peritoneal cavity of the abdomen).

The ingestion of caustic and corrosive substances generally produces immediate damage to the mucous membrane and the intestinal tract. Acids generally complete their damage within 1–2 min. Alkali, however, particularly solid alkali, may continue to cause liquefaction of tissue and damage for minutes to hours. Prehospital care is usually limited to airway and ventilatory support, intravenous fluid replacement, and rapid transport to an appropriate medical facility.

In cases of swallowed caustics and petroleum products, JRCALC[3] recommends the dilution of the product by oral administration of milk on scene wherever possible. Efforts to neutralize the ingested agent with other fluids such as fruit juice, lemon juice or vinegar are contraindicated. These fluids have the potential to induce intense heat-releasing (exothermic) reactions so may produce severe thermal burns.

Critical Thinking

What is a risk of administering milk or water to a patient with this type of ingestion?

Hydrocarbons

Hydrocarbons are a group of saturated and unsaturated compounds that are derived mainly from crude oil, coal or plant sources. Mixtures vary in their viscosity (resistance to flow) and in their volatility (ability to vaporize). These two attributes, along with other factors, determine the toxic effects of these agents. (Some of these other factors include surface tension, the presence of other chemicals in the product, total amount, and route of exposure.)

Hydrocarbons are found in many household products, including cleaning and polishing agents, spot removers, paints, cosmetics, pesticides, and hobby and craft materials. Baby oil is a hydrocarbon that is particularly dangerous if ingested. Hydrocarbons are also found in petroleum distillates (turpentine, kerosene, gasoline, lighter fluids, and pine oil products). In addition, a large group of halogenated hydrocarbons (carbon tetrachloride, trichloromethane, trichloroethylene, methyl chloride) and aromatic hydrocarbons (toluene, xylene, benzene) exist. Hydrocarbon poisonings are common, accounting for 7% of all ingestions in children under 5 years of age.[4]

The most important physical characteristic in the potential toxicity of ingested hydrocarbons is its viscosity. The lower the viscosity (the thinner the liquid), the higher the risk of aspiration and associated complications. For example, an ingested hydrocarbon product with a low viscosity, such as petrol or turpentine, rapidly spreads over the surface of the mouth and throat. The more volatile components become gases on contact with the warm mucous membranes. This exposure causes irritation, coughing, and possible aspiration. If aspiration occurs, it may allow a toxic amount of hydrocarbons to enter the lungs. Hydrocarbons with high viscosity (e.g. asphalt, grease, tar) are not aspirated or absorbed in the gastrointestinal tract, thus they do not have significant toxicity.

The clinical features of hydrocarbon ingestion vary widely depending upon the type of agent involved (Box 21-3). If the patient is not displaying symptoms on EMS arrival, the chances of serious complications are usually low. These patients are generally observed in the emergency department for several hours and often require no treatment. However, any patient suspected of hydrocarbon ingestion who coughs, chokes, cries or has spontaneous emesis on swallowing

Box 21-3

Clinical features of hydrocarbon ingestion

Immediate: up to 6 h

Gastrointestinal system
Abdominal pain
Belching
Irritation
Mucous membrane hyperaemia
Nausea and vomiting

Respiratory system
Cough and choking
Cyanosis
Dyspnoea
Inspiratory stridor
Tachypnoea

Neurological system
Coma
Fever
Lethargy
Malaise
Seizures
Systemic factors

Delayed: days to weeks

Gastrointestinal system
Diarrhoea
Hepatic toxicity

Respiratory system
Atelectasis
Bacterial pneumonia
Dyspnoea
Haemolytic and aplastic anaemias
Pulmonary oedema
Spontaneous haemorrhage
Sputum production
Systemic factors

should be assumed to have aspirated the hydrocarbon until proven otherwise. Hydrocarbon ingestion may involve the patient's respiratory, gastrointestinal, and neurological systems. The clinical features may be immediate or delayed. Emergency care for symptomatic patients who have ingested hydrocarbon products includes the following:

1. Ensure a patent airway. Provide adequate ventilatory and circulatory support as needed.
2. Identify the substance. Contact NPIS if required.
3. Initiate intravenous fluid therapy if required.
4. Monitor cardiac rhythm.
5. Transport the patient for physician evaluation.

Critical Thinking

Will the potential lethal effects of this ingestion always be visible on the scene?

Methanol

Methanol (wood alcohol) is a common industrial solvent and is obtained from the distillation of wood. Methanol is a poisonous alcohol found in a variety of products, including windscreen washer fluid, paints, paint removers, varnishes, canned fuels and many types of shellac (traditional wood finish). Methanol is a colourless liquid and has an odour that is distinct from that of ethanol, the form of alcohol in alcoholic beverages. Poisonings may result from intentional or unintentional ingestions, absorption through the skin, or inhalation. Examples include deliberate use of the agent by chronic alcohol-dependent people to maintain an inebriated state, unintentional ingestion resulting from misuse or distribution of methanol for ethanol (as in contraband liquor), and accidental ingestions in children.

Methanol itself is no more toxic than ethanol; however, its metabolites are extremely toxic. As the alcohol is absorbed, it is rapidly converted in the liver to formaldehyde. Within minutes the formaldehyde is converted to formic acid, causing massive metabolic acidosis. The accumulation of formic acid in the blood results in a group of symptoms relating to the CNS (depression), the gastrointestinal tract (pain, nausea, vomiting), the eyes (as little as 4 mL can cause blindness), and the development of metabolic acidosis. The onset of symptoms after ingestion ranges from 40 min to 72 h.

Critical Thinking

Do you think this could have been the origin of the expression 'blind drunk'?

The symptoms of methanol poisoning correlate with the degree of acidosis and may include the following:

- CNS depression
  - lethargy
  - confusion
  - coma
  - seizures
- Gastrointestinal tract
  - nausea and vomiting
  - abdominal pain
- Visual complaints
  - photophobia
  - blurred or indistinct vision
  - pupils that are dilated and sluggish to react to light
  - 'spots before the eyes'
  - 'snow-filled vision'
  - blindness
- Metabolic acidosis
  - shortness of breath
  - tachypnoea
  - shock
  - multisystem failure
  - death.

Emergency care for methanol poisoning

1. Supportive care: Secure a patent airway. Provide adequate ventilatory and circulatory support as needed. Adequate ventilation is essential to ensure adequate oxygenation, help correct the profound metabolic acidosis, and maximize respiratory excretion. Establish an intravenous line. The patient should be placed on a cardiac monitor to detect rhythm disturbances.
2. Correction of metabolic acidosis cannot be achieved by paramedics as it may require gastrointestinal decontamination, sodium bicarbonate administration, and possibly haemodialysis. Rapid transportation to hospital for physician evaluation is indicated.

Ethylene glycol

Ethylene glycol is a colourless, odourless, water-soluble liquid. Ethylene glycol is commonly used in windscreen de-icers, detergents, paints, radiator antifreeze and coolants. The accidental ingestion of ethylene glycol is common in young children because of the brilliant colours added to these preparations. Ingestion is also common due to the widespread availability of products containing ethylene glycol and the warm, sweet taste. The agent is commonly misused by alcohol-dependent people as a substitute for ethanol. Ethylene glycol poisoning occurs with ingestion of approximately 1–1.5 mL of the substance per kilogram, which is about 100 mL for adults although a dose of as little as 30 mL has been shown to be fatal.[5]

Early signs and symptoms of CNS depression are usually caused by the ethanol-like effects of ethylene glycol. However, toxicity from ethylene glycol, as from methanol, is caused by the build-up of glycolic and oxalic acids after metabolism. This build-up occurs mainly in the liver and kidneys and may affect the CNS and cardiopulmonary and renal systems. These acids also cause the development of hypocalcaemia (from the precipitation of oxalic acid as calcium oxalate). The signs and symptoms of ethylene glycol poisoning generally occur in three stages:

1. Stage one: CNS effects occurring 1 to 12 h after ingestion
   Slurred speech
   Ataxia (impaired ability to coordinate movement)
   Somnolence (condition of being sleepy)
   Nausea and vomiting
   Focal or generalized convulsions
   Hallucinations
   Stupor
   Coma
2. Stage two: Cardiopulmonary system effects occurring 12–36 h after ingestion
   Rapidly progressive tachypnoea
   Cyanosis
   Pulmonary oedema
   Cardiac failure
3. Stage three: Renal system effects occurring 24–72 h after ingestion
   Flank pain
   Cluster of urological symptoms (oliguria, crystalluria, proteinuria, anuria, haematuria, uraemia).

Critical Thinking

For what could the effects in stage one of ethylene glycol poisoning be mistaken?

Emergency care for ethylene glycol poisoning is similar to that used for methanol poisoning. The care includes the following:

1. Ensure a patent airway and provide adequate ventilatory and circulatory support as needed. Monitor the patient for dysrhythmias.
2. Consider intravenous fluid therapy to help maintain adequate urine output.
3. Anticipate the use of diazepam to control seizure activity.
4. Use of gastric lavage is indicated if the patient is seen within 1 h after ingestion, and activated charcoal has been shown to decrease gastrointestinal absorption of ethylene glycol by 50%. If possible, transport patient to hospital within 1 h to maximize the benefit of these interventions.
5. Definitive treatment may include haemodialysis and ethanol administration.

Isopropanol

Isopropanol (isopropyl alcohol) is a volatile, flammable, colourless liquid. It has a characteristic odour and bitter-sweet taste. Isopropanol is used in disinfectants, degreasers, cosmetics, industrial solvents, and cleaning agents. Common routes of toxic exposure to isopropanol include intentional ingestion as a substitute for ethanol, accidental ingestion, and inhalation of high concentrations of local vapour. Isopropanol is more toxic than ethanol but is less toxic than methanol or ethylene glycol. Fatalities have occurred after ingestion of 240 mL (70% isopropyl alcohol), although patients have survived ingestion of up to 1 L with supportive care.[6] In children, any amount of ingestion should be considered potentially toxic.

After ingestion, the majority of isopropanol (80%) is converted to acetone; the rest is excreted unchanged by the kidneys. The acetone is excreted by the kidneys and to a lesser extent by the lungs. Isopropanol poisoning affects several body systems, including the central nervous, gastrointestinal, and renal systems. The signs and symptoms often occur within 30 min after ingestion and include CNS and respiratory depression (isopropanol is two to three times more potent a CNS depressant than ethanol), abdominal pain, gastritis, haematemesis, and hypovolaemia. Isopropanol poisoning causes acids to build up in the blood (acetonaemia) and ketones to build up in the urine (ketonuria). However, no associated metabolic acidosis usually occurs unless the patient develops hypotension.

Emergency care for isopropanol poisoning is mainly supportive. Care includes airway and ventilatory support to ensure adequate respiratory elimination of acetone, fluid resuscitation as needed, and rapid transport to an appropriate medical facility, where dialysis may be necessary.

Metals

Infants and children are high-risk groups for unintentional iron, lead, and mercury poisoning. Their immature immune systems and increased absorption as a function of age contribute to this risk.

Iron poisoning

About 10% of the ingested iron (mainly ferrous sulphate) is absorbed each day from the small intestine. After absorption, the iron is converted and is stored in iron storage protein and then transported to the liver, spleen, and bone marrow for incorporation into haemoglobin. When ingested iron exceeds the ability of the body to store it, the free iron circulates in the blood and is deposited into other tissues. Most iron poisonings result from the ingestion of paediatric multivitamins by children less than 6 years of age.[7]

Unintentional or intentional ingestion of iron may be fatal. Ingested iron is corrosive to the lining of the gastrointestinal tract, so may produce gastrointestinal haemorrhage, bloody vomitus, painless bloody diarrhoea, and dark stools. Severe cases involve the ingestion of more than 20 mg/kg. In such cases, iron toxicity can produce cardiovascular collapse and death 12 to 48 h after ingestion.

Prehospital care includes supportive measures and rapid transport for physician evaluation and possible gastrointestinal decontamination to prevent further absorption. The use of activated charcoal generally is not recommended because it adsorbs iron poorly. Most patients with iron poisoning survive the episode and the long-term prognosis is favourable.

Lead poisoning

Metallic lead has been used by human beings for more than 5000 years and was widely used in paints until legislation recognizing the toxicity of lead paints was first introduced in 1921. Lead use in paint was severely curtailed in the 1960s although some use did continue until the 1980s. Some lead paints are still available for restoration purposes but their production, distribution and use are tightly regulated (Box 21-4). Children are the most common victims of lead poisoning, which may result from ingestion of lead-based paint chips and contaminated house dust. Lead toxicity in adults most commonly results from exposure by inhalation. If not detected early, children with high levels of lead in their bodies can suffer from damage to the brain and nervous system, behavioural and learning problems, hyperactivity, slowed growth, hearing problems and headaches. Even children who appear healthy can have dangerous levels of lead in their bodies. Adults can suffer from a number of problems, including the following:

- difficulties during pregnancy
- reproductive problems
- hypertension
- gastrointestinal disorders
- nerve disorders
- memory and concentration problems
- muscle and joint pain.

Most lead poisoning is slow in onset (from chronic ingestion or inhalation), eventually resulting in toxicity. The metal is excreted by the body slowly. Lead tends to accumulate in body tissues (mainly bone). Lead causes the most significant pathophysiology in the haematopoietic, neurological and renal systems; however, it also affects the reproductive, gastrointestinal, skeletal, hepatic and cardiovascular systems. Signs and symptoms of chronic exposure generally are non-specific and may include malaise, mental disturbances, incoordination, abdominal pain, diarrhoea and vomiting. If the intoxication is acute, anaemia, weakness or paralysis of the limbs, seizures and death may result. (If symptoms progress to include seizure and coma, the risk of death is high. Patients who survive are likely to sustain brain damage.) Prehospital care is focused on recognizing the potential for lead poisoning and transporting the patient for physician evaluation.

Box 21-4

Places where lead can be found

- Homes in the city, country, or suburbs
- Apartments, single-family homes, and private and public housing painted before the 1960s are most likely
- Soil around a home (soil contaminated from exterior paint, or other sources such as past use of leaded petrol in cars)
- Painted windows and window sills
- Doors and door frames
- Stairs, railings, and banisters
- Porches and fences
- Paint surfaces that have been scraped, dry-sanded, or heated (lead dust)
- Old painted toys and furniture
- The air after vacuuming or sweeping contaminated surfaces
- Food and liquid stored in lead crystal or lead-glazed pottery or porcelain
- Lead smelters or other industries
- Hobbies that use lead (e.g. making pottery or stained glass)
- Folk remedies (greta or azarcon used to treat an upset stomach)

Critical Thinking

Paramedics play a key role in the emergency management of lead poisoning. What other role can they play in the management of this problem?

Mercury poisoning

Mercury is the only metallic element that is liquid at room temperature. Mercury is used in thermometers, sphygmomanometers, and dental amalgam (dental fillings). Various compounds of mercury are also used in some paints, pesticides, cosmetics, drugs, and in certain industrial processes. All forms of mercury (except dental amalgam) are poisonous. Some, though, are absorbed into the body more readily than are others, thus are more dangerous.

Liquid mercury is highly volatile. Inhalation of mercury vapour is the most common route of this poisoning as mercury vapour is readily absorbed into the body via the lungs. It may cause shortness of breath and lung damage. Mercury may also be absorbed through the skin (causing severe inflammation) or intestines after ingestion (causing nausea, vomiting, diarrhoea, and abdominal pain). After mercury enters the body, it passes into the bloodstream and later builds up in various organs (mainly the brain and kidneys). This causes a wide range of symptoms that may include the following:

- malaise
- incoordination
- excitability
- tremors
- numbness in the limbs
- vision impairment
- nausea and emesis (symptoms of renal failure)
- mental status changes.

The prehospital care is mainly supportive. Following physician evaluation, patients are managed with gastrointestinal decontamination (if the ingestion was recent) and chelating agents (these chemically bind with mercury to form a complex). In severe cases, haemodialysis may be indicated.

Food poisoning

Food poisoning is a term used for any illness of sudden onset (usually associated with stomach pain, vomiting and diarrhoea) suspected of being caused by food eaten within the previous 48 h. Food poisoning can be classified as infectious (resulting from bacteria or virus), or non-infectious (from toxins or pollutants). Some foods can cause poisoning of either type; for example, shellfish such as mussels, clams and oysters may be contaminated by viruses or bacteria or by toxins or chemical pollutants in water.

Infectious (bacterial) types

One of the common types of bacteria responsible for food poisoning is *Salmonella*. This organism is found in many animals (especially poultry) and in human beings. *Salmonella* bacteria may be transferred to food from the excrement of infected animals or human beings or by food handling by an infected person. Other bacteria (e.g. strains of staphylococcal bacteria) cause formation of toxins. These toxins may be hard to destroy even with thorough cooking. Other bacteria that commonly cause diarrhoea are certain strains of *Escherichia coli* (traveller's diarrhoea) and *Campylobacter* and *Shigella* organisms.

Botulism is a rare but life-threatening form of food poisoning. It may result from eating improperly canned or preserved food that is contaminated with the bacterium *Clostridium botulinum*. This organism is found in soil and untreated water in most parts of the world, and is also harmlessly present in the intestinal tracts of many animals, including fish. Its spore-forming properties resist boiling, salting, smoking, and some forms of pickling. This allows the bacterium to thrive in improperly preserved or canned foods.

Botulinal toxin has the potential to be a biological weapon because it is made by a living organism (see Chapter 45). Botulism is associated with severe CNS symptoms that appear in a characteristic head-to-toe progression: headache, blurred or double vision, dysphagia, respiratory paralysis and quadriplegia. Death from respiratory failure occurs in about 70% of untreated cases. Pseudomembranous colitis (associated with long-term administration of certain antibiotics) is another life-threatening form of diarrhoea. It is often caused by *C. difficile*.

Infectious (viral) types

Two viruses often associated with food poisoning are the norovirus virus (common contaminant of shellfish) and the rotavirus. These agents may be responsible for illness when raw or partly cooked foodstuffs have been in contact with water contaminated by human excrement.

Non-infectious types

Non-infectious types of food poisoning may result from consuming mushrooms and toadstools. Food poisoning can also result from eating fresh foods and vegetables that are accidentally contaminated with large amounts of insecticide. Chemical food poisoning may result from eating food stored in a contaminated container (for example, this may be a container that was previously used to store poison). Chemical food poisoning may result from improperly preparing and cooking various exotic foods as well. Drugs or medications can also cause diarrhoea. Quinidine, certain antacids, some antibiotics, and stool softeners or laxatives may cause diarrhoea.

Management guidelines

The onset of signs and symptoms from food poisoning varies by cause and by how heavily the food was contaminated. As a rule, symptoms usually develop within 30 min in the case of chemical poisoning, 1–12 h in the case of bacterial toxins, and 12–48 h with viral and bacterial infections. General principles of the management for patients with suspected food poisoning include the following:

- Use precautions to avoid contamination of self and equipment.
- Ensure adequate airway, ventilatory, and circulatory support.
- Gather a complete history. This should include time and onset of symptoms, recent travel, the relation of symptoms to ingestion of a particular food, and effects on others who ate the same food. In addition, the paramedic should obtain information on the consistency, frequency, and odour of stool (including the presence of mucus or blood). Fever should be noted as well. Any patient history should include significant medical history, allergies, and use of medications.
- Consider intravenous therapy with a crystalloid solution in the presence of dehydration resulting from vomiting and diarrhoea.
- Transport the patient for physician evaluation.

Plant poisoning

Toxic plant ingestion is a frequently reported category of poisonings, second only to ingestion of cleaning substances.[3] The majority of these exposures occur in children under 6 years of age.

Critical Thinking

What features of a plant would make it attractive for children to eat?

Signs and symptoms

The signs of toxicity following the ingestion of major poisonous plants are predictable. They are categorized by the chemical and physical properties of the plant. Most signs and symptoms tend to be consistent with the type of major toxic chemical component in the plant; however, some differences exist. For example, anticholinergic crisis may result from ingestion of plants with certain alkaloid components (deadly nightshade). This produces tachycardia; dilated pupils; hot, dry skin; decreased bowel sounds; altered vision; and abnormal mental status. Cholinergic symptoms may result from the ingestion of certain mushroom species. This produces bradycardia, miosis, salivation, hyperactive bowel sounds, and diarrhoea. Nicotinic alkaloids (poison hemlock and delphinium) may at first act as stimulants, yet this is usually soon followed by depression and weakness. Most signs and symptoms appear within several hours after ingestion, but some symptoms may be delayed 1 to 3 days. Box 21-5 lists common poisonous plants. Paramedics should be familiar with common poisonous plant life in their response area.

Management

Several hundred species of green plants and several varieties of mushrooms in the UK contain toxic compounds. Identification of the plant is useful whenever possible but the inability to do so should not delay management. The paramedic could consult with the NPIS regarding appropriate emergency care but general principles of poison management also hold true for toxic plant ingestion:

1. Ensure adequate airway, ventilatory, and circulatory support.
2. Initiate intravenous fluid therapy as required.
3. Monitor the patient's vital signs and cardiac rhythm.
4. Obtain a sample of the suspected plant or mushroom (if possible).
5. Transport the patient for physician evaluation. Most patients are hospitalized for observation and treatment as indicated for the toxin involved. Dialysis has not been shown to be effective in removing most plant toxins.

Box 21-5

Common poisonous plants, trees and shrubs

House plants

Dieffenbachia
Hyacinth
Mistletoe
Narcissus
Oleander
Poinsettia

Flower-garden plants

Daffodil
Foxglove
Iris
Larkspur
Lily of the valley

Ornamental plants

Azaleas
Daphne
Jasmine
Rhododendron
Wisteria

Other plants

Buttercups
Nightshade
Water and poison hemlock

Trees and shrubs

Elderberry
Oaks
Wild and cultivated cherries

Poisoning by inhalation

The unintentional or intentional inhalation of poisons can lead to a life-threatening emergency. The type and location of injury caused by toxic inhalation depend on the specific actions and behaviours of the chemical involved.[8] Respiratory difficulty may not appear for several hours after exposure to toxic fumes and smoke, so all patients should be encouraged to be evaluated by a physician, including those who are asymptomatic.

Physical properties

The concentration of a chemical in the air and the duration of exposure help to determine the severity of inhalation injury. At low concentrations and with brief exposure, the chemical may be removed from the air before reaching the lungs. In contrast, large concentrations or prolonged exposure are more likely to cause contact with the lungs, which in turn is more likely to cause damage to lung tissue. As a rule, increasing the concentration of the chemical or the length of exposure increases the dose received.

Solubility of the inhaled chemical affects the amount of inhalation injury. For example, water-soluble chemicals such as chlorine and anhydrous ammonia can be converted to hydrochloric acid and ammonium hydroxide, respectively, when they contact moisture in the respiratory tract. This produces injury in the nasopharynx, oropharynx and conducting airways. In contrast, water-insoluble chemicals such as phosgene and nitrogen dioxide may have little effect on the upper airways but can produce severe damage to the alveoli and respiratory bronchioles.

Chemicals may be inhaled as gases and vapours, mists, fumes or particles. Gases and vapours mix with air and distribute themselves freely throughout the lung and its airways. Mists are liquid droplets dispersed in air and their toxic effects depend on droplet size (the larger the size, the greater the exposure). Fumes contain fine particles of dust dispersed in air. Large particles are likely to be trapped in the nasopharynx and conducting airways, whereas small particles (1–5 mm) are more likely to penetrate the lower airways.

Chemical properties

The ability of a chemical to interact with other chemicals and body tissue is called its reactivity. As a rule, highly reactive chemicals cause more severe and rapid injury than less-reactive chemicals. Four potential properties of chemicals that determine reactivity are the following:

1. *Chemical pH*: The likelihood for severe injury from alkaloid or acid exposure increases as the pH approaches its extremes: a pH of less than 2 for acidic substances and greater than 11.5 for alkaline substances.
2. *Direct-acting potential of chemicals*: Direct-acting chemicals are capable of producing injury without first being transformed or changed. An example is hydrofluoric acid, which causes severe corrosive burns on contact with mucous membranes of the upper airways.
3. *Indirect-acting potential of chemicals*: Indirect-acting chemicals must be transformed before they can produce injury. An example is phosgene. This is a gas that may cause acidic burns of the alveolar membranes after conversion to hydrogen chloride. (This process may take up to several hours.)
4. *Allergic potential of chemicals*: Some reactive chemicals bind with proteins to form structures that stimulate allergic reactions. For example, formaldehyde can cause severe asthmatic and anaphylactic reactions after even a small exposure. In general, the allergic potential of a chemical is related to its reactivity.

Critical Thinking

Do you think that situations involving toxic gas inhalation are likely to involve one patient or multiple patients? Why?

Classifications

Toxic gases can be classified in three categories: simple asphyxiants, chemical asphyxiants, and irritants/corrosives. Simple asphyxiants (methane, propane and inert gases) cause toxicity by displacing or lowering the amount of oxygen in the air. Chemical asphyxiants (carbon monoxide and cyanide) possess built-in systemic toxicity, which appears after absorption into the circulation. Irritants/corrosives (chlorine and ammonia) cause cellular destruction and inflammation as they come into contact with moisture.

General management

The general principles of managing patients who have inhaled poisons are the same as for any other hazardous materials incident (see Chapters 43 and 45). These principles include the following:

1. Scene safety.
2. Personal protective measures (protective clothing and appropriate respiratory protective apparatus).
3. Rapid removal of the patient from the poison environment.
4. Surface decontamination.
5. Adequate airway, ventilatory, and circulatory support.
6. Initial assessment and physical examination.
7. Irrigation of the eyes (as needed).
8. Intravenous line with a saline solution.
9. Regular monitoring of vital signs and cardiac rhythm by electrocardiogram.
10. Rapid transport to an appropriate medical facility.

Management of specific inhaled poisons

The specific inhaled poisons discussed in this section include cyanide, ammonia and hydrocarbons. Carbon monoxide poisoning is described in Chapter 30. Other gases associated with atmospheres with low oxygen levels and chemical and biological warfare are discussed in Chapters 43 and 45.

Cyanide

Cyanide refers to any of a number of highly toxic substances that contain the cyanogen chemical group. Because of its toxicity, cyanide has few applications although it is sometimes used in industry in electroplating, ore extraction, fumigation of buildings, and as a fertilizer. Cyanide has been used in gas chambers as a means of execution. Cyanide is one of the products of combustion from burning many products, including nylon and polyurethane, thus it is a hazard in fire environments.

Cyanide poisoning is rare but may result from the inhalation of cyanide gas; ingestion of cyanide salts, nitriles or cyanogenic glycosides (e.g. amygdalin, a substance found in the seeds of cherries, apples, pears and apricots, and the principal constituent of Laetrile); or the infusion of nitroprusside. Cyanide can also be absorbed across the skin. Regardless of the route of entry, cyanide is a rapidly acting poison that combines and reacts with ferric ions (Fe^{3+}) of the respiratory enzyme cytochrome oxidase to inhibit cellular oxygenation. The cytotoxic hypoxia produces a rapid progression of symptoms from dyspnoea to paralysis, unconsciousness and death (Box 21-6). Large doses are usually fatal within minutes from respiratory arrest.

After ensuring personal safety, emergency care for a patient with cyanide poisoning begins with securing an open airway and providing adequate ventilatory support with

Box 21-6

Early and advanced signs and symptoms of cyanide poisoning

Early effects

Agitation
Anxiety
Confusion
Dyspnoea
Hypertension with reflex bradycardia

Advanced effects

Acidosis
Dysrhythmias
Hypotension (may become intractable)
Lactic acidosis
Pulmonary oedema
Seizures
Coma

high-concentration oxygen. Oxygen displaces cyanide from cytochrome oxidase and increases the effectiveness of drug administration. If the poisoning occurred in an industrial setting, cyanide 'kits' containing dicobalt edentate should be available; these should be transported with the patient and not administered by the paramedic. If dicobalt edentate has been administered by medical personnel prior to EMS arrival, the paramedic should be aware of the potential for hypotension, tachycardia and vomiting.

Prehospital care for patients with cyanide poisoning includes:

1. Don personal protective equipment as needed. This will help to prevent rescuer contamination.
2. Remove the patient from the cyanide source. Rapid decontamination and removal of the patient's contaminated clothing is key.
3. Ensure a patent airway and provide adequate ventilatory support.
4. Administer high-concentration oxygen.
5. Initiate intravenous fluid therapy as required.
6. Closely monitor blood pressure and cardiac rhythm.
7. Rapidly transport the patient for physician evaluation.

Note

Hypotension should be anticipated as a side effect of antidote therapy. The patient should remain lying down, if possible, and the blood pressure must be monitored closely.

Ammonia inhalation

Ammonia is a toxic irritant that causes local pulmonary complications after inhalation. Exposure to ammonia vapours results in inflammation and irritation and, in severe cases, destruction of the mucosal tissue of all respiratory structures. This occurs when the ammonia vapour combines with water to create a highly caustic alkaline compound. Patients usually develop coughing, choking, congestion, burning and tightness in the chest, and a feeling of suffocation. These respiratory symptoms often go together with burning eyes and lacrimation. In severe cases, bronchospasm and pulmonary oedema may develop. In addition to the general management principles, emergency care may include positive-pressure ventilation and the administration of bronchodilators.

Hydrocarbon inhalation

The hydrocarbons that pose the greatest risk for injury have low viscosity, high volatility and high surface tension or adhesion of molecules along a surface. These characteristics allow hydrocarbons to enter the pulmonary tree, which causes aspiration pneumonitis. Inhalation of hydrocarbons creates the potential for systemic effects such as CNS depression and liver, kidney, or bone marrow toxicity.

Most hydrocarbon inhalations result from 'recreational use' of halogenated hydrocarbons (e.g. carbon tetrachloride and methylene chloride) or aromatic hydrocarbons (e.g. benzene and toluene). These agents may produce a state of inebriation or euphoria through 'sniffing' or 'huffing'. (These involve placing the solvent on a rag and inhaling the vapours through a plastic bag). The onset of these effects is usually rapid (typically occurring within seconds). It may be followed by CNS depression, respiratory failure, or cardiac dysrhythmias. Other signs and symptoms of hydrocarbon inhalation include the following:

- burning sensation on swallowing
- nausea and vomiting
- abdominal cramps
- weakness
- anaesthesia
- hallucinations
- changes in colour perception
- blindness
- seizures
- coma.

Emergency care for hydrocarbon inhalation is generally supportive and includes airway, ventilatory, and circulatory support; intravenous fluid therapy; vital sign and electrocardiogram monitoring; and transport for physician evaluation.

Poisoning by injection

Human poisonings from injection may result from drug misuse or abuse (described later in this chapter). They may also result from arthropod bites and stings, reptile bites and hazardous aquatic life. In contrast to most chemical compounds previously described, injected poisons are mixtures of many different substances. These mixtures may produce several different toxic reactions in human beings, thus the paramedic must be prepared to manage reactions in many organ systems at the same time.

Arthropod bites and stings

Arthropods are invertebrate animals with jointed legs, a segmented body, and an exoskeleton. About 900 000 species of arthropods exist throughout the world. Some arthropods bite, some sting, and a few bite and sting. Arthropod venoms are complex and diverse in their chemistry and pharmacology and may produce major toxic reactions in sensitized persons. Such reactions include anaphylaxis and upper airway obstruction. The various reactions to venoms are classified as local, toxic, systemic, and delayed[9] (Box 21-7).

Hymenoptera (wasps, bees, ants)

Hymenoptera is the name of a large, highly specialized order of insects that includes wasps, bees, and ants. Hymenoptera venom is used for defence and subjugation of prey. Medically important venoms are mixtures of protein or polypeptide toxins, enzymes, and other compounds such as histamine, serotonin, acetylcholine, and dopamine. Hymenoptera stings are most commonly inflicted on the head and neck, followed by the foot, leg, hand and arm. The mouth, pharynx and oesophagus may be stung when bees or wasps in soft drink or beer containers are swallowed accidentally.

A single wasp, bee, or ant sting in an unsensitized person usually causes instant pain followed by a wheal-and-flare

Box 21-7

Types of reactions to venoms

Local reaction

Marked and prolonged oedema at the sting site
Possible involvement of one or more neighbouring joints
Possible occurrence in the mouth or throat, producing airway obstruction
Severe local reactions that may increase the likelihood of future systemic reactions (controversial)
Symptoms that usually subside within 24 h

Toxic reaction*

Gastrointestinal disturbances
Diarrhoea
Light-headedness
Vomiting

Other symptoms
Convulsions (rare)
Oedema without urticaria
Fever
Headache
Involuntary muscle spasms
Symptoms that usually subside within 48 h
Syncope (common finding)

Systemic (anaphylactic) reaction†

Reactions that can progress to death within minutes

Immediate symptoms
Facial flushing
Generalized urticaria
Itching eyes or generalized itching

Subsequent symptoms
Bloody and frothy sputum production
Chest or throat constriction or both
Chills and fever
Cyanosis
Dyspnoea
Hypotension
Laryngeal stridor
Loss of bowel or bladder control
Loss of consciousness
Nausea and vomiting
Respiratory failure, cardiovascular collapse, or both
Shock
Wheezing

Delayed reaction‡

Serum sickness symptoms
Fever
Headache
Malaise
Polyarthritis
Urticaria

*Should be considered with a history of 10 or more stings.
†May occur in response to single or multiple stings.
‡Usually occurs 10–14 days after a sting.

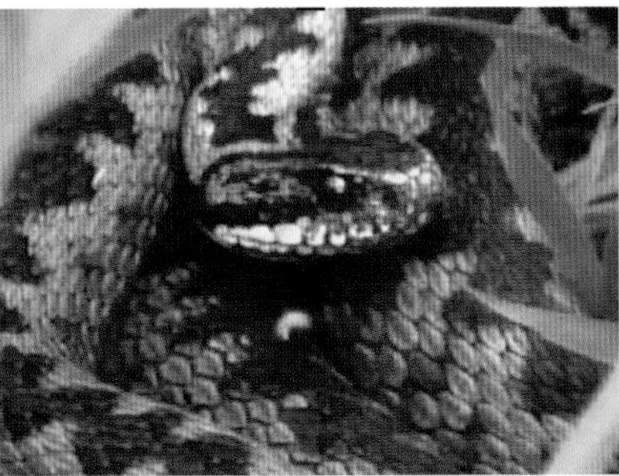

Figure 21-1 The adder.

reaction with variable oedema. Large local reactions can spread more than 15 cm beyond the sting site and can persist for more than 24 h. Anaphylaxis is the most serious complication of hymenoptera stings; in the UK, wasp and bee stings account for about 20 deaths due to anaphylaxis each year.[10] Persons with a history of allergic reactions to stings often wear medical alert identification and often carry an emergency kit that contains a preloaded syringe of adrenaline (epinephrine; Epi-Pen).

Management

The prehospital care for mild hymenoptera stings should include close watching for signs or symptoms of an allergic reaction. If an extremity is involved, immobilization and elevation of the affected extremity may shorten the duration of the reaction. If the history and physical findings are compatible with an allergic reaction, chlorphenamine should be administered in accordance with JRCALC guidelines.[3]

Honey bees (and other hymenoptera) often leave their stingers in the wound. If a stinger is present, it should be scraped or brushed off. Stingers should not be removed with forceps because squeezing the attached venom sac may worsen the injury. Severe allergic reactions should be managed as described in Chapter 18. Hypovolaemia (if present) should be treated in the conventional manner with a volume-expanding fluid.

Reptile bites

The adder (Figure 21-1) is the UK's only indigenous poisonous snake and fatalities are extremely rare (only 14 since 1876, the last being a 5-year-old in 1975).[11] Other exotic venomous snakes are kept legally by zoos, licensed individuals and research establishments, but may also be kept surreptitiously as macho pets.

Adder bites tend to occur between February and October, with peak incidence between June and August.

Adder bites

Local envenoming

Immediate sharp pain occurs followed by a sensation of tingling and local swelling that spreads proximally. Spreading pain, tenderness, inflammation (often described misleadingly as 'cellulitis', although there is no infection), and tender enlargement of regional lymph nodes are sometimes noticeable within hours. Reddish lines and bruising appear, and the whole limb may become swollen and bruised within 24 h, with involvement of the trunk and, in children, the whole body.[12]

Systemic envenoming

Dramatic anaphylactoid symptoms may appear within 5 min of the bite or may be delayed for many hours. These include nausea; retching; vomiting; abdominal colic; diarrhoea; incontinence of urine and faeces; sweating; fever; vasoconstriction; tachycardia; light-headedness; loss of consciousness; shock; angioedema of the face, lips, gums, tongue, throat, and epiglottis; urticaria; and bronchospasm.[12] These symptoms may persist or fluctuate for as long as 48 h in the absence of treatment. Hypotension is a most critical sign. It usually develops within 2 h and may resolve spontaneously, persist, recur or progress fatally.

Other exotic venomous snakes

If attending envenomation at a zoo or licensed premises, it is likely that information will be available on the action to take. If attending an incident involving an illegally owned snake, information may be less readily available. Safety is of paramount importance when dealing with this type of event and the paramedic should remain clear of the striking range of the snake (normally about the length of the snake). It is not essential to identify the snake involved but it may be helpful for later management and for obtaining advice from the NPIS.

Management of snake envenomation

Venom, like any drug or toxin, has absorption, distribution and elimination phases. Tissue damage increases as venom spreads into the lymphatics and blood. Emergency care is directed at retarding the systemic spread of the venom. Prehospital management of snake bites includes the following:

1. Stay clear of the striking range of the snake and move the patient to a safe area. If the snake has been killed before EMS arrival, it should be transported in a closed container to the emergency department with the patient. EMS personnel should make no attempt to capture or kill the snake; doing so may result in a paramedic being bitten. Identification of the snake is not absolutely necessary to manage the patient appropriately.
2. Provide adequate airway, ventilatory, and circulatory support to the patient as needed. Continually monitor vital signs and the electrocardiogram. Also establish an intravenous line in an unaffected extremity with a volume-expanding fluid on keep-open rate.
3. When practical, immobilize the bitten extremity in a neutral position. Immobilization by splinting may delay systemic absorption and may diminish local tissue necrosis. Every effort should be made to keep the patient at rest.
4. Prepare the patient for immediate transport to a proper medical facility.
5. Additional management of snake bites, such as incision and suction or use of a lymphatic-venous constriction band or pressure device, is controversial and potentially harmful. Application of ice or chemical cold packs should be avoided as their use may further damage tissue. In severe cases, administration of antivenin to neutralize the venom may be required but this is done in the hospital after the patient has been tested for allergies to the antivenin.

Critical Thinking

What strategies can you use to calm the emotional state of a patient who has sustained a snake bite?

Hazardous aquatic life

The marine animals most likely to be involved in human poisonings in UK coastal waters are the coelenterates. The specialized venom apparatuses of these animals are used for defence and for capturing prey. In addition to venom produced by the animal, aquatic life may contain other poisonous substances as a result of toxic ingestions. Exposures to hazardous aquatic life result from recreational, industrial, scientific and military oceanic activities.

Jellyfish (part of the coelenterate family)

The most common jellyfish in the UK is the moon jellyfish, a harmless jellyfish whose poison does not penetrate human skin. Recent increases in temperature have seen a proliferation in the hazardous Lion's mane jellyfish, and reports of Portuguese Man-o'-War jellyfish washed up on the south and south-west coast of England (Figure 21-2). Those species that carry venomous stinging cells (nematocysts) are known as Cnidaria. The nematocyst is venom filled and contains a long, coiled, hollow, thread-like tube that serves as a tiny hypodermic needle. Many types of nematocysts exist; an individual coelenterate may have more than one type. The severity of envenomation is related to the toxicity of the venom (which may contain various fractions), the number of nematocysts discharged, and the physical condition of the victim.

The Portuguese Man-o'-War is the largest jellyfish and its nematocyst-bearing tentacles may be up to 33 m long (100 feet). A single envenomation may involve several hundred thousand nematocysts. A swimmer who comes into contact with the tentacles of the jellyfish may suffer enough envenomation to produce systemic signs and symptoms.

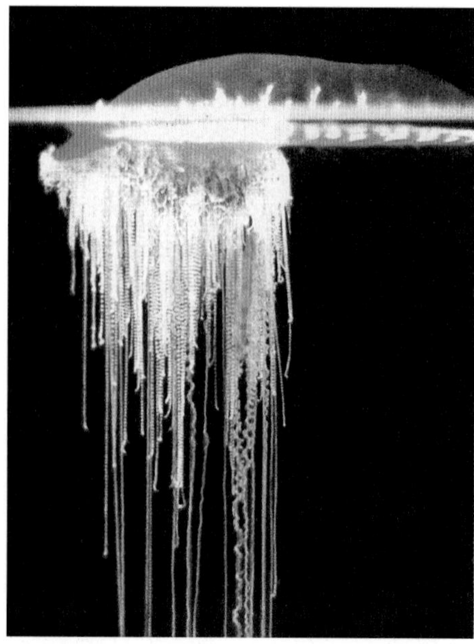

Figure 21-2 Portuguese Man-o'-War.

Nematocysts often remain embedded in the tissues of the victim. Detached tentacle fragments can retain their potency for months.

Management

Coelenterate envenomation ranges in severity from irritant dermatitis to excruciating pain, respiratory depression, anaphylaxis and life-threatening cardiovascular collapse. Envenomation is most often mild and usually characterized by stinging, paraesthesias, pruritus, and reddish-brown linear wheals or 'tentacle prints'. If a potent venom or a large body surface area is involved, systemic symptoms may include nausea, vomiting, abdominal pain, headache, bronchospasm, pulmonary oedema, hypotension and respiratory arrest. Emergency care is directed at stabilizing the patient and neutralizing the effects of the venom.

1. Stabilize the patient.
   - Provide adequate airway, ventilatory, and circulatory support as needed.
   - Continually monitor the patient's vital signs and electrocardiogram. Be prepared to provide advanced airway management if systemic reactions develop.
2. Counteract effects of the venom.
   - Remove visible tentacle fragments with forceps. Avoid touching the tentacles.
   - Immediately rinse the patient's wound with seawater. (Wet sand or freshwater usually causes the nematocysts to discharge their venom, thus are contraindicated.)
   - Continue to rinse until the pain is largely alleviated; consider analgesia in severe cases.
   - Transport the patient for physician evaluation.

Poisoning by absorption

Many poisons can be absorbed through the skin. Two compounds, organophosphates and carbamates, are responsible for a large number of skin-absorbed poisonings each year. Organophosphates and carbamates are commonly available for commercial and public use in the form of pet, home, and commercial insecticides. Organophosphates are also used in the development of military nerve agents such as sarin and soman (see Chapter 45). Because of the widespread availability of insecticides that contain organophosphate/carbamate compounds, paramedics must be aware of the nature of these chemicals, necessary precautions for personal safety, and the immediate management that may be required before symptoms or signs of illness occur.

Organophosphates and carbamates are highly toxic. In addition, they are well absorbed by ingestion, inhalation and dermal routes. Both classes have similar pharmacological actions, inhibiting the effects of acetylcholinesterase, an enzyme that degrades acetylcholine at nerve terminals. To review, acetylcholine is a cholinergic neurotransmitter for preganglionic autonomic fibres, somatic nerves to skeletal muscle, and many synapses in the CNS. When acetylcholinesterase is inhibited, acetylcholine accumulates at the synapses, resulting in a cholinergic 'overdrive'. The signs and symptoms resulting from cholinergic overdrive are seen in organophosphate and carbamate poisoning.

Box 21-8

Signs and symptoms of organophosphate or carbamate poisoning

Cardiovascular system

Bradycardia
Variable blood pressure (usually hypotensive)

Respiratory system

Bronchoconstriction
Dyspnoea
Rhinorrhoea
Wheezing

Gastrointestinal system

Cramps
Defecation
Emesis
Increased bowel sounds

Central nervous system

Anxiety
Coma
Convulsions
Dizziness
Respiratory depression

Musculoskeletal system

Fasciculations
Flaccid paralysis

Ophthalmological

Blurred vision
Lacrimation
Miosis
Rapidly changing pupil size

Skin

Diaphoresis

Other

Salivation
Urination

Signs and symptoms

Early signs and symptoms of organophosphate or carbamate poisoning may be non-specific, including headache, dizziness, weakness and nausea. As overstimulation and disruption of transmission in the central and peripheral nervous systems occur, signs and symptoms begin to develop. These signs and symptoms result from a wide range of physiological and metabolic problems (Box 21-8). The rapidity and sequence in which these signs and symptoms develop depend on the particular compound and on the amount and route of exposure. The onset of symptoms is probably quickest after inhalation. Onset is slowest (possibly delayed for several hours) after a primary skin exposure. A helpful mnemonic to recognize the signs of poisoning is SLUDGE. (This stands for salivation, lacrimation, urination, defecation, gastrointestinal upset and emesis.) Rapidly changing pupils with miosis are common with vapour exposure of organophosphates. Muscle twitching (fasciculations) can follow rapidly. Individual muscle twitching can result from liquid contact and local skin absorption at the site.

Critical Thinking

Consider a person who does not suspect poisoning. What condition might that person think he or she is suffering from with this clinical presentation?

Management

Emergency care begins with scene safety, personal protection, and decontamination procedures. The scene should be secured by qualified personnel. Personal protective actions include wearing protective clothing and using respiratory protection. The patient should be removed safely from the contaminated area as soon as possible. That way, the decontamination procedures can begin (see Chapter 43). After these measures, patient care can be started. The general principles of management for poisoning by absorption include respiratory support, drug administration, and electrocardiogram monitoring. Organophosphates and carbamates produce similar physiological effects. However, carbamates have a shorter duration of action, thus they have a more rapid decrease in their effect.

Respiratory support

Respiratory tract symptoms are usually first to appear after exposure to organophosphates or carbamates. In addition, respiratory paralysis may occur suddenly without warning. The need for advanced airway management and ventilatory support should be anticipated. Copious bronchial secretions may require suctioning; bronchoconstriction may also necessitate positive-pressure ventilation and positive end-expiratory pressure.

Drug administration

Drug therapy in organophosphate or carbamate poisoning is directed at blocking the effects of acetylcholine, separating cholinesterase from the chemical compound, and suppressing seizure activity (if present). The drugs currently used as antidotes include atropine and diazepam or lorazepam.

Drug therapy should be started only if the patient has two or more signs or symptoms of poisoning and/or respiratory distress is present.

Atropine reverses the muscarinic effects (bradycardia, bronchoconstriction, respiratory secretions and miosis) of moderate to severe organophosphate or carbamate poisoning. The drug competitively antagonizes the actions of acetylcholine, which results in a decrease in the hyperactivity of smooth muscles and glands. The drug is indicated to dry the patient's secretions and helps to decrease pulmonary resistance to ventilation. Potentially hypoxic patients may require the administration of large doses of atropine (see JRCALC guidelines). The electrocardiogram should be monitored for dysrhythmias (other than tachycardia) and supplemental oxygen should be given to minimize the risk of ventricular fibrillation. Atropine is the drug of choice for carbamate poisonings.

Note

As a rule, cholinergic poisoning causes the patient to be 'wet'. (This is manifested by profuse sweating, lacrimation, salivation, vomiting, diarrhoea and incontinence). However, anticholinergic poisoning generally causes the patient to be 'dry'. (This is manifested by dry, flushed skin, elevated temperature and urinary retention). Being keen to this 'wet vs. dry' symptomatology can be lifesaving for the poisoned patient. The wet-appearing patient will require atropine.

Diazepam may be indicated if seizures are present. The need for seizure control may arise before decontamination is complete; however, intravenous therapy should not be initiated in a patient in a contaminated area. When administering diazepam the paramedic should be alert to the risk of respiratory and CNS depression.

Critical Thinking

Consider that you give diazepam for seizures in this case. Will that eliminate the need for atropine?

Electrocardiogram monitoring

Electrocardiogram monitoring may reveal a variety of abnormalities, including idioventricular rhythms, multifocal premature ventricular contractions, ventricular tachycardia, torsades de pointes, ventricular fibrillation, complete heart block and asystole. These dysrhythmias usually occur in two phases. The first phase begins with a transient episode of intense sympathetic tone, which results in sinus tachycardia. This phase is followed by a period of extreme parasympathetic tone, which may manifest as sinus bradycardia, atrioventricular block, and ST segment and T wave abnormalities. Slow ventricular dysrhythmias that do not respond to the usual therapy may need to be treated with overdrive pacing (see Chapter 15).

SECTION II

Drug abuse

The term drug abuse refers to the use of prescription drugs for non-prescribed purposes. It also refers to the use of drugs that have no prescribed medical use (Box 21-9). Emergencies that result from drug abuse include adverse effects caused by the drug or impurities or contaminants mixed with the drug, life-threatening infections from intravenous or intradermal injection of drugs with unsterile equipment, injuries during intoxication, and drug dependence or withdrawal syndrome resulting from the habit-forming potential of many drugs (see Chapter 12).

Box 21-9

Drug abuse terminology

Drug abuse: Self-medication or self-administration of a drug in chronically excessive amounts, resulting in psychological and/or physical dependence, functional impairment, and deviation from approved social norms.

Drug dependence: Condition marked by an overwhelming desire to continue taking a drug for its desired effect, usually an altered mental activity, attitude, or outlook.

Physical dependence: An adaptive physiological state occurring after prolonged use of many drugs (discontinuation causes withdrawal syndromes that are relieved by re-administering the same drug or a pharmacologically related drug).

Psychological dependence: Emotional reliance on a drug. (Manifestations range from a mild desire for a drug to craving and drug-seeking behaviour to repeated compulsive use of a drug for its subjectively satisfying or pleasurable effects.)

Tolerance: A tendency to increase drug dosage to experience the same effect formerly produced by a smaller dose.

Withdrawal syndrome: A predictable set of signs and symptoms that occurs after a decrease in the amount of the usual dose of a drug or its sudden cessation.

Box 21-10

Illicit drug use in the United Kingdom

Prevalence of drug use: key findings from the 2002/2003 British Crime Survey

- Of all 16–59-year-olds, 12% had taken an illicit drug and 3% had used a Class A drug in the last year.
- This equates to around 4 million illicit drug users and around 1 million Class A drug users.
- Cannabis is the most frequently used drug – around 3 million 16–59-year-olds have used it in the last year (11%).
- People aged between 16 and 24 years are more likely than older people to have used drugs in the last year and in the last month – 28% had used at least one illicit drug in the last year.
- The use of Class A drugs in the last year among 16–24-year-olds has remained stable since 1996. Around 8% had used a Class A drug in the last year.
- Use of amphetamines and LSD in the last year has decreased and cocaine is the only drug where use has increased. There has been a decrease in ecstasy use since 2001–2002.
- The majority of people using drugs in the last year had only used one type of drug.

No single cause or set of conditions clearly leads to drug abuse. It is widespread among all socioeconomic, cultural and ethnic groups. Drug abuse is a major medical, social, and interpersonal problem that affects persons from all backgrounds and of all ages (Box 21-10). Because of the widespread use and misuse of drugs, the paramedic should maintain a high degree of suspicion. The paramedic should consider the possibility for a drug-related problem in any patient who has seizures, behavioural changes or decreased level of consciousness. In addition, consideration of the visibility, accessibility, and careful handling of all medications carried on an EMS vehicle should be a part of any EMS policy and procedure.

Box 21-11

Common agents involved in poisoning

Paracetamol
Cardiac medications
Drugs abused for sexual purposes/sexual gratification
Hallucinogens
Lithium
Metals (iron, lead, and mercury)
Monoamine oxidase inhibitors
Non-prescription pain medicines
Opioids
Salicylates
Sedative–hypnotics
Stimulants
Tricyclic antidepressants

Critical Thinking

Why might a patient (or their friends) delay calling for help in a situation involving drug overdose?

Toxic effects of drugs

EMS personnel often encounter persons who are suffering from the toxic effects of drugs. Toxicity may be the result of an overdose, a potential suicide, polydrug administration, or an accident (accidental ingestion, miscalculation, changes in drug strength). Box 21-11 lists the drugs discussed in this chapter.

Common drugs of abuse (along with their names and uses) vary widely in different geographical areas. Also, the drugs of abuse often change over time. Table 21-2 is a partial list of common drugs of abuse, their street names, and miscellaneous terminology relating to drug use.

General management principles

The following are general principles for managing drug abuse and the overdose that may result:

1. Ensure that the scene is safe. Be prepared for unpredictable behaviour from the patient as well. (Consider the need for help from the police.)
2. Ensure adequate airway, ventilatory, and circulatory support as needed.
3. Obtain a history of the event. (This should include the self-administration of other drugs that may have been taken by another route.) Obtain any significant medical or psychiatric history as well.
4. Identify the substance. Consult with NPIS if required.
5. Perform a full, focused physical examination. Continually monitor the patient's vital functions and electrocardiogram.
6. Start intravenous therapy and administer the proper drug antidotes such as naloxone if an opiate overdose is suspected. Pay special attention to the use of personal protective gear because many of these patients are at high risk of having an infectious disease.

Table 21-2 Commonly abused drugs and their street names

Substance	Examples of street names (may vary according to location)	Medical uses	Route of administration	Drug classification
Amfetamine	Black beauties, hearts, whizz	ADHD, narcolepsy	Injected, oral, smoked, sniffed	Class B; Class A if prepared for injection
Cocaine	Coke, charlie, snow, crack, flake	Topical local anaesthetic	Snorted, injected or smoked	Class A
Methamphetamine	Crystal meth, ice, speed	ADHD	Oral, snorted or injected	Class A
LSD	Acid, blotter, drops, flash, L, micro dot, paper mushroom	None	Oral	Class A
Amanita muscaria	Magic mushrooms, Liberties, magics, mushies, liberty cap, shrooms, Amani, agaric	None	Oral	Magic mushrooms that contain psilocin or psilocybin are classified as Class A drugs
Alkyl nitrates (Poppers)	Ram, Thrust, Rock Hard, TNT, Liquid Gold	Rarely used in medicine	Inhaled	Possession is not illegal but supply can be an offence
Ecstasy	E, pills, brownies, Mitsubishi's, Rolex's, Dolphins, XTC	None	Usually swallowed – may be smoked or snorted	Class A
Ketamine	Green, K, special K, super K, vitamin K	Short-acting, powerful anaesthetic	Injected	Class C
Methadone	Mixture, meth, linctus, physeptone	Opiate substitute for heroin in treatment of heroin addiction	Usually liquid that is swallowed. Can come in tablet or injectable form	Class A
Cannabis	Bhang, black, blast, blow, blunts, Bob Hope, bush, dope, draw, ganja, grass, hash, hashish, hemp, herb, marijuana, pot, puff, Northern Lights, resin, sensi, sinsemilla, shit, skunk, smoke, soap, spliff, wacky backy, weed, zero	Currently none but suggestion of possible benefit in the management of pain for sufferers of multiple sclerosis	Normally smoked but may be drunk as a tea or eaten as 'cannabis cookies'	Class B
Gamma hydroxybutyrate	GHB, Gabba, GBH, Liquid Ecstasy	None	Oral	Class C
Heroin	Brown, skag, H, horse, gear, smack	Opiate used for analgesia	Smoked, injected or snorted	Class A
Tranquillizers	Jellies, benzos, eggs, norries, rugby balls, vallies, moggies, mazzies, roofies, downers	Treat anxiety and depression	Oral, injection or suppository	Class C
Anabolic steroids	Roids. Product names include Sustanon 250, Deca-Durabolin, Dianabol, Anavar, Stanozolol	Anaemia and muscle weakness post surgery	Oral or injection	Class C

ADHD, attention deficit hyperactivity disorder.
Refer to Chapter 12 for details regarding the Misuse of Drugs Act.
Useful website: http://www.talktofrank.com/drugs.aspx?id=170

7. Rapidly transport the patient for physician evaluation and administration of activated charcoal where indicated.

When examining any patient suspected of abusing drugs, the paramedic should always look for track marks. (These may be in the antecubital space, under the tongue or on top of the feet). 'Body packing' is concealing packets of drugs in body cavities of the stomach, rectum and vagina. 'Body stuffing' is swallowing drugs to avoid arrest. The possibility of these should be considered when a person who abuses drugs appears ill for no apparent reason.

Critical Thinking

For what illnesses is the patient who uses intravenous narcotics at risk?

Opioid overdose

In the UK in 2003, heroin accounted for just over 18% of drug-related deaths where only one drug was indicated but 38% where more than one drug was found.[13] Pure heroin is a bitter-tasting white powder that is usually adulterated or 'cut' for street distribution. Heroin is cut with various agents such as lactose, sucrose, baking soda, powdered milk, starch, magnesium silicate (talc), procaine, quinine, and recently with scopolamine. A typical 'bag' is the single-dose unit of heroin and may weigh 100 mg. On average, heroin is only 20–30% pure. Other opioid drugs include morphine, hydromorphone, methadone, meperidine, codeine, oxycodone, and 'designer opiates' that have been chemically modified such as alpha-methyl fentanyl ('China white').

Depending on the preparation, these drugs may be taken orally, injected intradermally ('skin popping') or intravenously ('mainlining'), taken intranasally ('snorted') or smoked. All opioids are CNS depressants and can cause life-threatening respiratory depression. In severe intoxication, hypotension, profound shock, and pulmonary oedema may be present. Signs and symptoms of narcotic/opiate overdose include the following:

- euphoria
- arousable somnolence ('nodding')
- nausea
- pinpoint pupils (except with meperidine, hypoxia, or in combination with other types of drugs)
- coma
- seizures.

Antidote therapy

As described in Chapter 12, naloxone is a pure opioid antagonist effective for virtually all opioid and opioid-like substances. The drug reverses the three major symptoms of opioid overdose (respiratory depression, coma and miosis). Its use should be considered when there is respiratory depression, depression of cardiac function and CNS depression associated with intentional or accidental opioid overdose, and also in unconsciousness with respiratory depression of unknown cause where opioid overdose is a possibility. The patient's behaviour may be unpredictable when the effects of the drug are reversed and the patient experiences withdrawal symptoms, so it is recommended that naloxone be given by slow injection in order to restore airway reflexes and adequate breathing without fully awakening the patient.[14] The patient should be ventilated with a bag–mask prior to naloxone administration. If the patient does not respond to treatment with naloxone, intubation should be considered. (Note: In the absence of respiratory depression, the use of naloxone is controversial; seizure activity is a possible side effect of the drug.)

Note

Two other pure opioid antagonists are available. Naltrexone is an oral medication used in long-term programmes for opioid addiction. Nalmefene appears to be as effective as naloxone in acute opioid intoxications. Moreover, nalmefene has a longer duration of action (4–8 h) than naloxone.

Some opiates (e.g. heroin) have a longer duration than naloxone. Thus the patient must be monitored closely during antidote therapy as repeated doses of naloxone may be needed. In communities where abuse of naloxone-resistant opiates or the use of China white is common, larger initial doses of naloxone may be needed. The desired signs of reversal of opiate intoxication are adequate airway reflexes and ventilations, not complete arousal.

Naloxone can cause a withdrawal syndrome in opioid-dependent patients. Slowly administer a smaller dose of naloxone for these patients. Withdrawal can usually be managed by symptomatic and supportive care. Box 21-12 lists signs and symptoms of opioid withdrawal.

Box 21-12

Signs and symptoms of opioid withdrawal

Abdominal cramps
Anorexia
Cold sweats or chills
Diaphoresis
Diarrhoea
Fever
General malaise
Gooseflesh
Insomnia
Irritability
Nausea and vomiting
Pulmonary oedema
Severe agitation
Ventricular dysrhythmias
Tachycardia
Tremors

Sedative–hypnotic overdose

Sedative–hypnotic agents include benzodiazepines and barbiturates. These drugs are usually taken orally but may be diluted and injected intravenously. Taking these drugs with alcohol greatly increases their effects. Sedative–hypnotic drugs commonly are known as downers.

Benzodiazepines are among the best-known and most widely prescribed drugs used to control symptoms of anxiety, stress and insomnia. These drugs are sometimes used to manage alcohol withdrawal and to control seizure disorders as well. They promote sleep and relieve anxiety by depressing brain function and are often abused for their sedative effects. Individually, these drugs are somewhat non-toxic though they may accentuate the effects of other sedative–hypnotic agents. Common benzodiazepines are diazepam, nitrazepam and lorazepam.

Barbiturates are general CNS depressants that inhibit impulse conduction in the brainstem. These drugs were widely used to treat anxiety and insomnia but their addictive properties and potential for abuse have led to their replacement by benzodiazepines and other non-barbiturate drugs. Barbiturates that are commonly abused include phenobarbital, amobarbital and secobarbital.

Signs and symptoms of sedative–hypnotic overdose are chiefly related to the central nervous and cardiovascular systems. Adverse effects include excessive drowsiness, staggering gait and, in some cases, paradoxical excitability. In cases of severe toxicity the patient may become comatose, with respiratory depression, hypotension and shock. The pupils may be constricted. More often, though, they become

Box 21-13

Methamphetamine

Methamphetamine has become common in America and Asia. In crystal form (ice) it can be very strong, resulting in a quick, hard hit when smoked. This can often lead to intense paranoia and a very unpleasant comedown. It has not (yet) become common in the UK but there have been reports of it being sold as speed in places like Glasgow and in some clubs. Ice tends to be sold at £25 for a large rock. Common names for methamphetamine include meth, speed, crank, crystal, water or ice.

Once methamphetamine enters the body, it can produce skeletal muscle tremors, sleeplessness, and euphoria that can last up to 10 days. During these drug-induced sleepless 'binges,' users may become hostile and paranoid. This is followed by a 'crash' (an emotionally depressed state) that can last for several days.

fixed and dilated even in the absence of significant brain damage. Airway control and ventilatory management are the most important actions in managing significant sedative–hypnotic overdose. Flumazenil is a benzodiazepine antagonist that can be used to reverse the effects of benzodiazepines. The drug, however, can produce seizure activity and is contraindicated in patients who are prone to seizures and in those with tricyclic antidepressant overdose. It is generally only used to reverse benzodiazepine effects after procedural sedation and is not available for paramedic use.

Stimulant overdose

Commonly abused stimulant drugs are those of the sympathomimetic family (e.g. amfetamine sulphate, dexamfetamine, cocaine, methamphetamine) (Box 21-13).

Sympathomimetic drugs are often used to produce general mood elevation, improve task performance, suppress appetite and prevent sleepiness. Structurally, the amphetamines are similar to catecholamines (adrenaline and noradrenaline). Yet they differ in their more pronounced effects on the CNS. Adverse effects include tachycardia, increased blood pressure, tachypnoea, agitation, dilated pupils, tremors and disorganized behaviour. In severe intoxication the patient may exhibit psychosis and paranoia and may experience hallucinations. Sudden withdrawal or cessation of amphetamine use may result in a 'crash' stage. In this stage the patient becomes depressed, suicidal, incoherent or near coma. As a rule, these drugs are taken orally but they may be smoked or injected for a more rapid onset of action. Amphetamines are commonly known as speed or uppers.

Cocaine

Cocaine is a fine, white crystalline powder and, like heroin, street forms of cocaine are usually adulterated. They vary in purity from 25% to 90%; doses vary from near 0 to 200 mg. This form of cocaine is generally taken intranasally by snorting a 'line' containing 10–35 mg of the drug (depending on purity). After absorption through the mucous membranes, the effects of the drug begin within minutes. Peak effects occur 15 to 60 min after use, with a half-life of 1 to 2½ h. Cocaine is also used parenterally by the subcutaneous, intramuscular and intravenous routes; the intravenous route provides immediate absorption and intense stimulation (peak occurs within 5 min with a half-life of about 50 min). Speed-balling refers to an injection of a cocaine–heroin combination.

Freebase 'crack' cocaine is a more potent formulation of the drug. Crack is prepared by mixing powdered street cocaine with an alkaline solution and then adding a solvent such as ether. The combination separates into two layers, with the top layer containing the dissolved cocaine. Evaporation of the solvent results in pure cocaine crystals, which are smoked and absorbed via the pulmonary route. Cocaine in this form is called rock or crack because of the popping sound produced when the crystals are heated. Freebase cocaine is combined with marijuana or tobacco and is smoked in a pipe or a cigarette. The reactions are similar to those experienced in intravenous use, with equal intensity and effects.

Cocaine is a major CNS stimulant that causes profound sympathetic discharge. The increased levels of circulating catecholamines result in excitement, euphoria, talkativeness and agitation. The effects of the drug can cause significant cardiovascular and neurological complications such as cardiac dysrhythmias, myocardial infarction, seizures, intracranial haemorrhage, hyperthermia, and psychiatric disturbances. Cocaine overdose can occur with any form of the drug and any route of administration. The adult fatal dose is thought to be about 1200 mg (1.2 g), but fatalities from cocaine-induced cardiac dysrhythmias have been reported with single doses of as little as 25–30 mg.

Prehospital management of the cocaine-intoxicated patient may be difficult. Cocaine toxicity may range from minor symptoms to life-threatening overdose. Emergency care may require a full spectrum of basic and advanced life-support measures, including aggressive airway management, ventilatory and circulatory support, drug therapy (benzodiazepines are the mainstay of treatment initially in cocaine toxicity), and rapid transport to an appropriate medical facility. Paracetamol may be indicated if the patient has an elevated body temperature, and aspirin and GTN may be administered if the patient complains of chest pain.[14]

Phencyclidine overdose

Phencyclidine (PCP) is a dissociative analgesic that was originally used as a veterinary tranquillizer. The drug is still used in the US but is uncommon in the UK. Phencyclidine has sympathomimetic and CNS stimulant and depressant properties. It is a potent psychoactive drug illegally sold in liquid, tablet or powder form to be taken orally, intranasally, intravenously/intramuscularly, or with other drugs to be smoked (a 'Sherman'). Most tablets contain about 5 mg of PCP. As a rule, PCP in its powder form is purer (50–100% PCP). Chronic use can result in permanent memory impairment and loss of higher brain functions. The pharmacological effects are dose related and can be divided into low-dose and high-dose toxicity. Ketamine is a derivative of PCP and has identical actions.

Low-dose toxicity

In low doses (less than 10 mg), PCP intoxication produces an unpredictable state that can resemble drunkenness. The user may have a sense of euphoria or confusion, disorientation, agitation or sudden rage. An intoxicated patient often has a blank stare and a stumbling gait. The patient is often in a dissociative state. The patient's pupils are generally reactive. The patient may experience flushing, diaphoresis, facial grimacing, hypersalivation and vomiting. Nystagmus with a burst-like quality is characteristic of low-dose PCP use. In this range of toxicity, death is usually related to behavioural disturbances resulting from spatial disorientation, drug-induced immobility, and insensitivity to pain. This insensitivity to pain leads to bold acts of strength because the normal muscle activity limitation resulting from pain is inhibited.

Critical Thinking

Why does this type of drug intoxication put the patient at a high risk for injury?

In low-dose toxicity, sensory stimulation should be avoided, as verbal and physical stimuli will make the clinical symptoms worse. Violent and combative patients require protection from self-injury. Safeguards must also be provided for the emergency crew and bystanders. The paramedic should monitor the patient's vital signs and level of consciousness closely, and should observe the patient for increasing motor activity and muscle rigidity as well. These may precede seizures.

High-dose toxicity

Patients with high-dose PCP intoxication (more than 10 mg) may be in a coma, which may last from hours to several days. These patients are often unresponsive to painful stimuli. Respiratory depression, hypertension, and tachycardia may be present, depending on the dosage. In severe cases a hypertensive crisis causing cardiac failure, hypertensive encephalopathy, seizures and intracerebral haemorrhage may result. Prehospital care is directed at managing respiratory and cardiac arrest and status epilepticus and rapidly transporting the patient for physician evaluation.

Phencyclidine psychosis

Phencyclidine psychosis is a true psychiatric emergency; it may mimic schizophrenia. The psychosis is usually of acute onset but may not become apparent until several days after drug ingestion. Psychosis can occur after a single low-dose exposure to PCP and may last from several days to weeks. Signs and symptoms may range from a catatonic and unresponsive state to bizarre and violent behaviour. The patient appears agitated and suspicious and often experiences auditory hallucinations and paranoia. Appropriate management usually requires involuntary hospitalization, control of violent behaviour, and administration of antipsychotic agents. When dealing with these patients in the prehospital setting, personal safety is of prime importance; the police should be called upon for assistance.

Hallucinogen overdose

Hallucinogens are substances that cause perceptual distortions. The most common hallucinogen in use today is lysergic acid diethylamide (LSD). Other hallucinogens include mescaline, found in the buttons of the peyote cactus, which can be used legally in some religious settings; psilocybin mushrooms, found in the US and Mexico; marijuana, the active agent of the plant *Cannabis sativa*; morning glory plant; nutmeg; mace; and some amphetamines, such as methylenedioxymethamphetamine (Ecstasy) and 3,4-methylenedioxyamphetamine (MDEA Eve).

Depending on the agent, the effects of hallucinogens may range from minor visual to more serious complications (associated with LSD use). The more serious effects include respiratory and CNS depression (rare). Prehospital management is usually limited to supportive care, minimal sensory stimulation, calming measures, and transportation to a medical facility. After arrival at the emergency department, these patients are generally placed in a quiet environment for observation.

Tricyclic antidepressant overdose

Tricyclic antidepressants are commonly prescribed to help manage depression and certain pain syndromes. The drugs work by blocking the uptake of noradrenaline and serotonin into the presynaptic neurons and by altering the sensitivity of brain tissue to the actions of these chemicals. Serious tricyclic antidepressant toxicity results from sodium-channel blockade in the myocardium. Other toxicities include potassium efflux blockade and blockade of blood vessels, anticholinergic effects, and seizures. Commonly prescribed antidepressant drugs include the tricyclic antidepressants amitriptyline, imipramine, lofepramine and nortriptyline. The newer selective serotonin reuptake inhibitors such as fluoxetine, sertraline and paroxetine are chemically unrelated to tricyclic antidepressants. These are considered safe and effective compared with tricyclic antidepressants.

Early symptoms of tricyclic antidepressant overdose are dry mouth, blurred vision, confusion, inability to concentrate and, occasionally, visual hallucinations. More severe symptoms include delirium, depressed respirations, hypertension, hypotension, hyperthermia, hypothermia, seizures and coma (Box 21-14). Cardiac effects may range from tachycardia to bradycardia and various dysrhythmias caused by atrioventricular block. A prolonged QRS complex, a Glasgow Coma Scale less than 8, or both are characteristic findings that should alert the paramedic to a major toxicity with potentially serious complications. Sudden death from a cardiac arrest may occur several days after an overdose.

Prehospital management for major toxicity of a tricyclic antidepressant overdose is basic supportive care for the patient and rapid transport. Twenty-five percent of patients who ultimately die as a result of the overdose are alert and awake, and 75% have normal sinus rhythm when EMS personnel arrive.[14] Tachycardia, especially with a wide QRS

Box 21-14

Five signs of major tricyclic antidepressant toxicity

Cardiac dysrhythmias
Coma
Gastrointestinal disturbances
Hypotension or hypertension
Respiratory depression

complex greater than 100 ms, is an early sign of toxicity. Any patient with a history of tricyclic antidepressant ingestion should receive airway, ventilatory, and circulatory support; intravenous access; electrocardiogram monitoring; and rapid transport for physician evaluation. Treatment for specific problems (e.g. seizures and ventricular dysrhythmias) is complex, requiring a combination of alkalinization and anticonvulsants. In prehospital care, anti-arrhythmic agents should only be used if there is evidence of cardiovascular collapse; seizures should be managed with diazepam.[14] Rapid transport to the emergency department is the most prudent course of action.

Critical Thinking

How can you ensure rapid transport of these patients?

Lithium

Lithium is a mood-stabilizing drug that may be prescribed for the management of bipolar disorders (see Chapter 25). The drug has a narrow dosage range (low toxic-to-therapeutic dose ratio), thus lithium overdose is common. Patients who are prescribed lithium have frequent blood tests to monitor the level of lithium in the body.

Lithium helps to prevent mood swings by interfering with hormonal responses to cyclic adenosine monophosphate and by increasing the reuptake of noradrenaline. (This produces an anti-adrenergic effect.) As a result of these actions, lithium has many effects on the body. These include muscle tremor, thirst, nausea, increased urination, abdominal cramping, and diarrhoea. With toxic ingestion, signs and symptoms may include the following:

- muscle weakness
- slurred speech
- severe trembling
- blurred vision
- confusion
- seizure
- apnoea
- coma.

Prehospital care for patients with suspected lithium overdose should focus on airway management, ventilatory and circulatory support, and the control of seizure activity (if present). In-hospital care may include restoring intravascular volume, maintaining urine output, correcting hyponatraemia, and, sometimes, dialysis.

Cardiac medications

Cardiac drugs are a common cause of poisoning deaths in children and adults. The drugs responsible for the majority of these fatalities are digoxin, beta-blockers, and calcium channel blockers (Box 21-15). As in all other cases of poisoning, patients with toxic ingestion of cardiac drugs require high-concentration oxygen administration, intravenous access, and careful monitoring of vital signs and electrocardiogram.

Digoxin exerts direct and indirect effects on sinoatrial and atrioventricular nodal fibres. At toxic levels the drug can halt impulses in the sinoatrial node, depress conduction through the atrioventricular node, and increase sensitivity of the sinoatrial and atrioventricular nodes to catecholamines.[5] Digoxin also affects the Purkinje fibres and decreases the resting potential and action potential duration of the heart. Digoxin also increases automaticity, which can cause an increase in premature ventricular contraction formation. Unlike most cardiovascular drugs, digoxin can produce almost any dysrhythmias or conduction block. In addition to dysrhythmias, common signs and symptoms of digoxin toxicity include nausea, anorexia, fatigue, visual disturbances, and a variety of disorders of the gastrointestinal, ophthalmological and neurological systems. Oral overdoses are generally managed with activated charcoal and drugs to treat life-threatening dysrhythmias. Severe overdoses are managed with intravenous digoxin-specific Fab. This is a drug that decreases the morbidity and mortality associated with digoxin overdose.

Box 21-15

Toxic effects of common cardiac drugs

Digoxin

Atrial fibrillation
Atrial tachycardia
Bigeminal and multifocal premature ventricular contractions
First- and second-degree atrioventricular block
Sinus bradycardia
Ventricular tachycardia/ventricular fibrillation

Beta-blockers

Bradycardia
Hypotension
Respiratory arrest
Seizure
Unconsciousness
Ventricular tachycardia/ventricular fibrillation (rare)

Calcium channel blockers

Acute respiratory distress syndrome
Asystole
Atrioventricular dissociation
Coma
Confusion
Hypotension
Lactic acidosis
Mild hyperglycaemia/hyperkalaemia
Pulmonary oedema
Respiratory depression
Sinus arrest
Sinus bradycardia
Slurred speech

Critical Thinking

Why is it possible that this type of overdose would not be noticed immediately?

Beta-blockers are absorbed rapidly after ingestion. Toxicity impairs sinoatrial and atrioventricular node function, which leads to bradycardia and atrioventricular blocks. The associated depression in ventricular conduction and sodium channel blockade may cause the QRS complex to widen. Occasionally, patients become susceptible to ventricular dysrhythmias (rarely ventricular tachycardia or ventricular fibrillation). Other signs and symptoms include CNS and respiratory depression, hypotension, and seizures. Prehospital treatment for patients with beta-blocker overdose is largely supportive and managing hypotension and dysrhythmias. The in-hospital care may include infusions of glucagon and various catecholamines; haemodialysis may be necessary, depending on the particular agent involved.

Toxic ingestion of calcium channel blockers can lead to myocardial depression and peripheral vasodilatation with negative inotropic, chronotropic, dromotropic and vasotropic effects. Hypotension and bradycardia are early signs of toxicity. Overdose may result in serious dysrhythmias that include atrioventricular block of all degrees, sinus arrest, atrioventricular dissociation, junctional rhythm, and asystole. (Calcium channel blockers have little effect on ventricular conduction; ventricular dysrhythmias are uncommon.) Other signs and symptoms of calcium channel toxicity include nausea and vomiting, hypotension, and CNS and respiratory depression. In addition to airway, ventilatory, and circulatory support, emergency care may include the use of antidysrhythmics, vasopressors, and activated charcoal.

Monoamine oxidase inhibitors

As described in Chapter 12, monoamine oxidase inhibitors block the breakdown of monoamines (noradrenaline, dopamine, serotonin). These CNS transmitters are distributed throughout the body, with the highest concentration in the brain, liver, and kidneys. Monoamine oxidase inhibitors are prescribed as antidepressants, antineoplastics, antibiotics, and antihypertensives. Some monoamine oxidase inhibitors (e.g. the antidepressants phenelzine and tranylcypromine) have active metabolites. Signs of monoamine oxidase inhibitor toxicity are usually delayed and may present 6–24 h after ingestion. The duration of effects may also last for several days (Box 21-16). These effects include CNS depression and various neuromuscular and cardiovascular system manifestations.

The prehospital care is mainly supportive. Care includes airway, ventilatory, and circulatory support; cardiac medications as needed; and rapid transport for physician evaluation.

Box 21-16

Effects of monoamine oxidase inhibitor toxicity

- Agitation
- Bradysystolic rhythms
- Cardiovascular system manifestations
- Central nervous system depression
- Hallucinations
- Hyperreflexia
- Hypertension
- Hypotension with vascular collapse
- Neuromuscular system manifestations
- Nystagmus
- Rigidity
- Seizure
- Sinus tachycardia

Non-steroidal anti-inflammatory drugs

Non-steroidal anti-inflammatory drugs (NSAIDs) are a group of drugs that have an analgesic, anti-inflammatory and antipyretic action. They work by blocking the production of prostaglandins, which are chemicals that cause inflammation and trigger transmission of pain signals to the brain. NSAIDs are used widely to relieve symptoms caused by types of arthritis (rheumatoid arthritis, osteoarthritis, gout) and to treat back pain, menstrual pain, headaches, minor postoperative pain and soft tissue injuries. Common NSAIDs include diclofenac, fenoprofen, ibuprofen and naproxen. Ibuprofen and naproxen are available over the counter. They are promoted as safer and more effective than aspirin and paracetamol in the management of fever and mild to moderate pain.

Ibuprofen overdose

Ibuprofen is the most commonly ingested NSAID in overdose. The effects are usually reversible and are seldom life threatening. (However, significant toxicity may result in coma, seizure, hypotension, and acute renal failure.) Chronic and acute ingestion is usually more than 300 mg/kg. In such ingestion, common symptoms include mild gastrointestinal and CNS disturbances, which usually resolve within 24 h of ingestion. Other, less common effects include mild metabolic acidosis, muscle fasciculations, chills, hyperventilation, hypotension and asymptomatic bradycardia. Emergency care for patients who have ingested toxic amounts of ibuprofen consists of careful monitoring for secondary complications such as hypotension and dysrhythmias.

Salicylate overdose

Salicylates are widely available in prescription and over-the-counter products such as acetylsalicylic acid (aspirin), many cold preparations and oil of wintergreen (methyl salicylate), and in combination with some analgesics such as propoxyphene and oxycodone. Table 21-3 contains general guidelines for salicylate toxicity.

Table 21-3 Toxicity guidelines for salicylate

Toxicity	Amount ingested
Mild	Less than 150 mg/kg
Moderate to severe	150–300 mg/kg
Severe	More than 300 mg/kg
Fatal	More than 500 mg/kg

The process of toxicity with salicylate poisoning is complex. Toxicity includes direct CNS stimulation, interference with cellular glucose uptake, and inhibition of Krebs cycle enzymes that affect energy production and amino acid metabolism. The volume of distribution is dose dependent and usually small. With toxic ingestion, however, redistribution of the drug into the CNS occurs, which prolongs elimination of the drug from the body. Complications that may result from chronic or acute ingestion of salicylates include CNS stimulation, gastrointestinal irritation, glucose metabolism, fluid and electrolyte imbalance, neurological symptoms, and coagulation defects.

Central nervous system stimulation First, salicylates produce direct stimulation of the respiratory centre in the CNS, causing an increased rate and depth of respiration. This early respiratory alkalosis is followed by a compensatory elimination of bicarbonate ions by the kidneys, which produces a compensatory metabolic acidosis. Acids continue to build up from metabolism, leading to profound metabolic acidosis. Confusion, lethargy, convulsions, respiratory arrest, coma and brain death can occur in severe salicylate poisoning.

Critical Thinking

Would you predict a tachypnoea or bradypnoea in these patients? Why?

Gastrointestinal irritation Salicylates have irritant effects on the lining of the stomach. This can lead to nausea, vomiting, and haematemesis. They also can cause pylorospasm, which delays gastric emptying.

Glucose metabolism Interference with glucose uptake by the cells causes a build-up of serum glucose. Eventually, glucose in the cells is depleted. The patient shows signs of hypoglycaemia (particularly in CNS tissue). Patients who die from salicylate poisoning often have primary CNS tissue toxicity and severe cerebral oedema.

Fluid and electrolyte imbalance The total amount of body fluids is affected adversely by hypermetabolism. Fluid and electrolyte losses occur via gastrointestinal fluids, emesis, and renal clearance. Acid–base disturbances may result in hypokalaemia and hyperchloraemia. Cardiac dysrhythmias, including premature ventricular contractions, ventricular tachycardia and ventricular fibrillation, are possible.

Neurological symptoms Mild neurological effects are common. One example is tinnitus (common with salicylism on the cranial nerve VIII). Another common effect is lethargy. Severe intoxication may result in hallucination, seizure and coma.

Coagulation effects Salicylates alter normal platelet function. When taken in toxic amounts, they often lead to coagulation disorders, placing patients at an increased risk of significant bleeding. Patients who take anticoagulants are at even greater risk for haemorrhage after salicylate ingestion.

In addition to general supportive measures, prehospital care for salicylate poisoning may include the administration of intravenous glucose to manage hypoglycaemia. Definitive care includes in-hospital intensive care observation, continued support of vital functions, and perhaps haemodialysis.

Paracetamol overdose

Paracetamol is a commonly prescribed analgesic and antipyretic agent. Paracetamol is available in many prescription and non-prescription preparations (e.g. Anadin and Panadol). The widespread availability of paracetamol accounts for its high incidence in unintentional and intentional poisoning. Paracetamol is one of the 10 most commonly used drugs for intentional self-poisoning and is associated with significant morbidity and mortality. Paracetamol overdose can cause life-threatening liver damage from toxic metabolites if it is not managed within 16 to 24 h of ingestion. As few as 30 standard-size (325 mg) paracetamol tablets are toxic in an average adult. Paracetamol is also present in many drug combinations, including Solpadeine plus, Beechams Flu Plus, and Sinutab.

Acute paracetamol ingestion is doses of 140 mg/kg or greater. The toxic effects of such an ingestion can be classified in four stages (Box 21-17). The course of toxicity begins with mild symptoms that may be overlooked or masked by more dramatic effects of other agents, followed by temporary clinical improvement and, finally, peak liver damage. (If paracetamol was the only drug taken and a dangerously high dose was ingested, the first two stages may be asymptomatic.) If antidote management is started within 8 h of ingestion, full recovery should occur.

Critical Thinking

Do you think most laypersons realize that paracetamol overdose can be fatal?

Box 21-17

Stages of paracetamol poisoning

Stage I: Gastrointestinal irritability (0–24 h)

Anorexia
Diaphoresis
General malaise
Nausea
Pallor
Vomiting

Stage II: Abnormal laboratory findings (24–48 h)

Possible abdominal pain and tenderness in the right abdominal quadrant
Resolution of stage I symptoms

Stage III: Hepatic damage (72–96 h)

Dysrhythmias
Hepatotoxicity with significant increase in hepatic enzymes
Hypoglycaemia
Jaundice
Lethargy
Vomiting

Stage IV: Recovery (4–14 days) or progressive hepatic failure

Resolution of hepatic dysfunction
Lack of permanent effects in patients who recover

Note: The percentage of patients who recover in stage IV depends on the amount of paracetamol ingested and whether effective therapy (activated charcoal, acetylcysteine, or both) was given. Patients with serum levels in the hepatotoxic range have mortality rates up to 25% if untreated.

Emergency care includes respiratory, cardiac and haemodynamic support in critically ill patients. If ingestion is recent (within 1 h) and the patient is alert, administration of activated charcoal may be useful, in which case the patient should be transported rapidly to a suitable facility. Patients with progressive paracetamol toxicity require in-hospital administration of the antidote, *N*-acetylcysteine.

Drugs abused for sexual purposes/sexual gratification

Some drugs are abused for sexual purposes or for sexual gratification. These drugs are commonly classified by users as 'uppers', 'downers', and 'all-arounders' (those that have more than one primary effect). Box 21-18 gives a sampling of these drugs. As described before, uppers are CNS stimulants and downers are CNS depressants. The third category encompasses drugs such as anaesthetics and mood-altering agents, which may be taken alone or in combination to produce one or more of the following effects:

- a sense of euphoria
- excitation ('rush')
- relaxation ('blissed out')
- a loss of inhibition.

Each of these drugs has a different chemical structure, mechanism of action, and side effects, so the problems associated with their use can vary greatly. Signs and symptoms of abuse can range from mild nausea and vomiting to life-threatening respiratory depression, hypotension, methaemoglobinaemia, coma and death. The emergency care for these patients is mainly supportive. Care includes airway, ventilatory, and circulatory support, and rapid transport for physician evaluation. As with all other cases of patients who use mood-altering agents, personal safety is of primary importance.

Box 21-18

Uppers, downers and all-arounders

Uppers

Anabolic steroids
Coke/crack
Ecstasy
Speed/meth/crystal

Downers

Alcohol
Benzodiazepines (diazepam, temazepam, Rohypnol)
Gamma hydroxybutyrate (GHB)
Heroin

All-arounders

Cannabis/skunk
Ketamine
Lysergic acid diethylamide (LSD)
Poppers (alkyl nitrates)

SECTION III

Alcohol

Alcoholism and related illnesses continue to be a major problem in the UK. The alcohol-related death rate in the UK increased from 6.9 per 100 000 population in 1991 to 12.9 in 2005. The number of alcohol-related deaths has more than doubled from 4144 in 1991 to 8386 in 2005.[16] Among men who are victims of a fatal violent assault, alcohol has been found to play a role in 47% of all encounters; for women, the figure is 48%. Alcohol also figures in 30% of all fatal car accidents where men are the victims and alcohol misuse is related to at least 10% of the chronic disease burden. The cost to the NHS is up to £1.7 billion annually, of which £0.5 billion comes from the A&E budget.[17]

Critical Thinking

How many calls have you been on that involved patients intoxicated with alcohol? What kinds of calls were they?

Alcohol dependence

Alcohol dependence is a disorder characterized by chronic, excessive consumption of alcohol that results in injury to health or in inadequate social function and the development of withdrawal symptoms when the patient stops drinking suddenly. In 2007, the prevalence of alcohol dependence among people aged 16–64 years in England was higher among men than women, with 9% of men and 4% of women showing some signs of alcohol dependence. The prevalence of alcohol dependence was slightly lower for men in 2007 than in 2000, but there was no significant change for women.[18] Alcohol dependence should be considered a chronic, progressive, potentially fatal disease characterized by remissions, relapses and cures.

No single cause of alcohol dependence exists, although three causative factors are believed to interact in development of the illness. These are personality, environment (widespread social acceptance and availability of alcohol), and the addictive nature of the drug. In some cases, genetic and hormonal factors may also play a role in causing dependence. However, it is generally believed that any person, regardless of environment, genetic background, or personality traits, can become chemically dependent on alcohol when the drug is consumed for long periods.

The development of alcohol dependence can be divided into four main stages that merge imperceptibly. The time frame of these stages may range from 5 to 25 years, but the average is about 10 years. In the first stage, tolerance of the drug develops in the heavy social drinker. This allows a person to consume larger quantities of alcohol before experiencing its ill effects. On entering the second stage,

> **Box 21-19**
>
> **Alcohol 'proof'**
>
> Proof initially was based on a test in which gunpowder moistened with a distilled product was ignited. Ignition was 'proof' that the alcohol content of the product was at least 50%. Although the ignition test has been replaced with modern techniques to determine alcohol percentage, the term has been retained. A product containing 50% alcohol is considered 100 proof.

the drinker experiences memory lapses relating to events occurring during the drinking episodes. The third stage is characterized by loss or lack of control over alcohol; the drinker can no longer be certain of discontinuing alcohol consumption at will. The final stage begins with prolonged binges of intoxication. This is associated with mental and physical complications. Some drinkers halt their consumption for a brief time or permanently during one of the first three stages.

Ethanol

The active ingredient in all alcoholic beverages is ethanol, a colourless, flammable liquid produced from the fermentation of carbohydrates by yeast. All alcoholic drinks are rated based on their ethanol percentage. The alcohol content of beer and wine is measured as a percentage by weight or volume. Beers available in the UK usually contain between 2% and 6% alcohol by volume. Wines vary in ethanol content up to 14%. Distilled liquors are subjected to a rating process called proof (Box 21-19).

Metabolism

Eighty percent to 90% of ingested alcohol is absorbed within 30 min. (Twenty percent is absorbed in the stomach, the rest in the small intestine.) Once absorbed, the drug is distributed rapidly throughout the vascular space. Alcohol reaches virtually every organ system. About 3% to 5% of alcohol is excreted unchanged via the lungs and kidneys; the rest is metabolized in the liver to carbon dioxide and water. The actual rate at which alcohol is metabolized depends on individual variation (e.g. physical and mental state, body weight, and size). Metabolism also depends on whether the drinker is alcohol dependent. Alcohol is metabolized at a constant rate of about 20 mg/dL/h (in non-alcoholics) regardless of its concentration. The rate of metabolism may be increased in alcoholics.

Blood alcohol content

The alcohol content of blood is measured in terms of mass (milligrams) of alcohol per given volume of blood (millilitre). The time it takes for the alcohol concentration to peak in the blood depends on a number of factors, including the rate at which the alcohol is consumed, the amount of food present in the stomach before drinking, and physical characteristics of the drinker. Blood alcohol content is used widely to evaluate the CNS status of an intoxicated person, yet individuals differ greatly in how blood alcohol content relates to the degree of intoxication. The legal level for driving in the UK is 80 mg/100 mL of blood.

Medical consequences of chronic alcohol ingestion

Alcohol affects nearly every organ system of the body; thus, persons who consume large amounts of alcohol are at risk for a number of physical and mental disorders. Through a variety of direct and indirect mechanisms, alcohol causes multiple systemic effects, including neurological disorders, nutritional deficiencies, fluid and electrolyte imbalances, gastrointestinal disorders, cardiac and skeletal muscle myopathy and immune suppression. In addition, alcohol may affect a patient's ability to tolerate traumatic injury.

Neurological disorders

Alcohol is a potent CNS depressant. When consumed in moderate amounts, the drug reduces anxiety and tension. Alcohol gives most drinkers a feeling of relaxation and confidence. The clinical effects of alcohol depend on the dose. They progress predictably as the level of consumption increases and blood alcohol content rises. Initial feelings of well-being give way to impaired judgement and discrimination, prolonged reflexes, and incoordination and drowsiness. This ultimately may progress to stupor and coma. The long-term neurological effects of chronic alcohol abuse are similar to those of the ageing process. They include short-term memory deficit, problems with coordination, and difficulty with concentration and abstraction.

Nutritional deficiencies

Alcohol can satisfy the calorific requirements of the body for a brief time. It also decreases a drinker's appetite through an irritant effect on the stomach and satisfies the feeling of hunger. However, alcohol has no essential vitamins, proteins or fats, so alcohol-dependent persons may have a decreased dietary intake and malabsorption. This leads to multiple vitamin and mineral deficiencies. Clinical manifestations associated with these deficiencies include the following:

- altered immunity
- anorexia
- cardiac dysrhythmias
- coma
- irritability and disorientation
- muscle cramps
- paraesthesias
- poor wound healing
- seizures
- tremor and ataxia.

Fluid and electrolyte imbalances

After consuming alcohol, urinary output increases over and above that expected from the amount of fluid ingested. This diuresis results because alcohol blocks the secretion of antidiuretic hormone and can lead to dehydration and electrolyte imbalances.

Gastrointestinal disorders

The effects of alcohol on the gastrointestinal system can produce several types of alcohol-related illnesses and diseases. The alcohol-related gastrointestinal disorders most likely to initiate an EMS response include gastrointestinal haemorrhage, cirrhosis, and acute or chronic pancreatitis.

Gastrointestinal haemorrhage

Four primary causes of gastrointestinal haemorrhage in patients who drink alcohol are gastritis, ulcer formation, oesophageal tear (Mallory–Weiss syndrome) and variceal haemorrhage (see Chapter 19). Gastritis results from the toxic effects of ethanol on the gastric mucosa, which leads to diffuse or localized areas of erosion. In the chronic form of gastritis, blood may ooze continually from the mucosal lining, and ulcers may develop.

Oesophageal tears of the gastro-oesophageal junction, stomach or oesophagus usually follow severe or protracted vomiting or retching. The injury results when gastric contents are forced against an unrelaxed gastro-oesophageal junction. This produces a sudden increase in pressure and a mucosal tear with subsequent bleeding. The bleeding can be worsened by clotting abnormalities. Such abnormalities are common in patients with alcoholic liver disease.

Varices are a result of portal hypertension caused by cirrhosis. Any of these thin-walled, blood-engorged veins are subject to rupture and haemorrhage, but the most common site is the varices of the oesophagus. Bleeding oesophagogastric varices remain one of the most difficult conditions to manage. Severe blood loss through vomiting may require supportive care with controlled fluid resuscitation.

Cirrhosis

Cirrhosis of the liver is caused by chronic damage to liver cells, which results in inflammation and eventually necrosis. In the disease process, bands of fibrosis (scar tissue) develop and break up the normal structure of the liver. The distortion and fibrosis of the liver lead to portal hypertension and complications such as ascites, splenomegaly and bleeding oesophageal and gastric varices. In addition, cirrhosis may lead to hepatic encephalopathy, which is caused by the build-up of toxic metabolic waste products. These waste products would normally be detoxified by a healthy liver.

Acute or chronic pancreatitis

Alcohol is the most common cause of acute and chronic pancreatitis. The exact mechanism by which alcohol produces pancreatic inflammation is not clear although pancreatitis may be caused at least in part by activation of pancreatic proenzymes, obstruction of pancreatic ducts, and stimulation of enzymatic secretion. A direct toxic effect may result, as has been demonstrated for the liver. Chronic pancreatitis usually produces the same symptoms as the acute form (described in Chapter 19) but the pain may last from several hours to several days. The attacks also become more frequent as the condition progresses. Other effects of chronic pancreatitis include malabsorption (a result of a deficiency of pancreatic enzymes), electrolyte imbalances such as hypocalcaemia, and diabetes mellitus (caused by insufficient insulin production). Complications of pancreatitis are haemorrhagic pancreatitis, sepsis, and pancreatic abscess. These complications are associated with high mortality.

Cardiac and skeletal muscle myopathy

Cardiac and skeletal muscle damage is thought to result from a direct toxic effect of alcohol or its metabolites. The pathological changes associated with these alcoholic muscle syndromes include intracellular oedema, formation of lipid droplets, excessive cellular glycogen, and deranged sarcoplasmic reticula and mitochondria. In heart muscle, these changes result in a decreased force of contraction (negative inotropic effect), dysrhythmias, and a tendency to develop congestive heart failure. In skeletal muscle the major symptoms are weakness and muscle wasting.

Immune suppression

Long-term alcohol abuse renders the immune system less effective. Alcohol abuse suppresses bone marrow production of white blood cells. In addition, red blood cells and platelet production are often decreased. Alcohol has direct, specific effects on lung tissue. These effects may impair macrophage mobilization and mucociliary function. As a result, the ability of the body to fight pulmonary infection is lowered, making the alcohol-dependent patient more susceptible to viral and bacterial pneumonia. These infections may result from aspiration during alcoholic stupor or for other reasons. Although the exact cause is unknown, the incidence of cancer is increased in alcohol-dependent patients. This may also be related to immune suppression.

Critical Thinking

For what other pulmonary disease is the immune-suppressed alcohol-dependent patient at risk?

Trauma

Alcohol suppresses clotting factors that are produced in the liver. This blood-clotting deficiency makes alcohol-dependent patients prone to bruising and internal haemorrhage and adds to the frequency of subdural bleeding, even after relatively minor head trauma.

Alcohol emergencies

Several other conditions caused by consumption or abstinence from alcohol may require emergency care. These include acute alcohol intoxication, alcohol withdrawal syndromes, and disulfiram–ethanol reaction. Alcohol-induced ketoacidosis and hypoglycaemia were discussed in Chapter 17.

Acute alcohol intoxication

The ingestion of large amounts of alcohol over a short period may cause acute poisoning. The clinical features are similar to those induced by sedative–hypnotic agents and can be correlated to a degree with blood alcohol content. At toxic levels, hypoventilation (including respiratory arrest), hypotension and hypothermia may develop. The patient who has signs and symptoms of acute alcohol intoxication should be considered carefully for occult trauma and coexisting medical conditions such as hypoglycaemia, cardiac myopathy and dysrhythmias, gastrointestinal bleeding, polydrug abuse, and ethylene glycol or methanol ingestion. Because the patient is prone to injury and usually has other medical problems, the paramedic should never assume that an intoxicated patient is merely inebriated.

Management

A patient who is mildly intoxicated should be transported for physician evaluation. In most cases, management requires patient observation in the emergency department until the patient is sober. The paramedic should monitor the patient's vital signs and level of consciousness carefully en route. A thorough physical examination is warranted to rule out illness or injury masked by alcohol ingestion.

Care of the acutely intoxicated patient is aimed at protecting the patient from further injury and maintaining vital functions. If the patient is conscious and agitated, restraints may be necessary, in which case the police should be summoned. Once scene safety has been established, initial assessment and resuscitation should include the following:

1. Rapidly evaluate airway patency with spinal precautions. Assess the patient's ventilatory and haemodynamic status while obtaining a history. The patient's account of the event may be unreliable because of the alcohol ingestion.
2. Initiate intravenous therapy of 10% glucose if hypoglycaemia is likely or confirmed, and naloxone if opiate overdose is suspected.
3. Continually monitor the patient's airway and provide adequate ventilatory and circulatory support as needed. Be prepared to provide suction and aggressive airway management.
4. Monitor electrocardiogram for dysrhythmias.
5. Rapidly transport the patient for physician evaluation.

Alcohol withdrawal syndromes

A period of relative or full abstinence from alcohol may cause withdrawal in an alcohol-dependent individual. The severity of these syndromes depends on the magnitude of blood alcohol content (serum ethanol level), the length of time the level was maintained, the abruptness of cessation, the tissue tolerance to alcohol, and the general physical and psychological condition of the patient. The cause of alcohol withdrawal remains largely unknown. However, withdrawal is thought to result from CNS hyperexcitability (as the CNS depressant is removed). Biochemical changes such as respiratory alkalosis and hypomagnesaemia can also play a role. Alcohol withdrawal syndromes can be divided into four general categories: minor reactions, hallucinations, alcohol withdrawal seizures and delirium tremens.

Minor reactions

Minor reactions begin about 6–8 h after cessation or reduction of alcohol intake. These symptoms peak within 24–36 h but may persist for 10–14 days. When alcohol withdrawal is confined to minor reactions, the prognosis for full recovery is excellent with proper management. Minor reactions include the following:

- sudden and unexpected startle
- flushed face and diaphoresis
- anorexia
- nausea and vomiting
- insomnia
- general muscle weakness
- slight disorientation
- generalized tremor (worsened by agitation)
- mild tachycardia, hypertension, and hyperreflexia.

Critical Thinking

What kinds of feelings do you think the patient and the patient's family may be having during withdrawal reactions?

Hallucinations

Hallucinations usually occur 24–36 h after stopping the drinking of alcohol. Disorders of perception are common and may vary from auditory and visual illusions to frank hallucinations. The latter can produce agitation, fear, and panic. During this period, the patient may show signs of suicidal and homicidal tendencies, and minor reactions may be more pronounced. The prognosis for hallucinations is the same as for minor reactions with appropriate care.

Alcohol withdrawal seizures

Alcohol withdrawal seizures (or 'rum fits') usually occur 7–48 h after ethanol cessation. These seizures may occur singly or in groups of two to six. They are most often tonic–clonic and of short duration; status seizures are rare. Alcohol withdrawal seizures are associated with varying degrees of tremor, anorexia, hallucinations, and autonomic hyperactivity. This category of withdrawal may be self-limiting or may progress to delirium tremens with or without a lucid interval.

Because of the high drug tolerance level of the alcohol-dependent patient, seizure activity may require intravenous administration of large doses of diazepam. Diazepam may synergistically interact with any ethanol still in the patient's system, so should be used with caution; vital signs, respirations, and mental status should be monitored closely.

Delirium tremens (the DTs)

Delirium tremens is the most dramatic and serious form of alcohol withdrawal and affects about 5% of all alcohol-dependent patients hospitalized for withdrawal. Delirium tremens usually occurs 72–96 h after cessation of alcohol but it may be delayed up to 14 days. The syndrome is characterized by psychomotor, speech, and autonomic hyperactivity; profound confusion; disorientation; delusion; vivid hallucinations; tremor; agitation; and insomnia. A single episode may last 1–3 days and, with multiple recurrences, may last up to 1 month.

Autonomic hyperactivity is the most distinguishing feature of delirium tremens. Delirium tremens is characterized by tachycardia, fever, hypertension, dilated pupils and profuse diaphoresis. In severe cases, cardiovascular collapse may be present. Delirium tremens is a true medical emergency as it has a mortality rate as high as 15%. Associated alcohol-related illnesses such as pneumonia, pancreatitis, and hepatitis are frequent contributing causes of death.

Management

The care for patients with alcohol withdrawal syndromes is mainly supportive. After scene safety is ensured, the paramedic should monitor the patient's airway, ventilatory, and circulatory status carefully. Intravenous therapy should be started with a saline solution for rehydration where indicated. Pharmacological therapy may be indicated for an altered level of consciousness, dysrhythmias, or seizure activity. In addition, these patients need calm reassurance and frequent reorientation to the present. All patients with signs and symptoms of alcohol withdrawal syndrome require physician evaluation.

Disulfiram–ethanol reaction

Disulfiram (Antabuse) is a medication prescribed to some alcohol-dependent patients to help them abstain. The drug gives rise to extremely unpleasant systemic reactions after the ingestion of even a small amount of alcohol because it leads to accumulation of acetaldehyde in the body. Acetaldehyde produces ill effects on the gastrointestinal, cardiovascular and autonomic nervous systems. Acetaldehyde is the metabolic product that is thought to be responsible for the common 'hangover'. Patients who take disulfiram and then drink alcohol experience an unpleasant and potentially life-threatening physiological response. A disulfiram-like reaction also can occur in patients taking metronidazole for *Trichomonas* and other types of infection.

The disulfiram-ethanol reaction begins 15–30 min after the ingestion of two to five alcoholic drinks. The reaction continues for 1–2 h. The reaction causes the patient to experience vertigo, headache, vomiting, flushing (which may give the skin a 'lobster-red' appearance), dyspnoea, diaphoresis, abdominal pain and sometimes chest pain. More serious reactions include hypotension, shock and dysrhythmias. Sudden death, myocardial and cerebral infarction and cerebral haemorrhage have been reported after as little as one drink of ethanol in patients taking disulfiram.

Management

Prehospital care for a disulfiram–ethanol reaction involves airway, ventilatory and circulatory support; the administration of intravenous fluids to manage hypotension; pharmacological therapy as needed to manage dysrhythmias; and rapid transport for physician evaluation. Most patients recover from these episodes. Supportive care and in-hospital observation are usually all that are required.

SECTION IV

Management of toxic syndromes

As stated before, most poisoned patients require only supportive therapy to recover (Box 21-20). (This is regardless of the toxic agent.) Grouping toxic agents and physical findings into toxic syndromes, however, can give the paramedic an important clue to which type of poison or toxin is involved. This will aid the paramedic in remembering assessment and management strategies as well (Table 21-4). The five toxic syndromes presented in this chapter are the following.[15,19]

1. Cholinergic
2. Anticholinergic
3. Hallucinogenic
4. Opiate
5. Sympathomimetic.

Box 21-20

General management guidelines for the poisoned patient

1. Ensure scene and personal safety.
2. Provide adequate airway, ventilation, and circulation.
3. Obtain a thorough history, and perform a focused physical examination.
4. Consider hypoglycaemia in an unconscious or convulsing patient.
5. Administer naloxone to a patient with respiratory depression and suspected opioid ingestion.
6. If overdose is suspected, obtain an overdose history from the patient, family, or friends.
7. Consult with ambulance control or NPIS centre for specific treatment to prevent further absorption of the toxin (or antidote therapy).
8. Frequently monitor vital signs and electrocardiogram.
9. Safely obtain any substance or substance container of a suspected poison. Transport it with the patient.
10. Transport the patient for physician evaluation.

Note

Toxic syndrome classification does not consider how or why the toxin was introduced into the body. Thus the paramedic should consider route of entry in addition to specific treatments.

Cholinergics

Exposure to cholinergics is uncommon. However, it is important to recognize cholinergic poisoning so that lifesaving care can be started. Causative agents include pesticides (organophosphates, carbamates) and nerve agents (e.g. sarin and soman). Assessment findings include headache, dizziness, weakness, bradycardia, nausea, and a 'wet' presentation

Table 21-4 Toxicological syndromes

Common signs	Causative agents	Specific treatment
CHOLINERGIC ('WET' PATIENT PRESENTATION)		
Confusion, central nervous system depression, weakness, SLUDGE (salivation, lacrimation, urination, defecation, gastrointestinal upset, emesis), bradycardia, wheezing, bronchoconstriction, miosis, coma, convulsion, diaphoresis, seizures	Organophosphate and carbamate insecticides, nerve agents, some mushrooms	Atropine, pralidoxime (2-PAM chloride), diazepam or lorazepam, activated charcoal
ANTICHOLINERGIC ('DRY' PATIENT PRESENTATION)		
Delirium, tachycardia, dry, flushed skin, dilated pupils, seizures, and dysrhythmias (in severe cases)	Antihistamines, antiparkinson medications, atropine, antipsychotic agents, antidepressants, skeletal muscle relaxants, many plants (e.g. Jimson weed and *Amanita muscaria*)	Diazepam or lorazepam, activated charcoal, rarely physostigmine (Antilirium)
HALLUCINOGEN		
Visual illusions, delusions, bizarre behaviour, flashbacks, respiratory and central nervous system depression	LSD, PCP,* mescaline, some mushrooms, marijuana, Jimson weed, nutmeg, mace, some amphetamines	Minimal sensory stimulation and calming measures, diazepam or lorazepam if necessary
OPIOID		
Euphoria, hypotension, respiratory depression/arrest, nausea, pinpoint pupils, seizures, coma	Heroin, morphine, codeine, meperidine (Demerol), propoxyphene, fentanyl	Naloxone (Narcan), nalmefene (Revex)
SYMPATHOMIMETIC		
Delusions, paranoia, tachycardia or bradycardia, hypertension, diaphoresis; seizures, hypotension, and dysrhythmias in severe cases	Cocaine, amfetamine, methamphetamine, over-the-counter decongestants	Minimal sensory stimulation and calming measures, diazepam or lorazepam if necessary; manage dysrhythmias

*LSD, lysergic acid diethylamide; PCP, phencyclidine.

manifested by profound salivation, lacrimation, urination, defecation, gastrointestinal upset and emesis (SLUDGE). In severe cases, coma and convulsions may be present. In addition to airway, ventilatory, and circulatory support and decontamination, drug therapy may include administration of atropine and diazepam.

Anticholinergics

Exposure to anticholinergics is fairly common because so many medications and plants have anticholinergic properties. The signs and symptoms include tachycardia, dry, flushed skin, dilated pupils and facial flushing. This 'dry' patient presentation is usually managed with airway, ventilatory and circulatory support.

Hallucinogens

Common hallucinogens include LSD, PCP, peyote, mushrooms and mescaline. Depending on the agent and dose, signs and symptoms may include CNS stimulation and/or depression, behavioural disturbances, delusions, hypertension, chest pain, tachycardia, seizures and respiratory and cardiac arrest. Prehospital care for these patients is focused on ensuring personal safety and providing airway, ventilatory and circulatory support.

Opiates

The opiate syndrome carries a hallmark triad of depressed level of consciousness, respiratory depression and pinpoint pupils. Common causative agents include heroin, morphine, codeine, meperidine, oxycodone, hydrocodone and fentanyl. Drugs in this class are often mixed with alcohol or other drugs (e.g. benzodiazepines). This leads to increased respiratory depression, hypotension and bradycardia. Other signs and symptoms may include euphoria, nausea, pinpoint pupils and seizures. In addition to ensuring airway, ventilatory and circulatory support, drug therapy may include the administration of naloxone.

Sympathomimetics

The sympathomimetic syndrome usually results from acute overdose of amphetamines or cocaine. Signs and symptoms include elevated blood pressure, tachycardia, dilated pupils and altered mental status (including paranoid delusions). In severe cases, cardiovascular collapse can occur. Management consists of ensuring personal safety and providing airway, ventilatory and circulatory support.

Critical Thinking

Why is it important to be able to identify these toxic syndromes?

Summary

- A poison is any substance that produces harmful physiological or psychological effects.
- The toxic effects of ingested poisons may be immediate or delayed. This depends on the substance that is ingested. The main goal is to identify effects on the three vital organ systems most likely to produce immediate morbidity and mortality. These are the respiratory system, the cardiovascular system and the CNS. The goal of managing serious poisonings by ingestion is to prevent the toxic substance from reaching the small intestine. This limits its absorption.
- Strong acids and alkalis may cause burns to the mouth, pharynx, oesophagus and sometimes the upper respiratory and gastrointestinal tracts. Prehospital care is usually limited to airway and ventilatory support, intravenous fluid replacement and rapid transport to the appropriate medical facility.
- The most important physical characteristic in the potential toxicity of an ingested hydrocarbon is its viscosity. The lower the viscosity, the higher the risk of aspiration and associated complications. Hydrocarbon ingestion may involve the patient's respiratory, gastrointestinal and neurological systems. The clinical features may be immediate or delayed.
- Methanol is a poisonous alcohol found in a number of products. Methanol itself is no more toxic than ethanol yet its metabolites (formaldehyde and formic acid) are toxic. Ingestion can affect the CNS, the gastrointestinal tract and the eyes. Methanol can also cause the development of metabolic acidosis.
- Ethylene glycol toxicity is caused by the build-up of toxic metabolites, especially glycolic and oxalic acids, after metabolism. This occurs mainly in the liver and kidneys. This toxicity may affect the CNS and cardiopulmonary and renal systems and may result in hypocalcaemia.
- The majority of isopropanol (isopropyl alcohol) is metabolized to acetone after ingestion. Isopropanol poisoning affects several body systems, including the central nervous, gastrointestinal and renal systems.
- Infants and children are high-risk groups for accidental iron, lead and mercury poisoning. Their immature immune systems and increased absorption as a function of age contribute to this risk. Ingested iron is corrosive to gastrointestinal tract mucosa. Iron may produce lethal gastrointestinal haemorrhage, bloody vomitus, painless bloody diarrhoea and dark stools.
- Food poisoning is a term used for any illness of sudden onset (usually associated with stomach pain, vomiting and diarrhoea) suspected of being caused by food eaten within the previous 48 h. Food poisoning can be classified as infectious if it results from a bacterium or virus. Food poisoning can be classified as non-infectious if it results from toxins and pollutants.
- The toxic effects of major poisonous plant ingestions are predictable. They are categorized by the chemical and physical properties of the plant. Most responses are consistent with the type of major toxic chemical component in the plant.
- The concentration of a chemical in the air and the duration of exposure helps to determine the severity of an inhalation injury. Solubility also influences the extent of an inhalation injury. Highly reactive chemicals cause more severe and rapid injury than less reactive chemicals. Properties that determine chemical reactivity are chemical pH; direct-acting potential of chemicals; indirect-acting potential of chemicals; and allergic potential of chemicals.
- Cyanide refers to any of a number of highly toxic substances that contain the cyanogen chemical group. Regardless of the route of entry, cyanide is a rapidly acting poison. It combines and reacts with ferric ions of the respiratory enzyme cytochrome oxidase. This combination inhibits cellular oxygenation and produces a rapid progression from dyspnoea to paralysis, unconsciousness and death.
- Ammonia is a toxic irritant that causes local pulmonary complications after inhalation. In severe cases, bronchospasm and pulmonary oedema may develop.
- Hydrocarbon inhalation may cause aspiration pneumonitis. It also has the potential for systemic effects such as CNS depression and liver, kidney, or bone marrow toxicity.
- Simple asphyxiants cause toxicity by lowering ambient oxygen concentration. Chemical asphyxiants possess intrinsic systemic toxicity. This toxicity occurs after absorption into the circulation. Irritants or corrosives cause cellular destruction and inflammation as they come into contact with moisture in the respiratory tract.
- The general principles of managing inhaled poisons are the same as for any other hazardous materials incident.
- The only venomous snake indigenous to the UK is the adder. Adder venom can produce various toxic effects on blood and other tissues but is rarely fatal.
- Few marine animals around the coast of the UK are poisonous to humans although recent warmer weather has seen an increase in the number of hazardous Lion's mane jellyfish, and reports of Portuguese Man-o'-War jellyfish washed up on the south and south-west coast of England. A swimmer who comes into contact with the tentacles of the Portuguese Man-o'-War jellyfish may suffer enough envenomation to produce systemic signs and symptoms
- Organophosphates and carbamates inhibit the effects of acetylcholinesterase. A mnemonic aid that may help the paramedic to recognize this type of poisoning is SLUDGE.

Summary—cont'd

(This stands for salivation, lacrimation, urination, defecation, gastrointestinal upset, and emesis). The most specific findings, however, are miosis, rapidly changing pupils, and muscle fasciculation.

- General principles for managing drug abuse and overdose include scene safety; ensuring adequate airway, breathing, and circulation; history; substance identification; focused physical examination; initiation of an intravenous line where indicated; and rapid transport.
- Narcotics are CNS depressants. They can cause life-threatening respiratory depression. In severe intoxication, hypotension, profound shock, and pulmonary oedema may be present. Naloxone is a pure narcotic antagonist effective for virtually all narcotic and narcotic-like substances.
- Sedative–hypnotic agents include benzodiazepines and barbiturates. Signs and symptoms of sedative–hypnotic overdose are related chiefly to the central nervous and cardiovascular symptoms.
- Commonly used stimulant drugs are those of the amphetamine family. Adverse effects include tachycardia, increased blood pressure, tachypnoea, agitation, dilated pupils, tremors and disorganized behaviour. With sudden withdrawal, the patient becomes depressed, suicidal, incoherent, or near coma.
- Phencyclidine is a dissociative analgesic with sympathomimetic and CNS stimulant and depressant effects. In low doses, PCP intoxication produces an unpredictable state that can resemble drunkenness (and rage). High-dose intoxication may cause coma. This may last from several hours to days. Respiratory depression, hypertension and tachycardia may be present. Phencyclidine psychosis is a psychiatric emergency. It may mimic schizophrenia.
- Hallucinogens are substances that cause distortions of perceptions. Depending on the agent, overdose may range from visual hallucinations and anticholinergic syndromes to more serious complications, including psychosis, flashbacks, and respiratory and CNS depression.
- Tricyclic antidepressant toxicity is thought to result from central and peripheral atropine-like anticholinergic effects and direct depressant effects on myocardial function. A prolonged QRS complex, a Glasgow Coma Scale score less than 8, or both, should alert the paramedic to a major tricyclic antidepressant toxicity.
- Lithium is a mood-stabilizing drug. Toxic ingestion can include CNS effects that can range from blurred vision and confusion to seizure and coma.
- Cardiac drugs are a common cause of poisoning deaths in children and adults. The drugs responsible for the majority of these fatalities are digitalis, beta-blockers and calcium channel blockers.
- Monoamine oxidase inhibitors cause an accumulation of amine neurotransmitters (noradrenaline, dopamine, serotonin). Toxic effects include hypertension, tachycardia, tremors, seizures and hyperthermia.
- Non-steroidal anti-inflammatory drugs work by blocking the production of prostaglandins. The effects of overdose of ibuprofen are usually reversible, seldom life-threatening, and include mild gastrointestinal and CNS effects. Salicylate poisoning may cause CNS stimulation, gastrointestinal irritation, glucose metabolism, fluid and electrolyte imbalance, and coagulation defects.
- Paracetamol overdose may cause life-threatening liver damage. This results from formation of a hepatotoxic intermediate metabolite if it is not managed within 16 to 24 h of ingestion.
- Some drugs are abused for sexual purposes or for sexual gratification. These drugs commonly are classified by users as 'uppers', 'downers', and 'all-arounders' (those that have more than one primary effect). Problems associated with their use vary widely.
- Alcohol dependence is a disorder characterized by chronic, excessive consumption of alcohol that results in injury to health or in inadequate social function and the development of withdrawal symptoms when the patient stops drinking suddenly. Alcohol causes multiple systemic effects. These include neurological disorders, nutritional deficiencies, fluid and electrolyte imbalances, gastrointestinal disorders, cardiac and skeletal muscle myopathy, and immune suppression. Several conditions caused by consumption or abstinence from alcohol that may require emergency care are acute alcohol intoxication, alcohol withdrawal syndromes, and disulfiram–ethanol reaction.
- The most common toxic syndromes are cholinergic, anticholinergic, hallucinogen, opiate and sympathomimetic. Using these classifications allows the paramedic to group similar toxic agents together. Such classification allows the paramedic to remember more easily how to assess and treat the poisoned patient.

References

1. National Poisons Information Service on behalf of the Health Protection Agency. Burden of disease – poisoning, 2005. Online. Available http://www.hpa.org.uk/publications/2005/burden_disease/9_supporting_doc.pdf 10 February 2009
2. Karim A, Ivatts S, Dargan P, et al 2001 How feasible is it to conform to the European guidelines on the administration of activated charcoal within one hour of an overdose? Emerg Med J 18:390–392
3. Joint Royal Colleges Ambulance Liaison Committee 2006 UK Ambulance Service Clinical Guidelines v4. 2006. Online. Available http://jrcalc.org.uk/guidelines.html 10 February 2009

4. Rosen P, Barkin R 1998 Emergency medicine: concepts and clinical practice, 4th edition. Mosby, St Louis
5. Walder AD, Tyler CKG 1994 Ethylene glycol antifreeze poisoning; three case reports and a review of treatment. Anaesthesia 49(11):964–967
6. Olson K 2003 Poisoning and drug overdose. New York, Appleton & Lange
7. National Safety Council 2002 Injury facts. National Safety Council, Chicago
8. Borak J, Callan M, Abbott W, et al 1991 Hazardous materials exposure. Brady, Englewood Cliffs, NJ
9. Auerbach PS (ed) 1995 Wilderness medicine, 3rd edition. Mosby, St Louis
10. Warrell DA 2003 Taking the sting out of ant stings: venom immunotherapy to prevent anaphylaxis. Lancet 361(9362):979–980
11. Warrell DA 2005 Treatment of bites by adders and exotic venomous snakes. BMJ 331:1244–1247
12. Persson H, Irestedt B 1981 A study of 136 cases of adder bite treated in Swedish hospitals during one year. Acta Med Scand 210: 433–439
13. Ghodse H, Corkery F, Schifano A, et al Drug-related deaths as reported to participating Procurators Fiscal & Coroners in England, Wales, Northern Ireland, Scotland, Isle of Man, Guernsey, Jersey, annual report 2004 and npSAD Surveillance Report No. 13. London: St George's Hospital Medical School
14. National Safety Council 2002 Injury facts. National Safety Council, Chicago
15. Litovitz TL, Klein-Schwartz W, Rodgers GC 2001 Annual report of the American Association of Poison Control Centres Toxic Exposure Surveillance System. Am J Emerg Med 15:391–452
16. Office for National Statistics, General Register Office for Scotland, Northern Ireland Statistics and Research Agency. Alcohol-related deaths 1991–2005. Online. Available http://www.statistics.gov.uk/CCI/nugget.asp?ID=1091&Pos=2&ColRank=1&Rank=192 10 February 2009
17. Alcohol Concern 2002 Wasted: lives lost to alcohol. Alcohol Concern, London
18. The Information Centre for Health and Social Care. Statistics on Alcohol: England 2009. Online. Available at http://www.ic.nhs.uk/webfiles/publications/alcoholeng2009/Final%20draft%202009%20v7.pdf
19. US Department of Transportation, National Highway Traffic Safety Administration 1998 EMT-Paramedic national standard curriculum. Department of Transportation, Washington, DC

CHAPTER 22

Haematology

Chapter contents

Objectives

Upon completion of this chapter, the paramedic student will be able to:

1. Describe the physiology of blood and its components.
2. Discuss pathophysiology and signs and symptoms of specific haematological disorders.
3. Outline general assessment and management of patients with haematological disorders.

Key terms

anaemia A decrease in blood haemoglobin.

haematology The scientific study of blood and blood-forming organs.

haemophilia A group of hereditary bleeding disorders in which one of the factors necessary for blood coagulation is deficient.

Hodgkin's disease A malignant disorder characterized by pain and progressive enlargement of lymphoid tissue.

lymphoma A group of diseases that range from slowly growing chronic disorders to rapidly evolving acute conditions.

multiple myeloma A malignant neoplasm of the bone marrow.

polycythaemia A condition characterized by an unusually large number of red cells in the blood as a result of their increased production by the bone marrow.

sickle cell disease A debilitating and unpredictable recessive genetic illness that produces an abnormal type of haemoglobin with an inferior oxygen-carrying capacity.

Haematology is the study of blood and blood-forming organs. Dysfunction in the haematological system can affect other body systems, which results in a variety of clinical manifestations that characterize haematological disorders. Prehospital care for most patients with haematological disorders is mainly supportive. However, the paramedic's knowledge of these diseases enhances assessment skills and provides an understanding of the treatment these patients need.

Blood and blood components

Blood is composed of cells and formed elements surrounded by plasma. About 95% of the volume of formed elements consists of red blood cells (RBCs; erythrocytes), the remaining 5% consists of white blood cells (WBCs; leukocytes) and cell fragments (platelets) (Figure 22-1 and Table 22-1). The continuous movement of blood keeps the formed elements dispersed throughout the plasma, where they are available to carry out their chief functions:[1] (1) delivery of substances needed for cellular metabolism in the tissues; (2) defence against invading microorganisms and injury; and (3) acid–base balance.

All types of blood cells are formed within the red bone marrow, which is present in all tissues at birth. In the adult the red bone marrow is found primarily in membranous bone such as the vertebrae, pelvis, sternum, and ribs. Yellow marrow produces some white cells but is composed mainly of connective tissue and fat. Other blood-forming organs include the following:

- Lymph nodes, which produce lymphocytes and antibodies.
- The spleen, which stores large quantities of blood and produces lymphocytes, plasma cells, and antibodies.
- The liver, a blood-forming organ only during intrauterine life, which plays an important role in the coagulation process.

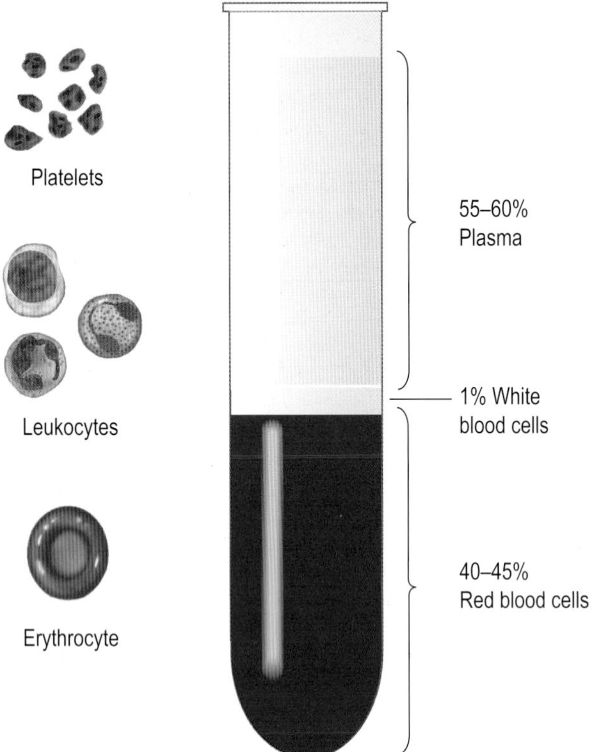

Figure 22-1 Blood will settle into three distinct, proportional layers when treated with salt. The transparent yellow layer at the top is plasma, the liquid portion of blood through which solid elements travel. White blood cells (WBCs) settle in the narrow white band in the centre, and red blood cells (RBCs), which give blood its crimson colour, fall to the bottom of the flask. Red blood cells outnumber white blood cells 600 to 1.

Plasma

Plasma, the clear portion of blood, is about 92% water. It contains three important proteins: albumin, globulins and fibrinogen. Albumin is the most plentiful protein and serves as the main contributor to blood colloid osmotic pressure. The globulins (alpha, beta and gamma) transport other proteins and provide immunity to disease. Fibrinogen is responsible for blood clotting. Plasma proteins perform various functions that include maintaining blood pH (acting as either an acid or a base); transporting fat-soluble vitamins, hormones, and carbohydrates; and allowing the body to digest them temporarily for food. Plasma also contains salts, metals and inorganic compounds.

Red blood cells

Red blood cells are the most abundant cells in the body. They are primarily responsible for tissue oxygenation. They appear as small rounded discs with nearly hollowed-out centres (Figure 22-2) and are comprised mainly of water and the red protein haemoglobin. RBC production continues throughout life to replace blood cells that grow old and die, are killed by disease, or are lost through bleeding. After RBC production occurs in the bone marrow, the new cell divides until there are 16 RBCs. The cells produce haemoglobin protein until the concentration of the protein becomes 95% of the dry weight of the cell. At this time, the cell expels its nucleus, giving the cell its characteristic pinched look. The new shape of the RBC increases the surface area of the cell and thus its oxygen-carrying potential. RBC have a lifespan of about 120 days. As the cells age, their internal chemical

Table 22-1 Cellular components of the blood

Cell	Structural characteristics	Normal amounts in circulating blood	Function	Lifespan
Erythrocyte (red blood cell)	Non-nucleated cytoplasmic disc containing haemoglobin	4.2–6.2 million/mm^3	Gas transport to and from tissue cells and lungs	80–120 days
Leukocyte (white blood cell)	Nucleated cell	5000–10 000/mm^3	Bodily defence mechanisms	See following times
Lymphocyte	Mononuclear immunocyte	25–33% of leukocyte count (leukocyte differential)	Humoral and cell-mediated immunity	Days or years, depending on type
Monocyte and macrophage	Large mononuclear phagocyte	3–7% of leukocyte differential	Phagocytosis; mononuclear phagocyte system	Months or years
Eosinophil	Segmented polymorphonuclear granulocyte	1–4% of leukocyte differential	Phagocytosis; antibody-mediated defence against parasites; allergic reactions; associated with Hodgkin's disease, recovery phase of infection	Unknown
Neutrophil	Segmented polymorphonuclear granulocyte	57–67% of leukocyte differential	Phagocytosis, particularly during early phase of inflammation	4 days
Basophil	Segmented polymorphonuclear granulocyte	0–0.75% of leukocyte differential	Unknown, but associated with allergic reactions and mechanical irritation	Unknown
Platelet	Irregularly shaped cytoplasmic fragment (not a cell)	140 000–340 000/mm^3	Haemostasis after vascular injury; normal coagulation and clot formation/retraction	8–11 days

From McCance KL, Huether SE 1998 Pathophysiology: the biologic basis for disease in adults and children, 3rd edition. Mosby, St Louis.

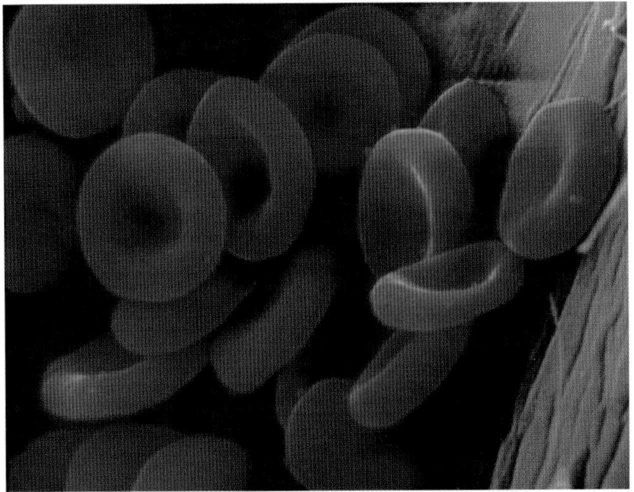

Figure 22-2 Mature erythrocytes.

> **Box 22-1**
>
> **Laboratory tests**
>
> Haematocrit is the fraction of the total volume of blood that consists of red blood cells (RBCs), normally about 45%. For example, a value of 46% implies that there are 46 mL of RBCs in 100 mL of blood. The normal haematocrit for males is 40–54%. In females, a normal haematocrit is 38–47%. A low haematocrit indicates anaemia, which may result from trauma, surgery, internal bleeding, nutritional deficiency (e.g. iron or vitamin B_{12}), bone marrow disease, or sickle cell disease. A high haematocrit may be caused by dehydration, lung disease, certain tumours, and disorders of the bone marrow.
>
> Haemoglobin is reported in grams per 100 mL of blood. The normal haemoglobin for males is 13.5–18 g/100 mL. In women, a normal haemoglobin is 12–16 g/100 mL.
>
> Reticulocyte count offers details about the rate of RBC production. A reticulocyte count of less than 0.5% of the RBC count usually indicates a slowdown in the process of RBC formation. A reticulocyte count greater than 1.5% usually indicates an acceleration of RBC formation.

machinery weakens; they lose elasticity; and they become trapped in small blood vessels in the bone marrow, liver, and spleen. They are then destroyed by specialized WBCs (macrophages). Most components of destroyed haemoglobin molecules are used again, although some are broken down to the waste product bilirubin.

Each RBC contains about 270 million haemoglobin molecules and each haemoglobin molecule carries four oxygen molecules. The normal amount of haemoglobin in blood is about 15 g/100 mL. This is normally a little higher in males than in females. The number of RBCs is about 4.2 to 6.2 million cells/mm^3 (Box 22-1).

White blood cells

WBCs arise from the bone marrow and are released into the bloodstream. They destroy foreign substances (e.g. bacteria

> **Box 22-2**
>
> **Clotting measurements**
>
> Clotting time is normally 7–10 min. The patient bleeds if the clotting time is prolonged and develops intravascular clots if the clotting time is less than normal. Prothrombin time (PT) measures the clotting time of plasma (the extrinsic clotting cascade). The PT test is used to monitor patients taking certain medications and to diagnose clotting disorders. The PT test specifically evaluates the presence of factors VIIa, V and X and of prothrombin and fibrinogen. A drop in the concentration of any of these factors will cause the blood to take longer to clot. A prolonged PT is considered abnormal. The PT test is used in combination with the partial thromboplastin time (PTT) to screen for haemophilia and other hereditary clotting disorders.
>
> The PTT uses blood to which a chemical has been added to prevent clotting before the test begins. The PTT measures the integrity of the intrinsic clotting cascade, which is affected by blood-thinning medications (e.g. heparin and warfarin). The PTT can help determine a possible cause of abnormal bleeding or bruising. An increased PTT in a person with a bleeding disorder may indicate that a clotting factor is missing or defective.

and viruses) and clear the bloodstream of debris. Leukocyte production increases in response to infection, which causes an elevated WBC count in the blood. Chapters 18 and 24 provide a discussion of the inflammatory process and the immune response.

The bone marrow and lymph glands continually produce and maintain a reserve of WBCs as there are not many in the healthy bloodstream (normal WBC count is about 5000 to 10 000 cells/mm^3). Monocytes make up about 5% of the total WBC count and increase with chronic infections. Lymphocytes account for about 27.5%, neutrophils about 65%, and eosinophils and basophils together about 2.5% of the total WBC count. A rise in the number of WBCs aids in the diagnosis of some diseases. An increased WBC count is specific for various illnesses such as bacterial infection, inflammation, leukaemia, trauma and stress.

> **Critical Thinking**
>
> What body functions are impaired if the white blood cell number or function is diminished?

Platelets

Platelets (thrombocytes) are small, sticky cells that play an important role in blood clotting. When a blood vessel is cut, platelets travel to the site and swell into odd, irregular shapes and adhere to the damaged vessel wall. Platelets plug the leak and allow other cells to stick to them to form a clot. However, if the damage to the vessel is too great, the platelets chemically signal the complex clotting process, the clotting cascade (described in Chapter 28). Platelets repair millions of ruptured capillaries each day. They often make the rest of the clotting cascade unnecessary (Box 22-2).

Specific haematological disorders

Haematological disorders presented in this chapter are anaemia, leukaemia, lymphomas, polycythaemia, disseminated intravascular coagulopathy, haemophilia, sickle cell disease and multiple myeloma.

Anaemia

Anaemia is a condition in which the amount of haemoglobin or erythrocytes in the blood is below normal. Precipitating causes of anaemia include chronic or acute blood loss, decreased production of erythrocytes, and increased destruction of erythrocytes.[2] One should note that anaemia is not a disease, rather, it is a symptom of a disease. Those at greatest risk are persons with chronic kidney disease, diabetes, heart disease and cancer; chronic inflammatory conditions such as rheumatoid arthritis or inflammatory bowel disease; and persistent infections such as human immunodeficiency virus (HIV). These conditions can cause anaemia by interfering with the production of oxygen-carrying RBCs. In the case of cancer and chemotherapy, anaemia can be caused by the treatment itself. Two common forms of anaemia are iron deficiency anaemia and haemolytic anaemia.

Iron deficiency anemia

Iron is the critical part of a haemoglobin molecule, giving it the ability to bind oxygen (Figure 22-3). The lack of iron in iron deficiency anaemia prevents the bone marrow from making sufficient haemoglobin for the RBCs. The RBCs produced are small, have a pale centre, and a reduced oxygen-carrying capacity. The most common cause of iron deficiency anaemia in adults is blood loss from menstrual bleeding or intestinal bleeding.[3] A diet that is low in iron is usually the cause of iron deficiency anaemia in children. Vitamin deficiencies, most commonly folic acid deficiency (one of the B vitamins), can also produce anaemia.

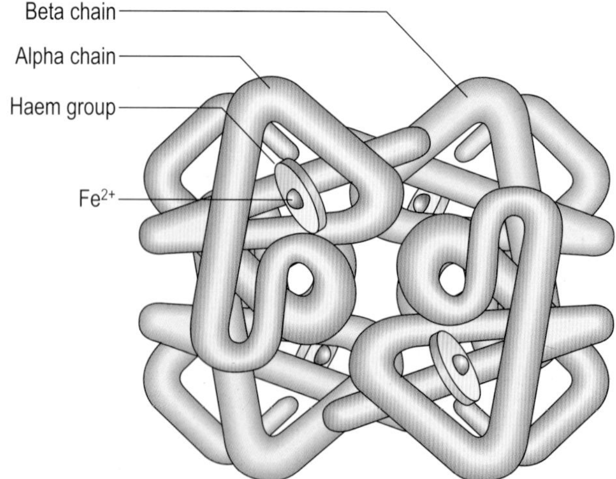

Figure 22-3 The four-chained haemoglobin molecule is made from more than 10 000 atoms. Yet when fully laden, the molecule will carry only four pairs of oxygen atoms. Haemoglobin is built around four atoms of iron that act like oxygen magnets. Each red blood cell holds 300 million of these vital protein molecules.

> **Critical Thinking**
>
> Can you predict the signs and symptoms of anaemia?

Haemolytic anaemia

Premature destruction of RBCs in the blood (haemolysis) causes haemolytic anaemia. This destruction can result from an inherited disorder inside the RBC or from a disorder outside the cell. The condition is usually acquired later in life.

Inherited disorders

Haemolysis can occur as a result of abnormal rigidity of the cell membrane. This rigidity causes the cell to become trapped in the smaller blood vessels (usually of the spleen) at an early stage of its lifespan. In these smaller blood vessels the RBC is destroyed by macrophages. This type of anaemia can occur from a genetic defect in the haemoglobin within the cell (e.g. sickle cell anaemia and thalassaemia). It can also occur from a defect in one of the enzymes in the cell that helps protect the cell from chemical damage during infectious illness. A deficiency of one of the enzymes, glucose-6-phosphate dehydrogenase, is common in African-Americans.

Acquired disorders

Acquired haemolytic anaemia results from one of three conditions:

1. Disorders in which normal RBCs are disrupted as a result of mechanical forces (e.g. abnormal blood vessel linings or blood clots).
2. Autoimmune disorders, which can destroy RBCs with antibodies that are produced by the immune system (e.g. an incompatible blood transfusion).
3. Conditions that can cause haemolytic anaemia when RBCs are destroyed by microorganisms in the blood (e.g. malaria).

Signs and symptoms of anaemia

All forms of anaemia share signs and symptoms. These signs and symptoms include fatigue and headaches, sometimes a sore mouth or tongue, brittle nails, and in severe cases, breathlessness and chest pain (Table 22-2). Other patient complaints are related to an abnormal decrease in the number of WBCs (leukopenia) or a reduction in platelets (thrombocytopenia) and may include the following:

- bleeding from mucous membranes
- cutaneous bleeding
- fatigue
- fever
- lethargy.

Diagnosis and treatment

The patient's signs and symptoms, patient history, and examination of the patient's blood through blood tests and bone marrow biopsy indicate a diagnosis of most forms of anaemia. For example, iron deficiency anaemia usually reveals RBCs that are smaller than normal, whilst haemolytic anaemia shows RBCs that are immature and abnormally shaped. Treatment should be indicated to correct, modify,

Table 22-2 Causes, signs and symptoms, and treatment for specific forms of anaemia

Form of anaemia	Causes	Signs and symptoms	Treatment
Iron deficiency anaemia	Insufficient intake of iron Gastrointestinal disorders (e.g. ulcer disease) External and/or internal bleeding Prolonged aspirin or NSAID therapy Gastrectomy (surgical removal of part or all the stomach	Those related to the underlying cause (e.g. bleeding) Those common to all forms of anaemia	Correction of the underlying cause Supplemental iron tablets or injections
Haemolytic anaemia	Genetic red blood disorder Autoimmune disorders Malaria and other infections	Jaundice Those common in other forms of anaemia	Splenectomy Immunosuppressant drugs Avoidance of drugs or foods that precipitate hemolysis Antimalarial drugs Blood transfusions

NSAID, non-steroidal anti-inflammatory drug.

or diminish the mechanism or process that is leading to defective RBC production or reduced RBC survival.

Note

A bone marrow biopsy specimen taken from the sternum or pelvis offers details about the various parts of blood. The specimen also provides information about the presence of cells foreign to the marrow. Bone marrow biopsy is useful in diagnosing many haematological disorders such as anaemia, leukaemia, and certain infections. A bone marrow transplant is sometimes used to treat these and other diseases.

Leukaemia

Leukaemia refers to any of several types of cancer in which an abnormal proliferation of WBCs occurs, usually in the bone marrow (Figure 22-4). The proliferation of leukaemic cells crowds and impairs the normal production of RBCs, WBCs and platelets. Leukaemia is more common in males than in females. Leukaemia is also more common in Caucasians than in African–Americans. In the UK in 2006 there were 7061 new cases of leukaemia registered.[4–6]

The exact cause of leukaemia is not known; however, genetics may play a role. Abnormal chromosomes associated with congenital disorders (e.g. Down syndrome) and HIV-type viruses are associated with a rare form of this disease. Other factors that may play a role in the development of leukaemia include exposure to radiation, viral infections, immune defects, and various chemicals in home and work environments.[2]

Classifications

Leukaemia can be classified as either lymphoid or myeloid, which denotes the type of WBC affected. It may also be categorized as either acute or chronic, reflecting the speed of progression. Almost all childhood leukaemias are of the acute form, meaning that they progress rapidly. Acute lymphoblastic (lymphoid) leukaemia (ALL) accounts for more than 80% of cases of childhood leukaemia; acute myeloid leukaemia (AML) accounts for the rest. AML is one of the most intractable blood cancers.

Chronic leukaemias progress slowly and tend to affect mainly middle-aged adults; indeed, chronic lymphoblastic leukaemia is largely unheard of in children.

In both lymphoid and myeloid leukaemia, abnormal WBCs are produced in such large amounts that they eventually accumulate in the vital organs (liver, spleen, lymph and brain). This impedes the function of these organs and leads to death. Chronic forms of leukemia can develop slowly over many years, and cases of disease are often discovered by chance during routine blood analysis.

Signs and symptoms

The proliferation of leukaemic cells or the resulting inadequate production of other normal blood cells makes the patient highly susceptible to serious infections, anaemia, and bleeding episodes. Signs and symptoms of leukaemia include the following:

- abdominal fullness
- bleeding
- bone pain
- elevated body temperature and diaphoresis
- enlargement of lymph nodes
- enlargement of the liver, spleen, and testes
- fatigue
- frequent bruising
- headache
- heat intolerance
- night sweats
- weight loss.

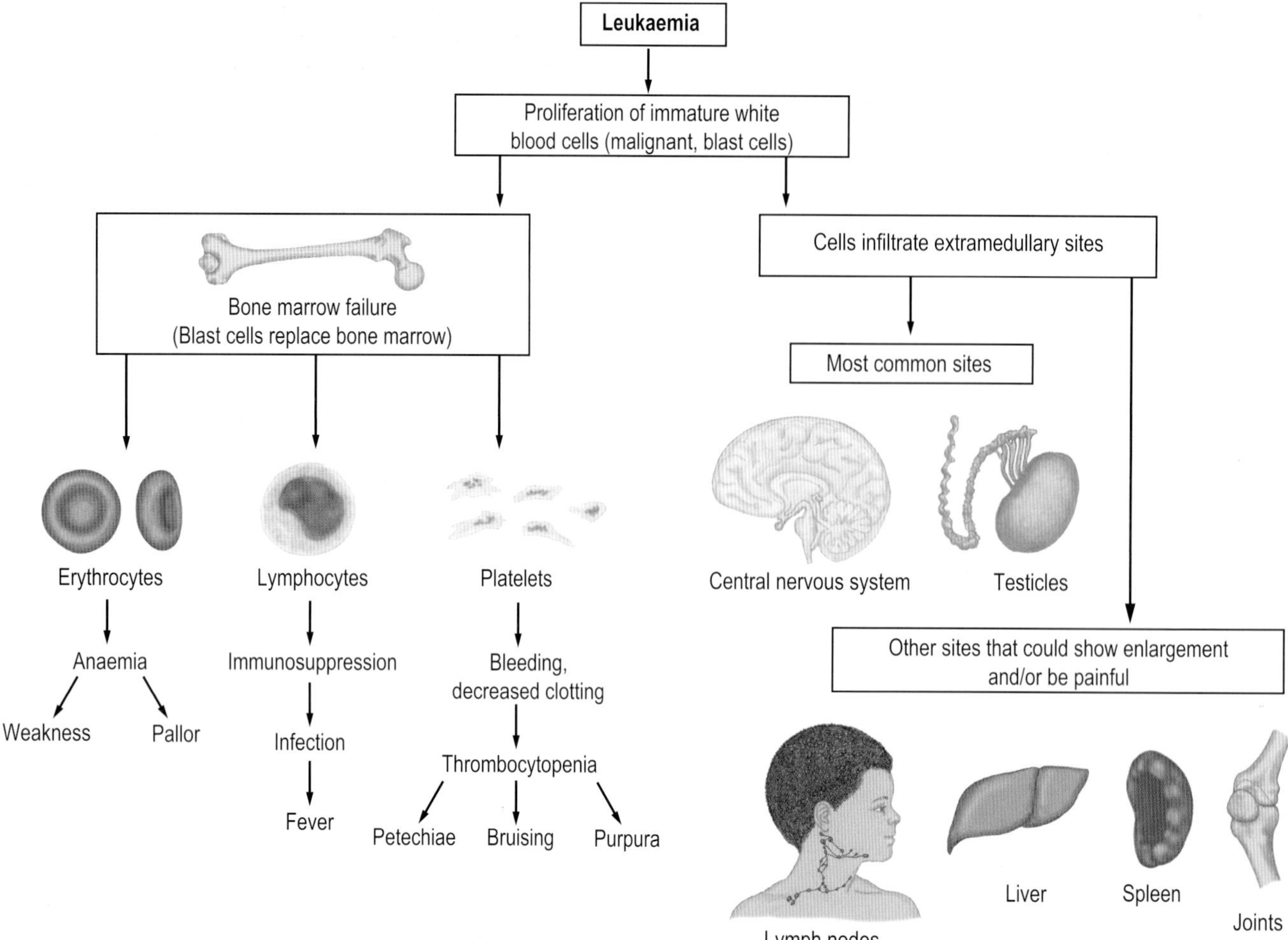

Figure 22-4 Pathophysiology of leukaemia.

> **Critical Thinking**
>
> If a child has a lot of odd bruises, what would you suspect if a diagnosis of leukaemia is not known?

Diagnosis and treatment

The diagnosis of leukaemia is confirmed by bone marrow biopsy. The severity of the disease is assessed by the degree of liver and spleen enlargement, anaemia, and lack of platelets in the blood. Treatment for acute leukaemia can include the transfusion of blood and platelets, antibiotic therapy to manage anaemia and infection, and the use of anticancer drugs and sometimes radiation to destroy the leukaemic cells. In some cases the leukaemia is treated with a bone marrow transplant (Box 22-3). Patients with chronic leukaemia can be managed effectively with medication. Many patients require no treatment in the early stages.

Lymphomas

Lymphoma is a general term applied to any neoplastic disorder of the lymphoid tissue. Hodgkin's disease is one type; all others, despite their diversity, are called non-Hodgkin's lymphomas. All lymphomas are malignant.

Hodgkin's disease

Hodgkin's disease is characterized by painless, progressive enlargement of lymphoid tissue found mainly in the lymph nodes and spleen (Figure 22-5). Left unchecked, these cancer cells multiply and eventually displace healthy lymphocytes, suppressing the immune system. Signs and symptoms include swollen lymph nodes in the neck, armpits or groin; fatigue; chills; and night sweats. Some patients also experience severe itching, persistent cough, weight loss, shortness of breath and chest discomfort.

Hodgkin's disease is a rare cancer of unknown cause that may have a heritable component. The disease is more common in males than in females, with a peak incidence in persons in their 20s and in persons between 55 and 70 years of age.[1] The disease is confirmed by the identification of Reed–Sternberg cells in lymph nodes or organs affected by the cancer. Treatment depends on the level of lymph node and organ system involvement (the stage of the disease) and can consist of radiation and chemotherapy with anticancer drugs. Hodgkin's disease is one of the most curable cancers.

Non-Hodgkin's lymphomas

Non-Hodgkin's lymphomas vary in their malignancy according to the nature and activity of the abnormal cells. At least

Box 22-3

Blood and marrow stem cell transplantation

A stem cell is a cell the daughter cells of which may give rise to other cell types. Some cells can develop into several different types of mature cells, including lymphocytes, granulocytes, thrombocytes, and erythrocytes. Stem cells reside in marrow and also circulate in the blood. They also circulate in large numbers in fetal blood. They can be recovered from umbilical cord and placental blood after childbirth. Stem cells can be harvested, frozen, and stored for future transplantation.

Stem cell transplantation is standard therapy for selected patients with leukaemia, lymphoma, and myeloma. The two major types of stem cell transplants are autologous and allogenic. An autologous transplant uses the patient's own marrow – the marrow is collected while the patient is in remission. The marrow may be treated with chemotherapy agents or antibodies to cleanse it of cancer cells that may be present in the marrow before it is given back to the patient. An allogenic transplant uses marrow from a donor, which is usually a brother or sister with the same tissue type. If a sibling is not available, a search of bone marrow registries for tissue-typed volunteers can be made for an unrelated donor. In addition to treating some cancers and other blood disorders, stem cells may play a key role in the future in treating diseases such as Alzheimer's, Parkinson's, and heart disease.

Adapted from The Leukemia and Lymphoma Society. Blood and marrow stem cell transplantation. http://www.leukemia .org/ all_page?item_id=5965.

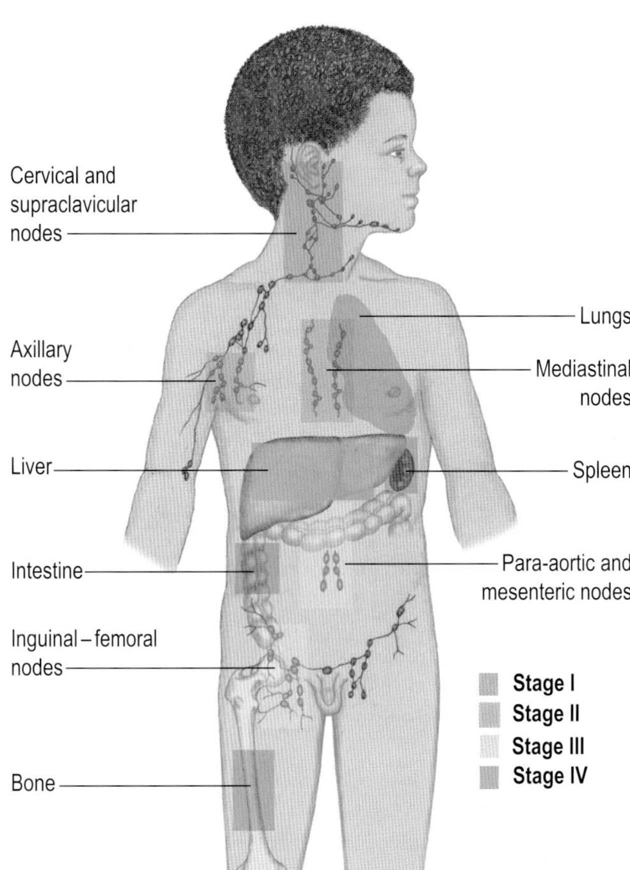

Figure 22-5 Pathophysiology of Hodgkin's disease.

10 types of non-Hodgkin's lymphoma have been identified. Each type is ranked as low, intermediate, or high grade based on how aggressively the disease behaves. Low-grade diseases usually progress slowly and tend not to spread beyond the lymphatic system. High-grade diseases can spread to distant organs within a few months. Signs and symptoms include painless swelling of one or more groups of lymph nodes; enlargement of the liver and spleen; fever; and, in rare cases, abdominal pain and gastrointestinal bleeding.

The cause of these cancers is largely unknown although one form, Burkitt's lymphoma, is strongly associated with infection by Epstein–Barr virus. This virus is commonly found in Africa. Other types have been linked to infection by HIV-type viruses and other conditions that affect the immune system (e.g. organ transplantation, radiation and chemotherapy, lupus, and rheumatoid arthritis). Treatment consists of radiation therapy, anticancer drugs, and sometimes bone marrow transplantation.

Polycythaemia

Polycythaemia is an increase in the total RBC mass of the blood. The condition may be a natural response to hypoxia (secondary polycythaemia) or it may occur for unknown reasons (primary polycythaemia). Polycythaemia can also result from dehydration (apparent polycythaemia) although the RBC production does not exceed the upper limits of normal.

Secondary polycythemia

Secondary polycythaemia can be naturally present in persons who live in or visit areas of high altitude, and occurs due to reduced air pressure and low oxygen. When the oxygen supply to the blood is reduced, the kidneys produce the hormone erythropoietin, which stimulates RBC production in the bone marrow to make up for the reduced oxygen supply. The result is an increase in the oxygen-carrying efficiency of the blood. The RBC numbers return to normal when the person returns to sea level. Secondary polycythaemia can also be present in heavy smokers. The disease can be caused by chronic bronchitis and conditions that increase erythropoietin production (e.g. liver cancer and some kidney disorders).

Primary polycythemia

Primary polycythaemia is also known as polycythaemia vera. Primary polycythaemia is a rare disorder of the bone marrow. In this disorder the increased production of RBCs causes the blood to thicken. This condition is primarily a disease of middle and older age[7] and can lead to several physiological problems that include the following:

- blurred vision
- dizziness
- generalized itching
- headache
- hypertension
- red hands and feet; red-purple complexion
- splenomegaly.

Other complications associated with primary polycythaemia include platelet disorders, which cause bleeding or clot formation; stroke; and the development of other bone marrow diseases (e.g. leukaemias). Treatment consists of phlebotomy (the slow removal of blood through a vein) and anticancer drug therapy. The therapy controls the overproduction of RBCs in the marrow.

Disseminated intravascular coagulopathy

Disseminated intravascular coagulopathy (DIC) (described in Chapter 28) is a complication of severe injury, trauma, or disease. DIC is a common abnormal clotting disorder and is most often seen in the critical care setting. It disrupts the balance among procoagulants, inhibitors, thrombus formation, and lysis. Signs and symptoms of DIC include dyspnoea, bleeding, and those associated with hypotension and hypoperfusion.

The pathophysiology of DIC involves loss of the fine homeostatic balance of thrombin generation. In addition, mechanisms fuelling and perpetuating the generation of thrombin are pathogenic in its dissemination. Also implicated are the concomitant activation of the inflammatory cascade and dysfunction of the endothelial microvasculature response.[8] DIC is characterized by free thrombin in the blood, fibrin deposits, and aggregation of platelets with subsequent haemorrhage caused by the depletion of clotting factors. The clinical consequences of these processes predispose the patient to multiple-system organ failure from bleeding and coagulation disorders caused by the following:

- loss of platelets and clotting factors
- fibrinolysis
- fibrin degradation interference
- small vessel obstruction, tissue ischemia, RBC injury, and anaemia from fibrin deposits.

Disseminated intravascular coagulopathy is confirmed through laboratory tests. Then the treatment is aimed at reversing the underlying illness or injury that triggered the event. In an effort to control the depletion of clotting factors, in-hospital care includes the replacement of platelets, coagulation factors, and blood. At the same time, attempts are made to manage the primary process.

Haemophilia

Haemophilia means 'love of blood'. Haemophilia is a group of inherited bleeding disorders (Box 22-4). Haemophilia A is due to a deficiency in factor VIII, a factor essential to the process of blood clotting (Table 22-3). Another less common form of haemophilia, caused by a deficiency of factor IX, is known as haemophilia B. This haemophilia is also known as Christmas disease (named after Steven Christmas, a 10-year-old boy first diagnosed with the disease in 1952). All types of haemophilia present with similar problems but the specific factor involved determines the severity of bleeding.

Bleeding from haemophilia can occur spontaneously or after only minor injury. It can also occur during some medical procedures (e.g. tooth extraction), and may occur anywhere in the body. Bleeding into joints, deep muscles, the urinary tract and intracranial sites are the most common. Head trauma is potentially life threatening and central nervous system bleeding is a leading cause of death for patients of all age groups with haemophilia.[9]

Box 22-4

Hereditary characteristics of haemophilia

Chromosomes from the mother link with an equal number from the father, and each pair determines the type of information that genes carry. Females have two X chromosomes. Males have an X and a Y chromosome. The mother passes on the X chromosome to her child, and the father passes on an X or a Y. Two X chromosomes produce a female child; an X and a Y produce a male child.

Haemophilia stems from an abnormal gene on the X chromosome. A female with an abnormal X chromosome is usually spared the disease because, although she received one abnormal X chromosome from one parent, the normal X chromosome passed on from her other parent counteracted the abnormal gene. However, she is a carrier of the disease and can pass it on to her children. A woman can have haemophilia only if her mother is a carrier and her father has haemophilia, which is rare. Affected males do not pass the defective gene to sons, but they pass it on to all of their daughters. A male, however, receives only one X chromosome. If his mother is a carrier, the male child will have a 50% chance of having haemophilia.

Table 22-3 Clotting factors and synonyms

Factor	Synonyms
I	Fibrinogen
II	Prothrombin
III	Thromboplastin
IV	Calcium
V	Proaccelerin
VI	None in use
VII	Serum prothrombin conversion accelerator
VIII	Antihaemophilic globulin
IX	Plasma thromboplastin component
	Christmas factor
X	Stuart factor
XI	Plasma thromboplastin antecedent
XII	Hageman factor
XIII	Fibrin-stabilizing factor

Haemophilia is controlled by infusions of concentrates of factor VIII, which can be administered by the patient. However, serious or unusual bleeding often calls for hospitalization. Persons with haemophilia are advised to avoid activities that may increase their risk of injury. Most patients with haemophilia are knowledgeable about their disease and seek emergency care only when problems and trauma-related issues arise.

Critical Thinking

Imagine that you are caring for a patient with haemophilia who has fallen 5 m (15 feet) from a ladder. This patient refuses care and transportation. What should you do?

Note

Factor VIII is made from large pools of donor blood. During the first few years of the acquired immunodeficiency syndrome epidemic, many persons with haemophilia and their sexual partners became infected with human immunodeficiency virus through factor VIII infusions. There are careful screening protocols for blood now. However, infusions still carry a minute risk of transmitting hepatitis B virus, hepatitis C virus, and HIV to factor VIII recipients. Another factor VIII product, recombinant factor VIII (Recombinate), is produced by inserting cloned factor VIII into animal tissues. Recombinate is not made from human plasma, is the purest form of factor VIII, does not transmit viral contamination, and is as effective as plasma-derived factor VIII.

Sickle cell disease

Sickle cell disease (also called sickle cell anaemia) is a debilitating and unpredictable recessive genetic illness. It mainly affects persons of African descent (less often, it affects persons of Mediterranean origin). In England, approximately 3000 babies carry the sickle cell trait annually[10] (Box 22-5) with a further 10 000 people estimated to be suffering from the disease in the UK.[11] Signs and symptoms of sickle cell disease include the following:

- delayed growth, development, and sexual maturation in children
- jaundice
- priapism in adolescent and adult males
- splenomegaly
- stroke.

Pathophysiology

Sickle cell disease produces an abnormal type of haemoglobin called haemoglobin S. This abnormal type has an inferior oxygen-carrying capacity. When haemoglobin S is exposed to low oxygen states, it crystallizes and distorts the RBCs into a sickle shape (Figure 22-6). The sickle-shaped cells are fragile and easily destroyed. They are also unable to pass easily through tiny blood vessels and block flow to various organs and tissues, which causes a vaso-occlusive sickle cell crisis that can be life threatening. As fewer RBCs pass through congested vessels, tissues and joints become starved for oxygen and other nutrients, causing excruciating pain. Other signs and symptoms of sickle cell disease are increased weakness, aching, chest pain with shortness of breath, sudden and severe abdominal pain, bony deformities, icteric (jaundice) sclera (Figure 22-7), fever, and arthralgia (joint pain) (Figure 22-8).

Critical Thinking

How do you think a patient with such chronic pain must feel at the beginning of a sickle cell crisis?

Sickle cell crisis can occur in any part of the body and varies in intensity from one person to the next and from one crisis to the next. Over time the crises can destroy the spleen, kidneys, gallbladder, and other organs. Sickle cell crisis may occur for no apparent reason but may also be triggered by conditions such as the following:

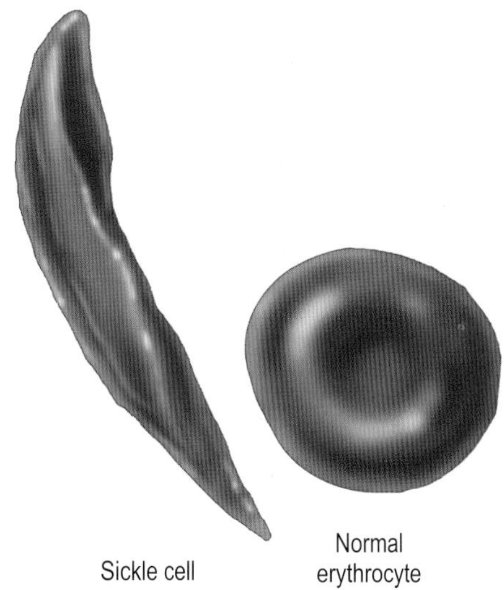

Figure 22-6 Sickle cell versus normal erythrocyte.

Box 22-5

Characteristics of sickle cell trait

A person must inherit two sickle cell genes – one from each parent – to develop sickle cell disease. When only one gene is present, the condition is known as sickle cell trait. Persons with sickle cell trait do not usually experience symptoms except occasionally under low-oxygen conditions (e.g. scuba diving or travelling at high altitudes). However, these persons can pass the gene, and possibly the disease, on to their children. If both parents have sickle cell trait, the child has a 25% chance of developing the disease, a 50% chance of having sickle cell trait, and a 25% chance of having neither. Genetic counselling should be considered for carriers of the disease who plan to become parents.

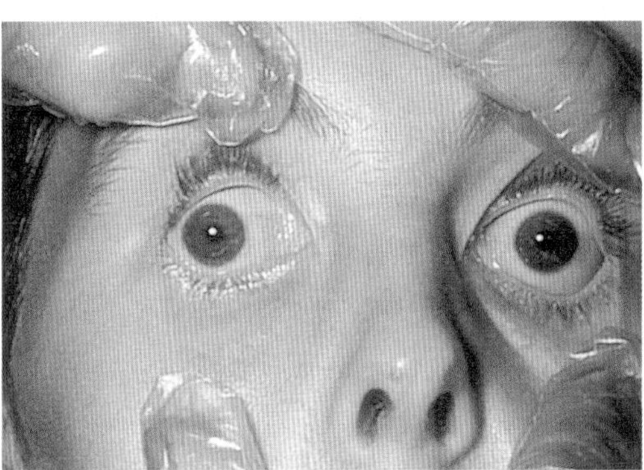

Figure 22-7 Jaundice of the sclera.

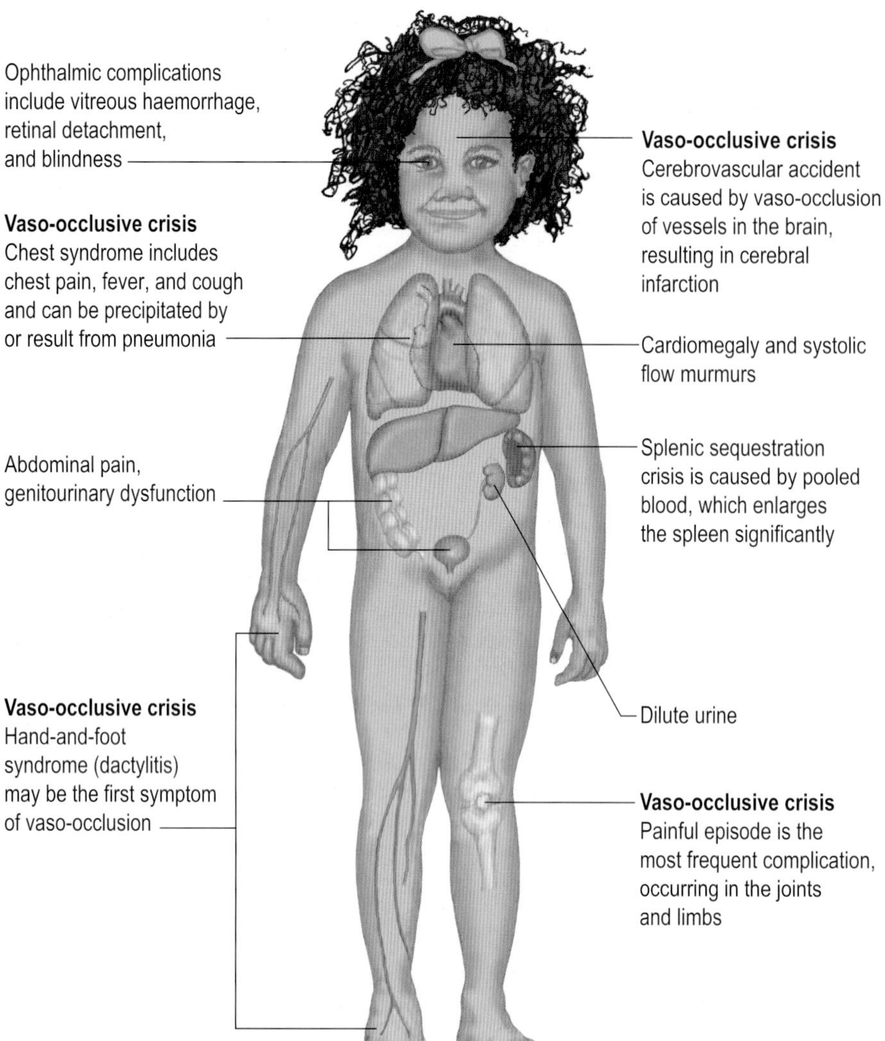

Figure 22-8 Pathophysiology of sickle cell disease.

- dehydration
- exposure to extremes in temperature
- infection
- lack of oxygen
- strenuous physical activity
- stress
- trauma.

Three less common types of sickle cell crisis are aplastic, haemolytic, and splenic sequestration. In aplastic crisis the bone marrow temporarily stops producing RBCs, whilst in haemolytic crisis the RBCs break down too rapidly to be replaced adequately. Splenic sequestration is usually a childhood difficulty that occurs when blood becomes trapped in the spleen. This causes the organ to enlarge and may possibly lead to death.

Management

At this time, no cure exists for sickle cell disease. Because of the eventual damage that occurs to the spleen, patients with sickle cell disease are at increased risk for septicaemia if infected by certain types of bacteria. Children with the disease should be current with all immunizations. When in crisis, these patients require prompt treatment with oxygen, intravenous therapy to manage dehydration, antibiotics to manage infection, and analgesics to manage pain. In severe cases a blood transfusion may be indicated to effect a temporary replacement of haemoglobin S. Blood transfusions may be advised during pregnancy to reduce the risk of a crisis, as a crisis can be fatal to the mother and fetus. Transfusions may also be advised before surgery because anaesthesia can be hazardous to those with the disease.

Multiple myeloma

Multiple myeloma is a malignant neoplasm of the bone marrow. The tumour, composed of plasma cells, destroys bone tissue (especially in flat bones) and causes pain, fractures, hypercalcaemia, and skeletal deformities. In myeloma the neoplastic cells produce large amounts of protein (M protein) that affect the viscosity of the blood. Masses of coagulated protein can build up within the tissues and impair function. Some patients with this disease die of kidney failure, which occurs because of the build-up of proteins that infiltrate the kidneys and block the renal tubules. In many ways, multiple myeloma resembles leukaemia; however, the plasma cell proliferation is generally confined to the bone marrow.

Critical Thinking

Which are the flat bones?

Other disorders associated with multiple myeloma include proteinuria, anaemia, weight loss, pulmonary complications from rib fracture, and recurrent infections from suppression of the immune system. Patient complaints associated with multiple myeloma may include weakness, skeletal pain, haemorrhage, haematuria, lethargy, weight loss, and frequent fractures.

Multiple myeloma rarely occurs before 40 years of age and then occurs increasingly with age. The disease is more common in males than in females and may have a heritable component.[1] Multiple myeloma is diagnosed through X-ray films, blood studies and tumour biopsy. Treatment consists of chemotherapy with anticancer drugs, radiation, plasma exchange, and bone marrow transplantation.

General assessment and management of patients with haematological disorders

As stated previously, most patients with haematological disorders are knowledgeable about their disease. Often they call emergency medical services to help manage a 'change' in their condition. They may also call to arrange for transportation to an emergency department for physician evaluation. The situations that invoke a call for emergency care vary by patient and disease. Common chief complaints can be classified by body system (Table 22-4).

Prehospital care

In many cases the prehospital care for a patient with a haematological disorder will be mainly supportive. As with any other patient care encounter, the paramedic should perform a general assessment, a focused history and focused physical examination. These measures will guide patient care and help to determine the appropriateness of emergency transport. Some patients with haematological disorders will have complex medical histories. When possible, these patients should be transported to their primary hospital (i.e. the hospital where they usually receive their medical care).

As referenced in Table 22-4, a patient with a haematological disorder may have a variety of complaints and physical findings. Some patient complaints may be vague (examples

Table 22-4 Chief complaints of patients with haematological disorders, classified by body system

Body system	Complaints	Possible causes
Central nervous system	Altered level of consciousness	Anaemia, sickle cell disease
	Increased weakness, numbness	Autoimmune disease
	Visual disturbances/loss of vision	Unilateral sensory deficits
Cardiorespiratory	Dyspnoea/crackles	Heart failure
	Anaemia	Bleeding disorders
	Haemoptysis	Pulmonary oedema
	Chest pain	Tachycardia
Integumentary	Prolonged bleeding	Haemolytic anaemia, polycythaemia
	Bruising	Sickle cell disease, liver disease
	Itching/petechiae	Jaundice
	Pallor	
Musculoskeletal	Bone or joint pain	Autoimmune disease
	Fracture	Haemophilia
Gastrointestinal	Abdominal pain	Haemolytic anaemia, viral disease
	Bleeding of the gums/gingivitis	Blood-clotting abnormalities
	Epistaxis	Autoimmune disease
	Generalized sepsis	
	Melaena/haematemesis	Ulceration
Genitourinary	Haematuria	Sickle cell disease, bleeding disorders
	Menorrhagia/amenorrhagia	
	Priapism	Infection
	Sexually transmitted disease	

include fever, fatigue, and headache), which can complicate the paramedic's assessment further. After ensuring adequate airway, ventilatory and circulatory status, the paramedic should assess vital signs and perform a physical examination. The paramedic should assess the patient's skin for colour and turgor, and note any cyanosis or jaundice, warmth or coolness, bruising, oedema or ulcerations. The paramedic should ascertain any new onset of fever, weakness, cough, rash, spontaneous bleeding (e.g. bleeding gums, epistaxis), vomiting or diarrhoea. Some haematological disorders can involve the ability of the blood to deliver enough oxygen to tissues; thus, the paramedic should question all patients with haematological disorders specifically about recent dizziness, syncope, difficulty breathing, and heartbeat irregularities.

Other key elements of the patient assessment and history include identifying existing haematological disease (including any family history of haematological disease), any significant medical history or recent injury, the patient's medication use (prescription and over-the-counter medications, herbal supplements), allergies, and alcohol or illicit drug use.

Based on the patient's condition, prehospital care measures may include oxygen administration, intravenous fluid replacement, the use of antidysrhythmics, and the administration of analgesics for pain management. Some of these patients will be gravely ill; calming and comfort measures for the patient and family should be provided.

Summary

- Blood is composed of cells and formed elements surrounded by plasma. About 95% of the volume of formed elements consists of RBCs (erythrocytes). The remaining 5% consists of WBCs (leukocytes) and cell fragments (platelets).
- Anaemia is a condition in which the amount of haemoglobin or erythrocytes in the blood is below normal. Two common forms of anaemia are iron deficiency anaemia and haemolytic anaemia. All forms of anaemia share signs and symptoms. These signs and symptoms include fatigue and headaches, sometimes a sore mouth or tongue, brittle nails, and, in severe cases, breathlessness and chest pain. Diagnosis is made by history and from blood tests and bone marrow biopsy.
- Leukaemia refers to any of several types of cancer in which an abnormal proliferation of WBCs occurs in the bone marrow. The proliferation of leukaemic cells crowds and impairs the normal production of RBCs, WBCs, and platelets. Leukaemia is classified as acute or chronic. The proliferation of leukaemic cells makes the patient highly susceptible to serious infections, anaemia, and bleeding episodes. The diagnosis is confirmed by bone marrow biopsy.
- Lymphoma refers to a group of diseases that range from slowly growing chronic disorders to rapidly evolving acute conditions. Hodgkin's disease is one type; all others are called non-Hodgkin's lymphomas.
- Polycythaemia is characterized by an unusually large number of RBCs in the blood as a result of their increased production by the bone marrow. Polycythaemia may be a natural response to hypoxia (known as secondary polycythaemia). Polycythaemia may also occur for unknown reasons (known as primary polycythaemia).
- Disseminated intravascular coagulopathy is a complication of severe injury, trauma, or disease. It disrupts the balance among procoagulants, thrombin formation, inhibitors, and lysis. Signs and symptoms of disseminated intravascular coagulopathy include dyspnoea, bleeding, and those associated with hypotension and hypoperfusion. The treatment is aimed at reversing the underlying illness or injury that triggered the event.
- Haemophilia A is caused by a deficiency of a blood protein called factor VIII. Haemophilia B is caused by a deficiency of factor IX. Bleeding from haemophilia can occur spontaneously, after even minor injury, or during some medical procedures.
- Sickle cell disease is a debilitating and unpredictable recessive genetic illness. It affects persons of African descent. Less often, it affects persons of Mediterranean origin. Sickle cell anaemia produces an abnormal type of haemoglobin called haemoglobin S. This abnormal type has an inferior oxygen-carrying capacity. Complications of sickle cell disease include episodes of severe pain, fatigue, pallor, jaundice, stroke, delayed growth, haematuria, priapism and splenomegaly.
- Multiple myeloma is a malignant neoplasm of the bone marrow. The tumour destroys bone tissue (especially flat bones). This causes pain, fractures, hypercalcaemia and skeletal deformities.
- In many cases of haematological disorders, the prehospital treatment is supportive. Treatment includes ensuring adequate airway, ventilatory, and circulatory support.

References

1. McCance KL, Huether SE 1998 Pathophysiology: the biologic basis for disease in adults and children, 3rd edition. Mosby, St Louis
2. US Department of Transportation, National Highway Traffic Safety Administration 1998 EMT-Paramedic national standard curriculum. US Department of Transportation, Washington, DC
3. Rosen P, Barkin R 1998 Emergency medicine: concepts and clinical practice, 4th edition. Mosby, St Louis
4. Office for National Statistics. Cancer statistics registrations, registrations of cancer diagnosed in 2006, England. Online. Available http://www.statistics.gov.uk/downloads/theme_health/MB1-37/MB1_37_2006.pdf 30 May 2009
5. Scottish Cancer Registry. Leukaemias, annual incidence 1985–2006. Online. Available http://www.isdscotland.org/isd/1538.html 30 May 2009
6. Welsh Cancer Intelligence and Surveillance Unit. Leukaemia factsheet. Online. Available http://www.wales.nhs.uk/sites3/Documents/242/Leukaemia1.pdf 30 May 2009
7. Messinezy M, Pearson TC 1997 Polycythaemia, primary (essential) thrombocythaemia and myelofibrosis. BMJ 314:587
8. Hock Toh C, Dennis M 2003 Disseminated intravascular coagulation: old disease, new hope. BMJ 327:974–977
9. Dietrich AM, James CD, King DR, Ginn-Pease ME, Cecalupo AJ 1994 Head trauma in children with congenital coagulation disorders. J Pediatr Surg 29(1):28–32
10. Hickman M, Modell B, Greengross P et al 1999 Mapping the prevalence of sickle cell and beta thalassaemia in England: estimating and validating ethnic-specific rates. Br J Haematol 104(4):860–867
11. Meremikwu M. Sickle cell disease. BMJ Clin Evidence. Online. Available http://www.clinicalevidence.com/ceweb/conditions/bly/2402/2402_background.jsp#REF5 10 February 2009

CHAPTER **23**

Environmental Conditions

Chapter contents

Objectives

Upon completion of this chapter, the paramedic student will be able to:

1. Describe the physiology of thermoregulation.
2. Discuss the risk factors, pathophysiology, assessment findings, and management of specific hyperthermic conditions.
3. Discuss the risk factors, pathophysiology, assessment findings, and management of specific hypothermic conditions and frostbite.
4. Discuss the risk factors, pathophysiology, assessment findings, and management of submersion and drowning.
5. Identify the mechanical effects of pressure on the body based on a knowledge of the basic properties of gases.
6. Discuss the risk factors, pathophysiology, assessment findings, and management of diving emergencies and high-altitude illness.

Key terms

acute mountain sickness A common high-altitude illness that results when an unacclimatized person rapidly ascends to high altitudes.

core body temperature The temperature of deep structures of the body as compared with the temperatures of peripheral tissues.

decompression sickness A multisystem disorder that results when nitrogen in compressed air converts back from solution to gas, forming bubbles in the tissues and blood.

drowning A mortal event in which a submersion victim is pronounced dead at the scene of the attempted resuscitation or within 24 hours after arrival in the emergency department or hospital.

frostbite A localized injury that results from environmentally induced freezing of body tissues.

heat cramps Brief, intermittent, and often severe muscular cramps that frequently occur in muscles fatigued by heavy work or exercise.

heat exhaustion A form of heat illness characterized by minor aberrations in mental status, dizziness, nausea, headache, and a mild to moderate increase in the core body temperature.

heat stroke A syndrome that occurs when the thermoregulatory mechanisms normally in place to meet the demands of heat stress break down entirely. As a result, the body temperature increases to extreme levels. Multisystem tissue damage and physiological collapse also occur.

high-altitude cerebral oedema The most severe form of acute high-altitude illness. It is characterized by a progression of global cerebral signs in the presence of acute mountain sickness.
high-altitude pulmonary oedema A high-altitude illness thought to be caused at least partly by an increase in pulmonary artery pressure that develops in response to hypoxia.
nitrogen narcosis An illness associated with scuba diving in which nitrogen becomes dissolved in solution as a result of greater than normal atmospheric pressure; also known as rapture of the deep or 'the bends'.
submersion An incident in which a person experiences some swimming-related distress that is sufficient to require support in the prehospital setting and transportation to a medical facility for further observation and treatment.
thermogenesis The production of heat, especially by the cells of the body.
thermolysis The dissipation of heat by means of radiation, evaporation, conduction, or convection.

Exposure to elements in the environment can produce many types of emergencies. Paramedics must be ready to recognize and manage these conditions. They can do this by becoming knowledgeable about the causative factors and by learning the pathophysiology of specific disorders.

Thermoregulation

A temperature centre in the brain regulates body temperature and is located in the posterior hypothalamus. It receives information from other areas of the brain (central thermoreceptors), as well as from the skin and some mucous membranes (peripheral thermoreceptors). Peripheral thermoreceptors are nerve endings, usually categorized as cold receptors or warm receptors; cold receptors are stimulated by low skin temperatures and warm receptors are stimulated by high skin temperatures. Information from these receptors is transmitted by the spinal cord to the posterior hypothalamus, which responds with appropriate signals to help the body reduce heat loss and increase heat production (cold receptor stimulation) or increase heat loss and reduce heat production (warm receptor stimulation).

Critical Thinking

The body has many more cold receptors than heat receptors. Why do you think this is so?

Central thermoreceptors are neurons that are sensitive to changes in temperature. These neurons react directly to changes in the temperature of the blood by sending messages to the skeletal muscle through the central nervous system (CNS). They affect vasomotor tone, sweating, and the metabolic rate through sympathetic nerve output to skin arterioles, sweat glands, and the adrenal medulla.

The thermoregulatory centre has a built-in set point, which maintains a relatively constant core body temperature (CBT) of 37°C (98.6°F). To maintain the best environment for normal cell metabolism (homeostasis), the body must keep the CBT about the same, even when external and internal conditions tend to raise or lower it. Body temperature can be increased or decreased in two ways; one way is through the regulation of heat production (thermogenesis) and the other way is through the regulation of heat loss (thermolysis).

Regulating heat production

The body can generate heat in response to cold, through mechanical, chemical, metabolic and endocrine activities. Several physiological and biochemical factors such as the person's age, general health, and nutritional status affect the direction and magnitude of these compensatory responses.

Heat is produced by cellular metabolism (oxidation of energy sources); every tissue contributes to this type of heat production. Skeletal muscles produce the largest amount of heat, particularly when shivering occurs; shivering is often associated with chattering of the teeth. Along with shivering, vasoconstriction occurs to conserve as much heat as possible. Shivering is the body's best defence against cold and can increase heat production by as much as 400%.

Critical Thinking

What fuels does the body need to increase heat production through the mechanism of shivering?

Endocrine glands also regulate heat production, through the release of hormones from the thyroid gland and adrenal medulla. An increase in the activity of sympathetic nerves that lead to adipose tissue increases the basal metabolic rate, which results in an increase in heat production. Box 23-1 presents examples of ways the body regulates heat production.

Regulating heat loss

Heat is lost from the body to the external environment through the skin, lungs, and excretions, with skin being the

Box 23-1

Compensatory mechanisms for regulating heat production

Mechanisms that decrease heat loss

Peripheral vasoconstriction
Reduction of surface area by body position (or clothing)
Piloerection (not effective in humans)

Mechanisms that increase heat production

Shivering
Increased voluntary activity
Increased hormone secretion
Increased appetite

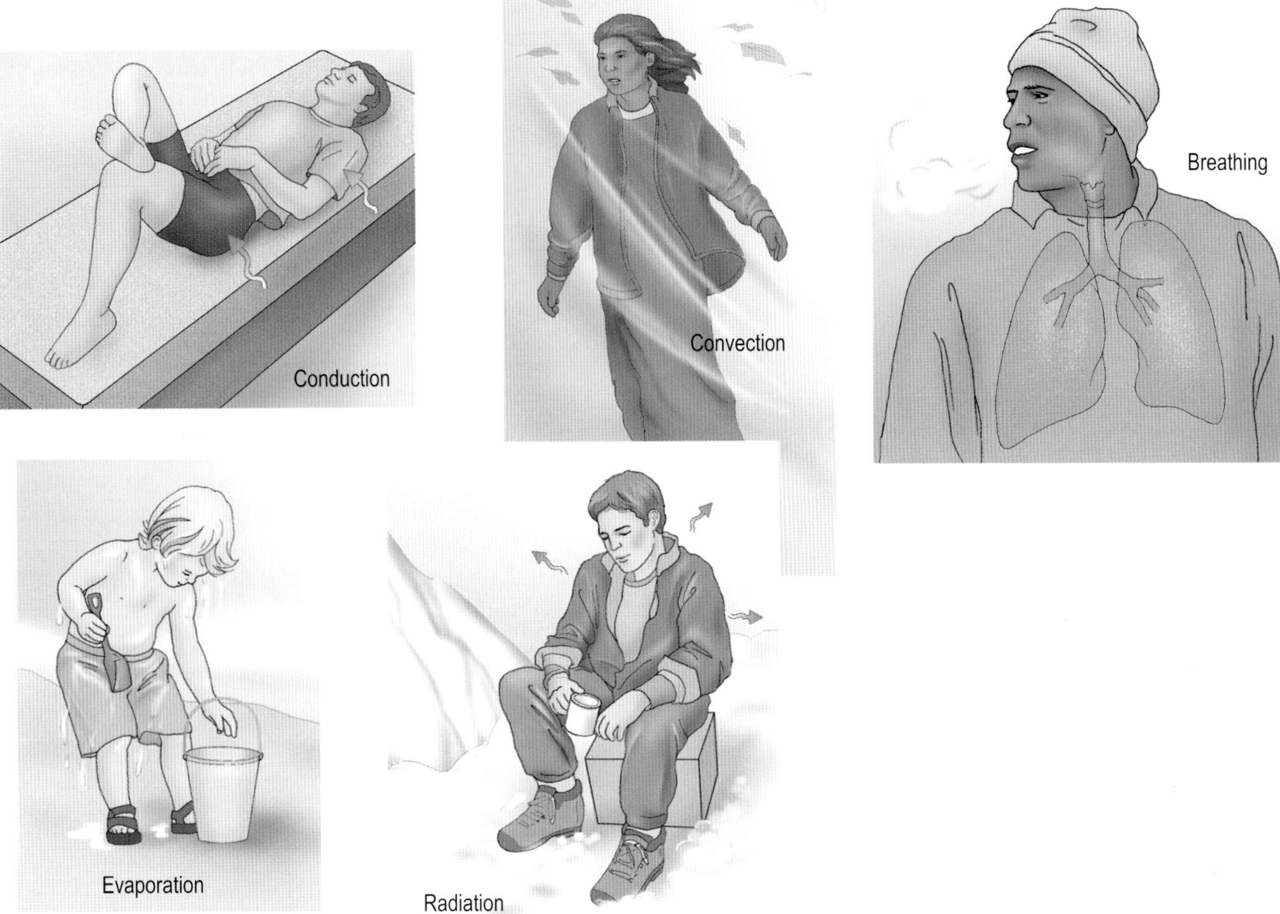

Figure 23-1 Mechanisms of heat loss.

most important of these in regulating heat loss. Radiation, conduction, convection, and evaporation are the major mechanisms of heat loss (Figure 23-1).

The surface of the human body constantly emits heat in the form of infrared rays; if the surface of the body is warmer than the environment, heat is lost through radiation (thermal gradient).

Conduction is the exchange of heat that occurs simply by transfer. Heat moves from a higher temperature to a lower temperature, causing body surface to lose or gain heat by direct contact with cooler or warmer surfaces, including air. If the ambient air temperature is lower than the skin temperature, body heat is lost to the surrounding air by conduction.

Convection is the process by which air or water next to the body is heated, moves away, and is replaced by cool air or water; the cool air or water then repeats the process. Convection can be greatly aided by external forces such as wind or fans and promotes conductive heat exchange by continuously maintaining a supply of cool air. Factors that contribute to the cooling effects of convection are the velocity of air currents and the temperature of the air; the windchill chart calculates the cooling effects of the ambient temperature based on thermometer readings and wind speed.

Critical Thinking

How does wearing the fully enclosed hazardous materials suit affect your body's ability to regulate temperature?

When fluid evaporates, it absorbs heat from surrounding objects and air. The temperature of the surrounding air and the relative humidity greatly affect the amount of heat lost as a result of evaporation of moisture from the skin or the respiratory tract. The relative humidity is 100% when the air is fully saturated with moisture. Sweating can markedly increase evaporative heat loss so long as the humidity is low enough to allow the sweat to evaporate. However, at humidity levels above 75%, evaporation decreases, and at levels approaching 90%, evaporation essentially ceases. Box 23-2 presents other examples of ways the body regulates heat loss.

External environmental factors

Some factors in the environment contribute to a medical emergency and may also affect rescue and transport. These elements include the climate, season, weather, atmospheric pressure and terrain. When the potential for an environmen-

Box 23-2

Compensatory mechanisms for regulating heat loss

Mechanisms that increase heat loss

Vasodilation of skin vessels
Sweating

Mechanisms that decrease heat production

Decreased muscle tone and voluntary activity
Decreased hormone secretion
Decreased appetite

Box 23-3

Drugs increasing risk of heat illness

Alcohol
Anaesthetics
Anticholinergics
Antihistamines
Amphetamines
Anti-Parkinson's drugs
α-adrenergic agonists
β-adrenergic antagonists
Benzodiazepines
Calcium channel blockers
Cocaine
Diuretics
LSD and PCP
Laxatives
Neuroleptics
Phenothiazines
Thyroid hormones
Tricyclic antidepressants

tal emergency exists, the paramedic must consider the following factors:

- localized prevailing weather norms and any deviations
- characteristics of seasonal variation in climate
- weather extremes (wind, rain, snow, humidity)
- barometric pressure (e.g. at altitude or under water)
- terrain that can complicate injury or rescue.

The patient's health also is a factor related to environmental stressors and can make other medical or traumatic conditions worse. Examples include the patient's age, predisposing medical conditions, use of prescription and over-the-counter medications (see Box 23-3), use of alcohol or recreational drugs, and previous rate of exertion.

Hyperthermia

Hyperthermia, or heat illness, results from one of two basic causes:

1. Temperature-regulating mechanisms are overwhelmed by high temperatures in the environment or, more commonly, by excessive exercise in moderate to extremely high temperatures.
2. Temperature-regulating centres fail, usually in older adults or in ill or incapacitated patients.

Either cause can result in heat illness such as heat cramps, heat exhaustion and heat stroke.

Heat cramps

Heat cramps are brief, intermittent and often severe muscular cramps that occur in muscles fatigued by heavy work or exercise; the primary cause of these cramps is sodium and water loss.

People who suffer from heat cramps sweat profusely and drink water without adequate salt. During times of high environmental temperatures, 1–3 L of water per hour can be lost through sweating. Each litre contains 30–50 mEq of sodium chloride; this water and sodium deficiency together causes muscle cramping. This normally occurs in the most heavily exercised muscles, including the calves and arms, although any muscle can be involved. The patient is usually alert, has hot, sweaty skin, tachycardia, and a normal blood pressure; the CBT is normal.

Heat cramps are easily managed. The patient should be removed from the hot environment and sodium and water should be replaced. In more serious cases, it may be necessary to commence an intravenous (IV) infusion of normal saline solution. Oral salt additives (e.g. salt tablets) can cause gastrointestinal irritation, ulceration and vomiting and should be avoided, but foods containing salt (such as a salty biscuit or snack) may be useful if the patient is not nauseous. Paramedics may consider rehydration fluids or sports drinks to replace lost electrolytes.

Heat exhaustion

Heat exhaustion is a more severe form of heat illness, characterized by changes in mental status (e.g. irritability and poor judgement), dizziness, nausea, headache, and mild to moderate elevation of the CBT up to 39 °C (103 °F). In severe cases, dizziness caused by significant intravascular volume loss, as well as fainting, may occur. This orthostatic dizziness occurs when the patient changes from a lying position to a sitting or standing position.

Like heat cramps, heat exhaustion more often is associated with a hot environment and results in profuse sweating. Loss of water and salt, electrolyte imbalance, and difficulty maintaining blood pressure contribute to the problem and this heat illness can be classified as water depletion or electrolyte depletion heat exhaustion. The patient shows signs of inadequate peripheral and cerebral perfusion. The person usually recovers rapidly when removed from the hot environment and given replacement fluids. Patients with significant fluid loss or who show a drop in blood pressure when they sit up or stand may require IV administration of normal saline solution. One factor to consider is that patients who are hot and take in significant amounts of water may become water intoxicated and electrolyte depleted, which leads to hyponatraemia. When sodium levels are critically low, cerebral oedema will develop and reduced levels of consciousness and convulsions become a concern. Heat exhaustion can progress to heat stroke if left untreated.

Heat stroke

Heat stroke occurs when the body's temperature-regulating mechanisms break down entirely; as a result of this failure, the body temperature rises to 41 °C (105.8 °F) or higher. This damages tissue in all the body systems and results in total body collapse. Increased body temperature caused by failure of the temperature-regulating mechanisms should not be confused with fever associated with a response to inflammation or infection. With fever, the effect on the hypothalamus is caused by endogenous pyrogens released by phagocytic leukocytes; antipyretic drugs can reverse these effects, returning the set point of the hypothalamus to normal.

Heat stroke is a true medical emergency with a possible mortality rate of 10%. The syndrome is classified into two types: classic heat stroke and exertional heat stroke.

Classic heat stroke occurs during periods of sustained high ambient temperatures and humidity and commonly affects the young, older adults, and those who live in poorly ventilated homes without air conditioning. An example is a young child left in an enclosed car on a hot afternoon or an older person confined to a hot room during a heatwave. Victims of classic heat stroke may also suffer from chronic diseases such as diabetes, heart disease, alcoholism or mental health disorders, which may predispose the individual to the syndrome. Many patients who are susceptible to classic heat stroke take prescribed medications for other conditions; for example, diuretics, antihypertensives, psychotropics (antipsychotics, antihistamines, phenothiazines) and anticholinergics. These drugs further impair a person's ability to tolerate heat stress and in these patients the illness develops from poor dissipation of environmental heat.

Note

The autoimmune neuropathy associated with diabetes can interfere with vasodilation, perspiration, and thermoregulatory input. Some cardiac drugs (e.g. diuretics and beta-blockers) can predispose a patient to dehydration, can interfere with vasodilation, and can reduce the body's ability to increase the heart rate in response to a volume loss.

In contrast to patients with classic heat stroke, patients with exertional heat stroke are usually young and healthy such as athletes and military personnel who exercise in the heat and humidity. In these situations, heat builds up more rapidly in the body than it can be dispersed into the environment. Preventive measures to reduce the risk of exertional heat illness for all age groups include the following:

- avoiding or limiting exercise in hot environments
- maintaining an adequate fluid intake
- achieving acclimatization, which results in more perspiration with a lower salt concentration, thereby increasing fluid volume in the body.

Clinical manifestations

As described previously, the temperature-regulating centres in the brain receive their information largely from the temperature of circulating blood in the deep and superficial veins and from the skin. In response to hypothalamic stimulation, a number of physiological events occur: (1) the respiratory rate quickens to increase heat loss through exhaled air; (2) cardiac output increases to provide more blood flow through skin and muscle to enhance heat radiation; and (3) sweat gland activity increases to enhance evaporative heat loss. These compensatory mechanisms require a normally functioning CNS to properly respond to the temperature extreme as well as a working cardiovascular system to move excess heat from the core to the surface of the body. Problems in either or both of these systems lead to a rapidly increasing CBT.

Central nervous system manifestations

The CNS manifestations of heat stroke vary. Some patients may be in frank coma whilst others may show confusion and irrational behaviour before collapse. Convulsions are common and can occur early or late in the course of the illness. Because the brain stores little energy, it depends on a constant supply of oxygen and glucose; decreased cerebral perfusion pressure results in cerebral ischaemia and acidosis and increased temperatures markedly increase the metabolic demands of the brain as well. The extent of brain damage depends on the severity and duration of the hyperthermic episode. Fever from illness (e.g. infection) and an increased CBT from heat stroke produce similar symptoms, especially in the central nervous system. The paramedic should obtain a thorough history (if available) so as to distinguish between the two syndromes. If unsure of the cause, the paramedic should treat the patient for heat stroke.

Critical Thinking

What other conditions can demonstrate the types of mental status changes seen with heat stroke?

Cardiovascular manifestations

A rise in skin temperature reduces the thermal gradient between the core and the skin, causing an increase in skin blood flow (peripheral vasodilation), which gives the skin a flushed appearance. About 25% of victims of exertional heat stroke have persistent sweating, which results from increased release of catecholamines. In classic heat stroke, sweating usually is absent, due to dehydration, drug use that impairs sweating, direct thermal injury to sweat glands, or sweat gland fatigue. Therefore the presence of sweating does not rule out the diagnosis and the cessation of sweating is not the cause of heat stroke.

Peripheral vasodilation results in decreased vascular resistance and shunting as the illness progresses. High-output cardiac failure is common, manifested by extreme tachycardia and hypotension, and cardiac output initially can be four to five times normal. However, as temperatures continue to rise, myocardial contractility begins to decrease and the central venous pressure rises. In any age group, the presence of hypotension and decreased cardiac output points to a poor prognosis.

Other systemic manifestations

Other systemic manifestations associated with heat stroke include pulmonary oedema (accompanied by systemic acidosis, tachypnoea, hypoxemia and hypercapnia), myocardial dysfunction, gastrointestinal bleeding, a reduction in renal function (secondary to hypovolaemia and hypoperfusion), hepatic injury, clotting disorders, and electrolyte abnormalities.

Imitators of heat stroke

Differentiating between heat stroke and other conditions may be difficult but must be undertaken: sepsis or other febrile illness, some CNS conditions, and poisoning with drugs such as atropine may mimic heatstroke. Equally, some drugs such as ecstasy (MDMA), antipsychotic medication (neuroleptic malignant syndrome) and anaesthetics (malignant hyperthermia) may result in hyperthermic episodes.

Management

Heat stroke almost invariably leads to death if left untreated. The factors most important to a successful outcome are rapid recognition of the heat illness, and rapid cooling of the patient, with initiation of basic life support (BLS) and advanced life support (ALS) measures. After ensuring an adequate airway and ventilatory (oxygen) and circulatory support, the paramedic should manage the patient with heat stroke as follows:

1. Move the patient to a cool environment and remove all the patient's clothing. Record the CBT; take and record the temperature at least every 5 min during the cooling process. This ensures adequate rates of cooling and also helps to prevent inadvertent (rebound) hypothermia. Rebound hypothermia can best be avoided by stopping the cooling measures when the patient's CBT reaches about 39 °C (102 °F).
2. Begin cooling by fanning the patient while keeping the skin wet and continue lowering the body temperature by this method en route to the hospital. If transport is delayed, spraying cool or tepid water (<16 °C [60 °F]) over the body surface with fanning of air is recommended or submersion in cool water may be beneficial although not always practicable. However, avoid submersion in iced water which can lead to shivering, frank shaking, peripheral vasoconstriction, and convulsions and act to increase the CBT as the body temperature is lowered. The use of cold packs in areas such as neck, axillae and groin may be helpful.
3. If hypovolaemia is present, give the patient an initial fluid challenge of 250 mL. In most patients the blood pressure rises to a normal range during the cooling process as large volumes of blood from the skin move back to the central circulation; rapid cooling directly improves cardiac output. Be very cautious with fluid replacement and closely monitor the patient for signs of fluid overload; the administration of too much fluid can cause pulmonary oedema, especially in older adults. The ECG must be monitored.
4. Administer medications as required. Depending on the patient's status and response to cooling methods, these drugs may include diazepam if the patient convulses and glucose to manage hypoglycaemia.

Hypothermia

Hypothermia (CBT less than 35 °C [95 °F]) can result from a decrease in heat production, an increase in heat loss, or a combination of these two processes.

Hypothermia can have metabolic, neurological, traumatic, toxic and infectious causes. However, it most often is seen in cold climates and in exposure to extremely cold conditions in the environment. Failure to recognize and properly treat hypothermia can increase the rate of morbidity and mortality.

Pathophysiology

Exposure to cold produces a chain of events in the body aimed at conserving core heat. Initially, immediate vasoconstriction in the peripheral vessels occurs. At the same time, the rate of metabolism by the CNS increases; the blood pressure and the heart and respiratory rates also increase dramatically. As cold exposure continues, muscle tone increases. The body generates heat in the form of shivering, which continues until the CBT reaches about 30 °C (86 °F), glucose or glycogen is depleted, or insulin is no longer available for glucose transfer. When shivering stops, cooling is rapid; a general decline then begins in the function of all body systems.

With continued cooling, respirations decline slowly; the pulse rate and blood pressure decrease; the blood pH drops; and significant electrolyte imbalances emerge. Hypovolaemia can develop from a shift of fluid out of the vascular space, with increased loss of fluid through urination (cold diuresis). After early tachycardia, progressive bradycardia develops; this does not often respond to atropine. Significant electrocardiograph (ECG) changes occur, including prolonged PR, QRS, and QT intervals; obscure or absent P waves; and ST-segment and T-wave abnormalities. In addition, the J point (Osborn wave) may be present at the junction of the QRS complex and ST segment (see Chapter 15) (Figure 23-2). These events generally are followed by cardiac and respiratory arrest as the CBT approaches 20 °C (68 °F).

The progression of clinical signs and symptoms of hypothermia is divided into three classes based on the CBT:[1] mild,

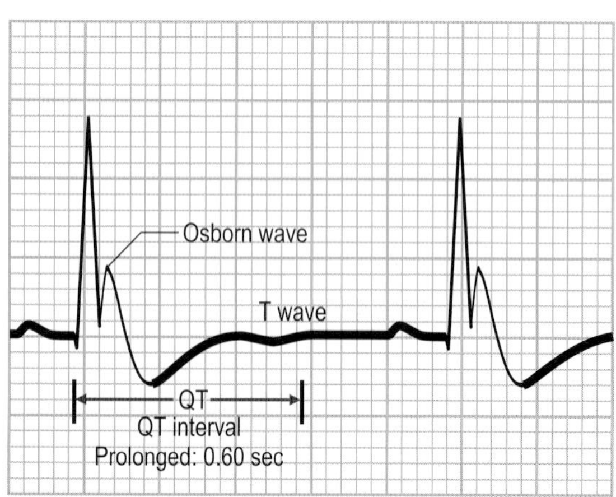

Figure 23-2 Osborn wave of hypothermia.

Table 23-1 Progression of clinical signs and symptoms of hypothermia

Classification	Core body temperature	Signs and symptoms
Mild	32–35°C (89.6–95°F)	Increased metabolic rate, maximum shivering, thermogenesis, Impaired judgement and coordination, slurred speech, apathy
Moderate	30–32°C (86–89.6°F)	Respiratory depression, myocardial irritability, bradycardia, atrial fibrillation, Osborn waves
Severe	<30°C (86°F)	Basal metabolic rate 50% of normal, loss of deep tendon reflexes, fixed and dilated pupils, spontaneous ventricular fibrillation

Often no reliable correlation is seen between clinical signs and symptoms and a specific core body temperature.

moderate, and severe. Mild hypothermia is classified as a CBT between 32° and 35°C (89.6° and 95°F); moderate hypothermia as a CBT between 30° and 32°C (86° and 89.6°F); and severe hypothermia as a CBT below 30°C (86°F). The signs and symptoms of the three classes of hypothermia are listed in Table 23-1.

Those at increased risk for developing unintentional hypothermia are outdoor enthusiasts (e.g. campers, hikers, hunters and fishermen), older adults, the very young, and individuals with concurrent medical or psychiatric illness. Thermoregulatory mechanisms also can be impaired by brain damage caused by trauma, haemorrhage, hypoxia, and CNS depression from drug overdose or intoxicants. Drugs known to impair thermoregulation include alcohol, antidepressants, antipyretics, phenothiazines, sedatives, and various pain medicines (including aspirin, paracetamol and non-steroidal anti-inflammatory drugs [NSAIDs]). Acid–base imbalances, such as those that occur during ketoacidosis, also can affect the body's ability to stabilize body temperature; this occurs when the imbalances cause a decrease in heat production or an increase in heat loss.

Critical Thinking

What group of people is especially vulnerable to hypothermia as a result of their environmental, medical and social situation?

Management

The first step in managing hypothermia is to maintain a high degree of suspicion for its presence. When the exposure is obvious (e.g. a victim involved in an avalanche or cold water immersion), diagnosis is simple. However, in some situations, signs and symptoms may be subtle (e.g. hunger, nausea, chills and dizziness). When hypothermia is suspected, the paramedic's immediate action is to extricate and evacuate the patient to a site of warm shelter; remove cold, wet clothing; prevent a further drop in the victim's CBT; survey for traumatic injuries; cover the patient with warm blankets and increase the temperature in the ambulance; and rapidly transport the patient for definitive care.

Rewarming techniques for managing patients with hypothermia are classified as passive, active external and active internal. Passive rewarming includes measures such as moving the patient to a warm environment, removing wet clothing and applying warm blankets. Active rewarming techniques refer to heating methods or devices such as radiant heat, forced hot air, warmed IV fluids, and warm water packs. Active internal rewarming is invasive; this type of rewarming is reserved for in-hospital care and include the administration of warmed, humidified oxygen; peritoneal and/or pleural lavage with warm fluids; use of oesophageal rewarming tubes; cardiopulmonary bypass (active core rewarming); and extracorporeal circulation (blood warming with partial bypass).

Note

Rewarming methods such as hot water immersion can cause hypotension from peripheral vasodilation (rewarming shock) and a sudden return of cold, acidotic blood and waste products to the body's core (afterdrop phenomenon). Therefore, active rewarming techniques in the prehospital setting generally are avoided unless patient transportation is to be delayed.

Mild hypothermia

In mild cases of hypothermia, removal of the victim from the cold environment and passive rewarming may be all that is necessary to manage the cold exposure. The paramedic can accomplish this by removing wet clothing (wet clothes allow five times as much heat loss as dry clothes) and wrapping the victim in a dry blanket to prevent further chilling and help retain his or her body heat. If the victim is conscious, warm drinks and sugar sources can support a gradual rise in CBT and help correct any dehydration present. Patients should not be given alcoholic beverages, which produce peripheral vasodilation and increase heat loss from the skin, or caffeine-containing beverages, which cause vasoconstriction and diuresis. These patients may be lethargic and somewhat dulled mentally but generally are oriented with no marked mental derangements.

Moderate hypothermia

At CBTs below 34°C (93°F), mental derangements are invariably present and include disorientation, confusion, and lethargy, proceeding to stupor and coma. Patients with moderate hypothermia usually have lost their ability to shiver, and their uncoordinated physical activity renders them unable to perform meaningful tasks. Management of patients with moderate hypothermia begins with ensuring adequate airway, ventilatory, and circulatory support and maintaining body temperature. The paramedic should first employ passive rewarming techniques and should not permit these patients to move about independently or physically exert themselves; even minor physical activity can bring about dysrhythmias, including ventricular fibrillation. External rewarming (e.g. heated blankets, forced air and warmed IV infusion), and rapid and gentle transportation for definitive care are indicated for these patients. Careful monitoring of the patient's mental status, ECG, and vital functions is crucial. Take care to avoid 'afterdrop', by applying the rewarming to the central areas.

Note

Paramedics should not delay urgent procedures in patients who are hypothermic. Airway management should begin with basic manual procedures (head-tilt, chin-lift) and slow ventilatory assistance. The use of oral or nasal adjuncts, including intubation, can induce ventricular dysrhythmias through vagal stimulus, and therefore, if required, the paramedic should perform these gently. All procedures should be performed gently while closely monitoring cardiac rhythm; these patients are prone to develop ventricular fibrillation.

Severe hypothermia

If the patient's CBT is below 30 °C (86.4 °F), he or she usually is unconscious. The patient should be gently moved to a warm environment if vital signs are present and the paramedic should commence passive and external rewarming, administer oxygen, and transport the patient to an appropriate medical facility.

If the patient with moderate to severe hypothermia is in cardiac arrest (VF or pulseless VT), CPR should be commenced and attempt defibrillation to a maximum of three attempts. If the patient does not respond to these shocks, further defibrillation attempts should be deferred until the CBT is >30 °C, and care should focus on effective CPR, rewarming the patient, and rapid transport to the emergency department. In-hospital active internal rewarming will be required for these patients. If a patient with severe hypothermia is pulseless, he or she may present with cyanosis, fixed and dilated pupils, and stiff and rigid muscles (simulating rigor mortis). Prolonged resuscitation can be beneficial in these patients, and CPR is indicated even if signs of death are present; resuscitation may be withheld, however, if the victim has obvious lethal injuries or if the body is frozen so that the nose and mouth are blocked by ice and chest compression is impossible. Practitioners normally will not presume a hypothermic patient to be dead until a near-normal CBT has been achieved and resuscitation efforts are still unsuccessful.

Special care considerations for patients with hypothermia

Prehospital care for patients with hypothermia should focus on airway, breathing, and circulation with some modification in approach. These modifications are listed below:

1. Pulse and respirations may be difficult to detect. These vital signs (including ECG readings) should be assessed for up to one minute to confirm the need for CPR. If there is any doubt as to the presence of a pulse, begin CPR immediately.
2. For unresponsive patients and those in arrest, endotracheal intubation is indicated. The intubation will serve two purposes: (1) it will enable provision of effective ventilation with warm, humidified oxygen (if available); and (2) it will isolate the airway to reduce the likelihood of aspiration. Caution must be exercised in the peri-arrest scenario that vagal stimulation is minimized.
3. The hypothermic heart may be unresponsive to cardiovascular drugs and drug metabolism is reduced, allowing for toxic accumulation of the drug in the peripheral tissues. For these reasons, IV drugs often are withheld when the CBT is less than 30 °C. If CBT is 30 °C, IV drugs may be given, but with double the time between doses.
4. Sinus bradycardia may be protective in severe hypothermia; this rhythm may maintain sufficient oxygen delivery when hypothermia is present and cardiac pacing usually is not indicated.

Frostbite

Frostbite is a localized injury resulting from environmentally induced freezing of body tissues. It often occurs in the lower extremities, particularly the toes and feet, and less often in the upper extremities (the fingers and hands). Frostbite also occurs on the ears, nose and other body areas not protected from environmental extremes.

Pathophysiology

Frostbite occurs as ice crystals form in tissue, causing macrovascular and microvascular damage and direct cellular injury. The freezing depth depends on the intensity and duration of cold exposure. Severe freezing can also occur in tissue exposed to volatile hydrocarbons at low temperatures.

Under most conditions of frostbite, ice crystals form in the extracellular tissue. This draws water out of the cells and into the extravascular spaces. As a result, the electrolyte concentration in the cell can reach toxic levels. The ice crystals can also expand and cause direct mechanical destruction of tissue; this leads to damage to blood vessels (particularly the endothelial cells), partial shrinkage and collapse of the cell membrane, loss of vascular integrity, local oedema, and disruption of nutritive blood flow. Ischaemia often produces the most damaging effects of frostbite.

When frozen tissue thaws, blood flow through the capillaries is initially restored; however, blood flow declines within minutes after thawing as the arterioles and venules constrict and release emboli, which travel through the small vessels. Progressive tissue loss results from thrombosis and hypoxia and the endothelium is damaged; this further damages the small vessels and causes the skin to die. The process of thawing and refreezing is more harmful to tissue than allowing the frostbitten part to remain frozen until it can be warmed with minimal risk of refreezing. In addition to extreme temperature, wind, and humidity, predisposing factors for frostbite include the following:

- lack of protective clothing
- poor nutrition
- pre-existing injury or medical or mental health illness
- fatigue
- decrease in local tissue perfusion
- tobacco use
- atherosclerosis
- tight, constrictive clothing
- increased vasodilation
- alcohol consumption
- use of medications
- history of previous cold injury.

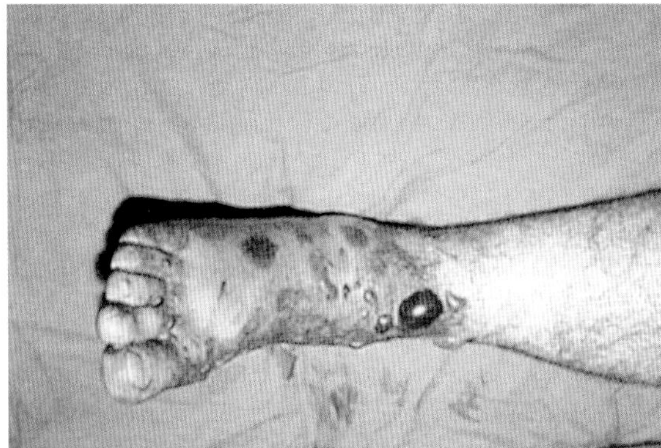

Figure 23-3 Oedema and blister formation 24 hours after frostbite injury in an area covered by a tightly fitting boot.

Classifications and symptoms

Cold injury may be subdivided into a number of classifications but usually cold injury is divided into two main categories: superficial frostbite (also known as frostnip) and deep frostbite. Superficial frostbite involves some minimal tissue loss, whereas in deep frostbite significant tissue loss occurs even with proper therapy. Superficial frostbite usually involves the dermis and shallow subcutaneous layers, whilst deep frostbite is associated with the subdermal layers and deep tissues.

Initial evaluation of the severity of the frostbite is difficult as the injury does not always reflect the underlying vascular changes. Regardless of the depth of injury, the area may appear to be frozen. Palpation may help the paramedic to distinguish between superficial and deep injury; with superficial injury, the underlying tissue springs back on compression, but in deep injury, the underlying tissue is hard and cannot be compressed.

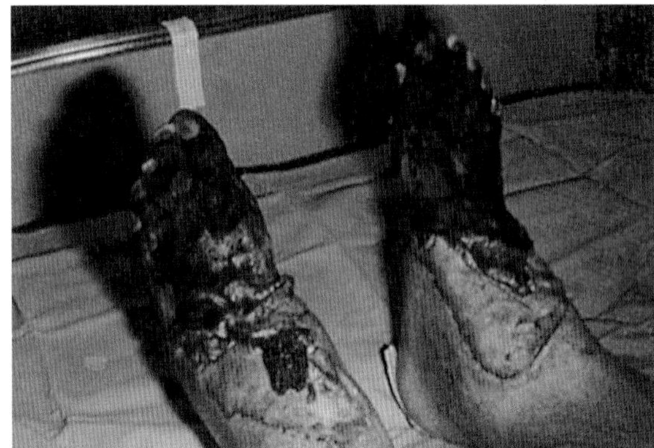

Figure 23-4 Gangrenous necrosis 6 weeks after a frostbite injury.

Superficial frostbite

In most patients with superficial frostbite, the initial symptoms are coldness and numbness in the affected area; these symptoms are followed by extreme pain (tingling and throbbing) during rewarming. After rewarming, oedema usually appears within 3 h, which is followed by the formation of vesicles within 3 to 24 h (Figure 23-3). The blisters begin to resolve within 1 week, after which the skin blackens into a hard eschar. Eventually the blackened tissue peels away (demarcation), revealing shiny, red skin beneath. This tissue is sensitive to heat and cold, and, for unknown reasons, the tissue remains unusually susceptible to repeated frostbite injury.

> **Note**
>
> Trench foot (immersion foot) is similar to frostbite but occurs at temperatures above freezing, due to conduction effects from feet that are wet. The signs and symptoms of this condition are similar to those of frostbite and include pain and the formation of blisters with rewarming. The paramedic should cover the affected area with sterile dressings and keep it dry and warm.

Deep frostbite

In deep frostbite the disrupted nutritional capillary flow is never restored to the damaged tissue. The affected area remains cold, mottled, and blue or grey after rewarming. During the first 9 to 15 days, severely frostbitten skin forms a black, hard eschar. In contrast to superficial frostbite, oedema is slow to develop. Deep blisters with purple, blood-containing fluid may appear within 1 to 3 weeks. Within 22 to 45 days, definite lines of demarcation develop between the eschar and viable tissue. In time, non-viable skin and deep structures mummify and slough (Figure 23-4).

Management

Prehospital care for frostbite is limited to supporting the patient's vital functions, elevation and protection of the affected extremity (jewellery should be removed), pain management, and rapid transport to a medical facility. Vigorous rubbing or massage is ineffective and potentially harmful. Partial, slow rewarming with blankets or other warm objects can worsen the injury, and if transport times are less than about an hour, it is better to provide supportive measures only and rapidly transport the patient. If the frostbite involves the patient's lower extremities, the person should not be allowed to walk. During transport, all restrictive and wet clothing should be removed from the patient and should be replaced with warm, dry clothing and blankets to guard against hypothermia. The paramedic should not allow the patient to consume alcohol or smoke tobacco. Rapid rewarming of the frozen part by immersion in hot water (at 35–40 °C is the most effective therapeutic measure for preserving viable tissue. However, because of the risk of refreezing and the practical difficulties involved, this method of rewarming is not recommended in the prehospital setting.

Submersion

Water-related incidents account for over 650 deaths per annum in the UK; there were around 435 accidental drownings in 2005 (of which 39 were under 14 years of age) with another 155 suspected suicides, and in 64 additional cases crimes were suspected, although specific statistics are difficult to confirm.[2] Additionally, near-drowning episodes occur many times more often; these submersion episodes may be precursors to a drowning event.

Classifications

Due to (historically) a wide variation in definitions of drowning, the Utstein definition and style of data reporting is now used, with the term drowning defined as: 'a process resulting in primary respiratory impairment from submersion/immersion in a liquid medium'. The definition further requires that a liquid–air interface be present at the entrance of the victim's airway, preventing the victim from breathing air. According to this definition, the victim may live or die after this process, but whatever the outcome, he or she has been involved in a drowning event. Victims of submersion incidents usually fall into one of two categories:

- conscious patients, such as non-swimmers, exhausted swimmers, river users who become trapped by roots or strong currents, individuals who fall overboard or off a dock, and motor vehicle crash victims who are trapped in submerged vehicles
- unconscious patients, such as those who suffer a stroke or cardiac arrest while swimming, and those who fall into water and die as a result of hypothermia.

Pathophysiology

Drowning begins with intentional or unintentional submersion. After submersion, the victim realizes he or she is in distress; an example of this is a non-swimmer who panics or a swimmer who tires out. Drowning begins with the conscious victim taking in several deep breaths; this is an attempt to store oxygen before breath-holding (Figure 23-5). The victim holds the breath until breathing reflexes override the breath-holding effort. As water is aspirated, laryngospasm occurs; laryngospasm and aspiration produce severe hypoxia, resulting in serious hypoxaemia and acidosis, which leads to cardiac dysrhythmias and loss of oxygen to the CNS. In 15% of fatal drownings, the laryngospasm is severe enough that very little fluid is aspirated (dry drowning); in the remaining 85% of fatal drownings, fluid enters the lungs (wet drowning). The physiological events that follow are partly determined by the type and amount of water aspirated. Regardless of the type of water aspirated, the pathophysiology of drowning is characterized by hypoxia, hypercapnia and acidosis, which result in cardiac arrest.

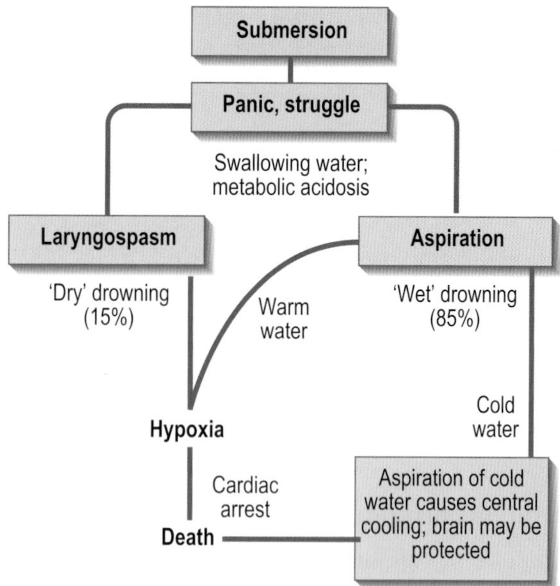

Figure 23-5 Progression of the drowning incident.

Critical Thinking

Do other swimmers or onlookers often 'hear' a person who is drowning?

Drowning can occur in almost any type of water. Victims of submersion aspirate salt water, fresh water, tap water or contaminated water (such as water containing sewage, chemicals, algae, bacteria or sand). In theory, different fluids have different effects; however, these differences are not clinically significant in prehospital care and should not be considered in the initial management of submersion patients. The single most important factors that determine outcome are the duration of submersion and the duration and severity of hypoxia.

Pulmonary pathophysiology secondary to drowning

Respiratory failure, lack of oxygen to the brain, and acidosis are the life-threatening complications of submersion. Hypoxia can result from the following factors:

- fluid in the alveoli and interstitial spaces
- loss of surfactant
- contaminant particles in the alveoli and tracheobronchial tree
- damage to the alveolar-capillary membrane and vascular endothelium.

Poor perfusion and hypoxemia lead to metabolic acidosis in most patients. In those who survive the incident, acute respiratory failure may occur; this includes the development of adult respiratory distress syndrome (ARDS), which reduces lung compliance and increases ventilation–perfusion mismatches and intrapulmonary shunting. The onset of symptoms can be delayed for as long as 24 h after the submersion.

In addition to pulmonary effects, submersion can affect other body systems. For example, cardiovascular problems such as dysrhythmias and decreased cardiac output can occur as a result of hypoxia and acidosis. CNS dysfunction and nerve damage result from cerebral oedema and anoxia. The paramedic also must be suspicious of spinal injury in drowning victims. Renal dysfunction is not a common complication. However, when it does occur, it can progress to acute renal failure; this is usually the result of hypoxic injury or haemoglobinuria, leading to acute tubular necrosis.

Factors that affect the clinical outcome

The following four factors can affect the clinical outcome of a submersion incident.

1. Temperature of the water. Submersion in cold water can have beneficial and negative effects although the relative contributions of hypothermia and the diving reflex are not clear. The rapid onset of hypothermia can serve a protective function; this is especially the case with brain viability in patients who have undergone prolonged submersion. This phenomenon is not fully understood but a contributing factor may be the mammalian diving reflex, a reflex stimulated by cold water which shunts blood to the brain and heart from the skin, gastrointestinal tract, and extremities. This reflex occurs in seals and lower mammals and also occurs in humans to some extent. Hypothermia may be organ protective and also contributes to neurological recovery after prolonged submersion, probably by reducing the metabolic needs of the brain. Hypothermia also may develop secondary to submersion and later heat loss through evaporation during attempts at resuscitation. In these cases, the hypothermia is not protective. The adverse effects of submersion in cold water include severe ventricular dysrhythmias.
2. Duration of submersion. The longer the time submersed, the less likely the patient is to survive. When rescue takes longer than 30 min, victims rescued from warm water in summer months usually do not survive. Submersion in cold water for up to 60 min has been associated with survival, including intact brain function; therefore, most patients rescued from cold water should receive resuscitation. Resuscitation is indicated unless physical evidence of death is present (e.g. putrefaction, dependent lividity and rigor mortis). Submersion victims who have spontaneous circulation and breathing when they reach the hospital usually recover, with good outcomes.[1]
3. Cleanliness of the water. Contaminants in water have an irritant effect on the pulmonary system that may lead to bronchospasm and consequent poor gas exchange. These can cause a secondary pulmonary infection with delayed severe respiratory compromise.
4. Age of the victim. The younger the patient or victim, the better the chance for survival.

Management

At the site of a submersion incident, the safety of the paramedic and other personnel is paramount; only personnel trained in water rescue should try to intervene. Depending on the type and duration of submersion, the patient's symptoms may vary; they may have no symptoms or may be in cardiac arrest. After gaining access to the victim, the paramedic should take spinal precautions while the victim is still in the water only if spinal injury is suspected (e.g. diving injury, obvious injury, alcohol consumption) as spinal injury in drowning victims in uncommon (<1%) and immobilization in the water is very difficult. The paramedic should begin rescue breathing (if needed) as soon as possible. The use of subdiaphragmatic thrusts to remove water from the airways is not recommended unless foreign body airway obstruction is suspected. Where possible, removal of the patient from the water in a horizontal position will minimize the hypotension and circulatory collapse that can occur post immersion.

After removing the patient from the water, the paramedic should evaluate the patient. An adequate airway should be maintained and ventilatory and circulatory support should be provided as needed; drowning victims may have suffered alveoli collapse (atelectasis) and the use of devices that can maintain positive end-expiratory pressure (such as automatic ventilators) may be of benefit. Other forms of initial patient care include administration of high-concentration oxygen, ECG monitoring, and establishment of an IV line. Patients who are in cardiac arrest should be managed with standard BLS and ALS protocols and rapidly transported to the hospital, although always consider the relevant modifications that apply if the patient is hypothermic; victims of submersion incidents often are at risk from immersion hypothermia; heat loss in water can be up to 32 times greater than in air. Hypothermia can make resuscitation more difficult and calls for special consideration with regard to gentle handling, the administration of drugs, and defibrillation. As with all other victims of hypothermia, the paramedic should remove the patient's wet clothing, and then dry the patient and wrap in blankets to conserve body heat. External warming and the administration of heated, humidified oxygen at the scene and during transport should be considered.

It is vital that all victims of drowning who require any form of resuscitation (including rescue breathing alone) should be transported to the hospital; even patients with no symptoms require transport for evaluation. Paramedics should monitor these patients carefully so as to recognize the aspiration pneumonia and hypoxia that can result from submersion and give oxygen which is the most important treatment needed by submersion victims.

Critical Thinking

What are the risks to rescuers on a call involving submersion victims?

Diving emergencies

Emergencies unique to pressure-related diving include those caused by the mechanical effects of pressure (barotrauma), air embolism and the breathing of compressed air (decompression sickness and nitrogen narcosis).

Note

The term scuba is actually an acronym. It stands for self-contained underwater breathing apparatus; this equipment allows divers to breathe underwater. Scuba gear typically consists of one or two compressed air tanks. These are strapped to the diver's back and connected by a hose to a mouthpiece.

Basic properties of gases

The weight of the atmosphere exerts a pressure of 1.01325 bar (101.325 kPa) of force at sea level. This weight is commonly referred to as 1 atmosphere of pressure (1 atm). Water weighs considerably more than air and can exert much more pressure; therefore hydrostatic pressure is much greater than atmospheric pressure. Consequently, at a depth of 10 m, the total pressure is 2 atm of pressure (1 atm from the air and 1 atm from the 10 m of water). This is referred to as absolute pressure or atmospheres absolute (ata). Every additional 10 m of seawater adds another 1 atm.

Laws pertaining to gases

Three laws of the properties of gases underpin all pressure diving-related emergencies (and some high-altitude illnesses). These are Boyle's law, Dalton's law and Henry's law. The following properties of gases can aid comprehension of these laws: increased pressure dissolves gases into the blood; oxygen metabolizes and nitrogen dissolves.

Boyle's law

Boyle's law states that, if temperature remains constant, the volume of a given mass of gas is inversely proportional to the absolute pressure; that is, when the pressure is doubled, the volume of gas is halved (compressed into a smaller space), and vice versa. This can be expressed by the equation $PV = K$, in which P is pressure; V is volume; and K is a constant. Boyle's law explains the 'popping' or 'squeezing' sensation in the ears that a person may feel when travelling by air. It is the basic mechanism for all types of barotrauma: trapped gases expand as pressure decreases. For example, when a diver uses a scuba tank of pressurized air, the lung volumes remain constant at various depths. If the diver ascends but does not exhale, water pressure decreases and the gas in the lungs expands; this greatly increases the pressure in the lungs.

Gas expands as pressure decreases; this fact applies to increases in altitude that occur during air transportation. For example, in a patient transported by air, gas can expand in the respiratory system, gastrointestinal system, or sinuses as altitude increases and pressure decreases in air volume. An example of this is an endotracheal tube cuff.

Dalton's law

Dalton's law states that the pressure exerted by each gas in a mixture of gases is the same pressure that the gas would exert if it alone occupied the same volume. On the other hand, the total pressure of a mixture of gases equals the sum of the partial pressures that make up the mixture. This law is expressed by the equation $P_t = PO_2 + PN_2 + P_x$, where P_t is the total pressure; PO_2 is the partial pressure of oxygen; PN_2 is the partial pressure of nitrogen; and P_x is the partial pressure of the remaining gases in the mixture.

To simplify, the air we breathe is about 80% nitrogen and 20% oxygen; that is, about 80% of the pressure of the air (i.e. the gas mixture) is exerted by the nitrogen in the mixture. About 20% of the pressure is exerted by the oxygen in the mixture. This means that at sea level, the pressure exerted on us by the nitrogen in the air is 80% of 1.01325 bar (101.325 kPa), or 0.88260 bar (88.260 kPa); the pressure from the oxygen is 20% of 1.01325 (101.325 kPa), or 0.20265 bar (20.265 kPa). Together, these account for the 1.01325 bar (101.325 kPa) of pressure at the surface. Even though the gas mixtures remain with normal percentages of nitrogen and oxygen, the partial pressures of these gases change at different altitudes above sea level or at depths below sea level. The principles of this law explain problems that can arise from the breathing of compressed air: gas expansion causes the partial pressure of oxygen to drop as gas molecules move farther apart, reducing the available oxygen.

Henry's law

Henry's law states that, at a constant temperature, the solubility of a gas in a liquid solution is proportionate to the partial pressure of the gas. This means that more gas can be dissolved into a liquid at a higher pressure, and less gas can be dissolved into the liquid when that pressure is released. For example, when a container of a carbonated beverage (pressurized with dissolved carbon dioxide gas) is opened, a 'pop' is heard and bubbles form on the liquid. This occurs because the pressure in the container is no longer great enough to hold the dissolved gas inside. Henry's law is expressed by the equation $\%X = P_x/P_t \times 100$, where $\%X$ is the amount of gas dissolved in a liquid; P_x is the partial pressure of the gas; and P_t is the total atmospheric pressure. This law explains why more nitrogen, which makes up almost 80% of air, dissolves in a diver's body as ambient pressure increases with descent; this dissolved nitrogen is released from the tissues on ascent as pressure decreases.

Barotrauma

Barotrauma is tissue damage. It results from compression or expansion of gas spaces when the gas pressure in the body or its compartments differs from the ambient pressure. The type of barotrauma depends on whether the diver is in descent or ascent. Barotrauma is the most common injury of scuba divers.

Barotrauma of descent

Barotrauma of descent (also known as squeeze) results from the compression of gas in enclosed spaces as the ambient pressure increases with descent under water. Air trapped in non-collapsible chambers is compressed. This leads to a vacuum-type effect that results in severe, sharp pain caused by the distortion; vascular engorgement; oedema; and haemorrhage of the exposed tissue (Box 23-4). As a rule, squeeze usually results from a blocked eustachian tube or from failure of the diver to clear (open) the eustachian tube with exhalation during descent. The ears and paranasal sinuses are most likely to be affected. Squeeze occurs in the ears, sinuses, lungs and airways, gastrointestinal tract, thorax, teeth (pulp decay, recent extraction sockets or fillings), or added air spaces (face mask or diving suit).

The management of barotrauma of descent involves slowly returning the diver to shallower depths. Prehospital care is mainly supportive. After the patient has been evaluated by a healthcare professional, definitive care may include bed rest with the head elevated, avoidance of strain and strenuous activity, use of decongestants and possibly antihistamines and antibiotics, and perhaps surgical repair.

Critical Thinking

What pre-existing illness can make a diver more susceptible to squeeze?

Barotrauma of ascent

Barotrauma of ascent occurs through the reverse process of descent ('reverse squeeze'). Assuming that the air-filled cavities of the body have equalized pressure during the diver's descent, the volume of air trapped in this pressurized space expands as ambient pressure decreases with ascent (Boyle's law). If air is not allowed to escape because of obstruction (e.g. breath-holding, bronchospasm, or mucus plug), the expanding gases distend the tissues surrounding them. The most common cause of this type of barotrauma is breath-holding during ascent; divers hold their breath because they are running out of air or because they panic. Making stops during the ascent allows more time for safe off-gassing. Many hyperbaric professionals advise a 3–5-min safety stop at 5–7 m for any dive. For dives below 20 m, another safety stop at 10 m may be of value. If possible, the paramedic should ask the diver about safety stops during ascent.

Note

Compressed gas at 10 m (2 atm) doubles in volume when the diver moves to the surface (1 atm). This is because the pressure is half of 10 m. The last 2 m of ascent have the greatest potential for volume expansion; this is considered the most dangerous depth.

Box 23-4

Signs and symptoms of diving-related conditions

Squeeze

Pain
Sensation of fullness
Headache
Disorientation
Vertigo
Nausea
Bleeding from the nose or ears

Pulmonary overpressurization syndrome (POPS)

Gradually increasing chest pain
Hoarseness
Neck fullness
Dyspnoea
Dysphagia
Subcutaneous emphysema

Air embolism

Focal paralysis or sensory changes (stroke-like symptoms)
Aphasia
Confusion
Blindness or other visual disturbances
Convulsions
Loss of consciousness
Dizziness
Vertigo
Abdominal pain
Cardiac arrest

Decompression sickness

Shortness of breath
Itch
Rash
Joint pain
Crepitus
Fatigue
Vertigo
Paraesthesias
Paralysis
Seizures
Unconsciousness

Nitrogen narcosis

Impaired judgement
Sensation of alcohol intoxication
Slowed motor response
Loss of proprioception
Euphoria

Problems from reverse squeeze are rare. However, pulmonary over-pressurization syndrome (POPS) can occur as a result of expansion of trapped air in the lungs and lead to alveolar rupture as well as leakage of air into areas outside the alveoli. The clinical syndromes associated with barotrauma of ascent include pneumomediastinum, subcutaneous emphysema, pneumopericardium, pneumothorax, pneumoperitoneum, and systemic arterial air embolism. Except for tension pneumothorax (a rare complication that may require needle or tube decompression) and air embolism, which may require hyperbaric recompression therapy, POPS usually requires only administration of oxygen, observation, and transport for evaluation by a physician.

Air embolism

Air embolism is the most serious complication of pulmonary barotrauma. It is a major cause of death and disability among sport divers. Divers risk this condition when they ascend too rapidly or hold their breath during ascent.

Air embolism results as the expanding air disrupts tissues and air is forced into the circulatory system. The air bubbles pass through the left side of the heart and become lodged in small arterioles, which occludes distal circulation. The syndrome usually manifests as the diver surfaces and exhales. Exhaling releases the high intrapulmonic pressure that resulted from lung overexpansion. With the decrease in intrathoracic pressure, bubbles advance into the left side of the heart and enter the systemic arterial supply, resulting in a dramatic presentation. The clinical manifestations depend on the site of systemic arterial occlusion. The most common presentation of air embolism is similar to that of stroke and includes vertigo, confusion, loss of consciousness, visual disturbances and focal neurological deficits.

Air embolism should be suspected if a diver suddenly loses consciousness immediately after surfacing. Paramedics should begin BLS and ALS measures, and the patient should be rapidly transported for recompression treatment. If endotracheal intubation is required, the balloon cuff of the ET tube should be filled with normal saline instead of air. This prevents inadvertent extubation during recompression; the patient should also be thoroughly evaluated for signs of POPS, such as a pneumothorax.

A patient suspected of having an air embolism should be transported in the left lateral recumbent position and, if not contraindicated by injury, the thorax should be elevated 15 degrees; some experts advise transporting the patient in a supine position, to avoid aggravating cerebral oedema that may develop. If air transport is to be used, the patient should be transported by an aircraft that is pressurized to sea level; the patient also can be transported by a rotary wing aircraft that flies at low altitude. This prevents existing intra-arterial air bubbles from expanding further. The flight altitude must be as low as possible if the internal cabin pressure cannot be maintained at sea level and, ideally, it should never be over 300 m above sea level.

Recompression

Management of a patient with an air embolism consists of rapidly increasing the ambient pressure (recompression). This is done in a hyperbaric oxygen chamber (Figure 23-6, Box 23-5) which allows for the delivery of oxygen at a higher than normal atmospheric pressure. The process is used to overcome the natural limit of oxygen solubility in blood and thus reduces the intravascular bubble volume and restores tissue perfusion. Slow decompression helps to prevent bubbles from reforming. In the UK there are a number of hyperbaric facilities able to treat dive-related emergencies; websites listing the various facilities available are in the further reading section.

Critical Thinking

Where is the nearest hyperbaric chamber in your area?

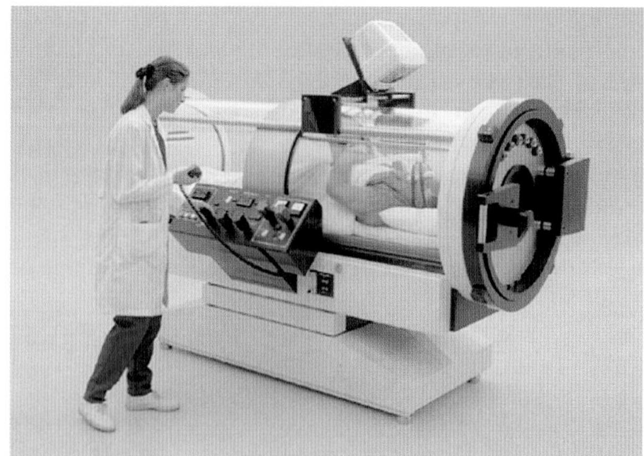

Figure 23-6 Hyperbaric oxygen chamber.

Box 23-5

Hyperbaric oxygen therapy

Altering the surrounding air pressure for medical treatment is a practice that dates back to the seventeenth century. At that time, 'fevers and inflammations' were treated in crude chambers that were pressurized using hand bellows. Today, hyperbaric oxygen therapy (HBOT) is carried out in single-person chambers. These are monoplace chambers. The treatment also can be done in larger multiplace chambers, which can house several patients and the attending hyperbaric healthcare workers. HBOT has proved to be effective in the treatment of a wide variety of medical disorders. These include air embolism and decompression sickness; carbon monoxide poisoning and smoke inhalation; carbon monoxide poisoning complicated by cyanide poisoning; clostridial myonecrosis (gas gangrene); crush injury, compartment syndrome, and other acute traumatic ischaemias; intracranial abscesses; and thermal burns. It also has been shown to enhance the healing of certain problem wounds.

Decompression sickness

Decompression sickness is also known as the bends, dysbarism, caisson disease and diver's paralysis. It is a multisystem disorder and results when nitrogen in compressed air (dissolved into tissues and blood from the increase in the partial pressure of the gas at depth) converts back from solution to gas, causing the formation of bubbles in the tissues and blood. The syndrome occurs when the ambient pressure decreases (Henry's law). The cause is an ascent that is too rapid and the balance between the dissolved nitrogen in tissue and blood and the partial pressure of nitrogen in the inspired gas cannot be reached.

The most significant effect of the nitrogen bubbles is occlusion of blood vessels, which impairs arterial venous flow. Because the bubbles can form in any tissue, lymphoedema (the accumulation of lymph in soft tissues), cellular distension, and cellular rupture also can occur; the net effect of all these processes is poor tissue perfusion and ischaemia. The joints and the spinal cord are most often affected.

The paramedic should suspect decompression sickness in any patient who has symptoms within 12 to 36 h after a scuba dive. These will be symptoms that cannot be explained by other conditions; an example is a patient with unexplained joint pain who had been diving within the previous 24 h. Prehospital care includes support of vital functions, administration of high-concentration oxygen, fluid resuscitation, and rapid transportation for recompression in an appropriate facility.

Nitrogen narcosis

Nitrogen narcosis ('rapture of the deep') is a condition in which nitrogen becomes dissolved in the blood and is caused by a higher than normal partial pressure of nitrogen. Dissolved nitrogen crosses the blood–brain barrier, producing depressant effects similar to those of alcohol; this can seriously impair the diver's thinking and lead to lethal errors in judgement. Symptoms of nitrogen narcosis usually become evident at depths of 25–35 m. At depths below 100 m, with standard air (an oxygen–nitrogen mixture), the diver loses consciousness. Nitrogen narcosis affects all divers, but experienced divers may tolerate it better. Helium–oxygen mixtures are used for deep dives to improve the nitrogen complication. The narcotic effects of nitrogen are reversed with ascent.

Nitrogen narcosis is a common factor in diving accidents, and it may be responsible for memory loss. Prehospital care is mainly supportive; the paramedic should assess the patient for injuries that may have occurred during the dive, and the patient should be transported for evaluation in hospital.

Note

Less common diving-related illnesses may result from oxygen toxicity (usually seen with prolonged exposure to oxygen or exposure to excessive concentrations of oxygen), breathing of contaminated gases, hypercapnia, and hyperventilation.

High-altitude illness

As high-altitude illness principally occurs at altitudes of approximately 2000 m or more above sea level, and the highest mountain in the UK is Ben Nevis at 1344 m, only a brief overview is provided. High-altitude illness is attributed directly to exposure to reduced atmospheric pressure (described previously), which results in hypobaric hypoxia. Activities associated with these syndromes include mountain climbing, aircraft or glider flight, riding in hot air balloons, and the use of low-pressure or vacuum chambers.

The high-altitude syndromes discussed in this chapter are acute mountain sickness (AMS), high-altitude pulmonary oedema (HAPO) and high-altitude cerebral oedema (HACO). Emergency care for all forms of high-altitude illness includes airway, ventilatory, and circulatory support and descent to a lower altitude. In addition, a physician should evaluate all patients with high-altitude illness. Strategies for preventing high-altitude illness include the following:

1. Gradual ascent (days).
2. Limited exertion.
3. Decreased sleeping at altitude.
4. High-carbohydrate diet.
5. Medications (all are controversial):
   - acetazolamide (to speed acclimatization and reduce the incidence of AMS)
   - nifedipine (used solely by those with a history of HAPO to prevent recurrence upon ascent)
   - steroids.

Exposure to high altitude can worsen chronic medical conditions such as angina pectoris, congestive heart failure (CHF), chronic obstructive pulmonary disease (COPD), and hypertension; this is the case even without apparent altitude sickness. These conditions can worsen as a result of a low partial pressure of oxygen, which means that less oxygen is inhaled with each normal respiratory volume.

Acute mountain sickness

AMS is a common high-altitude illness, occurring when an unacclimatized person ascends rapidly to high altitudes. The illness usually develops within 4 to 6 h of reaching a high altitude and reaches maximum severity within 24 to 48 h (Box 23-6). It abates on the third or fourth day after exposure with gradual acclimatization.

The physical findings with AMS vary and include tachycardia, bradycardia, postural hypotension and ataxia

Box 23-6

Signs and symptoms of high-altitude illness

Acute mountain sickness (AMS)

Headache (most common symptom) attributed to subacute cerebral oedema or to spasm or dilation of cerebral blood vessels secondary to hypocapnia or hypoxia
Malaise
Anorexia
Vomiting
Dizziness
Irritability
Impaired memory
Dyspnoea on exertion

High-altitude pulmonary oedema (HAPO)

Shortness of breath
Dyspnoea
Cough (with or without frothy sputum)
Generalized weakness
Lethargy
Disorientation

High-altitude cerebral oedema (HACO)

Headache
Ataxia
Altered consciousness
Confusion
Hallucinations
Drowsiness
Stupor
Coma

(impaired ability to coordinate movement); ataxia is a key sign of the progression of the illness. As AMS becomes severe, the victim may experience alterations in consciousness, disorientation, and impaired judgement. Coma may occur within 24 h after the onset of ataxia. Emergency care includes administration of oxygen and descent to as low an altitude as needed to achieve relief. Definitive treatment after evaluation in hospital may involve the use of diuretics to treat fluid retention associated with AMS, steroids to reduce associated cerebral oedema, and hyperbaric therapy.

High-altitude pulmonary oedema

HAPO is caused at least partly by increased pulmonary artery pressure that develops in response to hypoxia; the increased pressure results in the release of leukotrienes. These increase the permeability of pulmonary arterioles. The increased pressure also results in the leakage of fluid into the extravascular space. The initial symptoms of HAPO usually begin 24 to 72 h after the exposure to high altitudes with symptoms often preceded by vigorous exercise.

Physical findings in patients with HAPO include hyperpnoea, crackles, rhonchi, tachycardia and cyanosis. Emergency care includes administration of oxygen to increase arterial oxygenation and reduce pulmonary artery pressure and descent to a lower altitude. After evaluation by a physician, the patient may be hospitalized for observation.

Portable hyperbaric chambers (e.g. the Gamow bag and Gamow tent) are commercially available and reverse the effects of high-altitude pulmonary and cerebral oedema.

High-altitude cerebral oedema

HACO is the most severe form of acute high-altitude illness, characterized by a progression of global cerebral signs in the presence of AMS. These signs probably are related to an increase in intracranial pressure caused by cerebral oedema and swelling; therefore, the distinctions between AMS and HACO are inherently blurred. The progression from mild AMS to unconsciousness associated with HACO can occur quickly (i.e. within 12 h). However, it usually requires 1 to 3 days of exposure to high altitudes.

HACO must be managed promptly, because without treatment the syndrome rapidly progresses to stupor, coma, and death. As with other forms of high-altitude illness, emergency care focuses on airway, ventilatory, and circulatory support and descent to a lower altitude.

Summary

- Body temperature is governed by a thermoregulatory centre in the posterior hypothalamus. Body temperature can be raised or lowered in two ways: through the regulation of heat production (thermogenesis) and through the regulation of heat loss (thermolysis).
- Heat illness results from one of two basic causes. First, the normal temperature-regulating functions can be overwhelmed by conditions in the environment. These conditions can include heat stress. More often they involve excessive exercise in moderate to extreme environmental conditions. Second, the body's thermoregulatory mechanism can fail. This may occur in older adults or ill or debilitated individuals. Heat cramps are brief, intermittent, and often severe. They are muscular cramps that occur in muscles fatigued by heavy work or exercise. Heat exhaustion is characterized by minor aberrations in mental status, dizziness, nausea, headache, and a mild to moderate rise in the CBT (up to 39°C [103°F]). Heat stroke occurs when the temperature-regulating functions break down entirely, and the body temperature rises to 41°C (105.8°F) or higher. Temperatures this high damage all tissues and lead to collapse.
- Hypothermia (a CBT lower than 35°C [95°F]) can result from a decrease in heat production, an increase in heat loss, or a combination of these two factors. The progression of clinical signs and symptoms of hypothermia is divided into three classes based on the CBT: mild (CBT of 34–36°C [93.2–96.8°F]), moderate (CBT of 30–34°C [86–93°F]), and severe (CBT below 30°C [86°F]). Severely hypothermic patients have no vital signs, including respiratory effort, pulse and blood pressure.
- Frostbite is a localized injury. It results from environmentally induced freezing of body tissues. This freezing leads to damage to blood vessels. Ischaemia often produces the most damaging effects of frostbite. In deep frostbite this can include mummification and sloughing of non-viable skin and deep structures.
- Drowning is defined as a 'mortal' event. The victim is pronounced dead at the scene or within 24 hours after arrival in the ED. If death occurs after 24 hours, it is considered a drowning-related death.
- The three laws of the basic properties of gases that are involved in all pressure-related diving emergencies are Boyle's law, Dalton's law and Henry's law. Increased pressure dissolves gases into blood; oxygen metabolizes, and nitrogen dissolves.
- Barotrauma is tissue damage. It results from compression or expansion of gas spaces when the gas pressure in the body differs from the ambient pressure. The type of barotrauma depends on whether the diver is in descent or ascent. Air embolism is the most serious complication of pulmonary barotrauma. It is a major cause of death and disability among sport divers.
- High-altitude illness results from exposure to reduced atmospheric pressure, which results in hypoxia. Forms of high-altitude illness include acute mountain sickness, high-altitude pulmonary oedema and high-altitude cerebral oedema.

References

1. Soar J, Deakin C, Nolan J et al 2005 European Resuscitation Council Guidelines for Resuscitation 2005. Section 7. Cardiac arrest in special circumstances. Resuscitation 67 Suppl 1:S135–S170
2. National Water Safety Forum http://www.nationalwatersafety.org.uk/statistics/2005/index2.htm

Further reading

Auerbach PS 1995 Wilderness medicine, 3rd edition. Mosby, St Louis

Baskett P, Nolan J 2006 A pocket book of the European Resuscitation Council guidelines for resuscitation 2005. Mosby/Elsevier, Edinburgh

Biem J, Koehnecke N, Classen D, Dosman J 2003 Out of the cold: management of hypothermia and frostbite. Can Med Assoc J 168(3):305–311

Bledsoe B, Hertelendy A, Romig L 2003 Disorders of temperature regulation: prehospital implications. J Emerg Med Serv 28(3):36–50

Diving Diseases Research Centre http://www.ddrc.org/

Glazer J 2005 Management of heatstroke and heat exhaustion. Am Fam Phys 71(11):2133–2140

Hunt P, Smith J 2005 Heat illness. J Royal Army Medical Corps 151:234–242

Kempainen R, Brunette D 2004 The evaluation and management of accidental hypothermia. Resp Care 49(2):192–205

UK Hyperbaric Chambers http://www.ukdivers.com/info/hyperbaric.asp

Woods S 2001 Cold complications: assessment and management of hypothermic patients. J Emerg Med Serv 26(2):68–79

CHAPTER 24

Infectious and Communicable Diseases

Chapter contents

Objectives

Upon completion of this chapter, the paramedic student will be able to:

1. Identify general public health principles related to infectious diseases.
2. Describe the chain of elements necessary for an infectious disease to occur.
3. Explain how internal and external barriers affect susceptibility to infection.
4. Differentiate the four stages of infectious disease: the latent period, the incubation period, the communicability period, and the disease period.
5. Discuss principles of infection prevention and control.
6. Differentiate the three categories of infectious disease.
7. Describe the management and transportation of a patient infected with a category 3 infectious disease.
8. Describe the mode of transmission, pathophysiology, prehospital considerations, and personal protective measures to be taken for the human immunodeficiency virus (HIV), hepatitis, tuberculosis, meningococcal meningitis, and pneumonia.
9. Describe the mode of transmission, pathophysiology, signs and symptoms, and prehospital considerations for patients who have rabies or tetanus.
10. List the signs, symptoms, and possible secondary complications of selected childhood viral diseases.
11. List the signs, symptoms, and possible secondary complications of influenza, severe acute respiratory syndrome (SARS), and mononucleosis.
12. Discuss the paramedic's role in preventing disease transmission.

Key terms

carrier A person who harbours a disease yet does not exhibit signs of infection. This person may transmit infection to others.

communicability period A stage of infection that begins when the latent period ends and continues as long as the agent is present and can spread to other hosts.

communicable disease An infectious disease that can be transmitted from one person to another.

complement system A group of proteins that coat bacteria and help to kill them directly or assist in having them taken up by neutrophils in the blood or by macrophages in the tissues.

disease period A stage of infection that follows the incubation period; the duration of this stage varies with the disease.

exposure incident Any specific contact of the eyes, the mouth, other mucous membranes, or non-intact skin, or any parenteral contact, with blood, blood products, bloody body fluids, or other potentially infectious materials.

fomite An inanimate object which, when infected with a viable pathogen, can transfer the pathogen to a host.

Health Protection Agency An independent body that protects the health and well-being of the population. The Agency plays a critical role in protecting people from infectious diseases.

incubation period The stage of infection during which an organism reproduces; it begins with invasion of the agent and ends when the disease process begins.

infectious disease Any illness caused by a specific microorganism.

latent period A stage of infection that begins when a pathogenic agent invades the body and ends when the agent can be shed or communicated.

Emergencies that involve infectious and communicable diseases are common in the prehospital setting. They can pose a significant health risk to emergency medical services (EMS) providers. This chapter addresses the duties of the paramedic and EMS agencies in ensuring personal protection. It also presents the causes of infectious and communicable diseases, as well as special aspects of providing care for these conditions.

Introduction

An infectious disease is any illness caused by a specific biological organism such as bacteria, viruses, protozoa, worms, prions or fungi. A communicable disease is an infectious disease that can be passed from one person to another. Infectious (communicable) diseases involve interactions between microorganisms (bacteria, viruses, etc.), the patient, and the environment. Accordingly, they may affect entire groups of people as defined by location, age, socioeconomic status, and the relationships between the groups. Certain groups are at increased risk of infection (susceptible hosts) (Box 24-1).

Box 24-1

Persons at increased risk of infection

- Very young children
- The elderly
- Immunocompromised patients (e.g. patients with HIV)
- Patients with chronic illnesses (e.g. COPD, diabetes mellitus)
- Those with high-risk behaviours (e.g. shared needles, sexual promiscuity)
- Those receiving certain medications (e.g. steroids, cytotoxics)
- Those with a break in the body's defences (e.g. open wounds, intravenous cannulas, skin lesions)

Pathophysiology of infectious disease

Death due to infectious (communicable) disease has been declining since the early twentieth century[1] but infection still remains a significant cause of death. Deaths due to MRSA and Clostridium difficile are difficult to estimate but the number of mentions on death certificates may indicate where these infections contributed to the death. The number of death certificates in England and Wales mentioning *Staphylococcus aureus* infection increased each year from 2003 to 2006 but decreased slightly in 2007.[2] For Clostridium difficile, the trend has been worrying with a 565% increase in mentions since 1999.[3] The development and/or manifestations of clinical disease depend on several factors, including the virulence (degree of pathogenicity) of the infectious agent, the number of infectious agents (dose), the resistance (immune status) of the host, and the correct mode of entry.[4] These factors all rely on an intact chain of elements to produce an infectious disease (Figure 24-1). The elements of the chain include the following:[5]

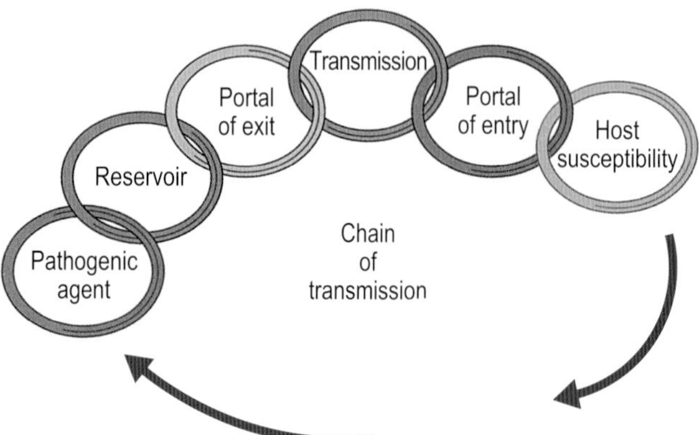

Figure 24-1 Chain of transmission for infection. The chain must be intact for an infection to be transmitted to another host. Transmission can be controlled by breaking any link in the chain.

- the pathogenic agent
- a reservoir
- a portal of exit from the reservoir
- an environment conducive to transmission of the pathogenic agent
- a portal of entry into the new host
- susceptibility of the new host to the infectious disease.

Even if all these elements are present, exposure does not necessarily mean that a person will become infected.

Pathogenic agent

Pathogens are organisms that can cause disease in the human host. They are classified according to shape (morphology), chemical composition, growth requirements, and viability. Pathogens rely on a host to supply their nutritional needs.

Box 24-2

Review of infectious agents and their properties

Bacteria

- Bacteria are prokaryotic (i.e. the nuclear material is not contained within a distinctive envelope).
- They can self-reproduce without a host cell.
- Signs and symptoms depend on the cells and tissues affected.
- Bacteria produce toxins (these are often more lethal than the bacterium itself).
- Endotoxins (chemicals, usually proteins) are integral parts of a bacterium's outer membrane and are constantly shed from living bacteria.
- Exotoxins are proteins released by bacteria that can cause disease symptoms by acting as neurotoxins or enterotoxins.
- Lysis of bacteria may result in the release of endotoxins.
- Bacteria can cause localized or systemic infection.

Viruses

- Viruses are living organisms without a nucleus.
- They must invade host cells to reproduce.
- Many cannot survive outside a host cell.
- Viruses may contain other microorganisms.

Fungi

- Fungi are eukaryotic (i.e. the nuclear material is contained within a distinct envelope).
- A protective capsule surrounds the cell wall to protect the organism from phagocytes.

Protozoa

- Protozoa are single-celled microorganisms.
- They are more complex than bacteria.

Helminths (worms [including tapeworms], roundworms)

- Helminths are pathogenic parasites.
- They are not necessarily microorganisms.

Some pathogens (e.g. certain bacteria) are metabolically equipped to survive outside a host, whilst others (e.g. certain viruses) can survive only in the human cell (Box 24-2). Some viruses, such as HIV and the hepatitis B virus (HBV), can survive for several hours outside a host, hence why blood products can be infectious.

Most bacteria are susceptible to certain drugs (antibiotics) that either kill the bacteria or inhibit their growth. Viruses, however, are more difficult to treat because they reside in cells for most of their life cycle and become intricately enmeshed in the host cell's deoxyribonucleic acid (DNA). Factors that affect a pathogen's ability to cause disease include the following:

- the ability to invade and reproduce in a host and the mode by which it does so
- the speed of reproduction, the ability to produce a toxin, and the degree of tissue damage that results
- potency
- the ability to induce or evade an immune response in the host.

Reservoir

Pathogens may live and reproduce in humans or other animal hosts. They may also live and reproduce in an arthropod, a plant, soil, water, food, or some other organic substance, or a combination of these reservoirs. When infected, the human host may show signs of clinical illness although the host may be an asymptomatic carrier (i.e. a person who can pass the pathogen to others without showing signs of illness). The life cycle of the infectious agent depends on three factors: the demographics of the host, genetic factors, and the efficacy of therapeutic interventions once infection has been established.

Portal of exit

The method by which a pathogenic agent leaves one host to invade another involves a portal of exit. The portal may be single or multiple, involving the genitourinary (GU) tract, intestinal tract, oral cavity, respiratory tract, an open lesion, or any wound through which blood escapes. The time during which an actively infectious pathogen escapes to produce disease in another host coincides with the period of communicability (described later in this chapter). This period varies with each disease.

Transmission

The portal of exit and the portal of entry determine the mode of transmission. This mode may be direct or indirect. Direct transmission results from physical contact between the source and the victim, such as oral transmission and transmission by airborne mucus droplets, faecal contamination, and sexual contact.

In indirect transmission, the organism survives on animate or inanimate objects (fomites) for a time without a human host. Diseases can be transmitted indirectly by air, food, water, soil or biological matter.

Portal of entry

The portal of entry is the means by which the pathogenic agent enters a new host. It may be ingestion, inhalation, percutaneous injection, crossing of a mucous membrane, or crossing of the placenta. The time it takes for the infectious process to begin in a new host varies with the disease and host susceptibility. Diseases differ in how long the exposure must be and how many pathogens are required to invade the new host. Exposure to an infectious agent does not always produce infection (Box 24-3).

Critical Thinking

Think of a precaution or intervention that could break each of the links in the chain of disease transmission.

Host susceptibility

Host susceptibility is influenced by a person's immune response (described in Chapter 18) along with several other factors. Some of these factors include the following:

Box 24-3

Methicillin-resistant *Staphylococcus aureus* (MRSA)

Staphylococcus (often referred to as Staph) *aureus* is a bacterium commonly carried on the skin and in the nose of healthy people. Sometimes staphylococcus can cause infection. Staph bacteria are one of the most common causes of skin infections in the UK.[6] Most infections are minor (e.g. pimples and boils) and can be managed without antibiotics. However, some infections, such as surgical wound infections, bone infections, pneumonia, septicaemia and others, are serious and may be resistant to penicillin-related antibiotics.

MRSA occurs more often in patients in hospitals and other healthcare facilities who are elderly or very sick; who have an open wound (e.g. bed sore) or an indwelling urinary catheter; or who are receiving intravenous (IV) therapy. Staphylococci and MRSA most often are spread by direct physical contact and not by airborne transmission. Spread may also occur through indirect contact by the touching of objects (e.g. towels, sheets, wound dressings, clothes) contaminated by the infected skin of a person with MRSA or staph bacteria. It is important for all healthcare providers to (1) use universal precautions; (2) practice good hand washing before and after each patient encounter; and (3) avoid contact with open wounds or material contaminated by wounds.

1. Human characteristics
   - Age
   - Gender
   - Ethnic group
   - Heredity
2. General health status
   - Nutrition
   - Hormonal balance
   - Presence of concurrent disease
   - History of previous disease
3. Immune status
   - Prior exposure to disease (conferring resistance)
   - Effective immunization against disease (conferring host immunity)
4. Geographical and environmental conditions
5. Cultural behaviours
   - Eating habits
   - Personal hygiene
   - Sexual behaviours.

Physiology of the human response to infection

The human body is regularly exposed to pathogens that can cause illness. Even so, most people do not succumb to infectious disease due to the protection conferred by external and internal barriers.

External barriers

The first line of defence against infection is the surface of the body, which is exposed to the environment. This includes the skin and the mucous membranes of the digestive, respiratory and GU tract. These areas are inhabited by an indigenous flora (agents that could produce disease if allowed access to the interior of the body). The surface of the body forms a continuous closed barrier between the internal organs and the environment (Figure 24-2).

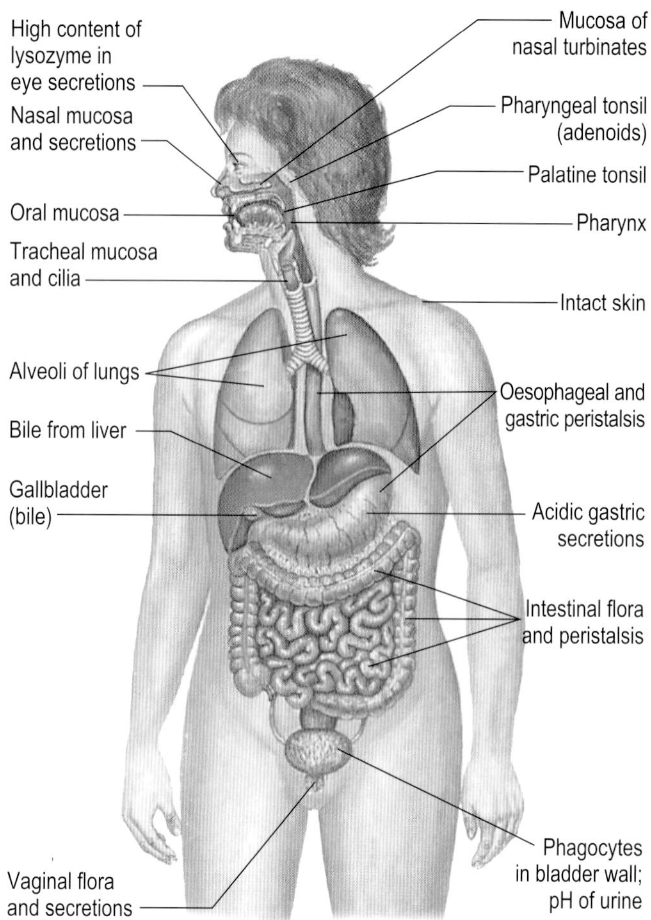

Figure 24-2 First line of defence: external barriers.

Flora

Nearly the whole body surface is inhabited by normal microbial flora. Microbial flora enhance the effectiveness of the surface barrier by interfering with the establishment of pathogenic agents. Indigenous flora compete with pathogens for space and nutrients and maintain a pH optimal for their own growth (this pH may be incompatible with that needed for many pathogenic agents to survive). Some flora also secrete germicidal substances and some are also thought to stimulate the immune system.

Resident (normal) flora play a key role in the body's defence; however, some indigenous flora can be pathogenic under certain conditions. For example, flora can cause infection when the skin or mucous membranes are interrupted or when flora are displaced from their natural habitat to another area of the body. (This is a common cause of urinary tract infection after catheterization of the bladder.)

Skin

Intact skin defends against infection in two ways. First, it prevents penetration, and second, it maintains an acidic pH level that inhibits the growth of pathogenic bacteria. In addition, microbes are sloughed from the skin's surface with dead skin cells, and oil and sweat wash microorganisms from the skin's pores.

Gastrointestinal system

The normal bacteria in the gastrointestinal (GI) system provide competition between colonies of microorganisms for nutrients and space and help prevent the growth of pathogenic organisms. In addition, stomach acid may destroy some microorganisms and deactivate their toxic products. The digestive system eliminates pathogens through faeces.

Upper respiratory tract

The sticky membranes of the upper airway protect against pathogens by trapping large particles. These particles may then be swallowed or expelled by coughing or sneezing. Coarse nasal hairs and cilia also trap and filter foreign substances in inspired air, so preventing pathogens from reaching the lower respiratory tract. In addition, the lymph tissues of the tonsils and adenoids allow a rapid local immunological response to pathogenic organisms that may enter the respiratory tract.

Genitourinary tract

The natural process of urination and urine's ability to kill bacteria help prevent infections in the GU tract. Antibacterial substances in prostatic fluid and the vagina also help prevent infection in the GU system.

Internal barriers

Internal barriers protect against pathogens when the external lines of defence cannot. Internal barriers include the inflammatory response and the immune response.

Inflammatory response

Inflammation is a non-specific local reaction to cellular injury that occurs in response to a microbial infection. When invasion occurs, this line of defence is activated. It works to prevent further invasion of the pathogen by isolating, destroying, or neutralizing the microorganism (Figure 24-3).

The inflammatory response is usually protective and beneficial; however, it may initiate destruction of the body's own tissue. It may be destructive if the response is sustained or directed against the host's own antigens. To review, the inflammatory response may be divided into three separate stages: first, cellular response to injury; second, vascular response to injury; and third, phagocytosis.

Cellular response to injury

Metabolic changes occur with any type of cellular injury. The most common primary effect of cellular injury is damage to the cell's aerobic metabolism and ATP-generating process (oxidative phosphorylation). This leads to a decrease in energy reserves which means that the sodium–potassium pump can no longer work effectively. The organelles in the cell begin to swell as sodium ions accumulate. This swelling, along with increasing acidosis, leads to further impairment of enzyme function and to further deterioration of the cell's membranes. In time, the membranes of the cellular organelles begin to leak. The release of hydrolytic enzymes by the lysosomes contributes further to cellular destruction and autolysis. As the cellular contents are dissolved by enzymes, the inflammatory response is stimulated in surrounding tissues.

Vascular response to injury

Localized hyperaemia (an increase in blood in the area) develops after cellular injury. This produces oedema. Leukocytes collect inside the vessels, where they release chemotactic factors (chemicals that attract more leukocytes to the area). These factors eventually migrate to the injured tissue.

Phagocytosis

Through phagocytosis, leukocytes engulf, digest, and destroy the invading pathogens. Circulating macrophages clear the area of dead cells and other debris. The ingestion of bacteria and dead cells (internal phagocytosis) releases chemicals that destroy leukocytes.

Immune response

The first two lines of defence against infection use the same mechanism to respond to all pathogens. However, the immune response is specific to individual pathogens. The immune system has four unique characteristics:

1. It has 'self–non-self' recognition; therefore it usually responds only to foreign antigens.
2. It produces antibodies that are antigen specific. That is, new antibodies can be produced in response to new antigens.
3. Some of the antibody-producing lymphocytes become memory cells. These cells allow for a more rapid response to repeat invasions by the same antigen.
4. The immune system is self-regulated. It activates only when a pathogen invades, which prevents healthy tissues from being destroyed. When this function goes awry, autoimmune disease can occur (e.g. rheumatoid arthritis, active glomerulonephritis and systemic lupus erythematosus). The immune system may require extrinsic regulation with drugs in patients with transplanted organs or severe autoimmune diseases.

Critical Thinking

Why would a person's internal defences be weakened after removal of the spleen?

The body's immune response to an invading pathogen depends partly on the size of the pathogen and partly on the body's ability to induce production of an antibody. Often, peripheral phagocytic cells encounter a pathogen first. However, circulating B and T cells are also scouting for pathogens (Box 24-4). Complex interactions occur among neutrophils, macrophages, and B and T cells. These cells assist each other in processing antigens that can recognize and destroy the invading pathogens.

Each B cell has a different antibody on its surface, which attaches to a specific antigen that has a complementary shape. When the B cell comes into contact with such an antigen it will bind with the antigen and commence a process that results in the production of large quantities of the specific antibody. Antibodies can also trigger the comple-

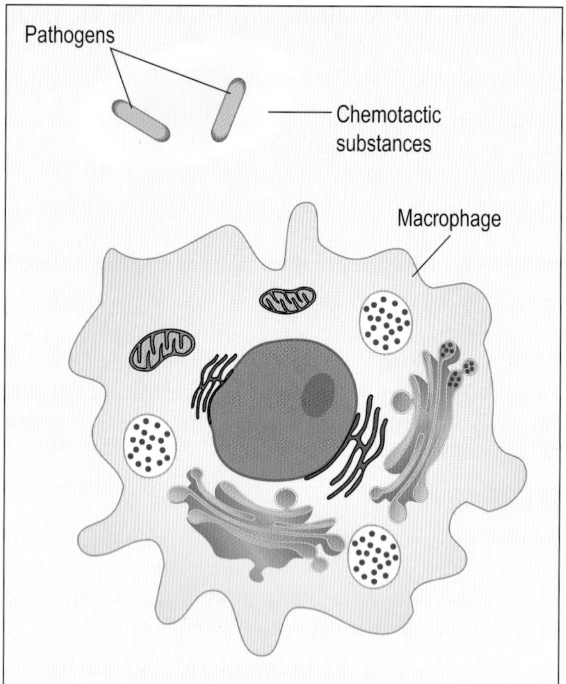

1. Injured area produces chemotactic exudate that attracts macrophages in area.

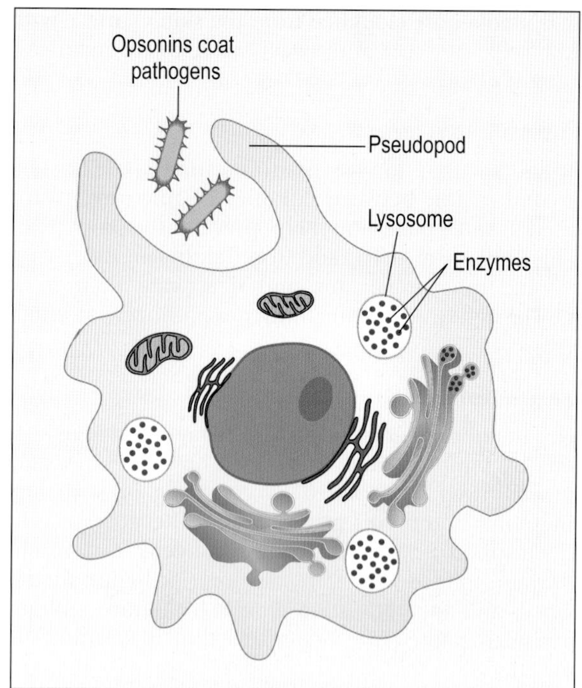

2. Opsonins facilitate phagocytosis.

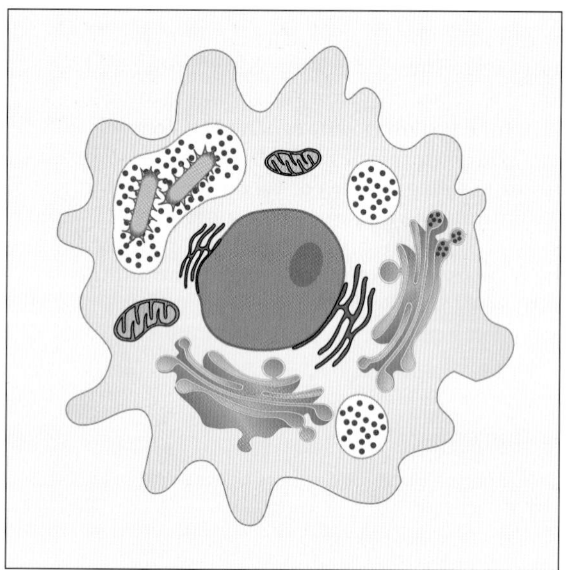

3. The engulfed pathogen becomes digested by enzymes in the lysosomes.

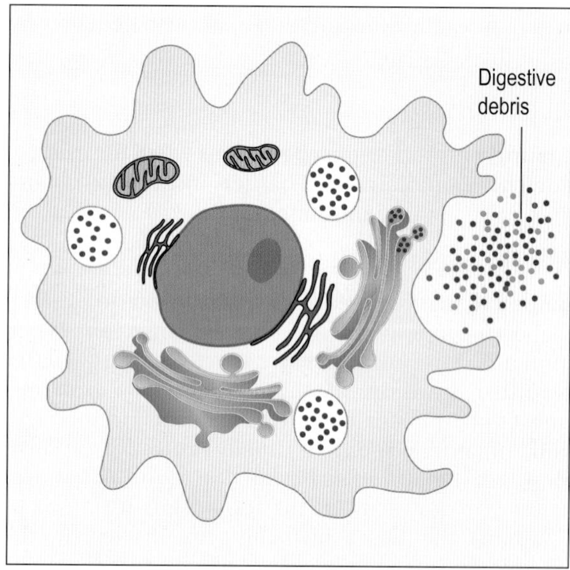

4. The macrophage expels debris after digestion is complete, including prostaglandins, interferon, and complement components. These elements continue the immune response.

Figure 24-3 Second line of defence: inflammatory response.

ment system, which is a group of proteins that increase blood vessel permeability, produce chemotaxis, increase the efficacy of phagocytosis, and destroy foreign cells by puncturing them. T cells not only process antigen for the B cells, they also include a subpopulation of 'killer cells'. These cells play a major role in cell-mediated immunity (Figure 24-4).

Both the humoral and cell-mediated types of immunity take time to work. Both require previous exposure to mobilize specialized white cells. In time, these white cells differentiate between antibodies. They then organize an attack on the foreign material. By comparison, the complement system recognizes and kills invaders on first sight. It does not take time to mobilize specialized responses.

Stages of infectious disease

The progression from exposure to an infectious agent to the onset of clinical disease follows specific stages. The duration of each stage and the potential outcomes vary, depending on the infectious agent and individual host factors. These stages are the latent period, the incubation period, the communicability period, and the disease period (Table 24-1). The risk of infection may be theoretical; that is, transmission is acknowledged to be possible but has not actually occurred. The risk of infection is considered measurable when infection is confirmed or deduced from reported data.

Box 24-4

Types of T cells

Sensitized T cells develop into distinct groups. Each group has a specific set of functions that coordinate the activity of other components of the immune system.

- Killer T cells (like B cells) are sensitized and stimulated to multiply by the presence of antigens on abnormal body cells. Unlike B cells, killer T cells do not produce antibodies.
- Helper T cells 'turn on' the activities of killer (cytotoxic) cells. They also control other aspects of the immune response.
- Suppressor T cells 'turn off' the action of the helper and killer T cells. This prevents them from causing harmful immune reactions.
- Inflammatory T cells stimulate allergic reactions, anaphylaxis, and autoimmune reactions.

Table 24-1 Stages of infectious disease

Stage	Begins	Ends
Latent period	With invasion	When the agent can be shed
Incubation period	With invasion	When the disease process begins
Communicability period	When the latent period ends	Continues as long as the agent is present and can spread to others
Disease period	Follows incubation period	Variable duration

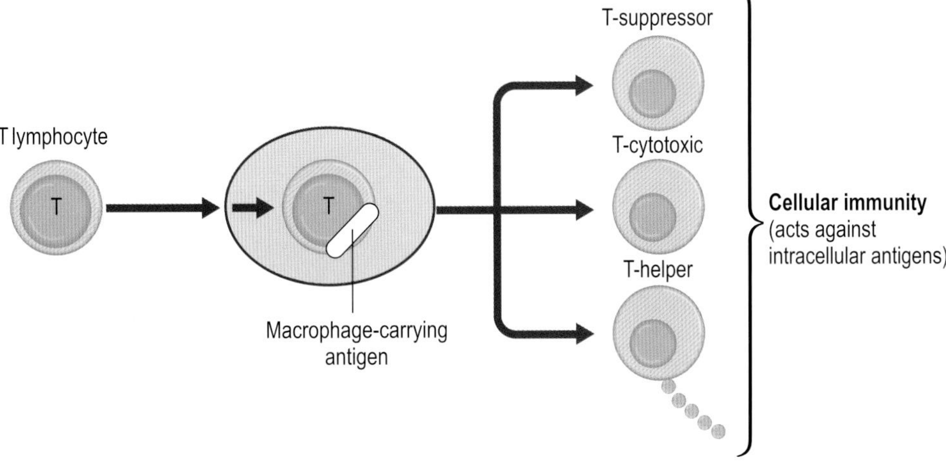

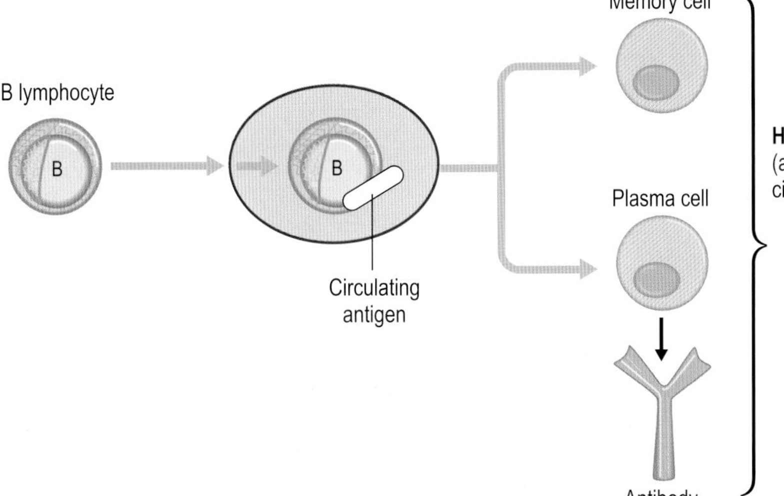

Figure 24-4 Cellular and humoral immunity. Cellular immunity results from activation of T cells through contact with intracellular organisms. Activated T cells differentiate and proliferate. Humoral (antibody-mediated) immunity results from the activation of B cells.

Latent period

The latent period begins when the pathogen invades the body. During this period, infection has occurred but the infectious agent cannot be passed to someone else or cause clinically significant symptoms. In some diseases (e.g. HIV), the latent period is quite stable and can last several years. In others (e.g. influenza), the latent period may last only 24 to 72 h. The latent period as a stage of infectious disease is distinct from a latent infection. A latent infection is an inactive infection that can still shed and produce symptoms; a latent disease is characterized by periods of inactivity either before signs and symptoms appear or between attacks. Herpes viruses are examples of pathogens that readily enter a latent stage. During this stage, symptoms disappear but may reappear at a later time upon reactivation of the latent infection.

Incubation period

The incubation period is the interval between exposure to the pathogen and the first onset of symptoms (Table 24-2). Like the latent period, the incubation period varies in length. It can range from hours to 15 years or longer, as is seen with some individuals with HIV infection. During the incubation period, the infectious organism reproduces in the host. The body is stimulated to produce antibodies specific for the disease or antigen. A person's blood may test positive (seroconversion) for exposure to the disease. A window phase, however, follows infection. In this phase, the antigen is present but there is no detectable antibody. A person whose blood is tested for disease-specific antibodies in the window phase may test negative, even when infection is present.

Communicability period

The communicability period follows the latent period. It lasts as long as the agent is present and can spread to other hosts. (Clinically significant symptoms from the infection may manifest during this period.) This stage is variable and is often the major determining factor in ease of transmission. The communicability period and the method of transmission can be altered in some diseases (e.g. tuberculosis, syphilis, gonorrhoea). This depends on the stage of the disease and the primary site of infection.

Disease period

The disease period follows the incubation period and varies in duration, depending on the specific disease. This stage may be free of symptoms or it may produce overt symptoms. These symptoms can arise directly from the invading organism or from the body's response to the disease. During the disease period, the body may be able to rid itself of the disease entirely; however, the organism may become incorporated and lie inactive inside certain cells (a latent disease). Several viruses (e.g. HIV and hepatitis) can lead to latent infection. The resolution of symptoms does not mean the infectious agent has been destroyed.

Critical Thinking

Which of the four stages of infectious disease can overlap? What problems can the overlap (or overlaps) pose?

Principles of infection prevention and control

The Department of Health has produced specific guidelines for infection control in prehospital care.[7] Paramedics should ensure that they are familiar with these guidelines and should implement them in everyday practice to minimize the risk of infection to themselves, their patients and their family and friends.

Ambulance staff may be exposed to blood-borne viruses such as hepatitis B (HBV), hepatitis C (HCV), and HIV whenever they come into contact with blood or body fluids. The most likely method of transmission of these viruses is by direct percutaneous inoculation of infected blood. This may occur as a result of needlestick injury, splashing of blood onto broken skin, or via mucous membranes and the eyes. In addition to blood, other bodily fluids may also contain pathogenic organisms. Examples include vomit, faeces, urine and sputum.

Note

It is not always possible to identify patients with infectious disease; therefore, paramedics should take precautions to prevent the spread of infection AT ALL TIMES.

Standard principles of infection control include:[8]

- hand washing and skin care
- personal protective equipment (PPE)
- safe handling and disposal of sharps
- waste management
- linen management.

Hand washing

Hands are the most common vehicle by which microorganisms are transmitted between healthcare workers and patients.[4] Resident flora have already been discussed and normally present minimal risk of cross-infection as they tend to live in the deeper skin layers and tend not to be pathogenic. Transient microorganisms do not normally reside on the skin but they are easily acquired and easily transmitted – effective hand washing removes these microorganisms and reduces the effect of cross-contamination. Hand washing should be carried out in accordance with the technique described by Aycliffe et al in 1978[9] (Figure 24-5):

- Remove jewellery (wedding rings excepted).
- Wet hands with water and then apply liquid soap/cleaning solution.
- Vigorously rub hands for 10–15 s; pay particular attention to tips of fingers, thumbs and between fingers.
- Rinse hands thoroughly and dry properly.

Regular use of hand creams will help to prevent dry skin and cracking, which will help to maintain an effective barrier against infection. The paramedic should use impermeable waterproof dressings to cover any cuts or abrasions whilst on duty, and should check these for integrity during the shift.

Table 24-2 Incubation and communicability periods of various infectious diseases

Incubation period	Communicability period
CHILDHOOD DISEASES	
Chickenpox 2–3 weeks (average 13–17 days)	Occurs 1 or 2 days before the onset of rash and until lesions have crusted over and not more than 6 days after the appearance of vesicles
Mumps 2–3 weeks (average 18 days)	Occurs 6 days before parotid symptoms to 9 days after; disease is most communicable 48 hours after parotid swelling develops
Pertussis 7–14 days, commonly 7–10 days	Occurs 7 days after exposure and lasts 3 weeks after onset; highly communicable in early stage before cough; not communicable after 3 weeks, although cough may be present
Rubella 14–23 days (average 16–18 days)	Occurs from 1 week before to 4 days after appearance of rash; infants with congenital rubella syndrome may shed virus for months after birth
Measles Commonly 10 days, 8–13 days until fever, 14 days until rash	Occurs a few days before the fever to 5 to 7 days after appearance of rash
Hantavirus 3 days to 6 weeks	No known human-to-human transmission
HEPATITIS VIRUS	
Hepatitis A virus (HAV) 15–50 days (average 28–30 days)	Usually occurs in latter half of incubation period and continues for several days after onset of jaundice
Hepatitis B virus (HBV) 45–180 days (average 60–90 days)	Occurs during incubation period and lasts throughout clinical course (carrier state may persist for years)
Hepatitis C virus (HCV) 2 weeks to 6 months (average 6–9 weeks)	Occurs 1 or more weeks before onset of symptoms and indefinitely during chronic and carrier states
Human immunodeficiency virus (HIV) Varies: 6–12 weeks from exposure to seropositivity, up to 20 years for symptomatic immune suppression and to diagnosis of acquired immunodeficiency syndrome (AIDS)	Is lifelong from presence of HIV in serum until death; degree of communicability may vary during course of HIV infection
Influenza 24–72 hours	Occurs 3 days after onset of symptoms; infection produces immunity to specific strain of virus, but duration of immunity varies
Meningitis 2–10 days	Varies; lasts as long as infectious agents remain in nasal and oral secretions; microorganisms disappear from upper respiratory tract within 24 h of antibiotic therapy
Mononucleosis 4–6 weeks	Prolonged; pharyngeal excretion may last for years; 15–20% of adults are carriers
Pneumonia 1–3 days	Occurs until organisms have been eliminated from respiratory discharges (24–48 h after antibiotic treatment)
Rabies Usually 2–16 weeks	Human-to-human transmission by bite, scratch, or aerosolization has not been documented; theoretical transmission from contact with secretions of infected person
Severe acute respiratory syndrome (SARS) 10 days	Information to date suggests that people are most likely to be infectious when they have symptoms, such as fever or cough. However, it is not known how long before or after symptoms appear that the disease can be transmitted
SEXUALLY TRANSMITTED DISEASES	
Chlamydia 5–10 days	Unknown
Gonorrhoea 2–7 days	Occurs for months if disease goes untreated
Herpes simplex virus (HSV) HSV-1 2–12 days	Occurs when lesions are present; virus is found in saliva as long as 7 weeks after recovery from lesions; transient shedding of virus is common
HSV-2 2–12 days (average 6 days)	Occurs in 7–12 days with lesion; transient shedding of virus in the absence of lesions probably occurs
Syphilis 10 days to 10 weeks (average 3 weeks)	Varies; occurs during primary and secondary stages and in mucocutaneous recurrences (2–4 years if disease goes untreated)
Tetanus 3–21 days, commonly 10 days	Not directly transmitted; recovery from tetanus does not confer permanent immunity
Tuberculosis (TB) 4–12 weeks after exposure or any time the disease is in a latent stage	Occurs as long as bacilli are present in sputum, sometimes intermittently for years

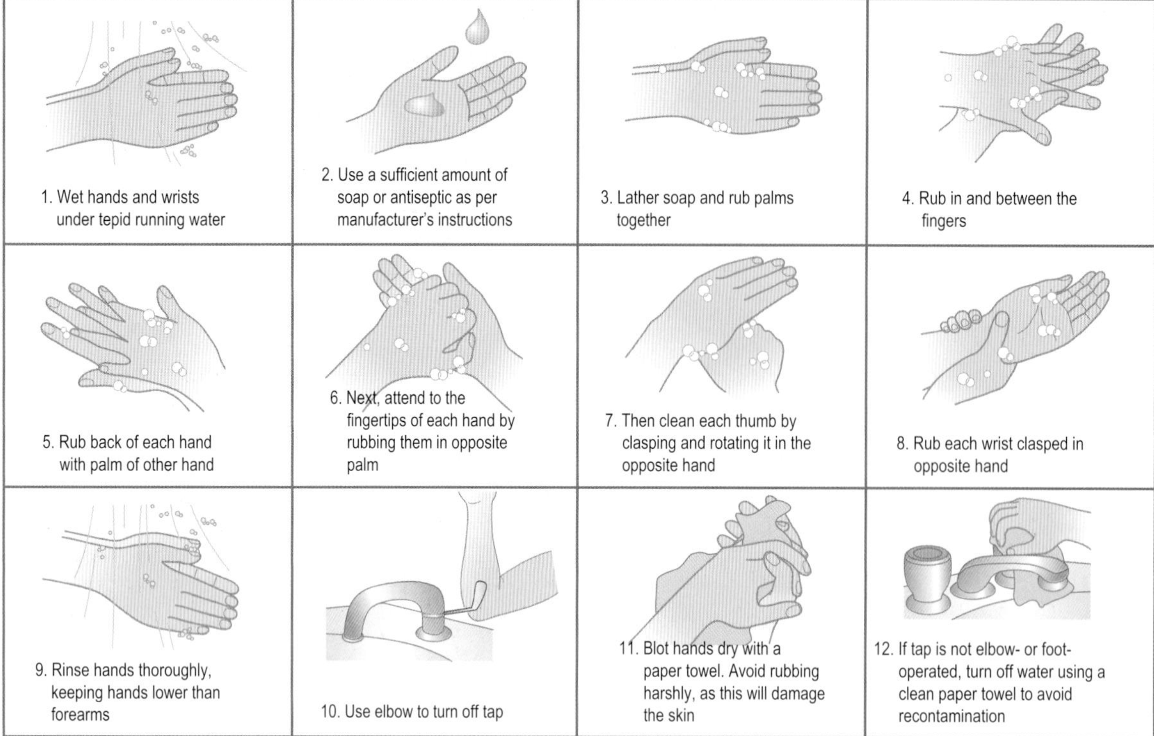

Figure 24-5 Hand washing. From Ayliffe GA et al 1978 A test for hygienic hand disinfection. J Clin Pathol 31:923.

Box 24-5

Determining the level of PPE required

Situation	PPE required
Exposure to blood/body fluids not anticipated	No protective clothing required
Exposure to blood/body fluids anticipated but risk of splashing is low (e.g. during intravenous cannulation)	Gloves and plastic apron
Exposure to blood/body fluids anticipated with high risk of splashing (e.g. serious trauma cases)	Gloves, plastic apron and eye/mouth/nose protection

Personal protective equipment (PPE)

The choice of PPE will be governed by the anticipated risk of exposure to body fluids during a given activity. Many of the activities carried out by a paramedic do not involve contact with body fluids and do not require the use of PPE, for example, taking a pulse, connecting ECG electrodes or taking a blood pressure. The paramedic should make a professional judgement as to the need for PPE and act accordingly (Box 24-5).

Disposable gloves

Disposable gloves should be fitted just prior to patient contact wherever contact with blood/body fluids is anticipated; they should not be worn whilst travelling to the job. In addition, the practice of driving back from a job with gloves still fitted is unacceptable as it will transfer blood/body fluids to the steering wheel, gear stick, handbrake, door handles, etc. In cases where the risk of puncture is high (e.g. when dealing with road traffic collisions where glass may be a hazard), the paramedic should consider wearing two pairs of gloves for extra protection.

The size and type of glove is also important. Gloves should be hypoallergenic, well-fitting, seamless and powder free. They should fit comfortably – not too tight that they become restrictive but not so loose that they impair the dexterity of the paramedic or get in the way during clinical procedures such as intravenous cannulation. The paramedic should also avoid writing patient details on gloves for hygiene reasons.

It is important to note that the wearing of gloves is not a substitute for hand washing; gloves should be changed after each procedure and hands should be cleaned following their removal.

Aprons

Disposable water-repellent aprons should be used where there is a possibility of clothing contamination from blood/body fluids. These are single-use and should be disposed of as clinical waste after use. The paramedic should always have a spare uniform available in the event of clothing contamination.

Facemasks

Facemasks are not frequently used in UK paramedic practice but they may confer protection against airborne infection and splashing against the face and mouth. Facemasks are recommended for use where there is a risk of blood/body fluid splashing into the mouth, if the patient is having recurrent episodes of coughing or sneezing, or during intubation of patients with suspected tuberculosis or meningococcal disease. A recommendation also suggests that a patient with an uncontrolled productive cough should be encouraged to wear a facemask to protect the healthcare worker.[8]

Facemasks should fit correctly with no gaps at the sides. The paramedic should avoid touching the mask once in situ and should not lift it up or down between episodes of close patient contact. Masks should be discarded into the clinical waste after each episode of use, or if they get wet.

Safe handling of sharps

Sharps include any article that can puncture or cut the skin, such as: needles, glass ampoules, razors and scalpels. All sharps should be handled safely in accordance with Trust policy to minimize the risk of exposure to blood-borne pathogens.

Clinical sharps should be single-use items that are stored either in the designated place on the vehicle or within response bags. The paramedic should wear disposable gloves when handling sharps and should dispose of the sharp directly into a properly assembled container (conforming to BS7320:1990/UN 3291 standards) immediately after use and at the point of use. There may be a temptation for the paramedic or an assistant to hold the sharps container whilst the paramedic is disposing of the sharp but this should be discouraged due to the risk of needlestick injury should the practitioner inadvertently miss the receptacle. It is important to note that it is the responsibility of the practitioner using the sharp to dispose of it safely and that sharps should not be passed from hand to hand or person to person. The drive to minimize time on scene for seriously ill or injured patients has led to recommendations in some areas that cannulation be attempted en route to hospital; the paramedic should only attempt cannulation in a stationary vehicle.

The risk of transmission of infection from needlestick injury is low but it is important to follow correct procedure in the event of sharp injury:[8]

- Encourage bleeding from the wound by gently squeezing; do not suck the wound.
- Wash the wound in soap and warm running water or with a disposable wipe if running water is not available.
- Do not scrub when washing.
- Cover wound with a sterile dressing.
- Safely dispose of any relevant sharps involved.
- Report the incident to the appropriate supervisor and complete an incident report form.
- Document details of the patient involved or source of injury (if known).

Within 1 h of the incident occurring, contact the Trust Occupational Health department for advice and post-exposure prophylaxis, including booster injections. If outside of normal Occupational Health working hours, this advice should be available from the local A&E department.

In the event of splash contamination involving eyes or mouth, irrigate eyes and mouth freely with water or saline and then seek advice as outlined above. The paramedic should ensure that they are familiar with their Trust Policy regarding post-exposure prophylaxis.

Waste management

The ambulance service is a producer of infectious waste, which falls within the requirements of the Hazardous Waste Regulations.[5,10,11] Healthcare waste can be subdivided into clinical and non-clinical waste. Clinical waste is defined as any waste which consists wholly or partly of:[12]

- human or animal tissue
- blood or bodily fluids
- excretions
- drugs or other pharmaceutical products
- swabs or dressings
- syringes, needles or other sharp instruments, which unless rendered safe may prove hazardous to any person coming into contact with it
- any other waste arising from medical, nursing, dental, veterinary, pharmaceutical or similar practice, investigation, treatment, care teaching or research, or the collection of blood for transfusion, being waste which may cause infection to any person coming into contact with it (The Controlled Waste Regulations 1992).

The key to the safe disposal of healthcare waste is to ensure that paramedics adhere to the system of segregation shown in Figure 24-6. Ambulance staff must make every attempt to dispose of clinical waste in the appropriate manner, but, where this has not been possible and waste has been left in a public place, the paramedic should contact the control centre and arrange for collection.

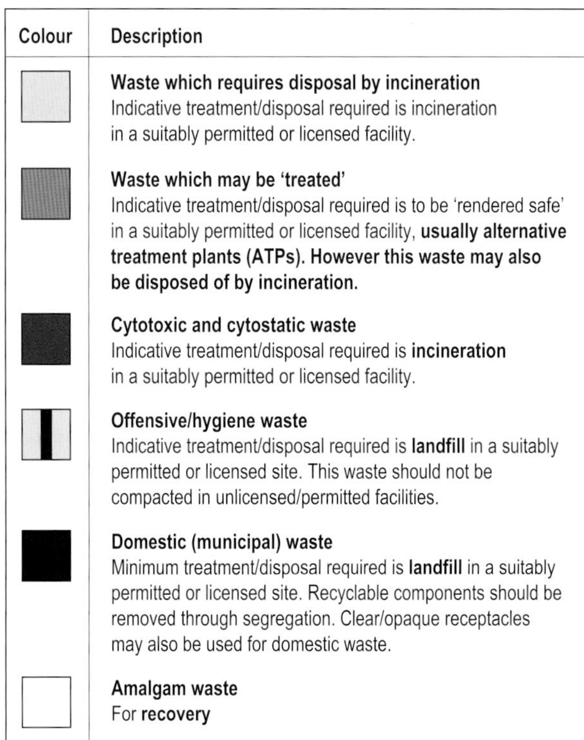

Colour	Description
	Waste which requires disposal by incineration Indicative treatment/disposal required is incineration in a suitably permitted or licensed facility.
	Waste which may be 'treated' Indicative treatment/disposal required is to be 'rendered safe' in a suitably permitted or licensed facility, **usually alternative treatment plants (ATPs). However this waste may also be disposed of by incineration.**
	Cytotoxic and cytostatic waste Indicative treatment/disposal required is **incineration** in a suitably permitted or licensed facility.
	Offensive/hygiene waste Indicative treatment/disposal required is **landfill** in a suitably permitted or licensed site. This waste should not be compacted in unlicensed/permitted facilities.
	Domestic (municipal) waste Minimum treatment/disposal required is **landfill** in a suitably permitted or licensed site. Recyclable components should be removed through segregation. Clear/opaque receptacles may also be used for domestic waste.
	Amalgam waste For **recovery**

Figure 24-6 Colour coding key to segregation of waste. From Safe Management of Healthcare Waste, Department of Health © Crown Copyright 2006.

Clinical waste should be:

- correctly bagged into yellow bags of suitable thickness
- double bagged where the exterior of the bag is contaminated, split or leaking
- kept in a rigid-sided holder with foot-operated lid
- inaccessible to children (as much as practicable)
- filled to a maximum of ¾ full
- sealed and labelled with tags identifying the Trust and base station.

Linen management

The risk of infection from soiled lined is low for a healthy paramedic provided that care is taken. The risks can be further minimized by:

- applying standard principles of infection control and prevention
- wearing disposable gloves and aprons when handling laundry
- removing PPE and washing hands before undertaking further duties.

Disposable linen is preferable for ambulance use but is not carried by all Trusts. All used items of disposable linen should be placed into a yellow bag and treated as clinical waste.

Non-disposable linen should only be used once and should be replaced after every patient. Linen may be exchanged at the receiving hospital or ambulance station according to local agreements. All used linen, irrespective of state, should be placed in a white bag (sometimes it may be contaminated with blood/body fluids), whilst infectious linen (contaminated with blood/body fluids from a known or suspected infectious patient) should be placed in a red soluble bag inside a red nylon bag. (NOTE: Check local procedures as some laundries may use different colour coding.) These bags should not be filled in excess of two-thirds capacity and should not be reopened once sealed.

Care of infected patients

Paramedics may not know if a patient is infected, so should apply standard principles for infection control at all times. It is expected that where a patient's infection status is known, it should be passed onto healthcare providers looking after the patient.

Classification of infectious disease

Infectious diseases are classified into three categories, depending upon the infection control precautions required:

Category 1: This encompasses infections where the risk of person-to-person spread is minimal; standard principles should be maintained.

Category 2: These infections carry a slightly higher risk of person-to-person spread but standard precautions should be effective.

Category 3: These infections are high-risk infections for which special precautions and procedures should be followed.

Examples of diseases in each of the categories can be found in Box 24-6.

Transportation of patients with category 3 infectious diseases

Diseases requiring category 3 precautions are extremely rare in the UK and are often suspected cases rather than confirmed diagnoses. The responsibility for transportation normally lies with the Ambulance Trust that covers the area in which the case has arisen, although there may be occasions where specialist support may be required from other Trusts. There are two high-security infectious disease units (HSIDU) in the UK, one located at Coppetts Wood Hospital in London, the other at Newcastle Upon Tyne Hospitals NHS Foundation Trust. These units have facilities to provide care up to intensive care standards but will only operate when a patient requiring HSIDU is identified. Since the mid-1970s,

Box 24-6

Categories of infectious disease

Category 1	Category 2		Category 3
Erysipelas (bacterial skin infection)	Anthrax	Infestations	Ebola
Glandular fever (infectious mononucleosis)	Chickenpox (Varicella)	Measles	Lassa fever
Influenza	Cholera	Meningitis	Marburg
Legionnaires' disease	Diphtheria	Meningitis and septicaemia	Plague (bubonic and zoonic)
Leptospirosis (Weil's disease)	Dysentery	Mumps	Smallpox
Leprosy	Encephalitis	Poliomyelitis	Viral haemorrhagic fever (VHF)
Malaria	Enteric fever	Rubella (German measles)	Yellow fever
MRSA	Food poisoning	Shingles	
Ophthalmia neonatorum	Gastroenteritis	Tuberculosis	
Scabies	Hepatitis B	Typhus	
Tetanus	HIV/AIDS		
Whooping cough			
Pose minimal or no risk of person-to-person spread – standard principles apply	Standard procedures apply unless additional measures are advised by hospital consultant		Requires special precautions and procedures

Coppetts Wood has treated seven cases of Lassa fever, one suspected case of Lassa fever, and one case of Ebola.[13] Specialist assistance may be available from either London Ambulance Service or the North East Ambulance Service who serve the HSIDUs.

Ambulance Trusts should ensure that they have staff trained and available for transferring category 3 patients and should have procedures in place for such an eventuality.

Preparation for transfer

Once a request for transportation has been received, ambulance control will designate a crew to undertake the case and an officer to escort the crew to the patient and then on to the receiving hospital. The officer helps with journey planning and carries clothes and personal belongings for the crew but s/he should have no direct contact with the patient. A crew of three may be required in cases where the patient has reduced mobility. In this case, one member of the team will undertake driving duties only and will not involve themselves in any part of the patient's care or handling. The crew should be directed to an appropriate point to pick up and don their PPE for the case; this will normally include:

- theatre greens/blues (remove all underwear and socks, otherwise they will be incinerated on completion)
- white boiler suit
- infectious disease suit with hood (worn over the boiler suit)
- double gloving (second glove should overlap the cuff of the boiler suit and be taped)
- white gumboots (boiler suit should be tucked inside the boots, infectious disease suit should be rolled down over the boots ready for taping)
- filter mask
- full-face anti-splash visor (placed over the hood and the filter mask).

Jewellery should be removed and handed to the escorting officer in a suitable storage container. Contact lenses should also be removed unless they are essential; if they are worn during the transfer, they will be decontaminated on completion, although it may be advisable to have a spare pair of lenses or glasses available.

Note

The appearance of a crew dressed in full protection suits may be disconcerting for the patient, so the paramedic should be prepared to offer reassurance and support to both the patient and relatives.

The vehicle

The vehicle should be checked for roadworthiness, fuel levels, etc., and all equipment not deemed to be essential should be removed from the vehicle and left on station for later collection (Boxes 24-7 and 24-8). If further equipment is specifically required for the patient, then this will be arranged between the control room and the duty officer.

Box 24-7

Essential equipment for category 3 infectious disease transfer

1 trolley stretcher
1 carrying chair
Manual handling aids appropriate to patient mobility
3 blankets (disposable if possible)
Disposable vomit bowls
Clinical waste bags
'Infectious for incineration' labels
Disposable gloves
Disposable plastic aprons
Tissue and paper handkerchiefs
Equipment to manage body fluid spillage
Drinking water flask and disposable cups
Disposable bed pans and urine bottles
Oxygen therapy equipment (sufficient for the journey)
Sharps box
Instructions for crew on category 3 infection control transfers

Adapted from IHCD Ambulance Basic Training, 1999. London IHCD.

Box 24-8

Additional items for storage in the cab

Cardiac monitor/defibrillator and pads
Bag–valve–mask and oxygen reservoir bag
Mechanical resuscitator
Primary response equipment pack (airway management equipment etc.)
Suction unit (charged)
Torch
Mobile telephone and contact numbers
Map books and specific directions (even if SATNAV fitted)
Patient report form and pens
Instructions on management of category 3 infection control transfers
Spare batteries for portable devices

Adapted from IHCD Ambulance Basic Training, 1999. London IHCD.

Collecting the patient and transportation

The crew should ensure that all protective clothing is correctly fitted prior to entering the patient's home or location. The patient should be asked to wear a facemask with respiratory filter and safety eyewear in order to minimize the risk to the crew. Moving and handling should be carried out as befits the patient's condition and all equipment should be removed from the location back to the ambulance. In a crew of three, the driver should maintain a distance from the patient and should endeavour to keep bystanders or onlookers away from the scene; the escorting officer may also help with this task.

During the journey, the crew should provide appropriate medical and emotional support for the patient but should avoid any unnecessary procedures or handling. It is essential that the crew who have been in contact with the patient do not leave the vehicle except for an emergency evacuation procedure. In the event of a breakdown, contact should be made with the escorting officer and control room; they will make arrangements to either repair the fault or tow the vehicle to its destination.

At the HISDU

The hospital staff or escorting officer will direct the crew to the appropriate entrance where the patient can be handed over. The crew will then take the vehicle to a decontamination area where it will be cleaned using hot water and detergent followed by agents specified for such use. All removable objects should be retaken off to facilitate cleaning of both the vehicle and the removed objects; all disposable equipment should be placed into a clinical waste bag. Clinical waste bags should be sealed and labelled with the patient's diagnosis clearly written on the label. Hospital staff will receive the clinical waste bags and make arrangements for their disposal.

The crew should then enter the HSIDU through the patient admission door and proceed to the 'dirty' changing room. There they should undress and place all items into a yellow clinical waste bag labelled as above. Items such as spectacles should be placed in a clear plastic bag for processing by hospital staff. Once undressed, the crew should proceed to shower and ensure that they wash thoroughly. It is the responsibility of each crew member to clean the shower and throw towels and paper footmats back into the 'dirty' area before moving to the 'clean' changing area. In the clean area, the crew should retrieve their clean uniform and get dressed before leaving the unit via the designated exit.

Transporting this category of patient is a daunting prospect, so the paramedic should consider counselling and further information from the Trust Occupational Health department. The receiving consultant will also advise on any subsequent medical surveillance or prophylactic therapy considered necessary.

Specific diseases

Human immunodeficiency virus

HIV is present in the blood and serum-derived body fluids (semen, vaginal or cervical secretions) of people infected with the virus. The disease is directly transmitted person to person through anal or vaginal intercourse, across the placenta, or by contact between infected blood or body fluids and mucous membranes or open wounds. It can also be transmitted indirectly through transfusion with contaminated blood or blood products, transplantation of tissues and organs, and the use of contaminated needles or syringes. The incidence of HIV is highest in people with the following risk factors:

- high-risk sexual behaviour
- intravenous drug abuse
- transfusion recipient between 1978 and 1985
- haemophilia or other coagulation disorders requiring blood products
- infant born to an HIV-positive mother.

Other factors that may affect susceptibility to HIV include concurrent sexually transmitted diseases (STDs), especially those that cause skin ulcerations.

Pathophysiology

HIV infection results from one of two retroviruses that convert genetic ribonucleic acid (RNA) to DNA after entering the host cell. The two types are known as HIV-1 and HIV-2. Once the retrovirus is inside the cell, the cell's genetic material is altered into a hybrid of part virus and part cell. The virus basically takes over the cell to make more viral particles. When enough of the viral particles have been produced, the host cell ruptures. This destroys the cell and releases the virus into the blood to seek new target cells. The cell receptor sought by HIV is a T cell that has molecules called CD4 on its surface (CD4 T cell). When HIV attaches itself to the CD4 molecule, it allows the virus to enter and infect the cells, damaging them in the process. The CD4 T-cell count is used to determine how active the disease is; a very low count suggests severe disease. These CD4 molecules are also found on the surface of certain nerve cells, and monocytes and phagocytes, which probably carry the disease to other parts of the body. Even though the body develops antigen-specific antibodies to HIV, these antibodies do not protect against HIV. Secondary complications are generally caused by opportunistic infections that develop as the immune system deteriorates. These infections include the following:

- pulmonary tuberculosis
- recurrent pneumonia
- *Pneumocystis carinii* pneumonia
- Kaposi's sarcoma
- wasting syndrome
- HIV dementia
- sensory neuropathy
- toxoplasmosis of the central nervous system.

Note

The two types of HIV (HIV-1 and HIV-2) are serologically and geographically distinct. However, they have similar epidemiological characteristics. HIV-1 is much more pathogenic than HIV-2. Most cases worldwide and in the UK are caused by HIV-1. HIV-2 seems to be more restricted to West Africa.[14] Some blood screening procedures test only for HIV-1.

Personal protection

Strict compliance with universal precautions is the only preventive measure healthcare workers can take against HIV. However, the chance of EMS personnel acquiring the infection through exposure to infected blood appears to be low. Up to December 2002, there had been 106 cases worldwide of healthcare workers in whom seroconversion was documented after occupational exposure to HIV from patients.[15] Five of these were cases in which transmission occurred in the UK.[16] HBV exposure is a much greater occupational hazard.[17] The risk to healthcare workers increases under the following circumstances:

1. The exposure involves a large amount of blood. This can occur when a piece of equipment is visibly contaminated with blood; when care of the patient involves placing a needle in a vein or an artery; and when the patient has deep injuries. The needle size

and type (hollow bore or suture) and the depth of penetration influence the volume transferred to the skin.

2. The exposure involves a patient with a terminal illness, possibly reflecting a higher dose of HIV in the late course of acquired immune deficiency syndrome (AIDS). The risk of exposure must be understood in terms of how the exposure occurred and what factors were involved. Although the potential may appear high, the probability actually may be quite low. Paramedics should follow Trust protocol for notification and reporting of significant exposures to any infectious disease.

Critical Thinking

Why would testing within 2 to 3 weeks of exposure be needed?

Post-exposure prophylaxis

If exposure is confirmed or suspected, the paramedic should immediately notify the duty officer (per protocol). This allows elective post-exposure prophylaxis (PEP) to begin. Information on primary HIV indicates that systemic infection does not occur immediately; this leaves a narrow window of opportunity in which post-exposure antiretroviral intervention may modify viral replication.[18] Antiretroviral agents from three classes of drug are currently licensed for first-line treatment of HIV infection, although zidovudine (an NRTI) is the only drug to date which has been studied and for which there is evidence of a reduction in risk of HIV transmission following occupational exposure.[19]

Note

There are three types of exposure in healthcare settings associated with significant potential to transmit HIV. These are: (i) percutaneous injury (from needles, instruments, bone fragments, significant bites which break the skin, etc.); (ii) exposure of broken skin (abrasions, cuts, eczema, etc.); (iii) exposure of mucous membranes, including the eye.[17] PEP should be offered as soon as possible where a significant exposure has occurred from a patient known to have HIV or considered to be at high risk of HIV. The recommended drugs for PEP starter packs are now: zidovudine 250 mg or 300 mg b.d. plus lamivudine 150 mg b.d. plus nelfinavir 1250 mg b.d. (or 750 mg t.d.s). It may still be worth considering PEP even if up to 2 weeks have elapsed since the exposure, as the early pathogenesis of HIV is still little understood. The paramedic should weigh up the balance of risks in their particular circumstances and should receive counselling regarding evaluation and treatment after an exposure.[20]

Psychological reactions to HIV

HIV is almost always a progressive disease with morbid late consequences. Throughout the course of the infection, patients are likely to feel and express anger about many aspects of their illness. These include pain, dying prematurely and without dignity, and the social rejection and prejudice that the person may experience. Patient care should include helping these patients feel that they can obtain acceptance and compassion from healthcare workers.

Although no vaccine exists for HIV, many clinical trials are underway. Despite current limitations, the progression of the illness can be delayed with drug therapy and other strategies. This allows time for access to new therapeutic options.

Hepatitis

As described in Chapter 19, hepatitis is a viral disease that produces pathological changes in the liver. The hepatitis viruses are divided into three main classes: hepatitis A (viral hepatitis), HBV (serum hepatitis), and hepatitis C (non-A/non-B hepatitis) (Table 24-3.)

Note

Hepatitis non-ABC is a fourth class of hepatitis caused by infection with the hepatitis D virus and the newer hepatitis viruses (E and G). The routes of transmission for these viruses are similar to those for the hepatitis B virus (HBV). They often are mistaken for HBV.

Hepatitis A virus

Hepatitis A is a disease acquired by ingesting HAV-contaminated food or drink or via the faecal/oral route. The virus localizes in the liver, reproduces, enters the bile, and is carried to the intestinal tract. From there it is shed in the faeces. (Faecal shedding usually occurs before the onset of clinical symptoms.) Antibodies (anti-HAV) develop during acute disease and also late in convalescence. Once infected, the person is immune to HAV for life. HAV is the only hepatitis virus that does not lead to chronic liver disease or a chronic carrier state. Many HAV infections are subclinical and often manifest with influenza-like symptoms. About 1 in 100 patients with HAV suffers from a fulminant infection that may require a liver transplant.[21]

Hepatitis B virus

Infectious HBV particles are found in blood and in secretions containing serum (e.g. oozing, cutaneous lesions). They also are found in secretions derived from serum (e.g. saliva, semen, vaginal secretions). Like other viral types of hepatitis, HBV affects the liver and causes the signs and symptoms described previously. The virus may produce chronic infection, which can lead to cirrhosis and other complications. Although HBV usually lasts less than 6 months, the carrier state may persist for years.

The effects of HBV vary from low-grade fever and malaise (influenza-like illness) with complete resolution of symptoms through to extensive liver necrosis that can lead to death. Other complications associated with HBV include coagulation defects, impaired protein production, impaired bilirubin elimination, pancreatitis, and hepatic cancer.

HBV is stable on environmental surfaces and can remain infective in visible blood for longer than 7 days.[8,22]

Critical Thinking

Why is information about exposure risks important to paramedics?

Table 24-3 The ABCs of hepatitis

	Hepatitis A (HAV)	Hepatitis B (HBV)	Hepatitis C (HCV)	Hepatitis D (HDV)	Hepatitis E (HEV)
Description	HAV is a virus that causes inflammation of the liver. It does not lead to chronic disease	HBV is a virus that causes inflammation of the liver. It can damage liver cells, leading to cirrhosis and cancer	HCV is a virus that causes inflammation of the liver. It can damage liver cells, leading to cirrhosis and cancer	HDV is a virus that causes inflammation of the liver. It infects only people with HBV	HEV is a virus that causes inflammation of the liver. It is rare in the UK. There is no chronic state
Incubation period	2–7 weeks (average 4 weeks)	6–23 weeks (average 17 weeks)	2–25 weeks (average 7–9 weeks)	2–8 weeks	2–9 weeks (average 40 days)
Transmission	By faecal/oral route, through close person-to-person contact or ingestion of contaminated food and water	Contact with infected blood, seminal fluid, vaginal secretions, and contaminated needles, including tattoo and body-piercing tools; infected mother to newborn; human bite; sexual contact	Contact with infected blood, contaminated intravenous (IV) needles, razors, and tattoo or body-piercing tools; infected mother to newborn; not easily spread through sexual contact	Contact with infected blood, contaminated needles; sexual contact with HDV-infected person	By faecal/oral route; in other countries, outbreaks associated with contaminated water supply
Symptoms	May have none; otherwise, the person may have light stools, dark urine, fatigue, fever, nausea, vomiting, abdominal pain and jaundice	May have none; some people have mild, flu-like symptoms, dark urine, light stools, jaundice, fatigue and fever	Same as for HBV	Same as for HBV	Same as for HBV
Treatment of chronic disease	Not applicable	Interferon and lamivudine, with varying success	Interferon and combination therapies, with varying success	Interferon, with varying success	Not applicable
Vaccine	Two doses may be given to anyone over 2 years of age	Three doses may be given to individuals of any age	None	HBV vaccine prevents infection with HDV	None
People at risk	Household members or those who have sexual contact with an infected person; those who live in an area where an HAV outbreak has occurred; travellers to developing countries; people who engage in anal/oral sex; injection drug users	Infants born to an infected mother; those who have sex with an infected person or multiple partners; injection drug users; emergency responders; healthcare workers; people who engage in anal/oral sex; hemodialysis patients	People who received a blood transfusion before 1992; healthcare workers; injection drug users; haemodialysis patients; infants born to infected mothers; those who have sex with multiple partners	Injection drug users; people who engage in anal/oral sex; people who have sex with an HDV-infected person	Travellers to developing countries, especially pregnant women
Prevention	Administration of immune globulin within 2 weeks of exposure; vaccination; washing hands with soap and water after using the toilet; using household bleach (10 parts water to 1 part bleach) to clean surfaces contaminated with faeces, such as changing tables; practising safe sex	Administration of immune globulin within 2 weeks of exposure; vaccination (provides protection for 18 years); cleaning up infected blood with household bleach; wearing protective gloves when touching blood; no sharing of razors, toothbrushes, or needles; practising safe sex	Cleaning up spilled blood with household bleach; wearing protective gloves when touching blood; no sharing of razors, toothbrushes, or needles; practising safe sex	Administration of HBV vaccine to prevent HBV infection; practising safe sex	Avoiding drinking or using water that may be contaminated

Pre-exposure prophylaxis

HBV is a serious concern to all healthcare workers. Blood is the most important potential source of HBV in the workplace and the risk of infection is directly proportional to the probability that the blood contains HBV, the recipient's immunity status, and the efficacy of transmission. Effective HBV vaccinations are available but they should not be viewed as an alternative to standard principles of infection control. The HBV vaccination schedule generally requires three doses over 6 months, although adults requiring rapid protection can have the vaccination at 0, 7 and 21 days. These are intramuscular (deltoid) doses. For the best protection against HBV, the series should be completed before an exposure occurs.

Post-exposure prophylaxis

Post-exposure prophylaxis may be indicated if an unvaccinated person or a person who has not completed the vaccination schedule is exposed to HBV. Before treatment, a blood test is performed to determine immunity to HBV. People who are not immune generally receive the HBV vaccine and hepatitis B immunoglobulin. (This is an antibody used in post-exposure treatment to provide passive immunity to HBV.)

Hepatitis C virus

Hepatitis C virus (HCV) is a blood-borne virus that causes a disease similar to HBV. The virus was associated with receipt of contaminated blood during transfusion before 1992. In 2006, the number of confirmed hepatitis C infections reported from laboratories in England rose to 8346; 10 per cent higher than in 2005.[22] Hepatitis C is the infection that most often results from needlestick and sharps injury.[23] Of healthcare workers who become infected, 85% become chronic carriers. About one-half to two-thirds of those infected with HCV develop chronic hepatitis; one in five suffers severe liver disease, such as cirrhosis and liver cancer. No vaccine is available for HCV.

Although HCV is transmitted in the same manner as other forms of hepatitis, it is not easily spread through sexual contact. Signs and symptoms of the disease, when they occur, are similar to those of other types of hepatitis. Most people infected with HCV are asymptomatic.

Signs and symptoms

Infection with any of the causative viruses may be symptomless. On the other hand, it may cause a typical hepatitis with an abrupt onset of flu-like illness that is followed by jaundice or dark urine, or both. A patient is most infectious during the first week of symptoms (see Table 24-2). Within 2 to 3 months of infection, the patient usually develops non-specific symptoms. These may include anorexia, nausea and vomiting, fever, joint pain, and generalized rashes. About 1% of patients hospitalized with HBV develop full-blown liver crisis and die.

Patient management and protective measures

The management of patients out of the hospital is mainly supportive. The goal is to maintain circulatory status and prevent shock. All healthcare workers involved in the patient's care must follow careful personal protective measures, including effective hand washing. It also involves proper care in the use of diagnostic and therapeutic equipment (e.g. high-level disinfection of laryngoscope blades) and appropriate disposal of sharps.

Tuberculosis

Each year, 8 million new cases of tuberculosis (TB) occur worldwide, and 3 million people die of the disease.[24] The prevalence of TB in England and Wales has been increasing over the last two decades, with 8417 cases reported in 2007 compared with 4659 in 1988, numbers and rates have remained stable since 2005.[25] The vast majority of cases of TB are found in London.[26] The trends in Scotland have been more stable over the last 20 years, whilst Northern Ireland has seen small increases. Whilst the incidence of TB has been declining in the white population, it has been increasing in all other ethnic groups. TB is also more prevalent where HIV/AIDS are epidemic; people with HIV and TB are 30 to 50 times more likely to become sick with TB than someone infected with TB who is HIV-negative.[27] Other factors include:

- immigration of people from areas with a high prevalence of TB
- transmission of TB in high-risk environments, such as prisons, homeless shelters, hospitals, and nursing homes
- deterioration of the TB public healthcare infrastructure.

Critical Thinking

Why is TB more prevalent in patients with HIV?

Pathophysiology

As described in Chapter 14, TB is a chronic pulmonary disease that is acquired through inhalation of a dried-droplet nucleus containing tubercle bacilli (*Mycobacterium tuberculosis, M. bovis,* or a variety of atypical mycobacteria). TB is passed mainly by infected persons coughing or sneezing the bacteria into the air. It can also be passed through contact with the sputum of an infected person. People who share the same air space as those with infectious TB are at highest risk for infection. Transmission may also occur by ingestion or through the skin or mucous membranes, although this is less common.

The pathology of TB is related to the production of inflammatory lesions throughout the body and to the ability of the TB bacillus to break through the body's natural defences. This leads to the formation of caseating granulomas (necrotic inflammatory cells) and TB cavities. These may cause chronic and debilitating lung disease. Susceptibility to mycobacterial infection is generally highest in children younger than 3 years of age; in adults older than 65; and in chronically ill, malnourished, and immunosuppressed or immunocompromised individuals. The infection may remain dormant for an indefinite time, often not causing disease, or it may lead to active, contagious disease.

TB is characterized by stages of early infection (frequently asymptomatic), latency, and a potential for recurrent post-primary disease (see Table 24-2). Signs and symptoms of TB include cough, fever, night sweats, weight loss, fatigue, and haemoptysis. The organ systems affected and the associated complications include the following:

1. Cardiovascular system
    - Pericardial effusions
    - Lymphadenopathy (cervical lymph nodes are usually involved)
2. Skeletal system
    - Intervertebral disc deterioration
    - Chronic arthritis of one joint
3. Central nervous system (CNS)
    - Subacute meningitis
    - Brain granulomas

4. Systemic miliary TB (extensive dissemination by the bloodstream of tubercle bacilli).

Paramedics should maintain a high degree of suspicion for TB in individuals with undiagnosed lung disease, especially patients who are HIV positive.

Patient care and protective measures

Paramedics should be aware of areas with a high incidence of active TB in their service region. (This information is reported by the local health authorities.) Prehospital care for patients with infectious TB is mainly supportive. As with any other infectious disease, universal precautions should be taken during patient care. This includes respiratory barriers for the patient and the paramedic. Surgical masks are insufficient for preventing inhalation of tuberculosis bacteria. However, they do reduce the number of droplet nuclei escaping from the patient. Therefore they should be placed on the patient during transport. NIOSH recommends that healthcare workers use particulate filter respirators (N-type respirators) when caring for patients with tuberculosis (Figure 24-7). Ambulance ventilation systems that include high-efficiency particulate air (HEPA) filtration and a non-recirculating ventilation cycle are another measure for preventing exposure to TB during patient transport. After each call, disinfection of all patient care equipment should be performed.

Treatment

If effective treatment is begun without delay, TB is usually curable. Multidrug-resistant TB is on the rise. For this reason, most patients with TB are started on a lengthy, four-drug regimen of isoniazid (INH), rifampin (RIF), pyrazinamide (PZA), and ethambutol (EMB) or streptomycin (SM) until the drug susceptibility results are known. (Patients who undergo preventive therapy should be monitored for drug side effects. They should be watched especially for signs and symptoms of hepatitis.) Sputum and cultures usually become negative 3 to 8 weeks after the start of therapy.

Meningococcal meningitis

Meningococcal meningitis is also known as spinal meningitis. It is inflammation of the membranes that surround the spinal cord and brain. Meningococcal meningitis can be caused by a variety of different bacteria, viruses, and other microorganisms (see Table 24-2). A major cause of bacterial meningitis is *Neisseria meningitidis*, which is spread by airborne pathogens. The usual mode of transmission is prolonged, direct contact with upper respiratory secretions (discharge from the nose and throat) from an infected person or carrier. Once inhaled, the bacteria invade the respiratory passages and travel by way of the blood to the brain and spinal cord. As the infecting agent spreads to more organs, it causes toxic effects in the involved organ system.

The throat's epithelial lining generally prevents the germ from invading the meninges and the cerebrospinal fluid. The total number of cases of meningococcal disease has been falling in the UK since the 1999–2000 epidemiological year, especially in serogroup C, following the introduction of vaccination into routine infant immunization.[28] The general trend in other strains of the disease is also encouragingly downwards but there is still a need for vigilance by the paramedic. The most common age group to be affected by meningococcal infection is the 1–4 year age group.[28]

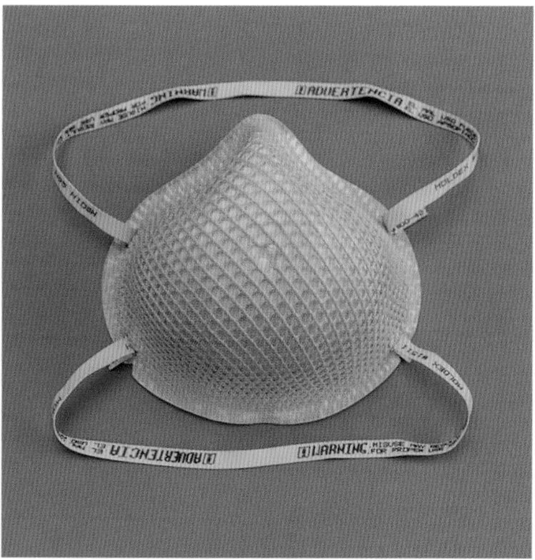

Figure 24-7 High-efficiency particulate air (HEPA) respirator.

Other infectious agents known to cause meningitis

Other common pathogens that cause meningitis include *Streptococcus pneumoniae* and *Haemophilus influenzae* type b (Hib), and some viruses. *S. pneumoniae* is the second most common cause of bacterial meningitis in adults, the most common cause of pneumonia in adults, and the most common cause of otitis media (middle ear infection) in children. This bacterium is spread by droplets, prolonged personal contact, or extended contact with linen soiled with respiratory discharges.

H. influenzae has the same mode of transmission as *N. meningitidis*. Vaccines for children were introduced in the 1980s. Before that time, *H. influenzae* was the leading cause of bacterial meningitis in children 6 months to 3 years of age. (These bacteria are also responsible for conditions such as paediatric epiglottitis, septic arthritis, and generalized sepsis.) This type of meningitis can be treated with antibiotics. However, 50% of infected children have lasting damage to the nervous system.

Viral meningitis (aseptic meningitis) is a syndrome generally associated with an existing systemic viral disease (e.g. enteroviral infection, herpes virus infection, mumps and, less commonly, influenza). Symptoms are similar to those of bacterial meningitis (described below); however, they are usually less severe. In most cases, viral meningitis is self-limited, and the patient recovers fully. The patient may experience muscle weakness and malaise during prolonged convalescence. Viral meningitis is not believed to be communicable.

Signs and symptoms

The signs and symptoms of meningitis depend on the patient's age and general health. In infants, for example, signs of meningeal irritation may be absent. On the other hand, they may include irritability, poor feeding or vomiting, a high-pitched cry, and fullness of the fontanelle. (Maternal antibodies generally protect neonates to 6 months of age.) In older infants and children, signs of meningitis may include malaise, low-grade fever, projectile vomiting,

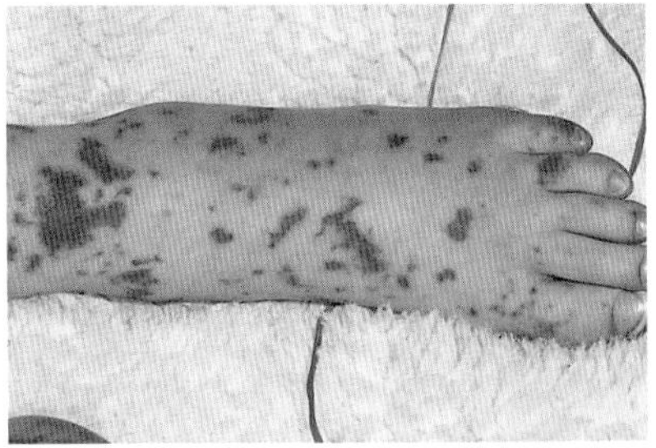

Figure 24-8 Petechial rash in meningococcal infection.

petechial rash (Figure 24-8), headache, and stiff neck from meningeal irritation (nuchal rigidity). Diagnostic signs of meningitis in older children include the Brudzinski sign (involuntary flexion of the arm, hip, and knee when the neck is passively flexed) and the Kernig sign (loss of the ability in a seated or supine patient to completely extend the leg when the thigh is flexed on the abdomen; the patient usually can extend the leg completely when the thigh is not flexed on the abdomen).

Critical Thinking

What does a petechial rash look like?

The risk of bacterial meningitis is most significant in neonates and in children 6 months to 2 years of age. However, infection should be suspected in any patient with fever, headache, stiff neck, altered mental status, or underlying health problems (e.g. recent neurosurgery, trauma or immunocompromise). If extensive meningeal involvement develops in a toxic or debilitated patient, the illness may be accompanied by acute adrenal insufficiency, convulsions, coma, and disseminated intravascular coagulation (Waterhouse–Friderichsen syndrome). In this case, death can occur in 6 to 8 hours. Other conditions and long-term complications associated with severe meningitis include blindness and deafness (from cranial nerve damage), arthritis, myocarditis, and pericarditis. Death can follow overwhelming infection.

Immunization and control measures

Vaccines are available for Hib, some strains of *N. meningitidis*, and many types of *S. pneumoniae*. The vaccines against Hib are very safe and highly effective. By 6 months of age, infants should have received at least three doses of Hib vaccine; a fourth dose ('booster') is recommended between 12 and 18 months of age. Vaccines to prevent meningitis caused by *S. pneumoniae* can also prevent other forms of infection arising from the bacterium. This vaccine is ineffective for children under 2 years of age; however, it is recommended for all people over age 65. It is also recommended for younger people with certain chronic medical problems.

Patient management and protective measures

Patient management focuses on ensuring an adequate airway and ventilatory and circulatory support. The paramedic must take protective measures when caring for patients who have signs and symptoms of meningitis. Universal precautions (with surgical masks on the patient) should be used during care and transport. The Ambulance Trust should have an exposure control plan for meningitis.

Early diagnosis and treatment of bacterial meningitis are essential. The diagnosis is usually confirmed by finding the bacteria in a sample of the patient's spinal fluid, which is obtained through a spinal tap (lumbar puncture). The disease is then treated using several antibiotics. Drugs to prevent the disease are available for those who may have intimate contact with the patient (e.g. family members).

Note

Meningitis is a true medical emergency. A chief goal of emergency care is administration of benzylpenicillin, which should be administered in the presence of a non-blanching rash and signs/symptoms indicative of meningococcal septicaemia.

Pneumonia

As described in Chapter 14, pneumonia is an acute inflammation of the bronchioles and alveoli. It can be spread by droplets and by direct and indirect contact with respiratory secretions (see Table 24-2). The organisms responsible for pneumonia may affect several body systems, including the respiratory system (pneumonia); the CNS (meningitis); and the ears, nose, and throat (otitis, pharyngitis media). The signs and symptoms of pneumonia include the following:

- sudden onset of chills, high-grade fever, chest pain with respirations, and dyspnoea
- tachypnoea and chest retractions (an ominous sign in children)
- congestion caused by the development of purulent alveolar exudates in one or more lobes
- a productive cough with yellow-green phlegm.

Susceptibility and resistance

Susceptibility to pneumonia is increased by processes such as smoking, pulmonary oedema, influenza, exposure to inhaled toxins, chronic lung disease, and aspiration of any form (post alcohol ingestion, near drowning, regurgitation caused by gastric distension from bag–valve–mask ventilation). Extremes of age also appear to increase susceptibility to the disease (e.g. elderly individuals and infants with a low birth weight and/or malnourishment). Other high-risk groups for pneumonia include people with the following conditions:

- sickle cell disease
- cardiovascular disease
- asplenia (congenital absence or surgical removal of the spleen)
- diabetes
- chronic renal failure (or other kidney disease)
- HIV
- organ transplantation
- multiple myeloma, lymphoma or Hodgkin's disease.

Patient management and protective measures

Prehospital care for patients with pneumonia includes providing airway support, oxygen, ventilatory assistance (as needed), intravenous (IV) fluids (as needed), cardiac monitoring, and transport for evaluation by a physician. Bacterial pneumonia is usually managed with analgesics, decongestants, expectorants, and antibiotic therapy. Patients generally do not need to be isolated from others. In hospitals, pneumonia patients may be isolated from other patients who may be more susceptible to infection.

> **Critical Thinking**
>
> Which locations in your area are at high risk for influenza outbreaks?

Measures for protecting healthcare workers include universal precautions and effective hand washing. Airway barriers should be used if TB is suspected. Immunizations exist for some causes of pneumonia, although they are not generally recommended for people who come in contact with patients who have the disease.

Tetanus

Tetanus is a serious, sometimes fatal, disease of the central nervous system. It is caused by infection of a wound with spores of *Clostridium tetani*. Tetanus spores live mainly in soil and manure but are also found in the human intestine. If the spores enter tissue (e.g. through a puncture wound or burn), they multiply and produce a toxin that acts on the nerves controlling muscular activity. (Dead or necrotic tissue is a favourable environment for *C. tetani*.) About 500 000 cases of tetanus occur worldwide each year, with a mortality rate of 45%. These deaths often occur from wounds that appear too trivial for medical evaluation. With the exception of 2003 and 2004 (12 and 22 cases respectively), there have been fewer than 10 reports of tetanus annually in England and Wales since 1994. It is extremely rare in children below the age of 15 years with only 3 cases reported since 1990.[29] The relatively low number of tetanus cases in the UK is a result of immunization of the general population with tetanus vaccines; by 2005–2006 95% of children in England were vaccinated by their 2nd birthday.[30]

Signs and symptoms

The most common symptom of tetanus is trismus (stiffness of the jaw); it is also known as lockjaw because of the accompanying difficulty in opening the mouth (Figure 24-9). Other symptoms include the following:

- muscular tetany (muscle spasms and twitching)
- painful muscular contractions in the neck, moving to the trunk
- abdominal rigidity (often the first sign in paediatric patients)
- painful spasms (contortions) of the face (risus sardonicus), which produce a grotesque smile
- respiratory failure.

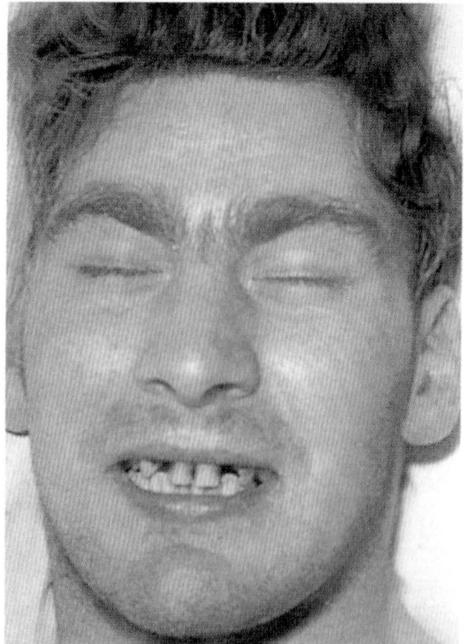

Figure 24-9 Trismus as a result of mild tetanus that developed 10 days after the individual received a benign-looking leg wound.

Patient management and protective measures

The prehospital care goals are to support vital functions. This may include aggressive airway management (intubation and surgical or needle cricothyrotomy). After evaluation by a physician and stabilization of the patient's condition, care for individuals with tetanus includes administration of antitoxin (tetanus immune globulin [TIG]) to provide post-exposure passive immunity, treatment to eliminate the toxin, active immunization with tetanus toxoid, and wound care. Most patients recover fully if they receive prompt treatment.

> **Critical Thinking**
>
> When a patient with an open skin wound refuses care, do you ever explain the risks of tetanus infection?

Rabies

Rabies (hydrophobia) is an acute viral infection of the central nervous system. The disease mainly affects animals but can be transmitted from an infected animal to a human through virus-laden saliva (e.g. by a bite or scratch). In the UK the last human death from indigenous classical rabies occurred in 1902, and the last case of indigenous terrestrial animal rabies was in 1922. Most cases of rabies in the UK now occur in quarantined animals, or in people infected abroad. Since 1946 there have been 22 deaths in people infected with rabies abroad.[31] Humans are highly susceptible to the rabies virus after exposure to saliva in a bite or scratch from an infected animal. Several factors govern the severity of infection, including the following:

- severity of the wound
- richness of nerve supply close to the wound
- distance from the wound to the CNS
- amount and strain of the virus
- degree of protection provided by clothing.

Signs and symptoms

The incubation period between a bite and the appearance of symptoms is generally from 2 to 8 weeks, but very variable. On some occasions incubation periods have been several months or more[31] (see Table 24-2). Initial symptoms include low-grade fever, headache, loss of appetite, hyperactivity, disorientation and, in some cases, seizures. Often the patient has an intense thirst, but any attempts to drink result in violent, painful spasms in the throat (hence the name hydrophobia). Eye and facial muscles may become paralysed as the disease progresses. Without medical intervention, the disease lasts 2–6 days, often resulting in death secondary to respiratory failure.

Patient management and protective measures

Physicians treat the signs and symptoms of the disease and provide respiratory and cardiovascular support (as needed). Patients are also treated with sedatives and analgesics. Thorough débridement of the wound without sutures (if possible) is indicated. This allows free bleeding and drainage. Human rabies immune globulin may be given to provide passive immunization. Also, a rabies vaccine (human diploid cell rabies vaccine) is given by injections spread over several weeks. (Injections are no longer given in the stomach.) Tetanus prophylaxis and antibiotics may be indicated for treatment of the bite wound.

If given within 2 days of the bite, immunizations almost always prevent rabies. Immunizations should be given for contact with open wounds or for exposure of mucous membranes to saliva. Immunizations should also be given to people with a high probability of contact with animal reservoirs (e.g. animal care workers, animal shelter personnel, and outdoor workers).

Rabies is a category 3 infectious disease (see section related to transportation of category 3 infectious disease cases).

Viral diseases of childhood

The childhood infectious diseases presented in this chapter include rubella (German measles), mumps (parotitis), chickenpox (varicella) and pertussis (whooping cough). These infectious diseases are preventable with immunization for chickenpox and with the triple immunization measles, mumps and rubella (MMR) vaccine. The incidence of these childhood diseases has declined because of widespread immunization of children. Immunization provides long-lasting immunity and is known to be 98–99% effective.

All healthcare workers should use personal protective measures when caring for children with viral infections. Protective immunization, effective hand washing, body substance isolation (BSI), and careful handling of linens, supplies, and equipment that may be contaminated are important in preventing the spread of these diseases.

Rubella

Rubella is a mild, febrile, and highly communicable viral disease caused by the rubella virus. It is characterized by a diffuse, punctate, macular rash (Figure 24-10). The disease is usually transmitted by direct contact with nasopharyngeal secretions or droplet spray from an infected person. It may also be passed transplacentally (producing active infection in the fetus) and by contact with articles contaminated with blood, urine or faeces. After inoculation, the virus invades the lymph system; from there it enters the blood and produces an immune response. The subsequent rash spreads from the forehead to the face to the torso to the extremities (lasting 3 days). Maximal communicability appears to be the first few days before and 5 to 7 days after the onset of the rash. Complications from the disease are rare. However, young females sometimes develop a self-limiting arthritis (see Table 24-2).

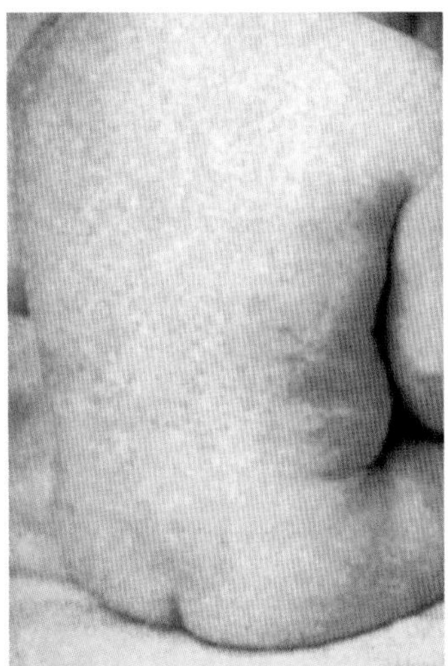

Figure 24-10 Acquired rubella (German measles) in an 11-month-old infant.

> **Critical Thinking**
>
> Is there any way a paramedic can avoid rubella other than being immunized against it?

Congenital rubella syndrome (CRS) affects approximately 90% of infants born to women who were infected with rubella during the first trimester of pregnancy.[32] The disease is associated with multiple congenital anomalies, mental retardation, deafness, and an increased risk of death from congenital heart disease and sepsis during the first 6 months of life. Infants with CRS shed large numbers of the virus in their secretions. The Department of Health recommends that all healthcare providers receive immunization with the MMR vaccine if they are not immune from previous rubella infection. This helps to reduce the risk of exposure to themselves and those they treat. Immunization is not recommended for pregnant women due to the theoretical risk that the vaccine could cause developmental defects. As a precaution, pregnant EMS providers should not be exposed to patients with rubella.

Mumps

Mumps is an acute, communicable systemic viral disease caused by the mumps virus. It is characterized by localized

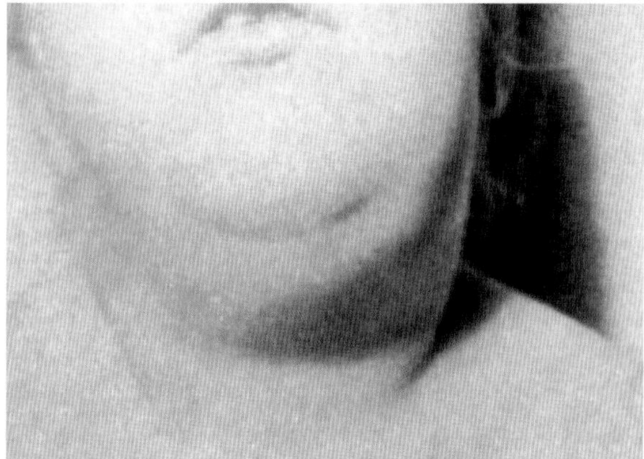

Figure 24-11 Submaxillary mumps in an infant.

oedema of one or more of the salivary glands (usually the parotid). The swelling may affect both or only one side of the neck (Figure 24-11). In some cases involvement of other glands also occurs. The virus is passed through direct contact with the saliva droplets of an infected person (see Table 24-2).

The virus invades and multiplies in the parotid gland or the upper respiratory passages. From there it enters the bloodstream and localizes in glandular or nervous tissue. The parotid, testes and pancreas are the most frequently involved glands. When mumps occurs after the onset of puberty, it may cause a painful inflammation of the testicle (orchitis) and testicular atrophy; however, sterility is rare. The intensity of symptoms in mumps varies; 30% of infections are asymptomatic. Immunity after recovery is lifelong. Placental transfer of antibodies sometimes occurs.

Critical Thinking

Why are some viral diseases of childhood still seen despite widespread immunization?

Chickenpox

Chickenpox is a common childhood disease caused by the varicella-zoster virus. (Varicella-zoster is a member of the herpes virus family.) It is highly contagious (see Table 24-2), infecting up to 90% of people who come into contact with the disease.[33] Transmission is through direct person-to-person contact, airborne droplet infection, or through contact with infected articles such as clothing and bedding. It is characterized by a sudden onset of low-grade fever, mild malaise, and a skin eruption that is maculopapular for a few hours and vesicular for 3 to 4 days, leaving a granular scab (Figure 24-12). At first, the skin lesions appear on the trunk and then usually progress to the extremities. The crops of skin eruptions (each associated with itching) are usually more abundant on covered areas of the body. The scalp, conjunctivae, and upper respiratory tract may also be affected. The appearance of crops of vesicles (fresh vesicles appearing while other lesions are scabbed) differentiates chickenpox from smallpox. (Smallpox has vesicles of the same age.) The disease is self-limited, so treatment is symptomatic. Complications may include secondary bacterial infections, aseptic meningitis, mononucleosis, and Reye's syndrome. Children with chickenpox should be isolated from schools, medical offices, emergency departments, and public places until all lesions are crusted and dry.

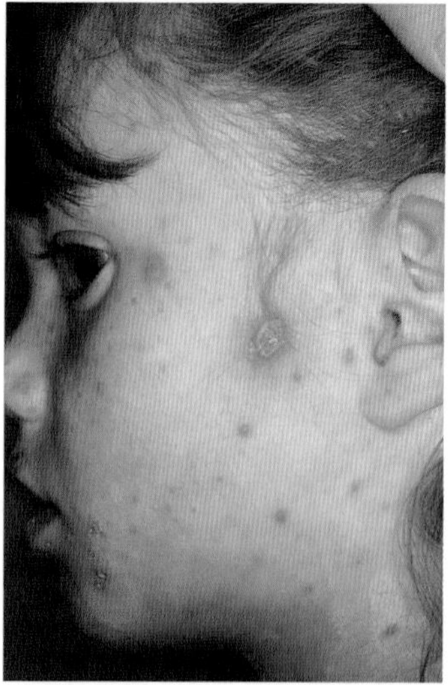

Figure 24-12 Chickenpox skin lesions.

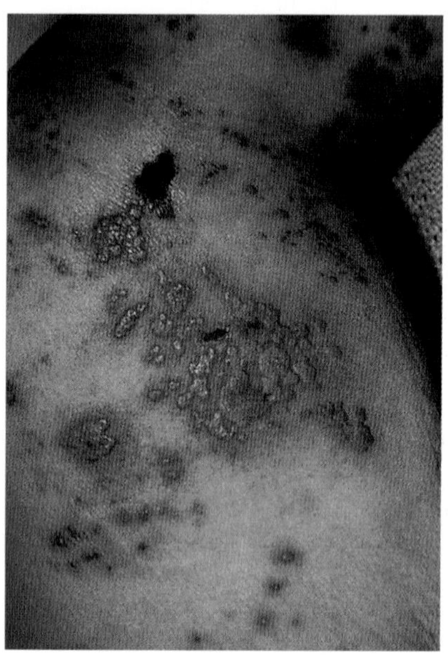

Figure 24-13 Vesicles associated with shingles.

After recovery, the virus is thought to remain in the body in an asymptomatic latent stage. (It is possibly localized in the dorsal root ganglia.) The virus may reactivate during periods of stress or immunosuppression, when it may produce an illness known as shingles. The vesicles associated with shingles appear on the skin area supplied by the sensory nerves of a single group or associated groups of dorsal root ganglia (Figure 24-13). Unlike chickenpox, shingles is not passed through respiratory droplets; however, it can cause chickenpox in susceptible individuals who come in contact with open skin lesions (lesions that are not yet scabbed).

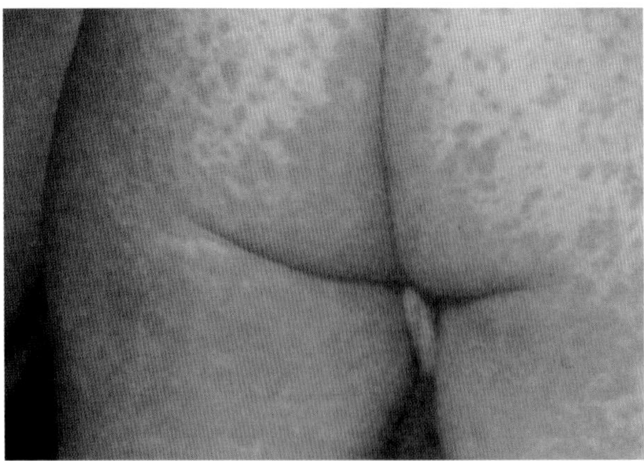

Figure 24-14 Measles rash on the third day.

Measles

Measles is an acute, highly communicable viral disease caused by the measles virus. It is characterized by fever, conjunctivitis, cough, bronchitis, and a blotchy red rash (Figure 24-14). The virus is found in the blood, urine, and pharyngeal secretions and is usually passed directly or indirectly through contact with infected respiratory secretions. The virus invades the respiratory epithelium and spreads via the lymph system. Measles may predispose a person to secondary bacterial complications such as otitis media, pneumonia, and myocarditis. The most serious life-threatening complication is subacute sclerosing panencephalitis (a slowly progressing neurological disease marked by loss of mental capacity and muscle coordination).

Early (prodromal) symptoms that mark the onset of disease include high fever, nasal discharge, conjunctivitis, photophobia, and cough (see Table 24-2). One or 2 days before the rash emerges, white spots are usually noted on the inside of the cheek (Koplik spots). The dermal rash begins a few days after respiratory tract involvement, spreading from the forehead to the face, neck, and torso, and eventually to the feet, usually by the third day. (The onset of the rash coincides with the production of serum antibodies.) The rash is red and maculopapular. Uncomplicated cases of measles usually last 6 days and recovery confers lifelong immunity.

Pertussis

Pertussis (whooping cough) is an infectious disease that mainly affects infants and young children (see Table 24-2). It is caused by *Bordetella pertussis* and is spread by direct contact with discharges from mucous membranes contained in airborne droplets. The disease causes inflammation of the entire respiratory tract. It also causes a subtle onset of cough that becomes paroxysmal in 1 to 2 weeks. This cough can last 1 to 2 months. The coughing episodes are violent (sometimes without an intervening inhalation), causing the high-pitched inspiratory 'whoop', and end with expulsion of clear mucus and vomiting. (The whoop is often not present in children younger than 6 months of age.) Before the introduction of pertussis immunization in the 1950s, the average annual number of notifications in England and Wales exceeded 100 000. In 1972, when vaccine acceptance was over 80%, there were only 2069 notifications of pertussis.[34]

The ability to spread pertussis is thought to be greatest before the onset of paroxysmal coughing. (This explains the need for BSI and surgical mask protection for the paramedic and the patient.) Pertussis commonly lasts 6–8 weeks even when treated with antibiotics, with severity of symptoms related to age. The most severe infections are usually in infants, and over 50% are hospitalized as a result. Morbidity and mortality is greatest in those aged less than 6 months of age. Infection with pertussis usually provides immunity, although immunity may diminish over time.

Other viral diseases

Other viral diseases easily transmitted during the course of patient care include influenza, severe acute respiratory syndrome (SARS), mononucleosis and herpes simplex type 1 (HSV-1) infection. As with all other contacts with patients who may have infectious disease, BSI precautions are indicated during patient care.

Influenza

As described in Chapter 14, influenza is a respiratory infection that is spread by influenza viruses A, B and C (see Table 24-2). The disease is popularly known as 'the flu' and is spread by virus-infected droplets that are coughed or sneezed into the air. Influenza usually occurs in small outbreaks or, every few years, in epidemics. Resistance is normally conferred after recovery, although this resistance is only to the specific strain or variant.

Signs and symptoms typically include chills, fever, headache, muscular aches, loss of appetite, and fatigue. These symptoms are followed by upper respiratory infection and a cough (often severe and drawn out) that lasts for 2 to 7 days. Patient management is mainly supportive. Mild cases of viral infection usually are not treated.

Severe cases (especially in the elderly and those with lung or heart disease) may result in secondary bacterial infection (e.g. *S. pneumoniae*). These cases can be fatal. Other viral respiratory diseases that can lead to bacterial complications include acute afebrile viral respiratory disease (excluding influenza) and acute febrile respiratory disease. Both diseases may cause illnesses in the upper and lower respiratory tract, including pharyngitis, laryngitis, croup, bronchitis, and bronchiolitis.

Flu vaccines contain killed strains of type A and type B virus that are known to be currently in circulation. These vaccines may help prevent infection. The flu vaccine is offered to certain groups of patients, including those over 65 years of age; those with chronic respiratory disease, chronic heart disease, chronic renal disease, chronic liver disease, diabetes requiring insulin or oral hypoglycaemic drugs, or immunosuppression, irrespective of age; and also to healthcare workers involved in the delivery of care and/or support to patients.

Zanamivir, oseltamivir and amantadine are licensed for the treatment of influenza in the UK and may be given to hospitalized patients.

Critical Thinking

Will you get the influenza vaccine? What influenced your decision?

Severe acute respiratory syndrome

As described in Chapter 14, severe acute respiratory syndrome emerged as a disease in China in November 2003. It has made thousands of people ill worldwide. SARS is caused by a new member of the coronavirus family (SARS coronavirus [SARS CO-V]). It appears to be spread by close person-to-person contact. This type of contact results in exposure to infectious droplets. It also is possible that SARS can be spread more broadly through the air or by other ways that are currently not known.

The illness usually begins with a fever over 38 °C (100.4 °F). The fever is sometimes associated with chills or other symptoms, including headache, a general feeling of discomfort, and body aches. Some people also experience mild respiratory symptoms at the outset. After 2–7 days, SARS patients may develop a dry, non-productive cough, which might be accompanied by or progress to hypoxaemia. In 10–20% of cases, patients require mechanical ventilation; the mortality rate for the disease is about 8%.[35]

Initial diagnostic testing for patients suspected of having SARS may include a chest X-ray, pulse oximetry, blood cultures, sputum culture, and testing for viral respiratory pathogens, notably influenza A and B and respiratory syncytial virus. Currently, there is no known cure or vaccine for the disease. More than 80% of patients with SARS improve on their own. Strict quarantine remains the most effective means of control.

Transport guidelines for possible SARS patients

If ambulance transfer is required for interhospital transfer, the control must be informed in advance and arrange for transportation of the patient using category 3 containment measures.[36]

Mononucleosis

Mononucleosis is caused either by the Epstein–Barr virus (EBV) or by cytomegalovirus (CMV). Both of these are members of the herpes virus family (see Table 24-2). Mononucleosis is spread from person to person via the oropharyngeal route and saliva (hence the name kissing disease). Most people with a healthy immune system are able to fend off the infection even after significant exposure. About 90% of people over age 35 have antibodies to CMV or EBV, probably the result of mild, childhood infection, often passed off as a common cold or the flu. Previous infection with EBV generally confers a high degree of resistance to future exposures.

Signs and symptoms appear gradually. They are characterized by fever (which may last for weeks), sore throat, oropharyngeal discharges, lymphadenopathy (especially posterior cervical), and splenomegaly with abdominal tenderness. About 10% of people also develop a generalized rash or darkened areas in the mouth that resemble bruises. Recovery usually occurs in a few weeks, although some people take months to regain their former level of energy. The patient may remain a carrier for several months after symptoms disappear. No immunization is available for mononucleosis.

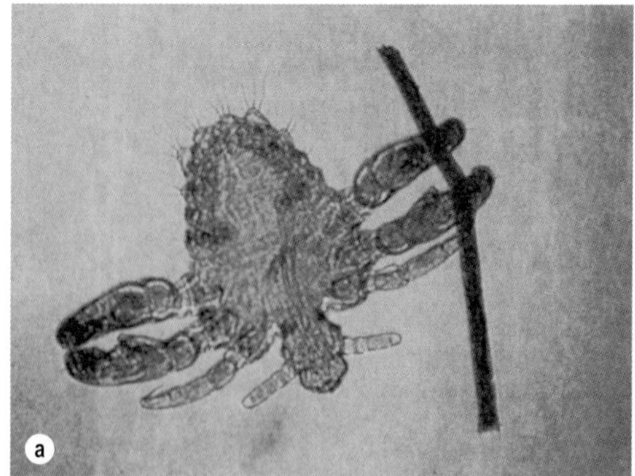

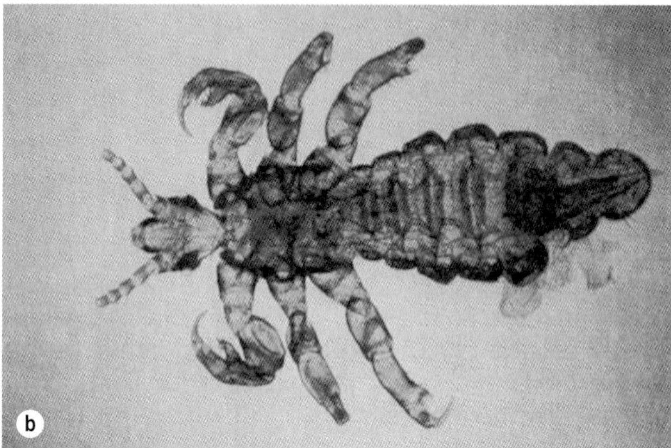

Figure 24-15 (a) The pubic, or crab, louse. (b) Male of the human head louse.

Infestations

Lice

Lice are small, wingless insects that are ectoparasites of birds and mammals. Most are host specific. Two of the species are human parasites: One is *Phthirus pubis*, the pubic, or crab, louse; the other is *Pediculus humanus*, which has two forms: *Pediculus humanus capitis* (the head louse) and *Pediculus humanus corporis* (the body louse, which was involved in outbreaks of epidemic typhus and trench fever in World War I) (Figure 24-15a, b). Lice have a three-stage life cycle. The eggs hatch in 7–10 days; the nymph stage lasts 7–13 days; and the egg-to-egg cycle lasts about 3 weeks.

Lice subsist on blood from the host and have mouths modified for piercing and sucking. During biting and feeding, secretions from the louse cause a small, red macule and pruritus. Long infestation periods may result in a decrease in pruritus and often a thick, dry, scaly appearance to the skin. In severe cases, oozing and crusting may be present. If sensitization to lice saliva and faeces occurs, inflammation may develop. Secondary infection may result from scratching of lesions. Lice spread through close personal contact, and sharing of clothing and bedding may result in outbreaks (e.g. at school, day care facilities and in families).

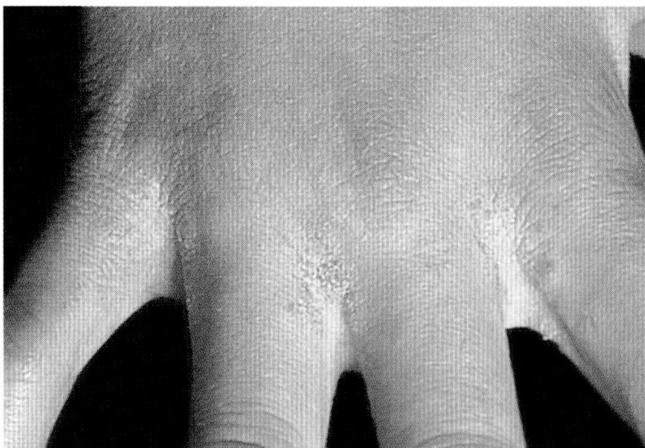

Figure 24-16 Common site of burrows in scabies.

Pubic lice have a distinctive appearance suggestive of miniature crabs. Grey–blue spots may be observed on the abdomen and thighs of infested patients. The eggs (nits or ova) are often evident on the shaft of pubic hairs. They are sometimes seen in the eyelashes, eyebrows and axillary hairs. Pubic lice are usually acquired during sexual activity or from unchanged bedding in which egg-infested pubic hairs have been shed. Although primary bite lesions are seldom evident, the patient normally complains of intense pruritus and pubic scratching.

Head lice have an elongated body with a head that is slightly narrower than the thorax. Each louse has three pairs of legs, which possess delicate hooks at the distal extremities. The white ova of head lice (usually one nit to a shaft) are easily mistaken for dandruff, but the nits cannot be brushed out. These parasites most frequently affect children.

Body lice are slightly larger than head lice and concentrate around the waist, shoulders, axillae, and neck. Body lice and their nits are usually found in seams and on the fibres of clothing. The lesions from their bites begin as small, non-inflammatory red spots, which quickly become papular wheals that resemble linear scratch marks (parallel scratch marks on the shoulders are a common finding). Head lice and body lice interbreed.

The treatment for all types of lice is designed to eradicate the parasites and nits and to prevent re-infestation. Patients are usually advised to wash all clothing, bedding, and personal articles thoroughly in hot water. The treatment of the lice may be with 'wet combing' or the use of insecticides depending upon the location of the lice.

Scabies

The human scabies mite (*Sarcoptes scabiei* var. *hominis*) is a parasite that completes its entire life cycle in and on the epidermis of its host. Scabies infestation resembles a lice infestation. However, scabies bites generally are concentrated around the hands and feet, especially in the webs of the fingers and toes (Figure 24-16). Other common infestation areas include the face and scalp of children, the nipples in females, and the penis in males. The scabies mite is usually passed by intimate contact or acquired from infested bedding, furniture, and clothing.

Scabies infestation is often manifested by severe nocturnal pruritus. However, it takes 4–6 weeks for sensitization to develop and itching to begin. The adult female mite is responsible for symptoms. After impregnation, she burrows into the epidermis to lay her eggs and then remains in the burrow for a life span of about 1 month. Although vesicles and papules form at the surface, they are often disguised by the results of scratching. In severe cases (e.g. Norwegian scabies), oozing, crusting, and secondary infection may result. Susceptibility is general; however, people with a previous exposure usually develop fewer mites on later exposures and experience symptoms earlier (within 1–4 days).

The treatment is similar to that prescribed for lice infestation. Symptoms may persist for longer than 1 month until the mite and mite products are shed with the epidermis. (Mites are communicable until all mites and eggs have been destroyed.) Re-infestation is common, therefore the patient should be re-examined if the itching has not abated after several weeks. Antibiotic therapy may be needed to treat secondary bacterial infection. Immunization is not available, so the paramedic should take protective measures against lice and scabies infestation as presented in Box 24-9.

Box 24-9

Protective measures against lice and scabies

1. Observe body substance isolation (BSI) and bag linen separately.
2. Spray the patient compartment of the ambulance with an effective insecticide. (Most commercial sprays contain effective pyrethrins, malathion, or carbamates.)
3. Spray the floor, stretcher, and immediate areas where the patient's head was positioned (lice do not jump great distances).
4. Remove all insecticide residues with an appropriate solution.
5. Wear gloves during all steps and wash hands thoroughly when finished.
6. To treat a lice or scabies infestation:
   - Use an appropriate body or hair pediculicide; repeat in 7 to 10 days.
   - Launder personal clothing in hot water in a washer and dry on high heat in the dryer (of questionable benefit).

Paramedic's role in preventing disease transmission

Paramedics will have to deal with patients who have infectious diseases. It is important for them to be vigilant about the consequences to themselves and to their patients and coworkers. Part of this professional duty in preventing the spread of disease is knowing when not to go to work. A healthcare worker should not go to work if the following conditions are present:

- fever
- diarrhoea
- draining wound or any type of wet lesion
- jaundice
- mononucleosis
- treatment with a medication and/or shampoo for lice or scabies
- strep throat (unless antibiotics have been taken for longer than 24 h)
- cold (unless the paramedic wears a surgical mask).

Healthcare workers should also ensure that their personal immunization status is current for MMR, hepatitis, DPT, polio, chickenpox and influenza.

Critical Thinking

Have you gone to school or work with any of these conditions?

Other considerations in disease prevention

When called to provide emergency care, paramedics should always approach the scene with caution. They must keep in mind that an uncontrolled scene increases the likelihood of transmission of body fluids. Body substance isolation guidelines should be observed at all times. These include wearing gloves, protective eyewear, a face shield and a gown (if splash or spray is possible) and wearing an appropriate particulate mask when airborne disease is suspected. As mentioned before, BSI is based on the premise that all body fluids, in any situation, may be infectious.

As a rule, if a patient has a cough, headache, general weakness, recent weight loss, nuchal rigidity or high fever, the paramedic should immediately suspect an infectious process. Regardless of the patient's infectious status, the paramedic should do the following:

- Provide the same level of care to all patients.
- Disinfect equipment and the patient compartment with the proper disinfectant solution.
- Practise effective hand washing.
- Report any infectious exposure to the Trust occupational health department.

Critical Thinking

Imagine that you are on a call and get a small splash of blood in your eyes. What do you think would prevent you from reporting it immediately so that your post-exposure care could begin?

Summary

- An infectious disease is any illness caused by a specific biological organism such as bacteria, viruses, protozoa, worms, prions or fungi. A communicable disease is an infectious disease that can be passed from one person to another.
- Pathogens are organisms that can cause disease in the human host; paramedics must be familiar with infection control guidelines and must take personal protective measures against exposure to these pathogens.
- The chain of elements needed to transmit an infectious disease includes the pathogenic agent, a reservoir, a portal of exit from the reservoir, an environment conducive to transmission of the pathogenic agent, a portal of entry into the new host, and susceptibility of the new host to the infectious disease.
- The human body is protected from infectious disease by external and internal barriers. These serve as lines of defence against infection. External barriers include the skin, GI system, upper respiratory tract, and genitourinary tract. Internal barriers include the inflammatory response and the immune response.
- The progression of infectious disease from exposure to the onset of symptoms follows four stages. These are the latent period, the incubation period, the communicability period, and the disease period.
- The human immunodeficiency virus is directly transmitted person to person. This occurs through anal or vaginal intercourse, across the placenta, by contact with infected blood or body fluids on mucous membranes or open wounds, through blood transfusion or tissue transplant, or by the use of contaminated needles or syringes. The virus affects the CD4 T cells. Secondary complications are usually related to opportunistic infections that arise as the immune system deteriorates. Progression of the disease can be divided into category A (acute retroviral infection, seroconversion, and asymptomatic infection); category B (early symptomatic HIV); and category C (late symptomatic HIV and advanced HIV). Paramedics should observe strict compliance with universal precautions for protection against HIV. Patient care should include helping these patients feel that they can obtain acceptance and compassion from healthcare workers.
- Hepatitis is a viral disease that produces pathologic changes in the liver. The three main classes of hepatitis virus are hepatitis A, hepatitis B and hepatitis C.
- Tuberculosis is a chronic pulmonary disease that is acquired through inhalation of tubercle bacilli. The infection is passed mainly when infected people cough or sneeze the bacteria into the air or by contact with sputum that contains virulent TB bacilli. The infection is characterized by stages of early infection (frequently asymptomatic), latency, and a potential for recurrent post-primary disease.
- Meningococcal meningitis is an inflammation of the membranes that surround the spinal cord and brain. It can be caused by bacteria, viruses and other microorganisms.
- Pneumonia is an acute inflammatory process of the respiratory bronchioles and alveoli. Bacteria, viruses and fungi can cause this disease.
- Tetanus is a serious, sometimes fatal, disease of the CNS. It is caused by infection of a wound with spores of the bacterium *C. tetani*. The most common symptom is trismus (difficulty opening the mouth).
- Rabies is an acute viral infection of the CNS. Humans are highly susceptible to the rabies virus after exposure to saliva from the bite or scratch of an infected animal.

Summary—cont'd

- Rubella is a mild, febrile, highly communicable viral disease. It is characterized by a diffuse, punctate, macular rash. The Department of Health recommends that all healthcare providers receive immunization if they are not immune as a result of previous rubella infection.
- Mumps is an acute, communicable systemic viral disease. It is characterized by localized unilateral or bilateral oedema of one or more of the salivary glands. Occasionally other glands are also involved.
- Chickenpox is highly communicable. It is characterized by a sudden onset of low-grade fever, mild malaise, and a maculopapular skin eruption that lasts for a few hours. This is followed by a vesicular eruption that lasts for 3–4 days, leaving a granular scab. The virus may reactivate during periods of stress or immunosuppression. At that time, it may cause an illness known as shingles.
- Measles is an acute, highly communicable viral disease caused by the measles virus. It is characterized by fever, conjunctivitis, cough, bronchitis, and a blotchy red rash.
- Pertussis is an infectious disease that leads to inflammation of the entire respiratory tract. It causes an insidious cough. The cough becomes paroxysmal in 1–2 weeks and lasts 1–2 months.
- Influenza is mainly a respiratory infection. It is spread by influenza viruses A, B and C.
- SARS is a viral illness first detected in 2003. It is spread by exposure to infected droplets. The illness begins with a fever and mild respiratory symptoms and can progress to respiratory failure and death.
- Mononucleosis is caused either by EBV or by CMV. Both of these are members of the herpes virus family.
- Herpes simplex virus is transmitted by skin-to-skin contact with an infected area of the body. The primary infection produces a vesicular lesion (blister) which heals spontaneously. After the primary infection, the virus travels to a sensory nerve ganglion. It remains there in a latent stage until reactivated.
- Lice are small, wingless insects that are ectoparasites of birds and mammals. During biting and feeding, lice secrete a substance that causes small, red macules and pruritus.
- The human scabies mite is a parasite. It completes its life cycle in and on the epidermis of the host. Scabies bites are usually concentrated around the hands and feet, especially in the webs of the fingers and toes.
- Part of the paramedic's professional duty with regard to infectious disease transmission is to know when not to go to work. Paramedics also have a duty to use the proper BSI precautions at all times.

References

1. Office for National Statistics. Mortality: circulatory diseases – leading cause group. ONS online. Available http://www.statistics.gov.uk/cci/nugget.asp?id=919 12 February 2009
2. Office for National Statistics. Health Statistics Quarterly, number 39. Autumn 2008. Online. Available http://www.statistics.gov.uk/downloads/theme_health/HSQ39.pdf
3. Office for National Statistics. Health Statistics Quarterly, number 37. Spring 2008. Online. Available http://www.statistics.gov.uk/downloads/theme_health/HSQ37.pdf
4. Wilson J 2006 Infection control in clinical practice. Baillière Tindall Elsevier, London
5. The Hazardous Waste (England and Wales) Regulations 2005. HMSO, London
6. Health Protection Agency. MRSA information for patients. Online. Available www.hpa.org.uk 12 February 2009
7. Department of Health. Reducing infection through effective practice in the pre-hospital environment. London, Department of Health. 2008
8. Ambulance Service Association and Health Protection Agency 2004 National Guidance and Procedures for Infection Prevention and Control. Ambulance Service Association, London
9. Ayliffe GA, Babb JR, Quoraishi AH 1978 A test for hygienic hand disinfection. J Clin Pathol 31:923–928
10. The Special Waste Amendment (Scotland) Regulations 2004. HMSO, London
11. The Hazardous Waste Regulations (Northern Ireland) 2005. HMSO, London
12. Department of Health 2006 Safe Management of Healthcare Waste. The Stationary Office, London
13. Coppetts Wood Hospital, the High Security Infectious Disease Unit. Online. Available http://royalfree.org.uk/default.aspx?top_nav_id=5&tab_id=453 12 February 2009
14. Health Protection Agency 2003 CDSC. HIV infections and AIDS in the United Kingdom: monthly report – May 2003 (HIV-2 and HIV infections acquired through sex between men updated). Commun Dis Rep 13(22)
15. Department of Health 2005 HIV Infected Health Care Workers: Guidance on Management and Patient Notification. Online. Available www.dh.gov.uk/publications 12 February 2009
16. Health Protection Agency 2005 Occupational transmission of HIV – summary of published reports. arch 2005 Edition (data to end of December 2002). Health Protection Agency, London. Online. Available http://www.hpa.org.uk/infections/topics_az/bbv/pdf/intl_HIV_tables_2005.pdf 12 February 2009
17. [Anonymous] 1991 Recommendations for preventing transmission of human immunodeficiency virus and hepatitis B virus to patients during exposure-prone invasive procedures. MMWR Morb Mortal Wkly Rep 40 (RR-8):1–9.
18. [Anonymous] 1998 Public Health Service guidelines for the management of health care worker exposures to HIV and recommendations for post exposure prophylaxis. MMWR Recomm Rep 47 (RR-7):1–33
19. Henderson DK 1999 Postexposure chemoprophylaxis for occupational exposures to the human immunodeficiency virus. JAMA 281:931–936
20. Department of Health 2004 HIV Post-Exposure Prophylaxis. Guidance

from the UK Chief Medical Officers' Expert Advisory Group on AIDS. Online. Available www.dh.gov.uk/publications 12 February 2009

21. Hepatitis International. Online. Available http://hepfi.org 12 February 2009
22. Health Protection Agency. Hepatitis C in England; The Health Protection Agency Annual Report 2007. London, HPA. 2007
23. [Anonymous] 1998 Recommendations for prevention and control of hepatitis C virus (HCV) infection and HCV-related chronic disease. MMWR Recomm Rep 47 (RR-19):1–39
24. Centers for Disease Control and Prevention 1999 TB facts for health care workers: tuberculosis – yes, it's still a problem. CDC, Atlanta
25. Health Protection Agency. Tuberculosis in the UK: Annual report on tuberculosis surveillance in the UK 2008. London, HPA. 2008
26. Health Protection Agency 2006 Focus on tuberculosis. Annual surveillance report 2006 – England, Wales and Northern Ireland. HPA, London
27. World Health Organization. Press Release WHO/21–23 April 2001
28. Health Protection Agency 2003 Enhanced surveillance of meningococcal disease, National Annual Report: July 2002–June 2003. Online. Available http://www.hpa.org.uk/infections/topics_az/meningo/ESMD_annual_report_0203.pdf 12 February 2009
29. Health Protection Agency. Tetanus Cases by Age Group and Year of Onset: England and Wales. 2008. Available online at http://www.hpa.org.uk/webw/HPAweb&HPAwebStandard/HPAweb_C/1195733758896?p=1191942149542
30. Health Protection Agency. Completed primary courses at two years of age: England and Wales, 1966–1977, England only 1978 onwards. Online. Available http://www.hpa.org.uk/infections/topics_az/cover/vaccine_uptake_data.htm 12 February 2009
31. Health Protection Agency. Topics – Rabies. Online. Available http://www.hpa.org.uk/infections/topics_az/rabies/menu.htm 12 February 2009
32. US Department of Transportation National Highway Traffic Safety Administration 1998 EMT-paramedic national standard curriculum. Department of Transportation, Washington, DC
33. Davies EG, Elliman DAC, Hart CA, Nicoll A, Rudd PT 2001 Manual of childhood infections, 2nd edition. WB Saunders, Royal College of Paediatrics and Child Health, China, pp. 240–244
34. Health Protection Agency. Topics – Pertussis. Online. Available http://www.hpa.org.uk/infections/topics_az/whoopingcough/gen_info.htm 12 February 2009
35. Centers for Disease Control and Prevention. Severe acute respiratory syndrome (SARS). Online. Available www.cdc.gov/niosh/topics/sars 12 February 2009
36. Health Protection Agency 2005 SARS – hospital infection control guidance. Online. Available http://www.hpa.org.uk/infections/topics_az/SARS/hosp_infect_cont.htm#trans 12 February 2009

CHAPTER 25

Assessment and Management of Behavioural and Mental Health Emergencies

Chapter contents

Objectives

Upon completion of this chapter, the paramedic student will be able to:

1. Explain what constitutes a behavioural emergency.
2. Identify potential causes for behavioural and mental ill-health.
3. List three critical principles that should be considered in the prehospital care of a patient with a behavioural emergency.
4. Outline key elements of the prehospital patient examination during a behavioural emergency.
5. Describe effective techniques for interviewing a patient during a behavioural emergency.
6. Differentiate key symptoms and management techniques for selected behavioural and mental health disorders.
7. Identify factors the paramedic must consider when assessing a suicide risk.
8. Formulate appropriate interview questions for determining suicidal intent.
9. Explain prehospital management techniques for a patient who has attempted suicide.
10. Describe the assessment of a potentially violent patient.
11. Outline measures that may be used to try to safely diffuse a potentially violent patient situation.
12. Explain variations in approach to behavioural emergencies in children.
13. Gain an overview of restraint for patients posing behavioural problems.
14. Explain variations in approach to behavioural emergencies in children.
15. Discuss the appropriate Sections of the Mental Health Act 1983.
16. Explain the main elements of the Mental Capacity Act 2005 and its implications for practice.

Key terms

affect An outward manifestation of a person's feelings or emotions.

anxiety A state or feeling of apprehension, uneasiness, agitation, uncertainty, and fear resulting from the anticipation of some threat or danger.

behavioural emergency A change in mood or behaviour that cannot be tolerated by the involved person or others and that requires immediate attention.

delusions Persistent beliefs or perceptions held by a person despite evidence that refutes them (i.e. false beliefs).

depression A mood disturbance characterized by feelings of sadness, despair and discouragement.

dyskinesia An impairment of the ability to execute voluntary movements; often an adverse effect of prolonged use of antipsychotic medications.

hallucinations The apparent perception of sights, sounds, and other sensory phenomena that are not actually present.

mania A mood disorder characterized by extreme excitement, hyperactivity, agitation, and sometimes violent and self-destructive behaviour.

mental status examination An evaluation tool that includes an assessment of appearance and behaviour, speech and language, emotional stability, and cognitive abilities.

paranoia A condition characterized by an elaborate, overly suspicious system of thinking.

psychosis Maladaptive behaviour involving major distortions of reality.

schizophrenia A group of disorders characterized by recurrent episodes of psychotic behaviour.

Behavioural and mental emergencies call for an approach that is different from those used for emergency medical or trauma calls. The paramedic has no scientific tools to use in assessing the situation. Also, no firm protocols can guarantee a positive outcome. Fortunately, most behavioural emergencies require only strong communication skills and supportive measures. These measures can prevent the crisis from escalating. Often, the paramedic's chief role is to provide understanding, compassion, and direction for people who are temporarily in turmoil. Emergency medical services (EMS) personnel must focus on helping and protecting these patients and do so until the patient is able to gain control or other therapeutic skills can be applied.

Understanding behavioural emergencies

One in four British adults experience at least one diagnosable mental health problem in any one year, and one in six experiences this at any given time.[1] In addition, one person in 250 will have a psychotic illness such as schizophrenia or bipolar affective disorder (manic depression), which suggests that mental illness is as common as asthma.[2]

There is no clear agreement on or ideal model for 'normal' behaviour. It is generally considered to be adaptive behaviour that is accepted by society. (This can vary by culture and ethnic group.) The concept of abnormal (maladaptive) behaviour is also defined by society as behaviour that:

- deviates from society's norms and expectations
- interferes with well-being and ability to function
- harms the individual or group.

Critical Thinking

Can you think of a time in your life when you, a family member, or a close friend had a behaviour that fit the definition of abnormal behaviour? How did it make you feel?

A behavioural emergency can be defined as a change in mood or behaviour that cannot be tolerated by the involved person or others and that requires immediate attention. Behavioural emergencies may range from a brief inability to cope with stress or anxiety to more intense situations in which patients may be dangerous to themselves and others. However, most people with mental illness function well on a daily basis. Common conditions such as depression, anxiety disorders and mild personality disorders are often effectively managed with medication and counselling in outpatient mental health centres. Ten common myths about mental illness are listed in Box 25-1. Most behavioural emergencies have a biological, psychosocial or sociocultural cause. In fact, mental illness may be the result of more than one of these factors (Figure 25-1).

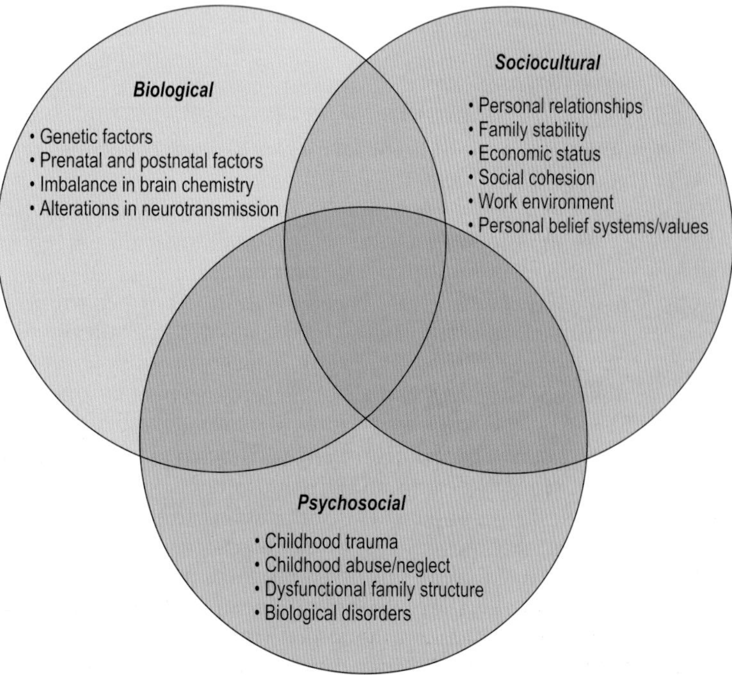

Figure 25-1 Common causes of behavioural emergencies.

Box 25-1

Top 10 myths about mental illness

Myth no. 1: Psychiatric disorders are not true medical illnesses like heart disease and diabetes. People who have a mental illness are just 'crazy'.

Fact: Brain disorders, like heart disease and diabetes, are true medical illnesses. Research shows that psychiatric disorders have genetic and biological causes. Also, these diseases can be treated effectively.

Myth no. 2: People with a severe mental illness, such as schizophrenia, are usually dangerous and violent.

Fact: Statistics show that the incidence of violence among people who have a brain disorder is not much higher than it is in the general population. Individuals suffering from a psychosis such as schizophrenia are more often frightened, confused and despairing than violent.

Myth no. 3: Mental illness is the result of bad parenting.

Fact: Most experts agree that genetic factors, along with other risk factors, lead to psychiatric disorders. In other words, mental illnesses have a physical cause.

Myth no. 4: Depression results from a personality weakness or character flaw. People who are depressed could just snap out of it if they tried hard enough.

Fact: Depression has nothing to do with being lazy or weak. It results from changes in brain chemistry or brain function. Medication and/or psychotherapy often help people to recover.

Myth no. 5: Schizophrenia means that the person has a split personality, and there is no way to control it.

Fact: Schizophrenia is often confused with multiple personality disorder. Actually, schizophrenia is a brain disorder that robs people of their ability to think clearly and logically. An estimated 2.5 million Americans have schizophrenia. Their symptoms range from social withdrawal to hallucinations and delusions. Medication has helped many of these people to lead fulfilling, productive lives.

Myth no. 6: Depression is a normal part of the ageing process.

Fact: It is not normal for older adults to be depressed. Signs of depression in older people include a loss of interest in activities, sleep disturbance and lethargy. Depression in the elderly often goes undiagnosed. Older adults and their family members need to recognize the problem and seek professional help.

Myth no. 7: Depression and other illnesses, such as anxiety disorders, do not affect children or adolescents. Any problems they have are just a part of growing up.

Fact: Children and adolescents can develop severe mental illnesses. In the US, 1 in 10 children and adolescents has a mental disorder severe enough to cause impairment. Yet only about 20% of these children receive treatment. Left untreated, these problems can get worse. Anyone who talks about suicide should be taken very seriously.

Myth no. 8: If you have a mental illness, you can will it away. Being treated for a psychiatric disorder means an individual has in some way 'failed' or is weak.

Fact: A serious mental illness cannot be willed away. Ignoring the problem does not make it go away, either. It takes courage to seek professional help.

Myth no. 9: Addiction is a lifestyle choice and shows a lack of willpower. People with a substance abuse problem are morally weak or 'bad'.

Fact: Addiction is a disease that generally results from changes in brain chemistry. It has nothing to do with being a 'bad' person.

Myth no. 10: Electroconvulsive therapy (ECT), formerly known as 'shock treatment', is painful and barbaric.

Fact: ECT has given a new lease on life to many people who suffer from severe and debilitating depression. It is used when other treatments such as psychotherapy or medication fail or cannot be used. Patients who receive ECT are asleep and under anaesthesia, therefore they do not feel anything.

From National Alliance for Research on Schizophrenia and Depression 2003 'Top 10 myths about mental illness based on a nationwide survey'. NARSD, Great Neck, NY.

Biological causes

Physical or biochemical disturbances in the brain may be inherited and can result in major changes in behaviour. In mental health care, biological disturbances are mental disorders that result from a physical (biochemical and organic) rather than a purely psychological cause. Examples include genetic factors, prenatal and postnatal factors (including infection, endocrine, metabolic and vascular disorders), an imbalance in brain chemistry, and alterations in neurotransmission. An example of a biological mental illness is schizophrenia (described later in this chapter). In this illness, specific genes have been identified that may influence the balance of chemicals in the brain. These chemicals are called neurotransmitters and are responsible for communication between the brain cells.

Organic causes of behavioural emergencies have been discussed throughout this text and include substance abuse, trauma, illness (e.g. diabetes, electrolyte imbalance), infections, tumours, and dementia (Box 25-2). It is important that the paramedic consider the possibility of these medical conditions in all behavioural emergencies.

Psychosocial causes

Psychosocial mental illness may have many causes. It is often related to an individual's personality type but may also be related to the person's ability to resolve situational conflict in life. For example, psychosocial mental illness may result from childhood trauma, child abuse or neglect, or a dysfunctional family structure that affects relationships with parents and siblings. Biological disorders (e.g. genetic factors and chemical imbalance) may contribute to psychosocial causes of mental illness.

Sociocultural causes

Sociocultural causes of mental illness are related to the way a person balances emotions, thoughts, and interactions in society. When this balance shifts rapidly, a person may expe-

Box 25-2

Common medical conditions that manifest as behavioural disorders

Metabolic disorders

Glucose, sodium, calcium, or magnesium imbalance
Acid–base imbalance
Acute hypoxia
Renal failure
Hepatic failure

Endocrine disorders

Thyroid disease
Parathyroid disease
Adrenal hormone imbalance

Infectious diseases

Encephalitis
Meningitis
Brain abscess
Severe systemic infection

Trauma

Concussion
Intracranial haematoma (especially subdural haematoma)

Cardiovascular disorders

Cardiac dysrhythmia
Hypotension
Transient ischaemic attack
Cerebrovascular accident (or stroke)
Hypertensive encephalopathy

Neoplastic diseases

Central nervous system tumours or metastases

Degenerative diseases

Dementia of the Alzheimer's type
Other dementias

Drug abuse

Alcohol
Barbiturates
Narcotics
Sedative–hypnotics
Amphetamines and other stimulants
Hallucinogens

Drug reactions

β-adrenergic blockers
Antihypertensives
Cardiac drugs
Bronchodilators
β-adrenergic agonists
Anticonvulsants

rience emotional turmoil, which may result in crisis. Factors that may be related to sociocultural causes of behavioural emergencies include personal relationships, family stability, economic status, social cohesion, work environment, and personal belief systems and values. Changes in behaviour caused by personal or situational stress are often linked to a specific event or series of events. Examples include environmental violence (e.g. war, riots, rape, assault), the death of a loved one, ongoing discrimination or prejudice, and economic and employment problems.

Assessment and management of behavioural emergencies

The initial assessment and management of a patient with a behavioural emergency are similar to those used in any other EMS response. These steps include ensuring scene safety, containing the crisis, giving proper emergency medical care, and transporting the patient to an appropriate healthcare facility.

Assessment

Paramedics should begin the assessment by creating a rapport with the patient. They can do this whilst gathering the information needed for immediate management of life-threatening conditions. On arrival, paramedics should survey the scene for any relevant details, to include evidence of substance abuse, a suicide attempt, or other clues that may shed light on the patient's state. The patient should be observed for emotional response, such as fear, anger, confusion, or hostility. Whilst providing patient care, the paramedic should focus the evaluation on the patient's level of cognitive functioning. This includes alertness, orientation, speech patterns, affect, and the way in which the patient interacts with friends, loved ones, and family members. When possible, the number of people around the patient should be limited. This helps to control the scene. Anyone who interferes with the scene or the patient assessment or who adversely affects the patient's condition should be removed from the area.

Other information can be volunteered by the patient, obtained from the patient interview, or provided by family members, bystanders, and first responders. The patient's family or caregiver should be interviewed about the patient's usual level of functioning, about recent stress in the patient's life, and about approaches that may help the paramedic to gain the patient's trust and cooperation. Information that should be obtained for a full background and history of the event include significant past medical history, medications the patient has taken (Table 25-1), past psychiatric problems, and any precipitating factors that may have contributed to the behavioural emergency.

Interview techniques

After managing any life-threatening illness or injury, the paramedic should interview the patient if possible. The paramedic should not ask for more details than are needed. A limited and supportive interview strengthens the paramedic's rapport with the patient and may also help to establish and maintain a relationship during the provision of patient care. Effective interview techniques include active listening, showing support and empathy, preventing interruptions, and respecting the patient's personal space by limiting physical touch (Box 25-3).

Table 25-1 Examples of drugs used to treat psychiatric disorders

Antipsychotic drugs

Group 1: chlorpromazine, levomepromazine (methotrimeprazine) and promazine. These tend to produce pronounced sedative effects and moderate antimuscarinic and extrapyramidal side effects.
Group 2: pericyazine and pipotiazine. This group is characterized by moderate sedative effects, marked antimuscarinic effects, but fewer extrapyramidal side effects than groups 1 or 3.
Group 3: fluphenazine, perphenazine, prochlorperazine and trifluoperazine. This group tends to produce fewer sedative effects, fewer antimuscarinic effects, but more pronounced extrapyramidal side effects than groups 1 and 2.

Other antipsychotics tend to resemble the group 3 phenothiazines and include:
Butyrophenones, e.g. benperidol and haloperidol
Diphenylbutylpiperidines, e.g. pimozide
Thioxanthenes, e.g. flupentixol and zuclopenthixol
Substituted benzamides, e.g. sulpiride

Newer antipsychotic drugs are referred to as 'atypical' drugs, and include:
amisulpride, aripiprazole, clozapine, olanzapine, quetiapine, risperidone and zotepine.
These drugs may be better tolerated than other antipsychotics as there are fewer extrapyramidal side effects. Further information regarding the prescribing of these drugs can be found in the 2002 National Institute of Clinical Excellence guidelines.[3]

Lithium

Lithium may be indicated in treatment and prophylaxis of mania, bipolar disorder, recurrent depression, and aggressive or self-mutilating behaviour.

Antidepressant drugs

These are most effective for treating moderate to severe depression associated with psychomotor and physiological changes such as loss of appetite and sleep disturbances. The first benefit is usually an improvement in sleep although therapeutic effects may not take place for up to 2 weeks. Those with sedative properties include:
amitriptyline, clomipramine, dosulepin (dothiepin), doxepin, mianserin, trazodone, and trimipramine.
Those with less sedative properties include:
imipramine, lofepramine and nortriptyline.

Monoamine oxidase inhibitors (MAOIs)

These drugs are used less frequently than other antidepressants due to their interactions with food and other medications. It is easier to prescribe MAOIs when other antidepressants have failed than vice versa. Examples include:
phenelzine, isocarboxazid and tranylcypromine (the most hazardous of the MAOIs).

Selective serotonin reuptake inhibitors (SSRIs)

This group of drugs selectively inhibit the reuptake of serotonin and include the following:
citalopram, escitalopram, fluoxetine, fluvoxamine, paroxetine and sertraline.

CNS stimulants

CNS stimulants include the amphetamines and related drugs such as methylphenidate. Methylphenidate and atomoxetine are used under close supervision in the management of attention deficit hyperactivity disorder (ADHD). Dexamfetamine (one of the amphetamines) may be used as an alternative when other drugs have not worked.

Anxiolytic drugs (anti-anxiety)

Benzodiazepine anxiolytics (previously termed incorrectly as minor tranquillizers) are useful in alleviating anxiety states and are the most commonly prescribed drugs for this condition. This group of drugs includes:
diazepam, alprazolam, chlordiazepoxide and clobazam (these have a sustained action); and lorazepam and oxazepam (shorter-acting).

Source: British Medical Association and Royal Pharmaceutical Society of Great Britain. British National Formulary 54. September 2007. Online. Available http://www.bnf.org.uk/bnf/ 13 February 2009

Mental status examination

A mental status examination (MSE) is an evaluation tool. It can help the paramedic during the patient assessment. Although many variations of an MSE are available, most include an assessment of appearance and behaviour, speech and language, cognitive abilities, and emotional stability.[4]

The following factors should be assessed in each of these areas.

Appearance and behaviour

- How does the patient look? Is the person neatly dressed and well groomed?

Box 25-3

Ten useful interviewing skills for behavioural emergencies

1. Listen to the patient in a caring, concerned, and receptive manner. Be aware of non-verbal cues such as eye contact, facial expression, and posture. These can reassure the patient that you are responding with empathy.
2. Elicit feelings as well as facts to help develop a more accurate impression of the patient. If the patient is anxious, encourage the person to share details relevant to that feeling.
3. Respond to the patient's feelings by acknowledging and labelling them. (For example, you might say, 'You seem angry'.) This may help validate and legitimize the patient's intense and sometimes overwhelming feelings.
4. Correct cognitive misconceptions or distortions. If a distorted sense of reality is producing fear or anxiety, offer a simple and correct explanation.
5. Explain to the patient the care the person can expect to receive upon arrival at the hospital.
6. Offer honest and realistic reassurance and support. Providing this support helps calm the patient and establishes rapport.
7. Ask effective questions. Ask closed-ended questions if you are seeking immediate information. For example, 'Are you thinking of hurting yourself?' and 'What medicines did you take?' Open-ended questions are appropriate after you have identified problems that require immediate attention. Such questions allow the patient to develop answers that usually help the paramedic more fully understand the problem.
8. Avoid leading questions that may lead the person to say things he or she did not intend.
9. Structure the interview to develop a pattern rather than allowing a natural flow of details. Histories or sequences of events in chronological order usually allow for a fuller understanding of the patient's problem. (This is particularly true for causal relationships.) This order also helps the patient to organize thoughts. Keep the patient's responses focused. This can be done by using comments such as 'What happened next?' and 'Was that before or after what you were just telling me about?'
10. Conclude the interview. After getting the relevant information, encourage the patient to describe other important events or feelings.

Modified from Bassuk EL 1983 Behavioural emergencies: a field guide for EMTs and paramedics. Little, Brown, Boston.

- Is the patient pleasant and cooperative or agitated?
- Is the patient's behaviour appropriate for the particular situation?
- What is the patient's body language?
- Do body movements or posture suggest tension, anxiety, hostility or aggression?
- Does the patient maintain eye contact during the patient interview?

Speech and language

- Is the patient's speech intelligible and normal in tone, volume, and rate?
- Does the tone of the patient's voice change?
- Is speech spontaneous, with ease of expression?
- Do the patient's words and sentences proceed in an orderly fashion?

Cognitive abilities

- Is the patient oriented to person, time, and place?
- Does the patient know who and where he or she is?
- Does the patient know who you are?
- Can the patient remain focused on your questions and conversation?
- What is the patient's attention span?
- Can the patient follow a series of short commands?
- Does the patient respond to directions appropriately?
- Are the patient's comments logical and presented in an organized fashion?

Emotional stability

- Is the patient aware of his or her environment?
- Can the patient describe or rate his or her mood using a scale of 1 to 10?
- Does the patient appear happy, sad, depressed, or angry?
- Is the patient's mood appropriate for the specific situation?
- Does the patient show mood swings or behaviours that indicate anxiety, depression, anger or hostility?
- Does the patient stay focused during the interview or stray quickly to related topics?
- Is the patient experiencing perceptual distortions or hallucinations?

Critical Thinking

Think about interviewing techniques that you've seen EMS crews use when caring for patients with behavioural emergencies. Were the techniques effective? Could the paramedics have improved their patient care by using any of the techniques listed in Box 25-3?

Difficult patient interviews

Some patients with behavioural or psychiatric disorders are difficult to interview. For example, a patient may refuse to talk to the paramedic. (This may be the case especially if the family requested EMS assistance without the patient's consent.) A patient may be extremely talkative and have disorganized speech. In addition, a patient may be confrontational. If a patient refuses to be interviewed, paramedics should speak to the patient in a quiet voice and should avoid questions that the patient may see as an 'interrogation'. Extra time should be allowed for the patient to respond. Patients who are too talkative need to have their attention focused on the interview. To do this, the paramedic can raise a hand or call the person's name. With a confrontational patient, additional help may be required to ensure scene safety.

Other patient care measures

After the initial assessment and history taking, the rest of the examination is determined by the patient; specifically, this means by the person's overall condition and the nature of the psychiatric problem. There may be a good reason to suspect an organic cause for the patient's condition. If so, a physical examination should be performed. Otherwise, patient care for a person with a behavioural emergency may be limited to maintaining an effective rapport with the patient during transfer to the hospital.

Specific behavioural and psychiatric disorders

More than 250 psychiatric conditions have been noted by mental health workers. In addition, some patients may have symptoms that are associated with more than one condition. The following are common classifications of mental disorders discussed in this chapter:

- cognitive disorders
- schizophrenia
- anxiety disorders
- mood disorders
- substance-related disorders
- personality disorders.

The World Health Organization International Classification of Diseases and Related Health Problems (ICD-10)[5] is used to classify diseases and other health problems recorded on many types of health and vital records. Chapter V encompasses Mental and Behavioural Disorders and these classifications are widely used by health professionals (except in the USA). Classes of psychiatric disorders include the following:

- organic, including symptomatic, mental disorders
- mental and behavioural disorders due to psychoactive substance use
- schizophrenia, schizotypal and delusional disorders
- mood (affective) disorders
- neurotic, stress-related and somatoform disorders
- behavioural syndromes associated with physiological disturbances and physical factors
- disorders of adult personality and behaviour
- mental retardation
- disorders of psychological development
- behavioural and emotional disorders with onset usually occurring in childhood and adolescence
- unspecified mental disorder.

Patient care for most behavioural emergencies is mainly supportive. It usually involves providing emotional support, assessing and managing coexisting emergency medical problems, and transporting the patient for evaluation by a physician. In some cases paramedics may need to take measures to protect the patient and others from harm. This includes the possible use of physical restraint (described later in this chapter).

Cognitive disorders

Cognitive disorders may have an organic cause (e.g. a disease process). They also may be a result of physical or chemical injury, such as trauma or drug abuse. All cognitive disorders result in a disturbance of cognitive functioning. This may manifest as delirium or dementia (see Chapter 39).

Delirium

Delirium is an abrupt disorientation of time and place. It usually involves delusions (false beliefs) and hallucinations (the individual appears to perceive sights, sounds, and other sensory phenomena that are not actually present). The symptoms vary according to an individual's personality, the environment, and the severity of the illness. Common signs and symptoms of delirium include inattention, memory impairment, disorientation, clouding of consciousness, and vivid visual hallucinations. Treatment of delirium is aimed at correcting the underlying physical disorder to reduce anxiety. Sedatives may be required to manage the patient. The exact occurrence rate of delirium is unknown, because it is often overlooked. However, some groups of people are more susceptible to delirium than others. These groups include the following:

- older adults
- children
- burns patients
- patients who have had major heart surgery
- patients who have had a previous brain injury (e.g. stroke)
- patients with acquired immunodeficiency syndrome (AIDS).

Dementia

Dementia is a clinical state characterized by loss of function in multiple cognitive domains. It is a slow, progressive loss of awareness of time and place and usually involves an inability to learn new things or to remember recent events. About 75 types of dementia have been identified (Box 25-4). However, most cases result from cerebrovascular disease (including stroke) and Alzheimer's disease (an irreversible, gradual loss of brain cells and shrinkage of brain tissue). Dementia is a major health problem in the UK because of the relatively long life spans of UK citizens. The disorder affects around 700 000 people in the UK, with the figure expected to rise to over 1 million by 2025.[6] Prevalence increases significantly with age; from 65–69 years the prevalence is 1.3%, rising to 32.5% in the 95 years and older group.[6] The personal habits of patients with dementia often deteriorate. Speech may become incoherent and many may appear to enter a 'second childhood'. These patients need total care for feeding, toileting and physical activities. Treatment of certain illnesses may help to slow the mental decline associated with this disease.

Delirium and dementia may be difficult to differentiate because both may cause disorientation and impaired memory, thinking and judgement. Dementia usually occurs in people without diminished alertness and appears slowly and worsens over time. Sleeping and waking problems occur less often in people with dementia than in those with delirium. People with dementia may have difficulty with short- and long-term memory, as well as impairment of judgement and abstract thinking. Delirium may sometimes occur at the same time as dementia, especially the case in older adults or people with chronic illnesses.

Box 25-4

Disorders causing dementia

Degenerative diseases

- Alzheimer's disease
- Pick's disease
- Huntington's disease
- Progressive supranuclear palsy
- Parkinson's disease (not all cases)
- Cerebellar degenerations
- Amyotrophic lateral sclerosis (ALS) (not all cases)
- Parkinson–ALS–dementia complex of Guam and other island areas
- Rare genetic and metabolic diseases (Hallervorden–Spatz, Kufs', Wilson's, late-onset metachromatic leukodystrophy, adrenoleukodystrophy)

Vascular dementia

- Multi-infarct dementia
- Cortical micro-infarcts
- Lacunar dementia (large infarcts)
- Binswanger's disease
- Cerebral embolic disease (flat, air, thrombus fragments)

Anoxic dementia

- Cardiac arrest
- Cardiac failure (severe)
- Carbon monoxide

Traumatic dementia

- Dementia pugilistica (boxer's dementia)
- Head injuries (open or closed)

Infectious dementia

- Acquired immune deficiency syndrome (AIDS)
- Opportunistic infections
- Creutzfeldt–Jakob disease (subacute spongiform encephalopathy)
- Progressive multifocal leukoencephalopathy
- Post-encephalitic dementia
- Behçet's syndrome
- Herpes encephalitis
- Fungal meningitis or encephalitis
- Bacterial meningitis or encephalitis
- Parasitic encephalitis
- Brain abscess
- Neurosyphilis (general paresis)

Normal pressure hydrocephalus (communicating hydrocephalus of adults)

Space-occupying lesions

- Chronic or acute subdural haematoma
- Primary brain tumour
- Metastatic tumour (carcinoma, leukaemia, lymphoma, sarcoma)

Multiple sclerosis

(some cases)

Autoimmune disorders

- Disseminated lupus erythematosus
- Vasculitis

Toxic dementia

- Alcoholic dementia
- Metallic dementia (e.g. lead, mercury, arsenic, manganese)
- Organic poisons (e.g. solvents, some insecticides)

From Alzheimer's Association. FYI: Disorders causing dementia. Online. Available http://www.alz-nca.org/aboutalz/fyi.php 5 June 2009

Critical Thinking

Besides auditory hallucinations, think of other sensory hallucinations that can occur in these patients.

Schizophrenia

Schizophrenia is a group of disorders characterized by recurrent episodes of psychotic behaviour. Although the exact cause of the disease has not yet been identified, it may result from a combination of genetics (a family history of schizophrenia often exists), chemical and hormonal changes, brain damage, street drugs and alcohol, childhood deprivation and abuse, and other stress factors.[7] Schizophrenia usually becomes apparent during adolescence or early adulthood (Box 25-5).[8]

Signs and symptoms of the illness appear slowly over time and become more pronounced and bizarre as the disease progresses. These patients often develop abnormalities of thought processing, thought content, perception, and judgement. Hallmarks of the disease are paranoia, delusions, and auditory hallucinations (e.g. hearing voices that insult or make demands) (Box 25-6.)

Box 25-5

Facts about schizophrenia

- Approximately 1 in 100 individuals will develop schizophrenia.[9]
- In men, schizophrenia usually appears in the late teens or early 20s.
- In women, schizophrenia usually appears in the 20s to early 30s.
- Schizophrenia affects men and women with equal frequency.
- Most people with schizophrenia suffer chronically throughout their lives.
- 5–13% of patients with schizophrenia die by suicide.[10]

Many patients with schizophrenia function quite well with drug therapy. Others function poorly between frank psychotic episodes. (These episodes are often the result of failure to comply with drug therapy.) Most patients must take antipsychotic drugs and agents that block the action of

Box 25-6

Responding to paranoia, delusions and hallucinations

1. First, assess whether the problem is troublesome or frightening to the person experiencing it. If not, ignoring it may be the best approach.
2. If a person seems to be hallucinating, leave the individual alone or approach slowly so as not to frighten the person. Respond with caution.
3. Don't try to argue or rationalize. Realize that hallucinations and delusions seem very real to the person who is experiencing them. Arguing does not build trust.
4. Offer reassurance and validation. You might say, 'I know this is troubling for you. Let me see if I can help.'
5. Check out the reality of the situation; maybe what the person sees or thinks is true.
6. Sometimes things in the environment may be misinterpreted (i.e. a glare or shadow in the window, a noisy furnace). These may be frightening. Explain the potential or actual misinterpretation (e.g. that the noise is the furnace turning on).
7. Modify the environment if necessary. (A mirror may become distracting or confusing; adding more lights may be helpful at night.)
8. Assess whether the person is having problems with hearing or vision. Resolving such problems can reduce the degree of disability.
9. Recall that whispering or laughing around the person may be misinterpreted.
10. Do not take any accusations personally.
11. Use distraction to try to pull the person's focus from the delusion or hallucination.
12. If the person asks you directly whether you see or hear something, be honest. However, don't struggle to convince or reason with the individual about what is real.
13. Try to respond to what the person may be feeling: insecurity, fear and confusion.
14. Rule out any illnesses or the use of any medicines that could be contributing to the problem.
15. Use tact and firmness in persuading a patient to be transported to the hospital.

Modified from the Alzheimer's Association handout. Hallucinations and delusions and understanding difficult behaviors; Anne Robinson, Beth Spencer, Laurie White (1989), Eastern Michigan University, Ypsilanti, MI.

dopamine for the rest of their lives. If the person takes these medications regularly, the obvious symptoms are usually controlled. However, the drugs may produce side effects, especially dyskinesia (abnormal muscular movements) and tremor.

Anxiety disorders

A certain amount of anxiety is useful. In fact, it is necessary for adapting constructively to stress (see Chapter 3). However, a patient who suffers from an anxiety disorder has a persistent, fearful feeling that cannot be consciously related to reality (Box 25-7).[9] This type of illness can be disabling and the patient may withdraw from daily activities. This is usually an unsuccessful attempt to avoid the episodes of intense activity. Severe anxiety disorders may manifest in a

Box 25-7

Facts about anxiety disorders

- The Office for National Statistics (ONS) estimates that 4.7% of adults experience generalized anxiety disorders not including depression, at any one time.
- Anxiety disorders are often complicated by depression, eating disorders, or substance abuse.
- Panic disorders are related to anxiety. According to the ONS study, 7 people per 1000 develop a panic disorder and this appears to be the same across all age groups and roughly the same for men and women.

panic disorder ('panic attack') with the following signs and symptoms:

- hyperventilation
- feeling of breathlessness or smothering
- blurred vision
- perioral and hand and foot paraesthesias
- fear of losing control
- fear of dying
- somatic complaints
- chest discomfort
- palpitations or tachycardia
- dyspnoea
- choking
- faintness
- syncope
- vertigo
- trembling and sweating
- urinary frequency and diarrhoea.

Patient management is mainly supportive. The paramedic should assure these patients that although they may feel as if they are dying, they are not. Also, the paramedic should assure them that effective treatment is available. Panic attacks may mimic a number of medical emergencies, including myocardial infarction; therefore any patient who shows the signs and symptoms described before should be fully assessed at the scene and transported for evaluation by a physician. Patients with anxiety disorders should not be left alone.

Phobia

A phobia is a type of anxiety disorder. A person with a phobia has transferred anxiety onto a situation or an object in the form of an irrational, intense fear, such as a fear of heights, closed spaces, water or other people. As the object or situation comes closer, the person's anxiety increases. If the crisis is allowed to continue, the patient's anxiety may escalate into a panic attack. These patients usually recognize that their fear is unreasonable; however, they cannot overcome the phobia. In some cases the phobia does not initiate the EMS response but becomes a secondary complication in emergency care. An example is a person who is phobic of water being trapped in a submerged car.

When caring for patients with a phobia, the paramedic should take care to explain each step of an emergency or rescue procedure. The key is a careful rehearsal with the patient, in which the paramedic explains exactly what care will be given and how it will be performed. In addition, the EMS crew should show patience and understanding of the phobia. They should assure the patient that no forceful steps will be taken to place the person into a position unwillingly.

Critical Thinking

Do you know someone with an intense fear of a situation or object? How does this person behave when subjected to the object of the phobia?

Obsessive–compulsive disorder

Obsessive–compulsive disorder (OCD) is a psychiatric disorder in which a person feels stress or anxiety about thoughts or rituals over which the individual has little control (Box 25-8).[11] The disorder can take many forms. These include excessive hand washing or showering, or upsetting thoughts (e.g. violence, vulgarities, harm to oneself or others). Obsessions may also involve special numbers, colours, single words or phrases, and sometimes melodies.

Although most adults realize to some degree that these obsessions and compulsions are senseless, they have great difficulty stopping them. Children with OCD may not realize that their behaviour is unusual. OCD affects men and women equally, can start at any age, and may have a heritable component. People with OCD often cleverly hide their condition from family, friends, and coworkers. Medications and behaviour therapy are often effective in controlling the symptoms of this disorder.

Post-traumatic stress disorder (PTSD)

The World Health Organization defines PTSD as 'a delayed or protracted response to a stressful event or situation (either short- or long-lasting) of an exceptionally threatening or long-lasting nature, which is likely to cause pervasive distress in almost anyone'.[12] The available estimates of PTSD stem mainly from large-scale studies from the US involving adults (Box 25-9);[13] it remains to be investigated whether these data apply to the UK and to children. The causative events are often life-threatening; e.g. events associated with military service or rape, and frequently result in repetitive, intrusive memories. Manifestations of this illness may include depression, sleep disturbances, nightmares, and survivor guilt. The syndrome is sometimes complicated by substance abuse.

EMS personnel and other emergency responders may be subject to this syndrome as a result of their work. Examples include responding to major incidents with a large number of injured people, the death of a coworker, a sudden infant death syndrome (SIDS) death, and the stress associated with responding to emergency calls (see Chapter 3).

Box 25-8

Facts about obsessive–compulsive disorder

- Between 1% and 2% of the UK population suffer from OCD.
- it can affect people of any age, from young children to older adults.
- OCD affects males and females with equal frequency.

Mood disorders

The term mood disorder is used to describe changes in emotions that a person experiences in life. (For example, these may include happiness, depression, fear and anxiety.) Two conditions commonly associated with mood disorders are depression and bipolar disorder, both of which are associated with an increased risk of suicide.[14–17]

Depression

Depression is a mood disturbance characterized by feelings of sadness, despair and discouragement. It is one of the most prevalent major psychiatric conditions, affecting 10–15% of the general population (Box 25-10).[1] Depression is usually episodic (episodes usually last longer than 1 month) with periods of remission. It may have a gradual or rapid onset and, at times, a clustering of episodes. The depressed patient may show feelings of hopelessness, extreme isolation, tenseness and irritability. In severe cases the depression may be followed by anhedonia (the inability to feel pleasure or happiness from experiences that ordinarily are pleasurable), insomnia or hypersomnia, weight loss (from diminished appetite) or gain, decreased libido, and deep feelings of worthlessness and guilt. The mnemonic 'IN SAD CAGES' identifies the major features of depression:[18]

Box 25-9

Facts about post-traumatic stress disorder (PTSD)

- About 5.2 million people in the US have PTSD during the course of a given year.
- PTSD can develop at any age, including childhood.
- PTSD is more common in women than men.
- About 30% of men and women who have spent time in a war zone experience this disorder.
- PTSD often occurs after violent personal assaults, such as rape, mugging or domestic violence; terrorism; natural or human-caused disasters; and accidents.
- Depression, alcohol or other substance abuse, or another anxiety disorder often accompanies PTSD.

Box 25-10

Facts about depression

- Depression is one of the most common mental illnesses, affecting nearly 1 in 6 people in the UK at some point in their lives.
- Women are more likely than men to report depressive illness.
- The percentage of men showing symptoms of depression in 2000 was 11%, a rise of 3% from 1993.
- Depression is a frequent and serious complication of heart attack, stroke, diabetes and cancer.
- Depression increases the risk of heart attack.
- Major depression is the leading cause of disability worldwide.

Interest
Sleep
Appetite
Depressed mood
Concentration
Activity
Guilt
Energy
Suicide

Depression is associated with an increased risk of suicide for all age groups (described later in this chapter). Care for depressed patients is directed at quietly talking to the patient about things that appear to be of interest and trying to gain responsiveness. Depression may be treated with antidepressant drug therapy (see Chapter 12), counselling, psychotherapy and, in a small number of cases, electroconvulsive therapy (ECT).

Bipolar disorder

Bipolar disorder is a biphasic emotional disorder in which depressive and manic episodes alternate (Figure 25-2). Mania is characterized by excessive elation, talkativeness, flight of ideas, motor activity, irritability, accelerated speech and, often, delusions that centre on personal grandeur. Bipolar disorders sometimes develop slowly over time; however, they may occur abruptly and may be brought on by a single event. The manic phase can be very brief or can last weeks to months. Compared with depression, mania is rare. The most frequent age for initial episodes is 20 to 35 years, with initial attacks of depression occurring about 10 years later (Box 25-11).[19–21] Many patients with bipolar disorder are treated with lithium. As described in Chapter 21, lithium has a narrow therapeutic index; a common illness, such as influenza with diarrhoea and or vomiting, can result in lithium toxicity.

Emergency care should consist of calm, firm emotional support and transport for evaluation by a physician. If this is the patient's first manic episode, the paramedic should consider the possibility of drug abuse. It is usually a good idea to keep sensory stimulation to a minimum. If the patient's condition allows, EMS transport should proceed without using the lights and sirens.

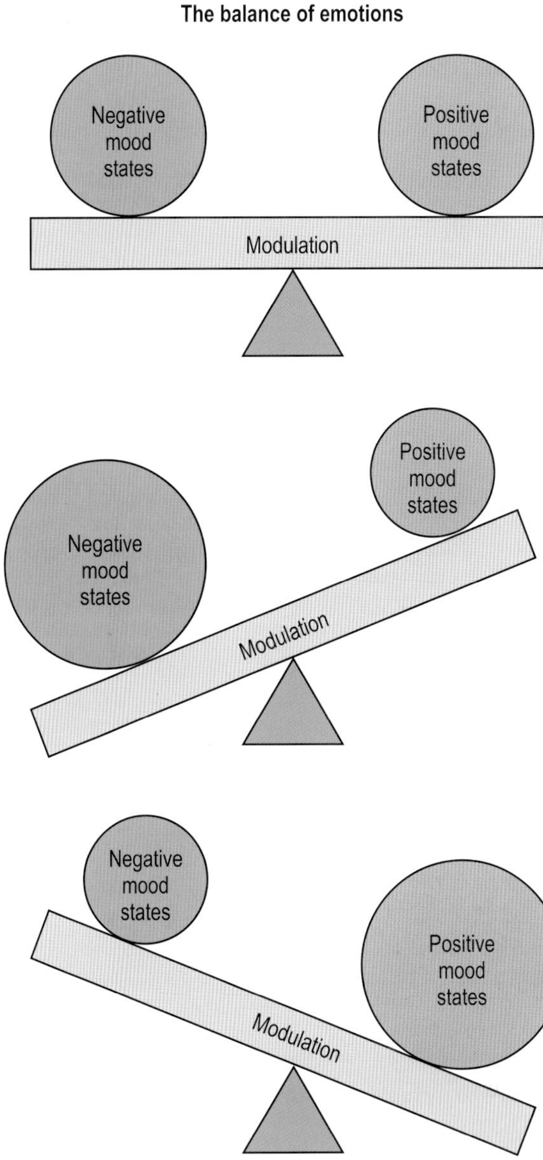

Figure 25-2 Bipolar disorder.

Critical Thinking

Do you think patients would be at higher risk for suicide during the depressive or the manic phase of bipolar disorder? Why?

Box 25-11

Facts about bipolar disorder

- Between 1% and 2% of the UK population is diagnosed with bipolar disorder.
- For those with bipolar disorder the suicide risk is much higher, at 15 times that of the general population.
- Men and women are equally likely to develop bipolar disorder.
- The annual cost of bipolar disorder to society has been estimated at £2 billion.

Suicide and suicide threats

A threat of suicide is a sign that a patient has a serious crisis that calls for immediate intervention. In many cases suicide attempts are a cry for help although they may be a form of direct or indirect communication. (They may be saying, 'I don't want to live' or 'I am angry with you'.) Other suicide attempts are an effort by the patient to manipulate relationships so that the patient is surrounded by people who are ready and willing to provide advice and support (Box 25-12). In assessing the risk of suicide, the paramedic should consider these eight facts:[22]

1. Suicide rates in both men and women continued to fall in 2007, reaching the lowest rates since 1991.
2. In 2007 the rate for men was 16.8 per 100 000 population (peak of 21.2 per 100 000 in 1998) and for women was 5.0 per 100 000 population.

Box 25-12

Myths about suicide

Myth: Talking about suicide or asking someone if they feel suicidal will encourage suicide attempts.

Fact: Serious talk about suicide does not create or increase risk; it reduces it. The best way to identify the possibility of suicide is to ask directly. Openly discussing someone's thoughts of suicide can be a source of relief for them and can be key to preventing the immediate danger of suicide.

Myth: People who talk about suicide never attempt or complete suicide.

Fact: People who feel suicidal often talk about their feelings and plans to friends or others. Listening to, validating, and acting to support a person in this circumstance, can save lives.

Myth: Suicide is illegal.

Fact: Suicide is not illegal. Even so, there are still legal questions in the UK, where suicidal individuals have been charged with Breach of the Peace, and even been made the subject of Anti-Social Behaviour Orders. 'A woman who has attempted suicide four times has been banned from jumping into rivers, canals or onto railway lines' (BBC, February 2005).

Myth: The only effective ways to help suicidal people come from professional therapists with extensive experience in this area.

Fact: You can help by identifying the potentially suicidal person and talking to them about it. Preventing suicide is everyone's business.

Myth: If somebody wants to take their life, they will, and there is nothing anyone can do about it.

Fact: Most people contemplating suicide do not want to die; they just want to stop the pain and difficulties they are experiencing. Although there are some occasions when nobody could have predicted a suicide, or intervened, in most cases there will have been a point in the process where a timely intervention might have averted the tragic outcome.

Myth: People who try to kill themselves must be mentally ill.

Fact: Most people have clear reasons for their suicidal feelings. Most people have thought of suicide from time to time. Though suicide is a tragic consequence of some mental health problems, around three out of four people who take their own lives have not been in contact with mental health services in the year before their death.

Myth: Some people are always suicidal.

Fact: Some groups, sub-cultures or ages are particularly associated with suicide. Whilst some groups, such as young men, seem to be at risk, suicide can affect anybody. Many people think about suicide in passing at some time or another. There isn't a 'type' for suicide, and whilst there are warning signs, they aren't always there. Whilst there is a risk of further suicide attempts, people who have had suicidal feelings or have made an attempt on their life move on.

Myth: Suicide is painless.

Fact: Most methods of suicide are extremely unpleasant. Some methods are violent, and catastrophic. Others are physically painful and drawn out.

Myth: A suicide in the elderly is less of a tragedy that the suicide of a teenager.

Fact: Any suicide is a tragedy for the individual, and the people around them. Saying 'at least they had had a good life' marginalizes the grief of those left behind after a suicide in later life.

Myth: When a suicidal person begins to feel better, the danger is over.

Fact: Often the risk of suicide can be greatest as depression lifts, or after a person appears to calm after a period of turmoil. This can be because once a decision to attempt suicide is made, people may feel they have a solution; however desperate it might be.

Myth: People who attempt suicide are merely looking for attention.

Fact: Often people who attempt suicide do not want to die. When a person decides to make an attempt on their life, it is often because all other options, including the means to communicate with other people more conventionally, are obscured by the pain the person feels.

Myth: Those around someone who has had a bereavement suicide shouldn't talk about it.

Fact: Ignoring loss is denying loss. It should not be given 'the silent treatment'.

See Me; Stigma and Suicide – Suicide Factsheet. Online. Available http://www.seemescotland.org.uk/images/pdfs/suicide.pdf

3. In 2007 there were 5377 suicides in adults aged 15 and over, 177 fewer than in 2006 (5554) and 940 fewer than in 1991 (6317).
4. Three-quarters of the suicides in 2007 were men, a constant statistic since 1991.
5. In the early 1990s the highest suicide rates in the UK were among men aged 75 and over. Rates in this age group have since decreased from 25.1 per 100 000 population in 1991 to 15.2 per 100 000 population in 2007.
6. Since 1997 the highest rates have been in men aged 15–44. In 2007 the rate for this age group was 17.6 per 100 000 population. Suicide rates among men aged 45–74 decreased from 17.3 per 100 000 population in 2006 to 16.0 per 100 000 in 2007.
7. Rates for women aged 75 years and over fell from 9.4 per 100 000 population in 1993 to 4.3 per 100 000 in 2007.
8. Since 2004 the highest suicide rates among women have been in those aged 45–74 and in 2007 the rate was 6.2 per 100 000 population. Suicide rates in women aged 15–44 have consistently been the lowest since 1991 and fell to 4.2 per 100 000 population in 2007.
9. Rates of suicide increase with deprivation.
10. Men use more violent means (guns, knives) than women (pills, razor blades).
11. About 60% of those who successfully commit suicide have a history of a previous attempt.
12. The more specific and detailed the suicide plan, the greater the suicide potential.

Other factors associated with suicide threats include the recent death of a loved one or loss of a significant relationship, a financial setback or job loss, chronic or debilitating illness, social isolation, alcohol or other drug abuse, depression, and schizophrenia. If a suicide attempt is suspected, the paramedic should discuss these intentions with the patient. Questions such as, 'Do you have thoughts about killing yourself or others?' or 'Have you ever tried to kill yourself?' are appropriate; many depressed patients are willing to discuss their suicidal (or homicidal) thoughts. During the patient interview, the paramedic should try to determine three important factors: (1) whether the patient has a plan (how and when the suicide will be done); (2) whether the plan is intended to be successful; and (3) whether the patient has the means or method to follow through with the plan.

Critical Thinking

How would you feel about asking a patient, 'Have you ever thought about killing yourself?'

When responding to a suicide attempt, paramedics should request police protection before approaching the scene. (Armed patients must be considered homicidal as well as suicidal.) After scene safety has been ensured and paramedics have gained access to the patient, the scene should be checked for the presence of dangerous objects (see Chapter 44).

The first priority in patient management is medical care. Unconscious patients should be managed with airway, ventilatory and circulatory support and rapid transport. If the patient is conscious, creating rapport as soon as possible is essential. The paramedic should conduct a brief interview to assess the situation and determine the need for and direction of further action. To help reduce the potential for suicide, paramedics can take the following six steps:

1. Provide support and honest assurance about the patient's well-being.
2. Provide for physical safety as well as emotional security. Establish protective limits and measures. This helps to prevent injury to the patient or others. It also conveys to these patients that the paramedic will help them control their behaviour until they can gain self-control.
3. Listen to the person, even if the speech seems bizarre, inappropriate, or unrealistic. Do not feel that every statement must be answered or that advice or opinions must be given. During the interview, acknowledge the patient's feelings; do not argue with the patient's wish to die. Explain alternatives to suicide that the patient may not have considered.
4. Determine the patient's support system or significant others when possible. Others may be better able to communicate with and calm the patient.
5. Encourage and reassure the patient during the crisis.
6. Transport the patient to the proper facility for emergency intervention.

Substance-related disorders

Some patients with a behavioural emergency may also be using alcohol or illegal drugs. This may cause difficulties during the physical examination. (Substance-related disorders are described in Chapter 21.) Often these patients are trying to 'self-medicate'. They are trying to improve their mood or lessen the anxiety associated with mental illness. Other patients self-medicate before receiving a diagnosis for their illness or before seeking professional help. Signs that may indicate alcohol or illicit drug use include a breath odour of alcohol, the presence of drug paraphernalia, and needle tracks on the extremities.

Personality disorders

Personality disorders are a large group of conditions distinguished by a failure to learn from experience or to adapt appropriately to changes. This failure results in personal distress and impairment of social functioning. These disorders may have an environmental component. They may also be genetic. Personality disorders become especially obvious during times of stress.

The symptoms of a personality disorder are usually first recognized in early adolescence. They continue throughout the person's life. The symptoms may vary in frequency and intensity. Generally, however, they are relatively constant. They usually affect most aspects of a patient's life. This includes thoughts, emotions, relationships and interpersonal skills, and impulse control. Personality disorders have been classified in a variety of ways. However, the following are three common disorders:

- Antisocial personality disorder: a long-standing pattern (after the age of 15) of disregard for the rights of others. It is often associated with irresponsible behaviour and a lack of remorse for wrongdoing.
- Borderline personality disorder: a pattern of unstable relationships, poor or negative self-image, mood swings, and poor impulse control. It may be associated with destructive and self-harming behaviours (e.g. suicide attempts, self-mutilation), an intense fear of abandonment, and displays of sudden anger.
- Narcissistic personality disorder: a pattern of grandiosity, need for admiration, and sense of entitlement. It often is associated with exaggerated achievements and fantasies about unlimited success, power, love, or beauty.

Many factors are associated with the development of a personality disorder. These may include unstable relationships during childhood, family violence, and childhood abuse or neglect. Treatment involves behaviour modification techniques, counselling, drug therapy, and individual psychotherapy.

Special considerations for patients with behavioural problems

In addition to caring for the immediate needs of patients with behavioural problems, paramedics may have to deal with complications arising from the situation or other factors affecting the patient. Among these factors are the patient's age and the possibility of violent behaviour. This section presents special considerations for paediatric patients, elderly patients and the potentially violent patient.

Critical Thinking

When responding to a behavioural emergency that involves a child or an adolescent, do you use the same safety guidelines that you use with an adult?

Behavioural problems in children

Young children who are victims of emotional crisis need to be managed with techniques that are different from those used to care for older children and adults. The following suggestions may be helpful to the paramedic in dealing with some children:

1. Gain the child's trust and try to convince the child that you are a friend who can help.
2. Make it clear that you are strong enough to be in control but will not hurt the child.
3. Keep the interview questions brief; the child's attention span may be extremely short.
4. Never lie; be honest.
5. Use all available resources to communicate (e.g. drawing pictures, telling stories).
6. Involve parents or caregivers in the interview or examination if appropriate.
7. Take any threat of violence seriously.

If the child's behaviour or physical condition makes restraint necessary, the paramedic should use only reasonable force (with sufficient help) to ensure the patient's safety and the safety of the EMS crew. Calming measures may fail to work. If so, wrapping the child in a full body blanket secured to the stretcher with straps often is sufficient during transport for evaluation by a physician. As with any method of restraint, the paramedic should monitor the child's airway and circulation and make sure that they are not compromised. Documentation should be thorough and complete.

Behavioural problems in elderly patients

Problem behaviour in an elderly patient can be a sign of a long-standing psychiatric disorder; a newly emerging psychiatric problem; a medical illness; substance abuse; drug non-compliance or drug interactions; and other factors (see Chapter 39). The following suggestions may be helpful to the paramedic in communicating with some elderly patients:

1. Identify yourself and speak at eye level to make sure the patient can see you.
2. Address the patient by surname (e.g. 'Mr. Jones' or 'Miss [or Mrs.] Smith') unless directed otherwise.
3. Speak slowly, distinctly, and respectfully.
4. Ask one question at a time and allow time for complete answers.
5. Listen closely.
6. Explain what you are doing and why.
7. Provide reassuring physical touch.
8. Be patient.
9. Permit family members and caregivers to remain with the patient if appropriate.
10. Preserve the patient's dignity.

Assessing the potentially violent patient

Only a small number of people with mental health problems are potentially violent. Nonetheless, assessment and management of the potentially violent patient should be part of an EMS protocol. The following four factors may help the paramedic determine the potential for a violent episode:[23]

1. Past history (Has the patient previously shown hostile, aggressive, or violent behaviour?)
2. Posture (Is the patient sitting or standing? Does the patient appear to be tense or rigid?)
3. Vocal activity (Loud, obscene, and erratic speech indicates emotional distress)
4. Physical activity (Is the patient pacing or agitated or protecting his or her physical boundaries?)

If any of these signs of potentially violent behaviour are present, paramedics should try to reduce the effect of the stress. However, they should avoid confrontation. Paramedics should prepare a way to cope with the crisis. This plan should reduce the potential for a life-threatening incident. It also should reduce the chance for psychologically damaging consequences.

Note

Paramedics should retreat from the scene in certain situations; for example, if they anticipate violence that would threaten their personal safety or the safety of the crew. They should wait for the police to ensure that the scene is safe.

Mental Health Act 1983

Severely disturbed patients who pose a threat to themselves or others may need to be restrained, transported, and hospitalized against their will. The Mental Health Act 1983[24] makes provision for the compulsory detention and treatment in hospital of those with mental disorder. The paramedic should be familiar with all relevant laws and their role in compulsory admittance of a patient.

Section 2

Section 2 provides the authority for someone to be detained in hospital for assessment for a period of 28 days. It requires an application by an approved social worker, which is based on medical recommendations by two doctors, one of whom must be approved under the Act. The social worker must have seen the patient within the last 14 days and should, wherever possible, consult the nearest relative. The 28-day period is intended to give sufficient time for an assessment of the person's mental health difficulties to be made. If continued detention is required, then Section 3 should be used.

The grounds for the application, as stated in the Act, are that the person is suffering from mental disorder of a nature or degree which warrants the detention of the patient in a hospital for assessment (or for assessment followed by medical treatment) for at least a limited period; and the patient ought to be so detained in the interests of his own health or safety or with a view to the protection of other persons.

Section 3

Section 3 provides the authority for someone to be detained in hospital for treatment for an initial period of 6 months. This Section may be renewed for a further 6 months and then for a year at a time.

The grounds for the application, as stated in the Act, are that the person:

- is suffering from mental illness, severe mental impairment, psychopathic disorder or mental impairment and his mental disorder is of a nature or degree which make it appropriate for him to receive medical treatment in a hospital; *and*
- in the case of psychopathic disorder or mental impairment, such treatment is likely to alleviate or prevent a deterioration of his condition; *and*
- it is necessary for the health or safety of the patient or for the protection of other persons that he should receive such treatment and it cannot be provided unless he is detained under this Section.

Section 3 will usually be implemented following a Section 2 when extended treatment is required, or where someone, and their mental health difficulties, are well known to the hospital. Therefore, a firm treatment plan, rather than open-ended assessment, can take place early in the period of detention. A Section 3 cannot normally be implemented if the nearest relative objects. Application is made by an approved social worker or the patient's nearest relative; the medical recommendations are the same as for Section 2.

Section 4

Section 4 is intended for emergency admissions, where if it were not for the extreme urgency, a Section 2 would be appropriate. A Section 4 requires only *one* medical recommendation, compared with *two* for a Section 2 and 3. An application has to be made based on that single medical recommendation. The grounds for application are the same as for Section 2 plus it must be stated that:

- it is of urgent necessity for the patient to be admitted and detained under Section 2, *and*
- that compliance with the usual Section 2 requirements (i.e. getting a second medical recommendation) would involve 'undesirable delay'.

The initial period of the order is 72 hours but this can effectively be converted to a Section 2 if a second medical recommendation is made.

Section 135

Section 135 enables an approved social worker to seek a warrant from a Justice of the Peace which will allow a police officer to enter premises (by force if necessary) in order to search for someone with mental health problems and take them to a place of safety. Section 135 has a duration of 72 hours, which cannot be renewed. The time starts from the moment the patient arrives at the place of safety and it is anticipated that any assessment will be carried out within the 72 hours and further provisions made as required.

NOTE: The police officer who attends, and, if necessary, breaks into premises in accordance with the warrant, must be accompanied by an Approved Social Worker and a doctor.

Section 136

Section 136 enables a police officer to remove someone from a public place and take them to a place of safety. The person must appear (to the police officer) to have a mental disorder and to be in 'immediate need of care or control'; *and* the police officer must think it necessary to take the person to a place of safety, in the interests of the person her/himself or for the protection of others. The duration of the Section is the same as for Section 135.

Place of safety

A place of safety is defined in the Act as one of the following:

- a hospital
- a police station
- a specialist residential or nursing home for people with mental health needs
- residential accommodation provided by a local social services authority
- 'any other suitable place, the occupier of which is willing temporarily to receive the patient'.

Restraint

Restraint techniques are not commonly used in the ambulance service and there is little clear guidance for paramedics. If violent behaviour must be contained, 'reasonable force' should be used to restrain the patient. It should be used as humanely as possible and with respect for the patient's dignity. In most cases the restraint duty (if needed) should be given to law enforcement personnel. As in all other aspects of healthcare, details of the incident should be carefully recorded for future reference. When dealing with a patient who may require restraint, the paramedic should do the following:

1. Provide a safe environment.
2. Gather a significant medical and psychiatric history.
3. Attempt to gain the patient's cooperation.
4. Be confident but not confrontational.

Critical Thinking

Have you ever seen an EMS crew member or a police officer lose control of his or her own behaviour when dealing with a violent patient? How did it affect the patient's physical or psychological state?

Restraint guidelines

The following guidelines can help paramedics to use restraint appropriately:

1. If the patient is homicidal, do not attempt restraint without assistance from law enforcement personnel. If the patient is armed, move everyone out of range and retreat from the scene. Wait for the police to arrive.
2. Remember that the patient may not be responsible for his or her actions.
3. When planning the restraining action, include a backup plan in case the initial attempt fails.
4. Make sure that adequate help is available. This means that at least four capable people should be available to help restrain an adult patient.
5. Keep in mind that the potential for personal injury and legal liability is always present.

Restraint techniques are not covered in this text; the paramedic should seek advice from her/his Trust with regards to the policies in place for restraining patients.

Mental Capacity Act 2005

The Mental Capacity Act 2005[25]provides a statutory framework to empower and protect vulnerable people who are not able to make their own decisions. It makes it clear who can take decisions, in which situations, and how they should go about this. It enables people to plan ahead for a time when they may lose capacity. The whole Act is underpinned by the following five key principles:

- A presumption of capacity – every adult has the right to make his or her own decisions and must be assumed to have capacity to do so unless it is proved otherwise.
- The right for individuals to be supported to make their own decisions – people must be given all appropriate help before anyone concludes that they cannot make their own decisions.
- That individuals must retain the right to make what might be seen as eccentric or unwise decisions.
- Best interests – anything done for or on behalf of people without capacity must be in their best interests.
- Least restrictive intervention – anything done for or on behalf of people without capacity should be the least restrictive of their basic rights and freedoms.

The Act enshrines in statute current best practice and common law principles concerning people who lack mental capacity and those who take decisions on their behalf. It sets out a single clear test for assessing whether a person lacks capacity to take a particular decision at a particular time and makes it clear that a lack of capacity cannot be established merely by reference to a person's age, appearance, or any condition or aspect of a person's behaviour which might lead others to make unjustified assumptions about capacity.

Everything that is done for or on behalf of a person who lacks capacity must be in that person's best interests. The Act provides a checklist of factors that decision-makers must work through in deciding what is in a person's best interests. This may be an issue for paramedics attending incidents involving patients deemed to lack capacity. It is worth noting that carers and family members gain a right to be consulted about treatment.

Where a person is providing care or treatment for someone who lacks capacity, then the person can provide the care without incurring legal liability. The key will be proper assessment of capacity and best interests. This will cover actions that would otherwise result in a civil wrong or crime if someone has to interfere with the person's body or property in the ordinary course of caring; for example, by giving an injection or by using the person's money to buy items for them.

Of particular interest to the paramedic is the definition of restraint. Section 6 of the Act defines restraint as the use or threat of force where an incapacitated person resists, and any restriction of liberty or movement whether or not the person resists. Restraint is only permitted if the person using it reasonably believes it is necessary to prevent harm to the incapacitated person, and if the restraint used is proportionate to the likelihood and seriousness of the harm.

It is clear that an act depriving a person of his or her liberty within the meaning of Article 5(1) of the European Convention on Human Rights does not exempt the paramedic from legal accountability.

The Act also allows a person to appoint an attorney to act on their behalf if they should lose capacity in the future; this would allow the attorney to make health and social care decisions on behalf of an incapacitated person. Statutory rules with clear safeguards confirm that people may make a decision in advance to refuse treatment if they should lose capacity in the future. Certain strict formalities need to be adhered to: the decision must be in writing, signed and witnessed, and there must be an express statement that the decision stands 'even if life is at risk'.

Summary

- A behavioural emergency is a change in mood or behaviour. This change cannot be tolerated by the involved person or others. It calls for immediate attention.
- Physical or biochemical disturbances can result in significant changes in behaviour. Psychosocial mental illness is often the result of childhood trauma, parental deprivation, or a dysfunctional family structure.
- Changes in behaviour caused by interpersonal or situational stress are often linked to specific incidents, such as environmental violence, the death of a loved one, economic or employment problems, or prejudice and discrimination.
- When dealing with behavioural emergencies, paramedics should contain the crisis. They also should provide the

Summary—cont'd

proper emergency care and transport the patient to an appropriate healthcare facility.

- During the patient assessment, an attempt should be made to determine the patient's mental state, name and age, significant past medical history, medications (and compliance), and past psychiatric problems, as well as the precipitating situation or problem.
- Effective interviewing techniques include active listening, being supportive and empathetic, limiting interruptions, and respecting the patient's personal space.
- All cognitive disorders result in a disturbance in thinking that may manifest as delirium or dementia.
- Schizophrenia is characterized by recurrent episodes of psychotic behaviour. This behaviour may include abnormalities of thought process, thought content, perception and judgement.
- Anxiety disorders may cause a panic attack. Anxiety disorders include phobias, obsessive–compulsive disorders, and post-traumatic stress disorder.
- Depression is an impairment of normal functioning. A person with depression may have feelings of hopelessness, worthlessness, and guilt, as well as loss of appetite and diminished libido.
- Bipolar disorder is a manic–depressive illness. In this illness, depressive and manic episodes alternate.
- Personality disorders are conditions characterized by failure to learn from experience or to adapt appropriately to changes. This results in personal distress and impairment of social functioning.
- A threat of suicide is an indication that a patient has a serious crisis. This crisis requires immediate intervention.
- Questions that determine the patient's plan, intent, and means to commit suicide should be asked.
- With a suicide attempt, the first step is to ensure the safety of the scene. The first priority in patient management is medical care. If the patient is conscious, it is crucial that paramedics develop a rapport with the individual as soon as possible.
- Assessment of a potentially violent patient should include past history of violence, posture, vocal activity and physical activity.
- When trying to defuse a situation involving a potentially violent patient, the paramedic should ensure a safe environment, gather the patient's history, try to gain the patient's cooperation, avoid threats, and explain the paramedic's role in providing care.
- Severely disturbed patients who pose a threat to themselves or others may need to be restrained.
- Reasonable force to restrain a patient should be used as humanely as possible. An adequate number of personnel is needed to ensure patient and rescuer safety during restraint. The risk of personal injury and legal liability is always present.
- Personal safety measures taken during a response to a behavioural emergency should include not allowing the patient to block the exit, keeping large furniture between the paramedic and the patient, working as a team, avoiding threatening statements, and using soft materials to absorb the impact of thrown objects.
- When caring for children with behavioural emergencies, the paramedic should attempt to gain their trust, tell them they won't be hurt, keep questions brief, be honest, involve the parents if appropriate, and take threats of violence seriously.
- Severely disturbed patients who pose a threat to themselves or others may need to be restrained, transported, and hospitalized against their will (Mental Health Act 1983).
- The Mental Capacity Act 2005 provides a statutory framework to empower and protect vulnerable people who are not able to make their own decisions.

References

1. Office for National Statistics 2000 Psychiatric morbidity among adults living in private households. ONS, London
2. Department of Health 1999 National Service Frameworks; Mental Health. Department of Health, London
3. National Institute for Health and Clinical Excellence 2002 Guidance on the use of newer (atypical) antipsychotic drugs for the treatment of schizophrenia. NICE, London
4. Seidel HM, Ball JW, Dains JE, Benedict GW, eds 2002 Mosby's guide to physical examination, 5th edition. Mosby, St Louis
5. World Health Organization 2006 International statistical classification of diseases and related health problems, 10th revision version for 2007. WHO, Geneva
6. Knapp M, Prince M et al 2007 Dementia UK: A report into the prevalence and cost of dementia prepared by the Personal Social Services Research Unit (PSSRU) at the London School of Economics and the Institute of Psychiatry at King's College London, for the Alzheimer's Society. Alzheimer's Society, London
7. The Royal College of Psychiatrists. Schizophrenia. Online. Available http://www.rcpsych.ac.uk/mentalhealthinformation/mentalhealthproblems/schizophrenia/schizophrenia.aspx#causes 12 February 2009
8. National electronic Library for Health. Mental health. Online. Available http://www.nelmh.org/page_view.asp?c=10&did=762&fc=001001004 13 February 2009
9. Office for National Statistics 2006 Mental health. ONS, London
10. Pompili M, Amador XF et al 2007 Suicide risk in schizophrenia: learning from the past to change the future. Ann Gen Psychiatry 2007(6):10
11. National Institute for Health and Clinical Excellence 2005 Treating obsessive–compulsive disorder (OCD) and body dysmorphic disorder (BDD)

in adults, children and young people. NICE, London

12. World Health Organization 1992 The ICD-10 classification of mental and behavioural disorders. World Health Organization, Geneva
13. National Institute of Mental Health 2001 The numbers count: mental illness in America, NIH Publication No. NIH 99-4584. National Institute of Mental Health, Bethesda, MD
14. Chen Y 1996 Lifetime rates of suicide attempts among subjects with bipolar and unipolar disorders relative to subjects with other axis I disorders. Biol Psychiatry 39(10):896–899
15. Fagiolini A 2004 Suicide attempts and ideation in patients with bipolar I disorder. J Clin Psychiatry 65(4):509–514
16. McElroy S 2006 Antidepressants and suicidal behavior in bipolar disorder. Bipolar Disord 8(5 Pt 2):596–617
17. Guze S 1970 Suicide and primary affective disorders. Br J Psychiatry 117(539):437–438
18. Salerno M 1994 Psychosocial disorders. In Millonig VL (ed.) Adult nurse practitioner certification review guide, 2nd edition. Health Leadership Associates, Potomac, MD
19. Gupta RD, Guest JF 2002 Annual cost of bipolar disorder to UK society. Br J Psychiatry 180:227–233
20. MIND. Understanding bipolar disorder. Online. Available http://www.mind.org.uk/Information/Booklets/Understanding/Understanding+manic+depression.htm#What_is_bipolar_disorder_manic_depression 13 February 2009
21. Harris EC, Barraclough B 1997 Suicide as an outcome for mental disorders. Br J Psychiatry 170:205–228
22. Office for National Statistics, General Register Office for Scotland, Northern Ireland Statistics and Research Agency. Online. Available http://www.statistics.gov.uk/CCI/nugget.asp?ID=1092&Pos=6&ColRank=2&Rank=1000
23. Judd R, Peszke M 1983 Psychological and behavioral emergencies. Top Emerg Med 4(4):7
24. House of Commons. The Mental Health Act 1983. The Stationery Office, London
25. House of Commons. The Mental Capacity Act 2005. The Stationery Office, London

PART SIX

CHAPTER **26**

Trauma Systems and Mechanism of Injury

Chapter contents

Objectives

Upon completion of this chapter, the paramedic student will be able to:

1. Describe the incidence and scope of traumatic injuries and deaths.
2. Identify the role of each component of the trauma system.
3. Predict injury patterns based on knowledge of the laws of physics related to forces involved in trauma.
4. Describe injury patterns that should be suspected when injury occurs related to a specific type of blunt trauma.
5. Describe the role of restraints in injury prevention and injury patterns.
6. Discuss how organ motion can contribute to injury in each body region depending on the forces applied.
7. Identify selected injury patterns associated with motorcycle and all-terrain vehicle collisions.
8. Describe injury patterns associated with pedestrian collisions.
9. Identify injury patterns associated with sports injuries, blast injuries, and vertical falls.
10. Describe factors that influence tissue damage related to penetrating injury.

Key terms

blunt trauma An injury produced by the wounding forces of compression and change of speed, both of which can disrupt tissue.

cavitation A temporary or permanent opening produced by a force that pushes body tissues laterally away from the track of a projectile.

kinematics The process of predicting injury patterns that can result from the forces and motions of energy.

penetrating trauma An injury produced by crushing and stretching forces of a penetrating object that results in some form of tissue disruption.

Trauma is a major cause of morbidity and mortality. The paramedic must have an appreciation of trauma systems. The paramedic must also be able to recognize mechanisms of injury. With these two abilities, the paramedic will be able to enhance patient assessment and emergency care.

Epidemiology of trauma

Unintentional injury is a devastating medical and social problem and is the leading cause of death among persons 10 to 39 years of age in the UK. Trauma accounted for over 16 000 deaths in the UK in 2004 and was responsible for greater mortality than any other single cause of death in those between 10 and 39 years.[1] Trauma deaths in all age groups were only exceeded by diseases of the circulatory system, diseases of the respiratory system, and diseases of the digestive system. The worrying trend is the disparity in the gender distribution of trauma deaths, with male deaths accounting for nearly 80% of trauma deaths in those between 10 years and 44 years. The number of road traffic accidents that resulted in injury has fallen since 1985 despite the increase in the amount of traffic on the roads; however, in 2007 there were still 247 780 casualties of all severities; 2946 people were killed, 27 774 were seriously injured and 217 060 were slightly injured.[2]

Phases of trauma care

Trauma care is divided into three phases. The three phases are pre-incident, incident and post-incident.[3] The pre-incident phase refers to the prevention of intentional and unintentional trauma deaths. Paramedics and other health-care professionals play a key role in this phase through public education and health promotion (For example, paramedics may educate the public in the use of personal restraint systems, motorcycle helmets, and the proper use of 999.)

The incident phase is the trauma event. The paramedic can assist in the prevention of many of these events through education and by practising personal safety. Thus, the paramedic's role in this phase is to 'practise what you preach' and teach by example. The paramedic can achieve this by driving safely and by using personal restraint systems whilst on and off duty. During the incident phase, the application of active (e.g. seat belts) and passive (e.g. air bags) systems can alter the outcome of a trauma event significantly.

The post-incident phase is when the paramedic uses his or her expertise and skills. (This is the delivery of emergency care to injured patients.) Important responsibilities for the paramedic in this phase include the following:

- scene survey and scene management
- performing lifesaving manoeuvres
- preparing the patient for transportation to an appropriate medical facility
- promptly transporting the patient to the appropriate medical facility (Box 26-1).

The factor most critical to any severely injured patient's survival is the length of time that elapses between the incident and definitive care[3] (Box 26-2).

Box 26-1

The golden hour

The first hour after severe injury is known as the golden hour and is a critical period. In this period, surgical intervention for the trauma patient can enhance survival and reduce complications. The paramedic must recognize patients who are in this group. The paramedic also must ensure that prehospital care does not delay patient transportation. The paramedic can best serve these patients through rapid assessment, stabilization of life-threatening injuries, and rapid transportation to an appropriate medical facility for definitive care.

Box 26-2

Prevention of trauma deaths

Deaths from trauma occur in three periods: immediate, early and late. Each period presents its own unique problems.[3]

Immediate

Immediate death occurs within seconds or minutes of the injury. Lacerations of the brain, brainstem, upper spinal cord, heart, aorta or other large vessels usually cause these deaths. Few if any patients in this category can be saved. Effective injury prevention programmes are the only way to reduce the number of these deaths.

Early

The second peak of death occurs within the first 2 to 3 h after injury. The causes of these deaths usually are major head injury, haemopneumothorax, ruptured spleen, lacerated liver, pelvic fracture or multiple injuries associated with significant blood loss. Most of these injuries can be treated with available techniques. However, the time lapse between injury and definitive care is critical.

Late

The third peak of death occurs days or weeks after the injury. These deaths most often result from sepsis, infection or multiple organ failure. Prehospital emergency care focused on early recognition and management of life-threatening injuries is critical to the prevention of late deaths from trauma.

Trauma systems

The eight components of a sophisticated trauma system are as follows:[4]

1. Injury prevention.
2. Prehospital care, including management, transportation, and trauma triage guidelines.
3. Emergency department care.
4. Interfacility transportation if needed.
5. Definitive care.
6. Trauma critical care.
7. Rehabilitation.
8. Data collection and trauma registry.

Critical Thinking

How can you learn more about the components of the trauma system during your career as a paramedic?

The paramedic should play a crucial role in the trauma system. This should involve injury prevention programmes; entering appropriate patients into the trauma care system; and taking part in data collection and research. Research is essential in the development of trauma care.

Transportation considerations

Determining the proper level of care and hospital destination is based on the patient's needs and condition. The determination may also be based on the advice of BASICS doctors or other medical staff on scene. First, the paramedic determines the level of care needed and the destination facility, and then the mode of transportation. (For example, the paramedic chooses between ground or air ambulance.)

Ground transportation

As a rule the paramedic should use ground transportation by ambulance if the appropriate facility can be reached within a 'reasonable time.' Reasonable time is defined by national standards (e.g. definitive care within 60 min after the injury for severe trauma) and local guidelines. Factors that affect the decision to use ground or air transportation include geographical location, topographical area, population, weather, availability of resources, traffic conditions and time of day.

Aeromedical transportation

The availability and use of aeromedical services varies throughout the UK. Aeromedical services can provide rapid response time, high-quality medical care, and rapid transportation to appropriate care facilities. Helicopters can also provide aerial surveillance of a medical scene and can provide transportation of additional personnel and equipment to the emergency scene. Paramedic crews should follow local protocol regarding the use of aeromedical services and consider air transportation in the following situations:

- The time needed to transport a patient by ground to an appropriate facility poses a threat to the patient's survival and recovery.
- Weather, road, or traffic conditions would seriously delay the patient's access to definitive care.
- Critical care personnel and equipment are needed to care for the patient adequately during transportation.

SECTION I

Kinematics

Energy

A transfer of energy from an external source to the human body causes injuries. The extent of injury is determined by three things: the type and amount of energy applied, how quickly the energy is applied, and the part of the body to which energy is applied.

Physical laws

Knowledge of four basic laws of physics is required to understand the wounding forces of trauma:

1. Newton's first law of motion. An object, whether at rest or in motion, remains in that state unless acted upon by an outside force.
2. Conservation of energy law. Energy cannot be created or destroyed; it can only change form. (Energy can take mechanical, thermal, electrical, chemical, and nuclear forms.)
3. Newton's second law of motion: Force (F) equals mass (M) multiplied by acceleration (a) or deceleration (d).

$$F = M \times a \quad \text{or} \quad F = M \times d$$

4. Kinetic energy: Kinetic energy (KE) equals half the mass (M) multiplied by the velocity squared (V^2).

$$KE = \tfrac{1}{2} M \times V^2$$

As the kinetic energy formula shows, velocity is much more critical than mass in determining total kinetic energy. For example, a car and its unrestrained 70 kg driver are travelling 100 kilometres per hour (28 metres per second) (60 mph). According to Newton's first law of motion, the car remains in motion until acted upon by an outside force. If the driver gradually applies the brakes, the friction of the brakes slowly converts the mechanical energy of the car to thermal energy (conservation of energy law); the energy transfer occurs gradually through the slow deceleration. If the car strikes a tree, though, and is stopped instantly, the tree, the car, and the driver absorb the mechanical energy. When the front of the car has stopped, the rear of the car continues forward until all of the energy of its motion is absorbed. The driver is travelling in the same direction and at the same speed as the car before impact, so, like the rear of the car, the driver continues forward. The driver suffers injuries in anatomical areas that strike the vehicle whilst the driver's organs continue to move and are damaged by internal impacts.

In this sequence the tree stops the motion of the front of the car. The steering column continues forward and stops against the dashboard. The driver's sternum stops against the steering column. The driver's chest cavity and its contents hit the sternum and are crushed from behind by the posterior thorax, deforming the entire chest. The kinetic energy in this example is calculated as follows:

KE = one half of the mass times the velocity squared, or

$$KE = \frac{1}{2} M \times V^2$$

$$KE = 70/2 \times 28^2$$

$$KE = 27\,440 \text{ joules or } 27 \text{ kJ (kilojoules)}$$

As shown in this calculation, the 70-kg driver travelling 60 miles per hour must change 27 kJ of kinetic energy into another form of energy when he or she stops. In addition (recall that force equals mass multiplied by acceleration – Newton's second law of motion): the 70-kg driver is moving forward in the car with about 1900 N (Newtons) of force (presuming the car stops in 1 s) when he hits the steering column. The energy of the motion of the body causes tissue destruction as this energy is absorbed into the body cells when the body stops. This example illustrates the principle. However, the actual total force is also determined by the true rate of deceleration, or '*g*' force, and several other factors. Lap and shoulder restraints and air bags increase the distance over which the body stops its movement, which can significantly decrease the deceleration force.

Critical Thinking

Can you apply these same four laws of physics to another traumatic situation, such as a fall onto concrete? What force is applied? What factors influence the kinetic energy?

Kinematics

Kinematics is the process of predicting injury patterns. Specific types and patterns of injuries are associated with certain mechanisms. In addition to individual factors (such as age) and protective factors (such as restraint systems, helmets, and air bags), the paramedic should consider the following when evaluating the trauma patient:

- mechanism of injury
- force of energy applied
- anatomy
- energy (for example, mass; velocity; distance; and thermal, electrical and chemical forms).

SECTION II

Blunt trauma

Blunt trauma is an injury produced by the wounding forces of compression and change of speed (usually deceleration). These forces can disrupt tissue. Direct compression is the pressure on a structure and is the most common type of force applied in blunt trauma. The amount of injury depends on the length of time of compression, the force of compression, and the area compressed. For example, compression of the thorax can lead to rib fracture or pneumothorax. Other compression injuries include contusions and lacerations of solid organs and rupture of hollow (air-filled) organs.

Acceleration is an increase in the velocity of a moving object; deceleration is a decrease in the velocity of a moving object. Both can produce major injury. For example, consider a car that comes to a stop abruptly. The occupant's body continues its constant velocity after the impact until it decelerates as a result of striking the steering wheel, restraint system, or dashboard. The external aspect of the body is stopped forcibly but the contents of the cranial, thoracic and peritoneal cavities remain in motion because of inertia. As a result, tissues can be stretched, crushed, ruptured, lacerated, or sheared from their points of attachment. Examples of injuries caused by a change of speed include concussion, cardiac or pulmonary contusion, organ laceration and aortic tear.

Motor vehicle collision

The various injuries produced by blunt trauma are illustrated best through examination of vehicle collisions. Forces that cause blunt trauma, however, can result from a variety of impacts. As described in the previous example, a vehicle collision involves three separate impacts as the energy is transferred. In the first impact, the vehicle strikes an object; in the second, the occupant collides with the inside of the car; and in the third, the internal organs collide inside the body. The injuries that result depend on the type of collision and the position of the occupant inside the vehicle. The injuries also depend on the use or non-use of active or passive restraint systems.

A vehicle collision is classified by the type of impact: head-on, lateral, rear-end, rotational and rollover. The forces of compression and change of speed produce predictable injury patterns in each type of collision.

Head-on (frontal) impact

Head-on collisions result when forward motion stops abruptly. (For example, one vehicle collides with another one travelling in the opposite direction.) The first collision occurs when the vehicle hits the second vehicle, resulting in damage to the front of the car. As the vehicle abruptly stops, the occupant continues to move at the speed of the vehicle before impact. The front seat occupant continues forward into the restraint system, steering column, or dashboard; this results in the second collision. The occupant who is not restrained usually travels in one of two pathways in relationship to the dashboard. The two pathways are down-and-under or up-and-over. The precise course of this pathway determines how the organs collide inside the body and the extent of tissue damaged.

In the down-and-under pathway the occupant travels downward into the vehicle seat and forward into the dashboard or steering column (Figure 26-1). The knees become the leading part of the body, striking the dashboard, and the upper legs absorb most of the impact. Predictable injuries include knee dislocation, patellar fracture, femoral fracture,

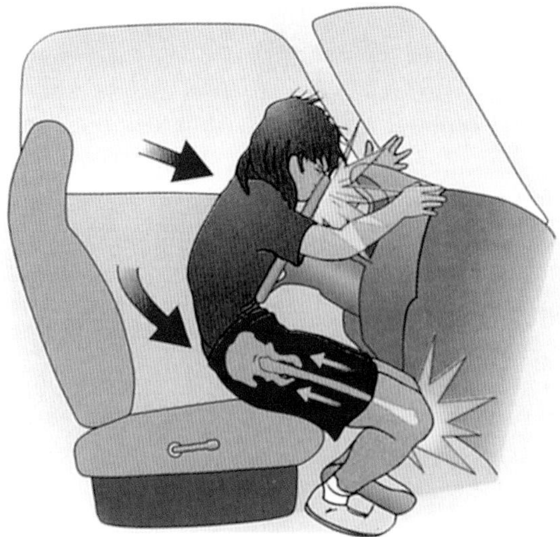

Figure 26-1 Down-and-under pathway.

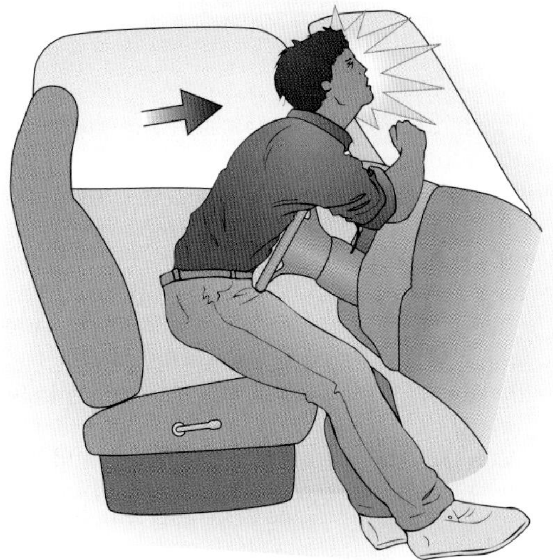

Figure 26-2 Up-and-over pathway.

fracture or posterior dislocation of the hip, fracture of the acetabulum, vascular injury and haemorrhage. After the initial impact of the knees into the dashboard, the body rotates forward. As the chest wall hits the steering column or dashboard, the head and torso absorb energy as indicated in the description of the up-and-over pathway.

Critical Thinking

How does the use of lap and shoulder restraints influence the patterns of injury described here?

In the up-and-over pathway the body in forward motion strikes the steering wheel. As this occurs, the ribs and underlying structures absorb the momentum of the thorax (Figure 26-2). Predictable injuries from this transfer of energy include rib fracture, ruptured diaphragm, haemopneumothorax, pulmonary contusion, cardiac contusion, myocardial rupture and vascular disruption (most notably aortic rupture).

If the abdomen is the point of impact, compression injuries can occur to the hollow abdominal organs, solid organs, and lumbar vertebrae. The kidneys, liver, and spleen are subject to vascular tears from supporting tissue. Such injuries may include the tearing of renal vessels from their points of attachment to the inferior vena cava and descending aorta. Predictable injuries include liver laceration, spleen rupture, internal haemorrhage, and abdominal organ incursion into the thorax (ruptured diaphragm).

If the head absorbs most of the impact, the cervical vertebrae take up the continued momentum of the body. Cervical flexion, axial loading and hyperextension (further described in Chapter 32) can result in fracture or dislocation of the cervical vertebrae. In addition, severe angulation of the cervical vertebrae can damage the soft tissues of the neck. This may cause spinal cord injury and spinal instability, even without fracture. Other predictable injuries include trauma to the brain (e.g. concussion, contusion, shearing injury and oedema) and disruption of vessels inside the head (intracranial vascular disruption), resulting in subdural or epidural haematoma.

Lateral impact

Lateral impact occurs when a vehicle is struck from the side. Injury patterns depend on whether the damaged vehicle remains in place or moves away from the point of impact. The external shell of a vehicle that remains in place after impact usually intrudes into the passenger compartment and usually directs force at the lateral aspect of the person's body. Predictable injuries result from compression to the torso, pelvis and extremities. Examples of these injuries include fractured ribs, pulmonary contusion, ruptured liver or spleen (depending on the side involved), fractured clavicle, fractured pelvis, and head and neck injury. Vehicles that have side-impact air bags can guard against injury in some lateral impacts.

If the damaged vehicle moves away from the point of impact, the occupant accelerates away from the point of impact and moves laterally with the car. The effects of inertia on the head, neck, and thorax produce lateral flexion and rotation of the cervical spine, which can result in neurological injury. Such movement can also result in tears or strains of the lateral ligaments and supporting structures of the neck. Injuries can occur on the side of the passenger opposite the impact as the occupant is propelled toward the other side of the car. If other occupants are in the vehicle, secondary collision with other passengers is likely.

Rear-end impact

A vehicle that is struck from behind rapidly accelerates, causing it to move forward under the occupant. The greater the difference in the forward speed of the two vehicles, the greater the force and damaging energy of the initial impact. For example, consider a vehicle that is going 50 mph and hits a stationary vehicle. The damaging energy is greater than when a vehicle going 50 mph hits a vehicle going 30 mph.

Thus, in forward collisions, the sum of the speeds of both vehicles is the velocity that produces damage. In rear-end collisions the difference between the two speeds is the damaging velocity.

Predictable injuries in rear-end collisions include back and neck injuries and cervical strain or fracture caused by hyperextension. The cervical portion of the spine is susceptible to secondary hyperextension caused by the rapid forward acceleration of the vehicle and subsequent relative rearward movement of the occupant. If the vehicle collides with an object in front of it, the paramedic should suspect injuries associated with frontal impact.

Rotational impact

Rotational impacts occur when an off-centre portion of the vehicle (usually the front quarter) strikes an immovable object or one that is moving more slowly or in the opposite direction. The part of the vehicle striking the object stops during impact. The rest of the vehicle continues in forward motion until the energy is transformed completely. The occupant moves inside the vehicle with the forward motion. The occupant usually is struck by the side of the car as the vehicle rotates around the point of impact. A rotational impact results in injuries common to head-on and lateral collisions.

Rollover accidents

In rollover crashes or collisions the person tumbles inside the vehicle. The occupant is injured wherever his or her body strikes the vehicle. The various impacts occur at many different angles, which can cause multiple-system injuries, so predicting injury patterns from rollover collisions is difficult. These crashes can produce any of the injury patterns that are associated with other types of collisions.

Restraints

In recent years, public awareness programmes and various laws have increased the use of personal restraints. The government has estimated that since seat belt wearing was made compulsory in 1983 it has reduced casualties by at least 370 deaths and 7000 serious injuries per year for front seat belts and 70 deaths and 1000 serious injuries for rear seat belts.[5]

A serious hazard to unrestrained occupants is ejection from the vehicle after impact. Among crashes in which a fatality occurred in 2000, only 10% of restrained passenger car occupants were ejected, compared with 22% of those who were unrestrained.[6,7] In addition, 1 of every 13 ejection victims suffers a spinal fracture, and ejected victims are killed six times more often than those who are not ejected.[3] The mortality rate among ejected victims is high. This results in part from the occupant being subjected to a second impact as the body strikes the ground or another object outside the vehicle.

Critical Thinking

How can you apply this knowledge about ejection statistics to your practice in each of the phases of trauma care (pre-incident, incident and post-incident)?

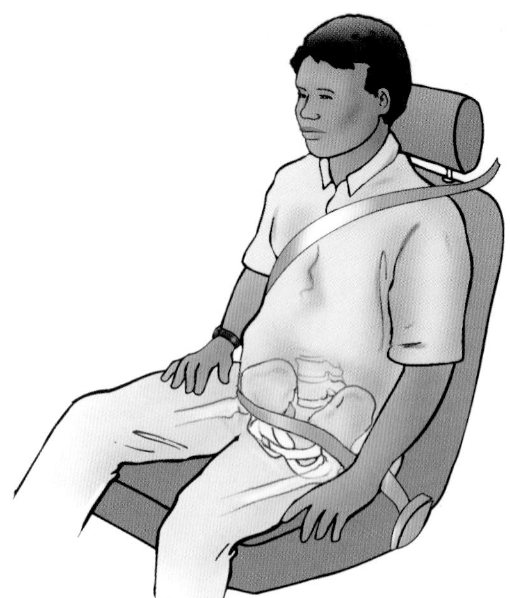

Figure 26-3 Properly positioned seat belt.

Four restraining systems are available in the UK. These are lap belts, diagonal shoulder straps, air bags and child safety seats. All of these restraints significantly reduce injuries. If they are used inappropriately, however, these protective devices can also produce injuries.

Lap belts

The lap-only belt is becoming less common in the UK although they are still found in the centre rear seat of many vehicles. A lap belt should be directed at a 45-degree angle to the floor between the anterior superior iliac spine and the femur (Figure 26-3). A lap belt worn tightly enough to stay in this position absorbs energy forces. The belt protects the abdominal cavity by transferring energy to the strong, bony pelvis.

If the lap belt is worn incorrectly above the anterior iliac spine, the forward motion of the body during impact is absorbed by vertebrae T12, L1, and L2. As the thorax is propelled forward, the abdominal organs are compressed between the vertebral column and the lap belt. This compression can cause injury to the liver, spleen, duodenum, and pancreas. A sign of these abdominal injuries is abrasions or a lap belt imprint over the abdomen.

Major injury can result even when a person uses a lap belt correctly. These injuries occur from angulation of the lumbar spine, pelvis, thorax, and head around the restraint system. Injuries also occur from failure of the restraint system to decrease the impact forces. Injuries that can occur during high-speed impacts include sternal fractures, chest wall injuries, lumbar vertebral fractures, head injuries and maxillofacial trauma.

Diagonal shoulder straps

Use of a shoulder strap helps absorb the forward motion of the thorax after impact. When a person wears the shoulder strap with the lap belt, the shoulder strap prevents the thorax, face and head from striking the dashboard, windscreen or steering column. Clavicular fracture can result from the position of the shoulder strap. Organ collision inside the body with resultant internal organ injury, cervical fracture, and spinal cord injury still can occur during high-speed impacts, even when personal restraint systems are used.

Air bags

Some vehicles are equipped with side-impact air bags to protect against lateral impacts. However, the more common air bag is a frontal air bag that inflates from the centre of the steering wheel and from the dashboard during frontal impact. These devices cushion the forward motion of the occupant when used with a lap and shoulder belt. Frontal air bags deflate rapidly. They are effective with initial frontal and near-frontal collisions, but are ineffective in multiple collisions, rear-impact collisions, and lateral or rollover impacts. These systems do not prevent movement in the down-and-under pathway, thus the occupant's knees may still be the point of impact, resulting in leg, pelvis and abdominal injuries.

An air bag can produce significant injury if it is deployed in proximity (25 cm or closer) to the occupant. Deployment in these situations can produce spinal fractures, hand and eye injury, and facial and forearm abrasions. The following groups are at higher risk of injury from air bag deployment:[8]

- infants and children less than 12 years of age
- adults of short stature (less than 5 ft 2 in)
- older adults
- persons with special medical conditions.

Most air bag injuries are minor cuts, bruises or abrasions and are far less serious than the head, neck, and chest injuries that air bags prevent. However, US research has identified 146 air bag-related deaths in relatively low-severity crashes.[8] Most of these deaths occurred as a result of the occupant being too close to the air bag when it deployed. This problem occurred more commonly in children, particularly those not being restrained adequately with lap/shoulder devices or child safety seats during pre-crash braking. To protect against injury from air bag deployment, the driver of the vehicle should be positioned at least 25 cm from the air bag cover; the front seat passenger should be positioned at least 45 cm away from the air bag cover; and children under 12 years of age should always ride in the back seat and be in the proper restraint device for their size.

Child safety seats

In 2007, 23 807 children below the age of 15 years were casualties on Britain's roads; 3090 of these were either killed or seriously injured.[9] Recent laws that came into force on 18 September 2006 require children who are passengers in a vehicle to use a child restraint. It has been estimated that the new law will save over 2000 child deaths or injuries every year,[10] although there are currently no statistics to demonstrate this. In the US, the National Safety Council reports that an estimated 4816 lives have been saved by child restraints from 1975 through 2000, with 316 lives saved in 2000 alone.

Child safety seats come in several shapes and sizes to accommodate the different stages of physical development. These seats include infant carriers, booster seats and toddler seats, which use a combination of lap belts, shoulder belts, full-body harnesses and harness-and-shield apparatus to protect the child during vehicle collision. Predictable injuries likely to occur even with the appropriate use of child safety seats include blunt abdominal trauma, change-of-speed injuries from deceleration forces, and neck and spinal injury. A large amount of misuse of child safety seats occurs. (For example, common issues include location, installation, and strapping.) Public education on the correct use of child safety seats is a key prevention measure. For information on transporting children in an ambulance, see Box 26-3.

Organ collision injuries

Organs can be injured as a result of movement caused by deceleration and compression forces. The paramedic must maintain a high degree of suspicion regarding injuries to organs, based on the principles of kinematics.

Deceleration injuries

When body organs are put into motion after an impact, they continue to move. They move in opposition to the structures that attach them to the body, thus there exists a risk of separation of body organs from their attachments. Injury to the vascular pedicle or mesenteric attachment can lead to brisk or exsanguinating haemorrhage.

Head injuries

When the head strikes a stationary object, the cranium comes to an abrupt stop. However, brain tissue inside the cranium continues to move until it is compressed against the skull (Figure 26-4). This movement can cause brain tissue to be bruised, crushed, or lacerated. Such movement can also cause blood vessels attached to the brain and skull to be torn, producing intracranial haemorrhage. Other injuries associated with deceleration of the head include central nervous system injury, caused by stretching of the spinal cord and its attachments, and cervical fracture.

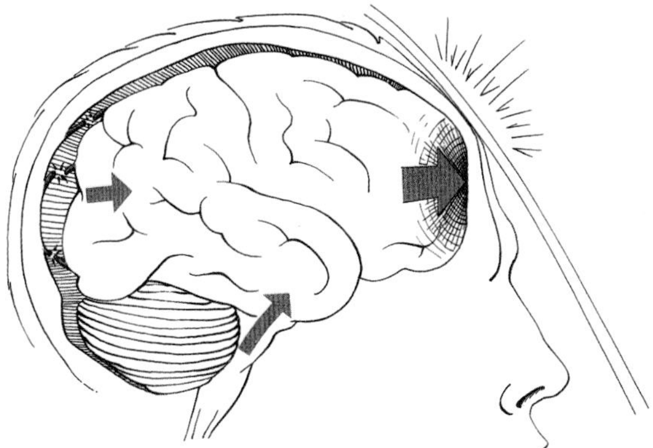

Figure 26-4 After cessation of forward motion of the skull the brain continues its motion, resulting in possible contusion and intracerebral haemorrhage.

Box 26-3

Transportation of children in an ambulance

Although no formal regulations have been established, it is recommended that child safety seats be available in emergency vehicles. In addition to practising safe driving in all patient transports, the paramedic should observe the following guidelines.*

The method or device used to secure children during transport must provide effective restraint without compromising the safety of others on board.

Younger children and infants who do not require spinal immobilization should be transported in child safety seats appropriate for their size. If an appropriate safety seat is not available, the paramedic should ask to borrow one from family members (preferably one that has not been in a motor vehicle collision).

Any time a child is secured to a device such as a safety seat or long-board, the paramedic must ensure that the device is secured to the stretcher.

For any patient where medically appropriate, position the patient on the stretcher with the back of the stretcher placed upright at least at a 45-degree angle. This angle optimizes transportation safety in the event of an impact or deceleration.

If the child is secured in a safety seat, the seat should be secured to the stretcher using at least two belts placed at a 90-degree angle to each other; that is, one strap oriented vertically, the other strap oriented horizontally, to secure the child seat to the upright stretcher. A child safety seat secured to the stretcher with the stretcher back in the upright position has performed well in the crash testing conducted to date.

Restraint systems applied to a flat stretcher are less secure in a crash. If a suboptimal restraint technique such as this must be used, the paramedic should notify the driver to exert additional caution during transport to minimize the risk.

Older children who do not require special positioning should be secured on a stretcher that has had the back elevated to an angle of at least 45 degrees.

The paramedic should use shoulder harnesses to restrain patients who must be immobilized in the supine position on a backboard and therefore cannot have the back of the stretcher elevated for protection. The paramedic should never secure the parent and child together on the stretcher. The paramedic also should never allow infants or young children to ride in the arms or lap of a parent or rescuer.

*The Centre for Paediatric Emergency Medicine 2004 Teaching resource for instructors in prehospital paediatrics for paramedics: safe transport of children. Online. Available http://cpem.med.nyu.edu/files/cpem/u3/trippals.pdf section 38, Safe Transport of Children

Thoracic injuries

The aorta is often injured by severe deceleration forces. The aorta is affixed at several points; proximally it is affixed by the aortic valve, in the descending portion of the aortic arch by the ligamentum arteriosum, and the descending aorta is attached to the thoracic spine. As the thorax hits a stationary object, the heart and aorta continue in motion. This motion is in opposition to their attachment at the lower end of the aortic arch so that the aorta may be sheared at the level of its ligamentum arteriosum attachment (Figure 26-5). Frank rupture of the aorta leads to rapid exsanguination. However, transection and dissection through to the internal lining (intima and media of the aorta) can tamponade, which can allow patients to arrive at an emergency department and survive the injury.

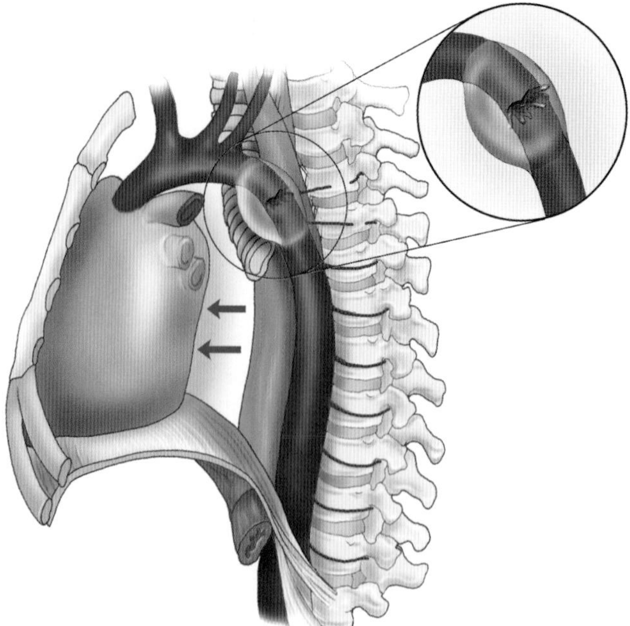

Figure 26-5 Shearing forces along the descending aorta move in opposition to the attachments at the lower end of the aortic arch.

Abdominal injuries

When deceleration forces are applied to the abdomen, intra-abdominal organs and retroperitoneal structures (most commonly the kidneys) are affected. The forward motion of the kidneys can shear them away from their vascular pedicle attachments (Figure 26-6). The forward motion of the small and large intestines can result in mesenteric tears. The downward and forward motion of the liver can cause separation at its midpoint from its vascular and hepatic duct pedicle. The spleen is restrained by the diaphragm and abdominal wall attachments such that forward motion of the spleen can result in a tear of the splenic capsule.

Compression injuries

Compressive forces can injure any portion of the body. This discussion is limited to injuries of the head, thorax, and abdomen.

Head injuries

Compression injuries to the head can result in open fractures, closed fractures, and bone fragment penetration (depressed skull fracture). Associated injuries include brain contusion and lacerations of brain tissue. Compression forces to the skull can also produce haemorrhage from fractured bone, meningeal vessels, or the brain itself. If facial structures are involved in the injury, soft tissue trauma and facial bone fractures can occur (see Chapter 31). The paramedic should also consider central nervous system injury,

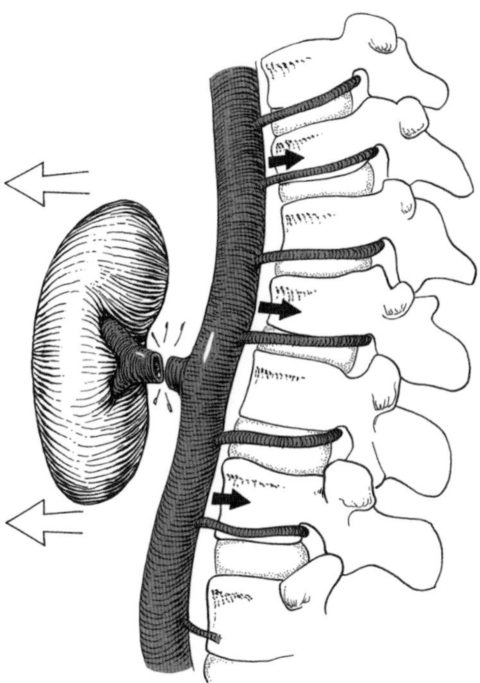

Figure 26-6 Forward motion of the kidney can cause separation at its midpoint from its vascular pedicle.

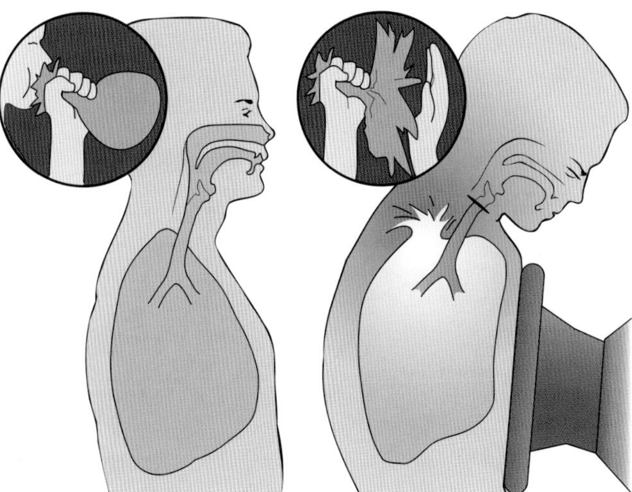

Figure 26-7 In a crash or collision, the lungs are similar to an air-filled paper bag held tightly at the neck and compressed with the other hand. Thoracic compression against the closed glottis causes the lungs to pop.

and assume cervical fracture when evaluating injuries to the head. Compression injury to the vertebral bodies can result in compression fracture, hyperextension and hyperflexion injury.

Thoracic injuries

Compression injury to the thorax often involves the lungs and heart. Associated injuries to external structures include fractured ribs and sternum, which can lead to an unstable chest wall, open pneumothorax, or both.

A serious lung injury that can occur from compression forces is called the paper bag effect. This injury occurs when increased intrathoracic pressure causes rupture of the lungs. For example, a driver of a car is threatened by an approaching vehicle. The driver notes the potential collision so instinctively takes a deep breath and holds it. This protective inhalation fills the lungs (paper bag) with air against the closed glottis and creates a closed container (Figure 26-7). As the thorax strikes the steering column, the inward motion of the chest wall causes an increase in lung pressure. This increased pressure results in alveolar rupture (as when a hand strikes the paper bag). This phenomenon is thought to be the cause of most pneumothoraces after vehicle trauma.[3] Penetration of a fractured rib through the pleura and laceration of the lung also contribute to pneumothorax after blunt trauma to the chest.

During compression injury to the thorax, the heart can become trapped between the sternum and the thoracic spine. Depending on the amount of energy applied, the compression of the contents of the abdomen and an increase in the pressure in the aorta, the aortic valve could rupture. Compression of the patient's heart between the sternum and the vertebral column can cause cardiac dysrhythmias, myocardial contusion, or atrial or ventricular rupture.

Abdominal injuries

Compression injuries to the abdominal cavity can have serious effects. Some of these effects include solid organ rupture, vascular organ haemorrhage, and hollow organ perforation into the peritoneal cavity. Common injuries include rupture of the bladder, especially if it is full, and lacerations to the spleen, liver and kidneys.

Just as the paper bag effect produces a pneumothorax in thoracic injury, compression of the abdominal cavity can cause increases in intra-abdominal pressure. This increase in pressure can exceed the tensile strength (resistance to lengthwise stretch) of the walls of hollow organs or the diaphragm. Predictable injuries include rupture or herniation of the diaphragm and rupture of hollow organs such as the gallbladder, urinary bladder, duodenum, colon, stomach and small bowel.

Other motorized vehicular collisions

Injuries from other motorized vehicular collisions include those involving motorcycles, all-terrain vehicles (ATVs), motorboats, water bikes, jet skis and farm machinery. This text deals with only motorcycles and ATVs because of their common recreational use and popularity. According to the Department for Transport, nearly 25 000 motorcycle riders and passengers were injured in 2005, 531 died from their injuries.[11]

Small motorized vehicles are thought to be more dangerous than other motor vehicles because they offer little protection to the rider. As with other types of motor vehicle collision, predictable injuries depend on the type of collision that occurs.

Motorcycle collision

Common motorcycle collisions result from impact that is head-on or at an angle. They also result from laying the motorcycle down.

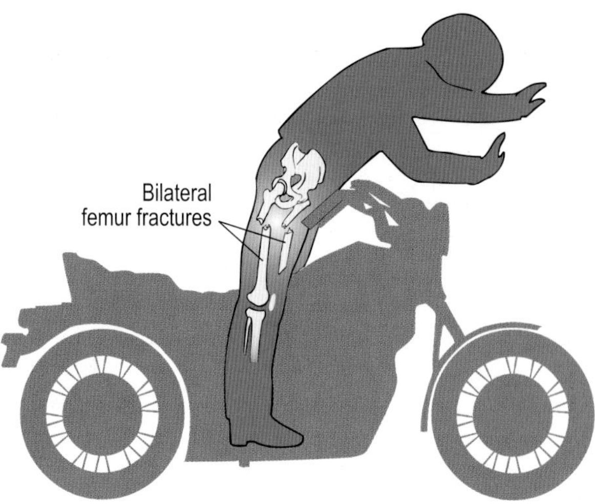

Figure 26-8 Head-on impact motorcycle collision.

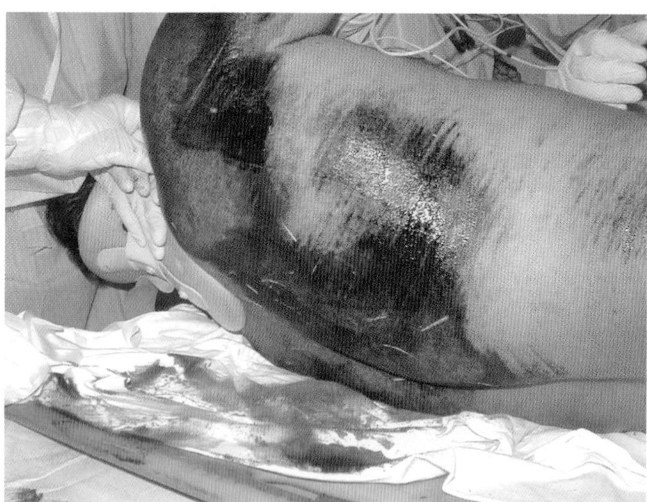

Figure 26-9 Road rash (abrasions).

Head-on impact

The centre of gravity of a motorcycle is above the front axle, forward of the rider's seat. When the motorcycle strikes an object that stops its forward motion, the rest of the bike and the rider continue forward until acted on by an outside force. Usually, the motorcycle tips forward, at which point the rider is propelled over the handlebars. Secondary impacts with the handlebars or other objects stop the forward motion of the rider. Predictable injuries caused by these secondary impacts include head and neck trauma and compression injuries to the chest and abdomen. If the feet remain on the foot rests during impact, the midshaft of the femur absorbs the rider's forward motion (Figure 26-8), which can result in bilateral fractures to the femur and lower leg. Severe perineal injuries can result if the rider's groin strikes the tank or handlebars of the motorcycle.

Angular impact

A motorcycle may strike an object at an angle. When this occurs, the rider is often caught between the motorcycle and the second object. Predictable injuries include crush-type injuries to the patient's affected side. Examples of such are open fractures to the femur, tibia and fibula, and fracture and dislocation of the malleolus.

Laying the motorcycle down

Professional racers and recreational riders often use the strategy of laying the motorcycle down before striking an object. This protective manoeuvre separates the rider from the motorcycle and the object and allows the rider to slide away from the bike. Predictable injuries include massive abrasions (road rash) and fractures to the affected side as the rider slides on the ground or pavement (Figure 26-9). These injuries can be severe but are usually less serious than those that occur from other types of impacts.

All-terrain vehicles

Injuries from crashes involving ATVs are different from those seen in motorcycle collisions. All-terrain vehicles have a higher centre of gravity than motorcycles and a large, flat front tyre that makes them difficult to steer. A specific balance different than that required for riding motorcycles or bicycles is necessary to keep the ATV from overturning.

A natural tendency is for the rider to put a foot down to support the ATV when stopping. This can lead to the rear tyre running over the rider's foot, catching the leg, and throwing the rider forward off the vehicle and onto his or her shoulder or crushing the rider. Predictable injuries from ATV collisions include extremity injury and fracture, clavicular fracture, and serious head and neck injuries.

Personal protective equipment

Protective equipment for riders of small motor vehicles includes boots, leather clothing, eye protection, and helmets. Helmets are structured to absorb the energy of an impact, thereby reducing injuries to the face, skull, and brain, and are estimated to be 29% effective in preventing fatal injuries.[1] Non-use of helmets increases head injuries by more than 300%.[6]

Pedestrian injuries

In 2005, over 33 000 persons were injured in auto–pedestrian collisions in Great Britain; of those injuries, 671 were fatal.[11] All collisions of this nature can cause serious injuries and require a high degree of suspicion for multiple-system trauma.

Three main mechanisms of injury (multiple impacts) exist in auto–pedestrian collisions. The first impact occurs when the bumper of the vehicle strikes the body, the second occurs as the pedestrian strikes the bonnet of the vehicle, and the third occurs when the pedestrian strikes the ground or another object.

Predictable injuries depend on whether the pedestrian is an adult or a child. Variations in the height of the pedestrian in relation to the bumper and bonnet of the car affect the injury pattern. The velocity of the vehicle is also a major factor although even low speeds can result in serious trauma because of the mass of the vehicle and the transfer of energy. Another consideration in evaluating an auto–pedestrian collision is the possibility the patient may have been hit by another vehicle.

Adult pedestrian

Most adult pedestrians who are threatened by an oncoming vehicle try to protect themselves by turning away from the vehicle. Therefore, injuries are often a result of lateral or posterior impacts. During the initial impact, the adult is usually struck by the vehicle bumper in the lower legs, which often produces lower-extremity fractures.

The second impact occurs as the pedestrian falls toward the bonnet of the vehicle. This impact can result in fractures to the femur, pelvis, thorax and spine. The impact can produce intra-abdominal or intrathoracic injury and, in addition, the head and spine can be injured if the victim strikes the bonnet or windshield.

The third impact occurs as the victim strikes the ground or is thrown against another object. This can result in serious damage to the hip and shoulder of the affected side as the body makes contact with the landing surface. Sudden deceleration and compression forces are associated with this impact and these forces can cause fractures, internal haemorrhage, and head and spinal injury.

Child pedestrian

Unlike adults, children tend to face the oncoming vehicle, making them vulnerable to a frontal impact. Because children are smaller than most adults, the initial impact of the vehicle occurs higher on the body, usually above the knees or pelvis. Predictable injuries from the initial impact include fractures to the femur and pelvic girdle and internal haemorrhage.

The second impact occurs as the front of the bonnet of the vehicle continues forward, making contact with the victim's thorax. The victim instantly is thrown backward, forcing the head and neck to flex forward. Depending on the position of the patient in relation to the vehicle, the child's head and neck may contact the bonnet of the vehicle. Predictable injuries include abdominopelvic and thoracic trauma, facial trauma, and head and neck injury.

The third impact occurs as the child is thrown downward to the ground or another landing surface. Because of the child's smaller size and weight, the child can fall under the vehicle and be dragged for some distance. The child can also fall to the side of the vehicle and be run over by the front or rear wheels. Predictable injuries consist of those previously described and may include traumatic amputation.

Other causes of blunt trauma

Other causes of blunt trauma include sports injuries, vertical falls, and blast injuries.

Sports injuries

Persons of all ages take part in sports. Sports that often are associated with injuries include contact sports, such as football, basketball, hockey and wrestling; high-velocity sports, such as downhill skiing, water skiing, cycling, rollerblading and skateboarding; racquet sports; and water sports, such as swimming and diving. Sports offer a range of health benefits but can also produce severe injury.

Injuries related to sports are caused by forces of acceleration and deceleration, compression, twisting, hyperextension and hyperflexion. The paramedic can use the general principles of kinematics to predict injuries by determining the following:

- What energy forces were transferred to the patient?
- To what part of the body was the energy transferred?
- What associated injuries should be considered as a result of the energy transfer?
- How sudden was the acceleration or deceleration?
- Was compression, twisting, hyperextension, or hyperflexion involved in the injury?

Critical Thinking

Injuries related to sports often occur outside. What other considerations will you have for patient care based on the environment?

If the patient used protective equipment, the paramedic should evaluate it to help determine the mechanism of injury. For example, the condition and structural stability of a helmet can provide clues as to the amount of energy transferred to the patient during the injury. Looking at the sporting equipment used by the patient may also provide clues, for example, structural deformities of a bicycle.

Blast injuries

Blast injury is damage to a patient who is exposed to a pressure field that is produced by an explosion of volatile substances. In recent years the number of blast injuries has increased due to the use of homemade bombs in social protests and terrorist activities. Other causes include exploding car batteries, industrial use of volatile substances, chemical reactions in clandestine drug laboratories, explosions in mining, and transportation incidents or crashes involving hazardous materials.

Critical Thinking

In all incidents related to blast injury, what is your first consideration on the scene?

Blasts release large amounts of energy in the form of pressure and heat. If this release of energy is confined in a casing (e.g. a bomb), the pressure ruptures the casing and ejects fragments of the housing at a high velocity. The remaining energy is transmitted to the surrounding environment and can severely injure bystanders. Blast injuries are

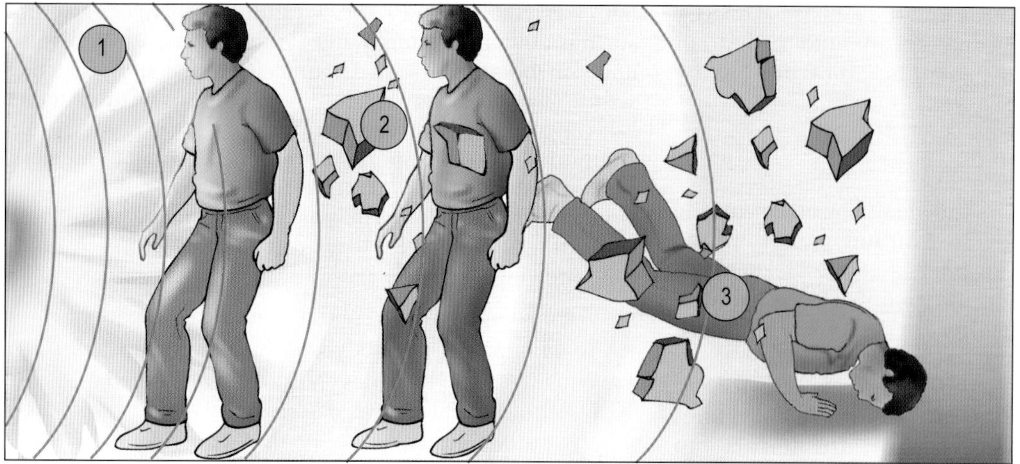

Figure 26-10 Three phases of injury occur during a blast. First, the pressure wave strikes the patient. Then, flying debris can produce injury. In the third phase, the patient is thrown and is injured after impact with the ground or other objects.

classified as primary, secondary, tertiary and miscellaneous (Figure 26-10).

Primary blast injuries

Primary blast injuries result from sudden changes in environmental pressure and usually occur in gas-containing organs. The most severe damage occurs when poorly supported tissue is displaced beyond its elastic limit. The organs and tissues most vulnerable to primary blast injury are the ears, lungs, central nervous system and gastrointestinal tract. Predictable damage to these areas includes hearing loss, pulmonary haemorrhage, cerebral air embolism, abdominal haemorrhage and bowel perforation. Thermal burns can also result from the release of energy in the form of heat. These injuries are likely to occur on unprotected areas that are close to the source of explosion (see Chapter 30). (For example, thermal burns might occur on the face and hands). In closed spaces, because of blast reflection, victims farther from the explosion may be injured as severely as those close to the explosion.

Secondary blast injuries

Secondary blast injuries usually result when bystanders are struck by flying debris. (Examples of such debris include glass, metal or falling mortar.) Obvious injuries are lacerations and fractures. Flying debris can also cause high-velocity missile-type injuries, especially if nails, screws or casing fragments are part of the debris.

Tertiary blast injuries

Tertiary blast injuries occur when victims are propelled through space by an explosion and strike a stationary object. These injuries are similar to those from vertical falls, or ejections from cars or small motor vehicles. In most cases, the sudden deceleration from the impact causes more damage than the acceleration through space because the deceleration is more sudden. Injuries from these forces include damage to the abdominal viscera, central nervous system and musculoskeletal system.

Miscellaneous blast injuries

Miscellaneous blast injuries result from radiation exposure and inhalation of dust and toxic gases (further described in Chapter 45). Predictable injuries include those to the eyes, lungs and soft tissues.

Vertical falls

Falls accounted for 2700 deaths in 2001[12] but were also a serious cause of morbidity. In predicting injuries associated with falls, the paramedic should evaluate three things: the distance fallen, the body position of the patient on impact, and the type of landing surface struck. Injuries associated with vertical falls are a result of deceleration and compression. More than half of all falls occur in homes; nearly 75% involve a person 65 years of age or older.

Falls from some levels are rarely associated with fatal injury. However, falls from distances greater than three times the height of an individual (4.5–6 m) are more likely to be associated with severe injuries. As a point of reference for these distances, the roof of a one-story house is about 5.5 m from the ground, and the roof of a two-story house is about 8.5 m from the ground.

Critical Thinking

What patients may be susceptible to serious injury from a fall that is from a low level?

Adults who have fallen more than 4.5 m usually land on their feet. A predictable injury from this vertical fall is bilateral calcaneus fractures. As the energy dissipates from the initial impact, the head, torso, and pelvis push downward and the body is forced into flexion. When this occurs, hip dislocations and compression fractures of the spinal column in the thoracic and lumbar areas are seen. About 10% of patients with calcaneal fracture have associated spinal fractures. If the patient leans forward or tries to break the fall with outstretched hands, bilateral Colles' fractures to the wrists (clinically evident by the so-called silver fork deformity) are likely.

If the distance fallen is less than 4.5 m, most adults land in the position in which they fell. For example, an adult who falls head-first strikes the landing surface with the head, arms, or both. Predictable injuries depend on the body part that strikes the landing surface and the route of transfer of energy through the body. The paramedic should suspect internal injuries if the trunk of the body is the initial impact area. The ability of the landing surface to absorb energy influences the severity of injury. For example, less damage is expected from a fall on a soft, grassy surface than from a fall on asphalt or concrete.

Children tend to fall head first, regardless of distance fallen or body position during the fall. This is because their heads are proportionally larger and heavier and, for this reason, children who experience a vertical fall are usually victims of head injury. Older adult patients sustain a high number of low-distance falls, often resulting in hip fracture.

SECTION III

Penetrating trauma

All penetrating objects, regardless of velocity, cause tissue disruption (penetrating trauma). This damage occurs as a result of two types of forces: crushing and stretching. The character of the penetrating object, its speed of penetration, and the type of body tissue it passes through or into determine which of the two mechanisms of injury predominates.

Cavitation

Cavitation is an opening produced by a force that pushes body tissues laterally away from the tract of a projectile. The amount of cavitation produced by a projectile is related directly to the density of tissue it strikes. Cavitation is also related to the ability of the body tissue to return to its original shape and position. For example, consider a person who receives a high-velocity blow to the abdomen. This person experiences abdominal cavitation at the moment of impact; however, because of the lower density of the abdominal musculature, the cavitation is temporary. (Cavitation lasts only a few microseconds.) Cavitation is temporary even in the presence of severe intra-abdominal injury (Figure 26-11).

Permanent cavities are produced by penetrating injuries in which the force of the projectile exceeds the tensile strength of the tissue. Tissues with high water density (e.g. liver, spleen, and muscle) or solid density (e.g. bone) are more prone to permanent cavitation. Certain injuries (e.g. a stab wound to the abdomen) can produce cavitations as tissues are displaced in frontal and lateral directions.

Ballistics

The energy created and dissipated by the object into surrounding tissues determines the effect of a projectile on the body. The paramedic should consider the principles of kinematics when dealing with injuries from penetrating trauma. To review, kinetic energy equals half the mass of an object multiplied by the square of its velocity. With reference to ballistic trauma, doubling the mass doubles the energy. However, doubling the velocity quadruples the energy. Therefore, a small-calibre bullet travelling at a high speed can produce more serious injury than a large-calibre bullet travelling at a lower speed. This is the case as long as the large-calibre bullet does not strike a major vessel or organ.

Damage and energy levels of projectiles

Injuries caused by penetrating trauma result from three energy levels; low, medium and high. This discussion considers hand-driven weapons as low-energy projectiles and bullets as medium- and high-energy projectiles.

Low-energy projectiles such as knives, needles, and ice picks cause tissue damage by their sharp, cutting edges (Figure 26-12). The amount of tissue crushed in these injuries is usually minimal because the amount of force applied in the wounding process is small. The more blunt the penetrating object, the more force that must be applied to cause penetration. The more force needed to cause penetra-

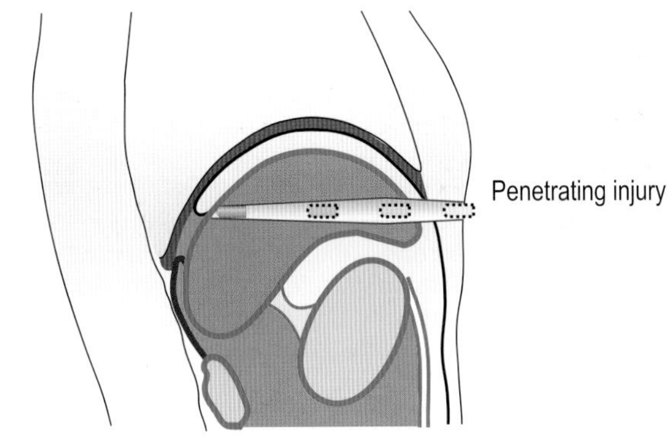

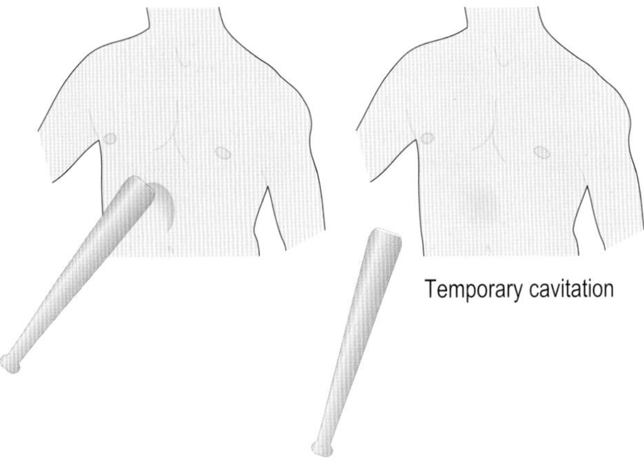

Figure 26-11 Permanent and temporary cavitation.

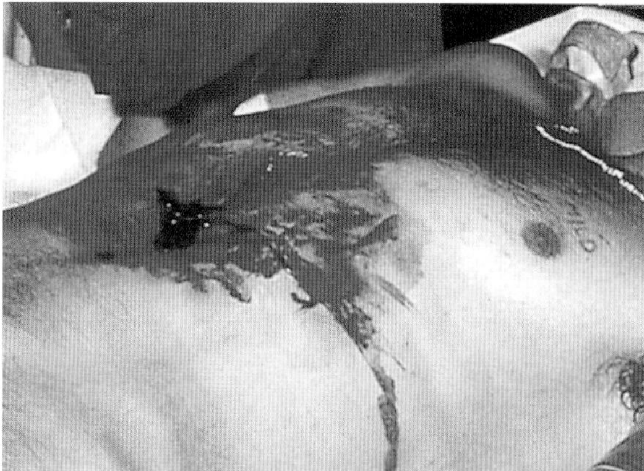

Figure 26-12 Stab wound in which a knife has pierced the liver and pancreas and entered the splenic vein.

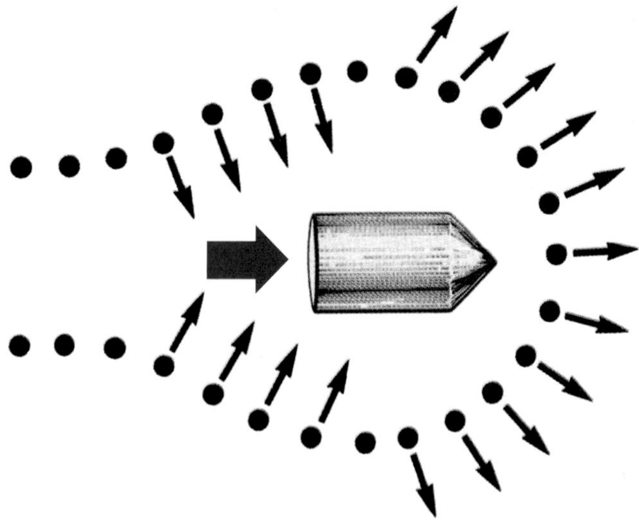

Figure 26-13 Bullet passing through tissue. Outward stretching of the permanent cavity as the tissue particles move away from the penetrating missile causes the temporary cavity.

tion, the more tissue crushed. The damage of tissue from low-energy injuries is normally limited to the pathway of the projectile.

When evaluating a patient with a stab wound, the paramedic should attempt to identify the weapon used to cause the wound. The paramedic should also consider the possibility of multiple wounds, embedded weapons, and hidden yet extensive internal damage to organs of the thorax and abdomen, and penetration of multiple body cavities. A high degree of suspicion of serious injury is also indicated for stab wounds to areas of the back and flank. These wounds may be associated with penetrating injuries to hollow organs and injuries to retroperitoneal organs, specifically the kidneys. Penetrating injuries of the thorax can involve the abdomen, just as abdominal injuries can involve the thorax.

Critical Thinking

Your patient has a stab wound in the midaxillary line, lateral to the left nipple. What organs may be affected by this mechanism? What else would you like to know about this injury?

Firearms can be labelled as medium- and high-energy weapons. Medium-energy weapons include handguns and some rifles. The injury tract produced by medium-energy weapons usually is two to three times the diameter of the projectile. Examples of high-energy weapons include military/assault rifles such as AR-15s, M-16s and AK 47/74s, and some hunting rifles. As with medium-energy injuries, the injury tract produced by high-energy weapons is usually two to three times the diameter of the projectile.

Wounding forces of medium- and high-energy projectiles

A firearm cartridge is composed of a bullet made of metal, gunpowder to propel the bullet, a primer to explode and ignite the gunpowder, and a cartridge case that surrounds these components. When the trigger is pulled, the metal hammer strikes the firing pin, which ignites the primer. The gunpowder ignites and forces the bullet to exit the cartridge case.

The mechanism of injury from firearms is related to the energy created and dissipated by the bullet into the surrounding tissues. When a firearm is discharged, several events affect this dissipation of energy and ultimately the wounding forces of the missile:

1. As the missile travels through air, it experiences wind resistance or drag. The greater the drag, the greater the slowing effect on the missile, therefore a firearm discharged at close range usually produces a more severe injury than the same firearm discharged at a greater distance.
2. As the missile travels through air, a sonic pressure wave spreads out behind the missile. Because the speed of sound in tissue is about four times the speed of sound in air, the sonic pressure wave jumps ahead and precedes the missile through the tissue. This pressure wave displaces tissue and sometimes stretches it dramatically.
3. The localized crush of tissue in the path of the missile and the momentary stretch of the surrounding tissue cause tissue disruption.

When a projectile strikes a body, tissue stretches at the point of impact to allow entry of the penetrating object (temporary cavitation). The energy of the projectile exceeds the tensile strength of the tissue, thus tissue crush occurs, forcing surrounding tissues outward from the path of the projectile (permanent cavitation). The differences in wounds caused by projectiles vary with the amount and location of crushed and stretched tissue (Figure 26-13). The wounding forces of a missile depend on the projectile mass, deformation, fragmentation, type of tissue struck, striking velocity, and range.[8]

Projectile mass

Tissue crush is limited by the physical size or profile of the projectile. If the missile strikes point first, the crushed area is no larger than the diameter of the bullet. If the missile is tilted as it strikes the body, the amount of crushed tissue is no larger than the length and longitudinal cross-section of the bullet.

Deformation
Some firearm missiles deform when striking tissue (e.g. expanding hollow- or soft-point hunting bullets). The points of these projectiles typically flatten on impact. The diameter of the bullet expands, creating a larger area of crushed tissue. Military use of these bullets in war is forbidden.

Fragmentation
Each piece of missile crushes its own path through tissue, causing extensive tissue damage. These fragments produce a larger frontal area than a single, solid bullet and disperse energy into the surrounding tissues rapidly. Tissues weaken from the multiple fragment tracts and increase the subsequent stretch of the temporary cavity. The higher the velocity, the more likely the bullet is to fragment. If a bullet fragments, there may be no exit wound.

Type of tissue struck
Tissue disruption varies greatly with tissue type. For example, elastic tissues such as the bowel wall, lung, and muscle tolerate stretch much better than non-elastic organs such as the liver.

Striking velocity
The velocity of a missile determines the extent of cavitation and tissue damage. Low-velocity missiles localize injury to a small radius from the centre of the injury tract. These missiles have little disruptive effect, pushing the tissue aside. High-velocity missiles produce more serious injuries because they lose more energy to the tissues and produce more cavitation.

Bullet yaw, or tumble, in tissue also contributes to cavitation and tissue damage. The centre of gravity of a wedge-shaped bullet is nearer to the base than to the nose. As the missile strikes body tissue, it slows rapidly. Momentum carries the base of the bullet forward; the centre of gravity becomes the leading part of the missile. This forward rotation around the centre of mass causes an end-over-end motion, which in turn produces more energy exchange and more tissue damage.

Range
The distance of the weapon from the target is a key factor in the severity of ballistic trauma. Air resistance (drag) slows the missile significantly; therefore, increasing the distance of the projectile from the target decreases the velocity at the time of impact.

If the firearm is discharged at close range (within 1 m), cavitation can occur from the combustion of powder and the forceful expansion of gases. The gas and powder can enter the body cavity and cause internal explosion of tissue. This is common with shotgun wounds. Internal explosion of tissue is less common with handguns because they produce a small amount of gas and create a small entrance wound. The expansion of only gas can cause extensive tissue destruction, especially in an enclosed area (e.g. the skull).

Note

Blanks are ammunition without projectiles. The explosion of gas explains how blanks can cause injury or death when fired at short range.

Shotgun wounds

Shotguns are short-range, low-velocity weapons that fire multiple lead pellets. These pellets are encased in a larger shell. Each pellet (there may be 9 to 400 or more, depending on pellet size and gauge of gun) is considered a missile capable of producing tissue damage. Each shell contains pellets, gunpowder, and a plastic or paper wad that separates the pellets from the gunpowder. This wad of unsterile material increases the potential for infection in shotgun wounds.

The energy transferred to body tissue and the tissue damage that results depends on several things: the gauge of the gun, size of the pellets, powder charge, and distance from the victim. For example, a 12-gauge, full-choke shotgun with number 6 shot (275 pellets) concentrates 95% of the pellets into a 7-inch circle at 10 yards (18 cm circle at 9 m). At close range a shotgun injury can create extensive tissue damage similar to that from a high-velocity missile weapon.

Entrance and exit wounds

The presence of entrance and exit wounds is affected by several factors, including range, barrel length, calibre, powder and weapon (Figure 26-14a–c). In general, an entrance wound over soft tissue is round or oval and may be surrounded by an abrasion rim or collar. If the firearm is discharged at intermediate or close range, powder burns (tattooing) may be present (Box 26-4).

Exit wounds, if present, are generally larger than entrance wounds because of the cavitational wave that occurs as the bullet passes through the tissues. As the bullet exits the body, the skin can explode, resulting in ragged and torn tissue. This splitting and tearing often produces a star-burst or stellate wound.

Box 26-4

Forensic considerations in managing gunshot wounds

Lifesaving procedures always take precedence over forensic considerations. However, the paramedic should not touch or move weapons or other environmental clues unless it is absolutely necessary for patient care. Other forensic considerations follow:

- Document the exact condition of the patient and wound appearance on arrival at the scene. This should include environment of the patient and body position in relation to objects and doorways.
- Disturb the scene as little as possible.
- If possible, cut or tear clothing along a seam to avoid altering tears made by a penetrating object.
- Avoid cutting through a bullet hole in the clothing.
- Do not shake clothing.
- Keep all clothing in a paper bag rather than a plastic bag that may alter evidence. Do not give clothing to the victim's family members.
- Save any avulsed tissue for forensic pathological examination.
- If the bullet is retrieved, place it in a padded container to prevent marring and secure the evidence until it is delivered to the authorities (obtain a receipt).

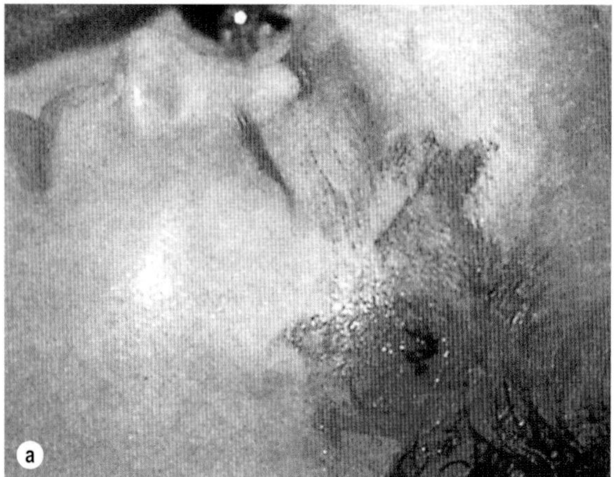

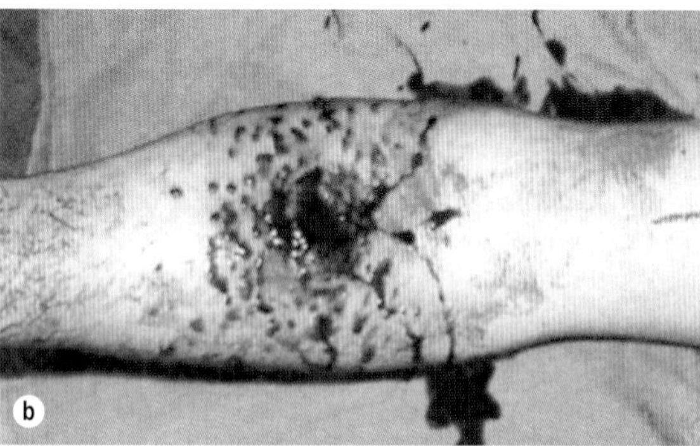

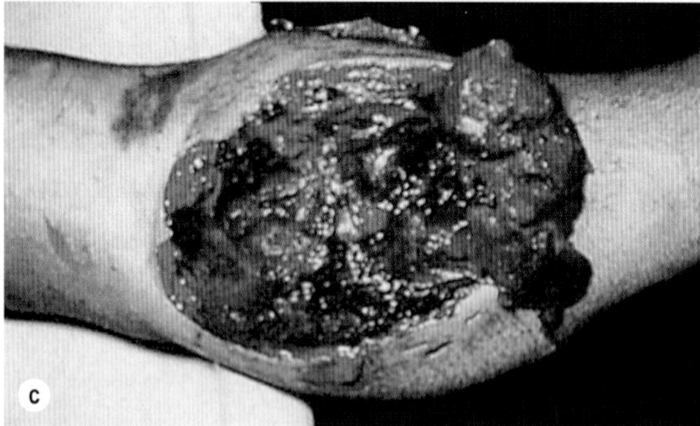

Figure 26-14 (a) The powder marks show that this .22-calibre bullet wound was inflicted at close range. (b) A short-range shotgun wound to the forearm. (c) Exit wound caused by a powerful shotgun fired at close range.

Critical Thinking

You locate an entrance wound but no exit wound on a patient who was shot. Does this mean that the injury is not serious?

If the muzzle is in direct contact with the skin at the time of firearm discharge, expanding gases can enter the tissue. These gases can produce crepitus. The burning gases can also produce thermal injury at the entrance site and along the injury tract.

Note

The paramedic should describe and document the appearance of all wounds. However, the paramedic should refrain from commenting or speculating on which is the entry or exit wound. Such speculation can result in the paramedic being served a subpoena. The paramedic may be subpoenaed to testify in court in an area that is beyond the scope of paramedic practice.

Special considerations for specific injuries

Locating ballistic injuries requires a thorough physical examination of the patient because the resulting trauma from high- and medium-velocity missiles is unpredictable. The impact of any projectile is critical in determining the type and severity of injury. Fractions of an inch can make a significant difference in the amount of trauma the patient suffers. These differences are often impossible to distinguish in the field.

Head injuries

Gunshot wounds to the head typically are devastating because of the direct destruction of brain tissue and subsequent swelling. Patients with head wounds often sustain severe face and neck injuries as well. These can result in major blood loss, difficulty in maintaining airway control, and spinal instability.

As a medium-energy projectile penetrates the skull, the energy is absorbed within the closed space of the cranium. The force of the injury compresses brain tissue against the cranial cavity, often fracturing orbital plates and separating the dura from the bone. Depending on the qualities of the missile, the bullet may not have enough force to exit the skull after penetration. This is what occurs with .22- and .25-calibre handguns. In these injuries the bullet follows the curvature of the interior of the skull. As it follows this curvature, it produces significant damage.

High-velocity wounds to the skull produce massive destruction. Pieces of the skull and brain typically are destroyed. At close range, high-velocity wounds result in part from the large quantities of gas produced by combustion of the propellant. If the weapon is held in contact with the head, the gas follows the bullet into the cranial cavity, producing an explosive effect.

Thoracic injuries

Gunshot wounds to the thorax can result in severe injury to the pulmonary and vascular systems. If the lungs are penetrated by a missile, the pleura and pulmonary parenchyma (the tissue of an organ, as distinguished from supporting and connective tissue) are likely to be disrupted, producing a pneumothorax. On occasion, the pulmonary defect allows air that cannot be expelled to continue to flow into the thoracic cavity. The subsequent increase in pressure can eventually cause collapse of the lung and a shift in the mediastinum to the unaffected side (tension pneumothorax).

Vascular trauma from penetrating injuries can result in massive internal and external haemorrhage. For example, if the pulmonary artery or vein, venae cavae or aorta is injured, the patient can bleed to death within minutes. Other vascular injuries from penetrating trauma to the thorax can result in haemothorax and, if the heart is involved, myocardial rupture or pericardial tamponade.

Penetrating injury can cause thoracic trauma in the absence of visible chest wounds. For example, a bullet can enter the abdomen and travel upward through the diaphragm and into the thorax. The paramedic should evaluate all victims of abdominal gunshot wounds for thoracic injury. Likewise, the paramedic should evaluate all victims of thoracic gunshot wounds for abdominal injury.

Abdominal injuries

Gunshot wounds to the abdomen usually require surgery to determine the extent of injury. Penetrating trauma can affect multiple organ systems, causing damage to air-filled and solid organs, vascular injury, trauma to the vertebral column and spinal cord injury. The paramedic should assume a serious injury when managing victims of penetrating abdominal trauma. This should be the rule even if a patient appears to be stable.

Extremity injuries

At times, gunshot wounds to the extremities are life threatening. Sometimes such wounds can result in lifelong disability. Special considerations with these injuries include vascular injury with bleeding into soft tissues and damage to nerves, muscles, and bones. The paramedic should evaluate any extremity that has sustained penetrating trauma for bone injury, motor and sensory integrity, and the presence of adequate blood flow (e.g. pulses and capillary refill).

Vessels can be injured by being struck by the bullet or by temporary cavitation. Either mechanism can damage the lining of the blood vessel, producing haemorrhage or thrombosis. Penetrating trauma can damage muscle tissue by stretching it as the muscle expands away from the path of the missile. Stretching that exceeds the tensile strength of the muscle produces haemorrhage.

Bone struck by a penetrating object can be deformed and fragmented. If this occurs, the transfer of energy causes pieces of bone to act as secondary missiles, crushing their way through surrounding tissue.

Summary

- Trauma is the leading cause of death among persons 10–39 years of age in the UK and is the fourth leading cause of death in the Western world.
- Trauma care is divided into three phases: pre-incident, incident, and post-incident.
- Components of the trauma system include injury prevention, prehospital care, emergency department care, interfacility transportation (if needed), definitive care, trauma critical care, rehabilitation, data collection, and trauma registry.
- Injuries are caused by a transfer of energy from some external source to the human body. The extent of injury is determined by the type of energy applied, by how quickly it is applied, and by the part of the body to which the energy is applied.
- Blunt trauma is an injury produced by the wounding forces of compression and change of speed, which can disrupt tissues.
- Four restraining systems are available in the UK. These are lap belts, diagonal shoulder straps, child safety seats and air bags. All of these significantly reduce injuries. However, if they are used inappropriately, these protective devices also can produce injuries.
- Organ injuries can result from sudden movement caused by deceleration and compression forces. The recognition of these injuries requires a high degree of suspicion. The paramedic must use the principles of kinematics.
- Small motorized vehicles such as motorcycles, all-terrain vehicles, motorboats, water bikes and farm machinery are considered to be more dangerous than other motor vehicles. They are more dangerous because they offer little protection to the rider. They offer minimal protection from the transfer of energy associated with collisions.
- All auto–pedestrian collisions can produce serious injuries. They require a high degree of suspicion for multiple-system trauma.
- Sports provide a variety of health benefits. However, they can also produce severe injury.
- Blast injury is damage to a patient exposed to a pressure field that is produced by an explosion of volatile substances. Blasts release large amounts of energy in the form of pressure and heat.
- Falls from greater than three times the height of a person (4.5–6 m) are associated with an increased incidence of severe injuries. In predicting injuries associated with falls, the paramedic should evaluate three things: the distance fallen, the body position of the patient on impact, and the type of landing surface struck.
- All penetrating objects, regardless of velocity, cause tissue disruption. The character of the penetrating object, its speed of penetration, and the type of body tissue it passes through or into determine whether crushing or stretching forces will cause injury.

References

1. Office for National Statistics 2004 Review of the Registrar General on deaths by cause, sex and age, in England and Wales. ONS, London
2. Department for Transport. Road Casualties Great Britain: 2007, Annual Report. Online. Available http://www.dft.gov.uk/pgr/statistics/datatablespublications/accidents/casualtiesgbar/roadcasualtiesgreatbritain20071 5 June 2009
3. National Association of Emergency Medical Technicians 2003 PHTLS: basic and advanced prehospital life support, 5th edition. Mosby, St Louis
4. US Department of Transportation, National Highway Traffic Safety Administration 1998 EMT-paramedic national standard curriculum. US Department of Transportation, Washington, DC
5. DETR 1997 Road safety strategy: current problems and future options. The Stationery Office, London
6. National Safety Council 2002 Injury facts. National Safety Council, Chicago
7. Kuehl A (ed) 1989 EMS medical director's handbook. Mosby, St Louis
8. McSwain N, Kerstein M 1987 Evaluation and management of trauma. Appleton-Century-Crofts, Norwalk, CN
9. Department for Transport 2008 Road Casualties Great Britain: 2007, Annual Report. The Stationery Office, Norwich
10. Department for Transport 2005 Compulsory seat belt/child restraint wearing in cars and goods vehicles. Online. Available http://www.dft.gov.uk/consultations/archive/2005/comsbcrw/compulsoryseatbeltchildrestr1198?page=5#1011 13 February 2009
11. Department for Transport 2006 Road Casualties Great Britain 2005. Department for Transport, London
12. Office for National Statistics 2005 Deaths, 2001 registrations: Death by age, sex and underlying cause. Office for National Statistics, London

CHAPTER **27**

Thoracic Trauma

Chapter contents

Objectives

Upon completion of this chapter, the paramedic student will be able to:

1. Discuss the factors and mechanism of injury associated with thoracic trauma.
2. Describe the mechanism of injury, signs and symptoms, and management of skeletal injuries to the chest.
3. Describe the mechanism of injury, signs and symptoms, and prehospital management of pulmonary trauma.
4. Describe the mechanism of injury, signs and symptoms, and prehospital management of injuries to the heart and great vessels.
5. Outline the mechanism of injury, signs and symptoms, and prehospital care of the patient with oesophageal and tracheobronchial injury and diaphragmatic rupture.

Key terms

Beck triad A combination of three symptoms that characterize cardiac tamponade: elevated central venous pressure, muffled heart sounds, and hypotension.

closed pneumothorax A collection of air or gas in the pleural space that causes the lung to collapse without exposing the pleural space to atmospheric pressure.

flail chest A chest wall injury in which three or more adjacent ribs are fractured in two or more places.

haemothorax The accumulation of blood and other fluid in the pleural space caused by bleeding from the lung parenchyma or damaged vessels.

open pneumothorax A chest wall injury that exposes the pleural space to atmospheric pressure.

pulmonary contusion Bruising of the lung tissue that results in rupture of the alveoli and interstitial oedema.

tension pneumothorax An accumulation of air or gas in the pleural cavity that can lead to collapse of the lung.

traumatic asphyxia A severe crushing injury to the chest and abdomen that causes an increase in the intrathoracic pressure. The increased pressure forces blood from the right side of the heart into the veins of the upper thorax, neck, and face.

Penetrating and blunt thoracic trauma account for 25–50% of all traumatic injuries.[1] Most patients can be managed without the need for surgery although a small number, 10–15%, require emergency thoracotomy.[1] Chest injuries are caused by blunt trauma, penetrating trauma, or both, and are often the result of motor vehicle crashes, falls from heights, blast injuries, blows to the chest, chest compression, gunshot wounds, and stab wounds. Thoracic trauma may be classified as skeletal injury, pulmonary injury, heart and great vessel injury, and diaphragmatic injury. (Anterior neck trauma is discussed in Chapter 31.)

Skeletal injury

Skeletal injuries may be caused by blunt or penetrating trauma. The injuries discussed in this chapter include clavicular fractures, rib fractures, flail chest and sternal fractures.

Clavicular fractures

The clavicle is the most commonly fractured bone although an isolated clavicular fracture is seldom a significant injury

(Figure 27-1). It is common in children who fall on their shoulders or outstretched arms, and in athletes involved in contact sports. Treatment usually involves applying a clavicle strap or a sling and swathe that immobilizes the affected shoulder and arm (see Chapter 34). These injuries usually heal well within 4 to 6 weeks.

Signs and symptoms of clavicular fractures include pain, point tenderness, and evident deformity. The subclavian vein or artery may be injured when the clavicle is broken. Bony fragments from the fracture may puncture a vessel, resulting in a haematoma or venous thrombosis, although this is rare.

Rib fractures

Rib fractures most often occur on the lateral aspect of the third through eighth ribs where they are least protected by musculature (Figure 27-2). Fractures are more likely to occur in adults than in children because younger patients have more resilient cartilage. Morbidity or mortality from rib fractures depends on the patient's age and the number and location of the fractures.

Critical Thinking

Why would you expect greater underlying pulmonary injury in a child versus an adult with rib fractures?

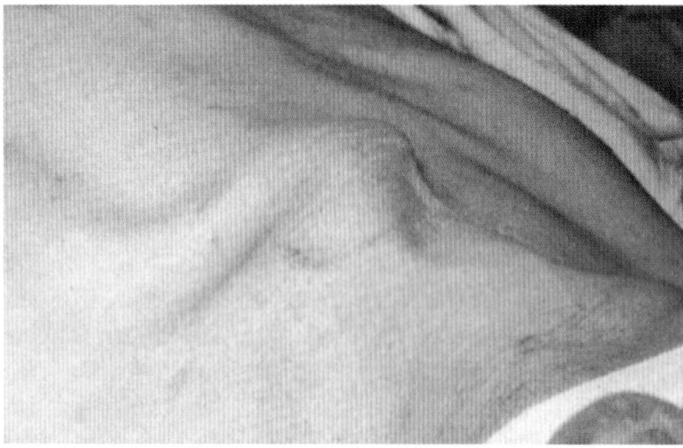

Figure 27-1 Fracture of the left clavicle seen from above the left shoulder.

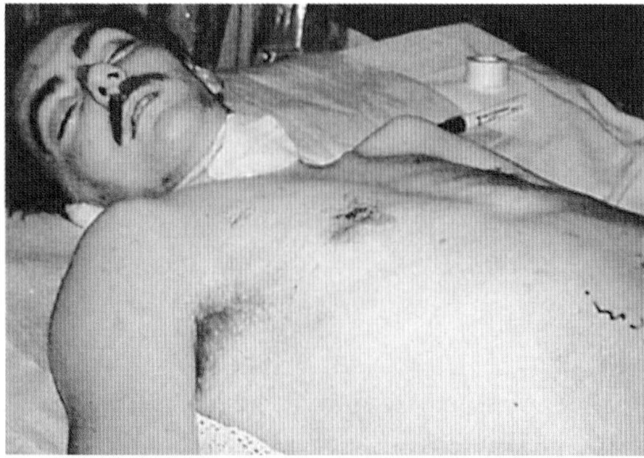

Figure 27-2 Chest wall asymmetry caused by rib fractures.

Simple rib fractures are usually very painful though rarely life-threatening. Most patients can localize the fracture by pointing to the area (this is confirmed by palpation). Sometimes movement or grating of the bone ends (crepitus) can be felt. Complications of rib fracture include splinting, which leads to atelectasis, and ventilation–perfusion mismatch (ventilated alveoli that are not perfused, or perfused alveoli that are not ventilated). The goal of treatment is to relieve the pain and counter the effects of hypoventilation. Analgesia may be achieved by splinting the patient's arm against the chest wall with a sling and swathe although circumferential splinting should not be used. Administration of analgesics as per guidelines may help but Entonox should be used with caution. Based on the mechanism of injury, the paramedic should consider the possibility of more serious trauma, such as closed pneumothorax and internal bleeding. Fractures to the lower ribs (eighth through twelfth) may be associated with injuries to the spleen, kidneys or liver.

Great force is required to fracture the first through third ribs due to their shape and the protection afforded by the scapulae, clavicles, and upper chest musculature. Fractures of the first three ribs may be associated with myocardial contusion, bronchial tears, and vascular injury.

Flail chest

A flail chest may occur when three or more adjacent ribs are fractured in two or more places (Figure 27-3a–c). This injury is not usually detected in the prehospital setting because of the muscle spasm that accompanies the injury. Within 2 h after the injury, however, the muscle spasm subsides and the injured segment of the chest wall may begin to move in a paradoxical (contrary) fashion with inspiration and expiration.

Note

In paradoxical breathing, part of the lung deflates during inspiration and inflates during expiration. This condition is commonly associated with chest trauma. An open chest wound or a rib cage injury is an example of this type of trauma.

Causes of flail chest include vehicle crashes, falls, industrial accidents, assault, and birth trauma. The mortality rate is relatively low in isolated unilateral flail chest although death rate rises significantly with associated injury. Around 28.5% of patients with critical injuries (Injury Severity Score >24) die, with advancing age also cited as a risk factor for mortality.[2]

During inspiration the diaphragm descends, which lowers the intrapleural pressure. The unstable chest wall is pushed inward by the negative intrathoracic pressure as the rest of the chest wall expands. During expiration, the diaphragm rises, and the intrapleural pressure exceeds atmospheric pressure, causing the unstable chest wall to move outward. Patients with flail chest may develop hypoxia because of the lung contusions that are often related to this injury. Bleeding from the alveoli and the lung tissue causes the contusion, which is associated with decreased vital capacity and vascular shunting of deoxygenated blood. Signs and symptoms of

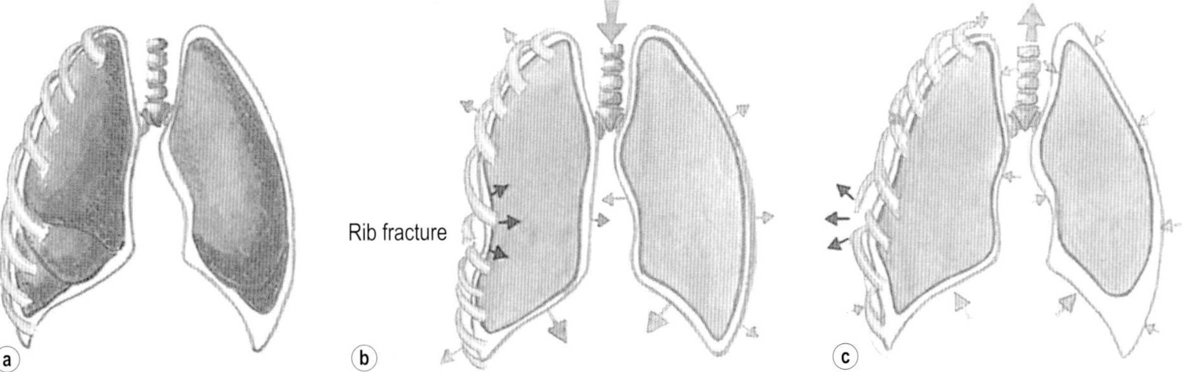

Figure 27-3 Flail chest. (a) Normal lungs. (b) Flail chest during inspiration. (c) Flail chest during expiration.

flail chest include tenderness and bony crepitus on palpation and paradoxical motion (a late sign).

Prehospital management of patients with flail chest includes assisting ventilation with positive pressure by means of a bag–mask device, use of high-concentration supplemental oxygen, and fluid replacement as needed. Field stabilization of the flail segment is controversial. In one method, the paramedic tries to splint the flail segment in the inward position with simple hand pressure, bulky dressings, or towels taped to the chest wall. This splinting can reduce vital capacity but may increase the efficiency of ventilation. A large percentage of patients with significant chest injury progress to respiratory failure requiring long-term ventilatory support and hospitalization. Prehospital use of positive end-expiratory pressure (PEEP) to keep alveoli open at the end of exhalation is not currently a part of JRCALC guidelines, as the procedure requires special equipment and training.

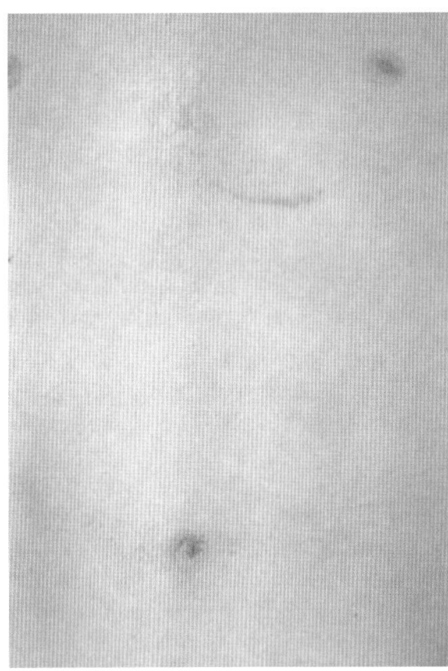

Figure 27-4 Well-marked band of spotty bruising caused by a steering wheel impact.

Critical Thinking

Why is positive-pressure ventilation the treatment of choice for this injury?

Sternal fractures

Sternal fractures are uncommon but serious. They usually result from a direct blow to the chest (e.g. striking a steering column or dashboard) or from a massive crush injury (Figure 27-4). Sternal fractures are usually very painful and may be associated with an unstable chest wall, myocardial injury, or cardiac tamponade. They occur in only 5–8% of patients with blunt chest trauma, yet the mortality rate is 25–45%.[3] Signs and symptoms include a history of significant anterior chest trauma, tenderness, and abnormal motion or crepitation over the sternum. Prehospital management includes maintaining a high degree of suspicion for associated injuries, airway maintenance, ventilatory support, electrocardiographic (ECG) monitoring and rapid transport to an appropriate medical facility. Associated injuries that often contribute to serious disability or death include the following:

- pulmonary and myocardial contusion
- flail chest
- vascular disruption of thoracic vessels (rare)
- intra-abdominal injuries
- head injury.

Pulmonary injury

Pulmonary injuries may be classified as closed pneumothorax, tension pneumothorax, open pneumothorax, haemothorax, pulmonary contusion and traumatic asphyxia. Any of these injuries can result in difficulty in breathing (respiratory insufficiency). Prehospital treatment must be directed at ensuring an open airway, providing support of ventilation and oxygenation, correcting immediately life-threatening ventilatory problems (e.g. tension pneumothorax), and rapid transport for definitive care.

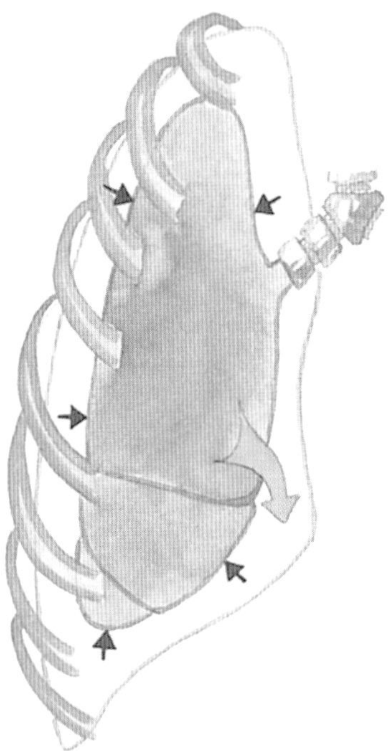

Figure 27-5 Closed (simple) pneumothorax.

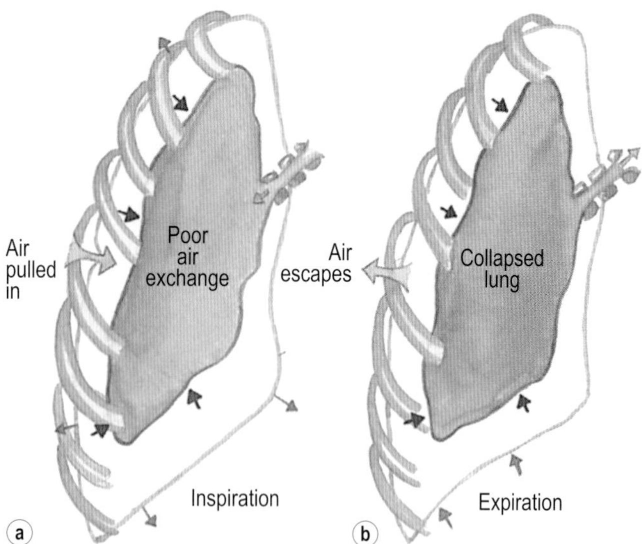

Figure 27-6 Open pneumothorax. (a) Air enters the pleural cavity during inspiration. (b) Air exits the pleural cavity during expiration.

Closed pneumothorax

A closed pneumothorax (simple pneumothorax) is caused by the presence of air in the pleural space. This air causes the lung to partly or totally collapse (Figure 27-5). A common cause of pneumothorax is a fractured rib that penetrates the underlying lung, although pneumothoraces may occur without rib fractures. They may be caused by excessive pressure on the chest wall against a closed glottis (paper bag effect; see Chapter 26). They may also be caused by rupture or tearing of the lung parenchyma and visceral pleura from no demonstrable cause (spontaneous pneumothorax). Closed pneumothorax occurs in 10–30% of patients with blunt chest trauma and in almost 100% of patients with penetrating chest trauma.[4]

Critical Thinking

How does high-flow oxygen promote faster resolution of a closed pneumothorax?

The signs and symptoms of a closed pneumothorax include chest pain, dyspnoea and tachypnoea. Breath sounds may be diminished or absent on the affected side. Treatment includes ventilatory support with high-concentration oxygen. The patient should be monitored carefully for signs of a tension pneumothorax, and transported in a semi-sitting position of comfort unless this position is contraindicated by the mechanism of injury. If the patient's respiratory rate is below 12 or above 28 breaths per minute, ventilatory assistance with a bag–valve–mask may be indicated.

Most healthy patients have large circulatory and ventilatory reserve capacities; therefore, closed pneumothoraces do not usually pose a threat to life. However, life-threatening consequences may develop if the pneumothorax is a tension pneumothorax, if it occupies more than 40% of the hemithorax, or if it occurs in a patient with shock or pre-existing pulmonary or cardiovascular diseases.

Open pneumothorax

An open pneumothorax develops when a chest injury exposes the pleural space to atmospheric pressure (Figure 27-6a, b). The severity of the injury is directly proportional to the size of the wound. When a chest wound is larger than the normal pathway for air through the nose and mouth, atmospheric pressure forces the air through the open wound and into the thoracic cavity during inspiration. As the air builds up in the pleural space, the lung on the injured side collapses and begins to shift toward the uninjured side. Very little air enters the tracheobronchial tree to be exchanged with intrapulmonary air on the affected side, which results in decreased alveolar ventilation and decreased perfusion. The normal side is also adversely affected because expired air may enter the lung on the collapsed side and is then rebreathed into the functioning lung with the next ventilation. This may result in severe ventilatory dysfunction, hypoxaemia and death unless the situation is quickly recognized and corrected.

Signs and symptoms of open pneumothorax include shortness of breath, pain, and a sucking or gurgling sound as air moves in and out of the pleural space through the open chest wound (thus the term sucking chest wound). Prehospital treatment of an open pneumothorax proceeds as follows (Figure 27-7):

1. Close the chest wound by applying an Asherman's chest seal or an adherent, non-permeable dressing taped on three sides to allow some air to escape;[5] this may allow spontaneous decompression of a developing tension pneumothorax. The paramedic should closely monitor for the development of a tension pneumothorax if the patient's dressing does not provide a venting mechanism.

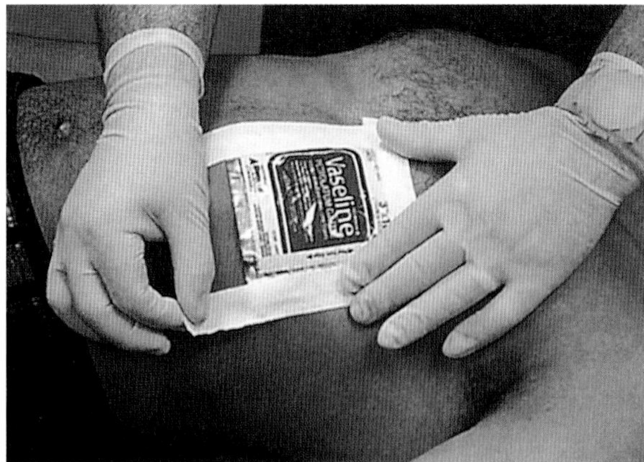

Figure 27-7 Sealing a chest wound.

2. Provide ventilatory support with high-concentration oxygen. Intubation may be considered but may also contribute to the pneumothorax.
3. Treat the patient for shock by administering crystalloid per guidelines.
4. Rapidly transport the patient to an appropriate medical facility.

Tension pneumothorax

When air in the thoracic cavity cannot exit the pleural space, a tension pneumothorax may develop (Figure 27-8). This is a true emergency that results in profound hypoventilation. Tension pneumothorax may result in death if it is not immediately recognized and managed.

When air is allowed to leak into the pleural space during inspiration and becomes trapped during expiration, the pleural pressure increases and produces a mediastinal shift. It further compresses the lung on the uninjured side and, in addition, it compresses the vena cava, so reducing venous return to the heart. This results in a decrease in cardiac output. The signs and symptoms of a tension pneumothorax include the following:

- anxiety
- cyanosis
- increasing dyspnoea
- tachycardia
- hypotension or unexplained signs of shock
- diminished or absent breath sounds on the injured side
- distended neck veins (unless the patient is hypovolaemic)
- unequal expansion of the chest (tension does not fall with respiration)
- subcutaneous emphysema
- tracheal deviation (a late sign).

Critical Thinking

Why might the neck veins be distended in a patient with a tension pneumothorax?

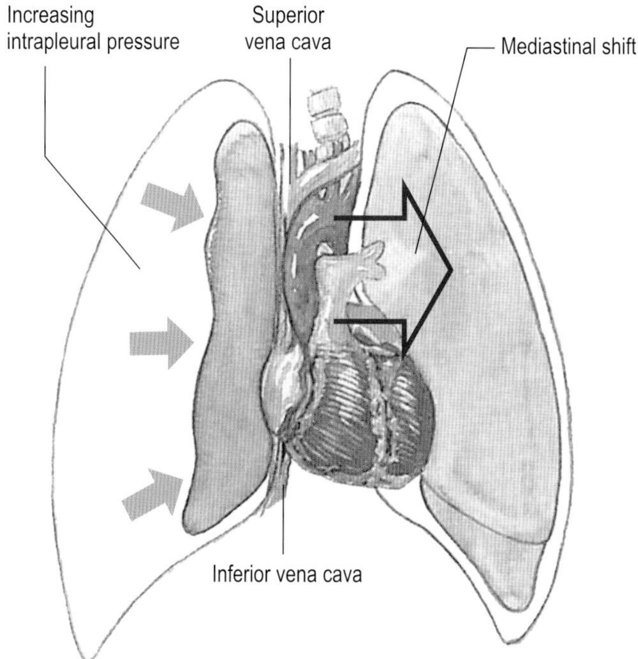

Figure 27-8 Tension pneumothorax.

Tension pneumothorax may be confirmed by X-ray films in the hospital setting; however, waiting for X-ray confirmation is less than optimal management. In the prehospital setting, a suspected tension pneumothorax should be managed aggressively. It is evidenced by increasing dyspnoea, compromised ventilation, tachycardia, tachypnoea, unilateral decreased or absent breath sounds, and hyperresonance on percussion. Emergency care is directed at reducing the pressure in the pleural space; that is, returning the intrapleural pressure to atmospheric or subatmospheric levels.

Note

The value of chest percussion in the prehospital setting is questionable. In the field, it should not be the only method used to identify a tension pneumothorax or haemothorax.[4] As a rule, hyperresonance on percussion points to the presence of air (pneumothorax); dullness on percussion points to the presence of blood and other fluid (haemothorax).

Tension pneumothorax associated with penetrating trauma

Sealing an open pneumothorax with an occlusive dressing may produce a tension pneumothorax. In such cases the increased pleural pressure can be relieved by momentarily removing the dressing. When the dressing is lifted from the wound, an audible release of air from the thoracic cavity should be noted. If this does not occur and the patient's condition remains unchanged, the paramedic should gently spread the chest wound open; this will allow the trapped air to escape. After the pressure has been released, the wound should again be sealed. The dressing may need to be removed more than once to relieve pleural pressure during transport. If the tension is not relieved with this procedure, thoracic decompression (needle thoracocentesis) should be performed.

Tension pneumothorax associated with closed trauma

A tension pneumothorax that develops in a patient with closed chest trauma must be relieved through thoracic decompression. This can be done with a large-bore needle or a commercially available thoracic decompression kit.

For needle decompression, a 14-gauge hollow needle or catheter is inserted into the affected pleural space, usually in the second intercostal space in the midclavicular line (Figure 27-9a–c). The needle should be inserted just above the third rib to avoid the nerve, artery, and vein that lie just beneath each rib. After insertion of the needle, an audible rush of air should be noted; this is pressure escaping from the pleural space (confirming the tension pneumothorax). At this point, the patient should show signs of improvement (i.e. the patient will be easier to ventilate, or the person's breathing will be less laboured). The needle or catheter should be secured in place with tape.

Critical Thinking

Put your finger on the point on your chest where a needle would be inserted for decompression of a tension pneumothorax. Is it easy to identify?

Haemothorax

A haemothorax is the accumulation of blood in the pleural space. It is caused by bleeding from the lung parenchyma or damaged vessels (Figure 27-10). If this condition is associated with a pneumothorax, it is called a haemopneumothorax. Blood loss may be massive in these patients; each side of the thorax can hold 30–40% (2500–3000 mL) of the patient's blood volume.[4] A severed intercostal artery can easily bleed 50 mL per minute; thus, patients with a haemothorax often have hypovolaemia and hypoxaemia.

As blood continues to fill the pleural space, the lung on the affected side may collapse. In rare cases the mediastinum may even shift away from the haemothorax, which would compress the unaffected lung. The resultant effects of respi-

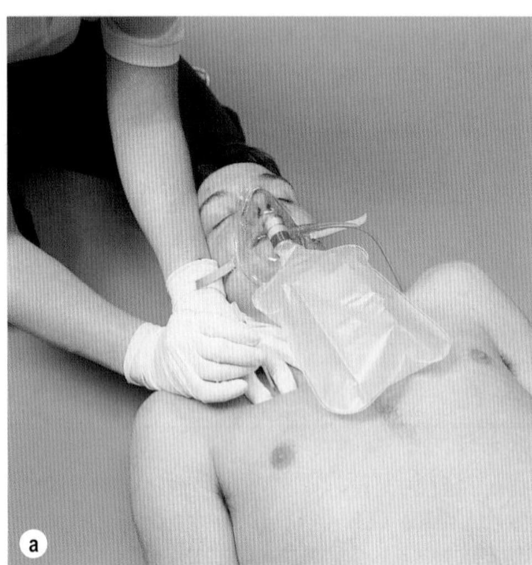

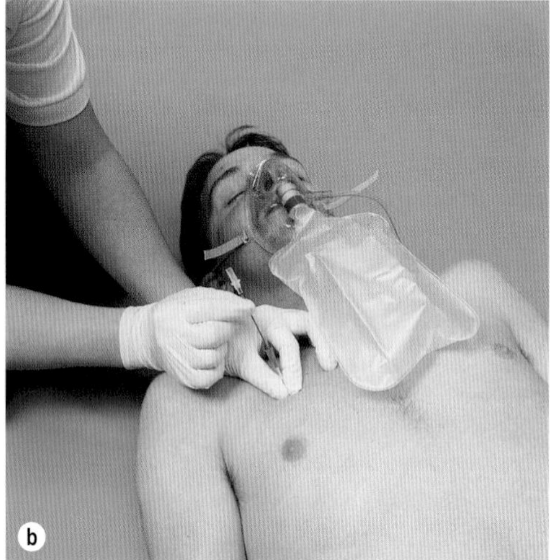

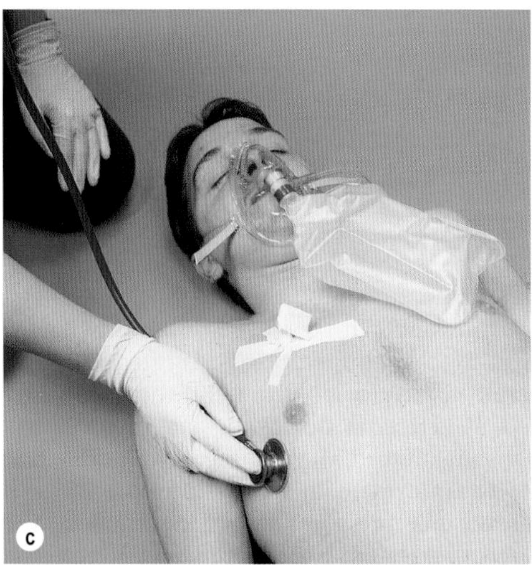

Figure 27-9 Needle decompression. (a) A 2-inch, 14- or 16-gauge hollow needle or catheter is inserted into the affected pleural space, usually in the second intercostal space in the midclavicular line. (b) After insertion of the needle, an audible rush of air should be noted as pressure escapes from the pleural space. (c) The catheter is secured in place with tape. Care is taken to prevent re-entry of air into the pleural space. The patient's respiratory status is monitored carefully.

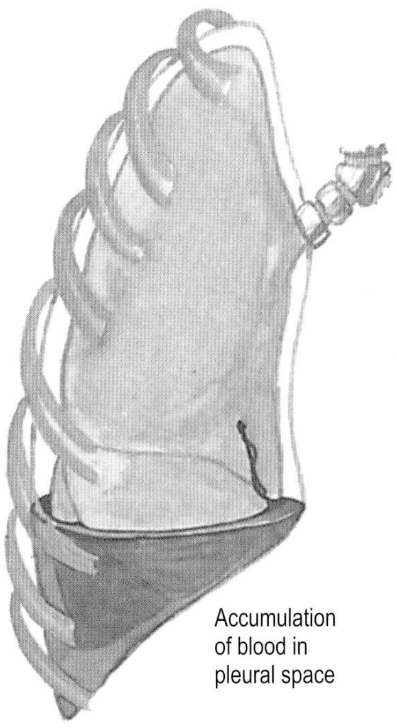

Figure 27-10 Haemothorax.

ratory and circulatory compromise are responsible for the following signs and symptoms:

- tachypnoea
- dyspnoea
- cyanosis (often not evident in haemorrhagic shock)
- diminished or decreased breath sounds (dullness on percussion)
- hypovolaemic shock
- narrow pulse pressure
- tracheal deviation to the unaffected side (rare).

Prehospital care for patients with a haemothorax is directed at correcting ventilatory and circulatory problems. This involves administration of high-concentration oxygen; ventilatory support with a bag-mask device, intubation, or both; administration of volume-expanding fluids to correct the hypovolaemia; and rapid transport to an appropriate medical facility. Haemothorax associated with great vessel or cardiac injury has a high mortality rate: 50% of these patients die immediately; 25% live for 5–10 min; and 25% may live longer than 30 min.[3]

Critical Thinking

Haemothorax is associated with a higher mortality rate than a simple (closed) pneumothorax. Why is that the case?

Pulmonary contusion

Pulmonary contusion is most often caused by rapid deceleration forces (such forces may be created by motor vehicle crashes and by injuries that result in a flail chest). These forces push the lung against the chest wall, resulting in rupture of the alveoli, with haemorrhage and swelling of the lung tissue. Pulmonary contusion is reported to be present in between 30% and 75% of patients with significant blunt chest trauma.[6]

During sudden inertial deceleration and direct impact, fixed and mobile parts of the lung move at varying speeds. The result is stretching and shearing of alveoli and intravascular structures (the inertial effect). This kinetic wave of energy is partly reflected at the alveolar membrane surface, the remainder causes a localized release of energy (the Spalding effect). Overexpansion of air in the lungs occurs after the primary energy wave has passed (implosion effect), then low-pressure rebound shock waves cause overstretching and damage to lung tissue. The combination of these events results in alveolar and capillary damage with bleeding into the lung tissue and alveoli. The contused area of the lung is unable to function properly after injury, therefore profound hypoxaemia may develop. The degree of respiratory complication is directly related to the size of the contused area.

The signs and symptoms of pulmonary contusion are subtle at first, so the condition should be suspected based on the kinematics of the event and the presence of associated injuries. Common signs and symptoms include the following:

- tachypnoea
- tachycardia
- cough
- haemoptysis
- apprehension
- respiratory distress
- dyspnoea
- evidence of blunt chest trauma
- cyanosis.

Critical Thinking

Will you always be able to distinguish between simple pneumothorax and pulmonary contusion in the prehospital setting? Why or why not?

Emergency care for pulmonary contusion includes ventilatory support and administration of high-concentration oxygen. Patients with associated injuries or pre-existing pulmonary or cardiovascular disease should be closely monitored in case ventilations need to be assisted with a bag–valve device, intubation, or both. Pulmonary contusions may be associated with a major chest injury although they generally heal spontaneously over several weeks.

Traumatic asphyxia

The term traumatic asphyxia is used to describe a severe crushing injury to the chest and abdomen (Figure 27-11). It results from an increase in intrathoracic pressure that forces blood from the right side of the heart into the veins of the upper thorax, neck, and face. The forces involved in this phenomenon may cause lethal injury, but traumatic asphyxia

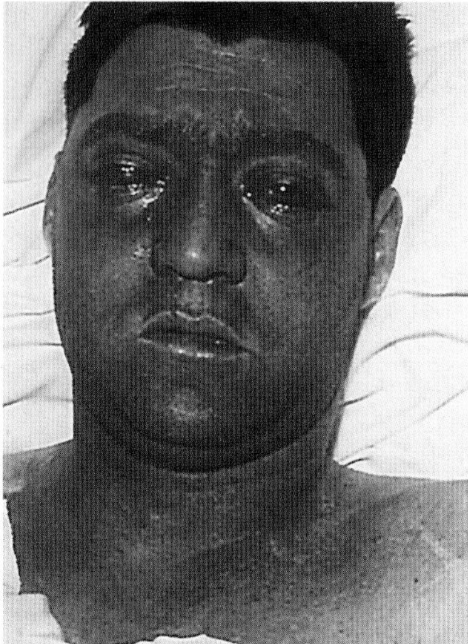

Figure 27-11 Discoloration of traumatic asphyxia, which results from forcible compression of the chest.

alone is not life-threatening[7] (although brain haemorrhages, seizures, coma and death have been documented to occasionally occur).

Signs and symptoms of traumatic asphyxia include reddish–purple discoloration of the face and neck (the skin below the area remains pink), jugular vein distension, and swelling or haemorrhage of the conjunctiva (subconjunctival petechiae may appear). Emergency care is directed at ensuring an open airway, providing adequate ventilation, and caring for associated injuries. The paramedic should be ready to manage hypovolaemia and shock when the compressive force is released.

Heart and great vessel injury

Trauma to the heart and to the great vessels (i.e. the aorta, pulmonary arteries and veins, and superior and inferior venae cavae) may be caused by the force of blunt or penetrating injuries. The injuries discussed in this section are myocardial contusion, pericardial tamponade, myocardial rupture, and traumatic aortic rupture.

Myocardial contusion

The clinical findings in myocardial contusion are often subtle and frequently overlooked for several reasons: (1) multiple injuries direct attention elsewhere; (2) often little evidence of thoracic injury is present; and (3) signs of cardiac injury may not be present on initial examination. Contusions to the myocardium are usually caused by a vehicle collision. In these cases the chest wall strikes the dashboard or steering column (sternal and multiple rib fractures are common). A deformed dashboard or steering column should alert the paramedic to the possibility of a cardiac injury. Blunt myocardial injury occurs in between 0% and 76% of blunt chest trauma victims, depending on whether the diagnosis was made clinically or at postmortem.[8]

Critical Thinking

How would you manage a cardiac rhythm disturbance resulting from a myocardial contusion?

The extent of injury may vary. The injury may be only a localized bruise or it may be a full-thickness injury to the wall of the heart with haemorrhage and oedema. Blood may accumulate in the pericardium (haemopericardium) as a result of a tear in the epicardium or endocardium. This, in turn, may result in cardiac rupture or a traumatic myocardial infarction. The fibrinous reaction at the contusion site may lead to delayed rupture or ventricular aneurysm.

Patients with a myocardial contusion may have no symptoms, or they may complain of chest pain similar to that seen with a myocardial infarction. Other signs and symptoms include ECG abnormalities, a new cardiac murmur, pericardial friction rub (late), persistent tachycardia, and palpitations. Emergency care for these patients is similar to that for myocardial infarction: oxygen administration, ECG monitoring, and pharmacological therapy for dysrhythmias and hypotension (see Chapter 15). Any intervention that increases myocardial oxygen consumption should be avoided.

Pericardial tamponade

Penetrating trauma (and, in rare cases, blunt trauma) may cause tears in the heart chamber walls. This allows blood to leak from the heart. If the pericardium has been torn sufficiently, blood leaks into the thoracic cavity and the patient rapidly dies from haemorrhage. Often, however, the pericardium remains intact. In such cases the blood enters the pericardial space, causing an increase in pericardial pressure. The increased pressure prevents the heart from expanding and refilling with blood, which results in a decrease in stroke volume and cardiac output. Myocardial perfusion decreases because of pressure effects on the walls of the heart, and decreased diastolic pressures. Associated ischaemic dysfunction may result in myocardial infarction. Pericardial tamponade occurs in fewer than 2% of patients who suffer chest trauma.[3]

Note

Penetrating injuries, such as those caused by some knife and gunshot wounds, may result in death from haemorrhage rather than tamponade. This happens when the wound is large enough that the pericardium cannot contain the blood in the pericardial space. Gunshot wounds have a higher mortality rate than stab wounds.[3]

At first, most patients with pericardial tamponade have peripheral vasoconstriction, so the diastolic blood pressure rises more than the systolic blood pressure, causing a decrease in pulse pressure. These patients manifest with tachycardia to compensate for the decrease in cardiac output. Up to this point, pericardial tamponade and haemorrhagic shock have similar signs, yet a key clinical finding often allows differentiation of the two forms of shock. This clinical finding was first described by Beck in 1935. It and two other clinical clues make up the Beck triad. The Beck triad is seen in only 30% of patients with pericardial tamponade.[3]

The Beck triad consists of elevated central venous pressure (evidenced by jugular vein distension), muffled heart sounds, and hypotension. The first element of the Beck triad, elevated central venous pressure, is the single best way to distinguish pericardial tamponade from haemorrhagic shock.[7] Other signs and symptoms of pericardial tamponade include the following:

- tachycardia
- respiratory distress
- narrow pulse pressure
- cyanosis of the head, neck, and upper extremities.

Note

Paramedics must keep in mind that problems other than pericardial tamponade can cause hypotension and elevated central venous pressure. The most common alternative causes are tension pneumothorax in trauma victims and cardiogenic shock. Patients with tamponade and haemorrhage may not have an elevated venous pressure at first.

Two other findings in pericardial tamponade may include pulsus paradoxus and electrical alternans. Pulsus paradoxus is a systolic blood pressure that drops more than 10–15 mmHg during inspiration compared with expiration (normally this drop is minimal). The excessive decline in systolic pressure occurs in cardiac tamponade when pleural pressure is reduced during inspiration. The reduction of pleural pressure provides some relief from the tamponade and causes the inspiratory fall in arterial flow and systolic pressure (pulsus paradoxus is difficult to measure in the prehospital setting). Electrical alternans refers to a change in the amplitude of a patient's ECG waveforms that decrease with every other cardiac cycle and is a rare finding in cardiac tamponade.

Pericardial tamponade is a true emergency. Pericardial blood must be removed in these patients and the bleeding must be stopped if the patient is to survive the injury. Prehospital management includes careful monitoring, oxygen administration, fluid replacement, and rapid transport to an appropriate medical facility. Treatment at the medical facility involves needle pericardiocentesis to remove blood from the pericardial sac. Removal of as little as 20 mL may drastically improve cardiac output.[3]

Myocardial rupture

Myocardial rupture occurs when blood-filled chambers of the ventricles are compressed with enough force to rupture the chamber wall, septum, or valve. The injury is nearly always immediately fatal, but death may be delayed for 2 to 3 weeks after blunt trauma.[3] Motor vehicle crashes are responsible for most cases of myocardial rupture, accounting for 15% of fatal thoracic injuries.[7] Other proposed mechanisms include the following:

- deceleration or shearing forces that disrupt the inferior and superior venae cavae
- upward displacement of blood (causing an increase in intracardiac pressure) after abdominal trauma
- direct compression of the heart between the sternum and vertebrae
- laceration from a rib or sternal fracture
- complications of myocardial contusion.

A significant mechanism of injury is often a factor in these cases. Also, signs and symptoms of congestive heart failure and cardiac tamponade are present. Prehospital care for these patients is mainly supportive and includes airway and ventilatory support and rapid transport for definitive care. It is crucial that paramedics consider the possibility of a tension pneumothorax in these patients. The signs and symptoms of tension pneumothorax mimic those of myocardial rupture with tamponade.

Traumatic aortic rupture

Traumatic aortic rupture is thought to be a result of shearing forces. These forces develop between tissues that decelerate at different rates. Common mechanisms of injury include rapid deceleration in high-speed motor vehicle crashes, falls from great heights, and crushing injuries. It has been estimated that one in six people who die in motor vehicle crashes has a rupture of the aorta.[7] Of these patients, 80–90% die at the scene as a result of massive haemorrhage. About 10–20% survive the first hour because the bleeding is tamponaded by the surrounding adventitia of the aorta and intact visceral pleura. Of these individuals, 30% have ruptures within 6 hours. For these reasons, rapid and pertinent evaluation and transport to an appropriate medical facility are critical. Aortic rupture is responsible for 15% of all deaths from blunt trauma.[3]

The usual site of damage to the aorta is in the distal arch. This is just beyond the takeoff of the left subclavian artery and proximal to the ligamentum arteriosum (Figure 27-12). The ligamentum arteriosum and descending thoracic arch are somewhat fixed, whilst the transverse portion of the arch is somewhat mobile. If shearing forces exceed the tensile strength of the arch, the junction of the mobile and fixed points of attachment may be partly torn. If the outer layer of tissue around the aorta remains intact, the patient may survive long enough for surgical repair.

Aortic rupture is a severe injury (the fatality rate is 80–90% within the first hour). Any trauma patient who has unexplained shock and an appropriate mechanism of injury (rapid deceleration) should be suspected of having a ruptured aorta. Blood pressure may be normal or elevated, with a significant difference between the two arms. In addition, upper extremity hypertension with absent or weak femoral pulses can occur in these patients (this is thought to result from compression of the aorta by the expanding haematoma). Other patients have hypertension because of increased activity of the sympathetic nervous system. About 25% of these patients have a harsh systolic murmur that can be heard over the pericardium or between the scapulae. In rare cases these patients may have paraplegia without a cervical or thoracic spine injury; this occurs as a consequence of decreased blood flow through the anterior spinal artery. The

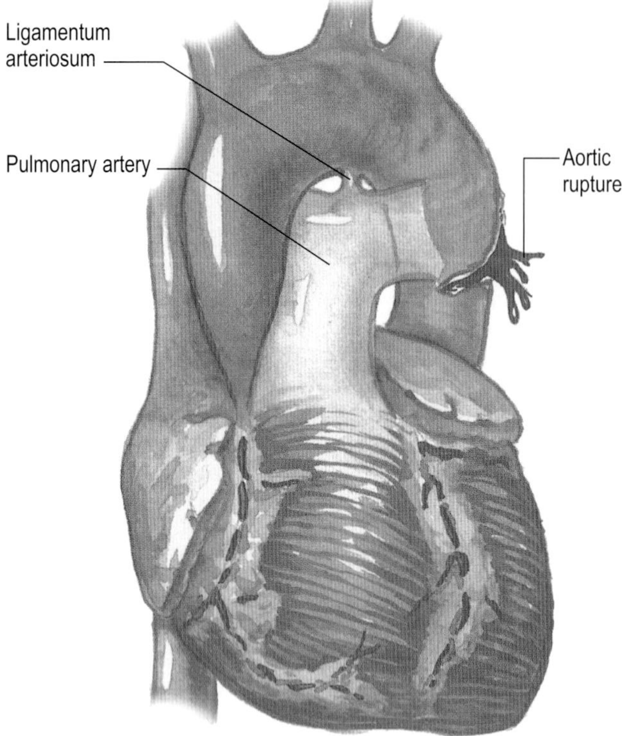

Figure 27-12 Aortic rupture.

anterior spinal artery is in the thoracic region and is composed of branches from the posterior intercostal arteries. These in turn are branches of the thoracic aorta.

Note

A difference in pulse quality between the arms and lower torso or between the left and right arms is sometimes detected with aortic rupture. Therefore, checking both radial and femoral pulses is important.[5]

Prehospital management of these patients includes alerting the hospital of the suspected rupture, administration of high-concentration oxygen, ventilatory support with spinal precautions, judicious fluid replacement (avoiding overhydration), and rapid transport for surgical repair.

Note

Fluid replacement should be limited in patients who have a stable blood pressure. This helps to prevent an increase in pressure in the remaining aortic wall tissue.

Penetrating wounds of the great vessels

Penetrating wounds of the great vessels usually involve injury to the chest, abdomen or neck. These wounds are often accompanied by massive haemothorax, hypovolaemic shock, cardiac tamponade, and enlarging haematomas that may cause compression of the vena cava, trachea, oesophagus, great vessels and heart. Prehospital care for patients with penetrating injury to the great vessels is directed at providing airway and ventilatory support, managing hypovolaemia with judicious fluid therapy, and rapid transport for definitive care.

Other thoracic injuries

Other injuries that may be associated with blunt or penetrating trauma to the thorax include oesophageal and tracheobronchial injuries (see Chapter 31) and diaphragmatic rupture.

Oesophageal and tracheobronchial injuries

Oesophageal injuries most often are caused by penetrating trauma (for example, these may be caused by projectile or knife wounds). They also can result from spontaneous perforation caused by cancer and from anatomic distortions caused by diverticula or gastric reflux, both of which can lead to violent vomiting.[3] Assessment findings may include pain, fever, hoarseness, dysphagia, respiratory distress and shock. If oesophageal perforation occurs in the cervical region, local tenderness, subcutaneous emphysema and resistance to neck movement may be noted. Oesophageal perforation that occurs lower in the thoracic region may result in mediastinal and subcutaneous emphysema, inflammation of the mediastinum and splinting of the chest wall.

Tracheobronchial injuries are rare, occurring in fewer than 3% of victims of blunt or penetrating chest trauma. However, the mortality rate for these injuries is over 30%.[3] Most injuries occur within 3 cm of the carina although they can occur anywhere along the tracheobronchial tree. Signs and symptoms of tracheobronchial injury include the following:

- severe hypoxia
- tachypnoea
- tachycardia
- massive subcutaneous emphysema
- dyspnoea
- respiratory distress
- haemoptysis.

Emergency care for patients with an oesophageal or a tracheobronchial injury is directed at providing airway, ventilatory and circulatory support, and rapid transport for definitive care at an appropriate medical facility.

Note

A tension pneumothorax that does not improve after needle decompression or the absence of a continuous flow of air from the needle after decompression should alert the paramedic to the possibility of a tracheobronchial injury.

Diaphragmatic rupture

The diaphragm is a sheet of voluntary muscle that separates the abdominal cavity from the thoracic cavity. Sudden compression of the abdomen (such as with blunt trauma to the trunk) results in a sharp increase in intra-abdominal pressure. When this occurs, the pressure differences may cause abdominal contents to rupture through the thin diaphragmatic wall and enter the chest cavity (Figure 27-13). Diaphragmatic rupture is detected more often on the left side than on the right side. However, rupture on either side may allow intra-abdominal organs to enter the thoracic cavity, where they may cause compression of the lung, resulting in reduced ventilation, decreased venous return, decreased cardiac output, and shock. Because of the mechanical forces involved, patients with diaphragmatic rupture often have multiple injuries.

Signs and symptoms of a ruptured diaphragm include abdominal pain, shortness of breath, and decreased breath sounds. If most of the abdominal contents are forced into the chest, the abdomen may have a hollow or empty appearance. Also, bowel sounds may be heard in the chest. Prehospital management includes oxygen administration, ventilatory support as needed (positive pressure may worsen the injury), volume-expanding fluids, and rapid transport with the patient in a supine position to an appropriate medical facility for surgical repair.

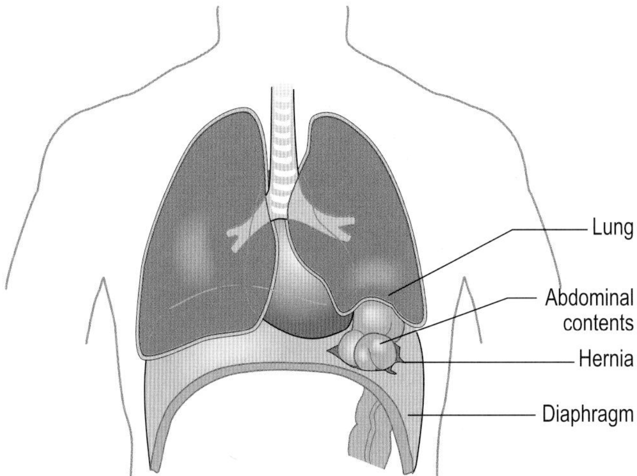

Figure 27-13 Diaphragmatic rupture. Sudden compression of the abdomen may increase intra-abdominal pressure, causing the abdominal contents to rupture through the thin diaphragmatic wall and enter the chest cavity.

Summary

- Thoracic injuries are caused by blunt or penetrating trauma. Such trauma is often caused by motor vehicle crashes, falls from heights, blast injuries, blows to the chest, chest compression, gunshot wounds, and stab wounds.
- Fractures of the clavicle, ribs or sternum, as well as flail chest, may be caused by blunt or penetrating trauma. Complications of skeletal trauma of the chest may include cardiac, vascular or pulmonary injuries.
- Closed pneumothorax may be life-threatening if (1) it is a tension pneumothorax, (2) it occupies more than 40% of the hemithorax, or (3) it occurs in a patient in shock or with a pre-existing pulmonary or cardiovascular disease. Open pneumothorax may result in severe ventilatory dysfunction, hypoxaemia, and death unless it is quickly recognized and corrected. Tension pneumothorax is a true emergency. It results in profound hypoventilation. It may result in death if it is not quickly recognized and managed. Haemothorax may result in massive blood loss. These patients often have hypovolaemia and hypoxaemia. Pulmonary contusion results when trauma to the lung causes alveolar and capillary damage. Severe hypoxaemia may develop. The degree of hypoxaemia is directly related to the size of the contused area. Traumatic asphyxia results from forces that cause an increase in intrathoracic pressure. When it occurs alone, it often is not lethal. However, brain haemorrhages, seizures, coma and death have been reported after these injuries.
- The extent of injury from myocardial contusion may vary. The injury may be only a localized bruise. However, it may also be a full-thickness injury to the wall of the heart. The full-thickness injury may result in cardiac rupture, ventricular aneurysm, or a traumatic myocardial infarction. Pericardial tamponade occurs if 150–200 mL of blood enters the pericardial space suddenly. This results in a decrease in stroke volume and cardiac output. Myocardial rupture is an acute traumatic perforation of the ventricles or atria. It is nearly always immediately fatal although death may be delayed for several weeks after blunt trauma. Aortic rupture is a severe injury. The mortality rate in the first hour is 80–90%. The paramedic should consider the possibility of aortic rupture in any trauma patient who has unexplained shock after a rapid deceleration injury.
- Oesophageal injuries most often are caused by penetrating trauma (e.g. projectile and knife wounds). Tracheobronchial injuries are rare (occurring in fewer than 3% of victims of blunt or penetrating chest trauma), but the mortality rate is over 30%. A tension pneumothorax that does not improve after needle decompression or the absence of a continuous flow of air from the needle after decompression should alert the paramedic to the possibility of a tracheobronchial injury.
- Diaphragmatic ruptures may allow abdominal organs to enter the thoracic cavity. There they may cause compression of the lung, resulting in reduced ventilation, decreased venous return, decreased cardiac output, and shock.

References

1. Hunt PA, Greaves I, Owens WA 2006 Emergency thoracotomy in thoracic trauma – a review. Injury 37(1):1–19
2. Borman JB, Aharonson-Daniel L, Savitsky B, Peleg K, the Israeli Trauma Group 2006 Unilateral flail chest is seldom a lethal injury. Emerg Med J 23:903–905
3. US Department of Transportation, National Highway Traffic Safety Administration 1998 EMT-paramedic national standard curriculum. US Department of Transportation, Washington, DC
4. National Association of Emergency Medical Technicians 2003 PHTLS: basic and advanced prehospital life support, 5th edition. Mosby, St Louis
5. Joint Royal Colleges Ambulance Liaison Committee 2006 UK Ambulance Service Clinical Practice Guidelines. JRCALC, London
6. Tyburski JG, Collinge JD, Wilson RF, Eachempati SR 1999 Pulmonary contusions: Quantifying the lesion on chest X-ray films and the factors affecting prognosis. J Trauma 46:833–838
7. Rosen P, Barkin R 2003 Emergency medicine: concepts and clinical practice, 5th edition. Mosby, St Louis
8. Bansal MK, Maraj S, Chewaproug D, Amanullah A 2005 Myocardial contusion injury: redefining the diagnostic algorithm. Emerg Med J 22:465–469

Further reading

Greaves I, Porter K, Garner J 2009 Trauma care manual. Oxford University Press, Oxford

CHAPTER 28

Haemorrhage and Shock

Chapter contents

Objectives

Upon completion of this chapter, the paramedic student will be able to:

1. Describe how to recognize signs and symptoms of internal or external haemorrhage.
2. Define shock.
3. Outline the factors necessary to achieve adequate tissue oxygenation.
4. Describe how the diameter of resistance vessels influences preload.
5. Describe the function of the components of blood.
6. Outline the changes in the microcirculation during the progression of shock.
7. List the causes of hypovolaemic, cardiogenic, neurogenic, anaphylactic and septic shock.
8. Describe pathophysiology as a basis for signs and symptoms associated with the progression through the stages of shock.
9. Describe key assessment findings to distinguish the aetiology of the shock state.
10. Outline the prehospital management of the patient in shock based on knowledge of the pathophysiology associated with each type of shock.
11. Discuss how to integrate the assessment and management of the patient in shock.

Key terms

disseminated intravascular coagulation A grave coagulopathy that results from the over-stimulation of the clotting and anti-clotting processes in response to disease or injury.

haemostasis The cessation of bleeding by mechanical or chemical means or by substances that arrest the blood flow.

pulse pressure The difference between systemic and pulmonic pressure.

Severe illnesses and trauma can threaten the normal internal environment of the body. During such events, the protective systems of the body try to compensate. They work to maintain cellular oxygenation. The paramedic must be able to integrate pathophysiological principles and assessment findings. This will help the paramedic to form a field impression and to implement a treatment plan for the patient with haemorrhage or shock.

Haemorrhage

Haemorrhage occurs when there is a disruption, or 'leak', in the vascular system. Sources of haemorrhage can be external or internal.

External haemorrhage

External haemorrhage results from soft tissue injury and accounts for over 1.2 million emergency department visits in the UK each year.[1] Most soft tissue trauma is accompanied by mild haemorrhage but does not usually pose a threat to life; however, it may carry major risks of morbidity and disfigurement. The seriousness of the injury depends on three factors: the anatomical source of the haemorrhage (arterial, venous, capillary), the degree of vascular disruption, and the amount of blood loss that the patient can tolerate.

Internal haemorrhage

Internal haemorrhage can result from a blunt or penetrating trauma, and may also result from acute or chronic illnesses. Internal bleeding that leads to an insufficient amount of circulating blood can occur in one of four body cavities: the chest, abdomen, pelvis and retroperitoneum. Internal haemorrhage is associated with higher morbidity and mortality rates than external haemorrhage. Signs and symptoms that can indicate significant internal haemorrhage include the following:

- bright red blood from mouth, rectum or other orifice
- coffee-ground appearance of vomitus
- melaena (black, tarry stools)
- haematochezia (passage of red blood through the rectum)
- dizziness or syncope on sitting or standing
- orthostatic hypotension (described later in this chapter).

> **Critical Thinking**
>
> Internal haemorrhage is associated with an increase in morbidity and mortality rates. Why do you think this is the case?

Physiological response to haemorrhage

The cessation of bleeding by chemical means is haemostasis. Clotting of blood is the initial response of the body to haemorrhage. This vascular reaction involves local vasoconstriction, formation of a platelet plug, coagulation, and the growth of fibrous tissue into a blood clot that permanently closes and seals the injured vessel. If haemorrhage is severe, these mechanisms can fail, which results in shock (hypoperfusion).

Shock

Shock is not a single event with one cause and one treatment; rather it is a clinical syndrome, which, if left untreated, may lead to death. Shock may be defined as:

> *acute circulatory failure with inadequate or inappropriately distributed tissue perfusion resulting in generalized cellular hypoxia.*[2]

Normal tissue perfusion requires an effective pump, an intact vascular system capable of constriction and dilatation, adequate circulating volume, and tissues able to extract and use oxygen and nutrients from the blood. If any of these components is impaired, blood flow to the tissues will become compromised, leading to tissue hypoxia, anaerobic metabolism and increased production of CO_2 and lactic acid. If left untreated, shock usually leads to death. The initial diagnosis is based upon clinical appreciation of inadequate organ perfusion and tissue oxygenation.

Shock can be classified into three main types:

- *Hypovolaemic shock*: loss of circulating volume from causes including haemorrhage, burns, diarrhoea, vomiting.
- *Cardiogenic and obstructive shock*: cardiogenic refers to a relative or absolute drop in cardiac output due to a primary cardiac disorder, whilst obstructive may be defined in terms of mechanical factors that interfere with filling or emptying of the heart and great vessels; e.g. tension pneumothorax, pericardial tamponade.
- *Distributive shock*: loss of vasomotor tone (neurogenic), presence of vasodilating substances in blood (anaphylactic), presence of inflammatory mediators (septic).

Hypovolaemic shock

Hypovolaemic shock is the most common clinical scenario in the prehospital environment and probably the most studied form of shock[3] and, as such, will be dealt with first. The body has many physiological responses to shock, knowledge of which is essential for its recognition and treatment.

Physiology of hypovolaemic shock

Compensatory mechanisms in shock involve many of the systems of the body, including the circulatory, respiratory and renal systems. The effect of haemorrhage on cardiac output and arterial pressure is illustrated in Figure 28-1.

Figure 28-1 illustrates that an average adult can lose around 10% of their blood volume without any adverse effects, but, as more blood is lost (10–25%) cardiac output falls but arterial blood pressure is maintained due to sympathetic-mediated increases in heart rate and vasomotor tone. Blood pressure can be maintained in the presence of a decrease in cardiac output for a short period of time. It is notable that cardiac output and tissue perfusion are compromised before evidence of hypotension can be detected.

Compensatory mechanisms

Within seconds of the onset of haemorrhage, the sympathetic-mediated responses of increased myocardial contractility, tachycardia, and vasoconstriction appear. Vasoconstriction largely affects the arterioles and veins – arteriolar vasoconstriction helps to maintain blood pressure by increasing vascular resistance, whilst venoconstriction mobilizes blood stored in the venous system. Remember that approximately 60% of blood is to be found in the venous system in normal health.[4] A further 350 mL of old blood can be mobilized from the liver.

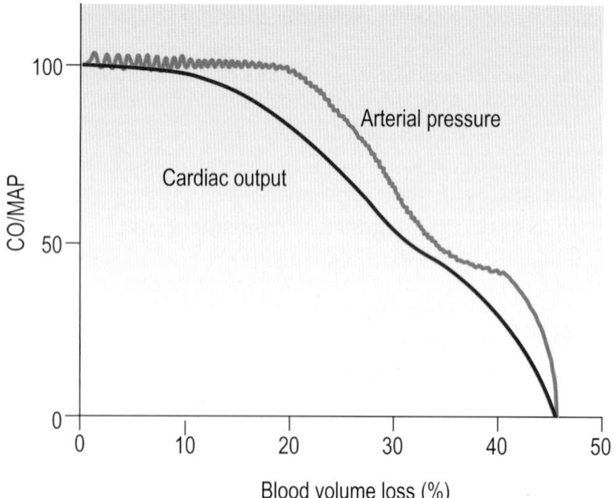

Figure 28-1 Effect of haemorrhage on cardiac output and arterial pressure. From Guyton AC, Hall JE 2005 Textbook of medical physiology, 11th edition. Elsevier Saunders, Philadelphia.

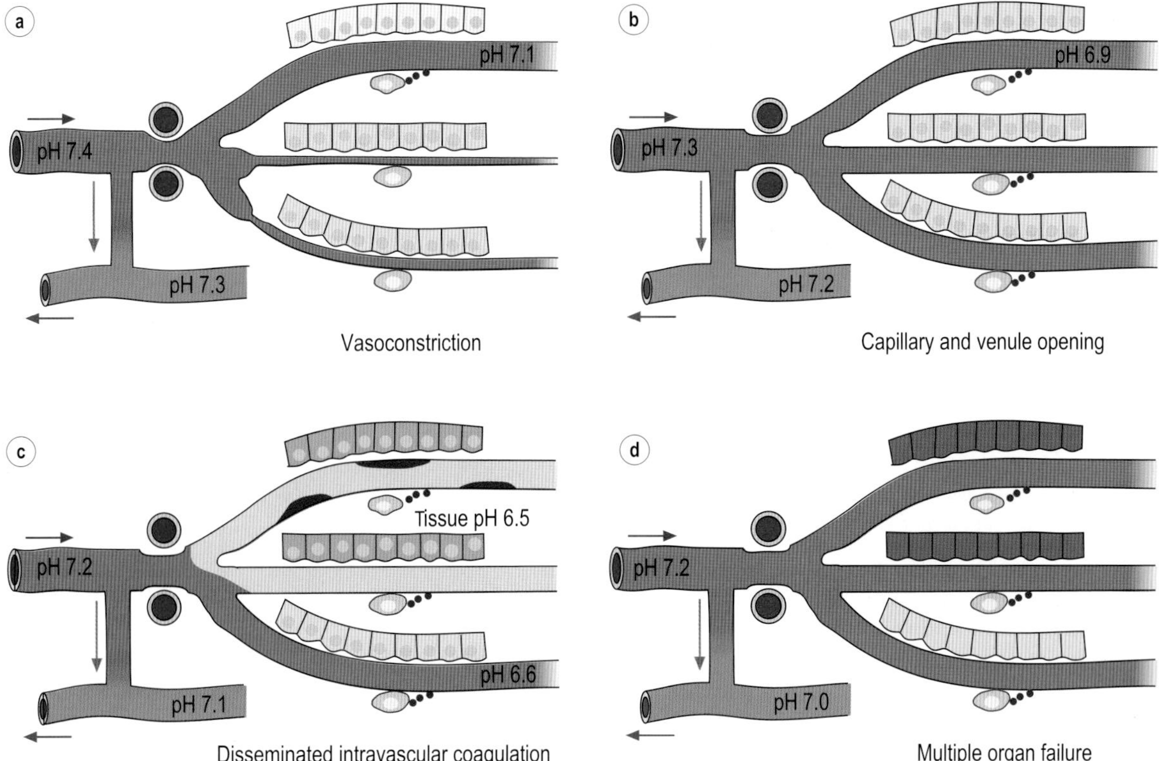

Figure 28-2 The effects of shock on the microcirculation.

During the early stages of shock, vasoconstriction causes a reduction in the size of the vascular compartment and an increase in systemic vascular resistance. If haemorrhage can be controlled at this stage, then this may be all that the body needs to do. However, if bleeding continues unhindered, then there will be further increases in heart rate, degree of contraction, and vasoconstriction. The vasoconstriction now targets the skin, skeletal muscles, kidneys and abdominal organs, which leads to anaerobic metabolism and production of lactic acid.

Further compensatory mechanisms work to restore blood volume by conservation of water and salts at the kidneys, reabsorption of interstitial fluid into the vascular compartment, and thirst. A decrease in renal blood flow activates the renin–angiotensin–aldosterone cycle, which enhances vasoconstriction and produces an increase in sodium and water reabsorption by the kidneys.

In addition to the cardiovascular response there will also be a respiratory response. Respiratory rate and depth will increase in an attempt to maximize oxygenation and eliminate CO_2, as well as trying to excrete the lactic acid generated by anaerobic metabolism.

All of these compensatory mechanisms can cope for short periods of time but have their limits. Prolonged activation of these mechanisms serves paradoxically to further injure the body. Intense vasoconstriction leads to a decrease in tissue perfusion, impairment of cellular metabolism, release of vasoactive mediators such as histamine, liberation of lactic acid, and cell death.[3] This means that once circulatory function has been re-established, the survival of the patient is going to be determined largely at a cellular level (Figure 28-2).

Trunkey (1983) suggested that deaths after trauma follow a trimodal distribution.[5] The first and largest peak, comprising 50% of the total, is seen immediately, or within seconds of injury; the second peak, 30% of deaths, occurs up to 4 h later, whilst the third group die after 4 h. Paramedics have generally seen their role as preserving the lives of those in the second category. What is becoming clearer is that the actions of paramedics in the early stages of care can influence the outcome of patients who survive the first hours and days after the insult.

Stages of hypovolaemic shock

The progression of hypovolaemic shock can be divided into four stages, although not all patients will present with the classic signs at each stage.

During stage I, the body is able to cope with the loss of blood and there are no serious effects. Stage II is the *compensatory stage* (Figure 28-3) – as the compensatory mechanisms are able to maintain arterial blood pressure despite the reduction in circulating blood volume. Stage III is the *decompensated stage* (Figure 28-4) where signs of falling blood pressure start to appear: blood pressure falls, there is a reduction in blood flow to the brain and heart, inflammatory responses lead to increased capillary permeability and leakage of fluid from the vasculature, and cellular damage occurs. Stage IV is considered to be *irreversible* (Figure 28-5). Although circulation may have been restored, the patient still goes on to die. The full mechanisms of this death are

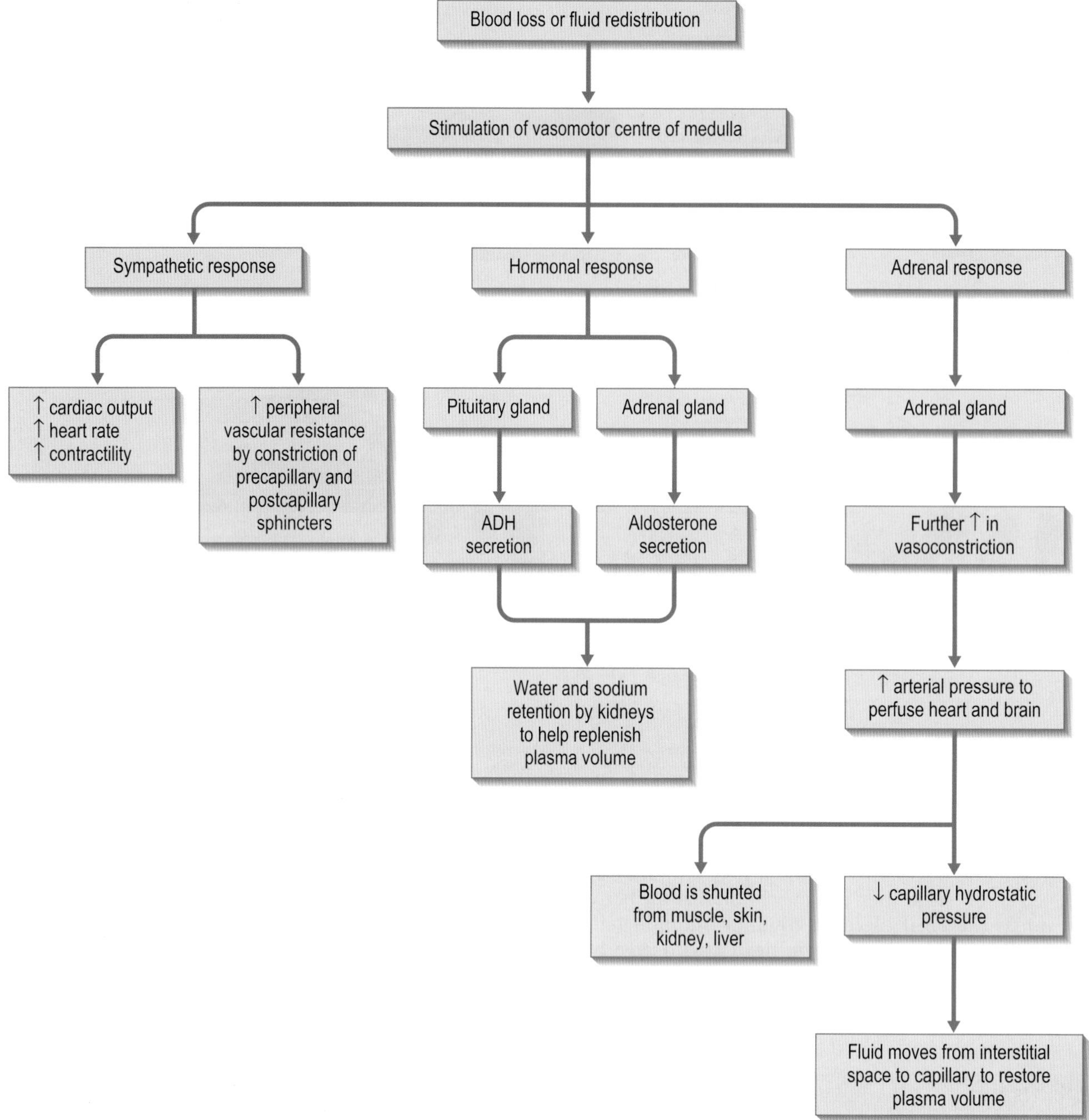

Figure 28-3 Compensatory shock. This stage of shock is reversible.

beyond the remit of this chapter but it is likely to be caused at the level of the microcirculation.

Table 28-1 shows the typical progression of shock through these stages.

Given that blood pressure is maintained until stage III, respirations, pulse rates and volumes, and capillary refill times are much more sensitive indicators of shock.

Caution

- The elderly tend to respond less well to haemorrhage than younger people and may display signs of shock in excess of the perceived blood loss.
- Young children compensate for longer but deteriorate more rapidly.
- Some very fit people compensate extremely well and may display few signs or symptoms even with significant blood loss. The lowest recorded resting heart rate belonged to five-time winner of the Tour de France, Miguel Indurain, at just 28 beats per minute.
- Some medications affect response to blood loss. Beta-blockers such as atenolol may blunt the normal tachycardia associated with haemorrhage.
- Those with pre-existing conditions such as ischaemic heart disease or pregnancy may be less able to cope with the effects of shock.
- Specific organ system affected.

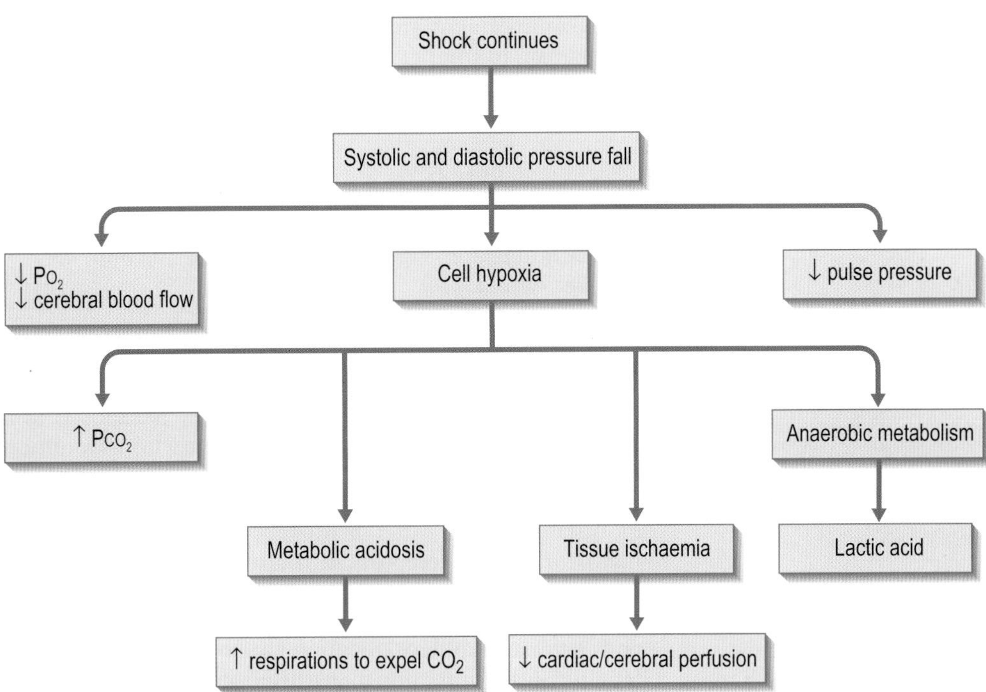

Figure 28-4 Decompensated shock. This stage of shock is reversible.

Table 28-1 Classification of stages of shock (adult)

Stage	Blood loss	Signs/symptoms	Urine output
I	Up to 750 mL (<15%)	Minimal – blood pressure normal, occasionally a tachycardia	Normal
II	750–1500 mL (15–30%)	Pale, tachycardia, narrowing pulse pressure, possible anxiety/aggression	20–30 mL/h
III	1500–2000 mL (30–40%)	Tachycardia >120 bpm, pallor, sweating, altered mental state (aggression, confusion, anxiety), hypotension, blood pressure does not drop until 30% of blood is lost	10–20 mL/h
IV	More than 2000 mL (>40%)	Tachycardia – weak and thready pulse, dramatic fall in systolic BP, narrowing pulse pressure, reduced level of consciousness	Negligible

Critical Thinking

What diseases can influence a patient's response to shock?

Obstructive shock

This term is used to describe shock that originates from mechanical obstruction of the flow of blood through the central circulation (great veins, heart or lungs),[3] and may also be referred to as cardiogenic shock. A number of conditions may cause obstructive shock and should be considered by the paramedic prior to intervention. Causes include tension pneumothorax, pericardial tamponade, dissecting aortic aneurysm, acute myocardial infarction, cardiac contusion, severe cardiac myopathy, or pulmonary embolism. The primary physiological result of obstructive shock is elevated right heart pressure and impaired venous return to the heart. Findings may include jugular venous distension (JVD), which helps differentiate it from hypovolaemic shock.

Cardiogenic shock affects around 5–10% of those hospitalized for acute myocardial infarction; the death rate is in excess of 80%.

Distributive shock

Distributive shock is characterized by loss of blood vessel tone, enlargement of the vascular space, and displacement of the vascular volume away from the heart and central circulation.[6] Expansion of the vasculature to this extent results in the failure of normal blood volume to fill the circulatory system. Venous return is also compromised, which precipitates a fall in cardiac output without a decrease in blood volume. This type of shock may be referred to as *normovolaemic* shock.

Loss of vessel tone may be caused by a decrease in sympathetic tone, or the presence of vasodilatory substances in the blood. It may also occur as a result of prolonged hypotension caused by haemorrhage, and forms part of the pathophysiology of irreversible hypovolaemic shock.

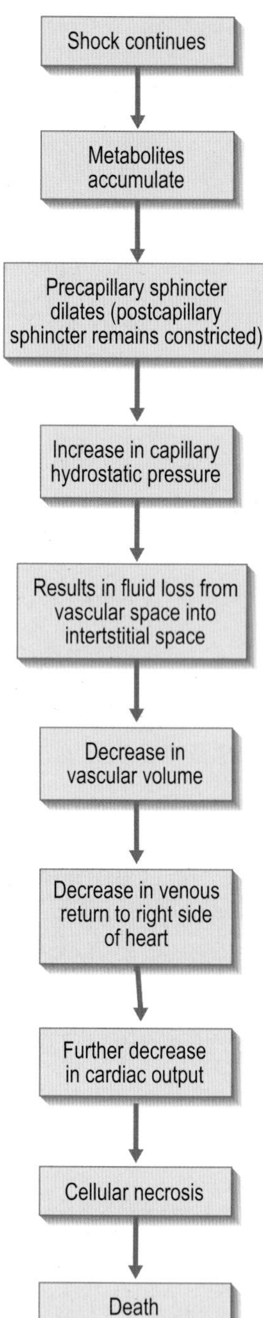

Figure 28-5 Irreversible shock. Regardless of fluid replacement and an initial favourable response in blood pressure, death will follow within 1 day to 3 weeks.

Three different shock states fall into the category of distributive shock:

Neurogenic shock

Neurogenic shock is also known as spinal cord or vasogenic shock. Neurogenic shock results from vasomotor paralysis below the level of injury, which leads to loss of vasomotor tone normally mediated by sympathetic nervous system. This results in a decrease in peripheral vascular resistance and an increase in the size of the container, so that normal intravascular volume is inadequate to fill the enlarged vascular compartment and perfuse the tissues. Because of the mechanism of injuries responsible for this syndrome, respiratory insufficiency, head injury, or both may be present.

> **Note**
>
> Fainting may be due to mild, readily reversible vasogenic shock. This shock can occur in the absence of injury. This shock results from bradycardia that produces a drop in cardiac output.

Anaphylactic shock

Anaphylactic shock occurs when the body is exposed to a substance that produces a severe allergic reaction. Common causes include antibiotic agents (especially penicillin), venoms and insect stings. The body responds to the release of histamine and other mediators. Histamine and other mediators act on receptors in the systemic and pulmonary microcirculation, and produce an effect on bronchial smooth muscle. Histamine causes arterioles and capillaries to dilate and increases capillary membrane permeability. Intravascular fluid leaks into the interstitial space and results in a decrease in intravascular volume. In addition, many of the mediators released cause constriction of the upper and lower airways, which creates the potential for complete airway obstruction (see Chapter 18).

Septic shock

Septic shock most often results from a serious systemic bacterial infection. Septic shock is thought to be caused by toxins that are a part of the microorganism (endotoxin – Gram-negative sepsis) or are released by the organism (exotoxin – Gram-positive shock). These toxins stimulate the release of complex vasoactive agents, which affect arterioles, capillaries and venules. They alter pressure in the microcirculation and increase capillary permeability. Septic shock can result from staphylococcal and streptococcal infections, pneumonia, postoperative infections, and infections from indwelling urinary catheters. Septic shock most often occurs in older adults (particularly nursing home residents), alcohol-dependent people, neonates, and patients who are immunosuppressed (e.g. patients with cancer, human immunodeficiency virus infection or sickle cell disease).

Management and treatment plan for the patient in shock

The management and treatment plan for the patient in shock focuses on assessment. The paramedic must assess oxygenation and perfusion of the body organs. The goals of the treatment plan are to ensure a patent airway, to provide adequate oxygenation and ventilation, and to restore perfusion.

Initial assessment

The initial assessment can help to identify whether cell perfusion is adequate. The following five-step description of the initial assessment focuses on evaluating the shock victim, but the paramedic should be aware of common objectives in evaluating any patient with other types of serious illness or injury:

1. Airway. The airway must be opened and patency must be maintained to ensure a pathway for adequate air movement. Follow a stepwise approach to airway management:
   - Consideration should be given to each procedure but steps may be omitted if deemed inappropriate.
   - All trauma patients should have high concentrations of O_2 administered.
2. Breathing. The respiratory pattern often reflects the adequacy of ventilation. Respiration can offer clues to the presence of shock; for example, if the patient is acidotic, the rate and depth of ventilation increase in an attempt to reduce carbon dioxide content of the blood and compensate for the metabolic acidosis.
3. Circulation. The paramedic should assess the patient's circulatory status. The first step is to check the patient for any uncontrolled arterial bleeding. In cases of external haemorrhage, applying direct pressure can almost always help to gain control (see Chapter 29 for ways to control external bleeding). This usually works until the patient can be taken to the emergency department for definitive care. Pressure dressings may also be applied to control haemorrhage. If the paramedic suspects internal bleeding, secure the airway, ensure adequate ventilation, and provide rapid transport to a proper facility. The paramedic should suspect internal bleeding in any trauma patient with signs of shock, especially trauma patients without evidence of external blood loss. Treatment for internal haemorrhage must be directed at definitive care to stop the bleeding, which is usually surgery, so rapid transportation to an appropriate facility is critical. Intravenous fluid therapy, if initiated in the field, should be performed en route to avoid a delay in definitive care.

Critical Thinking

Consider a patient with early signs and symptoms of shock. However, the patient's Sao_2 reading is normal. Should you administer oxygen?

The paramedic should evaluate the rate, character, and location of the patient's pulse as part of the circulatory assessment. Pulse rates increase fairly early in shock to help maintain adequate cardiac output. The contraction strength of the heart may also increase, although both of these attempts to maintain cardiac output may be negated by the decrease in preload. Tachycardia will not usually occur until the patient has suffered 10–15% volume depletion (relative to container size) as a result of blood loss or an increase in container size. The character of the pulse can be strong or weak and provides an estimate of the filling volume of the artery being palpated and an indirect measurement of systolic pressure.

Tissue perfusion can sometimes be estimated by evaluating the colour, moisture and temperature of the skin. These guidelines can be unreliable in patients who have been exposed to extremes of temperature, and those suffering from septicaemia or shock caused by neurological injury. An evaluation of the fingers and toes (the most distal points of circulation) is crucial as these areas may be the first to show inadequate tissue perfusion. If ambient temperatures are moderate and tissue perfusion is adequate, these areas will be pink, warm and dry.

The capillary refill test (described in Chapter 7) can offer useful details on the paediatric patient's tissue perfusion. These measurements should be used only as a guide, as accuracy of the test can be affected by the environment and by the patient's general health, age, and gender.

4. Disability. The evaluation of the patient's level of consciousness is crucial in assessing cerebral oxygenation. The patient can become restless, agitated and confused as cerebral ischaemia develops. In addition to shock, cerebral oedema and intracranial haemorrhage from head injury can compromise cerebral perfusion. Any significant change in the patient's behaviour or responses should be considered an indicator of a critical perfusion deficit to the brain. This is true whether the decrease in cerebral circulation is from shock or from an increase in intracranial pressure. The paramedic can measure the patient's level of consciousness with the AVPU (alert, verbal, painful, unresponsive) scale. Other evaluation methods are discussed in Chapter 31.

Note

Some practitioners believe that the level of consciousness and other indicators of adequate brain functions are the best way to determine appropriate blood pressure for the trauma patient. They contend that the brain is the organ most sensitive to changes in physiological state. The goals of this patient-focused method of shock management are to ensure that systolic pressure is at least 90 mmHg and that the patient has positive peripheral pulses and is awake or responsive to stimuli.[7]

5. Exposure of the body surfaces. The paramedic should expose the body surfaces in the initial assessment as indicated by situation or mechanism of injury. A visual inspection can reveal conditions that may be life-threatening that may otherwise be hidden by clothing.
6. Don't Ever Forget Glucose.

Differential shock assessment findings

Shock is assumed to be hypovolaemic until it is proved otherwise. However, assessment findings that can help the paramedic to differentiate between hypovolaemic shock and other causes of shock include the following:

1. *Cardiogenic shock.* The patient often has a chief complaint of chest pain, dyspnoea or extreme heart rates (tachycardia, bradycardia, other dysrhythmias). Some patients also show signs of congestive heart failure such as jugular vein distension (described in Chapters 15 and 27).
2. *Distributive shock* (neurogenic shock, anaphylactic shock, septic shock). The patient's history or situation may reveal a mechanism that suggests vasodilatation is

the cause of the shock state. Warm, flushed skin is a sign of distributive shock that would be unusual in the presence of hypovolaemic shock (especially in dependent areas). Those of neurogenic shock include a normal pulse rate (relative bradycardia).

3. *Obstructive shock* (caused by obstruction to blood flow). These patients are often victims of a major chest injury (usually a penetrating type of injury), or they reveal a history that is consistent with pulmonary embolism (for example, they have had recent surgery or a long bone fracture). Patients with cardiac tamponade or tension pneumothorax often have jugular vein distension, whilst those with tension pneumothorax almost always have decreased breath sounds on the affected side.

Detailed physical examination

As discussed, the first action is the initial assessment and management of any life-threatening conditions. The paramedic should then evaluate the patient further. A systematic approach offers a way to evaluate potentially life-threatening conditions and allows the paramedic to further assess the patient's perfusion status. This assessment should begin with baseline measurements of the patient's vital signs and evaluation of the patient's electrocardiogram.

Critical Thinking

Can blood donation cause a fluid deficit large enough to cause shock? If so, how is that fluid deficit managed?

The paramedic should expect the pulse rate to increase above normal limits after a fluid deficit of 10–15%. Some patients continue to have normal pulse rates even though a volume deficit of this extent exists; the patient's pulse rate should be only one factor in evaluating the patient's level of perfusion.

Bradycardia, which can result from hypoxaemia, existing neurological injury, increased vagal tone, pre-existing illness or prior medication use, can also indicate severe myocardial ischaemia – a primary cause of cardiogenic shock. Bradycardic rhythms often occur just before cardiac arrest. When a bradycardic rhythm is noted, the paramedic should optimize oxygenation by increasing the fraction of inspired oxygen and by assisting ventilations if needed.

The diastolic pressure at first rises as peripheral vascular resistance increases with increased vascular tone. These changes decrease the container size and serve to selectively shunt blood away from certain portions of the body. When the heart can no longer pump blood to keep the container full on the arterial side, the diastolic pressure begins to drop. The paramedic should expect this when blood loss is greater than 20–25% of normal circulating blood volume.

The systolic pressure falls when the heart can no longer pump enough blood to fill the container at the end of cardiac contraction. Systolic pressure is usually more sensitive to volume depletion than is diastolic pressure, therefore systolic pressure drops first. However, as the fluid deficit approaches 25%, systolic and diastolic pressures both begin to drop.

A fluid deficit can still exist even after the systolic pressure returns to normal following fluid replacement. Therefore fluid replacement initiated in the prehospital setting should continue until indicators of adequate tissue perfusion are present (e.g. improved skin colour, capillary refill of less than 2 s in paediatric patients, and normal pulse oximetry readings).

Resuscitation

Resuscitation of the shock victim is aimed at restoring adequate peripheral tissue oxygenation as quickly as possible. As previously stated, the paramedic accomplishes this by ensuring adequate oxygenation, maintaining an effective ratio of volume to container size, and rapidly transporting the victim to an appropriate medical facility.

Note

The over-resuscitation of trauma patients can occur. In patients with closed head injury or pulmonary or cardiac contusion, one must avoid fluid overload. Current guidelines should inform about fluid resuscitation for the shock patient.

Red blood cell oxygenation

Adequate oxygenation of red blood cells is required for adequate tissue oxygenation. For red blood cell oxygenation to be adequate, the patient must have a patent airway. Ventilation must also be supported with a high fraction of inspired oxygen. If needed, the paramedic can assist ventilation with positive pressure. In addition, any abnormality that interferes with adequate ventilation should be corrected (e.g. obstructed airway, pneumothorax, haemothorax, open chest wound, or unstable chest wall) (see Chapter 27).

Ratio of volume to container size

The second component necessary to maintain adequate oxygen-carrying capacity requires that the container be full of fluid. Currently the paramedic is not able to administer vasoconstricting drugs so cannot effectively treat distributive shock in the field. Volume replacement may be necessary in some patients but the use of fluids in prehospital management of serious trauma is a contentious issue.

Circulatory management

Circulatory problems should be managed immediately by

- Arresting external haemorrhage with the use of:
  - direct pressure
  - indirect pressure on proximal artery
  - tourniquet if exsanguinating
- Consider splinting:
  - major long bone fractures with various devices
  - pelvic fractures, e.g. triangular bandages, inverted Kendrick Extrication Device or pelvic straps.

Remember, uncontrolled or internal haemorrhage requires rapid transportation to an appropriate receiving centre.

Fluids

In prehospital care the most common emergency requiring fluid replacement is loss of volume caused by haemorrhage or dehydration. The type of fluid replacement needed depends on the nature and extent of the volume loss. The two main categories of fluids used in resuscitation are crystalloids and colloids, although UK paramedics no longer routinely use colloids. The paramedic should follow the recommendations for fluid resuscitation provided by JRCALC.

Crystalloids

Crystalloid solutions are created by dissolving crystals such as salts and sugars in water. These solutions do not have as much osmotic pressure as colloid solutions and can be expected to equilibrate more quickly between the vascular and extravascular spaces. Two-thirds of the infused crystalloid fluid leaves the vascular space within 1 h, so 3 mL of a crystalloid solution is needed to replace 1 mL of blood. Examples of crystalloid solutions are sodium lactate solution, normal saline, and glucose solutions in water.

Hypertonic solutions have higher osmotic pressure than that of body cells. They include 5% dextrose in 0.9% sodium chloride, 7.5% saline, and 5% dextrose in 0.45% sodium chloride. Hypotonic solutions have a lower osmotic pressure than that of body cells (e.g. distilled water and 0.45% sodium chloride).

Sodium lactate solution is currently the fluid of choice for resuscitating patients in shock.[8] The solution is well balanced and contains many of the chemicals found in human blood. Lactated Ringer's solution contains sodium chloride, small amounts of potassium and calcium, and 28 mEq of lactate, which can act as a buffer to neutralize acidity when metabolized by the liver. One-third of the infused solution remains in the vascular space after 1 h.

Normal saline contains 154 mEq/L of sodium but has no buffering capabilities. Although preferred by some physicians, the higher chloride content of normal saline is less desirable than the more balanced sodium lactate solution. As with sodium lactate, nearly one-third of the infused normal saline remains in the vascular space after 1 h. This makes it an equally effective volume expander. Studies have not shown superiority of one option over the other.

Glucose-containing solutions (e.g. 5% dextrose in water) have immediate volume expansion effects. However, the glucose leaves the intravascular compartment rapidly with a resultant free water increase. The volume-replacement benefits of glucose solutions only last 5–10 min while the glucose is metabolized. Thus use of 5% dextrose in water as a replacement fluid in volume deficits is inappropriate. Glucose solutions most often are used to maintain vascular access for administration of IV medications.

> **Note**
>
> Five percent dextrose in water is an isotonic solution. When administered, however, the dextrose molecules leave the circulation so rapidly that its effect is that of a hypotonic solution.

Colloids

Colloid solutions contain molecules (usually protein) that are too large to pass through the capillary membrane. These solutions exhibit osmotic pressure and remain within the vascular compartment for a considerable time. Examples of colloid solutions are whole blood, packed red blood cells, blood plasma, and plasma substitutes. Colloids are generally reserved for in-hospital use and are not recommended for prehospital management of shock.[9]

Plasma substitutes do not increase oxygen-carrying capacity by replacing red blood cells. They also do not improve clotting by the addition of plasma protein. Yet at times they are used to restore circulating blood volume as an emergency treatment for hypovolaemia caused by blood loss. Plasma substitutes such as dextran and hetastarch have osmotic properties similar to those of plasma, thus they stay in the intravascular space longer than crystalloid solution. Plasma substitutes do not carry the human immunodeficiency virus or hepatitis viruses, and do not require type and crossmatching before administration. Plasma substitutes do have some adverse effects, including increased bleeding tendencies and immune suppression. Emergency vehicles can carry plasma substitutes, but expense and storage issues make them impractical for general use in the prehospital setting.

> **Note**
>
> Oxygen-carrying blood substitutes (e.g. PolyHeme) are being studied. They may have future application in prehospital care for severely injured patients. These solutions contain haemoglobin from red blood cells (treated to destroy viruses). In addition, they are compatible with all blood types. They do not require refrigeration and can be stored up to several months.

Current research is looking into the administration of hypertonic saline dextran solutions in a single 250 mL bolus and suggests that early administration may down-regulate neutrophil–endothelial interaction; produce less capillary leak; less oedema; and better organ function. It also avoids the massive sodium and chloride overload associated with conventional fluid resuscitation. Results so far are encouraging and indicate that hypertonic saline and dextran needs to be administered early if it is to confer these advantages; if the evidence becomes overwhelming, the paramedic is in the ideal position to offer this treatment.

Fluid resuscitation in shock

The routine use of fluids in adult trauma patients is not currently supported by the literature, and has been shown to increase mortality in those with penetrating thoracic and abdominal trauma.[10]

Fluids may raise the blood pressure and cause dilutional coagulopathy, clot dislodgement, and fluid, sodium and chloride overload. Current thinking is that fluids should only be given when major organ perfusion is impaired. If there is visible external blood loss greater than 500 mL, fluid replacement should be commenced with a 250 mL bolus of crystalloid.[8]

The absence of central and peripheral pulses is an absolute indication for urgent fluid. If the patient has a carotid pulse but no radial pulse, then other clinical factors should also be considered before making a decision on fluid administration.

The presence of central pulses but absence of peripheral pulses is a relative indication for urgent fluid administration. Look for other indicators of tissue perfusion and visible or expected blood loss and base your decision on these findings.

If both central and peripheral pulses are present, there is no indication for immediate fluid resuscitation unless there are other signs of central hypoperfusion such as altered mental state, cardiac dysrhythmias, etc.[11]

Vital signs should be reassessed before any further fluid interventions are made.

Do not delay at scene for fluid replacement; wherever possible, cannulate and give fluid en route to hospital.

Theory of fluid flow

The flow of fluid through a catheter is related directly to its diameter (to the fourth power) and inversely related to its length. Therefore, a catheter with a large diameter has a much greater flow than a catheter with a small diameter; short catheters provide faster flow rates than longer catheters of equal diameter. Other factors that affect the flow of fluid include the diameter and length of the tubing, the size of the vein, and the viscosity and temperature of the IV fluid. (Temperature affects viscosity; warm fluids generally flow better than cold ones.) Pressure bags are available that pressurize the IV system to 300 mmHg to maximize the rate of fluid administration. Table 28-2 lists the maximum rate of fluid flow for various gauges of 2-inch Medicut catheters without pressure on the bag at a height of 1 m above the patient.[6] When aggressive fluid resuscitation is indicated, the paramedic should do the following:

- Use short, large-diameter catheters.
- Use warm fluids of low viscosity (if possible).
- Keep the tubing short, and pressurize the IV system.

Key principles in managing shock

The paramedic should follow these key principles as part of the plan for managing shock (Figure 28-6):

1. Establish and maintain an open airway.
2. Administer high-concentration oxygen and assist ventilation as needed.
3. Control external bleeding (if present).
4. If there is visible external blood loss greater than 500 mL, fluid replacement should be commenced with a 250 mL bolus of crystalloid. The IV administration of fluids in the prehospital setting should not delay patient transportation because crystalloid solutions cannot restore the oxygen-carrying capacity of blood. Generally, the patient is best served by rapid assessment, airway stabilization, immobilization and rapid transportation to an appropriate medical facility. JRCALC recommends that IV therapy for shock resuscitation be initiated en route to the hospital.[8]
5. Maintain the patient's normal body temperature. Patients in shock often are unable to conserve body heat and can become hypothermic easily. Be careful about over-warming the patient as this may induce peripheral vasodilatation, which will cause a fall in blood pressure.
6. In the absence of spinal or head injury and if hypovolaemia is suspected and ventilation is adequate, consider positioning the patient in the modified Trendelenburg position (legs elevated 35–45 cm).
7. Monitor cardiac rhythm and oxygen saturation.
8. Frequently reassess vital signs en route to the emergency department.

Table 28-2 Needle gauges and maximum fluid flow

Needle gauge*	Maximum fluid flow
18 Gauge	4.81 L/h or 80 mL/min
16 Gauge	7.45 L/h or 124 mL/min
14 Gauge	9.67 L/h or 161 mL/min

*Inside diameter.

Management of specific forms of shock

In addition to the general management appropriate for all shock victims, certain management guidelines are specific to each shock classification.

Hypovolaemic shock

The management of hypovolaemic shock is not considered complete until the volume is replaced and the cause or causes of shock are corrected. This includes crystalloid fluid replacement in cases of simple dehydration or volume replacement because of haemorrhage, definitive surgery, critical care support, and postoperative rehabilitation. The amount of fluid replaced in trauma is controversial and the paramedic should be guided by current best evidence and JRCALC guidelines.

Fluids should be administered according to best evidence and in keeping with current JRCALC guidelines. Aggressive fluid therapy may be warranted in certain circumstances but is not generally advocated in most cases of trauma. The short-term benefits that may be derived from aggressive fluid therapy in prehospital care are generally outweighed by the risks, especially in the presence of uncontrolled or internal haemorrhage. Fluid administration should be aimed at maintaining a radial pulse.

Cardiogenic shock

The key to achieving a good outcome in cases of cardiogenic shock is to undertake an organized approach that encompasses early diagnosis and treatment aimed at prompt initiation of therapy to maintain blood pressure and cardiac output.[12]

Therapy will vary according to the cause, so the paramedic should assess the patient to determine the most appropriate course of action. The most common cause of cardiogenic shock is myocardial infarction,[12] which requires rapid transportation to a centre with PCI facilities in accordance with local arrangements.[8] The use of fluids in the management of

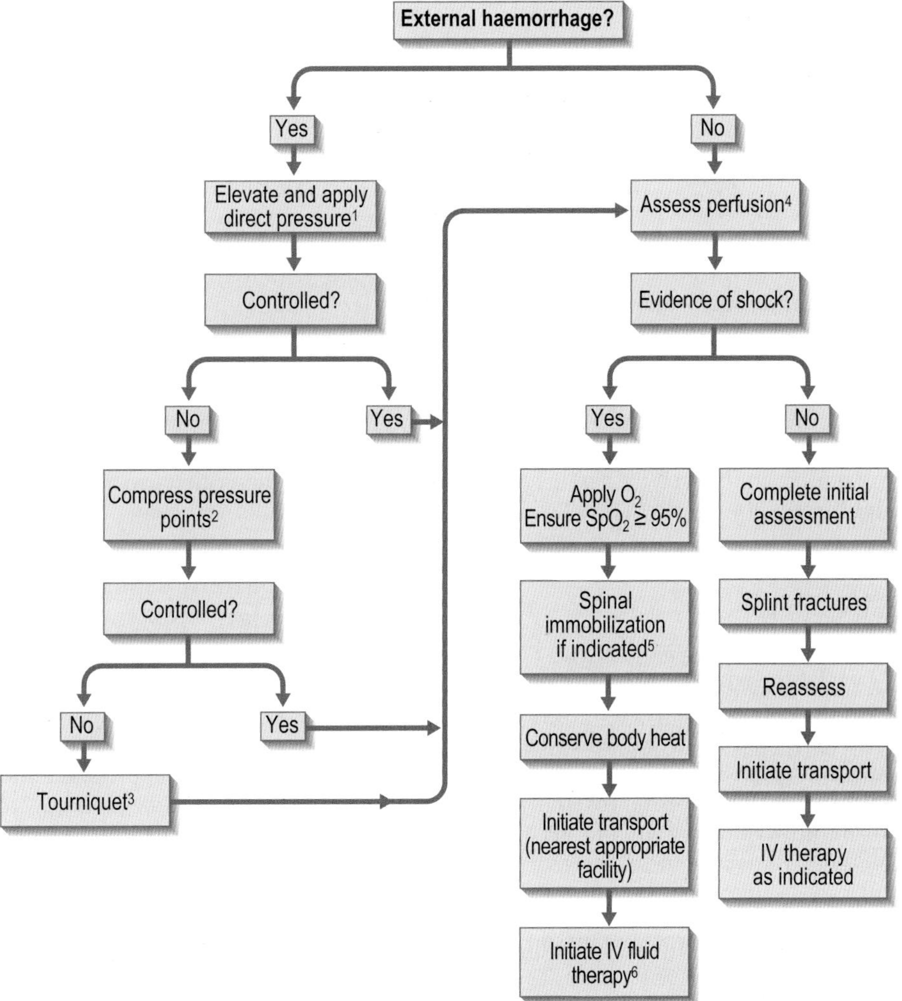

1 Elevation should be considered unless contraindicated by injuries
2 Apply pressure proximal to the bleeding site in one of the following locations: axillary artery, brachial artery, femoral artery, or popliteal artery
3 Tourniquet may electively be applied earlier in cases of catastrophic haemorrhage. Only appropriate arterial touniquets should be used or a manual blood pressure cuff inflated to above the systolic pressure
4 Assessment of perfusion includes presence,quality and location of pulses; skin colour, temperature and moisture; capillary refill time
5 See Chapter 32 for spinal immobilisation guidelines
6 Bleeding controlled:
- 250 mL boluses of IV crystalloid titrated against symptoms of shock
- In head injury, aim to maintain mean arterial pressure of 90 mmHg

Bleeding not controlled and **NO** penetrating injury to torso:
- 250 mL boluses of IV crystalloid titrated to ensure presence of RADIAL pulse. If RADIAL pulse present, do not administer fluids

Bleeding not controlled and penetrating injury to torso:
- 250 mL boluses of IV crystalloid titrated to ensure presence of CAROTID pulse. If CAROTID pulse present, do not administer fluids

Figure 28-6 Shock management algorithm.

cardiogenic shock is not advocated within the current guidelines and these should not be administered by paramedics in the prehospital phase of care.

Where there is evidence of an obstructive cause of cardiogenic shock, e.g. tension pneumothorax or pericardial tamponade (see Chapter 27), the paramedic should act accordingly.

Neurogenic shock

The management of neurogenic shock is similar to the management for hypovolaemia. However, the paramedic must take care during fluid therapy to avoid circulatory overload. Throughout the resuscitation phase, the paramedic should monitor the patient's lung sounds closely for signs of pulmonary congestion. In addition, patients in neurogenic shock may respond to the administration of vasopressors (e.g. dopamine), which are not currently used by paramedics. Atropine may be used if the patient is bradycardic but it is essential to rule out other potential causes first; e.g. severe hypovolaemia.

Anaphylactic shock

Intramuscular administration of adrenaline (epinephrine) is the treatment of choice in acute anaphylactic reactions (see Chapter 18). Depending on the severity of reaction, other treatment modalities can include oral, IV or intramuscular administration of antihistamines such as chlorphenamine. The paramedic can administer bronchodilators to treat bronchospasm and hydrocortisone to reduce the inflammatory response.

Crystalloid volume replacement may also be indicated. Crystalloids may compensate for the increased container size caused by vasodilatation resulting from histamine release during an anaphylactic reaction. Paramedics should anticipate the need for aggressive airway management in any allergic reaction (see Chapter 18).

Septic shock

With the exception of meningococcal septicaemia (see Chapter 24), septic shock usually takes some time to develop so is rarely seen in the prehospital phase. Depending on the patient's response to the infection, prehospital care may involve supplementary oxygen therapy, respiratory support, and fluid resuscitation if the transfer is likely to be delayed. If possible, the paramedic should obtain a thorough patient history, which will help to identify the cause of sepsis. Any immunocompromised group of patients has an increased risk of septic shock. Examples of such groups include those with human immunodeficiency virus infection, some cancer patients receiving chemotherapy, and patients with indwelling urinary or vascular catheters.

Integration of patient assessment and the treatment plan

The goals of prehospital care for the patient with severe haemorrhage or shock include rapid recognition of the event, initiation of treatment, prevention of additional injury, rapid transport to an appropriate medical facility by ground or air ambulance, and advanced notification of the receiving facility. The paramedic should follow guidelines established by local protocol and medical steering committees in determining the appropriate prehospital level of care for patients and in identifying the appropriate medical facility for patient transport.

Summary

- Shock is not a single event with one cause and one treatment; rather it is a clinical syndrome, which, if left untreated, may lead to death. It can be classified into three main types: hypovolaemic, obstructive and distributive.
- Shock may be defined as acute circulatory failure with inadequate or inappropriately distributed tissue perfusion resulting in generalized cellular hypoxia.
- Within seconds of the onset of haemorrhage, the sympathetic-mediated responses of increased myocardial contractility, tachycardia, and vasoconstriction appear. Vasoconstriction largely affects the arterioles and veins – arteriolar vasoconstriction helps to maintain blood pressure by increasing vascular resistance, whilst venoconstriction mobilizes blood stored in the venous system.
- Further compensatory mechanisms work to restore blood volume by conservation of water and salts at the kidneys, reabsorption of interstitial fluid into the vascular compartment, and thirst.
- Variations in the physiological response to shock can occur based on a number of factors. The patient's age and health are factors. The patient's ability to activate compensatory mechanisms plays a role. The specific organ affected is a factor as well.
- Obstructive shock is a term used to describe shock that originates from mechanical obstruction of the flow of blood through the central circulation (great veins, heart or lungs),[3] and may also be referred to as cardiogenic shock. Causes include tension pneumothorax, pericardial tamponade, dissecting aortic aneurysm, acute myocardial infarction, cardiac contusion, severe cardiac myopathy or pulmonary embolism.
- Distributive shock is characterized by loss of blood vessel tone, enlargement of the vascular space, and displacement of the vascular volume away from the heart and central circulation. Neurogenic, anaphylactic and septic shock all fall into this category.
- The management and treatment plan for the patient in shock focuses on assessment. The paramedic must assess oxygenation and perfusion of the body organs. The goals of the treatment plan are to ensure a patent airway, to provide adequate oxygenation and ventilation, and to restore perfusion. The initial assessment can help to identify whether cell perfusion is adequate.

References

1. Royal Society for the Prevention of Accidents, Home and Leisure Accident Statistics, 2002. Online. Available http://www.hassandlass.org.uk/ 16 February 2009
2. Hinds CJ, Watson D 1999 ABC of intensive care, circulatory support. BMJ 318:1749
3. Porth CM 2005 Pathophysiology, concepts of altered health, 7th edition. Lippincott, Williams & Wilkins, Philadelphia
4. Tortora GJ, Derrikson BH 2006 Principles of anatomy and physiology, 11th edition. Wiley, New York
5. Trunkey DD 1983 Trauma. Sci Am 249(2):20–27
6. Landry DW, Oliver JA 2001 The pathogenesis of vasodilatory shock. N Engl J Med 345:588–595
7. Criss E 1999 Trauma management in the new millennium. J Emerg Med Serv JEMS 24(12):34
8. Joint Royal Colleges Ambulance Liaison Committee 2006 UK Ambulance Service Clinical Guidelines. JRCALC, London
9. National Association of Emergency Medical Technicians 2003 PHTLS: basic and advanced prehospital trauma life support, 5th edition. Mosby, St Louis
10. Turner J, Nicholl J, Webber L, Cox H, Dixon S, Yates D 2000 A randomised controlled trial of prehospital intravenous fluid replacement therapy in serious trauma. Health Technol Assess 4(31):1–57
11. Revell M, Porter K, Greaves I 2002 Fluid resuscitation in prehospital trauma care: a consensus view. Emerg Med J 19:494–498
12. Hollenberg SM, Kavinsky CJ, Parrillo JE 1999 Cardiogenic shock. Ann Intern Med 131:47–59

CHAPTER **29**

Soft Tissue Trauma

Chapter contents

Objectives

Upon completion of this chapter, the paramedic student will be able to:

1. Describe the pathophysiological responses to soft tissue injury.
2. Discuss pathophysiology as a basis for key signs and symptoms, and describe the mechanism of injury and signs and symptoms of specific soft tissue injuries.
3. Outline management principles for prehospital care of soft tissue injuries.
4. Describe, in the correct sequence, patient management techniques for control of haemorrhage.
5. Identify the characteristics of general categories of dressings and bandages.
6. Describe prehospital management of specific soft tissue injuries not requiring closure.
7. Discuss factors that increase the potential for wound infection.
8. Describe the prehospital management of selected soft tissue injuries.

Key terms

abrasion A partial-thickness injury caused by scraping or rubbing away of a layer or layers of skin.

amputation A complete or partial loss of a limb caused by mechanical force.

avulsion A full-thickness skin loss in which the wound edges cannot be approximated.

compartment syndrome The result of a crush injury, usually caused by compressive forces or blunt trauma to muscle groups confined in tight fibrous sheaths with minimal ability to stretch.

crush injury Injury from exposure of tissue to a compressive force sufficient to interfere with the normal structure and metabolic function of the involved cells and tissues.

crush syndrome A life-threatening and sometimes preventable complication of prolonged immobilization; a pathological process that causes destruction, alteration, or both of muscle tissue.

haematoma A closed injury characterized by blood vessel disruption and swelling beneath the epidermis.

puncture wound An open injury that results from contact with a penetrating object.

rhabdomyolysis An acute, sometimes fatal, disease characterized by destruction of skeletal muscle.

The skin and its accessory organs are the primary cosmetic structures of the body. These structures perform many functions that are critical to survival. The paramedic must understand soft tissue trauma fully in order to assess life-threatening injury quickly. This understanding will also help the paramedic to intervene to promote normal healing and function.

Pathophysiology

Surface trauma can disrupt the normal distribution of body fluids and electrolytes, and can interfere with the maintenance of body temperature. The two physiological responses to surface trauma are vascular and inflammatory reactions, which can lead to healing, scar formation, or both. The extent and success of these responses are influenced by the amount of tissue that has been disrupted. Before exploring the haemostasis of wound healing, it may be advisable to review the normal anatomy and physiology of the integumentary system.

Haemostasis of wound healing

As described in Chapter 28, haemostasis is the initial physiological response to wounding. This vascular reaction involves vasoconstriction, formation of a platelet plug, coagulation, and the growth of fibrous tissue into the blood clot that permanently closes and seals the injured vessel.

In response to injury, severed blood vessels constrict and retract with the aid of the surrounding subcutaneous tissues. The vasoconstriction response is usually sustained for as long as 10 min, during which time blood coagulation mechanisms are activated to produce a blood clot. Platelets adhere to injured blood vessels and to collagen in the connective tissue that surrounds the injured vessel. As platelets contact collagen, they swell, become sticky, and secrete chemicals that activate other surrounding platelets. This process causes the platelets to adhere to one another and creates a platelet plug in the injured vessel. If the opening in the vessel wall is small, the plug may be sufficient to stop blood loss completely. For larger wounds, however, a blood clot is necessary to arrest the flow of blood (Figure 29-1).

Blood coagulation occurs as a result of a chemical process that begins within seconds of a severe vessel injury and within 1–2 min of a minor wound. Coagulation progresses rapidly; within 3–6 min after the rupture of a vessel, the entire end of the vessel is filled with a clot. Within 30 min the clot retracts and the vessel is sealed further. The blood-clotting mechanism is a complex process and includes the following three mechanisms:

1. Prothrombin activator is formed in response to rupture or damage of the blood vessel.
2. Prothrombin activator stimulates the conversion of prothrombin to thrombin.
3. Thrombin acts as an enzyme to convert fibrinogen into fibrin threads. These threads entrap platelets, blood cells, and plasma to form the clot.

The process of haemostasis is usually protective and is required for survival. In some instances, though, haemostasis can result in responses that threaten life and function. For example, blood clots that form in atherosclerotic vessels can lead to myocardial infarction or stroke (see Chapter 15).

Certain diseases or genetic factors that interrupt the clotting process (also referred to as the clotting cascade) can impair haemostasis and retard the process of clot formation. Examples include haemophilia, thrombocytopenia (low platelet count), and liver disease, which affects the production of clotting factors. Various drugs can also impair coagulation. Aspirin decreases platelet activity and warfarin suppresses the ability of the liver to make certain clotting factors. In any patient with impaired haemostasis, even minor trauma can result in uncontrollable and life-threatening haemorrhage.

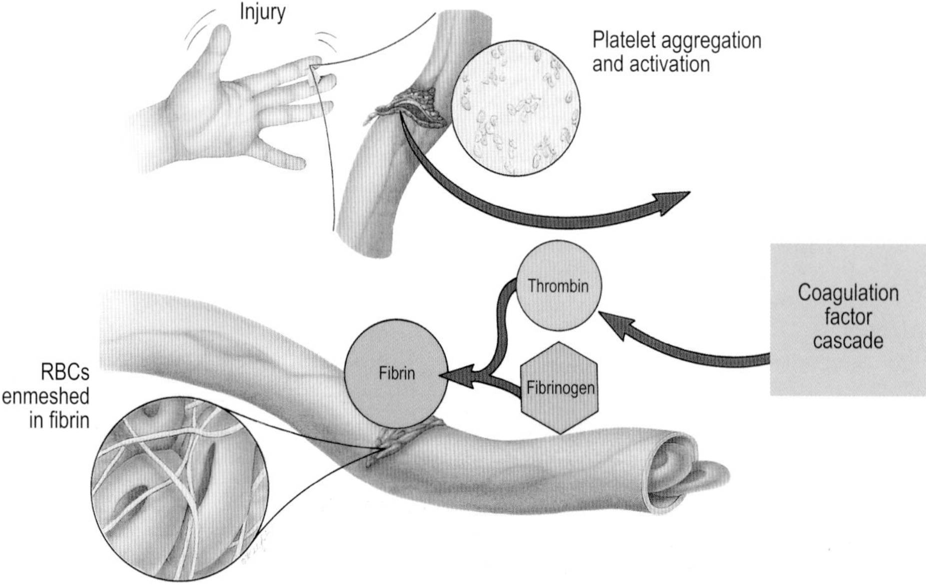

Figure 29-1 The complex clotting mechanism can be distilled into three basic steps: release of platelet factors at the injury site, formation of thrombin, and trapping of red blood cells in fibrin to form a clot.

Critical Thinking

List some drugs that may impair the normal clotting functions.

Inflammatory response

The release of chemicals from the injured vessel and various blood components (platelets, white blood cells) causes localized vasodilatation of arterioles, precapillary sphincters, and venules, increasing the permeability of the affected capillaries and vessels. Plasma, plasma proteins, electrolytes and chemical substances from the leaking venules accumulate in the extracellular space for about 72 h after the injury. Blood flow increases to the area of injury in order to supply the metabolic demands of the tissues during healing and results in the redness, swelling and pain associated with inflammation.

The transportation of granulocytes, lymphocytes, and macrophages to the injured area also increases local blood flow. These specialized cells prepare the wound for healing. They clear foreign bodies and dead tissue, and trigger neovascularization (new vessel formation). Within 12 h of the injury, new epithelial cells are regenerated (this is the epithelialization phase). These cells begin the process of healing through the re-establishment of skin layers (Figure 29-2).

Collagen is the main structural protein of most body tissues. The normal repair of tissues depends on collagen synthesis and deposition. In the healthy body, fibroblasts synthesize and deposit collagen within 48 h after injury. Collagen increases the tensile strength of the tissue although most injured tissue will not regain its full strength and function until at least 4 months later.[1]

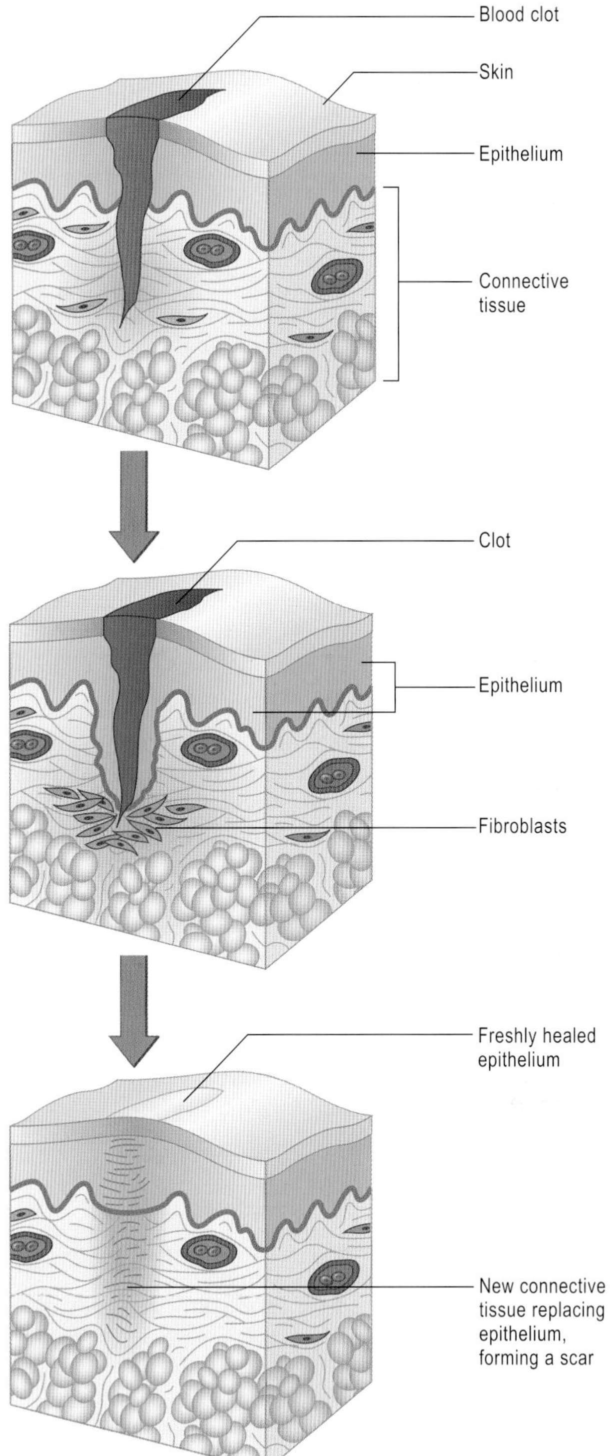

Figure 29-2 Healing of a minor wound.

Alterations of wound healing

Many factors can affect or alter wound healing. These include anatomical factors, concurrent drug use, medical conditions and disease, and wounds that are high-risk.

Anatomical factors

Some tissues of the body heal better and faster than others because of the body region and the amount of tension on the tissues (lines of tension). The elasticity of the skin and lines of tension vary in different areas of the body. Moreover, they are affected by muscular contraction and the body movements of flexion and extension, thus these factors affect wound healing and scar formation. For example, a soft tissue injury to the forearm generally heals better and faster than one over a joint. Other anatomical factors that may adversely affect wound healing and scar formation include oily skin and pigmentation.

Concurrent drug use, existing medical conditions and disease

Certain factors can delay or interfere with the normal wound-healing process through various mechanisms. For instance, a patient's concurrent drug use can interfere with or delay this process, as can certain pre-existing medical conditions. In addition, disease can delay or interfere with the process. Common drugs that can alter wound healing include corticosteroids, non-steroidal anti-inflammatory drugs (aspirin), penicillin, anticoagulants and antineoplastic agents. Medical conditions and diseases that can result in delayed healing include the following:

- advanced age (not in itself a medical condition)
- severe alcoholism
- acute uraemia

- diabetes
- hypoxia
- peripheral vascular disease
- malnutrition
- advanced cancer
- hepatic failure
- cardiovascular disease.

High-risk wounds

High-risk wounds have an increased potential for infection because of the location of the wound or the nature of the wounding force. Examples of high-risk wounds include those located on or near the hands, feet, and perineal areas. Wound forces that are associated with a high risk for infection include those produced by human and animal bites, foreign bodies, and injection (e.g. high-pressure grease guns). Other high-risk wounds are those contaminated with organic material or that have a significant amount of dead (devitalized) tissue, crush wounds, and any wounds in patients who are immunocompromised or who have poor peripheral circulation.

Abnormal scar formation

Abnormal scar formation can result in a keloid or hypertrophic scar. A keloid is the excessive accumulation of scar tissue that extends beyond the original wound borders and is more common in darkly pigmented patients. The scar is also more common in those who have injuries to the ears, upper extremities, lower abdomen or sternum. A hypertrophic scar has an excess accumulation of scar tissue within the original wound borders. This scar is more common in areas of high tissue stress such as the flexion creases across joints.

Wounds requiring closure

Although all serious wounds should be evaluated by a physician, the paramedic should expect the following types of wounds to require closure:

- wounds to cosmetic regions (e.g. face, lips and eyebrows)
- gaping wounds
- wounds over tension areas (e.g. joints)
- degloving injuries (described later in this chapter)
- ring finger injuries
- skin tearing.

Many techniques are used to close a wound, including suture, tape, staples and tissue adhesives.

Pathophysiology and assessment of soft tissue injuries

Soft tissue injuries are classified as closed or open. This classification depends on the absence or presence of a break in the continuity of the epidermis. Soft tissue wounds are often the most evident injury; however, they are generally considered low-priority injuries, unless life-threatening haemorrhage or associated airway compromise is present.

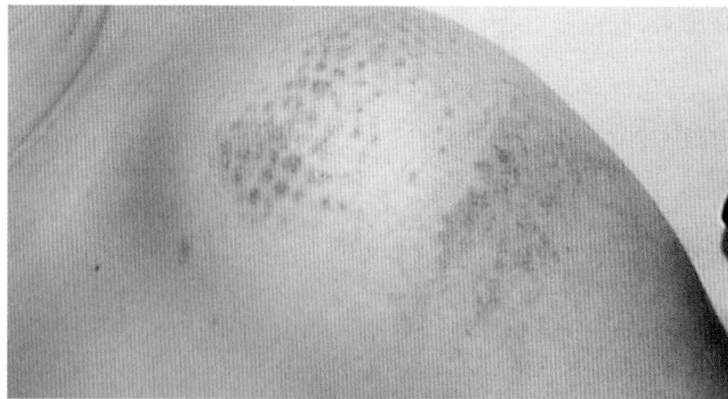

Figure 29-3 Spotty bruising on a well-padded part of the shoulder.

Closed wounds

Closed soft tissue injuries are usually associated with little blood loss. However, some of these injuries can cause significant haemorrhage in the cavities of the thorax, abdomen, pelvis, or soft tissues of the legs. This text classifies closed wounds as contusion, haematoma and crush injury.

Contusions and hematomata

Blunt trauma causes contusions and haematoma. A contusion is characterized by blood vessel disruption beneath the epidermis and results in swelling, pain, and ecchymosis (bruising) that can occur 24–48 h after the injury. A haematoma is a collection of blood beneath the skin and may occur with a contusion. However, the haematoma represents a larger amount of tissue damage and the disruption of larger vessels (Figure 29-3). These wounds are usually superficial, though they may be associated with underlying fractures, vascular involvement, and significant haemorrhage.

Crush injury

Crush injury can occur when a crushing force is applied to a body area (Figure 29-4) These injuries can be severe and may be associated with internal organ rupture, major fractures, and haemorrhagic shock. Overlying skin may remain intact with crush injury, even in the presence of severe injury and shock. Crush injuries are described further later in this chapter.

Critical Thinking

What are some mechanisms of crush injury?

Open wounds

Open soft tissue injuries are classified as abrasion, laceration, puncture, avulsion, amputation and bites.

Abrasion

An abrasion is a partial-thickness skin injury that is caused by the scraping or rubbing away of a layer or layers of skin (Figure 29-5). The wound usually results from friction with a hard object or surface, for example, abrasions occur in sports injuries and motorcycle crashes. Although these wounds are often superficial, they are painful and are at high risk for infection from contamination.

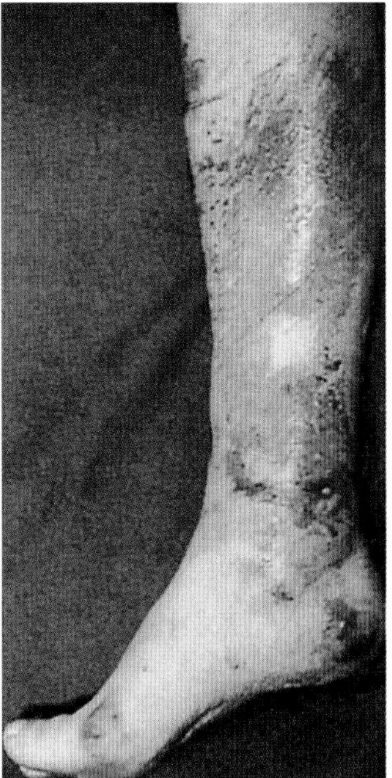

Figure 29-4 Appearance of a woman's leg after it had been run over by the wheel of a milk van.

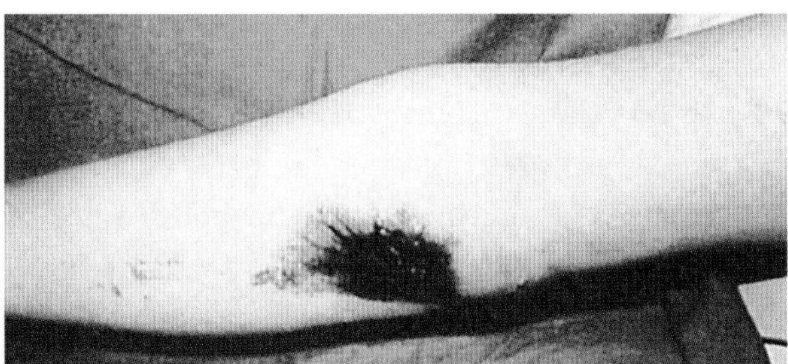

Figure 29-5 Deep abrasion caused by a fall from a bicycle.

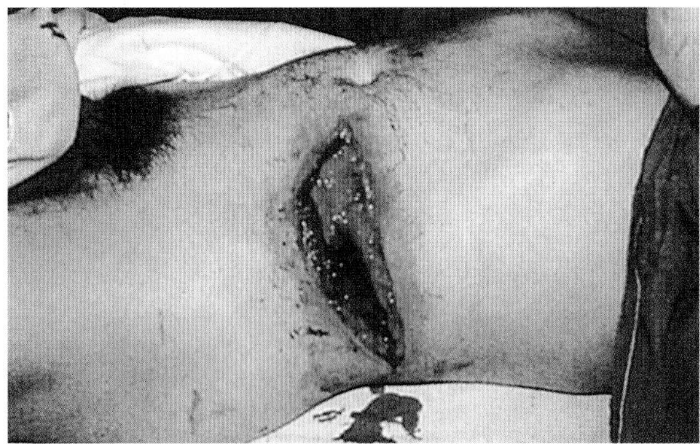

Figure 29-6 Large wound caused by a broken power saw.

Laceration

A laceration results from a tear, a split, or an incision of the skin (Figure 29-6). Lacerations are most often caused by a knife or other sharp object, resulting in a linear wound or incision. The sizes and depths of lacerations vary greatly depending on the injury sites and wounding mechanism. Lacerations can be sources of significant bleeding.

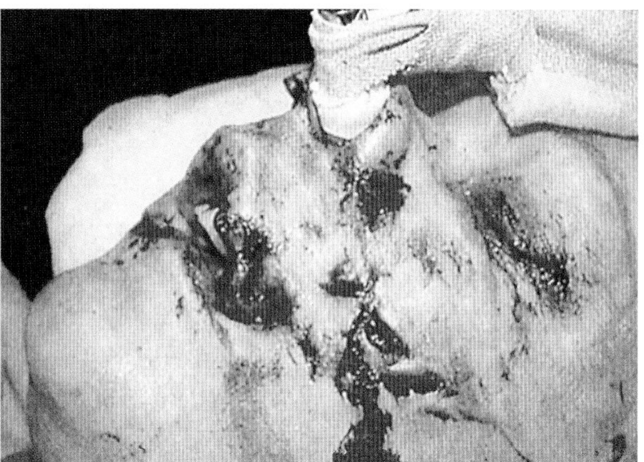

Figure 29-7 Puncture wounds caused by broken glass from a shattered windscreen.

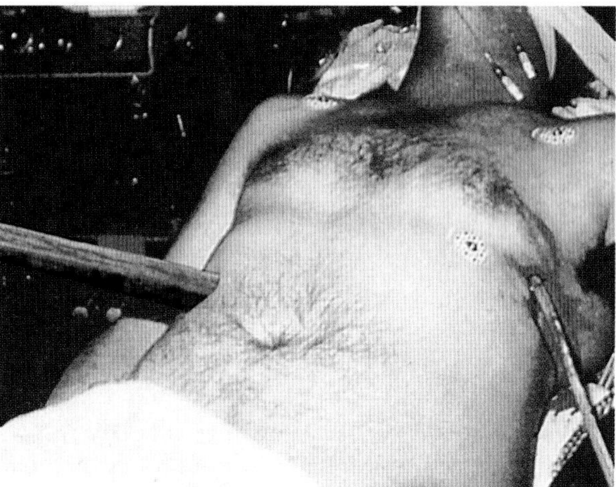

Figure 29-8 Piece of wood impaled in the right side of the chest, piercing the diaphragm and lacerating the spleen, stomach and liver.

Puncture

Contact with a sharp, pointed object commonly causes a puncture wound (Figure 29-7). (Examples of such objects include a wooden splinter, needle, staple, glass or nail.) The entrance wound is generally small yet these injuries may often be associated with deep penetration and injury to underlying tissues. Punctures can be hard to assess in the prehospital setting. Even an injury that appears to be minor can conceal a considerable amount of internal damage.

In some penetrating injuries, the object remains embedded or impaled in the wound (Figure 29-8). If this occurs to the chest or abdomen, severe bleeding can occur, as well as major underlying damage to internal organs. Examples include the following:

- chest injury
- pneumothorax (simple, open, tension)
- haemothorax
- pericardial tamponade
- penetrating heart wound

- rupture of the oesophagus, aorta, diaphragm, main stem bronchus
- abdominal injury
- hollow and solid organ damage
- peritonitis (bacterial, chemical)
- evisceration.

Critical Thinking

Why should a person always seek medical care to have a penetrating object removed?

The injection of a substance into the body under high pressure can also cause a puncture wound (Figure 29-9). (Examples include grease, paint, turpentine, dry-cleaning fluids and molten plastics.) These injuries often have life- or limb-threatening potential and require rapid surgical decompression and débridement. They are usually associated with minimal bleeding and may not appear serious. Numbness and blanching of the involved area often occur because of increased tissue pressure of the injected substance. Most patients with injection injuries are surgical emergencies and are at high risk for developing compartment syndrome. Definitive care for injection injuries usually requires surgery and hospitalization to prevent infection. Amputation may be needed if treatment is delayed.

Avulsion

An avulsion is a full-thickness skin loss (Figure 29-10) in which the wound edges cannot be approximated. Frequently involved body areas are the ear lobes, nose tip and fingertips. A common cause of avulsion injury is industrial equipment, such as meat slicers or sawing devices, but they may also be seen following domestic violence, such as human bites.

A degloving injury is a type of avulsion in which shearing forces separate the skin from the underlying tissues (Figure 29-11). A common cause of such an injury is industrial machinery. This machinery may entangle an extremity, producing circumferential tearing. Another common cause is finger jewellery that gets caught on a stationary object, which then produces a shearing of the soft tissue and possibly of the bone of the digit. Another common cause is machinery that entraps hair, resulting in scalp avulsion. Degloving injuries are sometimes associated with underlying skeletal damage and with massive loss of tissue in the affected area. Bleeding can be significant.

Amputation

Traumatic amputation involves a complete or partial loss of a limb by a mechanical force (Figure 29-12). The digits, lower leg, hand and forearm, and the distal part of the foot are most often injured in this way. Bleeding is a possible fatal complication of an amputation injury. In cases in which a complete amputation has occurred, injured arteries often retract so that haemorrhage may be less severe than in partial amputation injuries.

Bites

An animal or human bite wound is frequently a combination of puncture, laceration, avulsion and crush injury (Figure 29-13). The pressure from a bite can be as great as 2750 kPa and can involve deep structures such as tendons,

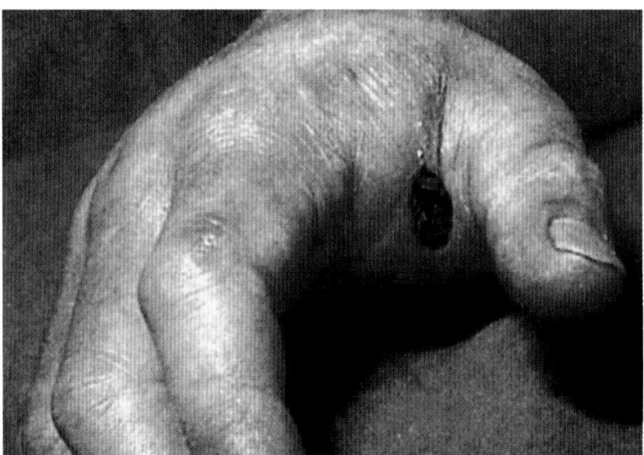

Figure 29-9 Injection of paraffin into the hand resulted in amputation of the index finger.

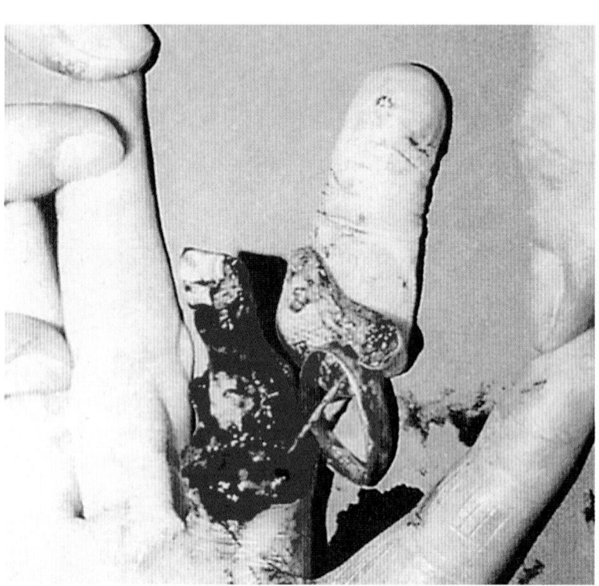

Figure 29-10 Ring avulsion injury.

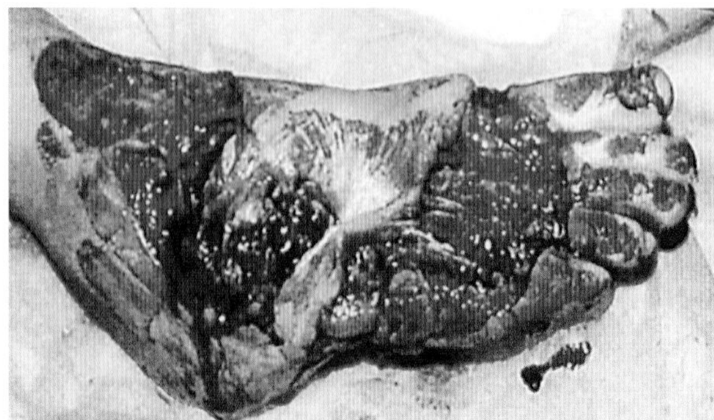

Figure 29-11 Degloving injury of the foot.

muscles and bones. Complications from bite wounds, particularly human bites, include abscesses, lymphangitis (inflammation of lymph vessels), cellulitis, osteomyelitis, tenosynovitis, tuberculosis, hepatitis B and tetanus. Although it is theoretically possible for a human bite to transmit human immunodeficiency virus, the potential for salivary transmission of the virus is remote.[2] Other less common complications of mammalian bites include the transmission of diseases such as actinomycosis and syphilis. All patients who have been bitten should seek physician evaluation.

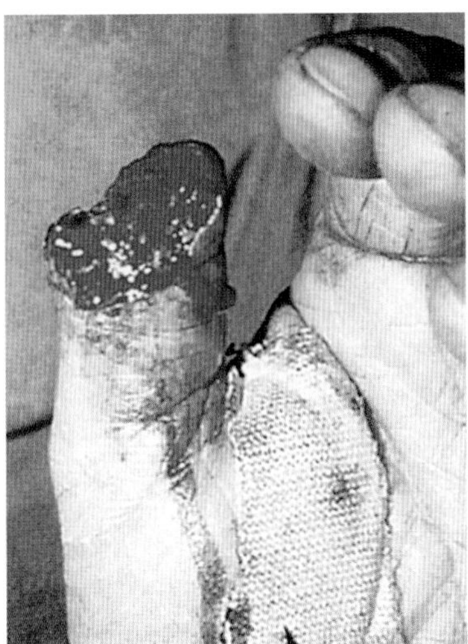

Figure 29-12 Amputation of the fingertip.

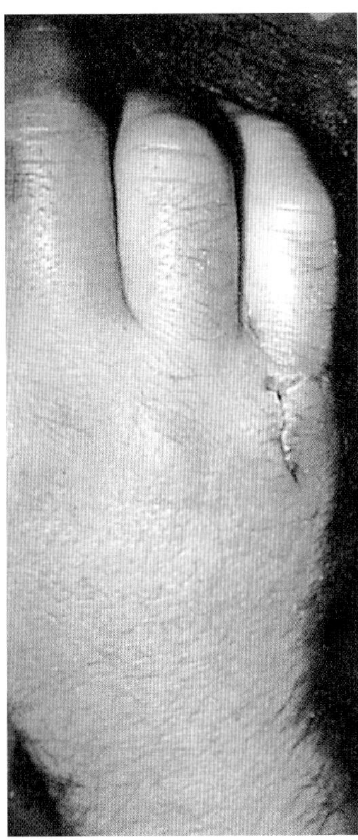

Figure 29-13 Human bite to the hand.

Critical Thinking

Consider that you are caring for a person who has sustained an animal bite. Aside from caring for the patient's wounds and documenting that care, what other concerns and responsibilities do you have?

Crush injury

Crush injury is one of the three injuries that occur when tissue is exposed to a compressive force. This force can be sufficient to interfere with the normal structure and metabolic function of the involved cells and tissues. The degree of injury produced by the crushing force depends on three things: the amount of pressure applied to the body, the amount of time the pressure remains in contact with the body, and the specific body region in which the injury occurs. A massive crush injury to vital organs can cause immediate death.

Crush injury usually involves the upper or lower extremities, torso or pelvis. Crush injury can result from entrapment under a heavy object, as in a building collapse, or from some other massive compressive force. Examples of situations that can cause crush injury include the following:

- collapse of masonry or steel structures
- collapse of earth (e.g. mud slides and earthquakes)
- motor vehicle crashes
- warfare injuries
- industrial incidents.

Compartment syndrome

Compartment syndrome is a result of crush injury and is a surgical emergency (Figure 29-14). Compartment syndrome usually results from compressive forces or blunt trauma to muscle groups confined in tight fibrous sheaths with minimal ability to stretch (below the knee, above the elbow). Other less common causes of compartment syndrome include the following:

- extreme exertional exercise
- low-level repetitive injury
- electrical injury

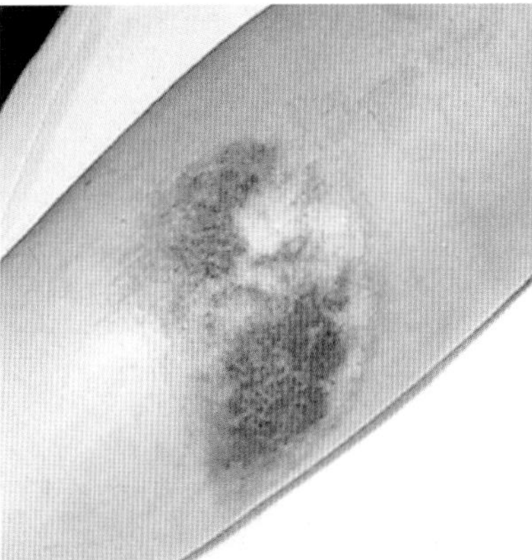

Figure 29-14 Appearance that can follow prolonged crushing, as when an unconscious person lies on a body part for several hours.

- haemorrhage into a compartment (e.g. coagulopathy among haemophiliacs)
- circumferential deep burns and electrical burns
- vascular occlusion
- high-pressure injection injuries
- immobility with the development of pressure necrosis (e.g. among alcoholics, drug addicts and victims of stroke).

Critical Thinking

Why would alcoholics, drug addicts and stroke victims be at risk for compartment syndrome?

Compartment syndrome develops as associated haemorrhage and oedema increase pressure in the closed fascial space (compartment). This results in ischaemia to the muscle, which causes further muscle cell swelling. The intra-compartmental pressure continues to rise and, as this occurs, circulation is compromised. Irreversible tissue damage from hypoxia develops within several hours to several days after injury. In addition to muscular damage, any nerves that travel through the compartment can undergo necrosis if the condition remains untreated. Signs and symptoms of compartment syndrome in an extremity include those of vascular insufficiency (the five Ps; Box 29-1). Other signs and symptoms that can indicate the presence of compartment syndrome include the following:

- pain seemingly out of proportion to injury
- pain on passive stretch (earliest finding)
- swelling (tautness of the compartment)
- tenderness to palpation
- weakness of the involved muscle groups.

The recognition of compartment syndrome calls for a high degree of suspicion based on patient history and mechanism of injury. Compartment syndrome is most often associated with tibial fracture of the lower leg yet may also occur with crush injury or fracture of the femur, forearm, or upper arm. Delayed treatment can result in nerve death, muscle necrosis, and crush syndrome.

Crush syndrome

Crush syndrome is a life-threatening and sometimes preventable complication of prolonged immobilization or compression. The syndrome is a pathological process that causes destruction or alteration of muscle tissue. Crush syndrome is rare and is most likely to occur in catastrophic events in which patient rescue and extrication are delayed beyond 4–6 h (examples of such events are mine or building collapses). The prehospital management of crush syndrome often determines patient outcome.

The exact mechanism of crush syndrome is unknown. The compressive forces of entrapment are believed to produce a pathological process that disrupts vascular integrity and causes loss of structure of the cell and the cell membranes. Patients with crush syndrome may appear stable for hours or days, as long as the compressive forces remain in place. But when the patient is released from the entrapment, three harmful processes occur at the same time that can lead to death:

1. Oxygen-rich blood returns to the ischaemic extremity and produces a pooling of intravascular volume into crushed tissue. This reperfusion reduces total circulating volume, which in turn often leads to shock.
2. With the return of oxygen-rich blood, various toxic substances and waste products of anaerobic metabolism are released into the systemic circulation, causing metabolic acidosis. High levels of intracellular solutes and water are released from damaged cells, resulting in hyperkalaemia, hyperuricaemia, hypocalcaemia and hyperphosphataemia.
3. Myoglobin is released from the damaged muscle cells of the injured extremity. Myoglobin is filtered through the kidneys (rhabdomyolysis) and results in acute renal failure.

Box 29-1

Five Ps of vascular insufficiency

1. Pain
2. Paresis (late finding)
3. Paraesthesia
4. Pallor (variable)
5. Pulselessness (late finding)

Blast injuries

As described in Chapter 26, severe injuries can result from an initial air blast, from flying debris, and from secondary contact with another object as the victim is thrown by the blast. Examples of situations that can result in blast injury include natural gas or petrol explosions, fireworks explosions and terrorist bombs. Scene and personal safety is of the highest importance; paramedics should not enter the scene where a blast injury occurred until the scene has been made safe by the authorities. (The appropriate authorities include, for example, police, fire service, specialized rescue teams, hazardous materials teams and other public service agencies.)

Injuries from blasts can be superficial or deep (Figure 29-15). The deep injuries can injure internal organs. Patients who suffer blast injury require rapid stabilization (airway and ventilatory support with spinal precautions; circulatory support) and rapid transportation for physician evaluation. Blast injuries and associated trauma can be hard to identify in the prehospital setting so these patients will need extensive evaluation in a centre equipped to manage trauma. Compression injuries that occur to air-filled organs include rupture of the eardrum, sinuses, lungs, stomach and intestines.

Critical Thinking

What injury do you suspect if a patient who has suffered a blast injury has a sudden onset of hearing loss?

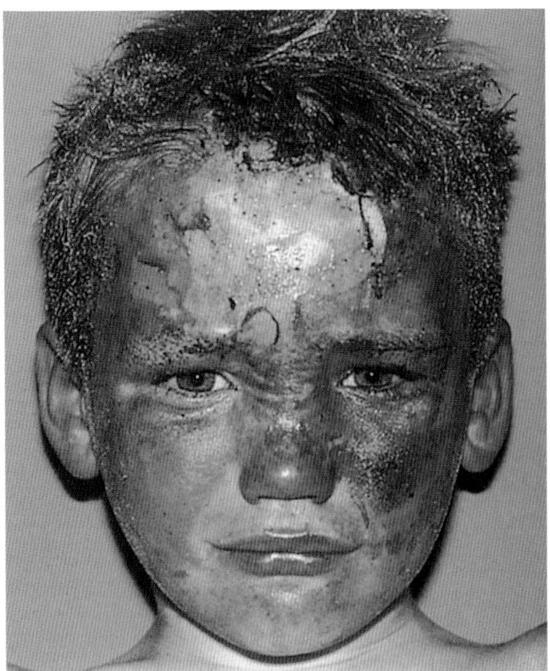

Figure 29-15 Blast injury to the face. His eardrums were normal. He was admitted because of the risk of swelling to his face and airway with potential airway obstruction.

Management principles for soft tissue injuries

Personal and scene safety is always the priority in any emergency response. If indicated, police and rescue personnel should assure the paramedic that the scene is safe for entry and that any perpetrators have been apprehended. Help from other public service agencies may also be needed if other types of dangers exist, e.g. hazardous materials or bombs.

Treatment priorities

The assessment of life-threatening injuries and resuscitation precedes evaluation and intervention of non-life-threatening soft tissue injuries. The paramedic should evaluate wounds that do not pose a threat to life later in the physical examination. General wound assessment should include a history of the wounding event and a careful examination of the injury. Figure 29-16 shows a treatment plan based on assessment findings for a patient with soft tissue injury.

Wound history

A wound history should include the following:

- time of injury
- environment where the injury occurred (risk of infection is greater in unclean environments)
- mechanism of injury and likelihood of concurrent or associated injuries
- volume of blood loss
- severity of pain
- medical history, including use of medications that may impair haemostasis
- tetanus immunization.

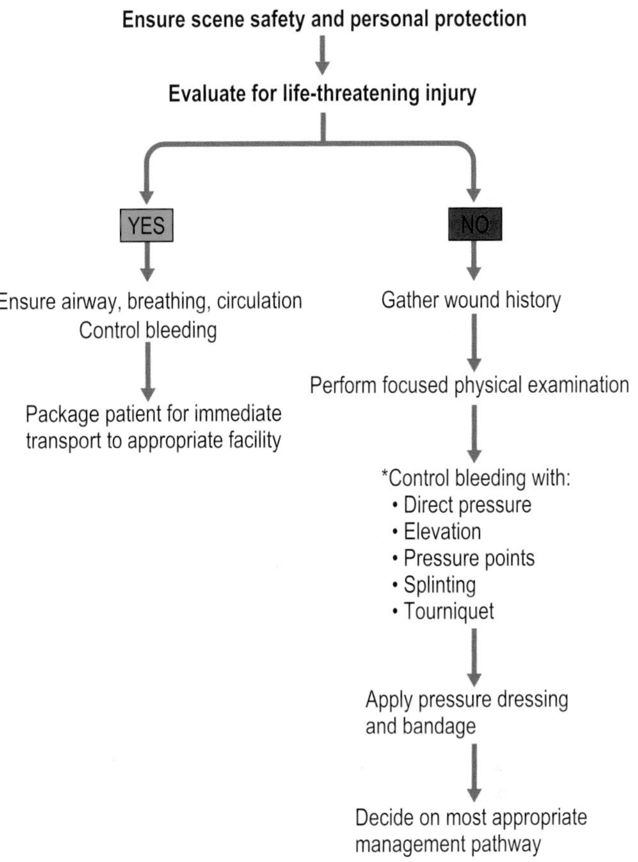

Figure 29-16 Treatment plan for a patient with soft tissue injury.

Physical examination

Physical examination of a wound should include the following:

- Inspection of the wound for bleeding, size, depth, presence of foreign bodies, amount of tissue lost, oedema and deformity.
- Inspection of the area surrounding the wound for damage to underlying structures, arteries, nerves, tendons or muscle.

> **Critical Thinking**
>
> Will you perform this physical examination on every wound in the prehospital setting?

- Assessment of sensory or motor function of the extremity.
- Evaluation of the perfusion status of the wound and tissue distal to the wound.
- Palpation of the injury and associated structures to evaluate capillary refill, distal pulses, tenderness, temperature, oedema and crepitus (if underlying bony injury is suspected).

Haemorrhage and control of bleeding

Blood loss is often associated with soft tissue injury and may result from damage to arteries, veins, capillaries, or a combination of these. Generally, arterial bleeding is characterized as bright red and spurting; venous bleeding is darker red and flowing; capillary bleeding is bright red and oozing. Differentiation among the types of vessel haemorrhage is often difficult so the main concern in haemorrhage, regardless of origin, is to control bleeding.

Methods of haemorrhage control include direct pressure, elevation, pressure point, immobilization by splinting, and rarely the use of tourniquets. As in any patient encounter in which contact with body fluids is likely, the paramedic must take personal protective measures.

Direct pressure

The paramedic can control external haemorrhage by applying direct pressure over the injury site (Figure 29-17a, b). Direct pressure controls most types of haemorrhage within 4–6 min. To maintain control, a pressure dressing can be applied over the site and held in place with an elastic bandage. The paramedic must continue direct pressure, even with a pressure dressing. Once the dressing has been applied, the paramedic should not remove it because removal can disrupt the fresh blood clot. If bleeding resumes and the dressing becomes soaked with blood, a second dressing should be applied on top of the first one and held in place with direct pressure until the bleeding is controlled.

Elevation

The paramedic can control or reduce venous bleeding in an extremity by elevating the extremity above the level of the heart (Figure 29-18). Elevation alone does not usually control haemorrhage but can supplement direct pressure.

Pressure point

Pressure-point control may become necessary if direct pressure and elevation have not controlled haemorrhage. The chosen artery must be proximal to the injury site and overlie a bony structure against which it can be compressed. Examples of pressure-point sites include the temporal artery to control bleeding from the scalp, the brachial artery to control bleeding from the forearm, and the femoral artery to control bleeding from the leg (Figure 29-19). Pressure-point control (Figure 29-20) should be maintained for at least 10 min. Continued compression of the pressure point may be needed during patient transport. The paramedic may need to combine techniques of direct pressure, elevation, and proximal pressure-point compression to control vigorous haemorrhage.

Critical Thinking

Why should the pressure point chosen to control haemorrhage be proximal to the injury?

Immobilization by splinting

Patient movement promotes the flow of blood and can disrupt the clot or increase vascular injury, thus patients should be immobilized whenever possible (Figure 29-21). Immobilization alone is not effective as a method to control bleeding and should be used as an adjunct.

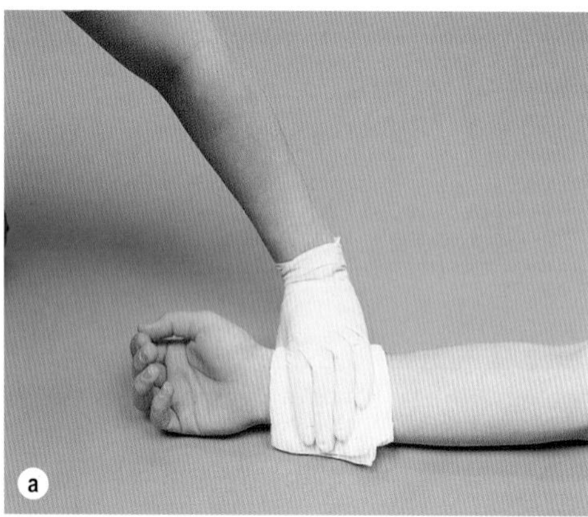

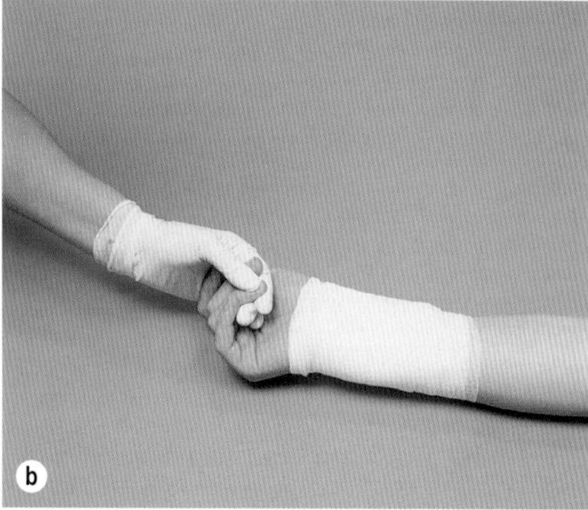

Figure 29-17 (a) Application of direct pressure to control haemorrhage. (b) Pressure dressing.

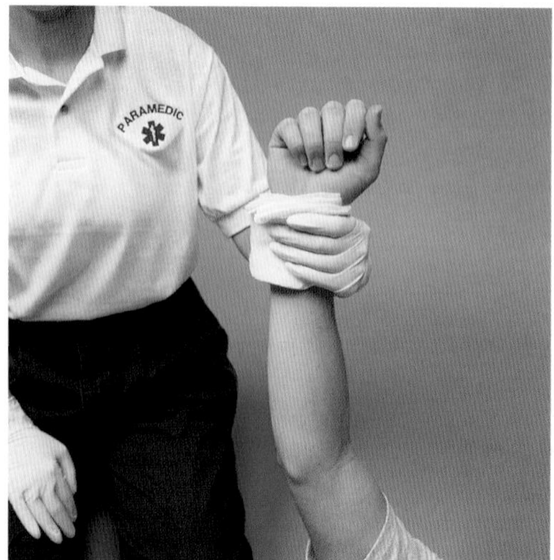

Figure 29-18 Elevation to control haemorrhage.

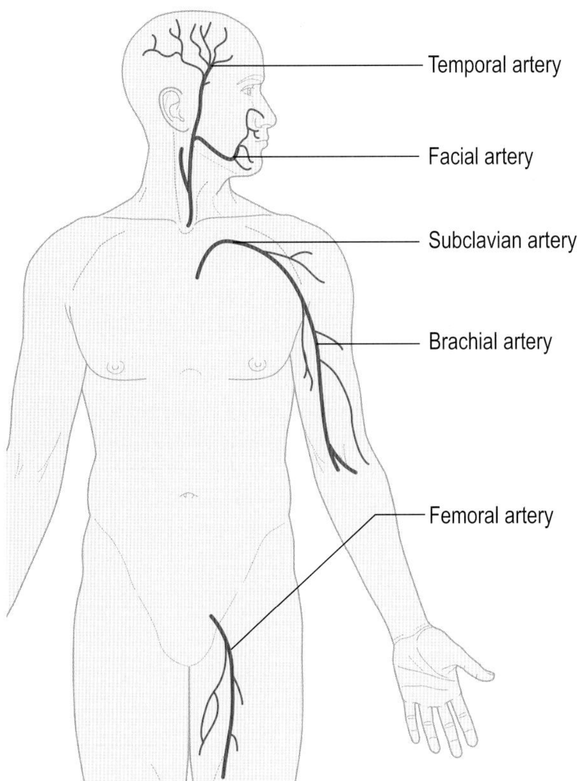

Figure 29-19 Arterial pressure points.

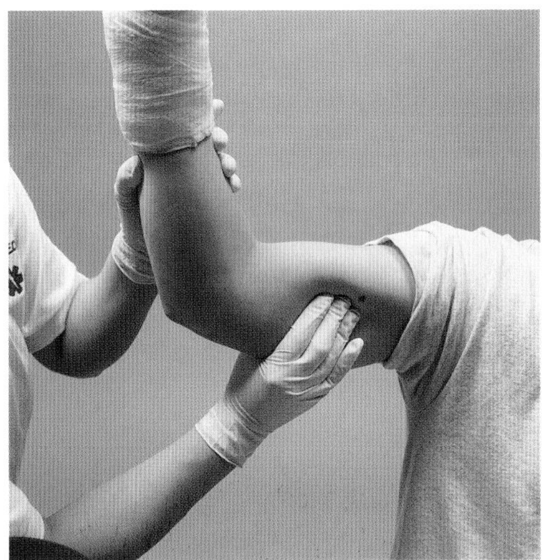

Figure 29-20 Pressure-point control.

Tourniquet

Tourniquets (Figure 29-22) work by compressing muscle and other tissues surrounding extremity arteries; this collapses the lumen of the artery and reduces distal blood flow. The tension required to achieve this is dependent upon the size of extremity[3] and the width of tourniquet.[4] The larger the circumference of the extremity, the greater the tension required whilst wider tourniquets tend to be more effective at stopping arterial flow at a given tension than narrow tourniquets.

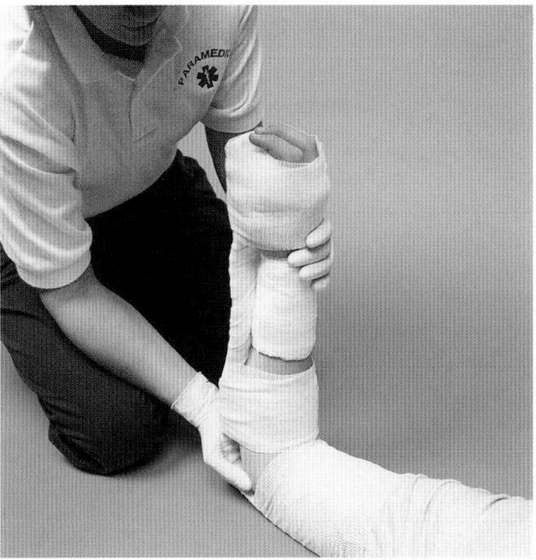

Figure 29-21 Immobilization by splinting to control haemorrhage.

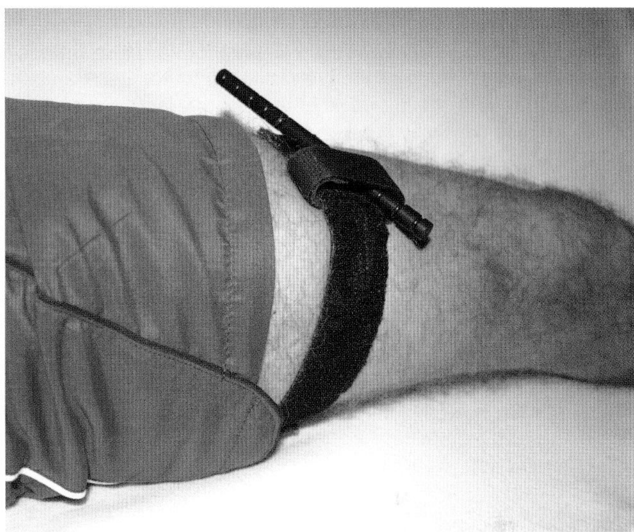

Figure 29-22 Combat application tourniquet in situ. Courtesy of N. Gregory.

There are many complications associated with tourniquet use, which have probably led to their demise in UK prehospital care (Box 29-2). However, recent advances in tourniquet design have led to a re-think and tourniquets are returning to the haemorrhage control armoury. Improvised tourniquets should not be used as they are likely to be ineffective and may cause further complications.

The stepwise approach to haemorrhage control outlined in Figure 29-16 should normally be followed but, on very rare occasions, immediate application may be necessary where:[5]

- there is extreme life-threatening limb haemorrhage, or limb amputation/mangled limb with multiple bleeding points
- life-threatening limb haemorrhage has not been controlled by simple methods
- the point of significant haemorrhage from a limb is not peripherally accessible due to entrapment
- there is a major incident or multiple casualties with extremity haemorrhage and lack of resources to maintain simple methods of haemorrhage control

Box 29-2

Complications associated with tourniquet use

- Duration of tourniquet use

  Tourniquet use leads to changes in muscle and nerve physiology with evidence of skeletal muscle stress and injury after 2 h.[6] Patients at advanced age, those with vascular diseases and traumatic injuries are at higher risk of complications, including nerve and muscle injury. Nerve injuries have been reported after only 30 minutes of tourniquet time whilst muscle, especially that directly beneath the tourniquet, has shown damage after 1 h. Actual myonecrosis seems to occur only after 3 h.[7]
- Increased venous bleeding

  An incorrectly applied tourniquet can increase bleeding by occluding venous return whilst not completely arresting arterial inflow.
- Post-tourniquet syndrome[8]
- Post-tourniquet syndrome related to tourniquet use in excess of 1.5–2 h was discovered in early surgical use. Damage to muscle, nerves and blood vessels causes weakness, paraesthesia, pallor, and stiffness. This tends to resolve after about 3 weeks. It is known that complications increase with prolonged use but, although releasing the tourniquet sounds like a sensible option, evidence suggests that incremental exsanguinations may occur and worsen the blood loss.[9]
- Ischaemia perfusion injury

  Acid–base changes may result from release of a tourniquet that has been in place for an extended period of time. Limb ischaemia leads to distal tissue lactic acidosis whilst release of the tourniquet leads to reperfusion and transportation of lactic acid and free radicals into circulation. The evidence for this is not clear.
- Pain

  There have been reports of 'excruciating pain'[10] with lower extremities having higher average times of pain tolerance than upper extremities (around 30 min).[11] Most patients will require analgesia.

- the benefits of preventing death from hypovolaemic shock by cessation of ongoing external haemorrhage are greater than the risk of limb damage or loss from ischaemia caused by tourniquet use.

Application (based upon the combat application tourniquet)

1. Place the tourniquet around the injured limb proximal to the wound and over the supplying brachial or femoral artery. Depending upon access to the injured limb, this can be achieved in one of two ways. Either insert a freely accessible limb through the loop of the self-adhering band or route the self-adhering band around the injured extremity. Feed the free-running end through the inside slit of the tourniquet buckle. This utilizes the friction adaptor buckle, which locks the band in place. Securely fasten the band back on itself.
2. Twist the windlass rod until bright red bleeding has stopped. DO NOT loosen the tourniquet once it has been tightened.
3. Lock the rod with the clip.
4. Secure the rod with the strap.
5. Note the time of the tourniquet application.

A video of the application process can be found at http://www.combattourniquet.com/index.php

Dressing materials used with soft tissue trauma

A variety of bandages and dressings are used in trauma care. The six general categories of dressings are as follows:

1. Sterile dressings are processed to eliminate bacteria. They should be used whenever infection of the wound is a concern.
2. Non-sterile dressings are not sterilized. They can be used when infection is not a prime concern.
3. Occlusive dressings do not allow the passage of air through the material. These dressings are useful in treating wounds of the thorax and major vessels where negative pressure can cause air to enter the body, resulting in a pneumothorax or air embolism, respectively (see Chapter 27).
4. Non-occlusive dressings allow air to pass through the material and are indicated for managing most soft tissue injuries.
5. Adherent dressings attach to the wound surface by incorporating wound exudate into the dressing mesh. Use of these dressings can sometimes assist in controlling acute bleeding.
6. Non-adherent dressings allow the passage of wound exudate and do not adhere to the wound surface. These dressings do not damage the wound when removed and are often used after wound closure.

Bandages hold dressings in place. Bandages are classified as absorbent, non-absorbent, adherent and non-adherent. Like dressings, bandages are sterile or non-sterile.

Complications of improperly applied dressings and bandages

Improperly applied dressings and bandages can harm the patient and can cause discomfort. Dressings that are applied too loosely often do not stop bleeding, whilst bandages that are applied too tightly can cause tissue ischaemia and structural damage to vessels, nerves, tendons, muscles, and skin.

Basic concepts of open wound dressing

The basic concepts of open wound dressing include the following steps:

1. Assess the wound for size, depth, location, and contamination.
2. Properly prepare the wound for dressing. Prehospital care is usually limited to cleaning the injured surface of gross contaminants by irrigation of the wound with sterile water or normal saline. Do not attempt extensive débridement in the prehospital setting. Apply

antibacterial ointment if the patient is not allergic (per guidelines).
3. Apply the appropriate dressing.
4. Secure the dressing in place with bandages or gauze wrappings.
5. Tape the loose ends of the bandage.

Management of specific soft tissue injuries not requiring closure

The paramedic encounters many minor open wounds that do not require closure or the evaluation of a physician. In these cases the paramedic provides basic first aid. The paramedic should also provide instructions for self-care to the patient.

Dressings and bandages

Depending on the nature and location of the patient's injury, dressings, bandages, and immobilization may be indicated to care for the wound properly. Figure 29-23a–j illustrates basic dressing and bandaging procedures for various wounds. Open wounds that always require physician evaluation include those with the following:

- neural, muscular or vascular compromise
- tendon or ligament compromise
- heavy contamination
- cosmetic complications (e.g. facial trauma)
- foreign bodies.

Patients with soft tissue injuries that pose a threat to life or limb require rapid assessment, stabilization, and rapid transportation for physician evaluation.

Evaluation

Local protocol may permit the paramedic to manage and release the patient with minor soft tissue injury to the patient's own care. Local protocol may also allow the paramedic to manage and refer the patient to the patient's GP, or an emergency care practitioner (ECP) for follow-up care. ECPs should be permitted to provide tetanus vaccine. Paramedics should consider giving written and verbal instructions regarding care to patients who will not be transported by ambulance for evaluation.

Tetanus vaccine

Tetanus is a serious and at times fatal disease. Tetanus is a disease of the central nervous system caused by the infection of a wound with spores of the bacterium *Clostridium tetani*. The patient can be protected against tetanus by periodic immunization with a tetanus vaccine. About half a million cases of tetanus occur across the world each year although only three were recorded in the UK in 2005.[12]

Adults receive a combined immunization against diphtheria and tetanus, and children receive vaccinations against diphtheria, pertussis (whooping cough), and tetanus routinely in the UK. After initial immunization during childhood, children receive booster vaccines every 5 to 10 years. Patients who have not been immunized against tetanus receive tetanus immune globulin because it confers instant immunity. During wound care, the paramedic should ascertain the patient's last tetanus immunization and should also determine any prior allergic reactions to tetanus preparations. Normal side effects from the vaccine include slight fever, sore injection site or minor rash. The tetanus vaccine is contraindicated in infants less than 6 weeks of age, in pregnant patients, and in those who are hypersensitive to the vaccine.

Critical Thinking

Why is it important for you to be knowledgeable about and to ask the patient about tetanus vaccination if the vaccine is not carried on your ambulance?

Patient instructions

Verbal and written instructions sometimes are referred to as a 'patient instruction sheet'. These instructions relate to wound care (Figure 29-24). Paramedics should give instructions to all patients who are not transported for physician evaluation. These instructions should include the following:

- protection and care of wounded area
- dressing change and follow-up
- wound cleansing recommendations
- signs of wound infection.

Wound infection

Infection is a common complication of soft tissue injury. It results from a break in the continuity of the skin and subsequent exposure to the non-sterile external environment. Most infections are minor. However, some can be serious. The goals of wound care are to prevent infection and protect from infection. Factors that influence the likelihood of infection include unclean wounds and wound mechanisms (e.g. wounds contaminated by soil, dirt or grease) and a patient's poor state of health. These factors can have both local and systemic complications and can affect the patient's general recovery.

Causes of wound infection

Many factors can cause wound infection. Nine of the most common factors are as follows:[13]

1. Time. The risk of infection can be reduced greatly if the wound is cleaned and repaired within 8 to 12 h after injury. Bacterial proliferation to a level that can result in infection can occur as early as 3 h after injury.
2. Mechanism. Lacerations caused by fine cutting forces resist infection better than crush injuries. High-velocity missile injuries can produce internal damage that may not be apparent for several days.
3. Location. Injuries of the foot, lower extremity, hand, and perineum have a higher-than-normal risk for infection.
4. Severity. The more tissue damage produced by the injury, the higher the risk for infection.
5. Contamination. The presence of foreign matter in a wound decreases resistance to infection. Of particular

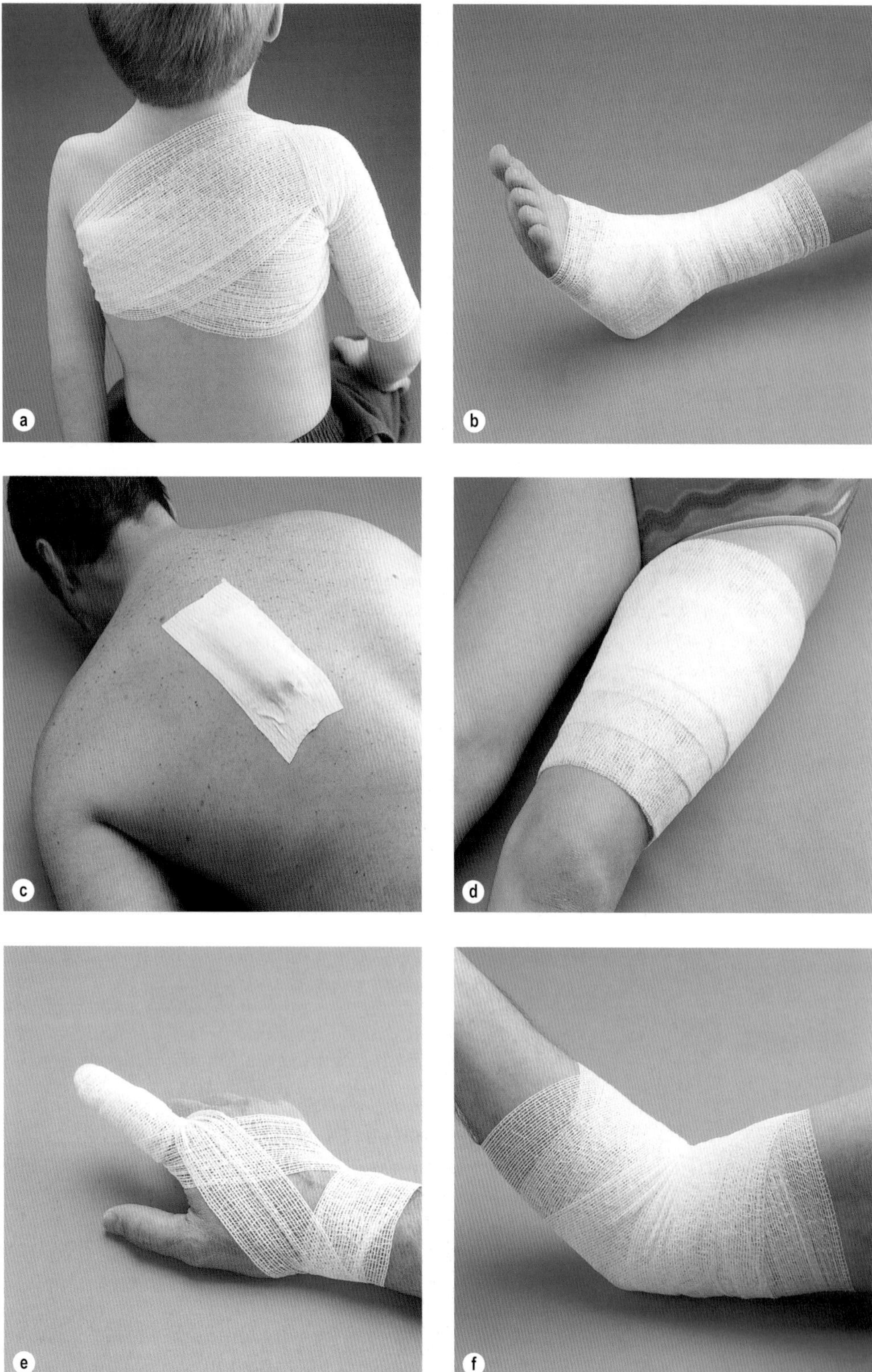

Figure 29-23 Types of dressings. (a) Shoulder dressing; (b) ankle dressing; (c) torso dressing; (d) thigh dressing; (e) finger dressing; (f) elbow dressing; (g) forehead dressing; (h) scalp dressing; (i) ear/mastoid dressing; (j) neck dressing.

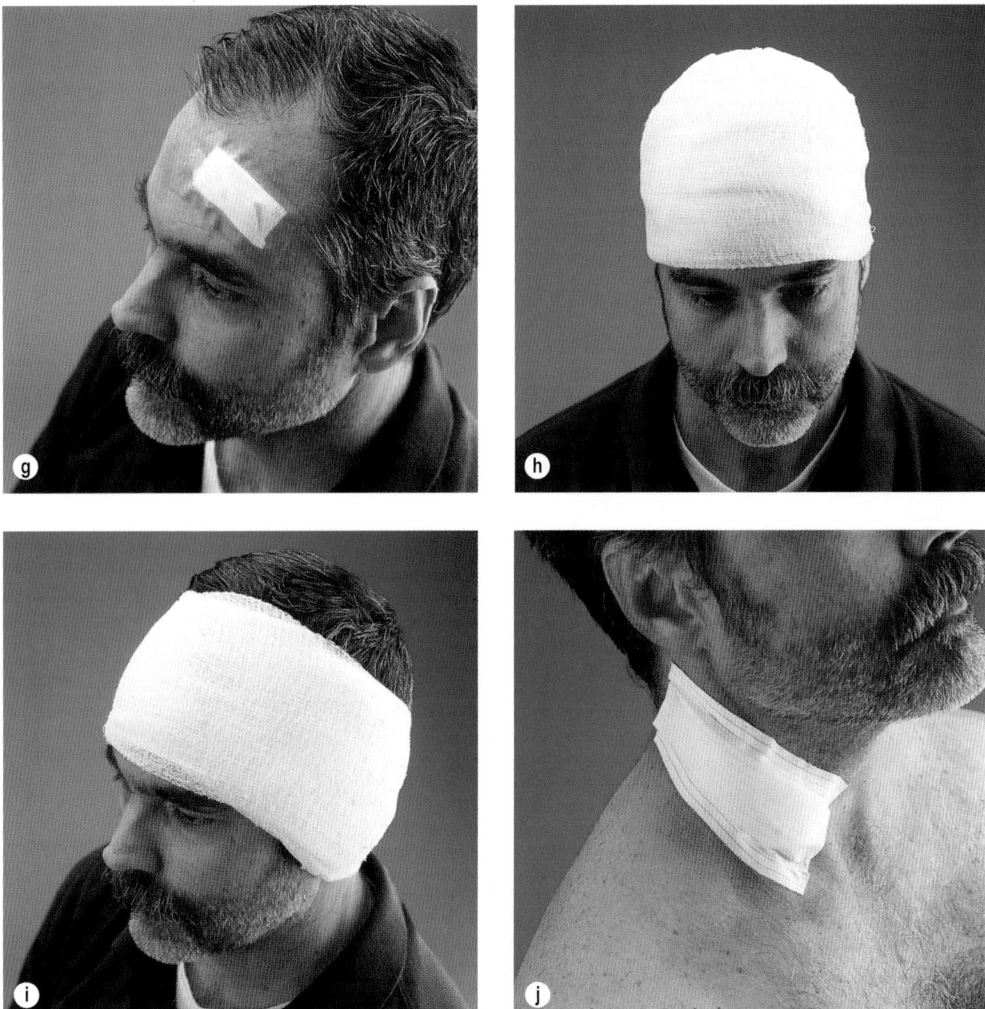

Figure 29-23, cont'd

concern are wounds contaminated by soil, saliva and faeces.

6. Preparation. Body, facial and head hair removed by clipping versus shaving is less likely to result in wound infection. Shaving can cause additional injury by abrading the skin and potentially moving skin flora into the larger wound.
7. Cleansing. Wound cleansing should be performed with normal saline and a high-pressure syringe.
8. Technique of repair. Wounds at high risk for infection (e.g. animal bites) may need to be cleaned, débrided, left open for 4–5 days, and then closed through traditional techniques.
9. General patient condition. Elderly patients and patients with concurrent illness or pre-existing disease (e.g. diabetes) are often less able to ward off infection.

Assessment of wound healing

A paramedic can assess a wound for proper healing by doing the following:

- Examine dressings for excess drainage. Change saturated dressings to prevent contamination of the wound.
- Examine wounds for early signs of infection or delayed healing. Inflammation, oedema and bloody drainage are normal during the first 3 days but should subside gradually as the wound heals.

Signs of wound infection include increasing inflammation or oedema, purulent drainage, foul odour, persistent pain, delayed healing and fever. If any of these is present, the paramedic should consider patient transport to the emergency department or refer the patient on for follow-up care if appropriate pathways are available.

Special considerations for soft tissue injuries

As stated before, assessment of life-threatening injuries and resuscitation precede evaluation of and intervention for non-life-threatening soft tissue injuries. After ensuring adequate airway, breathing, and circulatory status (with spinal precautions if indicated); controlling severe haemorrhage; and maintaining normal body temperature, the paramedic can proceed with wound care. Special considerations for specific wounds are described in the following sections.

WOUND CARE INSTRUCTION SHEET

Patient name: ______________________

1. Call your physician. He/she may have further instructions to offer for your care.
2. Keep the wound and dressing as dry as reasonably possible, since water aids bacterial growth.
3. Remove the dressing applied after 2 days.
4. Check for signs of infection:
   a. Swelling
   b. Excessive redness
   c. Pain
   d. Heat—either locally or systemically as reflected by a fever
   e. Excessive drainage from wounds
5. Reapply a sterile gauze dressing, taping it down at the edges. Repeat this every 2 days until the wound heals.
6. Wounds in areas of high mobility, such as around joints, are subject to excessive tension. Appropriate precautions should be taken to decrease the motion of the affected joint to assist in healing.

Other instructions: ______________________

Treatment rendered: ______________________

Tetanus: Yes / No Type: ______________________

I hereby acknowledge that I have read the instructions above, that they have been explained to me, that I understand them, and that I have received a copy of them.

I understand that I have had emergency treatment only and that I may be released before all of my medical problems are known and treated. I will arrange for the follow-up care as instructed.

Responsible Party's Signature ______________________ Relationship ______________________

Witness ______________________ Title ______________________

Original to Patient Care Report
Copy to Patient

Date/Time ______________________

Figure 29-24 Sample instruction sheet for wound care.

Penetrating chest or abdominal injury

Open wounds to the chest or abdomen must be covered properly with sterile and occlusive dressings. Open chest wounds can involve severe pulmonary injuries, which can include pneumothorax and tension pneumothorax (described in Chapter 27). Major complications of penetrating abdominal injury include haemorrhage from a major vessel or solid organ and perforation of a segment of bowel (see Chapter 33). The paramedic should observe the following guidelines in managing a penetrating wound to the chest or abdomen in which an impaled object is present:

1. Do not remove the impaled object; severe haemorrhage or damage to underlying structures can occur.

2. Do not manipulate the impaled object unless it is necessary to shorten the object for extrication or for patient transportation.
3. Control bleeding with direct pressure applied around the impaled object.
4. Stabilize the object in place with bulky dressings; immobilize the patient to prevent movement.

Avulsion

Prehospital management of avulsed tissue varies by protocol, but two guidelines generally apply:

1. If the tissue is still attached to the body, do the following:
   a. Clean the wound surface of gross contaminants with sterile saline.
   b. Gently fold the skin back to its normal position.
   c. Control bleeding, dress the wound with bulky pressure dressings, and maintain direct pressure.
2. If the tissue is completely separated from the body, do the following:
   a. Control the bleeding with application of direct pressure.
   b. Retrieve the avulsed tissue if possible, but do not delay transport to locate amputated body parts.
   c. Wrap the tissue in gauze, either dry or moistened with sodium lactate or saline solution (per guideline).
   d. Seal the tissue in a plastic bag.
   e. Place the sealed bag on crushed ice; never place tissue directly on ice.

Critical Thinking

Why should you use normal saline or sodium lactate solution instead of sterile water to wrap or clean avulsed tissue?

Amputations

As with other open wounds, haemorrhage control for amputation should be managed initially with direct pressure and elevation. The wound may require use of a tourniquet but this should be avoided if possible as the resultant damage can interfere with re-implantation attempts. An amputated limb should be retrieved and managed in the same manner as avulsed tissue.

Crush syndrome

Crush syndrome is complex and is difficult to diagnose and treat because of the many variables involved. These variables include the extent of tissue damage, duration and force of compression, patient's general health, and associated injuries. The management of crush syndrome is controversial and where suspected, support should be sought from BASICS doctors or other medical personnel.

Paramedics should consider possible crush syndrome when prolonged immobilization or compression occurs. The emergency care must be coordinated with rescue efforts, that way, the timing of the release from entrapment follows medical treatment, which will help to prevent hypovolaemic shock and crush syndrome. The steps in patient care management are as follows:[13]

1. Provide airway and ventilatory support. This includes high-concentration oxygen administration.
2. Maintain body temperature.
3. Hydrate the patient to manage hypovolaemia and to maintain urine output.
4. Use of arterial tourniquets before the release of a crushed limb can be beneficial. If intracompartmental pressure is greater than 40 mmHg, fasciotomy may be indicated to preserve the limb and cutaneous sensation. Performing a field fasciotomy carries an increased risk for infection and sepsis and should only be carried out by a medic trained in the procedure.
5. A physician may need to perform surgical amputation when extrication is impossible.
6. After extrication, care may include transporting the patient for hyperbaric oxygen treatment to restore tissue perfusion and to decrease tissue necrosis and muscle oedema. (Hyperbaric therapy is described further in Chapter 23.)

Summary

- The skin and its accessory organs are the main cosmetic structures of the body. These structures perform many functions that are critical to survival. The skin is composed of two distinct layers of tissue: the outer layer (epidermis) and the inner layer (dermis).
- Surface trauma can disrupt the normal distribution of body fluids and electrolytes and can interfere with the maintenance of body temperature. The two physiological responses to surface trauma are vascular and inflammatory reactions. These can lead to healing, scar formation, or both. Many factors can affect or alter wound healing.
- Soft tissue injuries are classified as closed or open. Classification is determined by the absence or presence of a break in the continuity of the epidermis. Closed wounds include contusions, haematoma, and crush injury. Open wounds are classified as abrasion, laceration, puncture, avulsion, amputation and bite.
- Assessment of life-threatening injuries and resuscitation precedes evaluation and intervention of non-life-threatening soft tissue injuries. General wound assessment should include a history of the event that caused the wound and a careful examination of the injury.
- Methods of haemorrhage control include direct pressure, elevation, pressure point, immobilization by splinting and tourniquets.

Summary—cont'd

- The general categories of dressings used in trauma care are sterile, non-sterile, occlusive, non-occlusive, adherent and non-adherent. The general categories of bandages are absorbent, non-absorbent, adherent and non-adherent.
- Depending on the nature and location of the patient's injury, dressings, bandages and immobilization may be indicated to care for a wound properly.
- The goals of wound care are to prevent infection and protect from infection. Factors that influence the likelihood of infection include unclean wounds and wound mechanisms and a patient's poor state of health.
- Special considerations for specific wounds include penetrating chest or abdominal injury, avulsion, amputations and crush syndrome.

References

1. Rosen P, Barkin R 2003 Emergency medicine: concepts and clinical practice, 5th edition. Mosby, St Louis
2. Rickman KM, Rickman LS 1993 The potential for transmission of human immunodeficiency virus through human bites. J Acquired Immune Deficiency Syndromes 6(4):402–406
3. Coupland RM, Molde A, Navein J 2001 Care in the field for victims of weapons of war: a report from the workshop organised by the ICRC on pre-hospital car for war and mine-injured. International Committee of the Red Cross, Geneva
4. Shaw JA, Murray DG 1982 The relationship between tourniquet pressure and underlying soft-tissue pressure in the thigh. J Bone Joint Surg Am 64(8):1148–1152
5. Lee C, Porter KM, Hodgetts TJ 2007 Tourniquet use in the civilian prehospital setting. Emerg Med J. 24:584–587
6. Heppenstall RB, Balderston R, Goodwin C 1979 Pathophysiologic effects distal to a tourniquet in the dog. J. Trauma 19(4):234–238
7. Patterson S, Klenerman L 1979 The effect of pneumatic tourniquets on the ultrastructure of skeletal muscle. J Bone Joint Surgery Br 61-B(2):178–183
8. Kam PC, Kavanagh R, Yoong FF 2001 The arterial tourniquet: pathophysiological consequences and anaesthetic implications. Anaesthesia 56(6):534–545
9. Clifford CC 2004 Treating traumatic bleeding in a combat setting. Mil Med 12;169(12 suppl):8–10
10. Hagenouw RR, Bridenbaugh PO, van Egmond J, Stuebing R 1986 Tourniquet pain: a volunteer study. Anesth Analg 65(11):1175–1180.
11. Sebesta J 2006 Special lessons learned from Iraq. Surg Clin North Am 86(3):711–726
12. Health Protection Agency. Epidemiological data – tetanus. Online. Available http://www.hpa.org.uk/infections/topics_az/tetanus/data.htm 16 February 2009
13. US Department of Transportation, National Highway Traffic Safety Administration 1998 EMT-Paramedic national standard curriculum. US Government Printing Office, Washington, DC

CHAPTER 30

Burns

Chapter contents

Objectives

Upon completion of this chapter, the paramedic student will be able to:

1. Describe the incidence, patterns, and sources of burn injury.
2. Describe the pathophysiology of local and systemic responses to burn injury.
3. Classify burn injury according to depth, extent, and severity, based on established standards.
4. Discuss the pathophysiology of burn shock as a basis for key signs and symptoms.
5. Outline the physical examination of the burned patient.
6. Describe the prehospital management of the patient who has sustained a burn injury.
7. Discuss pathophysiology as a basis for key signs, symptoms and management of the patient with an inhalation injury.
8. Outline the general assessment and management of the patient who has a chemical injury.
9. Describe specific complications and management techniques for selected chemical injuries.
10. Describe the physiological effects of electrical injuries as they relate to each body system, based on an understanding of key principles of electricity.
11. Outline assessment and management of the patient with electrical injury.

Key terms

eschar A scab or dry crust resulting from a thermal or chemical burn.

full-thickness burn A burn injury in which the entire thickness of the epidermis and dermis is destroyed; also known as a third-degree burn.

inhalation injury An upper and/or lower airway injury that results from thermal and/or chemical exposure.

Lund and Browder chart A method to estimate burn injury that assigns specific numbers to each body part and that accounts for developmental changes in percentages of body surface area.

partial-thickness burn A burn injury that extends through the epidermis to the dermis; considered a deep partial-thickness injury if it extends to the basal layers of the skin; also known as a second-degree burn.

rule of nines A method to estimate burn injury that divides the total body surface area into segments that are multiples of 9%.

superficial burn A burn injury in which only a superficial layer of epidermal cells is destroyed; also known as a first-degree burn.

The management of burns often poses a challenge for the paramedic. Understanding the long-term results of a serious burn injury is important. Appropriate prehospital management can reduce morbidity and mortality for burn patients.

Incidence and patterns of burn injury

Burns are a devastating form of trauma. They are associated with high mortality rates, lengthy rehabilitation, cosmetic disfigurement, and permanent physical disabilities. Each year, about 250 000 people are burnt in the UK. Of these, 175 000 attend accident and emergency departments and 13 000 will be admitted to hospital.[1] Around 1000 patients will have burns that are severe enough to warrant formal fluid resuscitation; half of these are children. On average, burns are responsible for 300 deaths per year in the UK.[1] Box 30-1 lists common complications that contribute to thermal injury deaths.

Morbidity and mortality rates from burn injury follow significant patterns regarding gender, age, and socioeconomic status. For example, the majority of fire fatalities affect men; the death rate from thermal injury is highest among children and older adults; and three-quarters of all fire deaths occur in the home, with the highest incidence in lower-income households.[2] It is believed that 90% of burn injuries are preventable through legislation and education; a key part of the professional role of the paramedic is community education, which should stress prevention as the most effective management of these injuries (see Chapter 3).

Major sources of burns

A burn injury is caused by contact between energy and living cells. The source of this energy may be thermal, chemical, electrical or radiation.

Thermal burns

The majority of burns are thermal and commonly result from flames, scalds, or contact with hot substances (frostbite is also a thermal injury and is addressed in Chapter 23). Studies have shown that surface temperatures of 44 °C do not produce burns unless exposure time exceeds 6 hours.[3] At temperatures between 44 °C and 51 °C, the rate of epidermal necrosis approximately doubles with each degree of temperature rise. At 70 °C or greater, the exposure time required to cause transepidermal necrosis is less than 1 s. The degree of tissue destruction depends on the temperature and on the duration of exposure. Factors that influence the ability of the body to resist burn injury include the water content of the skin tissue; thickness and pigmentation of the skin; presence or absence of insulating substances such as skin oils or hair; and peripheral circulation of the skin, which affects dissipation of heat. Anatomy and physiology of the skin should be reviewed in an appropriate anatomy and physiology textbook.

Box 30-1

Physiological and systemic complications of thermal injuries

Depending on the severity of thermal injury, physiological and systemic complications may include the following:

Acidosis
Anoxia
Dysrhythmias
Electrolyte loss
Fluid loss
Heart failure
Hypothermia
Hypovolaemia
Hypoxia
Infection
Liver failure
Renal failure

Critical Thinking

Based on these facts and your knowledge of lifespan development, who would you predict would have a deeper burn from the same energy source: an 18-year-old or a 75-year-old? Why?

Chemical burns

Chemical burns are caused by substances that are capable of producing chemical changes in the skin, with or without the production of heat. Heat may be generated during the burning process, yet the chemical changes in the skin, not the heat, produce the greatest injury. Chemical burns differ from thermal burns. With chemical burns, the topical agent usually adheres to the skin for prolonged periods, producing continuous tissue destruction. The severity of the chemical injury is related to the type of agent, its concentration and volume, and the duration of contact. Chemical agents that often cause burn injuries include acids and alkalis. These agents are found in many household cleaning products and organic compounds. Chemical burns are associated with high morbidity, especially when they involve the eyes. Inhalation injury (described later in this chapter) may also result from thermal and/or chemical exposure.

Electrical burns

Electrical injuries (including lightning injuries) result from direct contact with an electrical current. Electrical injuries can also result from arcing of electricity between two contact points near the skin. In a direct contact injury the current itself is not considered to have any thermal properties; the potential energy of the current, however, is changed into thermal energy. This transformation occurs when electricity meets the electrical resistance of biological tissue interposed between the entrance and exit sites. Arc injuries are localized at the termination of current flow and are caused by the intense heat or flash that occurs when the current 'jumps', making contact with the skin. Flame burn may also occur as a result of arcing if the heat generated ignites clothing or other fuel source near the patient.

> **Critical Thinking**
>
> Electrical energy is transformed to heat, causing tissue damage in a human being. Then why does an electrical cord not feel hot when you touch it?

Radiation burns

Radiation injury is caused by ionizing and non-ionizing radiation (described in Chapter 45). Burns may result from a high level of radiation exposure to a specific body area; however, radiation injuries make up a small percentage of burn injuries.

> **Critical Thinking**
>
> What industries in your area use radioactive materials? Is there a preplan for incidents at that site?

Local response to burn injury

Burn injury immediately destroys cells or so fully disrupts their metabolic functions that cellular death ensues. Cellular damage is distributed over a spectrum of injury; some cells are destroyed instantly, others are irreversibly injured. Some injured cells may survive if rapid and appropriate intervention is provided in the prehospital setting and in-hospital care.

Major thermal burns have three distinct zones of injury (Jackson's thermal wound theory). These zones usually appear in a bull's-eye pattern (Figure 30-1). The central area of the burn wound, which has sustained the most intense contact with the thermal source, is the zone of coagulation. In this area, coagulation necrosis of the cells has occurred, and the tissue is non-viable. The zone of stasis surrounds the critically injured area and consists of potentially viable tissue despite the serious thermal injury. In this zone, cells are ischaemic because of clotting and vasoconstriction. The cells die within 24 to 48 h after injury if no supportive measures are undertaken. At the periphery of the zone of stasis is the zone of hyperaemia; this zone has increased blood flow as a result of the normal inflammatory response. The tissues in this area recover in 7 to 10 days if infection or profound shock does not develop.

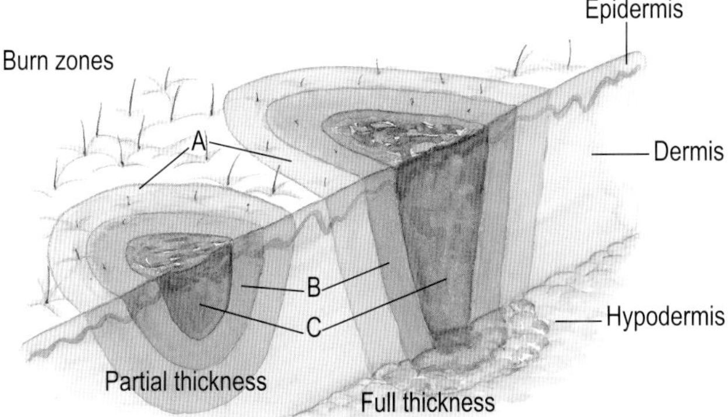

Figure 30-1 Three zones of intensity: (A) zone of hyperaemia (peripheral); (B) zone of stasis (intermediate); and (C) zone of coagulation (central).

Tissue damage from burns depends on the degree of heat and on the duration of exposure to the thermal source. As a rule, the burn wound swells rapidly because of the release of chemical mediators. These mediators cause an increase in capillary permeability and a fluid shift from the intravascular space into the injured tissues. The increased permeability is accentuated by injury to the sodium pump in the cell walls. As sodium moves into the injured cells, it causes an increase in osmotic pressure, which increases the inflow of vascular fluid into the wound. Finally, the normal process of evaporative loss of water to the environment is accelerated (5 to 15 times that of normal skin) through the burned tissue. In a small wound, these physiological alterations produce a classic local inflammatory response (pain, redness, swelling) without major systemic effects. If the wound covers a large area, however, these local tissue responses can produce effects throughout the body and life-threatening hypovolaemia.

Systemic response to burn injury

As local events occur at the injury site, other organ systems become involved in a general response to the stress caused by the burn. One of the earliest manifestations of the systemic effects of a large thermal injury is hypovolaemic shock. This hypovolaemic shock is known as burn shock (described later in this chapter). Burn shock is associated with a decrease in venous return, decreased cardiac output, and increased vascular resistance, and can lead to renal failure. Box 30-2 lists other systemic responses to major burn injury.

Classifications of burn injury

Burns must be assessed and classified (body surface area involvement and depth) as correctly as possible in the field. This will help to ensure the proper treatment and transport to the correct facility. It will also help to monitor the progression of tissue damage, although this is not usually possible in the prehospital setting because of the progressive nature of the injury. The amount of tissue damage may not be evident for hours or even days after a burn injury.

Depth of burn injury

Burns are classified in terms of depth as superficial, partial-thickness and full-thickness. Superficial and partial-thickness burns usually heal without surgery. This is the case, at least, if the burns are uncomplicated by infection or shock. Full-thickness burns usually require skin grafts.

Superficial burns

Superficial burns are also known as first-degree burns. These burns characteristically are painful, red and dry, and blanch with pressure (Figure 30-2). Superficial burns usually occur after prolonged exposure to low-intensity heat or a short-duration flash exposure to a heat source. In these burns, only a superficial layer of epidermal cells is destroyed. The cells slough (peel away from healthy tissue underneath the wound) without residual scarring. Superficial burn injuries usually heal within 2 to 3 days. Sunburn is an example of a superficial burn.

Partial-thickness burns

Partial-thickness burns are also known as second-degree burns. These burns may be divided into two groups: superficial partial-thickness and deep partial-thickness wounds. The superficial partial-thickness injury is characterized by blisters and is often caused by skin contact with hot but not boiling water or other hot liquids, explosions producing flash burns, hot grease and flame.

Box 30-2

Systemic responses to major burn injury

Pulmonary response
- Hyperventilation to meet increased metabolic needs

Gastrointestinal response
- Decrease in splanchnic perfusion that may lead to mucosal haemorrhage and transient adynamic ileus
- Vomiting and aspiration
- Stress ulcers

Musculoskeletal response
- Decreased range of motion from immobility and oedema
- Possible osteoporosis and demineralization (late)

Neuroendocrine response
- Increased amounts of circulating adrenaline and noradrenaline and transient elevation of aldosterone levels

Metabolic response
- Elevated metabolic rate, particularly with infection or surgical stress

Immune response
- Altered immunity, resulting in increased susceptibility to infection
- Depressed inflammatory response

Emotional response
- Physical pain
- Isolation from loved ones and familiar surroundings
- Fear of disfigurement, deformities, and disability
- Altered self-image
- Depression

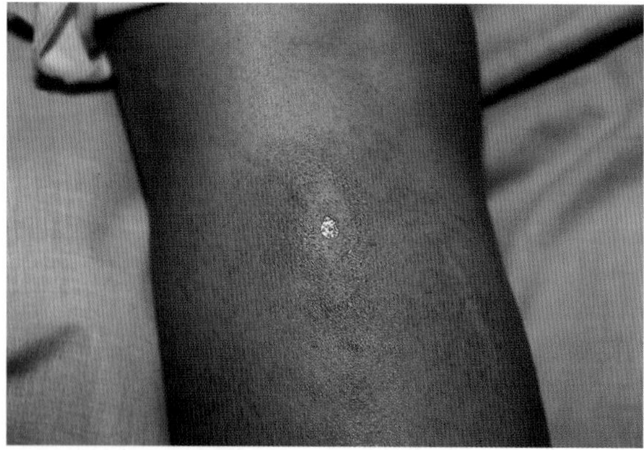

Figure 30-2 Superficial burn.

In superficial partial-thickness burns (Figure 30-3) injury extends through the epidermis to the dermis. However, the basal layers of the skin are not destroyed, and the skin regenerates within a few days to a week. Oedematous fluid infiltrates the dermal–epidermal junction, creating the blisters characteristic of this depth of wound. Intact blisters provide a seal that protects the wound from infection and excessive fluid loss (for this reason, blisters should not be broken in the prehospital setting). The injured area is usually red, wet and painful and may blanch when the tissue around the injury is compressed. In the absence of infection, these wounds heal without scarring, usually within 14 days.

If the depth of the partial-thickness burn involves the basal layer of the dermis, the burn is considered a deep partial-thickness burn (Figure 30-4). As with superficial partial-thickness burns, oedema forms at the epidermal–dermal junction. Sensation in and around the wound may be diminished because of the destruction of basal-layer nerve endings. The injury may appear red and wet or white and dry, depending upon the degree of vascular injury. Wound infection and subsequent sepsis and fluid loss are major complications of these injuries. If uncomplicated, deep partial-thickness burns generally heal within 3 to 4 weeks. Skin grafting may be needed to promote timely healing and minimize thick scar tissue formation. The formation of thick scar tissue may severely restrict joint movements and may cause persistent pain and disfigurement.

Full-thickness burns

In full-thickness burns (also known as third-degree burns), the entire thickness of the epidermis and dermis is destroyed; thus skin grafts are necessary for timely and proper healing

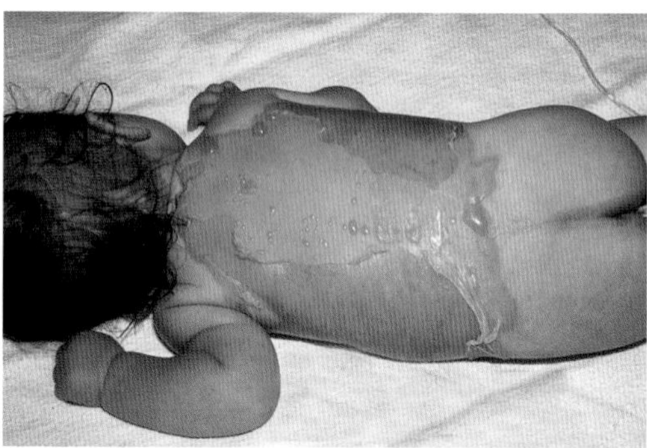

Figure 30-3 Superficial partial-thickness second-degree burn.

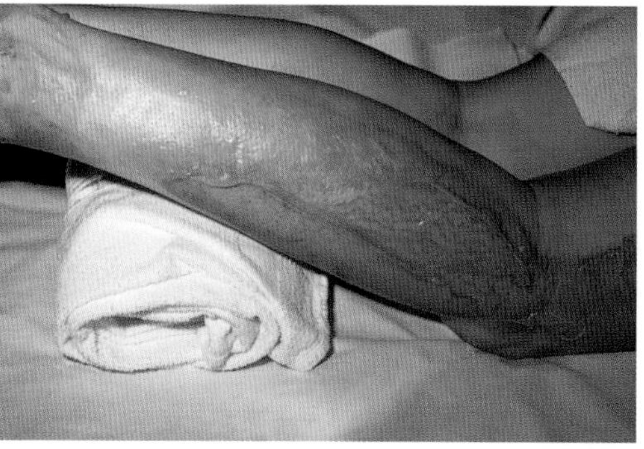

Figure 30-4 Deep partial-thickness burn.

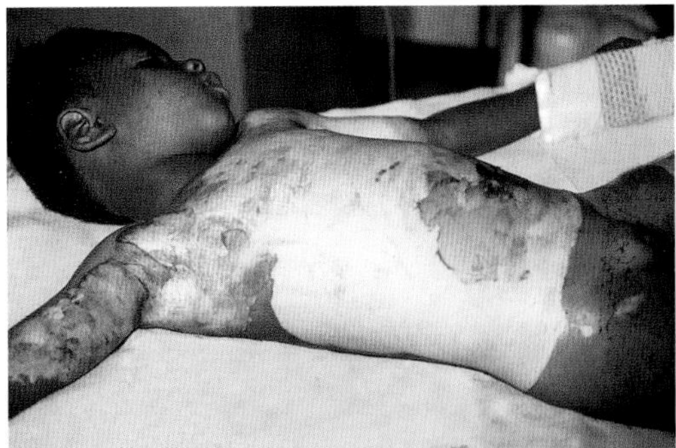

Figure 30-5 Full-thickness burn.

(Figure 30-5). The wound is characterized by coagulation necrosis of the cells, which gives the wound a pearly white, charred or leathery appearance. A definitive sign of a full-thickness burn is a translucent surface in the depths of which thrombosed veins are visible. Eschar, a tough, non-elastic coagulated collagen of the dermis, is present in these injuries.

Sensation and capillary refill are absent in full-thickness burns because small blood vessels and nerve endings are destroyed. This often results in large plasma volume loss, infection and sepsis. Natural wound healing may produce contracture deformity and severe scarring. Surgical intervention with skin grafting is necessary to close full-thickness wounds, minimize complications, and allow restoration of maximal function. Pain may be felt in neighbouring tissue that has been more superficially burnt.

Some burn classifications also describe a full-thickness injury (sometimes called a fourth-degree burn) that penetrates the subcutaneous tissue, muscle, fascia, periosteum or bone. These burns often result from incineration-type exposure and electrical burns in which the heat is great enough to destroy tissues below the skin.

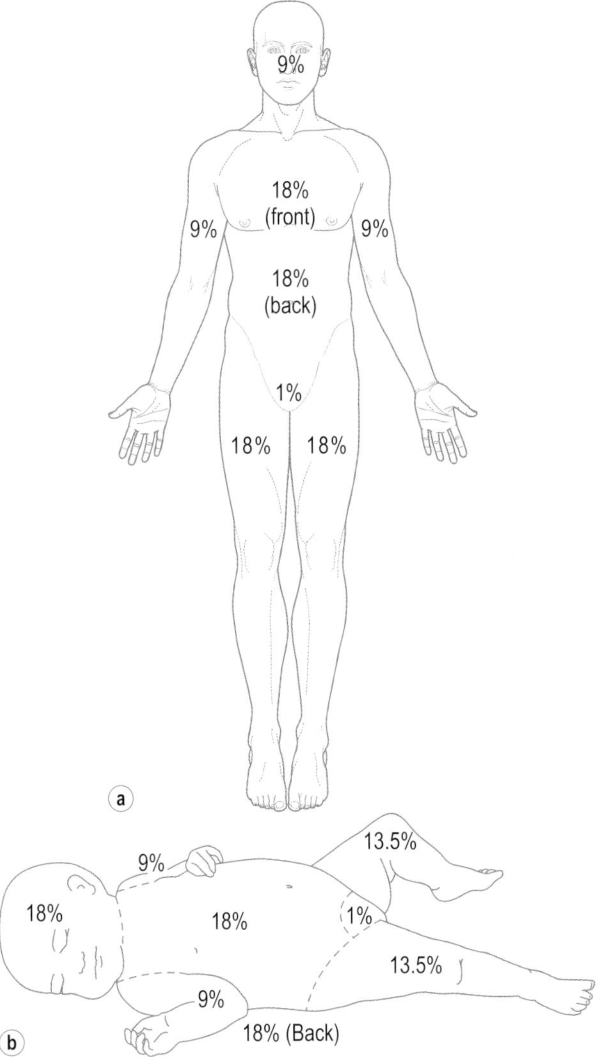

Figure 30-6 The rule of nines. (a) Adult. (b) Infant.

Extent and severity of burn injury

There are several methods to evaluate the extent of burn injury. Common methods include the serial halving method, rule of nines, and the Lund and Browder chart. The paramedic should use the method with which they are familiar but its use should never delay patient care or transport.

Serial halving

Ask 'Does the patient have 100% burns?', if not, 'Does the patient have 50% burns?' and so on, until an estimation is reached that reflects the area of the body affected. Erythema is not normally included in the evaluation of burns surface area as this may further complicate the process and delay transportation. Current UK guidelines recommend that paramedics do include erythema, as only a rough estimate is required and accurate evaluation is not possible in the early stages.[4]

Rule of nines

The rule of nines is commonly used in the prehospital setting. The measurement divides the total body surface area (TBSA) into segments that are multiples of 9%. This method provides a rough estimate of burn injury size and is most accurate for adults and children older than 10 years of age. Figure 30-6 explains the rule of nines.

Critical Thinking

Why is the calculation of body surface area different for children less than 10 years of age?

If the burn is irregularly shaped or has a scattered distribution throughout the body, the rule of nines is hard to apply. In these cases, burn size can be estimated by visualizing the patient's palm as an indicator of percentage (this is the rule of palms). The surface of the patient's palm equals about 1% of the TBSA.

Note

Only partial- and full-thickness burns are included when calculating total body surface area. For large burns, total body surface area may be calculated more easily by subtracting the percentage of unburned area from 100.

Age	0–1	1–4	5–9	10–14	15
A—½ of head	9½%	8½%	6½%	5½%	4½%
B—½ of one thigh	2¾%	3¼%	4%	4¼%	4½%
C—½ of one leg	2½%	2½%	2¾%	3%	3¼%

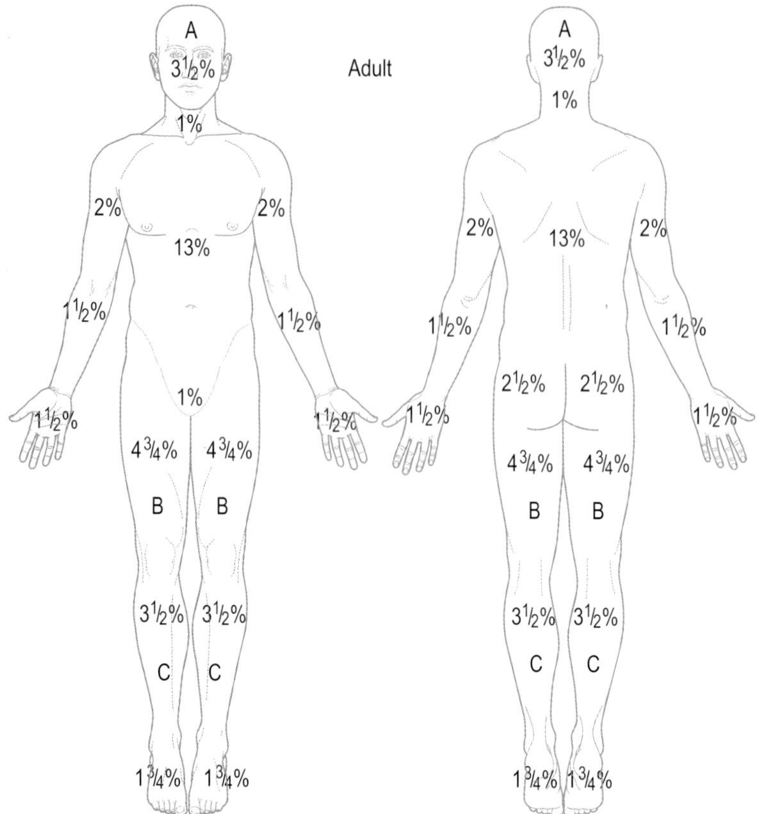

Figure 30-7 Lund and Browder chart.

Lund and Browder chart

The Lund and Browder chart (Figure 30-7) is a more accurate method of determining the area of burn injury because it assigns specific numbers to each body part. The chart is used to measure burns in infants and young children and allows for developmental changes in percentages of body surface area. For example, the adult head is 9% of TBSA, but the newborn head is 18% of TBSA.

Classification of burn severity

A method exists for classifying burn severity based on extent, depth and location of burn injury; age of the patient; aetiological agents involved; presence of inhalation injury; and coexisting injuries or pre-existing illness. Using these criteria, burn injuries are categorized as major, moderate and minor (Box 30-3).[5]

In determining severity, the paramedic must also consider factors such as the patient's age, the presence of concurrent medical or surgical problems, and the complications that accompany certain types of burns, such as those of the face and neck, hands and feet, and genitalia. For example, burns of the face and neck may cause respiratory compromise and may interfere with the ability to eat or drink. Burns of the hands and feet may interfere with ambulation and activities of daily living, whilst perineal burns present a high risk of infection because of the contaminants in this region, and may disrupt the normal patterns of elimination.

Burn centre referral criteria

The National Burn Care Review[6] published in 2005 identified local arrangements that allowed severe burn injuries to be taken from the scene directly to a burns unit, bypassing A&E departments that may be closer. Whilst this recognizes the benefits to the patient of prompt assessment and resuscitation, it does not allow for the possibility of associated non-burn injuries that the burn service may not be able to deal with. The review concluded that ad-hoc arrangements such as this were unsafe and that unless formally agreed by clinical stakeholders, burns victims should be transported to the nearest major A&E department. The paramedic is responsible for ensuring that s/he knows and understands the procedures that have been agreed in their Trust.

Box 30-3

Classification of burn severity

Major burns

1. Partial-thickness burns greater than 25% of body surface area (BSA) in adults or greater than 20% of BSA in children or the elderly.
2. Full-thickness burns greater than 10% of BSA.
3. All burns involving the face, eyes, ears, hands, feet, or perineum that may result in functional or cosmetic impairment.
4. Burns caused by caustic chemical agents.
5. High-voltage electrical injury.
6. Burns complicated by inhalation injury, major trauma, or poor-risk patients.

Moderate burns

1. Partial-thickness burns 15–25% of BSA in adults and 10–20% of BSA in children or the elderly.
2. Full-thickness burns 2–10% of BSA.
3. Not involving risk to areas of specialized function such as the face, eyes, ears, hands, feet, or perineum.

Minor burns

1. Partial-thickness burns less than 15% of BSA in adults or 10% of BSA in children or the elderly.
2. Full-thickness burns less than 2% of BSA.
3. No functional or cosmetic risk to areas of specialized function.

Pathophysiology of burn shock

As stated previously, shock can occur from large body surface area burns. Burn shock results from local and systemic responses to thermal trauma that lead to oedema and accumulation of vascular fluid in the tissues in the area of injury. Locally, a brief initial decrease in blood flow to the area occurs (this is the emergent phase), followed by a considerable increase in arteriolar vasodilatation. A concurrent release of vasoactive substances from the burned tissue causes increased capillary permeability, which in turn produces intravascular fluid loss and wound oedema (the fluid shift phase). The fluid shifts cause cardiovascular changes such as a compromised cardiac output, increased systemic vascular resistance, and reduced peripheral blood flow.

Note

Hypovolaemia caused by burn trauma is not usually seen in the prehospital setting. This is because burn oedema develops over the first several hours after the burn. A hypovolaemic patient with burns should be evaluated at the scene for other injuries as these other injuries may be responsible for the volume loss.

Hypovolaemia results from fluid loss in the injured tissues and fluid that evaporates from the body because of the loss of the skin. Despite the compensatory effort of the body to retain sodium and water, sodium is lost and potassium is released into the extracellular fluid. The blood becomes concentrated. In severe burns, red blood cells may burst (haemolyse). When combined with haemolysis, rhabdomyolysis, and subsequent haemoglobinuria and myoglobinuria seen with major burns and electrical injury, this hypovolaemic state can lead to renal failure. Impaired peripheral blood flow can further damage tissue and can result in metabolic acidosis.

The greatest loss of intravascular fluid occurs in the first 8–12 h, followed by a continued, moderate loss over the next 12–16 h. At some point within 24 h, the leaking of fluid from the cells greatly diminishes (this is the resolution phase). At this point, a balance between the intravascular space and the interstitial space is reached. Peripheral vascular resistance will increase in response to hypovolaemia and the resulting decrease in cardiac output. With volume replacement, cardiac output can increase to levels above normal (this is the hypermetabolic phase of thermal injury) (Figure 30-8).

Fluid replacement

Within minutes of a major burn injury, all capillaries in the circulatory system (not just those in the area of the burn) lose the ability to retain fluid. This increase in capillary permeability prevents the creation of an osmotic gradient between the intravascular and extravascular space. This change allows colloid solutions to equilibrate quickly across the capillaries and into the surrounding tissue. The process of burn shock continues for about 24 h, at which time the normal capillary permeability is restored.[7] Therefore, therapy for burn shock is aimed at supporting the patient's vital organ function through the period of hypovolaemic shock. Crystalloid solution (e.g. sodium lactate or normal saline) is considered the fluid of choice in initial resuscitation.

Several fluid resuscitation formulae consider body size and extent of burned body surface area. The paramedic does not need to know these formulae but should appreciate the complexity of the calculations and how administering fluids in the prehospital phase may complicate the calculations. Fluid resuscitation must be guided by regular monitoring of measures of haemodynamic function, including the patient's vital signs, respiratory rate, lung sounds, capillary refill, and, in some cases, urinary output. When determining the percentage of burn for fluid resuscitation, the paramedic should calculate only partial- and full-thickness burns.

Parkland formula

The Parkland formula for the total fluid requirement in 24 h is as follows:

- 4 mL × [total burn surface area (%)] × [body weight (kg)]
- 50% given in first 8 h
- 50% given in next 16 h.

Children receive maintenance fluid in addition, at an hourly rate of:

- 4 mL/kg for first 10 kg of body weight *plus*
- 2 mL/kg for second 10 kg of body weight *plus*
- 1 mL/kg for >20 kg of body weight.

A good worked example of this can be found in the ABC series of burns in the *British Medical Journal*.[8]

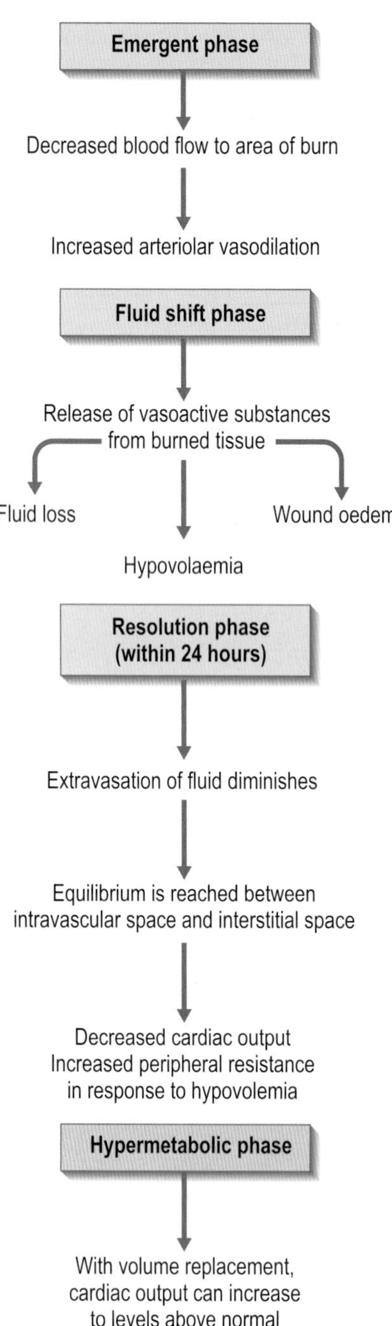

Figure 30-8 Phases of burn shock.

The amount and type of fluids required after the first 24 h are vastly different from those administered during the first 24 h. Fluid replacement is dictated by the patient's response to the burn and the treatment regimen.

Note

Fluid resuscitation in burn-injured persons is controversial. It is usually recommended that fluid resuscitation not be initiated in the prehospital setting if transport to a hospital can be accomplished within 30 min.[7] Transport should not be delayed to initiate intravenous therapy.

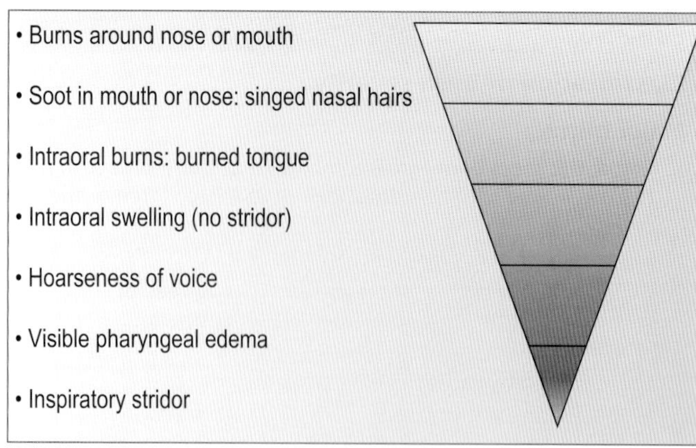

Figure 30-9 Probability of upper airway obstruction.

Assessment of the burn patient

As with any other trauma patient, emergency care for a burn patient begins with making sure the scene is safe and with an initial assessment. In this assessment the paramedic should recognize and treat injuries that pose a threat to life. In burn patients, however, the dramatic appearance of burns, the patient's intense pain, and the characteristic odour of burnt flesh may distract the paramedic from life-threatening problems. A confident assessment by the paramedic and direction of efforts away from the burn wound and toward the patient as a whole are crucial.

Initial assessment

The evaluation of the patient's airway is a major concern in the initial assessment, particularly for the patient with an inhalation injury (described later in this chapter). The paramedic should observe for stridor (an ominous sign that indicates the patient's upper airway is at least 80% narrowed), facial burns, soot in the nose or mouth, singed facial or nasal hair, oedema of lips and the oral cavity, coughing, inability to swallow secretions in the pharynx, hoarse voice, and circumferential neck burns. Airway management should be aggressive with these patients (Figure 30-9).

Critical Thinking

Consider a patient who has a large burn. Your initial assessment reveals that the airway is patent. Why should you perform frequent reassessment of the airway?

The paramedic should evaluate breathing for rate, depth, and the presence of wheezes, crackles or rhonchi, and should evaluate the patient's circulatory status by assessing the presence, rate, character, and rhythm of pulses; capillary refill; skin colour and temperature; pulse oximetry, which may be inaccurate in the presence of carbon monoxide; and obvious arterial bleeding.

The paramedic should determine the patient's neurological status by using the AVPU (alert, verbal, painful, unresponsive) scale and should carefully evaluate any deviations from normal for underlying cause. Abnormalities include hypoxia, decreased cerebral perfusion from hypovolaemia, and cerebral injury resulting from head trauma. After the initial assessment the paramedic should obtain a history of the event whilst performing the physical examination.

An accurate history from the patient or bystanders can help to determine the potential for inhalation injury, concomitant trauma, or pre-existing conditions that may influence the physical examination or patient outcome. When obtaining the patient history, the paramedic should ascertain the following information:

1. What is the patient's chief complaint (e.g. pain or dyspnoea)?
2. What were the circumstances of the injury?
   - Did the injury occur in an enclosed space?
   - Were explosive forces involved?
   - Were hazardous chemicals involved?
   - Is there related trauma?
3. What was the source of the burning agent (e.g. flame, metal, liquid, or chemical)?
4. Does the patient have any significant medical history?
5. What medications does the patient take (including recent ingestion of illegal drugs or alcohol)?
6. Did the patient lose consciousness at any time? (Suspect inhalation injury.)
7. What is the status of tetanus immunization?

Physical examination

At the start of the physical examination, the paramedic should obtain a full set of vital signs, to include blood pressure in an unburned extremity, if available. If all extremities are burned, the paramedic may place sterile gauze under the blood pressure cuff and attempt to auscultate a blood pressure. Patients with severe burns or pre-existing cardiac or medical illness should be monitored by electrocardiogram. Lead placement may need to be modified to avoid placing electrodes over burned areas (see Chapter 15). Field care and hospital destination are determined by the depth, size, location, and extent of burned tissue and the presence of associated illness or injury.

General principles in burn management

Goals for prehospital management of the severely burned patient include preventing further tissue injury, maintaining the airway, administering oxygen and ventilatory support, providing fluid resuscitation (per guidelines), providing rapid transport to an appropriate medical facility, using clean technique to minimize the patient's exposure to infectious agents, and providing psychological and emotional support. Patients with burns should also be evaluated for other types of trauma that pose a threat to life. Some will have additional injuries associated with the burn event. Examples include blunt or penetrating trauma sustained in automobile crashes, blast injury, and skeletal or spinal injury from attempts to escape the thermal source or contact with electrical current.

Stopping the burning process

The first step in managing any burn is to stop the burning process. This step must be achieved with the safety of the emergency crew in mind because it often occurs in proximity to the source that caused the burn. With superficial burns, the burning process can be terminated by cooling the local area with cold (but not ice-cold) water. Ice, snow or ointments should not be applied to the burn as they may increase the depth and severity of thermal injury. This may be due to extreme vasoconstriction, which can cause burn progression. In addition, ointments may impair or delay assessment of the injury when the patient arrives in the emergency department.

In cases of severe burns the paramedic should move the patient rapidly and safely from the burning source to an area of safety if possible. A person whose clothing is in flames or smouldering should be placed on the floor or ground and rolled in a blanket to smother the flames or should be doused with large quantities of the cleanest available water (Cold water to decrease skin temperature rapidly is preferred.) Contaminated water sources, such as lakes or rivers, should be avoided. These patients should never be allowed to run or remain standing. Running may fan the flame, and an upright position may increase the likelihood of the patient's hair being ignited.

Note

Those involved in fire safety and prevention advocate the system of Stop, Drop and Roll. The system was designed to teach children and adults that in the event of their clothing catches fire, they should: stop (do not run); drop (cover your face with your hands and drop to the ground in a prone position); and roll (to smother the fire until the flames are extinguished).

The paramedic should remove the patient's clothing completely whilst cooling the burn so that heat is not trapped under the smouldering cloth. If pieces of smouldering cloth have adhered to the skin, the paramedic should cut, not pull, them away. Melted synthetic fabrics that cannot be removed should be soaked in cold water to stop the burning process. After the burn is cooled, the paramedic should cover the patient who has a large body surface area injury with a clean, preferably sterile, sheet, over which blankets can be placed when ambient temperatures are low. The duration of cooling is controversial; cooling should continue at least until pain is relieved and probably for a total duration of 15 to 30 min,[8] although other sources suggest that it is rare to need more than 10 min.[4]

Airway, oxygen and ventilation

The paramedic should evaluate the adequacy of airway and breathing in all burn patients. If available, humidified high-concentration oxygen should be administered to any patient with severe burns and the paramedic should assist breathing as needed. If humidified oxygen is not available, non-humidified oxygen should not be withheld. If inhalation injury is suspected, observe the patient closely for signs of impending airway obstruction. Life-threatening laryngeal oedema may be progressive and may make tracheal intubation difficult if not impossible. The decision to intubate these patients should not be delayed and every effort should be made to intubate the patient's lungs with a normal (not smaller) size endotracheal tube. These patients are often hard to ventilate, even with an appropriately sized tube.

Circulation

The need for fluid resuscitation is based on three things: the severity of the injury, the patient's vital signs, and on transport time to the receiving hospital. Current guidelines advocate that fluid therapy should be commenced if an area greater than 25% TBSA is affected and the time from injury to hospital is likely to be in excess of an hour.[4] Where fluids are indicated, the following guidelines should be observed.

Crystalloid should be used in the following doses over the first 30 min from injury:[4]

Adult	1000 mL
Child 5–11 years	500 mL
Child <5 years	10 mL/kg

If intravenous therapy is to be performed, the paramedic should initiate it with a large-bore catheter in a peripheral vein in an unburned extremity (preferably the arm). If an unburned site is not available, leave cannulation until the patient is in hospital – do not delay transportation for cannulation. Secure the catheter with a dressing; tape may not adhere to the injured area as the tissue begins to leak fluid.

The administration of analgesia is an early intervention. Whilst cooling and covering the burn should provide significant pain relief, pharmacological agents may sometimes be indicated. The decision to administer and the choice of analgesia are based upon the paramedic's clinical judgement in accordance with current guidelines. Morphine may be indicated in some patients but be aware of the potential effect on respiratory and cardiac function in the compromised patient.

Critical Thinking

How should you administer pain medicine to a patient with a large burn? Why did you choose this route?

Special considerations

All burn injuries warrant good patient assessment and care; however, burns of specific body regions require special consideration. These include burns to the face and extremities and circumferential burns.

Burns of the face swell rapidly and may be associated with airway problems. The head of the ambulance stretcher should be elevated at least 30 degrees, if not contraindicated by spinal trauma, to minimize the oedema. If the patient's ears are burned, the paramedic should avoid use of a pillow, to minimize additional injury to the area.

If burns involve the extremities or large areas of the body, remove all rings, watches, and other jewellery as soon as possible. This will help to prevent vascular compromise with increased wound oedema. Frequent assessment of peripheral pulses is indicated along with elevation of the burned limb above the patient's heart if possible.

Critical Thinking

What life- or limb-threatening problems can develop from this swelling?

Burn injuries that encircle a body region can pose a threat to the patient's life or limbs. Circumferential burns that occur to an extremity may produce a tourniquet-like effect that may quickly compromise circulation and cause irreversible damage to the limb. Circumferential burns of the chest can severely restrict movement of the thorax, thereby significantly impairing chest wall compliance. If this occurs, the depth of respirations is reduced; tidal volume is decreased; and the patient's lungs may become difficult to ventilate, even by mechanical means. Definitive treatment for circumferential burns involves an in-hospital surgical procedure known as escharotomy. In this procedure, incisions are made through deep burns to reduce compartment pressure and allow adequate blood volume to flow to and from the affected limb or thorax.

Inhalation burn injury

Smoke inhalation injury has become the principal cause of death in burns patients,[9] and is responsible for more than 50% of fire deaths each year.[10] Prehospital considerations in caring for patients with inhalation injury include recognition of the dangers inherent in the fire environment, pathophysiology of inhalation injury, and early detection and treatment of impending airway or respiratory problems.

Smoke inhalation most often occurs in a closed environment such as a building, a vehicle, or an airplane. Such injury is caused by the accumulation of toxic by-products of combustion. Inhalation injury can also occur in an open space; therefore all burn victims should be evaluated for this injury. Dangers that contribute to inhalation injury in a fire environment are as follows:

- heat
- consumption of oxygen by the fire
- production of carbon monoxide
- production of other toxic gases.

Inhalation injury may occur in the absence of significant thermal injury from exposure to toxic gases (e.g. carbon monoxide).

Pathophysiology

Smoke inhalation and inhalation injury can produce a large number of complications. For this text, these complications are classified as carbon monoxide poisoning, inhalation injury above the glottis (supraglottic), and inhalation injury below the glottis (infraglottic).

Box 30-4

Physical effects of carbon monoxide blood levels

Carbon monoxide levels less than 10% do not usually cause symptoms; they are common in smokers, traffic police, truck drivers, and others who are exposed to carbon monoxide chronically. At carbon monoxide levels of 20% a healthy patient may complain of headache, nausea, vomiting, and loss of manual dexterity. At 30% the patient may become confused and lethargic, and electrocardiogram abnormalities may be present. At levels between 40% and 60%, coma may develop. Levels above 60% are often fatal. Tachypnoea and cyanosis are not usually present in these patients because arterial oxygen tension is normal. Patients with high carboxyhaemoglobin levels may have a skin appearance that is bright red. More commonly, though, the patient has normal or pale skin and lip coloration.

Carbon monoxide poisoning

Carbon monoxide is a colourless, odourless, tasteless gas produced by incomplete burning of carbon-containing fuels. Carbon monoxide does not harm lung tissue physically; however, it displaces oxygen from the haemoglobin molecule, forming carboxyhaemoglobin. The result is low circulating volumes of oxygen despite normal partial pressures. In addition, the presence of carboxyhaemoglobin requires that tissues be hypoxic before oxygen is released from the haemoglobin to fuel the cells. This condition is reversible.

Carbon monoxide has about 250 times the attraction to haemoglobin that oxygen has, so small concentrations of carbon monoxide in inspired air can result in severe physiological impairments, including tissue hypoxia, inadequate cellular oxygenation, inadequate cellular and organ function, and eventually death. The physical effects of carbon monoxide poisoning are related to the level of carboxyhaemoglobin in the blood (Box 30-4).

Note

As discussed in Chapter 13, the pulse oximeter is unreliable in determining effective oxygenation in a patient with carbon monoxide poisoning.

Treatment of the patient with carbon monoxide poisoning includes ensuring a patent airway, providing adequate ventilation, administering high-concentration oxygen, and possible pharmacological therapy (sodium thiosulphate) for severely poisoned patients. The half-life of carbon monoxide in normal room air is about 4 h but this can be reduced to 30–40 min if 100% oxygen and adequate ventilation are provided. The use of hyperbaric oxygen therapy may be recommended in treating carbon monoxide poisoning. The therapy promotes increased oxygen uptake by haemoglobin molecules that have not yet been bound to carbon monoxide. The paramedic should follow local guidelines.

In addition to carbon monoxide, other gases (e.g. cyanide and hydrogen sulphide) may be released when some materials are burned. The inhalation of these toxic gases can result in inhalation poisoning (e.g. thiocyanate intoxication), which may require pharmacological therapy (e.g. cyanide antidote kit).

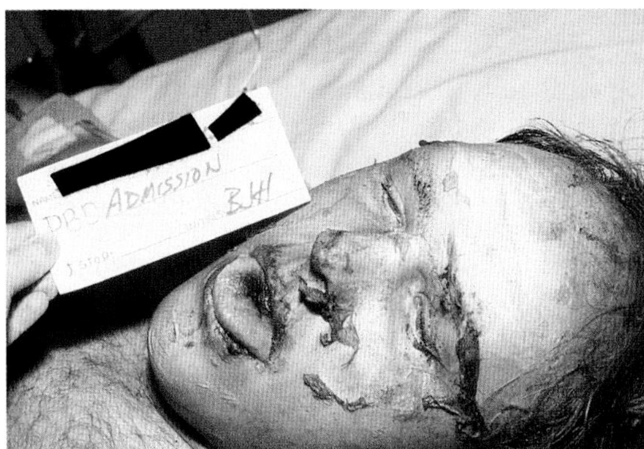

Figure 30-10 Inhalation injury.

Critical Thinking

Can carbon monoxide poisoning be ruled out if the patient does not have these signs or symptoms?

Inhalation injury above the glottis

The structure and function of the airway superior to the glottis makes it susceptible to injury if exposed to high temperatures. The upper airway is vascular and has a large surface area, which allows the upper airway to normalize temperatures of inspired air. Because of this design, actual thermal injury to the lower airway is rare. The upper airway sustains the impact of injury when environmental air is superheated.

Thermal injury to the airway can result in immediate oedema of the pharynx and larynx (above the level of the true vocal cords). This can progress rapidly to complete airway obstruction. Signs and symptoms of upper airway inhalation injury include the following (Figure 30-10):

- facial burns
- singed nasal or facial hairs
- carbonaceous sputum
- oedema of the face, oropharyngeal cavity, or both
- signs of hypoxaemia
- hoarse voice
- stridor
- brassy cough
- grunting respirations.

Prompt assessment of the airway is critical in these patients. The paramedic must establish and protect the airway. If impending airway obstruction is suspected, early nasotracheal or orotracheal intubation may be warranted because progressive oedema can make intubation hazardous if not impossible.

Inhalation injury below the glottis

The two main mechanisms of direct injury to the lung tissue (parenchyma) are heat and toxic material inhalation. Thermal injury to the lower airway is rare. One cause of such injury is the inhalation of superheated steam, which has 4000 times the heat-carrying capacity of dry air. Other causes include the aspiration of scalding liquids and explosions. These occur as the patient is breathing high concentrations of oxygen under pressure.

Most lower airway injuries in fires result from the inhalation of toxic chemicals. Such chemicals include the gaseous by-products of burning materials. Signs and symptoms of lower airway injury may be immediate, but more often they are delayed for several hours. Signs and symptoms include the following:

- wheezes
- crackles or rhonchi
- productive cough
- signs of hypoxaemia
- spasm of bronchi and bronchioles.

Prehospital care is directed at maintaining a patent airway, providing high-concentration oxygen and ventilatory support. This may include nasal or oral tracheal intubation and drug therapy with bronchodilators.

Chemical burn injury

Caustic chemicals are often present in the home and workplace; unintentional exposure is common. Three types of caustic agents are often associated with burn injuries; these are alkalis, acids and organic compounds. Alkalis are strong bases with a high pH and include hydroxides and carbonates of sodium, potassium, ammonium, lithium, barium and calcium. These compounds are commonly found in oven cleaners, household drain cleaners, fertilizers, heavy industrial cleaners, and the structural bonds of cement and concrete. Strong acids are in many household cleaners, such as rust removers and bathroom cleaners (**Figure 30-11**).

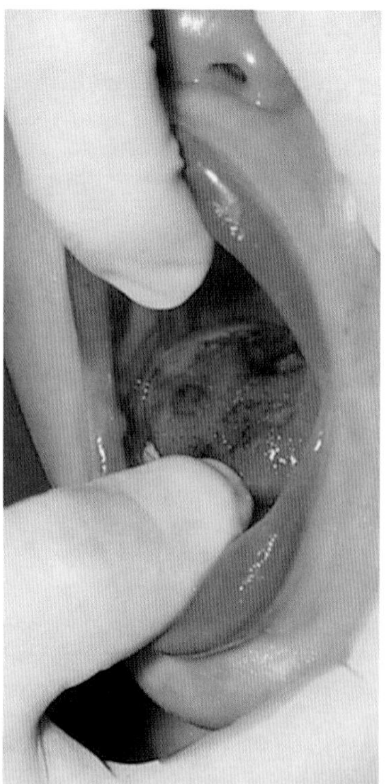

Figure 30-11 Intraoral chemical burns sustained by a boy who had ingested bleach.

Organic compounds are chemicals that contain carbon. Most organic compounds, such as wood and coal, are harmless chemicals, but several organic compounds produce caustic injury to human tissue. These compounds include phenols and creosote and petroleum products such as caustic soda. In addition to their role in producing chemical burns, organic compounds may be absorbed by the skin. Absorption in turn may cause serious systemic effects; the severity of chemical injury is related to the chemical agent, concentration and volume of the chemical, and duration of contact.

Assessment

While obtaining the patient history, the paramedic should collect facts regarding the exposure factors. When dealing with a chemical exposure, the paramedic should determine the following:

- type of chemical substance; if the container is available and can be transported safely, it should be taken to the medical facility
- concentration of chemical substance
- volume of chemical substance
- mechanism of injury (local immersion of a body part, injection, splash)
- time of contamination
- first aid administered before medical service arrival
- appearance (chemical burns vary in colour)
- pain.

Management

As with all burn injuries, the safety of the rescuers must be the first priority in managing the victim of chemical injury. (Police, fire service, and special rescue personnel may be needed to secure the scene before entry.) The paramedic must consider the use of protective gear before entering the scene. Depending on the scene and the chemical agent(s), decontamination may be required. Personal protection may include gloves, eye shields, protective garments, and appropriate breathing apparatus. A response to a hazardous materials incident requires special safety considerations and trained rescue personnel (see Chapter 43). The treatment of chemical injuries does not vary much from that of thermal burns during the initial assessment. Treatment is directed at stopping the burning process, which can best be achieved by the following:

1. Remove all clothing, including shoes. These can trap concentrated chemicals.
2. Brush off powdered chemicals.
3. Irrigate the affected area with vast amounts of water.
   (a) In otherwise stable patients, irrigation takes priority over transport. That is the case unless irrigation can be continued en route to the emergency department.
   (b) If a large body surface area is involved, a shower should be used for irrigation, if available.

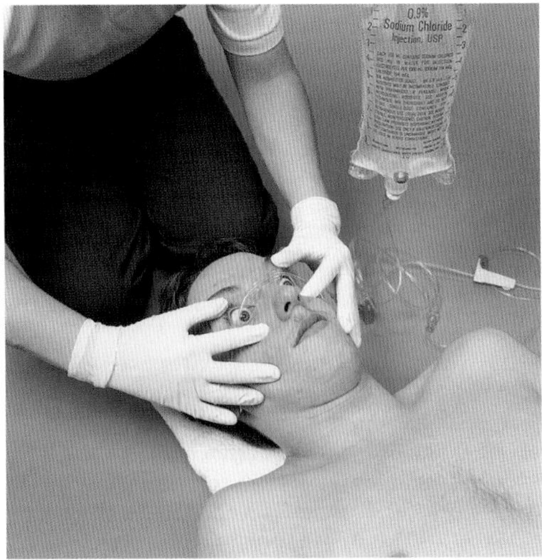

Figure 30-12 Use of nasal cannula for eye irrigation.

Chemical burn injury to the eyes

Chemical exposure to the eyes (e.g. from mace, pepper spray or other irritants) may cause damage ranging from superficial inflammation (chemical conjunctivitis) to severe burns. Patients with these conditions have local pain, visual disturbance, lacrimation (shedding tears), oedema and redness of surrounding tissues. Management guidelines include flushing the eyes with water. This can be done by using a mild flow from a hose, intravenous tubing or water from a container. (The affected eye should be irrigated from the medial to the lateral aspect to minimize the risk of flushing the chemical into the unaffected eye.) Irrigation should be continued during transport. If contact lenses are present, they should be removed. When retracting the lids to irrigate the eyes, take care to apply pressure only to the bony structures surrounding the eye and avoid applying pressure on the globe.

Consideration could be given to the use of a nasal cannula to irrigate both eyes at the same time. The cannula is placed over the bridge of the nose; the nasal prongs are pointing down toward the eyes. The cannula is attached to an intravenous administration set using normal saline or sodium lactate solution, and the fluid is run continually into both eyes (Figure 30-12). A chemical burn to the eye can be frightening for the patient and s/he may fear loss of sight from the injury. The paramedic should attempt to calm the patient before irrigating, as it may be uncomfortable. Reassurance often improves the patient's cooperation.

Use of antidotes or neutralizing agents

According to the American Burn Association, no agent has been found to be superior to water for treating most chemical burns.[11] Thus, the use of antidotes or neutralizing agents should be avoided in initial prehospital management of most burn injuries. Many neutralizing agents produce heat, which may increase injury when applied to the wound.

Specific chemical injuries

The main treatment for most chemical burns is copious irrigation with water. However, a number of chemical injuries call for further discussion and include those from petroleum, hydrofluoric acid, phenols, ammonia and alkali metals. Personal safety is a priority when working around any of these chemicals.

Petroleum

In the absence of flame, products such as petrol and diesel fuel can cause significant chemical burns if prolonged contact occurs. (This may occur, for example, with entrapment in a vehicle that is surrounded by spilled petrol.) At first, the injury may appear to be only a superficial or partial-thickness burn, though it may be a full-thickness injury. Systemic effects such as central nervous system depression, organ failure and death may result from the absorption of various hydrocarbons.

Hydrofluoric acid

Hydrofluoric acid is one of the most corrosive materials known. The acid is used in industry for cleaning fabrics and metals, for glass etching, and in the manufacture of silicone chips for electronic equipment. The hydrogen ion and fluoride ion are damaging to tissue. Fluoride hinders several chemical reactions that are required for cell survival and continues to penetrate and kill cells even when it is neutralized by binding to calcium or magnesium. Thus, endogenous or exogenous hydrofluoric acid has the potential to produce deep, painful, and severe injuries. If large body surface areas are involved, the patient may experience severe hypocalcaemia and even death. This is true with exposure to high concentrations of the acid also. Even the most minor-appearing wounds that involve hydrofluoric acid should be evaluated at an appropriate medical facility.

Irrigation of the exposed area with large amounts of water should be started immediately. On arrival in the emergency department, treatment may include subcutaneous injection of 10% calcium gluconate directly into the burn site.

Phenol

Phenol (carbolic acid) is an aromatic hydrocarbon. Phenol is derived from coal tar and is used widely in industry as a disinfectant in cleaning agents. Phenol is also used in the manufacture of plastics, dyes, fertilizers and explosives. Skin contact with phenol can result in local tissue coagulation and systemic toxicity if the agent is absorbed. A soft tissue injury from phenol exposure may be painless because of the anaesthetic properties of the agent. Minor exposures may cause central nervous system depression and dysrhythmias. Patients with significant exposures (10–15% TBSA) may require systemic support and should be observed carefully for signs of respiratory failure.

Wounds should be irrigated with large volumes of water.

Ammonia

Ammonia is a noxious, irritating gas and a strong alkali that is highly soluble in water. Ammonia is hazardous if introduced into the eye and may result in tissue necrosis and blindness. The patient with an ammonia burn to the eye will probably have swelling or spasm of the eyelids. These injuries must be irrigated with water or a balanced salt solution for up to 24 h.

Respiratory injury from ammonia vapours depends on two things: the concentration and duration of exposure. For example, short-term, high-concentration exposure usually results in upper airway oedema; however, long-term, low-concentration exposure may damage the lower respiratory tract. The initial care for patients with respiratory injury includes high-concentration oxygen administration, ventilatory support as needed, and rapid transport to an appropriate medical facility.

Alkali metals

Sodium and potassium are highly reactive metals that can ignite spontaneously. Water is generally contraindicated when these metals are imbedded in the skin because they react with water and produce large amounts of heat. Physically removing the metal or covering it with oil minimizes the thermal injury.

Electrical burn injuries

Electrical injuries account for 3–4% of burns unit admissions.[12] Good patient care and personal safety at the scene of an electrocution depends on understanding how electricity flows (current) through the body (Box 30-5).

Types of electrical injury

Three basic types of injury may occur as a result of contact with electric current. These are direct contact burns, arc injuries, and flash burns. Direct contact burns occur when electric current directly penetrates the resistance of the skin and underlying tissues. The hand and wrist are common entrance sites and the foot is a common exit site (Figure 30-13a, b).

Although the skin may initially resist current flow, continued contact with the source lessens resistance and permits increased current flow. The greatest tissue damage occurs directly under and adjacent to the contact points and may include fat, fascia, muscle and bone. Tissue destruction may be massive at the entrance and exit sites; however, injury to the area between these wounds is what poses the greatest threat to the patient's life.

Arc injuries occur when a person is close enough to a high-voltage source that the current between two contact points near the skin overcomes the resistance in the air, passing the current flow through the air to the bystander. Temperatures generated by these sources can be as high as 2000 °C to 4000 °C. The arc may jump as far as 3 m.

Flame and flash burn injuries can occur when the heat of electrical current ignites a nearby combustible source. Common injury sites include the face and eyes (welder's flash). Flash burns may also ignite a person's clothing or cause fire in the surrounding environment. No electrical current passes through the body in this type of burn.

Effects of electrical injury

Electrical injuries are often unpredictable, varying according to the parameters that have been described. Yet certain physiological effects should be expected by the paramedic crew.

The skin is almost always the first point of contact with electrical current. Direct contact and passage of the current

Box 30-5

Principles of electricity

Tissue damage produced by electric current is a function of six factors: amperage, voltage, resistance, type of current, current pathway and duration of current flow.

1. *Amperage*. Amperage is a measure of the current flow (intensity) per unit of time. One ampere is a passage of 1 coulomb of charge per second past any point in the circuit. Thus a 10-A flow means that 10 coulombs of electricity are passing a point per second.
2. *Voltage*. Voltage is a continuous force (tension) applied to any electric circuit that produces a flow of electricity. Volts are the driving force for electrical current. One V is the force needed to drive 1 A of current in a circuit with 1 ohm of resistance. High-voltage electrical injuries result from contact with a source of 1000 V or greater. High-tension accidents usually range from 7200 to 19 000 V. Yet they may involve current with as high as 100 000 to 1 million V.
3. *Ohm*. An ohm is a measure of the resistance of an electrical conductor. Electrical resistance is composed of four factors: (1) resistivity, the capacity of a material to resist current flow; (2) the size of the object pathway; (3) the length of the object pathway; and (4) temperature. Resistance to the flow of electricity varies greatly within the body because various tissues have different resistance to current flow. Tissue resistance to electrical flow in the body is highest in bone and decreases progressively through the fat, skin, muscle, blood, and nerve tissue.
4. *Type of current*. Two basic forms of electric current are in common usage: direct current (DC) and alternating current (AC). The type of current can influence patterns and severity of injury. Direct current flows in one direction only. Direct current often is used in industry; it is the type of current produced by batteries. Direct current commonly is used in electrosurgical devices and defibrillators and is characterized by high amperage and low voltage.
   Alternating current reverses the direction of flow at regular intervals (60-cycle current has 60 reversals per second). These alterations in current direction can cause tetanic muscle contractions. These contractions may 'freeze' the victim to the source until the current is terminated. Household current in the UK is generally alternating current and 230–240 V. Alternating current is a more common cause of electrical injury.
5. *Current pathway*. Electricity normally flows along a continuous pathway. This pathway is known as an electric circuit. The current pathway can be unpredictable. However, as a rule, low-voltage current (less than 1000 V) follows the path of least resistance. High-voltage current follows the shortest path. In either case, the greater the current flow, the greater the heat generated.
   The pathway of the current through the body is important because it gives a clue as to what anatomical structures are damaged. For example, if the current travels from one hand to the other, it may flow across the heart and provoke ventricular fibrillation or other dysrhythmias.
6. *Duration of flow*. Tissue injury results from the conversion of electrical energy into heat. The amount of heat produced is directly proportional to the square of the current strength multiplied by the resistance of the tissue multiplied by the duration of the current flow (Joule's law). Therefore injury is directly proportional to the duration of contact with the electrical source.

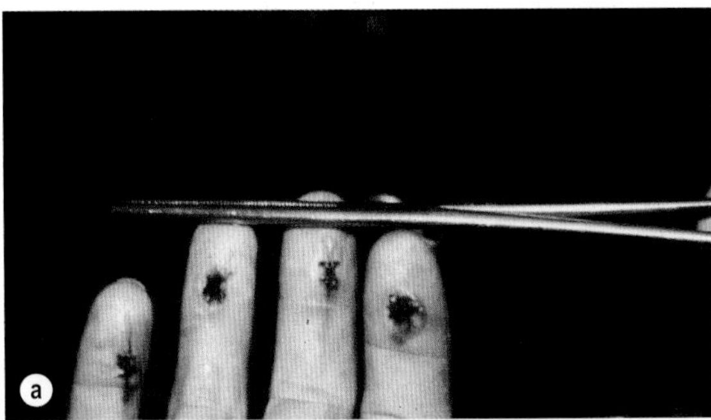

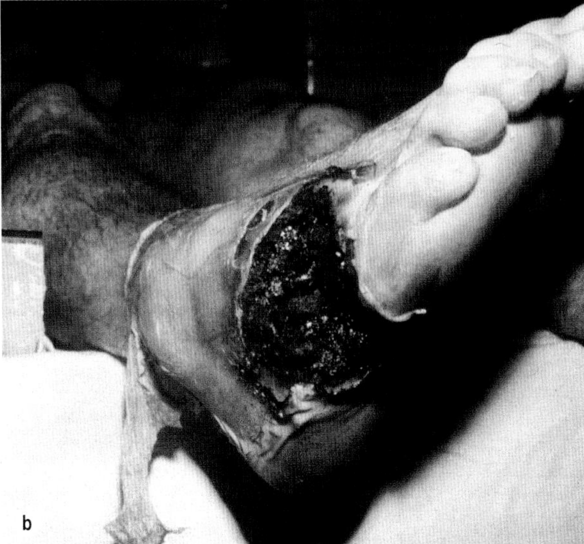

Figure 30-13 Direct contact burn. (a) Entry wound (hand). (b) Exit wound (foot).

through tissue may cause wide areas of coagulation necrosis. The entrance site is often a bull's-eye wound and may appear dry, leathery, charred or depressed. The exit wound may be ulcerated and may appear exploded; areas of tissue may be missing.

Oral burns are often seen in children younger than 2 years of age. These wounds are usually caused by chewing or sucking on a low-tension electrical cord. Oral burns may be associated with injury to the tongue, palate, and face.

Hypertension and tachycardia associated with a large release of catecholamines is a common finding in electrical injury. Electrical current may also cause significant dysrhythmias (including ventricular fibrillation and asystole) and damage to the myocardium as it passes through the body. If the patient suffers cardiac arrest and early rescue and resuscitation can be initiated, success rates are high.

Nerve tissue is a good conductor of electrical current, thus nerve tissue may often be affected in electrical injuries. Central nervous system damage may result in seizures or coma with or without focal neurological findings. Peripheral nerve injury may lead to motor or sensory deficits; these deficits may be permanent. If the current passes through the brainstem, respiratory arrest or depression, cerebral oedema, or haemorrhage may rapidly lead to death.

Electrical injury can cause extensive necrosis of blood vessels. This may not be evident upon the arrival of the medical services; however, such injuries can cause immediate or delayed internal haemorrhage or arterial or venous thrombosis and embolism with subsequent complications.

Damage within the extremities following an electrical burn is similar to crush injury (described in Chapter 29). Severe muscle necrosis releases myoglobin, whilst bursting of erythrocytes (haemolysis) releases haemoglobin. Both of these large molecules can precipitate in the renal tubules, producing acute renal failure. Decreased circulation and compartment syndrome in the affected extremity may lead to amputation. In the electrocuted patient, severe muscle spasms can produce bony fractures. These spasms may also produce dislocations, even at major joints. A patient may fall after an electrical shock, which may cause skeletal trauma, including damage to the cervical spine.

Acute renal failure is a serious complication that affects about 10% of significant direct-contact electrical injuries. Acute renal failure may result from a combination of myoglobin or haemoglobin precipitating out of solution in the renal tubules, disseminated intravascular coagulation caused by tissue damage, hypovolaemic shock, and direct current damage. Acute renal failure is not of immediate consequence in the prehospital setting, yet prompt fluid resuscitation and management of shock may have a positive impact on a number of these patients.

Ventilation may be impaired when electrical burns produce central nervous system injury or chest wall dysfunction. If the respiratory centre is disrupted, hypoventilation can lead to instant patient death. Contact with any alternating current sources has also been known to produce respiratory arrest and death from tetany of the muscles of respiration.

Conjunctival and corneal burns and ruptured tympanic membranes are common in some electrical injuries. Cataracts and hearing loss also may appear as late as 1 year after the event.

A number of other internal structures may be damaged from electrical injury. These structures include the abdominal organs and urinary bladder. Submucosal haemorrhage may occur in the bowel; various forms of ulceration are possible. Each patient requires a thorough physical assessment and a high degree of suspicion for associated trauma.

Assessment and management

Patient assessment should begin by ensuring that no hazards exist for the rescuers or bystanders. If the patient is still in contact with the electrical source, the paramedic should summon the electric company, fire service, or other specially trained personnel before approaching the patient. Once the scene is safe, the patient intervention may begin.

> **Critical Thinking**
>
> What will you do if you respond to a scene and there is a child still in contact with electrical current and who is having tetanic movements? A large crowd has gathered around and is screaming at you to help. The fire service is 3 min away. How will you feel?

Initial assessment

The initial assessment should proceed as it does for all other trauma patients, including immobilization of the cervical spine where appropriate. If the patient is not breathing, assisted ventilation should proceed immediately. The paramedic should consider early intubation because apnoea may persist for lengthy periods. A patient who is breathing should have a patent airway maintained using adjuncts as necessary and respirations should be supported with supplemental high-concentration oxygen. If the patient is in cardiac arrest, the paramedic should initiate resuscitation efforts according to protocol. If possible, the paramedic should obtain a history that includes the following:

- patient's chief complaint (e.g. injury or disorientation)
- source, voltage and amperage of the electrical injury
- duration of contact
- level of consciousness before and after the injury
- significant medical history.

Note

The source, voltage and type of current (alternating current versus direct current) is essential information for the attending physician to estimate internal damage from external wounds.

Physical examination

The physical examination should be thorough. The paramedic should search for entrance and exit wounds or any associated trauma caused by tetany or a fall. The paramedic should recall that there might have been multiple pathways of current, which would mean multiple wounds. All of the patient's clothing and jewellery should be removed, and the areas between the patient's fingers and toes examined for sites of entry or exit. The paramedic should carefully assess distal pulses, motor function and sensation in all extremities and document the findings to monitor for possible development of compartment syndrome. Entrance and exit wounds should be covered with sterile dressings and associated trauma should be managed appropriately.

Internal damage from electrical current may be much more significant than external wounds. Frequent reassessment is necessary because of the progressive nature of electrical injury. In addition, electrocardiogram monitoring should be implemented at the scene and continued during patient transport. As previously discussed, electrical injury may cause a variety of dysrhythmias, some of which can be lethal.

Management

Early administration of fluids is critical for patients with severe electrical injury. Fluid administration helps to prevent hypovolaemia and subsequent renal failure. If possible, the paramedic should establish two large-bore intravenous lines in the antecubital fossae, presuming the extremity has no entry or exit wounds. The fluid of choice is sodium lactate or normal saline without glucose. The flow rate should be determined by the patient's clinical status.

In the emergency department or during interhospital transfer, the patient's intravenous fluid rates will be regulated to maintain a urine output of 75–100 mL/h. This rate decreases the potential for renal damage caused by myoglobin. Emergency department management may include the administration of sodium bicarbonate to help maintain alkaline urine. Alkalinity in turn increases the solubility of haemoglobin and myoglobin and decreases the risk of renal failure.

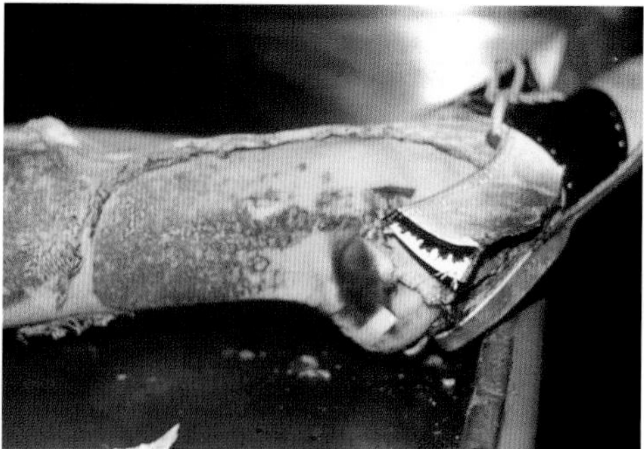

Figure 30-14 Lightning injury.

Lightning injury

Lightning strikes the earth about 7.4 million times each year but lightning injuries are uncommon in the UK. On average, 49 people are struck by lightning in the UK each year, 3 of who are killed.[13] Lightning can deliver direct current of up to 200 000 A at a potential of 100 million or more volts, with temperatures that vary between 8900 °C and 33 000 °C. Lightning injuries can occur from a direct strike or by a side flash (splash) between a victim and a nearby object that has been struck by lightning.

Lightning strikes produce tissue injuries that differ from other types of electrical injury because the pathway of tissue damage is often over rather than through the skin (Figure 30-14). The duration of the lightning is short (0.01–0.001 s), thus skin burns are less severe than those seen with other high-voltage current. In fact, full-thickness burns are rare. Common lightning burns are linear, feathery, and punctate (pinpoint). In addition, depending on the severity of the strike, the patient may suffer cardiac and respiratory arrest. These are the most common causes of death in lightning injuries.

Lightning injuries may be classified as minor, moderate or severe. The patients with minor lightning injuries usually are conscious but may be confused and amnesic. Burns or other signs of injury are rare and vital signs are usually stable.

The patients with moderate injury may be combative or comatose, and may have associated injuries from the impact of the lightning strike. Superficial and partial-thickness burns are common, as is tympanic membrane rupture. These patients may have serious internal organ damage so should be observed carefully for signs and symptoms of cardiorespiratory dysfunction.

Severe lightning injuries include those that cause immediate brain damage, seizures, respiratory paralysis, and cardiac arrest. The prehospital care is directed at basic and advanced life support measures and rapid transport to an appropriate facility.

Assessment and management

Like all other emergency responses, scene safety is the first priority. If the electrical storm is still in progress, all patient care should take place in a sheltered area. To prevent injury from subsequent lightning strikes, the paramedic crew should stay away from objects that project from the ground. Such objects include trees, fences and high buildings. The crew should also avoid areas of open water. If rescue attempts in an open area are necessary, the paramedic should stay low to the ground.

The prehospital management of lightning injuries is the same as for other severe electrical injuries. Initial patient care is directed at airway and ventilatory support; basic and advanced life support; patient immobilization; fluid resuscitation to prevent hypovolaemia and renal failure; pharmacological therapy (per protocol) to manage seizures and dysrhythmias (if present); wound care; and rapid transport to a proper facility.

Note

Cardiopulmonary resuscitation should be initiated immediately for patients who appear dead, because resuscitation is possible after lightning injury.

Summary

- Each year 250 000 people seek medical attention for burns in the UK. Morbidity and mortality rates from burn injury follow significant patterns regarding gender, age, and socioeconomic status. A burn injury is caused by an interaction between thermal, chemical, electrical, or radiation energy and biological matter.
- Tissue damage from burns depends on the degree of the heat and on the duration of exposure to the thermal source. As local events occur at the injury site, other organ systems become involved in a general response to the stress caused by the burn.
- Burns are classified in terms of depth as superficial, partial-thickness and full-thickness. The rule of nines or serial halving provides a rough estimate of burn injury size (extent) and is most accurate for adults and for children older than age 10. The Lund and Browder chart is a more accurate method of determining the area of burn injury. Severity of burn injury and burn centre referral guidelines are based on standards that take into account the depth, extent, and severity of the burn wound; the source of injury; patient age; presence of concurrent medical or surgical problems; and the body region that is burned.
- Shock after thermal injury results from oedema and accumulation of vascular fluid. These tissue changes occur in the area of injury and can produce systemic hypovolaemia if the burn area is large.
- Emergency care for a burn patient begins with the initial assessment. The goal is to recognize and treat life-threatening injuries.
- Goals for prehospital management of the severely burned patient include preventing further tissue injury, maintaining the airway, administering oxygen and ventilatory support, providing fluid resuscitation, providing rapid transport to an appropriate medical facility, using aseptic (clean) technique to minimize the patient's exposure to infectious agents, managing pain, and providing psychological and emotional support.
- Prehospital considerations in caring for patients with inhalation injury include recognition of the dangers inherent in the fire environment, pathophysiology of inhalation injury, and early detection and treatment of impending airway or respiratory problems.
- The severity of chemical injury is related to three things: the chemical agent, the concentration and volume of the chemical, and the duration of contact. Treatment is directed at stopping the burning process by using copious irrigation.
- Three types of injury may occur as a result of contact with electrical current: direct contact burns, arc injuries and flash burns. Once the scene is safe, patient intervention may begin. Internal damage from electrical current may be much more significant than external wounds.

References

1. Hettiaratchy S, Dziewulski P 2004 ABC of burns – introduction. BMJ 328(7452):1366–1368
2. National Safety Council 2001 Injury facts. National Safety Council, Itasca, IL
3. Achauer B 1987 Management of the burned patient. Appleton & Lange, Norwalk, CN
4. Joint Royal Colleges Ambulance Liaison Committee 2006 UK Ambulance Service Clinical Practice Guidelines. JRCALC, London
5. American Burn Association 1990 Hospital and prehospital resources for optimal care of patients with burn injury: guidelines for development and operation of burn centers. J Burn Care Rehabil 11:98–104
6. National Burn Care Review Committee Report 2005 Standards and strategy for burn care; a review of burn care in the British Isles. Online. Available http://jrcalc.org.uk/guidelines.html
7. Faldmo L, Kravitz M 1993 Management of acute burns and shock resuscitation. AACN Clin Issues Crit Care Nurs 4(2):351–366
8. Hettiaratchy S, Papini R 2004 ABC of burns: initial assessment and management of a major burn II – assessment and resuscitation. BMJ 329(19):101–103
9. Mushtaq F, Graham CA 2004 Discharge from the accident and emergency department after smoke

inhalation: influence of clinical factors and emergency investigations. Eur J Emerg Med 11(3):141–144

10. National Institute of General Medical Sciences, National Institutes of Health 1999 Trauma, burn, shock and injury: facts and figures. National Institute of General Medical Sciences, Bethesda, MD
11. American Burn Association 2001 Advanced burn life support provider manual. American Burn Association, Chicago, IL
12. Hettiaratchy S, Dziewulski P 2004 ABC of burns: pathophysiology and types of burns. BMJ 328(7453):1427–1429
13. Elsom D 2001 Deaths and injuries caused by lightning in the United Kingdom: analyses of two databases. Atmospheric Research 56(1–4):325–334

CHAPTER 31

Facial and Head Trauma

Chapter contents

Objectives

Upon completion of this chapter, the paramedic student will be able to:

1. Describe the mechanisms of injury, assessment, and management of maxillofacial injuries.
2. Describe the mechanisms of injury, assessment, and management of ear, eye, and dental injuries.
3. Describe the mechanisms of injury, assessment, and management of anterior neck trauma.
4. Describe the mechanisms of injury, assessment, and management of injuries to the scalp, cranial vault, or cranial nerves.
5. Distinguish between types of traumatic brain injury based on an understanding of pathophysiology and assessment findings.
6. Outline the prehospital management of the patient with cerebral injury.
7. Calculate a Glasgow Coma Scale, trauma score, Revised Trauma Score, and paediatric trauma score when given appropriate patient information.

Key terms

antegrade amnesia The loss of memory for events that occurred immediately after recovery of consciousness.

Battle's sign Ecchymosis over the mastoid process caused by a fracture of the temporal bone.

cerebral perfusion pressure A measure of the amount of blood flow to the brain calculated by subtracting the intracranial pressure from the mean systemic arterial blood pressure.

Cushing triad Increased systolic pressure, widened pulse pressure, and decrease in the pulse and respiratory rate, which result from increased intracranial pressure.

decerebrate posturing A position in which a comatose patient's arms are extended and internally rotated and the legs are extended with the feet in forced plantar flexion; usually observed in patients who have compression of the brainstem.

decorticate posturing A position in which the comatose patient's upper extremities are rigidly flexed at the elbows and at the wrists; usually observed in patients who have a lesion in the mesencephalic region of the brain.

intracerebral haematoma An accumulation of blood or fluid within the tissue of the brain.

Le Fort fracture: A fracture pattern that can be produced in the midface region.

mean arterial pressure The arithmetic mean of the blood pressure in the arterial portion of the circulation.

raccoon's eyes Ecchymosis of one or both orbits caused by fracture of the base of the sphenoid sinus.

retrograde amnesia The loss of memory for events that occurred before the event that precipitated the amnesia.

subarachnoid haematoma A collection of blood or fluid in the subarachnoid space.

Up to 1 million people a year in the UK attend an accident and emergency department because of head injury: 90% of these are classified as minor (Glasgow Coma Scale [GCS] of 15) or mild (13 or 14), 5% as moderate (9–12), and 5% as severe (3–8).[1] The categories of head trauma discussed in this chapter include maxillofacial trauma; ear, eye, and dental trauma; anterior neck trauma; and trauma to the skull and brain.

Maxillofacial injury

Fractures of the facial skeleton are most commonly seen following assault, road traffic collisions, falls and sporting injuries.[2] Fifty percent of maxillofacial injuries occur as a consequence of assault, and 50% of those cases will have raised alcohol levels.[3] However, it is important to remember that confusion may be the result of head injury or hypoxia. There is a 10–15% chance of cervical spine injury in unconscious patients with severe maxillofacial trauma.[3]

Soft tissue injuries

The face receives a rich vascular supply from the branches of the internal and external carotid arteries. As a result, soft tissue injuries to the face often appear to be serious (Figure 31-1a, b). With the exception of a compromised upper airway and the potential for heavy bleeding, damage to the tissues of the maxillofacial area is seldom life threatening. Depending on the mechanism of injury, facial trauma may range from minor cuts and abrasions to more serious injuries. The more serious injuries may involve extensive soft tissue lacerations and avulsions. If possible, the paramedic should obtain a thorough history from the patient to include mechanism of injury; events leading up to the injury; time of injury; associated medical problems; and allergies, medications, and last oral intake.

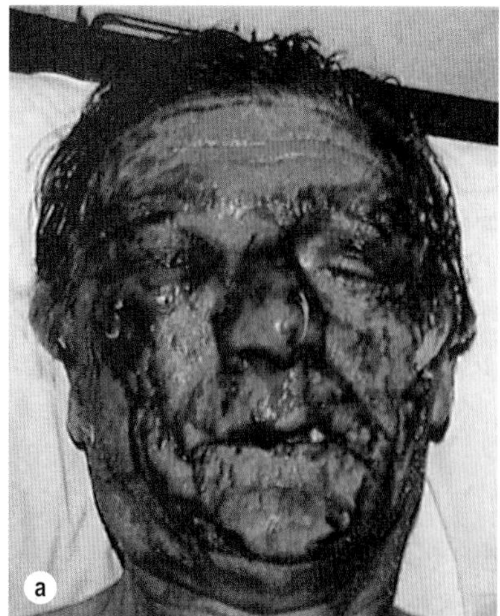

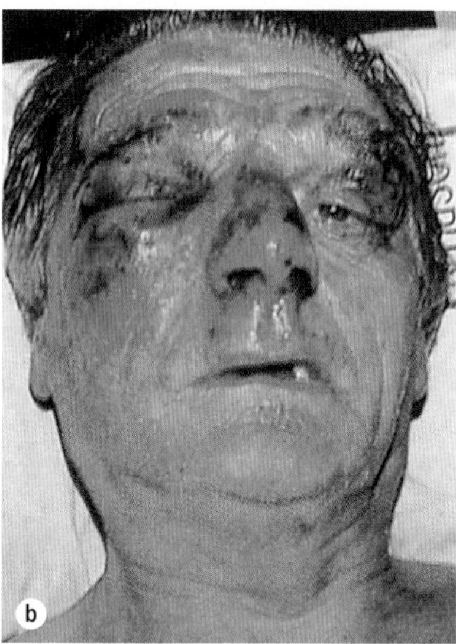

Figure 31-1 (a) Appearance of a patient after being attacked. (b) Appearance of same man after cleansing.

> **Critical Thinking**
>
> Why might it be difficult to obtain a history from a patient with this type of injury?

Management

The management of soft tissue injuries was described in Chapter 29. The key principles of wound management include the control of bleeding with direct pressure and pressure bandages. The paramedic should pay close attention to airway management, and should use spinal precautions if indicated by mechanism of injury (described in Chapter 32). Soft tissue injuries to the nose and mouth are common with facial injuries. The paramedic should assess the patient's airway for obstruction caused by blood, vomitus, bone fragments, broken teeth, dentures, and damage to the anterior neck. Suction may be needed to clear the patient's airway, and oral or nasal adjuncts, tracheal intubation, or cricothyroidotomy may be required to ensure adequate ventilation and oxygenation.

Facial fractures

Facial bones can withstand tremendous forces from the impact of energy but facial fractures are relatively common after blunt trauma. Blunt trauma injuries may be classified anatomically as fractures to the mandible, midface, zygoma, orbit and nose. Signs and symptoms of facial fractures include the following:

- asymmetry of zygoma prominences
- crepitus
- dental malocclusion
- discontinuity of the orbital rim
- displacement of the nasal septum
- ecchymosis
- lacerations and bleeding
- limitation of forward movement of the mandible
- limited ocular movements
- numbness
- pain
- swelling
- visual disturbances.

Fractures of the mandible

The mandible is the single facial bone in the lower third of the face. Because of its prominence, fractures to this bone rank second in frequency after nasal fractures. The mandible is a hemi-circle of bone and may break in multiple locations, often distant from the point of impact. Signs and symptoms specific to mandibular fractures include malocclusion (patients may complain that their teeth do not 'feel right' when their mouths are closed), numbness in the chin, and inability to open the mouth. The patient may have difficulty swallowing and may have excessive salivation. Patients with mandibular fractures require hospitalization.

Anterior dislocation of the mandible in the absence of fracture may occur as a result of blunt trauma to the face (rare), an abnormally wide yawn, and dental treatment requiring that the jaws remain open for long periods. In these cases, the condylar head advances forward beyond the articular surface of the temporal bone. The jaw-closing muscles spasm so that the mouth becomes locked in a wide-open position. The patient usually feels severe pain from the spasm and may experience anxiety and discomfort that perpetuate the spasm. Mandibular dislocations are reduced manually in the emergency department with the aid of a muscle relaxant or sedative or in the operating room with a general anaesthetic.

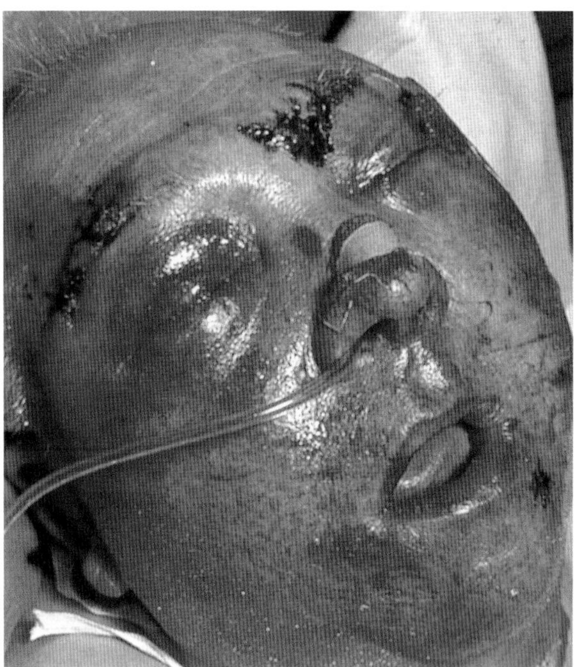

Figure 31-2 Fracture of the middle third of the face.

> **Critical Thinking**
>
> What will be your patient care priority with these patients?

> **Note**
>
> As described in Chapter 13, nasal airways are relatively contraindicated in patients who have fractures of the basal skull or facial bones. Cerebrospinal fluid leakage from the ear or nose should be allowed to drain freely. The paramedic should make no attempts to control cerebrospinal fluid leakage with direct pressure.

Fractures of the midface

The middle third of the face includes the maxilla, zygoma, floor of the orbit, and nose. Fractures to this region result from direct or indirect force (for example, fractures may result from blunt trauma to the mandible with the energy transmitted to produce fractures to the maxilla). These injuries are often associated with central nervous system injury and spinal trauma (Figure 31-2).

In 1901 a cadaver study undertaken by René Le Fort described three patterns of injuries (Le Fort fractures). These injuries occur in the midface region (Figure 31-3). The Le Fort I fracture involves the maxilla up to the level of the nasal fossa; the Le Fort II involves the nasal bones and medial orbits with a fracture line generally shaped like a pyramid; the Le Fort III results in craniofacial dislocation and involves all of the bones of the face. Depending on the severity of injury, different combinations of Le Fort fractures may be present.

Signs and symptoms specific to midface fractures include midfacial oedema, unstable maxilla, lengthening of the face (donkey face), epistaxis, numb upper teeth, nasal flattening, and cerebrospinal fluid rhinorrhoea (cerebrospinal fluid leakage caused by ethmoid cribriform plate fracture). Patients with midface fractures are at risk of having serious airway problems (particularly those with Le Fort II and III fractures), and will require urgent hospitalization. Because of the extent of the fractures, a risk exists of placing nasopharyngeal airways into the brain tissue.

Fractures of the zygoma

The zygoma (malar eminence) – commonly called the cheekbone – articulates with the frontal, maxillary and temporal bones. It is rarely fractured, due to its sturdy construction, but when fractures do occur, they are usually a result of physical assaults and vehicle crashes. Zygomatic fractures are often associated with orbital fractures and manifest similar clinical signs (Figure 31-4). The two are distinguished by X-ray examination. Signs and symptoms specific to zygomatic fractures include flatness of a usually rounded cheek area; numbness of the cheek, nose, and upper lip (particularly if an orbital fracture is involved); epistaxis; and altered vision.

Fractures of the orbit

The orbital contents are protected by a bony ring. The ring resembles a pyramid, with the apex pointed toward the back of the head. The bones of the walls, floor, and roof of the orbit are thin and are fractured easily by direct blows and transmitted forces. In addition, many orbital fractures are associated with other facial injuries, such as Le Fort II and III fractures.

A blowout fracture to the orbit can occur when an object of greater diameter than that of the bony orbital rim strikes the globe of the eye and surrounding soft tissue (Figure

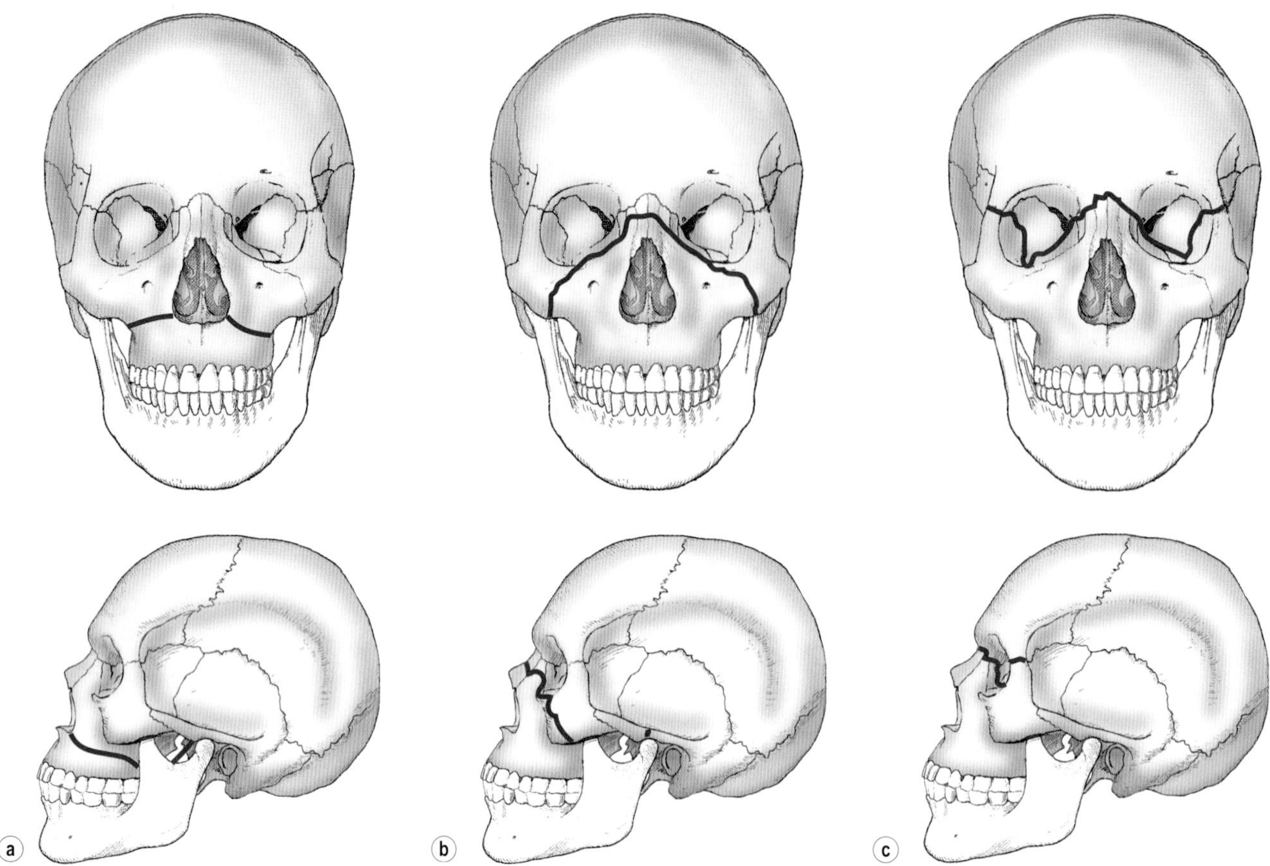

Figure 31-3 (a) Le Fort I facial fractures (lateral and frontal views). (b) Le Fort II fractures (lateral and frontal views). (c) Le Fort III fractures (lateral and frontal views).

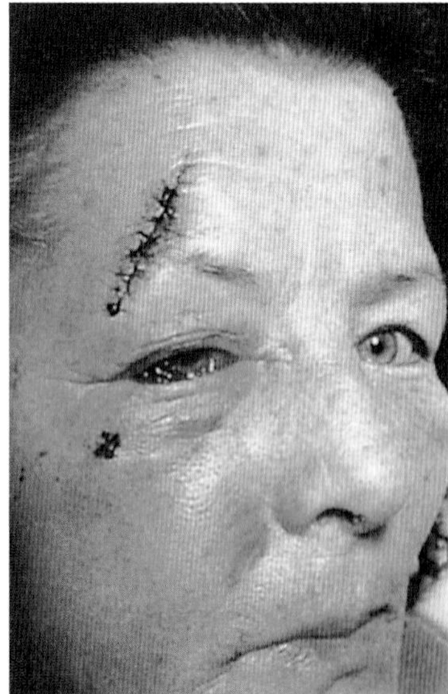

Figure 31-4 Fracture of the zygomatic bone.

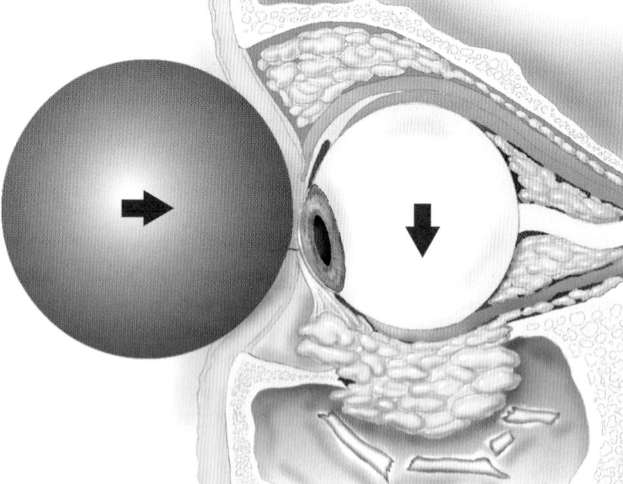

Figure 31-5 Artist's impression of a blowout fracture caused by the impact of a ball.

31-5). This impact pushes the globe into the orbit and in turn compresses the orbital contents. The sudden increase in intraocular pressure is transmitted to the orbital floor, which is the weakest part of the orbital structure. If the orbital floor fractures, the orbital contents may be forced into the maxillary sinus, where soft tissue and extraocular muscles may become trapped in the defect. Signs and symptoms of blowout fractures include periorbital oedema, subconjunctival ecchymosis, diplopia (double vision), enophthalmos (recessed globe), epistaxis, anaesthesia in the region of the infraorbital nerve (anterior cheek), and impaired extraocular movements.

Critical Thinking

How do you assess a patient's eye movement?

Orbital fractures are often associated with other fractures, including the Le Fort II and III injuries and those of the zygomatic complex. In addition, injury to the orbital contents is common and the paramedic should suspect such injury with any facial fracture.

Fractures of the nose

Of all the facial bones the nasal bones have the least structural strength and are fractured most frequently. The external portion of the nose, formed mostly of hyaline cartilage, is supported mainly by the nasal bones and the frontal processes of the maxillary bones. Injuries to the nose may result only in epistaxis and swelling without apparent skeletal deformity, or may depress the dorsum of the nose and displace it to one side. Fractures to the orbit may also be present. In children, even minimal displacement of nasal bones may result in growth changes and deformity.

Management of facial fractures

Facial fractures are associated with a high percentage of related cervical spine fractures[3] so the paramedic should assume that the spine has been injured and use spinal precautions. The paramedic should assess the patient's airway for obstruction caused by blood, vomitus, bone fragments, broken teeth, dentures, and damage to the anterior neck. Suction may be needed to clear the airway of debris and fluid. The paramedic may need to maintain the airway with an oral or nasal adjunct (midface or basal skull fractures are relative contraindications for nasal airways), tracheal intubation, or cricothyroidotomy if indicated.

Bleeding can usually be controlled by direct pressure and pressure bandages. Epistaxis may be severe and should be controlled by applying external pressure to the anterior nares. To prevent blood from draining down the throat, mild epistaxis is best controlled in the conscious patient by instructing the patient to sit upright or to lean forward (in the absence of spinal injury) whilst compressing the nares. An unconscious patient should be positioned on the side (if not contraindicated by injury). If bleeding is severe, the paramedic should evaluate the patient for haemorrhagic shock.

Critical Thinking

Why would you not want the blood to drain posteriorly?

Nasal and ear foreign bodies

The insertion of foreign bodies in the nose or ear is common in children. Foreign bodies may cause infection if they are not detected and removed. These patients may need to be transported for physician evaluation. The paramedic should remove a foreign body from the ear if it can be retrieved easily. As a rule, a foreign body in the nose should not be removed in the prehospital setting unless it is contributing to airway compromise or unless it can be removed easily without equipment.

Ear, eye and dental trauma

The ears, eyes, or teeth may be injured separately or along with other forms of head trauma. Injury to these regions may be minor, yet such injuries may result in permanent sensory function loss and disfigurement. Regardless of the severity, the paramedic should evaluate ear, eye and dental trauma and treat it only after identifying and managing life-threatening problems.

Ear trauma

Trauma to the ear may include lacerations and contusions, thermal injuries, chemical injuries, traumatic perforations, and barotitis.

Lacerations and contusions

Lacerations and contusions usually result from blunt trauma and are particularly common in victims of domestic violence (Figure 31-6a, b). These injuries are treated by direct pressure to control bleeding, whilst the application of ice or cold

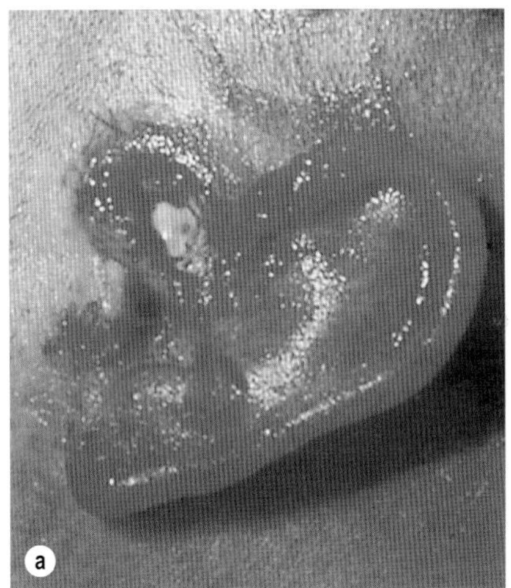

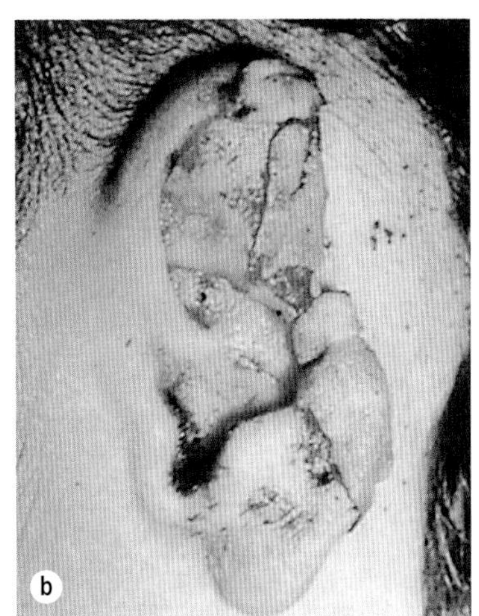

Figure 31-6 (a) Partially detached pinna. (b) Loss of rim.

compresses may decrease soft tissue swelling. If a portion of the outer ear (pinna) has been avulsed, the paramedic should retrieve the avulsed tissue if possible. It should be wrapped in moist gauze, sealed in plastic, placed on ice, and transported with the patient for surgical repair. Cartilage tears often heal poorly and are easily infected.

Thermal injuries

Thermal injuries may occur from prolonged exposure to extreme cold or from exposure of lesser duration to extreme heat. Contact with hot liquids or electrical currents can also lead to thermal injury. Prehospital treatment is usually limited to dressings to prevent contamination, and transportation for evaluation by a physician.

Chemical injuries

Strong acids or alkalis produce burns on contact. Emergency care consists of copious irrigation, after which the paramedic should bathe the ear and ear canal with saline or sterile water. The irrigation liquid should remain in the ear canal for 2–3 min. This should be repeated three or four times and afterward the ear dried and covered to prevent contamination. The patient should be transported for evaluation by a physician.

Traumatic perforations

The tympanic membrane can be perforated by objects such as a cotton-tipped applicator, and by changes in pressure. Pressure injuries may result from explosions (blast injuries) or scuba diving (barotrauma). These injuries usually heal spontaneously without treatment but physician evaluation is advised.

If the injury is caused by a penetrating object, the paramedic should stabilize the object in place and cover the ear to prevent further contamination. The inner or middle ear canal may have been contaminated (e.g. by swimming water or a foreign object), in which case antibiotic therapy is usually prescribed. Serious complications that may result from perforations include facial nerve palsy frequently accompanied by temporal bone fractures, hearing loss, and vertigo.

Barotitis

Barotitis occurs when a person is exposed to changes in barometric pressure great enough to produce inflammation and injury to the middle ear. Barotitis can result, for example, from flying at high altitudes and from scuba diving.

Gas pressure in the air-filled spaces of the middle ear normally equals that of the environment. Boyle's law states that at a constant temperature, the volume of gas is inversely proportional to the pressure. On ascent, gas expands; on descent, it contracts. Therefore when gases become trapped or partially trapped, they expand in direct proportion to the decrease in pressure. When trapped gas cannot reach equilibrium with environmental pressure, pain and the sensation of a blocked ear may develop. To equalize the pressure in the middle ear, the patient can be directed to bear down (Valsalva's manoeuvre), yawn, swallow and move the lower jaw. These methods may cause the eustachian tube to open, which will equalize the pressure in the middle ear cavity.

Eye trauma

In the UK in 2007–2008 there were 3539 episodes of admitted patient care as result of injury to the eye and orbit, accounting for 7402 bed days.[4] Common causes of eye injury are blunt and penetrating trauma from motor vehicle crashes, sport and recreational activities, and violent altercations; chemical exposure from household and industrial accidents; foreign bodies; and animal bites and scratches.

Evaluation

Acute eye injuries may be difficult to identify because a patient with normal vision may have a serious underlying injury. Symptoms requiring a high degree of suspicion include the following:

- obvious trauma with eye injury
- visual loss or blurred vision that does not improve with blinking, indicating possible damage to the globe, ocular contents or optic nerve
- loss of a portion of the visual field, indicating possible detachment of the retina, haemorrhage into the eye, or optic nerve injury.

Evaluation of eye injury should include a thorough history and measurement of visual acuity, pupillary reaction and extraocular movements. Assessing the patient's vision will be a rough estimation at best but the patient's vision will be re-evaluated in the emergency department under controlled circumstances.

> **Critical Thinking**
>
> Aside from trauma, what are some other causes of visual disturbances?

History

A thorough history should include the following information:

- exact mode of injury
- previous ocular, medical, and drug history, including cataracts, glaucoma, and presence of hepatitis or human immunodeficiency virus
- use of eye medications
- use of corrective glasses or contact lenses
- presence of ocular prostheses
- duration of symptoms and treatment interventions that may have been attempted before emergency medical services arrival.

Visual acuity

The measurement of visual acuity is usually the first step in any examination of the patient's eyes. (The exception is a chemical burn to the eye. In this case, irrigation should come before measurement of visual acuity.) The use a handheld visual acuity chart (e.g. Snellen chart) is uncommon in prehospital care, so the paramedic should use any printed material with small, medium, and large point sizes (e.g. an intravenous fluid bag). The paramedic should record the distance that the printed item was held from the patient's face (this does not have to be exact).

The paramedic should assess the vision of each eye separately whilst covering the other eye (no pressure should be applied). The injured eye should be tested first to allow for comparison with the uninjured eye. If the patient wears corrective lenses, the paramedic should measure acuity with lenses first and then without lenses. Illiterate or non-English-speaking patients require an alternative method of evaluation, which may include finger counting, hand motion, and presence or absence of light perception. Abnormal responses to any of these methods indicate significant loss of vision.

Critical Thinking

The assessment of visual acuity may be difficult on some calls. What factors in the prehospital setting may make it difficult?

Note

The two types of vision are central and peripheral. Central vision results from images falling on the macula of the retina. Peripheral vision is the ability to see objects that reflect light waves on areas of the retina other than the macula.

Pupillary reaction

Pupils should be black, round, equal in size, and should react to light in the same way and at the same time. Both eyes should constrict in response to light and dilate in response to dark. Abnormal pupillary responses after blunt trauma to the eye are common; they may be caused by tearing but more commonly are caused by direct trauma to the pupillary sphincter muscle. Abnormal responses may suggest a more serious injury involving the optic nerve or globe. Causes of pupil abnormalities in the absence of recent injury include drug use, cataracts, previous surgical procedures, ocular prosthesis, anisocoria (normal or congenital unequal pupil size), central nervous system disease, strokes and previous injury. The paramedic should document all of the patient's pupil abnormalities.

Extraocular movements

Extraocular muscles are responsible for movements of the globe or eyeball. Voluntary muscles are innervated by cranial nerves III, IV and VI. The muscles are attached to the outside of the eyeball and bones of the orbit and move the globe in any desired direction. Sympathetic nerves innervate involuntary eye muscles located within the eye; examples of involuntary eye muscles are the iris and the ciliary muscle. These muscles dilate and constrict the pupil and change the shape of the lens, respectively.

To evaluate the extraocular movement of the eyes (described in Chapter 9), the paramedic should instruct the patient to visually track the movement of an object (for example, a finger, pencil, or penlight). The paramedic should ask the patient to track the object up, down, to the right, and to the left. Abnormalities in movement may indicate orbital content oedema, cranial nerve injury, contusions or lacerations of extraocular muscles, or muscle entrapment in a fracture. Patients with limited or abnormal extraocular movements often complain of double vision in one or more directions of gaze. All findings should be documented.

Evaluation and management of specific eye injuries

Few eye injuries are truly urgent; however, all victims of ocular trauma should be evaluated by a physician. Some patients need specialized care by an ophthalmologist and should be conveyed to a facility with specialist physicians if available in the area. The paramedic needs to be aware of local procedures for managing eye injuries (Figure 31-7a–e).

Foreign bodies in the cornea, conjunctiva or eyelid usually cause the patient to complain of the sensation of something in the eye (especially when opening and closing the eyelids). If a foreign body is suspected, the paramedic should inspect the inner surface of the upper and lower lid and conjunctiva. The paramedic should remove the foreign body by gentle, copious irrigation with clear fluid (tap water, normal saline or sterile water would work).

Corneal abrasion occurs when the outer layers of the cornea are rubbed away. The injury often results from a foreign body scratching the cornea and is common in those who wear contact lenses. Patients with a corneal abrasion usually complain of pain and foreign body sensation under the upper eyelid, photophobia (abnormal light sensitivity), and sometimes a decrease in visual acuity. Often these signs and symptoms are delayed. The prehospital management of corneal abrasion is gentle irrigation with clear fluid and the application of a double patch to eyes to prevent the injured eye from moving when the uninjured eye moves, causing aggravation (Figure 31-8a–d). Corneal abrasions generally heal within 24–48 h.

Critical Thinking

Will the patient with a suspected corneal abrasion need to be evaluated by a physician?

Blunt trauma to the eye or its adjacent structures may result in a contusion injury, traumatic hyphaema (bleeding into the anterior chamber), or globe or scleral rupture. Box 31-1 lists the signs and symptoms of these injuries.

Blunt injury to the eye may be associated with other serious injuries. Such injuries include orbital fracture, vitreous haemorrhage and dislocation of the lens. The prehospital care should be limited to the control of any bleeding with gentle, direct pressure; protection of the eye with a metal shield or cardboard cup; and rapid transport for physician evaluation. If the paramedic suspects a traumatic hyphaema or globe or scleral rupture, the patient's head and spine should be immobilized. The paramedic should elevate the head of the spine board 40 degrees to decrease intraocular pressure and instruct the patient to avoid any activity that might increase intraocular pressure (e.g. straining and coughing).

Penetrating injury to the eye may be associated with embedded foreign bodies, lid avulsions, and lacerations to the lids, sclera or cornea. Penetrating globe injuries can damage retinal structures and can cause a loss of vitreous

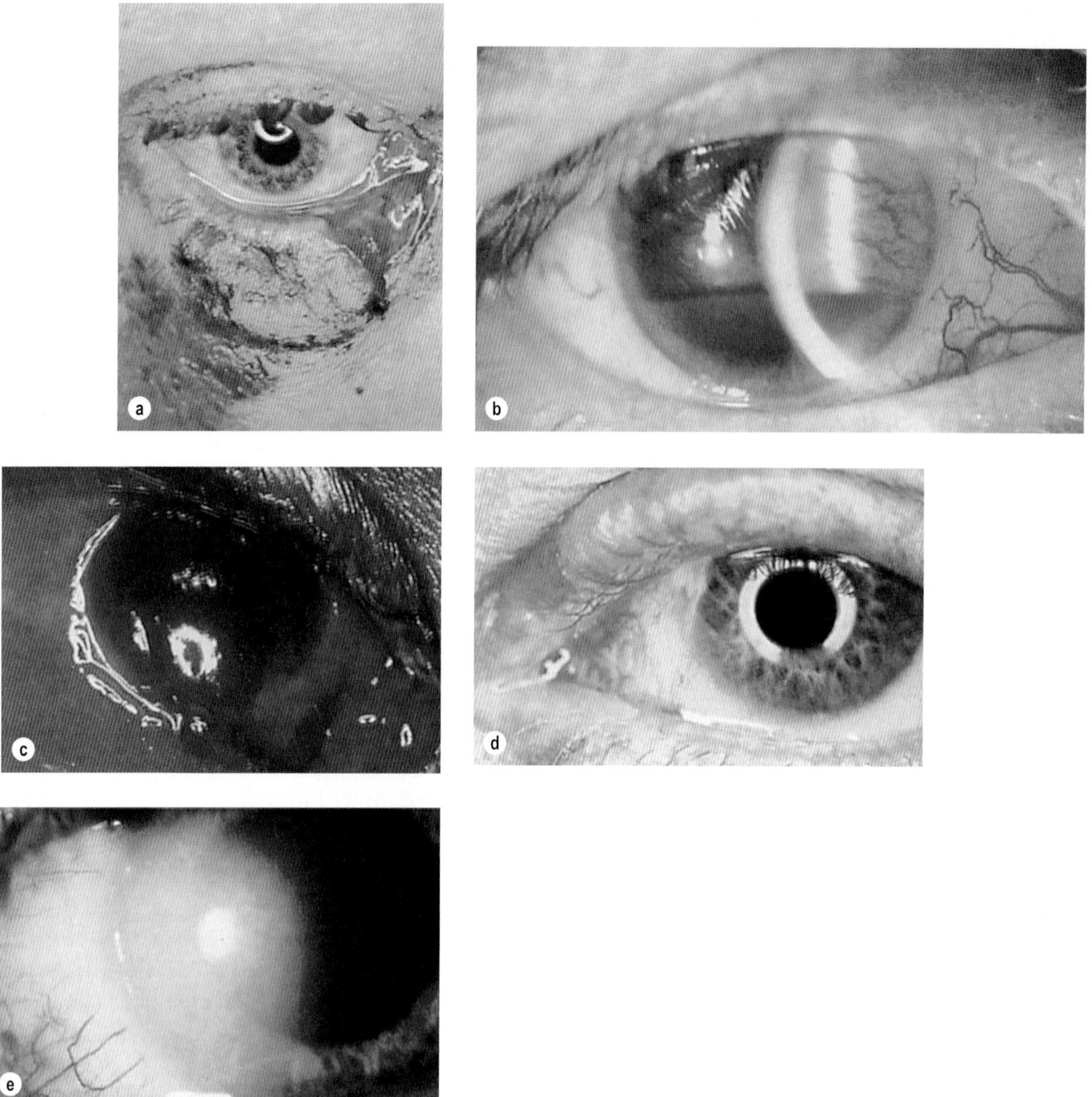

Figure 31-7 (a) Avulsion of lid. (b) Hyphaema. (c) Ruptured globe. (d) Acid burn. (e) Alkali burn.

humour and subsequent blindness. The paramedic should control any bleeding by gentle, direct pressure. The globe should be protected from dehydration or contamination from foreign material. One way is to cover the orbital area with plastic or damp, sterile dressings and an eye shield.

The paramedic should stabilize foreign bodies protruding from the eye and should cover these with a cardboard cup and secure the cup with tape. The unaffected eye should also be covered to prevent consensual movement. The paramedic should not attempt to remove the object; if needed, the penetrating object may be shortened for transport. Oxygen may be required in these cases.

Chemical injury to the eye (described in Chapter 30) may be associated with loss of corneal epithelial tissue, globe perforation, and scarring and deformation of eyelids and conjunctiva. These injuries are true emergencies that require immediate intervention. A chemical exposure generally mandates extensive, continuous irrigation of both eyes with a neutral fluid for 20 min before patient transport (if effective irrigation can be performed) and while en route to the emergency department.

Critical Thinking

How will you avoid contaminating the unaffected eye whilst irrigating?

Contact lenses

Contact lenses are of three general types: hard, soft hydrophilic and rigid gas-permeable. Hard lenses are microlenses that are sometimes prescribed for astigmatism (these lenses are rarely used today). Soft (hydrophilic) lenses are usually

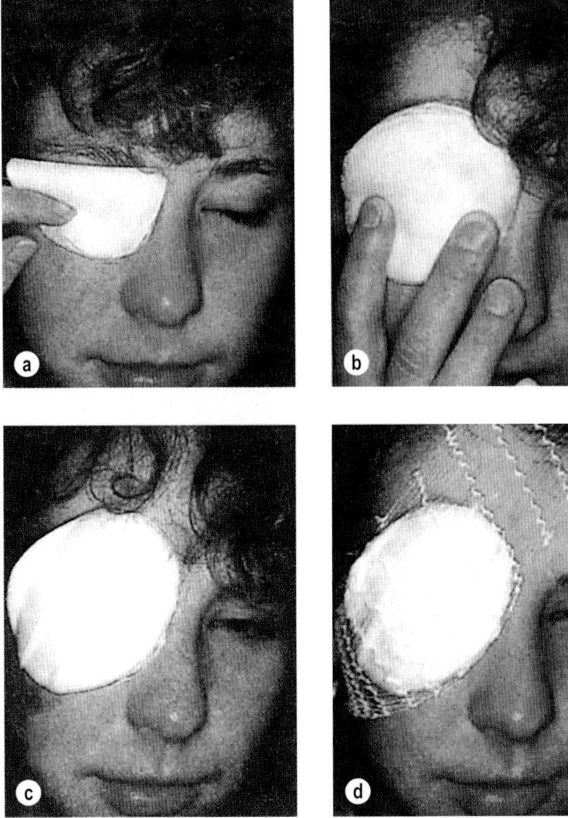

Figure 31-8 (a) A folded pad is placed over the closed eye. (b) A second unfolded pad is placed over the top of the first pad. (c) Tape is applied along the length of the pad. (d) The pads are secured firmly in place.

Box 31-1

Signs and symptoms of eye injuries

Contusion injury

Traumatic dilation or constriction of the pupil
Pain
Photophobia
Blurred vision
Tears of the iris (tear-shaped pupil)

Traumatic hyphaema

Traumatic dilation or, less commonly, constriction of the pupil
Decrease in visual acuity
Blood in the anterior chamber (may be visible with penlight)

Globe or scleral rupture

Decrease in visual acuity to hand movements or light perception
Lowered intraocular pressure (soft eye)
Pupil irregularity
Hyphaema

large in diameter (extending onto the conjunctiva) and may be designed for daily or extended wear. Rigid gas-permeable lenses are similar in size to microlenses and have low water content and high oxygen permeability.

As a rule, paramedics should not attempt to remove contact lenses in patients with eye injuries as this may cause more damage and may aggravate the injury. If management of an eye injury is complicated by the presence of contact lenses (e.g. chemical burns to the eyes), consideration should be given to their removal. If the patient is unable to remove the lenses, the paramedic may need to do so (Box 31-2).

Box 31-2

Removal of contact lenses

Removal of hard and rigid gas-permeable lenses

1. With gloved hands, separate the eyelids so that the margins of the lids are beyond the top and bottom edges of the lens.
2. Gently pass the eyelids down and forward to the edges of the lens.
3. Move the eyelids toward each other, forcing the lens to slide out between them.
4. Store the lens in a container with water or saline, and label the container with the patient's name. If a contact lens container is not available, store each lens in a separate container and label as left or right.
5. If lens removal is difficult, gently move the lens downward from the cornea to the conjunctiva overlying the sclera until arrival in the emergency department.

Note: Special suction cups are also available for the removal of hard and rigid contact lenses. This device should be moistened with saline or sterile water before contacting the lens.

Removal of soft lenses

1. With gloved hands, pull down the lower eyelid.
2. Gently slide the soft lens down onto the conjunctiva.
3. Using a pinching motion, compress the lens between the thumb and index finger.
4. Remove the lens from the eye.
5. Store the lens in a container (marked right or left) with water or saline, and label the container with the patient's name.

Dental trauma

The adult normally has 32 teeth. Each tooth consists of two sections: the crown, which projects above the gingiva (the portion of the oral mucosa surrounding the tooth), and the root, which fits into the bony socket (alveolus) of the maxilla or mandible. Three layers make up the hard tissues of the teeth: the enamel, the dentine (ivory), and the cementum. The soft tissues of the teeth include the pulp and the periodontal membrane (Figure 31-9).

The teeth and associated alveolar process may be injured alone or along with fractures of the jaw or facial bones. The two most common types of dental trauma involve fractures and avulsions of the anterior teeth. If a tooth is fractured, the paramedic should search the oral cavity carefully for tooth fragments. Removal of fragments reduces the risk of aspiration and obstruction of the airway. Lacerations and avulsions to the tongue and surrounding mucous membranes often occur with dental trauma. These injuries are often painful, they may bleed profusely, and they may compromise the patient's airway.

Tooth avulsions are common, and many teeth can be saved with proper emergency treatment.[5] Permanent teeth that have been avulsed have a good survival rate if reimplanted and stabilized within 1 h (deciduous teeth, or

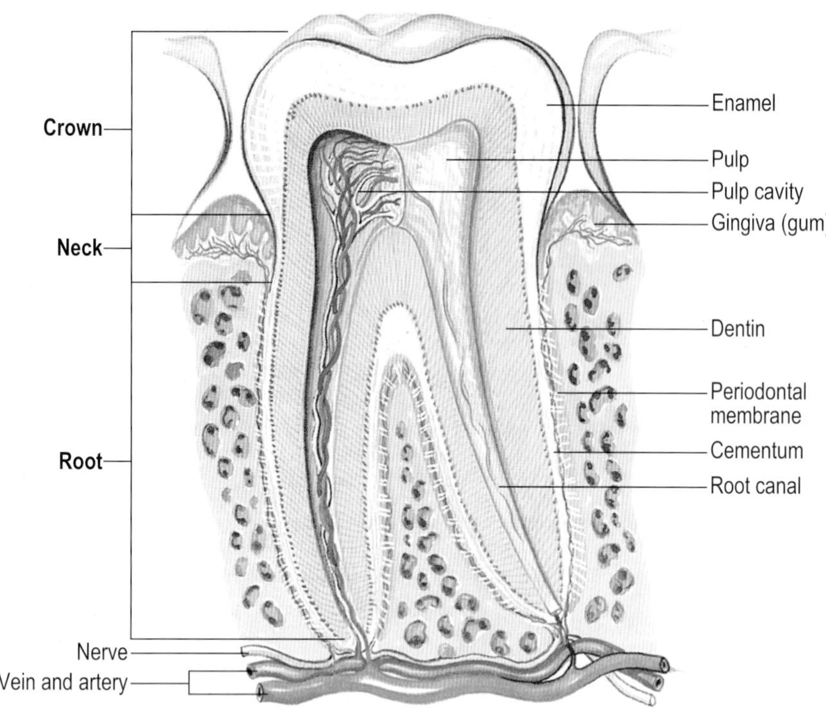

Figure 31-9 Longitudinal section of a tooth.

milk teeth, are not generally re-implanted as they may fuse to the bone, delaying formation and eruption of the permanent tooth). If the avulsed tooth has been out of the patient's mouth for less than 15 min, consider re-implanting the tooth into the original socket. The paramedic should take care not to re-implant the tooth backward and should handle the tooth from the crown side, not the root, to avoid damage to the periodontal ligament. If re-implantation is impossible, the tooth may be placed in a vessel containing cool fresh pasteurized milk, sodium chloride or contact lens solution and transferred to hospital with the patient. If the patient is cooperative, they may be able to hold the tooth in the buccal sulcus. Unsuitable and slightly damaging fluids include water (causes isotonic damage as a result of prolonged exposure), bleach, disinfectants and orange juice.[6] The paramedic should be cognizant of the risk of aspiration with an implanted tooth or a tooth held in the buccal sulcus, and should maintain vigilance.

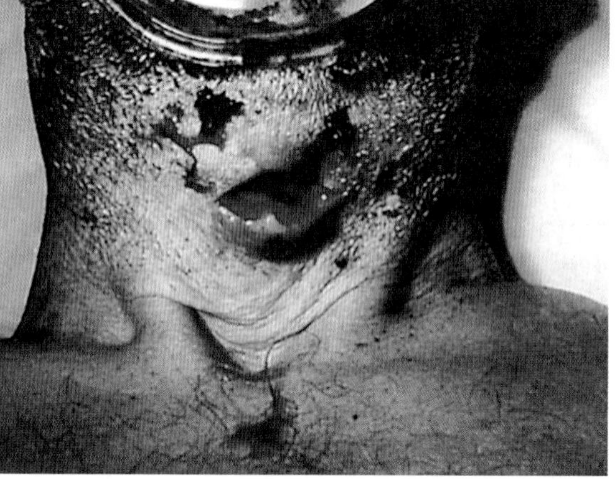

Figure 31-10 A self-inflicted stab wound that had entered the pharynx.

Anterior neck trauma

Anterior neck injuries are caused by blunt and penetrating trauma (Figure 31-10). These injuries may result in damage to the skeletal structures, vascular structures, nerves, muscles, and glands of the neck. Common mechanisms of injury to the anterior neck are as follows:

- strangulation injuries from clothing, jewellery, or personal equipment getting caught in machinery
- all-terrain vehicles and other small motor vehicles (clothesline injuries to the neck from running into wires, ropes or fences)
- blows to the neck
- contact sports (boxing, karate, basketball, football, hockey)
- hangings
- horseback riding
- hyperextension and hyperflexion injuries
- industrial injuries
- missile injury from firearms
- motor vehicle crashes
- neck striking dashboard or steering column
- sport and recreational activities
- stab wounds (knives, screwdrivers, ice picks)
- violent altercations
- water sports (jet skiing, water skiing).

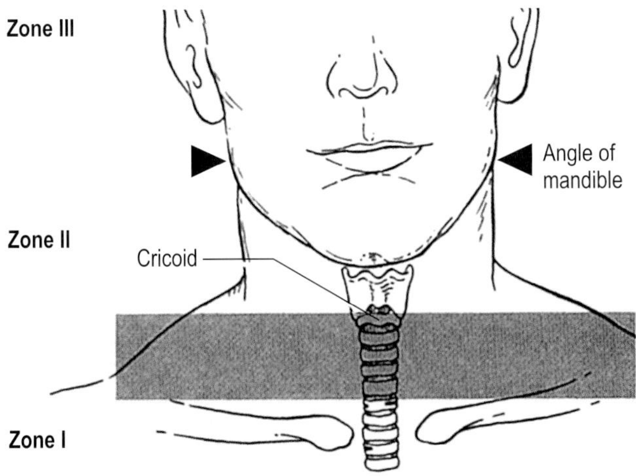

Figure 31-11 Zones of the neck. The junction of zone I and zone II is described variously as the cricoid cartilage or top of the clavicles.

With blunt and penetrating neck injuries, the paramedic should assume the patient has a cervical spine injury also. The paramedic must assume such injury until ruled out by clinical examination and radiography of the cervical region of the neck. X-ray examination alone does not rule out cervical spine injury (see Chapter 32).

Evaluation

For purposes of evaluating the trauma patient, the neck can be divided into three zones defined by horizontal planes (Figure 31-11).[7] Zone I represents the base of the neck. This zone extends from the sternal notch to the top of the clavicles or the cricoid cartilage. Injuries to this zone have the highest mortality rate because of the risk of injury to major vascular and thoracic structures (subclavian vessels and jugular veins, lungs, oesophagus, trachea, cervical spine, cervical nerve roots).

Zone II extends from the clavicles or cricoid cartilage cephalad to the angle of the mandible. The carotid artery, jugular vein, trachea, larynx, oesophagus and cervical spine are the vital structures in this zone. Because of the relative size of zone II, injuries to this zone are the most common. However, they have a lower mortality rate than zone I injuries.

Zone III is the part of the neck above the angle of the mandible. The risk of injury to the distal carotid artery, salivary glands, and pharynx is greatest in this zone.

Soft tissue injuries

Soft tissue injuries to the neck from blunt trauma often produce haematoma and associated oedema or direct laryngeal or tracheal injury. Both of these can result in airway compromise. Penetrating trauma may produce lacerations and puncture wounds with resultant vascular, laryngotracheal, or oesophageal injury. Blunt trauma may cause vascular injuries as well, although this is uncommon. As with all trauma victims, initial evaluation and resuscitation must begin with rapid assessment, control of the airway, and consideration for spinal injury.

Critical Thinking

Is prehospital airway control always possible in patients with anterior neck injuries?

Haematoma and oedema

Oedema of the pharynx, larynx, trachea, epiglottis and vocal cords may produce enough pressure in the neck tissues to obstruct the airway completely. If the airway is compromised (evidenced by dyspnoea, inspiratory stridor, cyanosis or changes in voice quality), the paramedic should consider endotracheal intubation with spinal precautions. Intubation stabilizes damaged areas of the neck, protects the airway, and provides a means for ventilatory support (a slightly smaller endotracheal tube may be needed to ensure passage through the airway).

Note

Crushed or severed airways can be blocked totally or partially by attempts at oral or nasal intubation. In these cases (if the patient is moving air), rapid transport with high-concentration oxygen is perhaps the most prudent course.

When direct intubation is impossible because of blood, vomitus (that cannot be removed by suction) or progressive oedema, a cricothyroidotomy or translaryngeal cannula ventilation (described in Chapter 13) may be indicated. Another measure that may help in treating oedematous airways includes the administration of cool, humidified oxygen. Yet another measure is the slight elevation of the patient's head (this can be done if it is not contraindicated by the injury).

Lacerations and puncture wounds

Lacerations and puncture wounds may be superficial or deep. Superficial wounds can usually be managed by covering the wound to prevent further contamination. Deep wounds are associated with more serious injuries to underlying structures and may require aggressive airway therapy and ventilatory support, suction, haemorrhage control by direct pressure, and fluid replacement. Signs and symptoms of significant penetrating neck trauma include the following:

- active bleeding
- dysphagia
- dyspnoea
- haematemesis
- haemoptysis
- hoarseness
- large or expanding haematoma
- mobility and crepitus
- neurological deficit (stroke, brachial plexus injury, spinal cord injury)
- pulse deficit
- shock
- stridor
- subcutaneous emphysema
- tenderness to palpation.

Critical Thinking

Why is rapid transport crucial when caring for a patient who has anterior neck injuries?

Vascular injury

Blood vessels are the most commonly injured structures in the neck; they may be injured by blunt or penetrating trauma. Vessels at risk of injury include the carotid, vertebral, subclavian, innominate and internal mammary arteries and the jugular and subclavian veins. Laceration of these major vessels can result in rapid exsanguination (death from extensive blood loss) if bleeding is not controlled.

Securing the airway (with spinal precautions) and providing adequate ventilatory support is the first priority. The next priority is to control haemorrhage. This can be achieved with constant, direct pressure. The paramedic should apply pressure only to the affected vessels to avoid completely obstructing blood flow to the brain. If bleeding cannot be controlled in this manner, it may be necessary to apply direct pressure with a gloved finger to the vessel.

Note

Under no circumstances should cervical vessels be clamped with haemostats in the prehospital setting. Doing so may traumatize critical vascular structures and may produce permanent nerve injury.

If the paramedic suspects a venous injury, the patient should be kept supine or in a slight head-down (Trendelenburg) position to help prevent air embolism (a rare but lethal complication). If the paramedic suspects air embolism, the patient should be placed in Trendelenburg (head-down) position and rotated toward the left lateral decubitus position; it is believed that this manoeuvre helps to trap air in the apex of the ventricle, prevents its ejection into the pulmonary arterial system, and maintains the output of the right ventricle. Fluid replacement for hypovolaemia should be guided by clinical findings and may include using large-bore catheters and isotonic crystalloid (sodium lactate solution or normal saline). If penetrating injury to the base of the neck (zone I) has occurred, upper extremity venous drainage may be compromised by the laceration. In this event, placement of a cannula in the upper limb on the affected side is not beneficial; IV access should be gained in the upper limb on the opposite side or in one of the lower limbs.

Laryngeal or tracheal injury

Injury from blunt or penetrating trauma to the anterior neck may cause fracture or dislocation of the laryngeal and tracheal cartilages, haemorrhage or swelling of the air passages. All of these injuries can compromise the airway and cause respiratory distress. Airway injury can lead to death in head and neck trauma patients, thus rapid and judicious control of the airway and prevention of aspiration are crucial. In addition, a high degree of suspicion for associated vascular disruption and oesophageal, chest, and intra-abdominal injury is a critical aspect of preventing death. Injuries that may be associated with laryngeal and tracheal trauma include the following:

- fracture of the hyoid bone resulting in laceration and distortion of the epiglottis
- separation of the hyoid and thyroid cartilages resulting in epiglottis dislocation, aspiration, and subcutaneous emphysema
- fractures of the thyroid cartilage resulting in epiglottis and vocal cord avulsion, arytenoid dislocation, and aspiration of blood and bone fragments
- dislocation or fracture of the cricothyroid resulting in long-term laryngeal stenosis, laryngeal nerve paralysis, and laryngotracheal avulsion
- fracture to the trachea resulting in tracheal avulsion, complete airway obstruction, and subcutaneous emphysema.

The prehospital management of laryngeal and tracheal trauma is controversial. These injuries may be seen as an indication for oral or nasal intubation, but intubation attempts may contribute to the potential for injury resulting from hypoxia during the procedure and further damage the airway structures. Alternative methods of airway management include the use of cricothyroidotomy and translaryngeal cannula ventilation, although these may also prove to be unsatisfactory.

Note

Airway procedures that involve entry through the neck are generally avoided in the field because of the associated risks. As a rule, these patients should be well ventilated with a bag–mask device and transported rapidly to the receiving facility for surgical tracheotomy. As described in Chapter 13, translaryngeal cannula ventilation is hazardous in the presence of complete airway obstruction. Incorrectly used, this technique does not provide adequate exhalation of gases and air. The technique may result in carbon dioxide retention and significant injury from high pressure developing in the chest and airways (barotrauma).

A stepwise approach to airway management is still the optimum clinical decision and, regardless of the method chosen, emergency care is directed at securing the airway with spinal precautions, providing adequate ventilatory support, controlling haemorrhage, treating for shock, and providing rapid transport to an appropriate medical facility for definitive surgical care.

Oesophageal injury

Oesophageal injuries should be suspected in patients with trauma to the neck or chest. Specific injuries that require a high degree of suspicion for associated oesophageal injury include tracheal fractures, penetrating trauma from stab or gunshot wounds, and ingestion of caustic substances.

Oesophageal injury is difficult to diagnose and may be overlooked as the paramedic focuses on more obvious injuries that pose a threat to life. Signs and symptoms may include subcutaneous emphysema, neck haematoma and bleeding from the mouth and nose.

Oesophageal perforation is associated with a high mortality rate resulting from mediastinitis caused by the release of gastric contents into the thoracic cavity. If not contraindicated by mechanism of injury, the paramedic should place the patient with a suspected oesophageal tear in a semi-Fowler position. (This is an inclined position. The upper half of the body is raised by elevating the head or stretcher about 30 degrees.) This position will help to prevent reflux of gastric contents.

Critical Thinking

Are these signs and symptoms so unique that you will be able to distinguish oesophageal injury as the cause, versus other kinds of traumatic conditions?

Head trauma

The anatomical components of the skull are the scalp, followed by the cranial vault, under which are the dural membrane, the arachnoid membrane, the pia and the brain substance. Injuries to the skull may be classified as soft tissue injuries to the scalp and skull fractures.

Note

All patients with head or neck trauma must be assumed to have a spinal injury. This must be the case until injury is ruled out by clinical examination and X-ray films in the emergency department. (Spinal precautions [including helmet removal] are presented in Chapter 32.) This text assumes that spinal precautions will be used for all patients with a significant mechanism of injury.

Soft tissue injuries to the scalp

The most common scalp injury is an irregular linear laceration. Like the face, the scalp is very vascular, thus scalp lacerations may bleed heavily (Figure 31-12). They may result in hypovolaemia, particularly in infants and children. Other, less frequent scalp injuries include stellate wounds, avulsions and subgaleal haematoma.

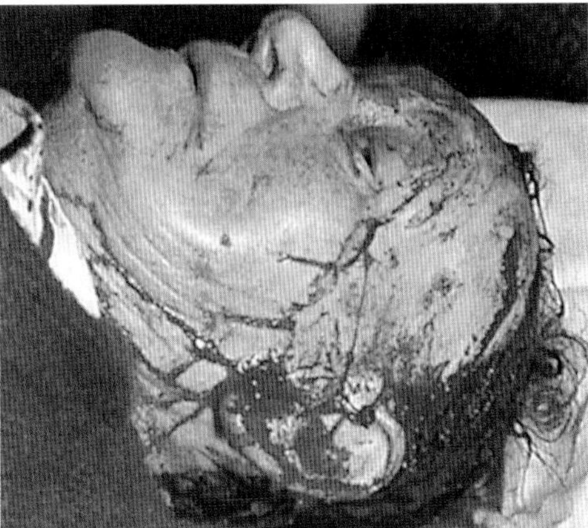

Figure 31-12 Even small wounds from the scalp can bleed profusely.

Management of soft tissue injuries to the scalp includes efforts to prevent contamination of open wounds, use of direct pressure or pressure dressings to decrease blood loss, and fluid replacement if needed. The potential for underlying skull fracture and brain and spinal trauma also exists with these injuries. Isolated scalp lacerations rarely produce life-threatening complications although they can result in excessive blood loss. If not contraindicated by injury, the paramedic should position all patients with head or facial trauma on a stretcher or spine board with the head elevated 30 degrees (semi-Fowler position).

Skull fractures

Skull fractures may be classified as linear fractures, basilar fractures, depressed fractures and open vault fractures (Figure 31-13a–d). Complications associated with these injuries are cranial nerve injury, vascular involvement (e.g. meningeal artery and dural sinuses), infection, underlying brain injury and dural defects caused by depressed bone fragments. As with all injuries to the head, the paramedic should consider the possibility of a spinal injury. Proper spinal precautions should be maintained.

Linear fractures

Linear fractures (seen as straight lines on X-ray film) account for 80% of all fractures to the skull.[4] Such fractures are not usually depressed. Linear fractures often occur without an overlying scalp laceration and, if an isolated injury, usually have a low rate of complication. If the fracture is associated with scalp laceration, infection is possible. Linear fractures that cross the meningeal groove in the temporal-parietal area, midline, or occipital area may lead to epidural bleeding from the middle cerebral artery.

Critical Thinking

Will you be able to detect linear skull fractures during a physical examination in the prehospital setting?

Basilar skull fractures

Basilar skull fractures are usually associated with major impact trauma. These injuries may occur when the mandibular condyles perforate into the base of the skull. More commonly, though, they result from an extension of a linear fracture into the floor of the anterior and middle fossae. Basilar skull fractures can be difficult to see on X-ray films. They are usually diagnosed clinically by the following signs and symptoms:

- ecchymosis over the mastoid process resulting from fracture to the temporal bone (Battle's sign) (Figure 31-14a)
- ecchymosis of one or both orbits caused by fracture of the base of the sphenoid sinus (raccoon's eyes) (Figure 31-14b)
- blood behind the tympanic membrane caused by fractures of the temporal bone (haemotympanum)

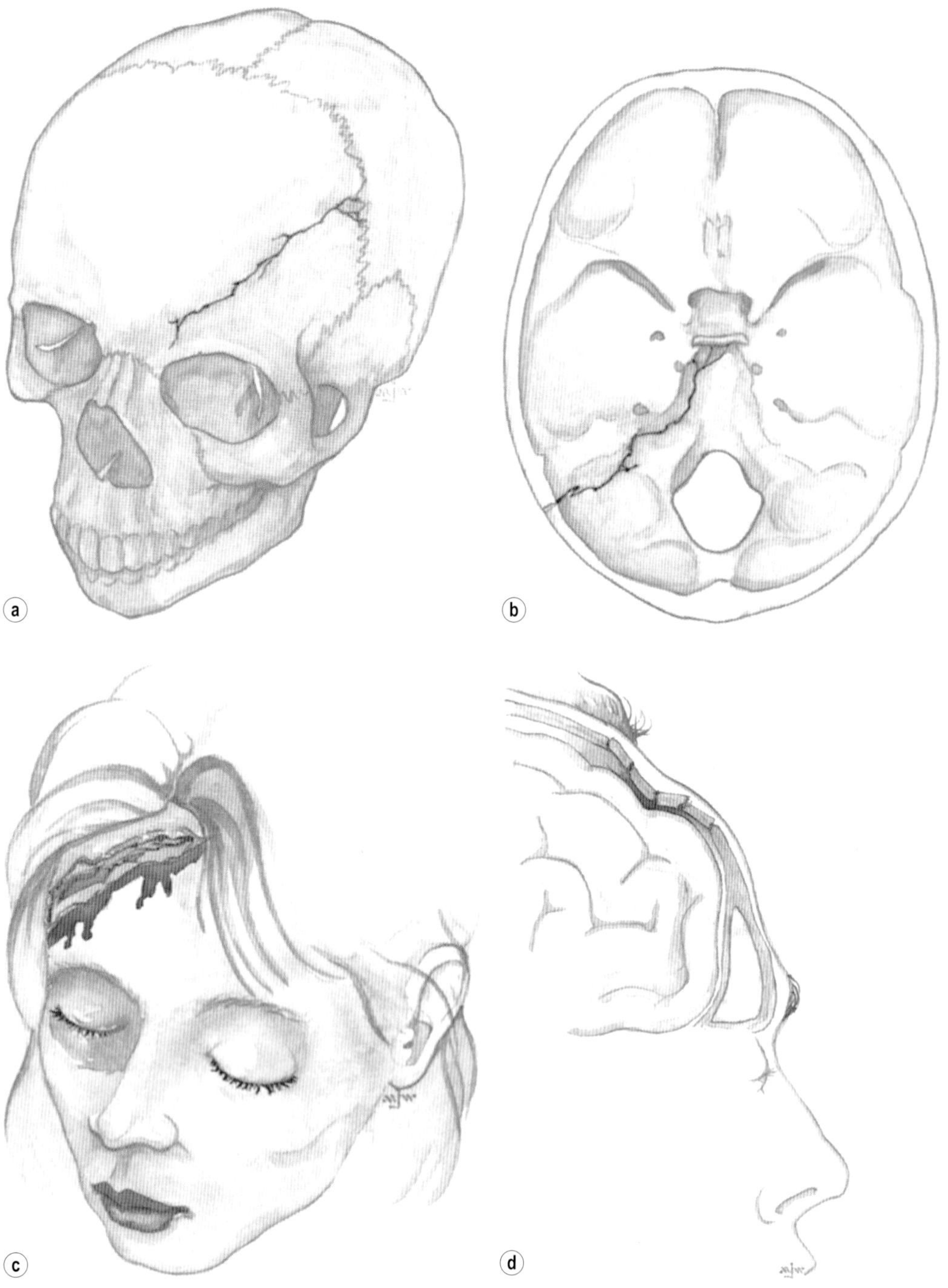

Figure 31-13 Skull fractures. (a) Linear skull fracture. (b) Basilar skull fracture. (c) Open vault fracture. (d) Depressed skull fracture.

- cerebrospinal fluid leakage, which can result in bacterial meningitis.

Note

Battle's sign and raccoon's eyes do not usually occur until some time after the injury. If they are present on the arrival of emergency medical services, the bruising is most likely the result of a prior injury.

Other complications associated with basilar skull fractures include cranial nerve injuries and massive haemorrhage from vascular involvement of the carotid artery. Treatment for basilar skull fractures includes bed rest, in-hospital observation and evaluation for hearing loss caused by acoustic nerve injury.

Depressed skull fractures

Depressed skull fractures usually result from a relatively small object striking the head at high speed and are commonly associated with scalp lacerations (Figure 31-15). The frontal and parietal bones are most often affected. Thirty percent of patients with depressed skull fractures are estimated to have associated haematomata and cerebral contusions.[4] If the depression is greater than the thickness of the skull, dural laceration is likely. Patients with depressed skull

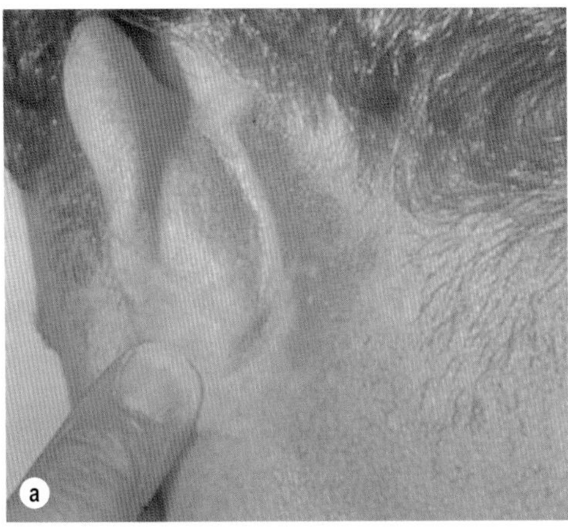

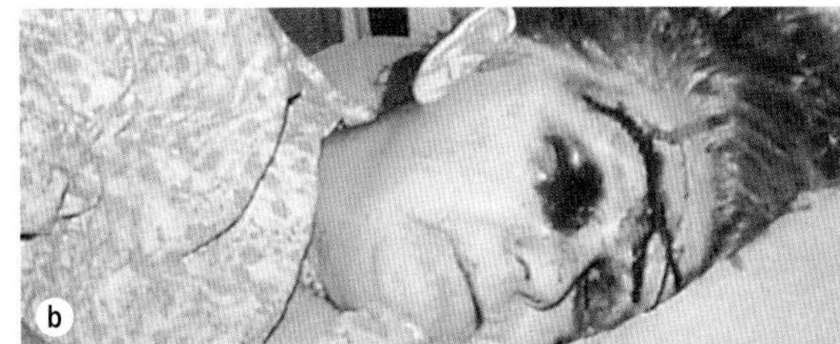

Figure 31-14 (a) Battle's sign. (b) Raccoon's eyes.

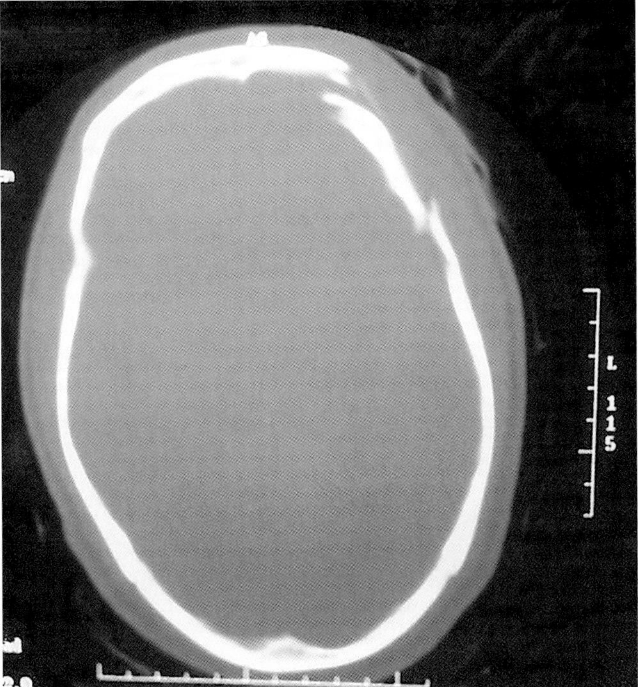

Figure 31-15 Head computed tomography scan showing a depressed skull fracture.

fractures often require surgical removal of the bone fragments (craniectomy).

Open vault fractures

Open vault fractures result when an opening exists between a scalp laceration and brain tissue (Figure 31-16). Because of the nature of these injuries and the force required to produce them, they are often associated with multiple trauma to other systems and have a high mortality rate. Exposure of brain tissue to the external environment may lead to infection (meningitis). Open vault fractures require surgical repair. Prehospital management is usually limited to spinal immobilization, ventilatory support, efforts to prevent contamination, and rapid transportation to an appropriate medical facility.

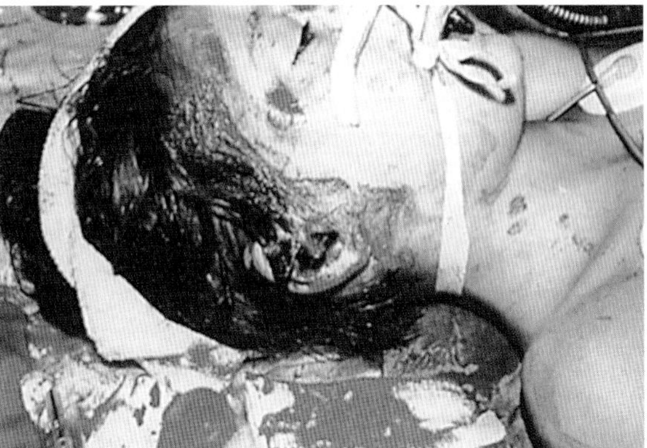

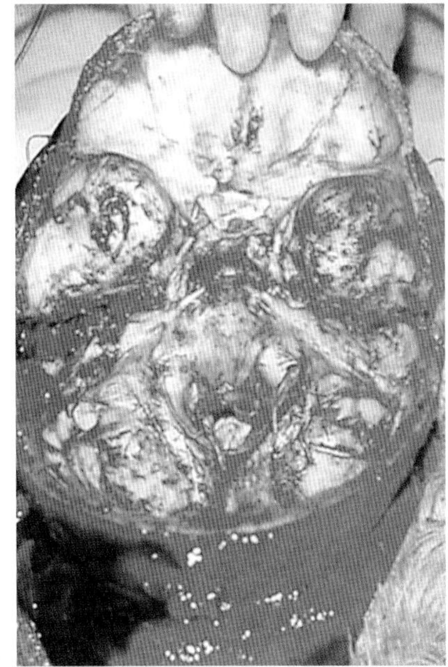

Figure 31-16 Severe fracture of the base of the skull.

Cranial nerve injuries

Twelve pairs of cranial nerves leave the brain and pass through openings in the skull called foramina. Injury to cranial nerves is usually associated with skull fractures. Signs and symptoms of common cranial nerve injuries are as follows:

Cranial nerve I (olfactory nerve)

- Loss of smell
- Impairment of taste (dependent on food aroma)
- Hallmark of basilar skull fracture.

Cranial nerve II (optic nerve)

- Blindness in one or both eyes
- Visual field defects.

Cranial nerve III (oculomotor nerve)

- Ipsilateral (same side), dilated, fixed pupil
- Especially compression by the temporal lobe
- Mimicking of direct ocular trauma.

Cranial nerve VII (facial nerve)

- Immediate or delayed facial paralysis
- Basilar skull fracture.

Cranial nerve VIII (auditory nerve)

- Deafness
- Basilar skull fracture.

Brain trauma

A brain injury is defined by the National Head Injury Foundation as 'a traumatic insult to the brain capable of producing physical, intellectual, emotional, social and vocational change'.[8] Traumatic brain injury can be divided into two categories: primary brain injury and secondary brain injury. Primary brain injury refers to direct trauma to the brain and to the associated vascular injuries that occurred from the initial injury. Secondary brain injury results from intracellular and extracellular derangements that were probably initiated at the time of the injury. These derangements may include: hypoxia, hypocapnia and hypercapnia from airway compromise; aspiration of gastric contents; thoracic injury; anaemia and hypotension from external and internal haemorrhage; and hyperglycaemia or hypoglycaemia that can injure ischaemic brain tissue further. The adverse effects of secondary brain injury can be minimized. They perhaps can be reversed, if they are recognized and properly managed in the prehospital setting. Brain injuries can be classified as mild and moderate diffuse injury, diffuse axonal injury, and focal injury.[9]

Mild diffuse injury (concussion)

Concussion is a fully reversible brain injury that does not result in structural damage to the brain. Concussion is caused by a mild to moderate impact to the skull, movement of the brain within the cranial vault, or both. Concussion occurs when the function of the brainstem (particularly the reticular activating system) or both cerebral cortices is disturbed temporarily. This results in a brief altered level of consciousness (usually less than 5 min). If the patient has been unconscious for more than 5 min, the paramedic should suspect a more serious injury caused by contusion or haemorrhage.

The loss of consciousness is usually followed by periods of drowsiness, restlessness and confusion, with a fairly rapid return to normal behaviour. The patient may have no recall of the events before the injury (retrograde amnesia). In addition, amnesia may exist after recovery of consciousness (antegrade amnesia). This short-term memory loss may produce anxiety and the patient may ask repetitive questions (e.g. 'Where am I? What happened?'). Other signs and symptoms of concussion are vomiting; combativeness; transient visual disturbances (e.g. light flashes and wavy lines); defects in equilibrium and coordination; and changes in blood pressure, pulse rate, and respiration (rare). After physician evaluation, treatment usually consists of in-hospital or home observation by a reliable observer for 24 to 48 h.

Critical Thinking

Consider the patient with a new onset of retrograde or antegrade amnesia. Why should the patient not be considered a reliable historian?

A concussion injury affects the patient most severely at the time of impact but is followed by improvement. Concussion is the most common and least serious type of brain injury. Any patient whose condition worsens over time or whose level of consciousness deteriorates rather than improves must be suspected of having a more serious injury. Therefore, documentation of baseline measurements of level of consciousness, memory status, and neurological function (e.g. Glasgow Coma Scale or AVPU [alert, verbal, painful, unresponsive] scale) in any victim of head injury is important.

Moderate diffuse injury

Moderate injuries are those that result in minute petechial bruising of brain tissue. The involvement of the brainstem and reticular activating system leads to unconsciousness. These injuries account for 20% of all severe head injuries and 45% of all cases of diffuse injury.[8] Often these patients will have basilar skull fracture. Most patients will survive the injury although permanent neurological impairment is common.

A patient with moderate diffuse injury will initially be unconscious, followed by persistent confusion, disorientation and amnesia of the event. During recovery, these patients often experience an inability to concentrate, frequent periods of anxiety, uncharacteristic mood swings, and sensorimotor deficits (e.g. an altered sense of smell). Patients with moderate diffuse injury are managed in the same way as those with concussion. Assurance of an adequate airway and tidal volume, and frequent reassessments of the level of consciousness are necessary. If possible, patients with head injury should be moved to a quiet, calm area and exposure to bright lights avoided as patients may be photophobic. Also, constant reorientation of the patient may be necessary.

Diffuse axonal injury

Diffuse axonal injury (DAI) is the severest form of brain injury. It results from brain movement within the skull from acceleration or deceleration forces, which cause shearing, stretching, or tearing of nerve fibres with subsequent axonal (nerve cell) damage. Diffuse axonal injury may be classified as mild, moderate, or severe. Mild DAI is associated with coma of 6–24 h and has a mortality rate of 16%.[4] Moderate DAI is more common and is distinguished by coma lasting more than 24 h and abnormal posturing (described later). The associated mortality rate of moderate DAI approaches 24%.[10]

Critical Thinking

Can a patient with a diffuse axonal injury die as a result of that injury?

Severe DAI was once known as a brainstem injury. Severe DAI involves severe mechanical shearing of many axons in both cerebral hemispheres extending to the brainstem. Severe DAI occurs in 16% of all severe head injuries and in 36% of all cases of DAI.[8] These patients are often unconscious for prolonged periods and may exhibit abnormal posturing and other signs of increased intracranial pressure (ICP). The prehospital care for these patients is focused on ensuring an adequate airway and tidal volume. Hypoxia must be prevented in all patients with head injury, to help avoid secondary injury to brain tissue.

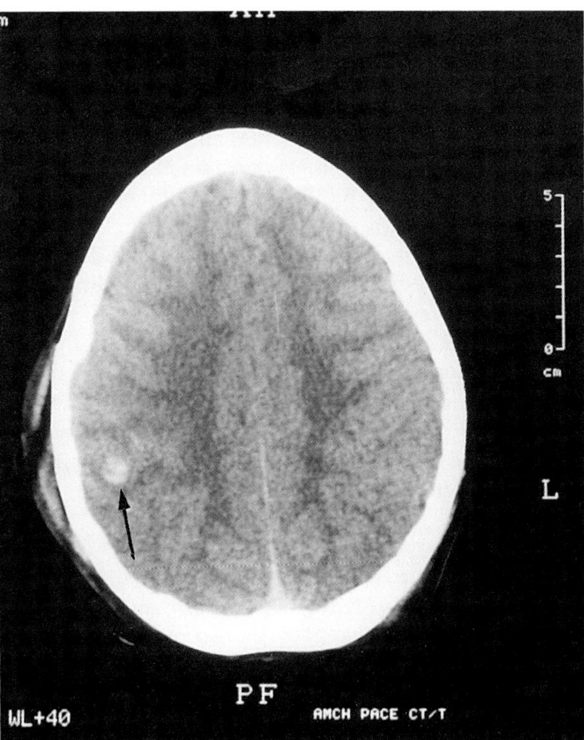

Figure 31-17 Head computed tomography scan demonstrating a cerebral contusion.

Focal injury

Focal injuries are specific, grossly observable brain lesions. Included in this category are lesions that result from skull fracture (previously described), contusion, oedema with associated increased ICP, ischaemia and haemorrhage.

Cerebral contusion

A cerebral contusion is bruising of the brain in the area of the cortex or deeper within the frontal (most common), temporal or occipital lobes (Figure 31-17). This bruising produces a structural change in the brain tissue and results in greater neurological deficits and abnormalities than are seen with concussions. These changes may include seizures, hemiparesis, aphasia and personality changes. If the brainstem is also contused, the patient may lose consciousness. In some cases, the comatose state may be prolonged and may last hours to days or longer. Of the patients who die from head injury, 75% have cerebral contusions at autopsy.[8]

If the applied force is sufficient to cause the brain to be displaced against the irregular surfaces of the skull, tiny blood vessels in the pia mater may rupture. The brain substance may be damaged locally at the site of impact (coup), or on the opposite, or contralateral, side (contrecoup). Contrecoup injuries are often caused by deceleration of the head such as may occur in a fall or motor vehicle crash.

As a rule, cerebral contusions usually heal without intervention and patients usually improve. However, the time to heal and level of improvement differ in these two conditions. The most important complication associated with cerebral contusion is increased ICP manifested by headache, nausea, vomiting, seizures, and a declining level of consciousness. These signs are usually delayed responses to the injury and are not often seen in the prehospital emergency setting.

Oedema

Major injuries to the brain often result in swelling of the brain tissue with or without associated haemorrhage. The swelling results from humoral and metabolic responses to injury. Swelling leads to considerable increases in ICP, which in turn can lead to decreased cerebral perfusion (described later) or herniation.

Ischaemia

Ischaemia can result from vascular injuries, secondary vascular spasm, or increased ICP. In any case, focal or more global infarcts can result.

Haemorrhage

The same forces that result in concussion and contusion may also cause serious vascular damage. This damage may result in haemorrhage into or around brain tissue and may cause epidural or subdural haematomata. The haematomata compress the underlying brain tissue, or produce intraparenchymal haemorrhage (bleeding directly into the brain tissue). This bleeding often results from cerebral contusions and skull fractures.

Cerebral blood flow

Although the brain accounts for only 2% of adult weight, 20% of total body oxygen use and 25% of total body glucose use are devoted to brain metabolism.[8] Oxygen and glucose delivery are controlled by cerebral blood flow.

Cerebral blood flow is a function of cerebral perfusion pressure (CPP) and resistance of the cerebral vascular bed.

Cerebral perfusion pressure is the difference between the mean arterial pressure (MAP) and the ICP (CPP = MAP – ICP). Normal mean arterial pressure ranges from 85 to 95 mmHg, whilst intracranial pressure is normally between 0 and 15 mmHg. Normal CPP is between 60 and 100 mmHg, with a perfusion pressure of 60 mmHg considered to be the critical minimum threshold. As ICP approaches mean arterial pressure, the gradient for flow decreases and cerebral blood flow decreases. That is, when ICP increases, CPP decreases. As CPP decreases, vessels in the brain dilate (cerebral vasodilatation), which results in increased cerebral blood volume (increasing ICP) and further cerebral vasodilatation. In most emergency medical services systems, CPP is not calculated because mean arterial pressure and ICP are not measured in the prehospital setting. However, maintaining a systolic blood pressure of at least 90 mmHg may help maintain adequate mean arterial pressure.[11]

Critical Thinking

What happens to the flow of oxygen to the brain, and carbon dioxide from the brain to the capillaries, when intracranial pressure is increasing and cerebral perfusion pressure is decreasing?

Vascular tone in the normal brain is regulated by carbon dioxide pressure (P_{CO_2}), oxygen pressure (P_{O_2}), and autonomic and neurohumoral control; P_{CO_2} has the greatest effect on intracerebral vascular diameter and subsequent resistance. For example, if P_{CO_2} is increased from 40 to 80 mmHg, cerebral blood flow is doubled. This results in increased brain blood volume and ICP.

Intracranial pressure

The normal range of ICP is 0–15 mmHg. When ICP rises above this level, the body has difficulty maintaining adequate CPP, usually because of an expanding mass or diffuse swelling. Cerebral blood flow is diminished when the CPP is not adequate. As the cranial vault continues to fill (because of brain oedema or expanding haematoma), the body tries to compensate for the decline in CPP by a rise in mean arterial pressure (Cushing reflex). Yet this increase in cerebral blood flow further elevates the ICP. As pressure continues to increase, cerebrospinal fluid is displaced to make up for the expansion. If unresolved, the brain substance may herniate over the edge of the tentorium. (This is one of three extensions of the dura mater that separates the cerebellum from the occipital lobe of the cerebrum.) Or it may herniate through the foramen magnum (Figure 31-18).

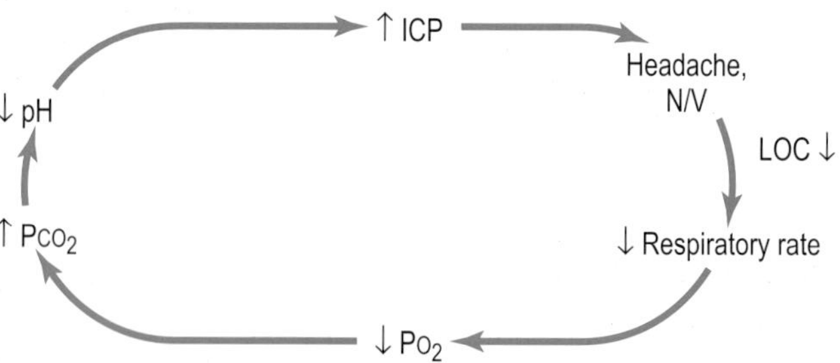

Figure 31-18 Effects of increased intracranial pressure.

Early signs and symptoms of increased ICP include headache, nausea and vomiting, and altered level of consciousness (Box 31-3). These signs and symptoms are eventually followed by increased systolic pressure, and widened pulse pressure, a decrease in the pulse and an irregular respiratory pattern (Cushing triad). As the volume continues to expand in the cranial vault, herniation of the temporal lobe of the brain through the tentorium may occur. The herniation causes compression of cranial nerve III, which produces a dilated pupil and loss of light reflex on the side of compression. The patient rapidly becomes unresponsive to verbal and painful stimuli and may exhibit the ominous signs of decorticate posturing (characterized by extension of the legs and flexion of the arms at the elbows). Alternatively, the patient may exhibit decerebrate posturing (characterized by extension of all four extremities) (Figure 31-19).

Critical Thinking

Why is cranial nerve III affected by this shift in brain tissue?

Respiratory patterns

As ICP continues to rise, abnormal respiratory patterns (described in Chapter 13) may develop. Respiratory abnormalities associated with increased ICP and significant brainstem injury include hypoventilation, Cheyne–Stokes breathing (which may accompany decorticate posturing), central neurogenic hyperventilation (which may accompany decerebrate posturing), and ataxic breathing. The clinical significance of decorticate (flexion) and decerebrate (extension) posturing and respiratory patterns are not of major

Box 31-3

Levels of increasing intracranial pressure

Cerebral cortex and upper brainstem

Blood pressure rises; pulse rate slows.
Pupils remain reactive.
Cheyne–Stokes respirations may be present.
Patient initially will try to localize and remove painful stimuli (eventually withdraws and flexion occurs).
All effects are reversible at this stage.

Middle brainstem

Wide pulse pressure and bradycardia are present.
Pupils become non-reactive or sluggish.
Central neurogenic hyperventilation develops.
Abnormal posturing (extension) occurs.
Few patients function normally with injury at this level.

Lower portion of brainstem/medulla

Pupil is 'blown' (fixed and dilated) on same side of injury.
Respirations become ataxic.
Patient will be flaccid.
Pulse rate is irregular.
QRS, S-T, and T wave changes will be present.
Blood pressure will fluctuate.
These patients generally do not survive.

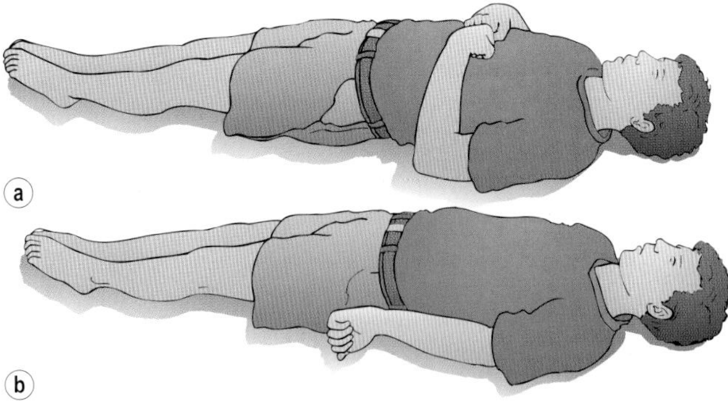

Figure 31-19 (a) Abnormal flexion (decorticate posturing). (b) Abnormal extension (decerebrate posturing).

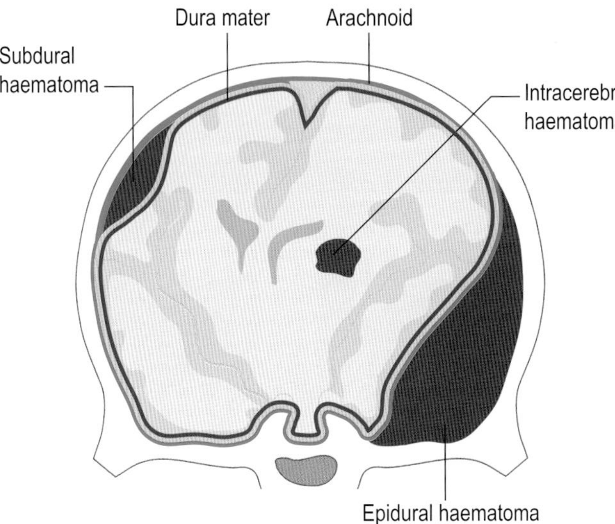

Figure 31-20 Varieties of intracranial haemorrhage.

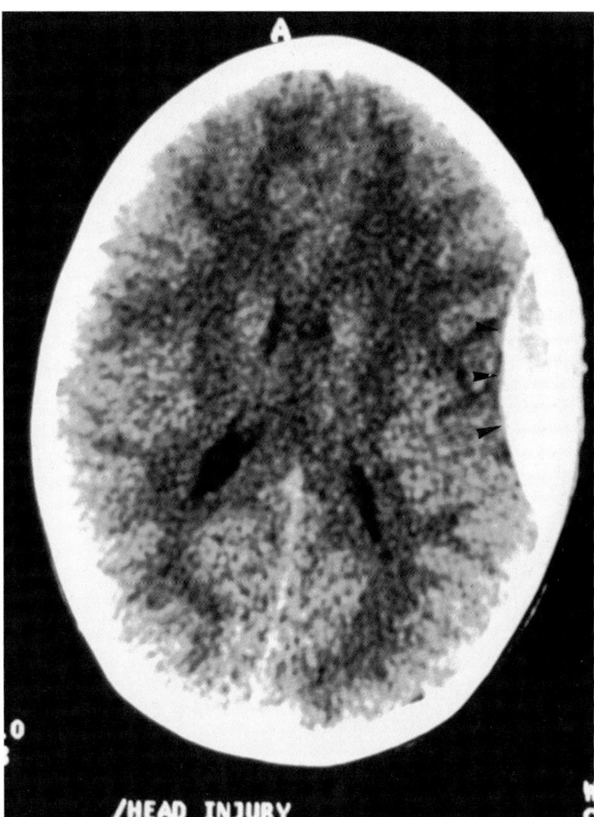

Figure 31-21 Head computed tomography scan showing an epidural haematoma.

clinical importance other than to identify the need for intervention and treatment (intubation and consideration of immediate neurosurgical intervention).

Note

Some motion of the limbs, albeit abnormal, is better than no motion of the limbs. (No motion indicates a worse level of neurological function.)

Types of brain hemorrhage

Traditionally, brain haemorrhages are classified according to their location as epidural, subdural, subarachnoid, or cerebral (intraparenchymal) (Figure 31-20).

Epidural haematoma

An epidural haematoma (accounting for 0.5–1% of all head injuries[4]) is a collection of blood between the cranium and the dura in the epidural space (Figure 31-21). The haematoma usually is a rapidly developing lesion. Usually the haematoma is associated with a laceration or tear of the middle meningeal artery. This haemorrhage often occurs as a result of a linear or depressed skull fracture in the temporal bone. Yet bleeding from other sites can produce epidural haemorrhage as well. If the source of haemorrhage is mostly venous, deterioration usually is not as rapid because low-pressure vessels bleed more slowly.

Fifty percent of patients with epidural haematoma have a transient loss of consciousness followed by a lucid interval in which neurological status returns to normal. (The remaining 50% of patients with acute epidural haematoma never recover consciousness.) The lucid interval usually lasts between 6 and 18 h during which time the haematoma enlarges. As ICP rises, the patient develops a headache with lethargy, decreasing level of consciousness, and contralateral hemiparesis. In the early stages of an epidural haematoma, the patient may complain only of headache and drowsiness. Definitive treatment includes immediate recognition and rapid transport to a proper facility for surgery. Common causes of epidural haematoma include low-velocity blows to the head, violent altercations, and deceleration injuries. About 15–20% of these patients die.[8]

Critical Thinking

What could account for delays in surgical treatment, causing subsequent death, in patients who have an epidural haematoma?

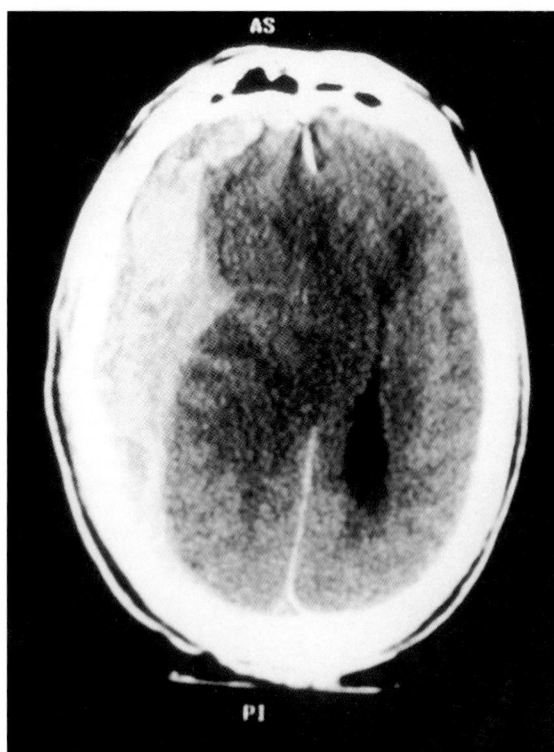

Figure 31-22 Head computed tomography scan showing an acute subdural haematoma.

Subdural haematoma

A subdural haematoma is a collection of blood between the dura and the surface of the brain in the subdural space (Figure 31-22). This injury usually results from bleeding of the veins that bridge the subdural space and is often associated with contusion or laceration of the brain. The haematoma often results from blunt head trauma and is commonly associated with skull fracture. Subdural haematomata are classified as acute (50–80% mortality rate), subacute (25% mortality rate), and chronic (20% mortality rate).[8] Classification depends on the time lapse between the injury and development of symptoms. As a general rule, if symptoms occur within 24 h, the haematoma is considered acute; between 2 and 10 days, subacute; and after 2 weeks, chronic. Subdural haematomata are more common than epidural haematomata.

Signs and symptoms of subdural haematoma are similar to those of epidural haematoma and, include headache, nausea and vomiting, decreasing level of consciousness, coma, abnormal posturing, paralysis, and, in infants, bulging fontanelles. These findings may be subtle because of the slow development of the haematoma in the subacute and chronic phases. Definitive care consists of surgery to remove the blood from the haematoma. Individuals at increased risk of developing subdural haematoma include older adults and patients with clotting deficiencies (e.g. alcoholics, haemophiliacs and persons who take anticoagulants) and patients with cortical atrophy (older adults, alcoholics).

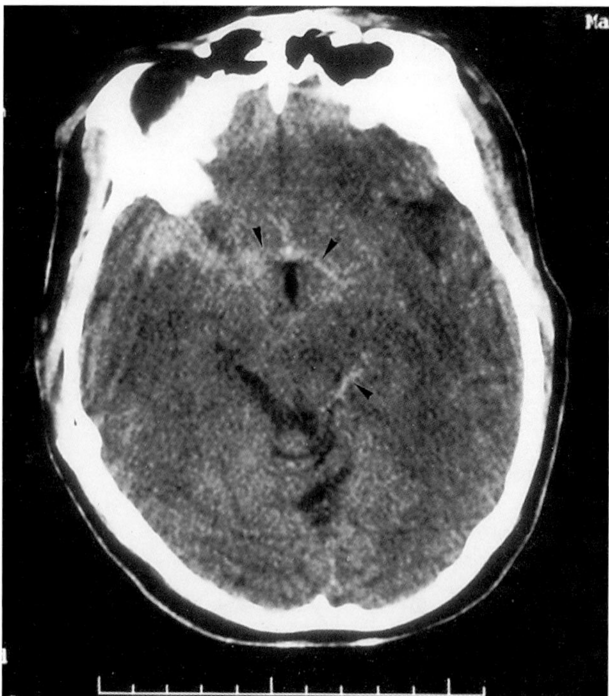

Figure 31-23 Head computed tomography scan showing a traumatic subarachnoid haemorrhage.

Subarachnoid haematoma

A subarachnoid haematoma refers to intracranial bleeding into the cerebrospinal fluid. This results in bloody cerebrospinal fluid and meningeal irritation (Figure 31-23). Bleeding that results from trauma, rupture of an aneurysm, or arteriovenous anomaly may extend into the brain if the force of the bleeding from the broken vessel is sudden and severe. Patients with this injury often complain of a sudden and severe headache. The headache initially may be localized but then spreads and becomes dull and throbbing (due to meningeal irritation). Other characteristics of a subarachnoid haemorrhage include dizziness, neck stiffness, unequal pupils, vomiting, seizures and loss of consciousness. Severe haemorrhage may result in coma and death. Permanent brain damage is common in those who survive.

> **Critical Thinking**
>
> What causes the vomiting, seizures, and loss of consciousness in a patient with subarachnoid haemorrhage?

Cerebral haematoma

An intracerebral haematoma may be defined as a collection of more than 5 mL of blood somewhere within the substance of the brain, most commonly in the frontal or temporal lobe.[8] This injury can result from multiple lacerations produced by penetrating head trauma (gunshot wound). The injury may also result from a high-velocity deceleration injury (automobile crash) in which vessels are torn as the brain moves across rough surfaces of the skull. Increased ICP can produce an intracerebral haematoma as the result of the brain being compressed.

Cerebral haematoma is often associated with subdural haemorrhage and skull fracture. Signs and symptoms may be immediate or delayed depending upon the size and location of the haemorrhage. Once symptoms appear, the patient usually deteriorates rapidly. The mortality rate after surgical evacuation of the haematoma (if possible) is more than 40%.[8]

Penetrating injury

Penetrating injuries to the brain are usually caused by missiles fired from handguns and stab wounds caused by sharp objects. Less often, penetrating trauma may result from falls and high-velocity vehicle crashes. Associated injuries include skull fracture; damage to cerebral arteries, veins, or venous sinuses; and intracranial haemorrhage. Complications include infection and post-traumatic epilepsy. Definitive care for these injuries requires neurosurgical intervention.

Assessment and neurological evaluation

Prehospital management of the patient with a head injury is determined by a number of factors, including the mechanism and severity of injury and the patient's level of consciousness. Associated injuries affect the priorities of emergency care.

Airway and ventilation

The initial step in treating all patients with head trauma is to ensure an open airway with spinal precautions. The next step is to provide adequate ventilation with high-concentration oxygen. Airway management may include oral or nasal adjuncts, LM(A) or tracheal intubation to maintain and protect the airway. Tracheal intubation and ventilatory support are usually recommended in all patients with head injuries who have a GCS score of 8 or less[8] (described later in the chapter), although this may not be achievable without sedation.

Critical Thinking

Imagine what a patient with a GCS score of 8 or lower would look like. Why should these patients be intubated? What if the GCS score improves rapidly?

Patients with head injuries are likely to vomit, so maintaining awareness of the risk and adopting proactive airway management techniques are essential to reduce the danger of aspiration and the associated complications. The patient should be secured to an appropriate immobilization device to allow for safe repositioning in the event of vomiting, and suction equipment with large-bore suction catheters should be available.

Ventilatory support should be focused on maintaining adequate oxygenation and optimizing cerebral perfusion. Capnography (where available) and pulse oximetry should be used to maintain oxygen saturation at a level of 95% or greater. Aggressive hyperventilation reduces carbon dioxide and can lead to secondary brain injury through cerebral vasoconstriction and a decrease in cerebral blood flow (routine prophylactic hyperventilation should be avoided).

Box 31-4

Indicators of herniation for hyperventilation

An unresponsive patient with the following:

Bilateral, dilated, unresponsive pupils *or* asymmetric pupils (>1 mm)

and

Abnormal extension (decerebrate) posturing *or* no motor response to painful stimuli

Box 31-5

Systolic blood pressure thresholds defining hypotension in head-injured patients

<65 mmHg in patients from birth to 1 year of age

<75 mmHg in patients 2–5 years of age

<80 mmHg in patients 6–12 years

<90 mmHg in patients 13 years or older

Source: Brain Trauma Foundation.

In the absence of capnography to guide ventilatory support, normal ventilations should be provided at 10 breaths/min for adults; 20 breaths/min for children; and 25 breaths/min for infants. With evidence of herniation (Box 31-4), the patient should be hyperventilated at the following rates: 20 breaths/min for adults; 30 breaths/min for children; and 35 breaths/min for infants. These rates should yield a P_{CO_2} of about 35 mmHg.[11]

Circulation

After the airway has been secured (maintaining spinal protection), support of the patient's cardiovascular function becomes the next priority. The paramedic should control major external bleeding and assess the patient's vital signs. Assessment establishes a baseline for future evaluations. A cardiac monitor will detect changes in rhythm (particularly bradycardia and tachycardia) that can occur with increasing ICP and brainstem injury. The blood pressure of every patient should be maintained at normal levels with fluid replacement (per guidelines). A single episode of hypotension doubles mortality and increases morbidity in the patient with traumatic brain injury.[11] The paramedic should administer intravenous fluids to support oxygen delivery and to avoid hypertension or limit hypotension to the shortest duration possible. Systolic blood pressure thresholds that can be used to define hypotension in head-injured patients are listed in Box 31-5.

Persistent hypotension from an isolated head injury is a rare and terminal event. The exception is head injury in infants and small children. Closed head injury in the adult does not produce hypovolaemic shock, thus a patient with head injuries who is also hypotensive should be evaluated for other injuries that could cause haemorrhage. The paramedic should also evaluate the patient for the possibility of neurogenic shock from spinal cord trauma. Infusion of isotonic fluids (sodium lactate or normal saline) may be indicated for haemorrhagic shock. However, these fluids should be used cautiously in patients with hypotension caused by neurogenic shock. In the latter patient group, vasopressors may be helpful in maintaining blood pressure but are not yet available to the paramedic. Neurogenic shock may be distinguished from haemorrhagic shock by the following:

- a relatively bradycardic response (e.g. a pulse of 80 with a blood pressure of 80 mmHg)
- skin that is often warm and dry (not cool and clammy)
- no evidence of significant blood loss or hypovolaemia
- paralysis and loss of spinal reflexes.

Neurological examination

Conscious patients should be interviewed to determine their memory status before and after the injury and to learn of significant medical history (e.g. heart disease, hypertension, diabetes, epilepsy, medication use, alcohol or other drug use, and allergies). The history should include the mechanism of injury and the events that led up to the injury (for example, the history may detail a loss of consciousness before or after the injury incident).

The paramedic should evaluate the motor skills of conscious patients to determine the patient's ability to follow commands and help the paramedic to note any paralysis. (Hemiparesis or hemiplegia, especially with a sensory deficit on the same side, indicates brain damage rather than spinal trauma.) If the patient is unconscious on emergency medical services arrival, the paramedic should interview bystanders about the history of the event. The paramedic should ask bystanders about the length of time the patient has been unconscious. The most important indicator of increasing ICP is deterioration in the patient's sensorium, thus the paramedic should evaluate the level of consciousness using the GCS every 5 min. A decrease of 2 points with a GCS score of 9 or lower is significant; it indicates significant injury.[11]

Critical Thinking

How reliable will the patient be regarding the duration of his or her loss of consciousness?

After the patient has been resuscitated and stabilized, the paramedic should assess the patient's pupils for symmetry, size, and reactivity to light. Abnormal pupillary responses may indicate an increase in ICP and cranial nerve involvement. Asymmetric pupils differ by more than 1 mm in size; dilated pupils are greater than or equal to 4 mm in adults; and a fixed pupil shows less than 1 mm change in response to bright light. (The paramedic should evaluate pupil size every 5 min.) Alcohol and some other drugs can cause abnormal pupillary reactions, but the reactions are commonly bilateral (except for certain eye drops, if placed in one eye). If the patient is conscious, the paramedic should also evaluate extraocular movement (see Chapter 9).

Note

The initial pupil evaluation and the GCS establish the baseline against which all subsequent neurological evaluations are compared.[11]

Fluid therapy

In the absence of hypotension, fluid therapy should be restricted in a patient with head injury to minimize cerebral oedema. If the patient is haemodynamically stable, the paramedic should consider establishing an intravenous line of crystalloid fluid to keep the vein open but should not delay on scene to achieve this. If significant hypovolaemia is present from another injury, the paramedic should give the patient a 250-mL isotonic fluid bolus in accordance with guidelines[12] and rapidly transport the patient to an appropriate facility. In this case, the injury causing hypovolaemia is usually more immediately life threatening than the head injury. The paramedic should remember that inadequate infusion will lead to reduced cerebral blood flow and will increase cerebral hypoxia.

Drug therapy

Prehospital use of drugs for the treatment of head injuries is controversial and they are currently not authorized for use by paramedics in the UK. Drugs that decrease cerebral oedema or circulating blood volume may include mannitol and hypertonic saline (both are controversial).

Note

The administration of glucose (dextrose 50%) is contraindicated in patients with head injuries unless hypoglycaemia is confirmed. Intravenously administered dextrose 50% may worsen cerebral damage.

Anticonvulsant agents such as diazepam are used to control seizure activity in head-injured patients. As a rule, these drugs are not used in the initial management of head injuries because of their sedating effects. Intravenously administered lidocaine has been shown to control increases in ICP that normally occur during endotracheal intubation.[8]

In addition, the use of sedatives and paralytics for some patients with head injuries may be indicated for airway management. These drugs may also be used to aid in the transport of combative patients (especially in aeromedical transport). The paramedic should follow local protocol and training regarding the use of these drugs.

Injury rating systems

Several injury rating systems are used to triage, guide patient care, predict patient outcome, identify changes in patient status, and evaluate trauma care in epidemiological studies and quality assurance reviews. (These also are known as indexes or scales.) These indexes are important to prehospital personnel as they aid in determining patient care needs with reference to hospital resources. Rating systems commonly used in emergency care include the Glasgow Coma Scale, trauma score, Revised Trauma Score, and paediatric trauma score.

Glasgow Coma Scale

The GCS evaluates eye opening, verbal and motor responses, and brainstem reflex function. The scale is considered one of the best indicators of eventual clinical outcome[8] and should be part of any neurological examination for patients with head injury (Table 31-1). A GCS score of 9 to 13 indicates moderate traumatic brain injury; a GCS score of 8 or less indicates a severe traumatic brain injury. (Note: The lowest possible score is 3; the highest possible score is 15.) Hypoxaemia and hypotension have been shown to affect GCS scoring negatively, thus GCS should be measured after the initial assessment. The score should be measured after a clear airway is established. Also, the GCS should be measured after necessary ventilation and circulatory resuscitation have been performed. Unresponsive patients with a GCS score of 3 to 8 should be transported to a trauma centre with traumatic brain injury capabilities.[11]

Trauma score/Revised Trauma Score

The trauma score was developed in 1980 to predict outcome for patients with blunt or penetrating injuries.

It is a physiological scoring system that uses GCS, systolic blood pressure and respiratory rate as markers of the trauma severity. A range of values for these physiological measurements is assigned a number between 0 and 4. These numbers are added to give a total between 0 and 12 (a score of 0 indicates the most critical; a score of 12 indicates the least critical) (Table 31-2). The trauma score may be used in the prehospital setting to determine which patients are transported to a trauma centre. A threshold of ≤4 has been proposed but this may be a little low. The scoring system is heavily weighted towards the GCS component to compensate for major head injury without multisystem trauma. Calculating the Revised Trauma Score en route to the receiving hospital also provides baseline measurements that can be helpful to the physician in managing the patient's care.

Paediatric trauma score

The paediatric trauma score grades six characteristics commonly seen in paediatric trauma patients. These are size (weight), airway, consciousness, systolic blood pressure, fracture and cutaneous injury (Table 31-3). The paediatric trauma score has a significant inverse linear relationship with patient mortality. A child with a paediatric trauma score less than 8 should be cared for in an appropriate paediatric trauma centre.[11]

Table 31-1 Glasgow Coma Scale

Criteria	Points assigned to score
EYE OPENING	
Spontaneous eye opening	4
Eye opening on command	3
Eye opening to painful stimulus	2
No eye opening	1
BEST VERBAL RESPONSE	
Answers appropriately (oriented)	5*
Gives confused answers	4
Inappropriate response	3
Makes unintelligible noises	2
Makes no verbal response	1
BEST MOTOR RESPONSE	
Follows commands	6
Localizes painful stimuli	5
Withdraws from pain	4
Responds with abnormal flexion to painful stimuli (decorticate)	3
Responds with abnormal extension to painful stimuli (decerebrate)	2
Gives no motor response	1
Total	___

From National Association of emergency medical technicians 2003 PHTLS basic and advanced prehospital trauma life support. Mosby, St Louis.
*It generally is agreed that a full verbal score of 5 should be assigned to a child less than 2 years of age who cries after stimulation.
Example: A head-injured patient with an eye-opening response to pain would be assigned a 2 (E2); with no verbal response would be assigned a 1 (V1); with decerebrate posturing would be assigned a 2 (M2). The Glasgow Coma Scale score for this patient would be 5.

Table 31-2 Revised Trauma Score

Variable	Score (points)	Start of transport	End of transport
A. VENTILATORY RATE			
10–29/min	4		
>29/min	3		
6–9/min	2		
1–5/min	1		
0	0		
B. SYSTOLIC BLOOD PRESSURE			
>89 mmHg	4		
76–89 mmHg	3		
50–75 mmHg	2		
1–49 mmHg	1		
No pulse	0		
C. GLASGOW COMA SCALE SCORE			
13–15	4		
9–12	3		
6–8	2		
4–5	1		
<4	0		
Trauma score total = A + B + C			

Adapted from Champion HR et al 1989 A revision of the trauma score. J Trauma 29(5):624.
Example: At the start of transport, a head-injured patient has spontaneous ventilations at 30 breaths/min (score of 3); a systolic pressure of 80 mmHg (score of 3); and a Glasgow Coma Scale score of 12 (score of 3); providing a Revised Trauma Score of 9. At end of transport, the patient has spontaneous ventilations of 18 breaths/min (score of 4); a systolic pressure of 62 (score of 2); and a Glasgow Coma Scale score of 7 (score of 2); providing a Revised Trauma Score of 8.

Table 31-3 Paediatric trauma score

Component	+2	+1	−1
Size (kg)	Child/adolescent >20 kg	Toddler 10–20 kg	Infant <10 kg
Airway	Normal	Assisted: O_2 mask, cannula	Intubated: endotracheal tube, cricothyroidotomy
Consciousness	Awake	Obtunded, lost consciousness	Coma, unresponsive
Systolic blood pressure	>90 mmHg	50–90 mmHg	<50 mmHg
	Good peripheral pulses	Carotid, femoral pulse palpable	Weak or no pulse perfusion
Fracture	None seen or suspected	Single closed fracture anywhere	Open or multiple fractures
Cutaneous	No visible injury	Confusion, abrasion, laceration <7 cm through fascia	Tissue loss, any gunshot wound or stab through fascia

From National Association of emergency medical technicians 2003 PHTLS basic and advanced prehospital trauma life support. Mosby, St Louis.

Patient size (weight) is one of the first parameters to assess. The smaller the child, the greater the risk for severe injury because of an increased ratio of body surface to volume. The risk is also greater because of the potential for limited physiological reserve.

The child's airway is scored by potential difficulty in management. Scoring is also judged by the type of care required to ensure adequate ventilation and oxygenation. Respiratory failure is the main cause of death in most paediatric patients. Aggressive management to control the airway should be started without delay.

As with adult patients, the most critical factor in assessing the central nervous system of a child is a change in the level of consciousness. Any change in the level of consciousness will reduce this score – no matter how brief the time.

The assessment of systolic blood pressure in the paediatric patient is critical because the circulating volume is notably less than the adult. Because of a normal child's healthy heart and excellent reserve capacity, children often do not show classic signs of shock until they have lost about 25% of their circulating volume. Any child who has a systolic blood pressure less than 50 mmHg is in obvious jeopardy.[13]

A child's skeleton is more pliable than that of the adult. It allows traumatic forces to be sent through the body and to the organs, thus a fracture in the paediatric patient is a sign that serious injury has occurred.

Like fractures, cutaneous injury in the paediatric patient is a potential contributor to mortality and disability. These injuries include open and visible wounds and penetrating trauma.

For example, a head-injured child who is 8 years of age weighs 34 kg (+2); has spontaneous respirations (+2); is unresponsive (−1); has a systolic pressure of 86 mmHg with palpable femoral pulses (+1); no visible fractures (+2); and an abrasion on the head with minimal bleeding (+1). The paediatric trauma score for this patient is 7.

Summary

- Major causes of maxillofacial trauma are motor vehicle crashes, home accidents, athletic injuries, animal bites, intentional violent acts, and industrial injuries.
- With the exception of compromised airway and the potential for significant bleeding, damage to the tissues of the maxillofacial area is seldom life threatening. Blunt trauma injuries may be classified as fractures to the mandible, midface, zygoma, orbit and nose.
- Injury to the ears, eyes or teeth may be minor or may result in permanent sensory function loss and disfigurement. Trauma to the ear may include lacerations and contusions, thermal injuries, chemical injuries, traumatic perforation and barotitis. Evaluation of the eye should include a thorough history. Evaluation should also include measurement of visual acuity, pupillary reaction and extraocular movements.
- Anterior neck injuries may result in damage to the skeletal structures, vascular structures, nerves, muscles and glands of the neck.
- Injuries to the skull may be classified as soft tissue injuries to the scalp and skull fractures. Skull fractures may be classified as linear fractures, basilar fractures, depressed fractures and open vault fractures.
- The categories of brain injury include diffuse axonal injury (DAI) and focal injury. DAI may be mild (concussion), moderate, or severe. Focal injuries are specific, grossly observable brain lesions. Included in this category are lesions that result from skull fracture, contusion, oedema with associated increased ICP, ischaemia and haemorrhage.
- The prehospital management of a patient with head injuries is determined by a number of factors. One factor is the mechanism of injury. A second factor is the severity of injury. A third factor is the patient's level of consciousness. Associated injuries affect the priorities of care.
- Several injury rating systems are used to triage, guide patient care, predict patient outcome, identify changes in patient status, and evaluate trauma care. Rating systems commonly used in emergency care include the Glasgow Coma Scale, trauma score/Revised Trauma Score, and paediatric trauma score.

References

1. Kay A, Teasdale GM 2001 Head injury in the United Kingdom. World J Surg 25:1210–1220
2. Haug RH, Prather J, Indresano AT 1990 An epidemiologic survey of facial fractures and concomitant injuries. J Oral Maxillofac Surg 48:926
3. Ceallaigh PO, Ekanaykaee K, Beirne CJ, Patton DW 2006 Diagnosis and management of common maxillofacial injuries in the emergency department. Part 1: Advanced life support. Emerg Med J 23:796–797
4. The Information Centre. Hospital Episode Statistics Primary diagnosis: 3 character, 2007–08. Online. Available http://www.hesonline.nhs.uk/Ease/servlet/ContentServer?siteID=1937&categoryID=203 6 June 2009
5. American Association of Endodontists 1998 Treating the avulsed permanent tooth. American Association of Endodontists, Chicago
6. Roberts G, Scully C, Schotts R 2000 ABC of oral health: dental emergencies. BMJ 321:559–562
7. Rosen P, Barkin R 2003 Emergency medicine: concepts and clinical practice, 5th edition. Mosby, St Louis
8. US Department of Transportation, National Highway Traffic Safety Administration 1998 EMT-Paramedic national standard curriculum. US Department of Transportation, Washington, DC
9. Hickey J 1997 The clinical practice of neurological and neurosurgical nursing, 4th edition. Lippincott, Philadelphia
10. Cardona V, Hurn PD, Bastnagel Mason PJ, et al (eds) 1994 Trauma nursing: from resuscitation through rehabilitation, 2nd edition. WB Saunders, Philadelphia
11. Gabriel E, Ghajar J, Jagoda A, et al 2002 Guidelines for prehospital management of traumatic brain injury, Brain Trauma Foundation. J Neurotrauma 19:111–174
12. Joint Royal Colleges Ambulance Liaison Committee. UK Ambulance Service Clinical Guidelines v4. 2006. Online. Available http://jrcalc.org.uk/guidelines.html 17 February 2009
13. National Association of Emergency Medical Technicians 2003 PHTLS: basic and advanced prehospital trauma life support, 5th edition. Mosby, St Louis

CHAPTER 32

Spinal Trauma

Chapter contents

Objectives

Upon completion of this chapter, the paramedic student will be able to:

1. Describe the incidence, morbidity, and mortality related to spinal injury.
2. Predict mechanisms of injury that are likely to cause spinal injury.
3. Outline the general assessment of a patient with suspected spinal injury.
4. Distinguish between types of spinal injury.
5. Describe prehospital evaluation and assessment of spinal cord injury.
6. Identify prehospital management of the patient with spinal injuries.
7. Distinguish between spinal shock, neurogenic shock, and autonomic dysreflexia syndrome.
8. Describe selected non-traumatic spinal conditions and the prehospital assessment and treatment of them.

Key terms

anterior cord syndrome A spinal cord injury usually seen in flexion injuries; caused by pressure on the anterior aspect of the spinal cord by a ruptured intervertebral disc or fragments of the vertebral body extruded posteriorly into the spinal canal.

axial loading Vertical compression of the spine that results when direct forces are transmitted along the length of the spinal column.

Brown–Séquard syndrome A hemitransection of the spinal cord. In the classic presentation, pressure on half of the spinal cord results in weakness of the upper and lower extremities on the ipsilateral (same) side and loss of pain and temperature sensation on the contralateral (opposite) side.

central cord syndrome A spinal cord injury commonly seen with hyperextension or flexion cervical injuries; characterized by greater motor impairment of the upper than lower extremities.

distraction A spinal injury that occurs if the cervical spine is stopped suddenly while the weight and momentum of the body pull away from it.

neurogenic hypotension Hypotension following spinal shock; caused by a loss of sympathetic tone to the vessels.

spinal shock A temporary loss of all types of spinal cord function distal to a cord injury.

subluxation A partial dislocation.

transaction A complete or incomplete lesion to the spinal cord.

Between 600 and 700 people sustain acute traumatic injuries to the spinal cord in the UK each year.[1] Injury to the spinal cord remains unrecognized in 4–9% of injuries.[2,3] Inadequate management of patients presenting with spinal cord injury has the potential to cause neurological deterioration, further functional disability, and litigation. Education in injury prevention, prehospital assessment, and proper handling and transportation of these patients can decrease morbidity and mortality.

Spinal trauma: incidence, morbidity and mortality

Most spinal cord injuries (SCIs) in the UK result from falls (45.5%) and road traffic accidents (39.2%). The next largest cause is sporting injuries (10.2%).[4] The majority of people who sustain spinal cord injury are active and less than 40 years old, although an increase in the number falls in older people is changing this profile.[5] The incidence of SCI is highest in men between the ages of 16 and 30 years.

Critical Thinking

Why do you think this group is at increased risk for spinal injuries?

Forty per cent of trauma patients with neurological deficit will have a temporary or permanent SCI. In addition to the devastating emotional and psychological impact on victims and their families, the annual cost to society is immense. Injury prevention strategies can have a positive effect on incidence, morbidity, and mortality associated with spinal trauma.

Traditional spinal assessment criteria

Assessment of suspected SCIs has traditionally focused on mechanism of injury (MOI). Spinal immobilization was required for two specific patient groups: (1) unconscious injury victims and (2) any patient with a motion injury. This MOI standard covers all patients with a potential for spinal injury, yet the standard is not always practical in the prehospital setting. The accuracy of prehospital assessment can be strengthened by applying clear, clinical guidelines (clinical criteria) for evaluating SCI, which includes the following signs and symptoms:

- altered level of consciousness (Glasgow Coma Scale score less than 15)
- spinal pain or tenderness
- neurological deficit or complaint
- anatomical deformity of spine
- evidence of alcohol or other drugs
- distracting injury
- inability to communicate.

Mechanism of injury/nature of injury

When determining MOI in a patient who may have spinal trauma, the paramedic can classify the MOI as positive, negative or uncertain.[6] This method, combined with the clinical criteria for spinal injury listed previously, can help the paramedic identify situations in which spinal immobilization is appropriate. When in doubt, full spinal precautions should be used (Figure 32-1).[7]

Critical Thinking

What are the disadvantages of immobilizing a patient on a long spine board?

Positive mechanism of injury

In a positive MOI, the forces exerted on the patient are highly suggestive of SCI and always call for full spinal immobilization. Examples of positive MOIs include the following:

- high-speed motor vehicle crashes
- falls from greater than three times the patient's height
- violent situations occurring near the patient's spine (e.g. blunt and penetrating injuries)
- sports injuries
- other high-impact situations.

Negative mechanism of injury

A negative MOI includes events in which force or impact does not suggest a likely spinal injury. In the absence of SCI signs and symptoms, negative MOI injuries do not require spinal immobilization. Examples of negative MOIs include the following:

- dropping an object on the foot
- twisting an ankle while running
- isolated soft tissue injury.

Uncertain mechanism of injury

At times, the impact or force involved in the injury is unknown or uncertain. Thus, clinical criteria must be the basis used to determine the need for spinal immobilization (Box 32-1). Examples of uncertain MOIs include the following:

- tripping or falling to the ground and hitting the head
- falls from 1–3 m
- low-speed motor vehicle crashes (fender benders).

Assessment of uncertain mechanism of injury

When evaluating the need for spinal immobilization in which the MOI is uncertain, the paramedic must ensure that the patient is reliable. A reliable patient is one who is calm, cooperative, sober, alert, and oriented. The following are examples of patients who would be considered unreliable:

- those who have acute stress reactions from sudden stress of any type
- those who have brain injury
- those who are intoxicated
- those who have abnormal mental status
- those who have distracting injuries
- those who have problems communicating.

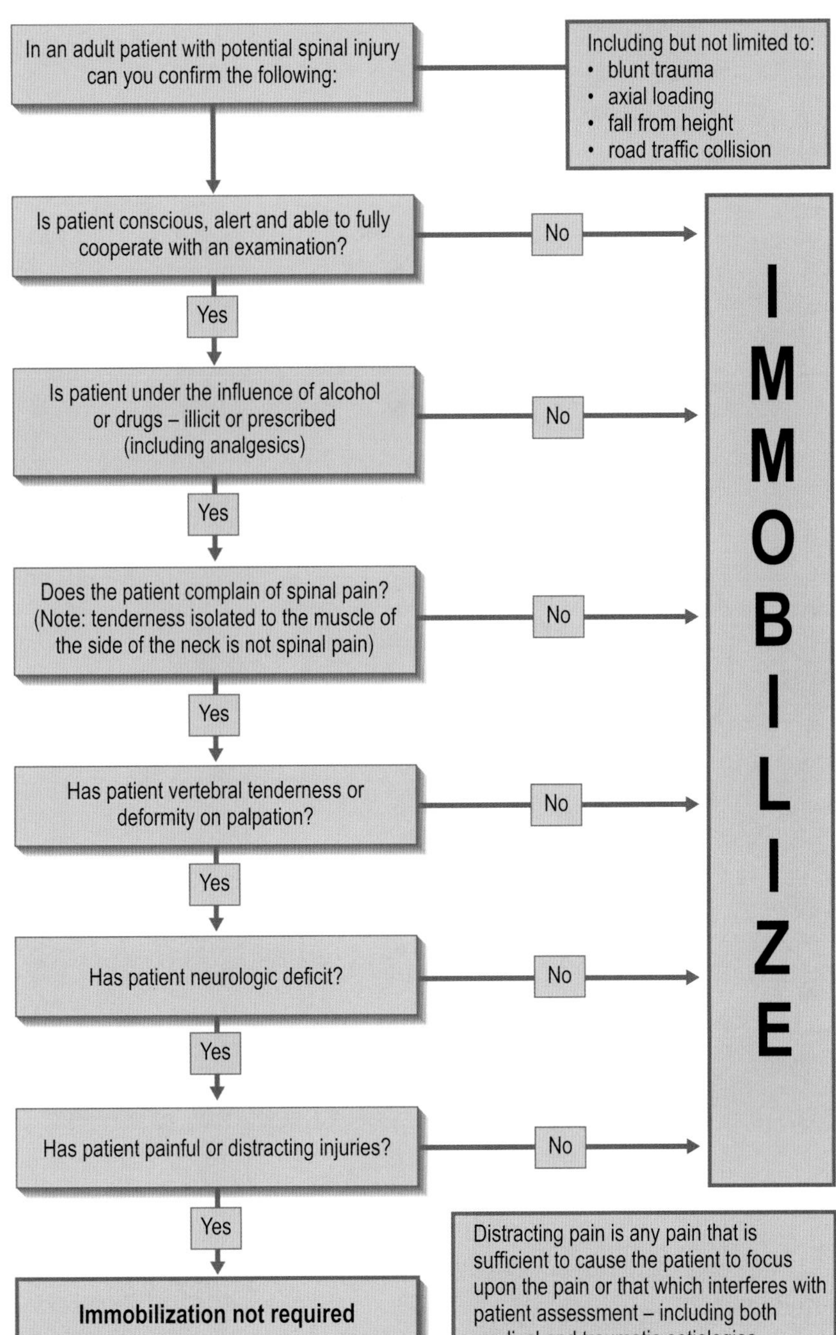

Figure 32-1 Indications for spinal immobilization. From the Joint Royal Colleges Ambulance Liaison Committee, UK Ambulance Service Guidelines, 2006.

Box 32-1

Clinical criteria versus mechanism of injury

Initial management is based solely on mechanism of injury.

Positive mechanism of injury requires spinal immobilization.

Negative mechanism of injury (without signs and symptoms) requires no spinal immobilization.

Uncertain mechanism of injury requires further clinical assessment and evaluation to determine need for spinal immobilization.

Critical Thinking

The reliability of a patient is not always easy to assess quickly in the prehospital setting. Why is this?

General assessment of spinal injury

Spinal injury most often results from the spine being forced beyond its normal range and limits of motion (Figure 32-2). The adult skull weighs 7–10 kg and sits on top of the first

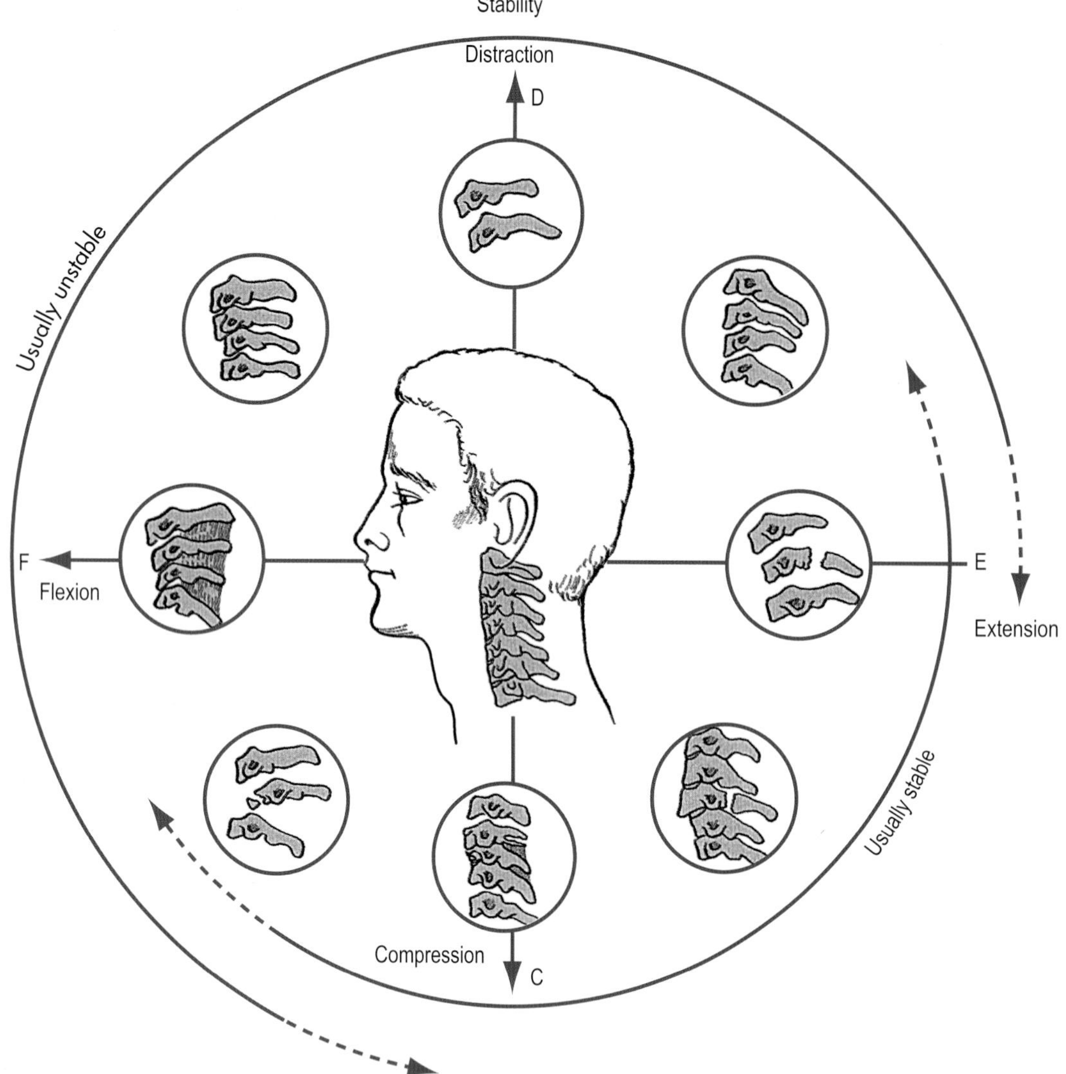

Figure 32-2 Mechanisms of cervical spine injury and fracture or dislocation. The mechanism of cervical injury (flexion versus extension) determines the type of cervical spine fracture or dislocation.

cervical vertebra (C1), or the atlas. The second cervical vertebra (C2), or the axis and its odontoid process, allow the head to move with about a 180-degree range of motion. Because of the weight and position of the head in relation to the thin neck and cervical vertebrae, the cervical spine is particularly susceptible to injury (27–33% of all SCIs occur in the C1 to C2 region).[8] Other spinal components that affect physiological limits of motion are the posterior neck muscles and the sacrum. The posterior neck muscles allow up to 60 degrees of flexion and 70 degrees of extension without stretching of the spinal cord. The sacrum is joined to the pelvis by immovable joints.

The specific MOIs that often cause spinal trauma are axial loading; extremes of flexion, hyperextension or hyper-rotation; excessive lateral bending; and distraction. These mechanisms may result in stable and unstable injuries depending upon the extent of damage to spinal structures and the relative strength of the structures remaining intact.

Axial loading

Axial loading (vertical compression) of the spine results when direct forces are sent down the length of the spinal column. Examples include striking the head against the windscreen of a car, shallow diving injuries, vertical falls, and being struck on the head or a helmet with a heavy object. These forces may produce compression fracture or a crushed vertebral body without SCI and most commonly occur from T12 to L2.[8]

Flexion, hyperextension and hyper-rotation

Extremes in flexion, hyperextension or hyper-rotation may result in fracture, ligament injury or muscle injury. Spinal cord injury is caused when one or more of the cervical vertebrae dislocate (subluxation) and are forced into the spinal canal. Examples of these motion extremes include rapid acceleration or deceleration forces from motor vehicle crashes, hangings, and midfacial skeletal or soft tissue trauma. Serious injuries are often the result of a combination of loading and rotational forces. These forces produce displacement or fracture of one or more vertebrae.

Lateral bending

Excessive lateral bending may result in dislocations and bony fractures to the cervical and thoracic spine. The injury occurs as a sudden lateral impact moves the torso sideways whilst initially the head tends to remain in place. The head is then pulled along by the cervical attachments. Examples of lateral bending include side or angular collisions from motor vehicle crashes and injuries from contact sports. The mechanism of this lateral force requires less movement to produce an injury than flexion or extension forces in frontal or rear impacts.

Distraction

Distraction may occur if the cervical spine is stopped suddenly while the weight and momentum of the body pull away from it. This force or stretching may result in tearing and laceration of the spinal cord. Examples of distraction include intentional or unintentional hangings (e.g. suicide or school yard or playground injuries).

Other mechanisms

Other less common mechanisms of spinal injury include blunt and penetrating trauma and electrical injury. The spinal cord, like the brain, may suffer concussions, contusions and lacerations. The spinal cord may develop haematomata and oedema in response to blunt trauma. Examples include spinal injuries that result from direct blows such as from falling tree limbs or other heavy objects.

Penetrating trauma to the spine may be caused by missile-type injuries or stab wounds to the neck, chest, or abdomen. These forces may result in laceration of the spinal cord or nerve roots over a wide area. At times, penetrating trauma may produce a complete transection (lesion). In addition, areas of oedema or contusion adjacent to the laceration may disrupt cord tissue.

Spinal trauma may occur from direct electrical injury or from violent muscle spasms that accompany electrical shock (described in Chapter 30).

Classifications of spinal injury

Spinal injuries may be classified as sprains and strains, fractures and dislocations, sacral and coccygeal fractures, and cord injuries. Regardless of the specific injury, all patients with suspected spinal trauma and signs and symptoms of SCI should be immobilized. Unnecessary movement should be avoided until injury to the spine or spinal cord can be excluded by clinical examination and radiography. An unstable spine can be ruled out only by radiography or lack of any potential mechanism for the injury. When deciding if a patient with potential spinal injury requires spinal immobilization, the paramedic should confirm the following:[9]

- The patient is conscious, alert and able to fully cooperate with examination.
- The patient is NOT under the influence of alcohol or drugs – illicit or prescribed (including analgesia).
- The patient has NO complaint of spinal pain (tenderness isolated to the muscles of the side of the neck is NOT spinal pain).
- The patient has neither vertebral tenderness nor deformity on palpation.
- The patient has NO neurological deficit.
- The patient has NO painful or distracting injuries – distracting pain is pain sufficient to cause the patient to focus upon that pain, or pain that interferes with patient assessment and can be traumatic or medical in origin.

If all of the above can be confirmed, then immobilization is not required.

Spinal injury (bony injury) can occur with or without SCI, but likewise, a patient may have SCI without bony injury. Spinal cord injury without radiological abnormality (SCIWORA) is a more common finding in children than in adults.

The damage produced by the injury forces can be further complicated by the patient's age (calcification from the ageing process), pre-existing bone diseases (osteoporosis, spondylosis, rheumatoid arthritis, Paget's disease), and congenital spinal cord anomalies (e.g. fusion or narrow spinal canal). Spinal cord neurons do not regenerate to any great extent, thus any injury to the central nervous system that causes destruction of tissue often results in irreparable damage and permanent loss of function. The role of the paramedic in protecting this critical area cannot be overemphasized.

Sprains and strains

Sprains and strains usually result from hyperflexion and hyperextension forces. A hyperflexion sprain occurs when the posterior ligamentous complex tears at least partially, which may also result in tears of the joint capsules. The sprain may allow partial dislocation (subluxation) of the intervertebral joints. Hyperextension strains are common in low-speed, rear-end car crashes and are commonly known as whiplash. Injury occurs as the person is thrown backwards against the posterior thorax during impact; this action damages anterior soft tissues of the neck.

Critical Thinking

How can the paramedic distinguish between cervical sprain/strain and spinal fracture in the prehospital setting?

With sprains and strains, local pain may be produced by spasms of the neck muscles and injury to the vertebrae, intervertebral discs and ligamentous structures. The pain is usually described as a non-radiating, aching soreness of the neck or back muscles. The discomfort often varies in intensity and with changes in posture.

On examination, a deformity of the spine may be palpable if dislocation (subluxation) has occurred. The patient may complain of associated point tenderness and swelling. Until the SCI is ruled out by X-ray examination, the paramedic should treat these patients as having unstable cervical spine injuries with a potential for damage to the spinal cord. After the diagnosis is confirmed, treatment of cervical sprain or strain is usually based on symptoms. Treatment may occasionally include a cervical collar to decrease neck movement, heat application, and analgesics.

Fractures and dislocations

The most frequently injured spinal regions in descending order are C5 to C7, C1 to C2, and T12 to L2.[8] Of these injuries, the most common are wedge-shaped compression fractures and teardrop fractures or dislocations. Neurological deficits associated with these fractures and dislocations vary with the location, and with the extent of injury. Although the spine and spinal cord are close to each other, the spine can be fractured without SCI and vice versa. In addition, spinal injuries at multiple levels are common.

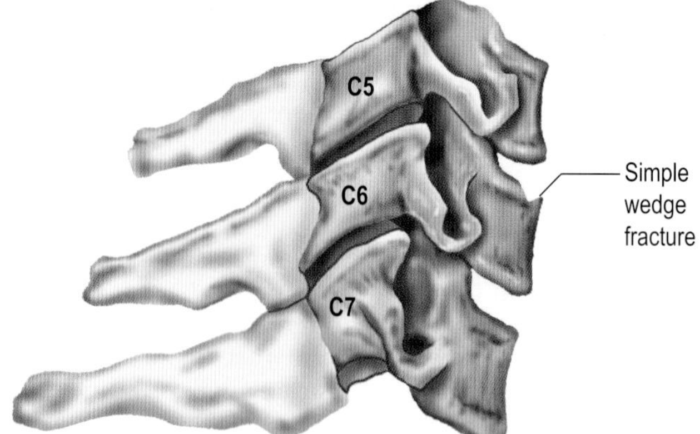

Figure 32-3 Lateral view of simple wedge fracture.

Critical Thinking

Look at an illustration of the spinal column. Why do you think these areas are susceptible to fractures?

Wedge-shaped fractures (Figure 32-3) are hyperflexion injuries that usually result from compressive force applied to the anterior portion of the vertebral body. This results in stretching of the posterior ligaments (these injuries often result from injuries and falls in industrial settings). These fractures usually occur in the mid or lower cervical segments or at T12 and L1; they generally are considered stable because the posterior ligaments are rarely disrupted totally.

Teardrop fractures and dislocations (Figure 32-4) are unstable injuries that result from a combination of severe hyperflexion and compression forces and are often seen in motor vehicle crashes. During impact, the vertebral body is fractured and the anterior–inferior corner of the vertebral body is pushed forward. Unlike simple wedge fractures, these fractures may be associated with neurological damage and are among the most unstable injuries of the spine. A number of other spinal injuries are associated with the mechanisms of flexion, extension, rotation and axial loading. Most of these are unstable and require careful immobilization.

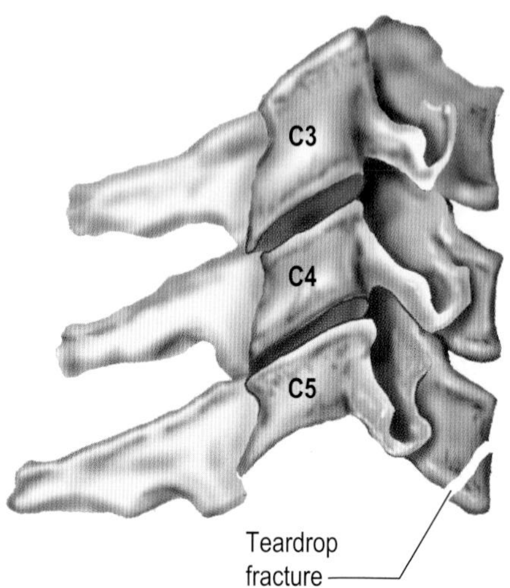

Figure 32-4 Lateral view of teardrop fracture.

Sacral and coccygeal fractures

The majority of serious spinal injuries occur in the cervical, thoracic, and lumbar regions. One reason for this is the location of the spinal cord and its termination in the adult spine at about L2. Another reason is the protection provided by the ring structure of the pelvis and the musculature of the buttocks and lower back. However, fractures through the foramina of S1 and S2 are fairly common and may compromise several sacral nerve elements. Such fractures may result in loss of perianal sensory motor function and may result in damage to the bladder and bladder sphincters.

The sacrococcygeal joint may also be injured as a result of direct blows and falls. Patients often complain that they have 'broken their tailbone' and often experience moderate pain from the mobile coccyx. Diagnosis is usually confirmed by a physician through a rectal examination.

Cord injuries

Spinal cord injuries may be classified further as primary and secondary injuries. Primary injuries occur at the time of impact, secondary injuries occur after the initial injury. This type of injury can include swelling, ischaemia, and movement of bony fragments. Like other tissues, the spinal cord can be concussed, contused, compressed and lacerated. All of these mechanisms can cause temporary or permanent loss of cord-mediated functions distal to the injury from compression or ischaemia. Bleeding from damaged blood vessels can also occur in the tissue of the spinal cord and may cause obstruction to spinal blood supply. The severity of these injuries depends on the amount and type of force that produced them and the duration of the injury.

Cord lesions

Lesions (transections) to the spinal cord are classified as complete or incomplete. Complete lesions are usually associated with spinal fracture or dislocation. Patients have total absence of pain, pressure and joint sensation accompanied with complete motor paralysis below the level of injury. Autonomic nervous system dysfunction may be associated with complete cord lesions depending upon the level of cord involvement. Manifestations of autonomic dysfunction include the following:

- bradycardia caused by loss of sympathetic autonomic activity
- hypotension caused by loss of vasomotor control and peripheral vascular resistance
- priapism
- loss of sweating and shivering
- poikilothermy (body temperature varying with ambient temperature)
- loss of bowel and bladder control.

Critical Thinking

Why should you immobilize a patient who already is showing signs and symptoms of a complete cord lesion?

The paramedic should be familiar with signs and symptoms of several incomplete spinal cord syndromes. Knowledge of these rare syndromes helps the practitioner understand the MOI and helps the paramedic to understand the potential for further injury. The three syndromes indicating incomplete lesions of the spinal cord are as follows:

1. *Central cord syndrome*: Central cord syndrome commonly occurs with hyperextension or flexion cervical injuries. The syndrome is characterized by greater motor impairment of the upper than lower extremities. Signs and symptoms of central cord syndrome are as follows:
   - paralysis of the arms
   - sacral sparing (the preservation of sensory or voluntary motor function of the perineum, buttocks, scrotum, or anus).
2. *Anterior cord syndrome*: Anterior cord syndrome is usually seen in flexion injuries. The syndrome is caused by pressure on the anterior aspect of the spinal cord by a ruptured intervertebral disc or fragments of the vertebral body forced posteriorly into the spinal canal. Signs and symptoms include the following:
   - decreased sensation of pain and temperature below the level of the lesion (including lesions of the sacral region)
   - intact light touch and position sensation
   - paralysis.
3. *Brown–Séquard syndrome*: Brown–Séquard syndrome is a hemitransection of the spinal cord. This syndrome may result from a ruptured intervertebral disc or the pushing of a fragment of vertebral body on the spinal cord. This often occurs after knife or missile injuries and, in the classic presentation, pressure on half of the spinal cord results in weakness of the upper and lower extremities on the ipsilateral (same) side. Pressure also results in loss of pain and temperature sensation on the contralateral (opposite) side.

Pharmacological therapy for incomplete cord injury

The benefits of pharmacological agents (glucocorticoids, naloxone, calcium channel blockers, GM-1 gangliosides and others) in the management of incomplete cord injury are controversial. These drugs are thought to provide some type of damage control following some SCIs. Some of the drugs are thought to work by reducing the toxicity of excitatory amino acids that cause cells to die; others, by encouraging the growth of new neurons or by reducing inflammation of the injured spinal cord and the bursting open of damaged cells.[6] Of these, only methylprednisolone is currently used routinely for human victims of SCI.[10]

Methylprednisolone is a synthetic steroid that reduces post-traumatic spinal cord oedema and inflammation and is routinely used in victims of SCI. Studies have found that patients treated with this drug within 8 h of injury show significant neurological improvement at 6 weeks compared with patients who were treated with a placebo.[9] There is currently no indication for the use of these drugs by paramedics in the UK.

Evaluation and assessment of spinal cord injury

Spinal cord trauma should be evaluated only after all injuries that pose a threat to life have been assessed and treated. As with any scenario of serious illness or injury, the paramedic's first priority must be scene survey (including ensuring personal safety) and assessment of the patient's airway, breathing, and circulation. The second priority is to preserve spinal cord function and avoid secondary injury to the spinal cord.

The primary injury to the spine occurs at impact, thus the critical role of paramedics is to prevent secondary injury. A secondary injury could result from unnecessary movement of an unstable spinal column, hypoxaemia, oedema or shock (which may reduce perfusion of the injured cord). These goals are best met by maintaining a high degree of suspicion for the presence of spinal trauma (based on scene survey, kinematics and history of the event), providing early spinal immobilization, and rapidly correcting any volume deficit through fluid replacement, and oxygen administration.

After any life-threatening problems found in the initial assessment have been treated, the paramedic should perform a neurological examination. This examination may be done in the field or en route to hospital if the patient's condition requires rapid transport. Any movement of the patient for performing a general or neurological examination must be accompanied by continuous, manual protection and in-line stabilization of the spine. Once the spine is stabilized, the paramedic should palpate the entire spine. Any report of pain on palpation indicates the need to immobilize the spine. Full documentation of the paramedic's findings provides an important baseline and will be useful for further assessment and evaluation of the patient in the emergency department. The components of the neurological examination include evaluation of motor and sensory findings and reflex responses.

Motor findings

The paramedic should question conscious patients about pain in the neck or back with and without palpation. The paramedic should also ask patients about their ability to move their arms and legs. If possible, the paramedic should test the strength and motion of all four extremities by asking the patient to flex the elbows (biceps, C6), extend the elbows (triceps, C7), and abduct/adduct the fingers (C8, T1). In unconscious patients, painful stimuli in the hands and lower extremities may initiate an involuntary muscle reflex unless the patient is in profound coma.

Upper extremity neurological function assessment

To test interosseous muscle function (controlled by T1 nerve roots), the paramedic should instruct the patient to spread the fingers of both hands. Instruct the patient to keep the fingers apart while the paramedic squeezes the second and fourth fingers. Normal resistance should be spring-like and equal on both sides.

To test the extensors of the hands and fingers (controlled by C7 nerve roots), the paramedic should instruct the patient to hold his or her wrists or fingers straight out and to keep them out while the paramedic presses down on the fingers. (The arm should be supported at the wrist to avoid testing arm function and other nerve roots.) The paramedic should feel moderate resistance with moderate pressure. Both sides of the patient should be evaluated if not contraindicated by injury.

Lower extremity neurological function assessment

To test plantar flexors of the foot (controlled by S1 and S2 nerve roots), the paramedic should place his or her hands at the sole of each foot and instruct the patient to push against the hands. Both sides should feel equal and strong.

To test dorsal flexors of the foot and great toe (controlled by L5 nerve roots), the paramedic should hold the patient's foot (with fingers on toes) and instruct the patient to pull the feet back or toward the nose; both sides should feel equal and strong.

Sensory findings

In conscious patients, sensory examination should be performed with light touch on each hand and each foot (while the patient's eyes are closed) to evaluate the ability to feel this type of stimuli (light touch is carried by more than one nerve tract). Sensation should be equal on both sides. The paramedic should also question the patient about weakness, numbness, paraesthesia or radicular pain (shooting pain that travels along a nerve).

If the patient cannot feel light touch or is unconscious, the paramedic may evaluate sensation by gently pricking the hands and soles of the feet. A sharp object that will not penetrate the skin is useful, for example, the end of a pen or broken cotton-tipped applicator can be used. One method of evaluation moves from head to toe; recording the level at which sensation stops or the unconscious patient ceases to respond to a painful stimulus by marking that location on the patient's skin with ink or a marker. Remember, it is best practice to gain consent before marking on a patient's skin. Another method is to begin the sensory assessment by moving from an area of no sensation to an area where sensation begins. The paramedic would note the area where sensation begins with ink or marker (these marks make it possible to compare sensory level accurately after repeated examinations). Lack of response to stimulation in the upper extremities indicates cord damage in the cervical region; failure of only the lower extremities to respond indicates cord injury in the thoracic region, lumbar regions, or both.

Critical Thinking

How will you respond to the patient who fearfully asks you, 'Why can't I move or feel my arms or legs?'

Dermatomes correspond to spinal nerves (Table 32-1), so the following four landmarks may be useful for a quick sensory evaluation in the prehospital setting:[6]

1. C2 to C4 dermatomes provide a collar of sensation around the neck and over the anterior chest to below the clavicles.
2. T4 dermatome provides sensation to the nipple line.
3. T10 dermatome provides sensation to the umbilicus.
4. S1 dermatome provides sensation to the soles of the feet.

Reflex responses

Reflex responses are seldom evaluated in the prehospital setting. However, some abnormal responses are observed easily and may indicate autonomic nerve injury. These responses include loss of temperature control, hypotension, bradycardia, priapism and a pathological reflex called Babinski's sign (the plantar reflex). This is a reflex movement in which the great toe bends upward when the outer edge of the sole of the foot is scratched (Figure 32-5). Babinski's sign (which may indicate a spinal cord lesion in the older child or adult) is a normal and expected response in children under 2 years of age.

Other methods of evaluation

A visual inspection of the spine may reveal the presence of injury and its level; for example, transection of the cord

Table 32-1 Common nerve root and motor/sensory correlation

Nerve root	Motor	Sensory
C3, C4	Trapezius (shoulder shrug)	Top of shoulder
C3 to C5	Diaphragm	Top of shoulder
C5, C6	Biceps (elbow flexion)	Thumb
C7	Triceps (elbow extension) Wrist/finger extension	Middle finger
C8, T1	Finger abduction/little finger adduction	Little finger
T4	Nipple	
T10	Umbilicus	
L1, L2	Hip flexion	Inguinal crease
L3, L4	Quadriceps	Medial thigh/calf
L5	Great toe/foot dorsiflexion	Lateral calf
S1	Knee flexion	Lateral foot
S1, S2	Foot plantar flexion	
S2 to S4	Anal sphincter tone	Perianal

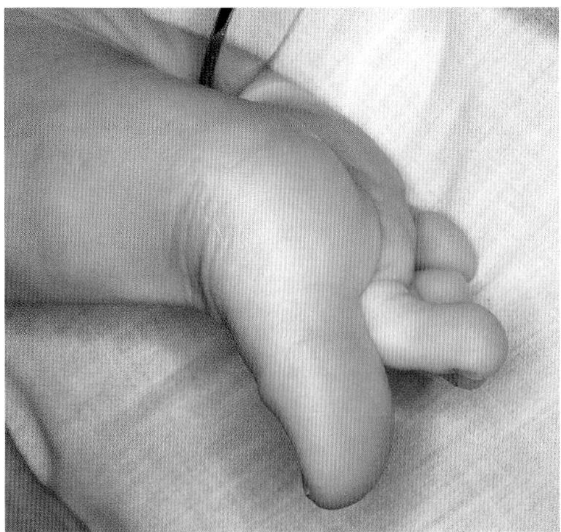

Figure 32-5 Babinski's sign: dorsiflexion of the great toe with or without fanning of the toes.

above C3 results in respiratory arrest. Lesions that occur at C4 may result in paralysis of the diaphragm although transections that occur at C5 to C6 usually spare the diaphragm, allowing diaphragmatic breathing. This occurs because the intercostal muscles are innervated sequentially between T1 and T11. As a result, intercostal muscle groups may be paralysed with cervical or thoracic spinal cord lesions below the level where diaphragmatic nerves are located (the higher the lesion, the greater the loss of intercostal muscle function).

The patient's body position may also offer clues about neurological injury; for example, a patient with a SCI at C6 may lie with the arms flexed at the elbows and wrists (the 'hold-up' position).

General management of spinal injuries

A significant spinal injury may be present even though the patient may show no signs of spinal injury. More than 50% of patients with cervical spinal injuries have normal responses to motor, sensory and reflex examinations,[10] thus if the paramedic suspects a spinal injury for any reason, the paramedic must protect the patient's spine. An estimated 15% of secondary SCIs are preventable with proper immobilization.[6] In addition, the patient's ability to walk does not rule out the need for spinal precautions. As previously stated, an unstable spine can be ruled out only by clinical examination, radiography, and the lack of any potential mechanism for spinal injury. General principles of spinal immobilization include the following:

1. The primary goal is to prevent further injury.
2. The spine should be treated as a long bone with a joint at either end (the head and pelvis).
3. The paramedic should always use complete spinal immobilization. (Splinting and isolation of a specific injury site is impossible. Having spine fractures in more than one location is common.)
4. Spinal immobilization begins in the initial assessment and must be maintained until the spine is immobilized completely on a suitable immobilization device.
5. The patient's head and neck must be placed in a neutral, in-line position unless contraindicated by condition or MOI. Neutral positioning allows for the most space for the spinal cord, thereby reducing cord hypoxia and excess pressure.

Spinal stabilization/immobilization techniques

As soon as a potential spine injury is recognized, the paramedic should manually protect the patient's head and neck. The basic principle to follow is that the head and neck must be maintained in line with the long axis of the body. If other injuries need treatment, the paramedic must maintain the patient's head and neck position without interruption.

A number of devices for immobilizing the spinal column are designed for prehospital use. When properly applied to patients who are sitting, standing or lying, these devices can provide adequate spinal protection. However, no device should be considered for use until the head and neck have been stabilized with manual in-line immobilization.

Note

All spinal immobilization techniques discussed in this text follow the guidelines recommended by the Prehospital Trauma Life Support Committee of the National Association of emergency medical technicians in cooperation with the Committee on Trauma of the American College of Surgeons.[9]

Manual in-line immobilization

Manual in-line immobilization can be done from almost any patient position and should be applied without traction to the head. Only enough tension should be applied to relieve the weight of the head from the cervical spine. After manual immobilization has been initiated, it must be continued until the head and spine are immobilized to a proper device (short spine board or vest, long spine board or vacuum mattress).

Contraindications for moving the patient's head to an in-line position follow. If any of these contraindications exist, all manual movement of the patient's head should stop at that point, and the head and neck should be stabilized in the position found. Contraindications include the following:

- resistance to movement
- neck muscle spasm
- increased pain
- the presence or increase in neurological deficits during movement (e.g. numbness, tingling, and loss of motor function)
- compromise of the airway or ventilation
- severe misalignment of the head away from the midline of the shoulders and body axis (rare).

Manual immobilization from the sitting or standing patient's side

1. Stand alongside the patient, holding the back of the head with one hand. Place the thumb and first finger of the other hand on each cheek, just below the zygomatic arch (Figure 32-6).

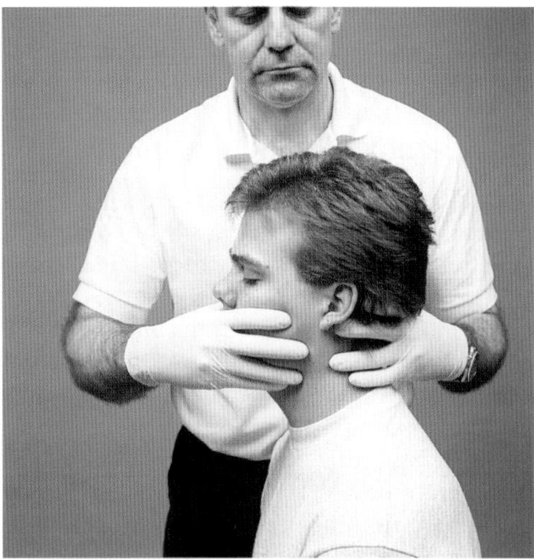

Figure 32-6 Manual in-line immobilization from the side.

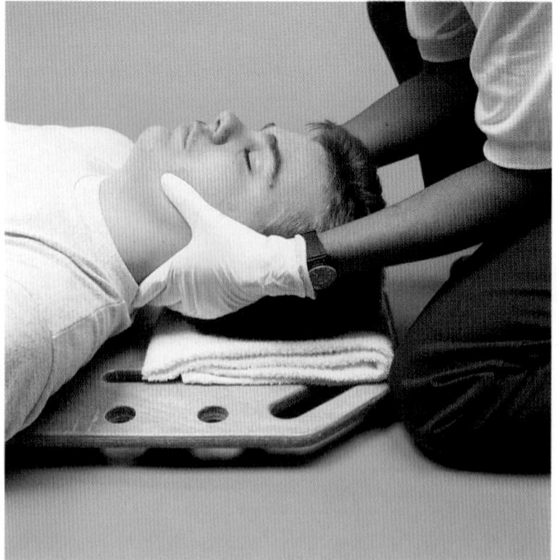

Figure 32-8 Manual in-line immobilization with a supine patient.

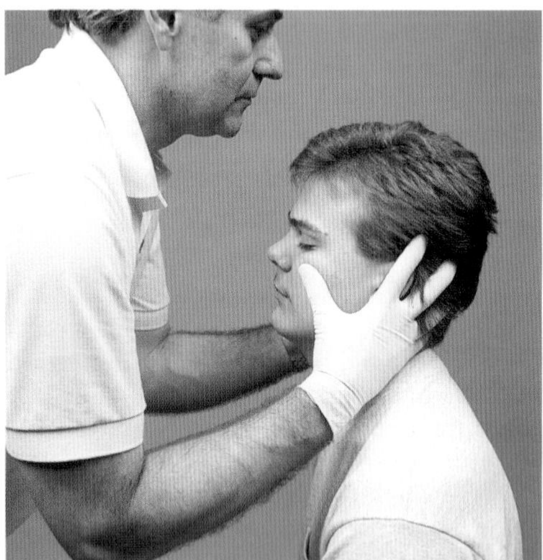

Figure 32-7 Manual in-line immobilization from the front.

2. Tighten the position of both hands without moving the head or neck.
3. Move the head to an in-line position if needed. Maintain this position by bracing the elbows against your torso for support.

Manual in-line immobilization from the front of the sitting or standing patient

1. Stand in front of the patient and place the thumb of each hand on the patient's cheeks, just below the zygomatic arch.
2. Place the little fingers of each hand on the posterior aspect of the patient's skull.
3. Spread the remaining fingers of each hand on the lateral planes of the head and increase the strength of the grip (Figure 32-7).
4. Move the head to an in-line position if needed. Maintain this position by bracing the elbows against your torso for support.

Manual in-line immobilization with a supine patient

1. Kneel or lie at the patient's head and place the thumbs of each hand just below the zygomatic arch of each cheek (Figure 32-8).
2. Place the little fingers of each hand on the posterior aspect of the patient's skull.
3. Spread the remaining fingers of each hand on the lateral planes of the head and increase the strength of the grip.
4. Move the head to an in-line position if needed. Maintain this position by bracing the elbows against your torso or ground surface for support.

Logroll with spinal precautions

Logrolling methods are used to move patients with a possible spinal injury although they are not recommended for use when moving supine patients onto a mechanical immobilization device – consider an orthopaedic stretcher to assist the move. It may be indicated for turning patients from a prone to a supine position, or for airway management in a potential spinal injury where the airway is at risk from profuse vomiting that cannot be controlled by suction. Logrolling from supine has been included for completeness as it may sometimes be necessary. Logrolling manoeuvres require at least four rescuers in order to provide adequate spinal protection. The position of the patient's arms during a logrolling manoeuvre may affect thoracic-lumbar motion and further compromise the stability of the spine. One method that may minimize lateral motion and help to maintain neutral alignment of the pelvis and legs is to position the patient with arms extended at the side. The patient's palms should be on the lateral thighs.

Logroll of the supine patient

The following steps should be used for logrolling of patients in the supine position (Figure 32-9a–c).

1. Rescuer 1 should be positioned at the patient's head. Rescuer 1 should provide in-line manual stabilization. Another rescuer should apply a rigid cervical collar and place a long spine board at the patient's side.

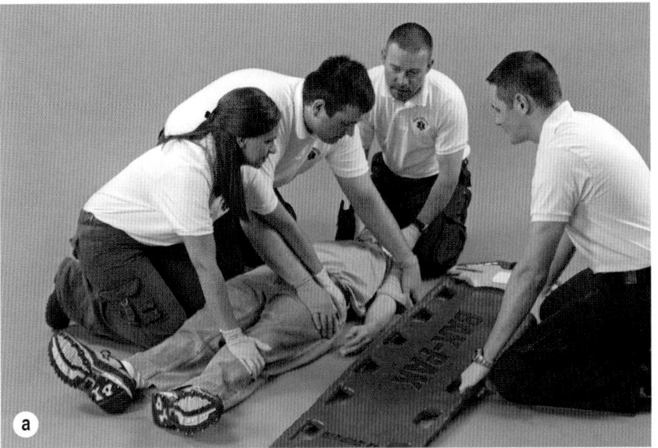

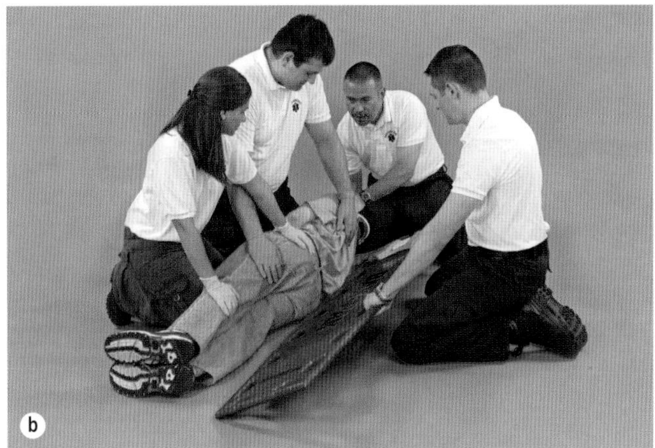

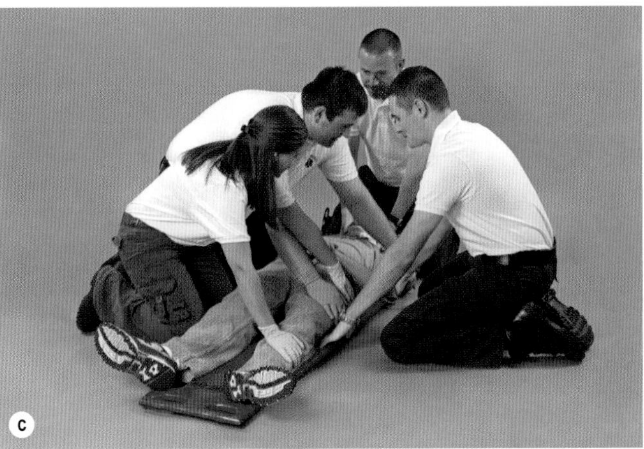

Figure 32-9 (a) To logroll a supine patient, Rescuer 1 is positioned at the patient's head, providing in-line manual stabilization. Rescuers 2 and 3 are positioned at the patient's midthorax and knees. (b) While maintaining immobilization, the rescuers slowly logroll the patient onto his or her side perpendicular to the ground in one organized move. Rescuer 4 positions the long spine board by placing the device flat on the ground or at a 30- to 40-degree angle against the patient's back. (c) In one organized move, the rescuers slowly logroll and centre the patient onto the long spine board.

2. Rescuers 2 and 3 should be positioned at the patient's midthorax and knees. The patient's arms should be extended at the sides, palms on lateral thighs. The legs should be brought together for neutral alignment.
3. Rescuer 2 grasps the far side of the patient at the shoulder and wrist. Rescuer 3 grasps the hips (just distal of the wrists) and both lower extremities at the ankles.
4. In one organized move, the rescuers slowly logroll the patient onto his or her side. At the same time, they slide the long board under the patient. In-line support of the patient's head must be maintained; this is achieved by rotating the head exactly with the torso to avoid flexion or hyperextension. In addition, the ankles must be elevated slightly to maintain lateral and anterior-posterior alignment.
5. Rescuer 4 positions the long board by placing the device flat on the ground or at a 30- to 40-degree angle against the patient's back.
6. In one organized move, the rescuers slowly logroll and centre the patient on the long spine board.

Logroll of the prone patient

The basic principles used in logrolling supine patients can be applied to a patient who is in a prone or semi-prone position. The procedure uses the same initial alignment of the patient's arms and legs. The rescuers have the same responsibilities for maintaining alignment. There are two major differences in this logroll manoeuvre. These are Rescuer 1's hand position during the logroll and the application of the rigid cervical collar, which can be applied only after the patient is in a supine position (Figure 32-10a–d).

1. Rescuer 1 places his or her hands in a position that provides in-line stabilization and that accommodates rotation of the patient with the torso.
2. In one organized move, the rescuers rotate the patient away from the direction of the initial prone position.
3. A rescuer places the long board on a flat surface or positions it between the patient's back and the rescuers at the patient's side.
4. In one organized move, the rescuers slowly logroll and centre the patient on the long spine board.
5. A rescuer applies a rigid cervical collar.

Mechanical devices

Spinal immobilization equipment covered includes rigid cervical collars, short spine boards, and long boards. This text presents only general principles of spinal immobilization by mechanical devices. The specific methods of applica-

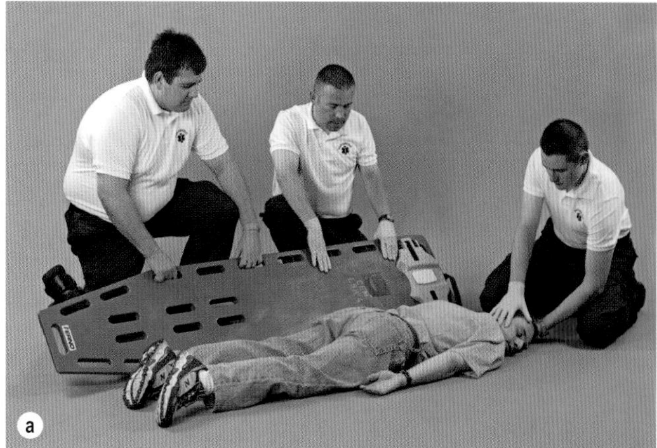
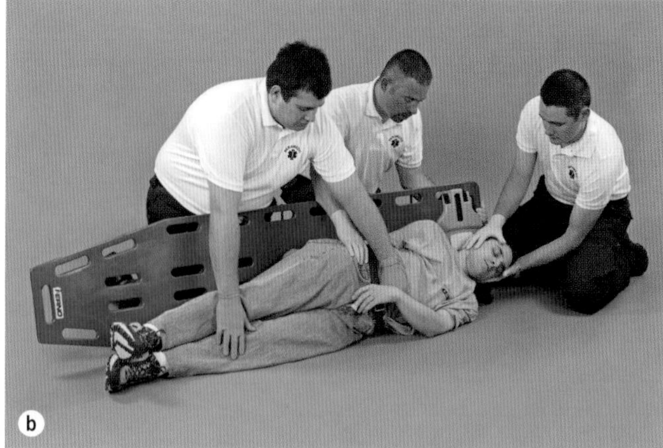
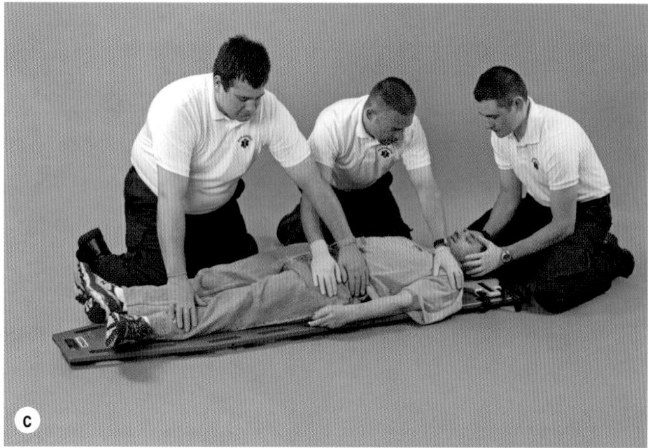
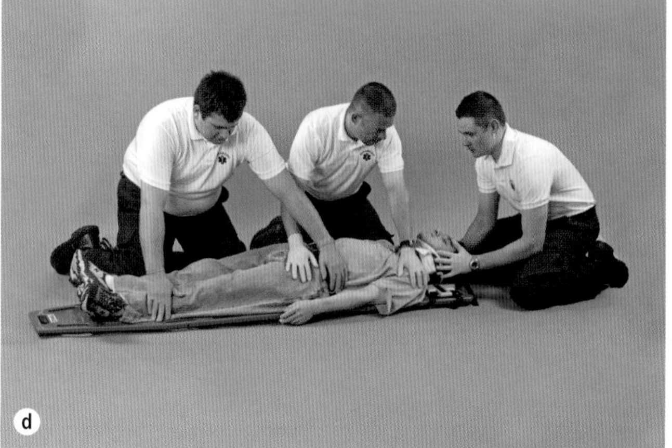

Figure 32-10 (a) Rescuer 1 places his or her hands in a position that provides in-line stabilization and that accommodates the rotation of the patient with the torso. Rescuer 2 positions the long spine board. (b) In one organized move, the rescuers rotate the patient away from the direction of his or her initial prone position. (c) In one organized move, the rescuers slowly logroll and centre the patient onto the long spine board. (d) Another rescuer then applies a rigid cervical collar.

tion vary by device; paramedics should become familiar with the equipment used in their locale and should follow the application guidelines of the manufacturer.

Rigid cervical collars

Rigid cervical collars are designed to protect the cervical spine from compression. These devices may reduce movement and some range of motion of the head but they do not provide adequate immobilization of the spine by themselves. These devices must always be used along with manual in-line stabilization or immobilization by a suitable device. To apply a rigid cervical collar, the paramedic should follow these general steps, which demonstrate the application of the Stifneck collar (Figure 32-11):

1. Rescuer 1 applies manual in-line immobilization from behind the patient and maintains this position throughout the procedure.
2. Rescuer 2 properly angles the collar for placement.
3. Rescuer 2 positions the collar bottom.
4. Rescuer 2 sets the collar in place around the patient's neck.
5. Rescuer 2 secures the collar with the Velcro straps.
6. Rescuer 1 spreads his or her fingers and maintains support until the patient is secured to a short or long spine board.

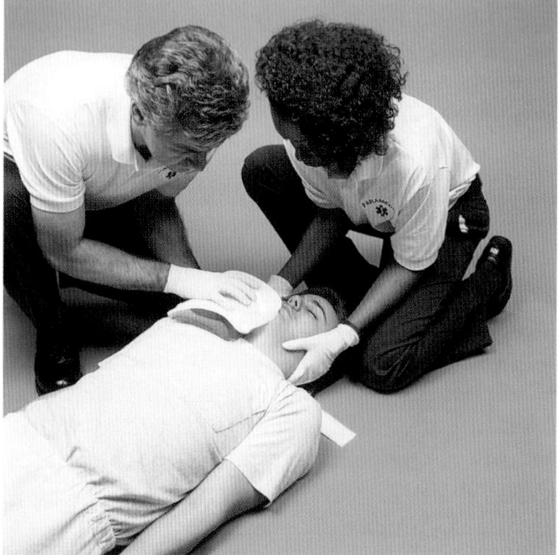

Figure 32-11 Rescuer 2 positions the collar and secures it with Velcro straps.

Rigid cervical collars come in a number of sizes (or they are adjustable) to accommodate the range of physical characteristics of patients. Choosing the proper size reduces flexion or hyperextension of the neck. The following guidelines apply to the use of rigid cervical collars:

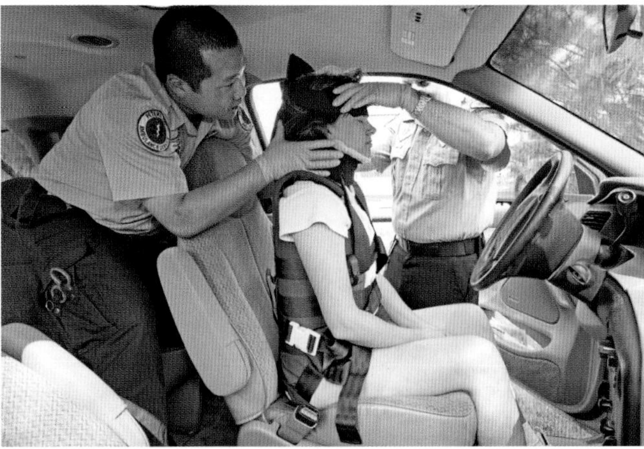

Figure 32-12 Application of the Kendrick extrication device.

- Rigid cervical collars must not inhibit the patient's ability to open the mouth nor must they inhibit the patient's ability to clear her or his airway in case vomiting occurs.
- Rigid cervical collars must not obstruct airway passages or hinder ventilation.
- Rigid cervical collars should be applied only after the head has been brought into a neutral in-line position.

Short spine boards

Short spine boards or other short spine extrication devices are used to splint the cervical and thoracic spine. They are available from a number of manufacturers and vary in design. In general, short spine boards are used to provide spinal immobilization when the patient is sitting or is in a confined space, and may be useful where other conditions preclude placing the patient in a supine position, e.g. respiratory compromise. After short spine board immobilization, the patient may be moved to a long board device for complete spinal immobilization. Examples of short spine boards include the plastic or synthetic half backboard, the Kendrick extrication device, the Oregon Spine Splint II, and the Hare extrication device. General principles of short spine board application, demonstrated with the Kendrick extrication device, are as follows (Figure 32-12):

Critical Thinking

When would the use of the short board not be indicated for spinal column immobilization?

1. After manual in-line immobilization and the application of a rigid cervical collar, place the short spine board device behind the patient. The board should be positioned snugly beneath the patient's axillae to prevent it from moving up the torso.
2. Immobilize the upper and middle torso by fastening the upper, middle, and lower chest straps. The upper strap can be relatively tight without impairing chest excursion. The middle and lower straps should be snug so that fingers cannot be slipped beneath the straps. Readjust as needed.
3. Position and fasten each groin strap separately, forming a loop. These straps prevent the Kendrick extrication device from moving up and the lower end from moving laterally.
4. Pad the device as needed and secure the head to the short spine board.
5. Carefully move the patient as a unit to a long board by rotating the patient and Kendrick extrication device onto the board. Hold the legs proximal to the knees and lift them during the transition.
6. Centre the patient on the long board, release the leg straps, and slowly lower the patient's legs to an in-line position.
7. Secure the patient and Kendrick extrication device to the long spine board, maintaining a neutral in-line position with the long axis of the body. Then slightly loosen the Kendrick extrication device chest straps.

Note

The use of a short spine board should be considered only if the patient's condition allows. If the patient is unstable because of life-threatening injury, the need for immediate resuscitation, or if the time required to apply the device would jeopardize the patient's life (e.g. a patient with a carotid pulse but absent radial pulse), the patient's head and neck should be stabilized with manual, in-line support, and the patient should be moved as a unit to a long spine board.

Rapid extrication

The steps required for rapid extrication may vary depending on the size and make of the vehicle. They may also vary based on the patient's location inside the vehicle. A general description of the steps required for rapid extrication are listed:

Three or more rescuers (Figure 32-13)

1. Rescuer 1 supports the patient's head and neck. Rescuer 1 uses manual in-line stabilization from behind the patient or from the patient's side. Rescuer 1 maintains this stabilization throughout the extrication process.
2. After a rapid initial assessment, Rescuer 2 applies a rigid cervical collar and positions a long board near the vehicle.
3. Rescuer 3 manually stabilizes and controls movement of the patient's upper and lower torso and legs during extrication.
4. The rescuers then rotate the patient in a series of short, controlled movements so that the patient's back faces the open doorway. Rescuer 2 exits the vehicle and assumes control of manual stabilization from outside the vehicle. Rescuer 1 assumes control of the patient's lower torso and legs. Each movement during the rotation of the patient should be coordinated, stopping so that the rescuers and the patient can be repositioned as needed to limit unwanted patient movement.
5. A rescuer should insert the foot end of the long board on the car seat at the patient's buttocks and should

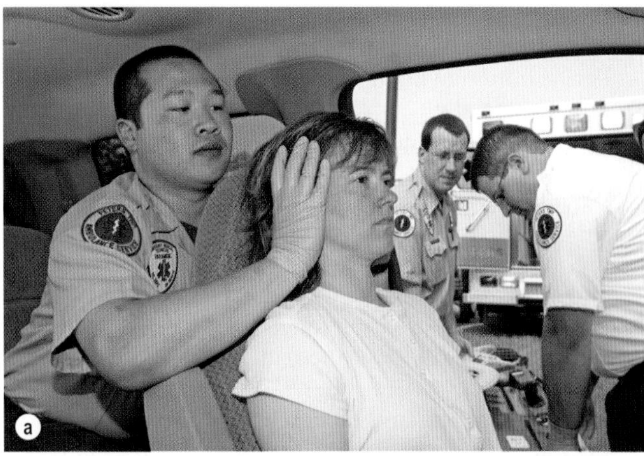

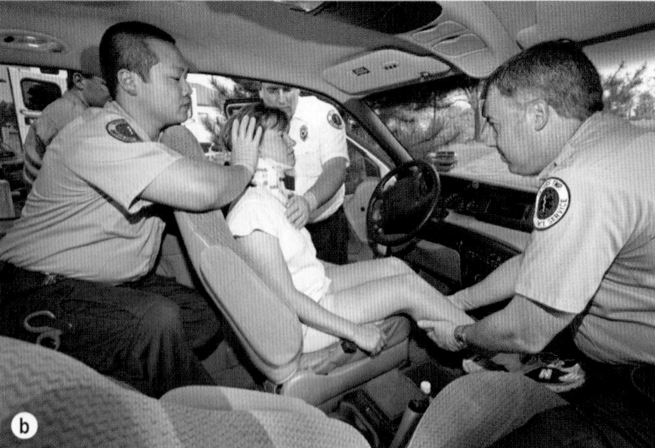

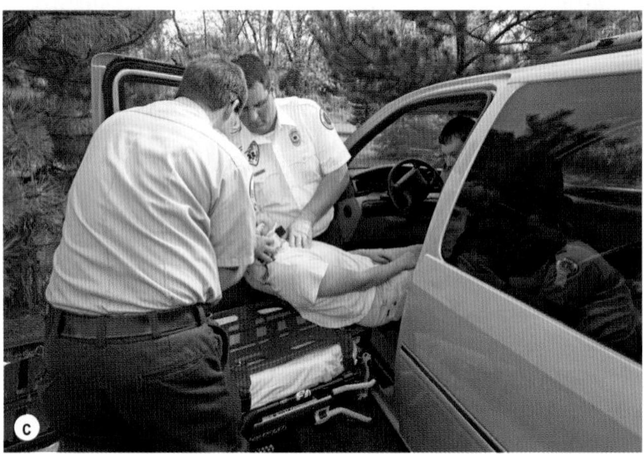

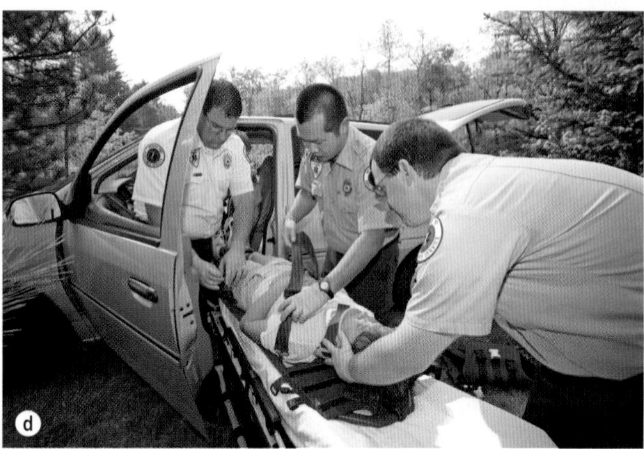

Figure 32-13 (a) Rescuer 1 supports the patient's head and neck and uses manual in-line stabilization throughout the procedure. (b) After a rapid primary assessment, Rescuer 2 helps support the patient's midthorax as Rescuer 3 frees the patient's lower extremities for extrication. (c) The rescuers carefully lower the patient onto the long spine board. (d) The rescuers centre and secure the patient on the long spine board.

position the head end on the ambulance stretcher. Rotation of the patient continues until the patient can be positioned onto the long board.

6. The rescuers centre and secure the patient on the long board as described later.

Two rescuers (Figure 32-14)

1. Rescuer 1 supports the patient's head and neck. Rescuer 1 uses manual in-line stabilization from behind the patient or from the patient's side and maintains this stabilization throughout the extrication process.
2. After a rapid initial assessment, Rescuer 2 applies a rigid cervical collar and places a pre-rolled blanket around the patient. Rescuer 2 places the centre of the blanket roll at the patient's midline on the rigid cervical collar. Rescuer 2 then wraps the ends of the blanket roll around the cervical collar and places them under the patient's arms. Rescuer 2 positions a long spine board near the vehicle.
3. Using the ends of the blanket roll, the rescuers rotate the patient in a series of short, controlled movements so that the patient's back faces the open doorway. Each movement during the rotation of the patient should be coordinated, stopping so that the rescuers and the patient can be repositioned as needed to limit unwanted patient movement.
4. Rescuer 1 takes control of the blanket ends, moving them under the patient's shoulders, and moves the patient by the blanket while Rescuer 2 controls the patient's lower torso, pelvis, and legs.
5. The rescuers centre and secure the patient on the long board as described next.

Long board with supine patient Like short spine boards, long boards are available in a variety of configurations. These include plastic and synthetic spine boards, metal alloy spine boards, vacuum mattress splints and scoop stretchers that must be used along with a long board. The following description of securing patients on a long board may be applied to any long spinal immobilization device.

Immobilization of the torso to a long board must be done before immobilization of the head; this will prevent angulation of the cervical spine. The torso must not be allowed to move up, down, or to either side. Straps should be placed at the shoulders or chest to avoid compression and lateral movement of the thorax, around the mid-torso, and across the iliac crest to prevent movement of the lower torso. The paramedic should take care not to tighten the straps to the point of reducing chest wall movement.

After immobilization of the torso, the head and neck should be immobilized in a neutral, in-line position. When most adults are placed on a long or short spinal device, a

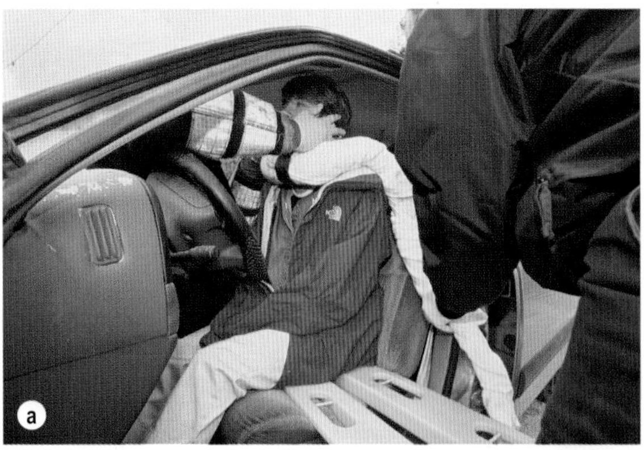
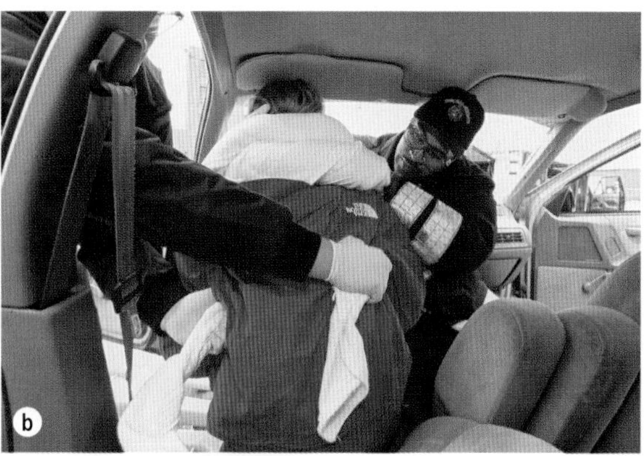
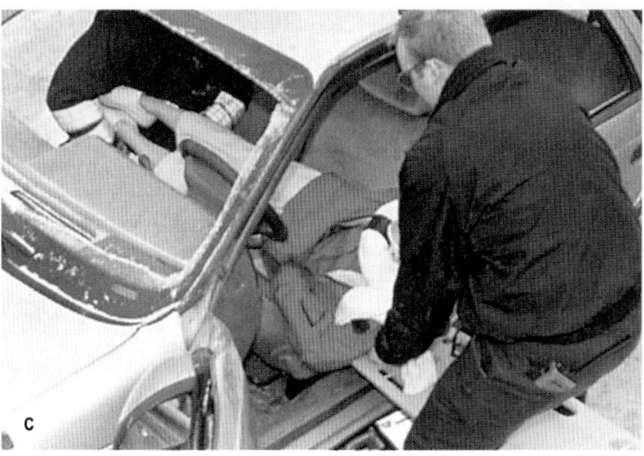

Figure 32-14 (a) Rescuer 1 supports the patient's head and neck and uses manual in-line stabilization throughout the procedure. (b) After assessment and application of a cervical collar, a rescuer positions the centre of a blanket roll at the patient's midline on the cervical collar. The rescuer wraps the ends of the blanket roll around the cervical collar and places them under the patient's arms. (c) The rescuers rotate the patient using the ends of the blanket roll until the patient's back faces the open doorway.

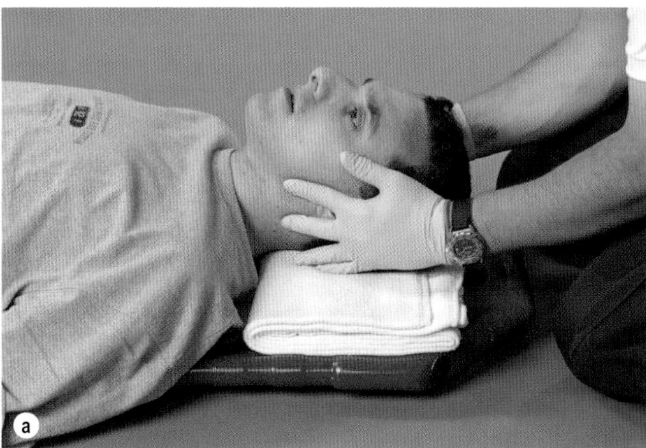
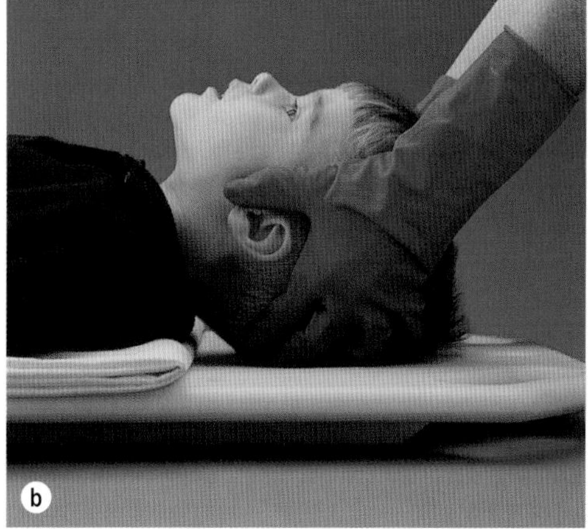

Figure 32-15 Padding requirements for adult (a) and paediatric (b) patients.

large space is produced between the back of the head and the spine board. Therefore non-compressible padding (e.g. commercial padding or folded towels) should be added (body shims). This can be done before securing the head (Figure 32-15a). The amount of padding required for in-line immobilization varies by patient and must be evaluated on an individual basis. Too little padding may cause hyperextension of the head, and too much padding may cause flexion; both may increase spinal cord damage. Children have proportionally larger heads than adults and may require padding under the torso to allow the head to lie in a neutral position on the board (Figure 32-15b). The padding (if needed) should be firm and should extend the full length and width of the torso from the buttocks to the top of the shoulders to prevent movement and misalignment of the spine.

The head is secured to the spinal device by placing commercial pads or rolled blankets on both sides of the head and securing them with the included straps, 2- to 3-inch tape strips, or a self-adhering firm wrap (elastic or gauze bandages do not prevent movement). The upper forehead should be

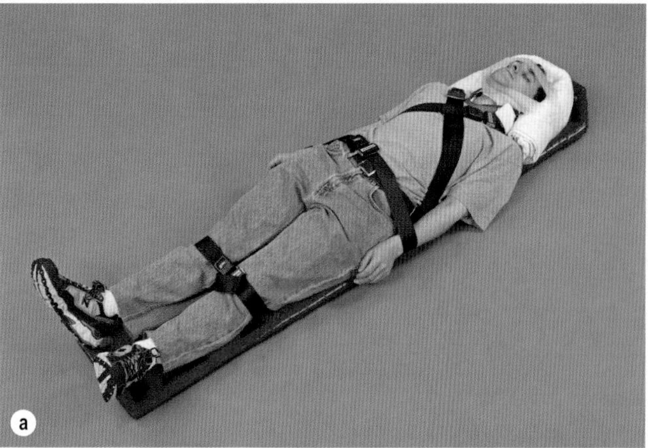

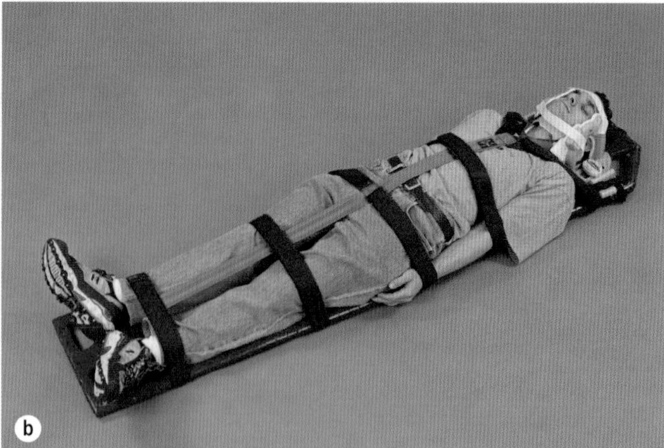

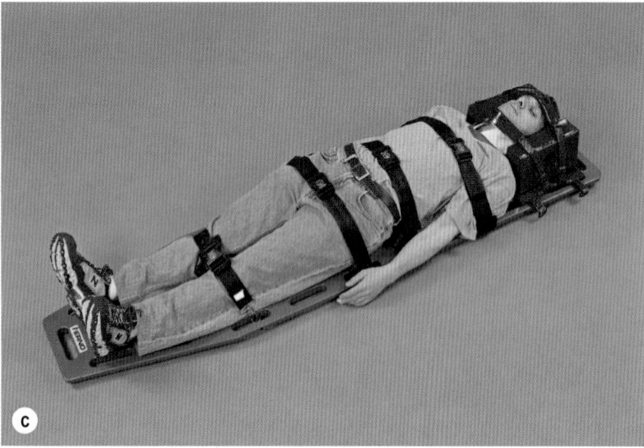

Figure 32-16 Long spine board immobilization (supine patient).

secured across the supraorbital ridge; the lower portion of the head should be secured across the anterior portion of the rigid cervical collar. Chin straps, sandbags, and intravenous bags are considered less optimal in immobilizing the head to a spinal device.

The patient's legs should be secured to the long board. Two or more straps can be applied above and below the knees. Towels, blankets, or suitable padding may be placed on both sides of the patient's lower legs. This will minimize movement and will help to maintain the patient's central position on the spinal device (Figure 32-16). A figure of eight should be used around the feet to restrict movement caused by acceleration and deceleration during transportation.

Before moving the patient, the patient's arms should be secured to the spinal device for safety. This is best achieved by placing the patient's arms at his or her side with the patient's palms facing the body. The arms should be secured with a separate strap placed across the forearms and torso.

Long board with standing patient Patients who are standing may be secured to a long spine board using the following technique (Figure 32-17):

1. Rescuer 1 applies manual in-line immobilization from behind the patient or in front of the patient and maintains this position throughout the procedure. Rescuer 2 applies a rigid cervical collar.
2. Rescuer 2 slides the long board behind the patient from the side and presses it against the patient.
3. Rescuers 2 and 3 stand on either side of the patient and insert the hand that is closest to the patient under the patient's armpit and grasp the nearest handhold of the backboard without moving the patient's shoulders. The rescuers grab the higher handhold on the board with their other hands and lower the patient and backboard to the ground whilst maintaining manual in-line immobilization.
4. Once on the ground, the rescuers secure the patient to the long backboard as previously described.

Immobilizing paediatric patients

As with adult patients, prehospital care of a paediatric patient with suspected spine trauma should be managed with manual in-line immobilization, a rigid cervical collar, and a long spinal immobilization device. Many different paediatric immobilization devices are available (Figure 32-18). If paediatric immobilization devices are not available, children may be secured on an adult long board (although a great deal of padding is needed to fill voids to prevent movement).

Helmet issues

The purpose of helmets is to protect the head and brain; helmets are not intended to protect the neck. The various types of helmet include full-face or open-face designs (used in motorcycling, cycling, in-line skating and other activities), and helmets designed for sports such as ice hockey and

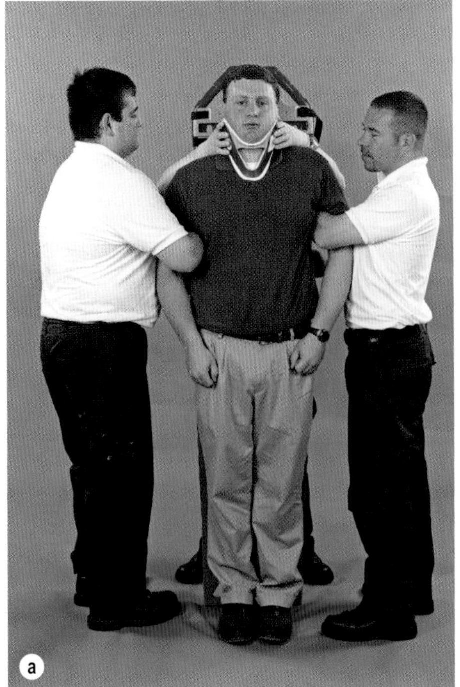
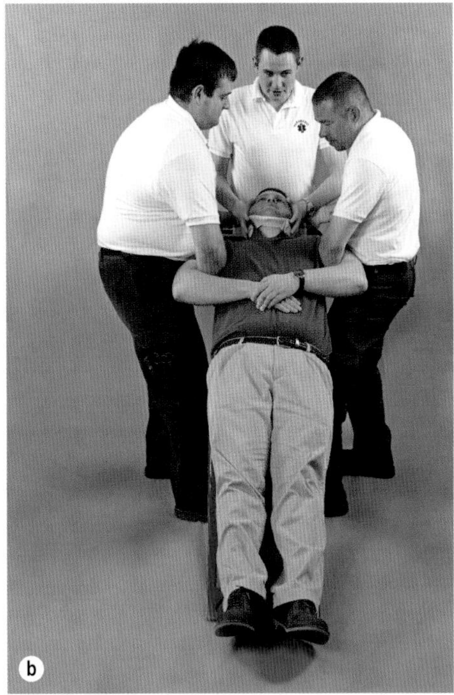

Figure 32-17 (a) While Rescuer 1 maintains manual in-line stabilization, Rescuers 2 and 3 support the patient. (b) In one organized move, the rescuers lower the patient to the ground onto the long spine board for further immobilization.

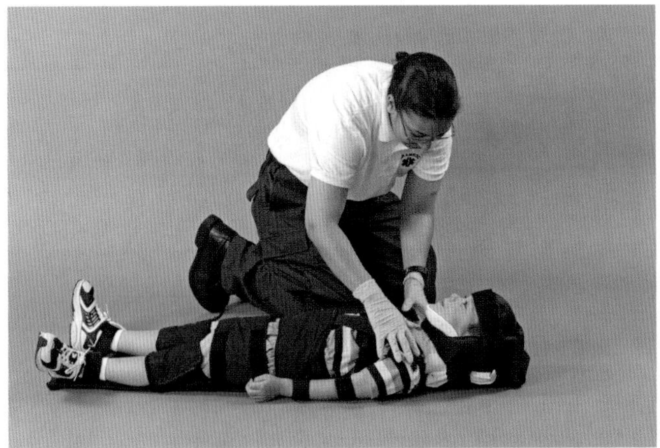

Figure 32-18 Infant and paediatric immobilization board.

motocross. Patients who are wearing full-face helmets must have the helmet removed early in the assessment process to allow the rescuers to assess and manage a patient's airway and ventilatory status. In addition, rescuers can look for bleeding, which may be hidden by the helmet, and they can move the patient's head from the flexed position caused by large helmets, into neutral alignment.

Helmet removal

The following steps in full-face helmet removal are recommended by the American College of Surgeons Committee on Trauma.[9]

1. Rescuer 1 immobilizes the helmet and head in an in-line position (Figure 32-19). Rescuer presses his or her palms on each side of the helmet with the fingertips curled over the lower margin of the helmet.
2. Rescuer 2 removes the face shield and chin strap, and assesses the patient's airway and ventilatory status.
3. Rescuer 2 grasps the patient's mandible by placing the thumb at the angle of the mandible on one side and two fingers at the angle on the other side. Rescuer 2 places his or her other hand under the neck at the base of the skull, taking over in-line immobilization of the patient's head.
4. Rescuer 1 carefully spreads the sides of the helmet away from the patient's head and ears and then rotates the helmet toward the rescuer to clear the patient's nose. Rescuer 1 then removes the helmet from the patient's head in a straight line. Just before removing the helmet from under the patient's head, Rescuer 1 assumes in-line immobilization by squeezing the sides of the helmet against the patient's head.
5. Rescuer 2 repositions his or her hands to support the head and to prevent it from dropping as the helmet is removed completely. This is accomplished by the rescuer placing a hand further up on the occipital area of the head and by grasping the maxilla with the thumb and first fingers of the other hand on each side of the nose. After securing this position, Rescuer 2 takes over in-line immobilization.
6. Rescuer 1 rotates the helmet about 30 degrees, following the curvature of the patient's head and completely removes the helmet by carefully pulling it in a straight line.
7. After removal of the helmet, Rescuer 1 applies in-line immobilization, and Rescuer 2 applies a rigid cervical collar.

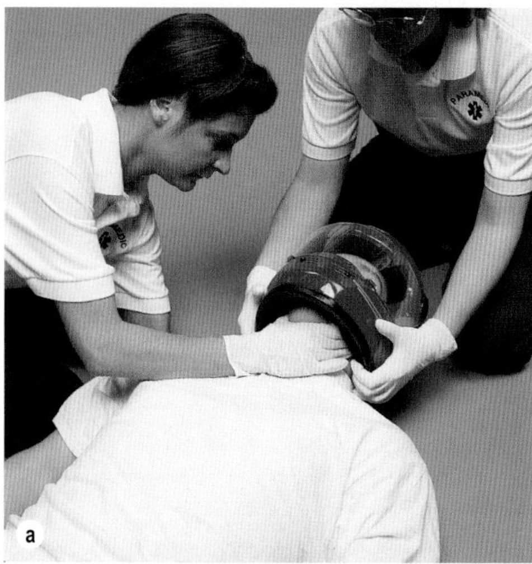

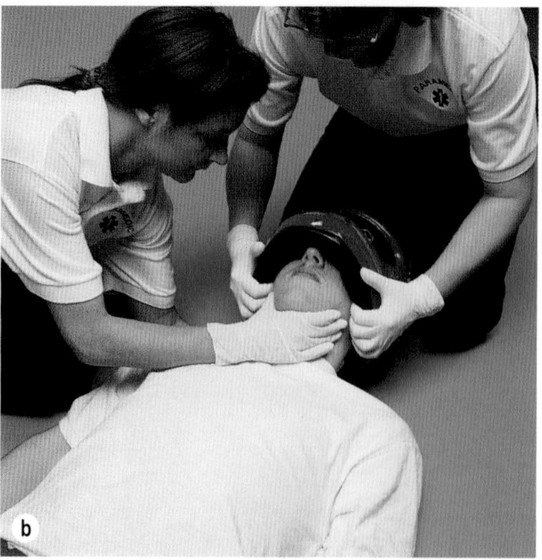

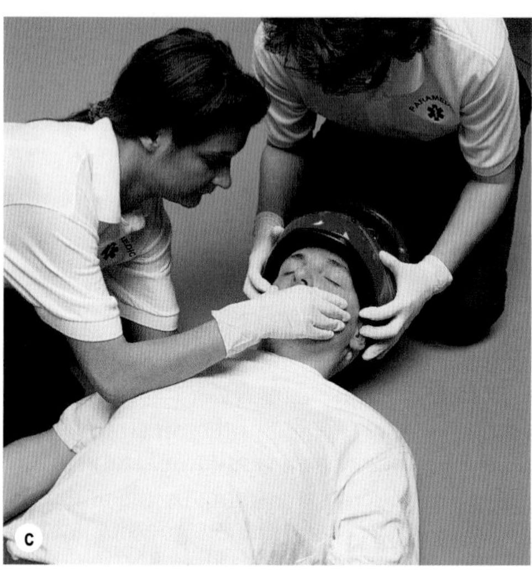

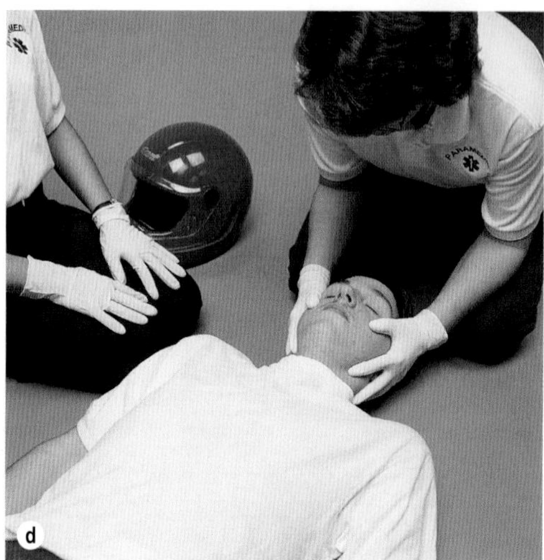

Figure 32-19 (a) Rescuer 1 immobilizes the helmet and head in an in-line position. Rescuer 2 grasps the patient's mandible by placing the thumb at the angle of the mandible on one side and two fingers at the angle on the other side. Rescuer 2 places the other hand under the patient's neck at the base of the skull, producing in-line immobilization of the patient's head. (b) Rescuer 1 carefully spreads the sides of the helmet away from the patient's head and ears. (c) Rescuer 1 then rotates the helmet toward the rescuer to clear the nose and remove it from the patient's head in a straight line. (d) After the removal of the helmet, Rescuer 1 applies in-line immobilization. Another rescuer applies a rigid cervical collar.

Note

A key point to remember during helmet removal is that in-line immobilization must be maintained throughout the procedure. Thus the rescuers should never remove their hands from the patient at the same time. In addition, the helmet must be rotated in one direction to clear the nose. The helmet must be rotated in the opposite direction to clear the back of the patient's head.

Spinal immobilization in diving incidents

Most diving incidents involve injury to the patient's head, neck, and spine. If the patient is still in the water when emergency medical services arrive, the patient should be managed as follows:

1. Ensure scene and personal safety – only rescuers trained in water rescue should enter the water (Figure 32-20).
2. Float a supine patient to a shallow area without unnecessary movement of the spine.
3. Approach a prone patient from the top of the head. Position one arm under the patient to support the head, neck and torso. Place the other arm across the patient's head and back, splinting the head and neck between the rescuer's arms. Carefully turn the patient to a supine position and quickly assess airway and breathing (the paramedic may initiate rescue breathing whilst in the water).
4. A second rescuer slides a long board or other rigid device under the patient's body while the first rescuer continues to support the patient's head and neck without flexion or extension. Apply a rigid cervical collar. Maintain manual in-line immobilization throughout the rescue.
5. Float the spinal immobilization device to the edge of the water and lift it out.
6. The patient should be immobilized completely on the long spine board as previously described.

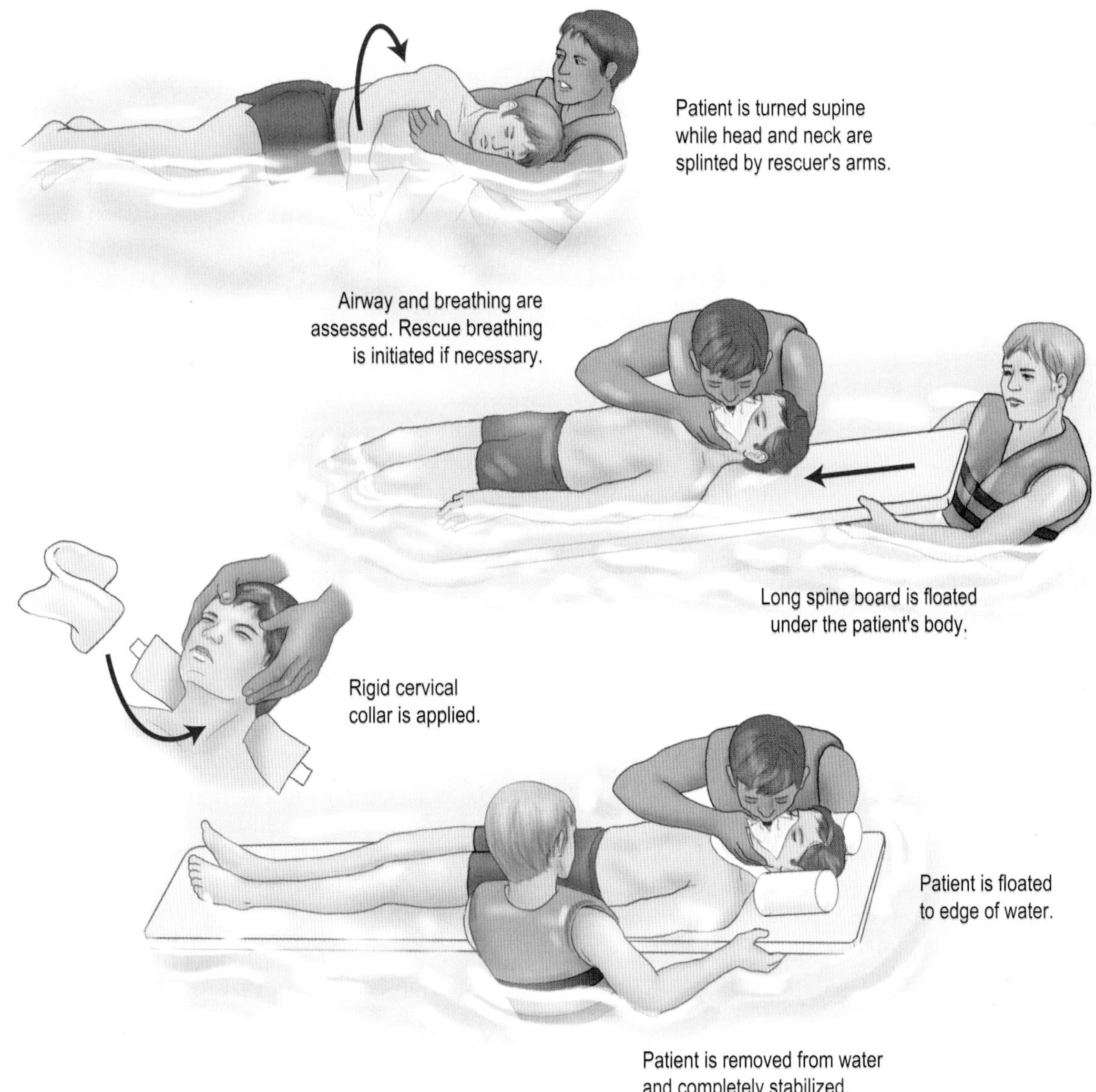

Figure 32-20 Extrication of a diving accident victim. Rescue breathing with barrier protection can begin in the water.

Cord injury presentations

Three cord injury presentations deserve special mention. These include spinal shock, neurogenic hypotension and autonomic dysreflexia syndrome.

Spinal shock

Spinal shock refers to a temporary loss of all types of spinal cord function distal to the injury. Signs and symptoms of spinal shock include flaccid paralysis distal to the injury site and loss of autonomic function, which may be demonstrated by hypotension, vasodilatation, loss of bowel and bladder control, priapism and loss of thermoregulation. Spinal shock does not always involve permanent, primary injury. The autonomic dysfunction usually resolves within 24 h although spinal shock may rarely last a few days to a few weeks. Careful handling of these patients to avoid secondary injury is crucial. Initial management includes full spinal immobilization, high-concentration oxygen administration, positioning the secured patient in a Trendelenburg position (elevating the foot end of the long board) providing it does not impair ventilation, and administering crystalloids intravenously (per guidelines).

Neurogenic hypotension

Neurogenic hypotension (neurogenic shock) following spinal shock results from the blockade of vasoregulatory fibres, motor fibres, and sensory fibres. This block produces a loss of sympathetic tone to the vessels or vasodilatation. Patients with neurogenic hypotension often have relative hypotension (a systolic blood pressure of 80–100 mmHg); warm, dry, and pink skin (from cutaneous vasodilatation); and relative bradycardia.

Neurogenic hypotension is rare and should not initially be presumed to be the cause of hypotension in the patient with a spine injury. The paramedic should consider other causes of hypotension, including internal haemorrhage, cardiac tamponade, and tension pneumothorax. If hypotension is severe, the paramedic should initiate shock management (per protocol).

Autonomic dysreflexia syndrome

Autonomic dysreflexia syndrome (sometimes known as autonomic hyper-reflexia) is an acute syndrome of excessive, uncontrolled sympathetic output that may occur in patients who have sustained injury to the spinal cord.[11] The condition is caused by retention of spinal reflex mechanisms in patients with injuries at T6 and above, but does not occur until there has been resolution of spinal shock and the return of autonomic reflexes return.[12] It is associated with patients who have injuries at T6 or above and is characterized by vasospasm, hypertension, skin pallor and gooseflesh associated with the piloerector response.[11] Triggers for the dysreflexic response include visceral distension (such as a full bladder), stimulation of pain receptors (e.g. through pressure ulcers or dressing changes), and visceral contractions (such as uterine contractions).[12] The syndrome results from a massive, uncompensated cardiovascular response that stimulates the sympathetic nervous system. The stimulation of sensory receptors below the level of cord injury causes the intact autonomic nervous system to respond with spasms of the arterioles. These spasms increase blood pressure and would ordinarily be moderated by another set of reflexes. However, due to the cord injury, moderating impulses are unable to reach their destination so vasodilatation is not possible and blood pressure continues to rise. The characteristics of this syndrome include the following:

- paroxysmal hypertension (up to 300 mmHg)
- pounding headache
- blurred vision
- sweating (above the level of injury) with flushing of the skin
- increased nasal congestion
- nausea
- bradycardia (30–40 beats/min)
- distended bladder or rectum.

The condition is a clinical emergency and may lead to convulsions, CVA, coma or death. The paramedic should bring the patient into an upright position to provoke an orthostatic reduction in blood pressure, and loosen tight or restrictive clothing or articles. The paramedic should look for any precipitating factors and eliminate them if possible. Blood pressure should be assessed every 2–5 min and the patient should be transported to hospital for further management.[11]

Non-traumatic spinal conditions

The non-traumatic spinal conditions to be discussed in this chapter include low back pain, degenerative disc disease, spondylosis, herniated intervertebral disc and spinal cord tumours.

Low back pain

It is estimated that 70% of the UK population experience some form of low back pain by the age of 60.[5] Low back pain usually affects the area between the lower rib cage and the gluteal muscles and often radiates into the thighs. About 1% of those with low back pain have sciatica – pain in the lumbar nerve root accompanied by neurosensory and motor deficits in the thigh and leg. Most low back pain is idiopathic, making a precise diagnosis difficult. Causes of this condition include the following:

- tension from tumours
- disc prolapse
- bursitis
- synovitis
- degenerative joint disease
- abnormal bone pressure
- inflammation caused by infection (e.g. osteomyelitis)
- fractures
- ligament strains.

Critical Thinking

What are some other medical conditions that may cause the patient to have a chief complaint of low back pain?

Risk factors associated with low back pain include occupations that require repetitive lifting, exposure to vibrations from vehicles or industrial machinery, and osteoporosis (elderly women report more symptoms than men).

Low back pain must come from innervated structures. However, deep pain and the way it is referred to other parts of the body vary by individual. Although the disc has no specific innervation, irritation of surrounding membranes that have pain receptors often occurs; especially in the presence of disc prolapse. The source of most low back pain occurs at L3, L4, L5, and S1. Other areas of abundant pain receptors are found in anterior and posterior longitudinal ligaments that are vulnerable to strains and sprains.

Degenerative disc disease

Degenerative disc disease is a common finding in persons older than 50 years of age. The causes of this condition include deterioration of the tissue of the intervertebral disc that occurs with ageing. The associated narrowing of the disc results in instability of the spine and can cause occasional low back pain.

Spondylosis

Spondylosis is a structural defect of the spine involving the lamina or vertebral arch. Spondylosis usually occurs in the lumbar spine between superior and inferior articulating surfaces; rotational stress fractures are common at the affected site. Heredity appears to be a key factor for this condition.

Herniated intervertebral disc

Herniated intervertebral disc (herniated nucleus pulposus) refers to a tear in the posterior rim of the capsule that encloses the gelatinous centre of the disc. Rupture of the disc is usually caused by trauma, degenerative disc disease, and improper lifting (most common). Men between the ages of 30 and 50 are most prone to develop this condition, with the most common injury sites being L5 to S1 and L4 to L5. (Herniated intervertebral disc may also occur in the cervical area at C5 to C6 and C6 to C7.) These injuries may have an immediate onset or may develop over months to years.

Spinal cord tumours

Tumours in the spinal cord may develop from cord compression, degenerative changes in bones and joints, or from an interruption in the blood supply to the cord. These tumours are classified by cell type, growth rate and structure of origin. Clinical manifestations depend on tumour type and location. The manifestations may include bilateral or asymmetrical motor dysfunction, paresis, spasticity, pain, temperature dysfunction, sensory changes, and other abnormalities.

Assessment and management of non-traumatic spinal conditions

As stated before, non-traumatic spinal conditions such as low back pain are difficult to diagnose. The assessment and management are based on the patient's chief complaint, the physical examination, and through the evaluation of associated risk factors. Signs and symptoms that are commonly seen with non-traumatic spinal conditions include the following:

- discomfort
- difficulty in standing erect
- pain with straining (e.g. coughing, sneezing)
- limited range of motion
- alterations in sensation, pain, and temperature
- upper extremity pain or paraesthesia that increases with motion
- motor weakness.

The management of patients with back pain in the prehospital setting is mainly supportive. Management focuses on decreasing the patient's pain and discomfort. Some patients are best managed with immobilization on a full long-board or vacuum-type mattress. Full spinal immobilization is not required unless the condition is a result of trauma. The in-hospital evaluation may include various testing such as computed tomography, electromyelography and magnetic resonance imaging.

Critical Thinking

How will the prehospital care differ for a patient who has signs or symptoms of one of these syndromes?

Summary

- Most SCIs are the result of motor vehicle crashes. Other causes are falls, penetrating injuries from acts of human violence and sport injuries.
- The paramedic can classify the MOI as positive, negative or uncertain. This classification is combined with the clinical guidelines for evaluating SCI, which include the following signs and symptoms: pain, tenderness, painful movement, deformity, cuts/bruises over spinal area, paralysis, paraesthesias and weakness. This system can help to identify cases in which spinal immobilization is appropriate.
- The spinal column is composed of 33 vertebrae. These are divided into five sections. The sections are 7 cervical, 12 thoracic, 5 lumbar, 5 sacral (fused), and 4 coccygeal (fused).
- The specific mechanisms of injury that frequently cause spinal trauma are axial loading; extremes of flexion, hyperextension, or hyper-rotation; excessive lateral bending; and distraction.
- Spinal injuries may be classified as sprains and strains, fractures and dislocations, sacral and coccygeal fractures, and cord injuries. The spinal cord may sustain a primary or a secondary injury. Lesions (transections) of the spinal cord are classified as complete or incomplete.
- With spinal injuries, the first priority is to evaluate and manage any threats to life. The second priority is to preserve spinal cord function, including avoiding secondary injury to the spinal cord. These goals are best met by maintaining a high degree of suspicion for the presence of spinal trauma, by providing early spinal immobilization, by rapidly correcting any volume deficit, and by administering oxygen.
- General principles of spinal immobilization include prevention of further injury; treating the spine as a long bone with a joint at either end (the head and pelvis); always using complete spinal immobilization; beginning spinal immobilization in the initial assessment and maintaining it until the spine is immobilized completely on the long immobilization device; and, placing the patient's head in a neutral, in-line position, unless contraindicated.
- Spinal shock refers to a temporary loss of all types of spinal cord function distal to the injury.
- Neurogenic shock produces a loss of sympathetic tone to the vessels. This causes relative hypotension; warm, dry, and pink skin; and relative bradycardia.
- Autonomic dysreflexia syndrome results from a massive, uncompensated cardiovascular response that stimulates the sympathetic nervous system. This response causes an increase in blood pressure and other symptoms.
- Some non-traumatic spinal conditions include low back pain, degenerative disc disease, spondylosis, herniated intervertebral disc, and spinal cord tumours. The management of patients with non-traumatic back pain in the prehospital setting is mainly supportive. The goal is to help patients decrease their pain and discomfort.

References

1. Wardrope J, Ravichandran G 2004 Risk assessment for spinal injury after trauma. BMJ 328:721–723
2. Ravichandran G, Silver JR 1982 Missed injuries of spinal cord. BMJ 284:953–956
3. Poonnoose PM, Ravichandran G, McClelland MR 2002 Missed and mismanaged injuries of spinal cord. J Trauma 53:314–320
4. Spinal Injuries Association. Annual report, 2007/2008. Online. Available http://www.spinal.co.uk/pdf/annual%20reports/report0708.pdf 8 July 2009
5. National Statistics 1998 Adults experiencing back pain: by age and total time suffered in previous 12 months, 1998. Online. Available http://www.statistics.gov.uk/STATBASE/xsdataset.asp?More=Y&vlnk=674&All=Y&B2.x=75&B2.y=5 17 February 2009
6. US Department of Transportation, National Highway Traffic Safety Administration 1998 EMT-Paramedic national standard curriculum. US Department of Transportation, Washington, DC
7. Joint Royal Colleges Ambulance Liaison Committee 2006 UK Ambulance service clinical practice guidelines. University of Warwick, JRCALC
8. Foundation for Spinal Cord Injury Prevention 1999 Spinal cord injury facts, Detroit. National Spinal Cord Injury Statistical Centre. Online. Available http://www.fscip.org/facts.htm
9. National Association of Emergency Medical Technicians 2003 PHTLS: basic and advanced prehospital life support, 5th edition. Mosby, St Louis.
10. Rosen P, Barkin R 2003 Emergency medicine: concepts and clinical practice, 5th edition. Mosby, St Louis
11. Blackmer J 2003 Rehabilitation medicine: autonomic dysreflexia. Can Med Assoc J 16(9):931–935
12. Porth CM 2005 Pathophysiology, concepts of altered health states. Lippincott, Williams & Wilkins, Philadelphia

CHAPTER **33**

Abdominal Trauma

Chapter contents

Objectives

Upon completion of this chapter, the paramedic student will be able to:

1. Identify mechanisms of injury associated with abdominal trauma.
2. Describe mechanisms of injury, signs and symptoms, and complications associated with abdominal solid organ, hollow organ, retroperitoneal organ, and pelvic organ injuries.
3. Outline the significance of injury to intra-abdominal vascular structures.
4. Describe the prehospital assessment priorities for a patient suspected of having an abdominal injury.
5. Outline the prehospital care of a patient with abdominal trauma.

Key terms

haematuria The abnormal presence of blood in the urine.
haemoperitoneum The presence of extravasated blood in the peritoneal cavity.
Kehr sign Pain in the left shoulder thought to be caused by referred pain secondary to irritation of the adjacent diaphragm.
peritonitis Inflammation of the serous membrane that covers the abdominal wall.

Abdominal trauma may not be easy to evaluate in the prehospital setting. It can cause many injuries to multiple organs. Physical findings may be absent, minimal, or exaggerated. Also, patients may have different perceptions of pain. Pain perception varies as a result of pre-existing conditions, shock, alcohol or other drug use, head injury, or other factors; therefore the paramedic must have a high degree of suspicion based on the mechanism of injury and kinematics. Death from abdominal trauma is usually a result of ongoing haemorrhage and the delay of surgical repair.

Note

Like most other types of trauma, many abdominal injuries can be prevented. An important prevention strategy is taking part in community programmes that promote safety. (For example, one could work to stress the importance of using personal restraints – see Chapter 3.)

Mechanisms of abdominal injury

Abdominal injury may result from blunt or penetrating trauma. Regardless of the organ injured, management is usually limited to securing the airway with spinal precautions, providing ventilatory support, providing wound management, managing shock with fluid replacement, and rapidly transporting the patient for definitive care (Box 33-1).

Blunt trauma

Blunt trauma to abdominal organs is usually caused by compression or shearing forces (see Chapter 26). Compression forces may cause the abdominal organs to be crushed between solid objects (e.g. between the steering column and the spinal vertebrae). Shearing forces may cause a tear or rupture of the solid organs or blood vessels; this occurs when the tissues are stretched at their points of attachment (stabilizing ligaments or blood vessels). The severity of injury is normally related to the degree and duration of force applied,

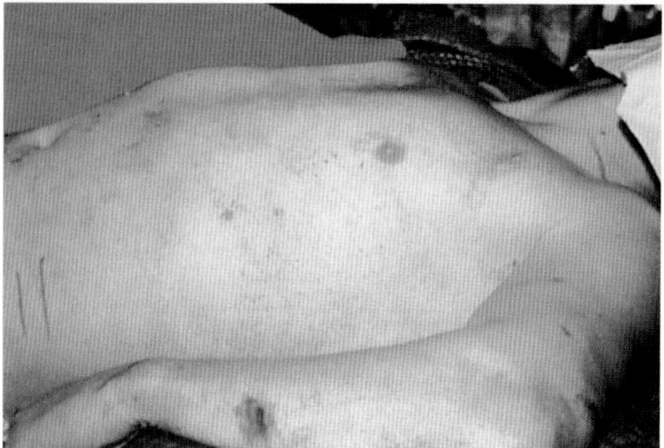

Figure 33-1 Marks of impact on the front-seat passenger in a car crash. The victim suffered rupture of the diaphragm and spleen.

Box 33-1

Prehospital care for abdominal injury

1. Secure the airway with spinal precautions.
2. Provide ventilatory support.
3. Provide wound management.
4. Manage shock with fluid replacement (per guidelines).
5. Rapidly transport the patient for definitive care.

and also to the type of abdominal structure injured (fluid filled, gas filled, solid or hollow). Blunt abdominal trauma may be caused by motor vehicle and motorcycle collisions (including injuries that result from the use of personal restraints), pedestrian injuries, falls, assaults, and blast injuries. The car is the major cause of blunt abdominal trauma (Figure 33-1). Automobile–automobile and automobile–pedestrian crashes have been cited as causes in 50–75% of cases, blows to the abdomen in about 15% of cases, and falls in 6–9% of cases.[1]

Critical Thinking

Young children are more susceptible to abdominal injuries than adults. Why?

Penetrating trauma

Penetrating injury may result from stab wounds, gunshot wounds, or impalement. Major complications of this type of trauma include haemorrhage from a major vessel or solid organ, and perforation of a segment of bowel. As a rule, injuries caused by penetrating trauma do not have as high a mortality rate as those caused by blunt trauma.[2]

Specific abdominal injuries

An abdominal injury may be classified as a solid organ, hollow organ, retroperitoneal organ, pelvic organ, or vascular injury (Figure 33-2a, b).

Solid organ injury

Injury to solid organs usually results in rapid and significant blood loss. The two solid organs most often injured are the liver and spleen, both of which are primary sources of life-threatening haemorrhage.

Critical Thinking

When does shock associated with injury to the liver or spleen develop?

Liver

The liver is the largest organ in the abdominal cavity. Because of its location, it is often injured by trauma to the eighth through twelfth ribs on the right side of the body (Figure 33-3). It may also be injured by trauma to the upper central part of the abdomen. Injury to the liver should be suspected in any patient with a steering wheel injury, lap belt injury, or history of epigastric trauma. After an injury to the liver, blood and bile escape into the peritoneal cavity, which results in the signs and symptoms of shock and peritoneal irritation (abdominal pain, tenderness, rigidity), respectively. The liver is damaged in about 19% of cases of blunt abdominal trauma and in about 37% of cases of penetrating trauma.[1]

Spleen

The spleen lies in the upper left quadrant of the abdomen and is slightly protected by the organs that surround it medially and anteriorly, and by the lower portion of the rib cage. Injury to the spleen is often associated with other intra-abdominal injuries. Splenic injury should be suspected in motor vehicle crashes and in falls or sports injuries involving an impact to the lower left chest or flank, or to the upper left abdomen. About 40% of patients with splenic injuries have no symptoms; however, the patient may complain of pain in the left shoulder (Kehr sign). This is thought to be caused by referred pain that occurs as a result of irritation of the adjacent diaphragm by a splenic haematoma or haemoperitoneum. The spleen is damaged in about 41% of cases of blunt abdominal trauma and in about 7% of cases of penetrating trauma.[1]

Hollow organ injury

Injuries to the hollow abdominal organs may result in sepsis, wound infection and abscess formation, particularly if trauma to the intestine remains undiagnosed for an extended period. With injuries to solid organs, haemorrhage is the major cause of symptoms. In contrast, injury to the hollow organs results in symptoms from spillage of their contents (this spillage results in peritonitis) (Box 33-2).

Stomach

Because of its protected location in the abdomen, the stomach is not often injured by blunt trauma. However, penetrating trauma may cause gastric transection or laceration. Patients with either of these injuries may show signs of peritonitis rather quickly as a result of leakage of acidic

Liver
Stomach
Pancreas
Duodenum
Transverse colon
Small intestine
Urinary bladder
Urethra
a

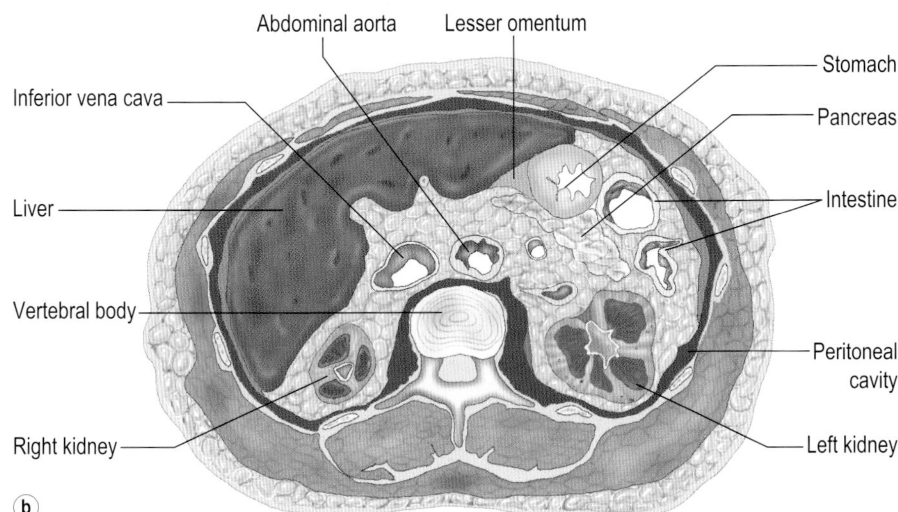

Figure 33-2 Hollow, solid, retroperitoneal and pelvic organs.

gastric contents. The diagnosis of injury to the stomach is usually confirmed during surgery or when nasogastric drainage returns blood. The stomach is damaged in about 1% of cases of blunt abdominal trauma and in about 19% of cases of penetrating trauma.[1]

Colon and small intestine

The colon and small intestine, like the stomach and duodenum, are more likely to be injured as a result of penetrating trauma than blunt trauma (for example, the injury may be caused by a gunshot wound to the abdomen or buttocks). However, the large and small bowel may be injured by compression forces in high-speed motor vehicle crashes. They may also sustain deceleration injuries associated with the wearing of personal restraints. Considerable force is required to cause an injury to the colon or small intestine; therefore other injuries are usually present. Peritoneal contamination with bacteria is a common problem. With blunt abdominal trauma, the colon is damaged in about 6% of cases and the small intestine in about 7% of cases. With penetrating abdominal trauma, the colon is damaged in about 16% of cases and the small intestine in about 26% of cases.[1]

Retroperitoneal organ injury

Injury to the retroperitoneal organs (kidneys, ureters, pancreas, duodenum) may occur as a result of blunt or penetrating trauma to the anterior abdomen, posterior abdomen (particularly the flank area), or thoracic spine. Haemorrhage

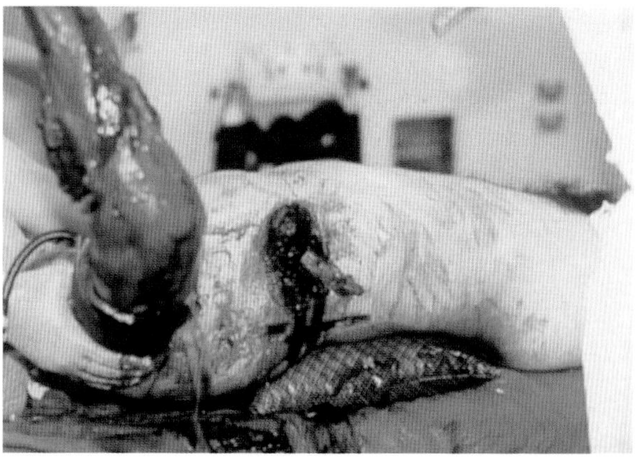

Figure 33-3 Liver injury visible beneath broken rib caused by high-speed vehicle crash.

Box 33-2

Peritoneal irritation

Peritonitis is usually acute and quite painful. It results from the spillage of enzymes, acids, and bacteria into the abdominal cavity, and may be delayed for hours or days after injury to a hollow viscus organ. The spillage causes chemical irritation of the peritoneum, which is the membrane that lines the wall of the abdomen and covers the abdominal organs (blood is not a chemical irritant to the abdomen). The pain of peritonitis is usually localized (via somatic nerve fibres); however, it may be diffuse. Signs and symptoms of peritonitis include the following:

- pain
- tenderness on percussion or palpation
- guarding, rigidity
- fever (if untreated)
- distension (a late finding).

Note: The adult abdomen can accommodate 1.5 L of fluid without the belly looking bloated (abdominal distension).

within the retroperitoneal area may be massive and generally is as a result of pelvic or lumbar fractures. Retroperitoneal structures are damaged in about 9% of cases of blunt abdominal injuries and in about 11% of cases of penetrating trauma.[1]

Note

Bruising of the flanks (Turner sign) or around the umbilicus (Cullen sign) indicates retroperitoneal haemorrhage (Figure 33-4). However, these signs are usually delayed 12 h to several days.

Kidneys

The kidneys are solid organs that lie in the retroperitoneal space. Injuries may involve contusion, fractures, and lacerations, resulting in haemorrhage, extravasation of urine, or both. Contusions are usually self-limiting and heal with bed rest and forced fluids. Fractures and lacerations are more severe and may require surgical repair.

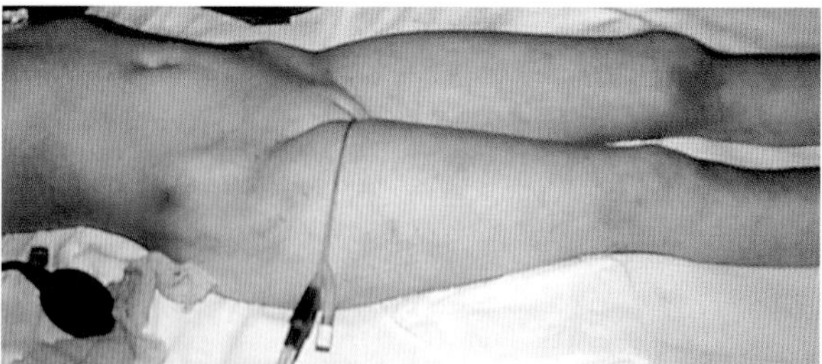

Figure 33-4 Bruising caused by rupture of the liver and right kidney.

Ureters

The ureters are hollow organs that are rarely injured by blunt trauma due to their flexible structure. When injury occurs, it is usually the result of penetrating abdominal or flank wounds (e.g. stab wounds, firearm injuries).

Pancreas

The pancreas is a solid organ that lies within the retroperitoneal space. Injury to the pancreas is rare. When it occurs, it is usually caused by compressive or penetrating forces on the upper left quadrant, as in steering wheel and bicycle handlebar impalement. The pancreas is more often injured by penetrating trauma (particularly firearms) than by blunt trauma.

Duodenum

The duodenum, which lies across the lumbar spine, is seldom injured. This is due to its location in the retroperitoneal area, near the pancreas. When great force from blunt trauma or a penetrating injury occurs, the duodenum may be crushed or lacerated. Injury to this organ is usually associated with concurrent pancreatic trauma; it is confirmed through surgery.

Pelvic organ injury

Injury to pelvic organs (bladder, urethra) usually results from motor vehicle crashes that cause pelvic fractures. Other, less frequent causes of pelvic organ injury are penetrating trauma, straddle-type injuries from falls, pedestrian injuries, and some sexual acts. The pelvis supports and protects multiple organ systems; therefore the risk of associated injury is high. The most common associated injuries are those to the urinary bladder and urethra. Fractures of the pelvis (Figure 33-5) are often associated with severe retroperitoneal haemorrhage. The mortality rate for pelvic fractures ranges from 6.4% to 19%.[1] (Pelvic fractures are further described in Chapter 34.)

Urinary bladder

The urinary bladder is a hollow organ that may be ruptured by blunt trauma, penetrating trauma or pelvic fracture. Rupture is more likely if the bladder is distended at the time of injury. With rupture, the integrity of the peritoneum may be disrupted and urine may enter the peritoneal cavity. Bladder injury should be suspected in inebriated patients who suffer trauma to the lower abdomen. Gross haematuria may be present and the patient may complain of being unable to void. The urinary bladder and surrounding structures are damaged in about 6% of cases of abdominal trauma.[1]

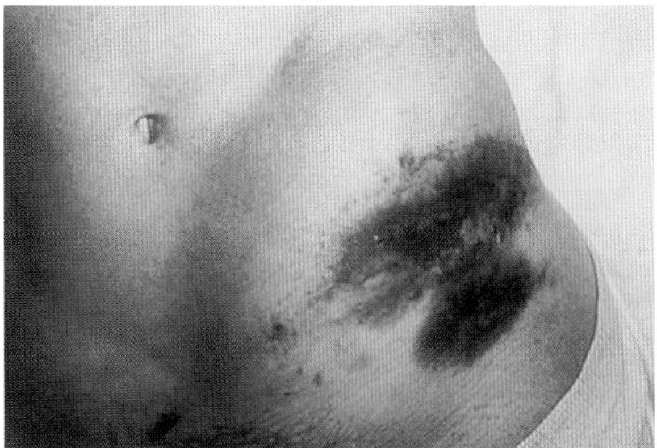

Figure 33-5 Massive swelling and bruising from a pelvic fracture.

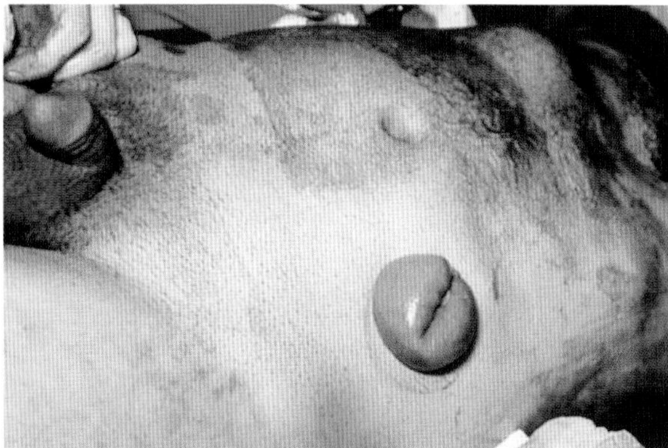

Figure 33-6 A loop of gut that emerged through a stab wound to the abdomen.

Urethra

A tear in the urethra occurs more often in men than in women. It usually occurs as a result of blunt trauma associated with pelvic fracture. The patient may complain of abdominal pain and of being unable to urinate. Blood at the meatus indicates urethral injury. An indwelling urinary catheter should not be used in these patients.

Vascular structure injuries

Injuries to arterial and venous vessels in the abdomen can be life threatening because of their potential for massive haemorrhage. These injuries are usually caused by penetrating trauma but may also be the result of compression or deceleration forces on the abdomen. As in solid organ injury, vascular injury is often marked by hypovolaemia. In some cases, vascular injuries are associated with a palpable abdominal mass. The major vessels most often injured are the aorta, the inferior vena cava, and the renal, mesenteric, and iliac arteries and veins. Injury to major vessels in the abdomen has a high mortality rate; immediate surgical repair is often required.

Critical Thinking

How can you attempt to manage shock when major vessels have been injured as a result of a severe pelvic fracture?

Assessment of abdominal trauma

The most significant sign of severe abdominal trauma is unexplained shock. The mechanism of injury and the classic presentation of hypovolaemia are important indicators. Other signs and symptoms that should alert the paramedic to the possibility of severe abdominal trauma are abdominal wall injuries (e.g. bruising and discoloration of the abdomen, abrasions) and the following:

- obvious bleeding
- pain and abdominal tenderness or guarding
- abdominal rigidity and distension
- evisceration (Box 33-3)

Box 33-3

Evisceration

Evisceration is the protrusion of an internal organ or the peritoneal contents through a wound or surgical incision, especially in the abdominal wall (Figure 33-6). The presence of an evisceration from abdominal trauma is generally associated with major abdominal injury. In the prehospital setting the wound is managed by covering the eviscerated contents with moist, sterile gauze or a dressing. This helps to prevent further contamination and drying. No attempt should be made to replace eviscerated organs into the peritoneal cavity; this would increase the risk of infection and complicate surgical evaluation of the injury.

- rib fractures
- pelvic fractures.

The absence of these signs and symptoms does not rule out an abdominal injury. The paramedic must maintain a high degree of suspicion based on the nature of the injury.

Management of abdominal trauma

Emergency care of patients with abdominal trauma is usually limited to two courses of action: (1) stabilizing the patient's condition and (2) rapidly transporting the patient to a hospital for surgical repair of the injury.

The following are the most important components of on-scene care:

- a thorough scene survey to identify forces involved in abdominal trauma
- rapid evaluation of the patient and the mechanism of injury
- airway maintenance with spinal precautions
- administration of high-concentration oxygen
- ventilatory support as needed
- reduction of haemorrhage by application of pressure
- fluid replacement with volume expanders
- cardiac monitoring.

En route to the hospital, a full physical examination and ongoing assessment can be performed. These procedures should include obtaining a focused history, vital sign assessment (and reassessment), and inspection, percussion and palpation of the abdomen (see Chapter 9). Auscultation of the abdomen for the presence of bowel sounds can establish a baseline measurement for hospital personnel. This assessment should never delay patient transport.

Critical Thinking

What functions of the pancreas may be disrupted after injury? What might be the effects of spillage of pancreatic juices into the abdominal cavity?

Summary

- Blunt trauma to abdominal organs usually results from compression or shearing forces.
- Penetrating injury may result from stab wounds, gunshot wounds, or impalement.
- The two solid organs most often injured are the liver and the spleen. Both of these organs are primary sources of death from haemorrhage. Injuries to the hollow abdominal organs may result in sepsis, wound infection and abscess formation.
- Injury to the retroperitoneal organs (kidneys, ureters, pancreas, duodenum) may cause massive haemorrhage.
- Injury to the pelvic organs (bladder, urethra) usually results from motor vehicle crashes that cause pelvic fractures.
- Injuries to abdominal vascular structures may be life threatening. This is due to their potential for massive haemorrhage.
- The most significant sign of severe abdominal trauma is unexplained shock.
- Emergency care of patients with abdominal trauma is usually limited to two courses of action: (1) stabilizing the patient's condition and (2) rapidly transporting the patient to a hospital for surgical repair of the injury.

References

1. Rosen P, Barkin R 1998 Emergency medicine: concepts and clinical practice, 4th edition. Mosby, St Louis
2. US Department of Transportation, National Highway Traffic Safety Administration 1998 EMT-paramedic national standard curriculum. US Department of Transportation, Washington, DC

Further reading

Emergency Nurses Association and Newberry L 2003 Sheehy's emergency nursing: principles and practice, 5th edition. Mosby, St Louis

Ferrera P, Colucciello S, Marx J et al 2001 Trauma management. Mosby, St Louis

National Association of Emergency Medical Technicians 2003 PHTLS: basic and advanced prehospital life support, 5th edition. Mosby, St Louis.

Roberts J, Hedges J 1998 Clinical procedures in emergency medicine, 3rd edition. WB Saunders, Philadelphia

CHAPTER **34**

Musculoskeletal Trauma

Chapter contents

Objectives

Upon completion of this chapter, the paramedic student will be able to:

1. Describe the features of each class of musculoskeletal injury.
2. Describe the features of bursitis, tendonitis and arthritis.
3. Given a specific patient scenario, outline the prehospital assessment of the musculoskeletal system.
4. Outline general principles of splinting.
5. Describe the significance and prehospital management principles for selected upper extremity injuries.
6. Describe the significance and prehospital management principles for selected lower extremity injuries.
7. Identify prehospital management priorities for open fractures.
8. Describe the principles of realignment of angular fractures and dislocations.
9. Outline the process for referral of patients with a minor musculoskeletal injury.

Key terms

DCAP-BTLS An acronym for wound assessment: deformity, contusions, abrasions, penetrations or punctures, burns, tenderness, lacerations, and swelling.

false movement An unnatural movement of an extremity, usually associated with fracture.

fracture A break in the continuity of bone or cartilage.

joint dislocation An injury that occurs when the normal articulating ends of two or more bones are displaced.

sprain A partial tearing of a ligament caused by a sudden twisting or stretching of a joint beyond its normal range of motion.

strain An injury to the muscle or its tendon from overexertion or overextension.

Musculoskeletal problems account for approximately 3.5 million emergency department attendances each year.[1] Trauma to an extremity is seldom life threatening. However, early recognition and management may prevent long-term disability

Note

Extremity trauma usually results from motor vehicle crashes, falls, acts of violence, and contact sports.[2] Prevention strategies include proper sports training (working with athletic trainers on the use of protective equipment), use of personal restraints, and fall prevention (e.g. high-rise window guards) (see Chapter 3).

Classifications of musculoskeletal injuries

The musculoskeletal system and associated neurovascular structures are made up of bones, nerves, vessels, muscles, tendons, ligaments and joints. Injuries that result from traumatic forces to these tissues include fractures, sprains, strains and joint dislocations. The paramedic should not attempt to differentiate these injuries in the prehospital setting. Patients suspected of having trauma to an extremity should be managed as though a fracture exists. Problems associated with musculoskeletal injuries include the following:

- haemorrhage
- instability
- loss of tissue
- simple laceration and contamination
- interruption of blood supply
- nerve damage
- long-term disability.

Critical Thinking

How could long-term disability result from a musculoskeletal injury?

Musculoskeletal injuries can result from direct trauma (e.g. blunt force applied to an extremity), indirect trauma (e.g. a vertical fall that produces a spinal fracture distant from the site of impact), or pathological conditions (e.g. some forms of arthritis or malignancy). Paramedics should consider kinematics when caring for a patient with a musculoskeletal injury. They should also carefully evaluate the scene (see Chapter 26).

Fractures

A fracture is any break in the continuity of bone or cartilage (Figure 34-1). It may be complete or incomplete, depending on the line of fracture through the bone. Fractures are also classified as open or closed, depending on the integrity of the skin near the fracture site (Box 34-1). Fractures of long bones may result in moderate to severe haemorrhage within the first 2 h. As much as 550 mL of blood may be released in the lower leg from a tibial or fibular fracture, 1000 mL of blood in the thigh from a femoral fracture, and 2000 mL of blood from a pelvic fracture.[3]

The head of long bones in children is separated from the shaft of the bone by the epiphyseal plate until the bone stops growing. Fractures that involve the epiphyseal plate are called epiphyseal fractures. These are serious injuries that may result in separation or fragmentation of the growth plate and permanent bending or deformity of an extremity (Figure 34-2).

Box 34-1

Classification of fractures

Open: A break in which a protruding bone or penetrating object causes a soft tissue injury.

Closed: A break in the bone that has not yet penetrated the soft tissue or skin.

Comminuted: A fracture that involves several breaks in the bone, resulting in multiple bone fragments.

Greenstick: A break in which the bone is bent but only broken on the outside of the bend (common in children).

Spiral: A break caused by a twisting motion.

Oblique: A break at a slanting angle across a bone.

Transverse: A break that occurs at right angles to the long axis of the bone.

Stress: A break (especially in one or more of the foot bones) caused by repeated, long-term or abnormal stress.

Pathological: A break resulting from weakness in bone tissue caused by neoplasm or malignant growth.

Epiphyseal: A break that involves the epiphyseal growth plate of a child's long bone; may result in permanent angulation or deformity and may cause premature arthritis.

Sprains

A sprain is a partial tearing of a ligament caused by sudden twisting or stretching of a joint beyond its normal range of motion (Figure 34-3). Two common areas for sprains are the knee and the ankle. Sprains are graded by severity (Box 34-2). A first-degree sprain has no joint instability as only a few fibres of the ligament are torn. Swelling and haemorrhage are minimal (repeated first-degree sprains can result in stretching of the ligaments). A second-degree sprain causes more disruption than a first-degree injury. The joint is usually still intact, but swelling and bruising are increased. In third-degree sprains the ligaments are completely torn. If third-degree sprains are accompanied by a dislocation, nerve or blood vessel compromise to the extremity is possible. Some second-degree sprains and most third-degree sprains have the same presentation as a fracture.

The application of ice to an injury during the first 24 h generally reduces pain and swelling. After that time, heat (e.g. warm soaks) is often prescribed to increase circulation.

Strains

A strain is an injury to the muscle or its tendon from overexertion or overextension. Strains commonly occur in the back and arms and may be accompanied by a significant loss of function. Severe strains may cause an avulsion of bone from the tendon attachment site.

Joint dislocations

A joint dislocation occurs when the normal articulating ends of two or more bones are displaced (Figure 34-4). Joints that often are dislocated are those of the shoulders, elbows,

Box 34-2

Grading of sprains by severity

First-degree sprain

No joint instability

Minimal swelling/haemorrhage

Second-degree sprain

Joint usually intact

Increased swelling/ecchymosis

Third-degree sprain

Total disruption of ligaments

Possible nerve or vascular compromise

Paediatric fractures are seldom complete breaks. Rather, children's bones tend to bend or buckle because of increased flexibility. This flexibility is due to a thicker periosteum and increased amounts of immature bone.

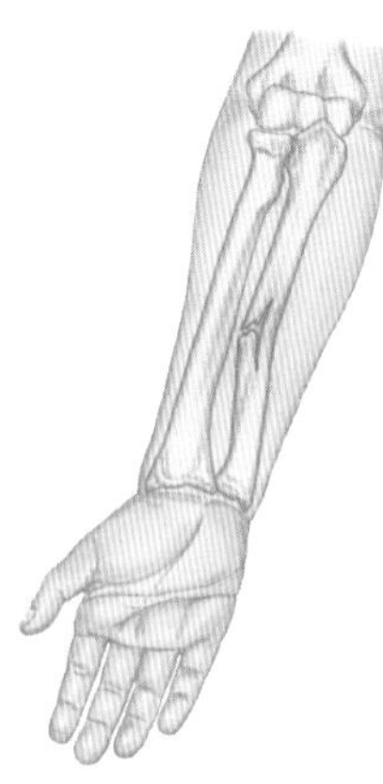

Greenstick

Break occurs through the periosteum on one side of the bone while only bowing or buckling on the other side. Seen most frequently in the forearm.

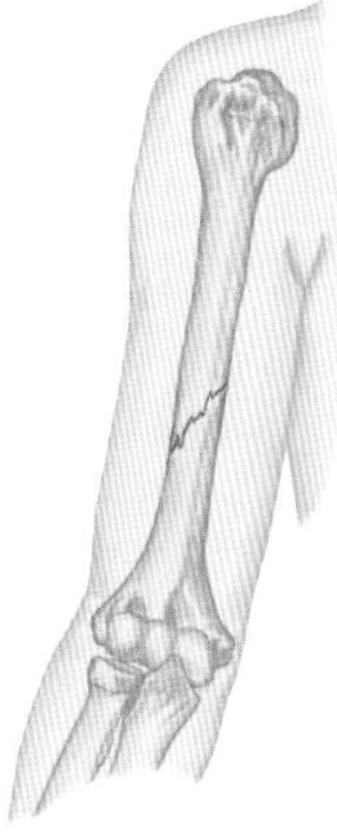

Spiral

Twisted or circular break that affects the length rather than the width. Seen frequently in child abuse.

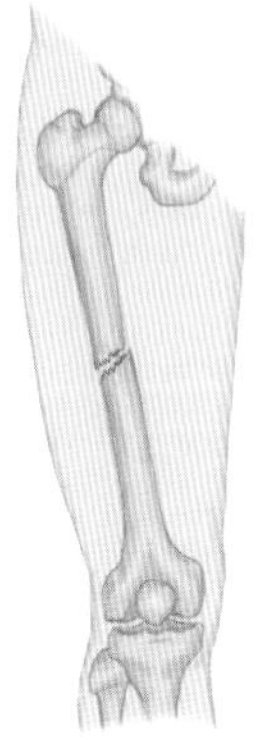

Oblique

Diagonal or slanting break that occurs between the horizontal and perpendicular planes of the bone.

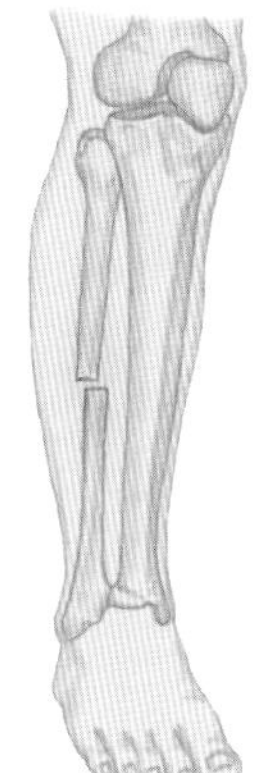

Transverse

Break or fracture line occurs at right angles to the long axis of the bone.

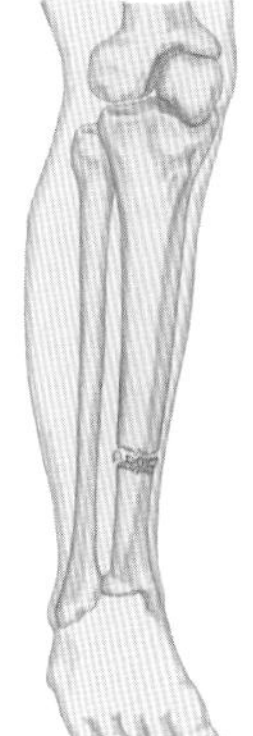

Comminuted

Bone is splintered into pieces. This is a rare occurrence in children.

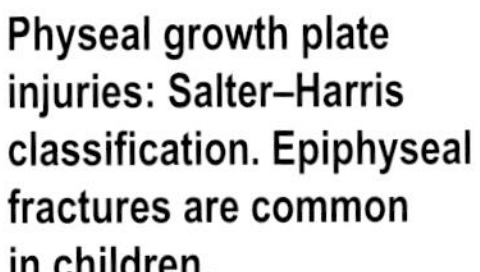

Physeal growth plate injuries: Salter–Harris classification. Epiphyseal fractures are common in children.

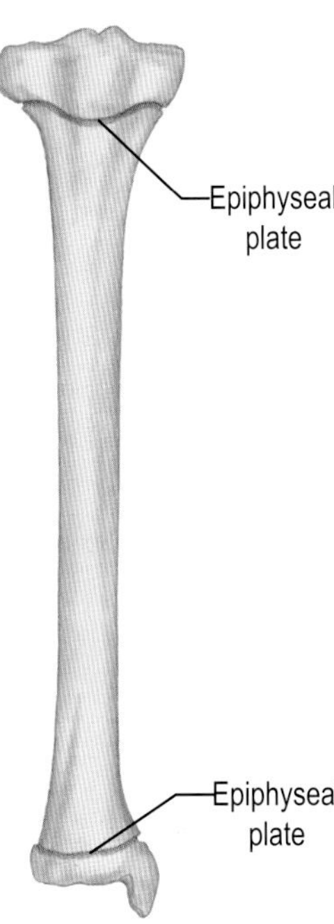

Type I

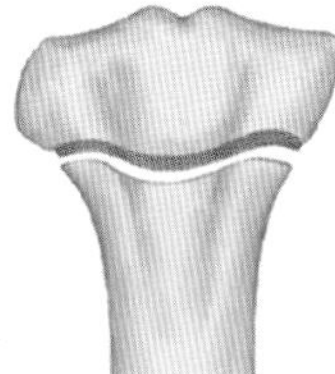

Epiphysis is completely separated from the metaphysis without fracture.

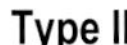

Type II

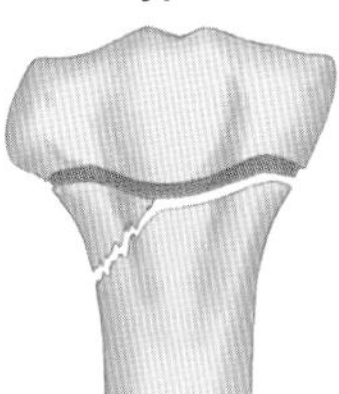

Transverse fracture extends through the separated epiphyseal plate, producing triangular break.

Type III

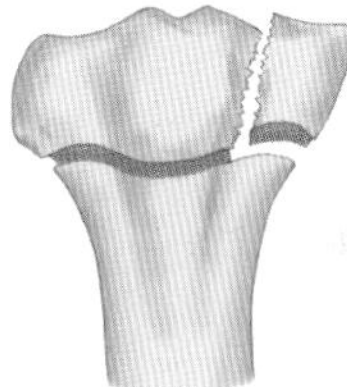

Fracture extends through part of the epiphyseal plate into the joint.

Type IV

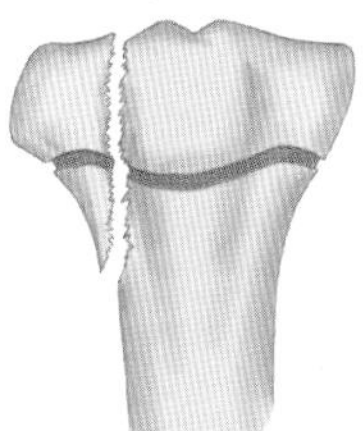

Fracture extends through the epiphyseal plate and through the metaphysis.

Type V

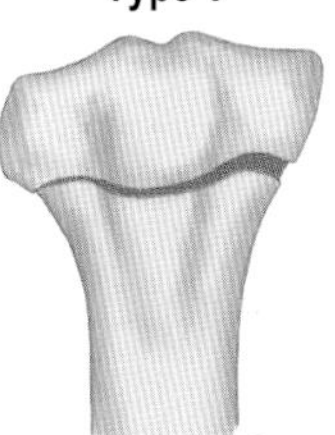

Epiphyseal plate is crushed, causing cell death in growth plate.

Figure 34-1 Bone fractures. Courtesy David J. Mascaro and Associates.

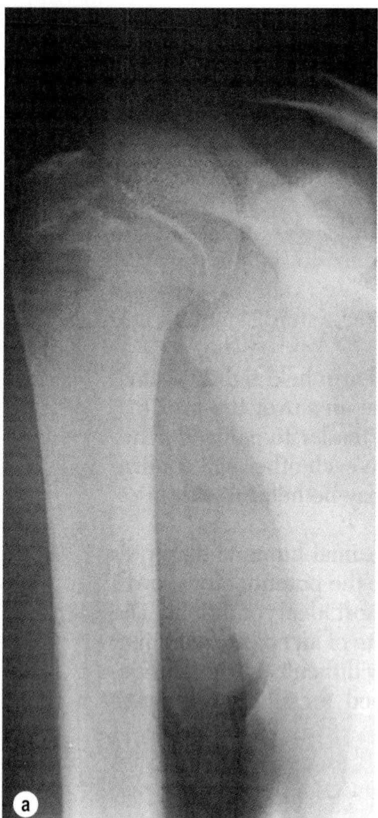

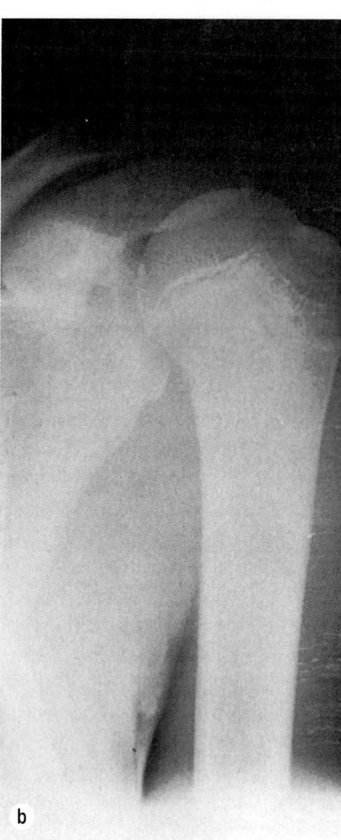

Figure 34-2 (a) Fracture of the proximal humeral epiphysis. Normal left side (b) is included for comparison.

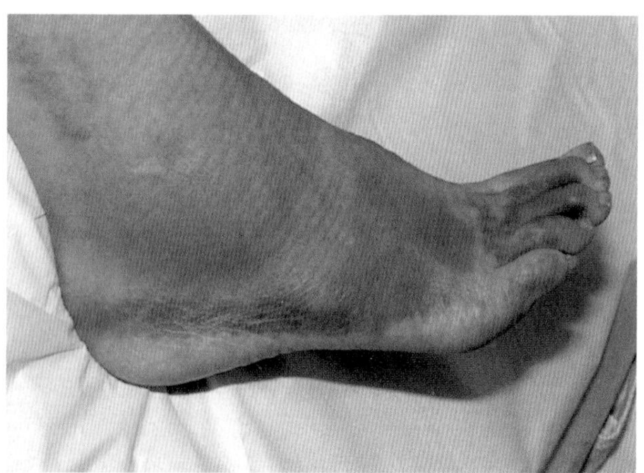

Figure 34-3 Swelling and bruising from a sprain of a lateral ligament.

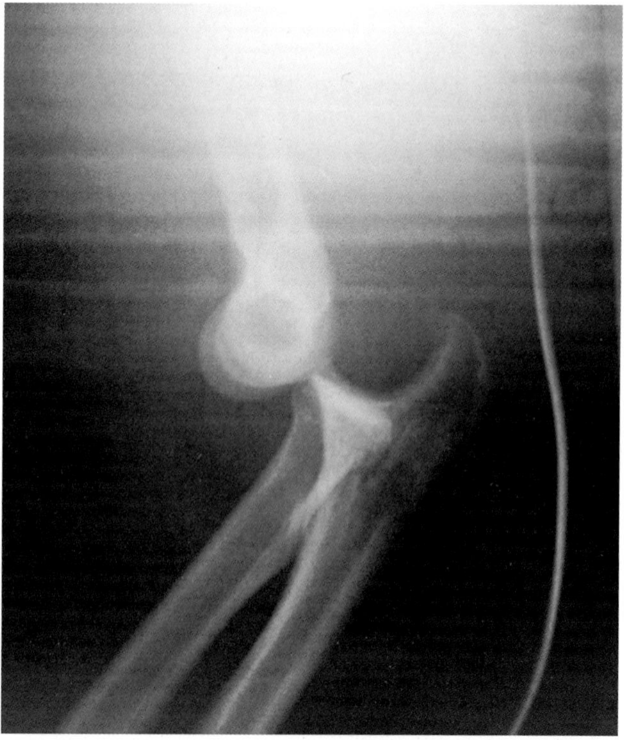

Figure 34-4 Posterior elbow dislocation. With kind permission from Derek Locke.

fingers, hips, knees, and ankles. Dislocation should be suspected when a joint is deformed or does not move with normal range of motion. A complete dislocation is called a luxation; an incomplete dislocation is called a subluxation. All dislocations can result in great damage and instability.

Critical Thinking

Why do dislocations have a high rate of vascular or nerve damage?

Inflammatory and degenerative conditions

Several inflammatory and degenerative conditions (Box 34-3) may manifest as or may be complicated by an extremity injury. These include bursitis, tendonitis, and arthritis.

Bursitis

Bursitis is inflammation of a bursa (a small, fluid-filled sac that acts as a cushion at a pressure point near joints). The most important bursae are around the knee, elbow and shoulder (Figure 34-5). The condition is usually a result of pressure (e.g. prolonged kneeling on a hard surface), friction, or slight injury to the membranes surrounding the joint. Management generally consists of rest, ice, and analgesics. The condition usually subsides after this treatment. In rare cases, bursectomy (surgical excision of a bursa) may be performed.

Tendonitis

Tendonitis is inflammation of a tendon, which is often caused by injury (Figure 34-6). Symptoms include pain, tenderness, and sometimes restricted movement of the muscle attached to the affected tendon (e.g. pain in the shoulder when the arm is raised above a certain angle). Management usually includes non-steroidal anti-inflammatory drugs (NSAID) and sometimes corticosteroid drugs that are injected around the tendon.

Box 34-3

Age-associated changes in bones

As a person ages, morphological changes occur in the bones. Some of the changes may increase the chance of injury or complicate the healing process. These morphological changes include the following:

- A decrease in the water content of the intervertebral discs (increasing the risk of herniation).
- Loss of about 1 to 2 cm (½ to ¾ inch) in height, resulting in a shortened trunk and the formation of an arc-shaped vertebral column that is prone to injury.
- Thoracic rigidity caused by ossification of costal cartilage (may lead to shallow breathing).
- Porous and brittle bones that are prone to fracture.
- Bone disorders (e.g. osteoporosis) that increase the risk of fracture.

Arthritis

Arthritis is inflammation of a joint. It is characterized by pain, swelling, stiffness and redness (see Chapter 39). The condition is not a single disease; rather, the term refers to joint disease (involving one or many joints) that can occur from a number of causes. Arthritis varies in severity from a mild ache and stiffness to severe pain and, later, joint deformity.

Osteoarthritis (degenerative arthritis) is the most common form of arthritis. It results from wear and tear on the joints and begins in middle age. The pain from this condition is generally managed with anti-inflammatory agents.

Rheumatoid arthritis is the most severe type of inflammatory joint disease. It is an autoimmune disorder in which the body's immune system acts against and damages joints and surrounding soft tissues. Many joints, most often those in the hands, feet and arms, become extremely painful, stiff, and deformed (Figure 34-7). Drugs used to treat this condition include NSAID to reduce pain and antirheumatic drugs

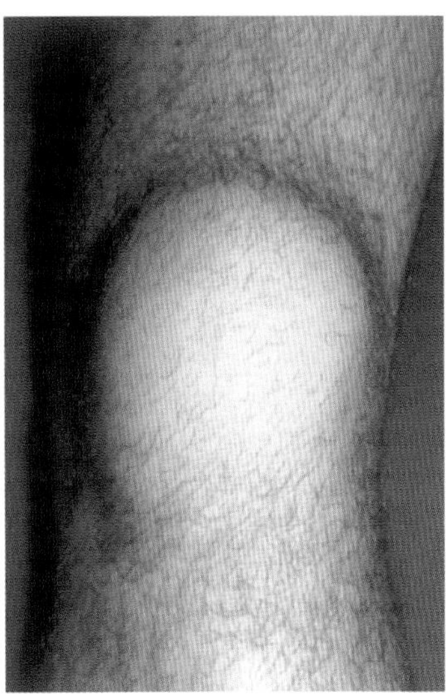

Figure 34-5 Prepatellar bursa (housemaid's knee).

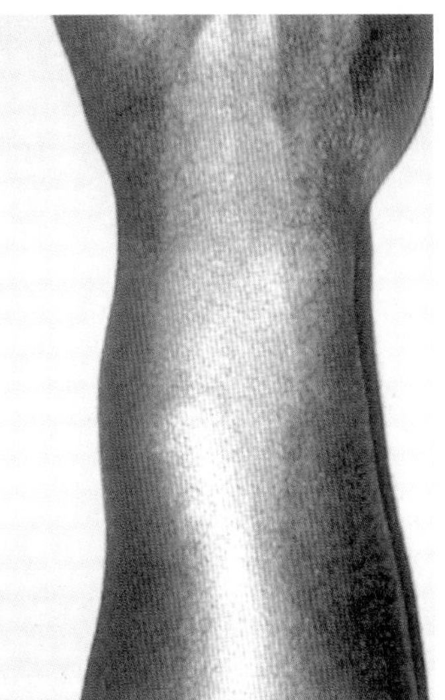

Figure 34-6 Swelling of the tendons over the radial side of the wrist.

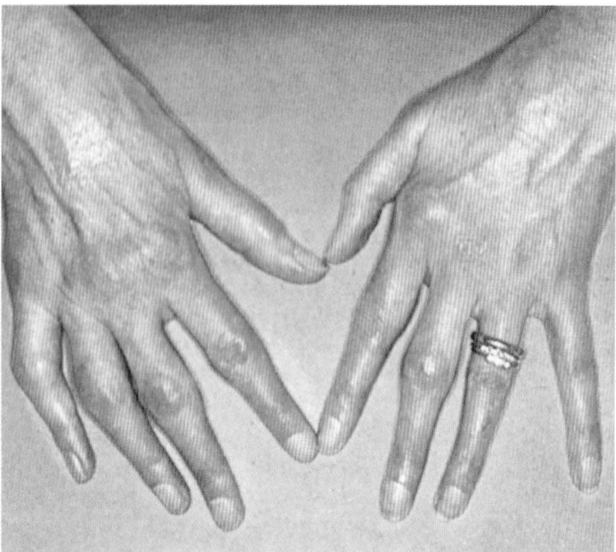

Figure 34-7 Rheumatoid arthritis.

and immunosuppressive agents to arrest or slow the progress of the disease.

Gouty arthritis is a form of joint disease in which uric acid builds up in joints in the form of crystals, causing inflammation. The first attack of this form of arthritis usually involves only one joint (e.g. the base of the big toe). This first attack usually lasts a few days but subsequent attacks may be more severe and may affect more joints (e.g. knee, ankle, wrist, foot, and small joints of the hand). Pain and inflammation from gouty arthritis are controlled with large doses of NSAID or corticosteroid injections. Other treatment may include drugs to prevent the formation of uric acid or to increase its excretion, and diet modifications.

Signs and symptoms of extremity trauma

The signs and symptoms of trauma to an extremity vary from subtle complaints of discomfort to obvious deformity or open fracture. Field evaluation should be rapid, assuming significant injury. Common signs and symptoms of extremity trauma include the following:

- pain on palpation or movement
- swelling, deformity
- crepitus
- decreased range of motion
- false movement (unnatural movement of an extremity)
- decreased or absent sensory perception or circulation distal to the injury (evidenced by alterations in skin colour and temperature, distal pulses and capillary refill).

Critical Thinking

How can a paramedic tell a serious sprain from a fracture in the prehospital setting?

Assessment of musculoskeletal injuries

For the purposes of musculoskeletal assessment, patients can be divided into four classes:

- those with life- or limb-threatening injuries or conditions including life- or limb-threatening musculoskeletal trauma
- those with other life- or limb-threatening injuries and only simple musculoskeletal trauma
- those with no other life- or limb-threatening injuries but with life- or limb-threatening musculoskeletal trauma
- those with only isolated injuries that are not life or limb threatening.

The paramedic should perform an initial assessment to determine whether the patient has any conditions that pose a threat to life. Such conditions must be dealt with first. Paramedics must never overlook musculoskeletal trauma but should never allow a frightful, but non-critical, musculoskeletal injury to distract from the priorities of care.

Evaluation of an injured extremity should always include checking the 'six Ps': pain, pallor, paraesthesia, pulses, paralysis, and pressure (Box 34-4). The paramedic should also evaluate an extremity's neurovascular status by assessing the distal pulse, motor function, and sensation (before and after movement or splinting). In addition, the paramedic should inspect and palpate the injured area for DCAP-BTLS:

Deformity
Contusions
Abrasions
Penetrations or punctures
Burns
Tenderness
Lacerations
Swelling.

If possible, the assessment should include comparison with the opposite, uninjured extremity. If trauma to an extremity is suspected, the extremity should be splinted.

Management

This text presents methods to immobilize fractures and dislocations for isolated extremity injuries. Again, seldom does trauma to an extremity pose a threat to life. Therefore patients with multiple-system traumatic injury should first be managed for conditions that compromise the airway, breathing and circulation (including internal and external haemorrhage in the extremities) and spinal stability. Rapid transport may be indicated by the patient's condition or mechanism of injury. If this is the case, injured extremities can be stabilized by fully immobilizing the patient on a long spine board (Figure 34-8).

General principles of splinting

The goal of splinting is immobilization of the injured body part, which helps alleviate pain; decreases tissue injury, bleeding, and contamination of an open wound; and simplifies and facilitates transport of the patient. The general principles of splinting are listed in Box 34-5.

Types of splints

A wide variety of splints and splinting materials are available. Splints can be broadly categorized as rigid splints, soft or formable splints, and traction splints.

The shape of a rigid splint cannot be changed, so the body part must be positioned to fit the splint's design. Examples of rigid splints include board splints, contoured metal and plastic splints, and some cardboard splints (Figure 34-9). Rigid splints should be padded before use to accommodate for shape and patient comfort.

Soft or formable splints can be moulded into a variety of shapes and configurations to accommodate the injured body part. Examples of soft or formable splints include pillows, blankets, slings and swathes, vacuum splints, some cardboard splints, wire ladder splints, and padded, flexible aluminium splints (Figure 34-10).

Traction splints are specifically designed for midshaft femoral fractures. These splints do not apply or maintain enough traction to reduce a femoral fracture but they provide enough traction to stabilize and align it. Examples include Thomas half-ring, Hare traction and Sager traction splints (Figure 34-11).

Box 34-4

Six Ps of musculoskeletal assessment

Pain or tenderness
Pallor (pale skin or poor capillary refill)
Paraesthesia (pins-and-needles sensation)
Pulses (diminished or absent)
Paralysis (inability to move)
Pressure

Box 34-5

General principles of splinting

1. Splint joints and bone ends above and below the injury.
2. Immobilize open and closed fractures in the same manner.
3. Cover open fractures to minimize contamination.
4. Check pulses, sensation and motor function before and after splinting.
5. Stabilize the extremity with gentle in-line traction to a position of normal alignment.
6. Immobilize a long bone extremity in a straight position that can be splinted easily.
7. Immobilize dislocations in a position of comfort; ensure good vascular supply.
8. Immobilize joints as found; joint injuries are aligned only if no distal pulse is felt.
9. Apply cold to reduce swelling and pain.
10. Apply compression to reduce swelling.
11. Elevate the extremity if possible.

Note: Immobilization requires a minimum of two rescuers.

Upper extremity injuries

Upper extremity injuries can be classified as fractures or dislocations to the shoulder, humerus, elbow, radius and ulna, wrist, hand, and finger (Figure 34-12a–i). Clavicular injury is discussed in Chapter 27. Most upper extremity injuries can be adequately immobilized with a sling and swathe.

Shoulder injury

Shoulder injuries are common in older adults due to a weaker bone structure, and often result from a fall on an outstretched arm. Patients with an anterior fracture or dislocation (accounting for 90% of cases) often have the affected arm and shoulder close to the chest (with the lateral aspect of the shoulder appearing flat instead of rounded). In addition a deep depression between the head of the humerus and the acromion laterally ('hollow shoulder') may be visible. Patients with posterior fracture or dislocation may be found with the arm above the head. Management of shoulder injuries includes the following:

1. Assessment of neurovascular status.
2. Application of a sling and swathe (Figure 34-13).
3. Application of ice.

Note

Ice should be placed in a plastic bag and applied for 20-min periods to the injury site. Refreezable packs of gelled solution are inefficient and should not be used.

Based on the position of the affected arm and shoulder, a makeshift splint may need to be devised to hold the injury in place. For example, with some fractures or dislocations, the paramedic may need to use a rolled blanket with a cravat at the centre. The blanket roll is positioned under the elevated arm and secured like a sling. The arm is then swathed to prevent movement. If the patient's arm is positioned above the head, it should be splinted in position. Alternatively, traction can be applied on the long axis of the arm to obtain a better position for immobilization.

Humeral injury

Upper arm fractures are common in older adults and children and are often difficult to stabilize. Radial nerve damage may be present if a fracture occurs in the middle or distal portion of the humeral shaft. A fracture of the humeral neck may cause axillary nerve damage whilst internal haemorrhage into the joint may be an added complication. Management includes the following measures:

1. Assessment of neurovascular status.
2. Realignment if vascular compromise is present.
3. Application of a rigid splint and sling and swathe (Figure 34-14) or splinting of the extremity with the arm extended.
4. Application of ice.

Elbow injury

Elbow injuries are common in children and athletes. They are especially dangerous in children as they may lead to

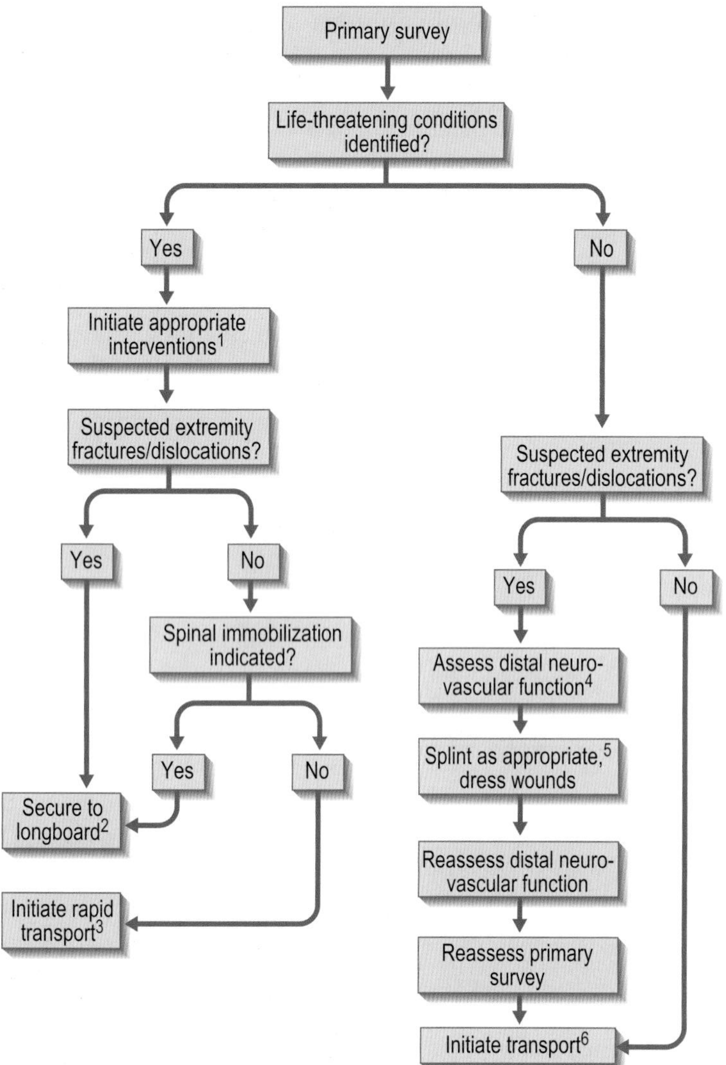

[1]Airway management, ventilatory support, shock therapy.

[2]Injured extremities are immobilized in anatomic position by securing to longboard.

[3]Transport to closest appropriate facility (trauma center, if available); assess distal neurovascular function and apply traction splint (if suspected femur fracture) as time permits.

[4]Assess perfusion (pulses and capillary refilling) and neurologic function (motor and sensory) distal to the suspected fracture or dislocation.

[5]Use appropriate splinting technique to immobilize suspected fracture or dislocation; if suspected midshaft femur fracture, apply traction splint.

[6]Transport to closest appropriate facility.

Figure 34-8 Evaluating extremity trauma.

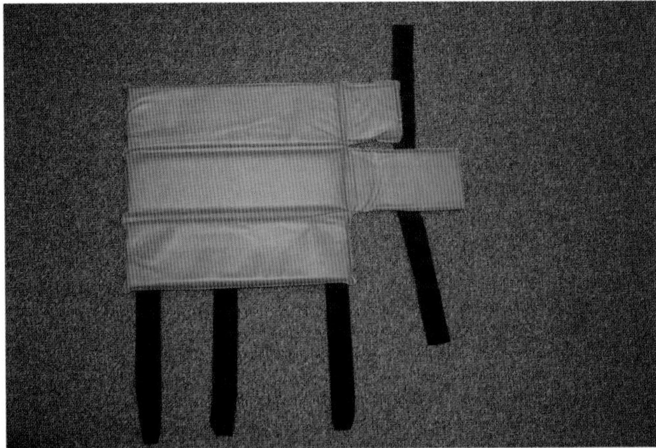

Figure 34-9 Rigid splints.

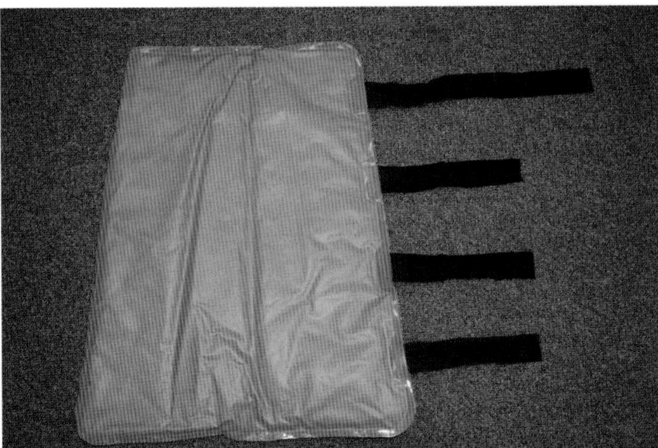

Figure 34-10 Formable splints (vacuum splint).

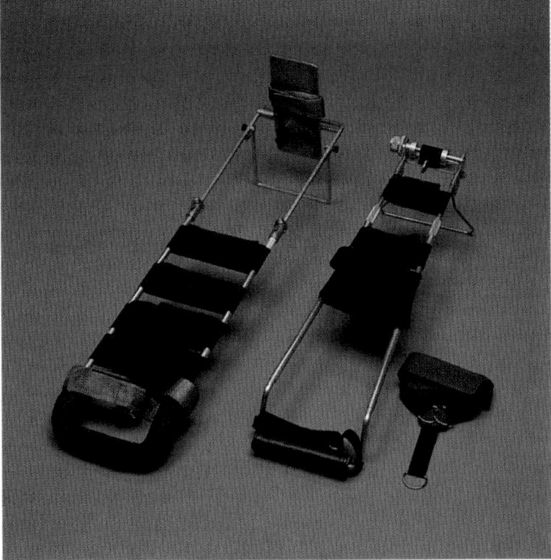

Figure 34-11 Traction splints.

ischaemic contracture (Volkmann contracture) with serious deformity of the forearm and a claw-like hand. The mechanism of injury usually involves falling on an outstretched arm or flexed elbow. Also, laceration of the brachial artery and radial nerve damage can occur. Management includes the following measures:

1. Assessment of neurovascular status.
2. Splinting in the position found with a pillow, blanket, rigid splint, or sling and swathe (Figure 34-15).
3. Application of ice.

Radial, ulnar or wrist injury

As with most other upper extremity injuries, injuries to the radius, ulna and wrist usually result from a fall onto an outstretched arm. Wrist injuries may involve the distal radius, the ulna, or any of the eight carpal bones. The most common wrist injury is a fracture with a 'silver fork' deformity of the distal radius with dorsal angulation (Colles fracture) (Figure 34-16). Forearm injury is common in both children and adults. Management includes the following measures:

1. Assessment of neurovascular status.
2. Splinting in the position found with rigid or formable splints or a sling and swathe (Figure 34-17).
3. Application of ice and elevation.

Critical Thinking

What effect does a cold pack have on musculoskeletal injuries?

Hand (metacarpal) injury

Injury to the hand often results from contact sports, violence (fighting) and work-related crushing injuries. A common metacarpal injury is boxer's fracture. This results from direct trauma to a closed fist, resulting in fracture of the fifth metacarpal bone (Figure 34-18). These injuries may be associated with haematomas and open wounds. Boxer's fracture is the most common metacarpal fracture, but any of the metacarpals can be fractured, depending on the mechanism of injury. Hand injuries should be splinted in the position of function (as with a hand grasping a ball). Rigid or formable splints (previously described for a radial, ulnar or wrist injury) may be used. Management includes the following measures:

1. Assessment of neurovascular status.
2. Splinting with a rigid or formable splint (pillow, blanket) in the position of function.
3. Application of ice and elevation.

Finger (phalangeal) injury

Injured fingers may be immobilized with foam-filled aluminium splints or tongue depressors. They may also be immobilized simply by taping the injured finger to an adjacent one ('buddy splinting') (Figure 34-19). Finger injuries are common; however, they should not be considered trivial. Fractures of the thumb and any open or markedly comminuted fractures of the hand or fingers are serious. Management includes the following measures:

1. Assessment of neurovascular status.
2. Splinting as previously described.
3. Application of ice and elevation.

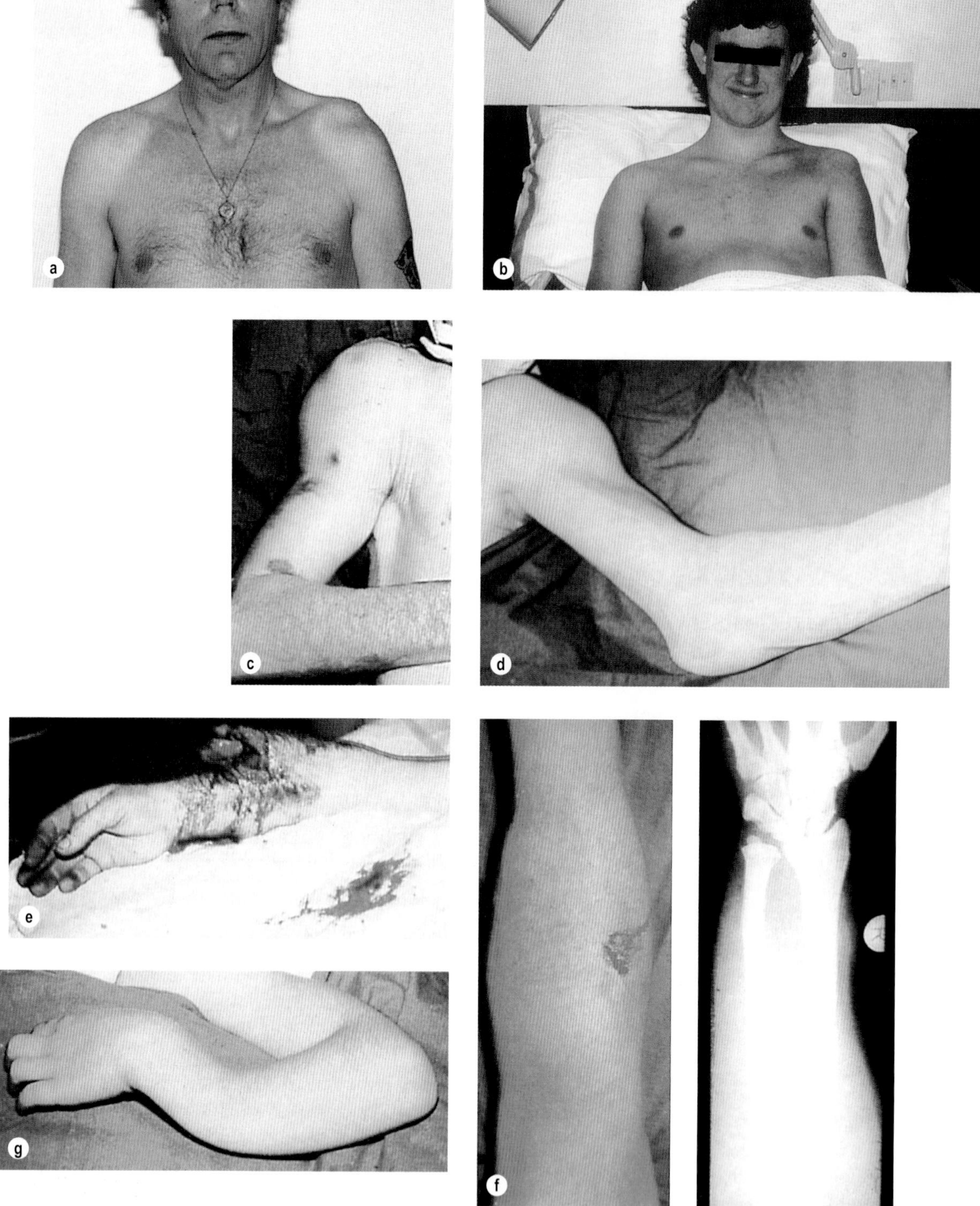

Figure 34-12 (a) Complete separation of the left acromioclavicular joint. (b) Anterior dislocation of the left shoulder. (c) Fracture of the proximal humerus. (d) Posterior dislocation of the elbow joint with marked deformity. (e) Severe open fracture of the forearm. (f) Penetration of the forearm caused by a nail gun. (g) Greenstick fracture with marked deformity.

Lower extremity injuries

Lower extremity injuries include fractures of the pelvis and fractures or dislocations of the hip, femur, knee and patella, tibia and fibula, ankle and foot, and phalanx (Figure 34-20). Compared with upper extremity injuries, lower extremity injuries are associated with greater forces and with greater blood loss. They are more difficult to manage in patients with multiple injuries, and they may be life threatening (e.g. femoral and pelvic fractures).

Pelvic fracture

As described in Chapter 33, blunt or penetrating injury to the pelvis may result in fracture, severe haemorrhage, and associated injury to the urinary bladder and urethra. The

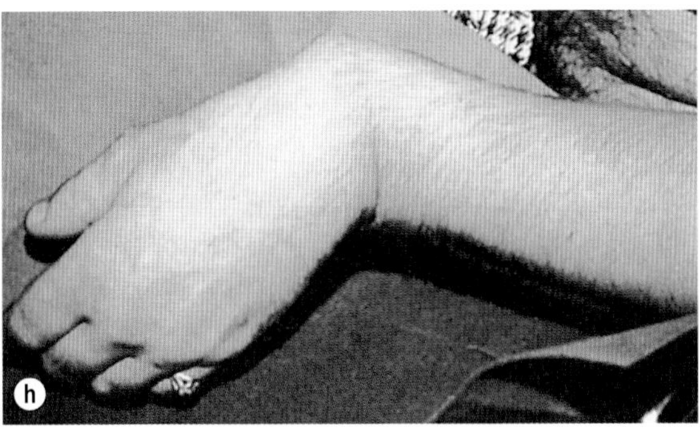

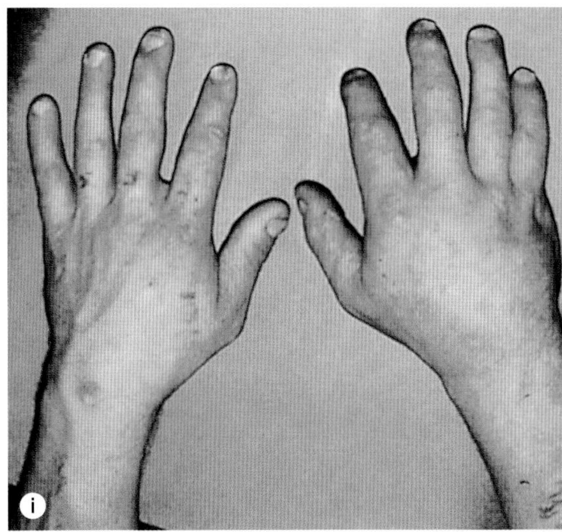

Figure 34-12, cont'd (h) Fracture of the distal radius. (i) Hand injury from a motorcycle crash.

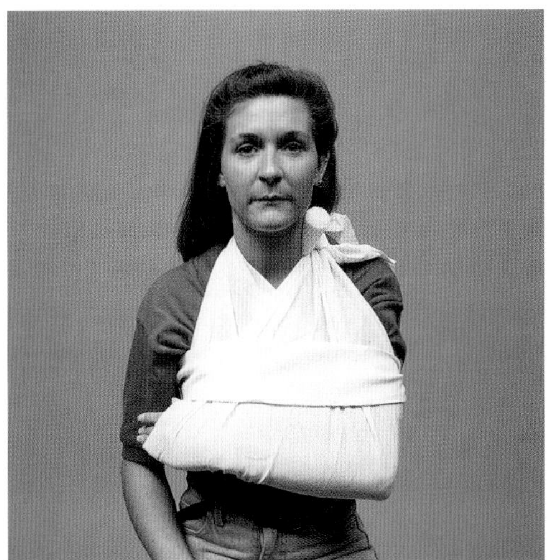

Figure 34-13 Immobilization of the shoulder.

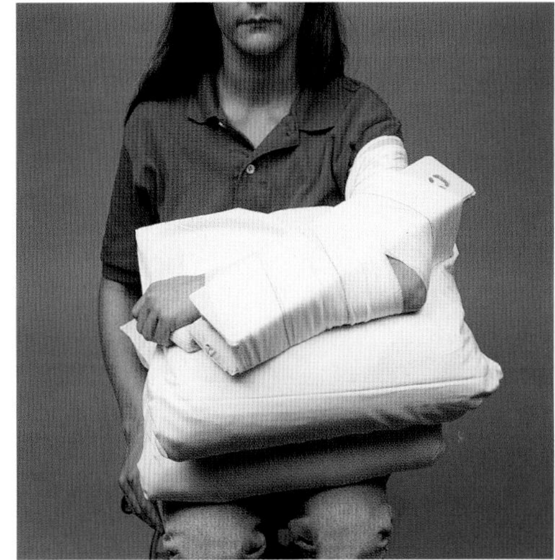

Figure 34-15 Immobilization of the elbow.

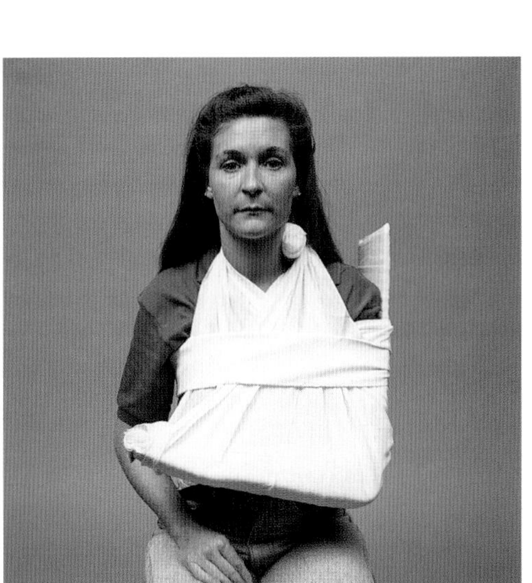

Figure 34-14 Immobilization of the humerus.

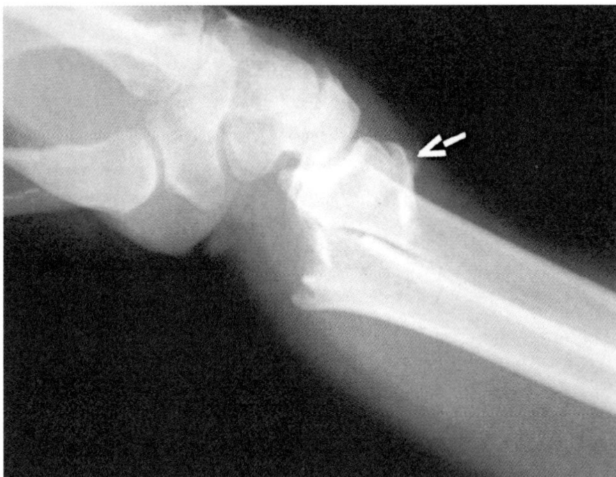

Figure 34-16 Colles fracture (arrow shows dorsal angulation of distal radius fragment).

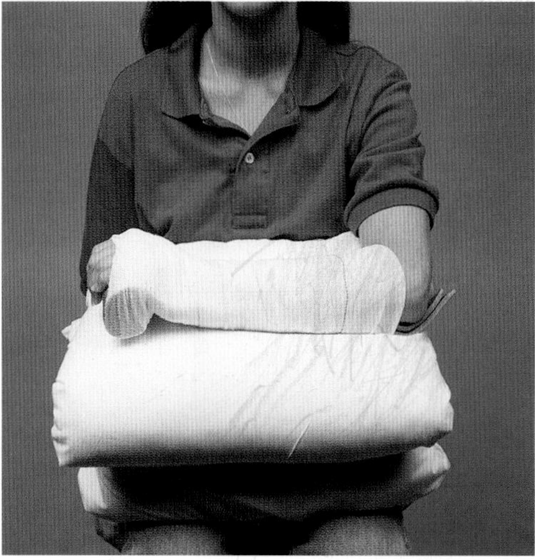

Figure 34-17 Immobilization of the forearm.

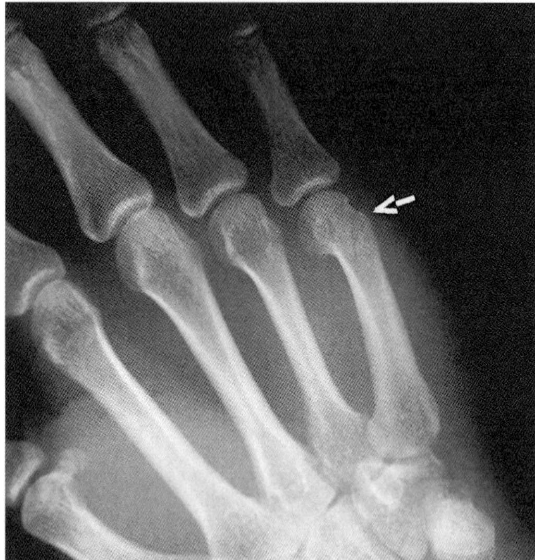

Figure 34-18 Boxer's fracture (arrow).

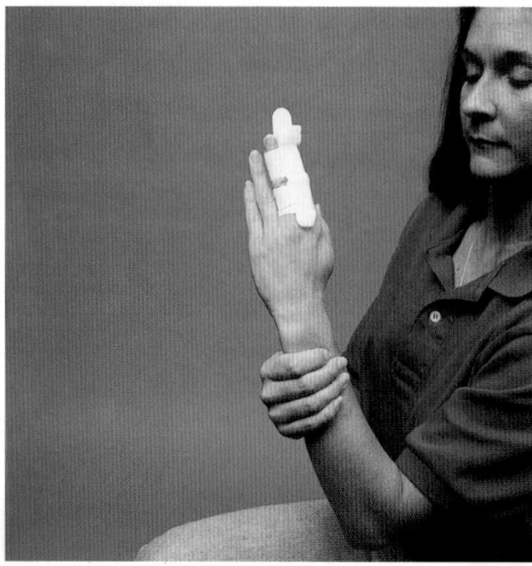

Figure 34-19 Immobilization of the finger.

pelvis is surrounded by heavy muscles and other soft tissues, so deformity may be difficult to see (Figure 34-21). In the alert, cooperative patient without distracting injury, the likelihood of pelvic injury should be assessed based on the mechanism of injury and the presence of pain in the pelvic area, including the lower back (assessing the sacroiliac joint), groin and hips. 'Springing' of the pelvis must NOT be undertaken as it is an unreliable test that may disturb developing clots and propagate further bleeding.[4] Where a history is unobtainable (e.g. an unconscious patient) and the mechanism of injury is indicative of pelvic injury, the paramedic should routinely immobilize the pelvis; palpation is not warranted. Trauma to the abdomen and pelvic area may be complicated by pregnancy (see Chapter 35). Management includes the following measures:

1. Administration of high-concentration oxygen.
2. Management for shock.
3. Full-body immobilization on a vacuum mattress or long spine board (adequately padded for comfort).
4. Regular monitoring of vital signs.
5. Rapid transport (essential).

Hip injury

Hip injuries commonly occur in older adults as a result of a fall. They commonly occur in younger patients as a result of major trauma. If the hip is fractured at the femoral head and neck, the affected leg is usually shortened and externally rotated. By comparison, with hip dislocation the affected leg is usually shortened and internally rotated (Figure 34-22). (Fractures closer to the head of the femur may manifest similar to an anterior hip dislocation, with a shortened and internally rotated leg.) Management includes the following measures:

1. Assessment of neurovascular status.
2. Splinting with a long spine board (Figure 34-23) and generously padding the patient for comfort during transport (slight flexion of the knee or padding beneath the knee may improve comfort).
3. Frequent monitoring of vital signs.
4. Consider fluid replacement with sodium chloride at a keep-open rate.

Femoral injury

Injury to the femur usually results from major trauma, such as may occur with motor vehicle crashes and pedestrian injuries. It may also occur as a result of child abuse.

Fractures of the femur result in powerful thigh muscle contractions, which cause the bone fragments to ride back and forth over each other. The patient generally has a shortened leg that is externally rotated, and midthigh swelling from haemorrhage, which can be life threatening (Figure 34-24). These fractures should be immobilized in the field with a traction splint. Management includes the following measures:

1. Administration of high-concentration oxygen.
2. Management for shock.
3. Assessment of neurovascular status.
4. Application of a traction splint (Figure 34-25).
5. Regular monitoring of vital signs.

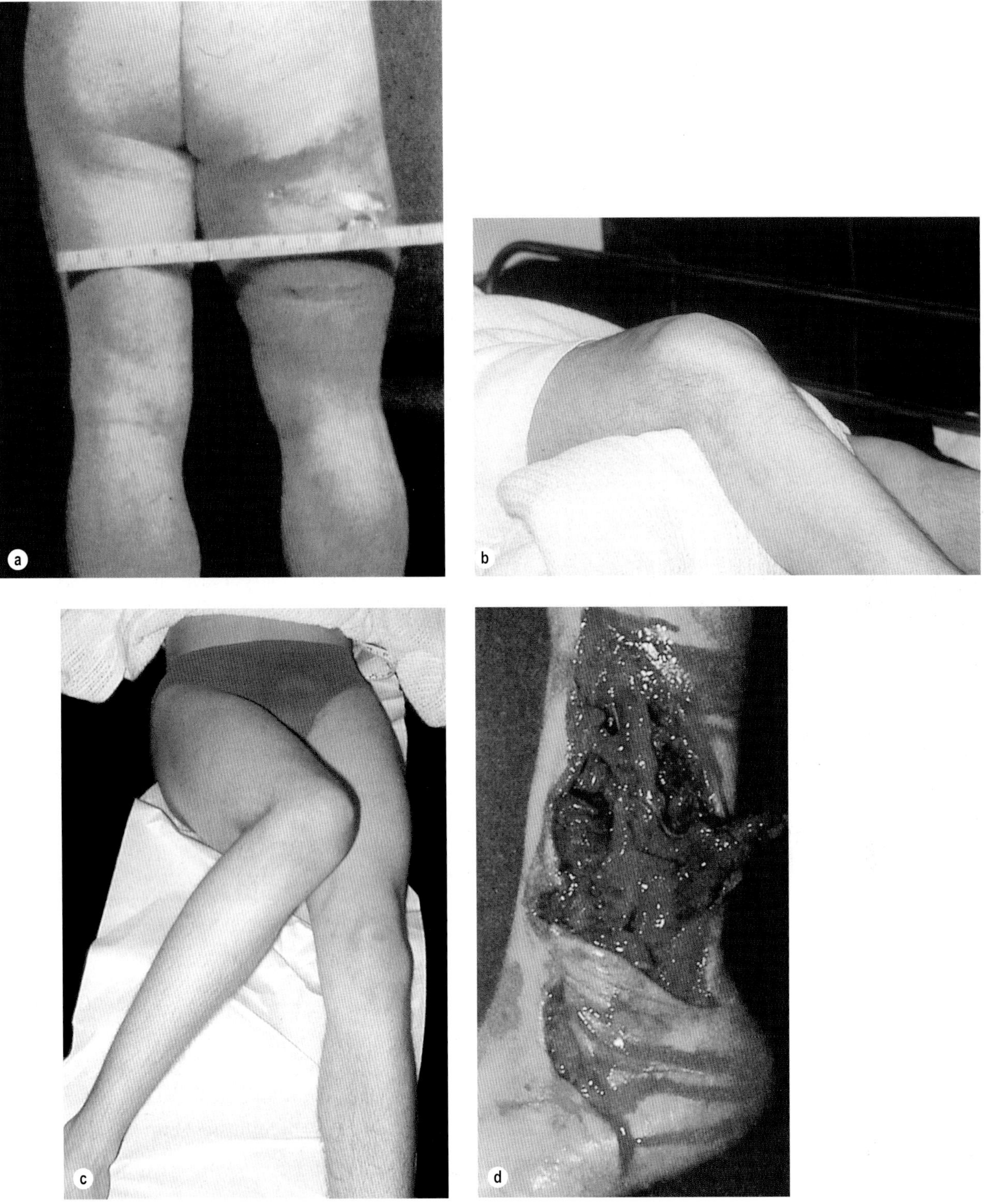

Figure 34-20 (a) The diameter of the right thigh represents an increase in volume of 2 to 3 L of blood. (b) Lateral dislocation of the right patella. (c) Posterior dislocation of the right hip. (d) Open fracture of the lower leg.

Note

Traction splints should be used only to immobilize midshaft femoral fractures. They should not be used with fractures of the lower third of the leg, pelvic fractures, hip injury, knee injury, or avulsion or amputation of the ankle and foot.

Knee and patellar injury

Fractures of the knee (supracondylar fracture of the femur, intra-articular fracture of the femur or tibia) and fractures and dislocations of the patella may result from motor vehicle crashes, pedestrian injuries, contact sports and falls on a flexed knee (Figure 34-26). The popliteal artery is close to the knee joint and may be damaged following injury to the

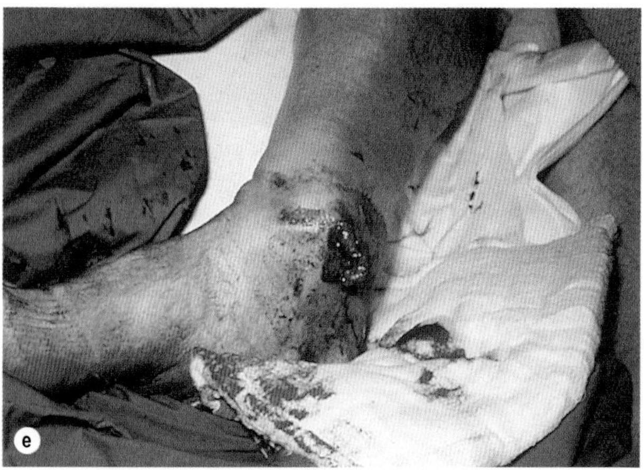
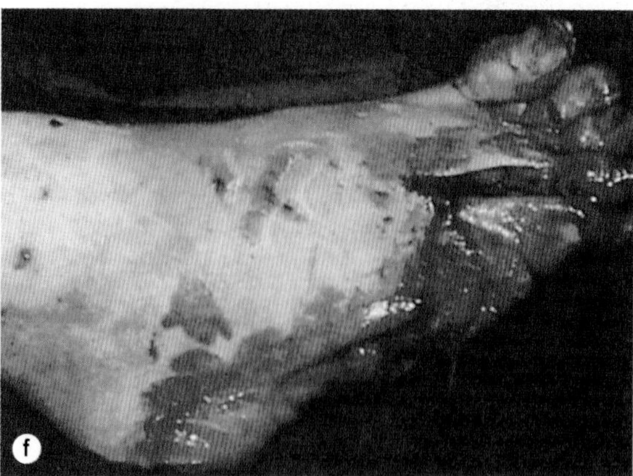

Figure 34-20, cont'd (e) Subtalar dislocation. (f) Foot that was run over by the wheel of a railway carriage.

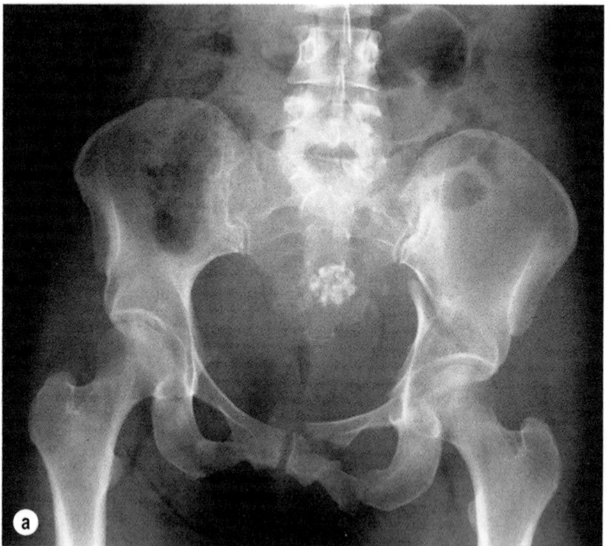
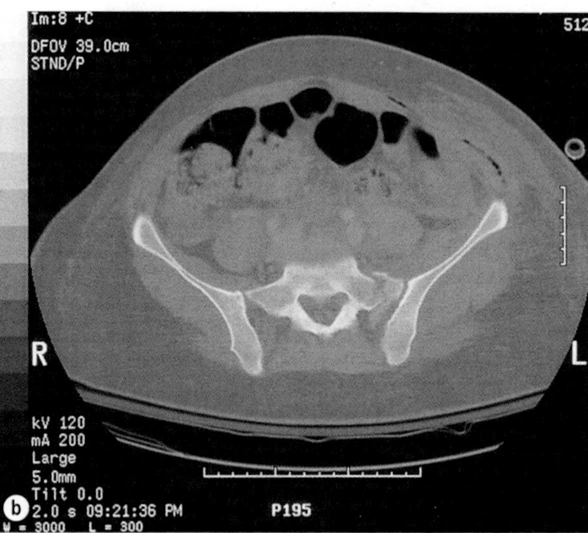

Figure 34-21 Lateral compression injury. (a) Anteroposterior projection demonstrating the characteristic horizontal anterior ring fracture and ipsilateral sacral crush fracture. (b) The sacral fracture is well visualized on the pelvic CT.

knee, particularly with posterior dislocations. Management includes the following measures:

1. Assessment of neurovascular status.
2. Splinting in the position found with a rigid or formable splint (Figure 34-27) that effectively immobilizes the hip and ankle (traction splints should not be used to immobilize a knee or patellar injury).
3. Application of ice and elevation, if possible.

Tibial and fibular injury

Injuries to the tibia and fibula may result from direct or indirect trauma. They also may result from twisting injury (Figure 34-28). If the injury is associated with the knee, popliteal vascular injury should be suspected. Management includes the following measures:

1. Assessment of neurovascular status.
2. Splinting with a rigid or formable splint (Figure 34-29).
3. Application of ice and elevation.

Foot and ankle injury

Fractures and dislocations of the foot and ankle may result from a crush injury, a fall from a height, or a violent rotating or twisting force (Figure 34-30). The patient usually complains of point tenderness. The person also often is hesitant to bear weight on the extremity. Management includes the following measures:

1. Assessment of neurovascular status.
2. Application of a formable splint, such as a pillow, blanket or air splint (Figure 34-31).
3. Application of ice and elevation.

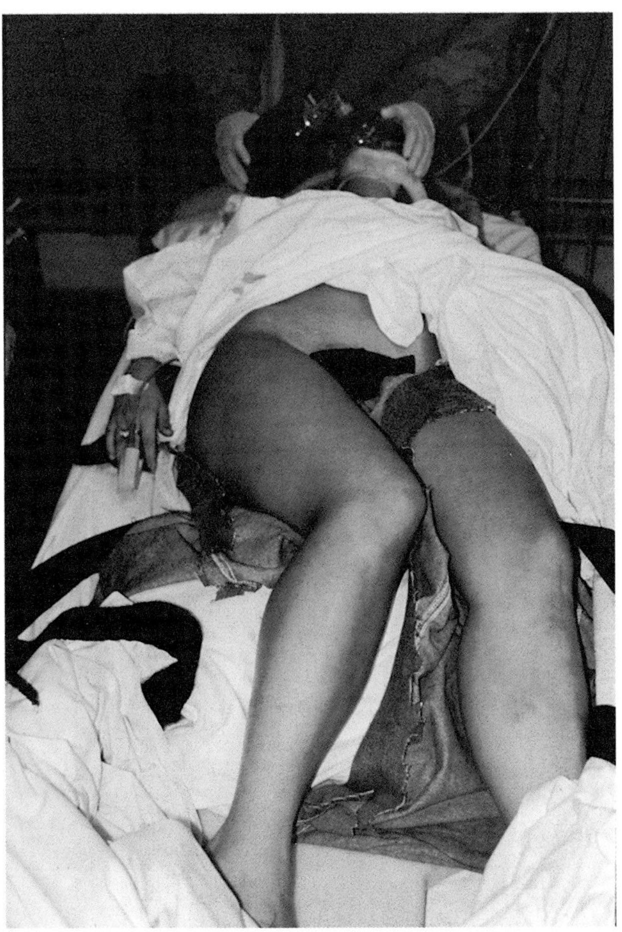

Figure 34-22 Young woman with internal rotation, adduction and shortening of right femur, consistent with her right posterior hip dislocation.

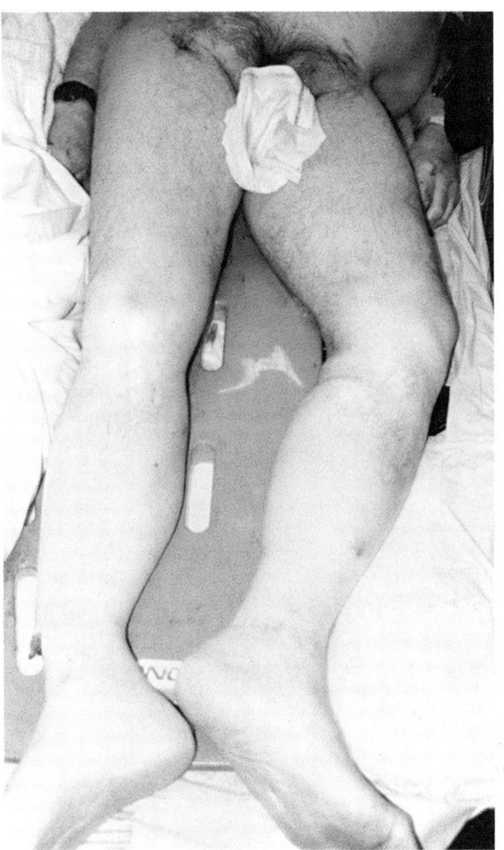

Figure 34-24 Young man with external rotation, abduction and shortening of the left femur, consistent with his midshaft fracture. Also note right tibia fracture.

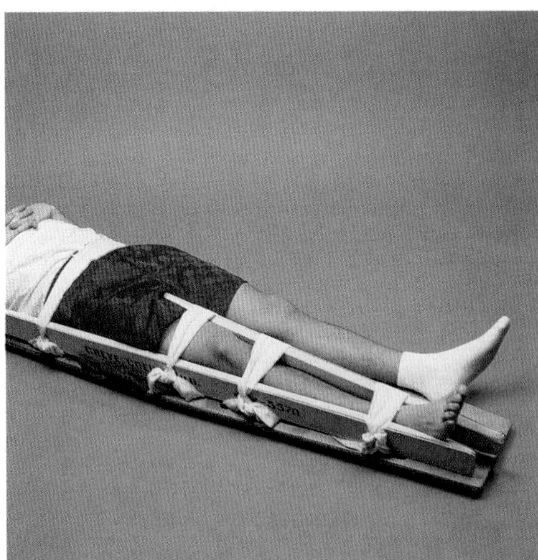

Figure 34-23 Immobilization of the hip.

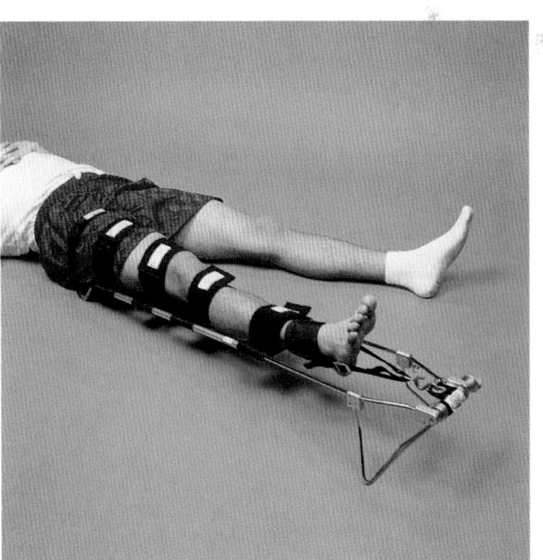

Figure 34-25 Application of a traction splint.

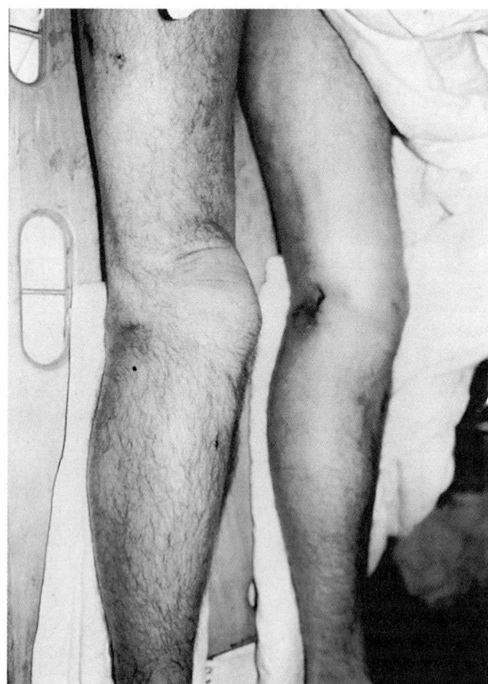

Figure 34-26 Right anterior knee dislocation with overriding of tibia on femur.

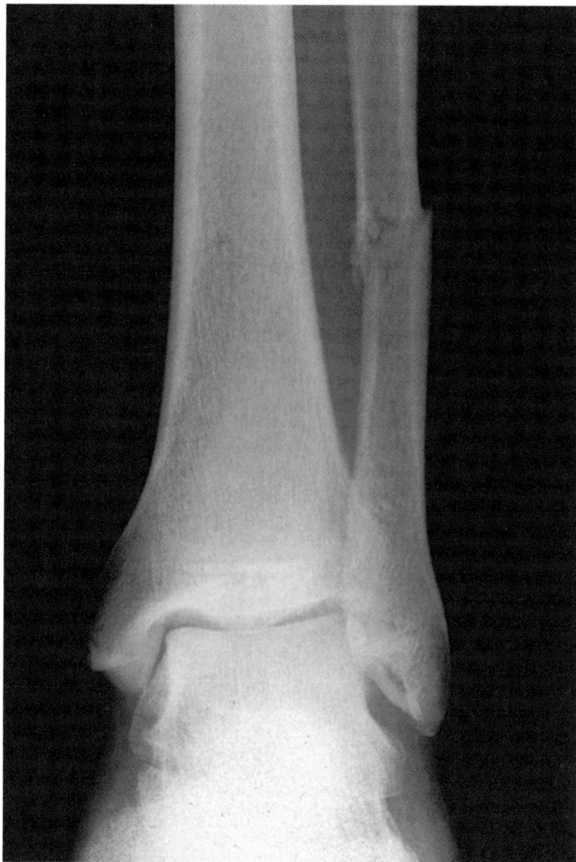

Figure 34-28 Isolated fibular shaft fracture. This patient sustained a direct blow to the lateral leg to produce this transverse fracture. A fracture in this location should arouse suspicion of associated injury to knee ligaments or ankle injury.

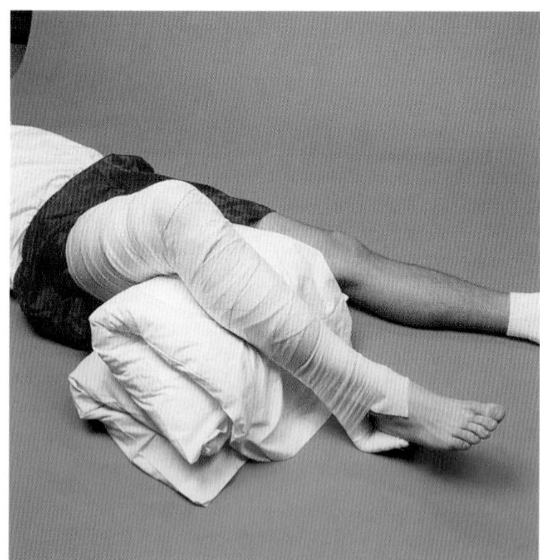

Figure 34-27 Immobilization of the knee.

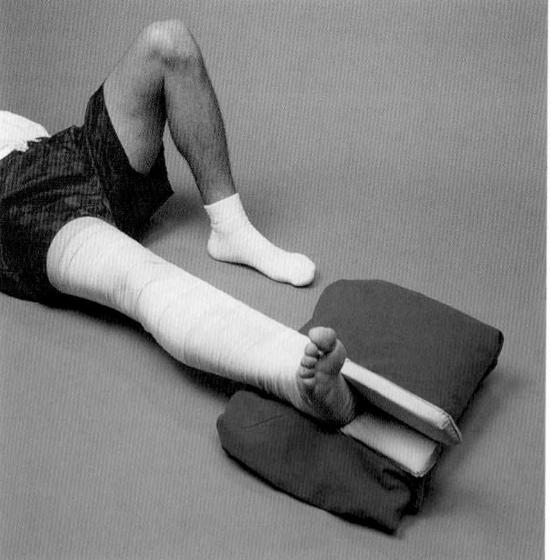

Figure 34-29 Immobilization of the lower leg.

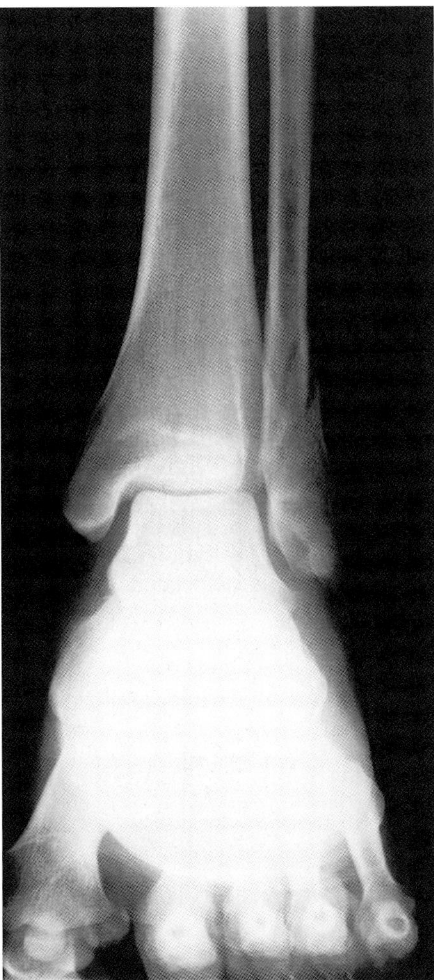

Figure 34-30 Weber B ankle fracture. The fracture lines extend obliquely from the mortise. The medial joint line (between medial malleolus and talus) is somewhat widened. This patient had deltoid ligament rupture and was later treated with surgery.

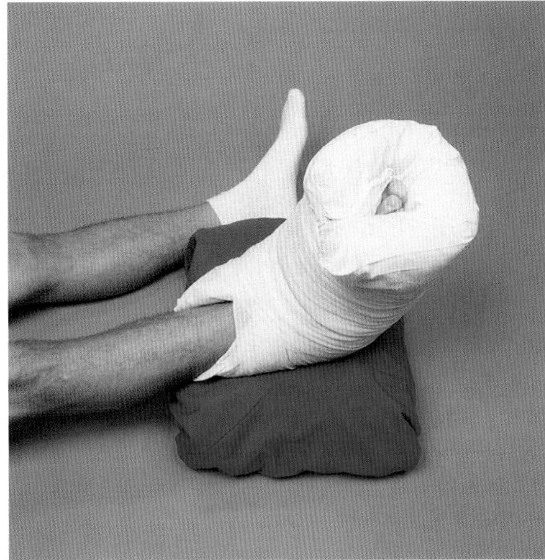

Figure 34-31 Immobilization of the foot and ankle.

Phalangeal injury

Toe injuries are often caused by 'stubbing' the toe on an immovable object. These injuries are usually managed by buddy taping the toe to an adjacent toe, which helps to support and immobilize the injury. Management includes the following measures:

1. Assessment of neurovascular status.
2. Buddy splinting.
3. Application of ice and elevation.

Open fractures

Patients with open fractures require special care and evaluation by the paramedic. Fractures may be opened in two ways: from within, as when a bone fragment pierces the skin, or from without (e.g. after a gunshot wound). An open fracture may also have made contact with the skin some distance from the fracture site. Although most open fractures are obvious because of associated haemorrhage, a small puncture wound may not be immediately apparent, and bleeding may be minimal. Therefore the paramedic must consider any soft tissue wound in the area of a suspected fracture to be evidence of an open fracture.

Open fractures are considered a true surgical emergency because of the potential for infection. It is generally agreed that open wounds associated with fractures should be covered with sterile, dry dressings. They should not be irrigated in the field or soaked with any type of antiseptic solution. Haemorrhage should be controlled with direct pressure and pressure dressings.

If a bone end or bone fragment is visible, it should be covered with a dry, sterile dressing and splinted. Bone ends that slip back into the wound during immobilization should be noted and reported to the receiving hospital so that the bone can be cleaned in surgery.

Straightening angular fractures and reducing dislocations

Angular fractures and dislocations may make it difficult to apply a splint. In some cases they also may make it difficult to extricate and transport a patient. Paramedics may need to attempt manipulation of a fracture or dislocation to aid transport or to improve circulation to the injured extremity.

Note

Limb-threatening injuries include knee dislocation, fracture or dislocation of the ankle, and subcondylar fractures of the elbow.[3] These serious injuries require rapid transport for evaluation by a physician.

Critical Thinking

Aside from narcotic analgesics, what other drugs may be indicated to relieve muscle spasm, provide anaesthesia and relax the patient while a dislocation or fracture is reduced?

As a rule, fractures and dislocated joints should be immobilized in the position of injury, and the patient should be transported as quickly as possible to the emergency department for realignment (reduction). However, if transport is delayed or prolonged, and if circulation is impaired, an attempt should be made to reposition a grossly deformed fracture or dislocated joint. The exception is the elbow. The elbow should never be manipulated in the pre-hospital setting. A grossly deformed fracture or dislocation elsewhere can often be realigned if required. This can usually be done without causing more damage or extreme discomfort to the patient. The injury should be handled carefully, and gentle, firm traction should be applied in the direction of the long axis of the extremity. If obvious resistance to alignment is felt, the extremity should be splinted without repositioning.

THE FOLLOWING TECHNIQUES SHOULD ONLY BE CARRIED OUT BY THOSE WHO HAVE BEEN TRAINED AND AUTHORIZED TO USE THE TECHNIQUES.

Specific techniques for specific joints

A brief description of specific techniques for realigning extremity injuries is provided in the following discussion.[3] Only one attempt at realignment should be made and should be done only if severe problems with nerve or vascular function are present (e.g. extremely weak or absent distal pulses). Manipulation (if indicated) should be performed as soon as possible after the injury. It should not be performed if the patient has other severe injuries. If not contraindicated by other injuries, the use of analgesics (e.g. morphine) for the realignment procedure should be considered. The paramedic should always assess and document pulse, sensation and motor function before and after manipulating any injured extremity or joint.

Finger realignment

1. Apply in-line traction along the shaft of the finger.
2. Continue with slow, steady traction until the finger is realigned and the patient feels relief from pain.
3. Immobilize the finger with a splint device or by buddy splinting.

Shoulder realignment

1. Attempt realignment only in the absence of severe back injury.
2. Check circulatory and sensory status.
3. Apply slow, gentle longitudinal traction, with countertraction exerted on the axilla.
4. Slowly bring the extremity to the midline. (Do not apply force.) Realign in the anatomical position while maintaining traction.
5. Immobilize with a sling and swathe.

Hip realignment

1. Apply in-line traction along the shaft of the femur with the hip and knee flexed at 90 degrees.
2. Continue with slow, steady traction to relax the muscle spasm. Successful realignment is indicated by a 'pop' into the joint, a sudden relief of pain, and easy manipulation of the leg to full extension.
3. Immobilize the leg in full extension with the patient positioned on a long spine board. Re-evaluate pulses and neurovascular status.
4. If full extension is not achieved, immobilize the leg at a flexion not to exceed 90 degrees with pillows or blankets. Place the patient supine.

Knee realignment

1. Apply gentle, steady traction while moving the injured joint into normal position.
2. Successful realignment is indicated by a 'pop' into the joint, resolution of deformity, relief of pain, and increased mobility.
3. Immobilize the leg in full extension (or slight flexion for comfort). Position the patient supine on a long spine board.

A knee dislocation should not be confused with a patellar dislocation (patellar dislocation is not a limb-threatening injury). An attempt should be made to reposition a dislocation of the knee into anatomical position if transport time is delayed or prolonged more than 2 h. This should be done even if distal circulation is normal. Realignment should not be attempted if the dislocation is associated with other severe injuries.[3]

Ankle realignment

1. Apply in-line traction on the talus while stabilizing the tibia.
2. Successful realignment is noted by a sudden rotation to a normal position.
3. Immobilize the ankle in the same manner as for a fracture.

Referral of patients with minor musculoskeletal injury

Some patients with a minor musculoskeletal injury (e.g. a minor sprain) do not require transport by emergency medical services. The decision not to transport is often made by an emergency care practitioner but may, on occasion, be made by a paramedic. To make this determination, the paramedic should follow these guidelines:

- Evaluate the need for immobilization.
- Evaluate the need for radiography. This is based on the patient's condition and the mechanism of injury.
- Evaluate the need for emergency department assessment versus the patient going to his or her general practitioner. This is based on the patient's condition and the mechanism of injury.
- Consider the need for medical advice prior to leaving the patient.

Patients who are not transported to the hospital should be given advice on how to care for the injury. (An instruction sheet should explain techniques for immobilization, elevation, cold, heat, rest, use of analgesics and indications for physician follow-up.) If any doubt exists about the seriousness of the patient's injury, the person should be transported to the emergency department for evaluation by a physician.

Critical Thinking

What should be documented for calls involving minor musculoskeletal injuries?

Summary

- Injuries that can result from traumatic force on the musculoskeletal system include fractures, sprains, strains and joint dislocations. Problems associated with musculoskeletal injuries include haemorrhage, instability, loss of tissue, simple laceration and contamination, interruption of blood supply, and long-term disability.
- Several inflammatory and degenerative conditions may manifest as or may be complicated by extremity injury. These include bursitis, tendonitis and arthritis.
- Common signs and symptoms of extremity trauma include pain on palpation or movement, swelling or deformity, crepitus, decreased range of motion, false movement, and decreased or absent sensory perception or circulation distal to the injury.
- Once the paramedic has assessed for life-threatening conditions, the extremity injury should be examined for pain, pallor, paraesthesia, pulses, paralysis and pressure. In addition, DCAP-BTLS should be evaluated for the injured extremity.
- Immobilization by splinting helps alleviate pain; reduces tissue injury, bleeding, and contamination of an open wound; and simplifies and facilitates transport of the patient. Splints can be categorized as rigid, soft or formable, and traction splints.
- Upper extremity injuries can be classified as fractures or dislocations of the shoulder, humerus, elbow, radius and ulna, wrist, hand and finger. Most upper extremity injuries can be adequately immobilized by application of a sling and swathe.
- Lower extremity injuries include fractures of the pelvis and fractures or dislocations of the hip, femur, knee and patella, tibia and fibula, ankle and foot, and toes.
- Most open fractures are obvious because of associated haemorrhage. However, a small puncture wound may not be initially apparent. In addition, bleeding may be minimal. The paramedic must consider any soft tissue wound in the area of a suspected fracture to be evidence of an open fracture. Open fractures are considered a true surgical emergency due to the potential for infection.
- Only one attempt at realignment should be made. This should be done only if severe neurovascular compromise is present (e.g. extremely weak or absent distal pulses) and if the practitioner is trained and competent in the techniques.
- The paramedic should evaluate the need for emergency department assessment versus having the patient see his or her general practitioner. This need is determined by the patient's condition and the mechanism of injury.

References

1. Fitzsimmons CR, Wardrope J 2005 The ABC of community emergency care: assessment and care of musculoskeletal problems. Emerg Med J 22:68–76
2. Rosen P, Barkin R 2003 Emergency medicine: concepts and clinical practice, 5th edition. Mosby, St Louis
3. US Department of Transportation, National Highway Traffic Safety Administration 1998 EMT-paramedic national standard curriculum. US Department of Transportation, Washington, DC
4. Lee C, Porter K 2007 The prehospital management of pelvic fractures. Emerg Med J 24:130–133

Further reading

Emergency Nurses Association and Newberry L 2003 Sheehy's emergency nursing: principles and practice, 5th edition. Mosby, St Louis

Ferrera PC, Colucciello S, Marx J et al 2001 Trauma management: an emergency medicine approach. Mosby, St Louis

National Association of Emergency Medical Technicians 2003 PHTLS: basic and advanced prehospital life support, 5th edition. Mosby, St Louis

Roberts J, Hedges J 2009 Clinical procedures in emergency medicine, 5th edition. WB Saunders, Philadelphia

PART SEVEN

CHAPTER **35**

Gynaecology

Chapter contents

Objectives

Upon completion of this chapter, the paramedic student will be able to:

1. Describe the physiological processes of menstruation and ovulation.
2. Describe the pathophysiology of the following non-traumatic causes of abdominal pain in females: pelvic inflammatory disease, ruptured ovarian cyst, cystitis, dysmenorrhoea, mittelschmerz, endometriosis, ectopic pregnancy, vaginal bleeding.
3. Describe the pathophysiology of traumatic causes of abdominal pain in females, including vaginal bleeding and sexual assault.
4. Outline the prehospital assessment and management of the female with abdominal pain.
5. Outline specific assessment and management for the patient who has been sexually assaulted.
6. Describe specific prehospital measures to preserve evidence in sexual assault cases.

Key terms

caesarean delivery A surgical procedure in which the abdomen and uterus are incised and the baby is delivered transabdominally.

dilation and curettage A gynaecological procedure that refers to widening of the uterine cervix and scrapping away of the endometrium of the uterus.

endometrium The mucous membrane lining of the uterus, which changes in thickness and structure with the menstrual cycle.

hysterectomy The surgical removal of the uterus.

menarche The first menstruation and commencement of the cyclic menstrual function.

menopause The cessation of menses.

menstruation The periodic discharge through the vagina of a blood secretion containing tissue debris from the shedding of the endometrium from the non-pregnant uterus.

ovulation The release of an ovum or secondary oocyte from the vesicular follicle.

sexual assault The forcible perpetration of an act of sexual contact on the body of another person, male or female, without his or her consent.

A number of disorders can occur in the female reproductive system. Some of these can lead to gynaecological emergencies. This chapter explains the causes of and emergency care for common problems associated with the female reproductive system.

Organs of the female reproductive system

The female reproductive organs include the ovaries, fallopian tubes, uterus, vagina, external genital organs and mammary glands. (Figure 35-1 provides a review of these structures.)

Menstruation and ovulation

Menstruation

Menstruation is the normal, periodic discharge of blood, mucus and cellular debris from the uterine mucosa. The normal menstrual cycle lasts about 28 days and occurs at more or less regular intervals from puberty to menopause (except during pregnancy and lactation). The average menstrual flow is 25–60 mL. The flow usually lasts 4–6 days and is fairly constant from cycle to cycle. The onset of menses (menarche) generally begins between ages 12 and 13. Menstruation ends permanently (menopause) at an average age of 47 years, although age may vary from ages 35 to 60 years (Box 35-1).

Follicle and oocyte development

By the fourth prenatal month, the ovaries contain about 5 million cells. From these cells, oocytes (immature ova) develop. At birth, there are about 2 million primary oocytes but these decline in number to 40 000 at puberty.[1] Of these primary oocytes, only about 400 will mature and ovulate during a woman's reproductive life. Oocytes are surrounded by a layer of cells (granulosa cells). The entire structure is known as a primary follicle (Figure 35-2).

The menstrual cycle is associated with hormonal changes. These changes stimulate some of the primary follicles to continue development and become secondary follicles. A secondary follicle continues to enlarge, which forms a lump on the surface of the ovary. The fully mature follicle is known as the vesicular, or graafian, follicle.

Ovulation

Cellular secretions of the graafian follicle cause it to swell more rapidly than can be accommodated by follicular growth. The follicle expands and ruptures, forcing a small amount of blood and follicular fluid out of the vesicle. Shortly after this initial burst of fluid, an oocyte escapes from the follicle. The release of this secondary oocyte is termed ovulation.

After ovulation the follicle is transformed into a yellow glandular structure called the corpus luteum. The cells of this structure secrete large amounts of progesterone and some oestrogen. If pregnancy occurs, the fertilized oocyte (zygote) begins releasing a hormone-like substance (chorionic gonadotropin). This substance keeps the corpus luteum

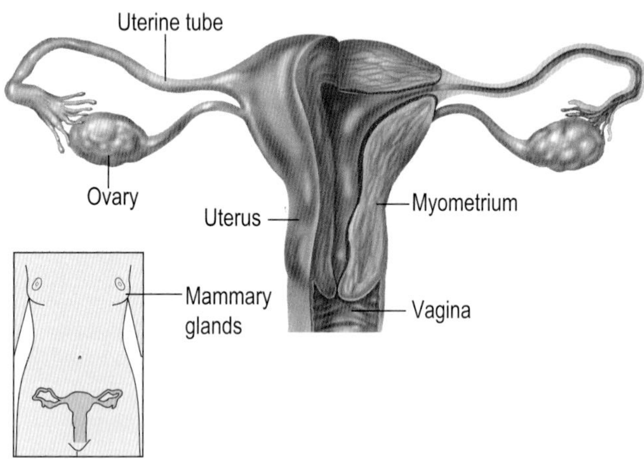

Figure 35-1 Female reproductive organs.

Box 35-1

Hysterectomy

Hysterectomy is the surgical removal of the uterus. In the financial year 2007/08 there were over 38 000 hysterectomies carried out in NHS hospitals in England.[8] Hysterectomy is most often performed to treat fibroid tumours that have caused symptoms and cancer of the uterus or cervix. Other indications for the surgery include heavy menstrual bleeding, endometriosis, pelvic inflammatory disease, and the removal of a prolapsed uterus, Depending on the type of hysterectomy, the surgery may be performed through the abdomen or vagina or laparoscopically.

In a *subtotal hysterectomy*, only the upper part of the uterus is removed; the cervix is not (the fallopian tubes and ovaries may or may not be removed). In a *total hysterectomy* (also called a complete hysterectomy), the body of the uterus, the cervix, the fallopian tubes and the ovaries are removed. If cancer is present or in advanced stage, a *radical hysterectomy* may be required, in which the pelvic lymph nodes and lymph channels are also removed. After a hysterectomy, women are unable to bear children, do not menstruate, and need no contraception.

Serious complications can occur from the surgery; these include blood clots, infection, adhesions, postoperative haemorrhage, bowel obstruction or injury to the urinary tract. In addition to the direct surgical risks, there may be long-term physical and psychological effects. Examples of such include depression and loss of sexual pleasure. If the ovaries are removed along with the uterus before menopause, the risk of developing osteoporosis and heart disease may be increased.

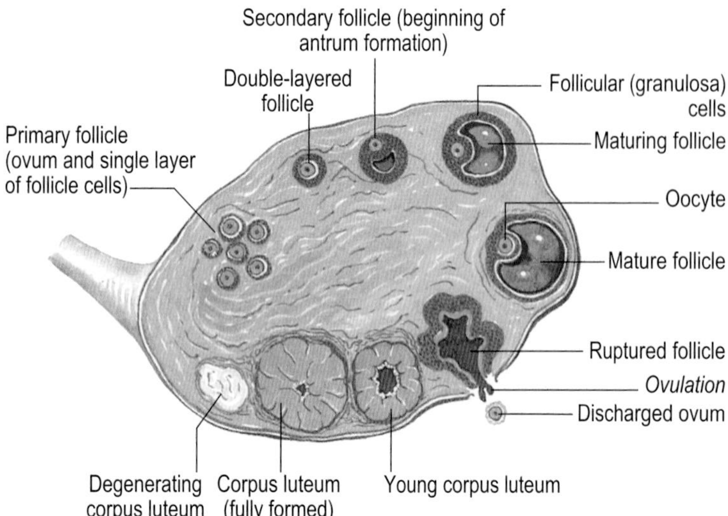

Figure 35-2 Diagram of ovary and oogenesis. Cross-section of mammalian ovary shows successive stages of ovarian (graafian) follicle and ovum development. Begin with the first stage (primary follicle) and follow around clockwise to the final stage (degenerating corpus luteum).

from degenerating. As a result, blood levels of oestrogen and progesterone do not decrease. Moreover, the menstrual period does not occur. In the absence of pregnancy the corpus luteum degenerates. The secondary oocyte passes out of the system with the menstrual flow.

Hormonal control of ovulation and menses

Hormones released from the hypothalamus and anterior pituitary control ovulation and menses. Follicle-stimulating hormone stimulates development of the follicle and stimulates the cells that produce oestrogen. Before ovulation, these cells release oestrogen and cause a surge in the pituitary production of luteinizing hormone. This initiates the ovarian cycle (and leads to ovulation), which in turn regulates the uterine cycle (Figure 35-3). Under the influence of the ovarian hormones, the lining of the uterus (endometrium) goes through two phases of development. These are the proliferative and secretory phases.

> **Critical Thinking**
>
> What could happen to the menstrual cycle if the hormonal balance was off?

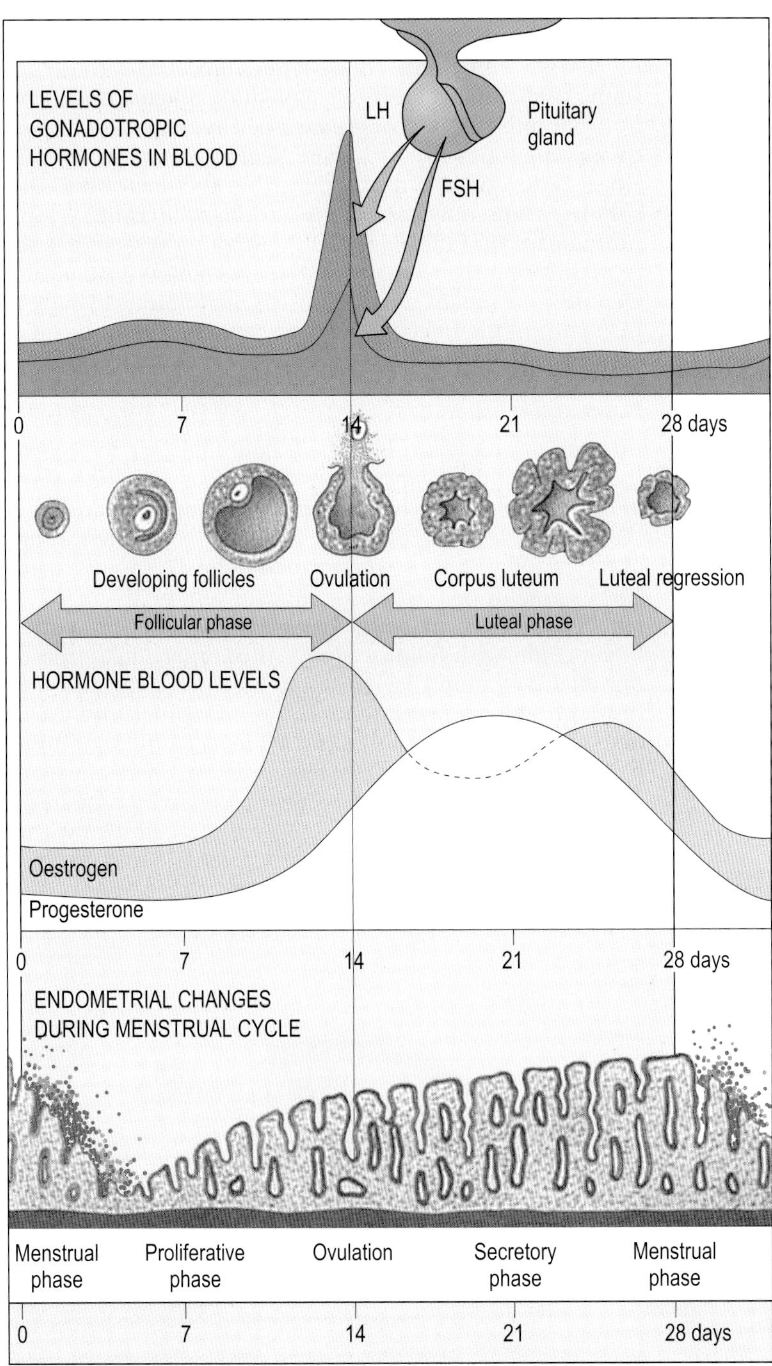

Figure 35-3 Human menstrual cycle. The interrelationship of pituitary, ovarian, and uterine functions throughout the usual 28-day cycle. A sharp increase in luteinizing hormone levels causes ovulation, whereas menstruation (sloughing of the endometrial lining) is initiated by lower levels of progesterone.

The proliferative phase starts and is sustained by increasing amounts of oestrogen, which is produced by the maturing follicle. Oestrogen stimulates the endometrium to grow and increase in thickness in order to prepare the uterus for implantation of a fertilized ovum. The secretory phase begins after ovulation and is under the combined influence of oestrogen and progesterone. During this phase, the endometrium is prepared for implantation of the fertilized ovum. Within 7 days after ovulation (about day 21 of the menstrual cycle), the endometrium is ready to receive the developing embryo if fertilization has occurred.

In the absence of fertilization, the ovum can survive only 6 to 24 h. After this time the hormone levels drop and the endometrium is shed as menstrual flow. This process usually takes place on day 28 of the cycle (about 14 days after ovulation). The oocyte is capable of being fertilized for up to 24 h after ovulation (see Chapter 36).

Specific gynaecological emergencies

Gynaecological emergencies are classified into three groups: non-traumatic, traumatic and sexual assault (Box 35-2). Regardless of the type of emergency, pregnancy should always be considered in any woman who is of child-bearing age. Pregnancy should be a possibility until determined otherwise by a physician.

Non-traumatic emergencies

In addition to gastrointestinal causes of abdominal pain (described in Chapter 19), acute or chronic infection involving a patient's uterus, ovaries, fallopian tubes and adjacent structures may be a source of severe abdominal pain. The scope of abdominal pain associated with the female reproductive system may range widely. Pain may be due to episodes of difficult menstruation but could also be from a haemorrhage from a ruptured ovarian cyst or ectopic pregnancy. These can pose a threat to life.

Pelvic inflammatory disease

The incidence of pelvic inflammatory disease (PID) is unknown as the disease cannot be reliably diagnosed from clinical signs and symptoms, and it can be asymptomatic.[2] Prevalence is estimated at 1.7% among women aged 16–46 years although this is believed to be an underestimate.[3] The disease results from infection of the cervix, uterus, fallopian tubes, and ovaries and their supporting structures (Figure 35-4). Pelvic inflammatory disease is often caused by sexually transmitted bacteria.

Infections from the vaginal area may travel up the vagina and infect the cervix (cervicitis). This can be followed by infection of the uterus proper (endometritis) and fallopian tubes (salpingitis). Finally, the supporting structures around the uterus and fallopian tubes (parametritis) may become infected. The infection may produce diffuse lower abdominal pain associated with low-grade fever (variable), vaginal discharge, and dyspareunia (pain with sexual intercourse). The inflammation often follows the onset of menstrual bleeding by 7 to 10 days. At that time the reproductive organs are vulnerable to bacterial infection because the lining of the uterus has been shed during menstruation.

Pelvic inflammatory disease is often accompanied by pain on ambulation, with the patient bent forward; taking short, slow steps; and often guarding the abdomen (the 'PID shuffle'). Consequences include secondary infertility, ectopic pregnancies, and tubo-ovarian abscesses. In severe cases the reproductive organs may need to be removed surgically. Definitive treatment usually consists of antibiotic therapy to help control the infection and prevent damage to the fallopian tubes.

Ruptured ovarian cyst

An ovarian cyst is a thin-walled, fluid-filled sac located on the surface of the ovary (Figure 35-5). They may be a cause of abdominal pain, which can be due to rapid expansion of the cyst, torsion that produces ischaemia, or acute rupture. The type of cyst most prone to rupture is known as the corpus luteum cyst, which develops when the tissue that is left behind after an ovum has been released (the corpus luteum) fills with fluid or blood. The corpus luteum develops after ovulation (day 14 of the 28-day cycle), thus most ruptures occur about 1 week before menstrual bleeding is due to begin. However, some patients with a ruptured ovarian cyst have vaginal bleeding or report a late or missed period at the time of rupture. Corpus luteum cysts can grow up to 6 cm across and usually go away on their own within a few months; however, rupture can cause internal bleeding and sudden pain.

Box 35-2

Classification of gynaecological emergencies

Non-traumatic abdominal emergencies

Cystitis
Ectopic pregnancy
Endometriosis
Endometritis
Mittelschmerz
Pelvic inflammatory disease
Ruptured ovarian cyst
Vaginal bleeding

Traumatic abdominal emergencies

Vaginal bleeding
Sexual assault

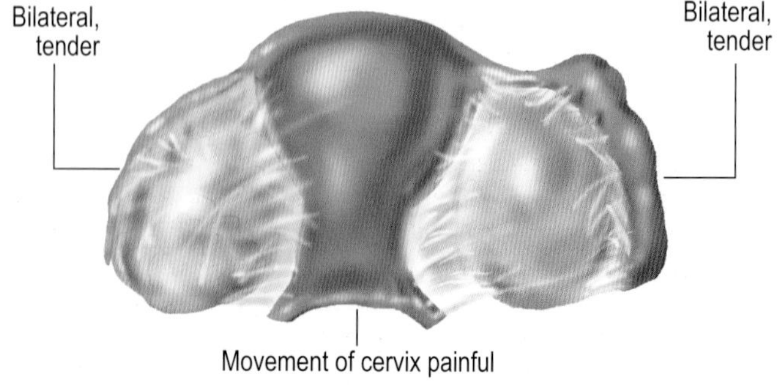

Figure 35-4 Pelvic inflammatory disease.

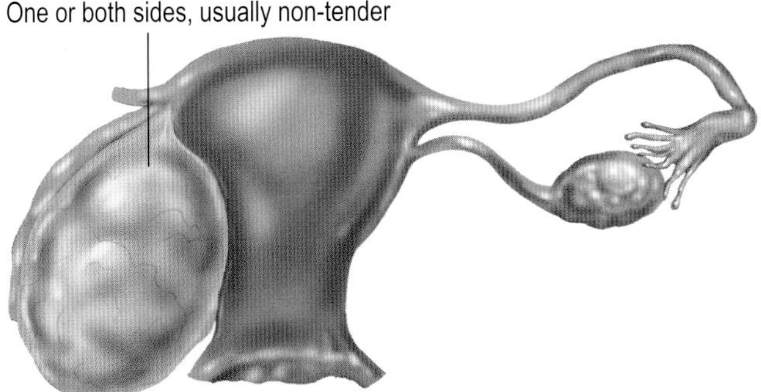

Figure 35-5 Ovarian cyst.

> **Critical Thinking**
>
> Consider a patient who you suspect has a ruptured ovarian cyst. How will you assess for the possibility of bleeding?

Pain from a ruptured ovarian cyst may be localized, one-sided lower abdominal pain but there may also be signs of peritonitis if massive haemorrhage has occurred. The onset of pain is often associated with minimal abdominal trauma, sexual intercourse or exercise.

Cystitis

Cystitis is inflammation of the inner lining of the bladder that is usually caused by a bacterial infection. Both sexes can develop infection although cystitis is more common in women. The main symptom of cystitis is a frequent urge to pass urine, with only a small amount of urine passed each time. Other signs and symptoms may include painful (burning) urination, fever, chills and lower abdominal pain. The urine may be foul smelling or contain blood. Prompt treatment of cystitis with antibiotics usually settles the infection within 24 h. Cystitis also can occur from structural abnormality of the ureters (common in children), or from compression of the urethra as well (e.g. an enlarged prostate gland in men). Finally, it can occur from indwelling urinary catheters.

Dysmenorrhoea and mittelschmerz

Many women experience pain during menstruation; this is called dysmenorrhoea. Dysmenorrhoea may also include headache, faintness, dizziness, nausea, diarrhoea, backache and leg pain. In severe cases, chills, vomiting and syncope can occur. The lower abdominal pains associated with dysmenorrhoea are thought to be related to muscular contraction of the myometrium (the muscular layer of the uterus). These muscle contractions are mediated by local prostaglandins. Other factors associated with dysmenorrhoea include infection, inflammation and the presence of an intrauterine contraceptive device.

Mittelschmerz is German for 'middle pain'. This pain may occur from the rupture of the graafian follicle and bleeding from the ovary during the menstrual cycle. Mittelschmerz is characterized by right or left lower quadrant abdominal pain that occurs in the normal midcycle of a menstrual period (after ovulation). The pain lasts about 24 to 36 h. The hormones produced by the ovary may also produce slight endometrial bleeding and low-grade fever. Dysmenorrhoea and mittelschmerz do not pose a threat to life; however, physician evaluation is required to rule out more serious causes of menstrual pain. Evaluation is also required to differentiate the pain from that of appendicitis.

Endometritis

Endometritis is inflammation of the uterine lining that usually results from infection. It is an occasional complication of childbirth, miscarriage, or gynaecological procedures such as dilatation and curettage (D&C). Symptom onset is 24–48 h after the procedure or miscarriage and may mimic the presentation of PID. Endometritis may affect the uterus and fallopian tubes and, if left untreated, it may result in sterility, sepsis, and death. Signs and symptoms of endometritis include fever, purulent vaginal discharge and lower abdominal pain. The treatment includes removal of any foreign tissue and antibiotic therapy.

Endometriosis

Endometriosis is an abnormal gynaecological condition characterized by endometrial tissue growing outside of the uterus. This ectopic endometrium responds to hormonal changes during the menstrual cycle, with subsequent bleeding, inflammation, and (if the ovaries are affected) the development of endometriotic ovarian cysts. The exact cause is unknown but the most widely accepted theory is that endometriosis occurs as a result of fragments of endometrium being regurgitated backward (retrograde menstruation) through the fallopian tubes into the peritoneal cavity. There the fragments attach and grow as small cystic structures.

Incidence of endometriosis peaks at around 40 years,[4] and is more common in women who defer pregnancy. Characteristic symptoms of endometriosis are pain (particularly dysmenorrhoea), painful defecation and suprapubic soreness. Other common symptoms include vaginal spotting of blood before the start of a period and infertility. After physician evaluation, treatment may consist of drug therapy with analgesics or hormones. Sometimes it may include surgery.

> **Critical Thinking**
>
> Why do you think these patients with endometriosis tend to be infertile?

Ectopic pregnancy

An ectopic pregnancy can be a life-threatening emergency. An ectopic pregnancy develops outside the uterus, most often in the fallopian tube. Most ectopic pregnancies are discovered in the first 2 months and are often found before the woman realizes she is pregnant. Signs and symptoms include severe abdominal pain and vaginal 'spotting'. If rupture occurs, internal haemorrhage, sepsis, and shock may develop. Once ectopic pregnancy is confirmed, it is treated with surgery. Surgery is performed to remove the developing fetus, placenta, and any damaged tissue at the site of the pregnancy. Ectopic pregnancy is common: occurring in 11.1 of every 1000 pregnancies.[5] Ectopic pregnancy should be considered in any female of reproductive age with abdominal pain. (Ectopic pregnancy is described further in Chapter 36.)

Vaginal bleeding

Vaginal bleeding refers to the loss of blood from the uterus, cervix or vagina, with the most common source of non-traumatic vaginal bleeding being menstruation. Possible causes of serious non-menstrual bleeding include the following:

- spontaneous abortion
- disorders of the placenta
- hormonal imbalances (especially menopause)
- lesions
- PID
- onset of labour.

The paramedic should never assume that vaginal haemorrhage is due to normal menstruation. Some causes of vaginal bleeding may be life threatening and may lead to hypovolaemic shock and death. (The vaginal passage of clots usually indicates bleeding at a rate greater than menstrual flow.)

Traumatic emergencies

Traumatic abdominal pain in a female patient is usually associated with vaginal bleeding or sexual assault.

Vaginal bleeding

Traumatic causes of vaginal bleeding are described in Chapter 33. Causes include straddle injuries, blows to the perineum, and blunt forces to the lower abdomen. Other causes include foreign bodies inserted into the vagina, injury during intercourse, abortion attempts, and soft tissue injuries resulting from sexual assault. Complications of vaginal bleeding that result from trauma may cause pelvic organs to rupture. This can lead to life-threatening hypovolaemia and shock. Treatment is the same as for other severe internal injuries and often requires surgical repair.

Assessment

Finding the cause of lower abdominal pain in females is difficult. Many gynaecological conditions produce common characteristics. For example, ruptured ectopic pregnancy, ruptured ovarian cyst, and PID can have identical presentations (Table 35-1). The goals of prehospital care are to rapidly identify the conditions that require urgent treatment and to transport rapidly for surgery. Prehospital care includes obtaining a history of the present illness (including a thorough gynaecological history); providing airway, ventilatory and circulatory support as needed; and transporting the patient for physician evaluation.

History of present illness and obstetrical history

The paramedic should obtain a history of the present illness to help better understand the patient's chief complaint (see Chapter 8). Important associated symptoms include the presence of fever, diaphoresis, syncope, diarrhoea, constipation and abdominal cramping. The interview should include a thorough obstetrical history to include (see also Chapter 36):

Critical Thinking

Will the patient always give you accurate information about whether she is pregnant? Why?

1. Pregnancy. The paramedic should determine the total number of pregnancies (gravida) the patient has had and the number of pregnancies that were carried to term (para).
2. Previous caesarean deliveries. A caesarean delivery is a surgical procedure. In a caesarean section the abdomen and uterus are incised and the baby is delivered through the abdomen. Caesarean delivery is usually done when maternal or fetal conditions might make vaginal delivery risky.
3. Last menstrual period. The paramedic should obtain information about the patient's last menstrual period. Questions to ask about the patient's last menstrual period include the following:
   - When did it start (the date)? When did it end (the duration)? Have the menstrual periods occurred regularly for the patient?
   - Was the last menstrual period normal for the patient? Was the menstrual flow heavier or lighter than other periods?
   - Was there any bleeding between periods?

Table 35-1 Characteristics of abdominal pain in gynaecological emergencies

	Onset	Location	Quality	Radiation	Vaginal discharge	Menstrual history
Ruptured ectopic pregnancy	Rapid (can become generalized)	Unilateral (can generalize)	Cramp-like, then steady	Shoulder (may indicate intraperitoneal bleeding)	Vaginal bleeding (75% of cases)	Amenorrhoea, 6 weeks or more since last period
Ruptured ovarian cyst	Sudden	Unilateral (can generalize)	Steady	Shoulder (may indicate intraperitoneal bleeding)	Possible vaginal bleeding	Usually 1 week before period
Pelvic inflammatory disease	Gradual (can become generalized)	Diffuse, bilateral	Steady ache	Right upper quadrant	Watery, foul-smelling discharge	Usually within 1 week after period

4. Possibility of pregnancy. Some patients may hesitate to disclose a possible pregnancy. They may not answer honestly a direct question such as 'Could you be pregnant?' If pregnancy is suspected (but not confirmed by the patient), the paramedic should ask specific questions about missed or late periods, breast tenderness, urinary frequency, morning sickness (nausea and/or vomiting), and unprotected sexual activity to determine the likelihood of a pregnancy.
5. History of previous gynaecological problems. The paramedic should identify previous gynaecological problems. Knowledge of these problems can be helpful to others who may be involved in the patient's care. Examples of previous gynaecological problems that are important to obtain during the patient history include infections, bleeding, dyspareunia, miscarriage, abortion, the need for a dilatation and curettage, and ectopic pregnancy.

Note

Dilatation and curettage is a gynaecological procedure. It refers to widening of the uterine cervix and scraping away of the endometrium of the uterus. The procedure is used for a variety of conditions, including diagnosing disease of the uterus, correcting heavy or prolonged vaginal bleeding, and emptying the uterus of the products of conception following delivery or abortion.

6. Present blood loss. If the patient is actively bleeding, the paramedic should ask questions about the colour (bright versus dark red blood), the amount of blood loss (estimated by the number of pads/tampons soaked per hour), and the duration of the bleeding episode.
7. Vaginal discharge. If the patient has a discharge, the paramedic should question her about the colour, amount and odour of the discharge. These findings may indicate the presence of infection, venereal disease or other illness.
8. Use and type of contraceptive. The use and type of contraception is a key part of the obstetrical history. For example, the use of birth control pills has been associated with hypertension and pulmonary embolus. Also, intrauterine devices can cause intrauterine bleeding and infection. Other methods of contraception include the withdrawal or rhythm method (which may increase the likelihood of pregnancy), the use of spermicides and condoms.
9. History of trauma to the reproductive system. The paramedic should question all patients about any injury to the reproductive tract. Such an injury may be responsible for vaginal bleeding or discharge. The paramedic should ask a sexually active patient whether pain or bleeding has occurred during or after intercourse.
10. Degree of emotional distress. The paramedic should evaluate the patient's emotional distress. Factors that may be responsible for a patient's emotional distress include personal health issues, depression, an unwanted pregnancy, and financial worries.

Physical examination

The paramedic should conduct a physical examination in a comforting and professional manner with consideration for the patient's modesty and privacy. The paramedic should be considerate of reasons for patient discomfort as well. When evaluating the potential for serious blood loss, the paramedic should assess the patient's skin and mucous membranes for colour, cyanosis or pallor. Vital sign assessment should include orthostatic measurements. Vaginal examination should not be undertaken by paramedics in the prehospital environment. The paramedic should auscultate and palpate the abdomen to assess for masses, areas of tenderness, guarding, distension and rebound tenderness (if time allows).

Management

Management includes support of the patient's vital functions and administration of oxygen as indicated. Intravenous access is not usually needed unless the patient is demonstrating signs of impending shock or has excessive vaginal bleeding. Many patients prefer to be transported in a left-lateral recumbent, knee–chest position, or they may prefer a hips-raised, knees-bent position for comfort. Vaginal bleeding should be controlled with the application of sanitary pads or trauma dressings. The vagina should never be packed with dressings or tampons. The paramedic should count the number of soaked pads and should record the number on the patient report form.

During transport, the paramedic should monitor the patient for the onset of serious bleeding. If this occurs or the patient's condition begins to deteriorate, consideration should be given to establishing an IV infusion in accordance with current JRCALC guidelines.[6] At this point, electrocardiograph and pulse oximetry monitoring are indicated. Analgesia should also be considered for abdominal pain.

Sexual assault

Sexual assault is a crime of violence that has serious physical and psychological implications. Anyone of either gender at any age can be sexually assaulted (see Chapter 40); however, women and girls are most often the victims. Police recorded 53 540 sexual offences in England and Wales in the year ending March 2008.[7] This represented a 7% drop over 2006–07 figures. Often, the paramedic is first to encounter these patients; tact, kindness, and sensitivity during the patient care episode is essential.

Critical Thinking

How do you feel about rape, and how would you manage a patient who has been raped?

Initially, the paramedic should care for a victim of sexual assault like any other injured patient. The first priority is to manage any injury that poses a threat to life. After that, though, the approach should be modified in reference to history taking and the physical examination. Before taking a history or performing an examination, the paramedic should move the patient to a private area. If possible, the patient should be interviewed and examined by a paramedic of the same sex. Every effort should be made to avoid disturbing the scene if the paramedic is called to the location of the assault.

History taking

As a rule, victims of sexual assault should not be questioned in detail about the incident in the prehospital setting. The history should be limited to the elements needed to provide emergency care. For example, questions regarding penetration, sexual history or practices are irrelevant to prehospital care; they only add to the patient's emotional stress. The patient should be allowed to speak openly and all information should be recorded accurately and thoroughly. Common reactions to sexual assault may range from anxiety to withdrawal and silence. Denial, anger and fear also are normal behaviour patterns.

Assessment

The physical examination should identify any physical trauma, outside the pelvic area, that needs immediate attention. To find facial fractures, human bites of the hands and breasts, long bone fractures, broken ribs, or trauma to the abdomen is not unusual. Consent should be obtained as for any other patient (see Chapter 2) but the paramedic should be aware that the patient may be distressed and may not consent to disclosure of details to other parties such as the police, or may refuse medical treatment. Where the patient is competent to refuse transport to hospital and does so, it is important for the paramedic to advise them to seek further medical assistance. All examination findings should be documented, including the patient's emotional state, condition of the patient's clothing, obvious injuries, and any patient care rendered. A non-judgemental and professional attitude is important. Feelings and prejudices about the victim or the assault should not affect the delivery of care.

Management

After managing life-threatening injury, emotional support is the most important patient care procedure one can offer a victim of sexual assault. The paramedic should provide a safe environment for the patient and should respond appropriately to the victim's physical and emotional needs. Paramedics also should be aware of the need to preserve evidence from the crime scene (further described in Chapter 44). Special considerations include the following:

- handle clothing as little as possible
- do not clean wounds unless absolutely necessary
- do not allow the patient to drink or brush teeth
- do not use plastic bags for blood-stained articles
- bag each clothing item separately
- ask the victim not to change clothes or bathe
- disturb the crime scene as little as possible.

Summary

- Menstruation is the normal, periodic discharge of blood, mucus and cellular debris from the uterine mucosa. Ovulation is the release of a secondary oocyte from the ovary.
- Pelvic inflammatory disease results from infection of the cervix, uterus, fallopian tubes and ovaries and their supporting structures.
- Ruptured ovarian cyst occurs when a thin-walled, fluid-filled sac located on the ovary ruptures. This can cause internal haemorrhage.
- Cystitis is inflammation of the inner lining of the bladder that is usually caused by a bacterial infection.
- Dysmenorrhoea is characterized by painful menses. It may be associated with headache, faintness, dizziness, nausea, diarrhoea, backache and leg pain.
- Mittelschmerz is German for 'middle pain.' This pain may occur from the rupture of the graafian follicle and bleeding from the ovary during the menstrual cycle.
- Endometritis is inflammation of the uterine lining. It is characterized by endometrial tissue growing outside of the uterus.
- An ectopic pregnancy is one that develops outside the uterus.
- Vaginal bleeding is the loss of blood from the uterus, cervix or vagina.
- Traumatic causes of vaginal bleeding include straddle injuries, blows to the perineum, blunt forces to the lower abdomen, foreign bodies in the vagina, injury during intercourse, abortion attempts, and soft tissue injuries from sexual assault.
- The goal of prehospital care of lower abdominal pain in the female is to obtain a history (including a gynaecological history); provide airway, ventilatory and circulatory support as needed; and provide transport for physician evaluation.
- Sexual assault is a crime of violence. It can have serious physical and psychological effects.
- Paramedics should be aware of the need to preserve evidence from a sexual assault crime scene.

References

1. Tortora GJ, Derrickson BH 2006 Principles of anatomy and physiology, 11th edition. John Wiley, New York
2. Ross J 2005 Pelvic inflammatory disease. Clin Evidence (14):2176–2182
3. Simms I, Stephenson JM 2000 Pelvic inflammatory disease epidemiology: what do we know and what do we need to know? Sexually Transmitted Infections 76(2):80–87
4. Johnson N, Farquhar C 2006 Endometriosis. Clin Evidence (15):2449–2464
5. Royal College of Obstetricians and Gynaecologists. Why Mothers Die 1997–99 – Report from the Confidential Enquiries into Maternal Deaths in the UK – December 2001. Online. Available http://www.cmace.org.uk/getattachment/8dccaef7-Oee9-4283-be46-fedbde83335a/Why-Mothers-Die-97-99.aspx
6. Joint Royal Colleges Ambulance Liaison Committee. UK Ambulance Service Clinical Guidelines v4. 2006. Online. Available http://jrcalc.org.uk/guidelines.html 18 February 2009
7. Kershaw C, Nicholas S, Walker A, eds. Crime in England and Wales 2007/08. Findings from the British Crime Survey and police recorded crime. Online. Available http://www.homeoffice.gov.uk/rds/pdfs08/hosb0708.pdf 17 June 2009
8. The Information Centre for Health and Social Care. Hospital Episode Statistics: Main procedures and interventions: 3 character, 2007–08. Online. Available http://www.hesonline.nhs.uk/Ease/servlet/ContentServer?siteID=19378 categoryID=205 17 June 2009

CHAPTER **36**

Obstetrics

Chapter contents

Objectives

Upon completion of this chapter, the paramedic student will be able to:

1. Describe the organization and function of the specialized structures of pregnancy.
2. Outline fetal development from ovulation through to adaptations at birth.
3. Explain normal maternal physiological changes that occur during pregnancy and how they influence prehospital patient care and transportation.
4. Describe appropriate information to be elicited during the obstetric patient's history.
5. Describe specific techniques for assessment of the pregnant patient.
6. Describe general prehospital care of the pregnant patient.
7. Discuss the implications of prehospital care after trauma to the fetus and mother.
8. Describe the assessment and management of patients with pre-eclampsia and eclampsia.
9. Explain the pathophysiology, signs and symptoms, and management of the processes that cause vaginal bleeding in pregnancy.
10. Outline the physiological changes that occur during the stages of labour.
11. Describe the role of the paramedic during normal labour and delivery.
12. Compute an Apgar score.
13. Describe assessment and management of postpartum haemorrhage.
14. Discuss the identification, implications, and prehospital management of complicated deliveries.

Key terms

abortion The termination of pregnancy from any cause before 24 weeks' gestation.

abruptio placentae A partial or full detachment of a normally implanted placenta at more than 24 weeks' gestation.

Apgar score The evaluation of a newborn's physical condition, usually performed 1 min and 5 min after birth, including heart rate, respiratory effort, muscle tone, reflex irritability, and colour.

crowning The phase at the end of labour in which the fetal head is seen at the opening of the vagina.

eclampsia A grave form of pregnancy-induced hypertension, characterized by convulsions, coma, proteinuria and oedema.

ectopic pregnancy A pregnancy that occurs when a fertilized ovum implants anywhere other than the uterus.

gestation The period from fertilization of the ovum until birth.

gravida The number of all current and past pregnancies.

para The number of past pregnancies that have remained viable to delivery.

parturition The process by which an infant is born.

placenta A highly vascular fetal–maternal organ through which the fetus absorbs oxygen, nutrients, and other substances and excretes carbon dioxide and other wastes.

placenta praevia Placental implantation in the lower uterine segment, partially or completely covering the cervical opening.

pre-eclampsia An abnormal disease of pregnancy characterized by the onset of acute hypertension after the 24th week of gestation.

uterine rupture A spontaneous or traumatic rupture of the uterine wall.

Childbirth is common in the prehospital setting. Most often, emergency medical services personnel only assist in this natural process by providing care for the mother and newborn. At times, though, obstetric emergencies can develop suddenly and may even become life threatening. The paramedic must be prepared to recognize and manage these events, and to assist in abnormal deliveries. The paramedic may wish to undertake a specialist course in the management of prehospital obstetric emergencies to supplement their initial training. One such course is provided by the Advanced Life Support Group, which is a charity dedicated to the training of lay and healthcare providers in life-saving techniques (http://www.alsg.org/en/?q=en/poet). This chapter presents the causes and treatment of obstetric emergencies and discusses the normal and abnormal events associated with childbirth.

Normal events of pregnancy

In a normal pregnancy, fertilization occurs in the fallopian tube. Fertilization takes place when the head of a sperm penetrates a mature ovum. After penetration, the nuclei of the sperm and ovum fuse and at this time the newly fertilized ovum becomes a zygote. The zygote undergoes repeated cell divisions as it passes down the fallopian tube. After a few days of rapid cell division, a ball of cells called a morula is formed, with cell differentiation between the inner layer of cells (blastocyst cells) and the outer layer of cells (trophoblast cells). Trophoblast cells attach to the endometrium lining of the uterus. Implantation begins within 7 days of fertilization and is completed when the trophoblast cells make contact with maternal circulation (this is about day 12). Trophoblast cells go on to make various life support systems for the embryo (placenta, amniotic sac, umbilical cord); blastocyst cells develop into the embryo itself (Figure 36-1).

Specialized structures of pregnancy

Specialized structures of pregnancy include the placenta, the umbilical cord, and the amniotic sac and its fluid. These structures provide nutrients for the developing embryo and are part of the fetal circulation.

Placenta

The trophoblast cells continue to develop and form the placenta for about 14 days after ovulation. The placenta is a disc-like organ composed of interlocking fetal and maternal tissues. It is the organ of exchange between the mother and fetus and is responsible for the following five functions:

1. Transfer of gases. The diffusion of oxygen and carbon dioxide through the placental membrane is similar to the diffusion that occurs in the lungs. Dissolved oxygen in maternal blood passes through the placenta into fetal blood due to a pressure gradient between the blood of the mother and fetus. However, as fetal carbon dioxide pressure (P_{CO_2}) builds up, a low pressure gradient of carbon dioxide develops across the placental membrane. The carbon dioxide then diffuses from fetal blood to maternal blood.

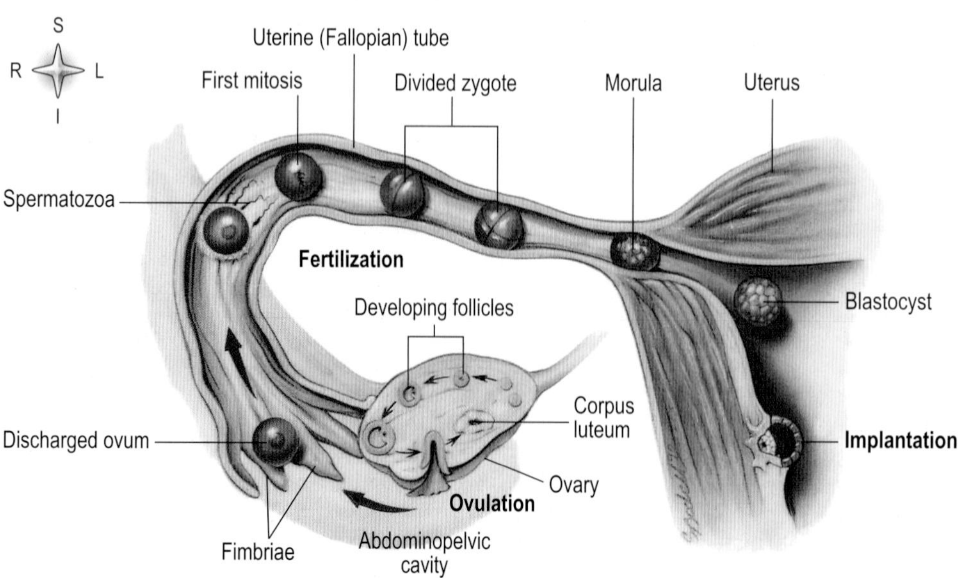

Figure 36-1 Fertilization and implantation. At ovulation the ovary releases an ovum, which begins its journey through the uterine tube. While the ovum is in the tube, a sperm fertilizes the ovum to form the single-celled zygote. After a few days of rapid cell division, a ball of cells called a morula forms. After the morula develops into a hollow ball (blastocyst), implantation occurs.

Critical Thinking

What happens to diffusion of gases if the mother becomes hypoxic?

2. Transport of nutrients. Other metabolic substrates required by the fetus diffuse into fetal blood in the same manner as oxygen. For example, glucose levels in fetal blood are about 20–30% lower than those in maternal blood, which results in a rapid diffusion of glucose to the fetus. Diffusion also transports other substrates, including fatty acids, potassium, sodium and chloride. The placenta also actively absorbs some nutrients from maternal blood.
3. Excretion of wastes. Waste products, such as urea, uric acid and creatinine, diffuse from fetal blood into maternal blood. They are excreted with the waste products of the mother.
4. Hormone production. The placenta becomes a temporary endocrine gland, secreting oestrogen and progesterone. By the third month of fetal development the corpus luteum (described in Chapter 35) on the ovary is no longer needed to sustain the pregnancy. Oestrogen, progesterone, and other hormones maintain the uterine lining, prevent the occurrence of menses, and stimulate changes in the pregnant woman's breasts, vagina, cervix, and pelvis that prepare her body for delivery and lactation.
5. Formation of a barrier. The placenta forms a barrier against some harmful substances and chemicals in the mother's circulation. The placental barrier is incomplete and only partially selective, so it does not fully protect the fetus. Certain medications easily cross the placenta, including steroids, narcotics, anaesthetics, and some antibiotics.

Umbilical cord

Deoxygenated blood flows from the fetus to the placenta through two umbilical arteries. Oxygenated blood returns through the umbilical vein. This system is independent of and separated from the maternal circulation. Other structures unique to fetal circulation are the ductus venosus, the foramen ovale and the ductus arteriosus. The ductus venosus is a continuation of the umbilical cord that serves as a shunt to allow most blood returning to the placenta to bypass the immature liver of the embryo. The ductus venosus empties directly into the inferior vena cava. The foramen ovale and the ductus arteriosus allow most blood to bypass the embryo's lungs. The lungs remain collapsed until birth.

The foramen ovale shunts about one-third of the blood that enters the right atrium directly into the left atrium. The blood that does pass into the right ventricle is pumped into the pulmonary trunk, where most of it passes through the ductus arteriosus into the aorta. The blood is then carried through the systemic circulation to fetal tissue. Blood is returned to the placenta via the umbilical arteries, which arise from the internal iliac arteries just past the bifurcation of the common iliac arteries. It is here that exchange of waste products and required materials takes place. At birth the various arteriovenous shunts close in most infants (Figure 36-2).

Amniotic sac and amniotic fluid

The amniotic sac is a fluid-filled cavity that completely surrounds and protects the embryo. Amniotic fluid originates from several fetal sources, including fetal urine and secretions from the respiratory tract, skin, and amniotic membranes. The fluid builds up rapidly and amounts to about 175 to 225 mL by the fifteenth week of pregnancy and about 1 L at birth. The rupture of the amniotic membranes produces the watery discharge at the time of delivery.

Fetal growth and development

The developing ovum is called an embryo during the first 8 weeks of pregnancy, and from 8 weeks until birth it is called a fetus. The period during which the fetus grows and develops within the uterus is known as gestation. Gestation usually averages 40 weeks from the time of fertilization to delivery of the newborn and is divided into 90-day periods called trimesters. Conception occurs about 14 days after the first day of the last menstrual period; thus the obstetrician can calculate fetal development with reasonable accuracy as well as the estimated delivery date. Rapid fetal growth and development characterize the period of gestation (Figure 36-3a–d and Box 36-1).

Adjustments of the infant at birth

Birth results in the infant's loss of the placental connection with the mother, which results in the loss of metabolic support. The infant's immediate need to obtain oxygen and excrete carbon dioxide is critical and requires changes in the fetal circulation that permit adequate blood flow through the lungs.

After a normal delivery by a mother who is not depressed with anaesthetics, a newborn usually begins to breathe spontaneously. This occurs when the chest exits the birth canal or with some external stimulation. At birth, surface tension of the viscid fluid that fills the alveoli holds the walls of the alveoli together. The newborn needs to create more than 25 mmHg of negative pressure to oppose the effects of this surface tension in order for the alveoli to open for the first time. The first breaths of the newborn can create as much as 50 mmHg of negative pressure in the intrapleural space. These powerful first breaths open the alveoli, which allows further respirations to occur with much less effort.

The ductus venosus, ductus arteriosus and foramen ovale bypass the immature liver and non-functional lungs of the developing fetus. Blood flow through the placenta ceases at birth. At that point, pressure in the aorta, left ventricle and left atrium increases, resulting in an increase in systemic vascular resistance. Also, pressure in the lungs decreases as they expand, which reduces the pulmonary arterial, right ventricular and right atrial pressures. As a result of these changes in pressure, the arteriovenous shunts close normally within a few hours after birth. They eventually close completely and are covered with a growth of fibrous tissue.

Critical Thinking

Do fetal heart tones sound normal if you auscultate them immediately after birth?

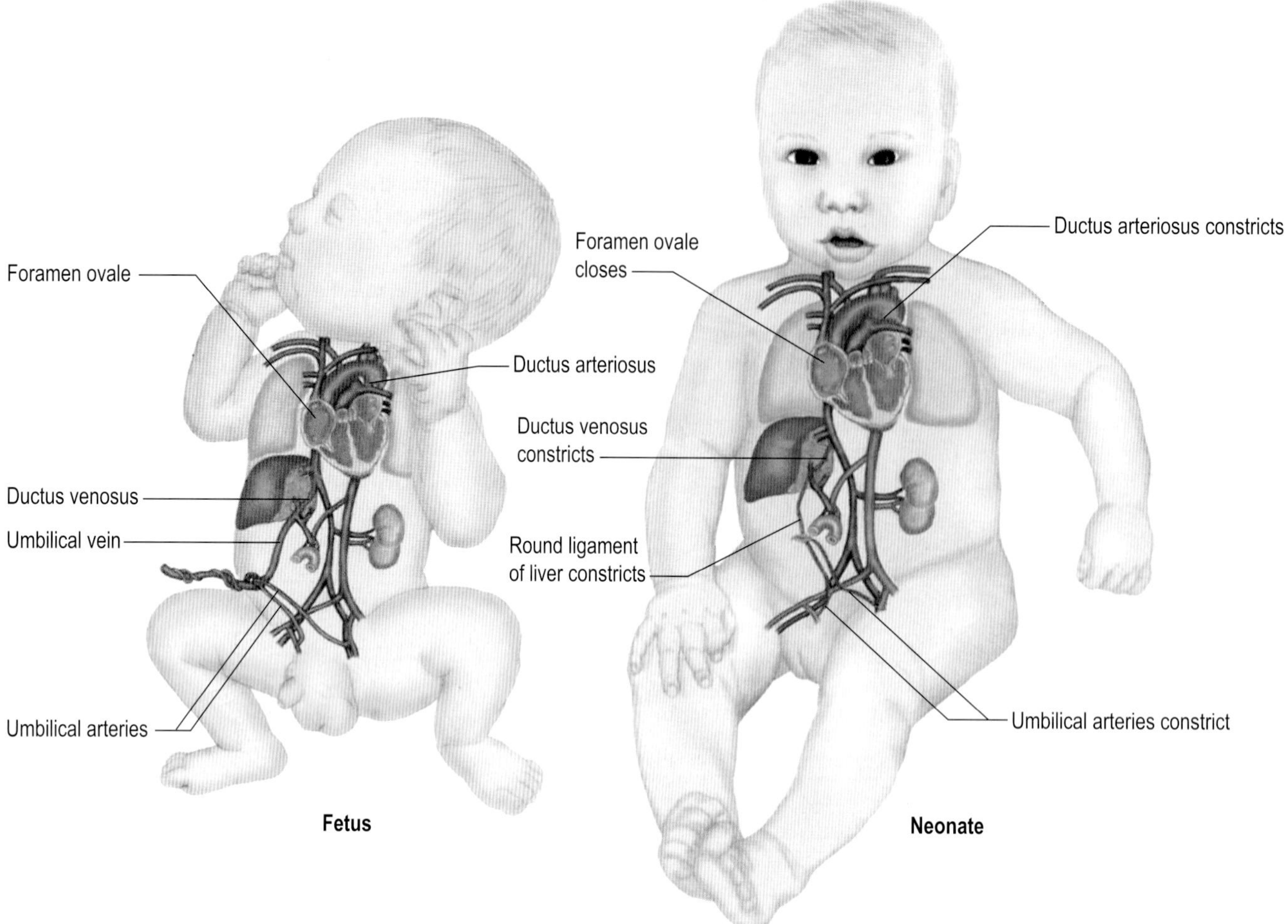

Figure 36-2 Fetal circulation and changes in circulation after birth.

Obstetric terminology

Pregnant patients are described by their gravid and parous states. The term *gravida* refers to the number of all of the woman's current and past pregnancies; *para* refers only to the number of the woman's past pregnancies that have resulted in a live birth. For example, a woman who is pregnant for the first time is gravida 1, para 0 (Box 36-2).

Patient assessment

The paramedic must be familiar with the normal physiological changes that occur in the pregnant woman. This will help the paramedic to assess a pregnant patient.

Maternal changes during pregnancy

Menstruation ceases in the pregnant woman and the uterus enlarges. The pregnant woman undergoes many other physical changes that affect the genital tract, breasts, gastrointestinal system, cardiovascular system, respiratory system and metabolism.

Genital tract

Uterus

- Uterine size increases from 70 g (non-gravid) to 1000 g by term.
- The uterus triples in size and weight by the second month of pregnancy.
- The uterus occupies the entire pelvic cavity. It may be palpated suprapubically by the third month of pregnancy.
- The uterus becomes an abdominal organ and the top of the uterus (fundus) reaches the level of the umbilicus by the fourth month of pregnancy.
- The uterine fundus recedes a little when the fetus descends into the pelvis. This occurs in the last trimester.

Cervix

Increased uterine blood and lymphatic flow cause pelvic congestion and oedema. This results in softening and bluish discoloration of the cervix (Chadwick's sign).

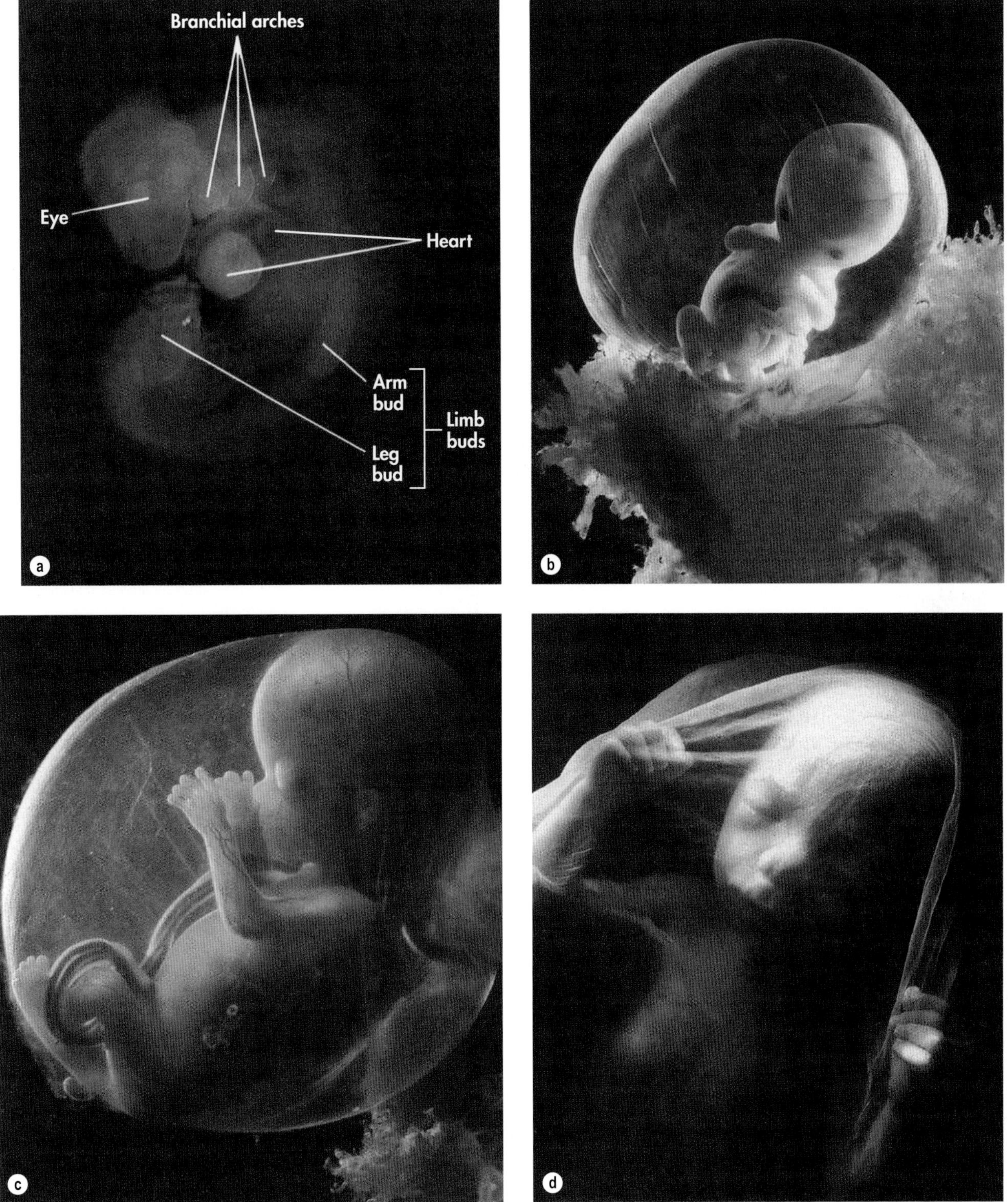

Figure 36-3 Human embryos and fetuses. (a) At 35 days. (b) At 49 days. (c) At the end of the first trimester. (d) At 4 months.

Box 36-1

Embryo and fetal development in utero for each lunar month (28 days)

First lunar month

Foundations form for the nervous system, genitourinary system, skin, bones, and lungs.

Buds of arms and legs begin to form.

Rudiments of eyes, ears, and nose appear.

Second lunar month

The head is disproportionately large because of brain development.

Gender differentiation begins.

The centres of bones begin to ossify.

Third lunar month

Fingers and toes are distinct.

The placenta is complete.

Fetal circulation is complete.

Fourth lunar month

Gender is differentiated.

Rudimentary kidneys secrete urine.

Heartbeat is present.

Nasal septum and palate close.

Fifth lunar month

Fetal movements are felt by the mother.

Heart sounds are perceptible with a fetoscope.

Sixth lunar month

The skin appears wrinkled.

Eyebrows and fingernails develop.

Seventh lunar month

The skin is red.

The pupillary membrane disappears from the eyes.

If born, the infant cries and breathes but frequently dies.

Eighth lunar month

The fetus is viable if born.

The eyelids open.

Fingerprints are set.

Vigorous fetal movement occurs.

Ninth lunar month

The face and body have a loose, wrinkled appearance because of subcutaneous fat deposits.

Amniotic fluid decreases somewhat.

Tenth lunar month

Skin is smooth.

Eyes are uniformly slate coloured.

The bones of the skull are ossified and nearly together at sutures.

Box 36-2

Obstetric terminology

Antepartum: the maternal period before delivery
Grand multipara: a woman who has had seven deliveries or more
Multigravida: a woman who has had two or more pregnancies
Multipara: a woman who has had two or more deliveries
Nullipara: a woman who has never delivered
Perinatal: occurring at or near the time of birth
Postpartum: the maternal period after delivery
Antenatal: existing or occurring before birth
Primigravida: a woman who is pregnant for the first time
Primipara: a woman who has given birth only once
Term: a pregnancy that has reached 40 weeks' gestation

Vagina

- The vagina develops a violet colour due to increased vascularity.
- The vaginal walls prepare for labour and the vaginal mucosa increases in thickness.
- Vaginal secretions increase. The pH decreases to about 3.5; this is due to increased production of lactic acid from glycogen in the vaginal epithelium. Acidic pH helps keep the vaginal area fairly free of pathogens.

Bladder

Frequency of urination increases due to the pressure of the expanding uterus on the bladder. Frequency disappears when the uterus rises out of the pelvis but returns once again when the fetal head engages in the pelvis near term.

Breasts

- The breasts become tender in the early weeks of pregnancy.
- The breasts increase in size as a result of hypertrophy of the mammary alveoli by the second month of pregnancy.
- The nipples become larger, more deeply pigmented, and more erectile early in pregnancy.
- As breast glands proliferate, they begin to secrete a clear fluid by the tenth week of pregnancy.

Gastrointestinal system

- Morning sickness and nausea may occur at any time. They usually begin by the sixth and abate by the fourteenth week of pregnancy. The cause of morning sickness is related to the high serum levels of chorionic gonadotropin in early pregnancy.
- The enlarging uterus displaces the patient's stomach and intestines upward and laterally. This may cause indigestion and can increase the risk for aspiration in unconscious patients.
- The liver is displaced backward, upward, and to the right.
- The tone and motility of the gastrointestinal tract decrease, leading to prolonged gastric emptying and relaxation of the pyloric sphincter. Heartburn and constipation are common.

Critical Thinking

Consider an unconscious pregnant woman who has sustained trauma. What are problems associated with these gastrointestinal changes?

Cardiovascular system

Heart

- Elevation of the diaphragm displaces the heart to the left and upward. Flat or negative T waves may be present in lead III on the electrocardiogram.
- Cardiac output increases by 30% by the thirty-fourth week of pregnancy.
- The pulse rate may increase 15 to 20 beats/min above baseline late in the third trimester (variable).
- Pulmonic systolic and apical systolic murmurs are common. This is because lowered blood viscosity and increased flow lead to turbulence in the great vessels.

Circulation

- Total blood volume increases by 30%. Plasma volume increases by 50%.
- Blood pressure decreases 10–15 mmHg during the second trimester. This is because of the reduction in peripheral resistance. Blood pressure gradually increases to pre-pregnancy levels toward term.
- The enlarged uterus interferes with venous return from the legs.
- Haemorrhoids, slight oedema of the ankles and varicose veins may be present.
- The supine position may cause the uterus to compress the inferior vena cava. This can produce decreased cardiac filling and decreased cardiac output (supine hypotension syndrome). The patient may become faint and hypotensive whilst lying on her back after the first or second trimester.

Blood

- Increased plasma volume results in a decrease in haemoglobin and haematocrit concentrations.
- The leukocyte count increases.
- Fibrinogen levels increase by 50% because of the influence of oestrogen and progesterone.

Respiratory system

- Tidal volume and minute ventilation increase by 30–40% in late pregnancy.
- Functional residual capacity decreases by about 25%.
- The respiratory rate may be normal but it often increases because of elevation of the diaphragm by the enlarged uterus.
- $P\text{CO}_2$ normally decreases. This is because of an increased respiratory rate. $P\text{CO}_2$ changes from 40 mmHg to 30 mmHg to provide a gradient for fetal carbon dioxide. This may cause dizziness and a sensation of shortness of breath for the pregnant woman.

Metabolism

- The mother experiences a normal weight gain of 9.1 kg (20 lb).
- Increased water retention produces an increase in pressure within the capillaries, which may result in oedema.
- The metabolic rate and caloric demand (especially for protein) increase.
- Glucose escapes into the urine because of increased glomerular filtration.
- Maternal gestational diabetes mellitus (GDM) may result from an impaired ability to metabolize carbohydrates. This usually is caused by a deficiency of insulin. Gestational diabetes mellitus is further described later in this chapter.
- Fetal demands for calcium and iron may deplete maternal stores if the patient does not supplement them through diet.

History

When obtaining a history from an obstetric patient, the paramedic should first gather details about the chief complaint. This complaint may not be related to the pregnancy. Paramedics should solicit information about the onset of signs and symptoms in confidence and should provide privacy for the physical examination. After ruling out life-threatening illness or injury, the paramedic should interview the patient to obtain relevant data, including the following eight points:

Note

Pregnancy may aggravate some pre-existing medical conditions such as diabetes, heart disease, hypertension and seizure disorders. Some medications (e.g. antihypertensive agents and oral hypoglycaemic drugs) used to manage these disorders cannot be taken by the mother during her pregnancy due to the potential harm to the fetus. Thus a thorough patient history is essential to help the paramedic anticipate care that may be required at the scene and during patient transport.

1. Obstetric history
   a. Length of gestation
   b. Parity and gravidity
   c. Previous caesarean delivery
   d. Maternal lifestyle (alcohol or other drug use, smoking history)
   e. Infectious disease status
   f. History of previous gynaecological or obstetric complications (e.g. eclampsia, GDM, premature labour or ectopic pregnancy).
2. Presence of pain
   a. Onset (gradual or sudden)
   b. Character
   c. Duration and evolution over time
   d. Location and radiation.
3. Presence, quantity, and character of vaginal bleeding.
4. Presence of abnormal vaginal discharge.
5. Presence of 'show' (expulsion of the mucus plug in early labour) or rupture of membranes.
6. Current general health and antenatal care (none, physician, nurse, midwife).
7. Allergies and medications taken (especially the use of narcotics in the last 4 h).
8. Maternal urge to bear down or sensation of imminent bowel movement, indicating imminent delivery.

Physical examination

The patient's chief complaint determines the extent of the examination. The goal in examining an obstetric patient is to rapidly identify acute life-threatening conditions and to identify imminent delivery. If delivery is near, the paramedic must take the proper management steps.

The paramedic should assess the patient's general appearance and skin colour. Pallor may indicate haemorrhage, whilst sunken cheeks, cracked lips or hollow eyes with a history of vomiting indicate dehydration. The paramedic should monitor the patient's vital signs frequently during the care and should recall that normal physiological changes in the pregnant patient can produce variations in vital signs. Examples of such are mild tachycardia, a slight fall in systolic and diastolic blood pressures, and an increase in respiratory rate. Orthostatic vital signs are important as they may indicate the early presence of significant bleeding or fluid loss.

The paramedic should examine the patient's abdomen for scars and gross deformities. The latter may be caused by a hernia or marked abdominal distension. Gentle palpation may reveal the presence of masses, enlarged organs, intestinal distension or a distended bladder, although these may be hard to recognize in late pregnancy. During the examination, it may be possible to discern peritoneal irritation, which may be diagnosed by the presence of tenderness, guarding, or rebound tenderness (rebound tenderness should not be undertaken by paramedics). If the patient is obviously pregnant, the paramedic may need to assess uterine size.

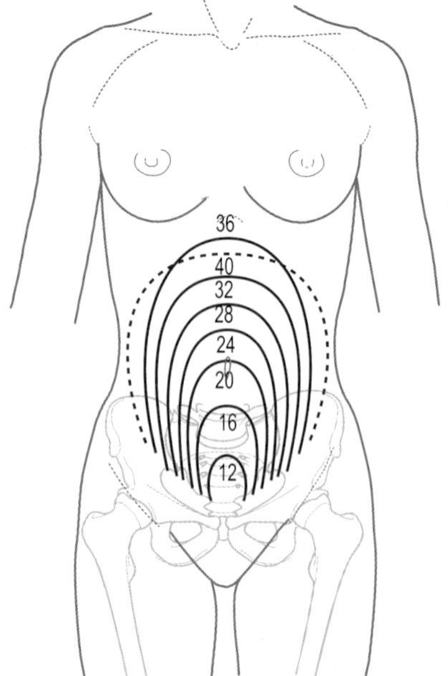

Figure 36-4 Changes in fundal height during pregnancy. Weeks 10 to 12: The uterus is within the pelvis, and fetal heartbeat can be detected with a Doppler probe. Week 12: The uterus is palpable just above the symphysis pubis. Week 16: The uterus is palpable just between the symphysis pubis and umbilicus. Week 20: The uterine fundus is at the lower border of the umbilicus. A fetal heartbeat can be auscultated with a fetoscope. Weeks 24 to 26: The uterus becomes ovoid, and the fetus is palpable. Week 28: The uterus is about halfway between the umbilicus and xiphoid process, and the fetus is easily palpable. Week 32: The uterine fundus is just below the xiphoid. Week 40: Fundal height drops as the fetus begins to engage in the pelvis.

Evaluation of uterine size

The uterine contour is usually irregular between 8 and 10 weeks' gestation. Thus, early uterine enlargement may not be symmetrical. Moreover, the uterus may be deviated to one side. The uterus is above the symphysis pubis at 12–16 weeks' gestation, around the level of the umbilicus at 24 weeks, and near the xiphoid process at term. Figure 36-4 shows changes in fundal height at the various weeks of gestation.

General management of the obstetric patient

If birth is not imminent, care for the healthy patient should be limited to basic treatment modalities (airway, ventilatory and circulatory support) and transportation for physician evaluation. In the absence of distress or injury, the patient should be transported in a comfortable position (usually left lateral recumbent). The paramedic may need to monitor the electrocardiogram, administer high-concentration oxygen, and monitor the fetus, based on patient assessment and vital sign determinations.

Complications of pregnancy

Complications associated with pregnancy can result from trauma, medical conditions, prior disease processes that the pregnancy can aggravate or mask, the pregnancy itself (vaginal or intraperitoneal haemorrhage), spontaneous abortion, or problems associated with labour and delivery. Often the patient with gynaecological or obstetric complaints is embarrassed, apprehensive, and, if pregnant, concerned about the unborn child. Tact, understanding, and a caring, supportive attitude from the paramedic are important when managing these patients.

Trauma during pregnancy

When a pregnant woman is severely injured, the fetus is at high risk for death. When the mother sustains life-threatening injuries, 40.6% of fetuses die, compared with only 1.6% in non-life-threatening cases.[1] Mortality related directly to the pregnancy itself is rare; accounting for 5.3 deaths per 100 000 maternities.[2,3] The anatomical and physiological changes of pregnancy can change the pregnant woman's response to injury, which may necessitate modified assessment, treatment, and transportation strategies.

Maternal injury

The causes of maternal injury in decreasing order of frequency are vehicular crashes, falls, and penetrating objects. These injuries can result in trauma to the gravid uterus as well as to the maternal bladder, liver, and spleen. In addition, an injury that results in a pelvic fracture can produce massive haemorrhage and damage to the fetal skull. As described in Chapter 26, the severity of any injury depends on many factors, including the involvement of multiple organ systems.

During pregnancy, the fetus is well protected within the uterus; amniotic fluid surrounds the fetus. This fluid serves as an excellent shock absorber and means that the fetus rarely experiences physical trauma except as a result of direct penetrating wounds or extensive blunt trauma to the maternal abdomen. The greatest risk of fetal death is from fetal distress and intrauterine demise caused by trauma to the mother or her death. Thus, when dealing with a pregnant trauma patient, the paramedic should promptly assess and intervene on behalf of the mother. Causes of fetal death from maternal trauma include death of the mother, separation of the placenta, maternal shock, uterine rupture, and fetal head injury.

Assessment and management

The priorities in assessing and managing a pregnant trauma patient are the same as for a non-gravid patient: adequate airway, ventilatory, and circulatory support with spinal precautions; haemorrhage control; rapid assessment, stabilization and rapid transportation to a medical facility. Resuscitating the mother is key to the survival of the mother and fetus; thus, during the first stages of assessing and managing, the mother's status should be the focus. Irrespective of severity, all pregnant trauma patients should be given high-concentration oxygen and transported for physician evaluation.

The examination should be thorough. The paramedic must detect, identify, and manage injuries that contribute to hypovolaemia or hypoxia. With the normal increase in maternal blood volume, the mother can lose greater volumes of blood before showing signs and symptoms of shock. A 30–35% reduction in blood volume can produce minimal changes in blood pressure but reduce uterine blood flow by 10–20%.[1] Given the reduced perfusion status of the uterus (and fetus), and the masking of blood loss, it is essential that fluids be considered earlier in the pregnant patient than the non-pregnant patient.[4]

Critical Thinking

How do you think the traumatized pregnant patient feels emotionally?

Special management considerations

Special considerations in managing the pregnant trauma patient include oxygenation, volume replacement and haemorrhage control. Labour is a complication of trauma in pregnancy so the emergency medical services (EMS) crew should be ready to manage delivery or spontaneous abortion.

Cardiac arrest can occur in pregnant women from a number of causes (Box 36-3) However, many cardiovascular problems associated with pregnancy are related to changes in anatomy that produce a decrease in the return of venous blood.[5] Key interventions to prevent cardiac arrest in a distressed or compromised pregnant patient include placing the patient in the left lateral position or manually and gently displacing the uterus to the left, administering 100% oxygen, and giving a fluid bolus. The key to resuscitation of the child is resuscitation of the mother. The mother cannot be resuscitated until blood flow to her right ventricle is restored.

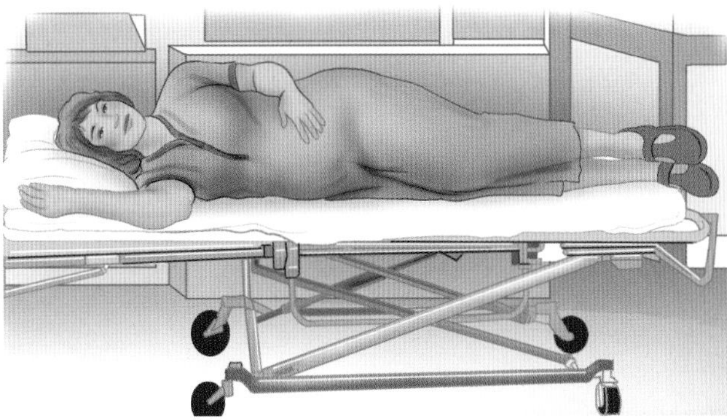

Figure 36-5 Patient positioning to displace the uterus.

Box 36-3

Causes of cardiac arrest associated with pregnancy

Events that occur at the time of delivery

Amniotic fluid embolism
Drug toxicity (e.g. because of magnesium sulphate or epidural anaesthetic)
Eclampsia

Events that occur from complex physiological changes associated with pregnancy

Aortic dissection
Congestive cardiomyopathy
Haemorrhage from a pregnancy-related pathological condition
Pulmonary embolism

If cardiac arrest occurs, the paramedic should follow adult basic life support guidelines with the following considerations:[4]

- Address the need for left lateral tilt of the torso to prevent compression or blockage of the vena cava. This can be achieved with wedge-shaped pillows that support the tilted torso during chest compression. It also can be achieved by using the angled backs of several chairs and the angled thighs of several rescuers to place the patient in the left lateral tilt position (Figure 36-5).
- Consider early intubation to protect from the increased risk of regurgitation.

An aggressive resuscitation effort is justified in patients who are near term. This can allow for a caesarean delivery at the emergency department. Fetal survival is good if the time between maternal death and delivery is less than 5 min, but prognosis is poor if the time is longer than 20–25 min. Alerting the emergency department staff of the possibility of the need for an emergency caesarean section is critical to neonatal survival.

Oxygenation

- Adequate maternal airway maintenance and oxygenation are essential to prevention of fetal hypoxaemia.
- Oxygen requirements are 10–20% greater than in the normal, non-pregnant patient. Fetal hypoxia may occur with even small changes in maternal oxygenation, therefore the paramedic should administer high-concentration oxygen.
- If available, pulse oximetry should be used to monitor oxygen saturation.

Volume replacement

- Signs and symptoms of hypovolaemia may not be present until a blood loss is large.
- Blood is shunted preferentially from the uterus to preserve maternal blood pressure.
- Bleeding may also occur inside the uterus, which can sequester up to 2000 mL of blood after separation of the placenta, with little or no evidence of vaginal bleeding.[1]
- Crystalloid fluid replacement is indicated, even when blood pressure remains normal.

Haemorrhage control

- External haemorrhage should be controlled the same as in a non-pregnant patient.
- Vaginal bleeding may point to placental separation or uterine rupture.
- Avoid a vaginal examination. It may increase bleeding and bring on delivery, especially if unsuspected placenta praevia is present (described later in chapter).
- Document the amount and colour of vaginal bleeding.
- Collect and transport any expelled tissue with the patient to the facility.

Transportation plans

Pregnant patients after 3–4 months' gestation should not be transported in a supine position because of the potential for supine hypotension. In the absence of suspected spinal injury, the patient should be transported in a left lateral recumbent position. If spinal injury is suspected, the patient should be prepared for transportation in the following manner:

1. Fully immobilize the patient on a long spine board.
2. After immobilization, carefully tilt the board on its left side by log-rolling the secured patient 30 degrees.[4]
3. Place a blanket, pillow, or towel under the right side of the board to move the uterus to the left side.

Critical Thinking

Are facilities in your community prepared to manage deliveries that are high risk?

Medical conditions and disease processes

Pregnancy can mask or worsen some medical conditions and diseases. These include acute appendicitis, acute cholecystitis, hypertension, diabetes, infection, neuromuscular disorders and cardiovascular disease. Two hypertensive disorders are specific to pregnancy. They are pre-eclampsia and eclampsia (toxaemia of pregnancy). Hypertensive disorders occur in about 5–7% of pregnancies in the UK and increase the risk to the mother and the fetus.[6]

Pre-eclampsia and eclampsia

Pre-eclampsia is a disease of unknown origin. It is defined as pregnancy-induced hypertension ≥140/90 mmHg developing after 20 weeks' gestation in a previously normotensive woman, in association with proteinuria. The pathophysiology of pre-eclampsia, which does not reverse until after delivery, is characterized by vasospasm, endothelial cell injury, increased capillary permeability and activation of the clotting cascade. The signs and symptoms of pre-eclampsia result from hypoperfusion to the tissue or organs involved (Box 36-4). Eclampsia is characterized by the same signs and symptoms with the addition of seizures or coma.

Factors predisposing to pre-eclampsia include nulliparity, advanced maternal age, chronic hypertension, chronic renal disease, vascular diseases such as diabetes and systemic lupus erythematosus, and multiple gestation. Pre-eclampsia is a clinical diagnosis that can be confirmed by postpartum renal biopsy. When pre-eclampsia is suspected, most patients are hospitalized or confined to bed rest at home until delivery.

Box 36-4

Signs and symptoms of pre-eclampsia

Cerebrum

Headache
Hyperreflexia
Dizziness
Confusion
Seizures
Coma

Retina

Blurred vision
Diplopia

Gastrointestinal system

Nausea
Vomiting
Right upper quadrant or epigastric pain and tenderness

Renal system

Proteinuria
Azotaemia
Oliguria
Anuria
Haematuria
Haemoglobinuria

Vasculature or endothelium

Hypertension
Oedema
Activation of the clotting cascade

Placenta

Abruptio placentae
Fetal distress

Management

Not all hypertensive patients have pre-eclampsia and not all pre-eclamptic patients have hypertension. The illness has many serious complications, so suspicion of pre-eclampsia or eclampsia should be high when hypertension is present in late pregnancy. If pre-eclampsia or eclampsia is suspected, prehospital care is directed at preventing or controlling seizures and treating hypertension.

Seizure activity in eclampsia is similar to generalized seizures of other causes. Seizure activity is characterized by tonic–clonic activity (described in Chapter 16) and often begins around the mouth in the form of twitching. Eclampsia may be associated with apnoea during the seizure. Labour can begin suddenly and progress rapidly. The regimen for managing severe pre-eclampsia is as follows:[7]

1. Place patient in 15–30° of left lateral tilt or the left lateral position. This helps to alleviate aortocaval compression.
2. Handle the patient gently, minimize stimulation (for example, darken the ambulance) and avoid use of sirens; this may help to avoid seizures. Administer high concentrations of oxygen and assist ventilation if required.
3. If the patient has continuous or recurrent fits, gain IV access. If not, gain IV access en route to hospital.
4. If available, administer magnesium sulphate per guidelines.
5. If magnesium sulphate is not available and the patient is in status, consider diazepam per guideline. Note: diazepam must not be used if the patient is not actually fitting as it will not prevent subsequent fits. Be aware that diazepam may:
   a. precipitate a fall in blood pressure
   b. jeopardize fetal circulation
   c. cause neonatal respiratory distress after delivery.
6. Closely monitor vital signs.
7. Provide smooth and rapid transportation to hospital.
8. DO NOT administer fluids as the patient is at risk of pulmonary oedema even with small boluses of crystalloids. If fluids are attached to the cannula, they should be flowing at a rate of no more than 80 mL/h.

Gestational diabetes mellitus

As stated before, GDM is caused by pregnancy. The condition occurs in between 3% and 5% of all pregnancies, affecting up to 40 000 women in the UK each year.[8] Gestational diabetes mellitus is thought to be related to an inability of the mother to metabolize carbohydrates. This may be caused by a deficiency of the mother's insulin or from placental hormones that block the action of the mother's insulin (insulin resistance). As a result, the mother's body is not able to produce or use all of the insulin it needs during the pregnancy. Excessive amounts of her glucose are transmitted to the fetus, where it is stored as fat. Treatment for GDM includes regular glucose monitoring, dietary modification, exercise, and, in some cases, insulin injections. The condition usually subsides after pregnancy but may return in later years or with future pregnancies.

Most women with GDM are aware of their condition through antenatal care and most have healthy pregnancies and healthy babies. Without treatment, however, mothers with GDM often have very large babies, which makes for a more difficult labour and delivery (with increased risk for fetal and maternal injury) and a longer recovery. In addition, children whose mothers had GDM are at higher risk for certain health problems. Examples of such are respiratory distress syndrome, obesity and related health issues as children or adults, and an increased risk for developing type 2 diabetes during their lifetime.

Management

Prehospital care for patients with GDM may include airway, ventilatory and circulatory support; glucose testing; and managing hypoglycaemia with IV fluids and glucose. (See Chapter 17.)

Vaginal bleeding

Vaginal bleeding during pregnancy can result from abortion (miscarriage), ectopic pregnancy, abruptio placentae, placenta praevia, uterine rupture or postpartum haemorrhage. Patients with vaginal bleeding have varying degrees of blood loss. Some require aggressive resuscitation.

Critical Thinking

As the mother loses blood from vaginal haemorrhage, what effect does that have on the fetus?

Abortion

Abortion is the termination of pregnancy from any cause before 24 weeks' gestation and is often referred to as miscarriage. (After 24 weeks, it is known as a preterm birth.) Abortion is the most frequent cause of vaginal bleeding in pregnant women and occurs in about 1 in 10 pregnancies. Box 36-5 lists common classifications of abortion.

Box 36-5

Classifications of abortion

Complete abortion: an abortion in which the patient has passed all of the products of conception.

Criminal abortion: an intentional ending of any pregnancy under any condition not allowed by law.

Incomplete abortion: an abortion in which the patient has passed some but not all of the products of conception.

Induced abortion: an abortion in which the pregnancy is terminated intentionally.

Missed abortion: the retention of the fetus in utero for 4 or more weeks after fetal death.

Spontaneous abortion: an abortion that usually occurs before the twelfth week of gestation (the lay term is miscarriage). (Predisposing factors include acute or chronic illness in the mother, abnormalities in the fetus, and abnormal attachment of the placenta. Often the cause is unknown.)

Therapeutic abortion: a pregnancy legally terminated for reasons of maternal well-being.

Threatened abortion: an abortion in which a patient has some uterine bleeding with an intrauterine pregnancy in which the internal cervical os is closed. A threatened abortion may stabilize and end in normal delivery or progress to an incomplete or complete abortion.

Most abortions occur in the first trimester, usually before the tenth week. The patient is often anxious and apprehensive and complains of vaginal bleeding. This bleeding may be slight or profuse. In addition, the patient may have suprapubic pain which may be referred to the lower back and described as cramp-like and similar to the pain of labour or menstruation. When obtaining a history, the paramedic should ascertain the time of onset of pain and bleeding, amount of blood loss (a soaked sanitary pad suggests 20–30 mL of blood loss), and whether the patient passed any tissue with the blood. If the patient passed tissue during bleeding episodes, the tissue should be collected and transported with the patient for analysis.

Management The paramedic should watch all first-trimester emergencies closely for signs of significant blood loss and hypovolaemia. The paramedic should measure vital signs (including orthostatic vital signs) often during transport. Depending on the patient's vital signs, IV fluid therapy may be indicated. All patients with suspected abortion should receive a high level of emotional support and should be transported for physician evaluation; oxygen may also be indicated.

Ectopic pregnancy

An ectopic pregnancy occurs when a fertilized ovum implants anywhere other than the uterus. Ectopic gestation occurs in 11.5 per 1000 pregnancies; it is the leading cause of first-trimester death and accounts for 4% of all maternal deaths in the UK.[6] Death from ectopic pregnancy usually results from haemorrhage.

Ectopic pregnancy has many causes. But most involve factors that delay or prevent the passage of the fertilized ovum to its normal site of implantation. Predisposing factors include pelvic inflammatory disease, adhesions from previous surgery, tubal ligation, previous ectopic pregnancy, and possibly the presence of intrauterine contraceptive devices. Thus, obtaining a full gynaecological history is key. Although the time from fertilization varies, most ruptures occur by 2 to 12 weeks' gestation.

The signs and symptoms of ectopic pregnancy are often difficult to distinguish from those of a ruptured ovarian cyst, pelvic inflammatory disease, appendicitis or abortion (hence the name the great imitator). The classic triad of symptoms includes abdominal pain, vaginal bleeding and amenorrhoea (absence of menstruation); however, vaginal bleeding may be absent, spotty or minimal, and amenorrhea may be replaced by oligomenorrhoea (scanty flow). The variable presentation of this type of pregnancy is one reason for its high-risk profile. Other symptoms of ectopic pregnancy include signs of early pregnancy. These include referred pain to the shoulder, nausea, vomiting, syncope, and the classic signs of shock.

Management A ruptured ectopic pregnancy is a true emergency that calls for initial resuscitation measures and rapid transportation for surgery. The patient may become unstable quickly. Where ectopic pregnancy is suspected, the paramedic should manage the patient like any victim of haemorrhagic shock – with airway, ventilatory and circulatory support and IV fluid resuscitation in accordance with current guidelines.

Third-trimester bleeding

Third-trimester bleeding occurs in 3% of all pregnancies and is never normal. The majority of bleeding episodes are a result of abruptio placentae, placenta praevia or uterine rupture. Table 36-1 differentiates among abruptio placentae, placenta praevia and uterine rupture.

Abruptio placentae Abruptio placentae is partial or full detachment of a normally implanted placenta at more than 20 weeks' gestation. It occurs in up to 1.8% of all pregnancies and produces perinatal mortality in between 4.4% and 67.3% of cases, depending upon the neonatal facilities and

Table 36-1 Differentiation of abruptio placentae, placenta praevia and uterine rupture

History	Bleeding	Abnormal pain	Abdominal examination
Abruptio placentae			
Association with toxaemia of pregnancy and hypertension of any cause	Single attack of scant, dark vaginal bleeding (often concealed) that continues until delivery	Present	Localized uterine tenderness
Labour			
Absent fetal heart tones (often)			
Placenta praevia			
Lack of association with toxaemia of pregnancy	Repeated 'warning' haemorrhages over days to weeks	Usually absent	Lack of uterine tenderness (usually)
Labour (rare)			
Fetal heart tones (usually)			
Uterine rupture			
Previous caesarean section	Possible bleeding	Usually present and associated with sudden onset of nausea and vomiting	Diffuse abdominal tenderness
Sudden cessation of labour			
Possible fetal heart tones			

the size of the abruption.[6] Predisposing factors to abruptio placentae include maternal hypertension, pre-eclampsia, multiparity, trauma and previous abruption.

Critical Thinking

Why is abruptio placentae associated with such a high fetal death rate?

The common presentation of abruptio placentae is sudden third-trimester vaginal bleeding and pain. The vaginal bleeding may be minimal but it is often concealed and disproportionate to the degree of shock. The more extensive the separation, the greater the uterine irritability, resulting in a tender abdomen and rigid uterus. Contractions may be present.

Placenta praevia Placenta praevia is placental implantation in the lower uterine segment, partially or completely covering the cervical opening. It complicates 0.5% of pregnancies[6] and has a higher incidence in preterm births. The condition is characterized by painless, bright red bleeding without uterine contraction. The bleeding may occur in episodes and may be slight to moderate. In addition, bleeding may become more profuse if active labour begins.

Placenta praevia is associated with increasing maternal age, multiparity, previous caesarean section and previous placenta praevia episodes. Recent sexual intercourse can lead to bleeding.

Uterine rupture Uterine rupture is a spontaneous or traumatic rupture of the uterine wall. It may result from reopening of a previous uterine scar (e.g. a previous caesarean section), a prolonged or obstructed labour, or direct trauma. Uterine rupture occurs in about 1 in 1500 deliveries in the UK and has a 5–15% maternal mortality rate and a 30% fetal mortality rate.[6]

Uterine rupture is characterized by sudden abdominal pain described as steady and 'tearing', active labour, early signs of shock (complaints of weakness, dizziness, anxiety), and vaginal bleeding, which may not be visible. On examination, the abdomen is usually rigid. The patient complains of diffuse abdominal pain and fetal parts may be felt easily through the abdominal wall.

Management The prehospital management of a patient with third-trimester bleeding is aimed at preventing shock. The paramedic should not try to examine the patient vaginally; doing so may increase haemorrhage and bring on labour. Emergency care measures should include the following:

1. Provide adequate airway, ventilatory and circulatory support as needed (with spinal precautions if indicated).
2. Place the patient in a left lateral recumbent position.
3. Begin transport immediately.
4. Initiate IV therapy with crystalloid fluid where indicated.
5. Apply a fresh perineal pad. Note the time of application to assess bleeding during transport.
6. Check fundal height. Document it for baseline measurement.
7. Closely monitor the patient's vital signs en route to the facility.

Labour and delivery

Parturition is the process by which the infant is born. Near the end of pregnancy the uterus becomes more and more irritable and exhibits occasional contractions. These contractions become stronger and more frequent until parturition begins. During and as a result of these contractions, the cervix begins to dilate. As uterine contractions increase, complete cervical dilatation occurs to about 10 cm; the amniotic sac ruptures; and the fetus, and shortly thereafter the placenta, are expelled from the uterus through the vaginal canal (Figure 36-6).

Stages of labour

Labour follows several distinct stages. The lengths of these stages vary depending on whether the mother is nullipara or multipara (Box 36-6). The paramedic should use the stages only as a guideline in assessing labour progression in the average pregnancy. About 2 to 3 weeks before the onset of active labour, the cervix undergoes the process of softening, effacement (thinning), and dilatation. At the same time, the uterus begins to become a contractile organ. Braxton Hicks contractions refer to irregular tightening of the pregnant uterus. These often begin in the first trimester and are usually benign and painless. They often subside with walking or other exercise. Many patients are not aware of Braxton Hicks contractions and may perceive them only as a slight uterine hardening. As the pregnancy continues, the contractions increase in frequency and duration. This heralds the onset of clinical labour. A great deal of individual variation exists in the perception and tolerance of uterine contractions. Some mothers experience somewhat painless contractions even with the onset of labour, whilst others are uncomfortable from the earlier and less intense Braxton Hicks contractions. In the former group, delivery may be more imminent than anticipated; members of the latter group may develop false labour several days to weeks before term.

Box 36-6

Stages of labour

Stage I (dilatation)

Onset of regular contractions to complete cervical dilatation

Average time: 8–12 h in primipara, 6–8 h in multipara

Stage II (expulsion)

Full dilatation of cervix to delivery of the newborn

Average time: 80 min in primipara, 30 min in multipara

Stage III (placenta delivery)

Immediately after delivery of the infant until expulsion of the placenta

Average time: 5–20 min

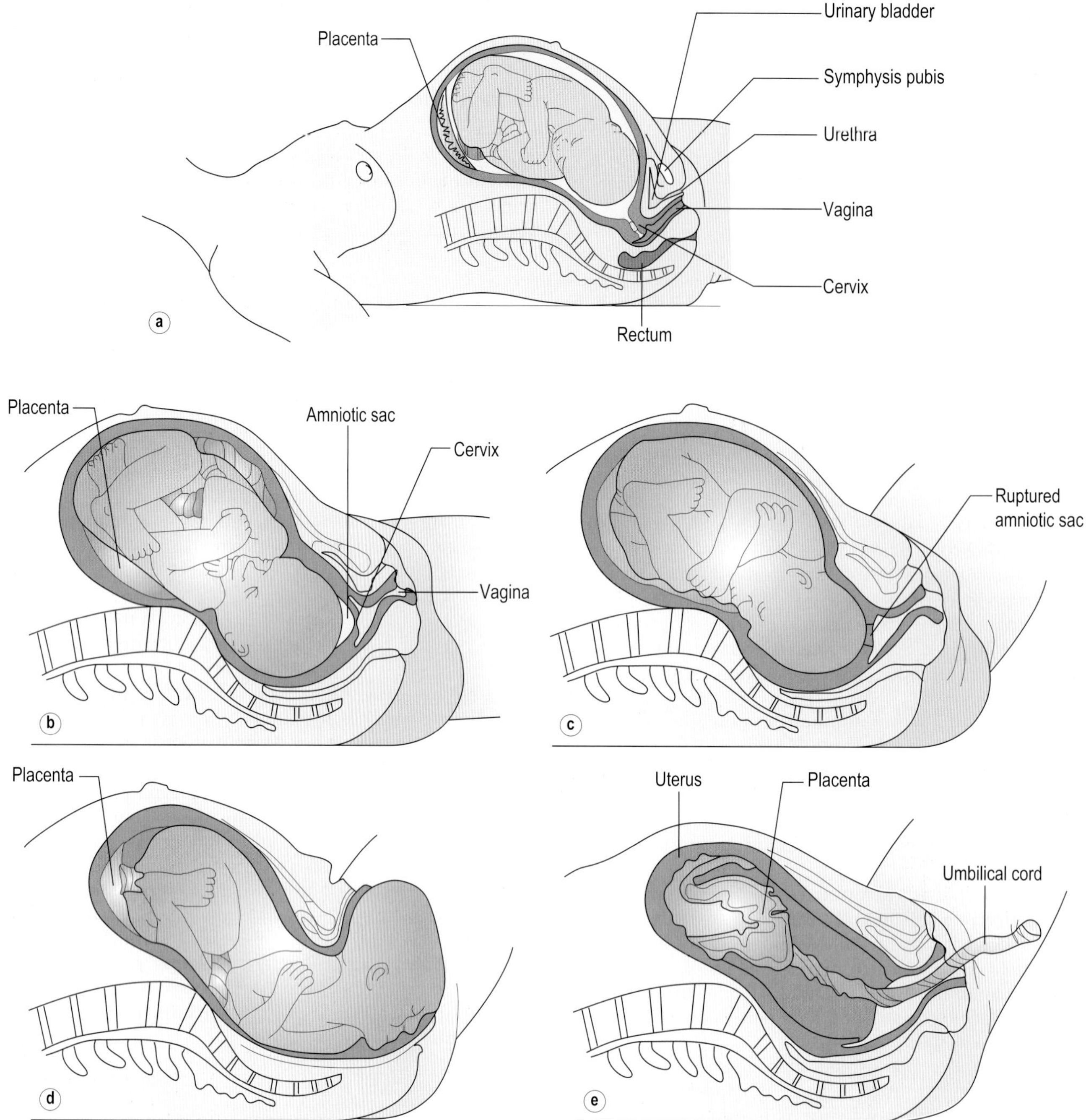

Figure 36-6 Parturition. (a) The relation of the fetus to the mother. (b) The fetus moves into the birth canal. (c) Dilatation of the cervix is complete. (d) The fetus is expelled from the uterus. (e) The placenta is expelled.

Labour begins with the infant's descent into the birth canal. The fetal descent is characterized by a relief of pressure in the upper abdomen and a simultaneous increase in pressure in the pelvis. During this stage a mucus plug (sometimes mixed with blood, thus the name bloody show) is expelled from the dilating cervix and discharged from the vagina. The mother may not notice these early changes as a sign of labour.

The first stage of labour begins with the onset of regular contractions and ends with full dilatation of the cervix. The uterine contractions generally occur at 5–15-min intervals. They are characterized by cramp-like abdominal pains. These pains radiate to the small of the back. As the uterus contracts, the cervix becomes soft and thinned (effaced). The less muscular lower segment of the uterus is pulled upward over the presenting part. The first stage usually lasts 8–12 h in the first-time mother. It usually lasts about 6–8 h in women who have had previous deliveries. In most pregnancies the amniotic sac ruptures (rupture of membranes) toward the end of the first stage of labour. Entonox should be offered during the first stage of labour, with inhalation commenced as soon as the mother feels the contraction, before the pain is fully established.

Critical Thinking

What comfort measures can you use during transportation for the patient who is in the first stage of labour?

The second stage of labour is measured from full dilatation of the cervix to delivery of the infant. During the second stage the fetal head enters the birth canal. The mother's pain and contractions become more intense and frequent (usually 2–3 min apart). Often the mother becomes diaphoretic and tachycardic during this stage, and experiences an urge to bear down with each contraction. In addition, she may express the need to have a bowel movement. (This is a normal sensation caused by pressure of the fetal head against the mother's rectum.) The presenting part of the fetus (usually the head) emerges from the vaginal opening. This process, known as crowning, indicates that delivery is imminent. The second stage of labour usually lasts 1–2 h in the nullipara mother and 30 min or less in the multipara mother.

The third stage of labour begins with delivery of the infant and ends when the placenta is expelled and the uterus has contracted. The length of this stage varies from 5 to 60 min, regardless of parity.

Signs and symptoms of imminent delivery

The following signs and symptoms indicate that delivery is imminent. With these, the paramedic should prepare for childbirth at the scene:

- Regular contractions lasting 45–60 s at 1–2-min intervals. Intervals are measured from the beginning of one contraction to the beginning of the next. If contractions are more than 5 min apart, there is generally time to transport the mother to a receiving hospital unless distances are great.
- The mother has an urge to bear down or has a sensation of a bowel movement.
- There is a large amount of bloody show.
- Crowning occurs.
- The mother believes that delivery is imminent.

If any of these signs and symptoms are present, the EMS crew should prepare for delivery. With the exception of cord presentation (described later in this chapter), the paramedic should not try to delay delivery. If complications are anticipated or an abnormal delivery occurs, a midwife and second crew should be requested (Figure 36-7).

Preparation for delivery

When preparing for delivery, the paramedic should try to provide an area of privacy. If birth becomes imminent on the way to hospital, the driver should pull in, park safely and inform ambulance control. If the crew have not left the home address, control should be contacted to arrange a midwife and second crew. The delivery area should be as clean as possible and should be covered with absorbent material to guard against staining and contamination by blood and faecal material.

The traditional position is for the mother to be placed on her back with her knees flexed and widely separated. Current thinking suggests that the mother should choose the position most appropriate to her and not be forced to lie on her back; many women who have attended antenatal classes may prefer to squat, kneel or be on all fours. If delivery occurs in a car, the mother should be instructed to lie on her back across the seat with one leg flexed on the seat and the other leg resting on the floorboard. A pillow or blanket, if available, should be placed beneath the mother's buttocks to aid in the delivery of the infant's head. The paramedic should evaluate the mother's vital signs for baseline measurements. It is not usual for the paramedic to administer maternal oxygen or to gain IV access for fluid administration and syntometrine; however, these skills may occasionally be required.

The mother should be coached to bear down and push during contractions and to rest between contractions to conserve strength. If the mother finds it difficult to refrain from pushing, the paramedic should encourage her to breathe deeply or 'pant' through her mouth between contractions. Deep breathing and panting help decrease the force of bearing down and promote rest.

Delivery equipment

Prehospital delivery equipment generally includes the following components (Figure 36-8):

- umbilical cord clamps
- quilted babywrap
- maternity pads
- umbilical cord scissors
- mucus extractor
- placenta tray/bowl
- incontinence sheets
- 10 × 10 cm gauze swabs
- plastic bag for placental transportation
- paper towel.

Personal protective measures should be used when assisting in a delivery. Sterile technique should be used when handling equipment.

Assistance with delivery

In most cases the paramedic only assists in the natural events of childbirth. The chief duties of the EMS crew are to prevent an uncontrolled delivery and protect the infant from cold and stress after the birth. The following are steps to be taken in assisting the mother with a normal delivery (Figure 36-9):

1. Don sterile gloves and other personal protective equipment.
2. When crowning occurs, apply gentle palm pressure to the infant's head to prevent an explosive delivery and tearing of the perineum. Instruct the mother to pant or puff, allowing the head to advance slowly with each contraction. If membranes are still intact, tear the sac with finger pressure to allow escape of amniotic fluid.
3. After delivery of the head, examine the infant's neck for a looped umbilical cord. If the cord is looped around the neck, gently slip it over the infant's head. If the cord is too tight, it is best to deliver the rest of

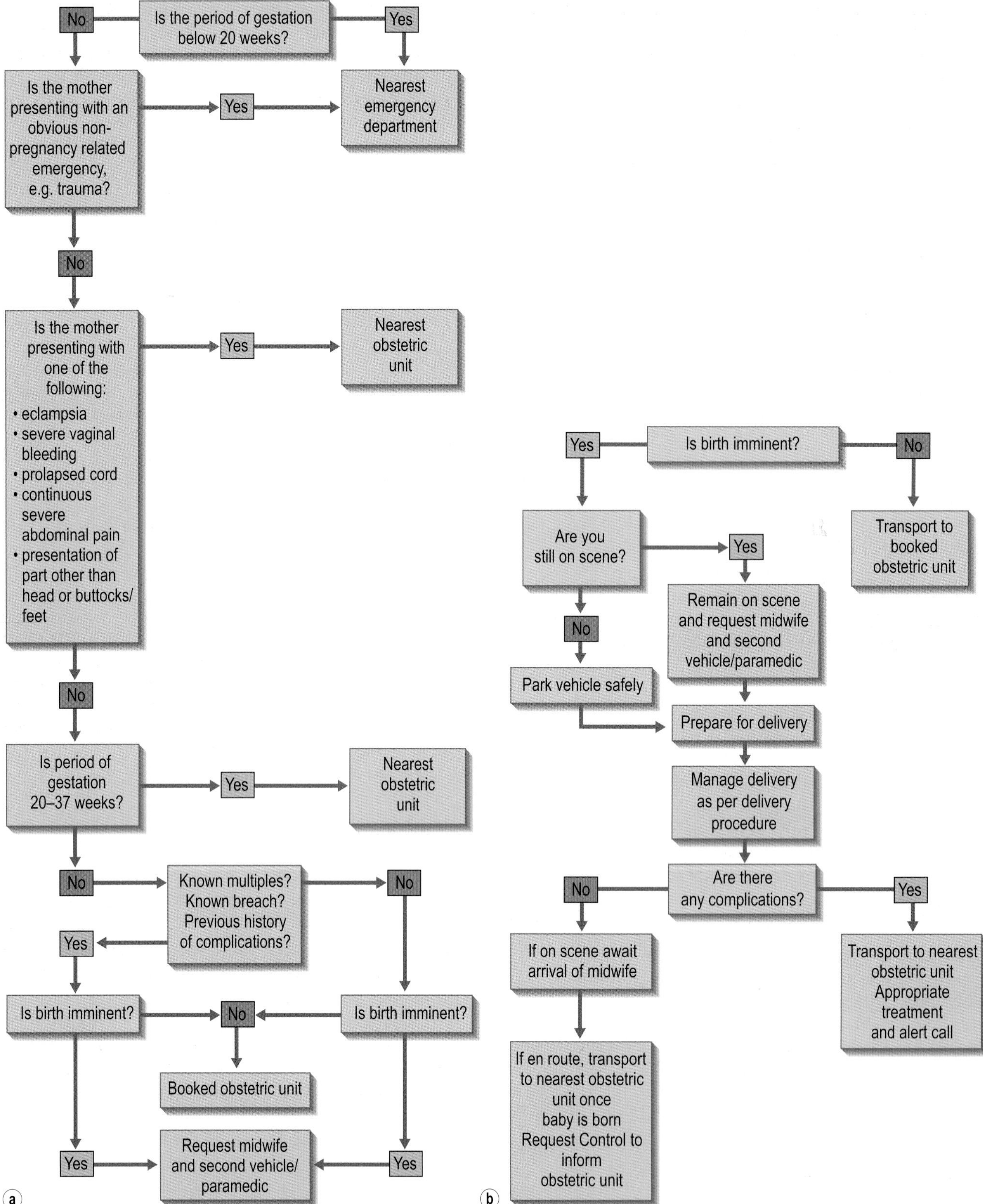

Figure 36-7 Decision-making algorithms. (a) Maternal assessment. (b) Delivery flowchart. Reproduced with permission of the Joint Royal Colleges Ambulance Liaison Committee.

the baby with the cord in situ – a tight cord will not prevent delivery of the baby.

4. Wipe any obvious mucus or secretions from the baby's mouth and nose. Consider suction (only the oral cavity), which should be performed after the head appears but before the next contraction as this should deliver the shoulders and chest. The birth canal prevents chest expansion and minimizes the risk of aspiration if suction is performed well before the first breath, which usually occurs on delivery of the chest and shoulders.
5. Support the infant's head as it rotates for shoulder presentation. Most babies present face down then rotate to the left so that the shoulders present in an anterior–posterior position.
6. With gentle pressure, guide the infant's head downward to deliver the anterior shoulder and then upward to release the posterior shoulder. The rest of the infant is delivered quickly by smooth uterine contraction.
7. Be careful to grasp and support the infant as he or she emerges. Use care because the infant is slippery. Hold the infant firmly with his or her head dependent to aid drainage of secretions. Maintain the infant's position at or slightly above the level of the mother's vagina; this will prevent over-transfusion or under-transfusion of blood from the umbilical cord.
8. Clear the infant's airway of any secretions with sterile gauze, and repeat suction of the infant's mouth if required.

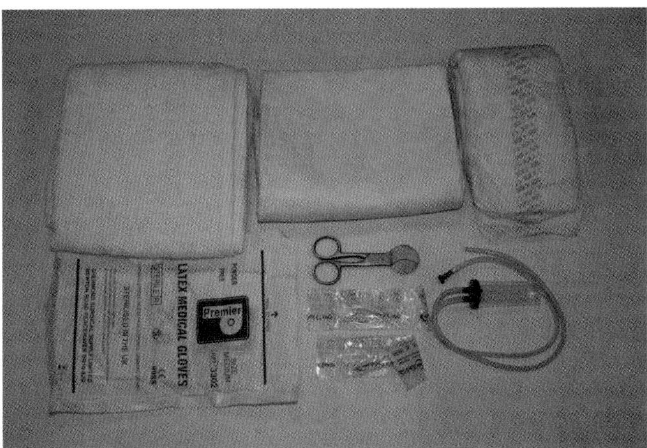

Figure 36-8 Prehospital delivery equipment.

9. Dry the infant with warm sterile towels. Remove the now wet towel and wrap the infant in dry towelling. It is especially important to cover the head to reduce heat loss.
10. Record the infant's gender and time of birth.

Critical Thinking

How do you think you will feel after delivering a healthy infant?

Evaluation of the infant

After delivery, the paramedic should dry and cover the newborn to prevent heat loss and should position the newborn on the side or with padding under the back, clear the airway, and provide tactile stimulation to initiate respirations. If there is no need for resuscitation, the paramedic should assign an Apgar score at 1 min and 5 min to evaluate the infant (Table 36-2).

Criteria for computing the Apgar score include appearance (colour), pulse (heart rate), grimace (reflex irritability to stimulation), activity (muscle tone) and respiratory effort. Each criterion is rated from 0 to 2 and the numbers added for a total Apgar score. The paramedic should never delay or interrupt resuscitation efforts to assign an Apgar score.

An Apgar score of 10 indicates that the infant is in the best possible condition, 7 to 9 indicates that the infant is slightly depressed (near normal), 4 to 6 indicates that the infant is moderately depressed, and 0 to 3 indicates that the infant is severely depressed. Most newborns have an Apgar score of 8 to 10 at 1 min after birth. Newborns with an Apgar score of less than 6 generally require resuscitation; however, the paramedic should not use the Apgar score to determine the need for resuscitation. (Neonatal resuscitation is presented in Chapter 37.)

Cutting the umbilical cord

After the paramedic delivers and evaluates the infant, the paramedic should clamp (or tie with umbilical tape) and cut the umbilical cord (Figure 36-10). The paramedic should take the following steps to manage the umbilical cord:

1. Securely apply two cord clamps approximately 3 cm ($1\frac{1}{2}$ inch) apart and approximately 15 cm (6 inch) from the umbilicus. Do not strip or milk the cord; doing so may lead to red blood cell destruction, polycythaemia, and hyperbilirubinaemia.

Table 36-2 The Apgar scoring system

Sign	0	1	2
Appearance (skin colour)	Blue, pale	Body pink, blue extremities	Completely pink
Pulse rate (heart rate)	Absent	<100/min	>100/min
Grimace (irritability)	No response	Grimace	Cough, sneeze, cry
Activity (muscle tone)	Limp	Some flexion	Active motion
Respiration (respiratory effort)	Absent	Slow, irregular	Good, crying

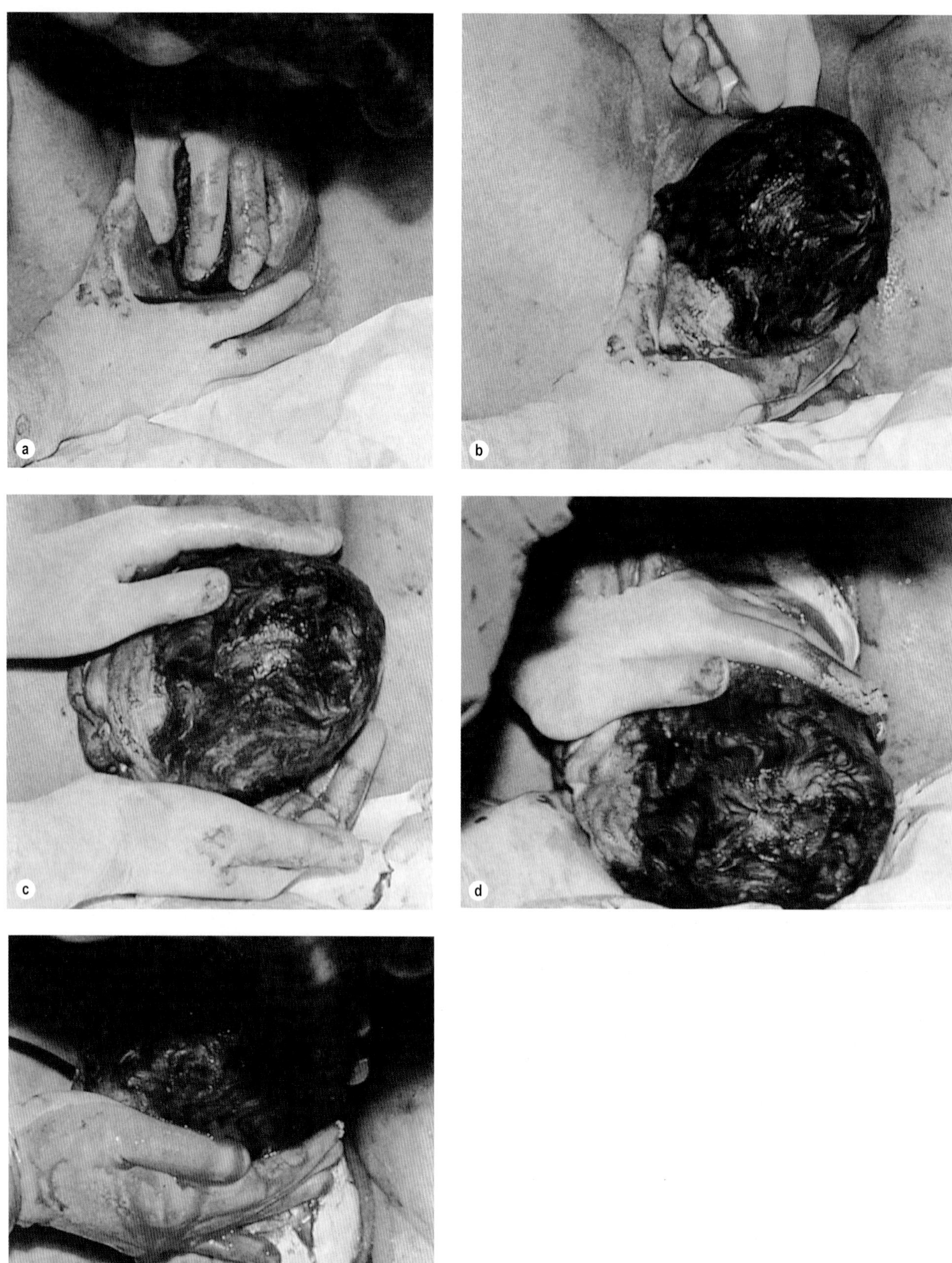

Figure 36-9 Normal delivery. (a) When crowning occurs, apply gentle palm pressure to the infant's head. (b) Examine the neck for the presence of a looped umbilical cord. (c) Support the infant's head as it rotates for shoulder presentation. (d) Guide the infant's head downward to deliver the anterior shoulder. (e) Guide the infant's head upward to release the posterior shoulder.

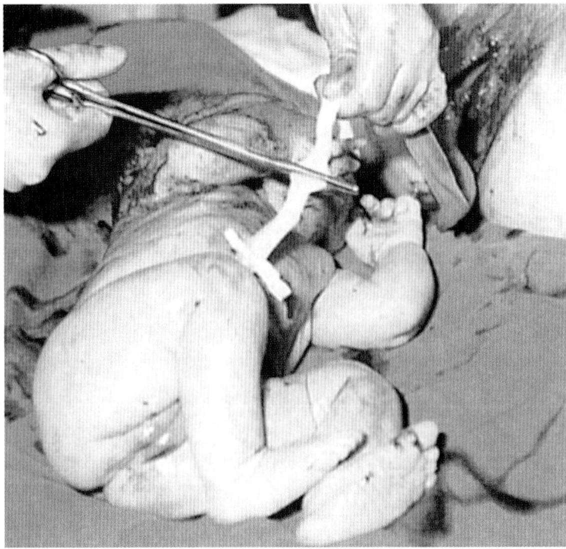

Figure 36-10 After delivery and evaluation of the infant, the paramedic clamps and cuts the cord.

2. Cut between the two clamps with sterile scissors or a scalpel.
3. Examine the cut ends of the cord to ensure that there is no bleeding. If the cut end attached to the infant is bleeding, clamp the cord proximal to the previous clamp and reassess for bleeding. Do not remove the first clamp.
4. Handle the cord carefully at all times because it can tear easily.
5. Ensure that the baby remains wrapped and then pass the baby to his/her mother.

Delivery of the placenta

The placenta is normally delivered within 20 min of the infant. Placental delivery is characterized by episodes of contractions, a palpable rise of the uterus within the abdomen, lengthening of the umbilical cord protruding from the vagina, and a sudden gush of vaginal blood (this should not exceed 200–300 mL).

As the placenta is delivered, the mother should be told to bear down with contractions. The paramedic should hold the placenta with both hands and twist the placenta gently as it is delivered to help it fully separate from the uterine wall. (Never pull on the umbilical cord to assist with placental delivery.) When the placenta is expelled, the paramedic should place it in a plastic bag or other container and ensure that it is either transported with the mother and infant to the receiving hospital, or available for inspection by the attending midwife. The placenta will be examined for abnormality and completeness, which is important as pieces of placenta retained in the uterus can cause persistent haemorrhage and infection.

After the delivery of the placenta, the paramedic should assess the perineum for tears. If tears are present, the paramedic should manage them by applying sanitary towels to the area and maintaining direct pressure. If the mother continues to bleed after the delivery of the placenta, initiate fundal massage to promote uterine contraction. Consider the need for fluid replacement and syntometrine where fundal massage does not control the haemorrhage. One ampoule containing 500 μg of ergometrine and 5 units of oxytocin in 1 mL should be administered via the intramuscular route. The paramedic should be familiar with JRCALC guidelines regarding the administration of syntometrine, including side effects and contraindications to administration.[3]

Postpartum haemorrhage

Postpartum haemorrhage is characterized by more than 500 mL of blood loss after the delivery of the newborn. Haemorrhage often occurs within the first few hours after delivery although it can be delayed up to 24 h. Postpartum haemorrhage occurs in about 5% of all deliveries. Haemorrhage often results from ineffective or incomplete contraction of the interlacing uterine muscle fibres. Other causes of postpartum haemorrhage include retained pieces of placenta or membranes in the uterus. Haemorrhage can also be caused by vaginal or cervical tears during delivery (rare). Risk factors associated with postpartum haemorrhage include uterine atony (lack of tone) from prolonged or tumultuous labour, grand multiparity, twin pregnancy, placenta praevia and a full bladder.

Management

Postpartum haemorrhage can occur in the prehospital setting after a field delivery or home delivery. The assessment and management are similar to those described for third-trimester bleeding. In addition, the paramedic should take the following six measures to encourage uterine contraction:

1. Control external haemorrhage. Manage external bleeding from perineal tears with firm pressure.
2. Massage the uterus. Palpate the uterus for firmness or loss of tone. If the uterus does not feel firm, apply fundal pressure by supporting the lower uterine segment with the edge of one hand just above the symphysis and massaging the fundus with the other hand. Continue massaging until the uterus feels firm. Re-evaluate the patient every 10 min; note the location of the fundus in relation to the level of the umbilicus, the degree of firmness, and vaginal flow.
3. Encourage the infant to breast-feed. If the mother and infant are stable, place the newborn to her breast to encourage breast-feeding. Stimulation of the breasts may promote uterine contraction.
4. Administer syntometrine per guidelines after ensuring that a second fetus is not present in the uterus. Commence fluid resuscitation as indicated by the patient's vital signs.
5. Do not attempt a vaginal examination. Also, do not attempt vaginal packing to control haemorrhage.
6. Rapidly transport the patient for physician evaluation.

Box 36-7

Factors associated with high risk of abnormal delivery

Maternal factors

- Maternal age: very young or very old
- Absence of antenatal care
- Maternal lifestyle: alcohol, tobacco, or drug usage
- Pre-existing maternal illness, including diabetes, chronic hypertension, or Rh sensitization
- Previous obstetric history of the following:
  Premature delivery or miscarriage
  Perinatal loss
  Previous malformed neonate
  Previous multiple births
  Previous caesarean delivery
- Intrapartum disorders:
  Pre-eclampsia
  Prolonged rupture of membranes
  Prolonged labour
  Abnormal presentation
  Abruptio placentae
  Placenta praevia

Fetal factors

- Lack of fetal well-being
- History of decreased fetal movement
- History of heart rate abnormalities
- Evidence of fetal distress
- Fetal immaturity: prematurity as established by dates, ultrasound, uterine size, amniocentesis
- Fetal growth: history of poor intrauterine growth or post-date delivery
- Specific fetal malformation detected by ultrasound: diaphragmatic hernia or omphalocele

Delivery complications

As stated before, most women have routine pregnancies. Prehospital deliveries seldom present any significant problems for the mother, newborn, or emergency crew. The delivery complications discussed in this chapter include cephalopelvic disproportion, abnormal presentation, premature birth, multiple gestation, precipitous delivery, uterine inversion, pulmonary embolus, and fetal membrane disorders. Box 36-7 lists factors that should alert the paramedic to anticipate an abnormal delivery.

Cephalopelvic disproportion

Cephalopelvic disproportion is a condition in which the newborn's head is too large or the mother's birth canal is too small to allow normal labour or birth. The mother is often primigravida and having strong, frequent contractions for a prolonged period. This condition requires a caesarean delivery to be performed because rupture of the uterus and fetal death are possible. Prehospital care is limited to maternal oxygen administration, IV access for fluid resuscitation if needed, and rapid transport to the receiving hospital.

Abnormal presentation

Most infants are born head first (cephalic or vertex presentation). But sometimes a presentation is abnormal. These include a breech presentation, shoulder dystocia, shoulder presentation and a cord presentation (prolapsed umbilical cord).

Breech presentation

In breech presentations the largest part of the fetus (the head) is delivered last. Breech presentation occurs in 3–4% of deliveries at term. Breech presentation is more frequent with multiple births and when labour occurs before 32 weeks' gestation. Categories of breech presentation include the following (Figure 36-11):

- Front or frank breech. The fetal hips are flexed and the legs extend in front of the fetus. The buttocks are the presenting part. Frank breech accounts for about 45–50% of breech presentations.
- Complete breech. The fetus has both knees and hips flexed. The buttocks are the presenting part. Complete breech accounts for about 10–15% of breech presentations.
- Incomplete breech. The fetus has one or both hips incompletely flexed. This results in presentation of one or both lower extremities (often a foot). Incomplete breech accounts for about 35–45% of breech presentations.

Critical Thinking

What resources can you use to assist in a delivery with an abnormal presentation?

Management

An infant in a breech presentation is best delivered in a hospital where emergency caesarean section provides an alternative to vaginal delivery. Sometimes, however, the paramedic must assist in a breech delivery. If delivery is imminent, the EMS crew should proceed as follows:[4]

1. If the mother is on a bed or sofa, encourage her to move to the edge to allow gravity to help the delivery; support the mother's legs.
2. Hands off, allow baby to deliver spontaneously. Do not touch the baby or umbilical cord until the body is free of the birth canal and the nape of the neck is visible. The only exception is if the baby's back rotates towards the floor, in which case the paramedic should gently support the baby by its pelvis and rotate the baby back towards the front (avoid pressure upon the neonate's abdomen).
3. Do not clamp or cut the cord until the head is delivered.
4. Once the body is born, gently lift the baby by its feet to facilitate delivery of the head; avoid pulling on the baby.
5. Be aware that the head often is delivered without difficulty after shoulder delivery. Be careful to avoid excessive head and spine manipulation or traction.

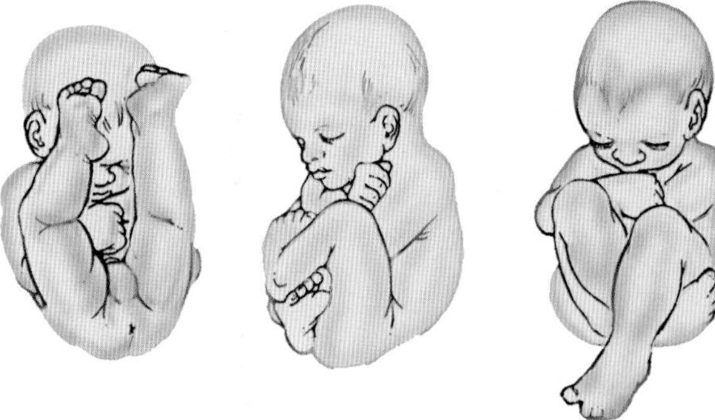

Figure 36-11 Types of breech presentation. (a) Front or back. (b) Complete. (c) Incomplete.

Once the baby has been born, it should be managed in the same way as for any other delivery. If any other body part is presenting (e.g. a foot, hand or arm) the mother should be transported immediately to the nearest obstetric unit with a pre-alert.

Shoulder dystocia

Shoulder dystocia occurs when the fetal shoulders are wedged against the maternal symphysis pubis, which blocks shoulder delivery. In this presentation the head delivers normally but then pulls back tightly against the maternal perineum. The incidence of shoulder dystocia is small but increases greatly with increasing birth weight. (Up to 10% incidence occurs with birth weights of 4.5 kg [10 lb] or more.) Complications include brachial plexus damage, fractured clavicle, and fetal anoxia from cord compression.

Management

Shoulder dystocia delivery calls for dislodging one shoulder and then rotating the fetal shoulder girdle at an angle into the wider part of the pelvic opening. Because the shoulder is pressing against the pelvis, there is a potential for cord compression; thus the paramedic should deliver the anterior shoulder immediately after the head. (This should be done before suctioning of the nares and mouth.) Several manoeuvres can help the paramedic successfully deliver an infant when shoulder dystocia arises. The following steps represent one approach to shoulder dystocia if the shoulders are not delivered within two contractions of the birth of the head:[7]

1. Call for assistance from on-duty midwife. It should be noted that if assistance is not readily available, the paramedic may take the decision to transport the patient before arrival of the midwife.
2. Position the mother in the McRobert's position (pillow under the head, knees drawn up to the chest and angled slightly outwards), or on 'all-fours'. This increases the diameter of the pelvis.
3. If the shoulders are not delivered following a further two contractions, move on to suprapubic pressure; this requires an assistant:
   - Identify which side the baby's back is facing.
   - Ask the assistant to move to the side of the baby's back.
   - Ask the assistant to hold their hands as if performing CPR and place the heel of the hand two fingerbreadths up from the symphysis pubis behind the baby's back.
   - The assistant should apply gentle to moderate pressure on the baby's shoulder, pushing downwards and away from them. This may help to dislodge and rotate the obstructed shoulder away from the symphysis pubis.
   - The paramedic should apply gentle downwards traction whilst suprapubic pressure is applied.

   If after two attempts the shoulders have still not delivered:

   - Ask the assistant to apply intermittent pressure by gently rocking backwards and forwards with the hands in the same position as before.
   - The paramedic should again attempt delivery whilst the assistant provides suprapubic pressure.

   If after two attempts the shoulders have still not delivered:

   - Ask the mother to adopt an 'all-fours' position. The mother's head needs to be as low as possible and there should be hip flexion with the bottom elevated as much as possible.
   - When the mother is in this position, attempt to deliver the shoulder nearest the maternal back first.

   If the shoulders have still not delivered, transport the mother as rapidly as possible to the nearest staffed obstetric unit, remembering to place the mother in left lateral tilt. Provide high-flow oxygen and consider IV access (DO NOT delay transportation in order to gain IV access).

   - Pre-alert receiving obstetric unit.
   - If delivery occurs, continue with resuscitative measures as needed.

Shoulder presentation

Shoulder presentation (transverse presentation) results when the long axis of the fetus lies perpendicular to that of the mother. This position usually results in the fetal shoulder lying over the pelvic opening. The fetal arm or hand may be the presenting part. This abnormal delivery occurs in only 0.3% of deliveries but occurs in 10% of second twins.

Management

Normal delivery of a shoulder presentation is not possible. The paramedic should provide the mother with adequate oxygen, ventilatory and circulatory support, and rapid transport to the hospital. A caesarean section is required whether the fetus is viable or not.

Cord presentation

Cord presentation occurs when the cord slips down into or out of the vagina after the amniotic membranes have ruptured. The umbilical cord is compressed against the presenting part of the fetus, which diminishes fetal oxygenation from the placenta. A prolapsed cord occurs in about 1 in every 200 pregnancies. Predisposing factors include breech presentation, premature rupture of membranes (described later), a large fetus, multiple gestation, a long cord and preterm labour.

Management

Fetal asphyxia can ensue rapidly if circulation through the cord is not re-established and maintained until delivery. If the paramedic can see or feel the umbilical cord in the vagina, the paramedic should take the following steps:

1. Position the mother with hips elevated as much as possible. The Trendelenburg or knee–chest position may relieve pressure on the cord, as will the lateral position with padding under the hips.
2. Administer oxygen to the mother.
3. Instruct the mother to pant with each contraction to prevent bearing down.
4. If possible, replace the cord in the vagina using two fingers. The cord should be handled as little as possible. If this cannot be achieved, apply moist sterile dressings to the exposed cord to minimize temperature changes that may cause umbilical artery spasm.
5. Transport the patient to the nearest obstetric unit as a matter of urgency (pre-alert is essential). The trolley cot should be used for transporting the patient although it may not always be possible to get the trolley to the patient's side. If necessary, the mother may be assisted to walk to the nearest point at which the trolley can be placed. Use of the carry chair should be avoided if at all possible; if it has to be used, the mother should be transported the shortest distance possible before transfer to the trolley.
6. Position the mother on her side with padding under the hips to raise the pelvis and reduce pressure on the cord.[4]
7. Administer entonox to reduce the urge to push during contractions.

Other abnormal presentations

Other abnormal presentations include face or brow presentation and occiput posterior presentation. In these presentations the infant's head is delivered face up instead of face down. Face-up presentations result in increased risks to the fetus because of difficult labour and delivery. Sometimes the fetus has other associated abnormalities. These presentations may require caesarean section, so early recognition of potential complications, maternal support and reassurance, and rapid transport for definitive care are the goals of prehospital management.

Premature birth

A premature infant is born before 37 weeks' gestation. Low birth weight (less than 2.5 kg [5.5 lb]) also determines prematurity, although the conditions are not synonymous. Premature deliveries occur in 6–9% of all pregnancies. After a preterm labour the newborn is at increased risk of hypothermia because of a large surface/mass ratio and for cardiorespiratory distress because the cardiovascular system is premature. Therefore these infants require special care and observation. If possible, the mother should be conveyed to her booked obstetric unit, but if birth is imminent, the paramedic should request a midwife and second vehicle. After delivery, prehospital management for a premature infant includes the following:

- Keep the infant warm. Dry the infant, wrap the infant in a warm dry blanket, place the infant on the mother's abdomen, and cover the mother and infant. Oxygen and resuscitation methods should be employed as necessary (see Chapter 37)
- Once born, utilize the second vehicle to transport the infant to the nearest obstetric or emergency department (depending upon local arrangements). The infant should be transported even if the midwife has not yet arrived.
- The crew should notify the receiving hospital of ETA and condition of the infant.
- The mother should then be transported to the same obstetric unit as the infant.

Multiple gestation

A multiple gestation is a pregnancy with more than one fetus. Twins occur in 1 in 80–90 births (Box 36-8), and triplets occur in 1 in 8000 births.[1] Multiple gestation places more stress on the maternal system and is accompanied by an increased complication rate. Associated complications include premature labour and delivery (30–50% of twin deliveries are premature), premature rupture of membranes, abruptio placentae, postpartum haemorrhage and abnormal presentation. A mother who has not had antenatal care is often unaware of her multiple pregnancy.

Critical Thinking

Do you have enough supplies on your ambulance to manage more than one delivery?

Delivery procedure

It is unusual for twins to be delivered out of hospital and, unless delivery is imminent, mothers should be transported to their booked obstetric unit. If delivery is in progress or commences on route to hospital, proceed with the principles of delivery as explained earlier. First-twin delivery is normally identical to single delivery with the same presentation. However, up to 50% of second-twin deliveries are not in a normal presentation position. Fetuses are smaller in

Box 36-8

Twin terminology

Fraternal twins result from the fertilization of two ova by two spermatozoa. Each fraternal twin has a separate placenta. Each also is separated by individual amniotic membranes. Fraternal twins are not identical in appearance. They are often of different gender.

Identical twins result from the fertilization of a single ovum. They may share a common placenta and amniotic sac or have separate placental structures. Identical twins are less common than fraternal twins. (They occur in one out of three twin conceptions.) Unlike fraternal twins, identical twins look alike, are of the same gender and are genetically identical.

multiple births; thus the breech presentation of the second twin does not usually pose any serious delivery issues.

After the delivery of the first twin, the paramedic should cut and clamp (or tie) the umbilical cord as usual. Within 5 to 10 min after delivery of the first twin, labour begins again. The delivery of the second twin usually occurs within 30 to 45 min. It is best practice to make arrangements to transport the mother and first baby to the obstetric unit once the first baby has been born and assessed. It is not necessary to wait for a midwife under these circumstances. If the second baby delivers en route to hospital, utilize both vehicles to transport mother and babies to hospital. If resuscitation is required, follow the guidelines discussed in Chapter 37. Usually both twins are born before the delivery of the placenta.

Infants in multiple births are often smaller than infants in single term births. The paramedic should give special attention to keeping these infants warm, well oxygenated, and free from unnecessary contamination as described for premature infants. Postpartum haemorrhage may be more severe after multiple births. Haemorrhage may require fluid resuscitation, uterine massage and syntometrine infusion to control bleeding.

Precipitous delivery

A precipitous delivery is a rapid spontaneous delivery with less than 3 h from onset of labour to birth. Delivery results from overactive uterine contractions and little maternal soft tissue or bony resistance. A precipitous delivery most often occurs in a mother who is grand multipara. It can be associated with soft tissue injury and uterine rupture (rare). Precipitous delivery has an increased perinatal mortality rate because of trauma and hypoxia. The main danger to the fetus during this kind of delivery is from cerebral trauma or tearing of the umbilical cord.

If the paramedic expects a precipitous delivery, the paramedic should try to prevent an explosive one. This can be achieved by providing gentle counter-pressure to the infant's head; however, the paramedic should not attempt to detain fetal head descent. After the delivery the paramedic should keep the infant dry and warm to prevent heat loss and should examine the mother for perineal tears. These tears often accompany a rapid birth.

Uterine inversion

Uterine inversion is an infrequent complication of childbirth. Yet uterine inversion is a serious condition. It occurs in about 1 in 2100 deliveries. With this condition the uterus turns inside out.

Uterine inversion may occur suddenly after a contraction. It may also appear with increased abdominal pressure caused by coughing or sneezing. However, uterine inversion is more often caused by medical personnel or a medical procedure (iatrogenic). It can result from excessive pulling on the umbilical cord and fundal massage. The risk is higher when the placenta has implanted high in the uterus. Uterine inversion is incomplete if the top of the uterus does not protrude through the cervix and complete if the entire uterus protrudes through the cervical opening. Signs and symptoms of uterine inversion include postpartum haemorrhage and sudden and severe lower abdominal pain. The haemorrhage may be profuse and hypovolaemic shock may develop quickly.

Management

Prehospital care for a patient with uterine inversion includes airway, ventilatory and circulatory support and rapid transportation for physician evaluation. Analgesia may be required if the patient is experiencing pain.

Pulmonary embolism

The development of pulmonary embolism during pregnancy, labour, or the postpartum period is one of the most common causes of maternal death. The embolus often results from a blood clot in the pelvic circulation (venous thromboembolism). Embolus is more often associated with caesarean section than vaginal delivery. The patient often has classic signs and symptoms including sudden dyspnoea; sharp, focal chest pains; tachycardia; tachypnoea; and sometimes hypotension. If the embolism occurs in the prehospital setting, emergency care should be focused on airway, ventilatory and circulatory support; electrocardiogram monitoring; and rapid transportation for physician evaluation (see Chapter 14).

Fetal membrane disorders

The fetal membrane disorders discussed in this chapter include premature rupture of membranes and amniotic fluid embolism. Another fetal membrane disorder, meconium staining, is described in Chapter 37.

Premature rupture of membranes

Premature rupture of the membranes is a rupture of the amniotic sac before the onset of labour. The condition is termed premature regardless of fetal age and occurs in about 1 in 10 pregnancies. At term, 70% of patients are in labour within 12 h of premature rupture of the membranes, and 85% are in labour within 24 h.[1] Signs and symptoms include a history of a trickle or sudden gush of fluid from the vagina. The paramedic should transport patients for physician evaluation. The medical facility will prepare for delivery if the patient begins labour. Delivery is required if an infection of fetal membranes is diagnosed (this is called chorioamnionitis).

Chorioamnionitis is linked to premature rupture of membranes occurring 24 h before labour begins. It can also occur with a prolonged labour. The infection is generally accompanied by maternal fever, chills and uterine pain. Infection is treated with antibiotics although the best treatment for this infection is the delivery of the fetus.

Amniotic fluid embolism

When amniotic fluid enters the maternal circulation during labour or delivery or immediately after delivery, an amniotic fluid embolism can occur. Probable routes of entry include lacerations of the endocervical veins during cervical dilatation, the lower uterine segment or placental site, and uterine veins at sites of uterine trauma. Particulate matter in the amniotic fluid (e.g. meconium, lanugo hairs and fetal squamous cells) forms an embolus and obstructs the pulmonary vasculature. Amniotic fluid embolism is rare, occurring in 1 in 20 000–30 000 deliveries.[6] The condition is most often seen in multiparous women late in the first stage of labour. Other conditions that can increase the incidence of this severe complication are placenta praevia, abruptio placentae and intrauterine fetal death. The maternal mortality rate is about 60–70%.[6]

The signs and symptoms of amniotic fluid embolism are the same as those described for pulmonary embolism. They may include cardiopulmonary arrest. These patients are managed with airway, ventilatory and circulatory support; fluid resuscitation; and rapid transportation.

Summary

- The placenta is a disc-like organ and is composed of interlocking fetal and maternal tissues. The placenta is the organ of exchange between the mother and fetus. Blood flows from the fetus to the placenta through two umbilical arteries. These arteries carry deoxygenated blood. Oxygenated blood returns to the fetus through the umbilical vein. The amniotic sac is a fluid-filled cavity. It completely surrounds and protects the embryo.
- The developing ovum is known as an embryo during the first 8 weeks of pregnancy. After that time and until birth it is called a fetus. Gestation (fetal development) usually averages 40 weeks from the time of fertilization to the delivery of the newborn.
- The pregnant woman undergoes many physiological changes that affect the genital tract, breasts, gastrointestinal system, cardiovascular system, respiratory system and metabolism.
- The patient history should include obstetric history; presence of pain; presence, quantity, and character of vaginal bleeding; presence of abnormal vaginal discharge; presence of bloody show; current general health and antenatal care; allergies and medicines taken; and maternal urge to bear down.
- The goal in examining an obstetric patient is to rapidly identify any acute life-threatening conditions. A part of this involves identifying imminent delivery. Then the paramedic must take the proper management steps. In addition to the routine physical examination, the paramedic should assess the abdomen, uterine size and fetal heart sounds.
- If birth is not imminent, the paramedic should limit prehospital care for the healthy patient. Care should be limited to basic treatment modalities including transport for physician evaluation.
- Causes of fetal death from maternal trauma include death of the mother, separation of the placenta, maternal shock, uterine rupture and fetal head injury.
- Pre-eclampsia occurs after 20 weeks' gestation. The criteria for diagnosis include hypertension, proteinuria and excessive weight gain with oedema. Eclampsia is characterized by the same signs and symptoms with the addition of seizures or coma.
- Vaginal bleeding during pregnancy can result from abortion (miscarriage), ectopic pregnancy, abruptio placentae, placenta praevia, uterine rupture or postpartum haemorrhage. Abortion is the termination of pregnancy from any cause before 24 weeks' gestation. Ectopic pregnancy occurs when a fertilized ovum implants anywhere other than the uterus. Abruptio placentae is partial or complete detachment of the placenta at more than 24 weeks' gestation. Placenta praevia is placental implantation in the lower uterine segment, partially or completely covering the cervical opening. Uterine rupture is a spontaneous or traumatic rupture of the uterine wall.
- The first stage of labour begins with the onset of regular contractions and ends with complete dilatation of the cervix. The second stage of labour is measured from full dilatation of the cervix to delivery of the infant. The third stage of labour begins with delivery of the infant and ends when the placenta is expelled and the uterus has contracted.
- One of the primary responsibilities of the EMS crew is to prevent an uncontrolled delivery. The other is to protect the infant from cold and stress after birth.
- Criteria for computing the Apgar score include appearance (colour), pulse (heart rate), grimace (reflex irritability), activity (muscle tone) and respiratory effort.
- More than 500 mL of blood loss after the delivery of the newborn is called a postpartum haemorrhage. It often results from ineffective or incomplete contraction of the uterus.
- Paramedics should be alert to factors that point to a possible abnormal delivery.
- Cephalopelvic disproportion produces a difficult labour because of the presence of a small pelvis, an oversized uterus or fetal abnormalities. Most infants are born head first (cephalic or vertex presentation). However, sometimes a presentation is abnormal. In breech presentation the largest part of the fetus (the head) is delivered last. Shoulder dystocia occurs when the fetal shoulders press against the maternal symphysis pubis. This blocks shoulder delivery. Shoulder presentation (transverse presentation) results when the long axis of the fetus lies perpendicular to that of the mother. The fetal arm or hand may be the presenting part. Cord presentation occurs when the cord slips down into the vagina or presents externally.
- A premature infant is born before 37 weeks' gestation.
- A multiple gestation is a pregnancy with more than one fetus. Multiple gestation is accompanied by an increased complication rate.

Summary—cont'd

- A precipitous delivery is a rapid, spontaneous delivery with less than 3 h from onset of labour to birth. The main danger to the fetus is from cerebral trauma or tearing of the umbilical cord.
- Uterine inversion is a rare and serious complication of childbirth. With this condition the uterus turns inside out.
- The development of pulmonary embolism during pregnancy, labour, or the postpartum period is one of the most common causes of maternal death.
- Premature rupture of the membranes is a rupture of the amniotic sac before the onset of labour, regardless of gestational age.
- An amniotic fluid embolism may occur when amniotic fluid enters the maternal circulation during labour or delivery or immediately after delivery.

References

1. Rosen P, Barkin R 1998 Emergency medicine: concepts and clinical practice, 4th edition. Mosby, St Louis
2. Confidential Enquiry into Maternal and Child Health 2004 Why mothers die 2000–2002 – Report on confidential enquiries into maternal deaths in the United Kingdom. CEMACH, London
3. National Statistics. Conceptions by age for March quarter 2004. Online. Available www.statistics.gov.uk
4. Joint Royal Colleges Ambulance Liaison Committee 2006 UK Ambulance Service Clinical Guidelines v4. 2006. Online. Available http://www2.warwick.ac.uk/fac/med/research/hsri/emergencycare/prehospitalcare/jrcacstakeholderwebsite/guidelines 29 February 2009
5. American Heart Association 2000 Guidelines 2000 for cardiopulmonary resuscitation and emergency cardiovascular care, International Consensus on Science. Circulation 102(8):247
6. Arulkumaran S, Symonds IM, Fowlie A 2004 Oxford handbook of obstetrics and gynaecology. Oxford University Press, Oxford
7. Advanced Life Support Group 2009 Prehospital obstetric emergency training. ALSG, Manchester
8. Lo JC, Feigenbaum SL, Escobar GJ, Yang J, Crites YM, Ferrara A 2006 Increased prevalence of gestational diabetes mellitus among women with diagnosed polycystic ovary syndrome: a population-based study. Diabetes Care 29(8):1915–1917

PART EIGHT

CHAPTER **37**

Care of the Newborn

Chapter contents

Objectives

Upon completion of this chapter, the paramedic student will be able to:

1. Identify risk factors associated with the need for neonatal resuscitation.
2. Describe physiological adaptations at birth.
3. Outline the prehospital assessment and management of the newborn.
4. Describe resuscitation of the distressed newborn.
5. Discuss post-resuscitative management and transport.
6. Describe signs and symptoms and prehospital management of specific newborn resuscitation situations.
7. Identify injuries associated with birth.
8. Describe appropriate interventions to manage the emotional needs of the newborn's family.

Key terms

antepartum The period before labour and delivery.
apnoea An absence of spontaneous respirations.
congenital anomalies Defects that occur during fetal development.
diaphragmatic hernia A herniation in the diaphragm caused by the improper fusion of structures during fetal development.
intrapartum The period during labour and delivery.
meconium staining The inhalation of meconium by the fetus or newborn; this can block air passages and result in failure of the lungs to expand or cause other pulmonary dysfunction.
neonate A baby in the first 28 days of life.
newborn A baby in the first few hours of life.
preterm baby A baby born before 37 weeks of gestation.

A small proportion of babies require resuscitation at birth and mostly this is confined to ventilation, with an even smaller proportion requiring a brief period of chest compressions.[1] This chapter addresses risk factors that may lead to the need for resuscitation in this patient group. It also describes initial patient care that may be required for the newborn.

Risk factors associated with the need for resuscitation

The vast majority of term newborns require no resuscitation beyond maintenance of temperature, suctioning of the airway, and mild stimulation. The incidence of complications, however, increases as birth weight decreases. In fact, resuscitation is required for about 80% of the 30 000 babies who weigh less than 1500 g (3.12 lb) at birth, whereas of those born beyond 32 weeks' gestation and in the context of normal labour, only 2 in 1000 (0.2%) appear to need resuscitation measures at delivery.

The average term newborn weighs about 3600 g (7.5 lb), with the baby's birth weight depending on a number of factors, which include the size and racial origin of the parents. For example, small parents tend to have small babies and Asian babies tend to be smaller than Caucasian babies. Newborn boys usually weigh about 225 g (8 oz) more than baby girls. Causes of low birth weight include premature birth, under-nourishment in the uterus, and certain maternal factors such as, for example, pre-eclampsia and cigarette smoking during pregnancy.

In addition to low birth weight, various antepartum (before labour and delivery) and intrapartum (during labour and delivery) risk factors may affect the need for resuscitation; these include the following[1] (the obstetric history is presented in Chapter 36):

Antepartum

- Multiple gestation
- Inadequate prenatal care
- Mother's age (less than age 16 or older than age 35)
- History of perinatal morbidity or mortality
- Post-term gestation
- Drugs/medications
- Toxaemia, hypertension, diabetes

Intrapartum

- Premature labour
- Meconium-stained amniotic fluid
- Rupture of membranes greater than 24 h before delivery
- Use of opiates within 4 h of delivery
- Abnormal presentation
- Prolonged labour or precipitous delivery
- Prolapsed cord
- Bleeding.

When any of the foregoing risk factors are present during delivery, the paramedic should prepare equipment and drugs that may be needed for newborn resuscitation (Box 37-1). The paramedic should also give consideration to the receiving hospital and if necessary confirm with them their ability to accept the newborn.

Box 37-1

Neonatal resuscitation equipment and drugs

In addition to a standard obstetrics kit, newborn resuscitation equipment should include the following:

- Suction equipment
  - Suction catheters (4, 6, 8, 10 and 12 French)
  - Meconium aspirator attachment
- Oropharyngeal airways: 000, 00
- Bag–valve–mask devices or similar with oxygen reservoir and oxygen supply
- Laryngoscope blades (straight, 0, and 1)
- Laryngoscope handles
- Endotracheal tube stylets
- Endotracheal tubes (2.5, 3.0, 3.5, 4.0)
- ET tube securing device or ties
- Laryngeal mask airways (1.0)
- $EtCO_2$ detector/devices/monitoring
- Medications and fluids
  - Adrenaline (epinephrine)1 : 10 000 (0.1 mg/mL)
  - Glucose 10%
  - Naloxone
  - Intravenous fluids: n/saline (0.9%)
- Orogastric/nasogastric tubes
- Multiple blankets/towels/towel roll/food wrap or plastic roll
- Umbilical vessel catheterization equipment
  - Umbilical catheters 3.5, 5 F
  - Gauze, gloves, scissors, tape or tie
  - Syringes (1, 2, 5, 10, and 20 mL)
  - Three-way tap

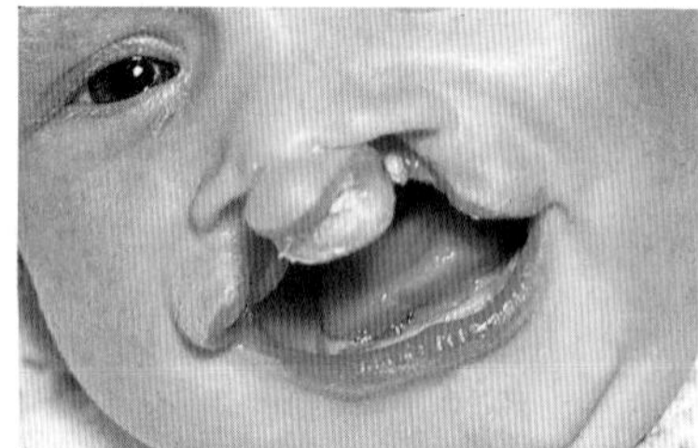

Figure 37-1 Cleft lip.

Critical Thinking

Does your ambulance have the right size equipment for resuscitation of the newborn?

Congenital anomalies

Congenital anomalies are defects that occur during fetal development, usually developing within the first trimester, and are present in about 2% of all births. These defects are responsible for nearly half of all deaths in newborns; therefore, the presence of congenital anomalies may be a factor in the need for newborn resuscitation. Congenital anomalies may be associated with genetics, hereditary factors, maternal infection, alcohol or other drug use during pregnancy, and other factors. Many types of congenital anomalies can occur; some of the more common include:

Choanal atresia: A bony or membranous occlusion that blocks the passageway between the nose and pharynx; it can result in serious ventilation problems in the newborn.

Cleft lip: One or more fissures that originate in the embryo; a vertical, usually off-centre split in the upper lip that may extend to the nose (Figure 37-1).

Cleft palate: A fissure in the roof of the mouth that runs along its midline; it may extend through the hard and soft palates into the nasal cavities.

Diaphragmatic hernia: The protrusion of a part of the stomach through an opening in the diaphragm (described later in this chapter).

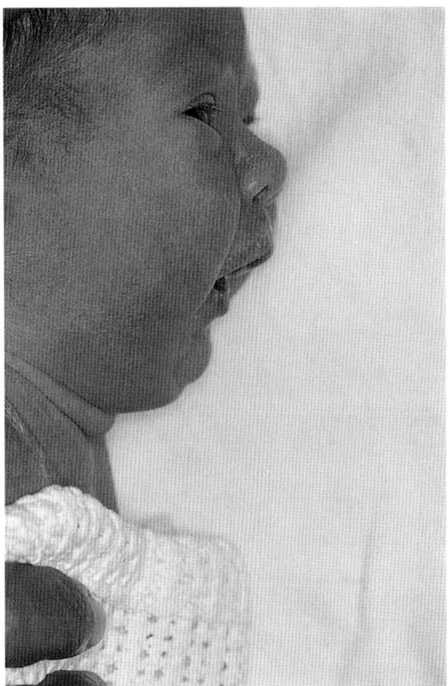

Figure 37-2 Pierre Robin syndrome.

Pierre Robin syndrome: A complex of anomalies including a small mandible, cleft lip, cleft palate, other craniofacial abnormalities, and defects of the eyes and ears (Figure 37-2).

Physiological adaptations at birth

At birth, newborns make three major physiological adaptations necessary for survival: (1) emptying fluids from their lungs and beginning ventilation; (2) changing their circulatory pattern; and (3) maintaining body temperature.[2]

During vaginal delivery, the newborn's chest usually is compressed and this forces fluid from the lungs into the mouth and nose. As the chest wall recoils, air is drawn into the lungs; the newborn takes the first breath in response to chemical changes and changes in temperature.

When the cord is cut and placental circulation shuts down, the circulatory system must function on its own. This involves the immediate and permanent closure of the pathways that allowed the fetus to receive oxygen without the use of lungs (described in Chapter 36). As the lungs expand with initial breaths, the resistance to blood flow in the lungs decreases and the newborn's blood begins to be oxygenated.

The newborn is sensitive to hypoxia; permanent brain damage will occur from prolonged hypoxaemia. Causes of hypoxia include compression of the cord, difficult labour and delivery, maternal haemorrhage, airway obstruction, hypothermia, newborn blood loss, and immature lungs in the premature newborn.

Newborns are at great risk for rapidly developing hypothermia due to their large body surface area in relation to weight, decreased tissue insulation, and immature temperature regulatory mechanisms and they should be delivered in

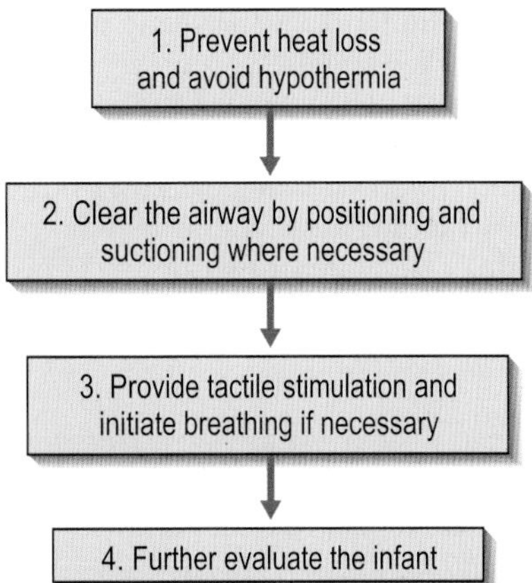

Figure 37-3 Steps in neonatal assessment and management.

a warm, draft-free area when possible; the cool, wet environment of an out-of-hospital birth increases the risk of heat loss for the newborn. Newborns try to conserve body heat through vasoconstriction and increasing their metabolism; this places them at risk for hypoxaemia, acidosis, bradycardia and hypoglycaemia.

Assessment and management of the newborn

The initial steps of assessment and management of any newborn are listed and described below. Following these steps enables the paramedic to immediately recognize a newborn in need of resuscitation. It also leads to efficient and effective emergency care delivery. The four steps in assessment and management of the newborn are (Figure 37-3):

1. Prevent heat loss and avoid hypothermia.
2. Clear the airway by positioning (and suctioning if required).
3. Provide tactile stimulation and initiate breathing if necessary.
4. Further evaluate the baby.

Note

Universal precautions (UP) are recommended during delivery of a newborn. Gloves and other appropriate protective barriers (including gowns and goggles) should be worn when handling the newborn or contaminated equipment.

Prevent heat loss and avoid hypothermia

Even healthy term newborns are limited in their ability to conserve heat when exposed to a cold environment and are subject to developing hypothermia; compromised newborns and preterm babies are even more vulnerable. Therefore, immediately after delivery, the baby's body and head should be dried to prevent evaporative heat loss and metabolic problems that may be brought on by cold stress. The act of drying also provides gentle stimulation, which may initiate respirations. Care should be taken to remove any wet coverings from the baby and cover with dry wrappings; the majority of heat loss can be prevented by covering the baby's head (which accounts for 20% of the newborn's body surface area). Consider wrapping vulnerable newborns in plastic food wrap (in this case without first drying) and, if feasible, place in the warmest possible area or under radiant heat.

Critical Thinking

What other measures can you take to warm the baby?

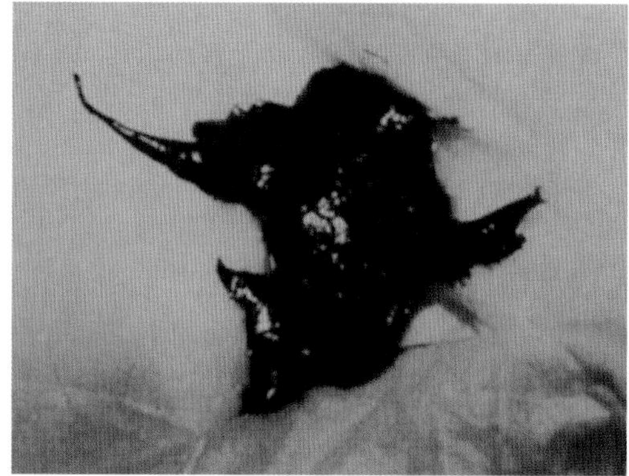

Figure 37-4 Meconium-stained birth.

Clear the airway by positioning and suctioning

After the newborn has been dried and covered, the next step is to establish an open airway, which is done by correctly positioning the baby (in neutral position); it may be necessary to supplement this in floppy babies with jaw thrust and insertion of a properly sized oropharyngeal (OP) airway. Care should be taken to prevent hyperextension or underextension, which may compromise the airway; placing a blanket or towel under the shoulders (thereby elevating the torso slightly) can help maintain the correct position.

Critical Thinking

Do babies breathe through their noses or mouths?

Once the baby has been properly positioned, the mouth and nose should be suctioned if there is actual matter blocking the airway (such as blood or other particles). Immediate suction (before other interventions) is only indicated if *thick* meconium in a non-vigorous baby is found; Vain et al 2004[3] found that meconium aspiration with the head still on the perineum ('intrapartum suction') does not prevent aspiration syndrome.[5] Suction should be applied using a 12–14 FG flexible suction catheter or a rigid tonsil tip catheter to suction with no greater than −100 mmHg vacuum. It is preferable to suction the mouth first, to prevent aspiration in case the baby gasps when the nose is cleared of secretions; each application of suction should last no more than 5 s to prevent hypoxia.

The paramedic should be careful to avoid deep or vigorous suctioning because stimulation of the posterior pharynx can produce a vagal response with resulting bradycardia, apnoea or both. The newborn's heart rate should be monitored during suctioning, and time should be provided during suction attempts for spontaneous ventilation. Like drying, suctioning provides a degree of tactile stimulation that initiates respirations.

Meconium staining

Meconium staining is the presence of fetal stool in the amniotic fluid and occurs in utero or intrapartum. The condition occurs in about 12% of all deliveries and causes a high morbidity risk. Meconium staining becomes more common in post-term and small-for-gestational-age newborns as well as in those babies who develop fetal distress during labour and delivery. Meconium staining is associated with increased perinatal mortality, hypoxaemia, aspiration pneumonia, pneumothorax and pulmonary hypertension.

The appearance of meconium depends on the amount of meconium particles and amniotic fluid. Meconium staining may appear as only a slight yellow or light green staining that is thin and watery or it may have a thick, pea-soup appearance that is dark green or black (Figure 37-4). When thick meconium is present in amniotic fluid, a chance exists that the particles will be aspirated into the baby's mouth, and potentially into the trachea and lungs, leading to partial or complete obstruction of the airways, and death can result from hypoxia, hypercapnia, and acidosis.

Note

Meconium can be used to test for maternal drug use. It has a greater sensitivity than urine and positive findings that persist longer. If time permits, a specimen should be collected and delivered to the emergency department.

If meconium (or evidence of infection) is observed but the newborn is vigorous (strong respiratory efforts, good muscle tone, and a heart rate greater than 100 beats per minute), no special care of the airway is required. If the newborn is not vigorous (absent or depressed respirations, decreased muscle tone, heart rate less than 100 beats per minute), endotracheal intubation and endotracheal suctioning is recommended immediately after birth.[4] The key indicator of the need for suction is how 'non-vigorous' the baby is, rather than how thick or tenacious the meconium appears. Because the presence of meconium can be determined only after the membranes have ruptured, it is critical that the paramedic crew have airway equipment available. Emergency care for these newborns includes the following steps (Figure 37-5):

1. Prepare the necessary equipment (e.g. intubation equipment, suction apparatus with 12 F or larger suction catheter, irrigation solution, gauze pads and bag/valve/mask device). Intubation equipment should include padding for patient positioning, stethoscope, number 0 and number 1 laryngoscope blades, ET tubes

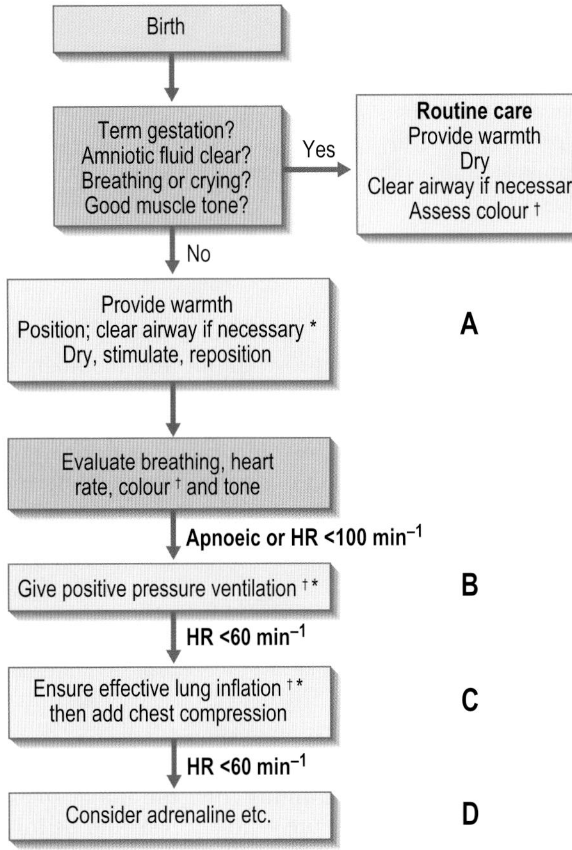

Figure 37-5 Newborn life support algorithm. Resuscitation Council (UK) 2005. From http://www.resus.org.uk/pages/nls.pdf page 2

(2.5, 3.0, 3.5, 4.0), stylet, meconium aspirator, and oxygen tubing. The procedure for endotracheal intubation is described in Chapter 13.

2. After delivery, clear the baby's airway and thoroughly suction the nose, mouth, and pharynx; remove residual meconium in the hypopharynx by suction under direct visualization.
3. Quickly intubate the trachea. Apply suction to the proximal end of the ET tube while withdrawing the tube. During intubation and suction, aim 100% oxygen toward the baby's face and monitor the fetal heart rate for bradycardia. If bradycardia develops, ventilate the baby's lungs using a bag device after suctioning, to prevent persistent bradycardia and hypoxia.
4. Repeat the intubation–suction–extubation cycle until no further meconium is obtained. Do not ventilate between intubations.
5. After tracheal suction is complete, continue resuscitative measures as needed. If respirations are adequate, manage the baby's airway in the normal fashion.

Provide tactile stimulation to initiate breathing

If drying and suctioning do not induce respirations in the baby, additional tactile stimulation should be provided. The two safe and appropriate methods of tactile stimulation are flicking the soles of the baby's feet and rubbing the baby's back.

Further evaluate the baby

Drying, positioning and stimulating are necessary in every baby at birth. These manoeuvres are used to clear the airway and initiate breathing. To further evaluate the baby the paramedic should follow these steps:

1. Observe and evaluate the baby's respirations. If they are normal (e.g. crying), continue the evaluation.
2. Evaluate the baby's heart rate by stethoscope or palpation of the pulse in the base of the umbilical cord (although the umbilical pulse can be unreliable at rates <100). If it is greater than 100 beats per minute, continue the evaluation.
3. Evaluate the baby's colour. Peripheral cyanosis (acrocyanosis) is common in the first few minutes of life and does not indicate hypoxaemia. If the baby's colour is normal or 'pinking up,' continue the evaluation with the Apgar score.

Apgar score

The Apgar score (described in Chapter 36) enables rapid evaluation of a newborn's condition at specific intervals after birth. It routinely is assessed at 1 and 5 min of age. Although the Apgar score is a useful tool to evaluate the newborn, it should not be used alone in determining the need for resuscitation. The Apgar evaluates appearance, pulse rate, grimace, activity, and respirations. A score of 7 to 10 is considered normal; a score of 4 to 6 identifies a moderately distressed baby who requires oxygen and stimulation; and a score less than 4 identifies a severely distressed baby who requires resuscitation.

Resuscitation of the distressed newborn

As described in Chapter 36, newborns who are full term; who have an airway that is clear of meconium or evidence of infection; who are breathing and crying; and who have good muscle tone, do not usually require resuscitation. If resuscitation is required because of inadequate respirations or heart rate, the baby will need one or more of the following interventions in sequence[4] (Figure 37-6).

1. Re-evaluate initial steps in stabilization (provide warmth, position, clear airway, dry, stimulate, reposition).
2. Provide ventilations.
3. Provide chest compressions.
4. Administer adrenaline (epinephrine) and/or volume expansion.

Note

The newborn should have regular respirations that are sufficient to improve colour and maintain a heart rate of greater than 100 beats per minute.

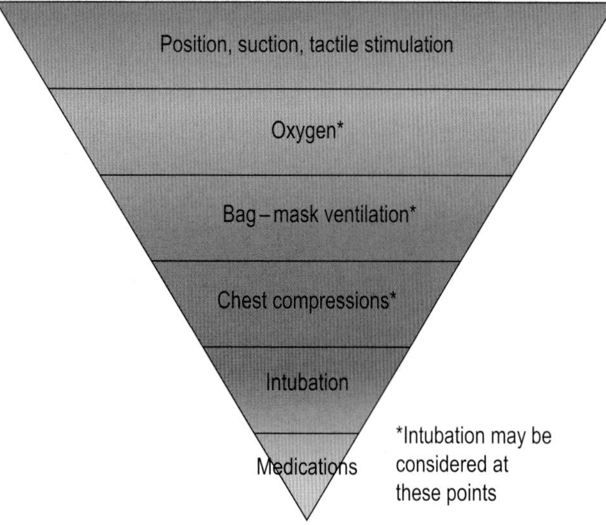

Figure 37-6 Inverted pyramid reflecting the approximate relative frequency of neonatal resuscitative efforts. Note that a majority of babies respond to simple measures.

The need to progress in sequence from one intervention to the next is based on the simultaneous assessment of the baby's respirations, heart rate, and colour. About 30 s should be allotted to complete each step; to re-evaluate; and to decide whether to progress to the next sequenced step in resuscitation.[4]

Re-evaluate initial steps in stabilization

The initial steps in stabilization should be re-evaluated. The paramedic should ensure that the baby is dry and warm; cold stress can increase oxygen consumption and impede effective breathing, and hypothermia can be associated with perinatal respiratory depression. Additional methods that can be used to warm a newborn include covering the baby in plastic wrap (food-grade, heat-resistant plastic), and placing the baby skin-to-skin with the mother and covering both with a blanket, but hyperthermia should be avoided. The goal is to achieve and maintain a normal body temperature for the newborn.

The head and neck of the newborn should be properly positioned (or repositioned) to ensure an open airway. In addition, the paramedic can make other attempts at stimulation to initiate breathing. If the baby is breathing but colour does not improve within 90 s after birth or if there is central cyanosis (blue colour of the face, trunk and mucous membranes), 100% supplemental oxygen should be given. Free-flow oxygen can be applied through a facemask and flow-inflating bag, an oxygen mask, or a hand cupped around the oxygen tubing (held 4–5 cm from the baby's nose). Using an oxygen flow rate of at least 5 L/min will provide 100% oxygen.[6] Oxygen therapy should be continued until mucous membranes are pink. The use of oropharyngeal airways in the newborn is rarely required except in conditions such as choanal atresia. Correct positioning is the key intervention required.

Note

Potential long-term hazards associated with 100% oxygen therapy in newborns, such as retinopathy, should not be a concern while providing emergency airway management in the prehospital setting. It is recommended, however, that administration of oxygen be guided by pulse oximetry.

Provide ventilations

As stated above, the newborn should have regular respirations that are sufficient to improve colour and maintain a heart rate greater than 100 beats per minute. Gasping, intercostal recessions, nasal flaring, grunting and apnoea indicate the need for assisted ventilations. Increasing or decreasing heart rate can also provide clues of improvement or deterioration in the newborn.

Note

Hypoxia is nearly always present in a newly born baby who requires resuscitation.

If respirations are inadequate (evidenced by persistent central cyanosis) or if the heart rate remains less than 100 beats per minute 30 s after administering the initial steps discussed above, positive-pressure ventilation should be initiated. The first five inflations should be given at a higher inflation pressure, which may need to be 30 cmH_2O or more to overcome the stiffness in the newborns lungs. Assisted ventilations should be provided at a rate of 40–60 breaths per minute, with a volume of approximately 8 mL/kg to achieve or maintain a heart rate greater than 100 beats per minute but ensuring no higher a rate which can lead to risks such as hypocapnia or pneumothorax.[4] Assisted ventilations can be delivered with a bag–valve–mask device with a safety device to prevent overinflation, a flow-inflating bag or with a T-piece (a valved, mechanical device designed to control flow and limit pressure).

Note

The lungs of a preterm baby can be easily injured by large-volume inflations immediately after birth. Therefore, high-pressures during assisted ventilations should be avoided with these newborns. Use caution when using bag–valve–mask devices; use a baby device with a volume of approximately 240 mL. High-inflation pressures may be evident by excessive chest wall movement. Once initially ventilated, babies should not require peak inflation pressure greater than 25 cmH_2O.

Endotracheal intubation

Endotracheal intubation may be indicated at several points during neonatal resuscitation. These include:[6]

- meconium staining is present and the newborn is not vigorous
- if bag–mask ventilation is ineffective or prolonged

- when chest compressions are performed
- when endotracheal administration of medication is desired (but the tracheal route is now thought ineffective unless high does are used)
- for special resuscitation circumstance, such as congenital diaphragmatic hernia, (described later) or extremely low birth weight (less than 1000 g).

Before the paramedic considers intubation or pharmacological therapy, two components of the resuscitation process should be re-evaluated:

1. Is chest movement adequate? Check for the adequacy of chest expansion and auscultate for bilateral breath sounds.
   a. Is the bag mask seal tight? A relatively large mask should be turned upside down for a better fit.
   b. Is the airway blocked from improper head position or secretions in the nose, mouth, or pharynx? Reassess head position and re-examine the airway for the presence of secretions.
   c. Is adequate ventilatory pressure being used? A bag mask pop-off valve may need to be disabled to allow for higher inspiratory pressures, especially for premature or meconium-aspiration delivery.[5]
   d. Is air in the stomach interfering with chest expansion? Consider nasogastric or orogastric decompression per protocol.
2. Is 100% oxygen being administered?
   a. Is the oxygen tubing attached to the bag and flowmeter?
   b. If using a self-inflating bag, is the oxygen reservoir attached?

A prompt increase in heart rate and chest wall movement after endotracheal intubation and administration of intermittent positive-pressure ventilation are the best indicators of correct tube placement. However, the paramedic should verify tube placement visually during intubation and by using primary and secondary confirmation methods (described in Chapter 13). Exhaled carbon dioxide detection is the recommended method of confirmation.[4] The laryngeal mask airway (LMA) may be used to establish an airway in a newborn if bag–mask ventilation is ineffective or tracheal intubation has failed.

Provide chest compressions

Chest compressions are indicated if the newborn's heart rate is less than 60 beats per minute despite attempts at positioning, airway opening, drying and stimulation and 30 s of adequate ventilation with supplemental oxygen. (The paramedic should ensure that assisted ventilations are effective before starting chest compressions.) As described in Chapter 29, chest compressions should be coordinated with ventilations at a ratio of 3 : 1 at a rate of 120 per minute, achieving 90 compressions and 30 breaths per minute.

> **Critical Thinking**
>
> Why would compressions be initiated when the baby still has a pulse?

The two thumb–encircling hands chest compression is the preferred technique for chest compressions for newly born babies and older babies when size permits. However, the two finger technique, the same as that used in paediatric chest compressions, is acceptable if there is a only a single rescuer. Compressions should be performed on the lower third of the sternum, with a depth of one-third of the anterior–posterior diameter of the chest and should be sufficiently deep to generate a palpable pulse.[4] Respirations, heart rate, and colour should be reassessed about every 30 s. Coordinated chest compressions and ventilations should continue until spontaneous heart rate is equal to or greater than 60 beats per minute.

Venous access: routes of drug administration

Gaining vascular access in the newborn may prove challenging but is sometimes required, for medication administration and fluid resuscitation. While IV or IM routes may be preferred for drug therapy in the newborn, other methods that may be considered include the endotracheal route (described in Chapter 12) and venous access though the umbilical cord (described below). Whilst theoretically possible, the IO route is not recommended in newborns as the small bones are fragile and the intraosseous space is small.

Accessing the umbilical vein

As described in Chapter 36, the umbilical cord contains three vessels: two arteries and one vein. The vein in the umbilical cord has a thin wall and is larger than the arteries. The arteries are thick walled and usually paired. The umbilical vein may be used up to 7 days post birth. To gain access to the umbilical vein, if within their scope of practice, the paramedic should take the following steps (Figure 37-7):

1. Set up intravenous line of normal saline with a three-way stopcock.
2. Select a 3.5 or 5 French umbilical catheter (which is pre-filled with normal saline).
3. Connect the catheter to the stopcock, and purge the air from the catheter.
4. Cleanse the umbilical stump and surrounding skin with antibacterial solution such as alcohol or similar.
5. Loosely tie umbilical tape around the cord near the body so that pressure can be applied to control bleeding.
6. Hold the umbilical stump firmly and trim (with a scalpel) the cord several centimetres above the abdomen.
7. Locate the umbilical vein (of which there is one and is large, thin walled) and insert the catheter until blood is freely obtained. Do not insert the catheter more than 4 to 6 cm. If the catheter is inserted farther, there is a risk of infusing solutions directly into the liver rather than the systemic circulation. Take care to avoid introduction of air emboli into the umbilical vein.

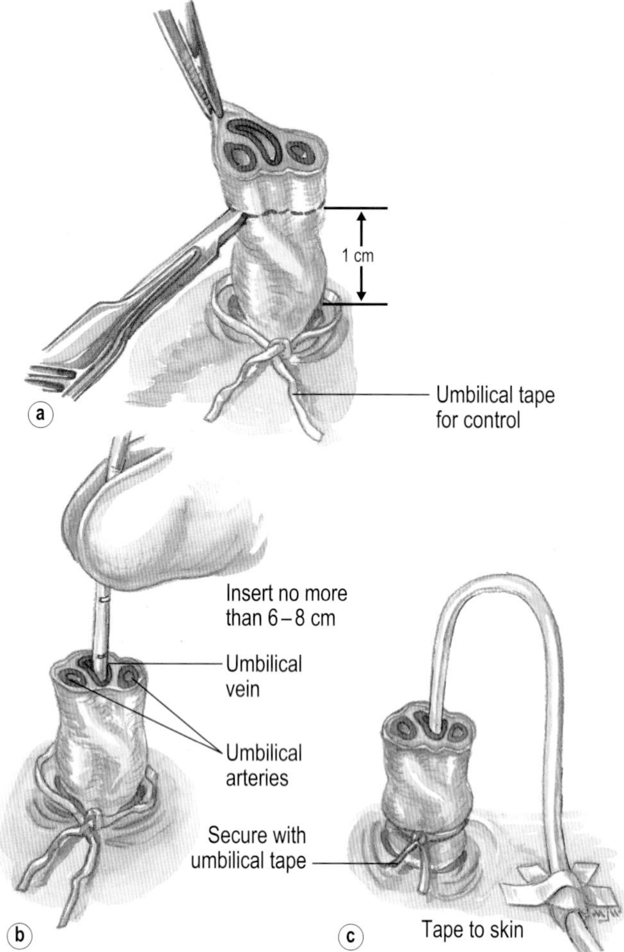

Figure 37-7 Umbilical vein cannulation procedure. (a) Identify the umbilical vein after trimming the cord. (b) Insert the umbilical catheter or angiocatheter into the vein. (c) Secure the base of the cord to hold the catheter in place and stabilize the catheter with tape.

8. Draw blood for a sample, if needed.
9. Start the infusion and regulate the fluid flow.
10. Secure the catheter in place with tape and cover with a sterile dressing.
11. Document the procedure.

The umbilical cord also may be cannulated by using a typical IV catheter. Insert the catheter-over-needle through the side of the proximal end of the cord into the vein and advance it upward through the translucent wall. Start the infusion, adjust the fluid flow, and secure the catheter in place with tape.

Administration of drugs or fluids

Drugs are rarely indicated in the resuscitation of the newly born baby and, as a rule, should be administered only if the heart rate remains below 60 beats per minute, despite adequate ventilation with 100% oxygen and effective chest compressions.[4] Drug therapy that may be indicated includes the administration of adrenaline (epinephrine), IV fluids, and, rarely, drugs such as naloxone (Table 37-1).

Note

Bradycardia in the newborn baby is usually the result of inadequate lung inflation or hypoxaemia. Therefore, establishing adequate ventilation is the most important step to correct it.

Important points for the paramedic to remember when administering drugs or fluids include:

1. The IV route is preferred for drug administration. All drugs should be given intravenously as soon as venous access is obtained. Whilst adrenaline (epinephrine) may be administered through the ET tube (at higher doses) while obtaining IV access, it is now felt to be ineffective. The IV dose of adrenaline (epinephrine) is 0.1–0.3 mL/kg of 1 : 10 000 (equates to 0.1–0.3 μg/kg) and should be flushed with saline.
2. IV fluids (normal saline is the preferred choice) should be considered when blood loss is suspected. They should also be considered if the baby appears to be in shock (pale skin, poor perfusion, weak pulse), and has not responded to other resuscitative measures. IV fluids should be given carefully (and calculated as 10–20 mL/kg) when resuscitating premature babies as rapid infusion of large volumes of fluids may cause haemodilution.
3. Naloxone is not recommended for initial resuscitation of newborns with respiratory depression. In addition, it should not be given to a newborn whose mother is chronically addicted, or has long-term exposure, to opioids, as doing so may precipitate convulsions in the baby. If naloxone is given, it should be administered only in cases of acute maternal exposure. The preferred route is IV or IM at 0.1 mg/kg. (Endotracheal administration in the newborn is not recommended.[4])

Post-resuscitation care

The three most common complications of the post-resuscitation period are endotracheal tube migration (including dislodgment), tube occlusion by mucus or meconium, and pneumothorax. These complications should be suspected in the presence of the following:

- decreased chest wall movement
- diminished breath sounds
- return of bradycardia
- unilateral decrease in chest expansion
- altered intensity to pitch of breath sounds
- increased resistance to hand ventilation.

Corrective management in the field for these post-resuscitative complications may include adjustment of the endotracheal tube (exhaled carbon dioxide devices are recommended for monitoring tracheal tube placement), re-intubation, and suction. Needle decompression to manage a suspected pneumothorax must be guided carefully by medical direction.

Table 37-1 Medication for newborn resuscitation

Medication	Dose/route	Concentration	Patient weight (kg)	Total (mL)	Precautions
Adrenaline (epinephrine)	10–30 μg/kg IV/IO	1:10 000	1 2 3 4	0.1–0.3 0.2–0.6 0.3–0.9 0.4–1.2	Give rapidly, repeat every 3–5 min
Atropine	20 μg/kg IV/IO	1 mg/10 mL	1 2 3 4	1.0 1.0 1.0 1.0	Minimum dose always 100 μg
		1 mg/5 mL	1 2 3 4	0.5 0.5 0.5 0.5	
IV fluids: normal saline	10 mL/kg IV/IO over 5–10 min		1 2 3 4	10 20 30 40	Reassess after each bolus
Naloxone	100 μg/kg IM	400 μg/mL	1 2 3 4	0.25 0.50 0.75 1.00	Repeat doses may be needed to prevent apnoea. Do not give if mother suspected of abusing opiates
Glucose	250 mg/kg IV	100 mg/mL (10% concentration)	1 2 3 4	2.5 5.0 7.5 10	Give if blood glucose <2.6 mmol/L, repeat if necessary

IM, intramuscular; IO, intraosseous; IV, intravenous.

Critical Thinking

How much movement would it take to dislodge an endotracheal tube from a newborn?

Neonatal transport

During transport of the newborn, it is important to maintain the baby's body temperature and prevent hypothermia as well as being critical to maintain oxygen administration and to support the baby's ventilations. In the initial prehospital phase of care, transport strategies usually are limited to providing a warm ambulance, free-flow oxygen administration, covering the baby's head, and applying warm blankets to prevent hypothermic complications. Specialized transport equipment such as isolettes and radiant heating units often are used for inter-hospital transfers and require special training. In the UK, several ambulance services have integrated neonatal retrieval teams using highly trained neonatal transport teams consisting of paramedics, nurses and medical practitioners (Figure 37-8).

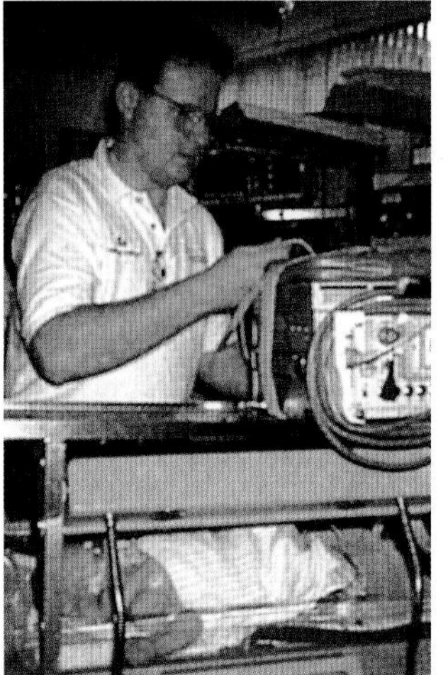

Figure 37-8 Neonatal transport.

Specific situations

Specific situations may call for advanced life support for the newborn. These situations include apnoea, diaphragmatic hernia, bradycardia, prematurity, respiratory distress and cyanosis, hypovolaemia, convulsions, fever, hypothermia, hypoglycaemia, vomiting and diarrhoea, and common birth injuries. While providing advanced life support in these and other situations, the paramedic must consider the emotional needs of the mother and family. When possible, the paramedic should explain what is being done for the baby and why a procedure is necessary.

Apnoea

Apnoea is an absence of spontaneous respirations, occurring most commonly in babies delivered before 32 weeks. Primary apnoea is controlled by P_{CO_2} levels and is a self-limiting condition and is common immediately after birth. Secondary apnoea is described as apnoea that exceeds 20 seconds without spontaneous breathing occurring, which can lead to hypoxaemia and bradycardia, is common in the preterm baby and often results from hypoxia or hypothermia. Secondary apnoea also may be caused by conditions that include maternal use of opioids or central nervous system depressants, prolonged or difficult labour and delivery, airway and respiratory muscle weakness, septicaemia, metabolic disorders, and central nervous system disorders.

Emergency care for a baby with prolonged apnoea begins with stimulating the baby to breathe. This is done by flicking the soles of the feet or rubbing the back. If needed, a bag–valve–mask device (with a disabled pop-off valve) should be used. The paramedic should use the least amount of pressure that produces adequate chest rise and suction secretions from the baby's airway as needed and maintain the baby's body temperature to prevent hypothermia. Endotracheal intubation and circulatory support may be required if central cyanosis persists despite adequate ventilations. Drug therapy that may be appropriate in managing some babies with prolonged apnoea includes dextrose (10% dextrose in water at 2.5 mL/kg) if hypoglycaemia is suspected or confirmed, and naloxone for reversal of respiratory depression in a newborn whose mother received opioids within 4 h of delivery.[4] (As discussed earlier, opioids antagonists should not be given to the baby if the mother is a drug abuser. Doing so may induce drug withdrawal in the newborn.) Apnoea that is treated early and aggressively normally results in a good outcome.

Diaphragmatic hernia

Diaphragmatic hernia is a rare condition occurring in 1 in 2200 live births. Herniation is caused by a malformation of the diaphragm during fetal development. It may occur on the left, right or both sides, but the left side is most common (90%), and leaves a hole in the diaphragm muscle. This allows abdominal organs such as the stomach, bowels, kidney, liver, and spleen to enter into the thorax, and the lung on the affected side cannot develop normally. This reduces lung capacity and can damage other organs, including the heart. Respiratory distress usually develops shortly after birth because the diaphragm cannot work properly and crowding of the lungs by other organs also may cause the lungs to collapse. Diaphragmatic hernia is a true emergency that requires surgical repair. Newborns who do not survive usually die during the first days or weeks of life; survival for the baby who requires mechanical ventilation in the first 18 to 24 h of life is about 50%. If there is no respiratory distress within the first 24 h of life, survival approaches 100%. Assessment findings may include the following:

- little to severe distress
- cyanosis unresponsive to ventilations
- diminished breath sounds on the left
- scaphoid (flat) abdomen
- the presence of bowel sounds in the chest
- displaced heart sounds to the right.

Prehospital care includes elevating the baby's head and thorax to assist with downward displacement of the abdominal organs, ensuring adequate oxygenation, providing ventilatory and circulatory support, and rapidly transporting the newborn to an appropriate hospital for definitive care. Further care may include the placement of an orogastric tube, with low periodic suction to improve ventilations. In some cases, tracheal intubation may be needed. The use of a bag device or aggressive positive-pressure ventilation, however, may worsen the condition as it may cause gastric distension; therefore the use of a bag device is contraindicated. If positive-pressure ventilation is required, this should be done via an endotracheal tube and care exercised with the inflation pressures, trying to keep below 25–30 cmH_2O.

Bradycardia

Bradycardia is described as a heart rate less than 100 beats/min. In the newborn, bradycardia most commonly is caused by hypoxia but may also result from increased intracranial pressure, hypothyroidism, and acidosis. Other risk factors include prolonged suctioning and the use of airway or any invasive procedures during resuscitation. Bradycardia is a minimal risk to life in newborns if it is corrected quickly.

The initial management for a newborn with bradycardia is to assess for upper airway obstruction. Such obstruction may be caused by airway secretions, foreign body, or the position of the tongue or soft tissues of the neck. Prehospital care to improve ventilation may include airway positioning, suction, positive-pressure ventilation with supplemental oxygen, and tracheal intubation. The paramedic should monitor ventilatory and circulatory status of the baby closely; this will determine the need for more advanced life support measures. Such measures may include chest compressions and drug therapy (described later in this chapter and in Chapter 12); however, use of drugs to reverse bradycardia should only be used when the measures described above have failed.

Prematurity

A premature baby refers to a baby who is born before 37 weeks' gestation; the weight of these newborns often is between 0.6 and 2.2 kg (1½ to 5 lb). Healthy premature babies who weigh greater than 1700 g have a survivability and outcome about equal to that of full-term babies; however, the mortality rate decreases weekly with gestation beyond the onset of fetal viability (currently around 23 to 24 weeks' gestation).[1] Premature babies have an increased risk for respiratory depression, hypothermia, and brain injury from hypoxaemia. They are also especially vulnerable to changes in blood pressure, intraventricular haemorrhage, and fluctuations in serum osmolarity. The degree of immaturity determines how the baby appears physically. However, most premature babies will have a large trunk, short extremities, less subcutaneous fat than full-term babies, and skin that appears translucent.

The prehospital care for premature babies is the same as for any other newborn. It may include airway, ventilatory, and circulatory support. The paramedic should attempt resuscitation if the baby has any signs of life. The paramedic must take special care to maintain the baby's body temperature and to prevent hypothermia. Examples include wrapping the baby in food-grade plastic film and the application of radiant heat.[4] Transport to a facility with special services for low-birth-weight newborns may be indicated.

Note

As with other newborns, concern for eye damage (retinopathy of prematurity) from long-term oxygen use in premature babies is not a factor in the emergency setting. Remember, hypoxaemia causes irreversible brain damage in these newborns; high-concentration oxygen must be used.

Box 37-2

Causes of neonatal convulsions

Developmental abnormalities
Drug withdrawal
Hypoglycaemia
Hypoxic–ischaemic encephalopathy
Intracranial haemorrhage
Meningitis or encephalopathy
Metabolic disturbances

Respiratory distress and cyanosis

Prematurity is the most common cause of respiratory distress and cyanosis in the newborn. These conditions occur most often in babies less than 1200 g (2½ lb) and 30 weeks' gestation; these problems may be related to the baby's immature central respiratory control centre. The centre is affected more easily by environmental and metabolic changes than that of the full-term baby. Other risk factors for respiratory distress and cyanosis in the newborn include multiple gestations, prenatal maternal complications, and babies born with the following conditions:

- birth defects
- central nervous system disorders
- diaphragmatic hernia
- lung immaturity
- lung or heart disease
- meconium or amniotic fluid aspiration
- metabolic acidosis
- mucus obstruction of nasal passages
- pneumonia
- primary pulmonary hypertension
- shock and sepsis.

Respiratory distress and cyanosis can lead to cardiac arrest in the newborn. The situation calls for immediate actions to improve breathing and support respirations. Assessment findings may include tachypnoea, paradoxical breathing, intercostal retractions, nasal flaring, expiratory grunting and central cyanosis. As described before, respiratory insufficiency in the newborn generally is managed with stimulation, positioning of the airway, prevention of heat loss and hypothermia, oxygenation and ventilation, suction, and intubation with ventilatory support (if needed).

Hypovolaemia

Hypovolaemia in babies may result from dehydration, haemorrhage, trauma or sepsis, or may also be associated with myocardial dysfunction. Signs and symptoms of hypovolaemia include mottled or pale colour, cool skin, tachycardia, diminished peripheral pulses and delayed capillary refill despite normal ambient temperature. Shock may be present despite a normal blood pressure. Prompt and effective treatment of early signs of compensated shock may prevent the development of hypotension (decompensated shock) and associated high morbidity and mortality. Prehospital care is always directed at ensuring adequate airway, ventilatory and circulatory support (including control of external haemorrhage) and providing rapid transport to an appropriate facility.

When signs of hypovolaemia are present, the paramedic should give a fluid bolus (10 mL/kg over 5–10 min of isotonic crystalloid) immediately after obtaining IV access. The paramedic should reassess the baby. If signs of shock persist, the paramedic should give a second 10 mL/kg bolus but fluids must always be administered carefully, in relation to the assessment findings.

Convulsions

Convulsions occur in a small percentage of newborns. When present, they are usually a sign of an underlying abnormality (Box 37-2). Prolonged convulsions or frequent convulsions may result in metabolic changes and problems with breathing and heart rate. They are more common in preterm babies, with an incidence rate of over 5% in babies with a birth weight of <1.5 kg, compared with less than 0.3% in those with a birth weight >2.5 kg.

Types of convulsions

Convulsions in newborns usually are fragmented and not well sustained. They have been classified as subtle convulsions, tonic convulsions, multifocal convulsions, focal clonic convulsions, and myoclonic convulsions.

Subtle convulsions involve eye deviation, blinking, sucking, swimming movements of the arms and pedalling movements of the legs. Apnoea may be present during subtle convulsions. Tonic convulsions usually involve extension of the limbs, and, less often, they involve flexion of the upper extremities and extension of the lower extremities. This type of convulsion is more common in babies who are premature. Tonic convulsion is more common especially in babies with intraventricular haemorrhage. Multifocal convulsions usually involve clonic activity in one extremity that may migrate randomly to another area of the body. This type of convulsion mainly occurs in full-term babies. Focal clonic convulsions involve clonic, localized jerking. They have been known to occur in full-term and premature newborns. Myoclonic convulsions involve flexion and jerking of the upper or lower extremities. These convulsions may occur on their own and may also occur in a series of repetitive jerking cycles.

Emergency care for managing neonatal convulsions includes providing airway, ventilatory, and circulatory support and maintaining the baby's body temperature. Drug therapy that may be prescribed by medical direction includes glucose (to treat hypoglycaemia after blood glucose assessment) and anticonvulsant agents such as benzodiazepines. Glucose solution (10% as a 2.5 mL/kg bolus), repeated as required to keep blood glucose values above 2.6 mmol/L, is indicated in hypoglycaemia. Convulsion activity is always considered pathological and rapid transport is indicated.

Fever

Fever in newborns is described as a rectal temperature greater than 38.0 °C (100.4 °F). Fever in newborns usually is a cause for concern and often is a response to an acute viral or bacterial infection. Fever also may result from a change in the baby's limited ability to control body temperature as well as an effect of dehydration. The rise in core temperature increases oxygen demands and increases glucose metabolism, which may lead to metabolic acidosis. Assessment findings may include mental status changes (e.g. irritability and somnolence), a history of decreased intake, rashes and petechiae, and warm or hot skin.

Note

Term newborns produce beads of sweat on their brow but not over the rest of their bodies. Premature babies generally have no visible sweat.

The prehospital care for febrile babies mainly is supportive. As a rule, cooling procedures and the use of antipyretics such as paracetamol and ibuprofen will be delayed until the child has arrived at hospital. Febrile convulsions usually affect children between 6 months and 5 years of age and therefore are not a concern in caring for the newborn (see Chapter 38). All febrile newborns require immediate transport for further assessment and management and these patients should be presumed to have systemic sepsis until it is proved otherwise.

Hypothermia

As described in Chapter 23, hypothermia is a core body temperature below 35 °C (95 °F). Hypothermia may result from a decrease in heat production, an increase in heat loss (through evaporation, conduction, convection, or radiation), or a combination of both. Newborns are sensitive to the effects of hypothermia because of their increased surface-to-volume ratio. This is especially the case when they are wet (e.g. after delivery). The associated increase in metabolic demand to maintain body temperature can cause metabolic acidosis, pulmonary hypertension, and hypoxaemia. Hypothermia also may be a sign of sepsis in the newborn. Assessment findings may include the following:

- pale colour
- cool skin (especially in the extremities)
- respiratory distress
- apnoea
- bradycardia
- central cyanosis
- acrocyanosis (cyanosis of the extremities)
- irritability (initially)
- lethargy (in the late stage)
- absence of shivering (variable).

The prehospital care for these patients may include provision of basic and advanced life support, depending on the severity of hypothermia, and prompt transport to an appropriate facility. Other therapeutic measures include ensuring that the baby is dry and warm, warming the hands before touching the newborn, and perhaps the administration of glucose to treat hypoglycaemia and IV therapy with warm fluids. The patient should be transported in a heated ambulance (24–26.5 °C [76–80 °F]).

Hypoglycaemia

A blood glucose measurement less than 2.6 mmol/L in the baby indicates hypoglycaemia (described in Chapter 17). The condition should be determined by blood glucose screening in all sick babies; in some cases, newborns are not symptomatic until blood glucose has dropped well below 2.6 mmol/L. Hypoglycaemia may be due to inadequate glucose intake or increased use of glucose. Risk factors associated with hypoglycaemia include asphyxia, toxaemia, being the smaller twin, central nervous system haemorrhage, and sepsis. Assessment findings may include the following:

- twitching or convulsion
- limpness
- lethargy
- eye rolling
- high-pitched crying
- apnoea
- irregular respirations
- cyanosis (possibly).

Note

Small babies and chronically ill children have limited glycogen stores; these may be depleted rapidly during stress events. If allowed to persist, hypoglycaemia can depress myocardial function and may have catastrophic effects on the brain as well.

The prehospital care is directed at ensuring adequate airway, ventilatory and circulatory support; maintaining body temperature; providing rapid transport; and consideration of IV administration of glucose 10% at 2.5 mL/kg IV. The paramedic should check the glucose level again if the baby fails to respond to initial resuscitative measures. All babies who do not respond normally and those who are hypoglycaemic and fail to respond to the glucose should be transported immediately to hospital.

Vomiting and diarrhoea

Occasional vomiting or diarrhoea is not unusual in the newborn. For example, vomiting mucus (that may be streaked with blood) is common in the first few hours of life. Also, five to six stools per day is considered normal, especially if the baby is being breast fed. Persistent vomiting and/or diarrhoea, however, should be considered warning signs of serious illness.

Box 37-3

Causes of vomiting in a newborn

Oesophageal atresia
Gastro-oesophageal reflux
Pyloric stenosis
Malrotation syndrome

Vomiting

Persistent vomiting in the first 24 h of life suggests an obstruction in the upper digestive tract or perhaps increased intracranial pressure (Box 37-3). Vomit that contains non-bile-stained fluid is a sign of anatomical or functional obstruction; this obstruction is at or above the first portion of the duodenum and a common cause can be pyloric stenosis. Vomiting also may indicate gastroesophageal reflux. Bile-stained vomit may result from obstruction below the opening of the bile duct. Vomit that contains dark blood usually is a sign of life-threatening illness. Assessment findings may include a distended stomach and signs of infection, dehydration, and increased intracranial pressure. The paramedic also should consider that the vomiting may be a result of drug withdrawal (from the mother's drug use).

The prehospital care requires maintaining an airway that is clear of vomit and ensuring adequate oxygenation. In severe cases, consideration is given to IV fluid therapy. Fluid therapy treats dehydration and any bradycardia that may develop from vagal stimulation. If possible, babies should be transported on their sides, which will help prevent aspiration.

Diarrhoea

Persistent diarrhoea can lead to serious dehydration and electrolyte imbalances in the newborn; the diarrhoea often is associated with a bacterial or viral infection. Other possible causes include the following:

- cystic fibrosis
- gastroenteritis
- intussusception (bowel 'telescopes' on itself)
- lactose intolerance
- neonatal abstinence syndrome (drug withdrawal)
- phototherapy (a treatment for hyperbilirubinaemia and jaundice in the newborn)
- rotavirus
- thyrotoxicosis
- poisons.

Assessment findings often include the presence of loose stools, increased number of stools (beyond the usual five to six per day in a newborn), decreased urinary output, and signs of dehydration. Treatment consists of supporting the baby's vital functions, IV fluid therapy at 10 mL/kg as per guidelines, and rapid transport to the receiving hospital.

Common birth injuries

Between 2 and 7 of every 1000 live births result in avoidable and unavoidable physical and anoxic trauma during labour and delivery. Of every 100 000 babies, 5–8 are estimated to die of birth trauma and 25 die of anoxic injuries (accounting for 2–3% of baby deaths).

An uncontrolled, explosive delivery (described in Chapter 36) is the greatest risk factor for birth injuries. Cranial injuries may include moulding of the head and overriding of the parietal bones, soft tissue injuries from forceps delivery, subconjunctival and retinal haemorrhage, subperiosteal haemorrhage and skull fracture. Intracranial haemorrhage can occur from trauma or asphyxia. Spine and spinal cord injury can result from strong traction or a lateral pull during delivery. Other birth injuries include peripheral nerve injury (such as a brachial plexus injury), liver or spleen injury, adrenal haemorrhage, clavicle or extremity fracture, and brain or soft tissue injury from hypoxia–ischaemia. The assessment findings vary by the nature of the injury but may include the following:

- diffuse, sometimes ecchymotic, oedematous swelling of the soft tissues of the scalp
- paralysis below the level of spinal cord injury
- paralysis of the upper arm with or without paralysis of the forearm
- paralysis of the diaphragm
- movement on only one side of the face when the newborn cries
- inability to move the arm freely on the same side of a fractured clavicle
- lack of spontaneous movement of an injured extremity
- hypoxia
- shock.

The goal of prehospital care for a baby with a birth injury is to support the newborn's vital functions. This can be done by ensuring adequate oxygenation, ventilation, and circulatory support and administering fluid or drug therapy (if indicated). These babies are high-risk newborns. They require rapid transport to a proper medical facility.

Neonatal resuscitation, post-resuscitation and stabilization

A newborn's heart generally is healthy and strong; however, disorders in the conduction system of the heart can and do occur. Most often the disorders occur as a result of hypoxaemia and respiratory arrest. The outcome for these babies is poor if interventions are not begun quickly. In addition, the likelihood for brain and organ damage is increased in babies who require resuscitation. The paramedic should continually assess and monitor newborns with respiratory distress for treatable causes of the distress.

Asystole and pulseless cardiac arrest are uncommon in the newborn. Like bradycardia, they usually are the result of hypoxia. Cardiac arrest also can be caused by primary and secondary apnoea, unresolved bradycardia, and persistent fetal circulation (persistent pulmonary hypertension). Assessment findings may include peripheral cyanosis, inadequate respiratory effort, and ineffective or absent heart rate. Risk factors associated with cardiac arrest in the newborn include the following:

- congenital malformations
- congenital neuromuscular disease

- drugs administered or taken by the mother
- intrapartum hypoxaemia
- intrauterine asphyxia.

Emergency care for newborns with asystole or pulseless arrest was described earlier in this chapter and includes airway, ventilatory and circulatory support; pharmacological therapy; and rapid transport to an appropriate medical facility.

Note

The decision to withhold resuscitation or to discontinue resuscitative efforts in the prehospital setting must be guided by medical direction. Babies without signs of life (no heart beat or respiratory effort) after 10 min of resuscitation show either a high mortality or severe neurodevelopmental disability. Therefore, after 10 min of continuous and adequate resuscitative efforts, the discontinuation of resuscitation may be justified if there are no signs of life.[4]

Critical Thinking

How will you feel if you deliver a critically ill or dead baby?

Psychological and emotional support

The paramedic must be aware of the normal feelings and reactions of parents, siblings, other family members, and caregivers while providing emergency care to an ill or injured child. (These events also are often highly charged and emotional for the emergency crew.) The paramedic should keep those at the scene abreast of all procedures being performed and inform family members of the necessity of the procedures.

Note

After delivery, the mother continues to be a patient herself. She still has certain physical and emotional needs.

As a rule, emergency responders should never discuss the baby's chances of survival with a parent or family member nor give false hope about the baby's condition, as so many variables can influence the outcome. The paramedic should assure the family that everything that can be done for the child is being done and that their baby will receive the best possible care during transport and at the hospital. The hospital will have support personnel who can assist family members and loved ones.

Summary

- When oxygenation and continued ventilations do not improve the baby's condition or the baby begins to deteriorate further, endotracheal intubation and administration of drugs may be required. The drugs most often used during neonatal resuscitation are adrenaline (epinephrine), IV fluids, and naloxone.
- Some of the more common congenital anomalies include choanal atresia, cleft lip, diaphragmatic hernia, and Pierre Robin syndrome.
- At birth, newborns make three major physiological adaptations necessary for survival: (1) emptying fluids from their lungs and beginning ventilation, (2) changing their circulatory pattern, and (3) maintaining body temperature.
- The first steps of newborn assessment and management are to prevent heat loss, clear the airway by positioning (and suctioning if required), provide tactile stimulation and initiate breathing if necessary, and further evaluate the baby.
- If resuscitation is required, the baby will need one or more of these interventions in sequence: re-evaluate initial steps in stabilization, provide ventilations, provide chest compressions, administer adrenaline (epinephrine) and/or IV fluids.
- The three most common complications during the post-resuscitation period are endotracheal position change (including dislodgment), tube occlusion by mucus or meconium, and pneumothorax. During transport of the newborn, it is important to maintain body temperature, oxygen administration, and ventilatory support.
- Specific situations that may require advanced life support for the newborn include meconium staining, apnoea, diaphragmatic hernia, bradycardia, premature babies, respiratory distress and cyanosis, hypovolaemia, convulsions, fever, hypothermia, hypoglycaemia, and vomiting and diarrhoea.
- Premature babies have an increased risk of respiratory suppression, hypothermia, and head and brain injury. In addition to low birth weight, various antepartum, and intrapartum risk factors may affect the need for resuscitation.
- Between 2 and 7 of every 1000 live births result in avoidable and unavoidable mechanical and anoxic trauma during labour and delivery.
- The paramedic should be aware of the normal feelings and reactions of parents, siblings, other family members and caregivers while providing emergency care to an ill or injured baby.

References

1. Birent D, Bingham R, Richmond S, et al 2005 European Resuscitation Council Guidelines for Resuscitation 2005. Section 6. Paediatric Life Support. Resuscitation 67(S1):S97–S133
2. McCance K, Huether S 2006 Pathophysiology: the biologic basis for disease in adults and children, 5th edition. Mosby, St Louis
3. Vain NE, Szyld EG, Prudent L et al 2004 Oropharyngeal and nasopharyngeal suctioning of meconium stained infants before delivery of their shoulders; multicentre, randomised controlled trial. Lancet 364:597–602
4. Resuscitation Council UK. Newborn life support. Online. Available http://www.resus.org.uk/pages/nls.pdf
5. American Heart Association 1995 Textbook of neonatal resuscitation. American Academy of Pediatrics, Dallas, TX
6. Eichelberger M, Ball J, Pratsch G, Clark J 1998 Pediatric emergencies, 2nd edition. Prentice-Hall, Englewood Cliffs, NJ

Further reading

Aehlert B 2007 Mosby's comprehensive pediatric emergency care (revised edition). Mosby, St Louis

Hoekelman R, Adam H, Nelson N, Weitzman M, Wilson M 2001 Primary pediatric care, 4th edition. Mosby, St Louis

CHAPTER 38

Paediatrics

Chapter contents

Objectives

Upon completion of this chapter, the paramedic student will be able to:

1. Identify the role of the emergency medical services in caring for paediatric patients.
2. Identify modifications in patient assessment techniques that assist in the examination of patients at different developmental levels.
3. Identify age-related illnesses and injuries in paediatric patients.
4. Outline the general principles of assessment and management of the paediatric patient.
5. Describe the pathophysiology, signs and symptoms, and management of selected paediatric respiratory emergencies.
6. Describe the pathophysiology, signs and symptoms, and management of shock in the paediatric patient.
7. Describe the pathophysiology, signs and symptoms, and management of selected paediatric dysrhythmias.
8. Describe the pathophysiology, signs and symptoms, and management of paediatric seizures.
9. Describe the pathophysiology, signs and symptoms, and management of hypoglycaemia and hyperglycaemia in the paediatric patient.
10. Describe the pathophysiology, signs and symptoms, and management of infectious paediatric emergencies.

11. Identify common causes of poisoning and toxic exposure in the paediatric patient.
12. Describe special considerations for assessment and management of specific injuries in children.
13. Outline the pathophysiology and management of sudden unexpected death in infancy (SUDI).
14. Describe the risk factors, key signs and symptoms, and management of injuries or illness resulting from child abuse and neglect.
15. Identify prehospital considerations for the care of infants and children with special needs.

Key terms

child abuse The physical, sexual, or emotional maltreatment of a child.

shunt A tube or device surgically implanted in the body to redirect body fluid from one cavity or vessel to another.

sudden unexpected death in infancy (SUDI) The unexpected and sudden death of an apparently normal and healthy infant that occurs during sleep.

Emergencies involving paediatric patients account for only a small percentage of emergency medical services responses; however, caring for these patients has unique challenges. The challenges are related to size, physical and intellectual maturation, and diseases specific to neonates, infants, and children. This chapter addresses the anatomical and physiological mechanisms of growth and development, medical emergencies common to children, and initial assessment and management strategies that often are critical in the patient's survival.

The paramedic's role in caring for paediatric patients

Paramedics play an important role in the prehospital care and interfacility transfer of infants and children, and also have a role in helping to reduce mortality and morbidity for children. They can become active participants in school, community, and parent education programmes and provide thorough documentation appropriate for prehospital trauma registries, epidemiological research, and surveillance. For paramedics, improvement of their knowledge and clinical skills is important. They can do this through continuing professional development (CPD) programmes that are specific to the paediatric age group. Examples of CPD programmes include

- Paediatric Advanced Life Support
- Prehospital Paediatric Life Support
- Paediatric Basic Trauma Life Support.

Other ways to enhance continuing education and clinical skills include reading textbooks and journals, Internet study, attending regional conferences and seminars, and working or volunteering at paediatric emergency departments, paediatric hospitals or a paediatrician's office.

Growth and development review

Children have unique anatomical, physiological and psychological characteristics that change during their development. The following is a review of growth and development by age group. Special considerations and approach strategies that must be taken into account when caring for paediatric patients are provided in Box 38-1.

Critical Thinking

How comfortable are you with the 'normal' well child?

Newborn (first few hours of life)

Assessment and care for the newborn is described in Chapter 37. The method most commonly used to evaluate the newborn is the Apgar score. Resuscitation of the newborn (if needed) should follow the recommendations established by the Resuscitation Council (UK) and published in the JRCALC guidelines for use by ambulance services.[1] To review, the newborn's heart rate during the first 30 min of life is between 120 and 160 beats/min and respirations are usually between 40 and 60 breaths/min. They average 30–40 breaths/min within a few minutes after delivery (Table 38-1). The full-term newborn normally weighs 3–3.5 kg (about 6–8 lb).

Neonate (first 28 days of life)

Total body weight in the neonate may decrease 5–10% during the first few days of life because of the excretion of extracellular fluid; this lost weight is regained by the second week of life and generally exceeds the newborn weight. Most infants gain an average of 175–225 g (6–8 oz) per week.

Neonates respond to a wide variety of stimuli and have a range of reflexes. Many of these reflexes are protective and

Table 38-1 Average vital signs by age group

Age	Pulse (per min)	Respirations (per min)	Blood pressure (mmHg)
Newborn	120–160	40–60	80/40
1 year	80–140	30–40	82/44
3 years	80–120	25–30	86/50
5 years	70–115	20–25	90/52
7 years	70–115	20–25	94/54
10 years	70–115	15–20	100/60
15 years	70–90	15–20	110/64

Note: Normal vital signs vary with age. Carry your JRCALC 'age per page' reminder chart to ensure accuracy. Do not depend on your memory in an emergency. Blood pressure in a child over 1 year may be estimated with the following formula: (age in years × 2) + 80 = typical systolic blood pressure. Example for a 3-year-old child: (3 × 2 = 6) + 80 = 86 mmHg.

Box 38-1

Developmental stages and approach strategies for paediatric patients

Infants

Major fears

Separation and strangers

Approach strategies

Provide consistent caretakers

Reduce parents' anxiety, because it is transmitted to the infant

Minimize separation from parents

Toddlers

Major fears

Separation and loss of control

Characteristics of thinking

Primitive

Unable to recognize views of others

Little concept of body integrity

Approach strategies

Keep explanations simple

Choose words carefully

Let toddler play with equipment (stethoscope)

Minimize separation from parents

Preschoolers

Major fears

Bodily injury and mutilation

Loss of control

The unknown and the dark

Being left alone

Characteristics of thinking

Highly literal interpretation of words

Unable to abstract

Primitive ideas about the body (e.g. fear that all blood will 'leak out' if a bandage is removed)

Approach strategies

Keep explanations simple and concise

Choose words carefully

Emphasize that a procedure will help the child be healthier

Be honest

School-age children

Major fears

Loss of control

Bodily injury and mutilation

Failure to live up to expectations of others

Death

Characteristics of thinking

Vague or false ideas about physical illness and body structure and function

Able to listen attentively without always comprehending

Reluctant to ask questions about something they think they are expected to know

Increased awareness of significant illness, possible hazards of treatments, lifelong consequences of injury, and the meaning of death

Approach strategies

Ask children to explain what they understand

Provide as many choices as possible to increase the child's sense of control

Reassure the child that he or she has done nothing wrong and that necessary procedures are not punishment

Anticipate and answer questions about long-term consequences (e.g. what the scar will look like and how long activities may be curtailed)

Adolescents

Major fears

Loss of control

Altered body image

Separation from peer group

Characteristics of thinking

Able to think abstractly

Tendency toward hyperresponsiveness to pain (reactions not always in proportion to event)

Little understanding of the structure and workings of the body

Approach strategies

When appropriate, allow adolescents to be a part of decision making about their care

Give information sensitively

Express how important their compliance and cooperation are to their treatment

Be honest about consequences

Use or teach coping mechanisms such as relaxation, deep breathing, and self-comforting talk

include those associated with breathing, eating, and stress or discomfort. Neonates sleep an average of 16–18 h per day, with sleep and wakefulness evenly distributed over 24 h. Breathing occurs mainly through the nose during the first month of life. The horizontal position of the ribs produces the characteristic diaphragmatic breathing in this age group. Although crying is common in the neonate, the crying gradually decreases throughout infancy. Persistent crying may indicate physiological distress. Illnesses that may be encountered in this age group are those that cause respiratory problems, jaundice, vomiting, fever, sepsis, meningitis, and problems of prematurity.

Infant (1–12 months)

Between 4 and 6 months of age, most infants have doubled their birth weight, tripling it within 9–12 months. In the first year of life the heart also doubles in size, the heart rate gradually slows, and weight and blood pressure begin to increase.

During infancy, major advances in physical and mental skills occur as the brain and nervous system gradually mature. By 12 months of age the development of mature nerves is nearly complete, and, along with muscle strength, enables many infants to stand and walk with little or no assistance. (Muscle weight in infants is about 25% of the entire musculoskeletal system.) Common illnesses typically affect the respiratory, gastrointestinal and central nervous systems and manifest as respiratory distress; nausea, vomiting and diarrhoea with dehydration; and seizures, respectively. Other illnesses that may be encountered in this age group include sepsis, meningitis, and sudden unexpected death in infancy (SUDI). In addition, the older infant (6–12 months of age) may experience bronchiolitis, croup, foreign body airway obstruction, and physical injury from sexual abuse, neglect, falls, and motor vehicle crashes.

Toddler (1–3 years)

Muscle mass and bone density increase during the toddler years. Most children gain an average of 2 kg (about 4 lb) each year. By age 2, much of the nervous system is fully developed and basic motor skills (e.g. balance and walking) and fine motor skills (e.g. stacking building blocks) become visible. In addition, most children are capable of controlling bladder and bowel function by 2–3 years of age. By 2 years of age, toddlers have developed unique personality traits, moods, and specific likes and dislikes. Basic language skills are mastered by age 3 but these skills continue to be refined throughout childhood. By 3 years of age, toddlers and preschoolers also begin to recognize the difference between the sexes and start to model themselves after persons of their own gender. Illnesses in this age group may cause respiratory distress (e.g. from asthma, bronchiolitis, foreign body aspiration or croup), vomiting and diarrhoea with dehydration, febrile seizures, sepsis and meningitis. Toddlers who are learning to walk are prone to falls and may also find themselves in dangerous environments without proper supervision or barriers (e.g. baby gates). Physical injuries also occur from poisonings from accidental ingestions, physical/sexual abuse, drowning, and motor vehicle crashes.

Preschool (3–5 years)

During the preschool years, children experience advances in gross and fine motor skills and develop peer relationships with other children near the same age and level of maturity. These relationships often begin with play that involves acting out fantasies or using imagination for new situations; all of which can lead to problem-solving skills and cognitive development. Illnesses and injuries that may be encountered in this age group include those mentioned before for toddlers. In addition, preschoolers are more likely to experience injuries from thermal burns and are also more likely to be victims of submersion incidents or drowning. Preschool children are curious and often have an urge to explore. Many have a minimal concept of danger.

School age (6–12 years)

The growth of school-age children is slower and steadier than during the infancy, toddler, and preschool years. Most children gain about 3 kg (6.6 lb) per year and average a yearly gain in height of about 6 cm (2½ inches). Most bodily functions reach adult levels in this age group. Two key areas of development during the school-age years include an increased ability to concentrate and learn quickly and the onset of puberty. Psychosocial development of school-age children varies by individual, but, as a rule, self-concept, moral traits and behaviour begin to emerge. During these years children spend more time with others outside their immediate family. Most illnesses in school-age children are caused by viral infection. Injuries become more common in this age group because of increased physical activity and include injuries from bicycle crashes, fractures from falls, and sport-related injuries.

Note

The UK compares well with other European countries in that it has the second lowest overall childhood injury death rate; however, mortality is only the tip of the iceberg. The lack of data on the incidence of injury, morbidity, and disability means that it is difficult to know the true size of the iceberg.[2]

Adolescent (13–18 years)

During adolescence, the final phase of change in growth and development occurs. Organs rapidly increase in size, blood chemistry values become nearly equal to adult levels, and growth of bone and muscle mass becomes nearly complete. Also, in adolescence, a person reaches reproductive maturity. The development of secondary sex characteristics in both sexes heralds a final period of rapid growth. Most boys gain an average of 20 cm (8 inches) in height before age 21, when growth usually stops. Growth in girls is less dramatic and is usually complete by age 18.

Along with the physical changes associated with adolescence, most teenagers begin to experiment with different identities as they begin to develop their personality into that of an adult. Many make dramatic moves away from parents and family members toward their peer groups. In their peer groups, they may experiment with alcohol and other drugs, sex, and extreme forms of behaviour. In addition to those physical injuries mentioned for younger age groups, situations that the paramedic may encounter in this age group (and that are not seen as often in other age groups) include behavioural emergencies associated with alcohol or other drugs use, eating disorders, depression, suicide and suicide gestures, sexually transmitted diseases, pregnancy, and sexual assault.

Anatomy and physiology review

As stressed throughout this text, physical differences in infants and children set them apart from the adult patient. The following is a review of anatomy and physiology by body region. Also included are special emergency care implications for the paediatric patient.

Head

A child's head is proportionally large and accounts for about 25% of the total body weight in newborns. Children also have a larger occipital region and a face that is small compared with the size of the head. Because of these anatomical features, a high percentage of blunt trauma in children involves the head and face. When using spinal stabilization for a child less than 3 years of age, a thin layer of padding under the child's shoulders may be needed to obtain a neutral position. A folded sheet placed under the occiput of a severely ill child over 3 years of age (or under the shoulders of a child less than 3 years of age) can help establish the 'sniffing' position needed to maintain the airway.

To accommodate for brain growth in the infant, the anterior fontanelle remains open for 9–18 months after birth. The anterior fontanelle is usually level or slightly below the surface of the skull. A tight or bulging fontanelle suggests increased intracranial pressure (ICP; as seen with meningitis); a sunken fontanelle indicates possible dehydration. The paramedic should assess the anterior fontanelle in infants and young children who are ill or injured. The fontanelle is best assessed when the child is upright and not crying.

Airway

The airway structures of children are narrower and less stable at all levels than those of adults. This makes the airways of paediatric patients more easily blocked by secretions, obstructions, and injury or inflammation. In addition, the larynx is higher (at the level of the cervical vertebrae C3 to C4) and more anterior, extending into the pharynx. The trachea is bifurcated at a higher level and the tracheal cartilage is softer and smaller in length and diameter. The cricoid ring is the narrowest part of the airway in young children. The jaw is proportionally small, and the tongue is proportionally large, which increases the likelihood of airway obstruction by the tongue in the unconscious child. The epiglottis in infants is omega shaped and extends into the airway at a 45-degree angle. The epiglottic folds also have softer cartilage and can become 'floppy', causing airway obstruction. As described in Chapter 13, and later in this chapter, management considerations for these patients include the following:

- placing a thin layer of padding under the shoulders to maintain a neutral position of the airway structures in children less than 3 years of age
- placing a folded sheet under the occiput to obtain a sniffing position in children over 3 years of age
- avoiding hyperflexion or hyperextension of the neck, which can obstruct the airway
- using suction to clear the airway of secretions and particulate matter
- modifying tracheal intubation techniques by ensuring a gentle touch to the soft tissue of the airway, which is easily injured and inflamed; using a straight blade that lifts the epiglottis; choosing an appropriately sized endotracheal tube (uncuffed for children under 8 years of age); and constantly monitoring the airway for proper endotracheal tube placement.

The paramedic should also remember that infants breathe mainly through the nose during the first month of life. Obstruction of the small nares by secretions can result in respiratory insufficiency. Assessment and suction of the nares as needed is important, especially in infants less than 6 months of age.

Chest and lungs

In infants and young children the chief support for the chest wall comes from muscles rather than bones. These chest muscles are immature and can fatigue easily. The use of these muscles for breathing requires higher metabolic and oxygen consumption rates than in older children and adults, which increases the paediatric patient's susceptibility to the build-up of lactic acid in the blood. The ribs of a child are more pliable and are positioned horizontally; the mediastinum is more mobile. Therefore the chest wall offers less protection to internal organs and allows for significant internal injury to occur without external signs of trauma (e.g. fractured ribs). Rib fractures are less common in children although they can occur.

The lung tissue of a paediatric patient is fragile. Because of this and the limited protection provided by the chest wall, pulmonary contusions from trauma and pneumothorax from barotrauma are common in this age group. When evaluating a paediatric patient who has suffered major trauma, the paramedic should remember that infants and children are diaphragmatic breathers and are prone to gastric distension; the mobile mediastinum may have a greater shift with a tension pneumothorax; and the thin chest wall easily transmits breath sounds which may complicate the assessment of a pneumothorax or endotracheal tube placement. As a result, auscultation of breath sounds from the axillary regions in addition to the anterior and posterior thorax often is helpful.

Abdomen

Like the chest wall, the immature muscles of the abdomen in a child offer less protection to internal organs. In addition, the abdominal organs are closer together, and the liver and spleen are proportionally larger and more vascular. These features mean that multiple organ injuries are more common following abdominal trauma, and that the liver and spleen are injured more often than in the adult patient.

Extremities

Bones in children are softer and more porous until adolescence. As long bones mature, hormones act on the cartilage in growing bones, replacing the soft cartilage with hard bones. The epiphyseal plate (growth plate) lengthens as bones develop, and bones thicken as new layers of bone are deposited on existing bone.

Due to the soft composition of bones in paediatric patients, the paramedic should initially consider all strains and sprains to be a fracture and should fully immobilize the extremity. In addition, paramedics should be wary of injuries to the growth plate that may disrupt bone growth. Careful technique during intraosseous infusion procedures is critical because improper insertion into the growth plate can affect future bone growth (see Chapter 12).

Skin and body surface area

The skin in children is thinner and more elastic than the skin of adults, and the child has less subcutaneous fat. The child has a larger body surface area–body mass ratio as well. These factors can affect injury and illness in children in several ways. For example, the thinner skin of a child allows for deeper injury to occur from heat or cold exposure. The lack of subcutaneous fat and the larger body surface area–body mass ratio also increase a child's likelihood of hypothermia, hyperthermia, and dehydration from fluid loss.

Respiratory system

Tidal volume is between 6 and 8 mL/kg in the spontaneously breathing child, and resting deadspace is about 33% of tidal volume (2 mL/kg).[3] When exercising, which is an imposed metabolic stress that the respiratory and cardiovascular systems must compensate for, the deadspace volume can decrease to about 20% of tidal volume in the healthy state. Disease may seriously impair the ability to recruit alveolar volume when increasing tidal volume, and so limit the ability to decrease the deadspace volume–tidal volume ratio.[3] Paediatric patients also have smaller functional residual capacity (therefore smaller oxygen reserves) and a metabolic oxygen requirement for normal breathing that is about double that of an adult. Because of these factors, hypoxia can develop rapidly in infants and young children. The paramedic should remember that muscles are the main support for the chest wall. These muscles can tire easily during respiratory distress, which in turn can lead quickly to respiratory arrest.

Cardiovascular system

Cardiac output is rate dependent in infants and small children (the faster the heart rate, the greater the cardiac output). Paediatric patients are not as able as adults to increase contractility of the heart or increase stroke volume. The circulating blood volume in paediatric patients is proportionally larger than in adults but the child's absolute blood volume is smaller. The ability of children to use vasoconstriction to decrease size of the vessels allows them to maintain blood pressure longer than adults. However, early intervention is required to prevent irreversible or decompensated shock. Special considerations in managing these patients include the following:

- Cardiovascular reserve is vigorous but limited.
- Loss of small volumes of fluid and blood can cause shock. In a 1-year-old child, for example, the loss of blood equivalent to a can of fizzy drink is sufficient to place the child in irreversible shock!
- A child may be in shock despite a normal blood pressure.
- Bradycardia is often a response to hypoxia.

As described in Chapter 28, hypotension is a late sign of shock in the paediatric patient. The assessment of shock must be based on clinical signs of tissue perfusion (e.g. level of consciousness, skin colour and capillary refill). The paramedic should suspect shock in any ill or injured child who has tachycardia and evidence of decreased perfusion.

Nervous system

Several factors associated with neurological development during childhood contribute to an increased risk of devastating brain injuries following direct trauma to the head. The developing neural tissue is fragile and less protected during early childhood due to the anterior and posterior fontanelles remaining open for a period of time. In addition, the child's brain and spinal cord are less well protected by the skull and spinal column. This allows for greater force to be transmitted to the brain and spinal cord, with resultant injury, even in the absence of spinal column injury.

Metabolic differences

The way in which children and adults expend energy differs in many ways. For example, infants and children have limited glycogen and glucose stores so their blood glucose levels may drop quite low in response to illness or injury, even without a history of diabetes mellitus. Paediatric patients can experience significant volume loss from vomiting and diarrhoea. Children are more prone to hypothermia because of their relatively high ratio of body surface area to mass; newborns and neonates do not have the ability to shiver to maintain body temperature. For these reasons, it is important to assess a severely ill or injured child for hypoglycaemia or hypoperfusion, to minimize heat loss, and to keep all children warm during treatment and transport.

Critical Thinking

Why it is important to know what injuries and illnesses are commonly seen in specific age groups?

General principles of paediatric assessment

Initial patient evaluation for children should include observing the patient and involving the parent or guardian in the assessment (see Chapter 7). The parent or guardian can often help make the child more comfortable during the assessment and can usually offer key details about the child's medical history. The parent may also know whether aspects of the child's behaviour or response are normal or abnormal.

Scene size-up

As with all other patient care, the paramedic should begin the physical assessment with a quick scene survey, noting any hazards or potential hazards. The paramedic should also note any visible mechanism of injury or illness; for example, the presence of pills, medicine bottles or household chemicals may indicate the possibility of toxic ingestion. Injury and a history that does not match or fit the mechanism of injury may indicate child abuse. In addition, the paramedic should observe the relationship between the parent, guardian, or caregiver and the child, and should determine the appropriateness of their interaction. For example, does the interaction demonstrate concern or is it angry or indifferent? Other important assessments the paramedic can make during the scene size-up include the orderliness, cleanliness and safety of the home and the general appearance of other children in the family.

> **Critical Thinking**
>
> Would you want to make a comment to the parents about an unsafe situation on the scene before transport? Why or why not?

Initial assessment

The initial assessment begins with the paramedic forming a general impression of the patient. This assessment should focus on the details most valuable for determining whether life-threatening conditions exist. The paediatric assessment triangle (Figure 38-1) is a paradigm that can be used to quickly assess a child (as well as an adult) and the need for immediate intervention. The assessment triangle has three components: appearance (mental status and muscle tone); work of breathing (respiratory rate and effort); and circulation (skin signs and skin colour). If the child's condition is urgent, care should proceed with rapid assessment of airway, breathing, and circulation; management; and rapid transport. If the child's condition is not urgent, care can proceed with a focused history and detailed physical examination.

> **Critical Thinking**
>
> Think about one abnormal finding in each area of the assessment triangle. Would that single finding influence your triage decision?

Vital functions

The AVPU scale (alert; responds to verbal stimuli; responds to painful stimuli; unresponsive) or the Modified Glasgow Coma Scale (Table 38-2) can be used to determine the child's level of consciousness and to assess for signs of inadequate oxygenation.

Airway and breathing

The child's airway should be patent, and breathing should proceed with adequate chest rise and fall. Signs of respiratory distress include the following:

- abnormal breath sounds
- absent breath sounds
- bradypnoea
- grunting
- head bobbing
- irregular breathing pattern
- nasal flaring
- tachypnoea
- use of accessory muscles.

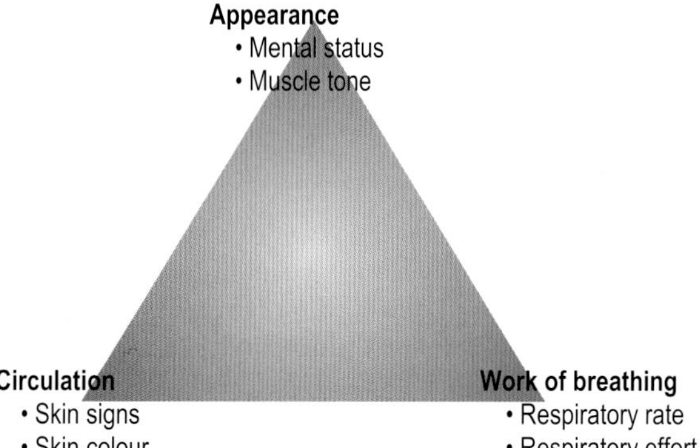

Figure 38-1 Paediatric assessment triangle.

Circulation

The paramedic assesses circulation by comparing the strength and quality of central and peripheral pulses, measuring blood pressure (in children over 3 years of age), evaluating skin colour, temperature, moisture, and turgor and capillary refill, and looking for visible haemorrhage. Table 38-1 provides normal vital signs for each age group.

Transition phase

The transition phase is included throughout assessment. This phase is used to allow the child to become more

Table 38-2 Paediatric modification of Glasgow Coma Scale*

Glasgow Coma Scale score	Paediatric modification
EYE OPENING	
≥4 years	*≤4 years*
4 Spontaneously	4 Spontaneously
3 To speech	3 To speech
2 To pain	2 To pain
1 No response	1 No response
BEST MOTOR RESPONSE	
≥4 years	*≤4 years*
6 Obeys commands	6 Obeys commands
5 Localizes pain	5 Localizes pain
4 Withdraws from pain	4 Withdraws from pain
3 Abnormal flexion (decorticate)	3 Abnormal flexion (decorticate)
2 Extensor response (decerebrate)	2 Extensor response (decerebrate)
1 No response	1 No response
BEST VERBAL RESPONSE	
≥4 years	*≤4 years*
5 Oriented and converses	5 Appropriate words/social smiles; fixes on and follows objects
4 Disoriented and converses	4 Cries but is consolable
3 Inappropriate words	3 Persistently irritable
2 Incomprehensible sounds	2 Restless, agitated
1 No response	1 Silent

*The Glasgow Coma Scale score is the sum of the individual scores from eye opening, best verbal response, and best motor response, using age-specific criteria. A Glasgow Coma Scale score of 13–15 indicates mild head injury; a score of 9–12 indicates moderate head injury; and a score of 8 or lower indicates severe head injury. In paediatrics it has been argued that a GCS of ≤5 rather than ≤8 should be used to indicate severe head injury.[4]

familiar with the paramedic crew and medical equipment (e.g. 'get to know you' conversations and playing with the stethoscope) (see Chapter 9). Use of this phase depends on the seriousness of the patient's condition; it is appropriate only for a conscious child who is not acutely ill. If the patient is unconscious or acutely ill, management should proceed quickly to emergency care and transport.

Focused history

When obtaining the focused history for an infant, a toddler or a preschool child, the paramedic may need to elicit information from the parent, guardian or caregiver. School-age and adolescent patients can provide most information by themselves. When appropriate to the complaint, the paramedic should question them in private (away from parents or family members) about sexual activity, pregnancy, alcohol or other drug use. The focused history can be obtained using the SAMPLE and OPQRST methods (described in Chapter 8). The paramedic should use these methods as appropriate for the patient's age. Important elements of the focused history are as follows:

1. Chief complaint
   - nature of illness or injury
   - the length (duration) of illness or injury
   - last meal
   - presence of fever
   - effects on behaviour
   - vomiting or diarrhoea
   - frequency of urination.
2. Medications and allergies.
3. Medical history
   - physician care
   - chronic illnesses.

Detailed physical examination

The paramedic should perform a detailed physical examination as described in Chapter 7. The examination should proceed from head to toe in older children but it should proceed from toe to head in younger children (under 2 years of age). Depending on the patient's condition, some or all of the following assessments may be appropriate:

- Pupils: Are they equal and reactive to light?
- Capillary refill (most accurate in patients under 6 years of age): Is it less than 2 s (normal) or delayed?
- Hydration: Does the skin show normal resiliency (skin turgor)? Are there tears and saliva? Are the fontanelles in the infant sunken or flat?

Note

When assessing a paediatric patient who is ill, it is important to note the presence or absence of fever, nausea, vomiting, diarrhoea, and frequency of urination.

If time allows and the patient's condition warrants, non-invasive monitoring of vital signs can provide more information. Examples include the use of pulse oximetry to measure perfusion and oxygen saturation, blood pressure assessment, and measurement of body temperature. In addition, all seriously ill or injured children should receive continuous electrocardiogram monitoring.

Ongoing assessment

Ongoing assessment is appropriate for all patients and should be performed throughout the patient care. The purpose of ongoing assessment is to monitor the patient for changes in respiratory effort, skin colour and temperature, mental status, and vital signs (including pulse oximetry measurements). Measurement tools (e.g. blood pressure cuffs and electrodes) should be appropriate for the size of the child. A key point to remember is that a child's condition can change rapidly; thus, vital signs should be assessed every 15 min in a child who is not critical. They should be assessed every 5 min in a child who is seriously ill or injured.

Critical Thinking

Why is ongoing assessment critical when caring for the young child?

General principles of patient management

The principles of patient care depend on the patient's condition. These principles may include basic airway management, advanced airway management, circulatory support, pharmacological therapy, non-pharmacological therapy, transport considerations, and psychological support and communication strategies.

Basic airway management

Basic and advanced airway management procedures for the paediatric patient are presented in detail in Chapter 13. These procedures may include manual positioning of the airway, removal of foreign body airway obstruction with chest or abdominal thrusts, suctioning secretions from the airway, providing supplemental oxygen, using oral or nasal airway adjuncts, and assisting ventilation with a bag–valve device.

Advanced airway management

Advanced airway management procedures may be needed when caring for a child who is acutely ill or seriously injured. These techniques include removing foreign body airway obstruction under direct visualization with Magill forceps, endotracheal intubation, or cricothyroidotomy (per service protocol) when other methods to maintain a patent airway have failed.

Circulatory support

Circulatory support may be required in an ill or injured child. In addition to providing basic life support with cardiopulmonary resuscitation, vascular access may be required for drug therapy and fluid resuscitation. Methods to obtain vascular access in paediatric patients are described in Chapter 12 and later in this chapter. These methods may include peripheral venous cannulation and intraosseous infusion.

Pharmacological therapy

At times, drug therapy will be required when caring for the paediatric patient. Examples include therapy for pain management, and patients with respiratory, cardiac, endocrinological or neurological conditions. Drugs that are used in paediatric emergencies are described later in this chapter but the paramedic should refer to the most up-to-date JRCALC guidelines for their authorized use in practice.

Additional therapy

Additional therapies are indicated depending on the type of illness or injury. These include spinal immobilization for trauma patients, haemorrhage control and bandaging and splinting, and electrical therapy (described later in this chapter). In addition, lowering body temperature with cooling methods or maintaining body temperature with blankets and warm clothing may be needed.

Transport considerations

As described in Chapter 26, some paediatric patients need transport to a specialty care medical facility. Examples of specialty care facilities are paediatric trauma centres, high-risk newborn care facilities, and paediatric burn centres. In addition to choosing a proper facility, the paramedic crew must consider the proper mode of caring for these patients. This includes deciding to provide rapid transport versus providing on-scene care and deciding on the use of ground or air ambulance.

Psychological support

It is important for the paramedic to provide psychological support to the paediatric patient and to the patient's family or caregivers. Paediatric emergencies are often emotionally charged events. Helpful strategies for approaching and communicating with paediatric patients and their caregivers are described in Chapter 6.

Specific pathophysiology, assessment and management

The conditions discussed in this section are respiratory compromise, shock, dysrhythmias, seizure, hypoglycaemia and hyperglycaemia, infection, poisoning and toxic exposure, trauma, SUDI, and child abuse and neglect.

Respiratory compromise

Respiratory problems can be caused by many conditions that affect the upper and lower airways. These include upper and lower foreign body airway obstruction, upper airway disease (croup, epiglottitis), and lower airway disease (asthma, bronchiolitis and pneumonia). Most cases of cardiac arrest in children occur because of respiratory insufficiency.[5] For this reason, respiratory emergencies call for rapid assessment and management. The severity of respiratory compromise may be classified as respiratory distress, respiratory failure and respiratory arrest.

The paramedic should try to calm and reassure a child with respiratory compromise and should not agitate the conscious patient or lay the child down (supine). Doing so may aggravate the airway condition and may even lead to life-threatening airway obstruction. When possible, allow the parent or other caregiver to stay with the child. The receiving hospital should be advised of the patient's status as soon as possible so that arrangements can be made for appropriate medical personnel.

Respiratory distress is the mildest form of respiratory compromise. Respiratory distress is evident by an increase in the rate and depth of breathing and by the use of accessory muscles to assist ventilation (Figure 38-2). These changes cause a slight decrease in arterial carbon dioxide levels in the blood as respiratory rate increases. As respiratory distress increases, the patient becomes exhausted and the PCO_2 gradually increases as the patient deteriorates. Signs and symptoms of respiratory distress include the following:

- a change in mental status from normal to irritable or anxious
- tachypnoea
- recession (indrawing of chest wall occurring whilst it expands during inspiration)
- nasal flaring (in infants)
- poor muscle tone
- tachycardia
- head bobbing
- grunting
- cyanosis that improves with supplemental oxygen.

If left untreated, respiratory distress may lead to respiratory failure.

Respiratory failure results from poor ventilation or lack of oxygenation and occurs when the heart and lungs do not exchange enough oxygen and carbon dioxide. This causes a decrease in PO_2 and an increase in PCO_2 (leading to respiratory acidosis). Signs and symptoms of respiratory failure include the following:

- irritability deteriorating to lethargy
- marked tachypnoea deteriorating to bradypnoea
- marked recession deteriorating to agonal respirations
- marked tachycardia deteriorating to bradycardia
- central cyanosis.

Respiratory failure in any patient is an ominous sign that can lead to respiratory arrest.

Respiratory arrest is the cessation of breathing. Good outcomes can be expected with early treatment, but failure to treat respiratory arrest will lead to cardiopulmonary arrest. Signs and symptoms of respiratory arrest include the following:

- unresponsiveness
- apnoea
- absent chest wall movement
- limp muscle tone
- bradycardia deteriorating to asystole
- profound cyanosis.

Providing ventilatory and circulatory support for patients in respiratory distress is critical. Airway interventions may include bag–valve–mask ventilation, endotracheal intubation, gastric decompression (if abdominal distension is impeding ventilation), needle decompression for

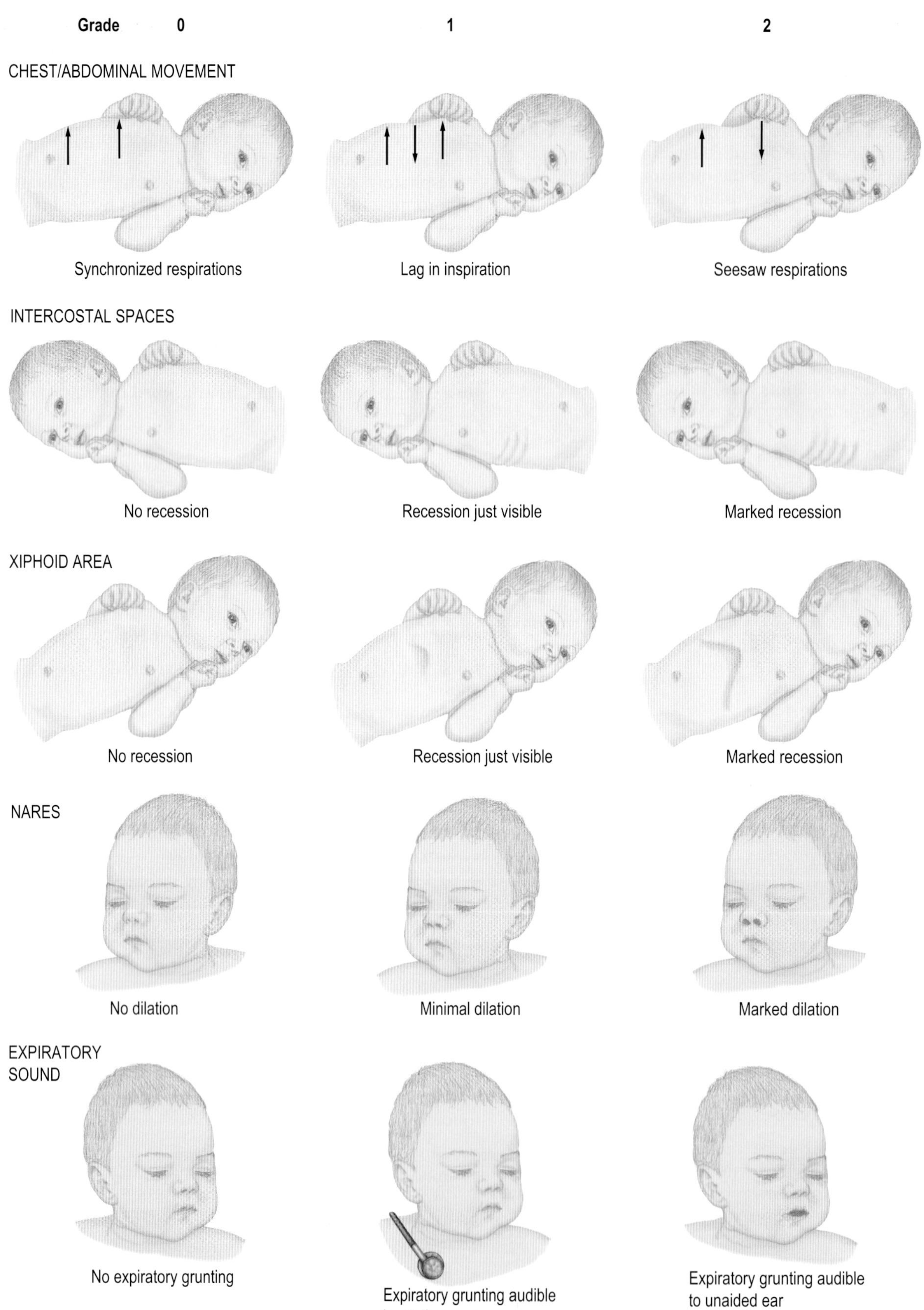

Figure 38-2 Assessment of respiratory distress. The Silverman–Andersen index is used to score the infant's degree of respiratory difficulty. The score for individual criteria matches the grade, with a total possible score of 10 indicating severe distress.

pneumothorax, and cricothyroidotomy for complete upper airway obstruction that cannot be relieved by other means. The success of emergency care is indicated by an improvement in the patient's colour and oxygen saturation, an improvement in the pulse rate, and an improved level of consciousness.

Upper and lower foreign body airway obstruction

Obstruction of the upper or lower airway by a foreign body may cause a partial or full obstruction. This usually occurs in toddlers and preschool children (1–4 years of age). Obstruction is often caused by food (hard sweets, nuts, seeds) or small objects (coins, balloons). The paramedic should suspect foreign body aspiration in an otherwise healthy child with sudden onset of respiratory compromise.

Signs and symptoms of airway obstruction include anxiety, inspiratory stridor, muffled or hoarse voice, drooling, pain in the throat, decreased breath sounds, rales, rhonchi, and wheezing. The child may have a history of choking (observed by an adult). If a full obstruction cannot be relieved with basic and advanced methods of clearing, tracheal intubation may be indicated. Full obstruction calls for immediate intervention to relieve the obstruction. Basic and advanced methods of clearing the airway are presented in Chapter 13.

If a child with a partial obstruction is conscious and has adequate movement of air, the paramedic should not agitate the child. Rather, the paramedic should provide continuous respiratory monitoring and immediately transport the child to the hospital. Agitation or attempts to relieve a partial obstruction may cause the foreign body to move, which may lead to full obstruction.

Croup

Croup (laryngotracheobronchitis) is a common viral infection of the upper airway. It usually occurs in children between the ages of 6 months and 4 years and is more prevalent during the late autumn and early winter months. Croup may involve the entire respiratory tract although the symptoms are caused by inflammation in the subglottic region (at the level of the larynx extending to the cricoid cartilage) (Figure 38-3).

A child with croup usually has a history of recent upper respiratory tract infection and a low-grade fever. The patient may have hoarseness, inspiratory stridor (from subglottic

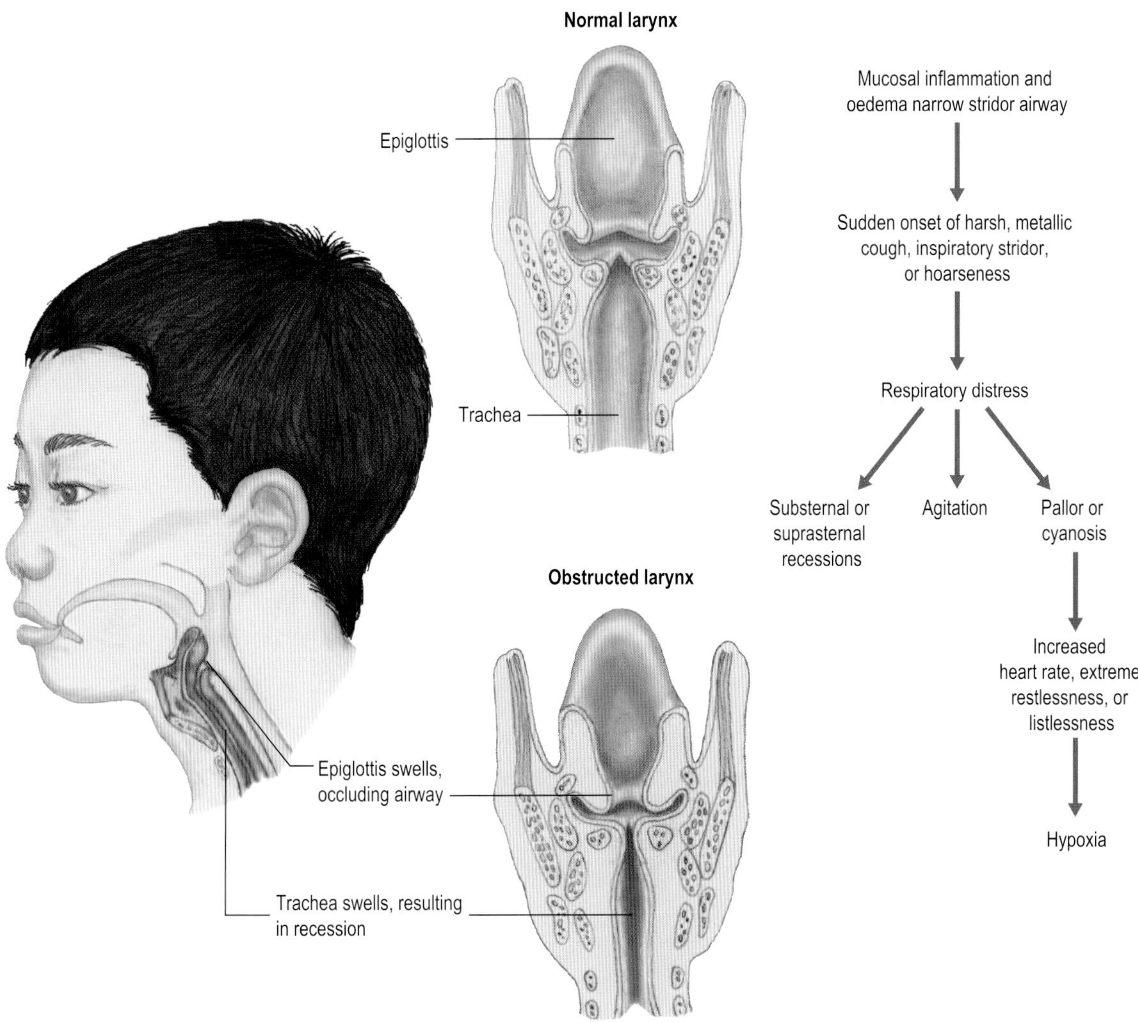

Figure 38-3 Pathophysiology of croup.

oedema), and a barking cough. Wheezing may be present if the lower airways are involved, but symptoms tend to occur mainly on inspiration. Most often, the emergency episode occurs at night after the child has gone to bed. On the arrival of the paramedics, a patient with severe croup may have all the classic signs of respiratory distress. The child may be sitting upright and leaning forward to aid breathing (variable), and nasal flaring, intercostal recession, and cyanosis (a late sign of respiratory insufficiency) may be present. Children with severe croup are at risk of serious airway obstruction from the narrowed diameter of the trachea.

Prehospital management of croup includes airway maintenance, administration of cool mist or humidified or nebulized oxygen (if available), and transportation in a position of comfort. Symptoms may improve dramatically in patients with croup after the child is exposed to cool, humidified air. (For example, this may occur after moving the patient from the residence to the emergency vehicle.) The paramedic should make all efforts to keep the child comfortable and at ease.

Table 38-3 Comparison of the symptoms of croup and epiglottitis

Characteristics	Croup	Epiglottitis
Occurrence	6 months to 4 years	3–7 years
Onset	Slow	Rapid
Comfortable position	Patient may lie down or sit upright	Patient prefers to sit upright
Cough	Barking cough	No barking cough; may have inspiratory stridor
Drooling	No drooling	Drooling, pain on swallowing
Temperature	Under 38°C	Over 38°C

Epiglottitis

Epiglottitis is caused by a bacterial infection of the upper airway and, although uncommon, it can progress rapidly and become life threatening. It most often affects children between 3 and 7 years of age although it can occur at any age. The bacterial infection causes oedema and occlusion from swelling of the epiglottis and supraglottic structures (pharynx, aryepiglottic folds and arytenoid cartilage). Epiglottitis is a true emergency that requires prompt, expert airway management.

Note

The *Haemophilus influenzae* type B (Hib) vaccine has dramatically reduced the number of cases of epiglottitis in children.[6] See Appendix 38-1 for recommended childhood and adolescent immunizations.

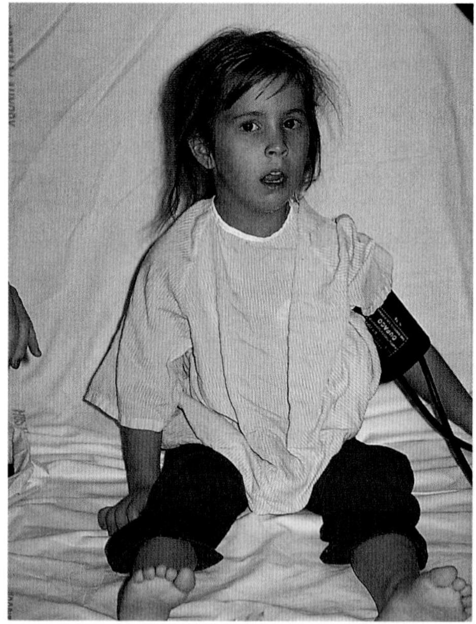

Figure 38-4 Acute epiglottitis at presentation.

The onset of epiglottitis is usually sudden. Typically, the child goes to bed without any symptoms but then wakes up complaining of a sore throat and pain on swallowing. The child may have fever, a muffled voice (from oedema of the mucosal covering of the vocal cords), and drooling from the pooled saliva that occurs because of difficult and painful swallowing (an ominous sign of impending airway obstruction). Differentiating epiglottitis from croup in the prehospital setting may be difficult. Table 38-3 lists the different characteristics of these illnesses.

On arrival, the paramedics usually find a child with epiglottitis sitting upright (Figure 38-4). Often the child is leaning forward with the head hyperextended (tripod position) to aid breathing. The tongue may be protruding, or the child may have inspiratory stridor. These children do not usually cry or struggle, because all of their attention and energy is being used to maximize air exchange. The child may be gasping or gulping for air and a characteristic inspiratory stridor may be present. Other classic signs of respiratory distress are usually present. The definitive care for epiglottitis is in-hospital intubation and parenteral antibiotic therapy.

Critical Thinking

What other childhood respiratory problems (traumatic and non-traumatic) can manifest with stridor?

Children with acute epiglottitis are in danger of full airway obstruction and respiratory arrest. Occlusion of the airway can occur suddenly and may be caused by minor irritation of the throat, stress, and anxiety. For these reasons, gentle handling of a child suspected of having epiglottitis is essential. The following guidelines should be observed:

- Do not try to lay the child down or to change the position of comfort.
- Do not try to visualize the airway if the child is still ventilating adequately.

- Alert the receiving hospital of the suspicion of epiglottitis. That way, the personnel and resources can be made available.
- Administer 100% humidified oxygen by mask (where available) unless it provokes agitation.
- Do not attempt vascular access.
- Have the correct-sized emergency airway equipment selected and ready.
- Transport the child to the hospital in the position of comfort.

If respiratory arrest occurs before arrival at the emergency department, intubation or cricothyroidotomy may be necessary. The paramedic should hyperventilate and pre-oxygenate the child's lungs with a bag–valve device before intubation and then endeavour to obtain intravenous (IV) access if time allows.

The paramedic should be prepared for a difficult intubation because the vocal cords are likely to be hidden by swollen tissues. An uncuffed endotracheal tube one to two sizes smaller than normal should be used. The paramedic should locate the opening to the larynx by looking for mucus bubbles in the cleft between the oedematous aryepiglottic folds and the swollen epiglottis – chest compressions during glottic visualization may produce a bubble at the tracheal opening. If intubation cannot be achieved and the child cannot be ventilated adequately by a bag–valve device, the paramedic may need to perform needle cricothyroidotomy. Often a child can be ventilated through the occlusive crisis of epiglottitis by bag–valve–mask ventilation using a tight facial seal. This may call for two persons – one to maintain the seal and the other to ventilate.

Asthma

Asthma (described in Chapter 14) is characterized by inflammation, bronchoconstriction and mucus production that obstruct the lower airways. Asthma results from autonomic dysfunction or exposure to sensitizing agents. The hallmarks of an acute exacerbation are anxiety, dyspnoea, tachypnoea, and audible expiratory wheezes with a prolonged expiratory phase. (A silent chest indicates impending respiratory failure.) Asthma is common among children over 2 years of age and affects 1.1 million children in the UK under 10 years of age.[7] An acute exacerbation may be triggered by infection, changes in temperature, physical exercise and emotional response.

Critical Thinking

What other signs or symptoms would lead you to believe that a child with asthma is decompensating?

The goals of prehospital management include ventilatory assistance (as needed), administration of humidified oxygen (where available), reversal of the bronchospasm, and rapid transport for evaluation and treatment. Severe asthma may be life threatening as the patient can progress rapidly to respiratory failure. The paramedic should be ready to begin aggressive airway management along with ventilatory and circulatory support. Depending on local protocol and prior medication use, drug therapy may include nebulizer therapy (salbutamol and ipratropium bromide) and hydrocortisone. The Joint Royal Colleges Ambulance Liaison Committee (JRCALC) suggests that the use of subcutaneous or intramuscular adrenaline (epinephrine) is not recommended in children.[1]

If the patient requires tracheal intubation, maintain low tidal volumes (5–8 mL/kg) to reduce the potential for barotrauma.

Table 38-4 Differentiation of bronchiolitis and asthma

Clinical features	Bronchiolitis	Asthma
Occurrence	Usually < 2 years	Any age
Season	Winter, spring	Any time
Family history of asthma	Usually absent	Usually present
Cause	Virus	Allergy, infection, exercise
Response to drugs	Some reversal of bronchospasm with β-agonists	Reversal of bronchospasm

Bronchiolitis

Bronchiolitis is a viral disease often caused by respiratory syncytial virus infection of the lower airway. It usually affects children under 2 years of age and often occurs in the winter months. Generally, bronchiolitis is associated with an upper respiratory infection and, like asthma, manifests with tachypnoea and wheezing. Bronchiolitis is sometimes unresponsive to therapy aimed at relieving bronchospasm. Table 38-4 lists key features that may aid in differential diagnosis.

Bronchiolitis is not generally serious and recovery is uneventful; however, it may sometimes become life threatening. Infants are at greater risk of developing respiratory failure from this condition because of the small diameter of the bronchioles. The prehospital care is aimed at providing ventilatory support with humidified oxygen and transporting the patient for evaluation by a physician.

Pneumonia

Pneumonia (described in Chapter 14) is an acute bacterial or viral infection of the lower airway and lungs involving the alveolar walls or the alveoli. Children with pneumonia may have a history of recent airway infection and may also have respiratory distress or failure (depending on the severity) and any of the following:

- decreased breath sounds
- fever
- pain in the chest
- rales
- rhonchi (localized or diffuse)
- tachypnoea.

Most children with pneumonia have only mild signs and symptoms and require no immediate treatment or airway support. However, when respiratory distress is present, stabilization of the airway is the highest priority. In severe cases, bronchodilators may be indicated. Assisted ventilations via a bag–valve device or intubation of the trachea also may be required.

Shock

As described in Chapter 28, shock is an abnormal condition characterized by inadequate delivery of oxygen to meet the metabolic demands of tissues. The condition may occur with increased, normal or decreased blood pressure. Shock is categorized as compensated (shock without hypotension) or decompensated (shock with hypotension) (Box 38-2).

Box 38-2

Signs and symptoms of compensated and decompensated shock

Compensated (reversible)

Cool, pale extremities
Decreased urinary output
Delayed capillary refill
Irritability or anxiety
Normal systolic blood pressure
Tachycardia
Tachypnoea
Weak peripheral pulses/full central pulses

Decompensated (often irreversible)

Absent peripheral pulses/weak central pulses
Cool, pale, dusky, mottled extremities
Hypotension
Lethargy or coma
Marked tachycardia or bradycardia
Marked tachypnoea or bradypnoea
Significantly decreased urinary output
Significantly delayed capillary refill

The paramedic must take into account a number of special considerations when caring for a child in shock. These include circulating blood volume, body surface area and hypothermia, cardiac reserve, respiratory fatigue, and vital signs and assessment.

Circulating blood volume

In children, blood volume accounts for 7–8% of total body weight, or 70–80 mL/kg of body weight. Although the percentage of circulating blood volume in a child is greater than that in an adult, a child's actual blood volume is considerably lower than an adult's. Therefore, a relatively small loss of blood may be devastating. For example, a blood loss of 100 mL in an adult is a 2% loss; a 100 mL loss in an infant is a 15–20% loss, resulting in shock.

A child with a blood or fluid deficit will maintain stable haemodynamics until all compensatory mechanisms fail (i.e. the blood pressure may be normal or only slightly decreased) (Table 38-5). At that point, shock progresses rapidly, with serious deterioration. These efficient compensatory mechanisms can mask a potentially life-threatening condition, thus the paramedic must hold a high degree of suspicion. The paramedic must actively search for shock as a cause of the patient's complaint or clinical presentation. Early recognition, stabilization (airway control, fluid replacement), and rapid transport to a proper facility are critical when caring for children in shock.

Critical Thinking

How comfortable are you with starting an intravenous infusion in an infant or young child?

Body surface area and hypothermia

Young children have a large body surface area in proportion to body weight. Their compensatory mechanisms (e.g. shivering) also are not well developed. Children in shock can quickly develop hypothermia from exposure and concurrent

Table 38-5 Classification of haemorrhagic shock in paediatric trauma patients based on systemic signs

System	Very mild haemorrhage (<15% blood volume loss)	Mild haemorrhage (15–25% blood volume loss)	Moderate haemorrhage (26–39% blood volume loss)	Severe haemorrhage (≥40% blood volume loss)
Cardiovascular	Normal or mildly increased heart rate	Tachycardia	Significant tachycardia	Severe tachycardia
	Normal pulse rate	Peripheral pulses may be diminished	Thready peripheral pulses	Thready central pulses
	Normal blood pressure	Normal blood pressure	Hypotension	Significant hypotension
	Normal pH	Normal pH	Metabolic acidosis	Significant acidosis
Respiratory	Normal rate	Tachypnoea	Moderate tachypnoea	Severe tachypnoea
Central nervous system	Slight anxiousness	Irritability, confusion	Irritability or lethargy	Lethargy
		Combative affect	Diminished pain response	Coma
Skin	Warm, pink colour	Cool extremities, mottling or pallor	Cool extremities, mottling	Cold extremities, pallor or cyanosis
	Brisk capillary refill	Delayed capillary refill	Prolonged capillary refill	Prolonged capillary refill
Kidneys	Normal urine output	Oliguria, increased specific gravity	Oliguria, increased blood urea nitrogen level	Anuria

metabolic acidosis, increased vascular resistance, respiratory depression, and myocardial dysfunction. Hypothermia makes resuscitation and drug therapy less effective. The paramedic should maintain the patient's body temperature by using blankets, covering the child's head with towels, and using warming devices for IV fluids.

Cardiac reserve

Infants and children already have high metabolic needs so they have less cardiac reserve than adults for stressful situations such as shock. An important step is to reduce the energy and oxygen requirements of a child in shock as much as possible. This can be done by providing ventilatory support, reducing anxiety and maintaining moderate ambient temperatures.

Respiratory fatigue

Respiratory muscle fatigue may lead to hypoventilation, hypoxaemia, and respiratory failure or arrest. Like other compensatory mechanisms of the child, respiratory compensation generally is at a maximum until it is depleted. At that time, deterioration can be sudden. For this reason, airway control and supplemental oxygen are essential in all children who are seriously ill or injured.

Vital signs and assessment

The paramedic must consider many factors when evaluating a child's vital signs. For example, blood pressure and pulse rate vary greatly with age, body temperature, and degree of agitation. The paramedic should measure vital signs as baseline assessments although they may be of limited value in assessing the circulation of a child in shock. The most effective assessment is constant monitoring of the child's mental and physical status and the response to therapy. The following nine evaluation components should be noted when assessing a child in shock:

1. Level of consciousness
   - Ability to make eye contact
   - Ability to recognize family members
   - Agitation
   - Anxiety
2. Skin
   - Capillary refill (in children under 6 years of age)
   - Colour
   - Moisture
   - Temperature
   - Turgor
3. Mucous membranes
   - Colour
   - Moisture
4. Nail beds
   - Capillary refill (in children under 6 years of age)
   - Colour
5. Peripheral circulation
   - Collapse
   - Distension
6. Cardiac
   - Electrocardiogram findings
   - Location of pulses
   - Quality of pulses
   - Rate
   - Rhythm
7. Respiration
   - Depth
   - Rate
8. Blood pressure (in children over 3 years of age and only if time permits)
9. Body temperature.

Note

Sustained tachycardia in the absence of obvious causes such as fever, pain and agitation may be an early sign of cardiovascular compromise. Bradycardia, however, may be a preterminal cardiac rhythm indicating advanced shock and often is associated with hypotension.[5]

Hypovolaemia

Common causes of hypovolaemia in children include dehydration resulting from vomiting and diarrhoea, and blood loss resulting from trauma or internal bleeding. Children are also at risk of intravascular volume depletion as a result of burns (see Chapter 30).

Dehydration

Profound fluid and electrolyte imbalances can occur in children as a result of diarrhoea, vomiting, poor fluid intake, fever or burns. Dehydration compromises cardiac output and systemic perfusion and occurs if the child loses the fluid equivalent of 5% or more of total body weight. For the adolescent, losses of 5–7% of total body weight can compromise perfusion (Figure 38-5). If allowed to progress, dehydration can result in renal failure, shock and death. The severity of the dehydration and fluid loss can be estimated from a history of the child's weight loss and the physical examination (Figure 38-6). Table 38-6 provides signs and symptoms related to degrees of dehydration.

Airway and ventilatory support (if needed) are the initial steps in treatment for the dehydrated child. Next, treatment is directed at replacing and maintaining blood volume and perfusion. Intravenous therapy should be initiated (per guidelines) with isotonic crystalloids such as 0.9% saline. Discussion surrounding the volume of fluids to be administered follows in the next section.

Critical Thinking

What are some ways to determine the child's weight for fluid and drug dosing?

Blood loss

As stated before, even a small amount of blood loss can be serious for the paediatric patient. After the paramedic secures the patient's airway, provides high-concentration oxygen, and achieves control of external haemorrhage (if present), consideration may need to be given to supporting the child's circulatory status with IV therapy (per guidelines).

As with other causes of hypovolaemia, volume replacement may be needed. Isotonic crystalloid solutions such as normal saline or sodium lactate solution should be used.

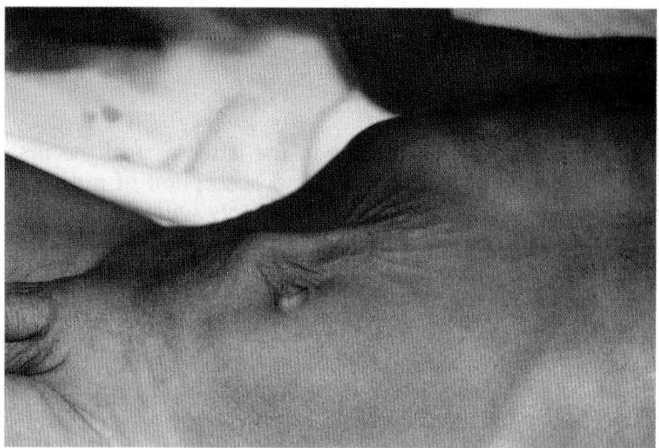

Figure 38-5 Severe dehydration.

Previously, a fluid bolus of 20 mL/kg has been recommended, but this is controversial given the move towards controlled hypotension in the adult patient. JRCALC currently recommends administration of boluses of 5 mL/kg of fluid until a response is observed,[1] but it is possible that further changes will occur as more evidence becomes available. The paramedic must keep up to date with current fluid management strategies. The child may show little response to the first bolus (for example, a slight improvement in colour and capillary refill and a decreased heart rate may be evident) (Figure 38-7). If this is the case or if the patient does not respond to the initial infusion, the paramedic should give a second bolus of 5 mL/kg.

Note

Establishing an intravenous line in a child through a peripheral vein (described in Chapter 12) can be difficult even in the most controlled settings. In some situations it may be advisable either to establish an intraosseous infusion for the child in shock or to rapidly transport to a proper facility without establishing venous access.

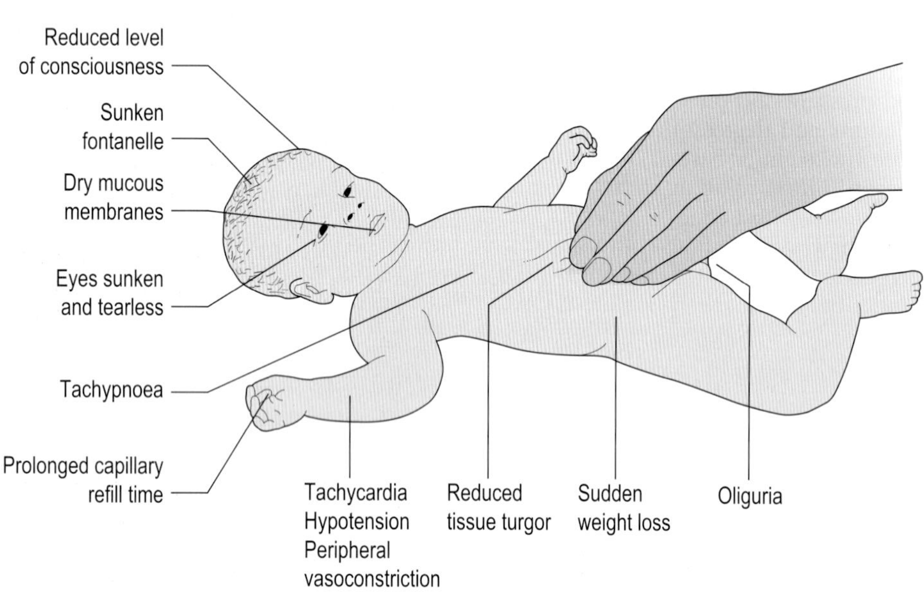

Figure 38-6 Clinical features of dehydration in an infant.

Table 38-6 Assessment of degree of dehydration

Clinical parameters	Mild	Moderate	Severe
Body weight loss (infant)	5% (50 mL/kg)	10% (100 mL/kg)	15% (150 mL/kg)
Skin turgor	Slightly decreased	Moderately decreased	Greatly decreased
Fontanelle (infant)	Possibly flat or depressed	Depressed	Significantly depressed
Mucous membranes	Dry	Very dry	Parched
Skin perfusion	Warm with normal color	Cool (extremities) Pale	Cold (extremities) Mottled or grey
Heart rate	Mildly tachycardic	Moderately tachycardic	Extremely tachycardic
Peripheral pulses	Normal	Diminished	Absent
Blood pressure	Normal	Normal	Reduced
Sensorium	Normal or irritable	Irritable or lethargic	Unresponsive

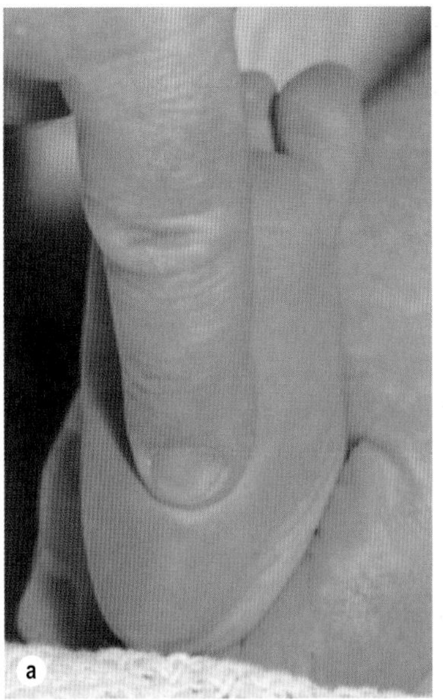

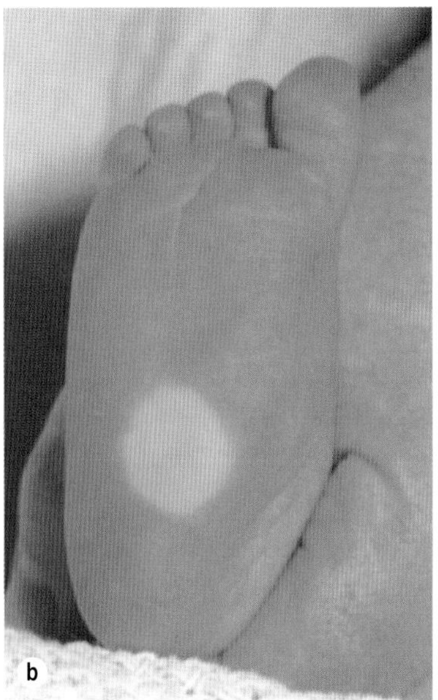

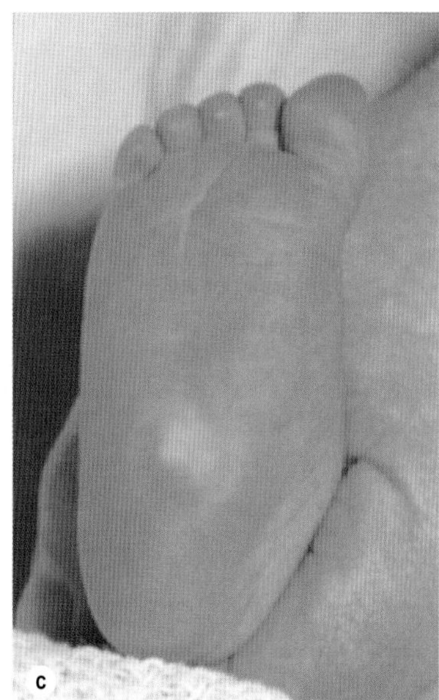

Figure 38-7 Capillary refill in a child in shock.

Distributive shock

As described in Chapter 28, distributive shock is used to refer to septic shock, neurogenic shock, and anaphylactic shock. This type of shock results in peripheral pooling because of loss of vasomotor tone. The vasodilatation that occurs causes the blood pressure to fall and allows plasma to leak from the vascular space. This type of shock is fairly uncommon in children.

Septic shock is usually caused by a systemic bacterial infection and is associated with illnesses such as meningitis and pneumonia. Toxins released by the pathogen affect arterioles, capillaries and venules, altering microcirculatory pressure and capillary permeability. These children usually appear very ill and may have signs and symptoms that include those of decompensated shock. Characteristic findings in septic shock include skin that is warm in the early stages, and skin that is cool in the late stages of the illness.

Neurogenic shock results from sudden peripheral vasodilatation caused by a traumatic injury. Most often this injury is to the spinal cord. The loss of sympathetic impulses and resultant vasodilatation increase the size of the vascular compartment such that the normal intravascular volume is not enough to fill the vascular compartment and to perfuse tissues. Characteristic findings in neurogenic shock include warm skin, bradycardia and impaired neurological function.

Anaphylactic shock occurs when a person is exposed to a substance that produces a severe allergic reaction (see Chapter 18). Common causes of allergic reactions include antibiotic agents, venoms and insect stings. The bodily response to the antigen causes a release of histamine, which results in peripheral vasodilatation and the leak of intravascular fluid into the interstitial space; this results in a decrease in intravascular volume. Characteristic findings in anaphylactic shock include vomiting and diarrhoea, hives, allergic rash, erythema, airway swelling and wheezing (from bronchoconstriction), and hypotension.

Emergency care for patients with distributive shock is directed at maintaining the patient's vital functions through airway, ventilatory and circulatory support, and rapid transport to an appropriate medical facility. Drugs may be indicated for distributive shock, including adrenaline (epinephrine), chlorphenamine, hydrocortisone, salbutamol, and possibly fluids for anaphylactic shock; the judicious use of fluids and consideration of atropine sulphate for neurogenic shock; and the use of benzylpenicillin for septic shock caused by meningococcal bacteria.[1] It is essential that paramedics use the 'age-per-page' guidelines in JRCALC to establish the correct dosage of drugs and fluids; guesswork is not acceptable.

Rhythm disturbances

As discussed in Chapter 37, most children have healthy hearts. When rhythm disturbances occur, they are usually the result of hypoxia, acidosis, hypotension or structural heart disease.[5] The most common dysrhythmias in paediatric patients are sinus tachycardia, supraventricular tachycardia, bradycardia and asystole. Ventricular tachycardia and ventricular fibrillation are uncommon in children but may occur in those suffering from tricyclic antidepressant overdose, hypothermia and with cardiac disease.[8] The recommended management for these dysrhythmias is outlined in Figures 38-8 and 38-9. Drug treatments and specific guidelines for use of airway equipment during paediatric life support can be found in the JRCALC guidelines.[1]

Dysrhythmias and basic and advanced life support procedures (including cardiopulmonary resuscitation) are addressed in Chapter 15. The reader should refer to that chapter for review. The following discussions outline the unique aspects of abnormal rhythms in children.[9]

Bradydysrhythmias

Clinically significant bradycardia is defined as a heart rate less than 60 beats/min (or a rapidly dropping heart rate)

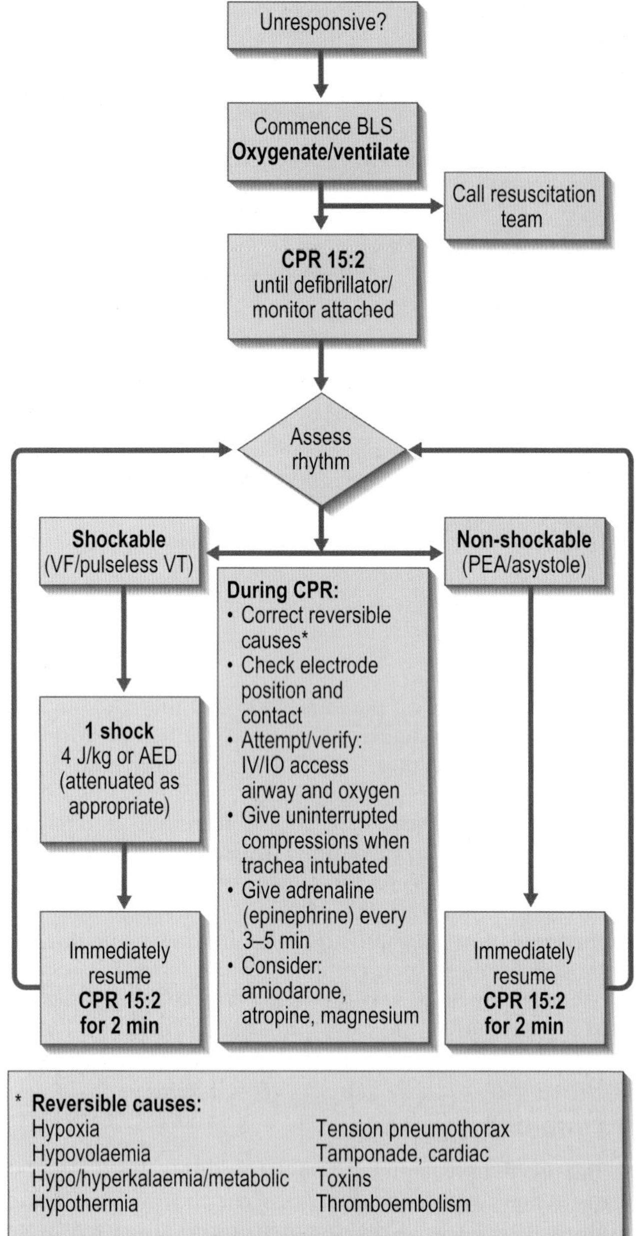

Figure 38-8 Paediatric advanced life support.

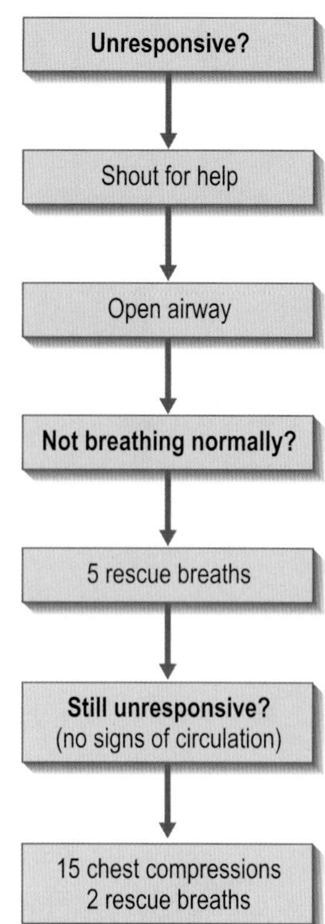

Figure 38-9 Paediatric advanced life support pulseless arrest algorithm. From The Resuscitation Council (UK).

associated with poor systemic perfusion. This bradycardia occurs despite adequate oxygenation and ventilation and is almost always a preterminal sign. Bradydysrhythmias may be caused by hypoxaemia, acidosis, hypotension, hypoglycaemia, central nervous system injury, or excessive vagal stimulation (e.g. from endotracheal intubation or pharyngeal suctioning). In infants and children, sinus bradycardia, sinus node arrest with slow junctional or idioventricular rhythm, and atrioventricular block are the most common preterminal rhythms. The paramedic should consider drug-induced causes (e.g. digitalis toxicity) and myocarditis with bradycardia caused by heart block. Infants and children with a history of heart surgery may have injury at the atrioventricular node or conduction system. This injury would produce sick sinus syndrome or heart block. All symptomatic bradycardias require treatment. Important electrocardiogram findings include the following:

- Heart rate is less than 60 beats/min.
- P waves may or may not be visible.
- QRS complex duration may be normal or prolonged.
- The P wave and QRS complex often are unrelated.

Treatment

The initial management of bradycardia should ensure that airway, breathing and circulation are adequate and the patient is receiving supplemental oxygen. If drug therapy is required, adrenaline (epinephrine) is the drug of choice. Atropine is only indicated for persistent bradycardia caused by heart block, increased vagal tone or organophosphate poisoning (all of which are uncommon in paediatric patients). In cases where bradycardia is caused by problems with the sinus node, external cardiac pacing may be life saving. External cardiac pacing is uncomfortable and its use in children is reserved for profound symptomatic bradycardia that does not respond to advanced life support and basic life support treatments. External cardiac pacing is not currently routinely available to UK paramedics.

Pulseless electrical activity

Pulseless electrical activity often precedes asystole. It is usually caused by prolonged periods of hypoxia, ischaemia, or hypercarbia. Reversible causes of pulseless electrical activity include the four Hs (hypovolaemia, hypoxaemia, hypothermia and hyperkalaemia) and the four Ts (tension pneumothorax, pericardial tamponade, toxins and thromboembolus) described in Chapter 15. Important electrocardiogram findings include the following:

- a slow, wide-complex rhythm
- the presence of some electrical activity (other than ventricular tachycardia/ventricular fibrillation) and the absence of a detectable pulse.

Treatment

Pulseless electrical activity is managed in the same way as asystole (Figure 38-9) with drug therapy (adrenaline [epinephrine]) and cardiopulmonary resuscitation. Defibrillation is not effective in the treatment of asystolic arrest. Reversible causes of the condition should be considered and corrected if possible. Identification and treatment of the underlying cause is the only true means of reversal of pulseless electrical activity. Early recognition and treatment of pulseless electrical activity that results in a return of a pulse before arrival in the emergency department is associated with improved chances for survival.

Supraventricular tachycardia

Supraventricular tachycardia is the most common non-arrest dysrhythmia during childhood and is the most common dysrhythmia that produces cardiovascular instability during infancy.[8] Two factors can help distinguish supraventricular tachycardia from sinus tachycardia caused by shock. They include patient history (e.g. dehydration or haemorrhage associated with shock) and heart rate. (Sinus tachycardia is usually less than 220 beats/min in infants, usually less than 180 beats/min in children, but usually greater than those rates with supraventricular tachycardia.) Important electrocardiogram findings in supraventricular tachycardia include the following:

- Heart rate is greater than 220 beats/min in infants and greater than 180 beats/min in children.
- The rhythm is usually regular because associated atrioventricular block is rare.
- P waves may not be identifiable, especially when the ventricular rate is high. If present, P waves are usually negative in leads II, III, and aV_F.
- QRS complex duration is normal in most children (<0.10 s). Supraventricular tachycardia with aberrant conduction (wide-complex supraventricular tachycardia) may be difficult to distinguish from ventricular tachycardia (but this form of ventricular tachycardia is rare in infants and children).

Treatment

Signs and symptoms during supraventricular tachycardia are affected by the child's age, duration of supraventricular tachycardia, prior ventricular function and ventricular rate. If the child is haemodynamically stable and cooperative, vagal manoeuvres such as blowing through a straw and carotid sinus massage may be successful in terminating the rhythm. Unstable supraventricular tachycardia is best managed with synchronized cardioversion or drug therapy, neither of which are routinely available to paramedics in the UK; the drug of choice is adenosine, which is not licensed for use by paramedics.

Wide-complex tachycardias with signs of compromised tissue perfusion and impaired level of consciousness require immediate care. The paramedic should treat these tachycardias as if they are ventricular tachycardia. Urgent treatment includes synchronized cardioversion (not available to UK paramedics) if pulses are present and defibrillation if pulses are absent.

Ventricular tachycardia and ventricular fibrillation

As stated before, ventricular tachycardia and ventricular fibrillation are uncommon in children. If present, the paramedic should consider causes of these dysrhythmias, which include congenital heart disease, cardiomyopathies, myocarditis, reversible causes (e.g. drug toxicity), metabolic causes (e.g. hypoglycaemia) and hypothermia. Important electrocardiogram findings include the following:

1. Ventricular tachycardia
   - Ventricular rate at least 120 beats/min and regular.
   - Wide QRS complex.
   - P waves that are often not identifiable.
2. Ventricular fibrillation
   - No identifiable P wave, QRS complex, or T wave.
   - Ventricular fibrillation waves that may be coarse or fine.

Note

A standard automated external defibrillate (AED) can be used in children over 8 years; purpose-made paediatric pads or programmes that attenuate the energy output of an AED are recommended for children between 1 and 8 years. If no such AED or manually adjustable machine is available, an unmodified adult AED can be used in children older than 1 year.[8] Currently, not enough evidence exists to support recommendation for or against the use of AEDs in children less than 1 year of age. For a lone rescuer responding to a child with no signs of circulation, 1 minute of cardiopulmonary resuscitation is still advised before any other action, such as activating emergency medical services or using an AED.

(Information from Samson RA et al 2003 Use of automated external defibrillators for children: an update – an advisory statement from the paediatric advanced life support task force, International Liaison Committee on Resuscitation. Circulation 107[25]:3250–3255.)

Treatment

Ventricular tachycardia with a pulse Haemodynamically stable ventricular tachycardia should be managed cautiously, with initial efforts aimed at determining the origin of the tachycardia. The paramedic should endeavour to obtain a full history, including relevant past medical history. Drug therapy is usually delayed until arrival in the emergency department,

Box 38-3

Terminating resuscitative efforts

Most children who have a cardiac arrest will not survive – even with a transient return of spontaneous circulation. Prolonged resuscitation is indicated, however, in infants and children with recurring or refractory ventricular fibrillation or ventricular tachycardia. Prolonged resuscitation is also recommended if the arrest resulted from toxic drug exposure, a primary hypothermic insult, or immersion.[1] In the absence of these conditions, paramedics may discontinue efforts if there is no spontaneous circulation despite 20 min of adequate and effective advanced life support interventions.[1] Family members are sometimes present during the resuscitation efforts. If this is the case, one person should be assigned to the family to answer questions and provide comfort measures.

where administration of amiodarone or procainamide may be considered. Ventricular tachycardia that produces a palpable pulse and signs of shock (low cardiac output, poor perfusion) requires immediate synchronised cardioversion.

Pulseless ventricular tachycardia and ventricular fibrillation Pulseless ventricular tachycardia and ventricular fibrillation are managed with immediate defibrillation, cardiopulmonary resuscitation, intubation with ventilatory support, and drug therapy. Infant paddles (4.5 cm) should generally be used during defibrillation for infants up to about 1 year of age or 10 kg. Adult paddles[8] (8–13 cm) should generally be used for patients older than 1 year of age or more than 10 kg (Box 38-3).

Critical Thinking

Are you comfortable using the paediatric paddles you will be using on the ambulance?

Post-resuscitation stabilization

The post-resuscitation phase begins after initial stabilization of the patient with shock or respiratory failure. It also includes the time after return of spontaneous circulation in a patient who was in cardiac arrest. The goals of post-resuscitation stabilization are as follows:[5]

- preserve brain function
- avoid secondary organ injury
- seek and correct causes of illness
- manage pain with analgesics (e.g. morphine)
- enable the patient to arrive at an appropriate care facility in the best possible physiological state.

Post-resuscitation stabilization includes stabilizing the airway and supporting oxygenation, ventilation, and perfusion; performing a thorough secondary assessment; and obtaining a medical history. This is best done en route to hospital to minimize on-scene delays. The paramedic should be sure to communicate to the family what has been done and how the patient is responding to care. The paramedic should also pre-alert the receiving hospital.

Seizure

A seizure (described in Chapters 16 and 37) is an episode of sudden abnormal electrical activity in the brain. It results in abnormalities in motor, sensory, or autonomic function, usually associated with abnormal behaviour, changes in level of consciousness, or both. Common causes of seizure in adults and children include non-compliance with a drug regimen for the treatment of epilepsy, head trauma, intracranial infection, brain tumour, metabolic disturbance, or poisoning. The most common cause of new onset of seizure in children is fever.

Febrile seizures

A febrile seizure is a seizure associated with fever but without evidence of intracranial infection or other definable cause; such seizures usually occur between the ages of 6 months and 5 years. About 2–5% of children under 7 years of age experience a febrile seizure. About 30% of those who have a seizure experience a recurrence. More than half of febrile seizures occur in children age 9–20 months, and in 60% of cases, a family history of febrile seizures is a factor.[10]

Febrile seizures are usually associated with an underlying viral infection (most often of the upper respiratory tract), gastroenteritis, otitis media or another febrile illness. The seizures usually occur in vulnerable patients during a rapid rise in body temperature. However, the intensity of the seizure is not related to the severity of the fever.

Febrile seizures may manifest with generalized tonic–clonic activity or they may have a more subtle presentation. As a rule, classic febrile seizures are of short duration (usually less than 5 min) and have an uncomplicated and short post-ictal period. Seizures that last longer than 20 min call for extensive investigation and should never be considered benign. Regardless of the suspected cause, all children who have suffered a seizure should be transported for evaluation by a physician per protocol.

Assessment and management

In most cases, the seizure has stopped before emergency medical services arrive, and in many instances, the child is in a postictal state. As in any emergency, the first priorities are airway management and ventilatory and circulatory support. This includes airway positioning, suctioning of the airway, and administration of oxygen. Repeated assessment of the adequacy of ventilation is necessary, with special emphasis placed on respiratory rate and depth. If the airway cannot be maintained with manual manoeuvres, airway adjuncts should be used.

After initial stabilization of the patient's condition, the paramedic should assess vital signs and obtain a history. Important elements of the history include the following:

- previous seizures
- number of seizures in this episode
- description of seizure activity
- presence of vomiting during the seizure (aspiration risk)
- condition of the child when first found
- recent illness
- potential for toxic ingestion
- potential head injury (as primary cause or secondary complication)

- significant medical problems
- recent headache or stiff neck (which may suggest meningitis)
- medication use and compliance with anticonvulsant medication.

During transport to the emergency department, the paramedic should monitor the child continuously and should be alert for recurrent seizures. The use of antipyretics is controversial but paracetamol may be indicated in the child who has ceased convulsing and has recovered consciousness (refer to JRCALC for dosage); this will reduce fever whilst en route to hospital. The paramedic should not apply ice or submerge the patient in cool bath in an effort to reduce fever.

Status epilepticus

Status epilepticus is continuous seizure activity that lasts 30 min or longer. It may be defined as a recurrent seizure without an intervening period of consciousness and is a true emergency. Status epilepticus can lead to hypotension and cardiovascular, respiratory and renal failure, in addition to permanent brain damage. Children in status epilepticus should be managed with the following initial interventions:

1. Provide adequate airway, ventilatory and circulatory support. Intubation for airway protection or mechanical ventilation is seldom needed and should be withheld unless the child fails to respond to the initial management.
2. Per protocol, obtain vascular access through an IV or intraosseous route. Measure the blood glucose level to screen for hypoglycaemia. If the value is less than 4 mmol/L, administer glucose 10%, (hypoglycaemia can be treated with an intramuscular injection of glucagon if IV or intraosseous access cannot be established, although this is not popular with paediatricians as it can cause vomiting in children). If seizures do not stop, administer diazepam either via the vascular access route or via the rectal route. The paramedic should ensure that they have checked dosages against guidelines.
3. Attach a cardiac monitor. Observe for rhythm or conduction abnormalities that may suggest hypoxia.

Diazepam

Diazepam breaks active seizures in 75–90% of cases.[11] The drug has a short duration of action (15 min) so may require repeat administration; the paramedic is not authorised to repeat paediatric doses, so should transport the patient to hospital rapidly in case further doses are required. The paramedic should also be prepared for sudden respiratory depression or hypotension when using this drug.

Hypoglycaemia

As described in Chapter 17, hypoglycaemia is an abnormally low concentration of glucose in the blood. In children, hypoglycaemia is usually the result of excessive response to glucose absorption, illness, physical exertion or decreased dietary intake. In diabetic children, hypoglycaemia is usually caused by too large a dose of insulin, a delayed or missed meal, or unusual or vigorous physical activity. The condition most commonly occurs in the prehospital setting in infants and children with type 1 diabetes, a disease that affects about 2 in 1000 young people below the age of 18.[12]

The signs and symptoms of hypoglycaemia can be classified as mild, moderate or severe. Mild symptoms include hunger, weakness, tachypnoea and tachycardia; moderate symptoms include sweating, tremors, irritability, vomiting, mood disorders, blurred vision, stomachache, headache and dizziness; and severe symptoms include decreased level of consciousness and seizure activity. This is an emergency that calls for prompt treatment with dextrose to prevent brain damage.

Prehospital care is directed initially at ensuring adequate airway, ventilatory and circulatory support. A blood glucose measurement should be obtained in any child with an altered level of consciousness that has no explainable cause. Conscious children who are mildly hypoglycaemic should receive an oral glucose solution or tablets. Unconscious children or those with moderate or severe hypoglycaemia require IV/intraosseous glucose or intramuscular glucagon administration. This should be followed by a repeat blood glucose measurement in 10–15 min. All children with signs and symptoms of hypoglycaemia should be transported for physician evaluation.

Hyperglycaemia

Hyperglycaemia is an abnormally high concentration of glucose in the blood that results from an absence or resistance to insulin. The low insulin level prevents glucose from entering the cells, which causes glucose to build up in the blood. If not treated, hyperglycaemia can lead to dehydration, diabetic ketoacidosis and coma. In children with type 1 diabetes, the condition is often the result of too small an insulin dose in relation to food intake, failure to take insulin, illness, or a malfunctioning insulin-delivery system (e.g. insulin pump).

The signs and symptoms of hyperglycaemia are classified as early or late. Early signs and symptoms include increased thirst (polydipsia), increased hunger (polyphagia), and increased urination (polyuria). (Weight loss is also considered an early sign of the illness.) Late signs and symptoms associated with dehydration and early ketoacidosis include weakness, abdominal pain, generalized aches, loss of appetite, nausea, vomiting, signs of dehydration (with the exception of urinary output), fruity breath odour, tachypnoea, hyperventilation and tachycardia. If untreated, Kussmaul respirations and coma may occur.

Children suspected of being hyperglycaemic should receive adequate airway, ventilatory and circulatory support, followed by glucose testing. These patients may require IV fluid therapy if signs of dehydration are present (Figure 38-10). The administration of insulin is an in-hospital procedure.

Critical Thinking

Why do you think type 1 diabetes may go undetected until a child is seriously ill?

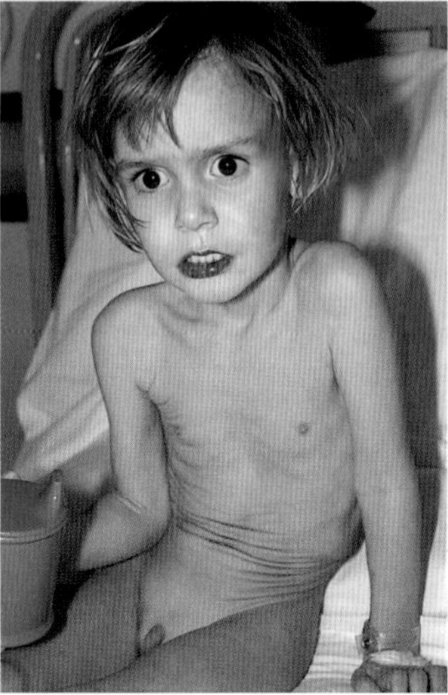

Figure 38-10 Severe dehydration and weight loss from diabetic ketoacidosis.

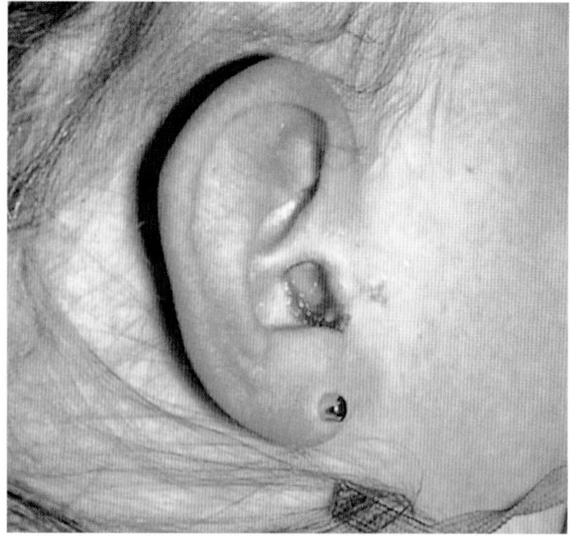

Figure 38-11 Otitis media.

Box 38-4

Signs and symptoms of infection in paediatric patients

Bulging fontanelle (infants)
Chills
Cool or clammy skin
Cough
Dehydration
Fever
Hypoperfusion
Hypothermia (neonates)
Irritability
Lethargy
Malaise
Nasal congestion
Poor feeding
Respiratory distress
Seizure
Severe headache
Sore throat
Stiff neck
Tachycardia
Tachypnoea
Vomiting or diarrhoea (or both)

Infection

Children with infection may have a variety of signs and symptoms. The symptoms depend on the source and extent of infection and the length of time since the patient was exposed (Box 38-4). Often the parent or caregiver provides a history of recent illness. (This may include, for example, fever, upper respiratory tract infection or otitis media [Figure 38-11].) When caring for any patient who may have an infectious disease, the paramedic must strictly adhere to infection control principles because of the unknown cause of the infection.

Most children with infection need only supportive care whilst being transported. However, in very sick children, support of the airway, ventilation and circulation may be needed. If signs of decompensated shock are present, IV therapy may be needed (per guidelines). Seizure activity may require the use of anticonvulsant agents. When possible, a child in stable condition should be transported in the child's position of comfort and in the company of the parent or caregiver.

Poisoning and toxic exposure

As discussed in Chapter 21, most poisoning in the UK involves children and is a major cause of preventable death in children under 5 years of age.

Common sources of poisoning (unintentional and intentional) include the following:[13]

- paracetamol
- alcohol
- anticholinergics
- aspirin
- barbiturates
- cold medicines
- corrosives
- digitalis, beta-blocker agents
- hydrocarbons
- narcotics
- organic solvents (inhaled)
- organophosphates
- sedatives
- vitamins (especially iron).

The signs and symptoms of poisoning vary depending upon the toxic substance and the length of time since the child was exposed. These signs and symptoms may include cardiac and respiratory depression, central nervous system stimulation or depression, gastrointestinal irritation, and behavioural changes. Emergency care should be directed first at ensuring adequate airway, ventilatory, and circulatory support. The paramedic should contact ambulance control and the National Poison Information Service (NPIS) for specific treatments. All pills, substances and containers associated with the poisoning should be transported with the child to the receiving hospital.

Critical Thinking

For what critical signs or symptoms of poisoning should you be alert?

Paediatric trauma

Blunt and penetrating trauma are major causes of injury and death in children.[9] These and other significant injuries often result from falls, motor vehicle crashes, pedestrian–vehicle collisions, drowning/submersion, penetrating injuries, burns, and abuse. The following common injuries highlight the value of injury prevention programmes (see Chapter 3):

- *Falls*: Falls are the single most common cause of injuries in children. Fortunately, serious injury or death from truly unintentional falls is uncommon; that is, unless the fall is from a significant height.

Critical Thinking

Why are children at risk for injuries related to falls?

- *Motor vehicle crashes*: Motor vehicle crashes are the leading cause of permanent brain injury, serious injury and death in children.
- *Pedestrian–vehicle collisions*: Pedestrian–vehicle collisions are an often lethal form of trauma in children. The initial injury is caused by impact with the vehicle (the impact usually occurs to the extremity or trunk). The child is often thrown from the force of the first impact, which causes additional injury (e.g. head and spine) upon a second impact with other objects. These objects may include the ground, another vehicle or nearby objects (see Chapter 26).
- *Drowning/submersion*: Drowning/submersion incidents are the third leading cause of death in children from birth to 4 years of age. The risk of drowning in the UK is small (0.8 per 100 000 population)[14] but the potential is high, especially given the recent upsurge in flash floods.
- *Penetrating injuries*: Penetrating injuries are a significant cause of trauma in children and occur especially during adolescence. Penetrating injuries that are intentional (e.g. from violent crime) are more common in inner cities; however, unintentional penetrating injuries in rural areas also occur. The risk of death from these injuries increases with the age of the patient. As with penetrating injuries to adults, the appearance of the external wounds cannot be used to determine the extent of internal injury in children.
- *Burns*: Burns are the leading cause of unintentional death in the home for children under 14 years of age. Survival from burn trauma is determined by the size and depth of the burn, the presence of inhalation injury, and the nature of other injuries that may have occurred during the event (see Chapter 30).

Critical Thinking

What types of situations cause burn injuries to children in the home?

- *Child abuse*: Injuries to children may result from physical abuse, sexual abuse, emotional abuse and child neglect. Physical abuse is often associated with lower socioeconomic status, domestic disturbances, younger-aged parents, substance abuse and community violence; however, physical abuse of children occurs in all levels of society. When caring for a child who may have been abused, thorough documentation of pertinent findings, treatment, and interventions are critical for legal purposes. (Physical abuse is described later in this chapter.)

Special considerations for specific injuries

Special considerations for managing paediatric injury are addressed in the chapters of Part Six. The following is a review of some of the more important elements in assessment and management for children with head and neck injury, traumatic brain injury, chest injury, abdominal injury, extremity injury, and burns.

Head and neck injury

1. Larger relative mass of the head and lack of neck muscle strength provide increased momentum in acceleration–deceleration injuries.
2. Fulcrum of cervical mobility in the younger child is at the C2 to C3 level (60–70% of fractures in children occur in C1 or C2).
3. Head injury is the most common cause of death in paediatric trauma victims.
4. Diffuse head injuries are common in children; focal injuries are rare.
5. Soft tissues, skull, and brain are more compliant in children than in adults.
6. Because of open fontanelles and sutures, infants up to 12 months of age may be more tolerant to increased ICP and can have delayed signs.
7. Subdural bleeding in an infant can produce hypotension (rare).
8. Significant blood loss can occur through scalp lacerations, and such bleeding should be controlled immediately.

9. The modified Glasgow Coma Scale (GCS) should be used for assessing infants and young children.

Traumatic brain injury

1. Early recognition and aggressive management can reduce mortality and morbidity.
2. Traumatic brain injury may be classified as mild (GCS score of 13–15), moderate (GCS of 9–12), or severe (GCS of 8 or lower).
3. Signs of increased ICP include elevated blood pressure, bradycardia, irregular respirations progressing to Cheyne–Stokes respirations, and bulging fontanelle in infants.
4. Signs of herniation include asymmetrical pupils and abnormal posturing.
5. Management
   a. Administer high-concentration oxygen for mild to moderate head injury (GCS score of 9–15).
   b. Consider intubation, and ventilate at normal breathing rate with 100% oxygen for severe head injury (GCS score of 3–8).

Critical Thinking

What are some early signs of increasing intracranial pressure in a child?

Chest injury

1. Chest injuries in children under 14 years of age are usually the result of blunt trauma.
2. Because of flexibility of the chest wall, severe intrathoracic injury can be present without signs of external injury such as rib fractures.
3. Tension pneumothorax is poorly tolerated and is an immediate threat to life.
4. Flail segment is an uncommon injury in children; when noted without a significant mechanism of injury, child abuse should be suspected.
5. Many children with cardiac tamponade have no physical signs other than hypotension.

Abdominal injury

1. Musculature is minimal and poorly protects the viscera.
2. Organs most commonly injured are the liver, kidneys and spleen.
3. Onset of symptoms may be rapid or gradual.
4. Because of the small size of the abdomen, palpation should be performed in one quadrant at a time.
5. Any child who is haemodynamically unstable without an obvious source of blood loss should be considered to have an abdominal injury until it is proved otherwise.

Extremity injury

1. Extremity injury is relatively more common in children than adults.
2. Growth plate injuries are common.
3. Compartment syndrome is an emergency in children.
4. Management includes the following:
   a. Control any sites of active bleeding.
   b. Perform splinting to prevent further injury and blood loss.
   c. An appropriate pelvic splint should be used for unstable pelvic fracture, especially with hypotension.

Burns

1. Burns may be thermal, chemical, or electrical.
2. Management priorities include the following:
   a. Prompt management of the airway is required because swelling can develop rapidly.
   b. If intubation is indicated, an endotracheal tube one-half size smaller than expected may be required.
   c. Suspect musculoskeletal injuries in electrical burn patients, and perform spine immobilization.

Trauma management considerations for paediatric patients

In addition to the general patient care guidelines appropriate for all injured persons, injured children require special consideration for airway control, immobilization techniques, fluid management and pain relief. The following discussion reviews the highlights of management guidelines presented in the chapters of Part Six.

Airway control

The airway of an injured child should be maintained in an in-line or neutral position. The sniffing position is appropriate for older children and adults. Padding may need to be placed under the shoulders in some children to help to maintain a neutral airway position. Jaw-thrust positioning and suctioning can be used to keep the airway open but endotracheal intubation may need to be considered when airway and ventilation remain inadequate. Cricothyroidotomy is rarely indicated for traumatic upper airway obstruction. High-concentration oxygen should be given to all patients.

All paramedics who provide care for infants and children must be able to provide effective oxygenation and ventilation using the bag–mask technique. Endotracheal intubation may sometimes be needed when caring for injured children although this will be a rare occurrence. When tracheal intubation is required, endotracheal tube placement should be confirmed by monitoring exhaled carbon dioxide, especially in children who have a pulse.

Immobilization

Spinal immobilization devices must be the right size for infants and children. Equipment that may be used includes the following:

- child safety seat
- long spine board
- padding
- paediatric immobilization device
- rigid cervical collar
- straps, cravats

- tape
- towel/blanket roll
- vest-type/short spine board.

The patient should be placed supine and immobilized in a neutral in-line position. This is achieved most effectively by using a backboard with a recess for the head or by using padding under the back from the shoulders to the buttocks.

Fluid management

Management of the child's airway and breathing takes priority over management of circulation. Circulatory compromise is less common in children than adults. When vascular access is indicated, the paramedic should consider the following:

- Large-bore IV catheters should be inserted into large peripheral veins.
- Transport should not be delayed to obtain vascular access.
- Intraosseous access in children can be used if IV access fails.
- An initial fluid bolus of 5 mL/kg of crystalloid should be given.[1] This will help to manage volume depletion.
- Vital signs should be reassessed and the bolus (5 mL/kg) repeated if needed to a maximum of 20 mL/kg;[1] vital signs that do not improve after 20 mL/kg indicate the need for rapid surgical intervention.

Pain relief

Injuries are often painful. Relief from pain should be a priority when providing care to an injured child (Box 38-5). Drugs that may be used to manage some forms of pain and to alter the emotional response in paediatric patients include morphine and nitrous oxide.[1] Morphine can be administered intravenously, intraosseously or orally. There is no evidence that metoclopramide is effective in relieving opiate-induced nausea and there is a high risk of dystonic reactions in younger people, therefore metoclopramide should not be administered in these circumstances. The use of the intranasal route for opiate administration is becoming more common in the hospital but is not yet authorized for paramedics.

Sudden unexpected deaths in infancy (SUDI)

Sudden unexpected death in infancy (SUDI) is a term that has now replaced use of sudden infant death syndrome (SIDS) and is defined as the sudden death of a seemingly healthy infant that remains unexplained by history and an autopsy. In the UK the rate has been falling steadily since the late 1980s and now occurs around 0.29 times for every 1000 live births (a fall from 0.61/1000 live births in 1995); however, the number of deaths where the cause was unascertained has increased 10-fold since 1995 and may be skewing the true SUDI figures.[15] In 2006, 143 deaths were attributed to SUDI in England and Wales[16] (Box 38-6).

SUDI occurs during periods of sleep. It usually occurs between midnight and 6 am. The typical age for SUDI is the first year of life, but most SUDI deaths (85%) occur within the first 6 months.[10]

The seasonal distribution for SUDI is October through March (in the northern hemisphere). The infant often has a history of minor illness, such as a cold, within 2 weeks before death. Classic signs that are usually present include lividity; frothy, blood-tinged drainage from the nose and

Box 38-5

Pain management

Pain management is important when caring for children. It should be considered when indicated to relieve pain associated with traumatic injury such as fractures and burns. Children do not always express their pain as clearly as adults. As a result, they are less likely to receive appropriate pain therapy in an emergency situation. Thus the paramedic should perform a systematic pain assessment. A memory aid for one type of pain assessment is QUESTT*:

Q: Question the child about his or her pain, using age-appropriate language.

U: Use pain rating scales (e.g. the Faces Pain Rating Scale for young children; a numeric pain scale from 0 to 10 for older children).

E: Evaluate the child's behaviour (e.g. facial grimace, rigidity, crying, and anxious behaviour).

S: Secure the parent or caregiver's involvement in assessing the child's pain. (The parent will have seen the child in pain or discomfort before and will be aware of subtle changes.)

T: Take cause of the pain into account (e.g. type of injury and expected intensity of pain).

T: Take action to provide comfort and to relieve pain (e.g. narcotic and non-narcotic drugs, comfort measures such as application of cold, elevation, and distraction techniques).

*Wong D, Hess C 2000 Clinical manual of paediatric nursing, 5th edition. Mosby, St Louis.

Box 38-6

Sleep positions and other factors that may reduce the risk of SUDI

This key publication, produced jointly by the Foundation for the Study of Infant Deaths and the Department of Health, outlines the key steps parents can take to reduce the risk of cot death including the advice to:

- Place your baby on the back to sleep.
- Cut smoking in pregnancy – fathers too!
- Do not let anyone smoke in the same room as your baby.
- Do not let your baby get too hot (or too cold).
- Keep baby's head uncovered – place your baby with their feet to the foot of the cot.
- The safest place for your baby to sleep is in a cot in a room with you for the first 6 months.
- Do not share a bed with your baby if you have been drinking alcohol, take drugs or if you are a smoker.
- If your baby is unwell, seek medical advice promptly.

Taken from the FSID website with permission: http://www.fsid.org.uk/reduce-risk.html

mouth; and rigor mortis. With most SUDI cases, no external signs of injury are found. Often evidence indicates that the baby was active just before the death (e.g. rumpled bed clothes, unusual position or location in the bed).

Pathophysiology

The cause of SUDI is unknown. Studies have failed to confirm a number of physiological, environmental, genetic, and social factors as causes. The studies have confirmed, however, that SUDI is not caused by external suffocation, regurgitation or aspiration of vomitus, hereditary factors, or allergies. Although no specific cause has been identified, a number of risk factors have been associated with the syndrome. These factors including the following:

- maternal smoking
- young maternal age (under age 20)
- infants of mothers who received poor or no prenatal care
- social deprivation
- premature births and low-birth-weight infants
- infants of mothers who used cocaine, methadone, or heroin during pregnancy.

SUDI is confirmed by excluding other causes of death.

Management

The main role of the paramedic is to offer emotional support for parents or other caregivers and loved ones. If the infant possibly could be viable, resuscitation should proceed as for any other infant in cardiac arrest. It is considered better for parents to know that resuscitation was started but not successful rather than being left wondering if anything could have saved their baby. Once resuscitation has been commenced, the paramedic should transport immediately to the nearest appropriate hospital with ongoing resuscitation. Where there is obviously no chance of successful resuscitation (e.g. rigor mortis), the paramedic will be left to manage possibly one of the most difficult situations in professional practice. The initial response of the paramedic (who is likely to be first on scene) will affect the family profoundly so it is imperative that the paramedic think before they speak. The paramedic should find out the name of the infant and use the name rather than referring to the baby as 'it'. If parents/carers wish to hold the baby, then this should be accommodated (unless there are signs of trauma) providing it does not interfere with clinical needs. It is advisable not to use a body bag in these situations. The infant should be conveyed to hospital and the paramedic should make facility for the parent(s)/carer to travel with their baby.

A variety of grief reactions should be expected from those who witness the event (parents, family members, neighbours, babysitters). These reactions may vary from shock and disbelief to anger, rage and self-blame. Where possible, arrangements should be made for a relative or neighbour to accompany the family to the hospital so that they are not left alone. Do not forget that other siblings may be in the house and will require care too.

SUDI victims may appear to have been abused or neglected. The mysterious nature of SUDI deaths and classic signs such as postmortem lividity and frothy fluid in the infant's nose and mouth give such appearance. Regardless of the circumstances, the paramedic should avoid comments or questions that may imply a suspicion of improper child care. Determining the cause of death is not the duty of the emergency medical services crew. (However, careful scene observation is crucial.) The paramedic should document all findings objectively, accurately and completely. Of particular importance is the description given by the parents/carer of the events leading up to their finding of the deceased infant as this may be valuable in later investigations.

The death of an infant has a powerful effect on all who are involved. Rescuers commonly have a range of emotional reactions after a SUDI death. Most emergency medical services provide counselling and formal debriefing programmes and it is likely that a Trust medical director or local paediatrician would be happy to discuss the event further if required. If these services are not available, the emergency medical services crew should discuss the event openly with others involved in the response (e.g. coworkers and police officers). This may help relieve normal feelings of anxiety and stress.

Critical Thinking

What factors do you think influence the reactions of each crew member to a SUDI death?

Child abuse and neglect

Safeguarding children

In 2008, 36 028 children were on child protection registers in the UK.[17] Sixteen per cent of children experience serious maltreatment by parents, of which one-third experience more than one form of maltreatment;[18] on average, one child is killed by their parent or carer every week in England and Wales.[19] *Working Together to Safeguard Children 2006*[20] states that 'safeguarding and promoting the welfare of children' means the process of:

- protecting children from maltreatment (i.e. abuse or neglect)
- preventing impairment of children's health and development
- ensuring that children are growing up in circumstances consistent with the provision of safe and effective care
- undertaking that role so as to enable children to have optimum life chances and to enter adulthood successfully.

'Child protection' is part of safeguarding and promoting welfare. The term child protection refers to the activity which is undertaken to protect specific children who are suffering, or at risk of suffering, significant harm. Although the police and social services have statutory responsibility to investigate suspicions or allegations of child abuse, the ambulance service has a responsibility to report all such concerns to social services. In situations where a child is believed to be at immediate risk, the case should be referred immediately to the police.

Elements of child abuse

Child abuse and neglect is the maltreatment of children by their parents, guardians, or other caregivers. Forms of maltreatment include infliction of physical injury (battered child syndrome, shaken baby syndrome), sexual exploitation, and infliction of emotional pain and neglect (medical neglect, safety neglect and nutritional deprivation). A number of factors come into play in the potential for child abuse. These include a caregiver with the potential to abuse, a child with particular characteristics that place him or her at risk for abuse, and an element of crisis.

Characteristics of abusers

Child abuse usually reflects a pattern of unstable behaviour and is typically not a single act of violence. In many cases the abuser is the child's parent, although other caregivers may be responsible; for example, other family members, a boyfriend of the child's mother, an unrelated babysitter, or a sibling of the abused child. In the case of physical abuse, most abusers tend to be unhappy, angry adults who are often under extreme stress. They are usually isolated and often they are incapable of using support agencies or an extended family in times of crisis. Often the abusers were the victim of physical or emotional abuse as children. Abusers come from all ethnic, geographical, religious, educational, occupational, and socioeconomic groups. Other factors that are characteristic of abusers include poverty and alcohol or other drug dependence.

Critical Thinking

Can you make a determination that someone is not an abuser if they do not fit this profile based on your prehospital assessment?

Characteristics of an abused child

Abused children often have certain characteristics that increase their risk for abuse. Common traits include demanding and difficult behaviour, decreased level of functioning (e.g. a child with a disability or preterm infant requiring extra parenting), hyperactivity, and precociousness with intellectual ability equal to or superior to the parent. Often the parent sees the abused child as 'special' or 'different' from other siblings. Other factors that tend to increase the potential for child abuse are age (the child is usually under 5 years old), gender (boys are involved more often than girls) and illegitimacy.

Crises that may precipitate abuse

Physical abuse or neglect can occur constantly during a child's life. More often, though, abuse and neglect are intermittent and unpredictable. The abuse is often brought on by stressors in the adult caregiver's life, especially when the caregiver expects the child to fill emotional needs created by the stress. Failure of the child to respond in an ideal way to the caregiver's needs may lead to abuse. Common crises associated with an episode of child abuse include the following:

- financial stress
- loss of employment
- eviction from housing
- marital or relationship stress
- physical illness in a child that leads to intractable crying
- death of a family member
- diagnosis of an unwanted pregnancy
- birth of a sibling.

History of injuries suspicious for abuse

Physical abuse or neglect is often hard to determine. The ultimate diagnosis usually begins with suspicions based on unexplained injuries, discrepant history, delays in seeking medical care, and repeated episodes of suspicious injuries. If at any time an injured child indicates that an adult caused him or her physical harm, the paramedic should take this report seriously and advise ambulance control. The paramedic should follow Trust policies for notifying social services as well. In many cases these accusations are true. The following are 15 indicators of possible abuse:[21]

1. Any obvious or suspected fractures in a child under 2 years of age.
2. Injuries in various stages of healing, especially burns and bruises.
3. More injuries than are usually seen in other children of the same age.
4. Injuries scattered on many areas of the body.
5. Bruises or burns in patterns that suggest intentional infliction.
6. Suspected increased intracranial pressure in an infant.
7. Suspected intra-abdominal trauma in a young child.
8. Any injury that does not fit the description of the cause.
9. An accusation that the child injured himself or herself intentionally.
10. Long-standing skin infections.
11. Extreme malnutrition.
12. Extreme lack of cleanliness.
13. Inappropriate clothing for the situation.
14. Child who withdraws from parent.
15. Child who responds inappropriately to the situation (e.g. quiet, distant and withdrawn).

Physical findings suggestive of abuse

Some physical findings, such as multiple, widely dispersed bruises, welts and burns, are suggestive of abuse. Such physical findings, along with a vague history or delays in seeking medical care for the child, should alert the paramedic to the possibility of abuse or neglect (Figure 38-12a–f).

Bruises (Table 38-7)

- Bruises that predominate on the buttocks or lower back are almost always related to punishment.
- Genital area or inner thigh bruises are often inflicted for toileting mishaps.
- Facial bruises or a number of petechiae on the ear lobe are usually caused by slapping.
- Bruises of the upper lip and labial frenulum are usually caused by forced feedings or from forcing a dummy into the mouth of a screaming infant.

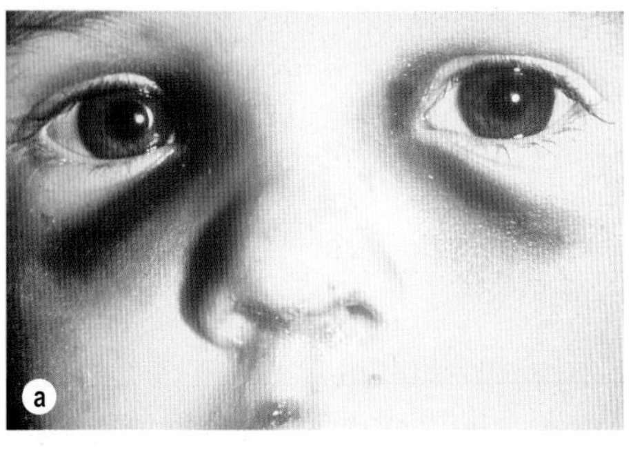

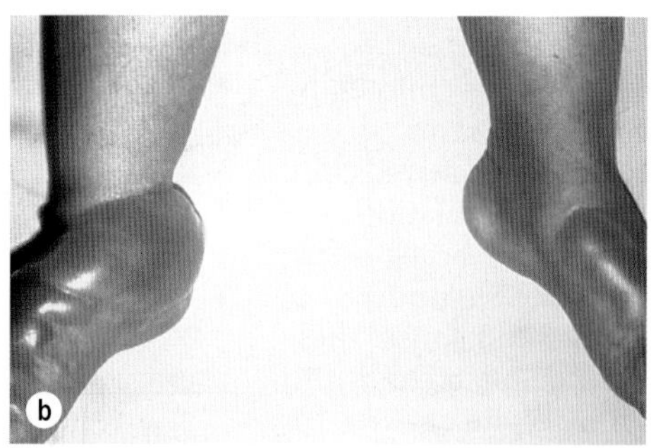

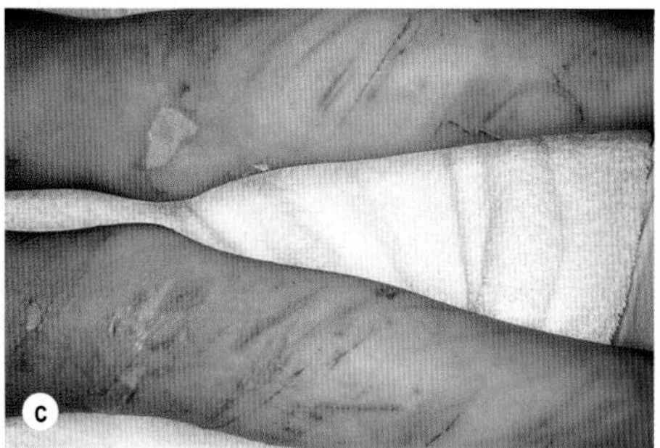

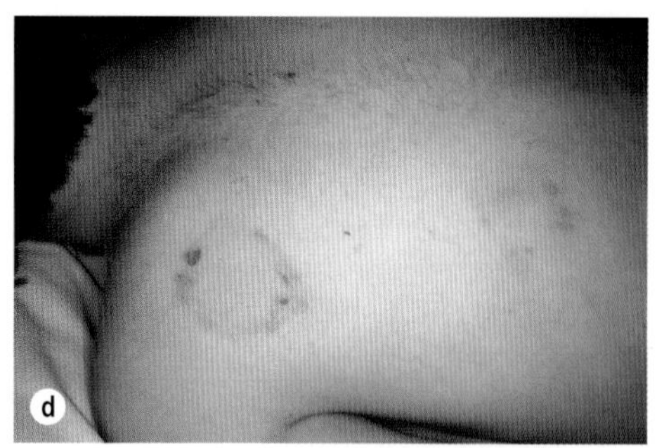

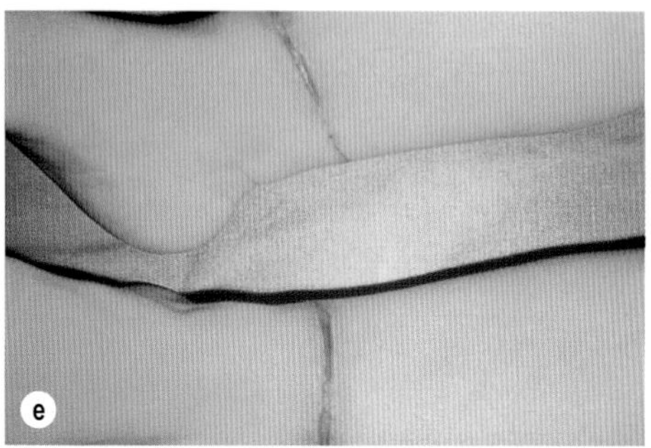

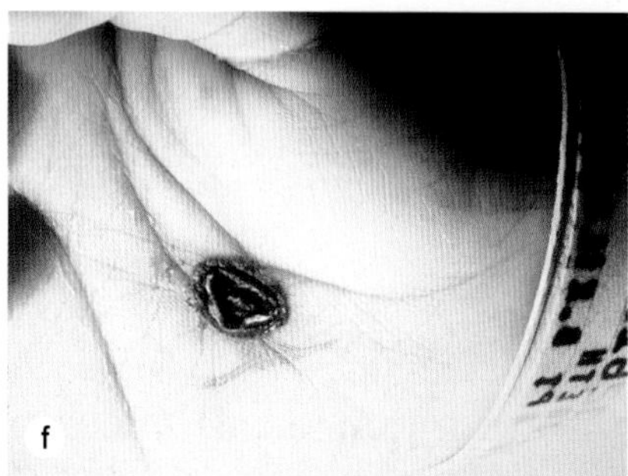

Figure 38-12 Cutaneous manifestations of child abuse. (a) 'Raccoon eyes,' or periorbital bruising, possible indication of anterior fossa skull fracture. (b) 'Dunking' burns of the feet. (c) Welts and abrasions to legs as a result of an electrical cord. (d) Human bites. (e) Fresh abrasions of restraint injury. (f) Fresh cigarette burn to palm.

Table 38-7 General guidelines for dating of bruises by colour

Colour of bruise	Age of bruise
Reddish blue or purple	Less than 24 h
Dark blue to purple	1–5 days
Green	5–7 days
Yellow	7–10 days
Brown	10–14 days or longer
Resolution	2–4 weeks

- Human hand marks resulting from squeezing are pressure bruises in shapes resembling fingertips, fingers, or the entire hand of the abuser.
- Human bite marks result in paired, crescent-shaped bruises and often contain individual teeth marks. The size of the arc distinguishes adult bites from child bites.

Critical Thinking

Consider an infant under 3 months of age. Based on the physical capabilities of this age group, where would you expect to see 'normal bruises'?

Welts

- Strap marks 2.5–5 cm (1–2 inches) wide are almost always caused by a belt.
- Bizarre-shaped welts or bruises usually are inflicted by a blunt object that resembles its shape (e.g. a toy or shoe).
- Choke marks may be seen on the neck.
- Circumferential bruising or abrasions on the ankles or wrists may be caused by rope, cord, or a dog leash.

Burns

- Cigarette burns often are found on the palms, soles or abdomen.
- A lighted cigarette, a hot match, or burning incense sometimes is applied to the hand to stop the child from sucking the thumb or to the genital area to discourage masturbation.
- Burns may be inflicted with lighters or other sources of open flame (e.g. a gas stove) to teach a child not to play with fire.
- Dry contact burns may result from forcibly holding a child against a heating device (e.g. a radiator, hot iron or electric hot plate).
- The most common hot-water burns or scalds occur from forcible immersion of the hands, feet, or buttocks in scalding water. These injuries often involve both

arms or both legs, or they may be circular burns restricted to the buttocks; such burns are incompatible with falling or stepping into a tub of hot water.

Other less visible injuries may indicate child abuse. These include brain injury, abdominal visceral injury, and bone fractures.

Subdural haematoma

Brain injury is the leading cause of death in battered children. The various pathological lesions include cerebral contusions, intraparenchymal haemorrhage, and subdural or even epidural haematomata. Subdural haematomata are among the most common injuries associated with intentionally inflicted head injury in children. They should be suspected in any young child who is in a coma or having convulsions. They should be suspected particularly if the child has no history of seizure disorder. In many cases, bleeding into the brain tissue occurs as a result of skull fractures or scalp bruises. These commonly result from a direct blow from a hand or by being thrown against a wall or door.

Subdural haematomata also can result from vigorous shaking of the child (shaken baby syndrome). The acceleration and deceleration forces on the brain associated with shaking cause tearing of the bridging cerebral veins. This leads to bleeding into the subdural space. Signs and symptoms of the shaken baby syndrome include retinal haemorrhages, irritability, altered level of consciousness, vomiting and a full fontanelle.

Critical Thinking

Why is it critical that your documentation be clear, objective, and complete in cases of suspected abuse?

Abdominal visceral injury

Intra-abdominal injuries are the second most common cause of death in battered children. These injuries usually are produced by a blunt force such as a punch or blow to the abdomen. Children with an abdominal injury often have recurrent vomiting, abdominal distension, absent bowel sounds and localized tenderness with or without abdominal bruising. Caregivers routinely deny a history of trauma to the child's abdomen in these cases.

Bone injury

More than 20% of physically abused children have a positive result on radiological bone survey from previous abusive episodes.[21] Injuries that may be obvious only through radiography include fractures of the ribs, lateral portion of the clavicle, scapula, sternum and extremities. Multiple fractures in various stages of healing are highly suspicious for physical abuse.

Injuries from sexual abuse

Sexual abuse of a child is a symptom of a seriously disturbed family relationship. Sexual abuse usually is associated with physical or emotional neglect or abuse. Often the sexually abusive adult received similar abuse as a child. The adult may justify this behaviour in his or her mind. Family relationships are complex, and silent complicity by at least one parent often is involved.

Injuries from sexual abuse may be physical and psychological. Sexual abuse may include vaginal intercourse, anal intercourse, oral–genital contact or molestation (fondling, masturbation or exposure). In many cases the victimized child is a girl and more than half of the victims are under 12 years of age at the time of the first offence. Many of these incidents are chronic and occur without force, thus an emergency medical services response is seldom initiated. If, however, a physical injury results from the abuse, emergency care may be summoned. Physical findings suggestive of sexual abuse include the following:

- pregnancy or venereal disease in a child 12 years of age or younger
- painful urination or defecation
- tenderness or lacerations to the perineal area
- bleeding from the rectum or vagina
- presence of dried blood, semen or pubic hair in the genital area of a child.

Emergency care for child victims of sexual abuse should be limited to managing injuries that pose a threat to life and giving emotional support during transport. These children undergo extensive interviews and examination by the emergency department physician and others. The paramedic should carefully document any statements made by the patient, family member, or caregiver. Any findings should be reported to medical direction. These children require compassionate support. A sexually abused child should never be made to feel that he or she is responsible for any of the abuse. The child also should not be given the impression that discussion of the event is inappropriate. If possible, a paramedic of the same sex should interview and care for the child.

Infants and children with special needs

Some infants and children are born with or develop conditions that pose special needs. These children may require special medical equipment to sustain life. Examples of these conditions include infants born prematurely, those who have altered functions from birth, and those who have chronic or acute disease of the lung, heart or central nervous system. Often these children are cared for at home by family and home health services. Many are dependent on special medical equipment such as tracheostomy tubes, home artificial ventilators, central venous lines, gastrostomy tubes, and shunts (see Chapter 41). The parents and other family members of a child with special medical needs are often 'experts' in caring for the child and maintaining the required medical equipment. Their knowledge, skills, and experience are invaluable. The paramedic should use the skills and expertise of the parents when managing these emergencies.

Critical Thinking

How can an emergency medical services agency prepare crews to care for these special needs children before a call is even received?

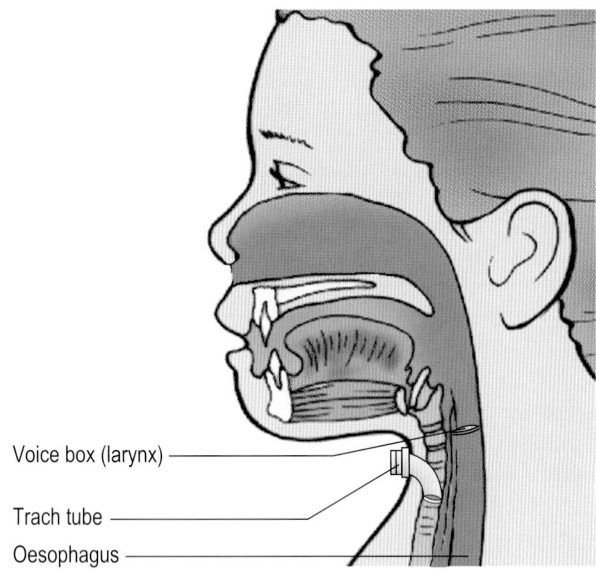

Figure 38-13 Paediatric tracheostomy tube.

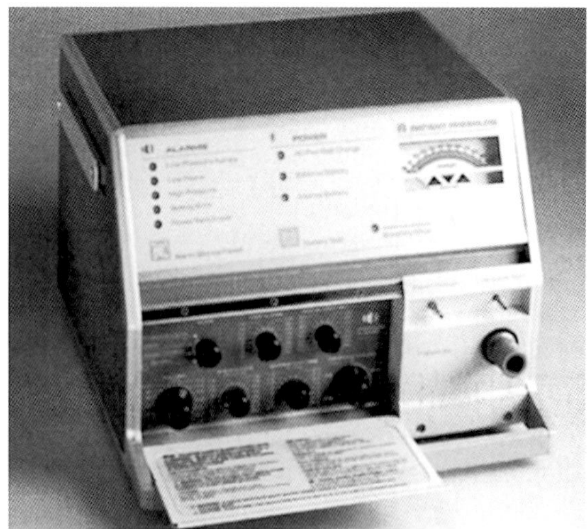
Figure 38-14 Home ventilator.

Table 38-8 Complications seen with home artificial ventilators

Complication	Possible cause
Airway obstruction	Bronchospasm, mucus or secretions, tracheostomy or endotracheal tube malfunction, patient cough, fear, anxiety
Barotrauma	
Pneumothorax	High-pressure volumes
Atelectasis	Improper deep breathing, pneumothorax
Cardiovascular impairment	Reduction in venous return to the heart caused by positive intrathoracic pressure, which compresses pulmonary circulation
Gastrointestinal	Swallowing air, gastrointestinal bleeding, gastric distension
Tracheal trauma	Cuff pressure on trachea
Respiratory infection	Bypass of natural defences of upper airway, poor aseptic technique
Oxygen toxicity	High concentration of oxygen over prolonged periods

Tracheostomy tubes

A patient with a complete tracheostomy has had the airway surgically interrupted so that the larynx is no longer connected to the trachea. Modern tracheostomy tubes are flexible and relatively comfortable for the patient. They have few associated risks (Figure 38-13). Complications that can occur with the tracheostomy tube include obstruction, air leak, bleeding, dislodgment and infection. All of these may lead to inadequate ventilation. (Bleeding around a tracheostomy usually occurs within 24 h of the surgery and is not commonly seen in the prehospital setting.) Aseptic technique and respiratory support are always high priorities in caring for these patients.

Management

The tracheostomy tube may become blocked or dislodged. In these cases, the paramedic must clear the tube with sterile water or saline or remove and reinsert it as described in Chapter 13. Tracheal suctioning (using sterile technique) may be required to remove secretions and mucus. If tracheal intubation becomes necessary in these patients, it must be performed via the stoma.

Note

Tracheal suctioning is a difficult procedure and is often traumatic for the patient. It can easily lead to hypoxia. Tracheal suctioning should be performed only when absolutely necessary and only for a period of 10–15 s. After that, high-concentration supplemental oxygen should be administered by mask to stoma or via a bag–valve–mask.

Home artificial ventilators

When a patient needs help breathing, the child may be put on a mechanical ventilator which simulates the normal movement of the diaphragm and thoracic cage. The type of home ventilator used depends on the patient's specific needs. Ventilators are classified by function based on the amount of air and pressure they are set to deliver during certain phases of the respiratory cycle (Figure 38-14). Complications can occur from malfunction of the machine and alarms, airway obstruction, and respiratory distress (Table 38-8).

Management

The many types of artificial ventilators work differently, so the paramedic should never try to troubleshoot a ventilator problem. The paramedic should not try to adjust the settings of the ventilator either. Rather, the emergency medical services crew should always treat the patient and not try to

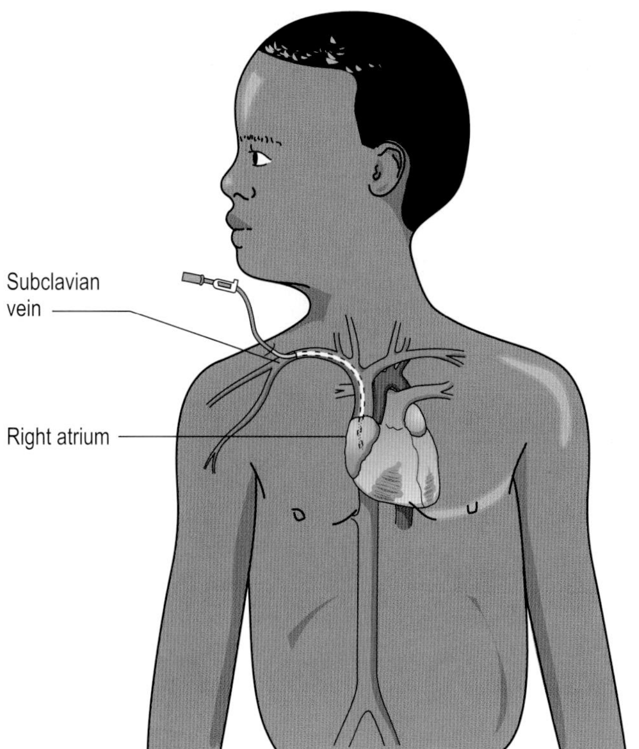

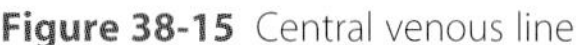
Figure 38-15 Central venous line.

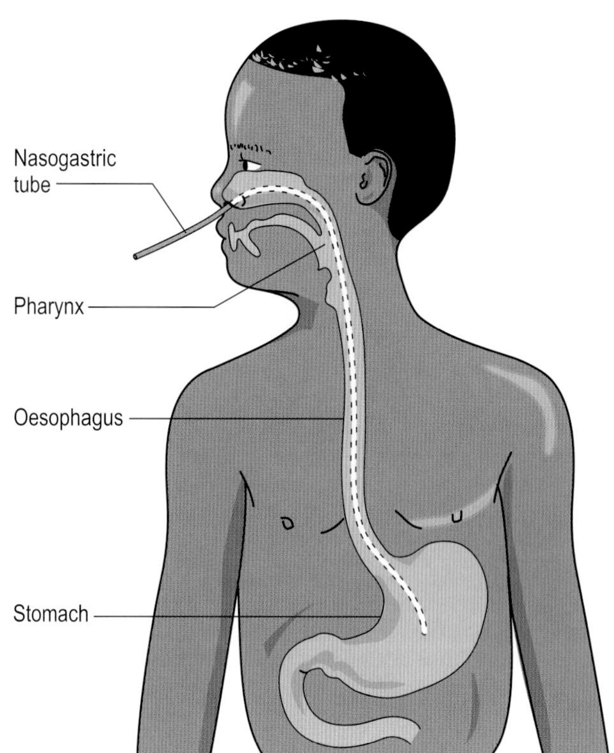

Figure 38-16 Nasogastric tube.

correct the malfunction of the machine. Steps in managing a patient with a home artificial ventilator problem are presented in Chapter 41.

Central venous lines

Some patients with chronic illnesses need prolonged and frequent access to venous circulation for drug or fluid therapy. This is made possible through vascular access devices. These devices are seen often in the prehospital setting in child and adult patients who are cared for in the home (Figure 38-15). These devices include surgically implanted medication delivery devices (e.g. Portacaths), peripheral vascular access devices (e.g. peripherally inserted central catheters, Intracath), and central venous access devices (e.g. Hickman and Groshong) (see Chapters 12 and 41). Complications that may occur with vascular access devices include a cracked line, air embolism, bleeding, obstruction and local infection. Patients with vascular access devices often have a serious illness such as cancer or acquired immunodeficiency syndrome. The effects of these illnesses may complicate the assessment and management of emergencies associated with central venous lines.

Management

A torn or leaking catheter (cracked line) may allow fluids or drugs to infiltrate into the surrounding tissues and can lead to an air embolism. A torn catheter is evidenced by leaking fluid, a complaint of a burning sensation, or swollen and tender skin near the insertion site. If a torn catheter is suspected, the paramedic should stop the infusion immediately and clamp the catheter between the tear and the patient. The patient who develops an altered level of consciousness (indicating a possible air embolism) should be positioned on the left side. The patient's head should be slightly lowered to help prevent the embolism from travelling to the brain. High-concentration oxygen, IV access, and rapid transport for evaluation by a physician are indicated. Any bleeding at the site should be controlled with direct pressure.

Occasionally, the lumen port becomes obstructed by a blood clot that disrupts the flow of fluids or drugs. (Signs and symptoms of obstruction include a sluggish flow and swelling and tenderness at the site.) When this occurs, the patient should be transported to the hospital so that the catheter can be cleared with thrombolytics or replaced. Attempts to clear a vascular access device require special training and should only be carried out by those trained to do so. The technique is described in Chapter 41.

Gastric tubes and gastrostomy tubes

A gastric tube (Figure 38-16) is used as a temporary measure to provide liquid feeding to a patient who cannot swallow or absorb nutrients (often used for feeding premature infants). The tubes are inserted through the nose or mouth into the stomach and can cause irritation to the nasal and mucous membranes. They are designed for short-term use.

A gastrostomy tube (Figure 38-17) provides a permanent route for gastric feeding in patients who usually cannot be fed by mouth (e.g. a patient with facial burns or paralysis). The tube is surgically placed into the stomach and can be

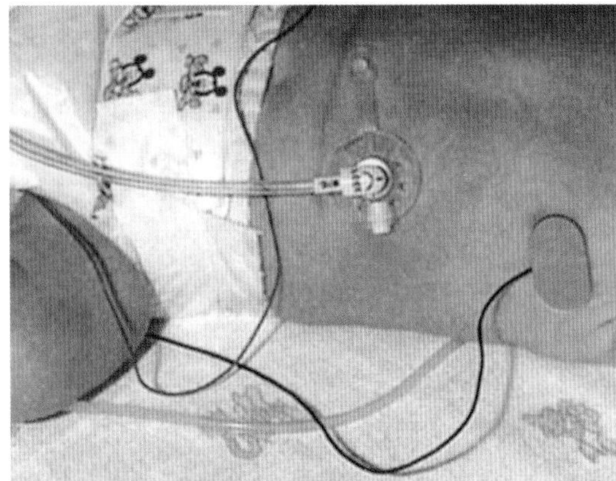

Figure 38-17 Gastrostomy tube.

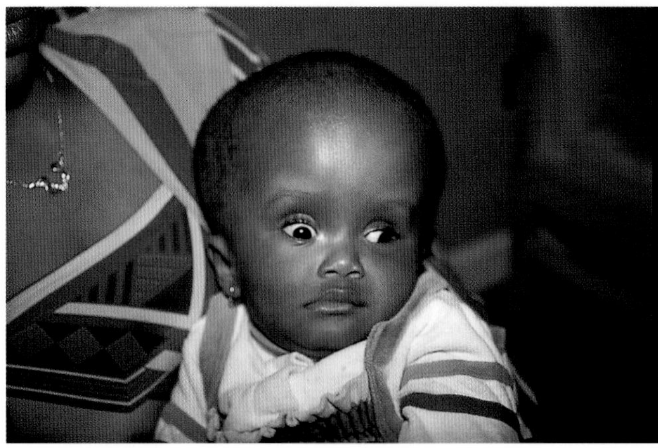

Figure 38-18 Untreated hydrocephalus.

visualized in the upper left quadrant of the abdomen. The opening (stoma) has a flexible, silicone 'button' (covered with a protective cap), which allows for regular feedings.

Management

Serious complications with gastric or gastrostomy tubes are rare and they seldom require emergency care. Potential complications include obstruction, pulmonary aspiration, gastrointestinal disturbances (vomiting and diarrhoea), irritation to the mucous membrane, and electrolyte imbalances. All of these can result in inadequate nutrition and fluid needs. Emergency care is mainly supportive and may include transport for evaluation by a physician. If not contraindicated, the patient will be most comfortable lying on the right side with the head elevated.

Shunts

A shunt is a tube or device that is implanted surgically in the body to redirect body fluid from one cavity or vessel to another. An example of a shunt is one used to relieve abnormal fluid pressures from excess cerebrospinal fluid around the brain in children with hydrocephalus (Figure 38-18).

The shunt for hydrocephalus consists of two catheters, a reservoir, and a valve to prevent backflow (Figure 38-19). The first catheter is inserted through the skull to drain fluid from the ventricles of the brain. The second catheter is passed into another body cavity (usually the abdomen or right atrium of the heart through the jugular vein), where the excess fluid is absorbed. The reservoir can usually be palpated over the mastoid area, just behind the ear.

Management

Complications from this procedure include the need for catheter replacement as the child grows (requiring several surgeries in the first 10 years of life), obstruction from clotted blood or fluid, and catheter displacement. Infection may occur within several weeks of surgical placement. The signs and symptoms of obstruction or displacement are those of increased ICP. They include the following:

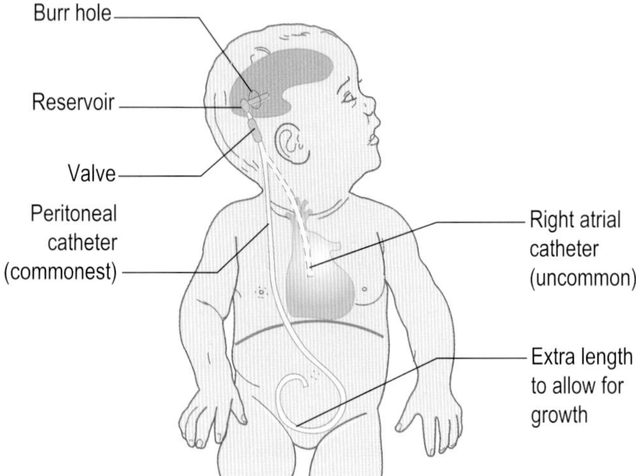

Figure 38-19 Ventricular shunt for drainage of symptomatic hydrocephalus.

- headache
- nausea and vomiting
- visual disturbances
- Cushing triad (elevated systolic pressure, irregular respirations, bradycardia).

Children who have complications from a ventricular shunt need emergency surgery to prevent brainstem herniation. The paramedic should first ensure adequate airway, ventilatory, and circulatory support for these patients. These patients are prone to respiratory arrest so need immediate transport to a proper facility for evaluation by a physician. If possible, the patient's head should be elevated during transport.

Summary

- Children have unique anatomical, physiological and psychological characteristics, which change during their development.
- Some childhood diseases and disabilities can be predicted by age group.
- Many elements of the initial evaluation can be done by observing the child. The child's parent or guardian also should be involved in the initial evaluation. The three components of the paediatric assessment triangle are appearance, work of breathing and circulation.
- Obstruction of the upper or lower airway by a foreign body usually occurs in toddlers or preschoolers. Obstruction may be partial or complete.
- Croup is a common inflammatory respiratory illness. It usually is seen in children between the ages of 6 months and 4 years. Symptoms are caused by inflammation in the subglottic region.
- Epiglottitis is a rapidly progressive, life-threatening bacterial infection. It causes oedema and swelling of the epiglottis and supraglottic structures. It often affects children between 3 and 7 years of age.
- Asthma is common in children over 2 years of age. Asthma is characterized by bronchoconstriction that results from autonomic dysfunction or sensitizing agents.
- Bronchiolitis is a viral disease frequently caused by respiratory syncytial virus infection of the lower airway; it usually affects children 6–18 months of age.
- Pneumonia is an acute infection of the lower airways and lungs involving the alveolar walls and the alveoli.
- Several special differences must be remembered when caring for a child in shock. These include circulating blood volume, body surface area and hypothermia, cardiac reserve and vital signs and assessment. A child in shock may appear normal and stable until all compensatory mechanisms fail. At that point, paediatric shock progresses rapidly, with serious deterioration.
- When dysrhythmias occur in children, they usually result from hypoxia or structural heart disease.
- The most common causes of seizure in adult and paediatric patients is non-compliance with a drug regimen for the treatment of epilepsy, in addition to head trauma, intracranial infection, metabolic disturbance or poisoning. The most common cause of new onset of seizure in children is fever.
- Hypoglycaemia and hyperglycaemia should be suspected whenever a child has an altered level of consciousness with no explainable cause.
- Children with infection may have a variety of signs and symptoms. These depend on the source and extent of infection and the length of time since the patient was exposed.
- Most poisoning events in the UK involve children. Signs and symptoms of accidental poisoning vary, depending on the toxic substance and the length of time since the child was exposed.
- Blunt and penetrating trauma is a chief cause of injury and death in children. Head injury is the most common cause of death in paediatric trauma patients. Early recognition and aggressive management can reduce morbidity and mortality caused by traumatic brain injury in children.
- Because of the pliability of the chest wall, severe intrathoracic injury can be present without signs of external injury. The liver, kidneys and spleen are the most frequently injured abdominal organs. Extremity injuries are more common in children than adults.
- Sudden unexpected death in infancy (SUDI) is the leading cause of death in UK infants under 1 year of age. It is defined as the sudden death of a seemingly healthy infant. The death cannot be explained by history and an autopsy.
- Child abuse and neglect is the maltreatment of children by their parents, guardians, or other caregivers. Forms of maltreatment include infliction of physical injury, sexual exploitation, and infliction of emotional pain and neglect.
- Some infants and children are born with or develop conditions that pose special needs. These children may require special medical equipment to sustain life. Often these children are cared for at home. Many are dependent on specialized medical equipment such as tracheostomy tubes, home artificial ventilators, central venous lines, gastrostomy tubes and shunts.

References

1. Joint Royal Colleges Ambulance Liaison Committee 2006 UK Ambulance Service Clinical Guidelines. JRCALC, London
2. Jarvis S, Court D 2001 The continuing global challenge of injury. The UK is lagging behind. BMJ 322(7302): 1557–1558
3. Lands LC 2006 Applying physiology to conventional mechanical ventilation. Paed Resp Rev 7(Suppl 1):S33–S36
4. Chung C-Y, Chen C-L, Cheng P-T, et al 2006 Critical score of Glasgow Coma Scale for pediatric traumatic brain injury. Pediatr Neurol 34(5):379–387
5. American Heart Association 2005 American Heart Association Guidelines for Cardiopulmonary Resuscitation. Circulation 112:(24 Suppl)
6. McVernon J, Slack MPE, Ramsay ME 2006 Changes in the epidemiology of epiglottitis following introduction of *Haemophilus influenzae* type b (Hib)

conjugate vaccines in England: a comparison of two data sources. Epidemiol Infect 134(3):570–572
7. Health Survey for England 2001; Joint Health Surveys Unit 2003; The Scottish Health Survey 1998; Joint Health Surveys Unit, 2000; Census 2001, Office for National Statistics: ONS. Online. Available www.statistics.gov.uk 20 February 2009
8. Resuscitation Council UK 2005 Resuscitation Guidelines 2005: Paediatric Advanced Life Support. Online. Available http://www.resus.org.uk/pages/pals.pdf 20 February 2009
9. Advanced Life Support Group 2005 Advanced paediatric life support. ALSG, London
10. Hoekelman R, Adam HM, Nicholas MN 2001 Primary paediatric care, 4th edition. Mosby, St Louis
11. Rosen P, Barkin R 1998 Emergency medicine: concepts and clinical practice, 4th edition. Mosby, St Louis
12. Diabetes UK 2006 Diabetes: State of the Nations 2006 Progress made in delivering the national diabetes frameworks. Online. Available www.diabetes.org.uk 20 February 2009
13. US Department of Transportation, National Highway Traffic Safety Administration 1998 EMT-Paramedic national standard curriculum. US Department of Transportation, Washington, DC
14. Royal Society for the Prevention of Accidents 2002 Drownings in the UK 2002. RoSPA, Birmingham
15. Office for National Statistics 2005 Investigation into sudden infant deaths and unascertained infant deaths in England and Wales, 1995–2003. Online. Available http://www.statistics.gov.uk/articles/hsq/HSQ27infant_death.pdf 20 February 2009
16. Office for National Statistics. Deaths by age, sex and underlying cause 2006. Online. Available http://www.statistics.gov.uk/downloads/theme_population/Table_2_Death_Registrations_Cause.xls 20 February 2009
17. Department for Schools, Children and Families. Referrals, assessments and children and young people who are the subject of a child protection plan, England – year ending 31 March 2008. Online. Available http://www.dcsf.gov.uk/rsgateway/DB/SFR/s000811/sfr24_2008.pdf 6 June 2009
Northern Ireland Statistics and Research Agency. Children order statistical bulleting 2008. Online. Available http://www.dhsspsni.gov.uk/children_order_statistical_bulletin_2008-final-2.pdf 6 June 2009
Scottish Government. Child protection statistics 2007/8, Tables 7 and 8. Edinburgh: National Statistics. Online. Available http://www.scotland.gov.uk/Publications/2008/09/23090901/0 6 June 2009
Data Unit Wales Dissemination Unit. Number of children and young persons on the Child Protection register 2007/08. Online. Available http://dissemination.dataunitwales.gov.uk/webview/index.jsp 6 June 2009
18. Cawson P 2002 Child maltreatment in the family: the experience of a national sample of young people. NSPCC, London
19. Home Office 2004 Crime in England and Wales 2002–3: Supplementary Volume 1, Homicide and Gun Crime. Home Office, London
20. HM Government 2006 Working together to safeguard children. Stationery Office, London
21. Touloukian R 1990 Paediatric trauma, 2nd edition. Mosby, St Louis

APPENDIX

When to immunize	Vaccine	How vaccine is given
2 months old	Diphtheria, tetanus, pertussis (whooping cough), polio and Hib (DTaP/IPV/Hib)	One injection
	Pneumococcal	One injection
3 months old	Diphtheria, tetanus, pertussis (whooping cough), polio and Hib (DTaP/IPV/Hib)	One injection
	Men C	One injection
4 months old	Diphtheria, tetanus, pertussis (whooping cough), polio and Hib (DTaP/IPV/Hib)	One injection
	Men C	One injection
	PCV	One injection
12 months old	Hib/MenC	One injection
Around 13 months old	Measles, mumps and rubella (MMR)	One injection
	PCV	One injection
3 years 4 months to 5 years old	Diphtheria, tetanus, pertussis (whooping cough) and polio (DTaP/IPV or dTaP/IPV)	One injection
	Measles, mumps and rubella (MMR)	One injection
13–18 years old	Tetanus, diphtheria and polio (Td/IPV)	One injection

By 4 months:	Three doses of DTaP/IPV/Hib Two doses of PCV and MenC
By 14 months:	A booster dose of Hib/MenC and PCV and the first dose of MMR
By school entry:	Fourth dose of DTaP/IPV or dTaP/IPV and the second dose of MMR
Before leaving school:	Fifth dose of Td/IPV

Source: Department of Health 2006 Immunisation against infectious disease. The Stationery Office, London

CHAPTER 39

Older Persons

Chapter contents

Objectives

Upon completion of this chapter, the paramedic student will be able to:

1. Explain the physiology of the ageing process as it relates to major body systems and homeostasis.
2. Describe general principles of assessment specific to older adults.
3. Describe the pathophysiology, assessment, and management of specific illnesses that affect selected body systems in the older person.
4. Identify specific problems with sensations experienced by some older patients.
5. Discuss effects of drug toxicity and alcoholism in the older adult.
6. Identify factors that contribute to environmental emergencies in the older patient.
7. Discuss prehospital assessment and management of depression and suicide in the older adult.
8. Describe epidemiology, assessment, and management of trauma in the older patient.
9. Identify characteristics of elder abuse.

Key terms

cataract A loss of transparency of the lens of the eye that results from changes in the delicate protein fibres within the lens.

continence The ability to control bladder or bowel function.

elder abuse The infliction of physical pain, injury, debilitating mental anguish, unreasonable confinement, or wilful deprivation by a caregiver of services that are necessary to maintain mental and physical health of a older person.

faecal impaction An accumulation of hardened faeces in the rectum or sigmoid colon that the person is unable to move.

gerontology The study of the problems of all aspects of ageing.

glaucoma A condition in which intraocular pressure increases and causes damage to the optic nerve.

incontinence The inability to control bladder or bowel function.

pressure ulcers Sores or ulcers in the skin over a bony prominence that occurs most frequently on the sacrum, elbows, heels, outer ankles, inner knees, hips and shoulder blades of high-risk patients, especially those who are obese, elderly, or suffering from chronic diseases, infections, injuries or a poor nutritional state.

retinopathy A group of inflammatory eye disorders often caused by diabetes, hypertension, and atherosclerotic vascular disease.

The 'greying' of UK society includes the prospect that the healthcare needs of older adults will continue to increase in all areas, which includes prehospital care. About 23% of the British population will be 65 years of age or older by the year 2031 and will represent around three-quarters of all ambulance transports. This chapter addresses anatomical and physiological changes that accompany the ageing process, special considerations in assessing and managing older patients, and common emergencies that may result from normal ageing and chronic illness.

Demographics, epidemiology and societal issues

More than 9.5 million Britons (16% of the UK population) are 65 years of age or older. The size of this group has increased during the last 100 years, and, at the same time, fertility rates in the UK have levelled out from a peak of 2.95 children per woman in the mid 1960s to a rate of 1.79 in 2005; this means in the future there will be fewer persons under 65 years of age to support the cost of healthcare and living expenses of those over 65 years of age. Additionally, the 'older old' are also increasing in number; in 2005 in the UK the 'over 85s' numbered around 1.2 million (around 2% of the population). Figures for the number of older people who are considered 'dependent' is also expected to grow from 2.5 million in 2001 to a little over 4 million in 2024, an increase of 57%.[1]

By the year 2031, it is projected that those over 65 years old will constitute 23% of the population and those over 85 years of age will constitute 3.8% of the population. This creates many challenges. Society will have to try to provide quality, cost-effective healthcare and support the increasing health and living expenses for the elderly. To meet the needs of this ageing population properly, society must achieve the following:[2]

- The public must become better educated about the needs of the elderly because caregiving often falls to families and friends.
- Current and new healthcare professionals must be educated on the special needs of the ageing population as they have unique qualities. These qualities distinguish them from younger populations; for instance, older persons have a higher level of adverse drug reactions and urinary incontinence, therefore healthcare professionals need special training to treat this population.
- The ageing of the UK population demands continued and expanded research efforts into long-term health conditions that affect the aged and their families.
- Healthcare professionals need to reform healthcare financing, delivery, and administrative structures to accommodate the predominance of long-term health conditions among the ageing population.
- Health care professionals must develop solutions for the long-term care needs of the growing ageing population. These solutions must address the emotional and financial needs of older adults and their families. They also must address the financial influence of long-term care in the UK.

Other key issues to consider in caring for the ageing population include legal ones such as advance directives, durable power of attorney, and 'do not resuscitate' orders, discussed in Chapter 2.

Box 39-1

Support and assistance services for the older patient

Community-based services
Home healthcare services
Hospice programmes
In-home services
Institutional services
Multipurpose centres
Nutrition services
Religious and pastoral services
National advisory councils
National ageing organizations (including voluntary groups) (e.g. Age Concern)

Living environments and referral sources

Many older Britons enjoy independent living and enjoy this lifestyle with the help of spousal or family support and health and social care support. Others live dependently in nursing care facilities, sheltered housing, and nursing homes and receive this help through local authorities as well as national programmes and agencies (Box 39-1). The paramedic should be familiar with the services in the community that offer assistance to the elderly.

Physiological changes of ageing

Gerontology is the study of the problems of all aspects of ageing; this process proceeds at different rates in different persons. In addition, organ systems age at differing rates within the individual. However, in certain areas, predictable functional declines occur in all persons with increasing age. As a rough guideline, these changes begin to occur at a rate of 5–10% for each decade of life after 30 years of age. The ageing process affects all body systems. However, the effects on specific organ systems particularly relevant to the older adult occur in the respiratory, cardiovascular, renal, nervous, and musculoskeletal systems (Table 39-1).

Critical Thinking

Consider your family members and friends who are in their 40s, 60s or 80s. What age-related changes have you noticed?

Respiratory system changes

Respiratory function in the older adult generally declines as the lung tissue ages. Reduced pulmonary capacity results from changes in lung and chest wall compliance. With ageing, the chest wall becomes stiffer as the bony thorax becomes more rigid and lung elastic recoil also decreases. Despite the loss of elasticity, which would tend to increase total lung capacity, total lung capacity remains the same. This is due to the opposing loss of chest wall compliance and weakened respiratory muscles. The diameter of the alveoli increase and the distal airways tend to collapse on expiration; these

Table 39-1 Physiological changes of ageing

Change	Result
Overall appearance	
Skin	
Loss of elasticity	Wrinkling, thinning of skin
Loss of collagen	Increased susceptibility to injury
Shrinking of sweat glands	Dryness
Pigment deposition	Age spots
Sun damage	Senile keratosis
Eyes	
Clouding of lens	Cataracts (decreased visual acuity) Poor peripheral vision
Pigment deposition	Arcus senilis (bluish circle that forms around the outer edge of the iris of the eye)
Cardiovascular system	
Increased internal thickening of arteries	Hypertension
	Increased risk of stroke or heart attack
	Varicosities and clots
	Dysrhythmias
Increased cholesterol deposits (atherosclerotic heart disease)	Coronary artery disease and peripheral vascular disease
Increased rate of cardiac hypertrophy	Decreased cardiac output
Decreased cardiac output	Loss of exercise tolerance
	Diminished activity
	Increased work to heart
	Increased risk of myocardial infarction
Pulmonary system	
Decreased elasticity	Diminished breathing capacity
Decreased compliance and surface area	Decreased maximal oxygen uptake
Decreased ciliary activity	Increased risk of infection/toxicity
Gastrointestinal tract	
Decreased hydrochloric acid production	Difficulty with digestion
	Food absorption problems and constipation
Delay in intestinal motility	Feeling full early, causing weight loss
Decreased saliva flow	Dry mouth, difficulty chewing
Fewer taste buds	Loss of food enjoyment, decreased appetite
Gum atrophy (shrinkage)	Tooth loss
Decreased liver function	Risk of toxicity from drugs
	Alcohol damage
	Loss of blood clotting
Central nervous system	
Decreased cortical cell count	Memory impairment (dementia)
Increased synapse time	Decreased complex learning
Decreased nerve conduction velocity	Slower psychomotor skills
	Increased reflex time, leading to risk of falling
Brain atrophy (shrinkage)	Prone to subdural haematomata
Vision	
Growth of lens	Decreased focusing ability
Cataract deposition	Hyperopia (farsightedness)
	Opacification of vision

Table 39-1 Physiological changes of ageing—cont'd

Change	Result
Decreased pupil size	Decreased acuity and colour perception
Loss of accommodation (focusing ability)	Decreased depth perception
	All cause increased risks of accidents and falls
Hearing	
Ossicle degeneration	Loss of high-frequency range of hearing
Atrophy (shrinkage) of auditory meatus	Loss of high-frequency range of hearing
Atrophy (shrinkage) of cochlear hair cells and auditory neurons	Decreased keenness and pitch discrimination
	Decreased sense of balance
	All cause increased risks of accidents and falls
Renal function	
Decreased glomerular function	Decreased renal clearance
Decreased renal blood flow	Increased risk of toxicity from all drugs and toxins processed in the kidneys
Genitourinary system	
Loss of bladder control	Urinary infections
Prostate enlargement	Tumours and urinary retention
Endocrine function	
Decrease in thyroid, ovarian and testicular function	Decreased energy, decreased metabolic rate
	Decreased heat/cold tolerance
	Decreased reproductive function
Increased insulin	Predisposition for hypoglycaemia
Musculoskeletal system	
Decreased muscle mass	Loss of strength
Increased joint/tendon breakdown	Arthritis, stiffness, loss of flexibility
	Increased risk of falls
	Loss of bone strength and size
Bone demineralization	Increased risk of fracture
Psychological/social	
Loss of physical function	Decreased activity
Loss of friends/family	Depression
Loss of social support	Increased isolation and anxiety
	Increased risk of suicide attempts
Immune system	
Loss of T cell function	Increased infection

From MedicAlert 1994 Older emergencies: an EMT teaching manual. MedicAlert Foundation, Turlock, CA.

changes lead to an increase in residual volume and a decrease in vital capacity. Consequently, by 75 years of age, vital capacity may decrease by as much as 50%, maximum breathing capacity by as much as 60%, and maximum work rate and maximum oxygen uptake by as much as 70%.

Arterial oxygen pressure (PaO_2) also slowly decreases with age but arterial carbon dioxide pressure stays the same (this is most likely related to the much greater reserve in carbon dioxide elimination than in oxygen absorption). At 30 years of age the PaO_2 of a healthy person breathing ambient air at sea level is about 12 kPa. At 70 years of age the expected PaO_2 is approximately 9.2 kPa. These findings, along with the normal decline in chemoreceptor function, produce a diminished ventilatory response to hypoxia and hypercapnia.

Other factors that affect the respiratory system are the loss of cilia in the airways and a diminished cough reflex and impaired gag reflex which impair the bodily defence against inhaled bacteria and particulate matter. The decline in these defence mechanisms makes infectious pulmonary diseases of the older adult more common and makes these infections harder to resolve.

Cardiovascular system changes

Cardiac function declines with age as a result of non-ischaemic physiological changes and the high incidence of atherosclerotic coronary heart disease. Differentiating changes that are solely due to ageing from those associated with ischaemia is difficult because coronary artery disease is so prevalent in the older adult. However, even with ageing alone, changes occur in the cardiovascular system that cause a decrease in cardiac function; these changes include a diminished ability to raise the heart rate even in response to exercise or stress, a decrease in compliance of the ventricle, a prolonged duration of contraction and a decreased responsiveness to catecholamine stimulation. Between 30 and 80 years of age, resting cardiac output decreases about 30%. Combined with the progressive increase in peripheral vascular resistance that occurs after 40 years of age, this decrease in cardiac output yields a significant drop in organ perfusion. Myocardial hypertrophy, coronary artery disease and haemodynamic changes predispose the older patient to dysrhythmias, heart failure, and sudden cardiac arrest when the cardiovascular system is placed under unexpected stress.

Changes also occur in the electrical conduction pathways of the heart. These changes occur as cells in the sinoatrial and atrioventricular nodes and the rest of the conduction system lose the ability to function. These physiological changes often lead to dysrhythmias which include chronic atrial fibrillation, sick sinus syndrome, and various types of bradycardia and heart blocks, which can contribute to the decline in cardiac output.

Critical Thinking

What lifestyle choices can slow down these physiological changes of ageing?

Renal system changes

Structural and functional changes in the kidneys occur during the ageing process. For example, renal blood flow falls an average of 50% between 30 and 80 years of age. This reduction in renal blood flow is associated with a proportional decrease in the glomerular filtration rate of about 8 mL/min per decade. Renal mass decreases by about 20% between 40 and 80 years of age. The steady decline in kidney function places the older patient at greater risk for renal failure from trauma, obstruction, infection, and vascular occlusion.

As the patient ages, significant impairment develops in renal concentrating ability, sodium conservation, free water clearance (diuresis), glomerular filtration and renal plasma flow. Hepatic blood flow decreases as well. This limits the effectiveness of liver metabolism. Decreases in kidney and liver function and loss of muscle and body water make the older patient more susceptible to electrolyte disturbances and more likely to experience problems with medications or drugs.

Nervous system changes

Although it was long thought that mental dysfunction in the older patient was caused solely by senility, it is now well known that intellectual functioning deteriorates selectively and may result from many organic causes. For example, beginning at about 30 years of age, the total number of neurons in certain cortical areas decreases gradually, so by 70 years of age, a 10% reduction in brain weight has occurred. These factors, decreased cerebral blood flow, and changes in the location and amounts of specific neurotransmitters probably contribute to changes in the central nervous system (CNS). The velocity of nerve conduction in the peripheral nervous system decreases with ageing as well, which may lead to changes in motor or position sense and delays in reaction time and motor responses. Other gradual changes in the patient's nervous system can result in decreased visual acuity and auditory keenness and changes in sleep pattern.

Toxic or metabolic factors that can affect mental functioning include the use of medications (e.g. anticholinergics, antihypertensives, antidysrhythmics and analgesics); electrolyte imbalances; hypoglycaemia; acidosis; alkalosis; hypoxia; liver, kidney and lung failure; pneumonia; congestive heart failure (CHF); cardiac dysrhythmias; infection; and the development of benign or malignant tumours.

Musculoskeletal system changes

As the body ages, muscles shrink, muscles and ligaments calcify, and intervertebral discs become thin. Osteoporosis is common in older patients (especially in women) and an estimated 68% of older patients show some degree of kyphosis (Figure 39-1); this is a humpback posture. These musculoskeletal changes result in a decrease in total muscle mass, a decrease in height of 3 to 5 cm, widening and weakening of certain bones, and a posture that impairs mobility and alters the balance of the body. As a result, falls are common. Moreover, the falls often are associated with significant morbidity and mortality.

Prevention strategies (described in Chapter 3) that can decrease injuries associated with falls include the following:

- using walking aids (e.g. zimmer frame or stick)
- removing scatter rugs and securing loose carpeting
- removing items that may cause tripping
- providing and using handrails
- ensuring adequate lighting
- removing clutter from the environment
- arranging furniture for walking ease
- using non-slip mats in the baths or shower
- providing handrails on baths, showers and commodes.

Critical Thinking

Consider a patient who has significant kyphosis. What aspects of care will you need to alter to immobilize the spine of this patient?

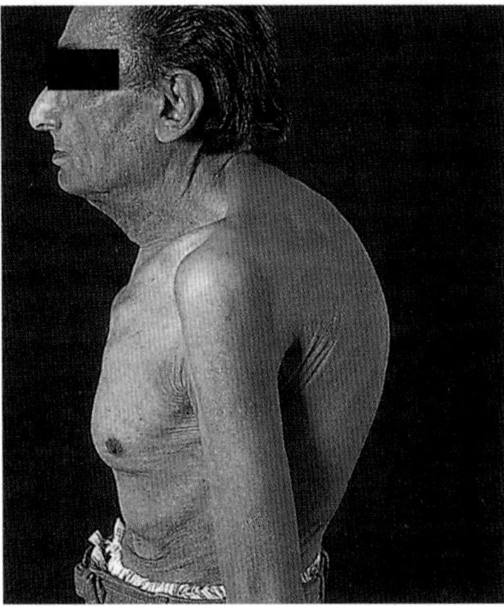

Figure 39-1 Kyphosis.

Other physiological changes

Other physiological changes that occur with ageing include changes in body mass and total body water, a decreased ability to maintain internal homeostasis, a decrease in the function of immunological mechanisms, nutritional disorders, and decreases in hearing and visual acuity.

As an individual approaches 65 years of age, lean body mass may decrease as much as 25%, and fat tissue may increase as much as 35%. These changes in body make-up can affect the dosage and frequency of administration of fat-soluble drugs; this is because there is more drug per weight of metabolically active tissue and a larger reservoir for build-up of the drug. In the same way, the decrease in total body water is likely to increase the concentration of water-soluble drugs.

The ability of the body to maintain normal temperature declines over time. The decline begins at about 30 years of age. Because of this, the older patient is at greater risk for cold- and heat-related conditions. These include hypothermia, heat exhaustion, and hyperthermia. Several factors contribute to the increased risk of thermoregulatory disorders, including impaired sympathetic nervous system function, causing decreased capacity for peripheral vasoconstriction, lowered metabolic rate, poor peripheral circulation, and chronic illness. Because of the decline in many body functions, including blood pressure, cardiac output, and temperature regulation, a specific illness or injury often puts the older patient 'over the edge'.

Ageing causes a decrease in primary antibody response and cellular immunity and elevations in the amount of abnormal immunoglobulins and immune complexes. These physiological changes increase the risk of infection, autoimmune disorders, and perhaps cancer. In addition, infections may not produce the usual signs and symptoms.

About one in eight deaths in older persons results from cancer. In younger patients, cancer often is the main or only disease from which they suffer, whereas older patients often have more than one disease and disability and signs/symptoms such as a change in bowel habits, rectal bleeding, malaise, fatigue, weight loss and anorexia may result from other conditions. Treatment with chemotherapy often results in immunosuppression, which increases the risk of infection and often masks the typical signs and symptoms associated with infection.

Many older patients consume less than the minimum daily requirement of most vitamins, which may be a result of loneliness and depression, decreased sensitivity to taste, decreased appetite, financial difficulties, physical infirmity, decreased vision, or a combination of these elements. All of these elements may act to reduce the motivation to shop for and prepare fresh food. Other factors associated with poor nutrition are poor dentition and reduced mastication, decreased oesophageal motility, frequent hypochlorhydria, and decreased intestinal secretions that reduce absorption. Older patients easily can become victims of malnutrition, which can cause dehydration and hypoglycaemia.

Critical Thinking

What effects can poor nutrition have on body function?

General principles in the assessment of the older patient

Normal physiological changes and underlying acute or long-term illness may make evaluation of an ill or injured older patient a challenge. In addition to the components of a normal physical assessment (described in Chapter 9), the paramedic should consider special characteristics of older patients that can complicate the clinical evaluation:

- Older patients are likely to suffer from more than one illness at a time.
- Long-term health problems can make assessment for acute problems difficult.
- Signs or symptoms of long-term illness can be confused with signs or symptoms of an acute problem.
- Ageing can affect an individual's response to illness or injury.
- Pain may be diminished or absent.
- The patient or paramedic can underestimate the severity of a condition.
- Social and emotional factors may have a greater influence on health in older patients than in any other age group.
- The patient fears losing autonomy.
- The patient fears the hospital environment.
- The patient has financial concerns about healthcare.

Patient history

Gathering a history from an older patient usually requires more time than with younger patients (see Chapter 8), and because of the patient's age, chronic illness and medication use, the older patient may have physical impediments such as hearing loss and visual impairment. Questioning a patient who is fatigued or easily distracted also may lengthen the interview process. The paramedic should use the following techniques when communicating with older patients:

- Always identify yourself.
- Speak at eye level to ensure that the patient can see you as you communicate.

- Locate a hearing aid, spectacles and dentures (if needed).
- Turn on lights.
- Speak slowly, distinctly and respectfully.
- Use the patient's surname, unless the patient requests otherwise.
- Listen closely.
- Be patient.
- Preserve dignity.
- Use gentleness.

Critical Thinking

Why should you ask older patients to bring all of their medications to the hospital?

Physical examination

When conducting the physical examination of an older patient, the paramedic should consider the following six points:

1. The patient may tire easily.
2. Older patients often wear many layers of clothing for warmth. This may hamper the examination.
3. Respect the patient's modesty and need for privacy unless it interferes with the care.
4. Explain actions clearly before examining all older patients; this is important with patients with diminished sight.
5. Be aware that the patient may minimize or deny their symptoms. Denial may be due to a fear of being bedridden or institutionalized or losing self-sufficiency.
6. Try to distinguish symptoms of long-term illness from acute problems.

If time allows, the paramedic should assess the older patient's immediate surroundings for evidence of alcohol or medication use (e.g. insulin syringes, 'vial of life' or MedicAlert or similar information), presence of food, general condition of housing, and signs of adequate personal hygiene. These and other observations help provide information to other healthcare professionals about the patient's general health and ability for self-care after release from the hospital.

The paramedic should question friends or family members who are present about the patient's appearance and responsiveness now versus the patient's normal appearance, responsiveness, and other characteristics. The paramedic also should discreetly ask about advance directives and initiation of care for the patient (described in Chapter 2). If these documents are available, the paramedic should obtain them and convey the information to medical direction. Finally, the paramedic should ensure gentle handling and padding for patient comfort if transport is needed.

System pathophysiology, assessment and management

The pathophysiology, assessment, and management of specific illnesses described in this section include those of the respiratory system, cardiovascular system, CNS, endocrine system, gastrointestinal system, integumentary system, musculoskeletal system and problems associated with special senses. Toxicology, environmental considerations, behavioural and mental health disorders, trauma, and elder abuse also are discussed in this section.

Respiratory system

Specific illnesses of the respiratory system that are common in older patients include bacterial pneumonia, chronic obstructive pulmonary disease and pulmonary embolism. These conditions are described in Chapter 14. They are presented here as a review.

Bacterial pneumonia

Pneumonia is a leading cause of death in the older age group and often is fatal in frail adults; older patients are more likely to develop bacteraemia. They also are more susceptible to several respiratory germs (e.g. Gram-negative bacilli) which, associated with the presence of long-term disease, impairs the ability of older adults to keep the respiratory tract clean. It also allows bacteria to grow in the throat that then may travel to or be aspirated into the lungs. Because of the decreased lung function, pneumonia often may be associated with respiratory failure. Risk factors for bacterial pneumonia include institutional environments, long-term illness and compromise of the immune system.

Unlike the younger patient with bacterial pneumonia, the usual clinical picture of fever, productive cough, pleurisy and signs of pulmonary congestion often is absent in the older patient; this atypical presentation is responsible for the common delay in diagnosis. The following are possible signs and symptoms:

- alterations in mental status
- cough
- fever (variable)
- shortness of breath
- tachycardia
- tachypnoea.

Older patients with pneumonia may be too weak to cough or produce sputum or may not be able to breathe deeply. Therefore breath sounds may be misleading because of pre-existing emphysema or chronic CHF. Tachycardia and tachypnoea often are the most reliable indicators of bacterial pneumonia in the prehospital setting.

Emergency care for older patients with bacterial pneumonia focuses on managing life threats, maintaining oxygenation, and providing transport for further evaluation as bacterial pneumonia is linked to a high rate of hospital admissions. Pneumonia generally is managed with antibiotics.

Critical Thinking

Why is the flu season linked to an increase in pneumonia in the elderly?

Chronic obstructive pulmonary disease

Chronic obstructive pulmonary disease (COPD) in the older patient is a major health problem in the UK. COPD is a common finding in the older patient with a history of smoking and is usually associated with various diseases that result in reduced expiratory air flow such as asthma, emphysema, and chronic bronchitis. An exacerbation of COPD often follows an acute respiratory infection that causes airway oedema, bronchial smooth muscle irritability and increased mucus secretion. These airway abnormalities may lead to factors associated with acute decompensation, including the following:

- limited air flow
- increased work of breathing
- dyspnoea
- ventilation–perfusion mismatching
- hypoxaemia
- respiratory acidosis
- haemodynamic compromise.

Signs and symptoms of COPD in the older patient include extreme anxiety, cyanosis, wheezing, and abnormal or diminished breath sounds associated with marked dyspnoea and the use of accessory muscles. Other signs and symptoms include dysrhythmias, paradoxical breathing, jugular vein distension, and decreased oxygen saturation levels via pulse oximetry. The paramedic should obtain a full history of the event, including a past history of intubation or steroid therapy. The paramedic also should be prepared for aggressive airway management. The care for a patient with COPD is aimed at correcting life-threatening hypoxaemia and improving air flow, and the use of airway and ventilatory support with supplemental oxygenation and the administration of bronchodilators is indicated. Failure to begin aggressive treatments to correct the acidosis and hypoxia from COPD can lead to a fast decline in the patient's condition.

Pulmonary embolism

Pulmonary embolism is a life-threatening cause of dyspnoea. In older adults this common condition is associated with venous stasis, heart failure, COPD, malignancy and immobilization. Most pulmonary emboli in older patients form in the veins of the legs and travel through the femoral veins to the inferior vena cava and the heart. The clinical presentation of pulmonary embolism often is misleading in older patients and frequently is misdiagnosed.

Signs and symptoms of pulmonary embolism may range from a presentation of left ventricular failure with sudden tachypnoea, unexplained tachycardia (a hallmark sign), and atrial fibrillation to signs and symptoms solely of the underlying venous thrombosis (calf discomfort without tenderness, mild calf or ankle oedema, increased warmth, and dilation of superficial veins in one foot or leg). Pulmonary embolism can cause CHF to develop. Pulmonary embolism also may be mistaken for bacterial pneumonia in older patients.

> **Critical Thinking**
>
> What other conditions have similar cardiovascular signs and symptoms?

Emergency care focuses on ensuring adequate airway, ventilatory and circulatory support, immobilizing and elevating an affected extremity and rapidly transporting the patient for physician evaluation. In-hospital care may include analgesics, bed rest, haemodynamic stabilization with intravenously administered fluids and vasopressors to support blood pressure, and efforts to prevent further embolization. Some patients may be given thrombolytics to dissolve the clot and anticoagulants to prevent further emboli.

Cardiovascular system

Cardiovascular disorders are described in Chapter 15. Specific disorders reviewed in this section include myocardial infarction, heart failure, dysrhythmias, abdominal and thoracic aneurysm, and hypertension.

Acute coronary syndrome and myocardial infarction

Chest pain as a symptom of acute coronary syndrome (ACS) becomes less frequent by 70 years of age and only 45% of patients over 85 years of age with ACS have this complaint. Lack of typical chest pain can cause ACS to go unrecognized in the older patient. The following are six major risk factors that the paramedic should evaluate when assessing a patient for ACS:

1. Previous ACS and infarction.
2. Angina.
3. Diabetes.
4. Hypertension.
5. High cholesterol level.
6. Smoking.

Some older patients have chest pain or discomfort. However, many complain only of vague symptoms. Examples of such include dyspnoea (the most common sign in patients over 85 years of age), abdominal or epigastric distress, and fatigue.

The mortality rate associated with acute infarction doubles after 70 years of age. For many older patients the event is totally 'silent' as a result of decreased visceral sensory function or a higher incidence of mental deterioration in this age group. Pain-free infarctions are almost always marked by an atypical complaint such as fatigue, breathlessness, nausea or abdominal pain and the paramedic must maintain a high index of suspicion for infarction in elderly patients with unusual warning signs or symptoms.

> **Critical Thinking**
>
> What hormonal change in older women increases their risk for heart disease?

Emergency care includes airway, ventilatory and circulatory support; oxygen administration and pain management therapy, thrombolytic therapy, if indicated, and management of serious dysrhythmias according to current guidelines; and rapid and smooth transportation for further evaluation.

Heart failure

Heart failure is more frequent in older patients. It also has a larger incidence of non-cardiac causes. Heart failure occurs when the ventricular output cannot meet the metabolic demands of the body. Heart failure often is caused by ischaemic heart disease, valvular heart disease, cardiomyopathy, dysrhythmias, hyperthyroidism and anaemia. The following are common signs and symptoms of heart failure:

- dyspnoea
- fatigue (often the first symptom of left-sided heart failure)
- orthopnoea
- dry, hacking cough progressing to productive cough with frothy sputum
- dependent oedema caused by right-sided heart failure
- nocturia
- anorexia, hepatomegaly, ascites.

Note

Differentiating among the causes of dyspnoea is difficult in the prehospital setting. However, such differentiation is important. If the patient has had acute episodes of heart failure in the past, the current emergency event also is likely to be heart failure – and a thorough patient history is important.

The emergency care is aimed at reversing the conditions associated with heart failure as soon as possible, which will help to prevent cardiac damage. In addition to oxygen administration and electrocardiograph monitoring, management may include intubation, intravenous (IV) therapy, and drug therapy (furosemide, nitrates and morphine).

Critical Thinking

How do furosemide, nitrates and morphine work to relieve the signs and symptoms of heart failure?

Dysrhythmias

The most common cause of dysrhythmias in the older patient is hypertensive heart disease. However, any condition that decreases blood flow to the heart can cause rhythm irregularities and the paramedic should consider the following:

- Premature ventricular contractions are common in most adults over 80 years of age.
- Atrial fibrillation is the most common dysrhythmia.
- Dysrhythmias may result from electrolyte imbalances or side effects of some medications as well as the effects of ageing (conduction defects and pacemaker site abnormalities).

In addition to the serious implications of some dysrhythmias, associated complications may include traumatic injury from falls that result from cerebral hypoperfusion, transient ischaemic attacks and heart failure. The paramedic should focus emergency care on ensuring adequate airway, ventilatory, and circulatory support; administering oxygen; and transporting the patient for further evaluation. The paramedic should manage serious dysrhythmias as described in Chapter 15.

Box 39-2

Signs and symptoms of abdominal and thoracic aneurysm

Absent or reduced pulses
Acute myocardial infarction
Chest pain
Diminished distal pulses
Heart failure
Hypotension
Low back pain or flank pain
Pericardial tamponade
Pulsatile, tender mass
Stroke
Sudden onset of abdominal or back pain
Syncope
Unexplained hypotension

Abdominal and thoracic aneurysm

Atherosclerotic disease is a common cause of abdominal and thoracic aneurysm. Abdominal aortic aneurysm affects about 2–4% of the UK population over 50 years of age. Acute dissecting aortic aneurysm is more common than abdominal aneurysm and is associated with a high mortality rate; signs and symptoms vary according to the site of rupture or extent of dissection (Box 39-2) but one way of assessing for thoracic dissection is to record blood pressure in both arms as a difference of >15 mmHg (systolic) is of concern. The patient may often present with very similar signs and symptoms, although the character of the pain in dissection is often tearing and sharp in nature.

The goals of prehospital care are relief of pain and immediate transport to a hospital. Airway, ventilatory, and circulatory support may be required if the patient's condition deteriorates. Other prehospital care measures include the following:

- gentle handling of the patient
- allaying anxiety
- high-concentration oxygen administration
- IV access and cautious use of fluid replacement if severe hypotension is present
- analgesia.

Hypertension

Older patients who have atherosclerosis also frequently have hypertension; associated risk factors for hypertension include advanced age, diabetes, and obesity. Hypertension is often defined by a resting blood pressure consistently greater than 140/90 mmHg; blood pressure greater than 160/95 mmHg doubles the mortality rate in men. Chronic hypertension is associated with many medical conditions, including the following:

- aneurysm formation
- blindness
- cardiac hypertrophy and left ventricular failure
- kidney failure
- myocardial ischaemia and infarction
- peripheral vascular disease
- stroke.

Hypertension in the older patient may only manifest in non-specific complaints such as headache, forgetfulness and general malaise; other signs and symptoms that may indicate chronic hypertension include epistaxis, tremors, and nausea and vomiting. Care is mainly supportive but the paramedic is in an excellent position to identify hypertension and provide advice to the patient (most importantly seeking advice from their GP). After physician evaluation, the patient with chronic hypertension often is managed with oral medications, dietary sodium reduction, weight loss, and exercise.

Note

The British Hypertension Society publishes guidelines for assessing and managing hypertension (http://www.bhsoc.org/default.stm). The 2004 guidelines identify blood pressure under 120/80 as optimal, with a pressure of <130/85 being normal. Mild hypertension is considered to exist when the systolic value is 140–159 and the diastolic is 90–99, and moderate hypertension when values are 160–179 systolic, 100–109 diastolic.

Nervous system

Neurological disorders were described in Chapter 16. Specific disorders described in this section for review include cerebral vascular disease, delirium, dementia, Alzheimer's disease and Parkinson's disease.

Cerebral vascular disease

Stroke is one of the leading causes of death in the developed world and a leading cause of brain injury in adults. It affects as many as 1 person in every 450 each year in the UK, with the majority affecting the population over 65 years of age. Moreover, it has a significant negative effect on lifestyle and ability to self-care after the initial episode. As described in Chapter 16 the neurological impairment is caused by an ischaemic or haemorrhagic interruption in the blood supply to the brain; associated risk factors for cerebral vascular disease in the older adult include smoking, hypertension, diabetes, atherosclerosis, hyperlipidaemia, polycythaemia and heart disease. Box 39-3 provides a review of the signs and symptoms of stroke and transient ischaemic attack.

Box 39-3

Signs and symptoms of stroke and transient ischaemic attack

Ataxia
Diplopia
Language disturbance
Monocular blindness
Numbness
Unilateral paralysis
Vertigo
Visual disturbance

Once the paramedic suspects stroke, time in the field must be minimized, in order that earlier therapy be commenced; less than 3 h from onset is recommended for fibrinolytic therapy. The paramedic should focus on managing the patient's airway, breathing, and circulation and on monitoring vital signs. Aside from supporting vital functions, the most important element of prehospital care for a stroke victim is identification of the patient with stroke and rapid transportation of the patient to an appropriate centre that can provide treatment within 1 h after arrival at the emergency department door.

The Department of Health (2006) have described several key ambitions for management and care of stroke patients which include the notion of a 'hub and spoke' care system, with specialist centres offering early scanning and care, within the key 3-h window. In some areas this will be easily achievable but in others less so. It will also require a change in procedure with the possibility of paramedics with suspected stroke patients bypassing a local A&E and taking a patient to a slightly more distant specialist centre.

Delirium

Delirium is an abrupt disorientation to time and place, which usually includes illusions and hallucinations. The patient's mind may 'wander', their speech may be incoherent and they may be in a state of mental confusion or excitement. Signs and symptoms vary according to personality, environment, and severity of illness; delirium commonly is a result of physical illness (associated with organic brain dysfunction) and may include the following:

- alcohol intoxication or withdrawal
- drug reactions
- fever
- metabolic disorders
- tumour.

Delirium can be life threatening and therefore requires emergency care. The condition may be reversible if it is diagnosed early but delirium can progress to chronic mental dysfunction. Prehospital care includes the following measures:

1. Ensure adequate airway, breathing and circulatory support.
   a. Manage hypoxia with oxygen.
   b. Manage hypotension with IV fluids if appropriate.
2. Reduce agitation and anxiety.
3. Avoid patient injury, and ensure personal safety.
   a. Restrain the patient if needed, per protocol.
   b. Sedate the patient as a last resort.

4. Consider hypoglycaemia or an opioids-induced state.
   a. Measure blood glucose level.
   b. Administer glucose or naloxone if appropriate.
5. Assess for CNS injury (e.g. trauma or stroke). Perform a careful neurological examination.
6. Look for signs of CNS infection (e.g. encephalitis).
7. Transport the patient for further evaluation.

Dementia

Dementia is a slow, progressive loss of awareness of time and place, with an inability to learn new things or recall recent events. Dementia is often a result of brain disease caused by strokes, genetic or viral factors, and Alzheimer's disease, and is generally considered irreversible. Dementia eventually results in full dependence on others as a result of the progressive loss of cognitive functioning. During the course of the disease, patients often try to cover up their memory loss, by confabulation (making up stories to fill gaps in memory). Sudden outbursts or embarrassing conduct may be the first clear signs of dementia and some patients eventually regress to a 'second childhood'; at that point, they need full care for their activities of living. Dementia is present in about 50% of nursing home residents and affects, to some degree, about 20% of those over 80 years of age.

Dementia can be difficult to differentiate from delirium in the prehospital setting. The key difference between the two is that delirium is new with rapid onset, and dementia is progressive (Table 39-2), so a history of the event from a reliable witness (e.g. friend or family member) is the best source of information; a history provided by the patient may be unreliable. If a good witness is not available, the paramedic should manage the patient for delirium that may be a life-threatening emergency.

Alzheimer's disease

Alzheimer's disease is a condition in which nerve cells in the cerebral cortex die and the brain substance shrinks. The disease is the single most common cause of dementia and is responsible for the majority of cases in persons over 75 years of age. Alzheimer's disease does not cause death directly; patients ultimately stop eating and become malnourished and immobilized and are prone to concurrent infections.

The cause of Alzheimer's disease is still not fully understood, although much current work into the process is underway; possible causes have been thought to include abnormalities in glutamate metabolism, chronic infection, toxic poisoning by metals, reduction in brain chemicals (e.g. acetylcholine), and genetics. Atherosclerosis is not a cause of Alzheimer's disease; the primary disorder is in the nerve cells, not the blood vessels.

Table 39-2 Differential diagnosis for delirium and dementia

	Delirium	**Dementia**
Onset	Abrupt	Gradual
Characteristics	Reduced attention span	Impaired recent memory
	Disorganized thinking	Regression
	Hallucinations	Poor judgement

Early symptoms of Alzheimer's disease mainly are related to memory loss, especially the ability to make and recall new memories (Box 39-4).

As the disease progresses, agitation, violence and impairment of abstract thinking occur; judgement and cognitive abilities begin to interfere with work and social relations. In the advanced stages of Alzheimer's disease, patients often become bedridden and totally unaware of their surroundings. Once the patient is bedridden, skin breakdown due to pressure sores, feeding problems, and pneumonia often shorten the patient's life.

No specific treatment exists for Alzheimer's disease and management mainly consists of nursing and social care for the patient and relatives; the paramedic manages patients with this disease the same as for dementia.

Parkinson's disease

As described in Chapter 16, Parkinson's disease is a brain disorder caused by degeneration of and damage to the part of the brain producing dopamine (substantia nigra) which causes dopamine shortage direct effects on smooth muscle contraction. This causes tremor, joint rigidity, and slow movement. Characteristic signs of Parkinson's disease are trembling (usually beginning in one hand, arm or leg), a rigid posture, slow movements, and a shuffling, unbalanced walk. If left untreated, the disease progresses over 10 to 15 years to severe weakness and incapacity. Parkinson's disease affects about 130 people per 100 000 population and is a leading cause of neurological disability in the over 60s.

The emergency care for these patients mainly is supportive. It includes airway, ventilatory and circulatory support, and transport for further evaluation. Parkinson's disease has no cure. However, counselling, exercise, special aids in the home, and drug therapy can improve the patient's morale, mobility and quality of life.

Box 39-4

The seven warning signs of Alzheimer's disease

1. Asking the same question over and over again.
2. Repeating the same story, word for word, again and again.
3. Forgetting how to cook, or how to make repairs, or how to play cards – activities that were previously done with ease and regularity.
4. Losing one's ability to pay bills or balance one's chequebook.
5. Getting lost in familiar surroundings, or misplacing household objects.
6. Neglecting to bathe or wearing the same clothes over and over again, while insisting that they have taken a bath or that their clothes are still clean.
7. Relying on someone else, such as a spouse, to make decisions or answer questions they previously would have handled themselves.

From Alzheimer's Disease Education & Referral Center: The seven warning signs of Alzheimer's disease. http://www.nia.nih.gov/Alzheimers/Publications/sevensigns.htm. Reprinted with the permission of the Suncoast Gerontology Center, University of South Florida. Revised September 1, 1999.

Endocrine system

Two common endocrine disorders often are seen in older patients; diabetes and thyroid disease (described in Chapter 17). The following is a review of these conditions.

Diabetes

About 20% of older adults have diabetes, and almost 40% have some impaired glucose tolerance. Type 2 (non-insulin-dependent) diabetes is most common in older patients and more common when the person is overweight. The following are associated risk factors in older adults for complications related to diabetes:

- decreased ability to care for self
- living alone
- concurrent illness
- decline in renal function
- polydrug use.

A combination of dietary measures, weight reduction, and oral hypoglycemic agents can usually keep type 2 diabetes under control; in most cases, insulin injections are not required for type 2 diabetes. However, if poorly controlled, diabetes can lead to complications such as retinopathy, peripheral neuropathy (ulcers on the feet are common), and kidney damage. Diabetic patients also have a higher-than-average risk for atherosclerosis, hypertension and other cardiovascular disorders, and for cataracts. Emergency care for diabetic patients is outlined in Chapter 17 and includes airway, ventilatory, and circulatory support; blood glucose measurement; IV glucose (if indicated and in the absence of cerebral damage); and transport for further evaluation.

Hyperglycaemic hyperosmolar non-ketotic coma, described in Chapter 17, is a serious complication of elderly type 2 diabetic patients, with a mortality rate of 20–50%. The paramedic often finds the type 2 diabetic patient comatose, but if awake, the patient may complain of profound thirst and frequent urination as a result of osmotic diuresis, leading to dehydration and electrolyte loss. Predisposing factors that make the older patient susceptible to hyperglycaemic hyperosmolar non-ketotic coma include infection, non-concordance with medications, polydrug use (polypharmacy), pancreatitis, stroke, hypothermia, heat stroke, and myocardial infarction. If the paramedic suspects hyperglycaemic hyperosmolar non-ketotic coma, the paramedic should ensure adequate airway, ventilatory, and circulatory support; should search vigorously for an underlying cause; should initiate IV fluid therapy; and should transport the patient rapidly for further evaluation.

Critical Thinking

What finding is present in the patient with diabetic ketoacidosis yet is absent in the patient with hyperglycaemic hyperosmolar non-ketotic coma?

Thyroid disease

Thyroid disease is more common in older patients and may be related to the ageing process. The classic signs and symptoms of thyroid disorders (e.g. fullness in the neck, goitre, muscle or joint pain) may not be present in the older patient so the paramedic should consider thyroid dysfunction in any older patient who is ill, especially if the cause of illness is unclear.

The older patient often attributes the signs and symptoms of hypothyroidism to 'growing old'; common complaints include weight loss, non-specific musculoskeletal complaints, and confusion. More serious conditions associated with this disorder include CHF, anaemia, hyponatraemia, depression, dementia, seizures and coma. Hyperthyroidism is less common than hypothyroidism in elderly patients; hyperthyroidism may result from medication errors (e.g. too many doses of a thyroid hormone replacement). Signs and symptoms of hyperthyroidism include weight loss, constipation, mental status changes, CHF, tachydysrhythmias and lethargy.

The emergency care is mainly supportive to ensure vital functions. The patient with thyroid disease will require further evaluation and possible treatment with various thyroid drugs, radioactive iodine treatments, and sometimes surgery. Severe complications from thyroid disease include thyroid storm and myxoedema coma (described in Chapter 17), which may be made worse in a patient who has heart disease.

Gastrointestinal system

Gastrointestinal emergencies (described in Chapter 19) are common in the older adult. The paramedic should always consider abdominal pain a serious complaint in a older patient. Life-threatening causes of abdominal pain in this age group include abdominal aortic aneurysm, gastrointestinal haemorrhage, ruptured viscus, dead or ischaemic bowel, and acute bowel obstruction. Specific disorders discussed in this section are gastrointestinal haemorrhage, bowel obstruction, problems with continence, and problems with elimination.

Gastrointestinal haemorrhage

Gastrointestinal bleeding most commonly affects patients between 60 and 90 years of age, with a mortality rate of about 10%. The older the patient, the higher the risk of death, due to the following:

- Older patients are less able to compensate for acute blood loss.
- They are less likely to feel symptoms and therefore seek treatment at later stages of disease.
- They are more likely to be taking aspirin or non-steroidal anti-inflammatory drugs, which places them at higher risk for ulcer disease and bleeding.
- They are at higher risk for colon cancer, intestinal vascular abnormalities, and diverticulitis.
- They are more likely to be on blood-thinning medications.

Signs and symptoms of gastrointestinal bleeding include vomiting of blood or coffee-ground emesis; blood-tinged stools or black, tarry stools; and weakness, syncope or pain. If the paramedic suspects or confirms bleeding in a patient with signs and symptoms of shock, the paramedic should begin measures to ensure adequate airway, ventilatory, and circulatory support. The paramedic also should transport the patient rapidly for definitive care.

Bowel obstruction

Bowel obstruction generally occurs in patients with prior abdominal surgeries or hernias and also in those with colonic cancer. Most complain of constipation, abdominal cramping and an inability to pass wind; other signs and symptoms can include protracted vomiting of food or bile and vomiting of faecal material. The patient's heart rate and blood pressure often are in normal ranges but the abdomen may be mildly distended and tender in all four quadrants; the pain is often variable.

The prehospital care mainly is supportive to ensure vital functions. After medical evaluation, patient care may include bowel rest, nasogastric suction and volume replacement. Some patients may need surgery to lyse the offending adhesions but this may result in a cycle of new scarring and obstruction. They also may need surgery for hernia repair (most often in men).

Problems with continence

Continence is the ability to control bladder or bowel function and requires anatomically correct gastrointestinal and genitourinary tracts, competent sphincter mechanisms, cognitive and physical function, and motivation. Some factors associated with continence are affected by age and include a decrease in bladder capacity, involuntary bladder contractions, decreased ability to postpone voiding, and medications that can affect bladder and bowel control. Incontinence of urine or bowel is abnormal at any age.

Urinary incontinence can vary in severity. It can be only mild incontinence (the escape of small amounts of urine) or it can be total incontinence, with complete loss of bladder control. Causes of urinary incontinence include injury or disease of the urinary tract, prolapse of the uterus, a decline in sphincter muscle control surrounding the urethra (common in the elderly), CNS injury or disease, pelvic fracture, prostate cancer and dementia.

Bowel incontinence in the older patient usually is the result of faecal impaction, which occurs when faeces lodged in the rectum irritate and inflame the lining. This allows faecal fluid and small faeces to pass involuntarily. Other causes of bowel incontinence include severe diarrhoea, injury to anal muscles (from childbirth or surgery), CNS injury or disease, and dementia.

All forms of incontinence usually are embarrassing for the patient. If incontinence is chronic, it can lead to skin irritation, tissue breakdown and urinary tract infection. Some cases are managed with surgery to restore sphincter function. Patients with mild cases often wear absorptive undergarments to relieve discomfort and embarrassment.

> **Critical Thinking**
>
> Consider the incontinent patient. How can you minimize the patient's embarrassment and discomfort?

Problems with elimination

Causes of difficulty in urination usually result from enlargement of the prostate (in men), urinary tract infection, urethral strictures, and acute or chronic renal failure. Difficulty in bowel elimination is often associated with diverticular disease, constipation and colorectal cancer. Problems with elimination can cause great pain and anxiety for older patients. The paramedic should take their complaints seriously; these conditions call for further evaluation to identify the cause and select the appropriate therapy.

Integumentary system

As we age, the skin gradually becomes dry, transparent and wrinkled. These integumentary changes are associated with a loss of elasticity, uneven pigmentation, and various benign and malignant lesions. In addition, ageing results in a gradual decrease in epidermal cellular turnover as well as a reduced rate of nail and hair growth. The associated loss of deep, dermal vessels and capillary circulation leads to common complaints such as dry, itchy skin; changes in thermal regulation; and skin-related complications. Some of these complications include the following:

- slow healing
- increased risk of secondary infection
- increased risk of fungal or viral infections
- increased susceptibility to abrasions and tears.

The paramedic should always be gentle with the skin of an older patient; for example, the use of aseptic technique during wound management, gentle placement and removal of electrocardiogram electrodes, and using careful taping procedures when securing IV cannulae or giving set tubing.

> **Critical Thinking**
>
> Consider an older patient who has a burn injury. How do these changes influence the patient's recovery?

Pressure ulcers

Pressure ulcers (also known as decubitus ulcers) are common in older patients (Figure 39-2) and often develop on the skin of patients who are bedridden or immobile. Most pressure ulcers occur in the lower legs, back, and buttocks, and over bony areas such as the greater trochanter or the sacrum. They often affect victims of stroke or other illnesses that result in a loss or change in the sensation of pain. Skin exposure to moisture (e.g. from incontinence), poor nutrition, and friction or shear also may be factors for developing pressure ulcers; other causes of pressure ulcers in older patients include vascular and metabolic disorders (e.g. venous stasis and diabetes), trauma and cancer.

Pressure ulcers result from tissue hypoxia; they generally start as red, painful areas that become purple before the skin breaks down, and then further develop into open sores. Once integrity of the skin has been breached, the sores often become infected, with a delay in healing. Pressure ulcers should be covered with sterile dressing using aseptic technique. The patient must be referred to further appropriate care.

Musculoskeletal system

Musculoskeletal changes occur as part of the ageing process; two musculoskeletal conditions that are common in older patients are osteoarthritis and osteoporosis.

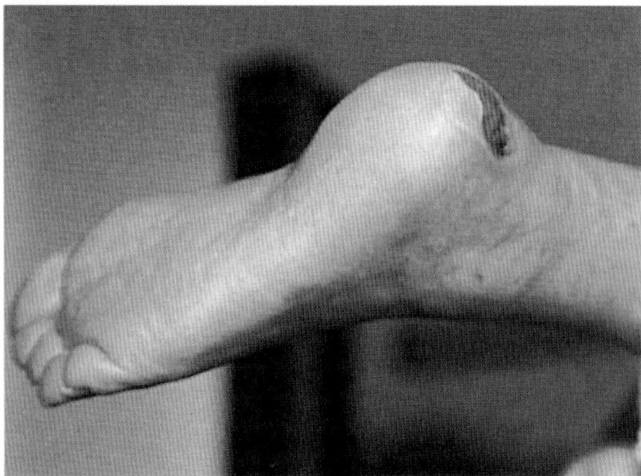

Figure 39-2 Pressure ulcer.

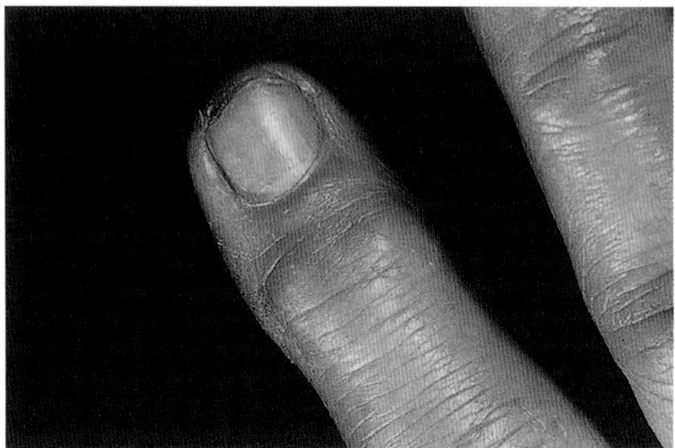

Figure 39-3 Osteoarthritis.

Osteoarthritis

Osteoarthritis is a common form of arthritis in older patients. It is a degenerative condition which results from cartilage loss and wear and tear on the joints (Figure 39-3). The condition leads to pain, stiffness, and sometimes loss of function of the affected joint, which becomes large and distorted from outgrowths of new bone (osteophytes) that tend to develop at the margins of the joint surface. Osteoarthritis evolves in the middle years and occurs to some extent in almost all persons over 60 years of age; although some people have no symptoms. After medical evaluation, treatment may include medications (analgesics, non-steroidal anti-inflammatory drugs, corticosteroids), physical therapy, and sometimes joint replacement surgery. Newer drugs (cyclooxygenase-2 inhibitors) such as celecoxib relieve the inflammation and pain associated with arthritis. These newer drugs have less risk of causing stomach irritation than traditional medications such as aspirin, non-steroidal anti-inflammatory drugs, and ibuprofen.

Osteoporosis

Osteoporosis is a natural part of ageing; it especially is common in older women after menopause, due to a decrease in the hormone oestrogen that helps maintain bone mass. Osteoporosis is present in most people by 70 years of age, by which time the density of the skeleton has diminished by one-third. Most persons with osteoporosis have some degree of kyphosis.

The loss of bone density causes bones to become brittle; consequently, they can fracture easily and this is often the first sign of osteoporosis. Typical sites for fractures are just above the wrist, at the head of the femur, and at one of several vertebrae (often a spontaneous fracture). Osteoporosis is treated with preventive measures such as a diet high in calcium, calcium supplements, exercise, and hormone replacement therapy after menopause (which is controversial).

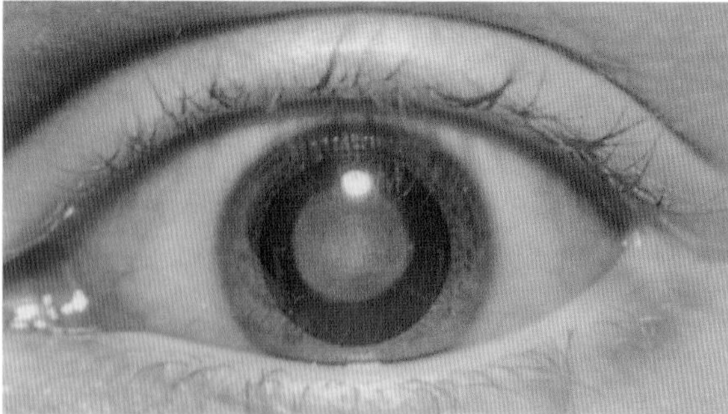

Figure 39-4 Appearance of an eye with a cataract.

Special problems with sensations

As persons age, they may experience problems with vision, hearing and speech.

Problems with vision

Vision changes begin to occur at around 40 years of age with a gradual loss over time. Vision impairments can severely limit daily activities with a loss of independence in older patients. The following are some effects of ageing on vision:

- reading difficulties
- poor depth perception
- poor adjustment of the eyes to variations in distance
- altered colour perception
- sensitivity to light
- decreased visual acuity.

Two common eye conditions that develop with age are cataracts and glaucoma. A cataract is a loss of transparency of the lens of the eye, resulting from changes in the delicate protein fibres within the lens (Figure 39-4). A cataract never causes full blindness, yet clarity and detail of an image progressively are lost. Cataracts usually occur in both eyes but in most cases one eye is affected more severely than the other. Almost everyone over 65 years of age has some degree of cataract; most persons over 75 years of age have minor visual deterioration from the disorder. Surgery to remove the cataract is a common procedure.

Glaucoma is a condition in which intraocular pressure increases, causing damage to the optic nerve. The result is nerve fibre destruction and partial or full loss of peripheral and central vision (Figure 39-5). Glaucoma may result from ageing (rarely seen before 40 years of age), a congenital abnormality, or trauma to the eye. Glaucoma is the most common major eye disorder in persons over 60 years of age

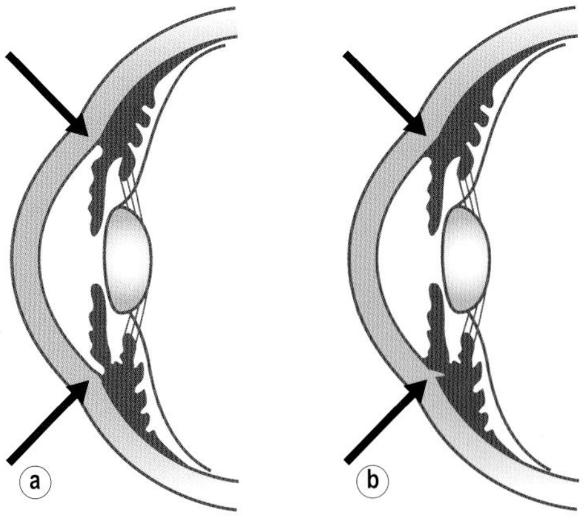

Figure 39-5 Glaucoma. (a) Open-angle glaucoma. The obstruction to aqueous flow lies in the trabecular meshwork. (b) Closed-angle glaucoma. The trabecular meshwork is covered by the root of the iris. From Stein HA, Slatt BJ, Stein RM 1988 The ophthalmic assistant: fundamentals in clinical practice. Mosby, St Louis.

and is a leading cause of preventable blindness. Symptoms of acute glaucoma include dull, severe, aching pain in and above the eye; fogginess of vision; and the perception of 'rainbow rings' (halos) around lights at night. Testing for glaucoma is part of most eye examinations in adults, and if detected early, the condition can be treated with oral medications and eye drops to relieve pressure.

> **Critical Thinking**
>
> Consider the patient who has glaucoma. What prehospital cardiac medication should not be given to this patient?

Problems with hearing

Not all older patients have hearing loss, though overall hearing tends to decrease with age. This results from degeneration of the hearing mechanism (sensorineural deafness). Ménière's disease (increased fluid pressure in the labyrinth), certain drugs, tumours, and some viral infections also can cause hearing problems. Hearing loss can interfere with the ability to perceive speech and it can limit the ability to communicate. Hearing aid devices and surgical implants sometimes can restore or improve hearing.

Tinnitus can occur as a symptom of many ear disorders. The noise in the ear (e.g. ringing, buzzing or whistling) sometimes may change in nature and intensity. However, in most cases it is present at all times with intermittent awareness by the person. Tinnitus is almost always associated with hearing loss, especially hearing loss that develops from ageing.

> **Critical Thinking**
>
> What common analgesic, when taken in excess, can cause tinnitus?

Problems with speech

Speech is the most often used method of communication. Common problems with speech in older patients often are associated with difficulty in word retrieval, decreased fluency of speech, slowed rate of speech and changes in voice quality. These disorders may occur from damage to the language centres of the brain (usually as a result of stroke, head injury or brain tumour), degenerative changes in the nervous system, hearing loss, disorders of the larynx, and poor-fitting dentures.

Toxicology

As described in Chapter 12, older patients are at increased risk for adverse drug reactions. This is the result of age-related changes in body composition, drug absorption, distribution, metabolism and excretion.

Age-related changes that affect absorption include increased gastric pH and decreased gastrointestinal motility; both of these may increase or decrease absorption of various drugs, depending on the chemical properties of the drug. Drug distribution may be affected by decreased cardiac output (e.g. as seen in CHF), decreased total body water, changes in the ratio of lean mass to fat, and increased body fat. Metabolic changes may result from decreased liver blood flow; diseases such as thyroid disease, CHF, and cancer; smoking; and drug interactions. Drug-induced metabolic changes are especially significant in the elderly; this is because they often take several different drugs for multiple diseases and conditions, which further increases their risk for adverse drug reactions. Renal function decreases with age in the majority of adults. This can lead to a build-up of drugs that normally are cleared through the renal system. In addition, the action of drugs affecting the CNS (e.g. benzodiazepines, anaesthetics and opiates) and the cardiovascular system (e.g. beta-blockers, calcium channel blockers and diuretics) often is altered in older adults. Because of these changes, drugs may not produce the desired effect or may cause major drug toxicity in older adults. Drugs that commonly cause toxicity in the older patient include the following:

- analgesics
- angiotensin-converting enzyme (ACE) inhibitors
- antidepressants
- antihypertensives
- beta-blockers
- digitalis
- diuretics
- psychotropics.

The adverse reactions associated with these and other drugs often result from 'accidents' or 'mishaps' in the prescribed drug regimen. Other common reasons for drug-induced illness in the older patient include dispensing errors, non-concordance, confusion, forgetfulness, vision impairment and the self-selection of drugs. In addition, older adults commonly have several prescriptions from more than one physician; improperly resume an old medication in addition to a newly prescribed one; or take prescribed medications along with over-the-counter drugs that may have synergistic or cumulative effects. Finally, changes in

Box 39-5

Symptoms of drug toxicity and adverse drug reactions in the older patient

Acute delirium
Akathisia
Altered vision
Bradycardia
Cardiac dysrhythmias
Chorea
Confusion
Constipation
Coma
Fatigue
Glaucoma
Hypokalaemia
Orthostatic hypotension
Paraesthesias
Psychological disturbances
Pulmonary oedema
Severe bleeding
Tardive dyskinesia
Urinary hesitancy

Box 39-6

Signs of substance abuse

Alcohol abuse

Anorexia
Confusion
Denial
Frequent falling
Hostility
Insomnia
Mood swings

Note: Ingestion of even small amounts of alcohol by the older patient can cause intoxication.

Other drug abuse

Altered level of consciousness
Falling
Hallucinations
Memory changes
Orthostatic hypotension
Poor coordination
Restlessness
Weight loss

Note: Individuals often have a history of alcohol and other drug abuse.

habits regarding alcohol, diet and exercise also can affect drug metabolism; these changes can increase the risk for adverse drug reactions. The emergency care for older patients with adverse drug reactions varies. Care may range from transport only to full advanced life support measures. Box 39-5 lists symptoms of drug toxicity and adverse reactions that can occur in the older patient.

Substance abuse

Substance abuse involving alcohol and other drugs is more common in the older population than might be expected, with men being more affected and alcohol rather than other drugs being the substance that is taken.

Substance abuse in the older patient often is attributed to severe stress as the primary risk factor. This stress may result from life changes such as age-related changes in health or appearance, loss of employment, loss of spouse or life partner, illness, malnutrition, loneliness, loss of independent living arrangements, and others. Box 39-6 lists signs of substance abuse.

If the paramedic suspects substance abuse, the paramedic should ask about this possibility with friends and family at the scene. The paramedic should ask them discreetly about the patient's alcohol or drug use. The cornerstones of therapy for these patients are identifying the problem and arranging referral for treatment. Treatment for the acutely intoxicated patient is described in Chapter 21 and may include resuscitative measures to manage the patient's airway, ventilation and circulation. In addition, the paramedic should carefully assess the older patient who has signs and symptoms of alcohol or other drug intoxication for hidden trauma injuries and any underlying medical conditions. These conditions may include hypoglycaemia, cardiomyopathy and dysrhythmias, gastrointestinal bleeding, polydrug/polypharmacy use (especially barbiturates and tranquillizers), and ethylene glycol or methanol ingestion.

Environmental considerations

Elderly patients are at risk for developing illness from extremes in the environment as a result of the ageing process and other factors (see Chapter 23). Two emergencies that relate to the environment are most common in older patients: hypothermia and hyperthermia.

Hypothermia

Patients who are younger often develop hypothermia from extremes in the environment; by contrast, an older patient may develop hypothermia while indoors. This may occur as a result of cold surroundings and/or an illness that alters heat production or conservation. This is due in part to the following characteristics of older adults:

- They are less able to make up for environmental heat loss.
- They have a decreased ability to sense changes in temperature.
- They have less total body water to store heat.
- They are less likely to develop tachycardia to increase cardiac output in response to cold stress.
- They have a decreased ability to shiver to increase body heat.

In addition to these physical changes, older patients are more prone to develop hypothermia as a result of socioeconomic factors. For instance, a fixed income may inhibit an older person from paying for the cost of properly heating and insulating his or her home and poor nutrition that results in a decrease in fat stores may contribute to hypothermia in older patients who live alone. The following are other medical causes of hypothermia in older patients:

- arthritis
- drug overdose
- hepatic failure
- hypoglycaemia
- infection
- Parkinson's disease
- stroke
- thyroid disease
- uraemia.

The signs and symptoms of hypothermia may be subtle. They may include an altered mental state, slurred speech, ataxia and dysrhythmias. In severe cases, coma without signs of life may be present. Hypothermia in the older patient carries a high mortality rate, with those aged over 85 years at greater risk. The paramedic should manage these patients as described in Chapter 23. Rapid and gentle transport for in-hospital rewarming and life support measures is crucial for the patient's survival.

Hyperthermia

Hyperthermia in the older patient is less common than hypothermia, yet hyperthermia carries a significant mortality rate. The condition most likely results from exposure to high temperatures. These temperatures most likely continue for several days (e.g. during a heat wave). As in hypothermia, older patients are unable to control body temperature even in moderate heat. Hyperthermia also may result from medical conditions such as hypothalamic dysfunction and spinal cord injury as well as certain medications (e.g. antidysrhythmics, beta-blockers and cyclic antidepressants). They do this by inhibiting heat dissipation, increasing motor activity, and impairing cardiovascular function.

As described in Chapter 23, hyperthermic illness may present as heat cramps, heat exhaustion or heat stroke. Emergency care includes removing the patient from the warm environment, cooling the patient, and ensuring the patient's vital functions through airway, ventilatory, and circulatory support. Rapid transport for further evaluation is indicated to manage the problems resulting from serious heat-related illness.

Behavioural and psychiatric disorders

Quite a number of older persons are expected to suffer from some kind of mental health illness as they grow older. In addition to the neurological disorders such as dementia and Alzheimer's disease, depression and suicide are common in older patients.

Depression

Depression is a serious illness that calls for specialist evaluation. In the older patient, depression can result from physiological and psychological causes such as cognitive disorders with physical causes (e.g. dementia) and various personality disorders such as schizophrenia, and occurs in around 1 in 16 older persons. Box 39-7 lists other physiological and psychological causes of depression in the older patient. The signs and symptoms of depression vary by individual. They may include the following:

Box 39-7

Common causes of depression in the older patient

Physiological

Dehydration
Electrolyte imbalance
Fever
Hyponatraemia
Hypoxia
Medications
Metabolic disturbances
Organic brain disease
Reduced cardiac output
Thyroid disease

Psychological

Fear of dying
Financial insecurity
Loss of a spouse
Loss of independence
Significant illness

- decreased libido
- deep feelings of worthlessness and guilt
- extreme isolation
- feelings of hopelessness
- irritability
- loss of appetite
- loss of energy (fatigue)
- recurrent thoughts of death
- significant weight loss
- sleeplessness
- suicide attempts.

Critical Thinking

What endocrine disorder can produce signs or symptoms that are similar to those of depression?

A major goal of care is to identify the patient who may be depressed, so that they can be evaluated by a specialist practitioner who can rule out medical illness, especially thyroid disease, stroke, malignancy, and dementia; or medication use (e.g. beta-blockers) that may be responsible for the patient's depression. After determining that there are no physical threats to life, the paramedic should try to establish a rapport with the patient who is depressed. The paramedic should encourage the patient to talk openly about feelings, especially any thoughts of suicide. The use of the suicide risk assessment tool may be helpful in determining level of risk. If possible, the paramedic should interview the family about the patient's mental health state and question family members about any history of depression in the patient.

Suicide

The rate of completed suicides for older patients is higher than that for the general population, and many of these persons visit their general practitioner or primary healthcare professional in the month before the suicide. Many may be suffering from their first episode of major depression, often only moderately severe, yet the depressive symptoms can go unrecognized and untreated. Importantly, the paramedic should be aware of the increased risk for suicide when evaluating older patients who are depressed. Clues and indicators for suicide in the older patient may be obtained through a patient history, risk assessment tools, or observations by friends and family. Some important indicators may include:

- Talking about or seemingly preoccupied with death and 'getting affairs in order'.
- Giving away prized possessions (e.g. family heirlooms, photographs, and keepsakes).
- Taking unnecessary risks (e.g. walking alone in unsafe areas or driving without personal restraints).
- Increased use of alcohol or other drugs.
- Non-adherence to a healthcare regimen (e.g. failure to take prescribed medications).
- Acquiring a weapon, especially firearms.

It is felt by most experts that there is no evidence that questions by the paramedic about suicidal thoughts and feelings increase the risk of suicide. Many depressed persons are willing to discuss their suicidal thoughts; therefore the paramedic should question the patient about suicidal thoughts if he or she suspects that the patient is at high risk. The following questions are appropriate for the paramedic to ask the patient:

1. Do you have thoughts about killing yourself?
2. Have you ever tried to kill yourself?
3. Have you thought about how you might kill yourself?

A number of suicides committed by older adults involve firearms, therefore the safety of those at the scene and the emergency medical services crew is a priority when caring for a patient with suicidal tendencies. When indicated, police support should be available at the scene. After assessing the risk for suicidal tendencies, the paramedic should transport the patient for further evaluation. While en route to the hospital, the paramedic should encourage the patient to discuss his or her feelings and reassure the patient that he or she can be helped through the crisis.

Trauma

Trauma is a leading cause of death for persons over 65 years of age, responsible for around a quarter of all UK trauma deaths. Major causes include road traffic collisions, falls and burns, and older persons have a higher mortality rate than other adults. Contributing factors that increase the severity of traumatic injury in older patients include the following:

- Osteoporosis and muscle weakness increase the likelihood of falls and fractures.
- Reduced cardiac reserve decreases the ability to compensate for blood loss.
- Decreased respiratory function increases the likelihood of adult respiratory distress syndrome.
- Impaired renal function decreases the ability to adapt to fluid shifts.

Vehicular trauma

There are approximately 5.5 million licence holders aged 65 years and over in the UK, with around 250 000 of those in the '85 years and over' age group. Most of these vehicle collisions are not related to high speed or alcohol but to errors in perception or judgement or to delayed reaction time. A large number of older adults are injured as drivers or passengers in moving vehicles, as well as others fatally injured as pedestrians.

The risk of death from multiple trauma is estimated to be three times greater at 70 years of age than at 20 years of age, because the older patient is more susceptible to serious injury from equivalent degrees of trauma. This patient also is less capable of an appropriate, protective physiological response. Prompt identification of injuries and sources of haemorrhage is critical in any trauma patient but is especially important in the older patient, as they have much less cardiac reserve and succumb more quickly to shock.

Head trauma

A head injury with loss of consciousness in older patients often has a poor outcome. The brain becomes smaller in size with age; this cerebral atrophy produces an increase in distance between the surface of the brain and the skull. As veins are stretched across this space, they more easily are torn, resulting in subdural haematomata. The extra space within the skull often allows a large amount of bleeding to occur before signs and symptoms of increased intracranial pressure are seen.

Critical Thinking

Consider older patients with head trauma. What home medications also can lead to an increased risk of intracerebral bleeding in these patients?

Older patients also are at high risk for injuries of the cervical spine because of the arthritic and degenerative changes associated with ageing. These structural changes lead to increased stiffening and decreased flexibility of the spine with narrowing of the spinal canal and make the spinal cord much more at risk for damage from fairly minor trauma.

Chest injuries

Any mechanism of injury that produces thoracic trauma in a older patient can be potentially lethal. The aged thorax is less elastic and is more susceptible to injury. The pulmonary system also has marginal reserve because of a reduced alveolar surface area, decreased patency of small airways, and diminished chemoreceptor response.

Injuries to the heart, aorta and major vessels are a greater risk to older patients than they are to younger patients. Again, this is due to decreased functional reserve in older patients as well as anatomical changes that make injury in these areas of greater significance. Myocardial contusion may be a complication of blunt injury to the chest. If severe, myocardial contusion may result in pump failure or life-threatening dysrhythmias. Rarely, cardiac tamponade occurs after blunt thoracic trauma. Cardiac rupture, valvular injury (e.g. flail valves) and aortic dissection also may occur with significant blunt chest injury. The first two entities are rare but rapidly fatal. When the mechanism of injury produces rapid deceleration, the paramedic should always consider the possibility of dissecting aortic aneurysm. Aortic dissections are often not immediately fatal, and proper evaluation and treatment can be lifesaving.

Critical Thinking

Consider the patient who has a dissecting aortic aneurysm. What specific signs and symptoms may the paramedic see in this patient?

In the older patient the heart cannot respond as effectively to increased demand for oxygen as in the younger person; this, coupled with a slowed conduction system, may cause ischaemia and dysrhythmias when the older patient has a significant trauma. These problems may occur even if the heart has not been damaged directly by the trauma. The paramedic should watch these patients' oxygenation and circulatory status closely.

Abdominal injuries

Abdominal injuries in older patients have more serious consequences than injuries to any other body area; often they are less obvious and call for a high degree of suspicion. The older patient is less likely to tolerate abdominal surgery well and is more likely to develop lung problems and infection following surgery.

Musculoskeletal injuries

The osteoporotic bones of older patients are more at risk for fractures and can fracture with even mild trauma. Pelvic fractures are highly lethal in this age group. They can cause severe haemorrhage and soft tissue injury. When assessing for skeletal trauma, the paramedic should recall that the older patient may have decreased pain perception; often these patients have amazingly little tenderness with major fractures. Even with proper care, the mortality rate for older patients with musculoskeletal injury is increased by delayed complications such as adult respiratory distress syndrome, sepsis, renal failure and pulmonary embolism.

Falls

Falls are a major cause of morbidity and mortality in older adults, with the majority of deaths due to falls being in the over-65 age group. About one-third of older adults living at home fall each year and up to 1 in 40 of these persons is hospitalized. A major cause of falls in older adults results from the use of prescribed sedative–hypnotics. These drugs affect balance and postural control. Some examples are diazepam and flurazepam.

Critical Thinking

Consider older patients who have fallen. What common problems may contribute to an increased death rate in these patients?

Fractures are the most common fall-related injuries, with hip fractures (fractured neck of femur) being the ones that most often result in hospitalization. In those who survive this injury, some will have significant subsequent problems with walking and moving about and may become more dependent on others for help. Falls that do not result in physical injury may lead to self-imposed immobility from the fear of falling again. When immobility is strict and prolonged, joint contractures, pressure sores, urinary tract infection, muscle atrophy, depression and functional dependency may result.

The paramedic should assume that any fall indicates an underlying problem until it is proved otherwise. The paramedic should try to uncover the medical, psychological and environmental factors that may have been responsible for the fall; the patient history should include a full review of all medical problems and medications. It also should include precise details of the fall, including the history of falling, time of fall, location, symptoms experienced, activity in which the victim was engaged, use of devices or walking aids, and presence of witnesses. The paramedic also should evaluate the patient's cardiovascular, neurological, and musculoskeletal systems.

Burns

A number of older adults die from fires and burns each year. The increased risk of morbidity and mortality from burn trauma in older adults is due to pre-existing disease, skin changes that result in increased burn depth, altered nutrition, and decreased ability to fight infection. The initial care and resuscitation of older patients with thermal injury follows normal practice but older burn patients need special approaches to fluid therapy to prevent damage to the kidneys. The patient's fluid status will need to be assessed in the initial hours after a burn injury by monitoring pulse and blood pressure, and striving to maintain a urine output of at least 50–60 mL/h.

Trauma management considerations

The priorities of trauma care for older patients are similar to those for all trauma patients. However, the paramedic should give special consideration to transport strategies and the older patient's cardiovascular, respiratory and renal systems.

Cardiovascular system

Special considerations for cardiovascular problems include the following:

- Recent or past myocardial infarction contributes to the risk of dysrhythmias and CHF.
- Adjustment of heart rate and stroke volume may be decreased in response to hypovolaemia.
- Older patients may need higher arterial pressures than younger patients for perfusion of vital organs. This is because of atherosclerotic peripheral vascular disease.
- Rapid IV fluid administration to older patients may cause volume overload. The paramedic must take care not to overhydrate these patients. Older adults as a group are more susceptible to CHF. However, hypovolaemia and hypotension are also poorly tolerated. The paramedic should consider hypovolaemia in any older patient whose systolic blood pressure is less than 120 mmHg. Tachycardia

Box 39-8

Signs and symptoms of elder abuse and neglect

Physical abuse

Bruises, black eyes, welts, lacerations and rope marks
Bone fractures, skull fractures
Open wounds, untreated injuries in various stages of healing
Sprains, dislocations, and internal injuries/bleeding
Broken eyeglasses/frames, physical signs of being subjected to punishment, and signs of being restrained
An elder's sudden change in behaviour
The caregiver's refusal to allow examination of an elder without the caregiver being present
An elder's report of being hit, slapped, kicked or mistreated

Abandonment

The desertion of an elder at a hospital, a nursing facility, or other similar institution
The desertion of an elder at a shopping centre or other public location
An elder's own report of being abandoned

Financial or material exploitation

Sudden changes in bank account or banking practice, including unexplained withdrawals of large sums of money by a person accompanying the elder
The inclusion of additional names on an elder's bank signature card
Unauthorized withdrawal of the elder's funds using the elder's automatic teller machine card
Abrupt changes in a will or other financial documents
Unexplained disappearance of funds or valuable possessions
Substandard care being provided or bills unpaid despite the availability of adequate financial resources
Discovery of an elder's signature being forged for financial transactions or for the titles of his or her possessions
Sudden appearance of previously uninvolved relatives claiming their rights to an elder's affairs and possessions
Unexplained sudden transfer of assets to a family member or someone outside the family
The provision of services that are not necessary
An elder's report of financial exploitation

Sexual abuse

Bruises around the breasts or genital area
Unexplained venereal disease or genital infections
Unexplained vaginal or anal bleeding
Torn, stained or bloody underclothing
An elder's report of being sexually assaulted or raped

Emotional or psychological abuse

Being emotionally upset or agitated
Being extremely withdrawn and non-communicative or non-responsive
Unusual behaviour usually attributed to dementia (e.g. sucking, biting or rocking)
An elder's report of being verbally or emotionally mistreated

Neglect and self-neglect

Dehydration, malnutrition, untreated or improperly attended medical conditions, and poor personal hygiene
Hazardous or unsafe living conditions/arrangements (e.g. improper wiring, no indoor plumbing, and lack of heat or running water)
Unsanitary or unclean living quarters (e.g. animal/insect infestation, no functioning toilet and faecal/urine smell)
Inappropriate and/or inadequate clothing, lack of the necessary medical aids (e.g. eyeglasses, hearing aids, and dentures)
Grossly inadequate housing or homelessness
An elder's report of being mistreated

Adapted from National Centre on Elder Abuse. The basics: major types of elder abuse. Online. Available http://www.ncea.aoa.gov/ncearoot/Main_Site/FAQ/Basics?Types_Of_Abuse.aspx.

may not occur if the patient takes beta-blockers. The paramedic should monitor lung sounds and vital signs carefully and frequently during fluid administration.

Respiratory system

Special considerations for respiratory problems include the following:

- Physical changes decrease chest wall compliance and movement. Thus they diminish vital capacity as well.
- PaO_2 decreases with age.
- Lower PO_2 at the same fractional inspired oxygen concentration occurs with each passing decade.
- All organ systems have less tolerance to hypoxia.
- Chronic obstructive pulmonary disease (common in older patients) requires that the paramedic carefully adjust airway management and ventilation support for appropriate oxygenation and carbon dioxide removal. High-concentration oxygen may suppress hypoxic drive in some patients. However, oxygen should never be withheld from a patient with clinical signs of cyanosis. The paramedic may need to remove the patient's dentures for adequate airway and ventilation management

Renal system

Special considerations for renal problems include the following:

- The kidneys have decreased ability to maintain normal acid–base balance. They have decreased ability to compensate for fluid changes as well.
- Kidney disease may decrease further the ability of the kidneys to compensate.
- Decreased kidney function (along with decreased cardiac reserve) places the injured older patient at risk for fluid overload and pulmonary oedema following IV fluid therapy.

Transportation strategies

Special considerations for transportation of older patients include the following:

- Positioning, immobilization and transport of an older trauma patient may require modifications to accommodate physical deformities (e.g. arthritis or spinal abnormalities).

- Packaging should include bulk and extra padding to support and give comfort to the patient.
- The paramedic can prevent hypothermia by keeping the patient warm.

Elder abuse

Elder abuse refers to the infliction of physical pain, injury, debilitating mental anguish, unreasonable confinement, or wilful deprivation by a caregiver of services that are necessary to maintain mental and physical health of an older person. Elder abuse has become more and more recognized as a growing problem in the UK, with varying estimates that it affects between 2% and 5% of that population.

Elder abuse takes many forms, including physical abuse, sexual abuse, emotional or psychological abuse, abandonment, financial or material exploitation, and neglect. Box 39-8 lists the signs and symptoms of each type of elder abuse as defined by the National Center on Elder Abuse (in the US).

The UK has strong guidelines on reporting of elder abuse and there is now more widespread understanding of the nature and extent of the problem. If the paramedic suspects abuse or neglect of an older adult, the paramedic may need to advise the receiving unit or contact the primary healthcare team, but most importantly the paramedic should follow the procedures that are established locally. Emergency care is aimed at managing injuries that pose a threat to life and transporting the patient for further evaluation. Action on Elder Abuse (http://www.elderabuse.org.uk/index.htm) provide a range of information on the topic.

Summary

- The ageing process proceeds at different rates in different persons. Respiratory function in the older adult generally is compromised. This is a result of changes in pulmonary physiology that go along with the ageing process. Cardiac function also declines with age. This is a result of normal physiological changes and the high incidence of coronary artery disease. Renal blood flow falls an average of 50% between 30 and 80 years of age. A gradual decrease in neurons, decreased cerebral blood flow, and changes in the location and amounts of specific neurotransmitters probably contribute to changes in the CNS. As the body ages, muscles shrink, muscles and ligaments calcify, and the intervertebral discs become thin. Other physiological changes that occur with ageing include changes in body mass and total body water, a decreased ability to maintain internal homeostasis, a decrease in the function of immunological mechanisms, nutritional disorders, and decreases in hearing and visual acuity.
- Normal changes with ageing and existing illnesses may make evaluation of an ill or injured older patient a challenge.
- Pneumonia is a leading cause of death in the older age group. It often is fatal in frail adults. COPD is a common finding in the older patient who has a history of smoking. The disease usually is associated with various other diseases that result in reduced expiratory airflow. Pulmonary embolism is a life-threatening cause of dyspnoea. Pulmonary embolism is associated with venous stasis, heart failure, COPD, malignancy and immobilization. All of these are common in older adults.
- A lack of the typical chest pain can cause MI to go unrecognized in the older patient. Heart failure is more frequent in older patients and has a larger incidence of non-cardiac causes. The most common cause of dysrhythmias in the older patient is hypertensive heart disease. Abdominal aortic aneurysm affects 2–4% of the UK population over 50 years of age. This aneurysm is most prevalent between 60 and 70 years of age. The incidence of hypertension in the older patient increases when atherosclerosis is present.
- Risk factors for cerebral vascular disease in the older adult include smoking, hypertension, diabetes, atherosclerosis, hyperlipidaemia, polycythaemia and heart disease.
- Delirium is an abrupt disorientation of time and place. Delirium is commonly a result of physical illness.
- Dementia is a slow, progressive loss of awareness of time and place. It usually involves an inability to learn new things or remember recent events. This condition often is a result of brain disease. Alzheimer's disease is the most common cause of dementia. Alzheimer's disease is a condition in which nerve cells in the cerebral cortex die and the brain substance shrinks.
- Parkinson's disease is a brain disorder. It causes muscle tremor, stiffness and weakness.
- About 20% of older adults have diabetes. Almost 40% have some impaired glucose tolerance. Hyperglycaemic hyperosmolar non-ketotic coma is a serious complication of elderly type 2 diabetic patients. It has a mortality rate of 20–50%. Thyroid disease is more common in older patients. It may not present in the classic manner.
- Gastrointestinal bleeding most often affects patients between 60 and 90 years of age. It has a mortality rate of about 10%. Bowel obstruction generally occurs in patients with prior abdominal surgeries or hernias. It also occurs in those with colonic cancer. Some older patients may have problems with continence or with elimination as well.
- Ageing results in a gradual decrease in epidermal cellular turnover. It also results in loss of deep and dermal vessels. Decreased capillary circulation leads to changes in thermal regulation and skin-related complications.
- Osteoarthritis is a common form of arthritis in older patients. It results from cartilage loss and wear and tear on the joints. The loss in bone density from osteoporosis

Summary—cont'd

causes bones to become brittle. These bones may fracture easily.

- As persons age, they may experience problems with vision, hearing and speech.
- Older patients are at an increased risk for adverse drug reactions. This is due to age-related changes in body make-up and drug distribution. It also is the result of changes in metabolism and excretion. Moreover, the risk for adverse drug reactions often stems from multiple prescribed drugs. Alcohol abuse is a common problem in older patients.
- The older patient may develop hypothermia while indoors. This may be the result of cold surroundings and/or an illness that alters heat production or conservation. Hyperthermia most likely results from exposure to high temperatures that continues for several days.
- Depression is common in older patients. It can result from physiological and psychological causes. The rate of completed suicides for older patients is higher than that for the general population.
- Trauma is a leading cause of death for persons over 65 years of age, responsible for around a quarter of all UK trauma deaths. Major causes include road traffic collisions, falls, and burns, and older persons have a higher mortality rate than other adults.
- Elder abuse is classified as physical abuse, emotional or psychological abuse, financial or material abuse, sexual abuse, abandonment and neglect.

References

1. National Statistics/Department of Work and Pensions. Focus on older people. Online. Available http://www.statistics.gov.uk/downloads/theme_compendia/foop05/Olderpeople2005.pdf
2. Modified from American Geriatrics Society Foundation for Health in Aging. 2000–2010 decade of health in aging: the challenge – the aging of the U.S. population. Online. Available http://www.healthinaging.org/thechallenge.html 3 November 2004

Further reading and resources

Action on Elder Abuse. Online. Available http://www.elderabuse.org.uk/index.htm

Bosker G, Schwartz G, Jones J, Sequeira M 1990 Geriatric emergency medicine. Mosby, St Louis

British Hypertension Society. Online. Available http://www.bhsoc.org/default.stm 21 February 2009

Hogan T 1994 Older emergencies. Medic Alert Foundation, Turlock, CA

Snyder D, Christmas C (eds) 2003 Older education for emergency medical services. American Older Society, National Council of EMS Training Coordinators, Sudbury, MA

Waters M 1999 Mental illness among elderly Americans expected to become a greater concern. APA Monitor. Online. Available http://www.apa.org/monitor/dec99/nl4.html 21 February 2009

CHAPTER **40**

Abuse and Neglect

Chapter contents

Objectives

Upon completion of this chapter, the paramedic student will be able to:

1. Define battering.
2. Describe the characteristics of abusive relationships.
3. Outline findings that indicate a battered patient.
4. Describe prehospital considerations when responding to and caring for battered patients.
5. Identify types of elder abuse.
6. Discuss legal considerations related to elder abuse.
7. Describe characteristics of abused children and their abusers.
8. Outline the physical examination of the abused child.
9. Describe the characteristics of sexual assault.
10. Outline prehospital patient care considerations for the patient who has been sexually assaulted.

Key terms

battering A form of domestic violence that establishes control and fear in a relationship through violence and other forms of abuse.

emotional abuse The infliction of anguish, pain or distress through verbal or non-verbal acts.

financial/material exploitation The illegal or improper use of funds, properties or assets.

neglect The refusal or failure of the caregiver to fulfil obligations or duties to a person.

patterned injuries Injuries that result from an identifiable object.

physical abuse The use of physical force that may result in bodily injury, physical pain, or impairment.

self-neglect A type of elder abuse; behaviours of an older adult that intentionally threaten personal health or safety.

sexual abuse Non-consensual sexual contact of any kind.

shaken baby syndrome A serious form of child abuse that describes injuries to infants that occur after being shaken violently.

Partner, elder, and child abuse are growing problems in the UK. Paramedics will encounter victims of domestic violence in their careers. Abuse and neglect can result in mental and physical illness as well as injury and even death. Education programmes for emergency medical services (EMS) personnel must include information about these violent crimes. This information includes identification of victims, special aspects of care, scene safety, and documentation requirements. This chapter addresses the types of abuse and neglect, the personality traits of those who abuse, and legal considerations in providing emergency care.

Domestic violence

Domestic violence is any incident of threatening behaviour, violence or abuse between adults who are or have been in a relationship together, or between family members, regardless of gender or sexuality.[1] It is a serious public health issue in the UK and the statistics are shocking (Box 40-1). For women between the ages of 19 and 44, domestic violence is the leading cause of morbidity; greater than cancer and motor vehicle accidents.[1] Eighty-nine percent of the victims

Box 40-1

Domestic violence: facts and statistics

- Domestic violence accounts for 15% of all violent incidents.
- One in four women and one in six men will be a victim of domestic violence in their lifetime with women at greater risk of repeat victimization and serious injury.
- 89% of those suffering four or more incidents are women.
- One incident of domestic violence is reported to the police every minute.
- On average, two women a week are killed by a current or former male partner.

Home Office. Domestic Violence Mini-Site.[2]

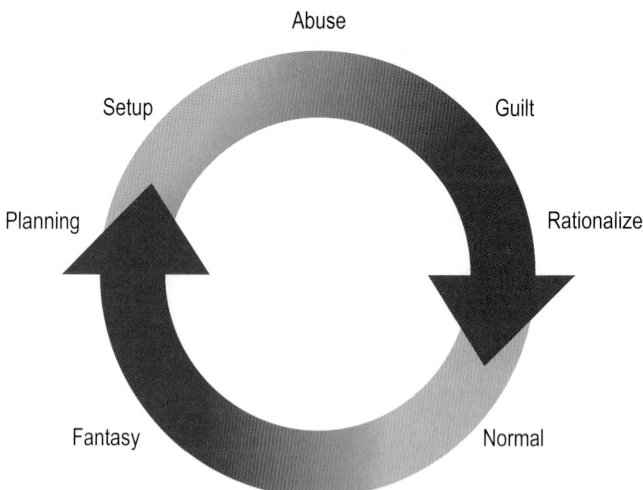

Figure 40-1 Cycle of violence. Reproduced with kind permission of Mid-Valley Women's Crisis Service.

who suffer sustained domestic violence are female, although domestic violence can affect the lesbian, gay, bisexual and transgender community and male victims.[1] Typical behaviours include intimidation, threats, psychological abuse and isolation, but these are rarely isolated events. Types of abuse and neglect include the following:

- *Emotional abuse*: Infliction of anguish, pain, or distress through verbal or non-verbal acts.
- *Financial/material exploitation*: Illegal or improper use of funds, properties or assets.
- *Neglect*: Refusal or failure of the caregiver to fulfil obligations or duties to a person.
- *Physical abuse*: Use of physical force that may result in bodily injury, physical pain, or impairment.
- *Sexual abuse*: Non-consensual sexual contact of any kind.

Half of those affected by domestic violence live with children under the age of 16 years,[3] many of whom are aware of the abuse that is occurring in the home. Abusers may involve children in the abuse in a range of ways, such as making them watch or encouraging them to be abusive towards their mothers. There is also a recognized overlap between domestic violence and child sexual and physical abuse.[4] Persons involved in abusive relationships often fail to see other options and often feel powerless to change.

Domestic violence may follow a cycle of phases[5] (Figure 40-1).

- *Abuse*: The abuser lashes out with aggressive or violent behaviour. The abuse is a power play designed to show the victim 'who is boss'.
- *Guilt*: After the abusive episode, the abuser feels guilt, but not over what they have done to the victim. The guilt is over the possibility of being caught and facing consequences.
- *Rationalization or excuses*: The abuser rationalizes what they have done. The abuser may come up with a string of excuses or blame the victim for their own abusive behaviour; anything to shift responsibility from themselves.
- *'Normal' behaviour*: The abuser does everything possible to regain control and keep the victim in the relationship. They may act as if nothing has happened, or may turn on the charm. This peaceful honeymoon phase may give the victim hope that the abuser has really changed this time.
- *Fantasy and planning*: The abuser begins to fantasize about abusing the victim again, spending a lot of time thinking about what the victim has done wrong and how they will be made to pay. Then the abuser makes a plan for turning the fantasy of abuse into reality.
- *Set-up*: The abuser sets up the victim and puts the plan in motion, creating a situation where the abuse can be justified.

Battered women

No accurate figures exist for the prevalence of domestic abuse in all its forms, as it is known to be grossly under-reported to authorities, such as the police, health service and social services.[6] There are many reasons why a woman may decide not to report domestic abuse; these include:

1. Personal fear or fear for her children.
2. Belief that the offender's behaviour will change (abusers often appear charming and loving after the battering incident).
3. Lack of financial and/or emotional support.
4. Belief that she is the cause of the violent behaviour.
5. Belief that battering is 'part of the marriage' and must be endured to keep the family together.

Women of all cultures, races, occupations, income levels and ages are battered by their husbands, boyfriends and lovers (opposite- and same-sex partners) (Figure 40-2).

Battered men

Women are the victims in 80% of cases;[7] men may also be victims of physical violence by a spouse or partner (from opposite- and same-sex relationships; Figure 40-3). Men report physical violence by a spouse or partner less often than women; this is probably as a result of humiliation, guilt, and/or fear to admit loss of control. In addition, society seems to be less empathetic toward battered men

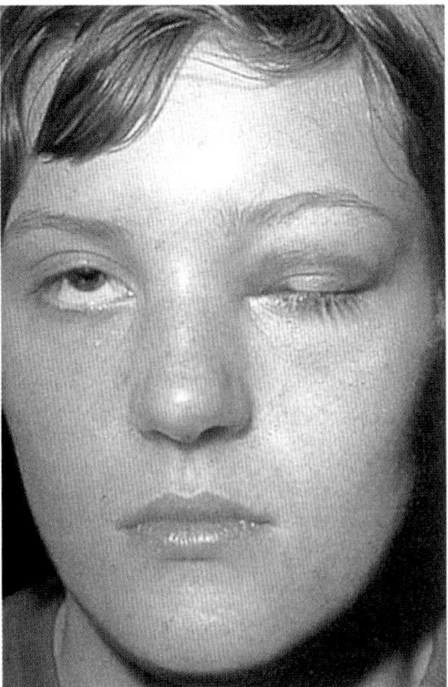

Figure 40-2 A woman struck in the face.

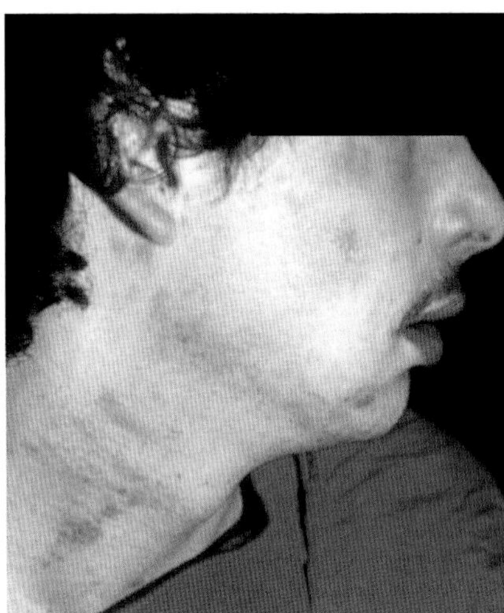

Figure 40-3 Soft tissue injury to the face from blows and to the neck from a firm grip.

than battered women and has allocated fewer resources for support.

Characteristics of people in abusive relationships

Certain personality traits may draw people into abusive relationships. The following are characteristics of one or both persons in an abusive relationship:[8]

1. Intense need for love and affection.
2. Low self-esteem.
3. Alcohol or other drug dependence.
4. Difficulty in finances, job security, and possible legal issues.
5. Background of physical, emotional or sexual abuse; abusers are often survivors of abuse.
6. Belief that abuse is demonstrating discipline.
7. Fear of being 'out of control'.
8. Uncontrolled temper, extreme jealousy, and insecurity.
9. Inability to set and enforce personal boundaries.
10. Unrealistic expectations of a relationship.
11. Difficulty in expressing anger.
12. Loyalty to the abuser that takes precedence over emotional or physical safety.
13. Repeated attempts to leave the relationship.
14. Clinical depression.
15. Suicidal ideation or attempts.

Identification of the victim of domestic violence

The paramedic may have difficulty identifying the battered patient. Often the description of the injuries may be incorrect, inaccurate, and protective of the attacker. Injuries that are unintentional often involve the extremities and the periphery of the body; however, injuries from domestic violence often involve contusions and lacerations of the face, head, neck, breast and abdomen. Bruises and lacerations may appear to be 'old' because many victims of abuse do not seek medical help for their injuries. Other clues of domestic violence are the following:

- excessive delays between injury and seeking treatment
- repeated requests for EMS assistance
- injuries during pregnancy
- substance abuse
- frequent suicide gestures.

Scene safety

The paramedic must ensure scene and personal safety in domestic violence events. If dispatch reveals that the scene involves domestic violence, the paramedic should call for police assistance. The EMS crew also should not enter the scene until it has been secured. If the paramedic does not suspect domestic violence until after arriving at the scene, the paramedic should remove the victim from the scene as soon as possible. Violence may be aimed at EMS personnel, especially if the abuser feels that the paramedic is giving too much empathy to the victim. Thus, the paramedic should not question the victim regarding possible violence and should be careful about displaying sympathy until the victim is in the ambulance or has been separated from the suspected batterer.

Care of the victim

All injuries should be managed according to standard protocols. The paramedic should direct special attention to the emotional needs of the victim. The abuser is often unwilling to allow the victim to give a history and may not want to allow the victim to be alone with EMS personnel. The paramedic should question the patient privately about the incident when possible.

Critical Thinking

If you suspect abuse, what can you say to invite the victim to talk about it?

The paramedic should obtain information about events that led to physical injury by using direct questions. Often the patient will avoid eye contact and be hesitant or evasive about details of an injury. Some may offer clues by saying, 'things haven't been going well lately', or 'there have been problems at home'. The paramedic should convey to the patient his or her awareness that the injuries may have resulted from battering. The patient may be relieved to know that someone else is aware of the abuse.

During the patient interview, the paramedic should be non-judgemental and avoid comments such as 'how awful' or 'why don't you leave?' The paramedic should listen carefully to the victim and offer emotional support. The patient should be encouraged to gain control of his or her life and to consider the best interests and needs of any children who may be involved in the abusive relationship. The paramedic should also provide access to community resources such as refuges, victim–witness assistance programmes, and other support agencies for abused victims and their families. Finally, the paramedic should discuss safety measures with the victim who elects not to be transported for evaluation. This may include helping the patient identify a quick way out of a dangerous situation (e.g. where to go and whom to call). It may also include providing an approved written list or a small card (that can be hidden easily from the abuser) of community resources. These may include shelters and hotline numbers.

Critical Thinking

How would you feel if you respond to a call in which a woman has been injured by a batterer but chooses not to leave?

Some patients who have suffered abuse eventually leave the abusive relationship. This is often made possible by health-care providers and support agency personnel who do the following:

- Treat the victim in a sensitive and sympathetic manner.
- Confirm that the victim is not at fault and does not deserve to be abused.
- Ensure the victim's safety.
- Become 'agents of change' in helping provide the support needed for the victim to leave the abusive environment.

Legal considerations

'Domestic violence' is not a specific crime under criminal law, but many forms of domestic violence are crimes, for example: assault, false imprisonment, criminal damage, harassment, attempted murder, rape. Statistics suggest that:[9]

- In 30% of domestic violence incidents reported to the police, no action is taken.
- In a further 38% of cases, they give a warning only.
- On average, 26% of reported incidents results in arrest – and just over a quarter of these lead to a charge (7% of all reported incidents).
- Perpetrators are often charged with crimes that are less serious than the original offence.
- 4% of reported incidents result in a conviction.
- Bindovers and fines are the most common sentences for perpetrators of domestic violence – and only 1 in 200 offenders receives a custodial sentence (0.5% of recorded incidents).

If early release from custody is likely, the patient must be made aware of this and should be encouraged to take personal safety precautions. EMS personnel are bound professionally to advise their control and command centre of their suspicions and observations about acts of violence.

Any act of physical abuse against a spouse, partner, elder or child is a crime, so the paramedic must treat the scene as a crime scene. Paramedics should be careful not to disturb the scene or destroy possible evidence. Documentation is key and should include a precise account of injuries, reported mechanisms of injuries, and a description of the behaviour of the victim and alleged abuser. Using body diagrams in the patient care report may be helpful. The paramedic should record the victim's own words in the narrative when possible and record the names of police officers and witnesses at the scene. These details are important in cases of litigation (see Chapter 11).

Elder abuse

Elder abuse (described in Chapter 39) is a prevalent medical and social problem in the UK. There is currently only limited research into the prevalence of the problem and the statistics used by the Government that suggest that 500 000 older people are being abused at any one time in the UK stem from work undertaken in 1992.[10] Approximately two-thirds of all elder abuse perpetrators are family members.[6] It has been suggested that in the UK the main perpetrator of abuse is the victim's partner, followed by a son.[11] Factors that contribute to elder abuse include the following:

- increased life expectancy
- physical and mental impairment
- decreased productivity
- increased dependence
- limited resources for care of the elderly
- economic factors
- stress of the middle-aged caregiver responsible for two generations.

Critical Thinking

Do you think that the problem of elder abuse will increase or decrease during your career in emergency medical services? Why?

Types of elder abuse

As described in Chapter 39, elder abuse is classified into four categories: physical abuse (Figure 40-4), psychological abuse, financial or material abuse, and neglect (active and passive) (Box 40-2). Self-neglect is another type of elder abuse, whereby the behaviours of an older adult intention-

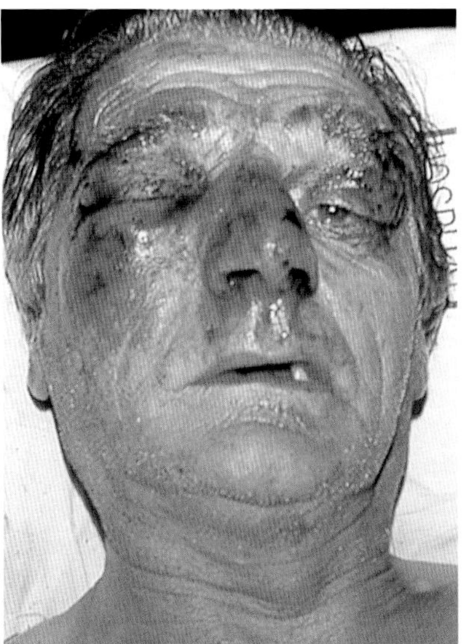

Figure 40-4 Injuries from facial blows to an older adult.

> **Box 40-2**
>
> **Types of elder abuse**
>
> **Physical abuse**
>
> Biting
> Hitting
> Physically restraining
> Sexually molesting
>
> **Psychological abuse**
>
> Causing fear
> Humiliating
> Insulting
> Intimidating
> Isolating
> Name calling
> Threatening verbally
>
> **Financial or material abuse**
>
> Forcing relocation from one dwelling to another
> Stealing or misusing money
> Stealing or misusing property
>
> **Neglect (active and passive)**
>
> Ignoring the person
> Withholding medication, food, exercise, companionship or bathroom assistance

ally threaten personal health or safety (such as poor nutrition and not taking prescribed drugs). Elder abuse is also classified by where it occurs. It occurs in domestic settings or in institutions.

Domestic settings

The average victim of elder abuse in domestic settings usually has multiple, chronic health conditions that make him or her dependent on others for care. Widows over 75 years of age carry the greatest risk of elder abuse. Neglect is the most common form of elder abuse in domestic settings; unexplained trauma is the most common finding. Evidence suggests that elder abuse is associated more with the personality of the abuser than with the burden of caring for a sick, dependent person.

Four major theories of causes of domestic elder abuse are as follows:[8]

1. Elder abuse occurs in settings where the caregiver is under a great amount of stress. This stress is a result of personal problems and/or a lack of knowledge about how to provide care to an older adult.
2. Mental and/or physical impairments common in many older adults make them more likely to be abused than older adults who are in good health.
3. A 'cycle of violence' often occurs in elder abuse. The cycle begins with ongoing tension. This tension escalates in a crisis in which abuse occurs. The abuse generally is followed by a period of calm, reconciliation, and denial, after which the cycle repeats.
4. Abusers of older adults often have more personal problems than non-abusers. (For example, they may have job insecurity and/or financial troubles.)

Older adults often are repeatedly abused by family members. The abusers most often are the children of the abused. Because of this familial relationship, many older adults do not report the abuse. Many also do not seek medical care for their injuries.

Institutional abuse

Individuals residing in residential nursing homes and other healthcare facilities are at risk of intentional harm, physical violence, verbal aggression or neglect from other residents and paid caregivers, staff, and professionals. Clues that may indicate institutional abuse include the following:

- burns caused by cigarettes, caustics, or acids
- caregiver who cannot explain the victim's condition adequately
- dehydration, malnutrition or pressure sores
- loss of weight
- open wounds, cuts, bruises, welts or discoloration
- unsanitary and unclean conditions (dirt, soiled bed, or faecal or urine odour)
- unusual behaviour by the victim (sucking, biting or rocking)
- victim who is begging for food
- victim who is emotionally upset or agitated
- victim who is extremely withdrawn and non-communicative
- victim with poor personal hygiene
- victim's sudden change in behaviour.

Legal considerations

Reporting of suspected elder abuse is imperative if the victim is to be removed from the source of the abuse. Each local authority has social workers specifically to deal with abuse or risk of abuse and they should be contacted through the appropriate channels where abuse is suspected. All findings should be documented carefully, the control centre should be notified, and established procedures and protocols should be followed.

Child abuse

A child is anybody under the age of 18 years, so although the term child will be used in this text, it is referring to children and young people. UK statistics on child abuse still make grim reading. Every 10 days in England and Wales one child is killed at the hands of their parent. In over 50% of all cases of children killed at the hands of another person, the parent is the principal suspect.[12] More than one third (36%) of all rapes recorded by the police are committed against children under 16 years of age,[13] and research by the National Society for the Prevention of Cruelty to Children (NSPCC) suggests that a significant minority of children are subjected to serious abuse or neglect.[14] Specific cases cause widespread condemnation and specific Government action, for example, the tragic case of Victoria Climbié in 2000 where local services had no fewer than 12 opportunities to intervene to protect her in the last 10 months of her life but failed to do so.[15] It is strongly recommended that paramedics access Lord Laming's report on the Victoria Climbié enquiry to read about the failings that led to her death (available online at http://www.victoria-climbie-inquiry.org.uk/).[16] Other key documents include 'Every Child Matters; Change for Children'[17] and 'Working Together to Safeguard Children'.[18]

There are four types of child abuse: neglect, physical abuse, emotional abuse and sexual abuse; it is not unusual for a child to be suffering from more than one form of abuse. Neglect is the most common category in the child protection registry in England, accounting for 43%.[19] Although difficult to define, it is reasonable to view neglect as 'the persistent failure to meet a child's basic physical and/or psychological needs resulting in serious impairment of heath and/or development'.[20] Physical abuse may involve acts such as kicking, punching, biting, suffocating, burning (e.g. with cigarettes), shaking or any other act that leads to physical harm. Emotional abuse is the persistent emotional maltreatment of a child, which may include being constantly put down or made to feel worthless. Sexual abuse is the act of forcing a child into performing sexual activities whether or not the child is aware of what is happening.[15]

Identifying a vulnerable child

Paramedics can play a vital role in identifying and protecting vulnerable children as they are able to pick up information that may not be available to other health professionals and social services. In cases of abuse that have ultimately led to the death of a child, three common failings have been found:[15]

- poor communication and information sharing amongst professionals
- inadequate training of staff
- failure to listen to children.

Paramedics may seek advice from a designated child protection nurse or doctor during normal working hours or from a senior officer in the service outside of these times. Where abuse is suspected, emphasis should be on shared professional responsibility and interprofessional communication.[21] It is usual to keep parents/guardians informed of the actions that need to be taken when safeguarding children although this may not be possible in the context of paramedic practice. It is usual for paramedics to conceal their concerns regarding the possibility of child abuse and this is even more important where expressing concerns to a parent/guardian may lead to a refusal to allow the child to attend hospital.

There are often tell-tale signs that a child is being abused and early detection may save a life or provide the facility for a child to be removed to a place of safety. Paramedics are well placed to identify children and young people who may be at risk of abuse and can act to safeguard their welfare. Although the characteristics of abusers are not related to social class, income or level of education, there are certain known factors that make a child more vulnerable:

- younger children (particularly infants), and children who have language or learning difficulties or physical disabilities[22,23]
- family and social factors such as poverty, homelessness, domestic violence, drug or alcohol abuse, parents with gambling addiction, history of animal abuse and mental health problems[16,18,24–26]
- children in care or in criminal justice settings.[27]

The signs of child abuse

The signs of child abuse will vary according to the type of abuse that is occurring. It is essential that paramedics are vigilant to all types of abuse and do not just look for signs of physical abuse. The following list suggests signs that the paramedic may look for, but it is by no means all-encompassing:[15,20]

- Evidence of poor physical care and inadequate hygiene, inappropriate dress or failure to seek appropriate health care.
- The child is left in unsafe situations or without medical attention.
- The child is constantly 'put down', insulted, sworn at or humiliated.
- A child's behaviour may also indicate that they have been abused. For example, the child may show fear of adults or a fear of certain adults when they approach them, display aggressive behaviour or deliberate self-harm and substance abuse.
- Physical signs such as hand-slap marks, bruising in unusual areas or unusual patterns, bruised eyes, bite marks.
- The history provided by the adult might be inconsistent with any injuries.
- The child may displays sexual behaviour that seems inappropriate for their age.
- The child may be growing up in a home where there is a history of domestic violence.

- The child may be living with parents or carers involved in serious drug or alcohol abuse.
- The parents may have unrealistic expectations and be overprotective of a child.
- The child may have repeatedly attended a healthcare organization with different types of injuries in a short period of time or presented in a variety of healthcare settings.

Action to be taken when abuse or risk of harm is suspected

Paramedics should follow normal patient assessment techniques for managing children but should pay particular attention to any inconsistencies in the history or any delays in calling for help. It is important that paramedics recognize their role in cases of suspected child abuse and do not overstep the boundaries of practice. The paramedic is there to report suspected cases but is not expected to be an expert in child protection. This means that questioning should be restricted to areas of necessity rather than questioning the child or probing into their suspicions as this may affect the credibility of the child as a witness at a later date. Any injuries identified should be managed in accordance with normal procedures.

It is important to remember that injuries during childhood are common and that most are unintentional and not the result of abuse. Distinguishing between an intentional and accidental injury can be challenging for the paramedic but the most important clues can be obtained by observing the child and his or her relationship with the parent or caregiver. The paramedic may obtain key clues by matching the history of the event to the injury. If the child volunteers the history of the event without hesitation and matches the history that the parent provides (and the history is suitable for the injury), child abuse is unlikely.

The following guidelines are adapted from the Joint Royal Colleges Ambulance Liaison Committee in a situation where it is suspected that a child has been abused and that child is the patient:[21]

1. If the parents/carers agree that the child is to be conveyed to hospital, the paramedic should not let the parents/carers know they are suspicious if this may result in refusal to go to hospital. The paramedic should hand over to the most senior member of nursing staff on duty and provide a copy of their documentation. A safeguarding children report form must be completed and a copy provided to the hospital. The handover and documentation should be done in private if possible. The paramedic should give full details of their concerns or suspicions to the receiving nurse, with a recommendation that the Child Protection Register be consulted.
2. The paramedic should inform ambulance control about the situation so that it can be reported. As soon as reasonably possible the crew should fax a copy of the safeguarding children report form to ambulance control. The paramedic should be careful to pass this information in a private location to avoid others overhearing the conversation. It is best to use a telephone rather than a two-way radio.
3. If parents/carers refuse to allow the child to be conveyed to hospital, the paramedic should inform ambulance control and complete a safeguarding children report form. Ambulance control will call the police and contact social services on the 24-hour emergency number, and will also arrange for an ambulance officer to attend the scene.

There may be an occasion where the child is not the patient but where a paramedic has suspicions or cause for concern about the well-being of a child on scene. In this scenario the paramedic should consider the implications of leaving the child. If the child is accompanying another person (e.g. a parent) who is being conveyed, the crew should inform staff at the emergency department of their concerns. If no-one is conveyed to hospital, and the crew leave the scene, they should contact ambulance control and inform them of the incident. A safeguarding children report form should be completed and faxed to ambulance control as soon as possible

In all cases, a safeguarding children report form should be completed. A copy MUST be left with the receiving hospital if the patient is conveyed, a copy MUST be faxed to ambulance control, and the original form MUST be retained with the patient report form for recording and archiving.

Common types of injuries

Common types of injuries associated with child abuse were described in Chapter 38. These injuries include the following:

- *Soft tissue injuries*: Soft tissue injuries are the most common injury seen in cases of child abuse and are often found in early abuse. They may present in various forms such as multiple bruises and ecchymosis, especially if bruises are extensive and are a mixture of old and new bruises. Defence wounds may be found on multiple body planes; these are often patterned injuries that result from an identifiable object. (For example, they might be bites, loop marks from a cord or belt [Figure 40-5], cigarette burns, or bristle marks

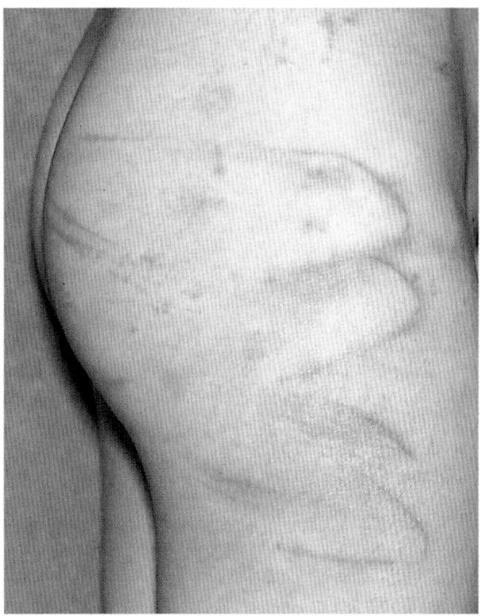

Figure 40-5 Patterned injury from being struck with a belt.

from a hairbrush.) In addition, scalds are a common form of abuse in the young and old (Figure 40-6). In addition, look in the mouth of babies as injuries to the frenulum are not uncommon following forced bottle-feeding (Figure 40-7).

- *Fractures*: Fractures are the second most common injury in cases of child abuse. They are often caused by twisting and jerking forces and may be of different ages (fresh and healed), indicating repeated injury. Rib fractures and multiple fractures are common findings.
- *Head injuries*: Head injury is the most common cause of death in cases of child abuse; and children who survive head injury often have permanent disability (Figure 40-8). Often there is a visible progression of injury that begins at the child's trunk and extremities and moves toward the head. Associated injuries include scalp wounds, skull fractures, subdural or subgaleal hematomata, and repeated concussions.

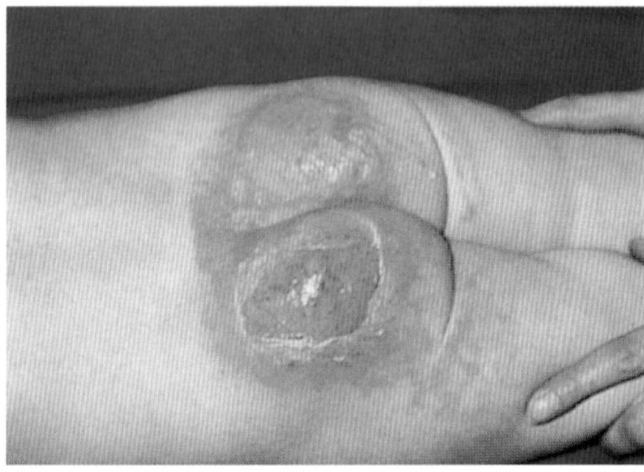

Figure 40-6 'Bath dipping' typically produces scalds on the buttocks and feet.

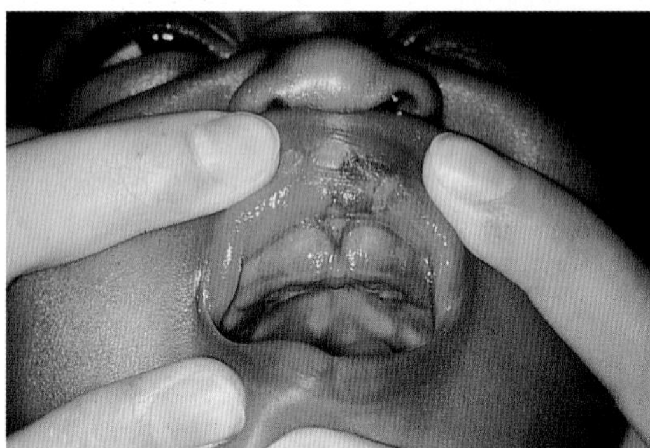

Figure 40-7 A torn frenulum that may have been caused by forced bottle-feeding.

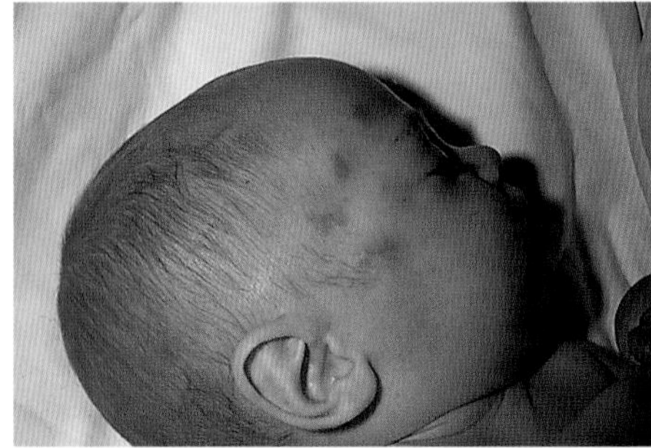

Figure 40-8 Multiple bruises on an infant's head from finger pressure.

- *Abdominal injuries*: Abdominal injuries in cases of child abuse are less common than those injuries just described; however, they are often serious. Blunt trauma to the abdomen may lead to rupture of the liver or may result in injuries to the intestines and mesentery.

Critical Thinking

How can you calm yourself after caring for a child killed by abuse before writing a patient care report that likely will be called to court?

Sexual assault

A report for the Home Office in 2004 estimated that in the 12 months prior to the report there were 190 000 incidents of serious sexual assault and an estimated 47 000 female victims of rape in the UK.[28] Sexual assault is not restricted to women; the same report suggested that 1.5% of men had been subjected to a serious sexual assault during their lives. In the year ending March 2007, police recorded 57 542 sexual offences in England and Wales.[29]

Legal aspects of sexual assault

In 2003, The Sexual Offences Act became law and described the following offences:[30]

- *Rape*: Rape is classified as penetration by the penis of somebody's vagina, anus or mouth, without their consent. Rape can be committed against men or women, but since it involves penile penetration it is only committed by men.
- *Assault by penetration*: Under this law, it is an offence to penetrate the anus or vagina of someone else with any part of the body or with an object, if the penetration is sexual and if the person does not consent.
- *Sexual assault*: This law covers any kind of intentional sexual touching of somebody else without their consent. It includes touching any part of their body, clothed or unclothed, either with your body or with an object.
- *Causing a person to engage in a sexual activity without consent*: This law covers any kind of sexual activity without consent. For instance it would apply to a woman who forces a man to penetrate her, or an abuser who makes their victim engage in masturbation.
- *Administering a substance with intent*: This law makes it a separate offence to give someone any substance – for instance spiking their drink – without their consent, and with the intention of stupefying them so that sexual activity can take place.

Legal considerations for providing care to a patient who has been sexually assaulted include the following:

1. Take steps to preserve evidence.
2. Discourage the patient from urinating or defecating, douching or bathing.

3. Do not remove evidence from any part of the body that was subjected to sexual contact unless necessary to provide urgent medical care.
4. Notify the police as soon as possible.
5. Be aware that there will be a 'chain of evidence' with specific requirements of proof.
6. Follow Trust procedures and established protocols.

Characteristics of sexual assault

Anyone can be a victim of sexual assault at any age. The highest incidence of sexual assault occurs in women who live alone in isolated areas. The victim often knows the assailant. Sometimes the victim feels shame and personal responsibility for the attack. The methods that the assailant uses to gain control over male and female victims include entrapment, intimidation and physical force. The assailant commonly uses threats of harm and a weapon to gain submission. Male victims are more likely to suffer significant physical trauma from sexual assault by other men than are female victims (Box 40-3). The following are common injuries that result from sexual assault:

- abrasions and bruises on the upper limb, head, and neck
- forcible signs of restraint (e.g., rope burns and mouth injuries)
- petechiae of the face and conjunctiva caused by choking
- broken teeth, swollen jaw or cheekbone, and eye injuries from being punched or slapped in the face
- muscle soreness or stiffness in the shoulder, neck, knee, hip or back from restraint in postures that allow sexual penetration.

Box 40-3

Five myths and misconceptions about sexual assault

Myth. All victims of sexual assault are women, and all perpetrators are men.

Fact. Most sexual assaults are perpetrated by men. However, men can be assaulted by other men. Sometimes women perpetrate sexual assaults against men and other women.

Myth. Rape is an impulsive act.

Fact. Fifty-eight percent to 71% of rapes clearly are planned.

Myth. Rape is motivated by sexual desire.

Fact. Rape is a crime of violence, motivated by anger and the desire for power and control.

Myth. Most women are raped by strangers.

Fact. Most women are victims of 'acquaintance rape' by a known, trusted assailant.

Myth. According to the law, a husband cannot be charged with rape against his wife.

Fact. The law stipulates circumstances in which the husband can be charged with rape against his wife.

Critical Thinking

How do you feel when you hear others say, 'That rape victim brought it on herself'?

Psychosocial aspects of care

The trauma of sexual assault creates physical and psychological distress. Victims may behave in various ways; some may be surprisingly calm and seem in control of their emotions whilst others may be agitated, apprehensive, distraught, or tearful. After managing all threats to life, the paramedic should proceed with care by providing emotional support to the victim. As described in Chapter 35, the paramedic should not question victims of sexual assault in detail about the incident in the prehospital setting. The paramedic should limit the patient history to what is required to provide care. The initial contact with the victim should include the following:

- non-judgemental and supportive attitude
- empathetic and sensitive comments
- quiet speech
- slow movements
- considerate gestures (ensure privacy and respect modesty).

The paramedic should move the patient to a safe and quiet environment as this will help to avoid further exposure and embarrassment. When possible, a paramedic of the same sex should provide care. If this is not possible, a chaperone should be present. The paramedic should not leave the patient alone and should ask for permission to call a friend, family member, or sexual assault crisis advocate. After the patient recovers from physical injury, the goal of treatment is for the patient to regain control of his or her life. Often this takes long-term counselling and support.

Child victims

Children are particularly vulnerable to sexual assault and usually have frequent contact with the assailant. Of the offenders themselves, about 30% are aged under 18,[31] approximately 99% are male,[32] and at least 75% are known to their victims as either a relative or a family friend.[33] Child sex offending is still a greatly under-reported crime, with research showing that 72% of sexually abused children do not tell anyone about what has happened at the time, and that 31% still have not told anyone by early adulthood.[34]

Assessment and patient care considerations

Assessment for child victims of sexual assault should proceed as described before for other victims. The assessment should include age-related considerations that are appropriate for all children. The paramedic should be aware of the following symptoms as they may indicate behaviour or physical manifestations as a result of sexual assault:

- abrupt behaviour changes
- sleep difficulties, sleep disorders and nightmares
- withdrawal from and avoidance of friends and family

- low self-esteem or desire to be invisible
- phobias related to the offender
- hostility
- self-destructive behaviours
- mood swings, depression and anxiety
- regression (e.g. bed-wetting)
- truancy
- eating disorders
- alcohol or other drug use.

The attitude and behaviour of adults, including healthcare providers, greatly influence a child's impression of the assault. The paramedic should try to lessen the emotional influence of the assault by reassuring the child that he or she is not responsible for the attack. The child should also be assured that he or she did nothing wrong. The paramedic also should encourage the child to talk openly about the assault and any concerns that he or she may have.

Legal considerations

The Sexual Offences Act 2003 contains a series of offences and tough punishments for perpetrators of sexual crime against children. Although it is perhaps not essential to know the definitions of each of these crimes, the paramedic should have an overview of the Act in order to further protect children. A key document is 'Children and Families: Safer from Sexual Crime. The Sexual Offences Act 2003'.[35] This provides an overview of the key laws related to children of different ages.

When managing suspected sexual crime against a child, the paramedic should follow the same procedures as for other forms of child abuse.

Summary

- Battering is the establishment of control and fear in a relationship through violence and other forms of abuse.
- Domestic violence follows a cycle. The phases include: abuse, guilt, rationalization, normality, planning and the set-up.
- The paramedic may have a hard time identifying a battered patient. Injuries from domestic violence often involve contusions and lacerations of the face, neck, head, breast and abdomen.
- The paramedic must ensure scene and personal safety in domestic violence events. The paramedic should manage physical injuries according to standard protocols but should direct special attention toward the emotional needs of the victim as well.
- Elder abuse is classified into four categories: physical abuse, psychological abuse, financial or material abuse, and neglect.
- Reporting of suspected elder abuse is a responsibility of paramedics.
- Most child abusers are known to the child. Abused children often exhibit behaviour that provides key clues about abuse and neglect. The paramedic should observe carefully the child under 6 years of age who is passive or the child over 6 years of age who is aggressive.
- If the child volunteers the history of the event without hesitation and matches the history that the parent provides (and the history is suitable for the injury), child abuse is unlikely.
- Injuries may include soft tissue injuries, fractures, head injuries and abdominal injuries.
- Sexual assault generally refers to any genital, anal, oral or manual penetration of the victim's body by way of force and without the victim's consent. The highest incidence of sexual assault occurs in women who live alone in isolated areas.
- After managing all threats to life, the paramedic should provide emotional support to the victim. The paramedic should deliver care in a way that preserves evidence.

References

1. Home Office 2005 Domestic Violence; A National Report. Home Office, London 2005
2. Home Office. Domestic Violence Mini-Site. Online. Available http://www.crimereduction.homeoffice.gov.uk/dv/dv01.htm 26 February 2009
3. Mirrlees-Black C 1999 Domestic violence: findings from a new British crime survey self-completion questionnaire. Home Office Research Study No. 191. Home Office, London
4. Mullender A 2000 Reducing domestic violence…what works? Meeting the needs of children. One of a pack of 12 briefing notes. Crime Reduction Research Series No.4. Home Office, London
5. Mid-Valley Women's Crisis Service. The cycle of domestic violence 2007. Online. Available http://www.mvwcs.com/cycledomesticviolence.html 26 June 2009
6. British Medical Association 2007 Domestic abuse. British Medical Association, London
7. Finney A 2006 Domestic violence, sexual assault and stalking: findings from the 2004/05 British Crime Survey. Home Office, London
8. US Department of Transportation, National Highway Traffic Safety Administration 1998 EMT-Paramedic national standard curriculum. US Department of Transportation, Washington, DC
9. Women's Aid. Criminal Law. Online. Available http://www.womensaid.org.uk/domestic_violence_topic.asp?section=0001000100220007§ionTitle=Criminal+Law 26 September 2008
10. Ogg J, Bennett G 1992 Elder abuse in Britain. BMJ 305:998–999
11. George M 2003 Elder abuse and its prevention. Care and Health 49(Nov 19):40–42
12. Home Office 2007 Homicides, firearms offences and intimate violence 2005/2006: supplementary volume 1 to Crime in England and Wales 2005/2006. Home Office, London
13. Walker A, Kershaw C, Nicholas S 2006 Crime in England and Wales 2005/06.

Home Office Statistical Bulletin (July 2006/12/06). Home Office, London
14. Cawson P et al 2000 Child maltreatment in the United Kingdom: a study of the prevalence of child abuse and neglect. NSPCC, London
15. Royal College of Nursing 2003 Safeguarding Children and Young People – Every Nurse's Responsibility. RCN, London (updated 2007)
16. HMSO 2002 The Victoria Climbié inquiry: report of an inquiry by Lord Laming. The Stationery Office, London. Online. Available http://www.victoria-climbie-inquiry.org.uk/finreport/finreport.htm 26 February 2009
17. HM Government 2003 Every child matters: change for children. The Stationery Office, London
18. HM Government 2006 Working together to safeguard children: a guide to interagency working to safeguard and promote the welfare of children. The Stationery Office, London
19. Department for Education and Skills 2006 Statistics of education. Referrals, assessments and children and young people on the child protection registers, England: Year Ending 31 March 2006 (Final). DfES, National Statistics
20. Turney D, Tanner K 2005 Understanding and working with neglect. Research in Practice: Every Child Matters Research Briefings 10:1–8
21. Joint Royal Colleges Ambulance Liaison Committee 2006 UK Ambulance Service Clinical Practice Guidelines version 4. 2006. Online. Available http://jrcalc.org.uk/guidelines.html 26 February 2009
22. Department of Health 2002 Safeguarding children in whom illness is fabricated or induced. The Stationery Office, London
23. Department of Health 2000 Safeguarding children involved in prostitution: supplementary guidance to 'Working together to safeguard children'. Department of Health, London
24. Cleaver H, Unell I, Aldgate J 1999 Children's needs – parenting capacity: the impact of parental mental illness, problem alcohol and drug use, and domestic violence on children's development. The Stationery Office, London
25. Christensen MH, Patsdaughter CA, St Germain M 2000 Mother–Bingo bonding: screening for gambling addiction in the NICU. Neonatal Network 19(7):7–11
26. Scottish Society for the Prevention of Cruelty to Animals 2001 Animal cruelty: family violence. SPCA, Edinburgh
27. Her Majesty's Inspectorate of Prison's for England and Wales 2002 Inspections of young offender institutions 2000 to 2002. Home Office, London
28. Home Office 2004 Domestic violence, sexual assault and stalking: Findings from the British Crime Survey. Home Office, London
29. Walker A, Kershaw C, Nicholas S. Crime in England and Wales 2005/2006. Online. Available http://www.homeoffice.gov.uk/rds/crimeew0506.html 26 February 2009
30. Home Office 2003 Adults: Safer from Sexual Crime. The Sexual Offences Act 2003. Home Office Communications, London
31. Fisher D, Beech A 2004 Adult male sex offenders. In Kemshall H, Mclvor G (eds) Managing sex offender risk. Research Highlights in Social Work 46. Jessica Kingsley Publishers, London, pp 25–47
32. Home Office 2006 Offender management caseload statistics 2005, Home Office Statistical Bulletin 18/06, Research, Development and Statistics. National Offender Management Service, London
33. Grubin D 1998 Sex offending against children: understanding the risk. Police Research Series Paper 99. Home Office, London
34. NSPCC 2006 Key child protection statistics: sexual abuse. NSPCC, London
35. Home Office. Children and Families: Safer from Sexual Crime. The Sexual Offences Act 2003. Online. Available http://www.homeoffice.gov.uk/documents/children-safer-fr-sex-crime?view=Binary 26 February 2009

Further reading

NSPCC. Child Abuse Information and Sexual Abuse Issues. Online. Available http://www.nspcc.org.uk/helpandadvice/whatchildabuse/whatischildabuse_wda36500.html 26 February 2009

CHAPTER **41**

Community Care: Patients with Long-Term Health Conditions, Palliative Care, Dialysis

Chapter contents

Objectives

Upon completion of this chapter, the paramedic student will be able to:

1. Discuss general issues related to the home healthcare patient.
2. Outline general principles of assessment and management of the home healthcare patient.
3. Describe medical equipment, assessment and management of the home healthcare patient with inadequate respiratory support.
4. Identify assessment findings and acute interventions for problems related to vascular access devices in the home healthcare setting.
5. Describe medical equipment, assessment, and management of the patient with a gastrointestinal or genitourinary crisis in the home healthcare setting.
6. Identify key assessments and principles of wound care management in the home healthcare patient.
7. Outline maternal/child problems that may be encountered early in the postpartum period in the home healthcare setting.
8. Describe medical therapy associated with hospice and comfort care in the home healthcare setting.

Key terms

bronchopulmonary dysplasia A chronic respiratory disorder characterized by scarring of lung tissue, thickened pulmonary arterial walls, and ventilation–perfusion mismatch; often occurs in infants who have long-term dependence on artificial ventilation.

colostomy A surgical opening into the large intestine.

failure to thrive The abnormal retardation of the growth and development of an infant resulting from conditions that interfere with normal metabolism, appetite and activity.

ileostomy A surgical opening into the small intestine.

obstructive apnoea A form of sleep apnoea involving a physical obstruction of the upper airways that can lead to pulmonary failure, chronic fatigue and cardiac abnormalities.

ostomy An artificial opening into the urinary tract, gastrointestinal tract or trachea; any surgical procedure in which an opening is created between two hollow organs or between a hollow viscus and the abdominal wall.

palliative care A unique form of healthcare primarily directed at providing relief to terminally ill persons through symptom management and pain management; also known as comfort care.

urosepsis Septic poisoning caused by retention and absorption of urinary products in the tissues.

The cost-driven allocation of healthcare resources and advances in technology have led to shortened hospital stays. This has also allowed many patients to be treated in the home setting. In September 2004, around 355 600 households received home healthcare services because of acute illness, long-term health conditions, personal preference, permanent disability or terminal illness.[1] Paramedics will likely play a key role in providing acute interventions to these patients.

Overview of home healthcare

Home care is defined as services that assist the client to function as independently as possible and/or continue to live in their own home.[1] Services may involve routine household tasks within or outside the home, personal care of the client, or respite care in support of the client's regular carers.

The aim of home healthcare in the UK is to reduce the number of emergency admissions for chronic conditions in a belief that patients with illnesses like asthma and heart disease could be better cared for by community nurses in their own homes. For example, patients with heart failure account for approximately 5% of acute medical admissions to hospital and 10% of bed occupancy. Readmission to hospital is a common problem, but the intervention of nurse-led community management programmes has been shown to lead to both improved compliance and reductions in hospitalizations in a number of different countries, including the UK.[2–4] The move towards this model of care has its origins in the Community Care Reforms of 1993, which set out to enable more people to continue to live in their own homes as independently as possible.

Advanced life support response to home healthcare patients

An increasing number of home healthcare patients have conditions related to diseases of the circulatory system as their primary diagnosis; including people with heart disease and congestive heart failure. Other common diagnoses of home healthcare patients include cancer, diabetes, chronic lung disease, renal failure/dialysis and hypertension. Thus it is likely that emergency responses for home healthcare patients will become increasingly common for ambulance services. Typical emergencies may include respiratory failure, cardiac decompensation, septic complications, equipment malfunction, and other conditions that worsen in the home healthcare setting (Box 41-1).

Box 41-1

Examples of home healthcare problems

Home care services requiring intervention by a home healthcare practitioner or physician

Acquired immune deficiency syndrome
Cardiopulmonary care
Catheter management/intravenous therapy infusion
Chemotherapy
Dermatological and wound care
Gastroenterological and ostomy care
Hospice care
Organ transplantation
Orthopaedic care
Pain management
Rehabilitative care
Specimen collection
Urological and renal care

Home healthcare problems requiring acute intervention

Acute cardiac events
Acute infections
Acute respiratory events
Gastrointestinal/genitourinary crisis
Hospice/comfort care
Inadequate respiratory support
Maternal/child conditions
Vascular access complications

Injury control and prevention in the home healthcare setting

The scientific approach to illness and injury prevention as a means to minimize morbidity and mortality is discussed in Chapter 3. Readers should refer to these areas to review primary prevention, acute care, and rehabilitation (tertiary prevention); their concepts; and their strategies.

Infection control

As with all other patient encounters, the paramedic should practise infection control in the home healthcare setting. Infection control includes using standard precautions and body substance isolation (or transmission-based precautions) when indicated. Practice should follow the guidelines set out by the Department of Health in 2008.[5] Equipment required in the home care setting may include:

Critical Thinking

What factors decrease the risks of spreading infection within a home healthcare setting versus a hospital?

- gloves – sterile and non-sterile
- aprons
- sleeve protectors
- shoe protectors
- protective suits
- mask
- goggles, glasses or face shield
- resuscitation mask
- specimen bags
- Health Protection Agency-approved disinfectant effective against hepatitis B virus, human immunodeficiency virus and tuberculosis
- soap and water
- disposable paper towels
- clinical waste bags and labels.

This text assumes that the proper personal protection will be used by paramedics. The nature of the emergency and the patient's condition will dictate what protection to use.

Types of home care patients

The need to reduce the costs of healthcare and technological advances in medicine have allowed many types of patients to receive home care. In the United States, many emergency medical services (EMS) agencies ask their communities to notify them when someone is on a complex home healthcare programme; this is not yet common practice in the UK and requires attention in order that these patients may receive the most appropriate emergency care. That way, a visit could be made to the home to allow EMS providers to become familiar with the patient's condition and special equipment before an emergency. Patients who may be being cared for at home include those with:

- pathological conditions of the airway causing inadequate pulmonary toilet or inadequate alveolar ventilation and/or oxygenation
- circulatory pathological conditions causing alterations in peripheral circulation (e.g. pressure ulcers, delayed healing or infection)
- gastrointestinal/genitourinary conditions requiring special devices such as ostomies, feeding catheters, and special equipment needed for home dialysis
- infection from cellulitis or systemic illness (e.g. sepsis)
- wounds that require care (e.g. surgical wound closure, decubitus wounds, and surgical drains).

Other patient groups the paramedic may encounter in the home healthcare setting include patients receiving hospice care, expectant or new mothers, patients with dementia or other conditions that require psychological support for the patient or family, patients receiving chemotherapy or home care for chronic pain, and patients with organ transplants or those who are waiting for organ transplantation (transport candidate).

General principles and management

Scene size-up

When paramedics arrive at the scene of a home healthcare patient, the scene size-up should include standard precautions, elements of scene safety, and an assessment of the patient's environment (environmental setting).

Standard precautions

As with all patient care, paramedics should use standard precautions to guard against communicable disease. Equipment that may be found in the home healthcare setting includes containers of medical waste, ostomy collection bags, tracheostomy tubes, sharps, soiled dressings, and other equipment (e.g. emesis basins, walking frames and wheelchairs) that may be contaminated with the patient's body fluids. In addition to personal precautions, the EMS crew should ensure that any infectious waste found in the home is contained properly. The waste should be disposed of per protocol.

Scene safety

Whenever an EMS response is made to a person's home, the paramedic should evaluate the scene for the presence of dangerous pets and for any home hazards (e.g. inadequate lighting, icy pathways or steep stair wells). For the safety of the EMS crew, the patient, and others at the scene, all potential hazards found in a home must be contained or remedied. For example, it may be necessary to request the police to help with unruly or hostile bystanders; and extra personnel and special equipment may be needed to help move a patient down a flight of steps for transport.

Environmental setting

The paramedic should assess the setting for the patient's ability to maintain a healthy environment. Examples include cleanliness of the home; evidence of basic nutritional support; and needs of heat, water, shelter, and electricity. The EMS crew should also note any signs of abuse or neglect. Other factors to note are the cleanliness and condition of any medical devices; examples include clean oxygen and ventilation equipment, and wheelchairs and hospital beds that are in good repair.

Patient assessment

The initial patient assessment should focus on illness or injury that poses a threat to life. The paramedic should take the appropriate measures as indicated (see Chapter 7). After the initial assessment, the paramedic should obtain a focused history and perform a physical examination. The paramedic should make use of any medical documents found in the home (e.g. patient records kept by home healthcare providers and 'do not resuscitate' orders). The paramedic should also gather information from family and healthcare professionals (e.g. a home care nurse or physical or respiratory therapist) who may be present at the scene. Critical findings should alert the paramedic to forego a detailed assessment and proceed with resuscitation measures and rapid transport for physician evaluation. If there are no critical findings, the paramedic should perform a physical examination that considers the possibility of medication interactions, compliance with the treatment regimen, and the possibility of dementia or a metabolic disturbance in a patient with an altered mental status.

A comprehensive assessment may include a physical examination using inspection, palpation, auscultation and percussion (as indicated by the patient's condition and chief complaint). The ongoing assessment should evaluate any changes in the patient's status while at the scene or en route to the hospital. These assessment strategies can aid in differential diagnosis, treatment, and direction of patient management.

Management and treatment plan

Depending on the patient's condition, the home healthcare treatment may need to be replaced with advanced life support measures. These measures may include airway, ventilatory and circulatory support, and pharmacological and non-pharmacological therapy (e.g. electrical therapy).

Some patients with acute illness or injury need to be transported to the hospital for evaluation. When transport is needed, the paramedic must give special consideration for patient packaging and for moving the patient's equipment. Examples include properly securing intravenous (IV) catheters, urinary catheters and feeding tubes; and ensuring available personnel to assist with moving patient care devices such as ventilation equipment. Family members at the scene are often well versed on the patient's medical devices and will usually be eager to help when asked by the EMS crew. If there is no family at the scene, the EMS crew should attempt to contact a family member or caregiver and advise this person of the patient's condition and hospital destination.

Other patients will only need home care follow-up by home healthcare practitioners, or they may need a referral to other agencies such as social services. The paramedic should follow guidelines and consult with ambulance control about referrals and the need for notifying private physicians or home healthcare agencies. Regardless of the need for EMS transport, the paramedic should document completely all findings and any care provided on the care report.

Critical Thinking

What feelings may a patient's family member (or caregiver) in the home setting have if there is a problem and the patient's condition worsens?

Specific acute home healthcare interventions

Acute home healthcare emergencies may occur from equipment failure or malfunction, drug reactions, complications related to home treatment and worsening medical conditions. This section discusses acute interventions for respiratory support, vascular access devices, gastrointestinal/genitourinary crisis, acute infections, maternal/child conditions, and hospice/palliative care.

Respiratory support

Many patients with respiratory diseases are discharged to community healthcare each year. These patients are at increased risk for airway infections. The progression of some respiratory diseases may also lead to an increased respiratory demand, making current support inadequate. Examples of chronic pathological conditions that require home respiratory support include the following:

- asthma
- awaiting lung transplant
- bronchopulmonary dysplasia
- chronic lung disease (more than 1 million patients in the UK)[6]
- cystic fibrosis
- infection causing exacerbation of condition
- sleep apnoea.

Acute interventions may be required for these patients. Any patient with respiratory distress should receive high-concentration oxygen and ventilatory support as a priority although care needs to be exercised in patients with chronic obstructive pulmonary disease (COPD). Problems that may lead to a request for EMS assistance include increased respiratory demand, increased bronchospasm, increased secretions, obstructed or malfunctioning respiratory devices, or improper application of medical devices to support respirations.

Oxygen therapy in the home setting

Three common ways to provide oxygen therapy in the home are compressed gas, liquid oxygen and oxygen concentrators. Compressed gas is oxygen stored under pressure in oxygen cylinders equipped with a regulator that controls flow rate. Liquid oxygen is cold and is stored in a container similar to a thermos. When released, the liquid converts to gas and is used like compressed gas. An oxygen concentrator is an electrically powered device that separates oxygen from air, concentrates it, and stores it (Figure 41-1). This system does not have to be resupplied and is not as costly as liquid oxygen. A cylinder of oxygen must be available as a backup in case of power failure.

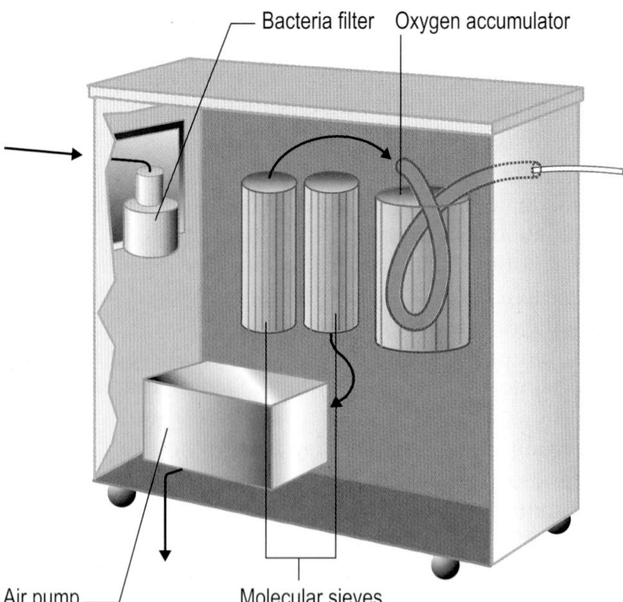

Figure 41-1 Oxygen concentrator.

Critical Thinking

What safety precautions for administering oxygen should be in place in the home setting?

Oxygen is delivered to patients via nasal cannulae, oxygen masks, tracheostomy collars (devices that deliver high humidity and oxygen to patients with surgical airways), and ventilators. Some patients may require continuous positive airway pressure (CPAP) delivered by ventilatory support systems through mask CPAP, nasal CPAP, or biphasic positive airway pressure (BIPAP). As described in Chapter 14, the BIPAP ventilatory support system (designed for mask-applied ventilation in the home) delivers two different levels of positive airway pressure. The system cycles spontaneously between a preset level of inspiratory positive airway pressure and expiratory positive airway pressure. The BIPAP ventilatory support system is intended only to augment the patient's breathing; it does not provide for total ventilatory requirements. The BIPAP system is used by some patients with sleep apnoea or chronic obstructive pulmonary disease.

Supportive ventilator management may be indicated to achieve the following:

- prevent nocturnal hypoxaemia caused by sleep hypoventilation in patients with neuromuscular disorders (e.g. muscular dystrophy or myasthenia gravis)

- prevent respiratory fatigue in patients with chronic obstructive pulmonary disease
- improve ventilation and oxygen saturation in patients with obstructive apnoea, a form of sleep apnoea involving a physical obstruction of the upper airways that can lead to pulmonary failure, chronic fatigue, and cardiac abnormalities.

Home ventilators

Home ventilators can be classified as volume ventilators, pressure ventilators, and negative-pressure ventilators. Most ventilators have a number of controls and ventilator settings. Box 41-2 describes some of these settings.

Volume ventilators (volume-preset) deliver a predetermined volume of gas with each cycle, after which inspiration is terminated. These types of ventilators deliver a constant tidal volume regardless of changes in airway resistance or compliance of the lungs and thorax. The volume remains the same unless very high peak airway pressures are reached, in which case, safety release valves stop the flow (Box 41-3; Table 41-1).

Pressure ventilators (pressure-preset) are pressure-cycled devices that terminate inspiration when a preset pressure is achieved. When the preset pressure is reached, the gas flow stops, and the patient passively exhales. These ventilators are most often used for patients whose ventilatory resistance is not likely to change.

Negative-pressure ventilators have settings for the respiratory rate and pressure of the negative force exerted. These devices use negative pressure to raise the rib cage and lower the diaphragm. This creates negative pressure within the lungs so that air flows into the lungs. Negative-pressure ventilators are often used for patients with healthy lungs who have a muscular inability to inhale. (For example, this may include patients with spinal cord injury or neuromuscular disease.) Examples of this type of ventilator are the 'iron lung' and plastic wrap, or poncho, ventilators.

Assessment findings

When caring for a patient who requires oxygen therapy, the paramedic should evaluate the patient's work of breathing,

Box 41-2

Standard initial ventilator settings

FiO_2 (fraction of inspired oxygen)	100%
Tidal volume	10–15 mL/kg body mass
Respiratory rate	10–15 breaths/min
Inspiratory flow	40–60 L/s
Sensitivity	12 cmH_2O
Sigh rate (optional)	1–2/min

Box 41-3

Ventilator alarms

Ventilators are equipped with alarms. These alarms signal that there are problems with ventilator function. There are alarms for loss of power, frequency alarms (indicating changes in respiratory rate), volume alarms (indicating low-exhaled volume or low/high minute-ventilation), and high-pressure alarms. If alarms are sounding, the paramedic should check for the following possible causes:

- kinks in endotracheal tube
- disconnected ventilator tubing or poor connections
- water in ventilator tubing
- excessive secretions
- pneumothorax
- patient anxiety.

After consulting with medical advice and If qualified to do so, acute interventions may include providing temporary ventilation assistance with a bag–mask device, repositioning the endotracheal tube, correcting poor ventilator tube connections, emptying water from tube or water traps, suctioning the airway, thoracic decompression, and possible sedation.

Table 41-1 Ventilator alarms

Alarm type	Causes	Interventions
High pressure	Increased secretions	Suction secretions from patient
High pressure	Kinked tubing	Unkink tubing
High pressure	Water in tubing	Disconnect tubing and allow it to drain
High pressure	Anxiety	Decrease anxiety by providing a calm environment
Low pressure	Disconnected tubing	Reconnect tubing
Low pressure	Cuff leak	Add 1 mL of air at a time to pilot balloon of tracheostomy tube
Low pressure	Tracheostomy tube out	Reinsert new tracheostomy tube
Oxygen	Insufficient oxygen supply	Manually ventilate patient and prepare for transport
Ventilator not operating	Power failure	Manually ventilate patient and prepare for transport

Note: A memory aid useful for identifying possible causes of ventilator malfunction is DOPE. This stands for displacement of the tube, obstruction of the tube, pneumothorax and equipment failure.

tidal volume, peak flow, oxygen saturation and quality of breath sounds. This assessment can be performed with visual inspection (chest rise and fall), peak flow meters, pulse oximetry and auscultation (described in Chapters 13 and 14). The paramedic should be alert for signs and symptoms of hypoxia, including the following:

- confusion and mental status changes
- cyanosis
- dyspnoea
- headache
- hypertension
- hyperventilation
- restlessness
- tachycardia.

Management

Management goals for a patient receiving oxygen therapy who requires acute intervention are to improve airway patency, ventilation, and oxygenation.

Improving airway patency

To improve airway patency, the paramedic first should reposition airway devices (e.g. facemasks and nasal cannulae) to ensure they are applied properly and are well fitted. The paramedic should clear secretions that obstruct airflow from the airway with suction. The paramedic should clear secretions from any airway device using sterile water. If needed, the home airway device should be replaced with a new device (Figure 41-2a–f) A tracheostomy tube that has become blocked and cannot be cleared may need to be replaced with another tracheostomy tube to ensure adequate ventilation. (Or the tube can be replaced temporarily with an endotracheal tube, see Chapter 13.)

Improving ventilation and oxygenation

If ventilation does not improve after providing a patent airway, the paramedic should remove the home ventilator care device. The paramedic then should assist the patient's ventilations with positive-pressure ventilation via a bag–valve–mask device and supplemental oxygen. Oxygen saturation should be monitored with pulse oximetry. The paramedic should also administer supplemental oxygen as needed to maintain oxygen saturation at 90% or higher. It should be possible to obtain medical advice from the patient's carers, who may advise adjusting the settings of a home care device or changing the flow rate of an oxygen delivery device to improve ventilation and oxygenation. Extra personnel may be needed to assist in moving the patient who has a ventilator device to the ambulance for transport for evaluation.

On some ventilators the inspiratory flow rate is determined by tidal volume, respiratory rate, and the inspiratory/expiratory ratio. (This ratio is generally 1:2. This allows for complete exhalation and prevents air trapping.) On other ventilators the flow rate is set independently. This allows for adjustment of air flow to the flow wave pattern that is most comfortable for the patient. If the patient is having difficulty with spontaneous breathing, an increase in the flow rate may be indicated. However, a higher flow rate means a shorter inspiratory time and usually a higher respiratory pressure because of increased resistance. A lower flow rate requires a longer inspiratory time with a decreased inspiratory pressure. The paramedic should always seek medical advice before changing the flow rate on any ventilator.

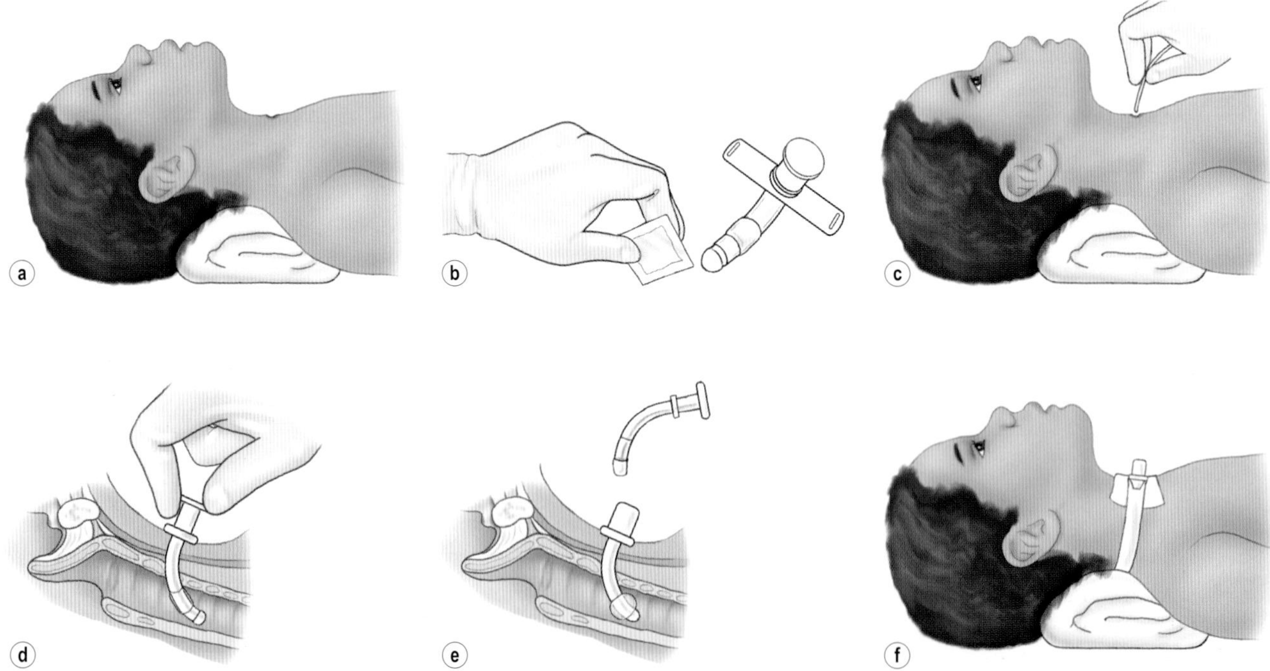

Figure 41-2 Replacement of a tracheostomy tube. (a) Position the child with padding under the shoulders. (b) Select a tube the same size or one size smaller than the one removed and moisten with sterile, water-soluble lubricant. (c) Suction the stoma and trachea before insertion of the new tube. (d) Insert the tube gently into the trachea with the curve pointing downward. (e) If the tube has an obturator, remove it; if it is a cuffed tube, inflate the cuff. (f) Assess for correct tube placement and secure the tube.

Psychological support and communication strategies

Difficulty breathing can be a horrifying experience for the patient, especially for a patient who depends on a ventilator. The paramedic crew should try to calm the patient and family and assure them that respirations will be supported adequately by other means whilst at the scene and during transport.

Some patients with tracheostomies have special valves attached to the tracheostomy tube ('talking trachs') that redirect exhaled air around the tracheostomy tube, through the vocal cords, and out of the mouth and nose to allow for normal speech. Loss of verbal communication is a major source of anxiety in patients who have tracheostomies. The ability to communicate with these patients will be based on the patient's cognition, level of consciousness, language, and fine and gross motor skills. Methods of communication may include signing and writing on notepads. The paramedic should enlist the help of family and other caregivers in communicating with the patient.

Vascular access devices

Many patients in the home care setting have indwelling vascular access devices (VADs). Vascular access devices are used to provide nutritional support, to administer medications, and are used for patients who need long-term vascular access; for example, patients receiving dialysis or chemotherapy. Those with indwelling vascular devices may experience problems, including the following:

- anticoagulation associated with percutaneous or implanted devices
- embolus formation associated with indwelling devices, stasis, and inactivity
- air embolus associated with central venous access devices
- obstructed or malfunctioning VADs
- infection at the access site
- infiltration and extravasation
- obstructed dialysis shunts.

Note

Congestive heart failure is a common reason for hospitalization although attempts are often made to manage these patients at home if possible. Thus paramedics may find patients with congestive heart failure receiving medications (e.g. dobutamine or furosemide) intravenously in the home setting.

Types

A variety of VADs are encountered in home healthcare patients. These include surgically implanted subcutaneous VADs, medication delivery devices (e.g. Mediports, as described in Chapter 12), peripheral VADs (e.g. peripherally inserted central catheters and midline catheters), central venous tunnelled catheters (e.g. Hickman, Groshong or Broviac), and dialysis shunts.

Assessment findings and acute interventions

Certain assessment findings may require acute interventions in patients with VADs. These findings include infection, haemorrhage, haemodynamic compromise from circulatory overload or embolus, obstruction of the vascular device, catheter breakage, and leakage of medication (e.g. chemotherapeutic agents) (Table 41-2).

Infection

Home healthcare patients who have VADs are generally instructed to examine the area for infection and to change the dressings around their device often. This is often done by family members and home healthcare practitioners. All types of dressings must be changed immediately if they become wet, soiled, contaminated, or unocclusive. A common problem of VADs is infection near the exit site, tunnel or port. Signs and symptoms of site infection include pain, redness, warmth, and purulence. Signs and symptoms of systemic infection (which may result from a site infection) include fever, tachycardia, general weakness, malaise, mental status changes, body aches and possibly septicaemia. If the patient has any evidence of systemic signs of infection, he or she should be transported to the hospital. General principles in managing the site infection are as follows:

1. Use aseptic technique when examining the line.
2. Clean the site with alcohol (per guidelines).
3. Apply antimicrobial ointment if guidelines state – this is controversial practice.
4. Cover site with transparent, sterile dressing.
5. Document the procedure and label the dressing with date, time and paramedic's initials.
6. Seek medical advice.

Critical Thinking

Will it always be possible to identify the catheter as the source of sepsis while on the scene?

Haemorrhage

Bleeding at the site of a VAD should be controlled by applying gentle, direct pressure with aseptic technique. These patients need to be transported for physician evaluation. Blood loss from a broken or dislodged VAD can be significant and the patient may need to be treated for haemorrhagic shock.

Haemodynamic compromise

Haemodynamic compromise may result from circulatory overload or embolus. Circulatory overload can develop from too much IV fluid delivered too fast. Signs and symptoms of circulatory overload include a rise in blood pressure, distended neck veins, pulmonary congestion (crackles and wheezes) and dyspnoea. If circulatory overload is suspected, the paramedic should do the following:

1. Slow the infusion to a keep-open rate.
2. Provide high-concentration oxygen.
3. Elevate the patient's head.
4. Maintain body warmth. This will promote peripheral circulation and ease the stress on the central veins.
5. Monitor vital signs.
6. Seek advice from patient's normal home care practitioners for patient management and disposition.

Table 41-2 Correcting common problems with venous access devices

Complication	Signs and symptoms	Prehospital interventions
Mechanical problems		
Clotted intravenous catheter	Interrupted flow rate, resistance to flushing and blood withdrawal	Attempt to aspirate the clot. If unsuccessful, seek medical advice
Cracked or broken tubing	Fluid leaking from the tubing	Apply padded haemostat above the break to prevent air from entering the line and change the tubing (seek medical advice)
Dislodged catheter	Catheter out of the vein	Apply pressure to the site with a sterile gauze pad
Too-rapid infusion	Nausea, headache, lethargy, dyspnoea	Adjust the infusion rate, and if applicable, check the infusion pump. Contact medical support about need to transport
Other problems		
Air embolism	Apprehension, chest pain, tachycardia, hypotension, cyanosis, seizures, loss of consciousness and cardiac arrest	Clamp the catheter; place the patient in a steep, left lateral Trendelenburg position; give oxygen as required; if cardiac arrest occurs, begin cardiopulmonary resuscitation
Extravasation	Swelling and pain around the insertion site	Stop the infusion and assess the patient for cardiopulmonary abnormalities; request further medical advice.
Phlebitis	Pain, tenderness, redness, and warmth	Apply gentle heat to the area; elevate insertion site if possible
Pneumothorax and hydrothorax	Dyspnoea, chest pain, cyanosis, and decreased breath sounds	If signs and symptoms of tension pneumothorax are present, consider needle decompression; rapid transport is indicated
Septicaemia	Red and swollen catheter site, chills, fever	Transport for physician evaluation
Thrombosis	Erythema and oedema at the insertion site; ipsilateral swelling of the arm, neck, face and upper chest; pain at the insertion site and along the vein; malaise; fever; tachycardia	Apply warm compresses to insertion site; elevate affected extremity; transport patient
Haemorrhage	Bleeding at site of venous access device or from broken device	Apply pressure to site; clamp venous access device and treat for shock

Displacement of a surgically implanted catheter or port is rare. However, an embolus that occurs from air, thrombus, or plastic or catheter tip entering the circulation can develop (Box 41-4). Signs and symptoms of an embolus include hypotension; cyanosis; weak, rapid pulse; and loss of consciousness. A patient suspected of having an embolism should be managed as follows (described in Chapter 12):

1. Stop the IV infusion.
2. Position the patient on the left side with the head down (in an attempt to keep the embolus in the right side of the heart).
3. Administer high-concentration oxygen.
4. Transfer to hospital for physician evaluation – consider seeking medical advice before moving the patient.

If a plastic or catheter tip embolism is suspected, a suggestion is to apply a constrictive band to prevent further movement. There is no evidence to support this technique as it is likely that the embolus will move rapidly away from the infusion site and it may not be possible to apply sufficient pressure using a venous tourniquet; however, it may be worth trying if the case presents.

Box 41-4

Causes of embolus formation

Air embolism

Intravenous fluid containers that run dry
Air in intravenous tubing
Loose connections in catheter tubing
Catheter tears and breakage

Thrombus

Clot formation from inactivity or stasis

Plastic or catheter tip migration

Plastic or catheter fragment from tugging or shearing forces
Wire from central line placement

Obstruction of the vascular device

An indwelling vascular device may become obstructed and disrupt the flow of fluids and medications. When this occurs, immediate intervention is needed. The device must be cleared by irrigation or the administration of fibrinolytic agents. The paramedic should seek medical advice before trying to clear an obstruction from a VAD and the most experienced paramedic should perform any procedure.

Flushing and irrigation Vascular access devices and medication ports need regular irrigation with normal saline and/or heparin. The frequency of irrigation depends on the specific device and on the frequency of medication administration. The paramedic should follow these steps:

1. Explain the procedure to the patient.
2. Prepare prescribed irrigation solutions (normal saline or normal saline and heparin).
3. Clean the injection cap(s) with an antiseptic and alcohol wipe (per protocol) and allow to air dry.
4. Release the clamp from the catheter (if present).
5. Irrigate the lumen with an appropriate volume of solution using a 10 mL syringe (no faster than 0.5 mL/s). If resistance is persistent, stop the irrigation, or the catheter may rupture. Note: The paramedic must never try to force or dislodge a clot or other obstruction. Fibrinolytic agents may be required, which is beyond the current scope of practice. The application of force could dislodge the obstruction and cause it to enter the circulatory system.
6. If resistance is met, the device may need resiting – the paramedic may consider contacting the patient's home care team to seek advice about the best course of action; this may necessitate transporting the patient to an appropriate medical facility.

Anticoagulant therapy At times, a medication port or other vascular device may require declotting with fibrinolytic agents (t-PA). Flushing with fibrinolytic agents should be performed by specialized personnel. An X-ray may be needed prior to administration of these agents.

Other complications

Advice from online medical support may include aspirating blood from the CVAD. If you are unable to aspirate blood, or the patient or family reports that the length of the catheter that was visible has changed, do not administer fluid or drugs through it. The patient will need transport for further evaluation.

A decrease in the length of catheter coupled with a sudden onset of tachycardia can mean that the catheter has moved into the right atrium. If the patient hears bubbling in the ear when the catheter is flushed, or has a sudden earache on the side of the body where the catheter is inserted, the catheter may have advanced into the jugular vein. In all of these situations, an X-ray will be needed to determine the location of the catheter.

Catheter damage

A damaged (e.g. cracked or torn) catheter can allow fluids or medications to infiltrate into the surrounding tissues, which can lead to an air embolism. Signs and symptoms of a damaged catheter include leaking fluid, complaint of a burning sensation, or swollen and tender skin near the insertion site. If catheter damage is suspected, the infusion should be stopped immediately. The catheter should be clamped between the crack or tear in the catheter and the patient. These patients are managed with high-concentration oxygen, IV access through a peripheral vein, and transport for physician evaluation. A patient who develops an altered level of consciousness (indicating a possible air embolism) should be positioned on the left side. The head should be slightly lowered. This positioning will help to prevent the embolism from travelling to the brain.

Box 41-5

Medical therapy found in the home setting for patients with gastrointestinal/genitourinary disease

Devices for gastric/intestinal emptying or feeding

Colostomy
Feeding tube
Nasogastric tube
Percutaneous endoscopic gastrostomy tubes, jejunostomy tubes, gastrostomy tubes

Devices for the urinary tract

External urinary catheters (e.g. condom catheter or Texas catheter)
Indwelling urinary catheter (e.g. Foley catheter or Coudé catheter)
Surgical urinary catheters (e.g. suprapubic catheters)
Urostomy

Gastrointestinal/genitourinary crisis

Many patients with diseases of the digestive or genitourinary system are discharged to home healthcare each year. Some of these patients have medical devices such as urinary catheters or urostomies, indwelling nutritional support devices (e.g. percutaneous endoscopic gastrostomy tube or gastrostomy tube), colostomies, and nasogastric tubes (Box 41-5). Acute interventions that may be required for these patients can result from urinary tract infection (UTI), urosepsis, urinary retention, and problems with gastric emptying or feeding.

Urinary tract infection, urosepsis and urinary retention

Urinary tract infection

Urinary tract infection is common, occurring in all age groups and both sexes (see Chapter 20). The organisms most often associated with UTI are Gram-negative organisms normally found in the gastrointestinal tract. These include *Escherichia coli*, *Klebsiella*, *Proteus*, *Enterobacter* and *Pseudomonas*. These are frequently introduced from the hands of healthcare personnel at the time of bladder catheterization.[7] (Sterile technique during these procedures is crucial.) Other factors that increase the risk of UTI include the following:

- obstructions (e.g. urethral strictures, calculi, tumours or blood clots)
- trauma (e.g. abdominal injury, ruptured bladder, or local trauma related to sexual activity)
- congenital anomalies (e.g. polycystic kidneys, horseshoe kidney, or spina bifida)
- abdominal or gynaecological surgery
- acute or chronic renal failure
- immunocompromised state (e.g. patients with human immunodeficiency virus or older adults)
- postpartum state
- ageing changes, particularly in women.

If UTI is allowed to progress, it may lead to septic complications (urosepsis). This disease is managed with antibiotics.

Urinary retention

Urinary retention may result from urethral stricture, inflammation, enlarged prostate, central nervous system dysfunction, foreign body obstruction, and use of certain drugs, such as parasympatholytic or anticholinergic agents. These patients need to be evaluated by a physician to determine the cause of the retention. If the cause is not easily correctable, the patient may need to be hospitalized.

Some patients may require bladder catheterization with an indwelling Foley catheter device. This procedure may be indicated to empty the bladder of a patient with urinary retention or replace an indwelling urinary catheter that is not functioning. Bladder catheterization is an invasive procedure so carries some associated risks. These include the introduction of bacteria, which may lead to UTI; haematuria; and the creation of a false urethral passage, which may result in significant blood loss and the need for surgical repair. Special training is required to perform bladder catheterization.

Indwelling Foley catheter insertion To insert a Foley catheter, the paramedic should prepare the required equipment (e.g. Foley catheter insertion set). The paramedic should also follow closely the recommendations of the manufacturer (Box 41-6). Steps in bladder catheterization for male and female patients are described in this section. Most patients will be anxious and frightened of the procedure so it is especially important that the paramedic provide a full explanation of the procedure, reassure the patient, and make every effort to ensure privacy.

Critical Thinking

What measure should you take to protect yourself legally when inserting a Foley catheter into a patient in a home?

Male catheterization (Figure 41-3)

1. Explain and discuss the procedure with the patient.
2. Wash hands.
3. Assist patient into supine position with the legs extended and remove the patient's pants and undergarments – keep the patient covered until all equipment is prepared.
4. Wash hands using bactericidal soap and water.
5. Put on a disposable apron.
6. Open the catheterization set using sterile technique.
7. Wash hands and don sterile gloves.
8. Place one sterile drape under the patient's penis and another above the penis to cover the abdomen.
9. Open a package of antiseptic solution and saturate sterile sponges (or cotton balls).
10. Attach the syringe to the catheter and test the balloon to make sure it inflates.
11. Open a package of water-soluble lubricant and lubricate the first several inches of the catheter.
12. Grasp the patient's penis with one hand and retract the foreskin (if present).
13. With the other hand, cleanse the glans with a sterile sponge (maintaining hand sterility) and then discard the sponge. Repeat the procedure.
14. Raise the shaft of the penis upright to straighten the penile urethra and pass the tip of the catheter through the meatus.
15. Continue passing the catheter with gentle, steady pressure, advancing the catheter 15–25 cm or until urine flows out the distal end of the catheter. Once urine appears, advance the catheter another 5 cm. If mild resistance is felt at the external sphincter, slightly increase traction on the penis and continue with steady, gentle pressure on the catheter. If significant resistance is met, withdraw the catheter and consult with medical direction.
16. Attach the syringe to the catheter and inflate the balloon with 3–5 mL of sterile saline.
17. Gently pull back on the catheter until the balloon rests against the prostatic urethra. (Resistance will be encountered.) Reposition the retracted foreskin of an uncircumcised patient. Attach the drainage bag to the catheter.
18. Run the catheter tubing along the patient's leg and tape the connecting tubing to the patient's thigh. Do not place any tension on the catheter.

Box 41-6

Necessary equipment for bladder catheterization

Personal protective equipment
Catheter pack
Appropriate catheter
Sterile gloves
Local anaesthetic lubricating gel
Universal specimen container
Normal saline for cleaning
Sterile water, syringe and needle
Bactericidal alcohol hand rub
Apron
Drainage bag and stand

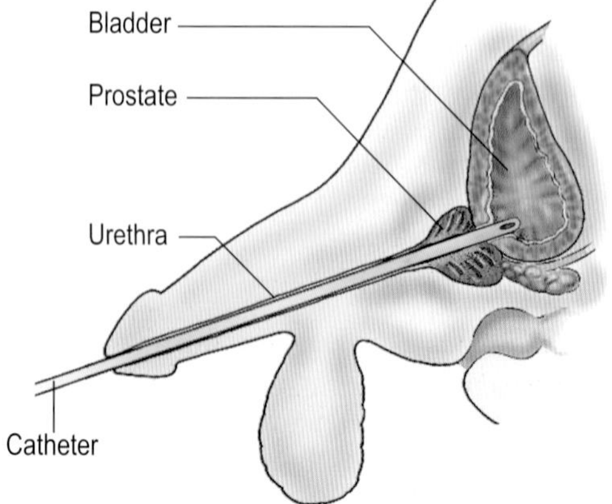

Figure 41-3 Male catheterization.

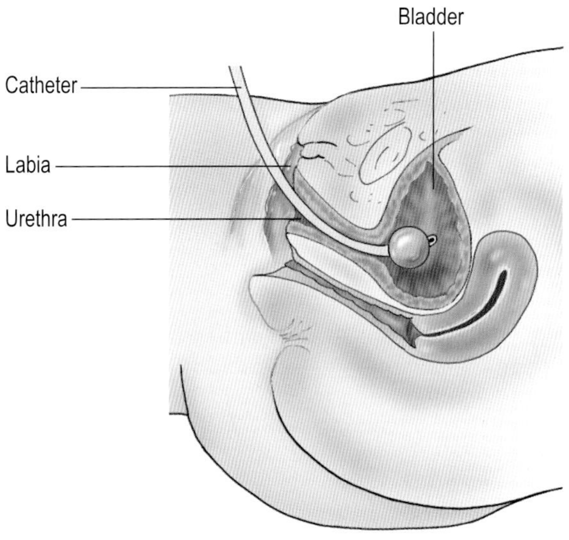

Figure 41-4 Female catheterization.

19. Attach the collection bag to the bed or stretcher at a level below that of the patient to facilitate drainage by gravity.
20. Record urinary output on a fluid chart.
21. Make patient comfortable and ensure that he is dry.
22. Dispose of equipment according to local policy.
23. Wash hands.
24. Record the insertion of urinary catheter in the patient's notes. Include: date and time of catheterization, catheter type, length, balloon volume, batch number and manufacturer, any problems occurring.

Female catheterization (Figure 41-4)[8]

1. Explain the procedure to the patient.
2. Ensure privacy and adequate lighting.
3. Assist the patient into a supine position with knees bent and feet comfortably apart.
4. Place protective sheeting under the patient's buttocks.
5. Wash hands with a bactericidal soap.
6. Put on a disposable apron.
7. Open the catheter pack to act as a sterile field in which to place all other equipment, using an aseptic technique.
8. Uncover the patient ensuring exposure of the vulva.
9. Clean hands with an alcohol rub and apply two pairs of sterile gloves.
10. Arrange sterile towels to cover surrounding areas.
11. Separate the labia majora and cleanse with gauze swabs soaked in cleansing solution; firstly the labia majora, then the labia minora, identifying the urethral meatus. Always swab from front to rear in single strokes, to minimize the risk of infection.
12. Insert the nozzle of the anaesthetic gel gently into the urethra and slowly instil 6–10 mL of gel. Warn the patient that the gel may cause some stinging. Remove the nozzle and discard the tube. NB Allow a minimum of 5 min to elapse before catheterization.

Table 41-3 Feeding tubes: types and placement

Type of tube	Placement
Nasogastric	Passed via nose into stomach
Nasointestinal	Passed via nose into intestine
Oesophagostomy	Passed into the oesophagus tube though a surgically created opening in the anterior neck
Gastrostomy	Passed directly into the stomach through an opening created in the abdominal wall
Jejunostomy, percutaneous endoscopic gastrostomy	Passed into the jejunum through an opening created in the abdominal wall

13. Discard first pair of sterile gloves.
14. Place the catheter in the sterile receiver between the patient's legs.
15. Hold the catheter in the dominant hand.
16. Remove the perforated end of the plastic cover and introduce the catheter tip into the urethral orifice in an upward and backward motion for 5–6 cm.
17. Once urine starts to flow, advance the catheter a further 5 cm to ensure the balloon is in the bladder. NB If the patient experiences undue pain or there is excessive resistance, stop and seek medical advice.
18. Inflate the balloon with 10 mL of sterile water according to manufacturer's guidelines. NB If the patient experiences pain while inflating the balloon, it may still be in the urethra. Deflate and advance the catheter a further few centimetres.
19. Withdraw the catheter until resistance is felt.
20. A urine specimen may be collected in a sterile container for microbiology at this stage.
21. Connect to an appropriate closed drainage system.
22. Record urinary output on a fluid chart.
23. Make patient comfortable and ensure that she is dry.
24. Dispose of equipment according to local policy.
25. Wash hands.
26. Record the insertion of urinary catheter in the patient's notes. Include: date and time of catheterization, catheter type, length, balloon volume, batch number and manufacturer, any problems occurring during the procedure and gel used.

Problems with gastric emptying or feeding

Gastric tubes used in the home healthcare setting are devices that are inserted into the stomach or intestines. They are used to remove fluids and gas by suction or gravity, to instil irrigation solutions or medications, and to administer enteral feedings (Table 41-3). Two common problems with gastric tubes are aspiration of gastric contents and malfunction of gastric devices.

Aspiration of gastric contents

Aspiration of gastric contents may occur in the home healthcare patient as a result of a non-patent gastric tube, improper nutritional support via a feeding tube, or patient positioning with these medical devices. The patients at greatest risk for aspiration of tube feedings are those who

- are unconscious
- are confused
- are seriously debilitated
- are older adults
- have tracheostomies or large-bore feeding tubes
- have impaired gag reflexes
- cannot sit upright.

The paramedic should monitor patients with feeding tubes closely for signs of increased respiratory effort. Lung sounds should be clear on auscultation. Respiratory difficulty or tachypnoea may indicate developing aspiration pneumonitis. Other problems that can occur in patients with feeding tubes include diarrhoea, choking, irritable bowel syndrome, and bowel obstruction.

Obstruction or malfunction of gastric devices

A gastric device may become obstructed or malfunction for different reasons. For example, there may be a kinked or clogged tube, or a surgically implanted feeding tube may become displaced. Acute interventions that may be required include unkinking a tube, irrigating a clogged tube, and reinserting a displaced tube (if qualified and authorized to do so) (Table 41-4). When transporting a patient with a gastric device, the paramedic must ensure patient comfort and should position the device to allow for proper drainage and to prevent reflux.

Ostomies

An ostomy is a temporary or permanent artificial opening into the urinary tract, gastrointestinal tract, or trachea. (An ileostomy is an opening into the small intestine; a colostomy is an opening into the large intestine.) The bowel usually discharges liquid or solid faeces into the bag (pouch) once or twice a day; the bag then is changed. Potential complications associated with ostomies include infection, haemorrhage, obstruction, and stomal problems (e.g. necrosis, retraction, stenosis and prolapse).

Colostomy irrigation, ostomy care, and pouch changes are usually performed for home healthcare patients by the patients themselves, family members and home healthcare practitioners. These procedures require special training and are not usually considered an acute intervention for paramedic practice. Bowel perforation and significant fluid/electrolyte imbalances may accidentally occur from colostomy irrigation performed by the patient or caregiver.

Assessment and management of patients with gastrointestinal/genitourinary crisis

The paramedic should evaluate a patient with gastrointestinal/genitourinary complaints by obtaining a focused history and performing a physical examination to determine the need for immediate transport for physician evaluation. Depending on the patient's chief complaint, the physical examination may include assessment for the following:

Table 41-4 Managing tube-feeding problems*

Complication	Interventions
Aspiration of gastric secretions	Discontinue feeding immediately
	Perform tracheal suction of aspirated contents if possible
	Notify the doctor
	Check tube placement before feeding to prevent complications
Tube obstruction	Flush the tube with warm water. If necessary, replace the tube
	Flush the tube with 50 mL of water after each feeding to remove excess sticky formula, which could occlude the tube
Nasal or pharyngeal irritation or necrosis	Provide frequent oral hygiene using mouthwash or lemon-glycerin swabs. Use petroleum jelly on cracked lips
	Change the position of the tube. If necessary, replace the tube
Vomiting, bloating, diarrhoea or cramps	Reduce the flow rate
	Warm the formula
	For 30 min after feeding, position the patient on the right side with the head elevated to facilitate gastric emptying
	Notify the doctor. The doctor may want to reduce the amount of formula being given during each feeding
Constipation	Provide additional fluids if the patient can tolerate them
	Administer a bulk-forming laxative
	Increase fruit, vegetable, or sugar content of the feeding

*This table lists some interventions that the nurse, paramedic, patient, or caregiver may use to solve home tube-feeding problems.

- abdominal distention
- abdominal pain
- aspiration
- fever
- intestinal obstruction
- peritonitis
- urinary tract infection
- urinary retention.

Acute infections

Home healthcare patients with acute infections have an increased death rate from sepsis and severe peripheral infections. They may also have a decreased ability to perceive pain or perform self-care. Patients with chronic diseases, poor nutrition, or an inability to perform self-care are at increased risk for infection and impaired healing. Conditions that may result in the need for acute interventions in the home healthcare population include the following:[9]

- airway infections in the immunocompromised patient
- delayed healing and increased peripheral infection from poor peripheral perfusion
- skin breakdown and peripheral infections from immobility or sedentary lifestyle
- infection and sepsis from implanted medical devices
- wounds and incisions
- abscesses
- cellulitis.

Box 41-7

Sampling of wound care devices found in home healthcare patients

Dressings and wound packing material

Combination dressings
Cotton dressings (gauze)
Exudate absorptive dressings
Foam dressings
Hydrocolloid dressings
Hydrogel dressings
Hydrophilic powder dressings
Impregnated cotton dressings
Paste bandages
Transparent film (adhesive or non-adhesive)

Drains

Jackson–Pratt drains
Penrose drains

Wound closure techniques

Skin adhesive
Staples
Sutures
Tape
Wires

Open wounds

Patients with open wounds who are discharged to home healthcare may have a variety of dressings, wound packings, and drains that permit drainage of fluid or air. They may also have a variety of wound closure devices (Box 41-7). (Dressings, packings and wound closure devices can become contaminated; drains can become occluded or displaced.) Wound healing greatly depends on wound management. The patient must be made aware of the importance of taking all prescribed medications (especially antibiotics) and should also be informed of the importance of completing all wound care procedures. Wound repair is generally believed to be enhanced by the following:

- moist environment
- wound bed free of necrotic tissue, eschar, and environmental contamination or infection
- adequate blood supply to meet metabolic demands for tissue generation
- sufficient oxygen and nutrition for cellular metabolism and tissue generation.

General principles in wound care management

Wound care requires assessment of the wound and the surrounding tissues. It also requires evaluation for infection or sepsis. General principles in wound care management include an assessment for the following:[10]

1. Assess the patient to include:
   Factors that may impede healing – e.g. concurrent medical conditions or medications being taken.
2. Assess the wound:
   Measure wound location, size and shape.
   Consider whether the wound is healthy for the stage of healing. Assess colour of the wound bed; a red or pink granular wound bed indicates healing; a green, yellow or black wound bed suggests infection or necrosis (tissue death).
   Drainage. Clear or blood-tinged drainage is common in a healing wound. Green or yellow drainage suggests infection.
   Wound odour. A sweet smell may indicate decay. A foul smell may indicate infection.
   Surrounding skin. The paramedic should assess the skin for redness, inflammation, or signs of tissue breakdown.

If the dressing is wet or contaminated, the paramedic should change it after wound evaluation. Consider cleaning the wound with normal saline and/or antiseptic solution before redressing it (seek advice if unsure). The débridement of necrotic tissue may be required. Mechanical débridement is achieved by gently rubbing the tissue with a gauze pad moistened with sterile, normal saline. Some patients may need transport for physician evaluation if severe infection or sepsis is suspected.

Maternal/child conditions

The vast majority of births in the UK take place in NHS hospitals but new mothers are likely to return home within 2–4 days of delivery.[11] Problems that may be encountered when mothers return to the home healthcare setting include:

- postpartum pathophysiologies (e.g. haemorrhage, infection and pulmonary embolism)
- postpartum depression
- septicaemia in the newborn
- infantile apnoea
- failure to thrive
- sudden infant death syndrome.

Postpartum pathophysiologies

Postpartum pathophysiologies include haemorrhage, infection and pulmonary embolism. (Acute interventions for these patients are presented in Chapter 36.) Postpartum haemorrhage occurs in about 5% of all deliveries and usually takes place within the first few hours after delivery, but it can be delayed up to 6 weeks.[12] Causes of postpartum haemorrhage include incomplete contraction of uterine muscle fibres, retained pieces of placenta or membranes in the uterus, and vaginal or cervical tears during delivery (which are rare).

Postpartum infection affects 2–8% of all pregnancies. (The most common infection is endometritis.) The condition occurs when bacteria grow and invade the uterus or other tissues along the birth canal. The symptoms usually develop on the second or third day after delivery, with fever and abdominal pain being the most common signs of infection.

Pulmonary embolism during pregnancy, labour or the postpartum period is one of the most common causes of maternal death. The embolus often results from a blood clot in the pelvic circulation but is more commonly associated with caesarean section than with vaginal delivery.

Critical Thinking

A mother is having a postpartum complication that requires urgent transport. What will you do with the baby if they are home alone?

Postnatal depression

Postnatal depression affects 10–15% of mothers.[13] The depression is most likely caused by a combination of sudden hormonal changes and psychological and environmental factors. It is important to distinguish postnatal depression from 'baby blues', the brief episode of misery and tearfulness that affects at least half of all women following delivery, especially those having their first baby. It is also important that the term postnatal depression should not be used as a generic term for all mental illness following delivery.[11] Risk factors for postpartum depression are similar to those for non-postnatal depression and include the following:[11]

- past history of psychopathology and psychological disturbance during pregnancy
- low social support
- poor marital relationship
- recent life events
- 'baby blues'.

Box 41-8

Signs and symptoms of postpartum depression

Anxiety
Change of appetite (loss of appetite or overindulgence)
Desire to leave or feelings of being trapped
Difficulty making decisions
Excessive concern or lack of concern for baby
Fantasies of disaster or bizarre fears
Fatigue or exhaustion
Fear of harming self or baby
Forgetfulness or memory loss
Hatred of spouse, self, or baby
Hopelessness
Hostility
Inability to care for baby
Increased alcohol consumption or other drug use
Irritability
Lack of interest in previously enjoyed activities
Lack of sexual interest
Loss of hope
Panic attacks
Rapid mood swings
Severe sleep disturbance
Unexplainable crying (in joy or sadness)

Recognizing and treating postpartum depression is important. The depression can interfere with the bonding between the mother and infant and can seriously affect the mother's ability to care for her newborn (Box 41-8). Many women with postpartum depression fear they will harm their babies. They often feel ashamed and guilty for these feelings. Sensitivity to the possibility of depression is crucial. Such sensitivity also is necessary for successful diagnosis and treatment. (Interventions for depression are presented in Chapter 25.)

Septicaemia in the newborn

Healthy newborns are vulnerable to several conditions that can require hospital treatment (see Chapters 37 and 38). Examples include jaundice that results from physiological immaturity of bilirubin metabolism, dehydration that can lead to serious electrolyte abnormalities, and sepsis. In addition, neonates are highly susceptible to infection because of diminished non-specific (inflammatory) and specific (humoral) immunity.

Septicaemia in the newborn is usually caused by group B streptococci, *Listeria monocytogenes*, or Gram-negative enteric organisms (especially *Escherichia coli*).[14] Signs and symptoms of sepsis may be minimal and non-specific. ('In the newborn, anything can be a sign of anything.')[9] Examples of signs and symptoms of sepsis in the newborn include the following:

- temperature instability
- respiratory distress
- apnoea
- cyanosis
- gastrointestinal changes (e.g. vomiting, distention, diarrhoea and anorexia)
- central nervous system features (e.g. irritability, lethargy and weak suck).

Risk factors for sepsis include prematurity, prolonged rupture of membranes, and chorioamnionitis (an inflammatory reaction in the amniotic membranes caused by bacteria in the amniotic fluid). The diagnosis is generally confirmed after physician evaluation by a positive blood, urine, or cerebrospinal fluid culture.

Infantile apnoea

Apnoea is defined as the cessation of breathing for more than 20 s or the cessation of breathing for less than 20 s if it is accompanied by bradycardia or oxygen (O_2) desaturation.[15,16] The condition is primarily a disorder of prematurity and is usually secondary to immaturity of central nervous system respiratory control.[17] This is described as an apparent life-threatening event (ALTE) and poses problems for the attending clinician as the infant may appear well by the time of arrival. ALTE was defined in 1986 as 'an episode that is frightening to the observer and that is characterized by some combination of apnoea (central or occasionally obstructive), colour change (usually cyanotic or pallid but occasionally erythematous or plethoric), marked changes in muscle tone (usually marked limpness), choking or gagging'.[18]

Primary causes of infantile apnoea include the following:[19]

- Idiopathic central apnoea: often presumed to be immaturity of the respiratory centre and a weak respiratory response to hypercapnia.
- Gastrointestinal: gastro-oesophageal reflux disease.
- Respiratory: lower respiratory tract infections such as pertussis and respiratory syncytial virus infection, pneumonia.
- Central nervous system: seizures, head injury, hydrocephalus, encephalitis.
- Cardiovascular system: arrhythmias, cardiomyopathies.
- ENT: ENT infection, anatomical airway obstruction.
- Other: hypoglycaemia, hypocalcaemia, poisoning.

The paramedic must assess the presence of apnoea carefully and document it. Most infants with the diagnosis of apnoea will be hospitalized and observed closely using electronic apnoea monitoring devices. These devices detect changes in thoracic or abdominal movement and heart rate. Managing apnoea in these patients may include the home healthcare use of apnoea monitors, oscillating waterbeds, and CPAP with supplemental oxygen. Some patients may also be prescribed respiratory stimulants (e.g. doxapram or methylxanthines).

Failure to thrive

Failure to thrive is an abnormally slow rate of growth and development of an infant. It results from conditions that interfere with normal metabolism, appetite, and activity. Causative factors include the following:

- chromosomal abnormalities
- major organ system defects that lead to deficiency or malfunction
- systemic disease or acute illness
- physical deprivation (primarily malnutrition related to insufficient breast milk, poverty, or poor knowledge of nutrition)
- various psychosocial factors (e.g. maternal deprivation).

Failure to thrive can result in permanent and irreversible retardation of physical, mental, or social development. Any suspicions of failure to thrive should be documented carefully and the incident reported in accordance with safeguarding children procedures (Chapter 38).

Hospice/palliative care

In the UK, 2005/06 minimum data set returns from service providers showed that 39 000 new patients were admitted to in-patient units, 20 000 entered into day care and a further 101 000 new patients were supported in home care.[20] Hospice services include supportive social, emotional, and spiritual services for the terminally ill as well as providing support for the patient's family. Hospice care relies on the combined knowledge and skill of a team of professionals. This team includes physicians, nurses, medical social workers, therapists, counsellors, chaplains, and volunteers. These people work together to provide a personal plan of care for each patient and family. The need for hospices is likely to continue to rise because of an ageing population.

Palliative care

Palliative care is a unique form of healthcare that is mainly directed at providing relief to terminally ill people through symptom management and pain management. This specialty focuses on the needs of the patient and family when a life-threatening illness such as cancer or acquired immunodeficiency syndrome has reached the terminal stage. A chief goal of palliative care is to improve the quality of a person's life as death approaches and to help patients and their families move toward this reality with comfort, reassurance, and strength. Palliative care is not focused on death; it is about specialized care for the living. Well-rounded palliative care programmes also address mental health and spiritual needs. Palliative care may be delivered in hospices, home care settings, and hospitals. Medical needs vary depending on the disease that is leading toward death, so specialized services exist to meet the needs of specific patient groups (Box 41-9).

Emergency medical services should work closely with the families and physicians of terminally ill patients in private homes and hospice programmes so that they will make the best use of the EMS system. (For instance, they will know when to call 999.) Even though resuscitation may not be indicated, EMS may be needed to manage pain, treat acute medical illness or traumatic injury, and provide transport to a hospital. If the patient is not to receive medical intervention to prolong life, the paramedic should provide measures of comfort to the patient. In addition, the paramedic should provide emotional support to family members and loved ones (see Chapter 3).

Hospice care in the home setting

A patient receiving hospice care may be receiving medication delivery for the relief of pain (e.g. narcotic infusion devices). The patient will also have medical and legal documents such as 'do not resuscitate' orders and advance directives (see Chapter 2). The paramedic should discuss any concerns about effective pain management, overmedication, or interpreting medical or legal documents with ambulance control. It is important to note that not all patients who receive hospice care have 'do not resuscitate' orders (Box 41-10).

Box 41-9

Essential elements of a palliative care programme

Palliative care is an accepted specialty of medicine and nursing that concentrates on the total care of patients suffering from any form of terminal illness. Its development, as part of the healthcare services, is a recognition that dying is a normal consequence of living. The support of health professionals and use of modern medical technology can relieve much of the distress normally associated with dying. Essential elements of a palliative care programme are the following:

1. The coordination of care for patients with a terminal illness, at home or in hospital, by a distinct service.
2. The unit of care is the patient and the patient's family, who have the right to make choices and decisions based on an understanding of the illness and to have those decisions respected.
3. The care is provided by an interdisciplinary team.
4. The care is coordinated and delivered by specifically selected and trained nurses.
5. The service is directed by a physician.
6. The emphasis is on control of symptoms, be they physical, social, or emotional.
7. The services are available on a 24 hours a day, 7 days a week, on-call basis.
8. The programme must be sensitive to differences in faith and culture and must incorporate the patients' beliefs into decisions on their care.
9. Following the death of a patient, the programme should ensure that grief support is available for the family. This may be provided by the programme itself or by other community services.
10. There is a system of structured staff support and communication.
11. The programme is integrated and coordinated with other services, and continuity of care for the patient is provided.
12. Evaluation of the programme and its services must be regular. This evaluation may extend into the area of research.
13. The programme will provide education for its own staff, other healthcare providers, and the public.

From Essential elements of a palliative care program, Health Canada, Minister of Public Works and Government Services, 2000, Ottawa, Canada.

Box 41-10

Bill of rights and responsibilities for terminally ill patients

A. Personal dignity and privacy

1. You have the right to considerate, respectful service and care, with full recognition of your personal dignity and individuality, without regard to gender, age, ethnicity, income level, lifestyle, educational background or spiritual philosophy.
2. You have the right to be dressed as you wish and not to be disrobed or uncovered any longer than necessary for your care.
3. You have the right to privacy and the assurance of confidentiality when receiving care, to refuse visitors or persons not directly involved in your care, and to choose who will receive information about your condition.
4. You have the right to request the presence of a person of your choice during interactions with healthcare professionals.
5. You have the right to experience all emotions, including anger, sadness, confusion, guilt, depression, impatience, fear and loss.
6. You have the right to have your end-of-life choices respected by healthcare professionals, including continuing or discontinuing treatment or requesting medications to self-administer for a hastened death.
7. You have the right to die with your loved ones present and to request the presence of a healthcare professional, if desired.
8. You have the responsibility to treat your caregiver with respect and to follow their directions when consistent with your wishes.
9. You have the responsibility to make certain that your right to privacy and confidentiality is clearly understood by all parties involved in your care and to communicate to your healthcare providers when you feel that your rights to privacy and confidentiality are in jeopardy.

B. Informed participation

1. You have the right to honest, accurate, and understandable information about your current diagnosis and prognosis; the recommended treatment and what it is expected to do; the possibility of success; and the possible risks of complications and side effects, including the probability of their occurrence.
2. You have the right to be informed about alternative forms of treatment, including hospice and home care, and to participate in all decisions affecting your care.
3. You have the right to request and receive a second opinion. When curative care is no longer indicated or desired, you have the right to access palliative care, including pain medication in whatever dosage or schedule you deem necessary to alleviate pain and suffering, even at the risk of hastening death.
4. You have the right to make your own decisions regarding what constitutes your human dignity, as long as you are mentally competent and continue to have basic decision-making capacity. You will be considered mentally competent if you can understand the nature of your condition, the treatment alternatives available, the likely outcomes of treatment versus non-treatment, and can accept responsibility for your decisions.
5. You have the right to access information in your medical record and to know if your healthcare providers believe that your condition or course of disease will result in death. This information may be needed to make informed decisions about your future.
6. You have the right to forgo eating and drinking naturally in order to permit the process of dying to proceed unencumbered.
7. You have the right and responsibility to complete a directive to physicians (living will).
8. You have the right and responsibility to execute a durable power of attorney for healthcare so that someone you choose can make healthcare decisions for you, if needed.

Box 41-10

Bill of rights and responsibilities for terminally ill patients—cont'd

C. Competent care

1. You have the right to competent medical, nursing, and social services care.
2. You have the right to choose your personal physician and to change your physician at any time.
3. You have the right to know who is responsible for coordinating and supervising your care and to know how to contact that person.
4. You have the right to be informed about who owns and controls the agency or facility involved with your care and the right to referral to institutions, facilities, and practitioners who can provide the care you need.
5. You have the responsibility to choose a primary care physician who is able and willing to carry out your wishes.
6. You have the responsibility to communicate your end-of-life wishes to family, friends, and healthcare providers.

From Compassion In Dying Federation, Portland, Oregon.

Summary

- An increasing number of home healthcare patients have conditions related to diseases of the circulatory system as their primary diagnosis; including people with heart disease, including congestive heart failure. Other common diagnoses of home healthcare patients include cancer, diabetes, chronic lung disease, renal failure/dialysis and hypertension. Typical EMS calls to a home healthcare setting may include respiratory failure, cardiac decompensation, septic complications, equipment malfunction and other medical problems.
- After arrival at the scene of a home healthcare patient, the scene size-up should include standard precautions, elements of scene safety and environmental setting. The initial assessment should focus on illness or injury that poses a threat to life. The paramedic should take appropriate measures as indicated.
- Patients with diseases of the respiratory system being cared for at home are at increased risk for airway infections. In addition, the progression of their illnesses may lead to difficulty breathing, making current support equipment inadequate.
- Assessment findings that may require acute interventions in patients with VADs include infection, haemorrhage, haemodynamic compromise from circulatory overload or embolus, obstruction of the vascular device, and catheter damage with leakage of medication.
- Patients with diseases of the digestive or genitourinary system may have medical devices such as urinary catheters or urostomies, indwelling nutritional support devices (e.g. percutaneous endoscopic gastrostomy tube, or gastrostomy tube), colostomies and nasogastric tubes. Acute interventions required for these patients can result from UTI, urosepsis, urinary retention, and problems with gastric emptying or feeding.
- Home healthcare patients with acute infections have an increased death rate from sepsis and severe peripheral infections. Many also have a decreased ability to perceive pain or perform self-care.
- Maternal/child conditions that one may encounter in the home healthcare setting during the postpartum period include postpartum haemorrhage, infection, pulmonary embolism, postpartum depression, septicaemia in the newborn, infantile apnoea and failure to thrive.
- Hospice services include supportive social, emotional, and spiritual services for the terminally ill. They also provide support for a patient's family. Palliative care is directed mainly at providing relief to a terminally ill person. They do this through symptom and pain management.

References

1. National Statistics. Community Care Statistics 2004: Home care services, England. Online. Available http://www.dh.gov.uk/en/Publicationsandstatistics/Publications/PublicationsStatistics/DH_4111548 26 February 2009
2. Rich MW, Beckham V, Wittenberg C et al 1995 A multidisciplinary intervention to prevent the readmission of elderly patients with congestive heart failure. N Engl J Med 333:1190–1195
3. Stewart S, Vandenbroek AJ, Pearson S et al 1999 Prolonged beneficial effects of a home-based intervention on unplanned readmission and mortality among patients with congestive heart failure. Arch Intern Med 159:257–261
4. Blue L, Lang E, McMurray JJV et al 2001 Randomised controlled trial of specialist nurse intervention in heart failure. BMJ 323:715–718
5. Department of Health 2008 Reducing infection through effective practice in the pre-hospital environment. HMSO, London
6. Meldum M, Rawone R, Curran A, Fishwick D 2005 The role of occupation in the development of chronic obstructive pulmonary disease (COPD). Occup Environ Med 62:212–214
7. Hart S 2008 Urinary catheterisation. Nursing Standard 22(27):44–48
8. Dougherty L, Lister S (eds) 2008 The Royal Marsden Hospital Manual of Clinical Nursing Procedures. Wiley-Blackwell, Oxford
9. US Department of Transportation, National Highway Traffic Safety Administration 1998 EMT-Paramedic national standard curriculum. US

Department of Transportation, Washington, DC

10. Rice R 1995 Handbook of home health nursing procedures. Mosby, St Louis
11. Office for National Statistics 2005 Birth statistics. Review of the Registrar General on births and patterns of family building in England and Wales, 2005. Office for National Statistics, London
12. Rosen P, Barkin R 1998 Emergency medicine: concepts and clinical practice, 4th edition. Mosby, St Louis
13. Scottish Intercollegiate Guidelines Network 2002 Postnatal depression and puerperal psychosis. Online. Available http://www.sign.ac.uk/guidelines/fulltext/60/index.html 26 February 2009
14. Hoekelman R 1997 Primary pediatric care, 3rd edition. Mosby, St Louis
15. American Academy of Pediatrics, Committee on Fetus and Newborn. 2003 Apnea, sudden infant death syndrome, and home monitoring. Pediatrics 111(4 Pt 1):914–917
16. Finer NN, Higgins R, Kattwinkel J, Martin RJ 2006 Summary proceedings from the apnea-of-prematurity group. Pediatrics 117(3 Pt 2):S47–S51
17. Dison KR, Ashtyani H 2004 Diagnosis and treatment of apnea of infancy in apparent life threatening events. Chest 126(4):1002S
18. [Anonymous] 1987 National Institutes of Health Consensus Development Conference on Infantile Apnea and Home Monitoring, Sept 29 to Oct 1, 1986. Consensus statement. Pediatrics 79(2):292–299
19. McGovern MC, Smith MBH 2004 Causes of apparent life threatening events in infants: a systematic review. Arch Dis Child 89(11):1043–1048
20. National Council for Palliative Care 2007 Minimum data sets, project updates including 2005/06 data. NCPC, London

PART NINE

CHAPTER **42**

Major Incidents

Chapter contents

Objectives

Upon completion of this chapter, the paramedic student will be able to:

1. Identify the components of an effective major incident system.
2. Outline the activities of the preplanning, scene management, and post-incident follow-up phases of an event.
3. List command responsibilities during a major incident response.
4. Identify situations that may be classified as major incidents.
5. Given a major incident, describe the various staff roles and responsibilities that would need to be established.
6. List common problems related to major incidents.
7. Outline the principles of triage.
8. Identify resources for the management of critical incident stress.

Key terms

CHALETS Mnemonic for providing a report to control.

major incident An event for which available resources are insufficient to manage the nature of the emergency.

mass casualty incident An event for which available resources are insufficient to manage the number of casualties.

MERIT Mobile Emergency Response Incident Team. A mobile medical team sent to the site of a major incident/emergency.

METHANE Mnemonic for providing a report to control (situation report when first on scene).

mutual aid An agreement with neighbouring emergency agencies to exchange equipment and personnel when necessary.

sectors Smaller areas within an inner cordon with groups of staff managed by a Bronze Forward Incident Officer.

triage To sort: the process of assessing severity of injury to determine most appropriate action and clinical management.

Background

In the past, the management of a major incident often involved a number of different agencies. For example, ambulance and emergency medical services (EMS) agencies, the fire service and rescue, police, and others may have responded. Each of these agencies operate independently, and historically there have been times when inter-service organization and personnel accountability were less than optimal, making it difficult to determine who was in charge of the scene as well as making it difficult to determine which emergency services were needed or were being provided.

The experience of various major incidents of the last century and the early years of this century has shaped how services respond. Terrorist acts in various parts of the British Isles since the late 1960s, in Northern Ireland as well as on the mainland, collisions and incidents on various forms of transport such as rail crashes (Harrow, Moorgate, Clapham, Paddington, Potters Bar and Hatfield), air crashes (such as Staines, Manchester and Kegworth), disasters such as the Bradford football stadium fire, the football disaster at Hillsborough and the fire at King's Cross Station, and natural disasters such as flooding that have become a frequent occurrence over the past decade are just a few of the many scenarios that have provided both challenges and experience to all of the services that become involved. The earliest incidents are often acknowledged to have been managed in a much less coordinated way than might occur today; indeed, at Harrow in 1952, the local services were overwhelmed and the American Air Force was one notable organization locally that provided much needed resources, as well as having a plan and more coordinated response which allowed delivery of equipment and supplies to the scene and most importantly a command structure that allowed some degree of order. They also had devised methods of recording details of casualties and the care given (for example if morphine had been given).

Even if well planned for and however many mock exercises are undertaken, major incidents still can be chaotic, difficult to manage and very draining on staff and resources, in many different ways. These incidents can overwhelm, or at best put under severe pressure, the normal structures and processes in place even though adequate preparedness has been undertaken, and so, it must be borne in mind that things will not always run smoothly. However, by following a structured response and having clearly designated roles and responsibilities, many of the difficulties encountered can be minimized and the best possible outcome to an often sudden occurrence can be obtained.

Definition of a major incident

In 2005 the Department of Health updated its Emergency Planning Guidance (EPG), with detailed guidance about how organizations in the NHS should prepare for major incidents.

It defines a major incident as

any occurrence that presents serious threat to the health of the community, disruption to the service or causes (or is likely to cause) such numbers or types of casualties as to require special arrangements to be implemented by hospitals, ambulance trusts or primary care organisations (Department of Health, 2005, Emergency Planning Guidance).

It furthers suggests the broad range of incidents that may put pressure on services, other than the traditional notion of a major incident (the 'Big Bang' type incident described above): for example, major chemical leaks, preplanned events that require emergency planning and preparedness, and possible developing disease epidemics all require a response that cannot be handled routinely and that require special arrangements.

The Civil Contingencies Act (CCA) in 2004 has brought about the term 'emergency' and many organizations are using this term rather than the word 'incident'. It describes an emergency as

an event or a situation which threatens serious damage to human welfare in a place in the UK, the environment of a place in the UK, or war or terrorism which threatens serious damage to the security of the UK.

The development of the CCA followed a number of national civil emergencies (such as the foot and mouth outbreak and severe flooding in several parts of the country) and was a result of the review of the emergency planning arrangements in force at the time. It was felt that modern civil protection required updating and the Act was the end result of this work.

In short it provides a framework for civil protection in the UK and is in two main parts: part 1 emphasizes local arrangements for civil protection, whereas part 2 focuses on emergency powers and special legislative measures on a more macro level. EMS/ambulance services are considered to be a category 1 responder (along with services such as police and fire/rescue).

Preparation and planning (emergency preparedness)

The Department of Health makes very clear the requirement for all NHS organizations to provide adequate resources and planning in anticipation of these events and also makes the point that a major incident for one organization may not be so for another. Local conditions and circumstances will influence what constitutes a major incident; a major structural fire at a chemical plant with no casualties will be a major incident for fire and rescue but not necessarily for the ambulance service; equally, the collapse of a fairground ride may yield 10 or 20 casualties, putting strain on local ambulances services but not necessarily such a major input will be required from the fire and rescue service. Geography, environment and the involvement of utilities and other infrastructure also influence the specific nature of the event.

Overall, the objective of the NHS at a national level is:

to ensure that the NHS is capable of responding to major incidents of any scale in a way that delivers optimum care and assistance to the victims, that minimizes the consequential disruption to healthcare services and that brings about a speedy return to normal levels of functioning; it will do this by enhancing its capability to work as part of a multi-agency response across organizational boundaries (Department of Health 2005).

It can be considered there are several stages to planning for a major incident: Assessment, Prevention, Preparation, Response and Recovery.

First, there is risk assessment, where the plans are made by the NHS that are appropriate and consider all relevant risks. The next stage is maintenance of plans to prevent the emergency as well as reducing or limiting the effects. The third stage is the actual preparation, which can include the process of writing the plan, as well as testing through exercises and training. The fourth stage is the actual response should an incident or emergency occur, and the fifth stage is the recovery and restoration, which includes business continuity management, the smooth running of the service during and after the event.

Ambulance service major incident plans

EMS and the ambulance service as part of the NHS has special responsibilities; it is clear that in many major events EMS is a 'gateway' to the healthcare network and as such will be responsible for the initial alerting, activation and management of NHS resources that are required in a major emergency. At a strategic level, EMS responsibilities include preservation of life and limb, implementation of a control/communications function to coordinate on site NHS and other health resources, initiate triage, treat and convey casualties, maintain core activity and the other day-to-day activity of the service as far as possible and to make provision for conveying the Medical Emergency Response Team (MERIT) if required. There are very specific responsibilities and roles (discussed below) that EMS will undertake that are contained in the services own major incident/major emergency plan. This plan is authorized by the Chief Executive of the Ambulance Trust.

There are certain criteria that plans must meet: for instance they must clearly define the process of declaration of a major incident/emergency, state the roles and responsibilities of the first personnel on scene as well as subsequent personnel, identify how the control and communications systems will operate (with other services, media, etc.), be clear about the provision of casualty management and consider special circumstances such as mutual aid or CBRN incidents. Action cards are provided to allow staff an 'aide-memoire' and ensure that a systematic approach to an incident is taken.

NHS organizations including EMS (and other services such as police and fire/rescue) utilize a formal structure to ensure appropriate levels of command. These are Strategic, Tactical and Operational, often known as Gold, Silver and Bronze respectively.

Gold Command refers to the individual overall in charge of the organization and its response to an emergency. This may be the Chief Executive or another senior member of staff such as a Director who will liaise with their counterparts in the various organizations who become involved in the response. They will provide the overall strategy for the incident response and have the power to delegate responsibilities and functions down to the tactical command (Silver). Gold staff are off site and based usually at the headquarters or similar location.

Silver Command is considered tactical and those tasked with this role are on-site providing the plan that EMS needs to undertake to achieve the strategic direction identified by Gold. Silver oversees but does not become directly involved in the operational response to an incident.

Operational (Bronze) response by contrast is hands on and provides the main operational input to an incident. There will be several Bronze officers in a very large or protracted incident (for instance Bronze Triage, Bronze Marshalling, Bronze Clearing, Bronze Forward Incident Officer/Ambulance Officer) and these staff will be within the inner cordon. In large or geographically widespread incidents, there may be more than one Bronze Ambulance Incident Officer.

Specific responsibilities and posts

EMS/ambulance services will use a number of staff to fulfil key roles. In some smaller incidents it is possible that roles will be merged but in most cases specific roles are allocated to specific individuals. Most services use similar terminology but it is essential paramedics are familiar with their own service plan and how it would operate.

Incident site cordon

Depending on the nature of the incident different cordons will be set up. Normally, two cordons (an inner and outer) will be formed, the outer cordon being controlled by police and only nominated personnel will be allowed in. This would be as far as any non-authorized personnel and members of the public might be able to get. Inside the outer cordon an inner cordon will be set up, which is often controlled by Fire and Rescue; this is immediately around the site of the incident (in larger-scale incidents where there are several sectors there may be more than one inner cordon). Inside the inner cordon only personnel directly involved in the scene will be allowed. Although an oversimplification, in practice Silver staff and functions are adjacent to but inside the entrance to the outer cordon and the Bronze staff and functions (such as casualty clearing and ambulance parking and loading) closer to the inner cordon perimeter between the outer and inner cordons, with other Bronze staff working inside the inner cordon. In some cases, to ensure the functions of the emergency services are not hampered, a further outer cordon may be implemented. Each situation is different and will be handled accordingly.

Incident site posts

A number of incident site posts will be set up. These may include:

- Joint Emergency Service Control Centre (Silver function): This will be the ambulance service control vehicle which ideally will be parked in close proximity to the control vehicles of the other services and from which the Silver command staff can liaise with other Silver staff.
- Ambulance Control Point: The location at which the communications vehicle is parked. In the early stages of the incident this will often be the first ambulance on scene.
- Ambulance Loading Point: This is where triaged casualties are placed on ambulances (and possibly other vehicles) to be conveyed to receiving units. It is under the control of the ambulance loading officer.
- Ambulance Rendezvous Point: A point a short distance away from the site of the incident where ambulances can be staged and then fed into the scene as required.
- Ambulance Parking Points: An area at the incident site where vehicles are parked or held prior to use, near to but not at the ambulance loading point.
- Body Holding Area and Temporary Mortuary: An area under police control where the deceased are placed for a short period of time, until transfer to a temporary mortuary.
- Casualty Clearing Station: The area where the triage sort is undertaken and casualties are further managed prior to being conveyed off the site.
- Forward Control Point: An area close to the scene where the Bronze Incident Officer(s) can direct operations with mobile communications.
- Staff Rest Point: In protected incidents there may be a need for some sort of rest/rehabilitation point to be set up or arrangements for fatigued staff to be stood down for a short while to be replaced by fresh staff. This may

be close to the site or away from site at an established location such as an ambulance station.

There are a number of functions that nominated staff will perform, which include the following.

Silver

Silver staff are usually on site but work away from the core of the incident, usually inside the outer cordon.

- Ambulance Incident Commander (AIC): Is overall in charge of ambulance staff on site and ensures that the service response is appropriate. They maintain a liaison function with other Silver Commanders from police and fire/rescue for example.
- Medical Incident Commander (MIC): Also acts in conjunction with Ambulance Incident Commander and is responsible for the deployment of doctors operating on scene at a Bronze level.
- Ambulance Tactical Advisor (Silver Advisor): This will often be the emergency planning officer, who will have a detailed knowledge of the service's major incident policy as well as CBRN and other specialty plans. They will work closely with the Silver AIC.
- Communications Manager (Silver Control): on site: Again, working closely with the Silver AIC will ensure that communication systems are operative and will provide a link between the control room and the communications service provided on site. In many cases, services provide a speciality control vehicle for such a function which may house other Silver staff.

Bronze

Bronze staff will work within the inner cordon.

- Forward Incident Officers (Ambulance Incident Officer and Medical Incident Officer): These staff are usually middle managers or supervisors who manage and oversee the medical activities provided by the various teams of staff on the incident site. In larger incidents there may be several Bronze Incident Officers who each have a sector to manage. The teams on the ground dealing directly with the casualties will undertake a triage sieve to determine which casualties are removed first to the casualty clearing station.
- Ambulance Casualty Clearing Officer: They are tasked with setting up and maintaining a casualty clearing station using a triage system (triage sort) to determine which casualties will be removed from the site first.
- Ambulance Decontamination: Where appropriate for certain incidents, the decontamination of casualties and the use of the ambulance decontamination teams will fall under this individual's responsibility.
- Ambulance Loading: Ensures that adequate access and egress for ambulance transport is available and maintained and is responsible for the safe loading of casualties and transport off site.
- Ambulance Marshalling/Parking: Works to marshal and control ambulance transport and staff entering the site.
- Ambulance Rendezvous: Appointed to oversee the designated rendezvous point and from there forwards vehicles and staff to the Bronze Marshalling/Parking.
- Ambulance Equipment Officer: Responsible for coordinating equipment and supplies on site, where necessary may create equipment dumps, from which staff can withdraw supplies as needed.
- Ambulance Safety: Is responsible for overseeing the safety of all ambulance staff on site and works closely with fire/rescue as well as other agencies' safety officers.
- Ambulance Triage: May be a medical officer or a senior ambulance paramedic who has responsibility for determining which casualties leave the site for the casualty clearing station first.
- Hospital Ambulance Liaison Officer (HALO) and Hospital Ambulance Liaison Control Officer (HALCO): Based at the receiving hospital(s) and are tasked with maintaining communications between the ambulance service and the hospital as well as recording details of casualties taken into the hospital by the service.

Military and voluntary aid societies' assistance

In some cases the military will offer assistance and this will be coordinated initially via Silver and Gold Command only.

The voluntary aid societies such as the Red Cross, St John, St Andrews and Women's Royal Voluntary Service (WRVS) may become involved and will work closely under the supervision of the statutory services already present. In many areas, locally prearranged plans exist that clearly identify the remit of those services should a major incident/emergency occur.

Helicopters may also be utilized and the decision to task an aircraft to the scene will be made at Silver Command level. If several helicopters are deployed, then an officer responsible for Air Support is allocated, probably a crew member of the first helicopter on scene.

Declaring a major incident

Declaring a major incident is a critical phase of the response. If an EMS unit is dispatched to a scene that has this potential, the crew should be advised that they are responding to a possible major incident or mass casualty incident (MCI). In this case, the standard message used to other parts of the NHS and outside will be 'Major incident – standby'. This information allows other services to be contacted and allows organizations to make arrangements in advance of any confirmation and others can be placed on standby. It also allows time for determination of the availability of other resources; local hospitals also can be alerted. Invariably, multiple resources including duty officers will be sent at the same time and the first crew on scene will confirm on arrival the extent and nature of the incident. In the early stages a decision is made about the incident and a decision made to activate the next phase, which is 'Major incident declared – activate plan' or, if no major incident is found, 'Major incident – cancelled', which will allow standing down of some or all of the deployed resources. As described later, the roles of the first crew/officers on scene are very specific as the receiving hospitals need information on the number of patients and the severity of injuries as soon as possible; that way, they can begin to prepare for the patients' arrival. Other agencies require detailed information to allow them to implement their own plans and resources/response and to allow the implementation of differing levels of command and communications.

Classification

There are a number of commonly used classifications for major incidents and emergencies. Their use simply gives a context to the way the incident might be managed and acknowledges the fact that every incident is different.

Simple major: This is where the infrastructure (such as utilities, roads, communications, etc.) around the incident remains in place and is not affected by the incident; for example a coach crash would be considered to be such as it is likely to be self-contained and localized to the site of the incident.

Compound major: This is an incident where some of the local infrastructure is affected: for instance, a chemical leak might contaminate a water supply or an explosion might affect a major road or rail network.

Compensated: This is where an incident can be managed with local resources: the definition of 'local' will vary and it will depend on the type of service provided; an urban EMS system is arguably better equipped and able to handle a major emergency with locally available resources than is a rural EMS system, which is likely to be more quickly put under pressure.

Uncompensated: This is an incident which puts an unmanageable burden on local resources that has to be supported by additional services and resources from outside the locality.

CSCATTT

This is a mnemonic that describes the structured approach to a major incident/emergency. These components are described widely elsewhere in this chapter.

C: Command and Control: Appointment of various roles and posts in the Silver and Bronze structures.

S: Safety: Reminds all involved of the varied safety issues that must be addressed.

C: Communications at scene, with hospitals and with other agencies. The allocation of communications equipment and a communications vehicle or post is essential for the smooth running of a major incident/emergency.

A: Assessment: An assessment of the scene by the first crew, using METHANE, then regular updates from scene to other agencies and to Gold command.

T: Triage: This is the assessment of patients and determination of clinical need using triage sieve and triage sort methods. Triage cards or labels will be utilized.

T: Treatment: Teams on the incident site will provide treatment to those injured, using the triage categories to guide them. Basic care is given first, then more advanced interventions will be undertaken as resources become available. Medical teams (MERIT) will work closely with other EMS staff to provide this care under the guidance of Bronze officers.

T: Transport: The utilization of appropriate and adequate transport resources to get equipment and staff to scene and remove casualties away from scene to receiving units.

Response of first on scene

The roles of the first EMS staff on scene are very clear. There is a temptation to start assessing and treating casualties; however, the important thing is that early reporting back allows the activation of the major incident/emergency plan which will ensure additional resources are sent promptly to the scene. An early situation report ('sit rep') is vital for any incident which has a number of casualties likely to put strain on the service or where it is considered that a major incident/emergency has occurred. It also allows the crew to determine if the scene is safe; whatever the pressure, staff should not enter until the scene is determined to be safe. It is also vital to remember to utilize normal universal precautions and wear protective headgear and reflective jackets, etc.

The mnemonics METHANE and CHALETS are often used to provide initial situation reports to control about an incident. METHANE is often the preferred method although either will provide important information and paramedics must be guided by their own service protocol.

METHANE

M: Major incident standby or declared.

E: Exact location of the incident, using map references if possible.

T: Type of incident with brief details of types and numbers of vehicles, trains, buildings, aircraft, etc.

H: Hazards present and potential.

A: Access. Best access routes for emergency vehicles and suitable provisional rendezvous points (RVPs).

N: Numbers, approximately, of casualties – dead, injured and uninjured.

E: Emergency services present and required, including local authorities. Consider MERIT, special equipment and services, i.e. HEMS, BASICS doctors, etc. Request number of ambulance resources required.

CHALETS

C: Casualties

H: Hazards

A: Access

L: Location

E: Emergency services

T: Type

S: Safety of all personnel is paramount.

Initial crew on scene

- Do not treat casualties or begin rescue attempts but assess situation and inform control.
- Driver of the first ambulance at the scene, finding that a major incident/emergency may have occurred, will inform the Ambulance Control as soon as practicable using METHANE. He/she should remain in radio contact with the Ambulance Control Centre.
- The attendant will make a *brief* reconnaissance, liaise with any other services at the scene and give a situation

report to the Ambulance Control Centre via their colleague based at the vehicle.

- Until the arrival of a Senior Manager, the attendant in consultation with other services present such as Police and Fire Officers will if able:
  - Set up an Ambulance Control Centre Point.
  - Set up a Rendezvous Point and establish access and egress (an Ambulance Parking Point).
  - Set up a casualty clearing station.
- Until the arrival of more senior staff/managers/supervisors, crews will assume responsibility for the ambulance aid given at the scene and the triage of casualties. Evacuation should only take place in the event of a hazardous environment being present. The first crew will not, however, undertake the treatment of casualties themselves and should act as temporary ambulance incident officers.

Subsequent crews

Other crews directed to the scene should:

- Locate the designated Ambulance Parking or Rendezvous Point, and report immediately on the radio to the Ambulance Control Centre Point for instruction and work under the direction of those staff already on scene and in charge. Do not work independently.
- Ideally, drivers should remain in the vehicles at the rendezvous point or ambulance parking point, waiting to move up to the loading points, but in reality this is often impracticable as all staff will be needed to help assess and treat/transport casualties. Care must be taken to leave the vehicle with the keys in, parked in an appropriate location and consider the drain on equipment if the engine is turned off; consider the need to leave the engine running (be aware of safety and security issues though and perform a dynamic risk assessment at the time).
- All attending personnel should report to the designated Ambulance Control Centre Point for instructions.
- Only the designated Ambulance Control Centre Point (first vehicle on scene) will keep their blue lights on. Drivers of subsequent vehicles should switch off their blue lights at the Ambulance Rendezvous Point and the Ambulance Parking Point. On arrival of the Communications Vehicle, this will take over as the Ambulance Control Centre Point and will show a green flashing light (at this point the initial ambulance will turn off blue lights).
- Whilst at the scene, all messages should be passed to the Ambulance Control Centre Point on the channel dedicated for the purpose (usually the Emergency Reserve Channel) unless otherwise instructed.
- Treatment at the scene will be limited to managing primary survey positive complaints such as airway and control of bleeding and pain relief etc. There is little time for intricate and detailed care and some compromises in clinical care are occasionally necessary.
- Casualties will be triaged for evacuation and loaded in accordance with instructions of the officer delegated to carry out this function. This person will be the bronze triage office or another bronze officer or bronze medic assigned the role.
- On leaving the incident, crews should advise the Ambulance Control Centre Point (ACP) and then revert to the designed channel and inform the Ambulance Control Centre of the number and triage categories of patients carried, their destination and then proceed as directed.
- All casualties should be suitably labelled before arrival at the receiving hospital. It may not always be possible for crews to record details of patients carried and therefore a general description should be made (e.g. male in his teens, female elderly). Where possible however, obtain as much detail of the casualties as is possible as this will be required by the HALO.
- Wherever possible, crews should recover equipment or obtain replacements before leaving hospital by liaising with a designated Ambulance Liaison Officer (HALO) if one is available.
- On becoming available at hospital, inform the Ambulance A&E Control Centre via the HALO and await further instructions. Crews should not automatically return to the incident and may be dispatched to other calls in the area and not returned to the incident site.

Communication skills and systems play a vital role in the smooth running of any incident. It is worth remembering that:

- Radio traffic must be clear, concise, and in plain English.
- Messages should be given thought and prepared before transmission.
- The speaker should clearly identify the unit number, designation (such as bronze medic 1) or call sign as appropriate.
- All radio traffic should be minimized.
- Face-to-face communication is preferable in some circumstances.

Triage

Triage is 'to sort'. The whole purpose of triage is to maximize the response to the emergency with the resources available at the time and focusing efforts on those who may survive, and making the difficult decision, in some large incidents, to leave those who are dying and who are highly unlikely to survive.

Two forms of triage exist in the UK: triage sieve and triage sort (see Figures 42-1 and 42-2). Triage sieve is the initial triage done at the incident site where the casualties are first located and the triage sort is undertaken at the casualty clearing station; further triage may be undertaken later but this is usually away from the incident site and at the receiving unit. The triage sieve gives Silver command some notion of the numbers involved and the severity of injuries etc. and allows the continued response to be accurately formulated. In the US, the triage sieve and sort are replaced by primary and secondary triage categories.

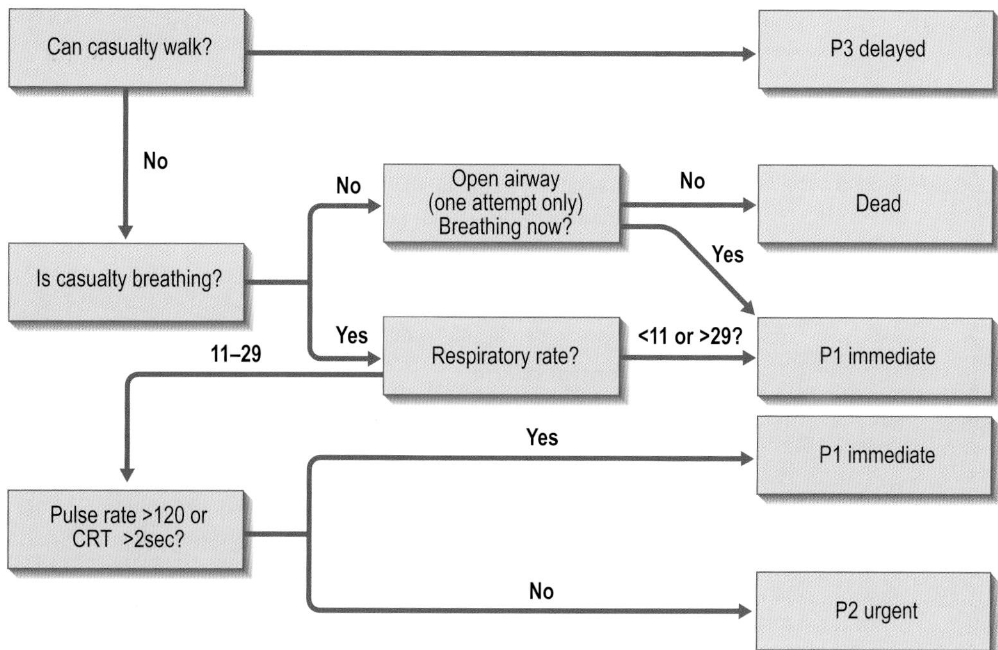

Figure 42-1 Triage sieve.

Triage categories

There are many different labelling systems: Cruciform, METTAG, START and others all use similar principles; a colour-coded system and to prioritize the highest-acuity patient with a 1 (Figure 42-3).

One concern is that triage labels may not arrive on site promptly and there have been cases in the past when crews have made improvised arrangements for the labelling of casualties.

Generally, triage categories are universal and adopted by the military (such as NATO) as well as for civilian use:

Priority One: P1: Immediate: Red colour: these patients are the highest acuity and require interventions and conveyance first. These patients are likely to have severe multiple trauma, severe shock and/or be primary survey positive.

Priority Two: P2: Urgent: Yellow colour: those patients whose injuries are not so serious but will still require urgent interventions. These patients may have multiple injuries but limited perhaps, for example, to limbs and do not have immediate problems with their primary survey. They require definitive medical care within 2 to 4 h.

Priority Three: P3: Delayed: Green colour: those with minor injuries or who are uninjured ('walking wounded'). These patients may have, for example, soft tissue injuries, minor burns and so on. Treatment in these patients can safely be delayed for a number of hours.

Priority Four: P4: Dead: Expectant: White or black colour (varies by system and country): those who are injured beyond help or who are obviously dead. The use of this category is usually confirmed by the senior staff (e.g. Silver) on scene as there are implications of a legal and ethical nature.

> **Note**
>
> The use of the triage sieve will allow the allocation by staff of one of the above categories P1–P3 (Table 42-1).

Once in the casualty clearing station, more definitive assessment and treatment can be made and the triage sort is used for this purpose. More specific clinical parameters are used and a numerical weighting is given to the score.

Transportation of patients

The way patients are transported depends on their triage priority and situation. Ambulances typically are used. However, buses and other vehicles such as non-emergency ambulances may be used to transport a large number of stable patients. Air ambulances are usually reserved for the transport of patients in critical condition.

Post-incident issues

However well planned, rehearsed and prepared for, major incidents and emergencies will always present with operational and logistical difficulties (Box 42-1). Common problems in the past have included:

- failure to adequately provide widespread notification of the event
- failure to provide rapid initial assessment of scene and a situation report
- failure to move, collect, and organize patients quickly in a treatment area
- failure to provide proper triage
- provision of overly time-consuming care

Triage sort

Step 1	Calculate the Glasgow Coma Score	
A	**Eye opening**	
	Spontaneous	4
	To voice	3
	To pain	2
	None	1
B	**Verbal response**	
	Oriented	5
	Confused	4
	Inappropriate	3
	Incomprehensible	2
	No response	1
C	**Motor response**	
	Obeys commands	6
	Localizes	5
	Pain withdrawal	4
	Pain flexion	3
	Pain extends	2
	No response	1
GCS = A+B+C		

Step 2	Calculate the triage sort score	
X	**GCS**	
	13–15	4
	9–12	3
	6–8	2
	4–5	1
	3	0
Y	**Respiratory rate**	
	10–29	4
	>29	3
	6–9	2
	1–5	1
	0	0
Z	**Systolic blood pressure**	
	>90	4
	76–89	3
	50–75	2
	1–49	1
	0	0
Triage score = X+Y+Z		

Assign triage priority	
	12 = Priority 3: Green
	11 = Priority 2: Yellow
	≤10 = Priority 1: Red

Figure 42-2 Triage sort.

Box 42-1

Common failures seen in the incident command system

Incident command failures

To establish a structured, unified command

To establish the various points such as casualty clearing and ambulance loading points

To request additional resources early

To delegate authority

To wear identification tabards

Control failure

To coordinate the response of on-duty and off-duty emergency personnel to the scene

Communications failures

To designate a single radio channel for major incidents/emergencies (mostly the Emergency Reserve Channel (ERC) will be used unless local policy determines otherwise

To adopt standard operating procedures that limit radio traffic during incident operations

Operation failures on site

To establish an ambulance control point

To select a large or easily accessible casualty clearing station and other points on the incident site

To frequently ensure specialized equipment and personnel are available as required

General failures on site

To provide adequate progress reports to command

To become involved in physical tasks, such as carrying stretchers when not tasked to do so

To control the perimeter (police and fire/rescue)

To advise command of available personnel

To triage and tag patients appropriately

To treat patients where they are found (as opposed to stabilizing them and moving them to a treatment area) (rescuers)

To provide adequate safety precautions

Treatment group failures

To collect patients into an organized treatment area (casualty clearing station)

To establish a sufficiently large treatment area (casualty clearing station)

To organize the treatment area and monitor patients

To effectively coordinate ambulance transport with the ambulance loading officer

Transportation failures

To establish adequate access and egress routes for vehicles

To have adequate personnel to assist in transportation

To alert or update hospitals

To advise hospitals when the last patient has been transported

Supply failures

To plan for the medical supply needs of mass casualty events

To provide rapid transport of supplies to the scene

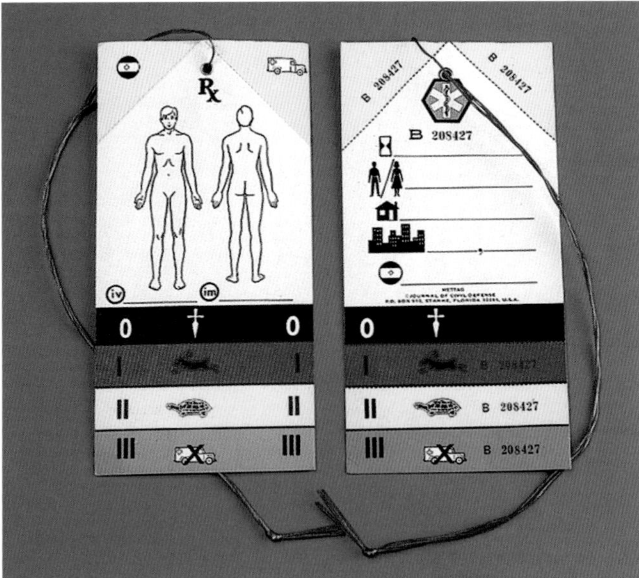

Figure 42-3 METTAG card.

Table 42-1 International colour-coding and priorities

Patient	Status colour code	Priority
Immediate	Red	Priority no. 1 (P1)
Urgent	Yellow	Priority no. 2 (P2)
Delayed	Green	Priority no. 3 (P3)
Deceased/expectant	Black (or white)	Priority no. 4 (P4)

- transport of patients prematurely
- improper use of staff on the incident site (or operating outside of designated roles)
- failure to distribute patients to appropriate receiving hospitals (hospitals will have a limited capacity in some circumstances)
- failure to communicate with local hospitals regarding patient flow and hospital capacity
- lack of proper preplanning and of adequate training for all staff.

On this last point, current UK legislation mandates that major incident and emergency plans are tested by several means:

- communications-type exercise twice a year
- table-top exercise once per year
- live exercise once every 3 years unless the service has tested the plan due to its activation at an actual major incident or emergency.

Critical incident stress management

Critical incident stress is a potential hazard for rescue personnel. For this reason, critical incident stress debriefings often are conducted after a major emergency or incident. Basic types of services that might be made available include the following:

- preincident stress training for all personnel
- on-scene support for obviously distressed personnel
- individual consults when only one or two rescuers are affected by an incident
- defusing services immediately after a large-scale incident
- mobilization services after a large-scale incident
- critical incident stress debriefing 24 to 72 h after an event for any emergency personnel involved in a stressful incident
- follow-up services to ensure that personnel are recovering
- specialty debriefings to non-emergency groups when no other timely resources are available in the community
- support during routine discussions of an incident by emergency personnel
- advice to command staff during large-scale events.

Other approaches that can aid stress management include occupational health-related support, including counselling, pastoral services, and periodic stress evaluations.

Summary

- The formalized approach should be adopted in response to a major incident or emergency. It should be flexible and adaptable to the many differing types of incident that may occur.
- All potential responding services must agree to the preplanning and preparedness work. The preplanning must address common goals and the specific duties of each group.
- The first EMS/ambulance vehicle and crew to arrive at the scene should make a quick and rapid assessment of the situation. The crew must immediately establish radio contact with the control room and use METHANE or similar to activate additional units.
- Common facilities that need to be established include casualty clearing, ambulance control point and ambulance parking and loading. An equipment dump may also be needed. Bronze officer will manage small groups of staff who will give care and manage the casualties, removing them to the casualty clearing station. Others will staff ambulances which will convey patients from the casualty clearing station to appropriate hospitals. An ambulance parking point is used in large

Summary—cont'd

incidents to prevent vehicle congestion and delays in response.

- Problems of mass casualty incidents and incident command systems stem from numerous issues related to communication, resource allocation, and delegation.
- Triage is a method used to categorize patients for priorities of treatment. Triage sieve is a rapid assessment and focuses on the patient's ability to walk, respiratory effort, and pulse rate/perfusion. Various label systems used to categorize patients during triage include Cruciform, METTAG and SMART.
- Critical incident stress debriefing is part of a critical incident stress management programme. Such debriefing should be part of post-disaster standard operating procedures.

Further reading

Ambulance NHS Trust Major Incident Plans: available to staff employed by that trust only

Civil Contingencies Act 2004. Online. Available http://www.opsi.gov.uk/Acts/acts2004/ukpga_20040036_en_1 26 February 2009

Department of Health: Emergency Preparedness Division 2005 The NHS emergency planning guidance 2005. Department of Health, London

Department of Health 2007 Strategic command arrangements for the NHS during a major incident. Department of Health, London

UK resilience. The Government's website on civil contingencies. http://www.ukresilience.gov.uk/

CHAPTER 43

Hazardous Substances Incidents

Chapter contents

Objectives

Upon completion of this chapter, the paramedic student will be able to:

1. Define hazardous substance terminology.
2. Identify legislation about hazardous substances that influences emergency healthcare workers.
3. Describe resources to assist in identification and management of hazardous substance incidents.
4. Identify the protective clothing and equipment needed to respond to selected hazardous substance incidents.
5. Describe the pathophysiology, signs and symptoms of internal damage caused by exposure to selected hazardous substances.
6. Identify the pathophysiology, signs and symptoms, and prehospital management of selected hazardous substances that produce external damage.
7. Outline the prehospital response to a hazardous substance emergency.
8. Describe medical monitoring and rehabilitation of rescue workers who respond to a hazardous substance emergency.
9. Describe emergency decontamination and management of patients who have been contaminated by hazardous substances.
10. Outline the eight steps to decontaminate rescue personnel and equipment at a hazardous substance incident.

Key terms

decontamination The process of making patients, rescuers, equipment, and supplies safe by eliminating harmful substances.

hazard warning diamond A diamond mark is used to identify the nature of the substance, for example radioactive material or compressed gases. If there is more than one hazard being carried, the diamond has an exclamation mark to identify a multi-load of mixed hazards.

hazard warning panels Wagons and containers carrying dangerous goods in bulk and tank wagons and tank containers must display hazard warning panels. The hazard warning panel has five sections on a bright orange background and provides information on the nature of the hazard. Vehicles from outside the UK will carry an orange placard known as the ADR plate.

primary contamination Exposure to a hazardous substance that is harmful only to the person exposed and that poses little risk of exposure to others.

secondary contamination Exposure to a hazardous substance whereby liquid and particulate substances are transferred easily to others by touching.

Transport Emergency Cards (Tremcards) This is a standard A4 card in red and black issued for each hazardous chemical that a vehicle is conveying. It provides EMS with vital information concerning the nature of the substance.

Hazardous substances

The term *hazardous substances* is very broad and can include chemicals, biological agents such as bacteria and other microorganisms, carcinogens and naturally occurring grain dust. Other hazardous substances can be found within the workplace and include adhesives, paints and cleaning agents, as well as substances generated during work, such as fumes from soldering or welding. All these substances have the potential to cause harm to human health and the environment.

Hazardous substance incidents create added responsibilities for emergency service providers. The primary role of ambulance services is to alert, mobilize and coordinate all primary NHS resources necessary to deal with any incident at the scene. This is achieved by planning, preparing and responding to all types of major incidents such as naturally occurring incidents (otherwise known as hazards) or hostile or deliberate acts (otherwise known as threats) that cause infrastructure failure and/or mass casualties.[1]

With any large incident there are specialized roles and responsibilities. This section will explore the main roles and responsibilities of the UK ambulance services. The most important roles are to save lives, in conjunction with other emergency services, and to ensure scene safety. Other responsibilities include instigating the command and control structure, coordination of the NHS communications on site, and alerting the main receiving hospitals for receipt of the injured. In addition, staff need to instigate a triage process after which casualties will be treated and transported to hospital as appropriate. Transportation will also be required to convey the medical emergency response incident team to the scene.[1]

The ambulance services have a responsibility to provide clinical decontamination of casualties and support mass decontamination; they protect the health, safety and welfare of all health service personnel on site.[1]

Everyday life within the ambulance service must continue and therefore adequate emergency cover must be maintained to minimize the disruption of the normal work of the service. Assistance from the voluntary aid societies may be requested and the ambulance services will coordinate their requirements and movements.

Scope of hazardous substances

A hazardous substance has been defined in the UK as any substance which is listed as dangerous for supply because it is very toxic, toxic, harmful, corrosive or irritant.[2] In the USA the definition is perhaps more broadly defined as any substance or material capable of posing an unreasonable risk to health, safety and property.[3] Over 49 million tonnes are transported around the UK on an annual basis,[4] and approximately 4 billion tonnes are shipped within the US.[5] Society as a whole is extremely dependent upon chemicals for use in daily life. The magnitude of chemical utilization is underlined by the fact that over 25 million chemicals exist within the 'universe of chemicals', 70 000 of which are in regular use. Within the US, emergency responses to vehicle crashes are common; thus, the potential for exposure to hazardous substances is great. Statistics for the UK illustrate that 1.3 million people, including 340 000 children, lived within 1 km of the 152 uncontained chemical incidents recorded from July to December 2005. The statistics suggest that, on average, one in every four people living in the proximity of a chemical incident is a child.[6] In 2005 there were 191 cases (18%) in which the chemical involved was unknown. Encouragingly there has been a 59% reduction in the rate of chemical accidents since 1987.[7]

> **Critical Thinking**
>
> Consider the industries in your area. Do any of these have the potential for a hazardous substance exposure?

Injury or illness may also result from exposure to household chemicals, pesticides and industrial toxins. EMS crews should be aware of how to manage such cases or know where to access or find the necessary information.

- An estimated 27 000 industrial workers in the UK are exposed to respiratory irritants each year.
- UK statistics highlight that approximately 3400 people will experience symptoms of chemical incident toxicity and there will be approximately eight fatalities per annum which are directly related to chemical exposure.
- The records for 2005 show pesticide poisoning accounts for 1% of all chemicals involved in incidents.
- Fire-related deaths as a result of inhalation of toxic products of combustion is the most frequently reported chemical cause of death, equating to 272 incidents, or 27%, in 2005.

Laws and regulations

In recent years much focus has been placed on the handling of hazardous materials. A series of major incidents have attracted the attention of employee and citizen groups and also the attention of local and national government officials. Some of these incidents include the Buncefield oil depot explosion in the UK (2005); chemical factory fire in Cheltenham (2006); the union carbide disaster in Bhopal, India (1984); the Chernobyl nuclear accident in the Soviet Union (1986); the Three Mile Island incident in the United States (1979); and the criticality accident in Tokaimura, Japan (1999). Threats and acts of bioterrorism (e.g. the sarin gas attack on Tokyo subways in 1995) have added to the concerns. There have been several types of chemical incidents in the UK; in 2005, 21% were within the industrial sector, 15% within the commercial sector and 19% within the residential sector.[6]

This attention has resulted in more laws and regulations, which have helped to ensure stricter control of hazardous materials. The principal legislation in the UK is:

- The Control of Major Accident Hazards Regulations 1999 (COMAH), which regulates the operators of sites that hold dangerous substances in large quantities above specified thresholds.
- The Chemicals (Hazard Information and Packaging for Supply) Regulations 2002 (CHIP), ensures people are supplied with the information they need to protect themselves from chemicals.

- The Control of Substances Hazardous to Health Regulations 2002 (COSHH), requires employers to control exposure to hazardous substances and protect employees and others who may be exposed.
- The Carriage of Dangerous Goods by Road Regulations 2004 (CDGR), which places a duty upon everyone involved in the carriage of dangerous goods to minimize the risks of incidents.
- The Dangerous Substances in Harbour Areas Regulations 1987.
- The Merchant Shipping (Dangerous Goods and Marine Pollutants) Regulations 1997.
- The Health and Safety at Work Act 1974.

Note

UK legislation places a requirement on Local Government, National Government and Industry to have in place emergency plans and to report incidents involving hazardous materials.

Definition of a chemical incident: An acute event in which there is, or could be, exposure of the public to chemical substances which cause, or have the potential to cause, ill health. In 2005, the Health Protection Agency (HPA) recorded 1040 chemical incidents in England and Wales, in which 27 000 people were exposed, 3000 of whom exhibited symptoms of exposure. Fourteen per cent of these incidents resulted in evacuation of the local population.[6]

Identification of hazardous substances

Two methods can be used to identify such substances. The first is informal product identification; the second is formal product identification. (The second method involves placards, shipping papers, and other Hazmat information resources.)

Informal product identification

Arriving emergency personnel may be able to determine the presence and type of hazardous substances at the scene. Informal methods of identification include the following:

- visual inspection of the scene from a safe distance before entering the site
- verbal reports by bystanders or other responsible individuals
- occupancy type, such as fuel storage, chemical or pesticide plant
- tankers with identifiable Hazchem labels; if you can read it you are probably too close
- vehicle types (named carriers or company)
- incident location (probable location for presence of hazardous substances)
- location within a building – offers warning sign of what is stored in that area
- visual indicators (vapour clouds, smoke, leakage)
- container characteristics (size, shape, colour, deformed containers)

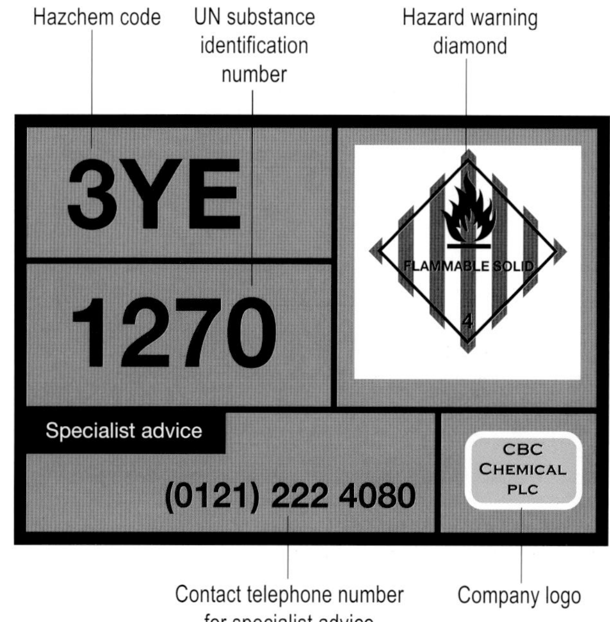

Figure 43-1 United Kingdom Hazardous Information Service panel (UKHIS panel).

- senses (peculiar smell)
- signs and symptoms of victims of exposure.

These informal ways of identifying a product should be used as a quick means to determine the presence of any hazardous substances. The paramedic should always identify a product formally before taking any action that may pose a threat to the safety of responders.

Note

Personal safety is the primary priority when responding to a hazardous substances incident. If the scene is not safe, the emergency medical services crew should not enter or should retreat until it has been made safe by appropriately trained personnel.

Formal product identification

Traditionally, hazardous substances have been labelled by one or more of the following systems:

1. *Hazard warning panels*: The Carriage of Dangerous Goods by Road and Rail Regulations requires that each vehicle/carriage should display a composite hazard warning panel, which is also known as a United Kingdom Hazardous Information Service panel (UKHIS panel). See Figure 43-1.[8] Hazard warning panels are mounted and are clearly visible whichever way the vehicle is facing. Panels can be found on the rear of the vehicle, on both sides and in some cases at the front.
2. *United Nations number* (UN number): This number is exclusive to the substance being conveyed and is used worldwide. Should more than one substance be carried, a multi-load panel will be displayed separately on each

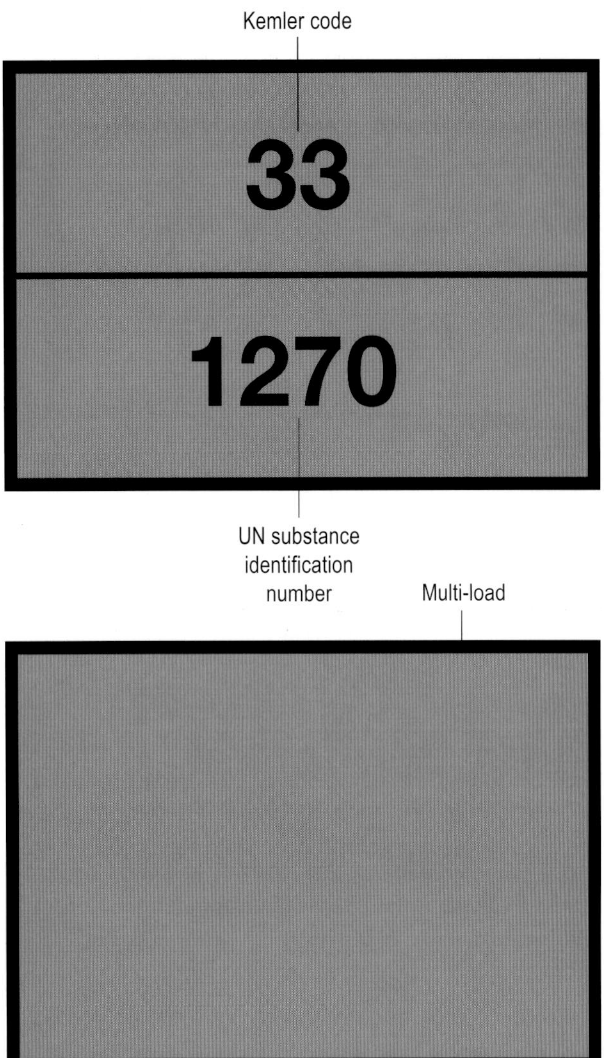

Figure 43-2 ADR and multi-load panel.

tank compartment and UN numbers displayed for each individual substance. EMS crews must communicate these numbers to ambulance control when providing an update or requesting other services.

3. *Hazchem code*: The fire services mainly use this system to interpret emergency action codes. See Figure 43-1. The code does not identify the contents of the vehicle; its purpose is to indicate the basic method of dealing with the incident, such as how to contain spillages, prevent the risk of explosion and to determine if the vicinity of the incident needs to be evacuated. Clearly, personal protection and safety are paramount.[9]
4. The international operations – *ADR*: The transport of dangerous goods between most European countries is governed by an agreement known as ADR (*Accord Dangereuse Routiers*). The purpose of this agreement is to ensure that dangerous goods transported across European frontiers comply with uniform conditions concerning the marking of vehicles. The ADR warning panel is orange in colour, with black lettering and will be found at the front and rear of the vehicle. The plate contains the hazard identification code, also called the Kemler code, and the UN substance identification number. Blank orange plates with no lettering or numbers indicate that the vehicle is carrying a multi-load which is dangerous in nature. The package goods regulations will require each substance to be clearly marked and identifiable. See Figure 43-2.
5. *Transport Emergency Cards* (Tremcards) (Figure 43-3): Companies conveying dangerous or hazardous substances must meet their obligation to provide written instruction on the action to be taken in case of emergency, in the form of an A4 sized card in red and black. Tremcards are issued for each substance conveyed and describe:
   - the chemical name of the substance
   - its appearance and chemical properties
   - the hazards inherent in its use
   - details of the actions necessary in the event of fire or spillage
   - appropriate precautions and first aid treatment to be taken.
6. *Hazard warning diamonds*: The diamond marking is an international pictogram which indicates visually the nature of the substance. If there is more than one hazard the diamond will carry an exclamation mark (!) to indicate the load is of multiple mixed hazards. See Figure 43-4a–e for examples of hazard warning diamonds.
7. *Transport by sea*: The carriage, loading, unloading and storage of dangerous goods is controlled by the Dangerous Substances in Harbour Areas Regulations 1987. Duties are imposed upon companies, personnel and harbour authorities to regulate the activities of ships. Transporting of dangerous goods by sea is regulated by the Merchant Shipping (Dangerous Goods and Marine Pollutants) Regulations 1997.[10]

Other sources of information on hazardous substances include:

National Poisons Information Service (NPIS) is a clinical toxicology service for healthcare professionals working in the NHS. It is a service commissioned by the Health Protection Agency (HPA) and supported by the Department of Health. The information service is made up of a two-tier consultant-led service operating from five regional poisons information service units throughout the UK. This service provides 24-h information and advice, supplying poisons information necessary for the diagnosis, treatment and management of cases which are clinically more complex. Ambulance services have a direct link to TOXBASE and crews should contact their control when information is required. TOXBASE is the primary clinical toxicology database of NPIS and all units contribute to and authenticate the content of TOXBASE; it represents the most authoritative source of information available.

Specialist advice centres: A telephone number of the specialist advice centre is displayed on the hazard warning panel. EMS crews must be aware of the

Cefic Tremcard - Instructions in Writing [THIS IS A SAMPLE TREMCARD ONLY - NOT FOR COMMERCIAL USE]

NCEC-SAMPLE

Class	5.1
HI No	58
PG	II
UN	1463

LOAD

Oxidising solid, corrosive

Name of substance(s): EXAMPLE TREMCARD

- Coloured solid.
- Usually with perceptible odour.
- Soluble in water.

NATURE OF DANGER

- Promotes combustion (oxidising agent)
- Not itself combustible but assists fire in burning materials.
- May react with combustible substances creating fire or explosion hazard and formation of toxic fumes. Heating will cause pressure rise with risk of bursting and subsequent explosion.
- Corrosive.
- Causes severe damage: to eyes.
- May be harmful by contact, inhalation or ingestion.

PERSONAL PROTECTION

- Goggles or face shield.
- Light protective clothing.
- Protective gloves.
- Protective footwear.
- Eyewash bottle with clean water.

INTERVENTION EQUIPMENT

- Broom.

GENERAL ACTIONS BY THE DRIVER

- Stop the engine.
- No naked lights. No smoking.
- Mark roads with self-standing warning signs and warn other road users or passers-by.
- Keep public away from danger area. Keep upwind.
- Notify police and fire brigade as soon as possible.

ADDITIONAL AND/OR SPECIAL ACTIONS BY THE DRIVER

- Any action only if without personal risk.
- Stop leaks if without risk.
- Sweep up spilled substance but avoid making dust.
- Do not absorb in sawdust or other combustible materials.
- Avoid direct contact with substance.
- If substance has entered a water course or sewer or been spilt on soil or vegetation, inform police.

FIRE (information for the driver in case of fire)

- Do not attempt to deal with any fire involving the load.

FIRST AID

- If substance has got into the eyes, immediately wash out with plenty of water. Continue treatment until medical assistance is provided.
- If clothing is burning extinguish with copious amount of water. Remove loose clothing, but do not attempt removal if adheringto skin. Cover affected areas with well wetted cloths. Remove to hospital immediately, maintaining cloths wetted at all times. Even ifcontaminated clothing is not burning drench with water immediately. Remove clothing and drench affected skin with plenty of water till all taces of substance have been removed.
- Apply artificial respiration only if patient is not breathing or under medical supervision. Do not use mouth-to-mouth respiration if victim ingested or inhaled the substance.
- Seek medical treatment when anyone has symptoms apparently due to inhalation, swallowing or contact with skin or eyes.

SUPPLEMENTARY INFORMATION FOR EMERGENCY SERVICES

- Keep container(s) cool by spraying with water if exposed to fire.
- Extinguish with waterspray, foam or dry chemical.
- When collecting do not use iron containers but use plastic, aluminium or stainless steel containers. Do not seal.

Additional information

EMERGENCY TELEPHONE: +44 (0)870 190 6621

National Chemical Emergency Centre
J Wing, Building 329, Harwell, DIDCOT, Oxfordshire OX11 0QJ UK
www.tremcards.com www.the-ncec.com

© Cefic Prepared by Cefic from the best knowledge available; no responsibility is accepted that the information is sufficient or correct in all cases. [THIS IS A SAMPLE TREMCARD ONLY]

Cefic TEC(R) - 51GOC2-I+II+III

APPLIES ONLY DURING ROAD TRANSPORT ENGLISH

0001 15-APR-2005

Cefic Revision 04/2003 Issue: ADR 2005.0 (DEMO)

Figure 43-3 Transport Emergency Card.

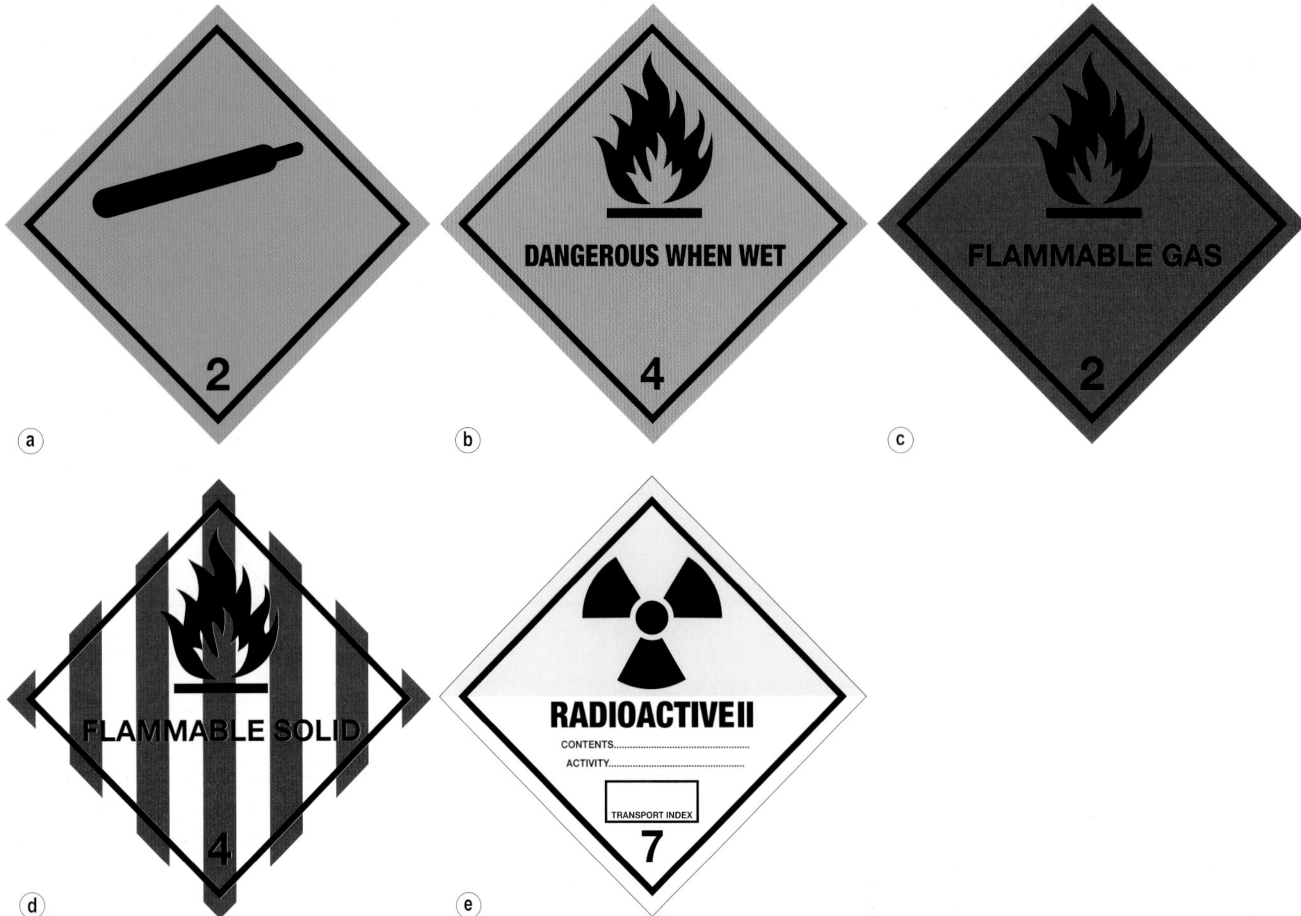

Figure 43-4 Hazard warning diamonds. (a) Compressed gas. (b) Dangerous when wet. (c) Flammable gas. (c) Flammable solid. (e) Radioactive 2.

number whilst communicating with ambulance control. As well as providing advice by telephone, a company may dispatch a team of experts to the incident if considered necessary.[11]

REACH: In June 2007 REACH was launched as the new European system for the registration, evaluation, authorization and restriction of chemicals. The REACH process is a single system that replaces a patchwork of European directives and regulations and will provide information on chemicals and technical and scientific advice from an extensive database with a single point of entry.[12]

Tanker drivers: Tanker drivers should have knowledge of the substances carried and Tremcards are frequently kept with the driver in the cab of the vehicle. The driver is responsible for the safe loading and security of the load during transit and many have been trained to give immediate care to casualties of incidents involving hazardous substances.

Chemsafe procedure: The Chemical Industries Scheme for Assistance in Freight Emergencies (Chemsafe) recognizes that the emergency services may urgently require more detailed advice or help either by telephone or at the scene. The system works to ensure that vehicles are clearly labelled with a specialist telephone advice centre number but also it provides assistance when the manufacturer or trader is unknown or the product is unidentified. The National Chemical Emergency Centre (NCEC) at Harwell provides advice to the emergency authorities on the chemical hazards of a product involved in any incident.

The Fire Service chemical database (CHEMDATA) is an invaluable tool. It is used in times of emergency when rapid access to relevant chemical information is required and is critical to making the right decisions. CHEMDATA provides information that allows operational staff to make confident and rapid decisions by providing reliable information on substances.[13]

Personal protective clothing and equipment

The potential for injury from exposure to hazardous substances is related to the toxicity, flammability, and reactivity of a particular substance. Use of the right protection is crucial for anyone dealing with hazardous substances. This includes the use of the proper respiratory protection and personal protective equipment (PPE).

Protective respiratory devices

EMS crews should always be aware of the potential for damage to the respiratory system from any unknown haz-

Box 43-1

Forms of chemical intrusion

Degradation: The physical destruction or decomposition of a clothing material caused by exposure to chemicals, use, or ambient conditions.

Penetration: The flow of a hazardous liquid chemical through zippers, stitched seams, pinholes, or other imperfections in a material.

Permeation: The process by which a hazardous liquid chemical moves through a material on a molecular level.

ardous substance. When dealing with such incidents it is best practice to protect the respiratory system by either using air purification devices or respiratory equipment that supplies clean air (atmosphere supplying device).

Classifications of protective clothing

There are three broad types of protective clothing: disposable, limited use and reusable. The clothing is made from a variety of materials that are designed specifically for certain chemical exposures. EMS crews must practise using this type of clothing within a simulated and safe environment prior to using it in emergency situations. Examples of this material include Tyvek®; Tychem®; nitrile rubber and Teflon®. No single material is compatible with all chemicals but they must all comply with the relevant European standards; the manufacturer's guidelines and recommendations must also be followed. Box 43-1 shows the various forms of chemical intrusion. Protective clothing is categorized in several ways. The classifications defined by the Home Office and the NHS are as follows:

- *Level 1*: This provides the highest level of skin, respiratory, and eye protection. Personnel entering the *hot zone* will be provided with Level 1 equipment which consists of a gas-tight suit that is designed to protect the wearer from hazardous substances. These substances include gaseous, liquid or solid contaminants, and radiation particles. It must be worn in conjunction with STOPCAB which is also protected under the suit. Personnel are also provided with chemical-resistant outer and inner gloves, an undersuit hard hat (optional), and a disposable protective suit (including gloves and boots) which may be worn over a totally encapsulating suit.
- *Level 2*: The second level of PPE is the Civilian Responder 1 (CR1) suit, which is the Home Office standard issue protection suit for attending CBRN incidents. This suit is structured to provide incremental levels of protection and is worn in conjunction with an air purification respirator. Each incremental layer performs an individual function as well as integrating with other layers to provide protection against a wide range of toxic industrial chemicals and weapons of mass destruction contaminants.
- *Level 3*: This is a short-term level of protection used for emergency working and is generally provided to those members of staff who are involved in casualty decontamination and *warm zone* working. It is usually a one-piece suit manufactured from DuPont Tychem®. It incorporates a powered respirator and filters for air supply, and provides high barrier protection against infiltration by most inorganic and organic chemicals. Staff members with a limited level of training can use this type of suit.

CBRN escape hoods

The chemical protective hood is designed for first responders who might be caught up in a CBRN or Hazmat incident, as they are most likely to be the first emergency responders to the scene. The hood improves the current PPE and is worn if the responder finds themselves in a contaminated environment. It provides approximately 20 min of protection, which enables the individual to get to a safe area.[14]

Critical Thinking

What level of patient care do you think you will be able to provide when wearing each of the levels of hazardous substance PPE?

Regardless of the type of PPE used during a Hazmat incident, all avenues through which hazardous substances can enter the body must be protected. The following points should be of particular concern to any rescuer involved in a Hazmat response:

- Protective clothing should not be affected adversely by the hazardous substances involved.
- Protective clothing should seal all exposed skin.
- Contact with the hazardous substances should be of the absolute minimal duration required.
- Protective clothing and equipment should be decontaminated properly or discarded properly.
- The safety standards and methods for cleaning and disposing of clothing and equipment should be strictly followed.
- Contaminated patient clothing should be left at the scene. It should not be transported with the patient in order to limit the contamination of the ambulance.

Health hazards

Hazardous substances may enter the human body by inhalation, ingestion, injection, and absorption (see Chapter 21). Entry by means of any of these routes may result in internal and external damage to the rescuer. Exposure to dangerous substances may affect the body in several different ways. It may produce numerous injuries or illnesses.

Exposure to poisons can produce acute toxicity, delayed toxicity, and local and systemic effects. How the body responds depends on the concentration of the chemical to which the body is exposed (also called the dose response). The paramedic should also be aware that drug treatment can result in synergistic effects; thus all treatment methods should be guided by medical personnel, a poison control centre, or other appropriate authority.

Internal damage

Internal damage to the human body from exposure to hazardous substances may involve the respiratory tract, the central nervous system, or other internal organs. Some substances damage cells on contact; others have a more direct effect on specific organs (target organs), such as the kidneys and liver.

Depending on the hazardous substances, the physical injury may vary, ranging from minor irritation to more serious complications. The more serious ones may include cardiac and respiratory compromise, arrest and death. Chronic illness (e.g. chronic obstructive pulmonary disease) and various forms of cancer may also result. Some substances can cause abnormal fetal development and changes in gene structure. For example, penetrating radiation can lead to cell and chromosomal changes and can cause genetic changes, cell death and sterility.

Irritants

Respiratory problems are a common complaint of rescuers and patients who have been exposed to hazardous substances. Chemical irritants emit vapours that affect the mucous membranes of the body, such as those found on the surface of the eyes, nose, mouth and throat. As these irritants combine with moisture, acidic or alkaline reactions may occur. Exposure to these irritants may result in damage to the upper, lower, and deep respiratory tract. Examples of chemical irritants are hydrochloric acid, halogens, and ozone. Self-defence chemical sprays used by some civilians and police officers are common and present a hazard to responders. These irritant sprays include chloroacetophenone, orthochlorobenzalmalononitrile, and capsicum oleoresin and produce excessive tears in the eyes.

Asphyxiants

Asphyxiants are gases. They displace the oxygen in the air and also dilute the oxygen concentration of the air. Examples of simple asphyxiants are carbon dioxide, methane and propane. Other gases not only displace oxygen in the air but also interfere with tissue oxygenation; these are referred to as blood poisons or chemical asphyxiants. They tend to interrupt the transport or use of oxygen by tissue cells. Through various mechanisms, these toxic gases deprive body tissue of needed oxygen. Examples include hydrogen cyanide, carbon monoxide and hydrogen sulphide.

Nerve poisons, anaesthetics and narcotics

Nerve poisons, anaesthetics and narcotics act on the nervous system. They change the ability of the brain to regulate the heart and the respiratory system, as well as interfere with the ability to transmit nerve impulses to the heart and lungs.

Nerve poisons were developed by the military, and are often referred to as war gases, nerve gases or nerve agents (see Chapter 45), with similar substances used in solid pesticides. Exposure to these chemicals may result in fatal complications. Examples of these poisons include carbamates, organophosphates, parathion and malathion. Anaesthetics and narcotics are less hazardous than nerve poisons. However, exposure to large or continuous amounts may result in unconsciousness or death. Examples include ethylene, nitrous oxide and ethyl alcohol.

Hepatotoxins

Hepatotoxins are substances that damage the liver. As these poisons build up in the body they can destroy the ability of the liver to function. Examples include chlorinated and halogenated hydrocarbons.

Cardiotoxins

Cardiotoxins are hazardous substances that can cause myocardial ischaemia and dysrhythmias. Examples include some nitrates and ethylene glycol. Acute myocardial infarction and sudden death have been reported in healthy young persons who were exposed to these substances. Short-term exposure to fluorocarbons and other halogenated hydrocarbons has also been known to cause cardiac abnormalities.

Nephrotoxins

Nephrotoxins are hazardous substances that are especially destructive to the kidneys. Examples include carbon disulphide, lead, high concentrations of organic solvents, and inorganic mercury. Exposure to carbon tetrachloride used as a solvent for dry cleaning or fire-extinguishing agent can damage the kidneys.

Neurotoxins

Neurological and behavioural toxicity may result from exposure to hazardous substances such as arsenic, lead, mercury, and organic solvents, and in some cases, cerebral hypoxia may occur as a result of decreased oxygen in the blood.

Haemotoxins

Haemotoxins are hazardous substances that may cause the destruction of red blood cells and such destruction can result in haemolytic anaemia (see Chapter 22). Substances that can produce haemolytic anaemia include aniline, naphthol, quinones, lead, mercury, arsenic and copper. Pulmonary oedema, and cardiac and liver injury may also be caused by haemotoxin exposure.

Carcinogens

Carcinogens are cancer-causing agents. Many hazardous substances are carcinogenic or described as suspected carcinogens. The exact amount of hazardous substance exposure required for cancer to develop is unknown; however, short-term exposure to specific agents is known to produce long-term effects. Disease and complications have been reported 20 years after exposure to hazardous substances.[17]

Particular interest to rescuers involved in fire fighting, is that all fossil and organic fuels when burned produce dioxins, with many of the dioxins being carcinogens. (For example, burning wood produces carcinogenic formaldehyde.) Positive-pressure breathing apparatus is the most important piece of protective equipment to protect against these carcinogenic vapours and respiratory poisons. All rescuers should avoid exposure to smoke or clouds of fumes as a standard practice in scene safety.

Note

An important sign of a critical exposure is several persons having the same symptoms at the same time. Any time two or more members of the team report that they 'feel' similar symptoms, the team should suspect a toxic gas or agent. EMS responders should always report back to control immediately the onset of symptoms becomes apparent. In turn control will inform all other emergency services attending the incident.

General symptoms of exposure

Health effects from exposure to hazardous substances vary by individual. They also depend on the chemical involved, the concentration of the chemical, the duration of exposure, the number of exposures, and the route of entry (inhalation, ingestion, injection, absorption). In addition, a person's age, gender, general health, allergies, smoking habits, alcohol consumption, and medication use can influence those persons affected

Various symptoms may result from exposure to hazardous substances. Some symptoms may be delayed or masked by common illnesses such as influenza or by smoke inhalation. If any of the following symptoms is present after exposure to hazardous substances, the rescuer or patient should seek immediate medical attention:

- changes in skin colour or blushing
- chest tightness
- confusion, light-headedness, anxiety, dizziness
- coughing or painful respiration
- diarrhoea and involuntary urination or defecation (or both)
- dim, blurred, or double vision; photophobia
- loss of coordination
- nausea, vomiting, abdominal cramping
- salivation, drooling, rhinorrhoea
- seizure
- shortness of breath, burning of the upper airway
- tingling or numbness of extremities
- unconsciousness.

Critical Thinking

Two rescuers complain of similar symptoms on the scene of a rescue that may involve hazardous substances. What actions should be taken immediately?

External damage

Body surface tissue may be injured by hazardous substances and many substances have corrosive properties. Numerous substances can become corrosive when mixed with water, and exposure to these substances may produce chemical burns and severe tissue damage. Examples include hydrochloric acid, hydrofluoric acid, and caustic soda.

Soft tissue damage

Corrosives are acids or bases (alkaline). Exposure to either may cause pain on contact; however, alkalis generally burn more extensively than acids. Exposing human tissue to a base corrosive such as sodium hydroxide may result in a breakdown of fatty tissue (liquefaction) that produces a greasy or slick feeling to the skin. These signs should alert the rescuer to decontaminate immediately and seek medical attention. Unless the substance is identified, decontamination should begin by brushing off the dry powder and flushing the skin with copious amounts of water. Different areas of the skin absorb chemicals at different rates and paramedics should never try to neutralize an acid or base; doing so could produce great heat and cause further burns. The area should be flushed copiously with flowing water, and the patient should be transported for care. Rescuers should be aware of possible fumes that result from the decontamination of a wound site.

Cryogenics are refrigerant liquid gases that can freeze human tissue on contact. These liquids vaporize as soon as they are released from their containers, which may cause tissue damage. Paramedics should take extreme caution when dealing with this type of incident as they can produce freeze burns, frostbite and other cold-related injuries. Examples include freon, liquid oxygen, and liquid nitrogen.

Chemical exposure to the eyes

Chemical exposure to the eyes (described in Chapter 30) may cause damage. The damage may range from superficial inflammation to severe burns. Patients with these conditions have local pain, visual disturbance, tearing, oedema and redness of surrounding tissues. Basic management guidelines include flushing the eyes with flowing water; however, care should be taken to prevent the water from contaminating the unaffected eye. Sterile water should be used for irrigation wherever possible. Methods of irrigation include use of an irrigation lens (if provided), or continuous flow can be achieved by using an intravenous giving set. A rapid assessment of visual acuity is important although this should not delay flushing or irrigation of the eyes.

Response to hazardous substance emergencies

Not all Hazmat incidents are large-scale events; a single event involving only one patient may require a full Hazmat response. Rescuer safety, the type and degree of the potential hazard, the involvement of other agencies, and protection for the general public all require consideration. Preplanning and early coordination of activities in these major incidents is important so the paramedic should provide continuous situation reports to control and ensure good liaison with other emergency services.

The first rescue personnel to arrive at the scene of a Hazmat incident may not be the most qualified or best equipped. However, most communities look to the first professional on scene to provide immediate safety and direction. The first crew on scene will remain the point of contact until other emergency service resources arrive, therefore the EMS crew must be capable of the initial management of Hazmat incidents.

Hazard and risk assessment

Whatever the incident, the EMS crew should be thinking about a hazard and risk assessment en route to the scene. All UK EMS personnel are trained in how to respond to Hazmat situations and what to do if they are first crew on scene. In Hazmat incidents, hazards are the chemical properties of a material that may cause danger or peril (Box 43-2). Risk refers to the possibility of suffering harm or loss. Risk levels vary and are influenced by several factors, including the following[15] (Figure 43-5):

- hazardous nature of the material involved
- worst-case scenario situations
- quantity of the substances involved
- weather conditions that might affect the scene adversely
- containment system and type of stress applied to the container
- proximity of exposures (e.g. schools, nursing homes, and shopping centres)
- level of available resources
- lead time for mutual aid.

A hazard and risk assessment also includes consideration of the potential hazards to the public and environment, the potential risk of primary contamination to patients, and the potential risk for secondary contamination to rescuers (Box 43-3).

If the product can be identified through Hazmat references, the EMS crew should familiarize themselves with potential health hazards, recommended PPE, initial first aid, and the 'safe distance' factor as outlined in the reference guides. Crews must maintain radio contact with control and provide situation reports on a frequent basis. All radio contact with control and communications with other emergency services must be documented on a log sheet. Most emergency response guides (Tremcard) offer only general management actions. After formal product identification, the appropriate Hazmat agencies (e.g. NPIS and the National Chemical Emergencies Centre) can give more exact information.

Approaching the scene

The paramedics should approach the scene cautiously from uphill and upwind. The EMS crew should be alert to environmental clues such as wind direction, unusual odours, leakage and vapour clouds. Other environmental clues that are good indicators for the presence of hazardous substances include affected or afflicted wildlife and plant life (e.g. dead birds and wilted or discoloured plants). Emergency vehicles should never be driven through leakage or vapour clouds or smoke. In addition, personnel should not enter the incident area until it has been determined to be safe. All ambulance services within the UK have their own guidelines for dealing with such incidents, and staff are encouraged to keep themselves up to date with the ever-changing nature of major and incidents involving hazardous materials. In addition to these guidelines, rescuers should do the following:[16]

Box 43-2

Hazardous materials terminology and definitions

Toxicological terms used to determine toxicity of a compound

IDLH (immediately dangerous to life and health): Any atmosphere that poses an immediate hazard to life or that produces immediate, irreversible debilitating effects on health.

LD_{50} (lethal dose, 50% kill): The amount of a dose that, when administered to laboratory animals, kills 50% of them.

PEL (permissible exposure limit): The maximum time-weighted concentration at which 95% of exposed, healthy adults suffer no adverse effects over a 40-hour workweek.

ppm/ppb: Parts per million/parts per billion.

TLV-C (threshold limit value–ceiling level): The maximum concentration that should not be exceeded even instantaneously.

TLV-STEL (threshold limit value–short-term exposure limit): A 15-minute, time-weighted average exposure that should not be exceeded at any time nor repeatedly more than 4 times a day, with 60-minute rest periods required between each STEL exposure.

Specific terminology for medical hazardous materials operations

Alpha radiation: Large radioactive particles that have minimal penetrating ability.

Beta radiation: Small radioactive particles that can penetrate subcutaneous tissue and usually enter the body through damaged skin, ingestion, or inhalation.

Boiling point: The temperature at which a liquid changes to a vapour or a gas; the temperature at which the pressure of the liquid equals atmospheric pressure.

Flammable/exposure limits: The range of gas or vapour concentration that will burn or explode if an ignition source is present.

Flash point: The minimum temperature at which a liquid gives off enough vapours to ignite and flash-over but not to continue to burn without additional heat.

Gamma radiation: The most dangerous form of penetrating radiation, which can produce internal and external hazards.

Ignition temperature: The minimum temperature required to ignite gas or vapour without a spark or flame being present.

Specific gravity: The weight of a material as compared with the weight of an equal volume of water.

Vapour density: The weight of a pure vapour or gas compared with the weight of an equal volume of dry air at the same temperature and pressure.

Vapour pressure: The pressure exerted by the vapour within the container against the sides of a container.

Vapour solubility: The ability of a vapour to mix with water.

From Noll G et al 1988 Hazardous materials: managing the incident. Fire Protection Publications, Stillwater, OK.

- Approach cautiously. Resist the urge to rush in; you cannot help others until you know what you are facing.
- Identify the hazards. Placards, container labels, shipping papers, and knowledgeable persons on the scene are valuable sources of information. Evaluate all of them and then consult the appropriate resources (e.g. Chemsafe, control fire service personnel) before

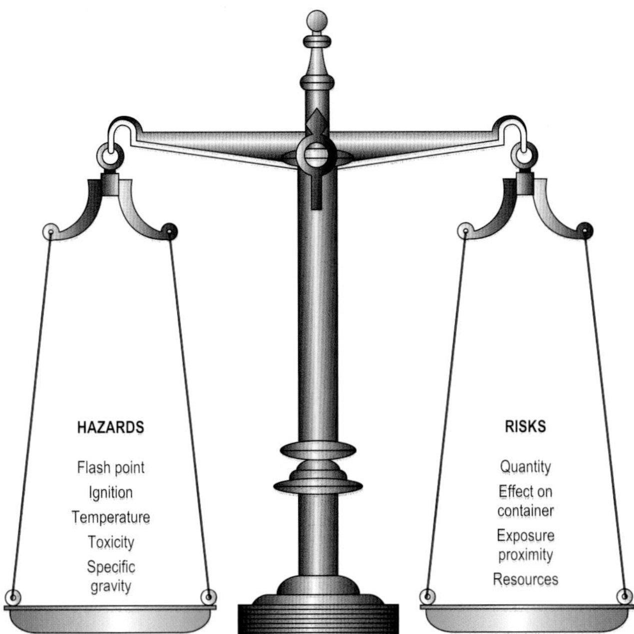

Figure 43-5 Hazards versus risk.

Box 43-3

Types of contamination

Primary contamination

Exposure to substance
Substance only harmful to exposed person
Little chance of exposure to others

Secondary contamination

Exposure to substance
Liquid and particulate substances easily transferred by touching

you place yourself or others at risk. As more accurate, material-specific information becomes available, your response becomes more appropriate for the situation.

- Secure the scene. Without entering the immediate hazard zone, do what you can to isolate the area and ensure the safety of persons and the environment. Move and keep persons away from the scene and the perimeter. Allow enough room to move and remove your own equipment.
- Obtain help. Advise your headquarters to notify responsible agencies and call for assistance from trained experts through ambulance control and Chemsafe.
- Decide on site entry. Any efforts you make to rescue persons or protect property or the environment must be weighed against the possibility that you could become part of the problem. Enter the area with the appropriate protective gear (if trained to do so). Above all, do not walk into or touch spilled material. Avoid inhaling fumes, smoke and vapours, even if no hazardous materials are known to be involved. Do not assume that gases or vapours are harmless because of lack of smell.

Critical Thinking

Which of these guidelines would it be easy for the first arriving crew to miss?

Control of the scene

The first professionals to arrive at the scene have several responsibilities. Its members must detect and identify the materials involved, assess the risk of exposure to rescue personnel and others, consider the potential risk of fire or explosion, gather information from on-site personnel or other sources, and confine and control the incident. If the incident comprises a major incident, a command post should be established and the major incident plan followed (see Chapter 42).

Safety zones

After the presence of the hazardous substance has been confirmed, the scene should be separated into hot, warm, and cold zones (Figure 43-6). These zones should have access and egress corridors between them. Corridors provide control points. They also allow responders working in the zones to know where they should exit and enter for decontamination, accountability, and debriefing. Safety zones should be established and enforced early in the incident (Box 43-4). The control centre and responding units should be advised of the location of the hot zone and safe approach directions.

The hot zone is the area of the incident that includes the hazardous substance, which includes any surrounding area that may be exposed to gases, vapours, mist, dust or runoff. All EMS crews and vehicles should be stationed outside this zone. Anyone entering this zone must wear high-level personal protective equipment (PPE). Only specially trained EMS personnel (e.g. Hazardous Area Response Teams [HART]) should attempt patient care activities in this area. Some EMS agencies and incident command system structures refer to the hot zone as the exclusion zone, a restricted area, or the red zone.

The warm zone is a larger, buffer area that surrounds the hot zone with 'cold' and 'hot' end corridors. Although protective clothing is required, it is usually considered a safer environment for workers. However, if the hot zone becomes unstable, the warm zone may be exposed to the hazardous substances. This zone is where most EMS activities, such as decontamination and patient care activities, are performed. Some agencies refer to this zone as the limited-access zone, the containment reduction corridor, or the yellow zone.

The cold zone is the area that encompasses the warm zone. The cold zone is also restricted to emergency personnel. This area is usually considered safe, requiring only minimal protective clothing. The cold zone contains the command post and other support agencies necessary to control the incident. This area is referred to by some agencies as a support zone or the green zone.

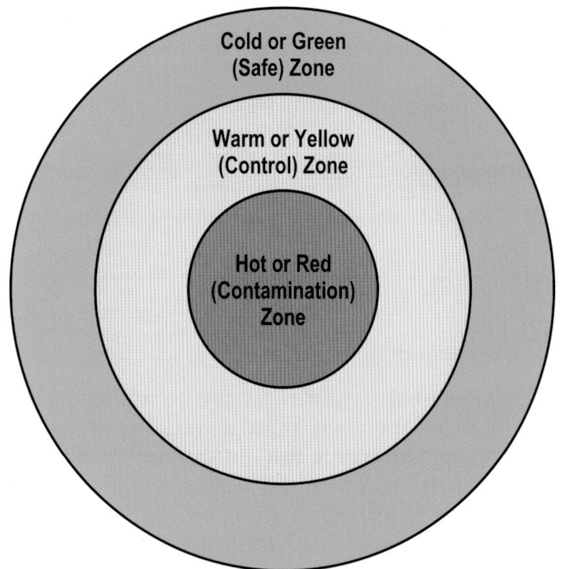

Hot or Red (Contamination) Zone

- Contamination is actually present
- Personnel must wear appropriate protective gear
- Number of rescuers limited to those absolutely necessary
- Bystanders never allowed

Warm or Yellow (Control) Zone

- Area surrounding the contamination zone
- Vital to preventing spread of contamination
- Personnel must wear appropriate protective gear
- Life-saving emergency care and decontamination are performed

Cold or Green (Safe) Zone

- Normal triage, stabilization, and treatment are performed
- Rescuers must shed contaminated gear before entering the cold zone

Figure 43-6 Zones at a Hazmat incident.

Box 43-4

Hazardous materials zones

Hot zone

Contamination present
Site of incident
Entry with high-level personal protective equipment
Entry limited

Warm zone

Buffer zone outside hot zone
Contains decontamination corridor with 'hot' and 'cold' end

Cold zone

Safe area
Staging area for personnel and equipment
Site of medical monitoring
One end of corridor

Medical monitoring and rehabilitation

The safety of EMS crews is of high priority in any emergency and situations that involve hazardous substances are among the most dangerous. Whilst medical monitoring programmes are not mandatory, they should be part of any EMS/Hazmat system and all Hazmat incidents.

Current UK ambulance services require any personnel who wish to be part of the HART team to have medicals prior to undertaking their training. This is to ensure that staff are fit and healthy to work in chemical protection suits in such hazardous situations.

Health and Safety legislation requires a medical examination for members of Hazmat response teams who may have been exposed to hazardous substances during an emergency. Other elements of Hazmat medical monitoring programmes may include any needed medical care, record keeping, and periodic review of the surveillance programme.

It is the responsibility of individuals to highlight any sudden medical illnesses that they are experiencing that may prevent them from entering the scene of a Hazmat incident. In certain circumstances, it is customary to establish the responders' vital sign readings prior to entering a hazardous incident; this will help detect signs and symptoms of deterioration and fatigue throughout the event. Chemical protection suits protect but also prevent cooling through evaporation, conduction, convection, or radiation. Heat-stress factors are affected by the prehydration of the rescuer, degree of physical fitness, ambient air temperature, and the degree and duration of physical activity. The parameters of the presuit evaluation should include the following:

- temperature, pulse, respiration and blood pressure measurements
- cardiac rhythm
- body weight
- cognitive and motor skills
- hydration
- significant recent medical history (e.g. medications or illnesses).

After entry into the hazardous area, medical monitoring should note the amount of time a rescuer has been in protective clothing. Rescuers should be observed for any signs of heat-related illness or exposure. If illness or injury occurs to any team member, all entry team members should be removed from the hot zone for treatment. A backup team should be ready to assist the entry team members in the hot zone at all times.

After the incident, rescue personnel should be re-evaluated in the 'rehab sector'. They should be re-evaluated using the same parameters as in the presuit examination in order to determine the rescuer's ability to re-enter the operation if needed. As a rule, rescuers are not allowed to re-enter the site until vital signs and hydration are normal. Please refer to local policy to ensure accuracy.

Critical Thinking

What types of incident will HART teams enter that may create a medical emergency? How would you as the EMS crew deal with this?

Documentation

Documentation has to include a detailed account of the nature of the incident and comprehensive records are essential as part of Hazmat medical monitoring and rehabilitation. At a minimum, records should include the following:

- the hazardous substance
- the toxicity and danger of secondary contamination
- use of appropriate PPE and any permeation ('breakthrough') that occurred
- the level of decontamination performed or required
- use of antidotes and other medical treatment
- the method of transportation and destination.

Baseline statistics from pre-entry and post-entry screenings should also be included in the records; pre-printed forms may be available for this.

Emergency management of contaminated patients

Decontamination is not an automatic or inevitable response to incidents involving hazardous chemicals. The decision on whether or not to initiate decontamination procedures will depend on the assessment of the nature of the incident by the first responder. If the first responder confirms the need for decontamination, it is usual for all casualties, whether injured or not, to receive decontamination at the scene if they are suspected of being contaminated.

Cross-contamination is a potential risk and it is particularly important to protect healthcare staff, other patients and the healthcare facilities from this. NHS hospitals within the UK have decontamination resources and are responsible for the treatment and care of self-presenting patients. However, the Ambulance Service and Fire Service have arrangements in place to collaboratively support hospital services with clinical or mass decontamination.

Security of these facilities will remain the responsibility of the police.[17]

The primary focus is to remove the contaminated persons from the area of greatest contamination, which is usually to the open air and upwind of the incident. A priority will be to remove contaminated clothing carefully, preferably from head to foot, to reduce the risk of inhalation and spread of any contaminant. Special care must be taken to ensure there is no spread of contamination from clothing to exposed skin.

Non-injured patients or potential witnesses or suspects may require decontamination but they should be able to remove their own clothing and self-decontaminate under supervision.

Personal clothing and property, which may or may not be contaminated, should, wherever possible, be recorded and linked to an individual. Such material may contain valuable intelligence or evidence and the continuity of its recording is vital. People who have had personal articles such as spectacles or hearing aids removed from them need reassurance and support. In circumstances where decontamination exceeds the rate at which the rinse–wipe–rinse method can be applied, mass decontamination (MD) may be an alternative.

Removal of casualties from the inner cordon and the hot zone

Trained personnel using appropriate levels of personal protection should conduct the removal of casualties who are either mobile or capable of being removed from the inner cordoned area. Prioritizing order of evacuation and rescue is the responsibility of designated EMS crews and will be dependent on the complexity of the situation and availability of resources. Entrapped casualties may have to be partially decontaminated in situ by removing clothing and decontaminating exposed skin areas, depending on the nature of the incident.[17]

Dealing with non-ambulant casualties

Non-ambulant casualties who have been removed from the hot zone are taken to the decontamination point, where limited clinical support and decontamination can start concurrently. Priority should be given to the decontamination of the face and mouth to allow for early resuscitation to take place before disrobing.

Ambulant casualties using the guided self-decontamination method

Ambulant contaminated casualties should remain within the inner cordon, but outside the hot zone, until they have been decontaminated. The majority of contamination will be contained on clothing and casualties should be encouraged to remove top layers of clothing down to their underwear, which should also be removed if contamination is suspected. Removed clothing should be treated as hazardous waste and should be double bagged and placed in a controlled area, in accordance with the rules concerning continuity of evidence.[17]

Showering

The correct percentages of detergent should be mixed before being used via temporary showers in the form of spray jets, hose reels or flat fan sprays; this may not be feasible to do and plain water should be used as an alternative. Casualties who have undergone decontamination will need further clinical assessment and may need further treatment.

Dangers

Where the incident involves radiological or nuclear material, special consideration should be given to minimize the exposure of pregnant casualties and carers. It is however a principle of the treatment of casualties contaminated with radioactivity that life-saving treatment takes precedence over decontamination. Health plans therefore include arrangements for ambulance transport of contaminated casualties with serious injuries, without exposing ambulance crews to significant risk.[17]

The decontamination process must be adequately controlled from the outset to avoid public disorder. Risks from secondary devices, confused, violent or rowdy victims, undetected perpetrators attempting to escape, prisoners under arrest, and police/military weaponry can be a problem to CBRN responders when dealing with a MD incident.

Decontamination will be based on the need to preserve life, evidence and the availability of resources. People suspected of being involved in a serious crime are detained at a CBRN scene, and will be under escort and should not normally be decontaminated through facilities used by others. The exception to this would be where life is threatened.

Dealing with fatalities

When EMS crews are dealing with the dead at major incidents or CBRN incidents, respect and dignity for the remains should be upheld. The dead should where practicable be left in situ during the immediate response, unless they are a hazard to the living and the management of the incident. HM Coroner will be responsible for identifying the deceased and determining how, when and where death occurred. In the event of a CBRN incident both HM Coroner and the police will be key members of the Identification Commission and will be an important element in managing any mass fatality incident.[17]

Mass and emergency decontamination and its definition

Mass decontamination (MD) is the procedure to be used by the Fire and Rescue Service, they will be drafted in when the number of people requiring decontamination exceeds, or threatens to overwhelm, the existing capacity of the NHS and/or the Ambulance Service. The Fire Service can initiate MD procedures prior to the arrival of other health professionals or where specialist NHS resources are not readily available. This may involve improvisation of equipment available until specialist facilities can be deployed. Basic triage is established by collaboration of the Ambulance and Fire Service and should be carried out with due regard to any attendant risks such as thermal shock, hypothermia and further injury (Figure 43-7).[17]

Location and equipment

In normal circumstances MD will be undertaken at the inner cordon, but this can change in the event of trapped casualties where MD will take place within the inner cordon. Such a decision should consider all operational requirements and clinical advice.

The decontamination point siting should take account of wind direction and topography. A check should always be made around the decontamination point for secondary devices in the event of terrorist incidents.

Disrobe and re-robe packs

The Fire Service is equipped with mobile MD units which include disrobe and re-robe packs and are normally positioned spanning the inner cordon. The MD process will include disrobing, showering and re-robing and a facility to seal and uniquely number clothing and property. The storage and/or release of this property is determined by the police.[17]

The rinse–wipe–rinse method of casualty decontamination[17]

The effective application of the rinse–wipe–rinse method requires the following equipment:

- water (preferably lukewarm)
- a bucket or other container (5–10 L capacity)
- liquid soap
- a sponge or soft brush.

Procedures

- For contamination by industrial chemicals, suspected chemical weaponry, biological agents or other unidentified substances, make up a solution of 0.5% soap in lukewarm water (5 mL of soap per litre of water or about three squirts of liquid soap into a bucket of water).
- Having removed the contaminated person's clothes, rinse the affected areas with the soap solution. This first rinse helps to remove particles and water-based chemicals, such as acids and alkalis. Rinse from the head downward.
- The rinse should be applied to contaminated areas of skin only, to avoid spread to uncontaminated areas. Wipe the affected areas with a wet sponge or soft brush, which helps to remove organic chemicals and petrochemicals that adhere to the skin.
- Rinse for a second time, (this is particularly important where it is known that the contaminant comprises primarily biological material) and dry the skin with a clean towel.
- This process should not take more than 3–5 min and you may need to repeat the rinse–wipe–rinse procedure if obvious skin contamination remains.
- It may not be possible to guarantee total decontamination of a casualty at the end of this procedure, and EMS crews should remain cautious and observe for ill effects in the decontaminated patients, persons or staff.
- Persistent chemical weaponry (CW) agents are poorly soluble in water. The wipe stage is necessary to assist in their removal.
- The rinse water itself will be contaminated, hazardous, and a potential source of further contamination, and therefore new brushes and sponges must be used for each patient.

Notes on the use of hot and cold water

The use of cold water may be preferable, depending on the nature of the contamination. However, certain people are more susceptible to hypothermia than others, examples include the old, frail, infants and traumatized casualties, and in this situation warm water should be used.[17]

Advantages of using cold water

- Readily available
- Rapid decontamination
- Vasoconstriction (closure of pores of skin, reducing chemical absorption).

Disadvantages of using cold water

- Hypothermia
- Thermal shock.

Advantages of using warm water

- Reduces possibility of hypothermia and thermal shock.

Disadvantages of using warm water

- Does not help dissolve some chemical weapon material
- It increases blood flow to the skin thereby increasing the skin absorption of material
- May not be readily available.

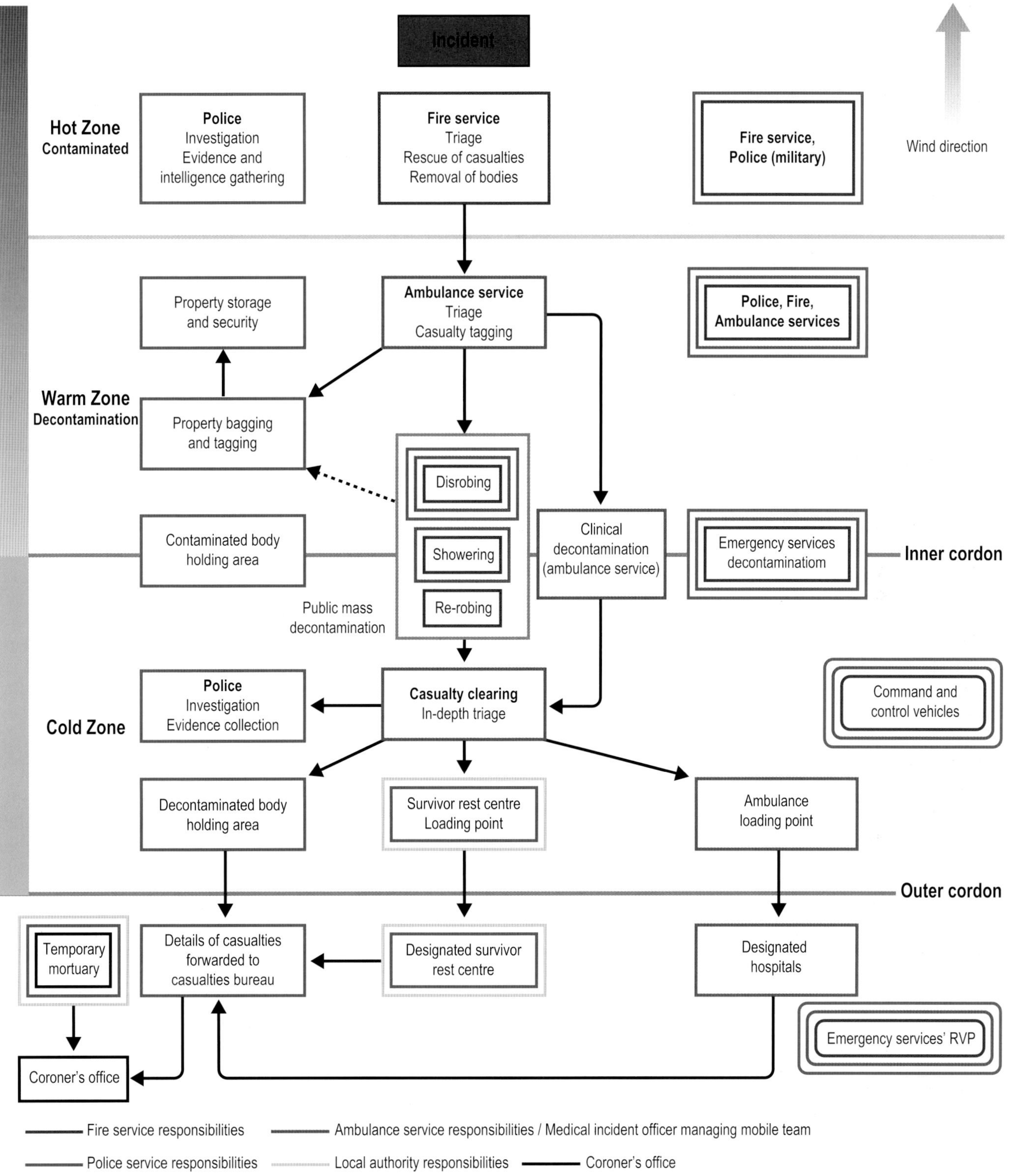

Figure 43-7 CBRN decontamination diagram.

Critical Thinking

Can water turn some compounds caustic? In cases where water is not available what would you consider? Would you consider using dry decontaminants? If so, why?

EMS crews must not wash or dispose of clothing or equipment at home. This helps to avoid exposing family members and contaminating home articles. You must follow local procedure regarding disposal or decontamination of equipment and clothing.[17]

Signs and symptoms of a generic chemical incident

- Coughing
- Difficulty in breathing
- Eye irritation
- Skin irritation/burns
- Nausea and vomiting
- Convulsions/unconsciousness.

Signs and symptoms of low doses of nerve agents

- Pupil constricted
- Headache and eye-pain
- Difficulty in breathing
- Tightness of chest.

Signs and symptoms of high doses of nerve agents

- Excessive secretion from the mouth
- Difficulty breathing and coughing
- Convulsions
- Incontinence of urine and defecation
- Running eyes and sweating
- Muscular weakness and tremors
- Stomach cramps and vomiting
- Collapse and death may occur.

Signs and symptoms of doses of mustard agents

Mustard agent gives no immediate effect on contact and consequently a delay of between 2 and 24 h may occur before pain is felt and the victim becomes aware. Mustard attacks the skin, eyes, lungs and gastrointestinal tract.

- Aching eyes and excessive tears
- Irritation of the mucous membranes
- Loss of sight (may be temporary)
- Vomiting and diarrhoea
- Inflammation of the skin
- Hoarseness, coughing and sneezing
- Blisters on the skin
- Severe respiratory difficulties.

Signs and symptoms of a radiological incident

There are five primary routes of exposure to radioactive materials (RM):

- absorption – contact between RM and the skin or eyes
- injection – through breaks in the skin
- external irradiation – where gamma and/or beta radiation particles penetrate the skin
- inhalation – through RM breathed into the lungs
- ingestion – through contaminated food and/or water.

Signs and symptoms of exposure to radiological material

The effects of radioactive contamination relate to the type of radiation, the dosage, the length of time in the contamination and exposed parts of the body to the material. Manifestation of symptoms can take days or weeks, and whilst some victims may not display severe symptoms at the time, cancer or leukaemia may develop decades later.

- Nausea, vomiting and diarrhoea
- Dehydration
- Hair loss and ulcers
- Skin burns and blistering
- Swelling
- Bleeding.

Cultural, religious and diversity issues

Police, local authorities and other organizations will be responsible for ensuring that the religious and cultural requirements of different communities and social groups and the special needs of individuals are met. Primary consideration in a CBRN incident is health and safety. If mass decontamination procedures become necessary, saving life or alleviating suffering will take precedence over diversity issues. Cultural considerations may include: enough female medical staff to deal with respective medical treatments facilitation of personal hygiene, and toilet needs. Further consideration needs to be given to dietary requirements, provision of separate areas for men and women, especially if overnight stays are envisaged, and having interpreters on site or on call. Arrangements should be made for ensuring places are set aside for personal worship with sensitivity to various cultural attitudes and requirements for dealing with death, burial and bereavement.[17]

Critical Thinking

What type of hazardous materials response resources does your community have?

Preparing the ambulance for patient transfer

Contamination of ambulances and equipment can be minimized by preparing the vehicle before transporting a partly decontaminated patient. These measures include using as much disposable equipment as necessary. They also include removing all items from cabinets that will not be needed for patient use.

Summary

- A hazardous material is any substance or material that is capable of posing an unreasonable risk to health, safety, and property.
- There are numerous laws and regulations relating to the transport, storage, and handling of hazardous substances. UK legislation places a requirement on Local Government, National Government and Industry to have in place emergency plans and to report incidents involving hazardous materials.
- Two methods are used to identify hazardous materials. One is informal product identification. (This includes visual, olfactory and verbal clues.) The other is formal product identification. (This includes, for example, placards and shipping papers.) Resources for Hazmat reference include the National Poisons Information Service, Specialist Advice Centres, the National Chemical Emergency Centre and CHEMDATA.
- Use of proper protection is crucial for anyone dealing with hazardous materials. This includes using the proper respiratory devices and wearing protective clothing. This clothing is made of a variety of materials. The clothing is designed for certain chemical exposures, thus the paramedic must follow the manufacturer's guidelines.
- Hazardous materials may enter the body through inhalation, ingestion, injection and absorption. Internal damage to the human body from Hazmat exposure may involve the respiratory tract, central nervous system, or other internal organs. Chemicals producing internal damage include irritants, asphyxiants, nerve poisons, anaesthetics, narcotics, hepatotoxins, cardiotoxins, nephrotoxins, neurotoxins and carcinogens.
- Exposure to hazardous materials may result in burns and in severe tissue damage.
- The first agency to arrive at the scene of a Hazmat incident must detect and identify the materials involved, assess the risk of exposure to rescue personnel and others, consider the potential risk of fire or explosion, gather information from on-site personnel or other sources, and confine and control the incident.
- A Hazmat medical monitoring programme may include medical examination for members of Hazmat response teams, providing medical care, record keeping, and periodic evaluation of the surveillance programme.
- The primary goals of decontamination are to reduce the patient's dosage of material, decrease the threat of secondary contamination, and reduce the risk of rescuer injury.
- Rescuers should follow strict protocols for proper decontamination of themselves, their clothing, and any contaminated equipment.

References

1. Department of Health 2005 The NHS emergency planning guidance 2005; underpinning materials; the Ambulance Service. Department of Health, London
2. Health and Safety Executive. What is a hazardous substance? Online. Available http://www.hse.gov.uk/coshh/detail/substances.htm 25 June 2009
3. General Services Administration, National Archives and Records Service, Office of the Federal Register 1981 Code of federal regulations, 49 CFR, 173.500, parts 100–177. General Services Administration, Washington, DC
4. Health Protection Agency, Chemical Hazards and Poisons Division 2007 Chemical incident management. HPA, London
5. Dickinson E (validated by International Fire Service Training Association) 1999 Fire service emergency care. Brady/Prentice Hall, Upper Saddle River, NJ
6. Health Protection Agency 2005 Chemical incidents in England and Wales 2005. HPA, London
7. Chemical Industries Association 2006 Facts and figures UK chemical industry. Chemical Industries Association, London
8. The carriage of dangerous goods & use of transportable pressure equipment regulations 2007; SI 568. HMSO, London
9. Fire Services Examinations Board 2006 Handbook for candidates taking statutory promotion examinations.
10. Department for Transport 2007 National carriage of dangerous substances. DFT, London
11. HSE Consignment procedures (including marking, labelling and placarding). 2006
12. HSE 2007 About REACH. Online. Available www.HSE.gov.uk/reach 26 February 2009
13. National Chemical Emergency Centre 2007 Chemdata; Clear, concise advice for Hazmat incidents. Online. Available http://the-ncec.com/chemsafe/ 26 February 2009
14. Home Office 2006 CBRN news. Home Office, London
15. Noll G et al 1988 Hazardous materials: managing the incident. Fire Protection Publications, Stillwater, OK
16. US Department of Transportation 2000 North American emergency response guidebook. US Department of Transportation, Washington, DC
17. Home Office 2004 The decontamination of people exposed to chemical, biological, radiological or nuclear (CBRN) substances or material. Strategic National Guidance, 2nd edition. Home Office, London

CHAPTER 44

Crime Scene Awareness

Chapter contents

Objectives

Upon completion of this chapter, the paramedic student will be able to:

1. Describe general techniques for determining whether a scene is violent and choosing the appropriate response.
2. Outline techniques for recognizing and responding to potentially dangerous residential calls.
3. Outline techniques for recognizing and responding to potentially dangerous calls on the highway.
4. Describe signs of danger and emergency medical services (EMS) response to violent street incidents.
5. Identify characteristics of and EMS response to situations involving gangs, clandestine drug laboratories, and domestic violence situations.
6. Outline general safety tactics that EMS personnel can use if they find themselves in a dangerous situation.
7. Describe special EMS considerations in the provision of tactical patient care.
8. Discuss EMS documentation and preservation of evidence at a crime scene.

Key terms

avoidance The act of keeping away from someone, something, or a situation, or of preventing the occurrence of something; it requires the paramedic to be continually aware of the scene by remaining observant and being knowledgeable about warning signs that may indicate a dangerous situation.

concealment A means of keeping out of sight; it does not provide ballistic protection.

cover A type of concealment that hides the body and offers ballistic protection.

crime scene A location where any part of a criminal act has occurred, or a location where evidence relating to a crime may be found.

distraction A self-defence measure in which a diversion is created to draw a person's attention.

evasive tactics To avoid something or someone. A self-defence measure in which an aggressor's moves and actions are anticipated, and unconventional pathways are used during retreat for personal safety.

tactical EMS Emergency medical services provided by EMS personnel who are prepared and trained to provide prehospital emergency care in tactical environments.

tactical patient care Patient care activities that occur inside the perimeter, or hot zone, of a dangerous scene.

tactical retreat Requires immediate and decisive action by leaving the scene when danger is observed or when violence or indicators of violence are displayed.

Many violent crimes require an EMS response, and, on many occasions, EMS crews arrive at the scene before police personnel. Awareness and avoidance of dangerous situations are issues of concern for responders within the UK. National statistics shows violent crime has remained stable.[1] However, the National Audit Office 2003 (NAO) reported 95 500 violent or abusive incidents against National Health Service (NHS) personnel in 2002, a 30% increase from 1999. Street gangs, threat groups, domestic disputes, and drug users are also on the rise within the UK.[1,2]

Personal safety and crime scene awareness must therefore be a high priority on every call of this nature.

Critical Thinking

Why isn't it always possible to identify a dangerous scene before arriving at the scene?

Approaching the scene

For paramedics and other responders, determining personal safety is a basic part of analysing a scene. Every year some people die trying to save the lives of others, many others are hurt, and almost all emergency personnel will be able to recall a lucky escape from some kind of injury.[3] Scene safety begins prior to the paramedic's arrival at the scene. The paramedic needs to be aware of the excitement and anxiety that can create the 'red mist' or 'tunnel vision effect'.[3] The details provided by the control centre can supply key information about the scene and the nature of the incident; however, the initial information may have changed so it is important to remember that safety is dynamic and needs to be continually reassessed.[4] It is crucial when ensuring personal safety to identify and respond to potential dangers before they develop. Further types of information may be available from the control centre although this should be viewed as a two-way communication whereby the control centre is kept up to date with the ever-changing environment of the scene. Information that may be available includes known locations of unsafe scenes (e.g. through computer-aided dispatch systems) and/or the presence of the following:

- large crowds
- people under the influence of alcohol or other drugs
- on-scene violence
- weapons.

Other information can sometimes be gathered en route to the scene from crew members and other responders monitoring the call. Some of these people may have had previous experience with a particular area or address. Scene safety relates to paramedics looking from the outside inwards[3] and they should be aware of additional inherent hazards that may exist at the scene. Examples include natural disasters, fallen power lines, busy roads, toxic substances, the potential for fire, dangerous pets, and vehicle hazards and dangers. The paramedic should be vigilant and be prepared to report on or deal with terrorism, particularly since the events of 9/11 in the US. If the scene is not safe, the paramedic should retreat to a safe location, stay in contact with control, and await the arrival of police or other appropriate emergency services.

When responding to a scene with a potential for danger, the paramedic should begin observation several streets from the scene. They should also use audible and visual warning (AVW) devices that are appropriate for the call. For example, responding with AVW devices to an urban scene may draw a crowd of bystanders; lights generally are required for safety at highway scenes. When possible, joint fire–EMS–police responses should be defined through preplanning (e.g. fire–EMS response with full use of AVW devices; police responding without AVW devices and at normal speed).

Scene safety considerations for all types of danger must continue throughout the EMS response. A scene that has been made safe can become unsafe, even when the police are present. This can happen if violence resumes, crowds gather or turn violent, or other people enter the scene. EMS providers could be subject to violence against them as they may be mistaken for police officers mainly due to confusion regarding identity of the uniform worn. The paramedic crew must be familiar with local protocols when intervening in violent situations and must also have a strategic escape plan ready.

Scenes known to be violent

If the scene is known to be violent, the paramedic should remain at a safe, out-of-sight distance from the area ('out of sight – out of scene'). They should remain at this distance until the area has been secured by the police. Remaining at a safe standby area away from a violent scene is important for several reasons:

- If paramedics can be seen, people will come to them.
- Entering an unsafe scene adds one or more potential victims.
- Paramedics may be injured or killed.
- Paramedics may be taken hostage.
- Paramedics may become additional patients in a scene that is already a multiple casualty incident.

It must be stressed that if the scene is unsafe, the paramedic should retreat to a standby point and wait for the resource personnel who can provide scene safety.

Dangerous residence

A response to a residence is an everyday occurrence for most EMS providers. However, even calls that appear routine require scene safety awareness. This should begin before the paramedic leaves the emergency vehicle. Warning signs of danger in residential areas include the following:

- a history of problems or violence
- a known drug or gang area
- loud noises (e.g. screams, items breaking, possible gunshots)
- seeing or hearing acts of violence
- the presence of alcohol or other drug use
- the smell of chemicals or the presence of empty chemical containers
- evidence of dangerous pets (e.g. exotic snakes and reptiles, breeds of dogs that are often trained to be vicious)
- unusual silence or darkened residence.

If any of these or other warning signs are present, the paramedic should retreat from the scene and call for police assistance.

When approaching a suspicious residence, the paramedic should choose tactics that match the threat or situation. For example, they should not use AVW devices; they should take

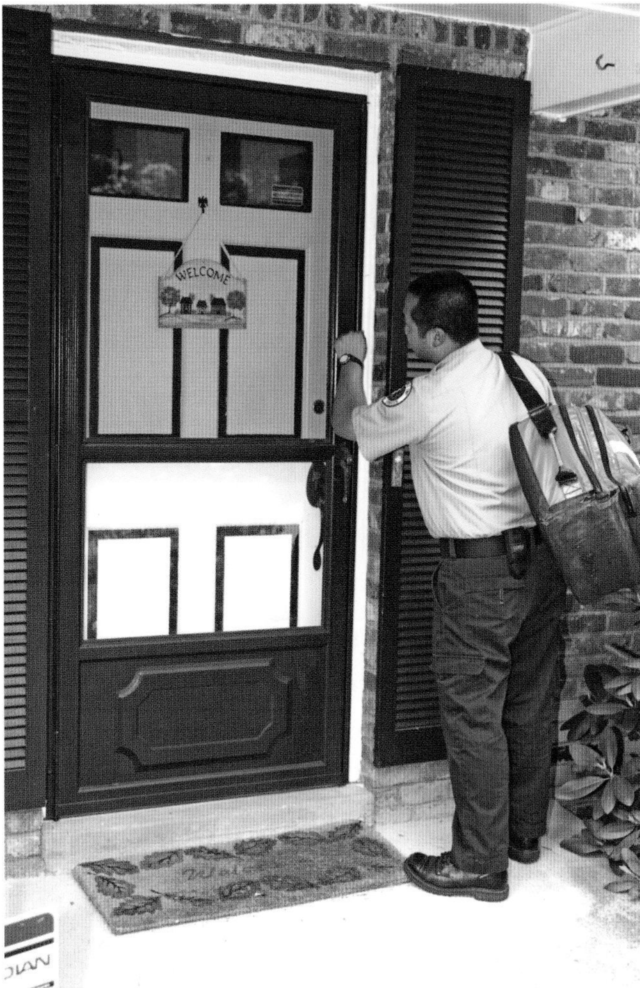

Figure 44-1 If danger from inside a residence is suspected, paramedics should stand on the side of an entry door opposite the hinges (i.e. the doorknob side).

unconventional pathways (rather than using the pavement for example); and they should not stand in front of the ambulance lights (backlighting). In addition, paramedics should listen for sounds indicating danger before announcing their presence or entering the home. They should stand on the side of the entry door opposite the hinges (doorknob side) (Figure 44-1). If danger becomes evident, the first responder or EMS crew should immediately retreat from the scene.

Dangerous road encounters

As with calls to residences, a response to a traffic incident should never be considered routine. Such calls involve inherent dangers associated with traffic flow, emergency vehicle positioning, and extrication. Also, the danger of violence may exist. For example, a vehicle's occupants may be armed, wanted, or fleeing criminals. Occupants within a vehicle may be under the influence of alcohol or drugs and exhibiting signs of abusive or violent behaviour because of an altered mental state.

The paramedic will have to deal with incidents on a variety of road structures; in the UK there are single, dual and three-lane carriageways to contend with. All of these have varying road speeds and each has its own particular hazard; therefore, the approach to a vehicle may vary depending on which lane the incident has occurred in.

Box 44-1

Street-smart safety tips

- When working on a road or street always wear reflective clothing and make sure you can leave the scene quickly and safely if required.
- At night time, use the ambulance lights to illuminate a vehicle's interior.
- If a passenger in the car is adjusting the side or rear view mirror as you approach, retreat to safety. (This is a sign of danger.)
- Open or unlatched boots may indicate that people are hiding or have been restrained in the compartment. If the boot is slightly open, slam it shut without opening it further.
- Retreat to the ambulance (or another place of safety) at the first sign of danger.

Critical Thinking

Where would you park your vehicle if you were responding to an incident in the second lane of a three-lane carriageway and why?

For approaching a vehicle, a one-person approach is recommended.[5] This allows the person who remains in the ambulance to notify control of the situation, location and registration number of any suspicious vehicles. (Because the ambulance is elevated, it provides greater visibility.) At night, the ambulance's lights should be used to illuminate the interior of the vehicle. They can also be used to illuminate the surrounding area (Box 44-1).

The paramedic who approaches the car should do so from the passenger side of the vehicle. This provides protection from vehicular traffic on single carriageway roads. Furthermore, it is usually the opposite approach a driver would expect from police. As another safety precaution, the paramedic should not walk between the ambulance and the other vehicle, to avoid being trapped and injured if the vehicle reverses or rolls back. The paramedic should walk around the rear of the ambulance to reach the passenger side of the vehicle.

Car posts A, B, and C (see Chapter 43) may provide the best ballistic protection. The paramedic should observe for unusual activity in the rear seat. He or she should not move forward of the post nearest the threat unless no threats exist in these areas. The paramedic should observe the front seat from behind post B. He or she should move forward only after making sure it is safe to do so (Figure 44-2). If signs of danger are present (e.g. weapons, suspicious behaviour or movements in the vehicle, arguing or fighting among passengers), paramedics should immediately retreat to a safe standby area. From that area, they should request the help of the police.

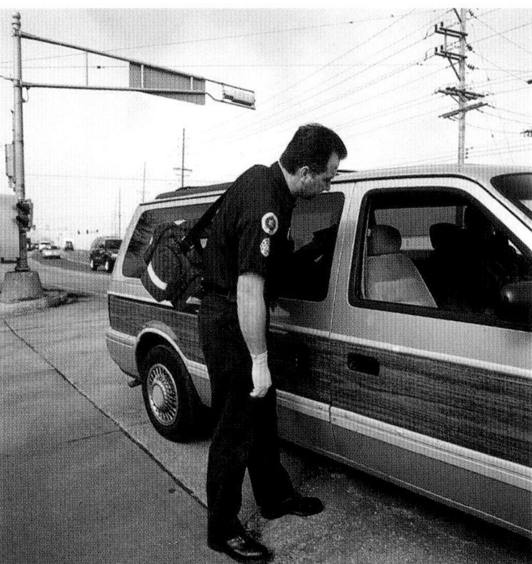

Figure 44-2 In approaching a car with potentially dangerous occupants, paramedics should observe the front seat from behind post B. They should move forward only after ensuring their safety.

Critical Thinking

In your community, what type of EMS calls routinely merit a police response?

Violent street incidents

Murder, assault and robbery are common occurrences in the UK. Many of these crimes involve dangerous weapons. Violence may be directed toward EMS personnel from perpetrators at the scene or who return to the scene. The violence may even come from injured and distraught patients. In addition, dangerous crowds and bystanders can quickly become large in number and volatile. They may direct violence toward everyone and everything in the surrounding area. Warning signs of potential danger in violent street incidents include the following:

- voices that become louder, escalating in tone
- pushing and shoving
- hostility toward people at the scene (e.g. perpetrator, police, victim)
- a rapid increase in the size of the crowd
- the use of alcohol or other drugs by people at the scene
- inability of the police to control the crowd.

Paramedic crews should constantly monitor crowds and retreat from the scene if necessary. The location and careful parking of the emergency vehicle is important for personal safety. The paramedic should position the ambulance so that it cannot be blocked by other vehicles (allowing for easy retreat from the scene). When possible and when it is safe to do so, the patient should be removed from the scene as the crew retreats (this may eliminate the need to return to the scene).

Violent groups and situations

Gang culture is growing in the UK, with increasingly young people joining gangs, often carrying real or imitation fire arms or knives, both for protection and as part of their image. Gang culture has long been association with the United States but reports of gangs in the UK are showing increasing similarity with those in the US (Box 44-2).[6] Most gangs and other threat groups operate through intimidation and extortion (Box 44-3).

Box 44-2

Short history of gangs

Modern-era gangs are growing in the UK. Most major cities in the UK have increasing numbers of gang members with signs that gang activity is becoming more organized. Gangs have their own hierarchy and fall into three principal groups. (1) Peer groups – small unorganized groups who share a common history and territory, they are mostly involved in low-level crime. (2) Gangs mostly comprised of groups of street-based young people; the group tends to have a name and crime and violence makes up an essential part of their identity. (3) Organized criminal groups, groups of individuals whose principal occupation is the involvement in crime for personal gain. They frequently operate in the illegal marketplace and violence is an essential part of protecting their identity. Gang membership often is a lifetime commitment.

Box 44-3

Some gangs and other threat groups found within the UK

Bloods
Crips
Hell's Angels
Skinheads
Outlaws
Yardies
Gangs with religious affiliations
Jamaican drug gangs
Chinese drug gangs

Plus many other gangs which have been developed to deal in crime, extortion and prostitution.

Gang characteristics

Gangs often share an identity based on either: age, location, ethnicity, peer networks or blood relationships. Gangs tend to be hierarchical communities with common interests and shared purposes. Research carried out in Manchester and Birmingham suggests that gangs consist of key individuals surrounded by ordinary members.[6] The gang may choose a name, logo, specific colour or method of dress to identify its own members and counterparts.

A distinction must be made between street gangs and criminal gangs; a gang may simply be defined as an informal group of people who regularly meet and do things together. Alternatively, a gang can be seen as an organized group of criminals or disorderly young people.[7] The paramedic must distinguish gangs from social street groups very quickly; gangs can be identified by their willingness to use deadly violence, the importance of defending territory, and their non-transitory nature. Organized gangs are usually territorial, and are usually made up of all male or all female.[6] Gangs also operate by creating an atmosphere of fear in a community.

Britain's first Los Angeles-style 'gang squad' is being set up in Manchester to tackle the growing menace of organized groups of violent youths; the rationale for the squad is the belief that up to 500 active gang members exist in Manchester alone. The rising violence is graphically illustrated by the shooting, in 2006, of a 15-year-old boy who was caught in the crossfire of a turf war.[8]

Critical Thinking

In addition to consulting police sources and familiarizing yourself with gang markings, dress and colours, it is important to know if you have gangs operating within your community. How can you obtain information about gang activity in your community?

Graffiti and clothing

The most common form of graffiti is 'tagging', which is where gangs or individuals compete for territory or marking territorial boundaries (known as turf). This allows gang members to leave their special mark or name tag and is probably the most visible sign of criminal gang activity. The term graffiti refers to drawings, patterns, scribbles, messages or 'tags' that are painted, written or carved on public walls, neighbourhood parks, retaining walls, spaces and any other prominent structure that is paintable.[9]

Gang-related clothing is often unique and specific to a group. It is worn to identify affiliation and rank. Common gang-related clothing and styles are listed in Box 44-4.

Box 44-4

Gang clothing and styles

Male

- Shaved, bald head or extremely short hair
- Tattoos (variable) and jewellery
- Bandanas
- White, oversized T-shirt that is creased in the middle
- White, athletic-type undershirt
- Polo-type knit shirts (oversized), usually worn buttoned to the top and not tucked in; other types of oversized shirts
- Oversized Dickie, Ben Davis or Solos trousers
- Trousers worn low, or 'sagging', and cuffed inside at the bottom or dragging on the ground
- Baseball caps worn backward (usually black and sometimes having the gang's initials)
- Cut-off, below-the-knee short trousers worn with knee-high socks
- A predominance of dark or dull clothing or clothing of one particular colour
- Black stretch belt with chrome or silver gang initial belt buckle
- Clothing: a mixture of gang colours, black and silver, or white

Female

- Exaggerated use of mousse, gel or baby oil in the hair
- Tattoos (variable) and jewellery
- Black or dark clothing and shoes
- Black oversized jackets, sweatshirts or athletic football jerseys
- Oversized shirts worn outside of trousers
- Oversized T-shirts
- Dark jackets with lettering (cursive or Old English style)
- Baggy, long trousers that drag on the ground
- Heavy makeup, dark and excessive eye shadow, shaved eyebrows, dark lipstick, dark fingernail polish
- Tank tops or revealing blouses
- Stretch belt with initial on belt buckle

Safety issues in gang areas

Common gang activities include fighting, vandalism, armed robbery, weapon offences, vehicle theft, battery and drug dealing. Not all gang members are engaged in illegal activities. The criminal activity is usually committed for monetary benefit, either for the gang in general or for a single member. Violent acts from gangs are highly likely. Because the uniforms of EMS personnel often look like those of police, paramedics must be very cautious about personal safety when working in gang areas.

Clandestine drug laboratories

As described in Chapter 21, the illegal manufacture of drugs can pose major hazards for emergency providers. In some clandestine laboratories, drugs are created from chemical precursors (e.g. lysergic acid diethylamide [LSD], methamphetamine). (This is known as synthesis.) Also, a drug's form can be changed. (This is known as conversion.) For example, cocaine hydrochloride may be changed to a base form. The processes of drug synthesis and conversion can produce low-oxygen atmospheres, or they may also create highly explosive and toxic gases (e.g. phosgene). These gases can readily be absorbed through the skin in amounts that can be fatal. Some of the chemicals involved in creating illicit drugs are corrosive and carcinogenic.[10] Toxic solvents involved in drug-making processes can also lead to laboratory explosions and exposure to dangerous chemicals.

Booby traps are another danger associated with clandestine drug laboratories; these can maim or kill an intruder. People who operate these laboratories are sometimes armed or otherwise violent. Clandestine laboratories are usually located in an area that ensures privacy. They are generally well ventilated and there may be powerful lights on all day or night in places such as the attic, roof space or cellar. They also usually have access to water, electric and gas utilities, which are required for the drug-making process. Regular activity at extremely late hours coupled with noise and visitors between midnight and dawn are frequently signs of clandestine drug activity. Younger people tend to act as lookouts and may be seen hanging around the property during heavy traffic periods. Other obvious signs include people exchanging small packets for cash, and syringes or other paraphernalia associated with drug abuse in the neighbouring vicinity.

Critical Thinking

What type of calls might EMS crews respond to at a drug laboratory?

The paramedic should be alert for signs of illegal drug manufacture when responding to a scene, particularly in areas where this activity is known to be commonplace. The signs may include strong unpleasant or chemical odours that resemble ammonia or cat urine, which drug producers will try to disguise with deodorizers or air fresheners. Visual sightings include the presence of chemical equipment (e.g. glassware, chemical containers, heating mantles and burners), large amounts of powder, Duracell-type battery cases cut up, and excessive amounts of coffee filters with red staining.[10] If a drug laboratory is identified, the EMS crew should:

1. Leave the area at once.
2. Notify control for police presence and request any appropriate agencies and personnel.
3. Initiate an incident management system and Hazmat procedure per protocol.
4. Help the police to evacuate the surrounding area in an orderly fashion (to ensure public safety).

Note

EMS crews should never touch anything found in or around a drug laboratory. Only specially trained personnel should try to alter drug-making equipment or stop chemical reactions in a drug laboratory.

Domestic violence

Domestic violence (DV) can be defined as any incident of threatening behaviour, violence or abuse (psychological, physical, sexual, financial or emotional) between adults, aged 18 or over, who are or have been intimate partners or family members, regardless of gender and sexuality.[11]

DV is a huge problem for society. In the UK:

- It accounts for around 15% of all violent crime.
- It will involve one in four women and one in six men at some time in their lives.
- It has the highest rates of repeat victimization.
- Two women are murdered as a result of DV each week, accounting for 35% of all murders.[12]

DV is clearly linked with sporting events and alcohol, which is something that all agencies need to be aware of and include in their strategic planning for such events.[12]

Possible signs and symptoms of domestic violence and abuse may include the following:

Physical

- stress-related ailments – headaches, irritable bowel syndrome
- sexually transmitted diseases (STD)
- repeated terminations of pregnancy
- bruises on the body and/or injuries to face, head or neck
- multiple injuries in different stages of healing
- burns – cigarette and/or rope burns
- hair loss consistent with hair pulling
- unexplained injuries or those inconsistent with explanations
- unusual or unsanitary living conditions or personal hygiene.

Behavioural

- frequent visits to emergency department and partner answers questions directed to patients
- patient appears fearful, evasive, ashamed or embarrassed
- use of alcohol and drugs and/or frequent use of pain medication
- eating disorders.

Psychological and emotional

- depression, anxiety and/or panic attacks
- self-harm and/or attempted suicide.[13]

EMS personnel who respond to a scene of domestic violence should be aware that acts of violence may be directed toward them by the perpetrator. Safety is paramount and the paramedic should take all necessary safety precautions. Once the scene is considered safe, the paramedic should treat the patient's injuries. Health professionals can make an important contribution to tackling DV. In order to achieve this, the mnemonic RADARR may be useful:[13]

R Routine enquiry
A Ask direct questions
D Document findings safely
A Assess the patients safety
R Resources, provide information on resources available
R Respect the patient's choices.

The paramedic should follow their own ambulance service protocols or guidance regarding the notification of DV incidents. To help ensure scene safety for the crew and the abused person, paramedics should not be judgemental about the relationship, and should not direct accusations toward the abuser. When appropriate, paramedics should supply the victim with phone numbers for domestic violence hotlines, community support programmes, and available shelters.

Safety tactics

The aim of tactical EMS is to accomplish the task without injury or death resulting from the team's intervention. Preservation of the life and safety of the team members, hostages, bystanders and victims is paramount.[14] Tactics that help ensure personal safety include avoidance, tactical retreat, cover and concealment, distraction and evasive manoeuvres. Many programmes in the UK teach tactics for safety and patient care. Some EMS providers are specially trained and equipped to work in tactical police enforcement settings (Box 44-5).

Box 44-5

Tactical EMS

The term tactical EMS (TEMS) refers to EMS personnel who are specially trained and equipped to provide prehospital emergency care in police tactical firearms settings. Such settings may include hostage-barricaded situations, high-risk search warrants, and other adverse situations involving police and/or rescue operations in which standard EMS units may be inappropriate.

The concept of training emergency medical technicians (EMTs) and paramedics in TEMS is still in its infancy in the UK. Forward-thinking police services have adopted TEMS programmes as a way to increase the safety of their tactical firearms unit, officers, and the innocent hostage or bystander.

The overall aim of the tactical paramedic is to provide healthcare to members of the public and the tactical teams on an ongoing basis. This is achieved by the ability to:

- assess and plan for preventive medicine needs in sustained operations
- provide preventive medical care in sustained operations
- recognize and treat unique wound patterns resulting from deliberate interpersonal aggression
- use medical care skills appropriate to hostile and austere environments
- explain medical and physiological parameters that lead to performance decrement and implement plans that minimize those effects
- develop and apply injury control strategies
- access and analyse medical information and make a medical threat assessment
- apply special police principles to the delivery of medical care.

Avoidance

Avoidance is always preferable to confrontation. To practise avoidance, paramedics must continually be aware of the scene. They can stay aware by being observant and by being knowledgeable about warning signs that may indicate a dangerous situation. In addition, they must be knowledgeable about tactical responses for avoiding danger or for dealing with danger that cannot be avoided. Frequently EMS crews will be asked to standby at a safe location until the scene has been rendered safe. Crews should not enter the scene until advised to do so by control or the police.

Tactical retreat

Tactical retreat means leaving the scene when danger is observed or when violence or indicators of violence are displayed. Tactical retreat requires immediate and decisive action. Retreat on foot or by vehicle (in a calm, safe manner) involves choosing the mode and route of retreat that provides the least exposure to danger. During tactical retreat, the paramedic should be aware that the risks they faced are now located behind them. They must stay alert for associated dangers. Of course, the required distance from danger for a safe tactical retreat must be guided by the nature of the incident. In general, a safe distance must:

- protect the crew from any potential danger
- keep the crew out of the immediate line of sight
- protect the crew from gunfire (i.e. provide cover)
- keep the crew far enough away to give them time to react if danger reappears.

Critical Thinking

Could the EMS crew be charged with abandonment if they make a tactical retreat and leave the patient?

Once tactical retreat has been achieved, the paramedic must notify other responding units and agencies of the danger. They notify other units using interagency EMS and police standard operating procedures and agreements. (Interagency procedures that deal with violent situations should be established in the preplanning stages. That way, each agency is aware of its specific duties.)

Documentation is also essential to reducing liability if injuries or deaths occur. Thorough documentation should include observations of danger at the scene; who was notified of the danger; actions at the scene; and accurate times that retreat or return to the scene occurred. Tactical retreat for appropriate circumstances is not considered patient abandonment.[14]

Cover and concealment

Cover and concealment provide protection from injury; cover involves large, heavy structures and thus provides ballistic protection that can shield the body. Examples include large trees, telephone poles, and a vehicle's engine block. Concealment offers little or no ballistic protection; for example, bushes, wallboards, and the doors of vehicles. Cover and concealment should be integrated into tactical retreat or used when the EMS crew is pinned down (e.g. by gunfire) or in other dangerous settings. Be aware of signs of violence and aggression from individuals who are at the scene when you arrive (see Box 44-6).

When the need for cover or concealment arises, paramedics should:

- constantly be aware of their surroundings
- place as much of the body as possible behind adequate cover
- constantly look for ways to improve protection and location
- be aware of reflective clothing (e.g. trim, badges) that may draw attention or serve as a target.

Critical Thinking

What parts of your ambulance provide cover?

Tactical patient care

The term tactical patient care describes patient care activities that occur inside the scene perimeter, which is known as the hot zone. The provision of emergency medical services in the hot zone requires special training and authorization. Within the hot zone the EMS crew are likely to encounter the use of body armour, tactical uniform, compact and functional

Box 44-6

Warning signs of possible violent aggression and self-defence measures

People who are about to escalate to violence often give subtle warning signs of this development. Such a person may:

- conspicuously ignore emergency responders
- be verbally abusive
- invade the responder's personal space
- shift the body weight from side to side or foot to foot (boxer stance)
- clench the fists
- tighten the muscles (e.g. have stiff arms and/or shoulders)
- maintain eye contact by staring.

Sometimes escape is impossible, and paramedics may be caught in a dangerous situation. (For example, they may be held as a hostage.) In such cases, paramedics should:

- remain as calm as possible
- avoid any confrontation
- play an active role with the captor in resolving the incident
- focus on a peaceful resolution and escape.

equipment, and, in some operations, work with police who are issued with personal defensive weapons.

Body armour

Some EMS crews within the UK are provided with soft body armour (also known as stab-proof vests). These offer protection from some blunt and penetrating trauma. This equipment is effective against most knives; however, it does not provide protection from high-velocity rifle bullets or thin or dual-edged weapons (e.g. ice picks). Like all other protective clothing, body armour is effective only when it is properly worn and in good condition. This armour may carry an expiration date that should be observed. Wet or worn vests do not provide optimum protection. A type III or higher level of protection is generally recommended for tactical EMS providers.

When wearing body armour, paramedics should take care not to develop a false sense of security. A general rule is, never try a manoeuvre that would not normally be done without body armour. Also, paramedics should keep in mind that body armour does not cover the entire body. Severe injury can still result from the forces of blunt trauma (in the absence of penetration) even when the vest is properly worn.

Zones within the tactical arena

There are three zones within a tactical incident area that EMS crews should be aware of. The most dangerous is the hot zone, where care is performed under fire or within the line of fire. When there is a need to remove a casualty from the area safely, the care of patients in the hot zone is the responsibility of the tactical police team, who will move the patient to the warm zone. Often the only immediate options in this situation are self-care and self-rescue.[14]

EMS care in the hot zone

Patient care in dangerous settings involves a number of special concerns. Within the hot zone, care normally requires the paramedic to make a remote assessment of the patient; this can be achieved by asking the following questions:

- Are his wounds survivable?
- Can I tell his skin colour?
- Is he breathing?
- Is there active bleeding?
- Is there movement?
- Are limbs bent at an odd angle?

The warm zone

The next zone is referred to as the warm zone, where tactical field care of the patient is provided. The purpose of warm zone care is to allow the paramedic to perform a risk-versus-benefit analysis, and to provide advanced emergency medical care to permit safe evacuation as soon as possible. Interventions that are required should be as rapid as possible and the paramedic should be prepared to abandon tactical field care if the warm zone becomes hot.

The cold zone

The third zone is known as the cold zone, where no current risk of injury to EMS personnel is evident, but paramedics should remain vigilant at all times as the situation can change and the need for rapid retreat could become evident.

Cold-zone care is where casualty evacuation is performed; it encompasses standard prehospital care procedures and allows the EMS crew to perform further assessment and management of the patient as required.

The role of the tactical paramedic

The provision of EMS care in tactical situations calls for special training and authorization. The overall aim of the tactical paramedic is to provide healthcare to members of the tactical teams on an ongoing basis. This is achieved by:

- wearing personal protective gear
- delivery of advanced tactical medical care
- operational medical support planning
- medical planning/intelligence
- barricade medicine (remote care)
- maximizing team operational health status
- management of multiple casualties and triage in potentially hostile environments
- police canine emergency care.

Any movement of patients within these unpredictable areas will be coordinated by the incident commander. Often, tactical EMS providers work under protocols and standing orders that are different from those of 'standard' EMS practice.

EMS at crime scenes

The safety and physical well-being of all individuals in and around the crime scene are the initial responsibility and first priority of any responding officer or EMS crew. After controlling any dangerous situation it is vital to ensure that medical attention is provided to injured persons whilst minimizing contamination of the scene.

Patient care is the paramedic's top priority, even at crime scenes. However, evidence can be protected during patient care if the paramedic is careful not to disturb the scene unnecessarily and does not destroy evidence. For example, paramedics should be observant of the scene and surroundings; they should touch only what is required for patient care; and they should wear latex gloves for infection control and to avoid leaving additional fingerprints at the scene.

What is a crime scene?

A crime scene is a location where any part of a criminal act has occurred. It can also be a location where evidence relating to a crime may be found. Important physical evidence that may be found at a crime scene includes fingerprints, footprints, and blood and other body fluids. Fingerprints and footprints are unique to an individual and no two people have identical prints. These ridge characteristics are often left behind on a surface, along with oil and moisture from the skin. Blood and other body fluids can be tested for deoxyribonucleic acid (DNA) and ABO blood typing, which also have characteristics that may be unique to the individual. In addition, particulate evidence (e.g. hair, carpet and clothing fibres) can provide useful information and is considered valuable at a crime scene.

The paramedic's observations at a crime scene are important and should be documented carefully on the clinical report form. For example, victims' positions, their injuries, and conditions at the scene may be helpful to police in solving the crime. Documentation should also include any statements made by the patient or other people at the scene and any dying declarations. Paramedics should be careful to:

- record their observations objectively
- record patients' or bystanders' words in quotes
- avoid personal opinions that are not relevant to patient care.

Paramedics must keep in mind that patient care reports are legal documents and may be used in court. Other measures that aid crime scene preservation are listed in Box 44.7.

Critical Thinking

If the main goal is caring for the patient, why should a paramedic be concerned about preserving evidence?

Note

A *dying declaration* is a statement(s) made by a person who believes he or she is about to die and should be passed on either in writing or verbally. A dying declaration is considered credible and trustworthy based upon the general principle that most people who know they are going to die will not tell a lie. Dying declarations may be used in a court of law as evidence if the patient's death is connected with a charge of murder or manslaughter. Should you believe there are legal implications in the declaration, then you should record an accurate account which, where possible, should be witnessed. The statement may relate to personal wishes at the time of death, personal feelings, or concern about their property. More importantly it may raise concerns about the cause or circumstance surrounding his or her impending death. An example is an assault victim who makes a dying declaration implicating a certain person as being his or her attacker.

Box 44-7

Considerations for crime scene preservation

Paramedics should observe the following rules when called to a known or a possible crime scene:

1. Do not approach a crime scene until it has been secured for your safety.
2. Park your vehicle in a safe location and try to park in a way that affords you easy egress from the scene and avoids reversing. When parking, avoid possible contamination of skid marks, tyre prints, or other evidence.
3. Survey and assess the scene before proceeding to the victim.
4. Try to approach the victim from a route different from the assailant's probable route. If the assailant is still present, do not approach until safe to do so.
5. Follow the same path to and from the victim.
6. Avoid stepping on bloodstains or spatter if possible.
7. Whilst performing your assessment and treatment, try not to disturb the victim and the victim's clothing.
8. When cutting clothing from a victim, try to do it in a way that preserves the points of wounding.
9. Report your actions and any disturbances you make to the crime scene investigator.
10. Keep all unnecessary people away from the victim.
11. Do not smoke or eat at the crime scene.
12. Do not touch any evidence if at all possible.
13. Make no comments to bystanders about the situation.
14. Save the victim's clothes and personal items in a bag. The bag should be labelled, sealed, and turned over to police.
15. Be alert to any dying declarations the patient makes.
16. Keep accurate, detailed records.
17. Keep in mind that police are in charge of the crime scene; you are in charge of the patient.

Modified from Vollrath R 1995 Crime scene preservation: it's everybody's concern. J Emerg Med Serv 20(1):53.

Summary

- A key point in ensuring scene safety is to identify and respond to dangers before they occur. If the scene is known to be violent, the EMS crew should remain at a safe distance and out of sight of the area, until they are given the all clear to approach by the police.
- Calls to residential areas should be approached with caution. Paramedics should listen and look for warning signs of violence before and during their attendance and should retreat from the scene if danger becomes evident.
- A response to a traffic incident may involve dangers associated with pedestrians, traffic and extrication. However, the incident may present danger from the occupants of a vehicle who are armed, wanted or fleeing felons, intoxicated or drugged, or may be violent or abusive because of an altered mental state.
- Paramedics should be vigilant when attending violent street incidents and should know their exit routes to allow retreat from the scene if necessary.
- Gang culture is a growing problem in the UK and sometimes the members will carry knives or firearms and can be involved in violent criminal activities. EMS personnel wear uniform and could be mistaken for police officers so should be very cautious about personal safety when working in known gang areas.
- Clandestine laboratories can produce explosive and toxic gases. Other risks include armed or violent occupants and booby traps that can maim or kill an intruder.
- EMS personnel who respond to a scene of domestic violence should remain non-judgemental but keep alert for any acts of violence toward them by the perpetrator and should take all safety precautions.
- Safety tactics for EMS intervention should result in the accomplishment of the task without injury or death. Tactical safety includes avoidance, tactical retreat, cover and concealment, and distraction and evasive manoeuvres.
- The term tactical patient care refers to care that occurs inside the scene perimeter (the hot zone) by specially trained and authorized EMS crews and police. The care and removal of patients within the hot zone is normally the responsibility of the police, who will move patients to a safer area for treatment by EMS crews. Paramedics should be aware of the dangers that can arise in any of the zone areas and vigilance should be maintained.
- The paramedic's observations at a crime scene are important and should be carefully documented. Paramedics should try to protect evidence while caring for the patient. This can be done by not destroying evidence and by taking care not to disturb the scene unnecessarily.

References

1. Home Office 2006 Crime in England & Wales 2005/6. A summary of the main statistics. Home Office, London
2. Centre for Social Justice 2009 Dying to belong: an in-depth review of street gangs in Britain. Centre for Social Justice, London
3. Calland V 2006 A brief overview of personal safety at incident sites. Emerg Med J 23:878–882
4. Fisher J, Brown S, Cooke M (eds) 2006 UK Ambulance Service Clinical Practice Guidelines. JRCALC, London, section 4, p 1
5. US Department of Transportation National Highway Traffic Safety Administration 1998 EMT-Paramedic National Standard Curriculum. US Department of Transportation, Washington, DC
6. Bennett T, Holloway K 2004 Gang membership, drugs and crime in the UK. Br J Criminol 44:305–323
7. Compact Oxford English Dictionary. Online. Available http://www.askoxford.com 19 June 2009
8. Bennetto J 2006 The Independent, 12 September 2006. The Independent News and Media Limited, London
9. Northampton Borough Council 2007 Dealing with graffiti. Online. Available www.Northampton.gov.uk 8 August 2007
10. Lancashire Constabulary 2006 Keeping illegal drugs out of rental properties. Crime Stoppers
11. The Association of Police Officers 2004 Guidance on investigating domestic violence 2004. Home Office, London
12. Home Office 2006 Lessons learned from the domestic violence enforcement campaigns 2006; Police And Crime Standards Directorate. Home Office, London
13. Taket A 2004 Tackling domestic violence; the role of health professionals, 2nd edition. Home Office, London
14. Woollard M 2005 Tactical EMS: supporting police firearms teams. In: Contemporary issues in trauma care; 8th International Trauma Care Conference, Telford, June 2005

CHAPTER **45**

Chemical, Biological, Radiological and Nuclear (CBRN) Incidents

Chapter contents

Objectives

Upon completion of this chapter, the paramedic student will be able to:

1. List the main CBRN agents of concern.
2. Identify actions, signs and symptoms, methods of distribution and management of chemical agents.
3. Identify actions, signs and symptoms, methods of distribution and management of biological agents.
4. Identify actions, signs and symptoms, methods of distribution and management of radiological and nuclear material.
5. Identify measures to be taken by paramedics who respond to incidents with suspected CBRN involvement.

Key terms

anthrax An acute infectious disease caused by the spore-forming bacterium *Bacillus anthracis*.

bioterrorism The use of biological agents, such as pathogenic organisms or agricultural pests, for the express purpose of causing death or disease, to instil a sense of fear and panic in the victims, and to intimidate governments or societies for political, financial, or ideological gain.

CBRN(E) An acronym used for agents that may be used deliberately to cause harm: chemical, biological, radiological, nuclear (and explosives).

chlorine A poisonous, yellow–green gas.

FFP Classification of face protection against particulate material. FFP3 is the highest specification.

Hazmat Hazardous material that may cause harm if released accidentally.

hot zone Areas of high concentration of hazardous/CBRN materials causing primary contamination.

NBC An older acronym for nuclear, biological and chemical weapons, now replaced by CBRN.

phosgene A poisonous gas that appears as a greyish white cloud and smells of newly mowed hay.

plague A disease caused by the bacterium *Yersinia pestis*, found in the fleas of rodents (e.g. chipmunks, prairie dogs, ground squirrels, and mice) and in many areas around the world – not normally seen in Europe.

PPE Personal protective equipment.

ricin A potent protein cytotoxin derived from the beans of the castor plant (*Ricinus communis*).

riot control agents Chemicals that can produce sensory irritation or disabling physical effects that disappear within a short time after termination of exposure.

sarin A clear, colourless, and tasteless volatile nerve agent that has no odour in its pure form; may be used as a nerve agent.

soman A clear, colourless, tasteless nerve agent with a slight camphor odour.

tabun A clear, colourless, tasteless nerve agent with a faint fruity odour.

tularaemia A serious illness that is caused by the bacterium *Francisella tularensis* found in animals (especially rodents, rabbits and hares).

vesicants Chemicals with severely irritating properties that produce fluid-filled blisters on the skin and damage to the eyes, lungs, and other mucous membranes.

viral haemorrhagic fevers A group of illnesses caused by several distinct families of viruses that include arenaviruses, filoviruses, bunyaviruses and flaviviruses.

VX A thick, amber-coloured, odourless nerve agent that resembles motor oil.

warm zone Areas where there is potential of secondary contamination from casualties or equipment coming out of the hot zone.

weapons of mass destruction (WMD) Large conventional biological, nuclear, incendiary, chemical or explosive weapons (B-NICE).

International conventions have long prohibited the use of chemicals and biological warfare (CBW) agents during war and bar any country from making or acquiring biological weapons (BW). However, a number of countries and terrorist groups maintain or seek to acquire them. This chapter serves as an overview of CBRN and provides general guidelines for emergency response.

Note

CBRN is an acronym that can be used for identifying the four categories of agents/materials that are likely to be deliberately released. It stands for chemical, biological, radiological and nuclear – explosives may also be included (CBRN(E)). There is some overlap with hazardous materials as some toxic industrial hazards (TIH) may be deliberately released.

History of CBRN (NBC) weapons

The use of CBRN agents as weapons has occurred throughout history, dating back to antiquity with poisoned tipped arrows. In 184 BC Hannibal ordered that pots filled with venomous snakes be thrown onto the decks of enemy ships (Box 45-1). Many countries, including the UK, the former Soviet Union, Canada, and the US, have agreed to non-proliferation treaties to stop research and development into chemical and biological weapons; however, some countries continue to have CBRN capability or research programmes. In addition, some terrorist organizations have active programmes to acquire CBRN weapons for use against military and civilian populations. Recent CBRN events include the sarin attack on the Tokyo subway (1995), the US 'anthrax letters' (2001) and the use of radioactive polonium-210 against an individual in London (2006). The threat of a CBRN attack depends on the *intent* of terrorist cells to use such devices and their *capability*. Acts of terrorism can pose significant risk to civilian populations. The use of CBRN agents may cause mass casualties and overwhelm medical resources, require decontamination to take place, require isolation of contagious cases, or require additional mental health services to deal with a proportional increase in 'worried well' casualties as a reaction to a CBRN event. In addition, the threat of a CBRN attack may compromise a conventional prehospital response to an explosive incident, which may lead to an unnecessary delay in life-saving interventions and preventable deaths.

Box 45-1

Timeline of CBRN weapons

Early examples

- Hercules dips his arrows into the toxic blood of the decapitated Hydra.
- Hannibal uses snake-filled pots catapulted onto the Roman fleet.
- The Tartar army catapult bodies of plague victims into the city of Kaffa in 1346.
- The British army provided the Delaware Indians in 1763 with blankets that had been used by smallpox patients.

World War I

- Chlorine, phosgene, cyanide and mustard gas used by the main protagonists.
- The pandemic flu outbreak of 1918–1919 kills more people worldwide than throughout World War I.

World War II

- The Japanese use germ warfare against the Chinese by scattering plague-infected fleas by airplane.
- The Japanese experiment with biological agents on prisoners of war.
- The British perform trials with anthrax off the coast of Scotland.
- An air raid on a US ship releases mustard gas in Bari harbour.
- First detonation of a nuclear weapon over Hiroshima, shortly followed by a second on Nagasaki.

Post-World War II

- Georgi Markov is assassinated with an umbrella-delivered pellet containing ricin.
- An accidental release of anthrax spores occurs from a BW facility in the Soviet Union in 1979 and was masked as a natural outbreak.
- Iraq uses chemical weapons against the Iranians and its own Kurdish minority.

Last 20 years

- The Aum Shinrikyo cult release nerve agent in Japanese cities in 1994 and 1995.
- A religious group contaminate salad bars with salmonella to influence a local election.
- Anthrax in letters attacks in 2001, closely following the 11 September attacks.
- Alexander Litvinenko is killed in London following exposure to the radioisotope polonium-210.
- Chlorine tanks are blown up in Iraq by insurgents in 2007.

Methods of dissemination

Most CBRN agents need some form of delivery mechanism, which may be *overt* or *covert*. Overt methods include the use of explosive and other dispersal devices such as an aerosol system. Equipment that may be used to disseminate aerosols include crop-spraying planes for open spaces, aerosol-generating devices for enclosed areas (e.g. underground systems and enclosed shopping centres), ventilation systems in buildings, and contamination of items in the environment with fine powders that are aerosolized easily when disrupted (this is what occurred with the anthrax cases in the US in 2001, which were caused by opening contaminated mail). Explosive devices, such as a radioactive dirty bomb, have the potential to cause conventional injuries and CBRN exposure, *combined injuries*.

Covert methods of CBRN release include the contamination of water or food supplies and lend themselves more to biological and radiological agents. Covert agents may also have a longer latency or incubation period, which means that some releases may be mistaken for natural events. This was true in the case of the Oregon salmonella outbreak of 1984 that was later found to be a deliberate contamination of local salad bars. Overt methods are likely to lead to the 'big bang' type of major incident whilst a covert release is more likely to cause a 'rising tide' type.

Note

Why would aerosolized agents of mass destruction pose a great risk to first responders?

Routes of exposure

There are a number of ways that CBRN agents can penetrate the body; inhalation, ingestion and percutaneous. Some routes are quicker than others for producing systemic effects. Other routes are more resistant to some forms of exposure (intact skin resists biological agents).

- *Inhalation* – agent (gas, vapour, particles and smoke) breathed in (cyanide gas, carbon monoxide, chlorine, inhalational anthrax).
- *Ingestion* – agent (liquid, solid) eaten or drank (cyanide salts, intestinal anthrax, salmonella).
- *Percutaneous* – Absorption through the skin (percutaneous) can be split into three types (inoculation, wound, transcutaneous).
  - *Inoculation* – any penetration of the skin to introduce the agent (liquid, solid). An example of this was the ricin-loaded pellet used to kill Georgi Markov in 2003, the weapon being disguised as an umbrella. Medics routinely inoculate patients when giving intramuscular injections and malaria is transmitted by this route.
  - *Wound* – any contamination after the skin has been broken, mainly by live biological agents (tetanus, MRSA). There is some overlap with inoculation depending upon the wound size and primary intent of the weapon.
  - *Transcutaneous* – agent (liquid, solid) is absorbed through the skin without initially breaking it. This includes VX (causing no skin damage), mustard, acids and alkali (causing blistering wounds).
- *Ocular* – agents (gas, vapour) may have a local effect on the eye, although there may not be any significant systemic absorption. A good example of this is low-level nerve agent exposure causing pinpoint pupils (miosis) only. Ocular injuries may also need specific management and follow-up (mustard casualties).

Classification of CBRN agents

There are several classification systems for CBRN agents. Some classification systems date back to the early twentieth century and are based upon the initial presenting complaint before the true pathophysiology was known; examples include choking (chlorine) and blood agents (cyanide) although these terms are misleading.

Using an all-hazards approach, most agents can be categorized into one of three groups:

- *lethal* (cyanide, nerve agents, anthrax, plague, high-dose radiation)
- *damaging* (mustard gas, low-dose radiation)
- *incapacitating* (CS, LSD, salmonella, tularaemia).

However, toxicity is also associated with some of the drugs used as antidotes (atropine) in the management of CBRN casualties as well as trauma; a fourth group is therefore included:

- *iatrogenic* (antidotes).

Physical properties

The physical properties of CBRN agents are very important because of the risk to medical staff if responding on scene or if casualties may potentially be contaminated.

- *Non-persistent. Gases* (hydrogen cyanide, carbon monoxide) and *volatile liquids/vapours* are unlikely to remain and are called non-persistent. There may only be a limited requirement for decontamination.
- *Persistent.* Some agents are more persistent and include the less volatile liquids (mustard/VX nerve agent) and particulate/dry material (asbestos/anthrax spores/radioactive debris). These agents require decontamination and the actual method used depends upon the physical properties of the agent. The urgency of decontamination depends upon the toxicity of the substance, risk of transcutaneous absorption (VX) and state of the patient.

Contamination/contagious (two Cs)

All CBRN hazards have the potential to cause contamination. The extent of the contamination depends on the physical properties of the agent and its presentation (persistent/non-persistent). Contamination can be *external* and *internal* as well as *wound contamination*. Internal contamination may be due to *inhalation, ingestion, inoculation* (breaks the skin), *transcutaneous* (through intact skin) and *wound contamination*. Once an infection has been established, some live biological agents will self-replicate so have the potential to be spread by person-to-person contact; this status is known as *contagious*.

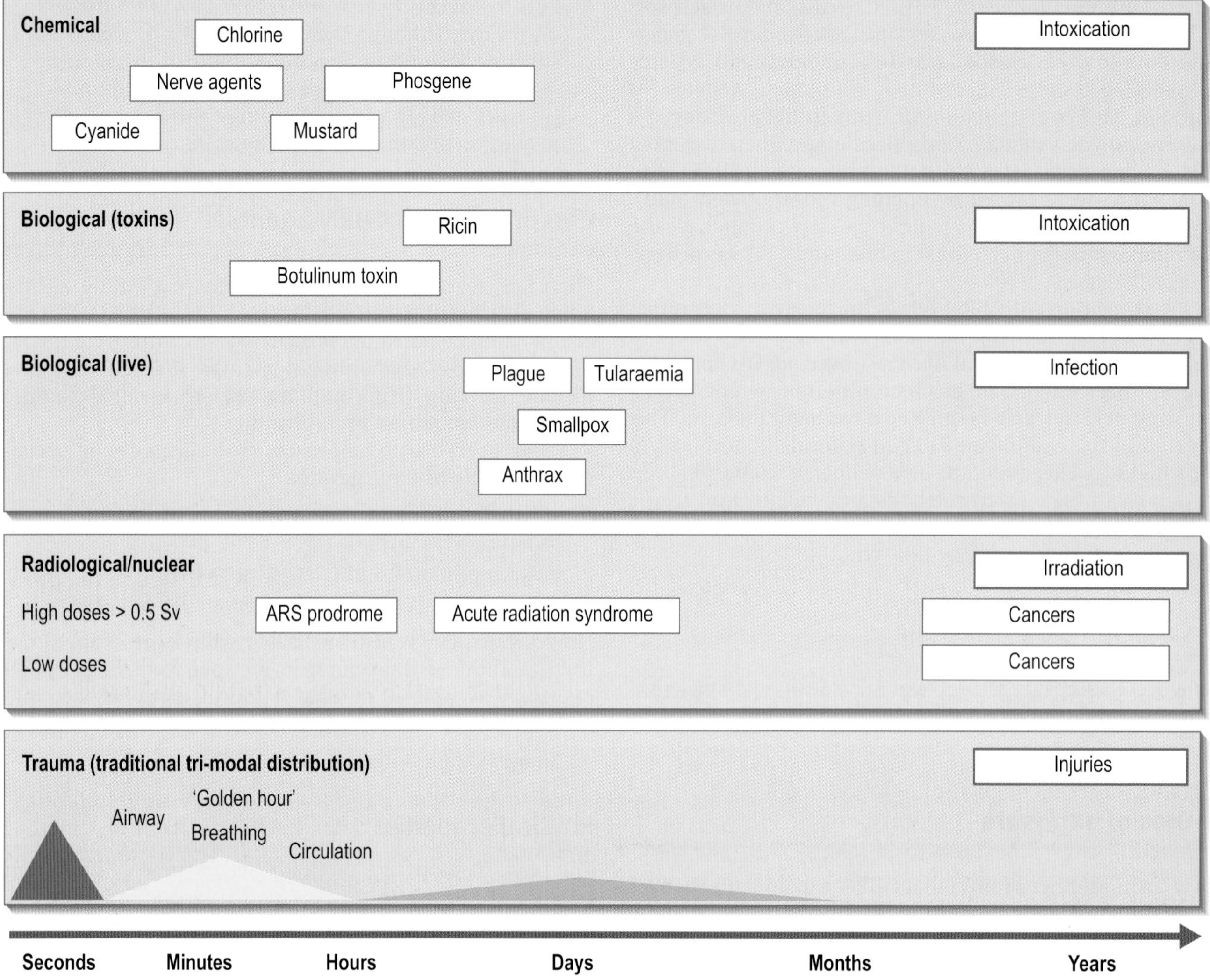

Figure 45-1 Onset of effects from CBRN agents and trauma. (© S.A. Bland.)

Effects of exposure (four Is)

The effects from CBRN agents can be summarized using the four Is. When assessing a casualty or incident scene where there may be a CBRN threat, consider potential clinical signs that may suggest there has been a significant exposure.

- *Intoxication* (chemical and biological [toxins])
- *Infection* (biological [live agents])
- *Irradiation* (radiological/nuclear)
- *Injuries* (trauma).

The onset of symptoms is dependent upon the type of CBRN agent. Generally, the more complex the agent, the longer the latency or, in the case of live biological agents, incubation period. This is shown in Figure 45-1.

Specific chemical threats

Specific chemicals that may be used in war or acts of terrorism include nerve agents, cyanides, pulmonary agents (chlorine/phosgene) and blister agents (mustard/lewisite). There is some overlap with toxic industrial chemicals (chlorine, phosgene, cyanide, carbon monoxide). Some signs and symptoms may also overlap or be confused with pharmacological agents including morphine and atropine. In order to assist with diagnosis, a summary of clinical signs is given in Table 45-1 and a summary of suggested antidotes is given in Box 45-2.

Nerve agents

Nerve agents were used in the Iran/Iraq War in the 1980s and also against the Kurdish population in northern Iraq. They were also used in terrorist attacks in Japan in 1995. They are highly toxic and rapidly acting. Nerve agents are based on organophosphate pesticides, but with greater potency and can be delivered as vapours (see Chapter 21). Nerve agents inhibit the enzyme acetylcholinesterase causing a cholinergic crisis. This is due to overstimulation of voluntary muscles, central nervous system and elements of the autonomic system, predominantly parasympathetic. The severity of intoxication caused by nerve agents depends on the amount, route, and length of exposure. Mildly or moderately exposed persons usually recover fully, whilst severely exposed persons are not likely to survive in the absence of

Table 45-1 CBRN quick look

	Nerve agent	Cyanide	Methaemoglobin	Pulmonary agents	Mustard/lewisite	Botulism	Atropine	Opiate
Respiration	↑↑	↑↑/↓	↑	↑↑	↑	↓	N/↑	↓
Pupils	Pinpoint	N/dilated	N	N	N/red	Dilated	Dilated	Pinpoint
Skin	Sweaty	Pink or cyanosed	Cyanosed	N or cyanosed	Erythema	Dry	Dry	N
Secretions	↑↑	N	N	↑	N/↑	↓	↓	N
Other	Fasciculation Fitting	Sudden onset	Chocolate blood		Mustard (delayed)	Paralysis, no CNS effects	CNS effects	CNS effects

N = Normal

Box 45-2

Summary of antidotes

Nerve agent

- ComboPen IM (atropine 2 mg, pralidoxime 500 mg, diazepam 5 mg equiv.)
- Atropine 2 mg IV, repeat to effect
- Pralidoxime (30 mg/kg) 2 g IV (other oximes: obidoxime, HI-6)
- Diazepam 5 mg IV, repeat to effect

Cyanide

- High-flow oxygen
- Dicobalt edetate 300 mg IV, followed by glucose 50% 50 mL IV, repeat once
- Sodium nitrite 300 mg IV over 5–20 min, followed by sodium thiosulphate
- Sodium thiosulphate 12.5 mg IV over 10 min (may be used alone)

Methaemoglobin formers

- High-flow oxygen
- Methylene blue 1–2 mg/kg IV

Chemical burns/vesicants (blister)

- IMMEDIATE DECONTAMINATION
- Mustard: no antidote
- Lewisite: British Anti-Lewisite (BAL), chelating agents
- Hydrofluoric (HF) acid: calcium gluconate (top)/calcium chloride (IV)

Atropine overdose

- Rest, sedation
- Consider physostigmine

Opiate

- Naloxone 0.4–2 mg IV, repeat to effect

advanced medical support and early antidote therapy. The nerve agents discussed in this chapter are sarin, soman, tabun and VX.

Critical Thinking

Would you expect a fast or slow heart rate if the patient has been exposed to a nerve agent?

Sarin

Sarin (also known as 'GB') is a clear, colourless and tasteless liquid that has no odour in its pure form. Sarin evaporates into a vapour (gas) and spreads into the environment. Symptoms may begin within minutes to hours after exposure. They may include headache, excessive secretions, chest pain/tightness, abdominal cramps, wheezing, fasciculations, seizure and respiratory failure that may lead to death. Because it is a vapour, early symptoms include dimmed vision due to pinpoint pupils.

Soman

Soman (also known as 'GD') is a clear, colourless, tasteless liquid with a slight camphor odour similar to the smell of Vicks Vapo-Rub or a rotting fruit odour. Compared with other nerve agents, soman is more volatile than VX but less volatile than sarin. (The higher the volatility of a chemical, the more likely it will evaporate and disperse into the environment.) Persons can be exposed to the vapour even if they do not come in contact with the liquid form. Symptoms may begin within seconds to hours after exposure and are similar to those caused by sarin.

Tabun

Tabun (also known as 'GA') is a clear, colourless, tasteless liquid with a faint fruity odour with similar physical properties and toxic effects to the previous nerve agents described.

VX

VX is a thick, amber-coloured, odourless liquid. It resembles motor oil and is more potent than the previous nerve agents described; a lethal dose being as small as a pinhead applied to the skin. VX is considered to be much more toxic when absorbed through the skin (percutaneous). VX is primarily a liquid exposure hazard although if heated to very high temperatures, it can turn into small amounts of vapour. Following release of VX, persons can be exposed through skin contact, eye contact, or inhalation. VX can also be released into the water, which allows for exposure by ingestion or absorption. Symptoms will appear within a few seconds after exposure to the vapour form of VX. They will appear within a few minutes to up to 18 h after exposure to the liquid form. Signs and symptoms of exposure are the same as for other nerve agents.

Treatment

Treatment for exposure to nerve agents consists of rapid extrication from the contaminated area ('hot zone') and decontamination. Treatment also consists of supporting management with basic airway manoeuvres and suction. The patient's clothing should be removed and decontaminated by trained personnel. A person's clothing and other contaminated surfaces can 'off-gas' and release nerve agent for up to 30 min after exposure, so secondary contamination is possible. *Atropine* and *pralidoxime* are the antidotes of choice. Atropine blocks the parasympathetic effects of the cholinergic crisis while pralidoxime works directly on the interaction of the nerve agent with the enzyme acetylcholinesterase. Large doses of atropine may be required and is not limited to the 3 mg recommended for cardiac arrest. Diazepam or other benzodiazepines may be indicated if seizures are present. The paramedic should seek medical advice before administering these drugs if only muscle twitching is present. Caring for patients who have been exposed to a nerve agent should be guided by medical advice, a poison control centre, or other authority.

Cyanides

Cyanide either in its non-persistent gaseous form or as a cyanide salt may be used by terrorists as well as occasionally used in suicide. Cyanide acts by inhibiting intracellular respiration within the mitochondria, which leads to the failure to utilize oxygen and therefore aerobic respiration causing the production of lactic acid. This precipitates rapid organ dysfunction, especially brain and heart. Symptoms and signs include dizziness, nausea, sudden collapse, hyperventilation, seizures, apnoea, coma, dysrhythmias and death. The lack of tissue oxygen extraction leads to arterialization of venous blood and an initial pink skin colour. Subsequent acidaemia causes oxygen dissociation, desaturation and an observed cyanosis. The key feature of cyanide toxicity is the rapidity of onset. Other agents and drugs to consider include carbon monoxide, hydrogen sulphide (bad-egg gas), methaemoglobin formers, including nitrates and nitrites, and the absence of an oxygen environment (anoxia).

Treatment

Treatment for exposure to cyanide includes ventilation of the area, rapid extrication of the casualty from the contaminated area ('hot zone') and oxygen administration. Decontamination may not be required if the casualty has been exposed to hydrogen cyanide gas. Antidote treatment depends on availability and there is regional variation. The traditional antidote regimen uses two antidotes, *sodium (amyl) nitrite* and *sodium thiosulphate*. The nitrite causes a mild methaemoglobinaemia and draws the cyanide back into the intravascular space (bloodstream), this then allows cyanide to be detoxified by the thiosulphate catalysed by the liver enzyme rhodanase. The other antidotes use cobalt, which cyanide has a greater affinity for, to directly bind and detoxify. The two antidotes in this group are *dicobalt edetate* and *hydroxocobalamin (vitamin* B_{12a}*)*. Unfortunately all the cyanide antidotes have some side effects and should be used with caution. Dicobalt edetate has a more severe side-effect profile in the absence of cyanide and therefore the diagnosis of cyanide poisoning should be certain and where possible supported with detection equipment or a high clinical suspicion.

Pulmonary agents

Pulmonary agents were the first chemical warfare agents to be used in World War I. In addition, the two main agents, *chlorine* and *phosgene*, are toxic industrial chemicals and are widely available worldwide. The use of these gases for acts of terrorism is therefore a possibility.

Chlorine is a yellow–green gas often associated with water purification. Chlorine gas can be pressurized and condensed into a liquid form that can be shipped and stored. When liquid chlorine is released, it quickly vaporizes into a gas that is heavier than air and stays close to the ground. Persons exposed to chlorine gas are likely to experience an immediate effect of sore throat and eyes as it reacts with moisture to form hydrochloric acid. Like other gases, the severity of poisoning depends on the concentration, route and duration of exposure. Signs and symptoms may include cough, chest pain, burning sensation in the nose, eyes, or throat, watery eyes, blurred vision, dermal burns from skin contact, and shortness of breath. Pulmonary oedema can develop within hours following inhalation of the gas.

Phosgene is a poisonous gas that appears as a greyish white cloud and smells of freshly mowed hay. With cooling and pressure, the gas can be condensed into a liquid that can be shipped and stored. When liquid phosgene is released, it quickly vaporizes into a gas that is heavier than air and stays close to the ground. Unlike chlorine there may be no immediate effects during exposure. Inhaled phosgene damages the lungs but classically with a latency period of up to 24 h. Symptoms include cough and laboured breathing. Pulmonary oedema with frothy sputum production may develop and is generally more severe than that caused by chlorine. The effects are thought to be inflammatory mediated rather than as a direct effect on lung tissue. Cutaneous exposure to the gas can result in skin or eye injury, including cold injuries. In addition to the signs and symptoms noted previously for chlorine exposure, phosgene poisoning may cause hypotension and heart failure. In lethal doses, death can occur rapidly within 48 h. During World War I, phosgene accounted for the majority of chemical warfare deaths.

Treatment

No antidotes exist for chlorine or phosgene poisoning. Treatment for exposure to these gases consists of removing the casualty from the contaminated zone as soon as possible and providing supportive medical care. All patients should be moved to an area of fresh air and to the highest ground possible (if exposure occurred in an open air space). The patient's clothing should be removed; however, only limited decontamination is required as the hazard is gaseous.

Blister agents

Blister agents or vesicants are chemicals with highly damaging local effects; some agents also have systemic effects. Symptoms of exposure may be delayed until hours after exposure. The major chemicals in this category are sulphur mustard, nitrogen mustard and lewisite. Phosgene oxime (not to be confused with phosgene gas) is also a theoretical hazard but is not discussed in detail.

Mustard is an oily liquid that comes in a variety of colours ranging from brown to yellow. It may smell like garlic, onion, horseradish or mustard itself. Symptoms from mustard exposure are delayed (hours). Although widely used in World War I and during the Iran/Iraq War, it has a relatively low mortality rate (~4%) but caused significant casualty numbers and morbidity. Body regions affected include moist areas such as the armpits and groins, as well as the eyes. Systemic features include white blood cell depression and potential secondary infections due to immunosuppression.

Lewisite is an oily liquid that is more volatile than mustard and smells like geraniums in its gaseous state. Unlike mustard, lewisite causes immediate pain on contact. There is a significant risk of death due to the absorption of arsenic, which causes multiorgan failure.

Treatment

After ensuring personal safety (including the use of appropriate personal protective equipment, PPE), the initial management of the patient should be immediate extrication and decontamination as mustard binds rapidly to tissue. Basic airway management is important with ventilatory and circulatory support as needed. All skin exposures should be treated with conventional burn care. Lewisite has a specific treatment, the chelating agent dimercaprol, also known as British Anti-Lewisite. Other chelating agents that bind directly with the metal ions of arsenic can also be considered.

Biological agents

Biological agents can be classified as *live* (bacterial, viral, fungal, chlamydial and rickettsial) or *toxin*. A toxin can be considered to be a chemically active agent of biological origin. It therefore does not self-replicate and is non transmissible, although decontamination may be required. Biological toxins may be derived from microbes, animal or plant origin. Examples include botulinum, snake/scorpion venom and digitalis from foxglove. Toxins will generally have a shorter *latency* period (hours–days) compared to the *incubation period* of a live agent, which may be up to weeks and in some cases months (viral hepatitis, HIV). Some live agents will also produce toxins as part of the infection (tetanus, anthrax, botulinum). However, some toxins can be used and spread without needing a live agent (botulinum, ricin, staphylococcal toxin).

Biological agents can be categorized as *lethal* or *non-lethal, transmissible* or *non-transmissible*. *Pathogenicity* is used to describe live agents that have the ability to cause disease (pathogen). *Transmissibility* reflects the ability of a live agent to spread from person to person. *Infectivity* differs from transmissibility as it reflects the ease with which an agent can establish an infection. For example, tularaemia is extremely infectious, requiring only 10–50 organisms, while anthrax spores require 10^4–10^5 spores to establish an infection. However, both are virtually non-transmissible directly from an infected patient. Some patients may therefore be infected but not infectious/contagious. Malaria is another important disease that is not transmissible from human to human and requires an animal *vector*, in this case the mosquito.

Box 45-3

Biological agents threats

Category A

Anthrax (*Bacillus anthracis*)
Botulism (*Clostridium botulinum* toxin)
Plague (*Yersinia pestis*)
Smallpox (variola major)
Tularaemia (*Francisella tularensis*)
Viral haemorrhagic fevers (filoviruses [e.g. Ebola and Marburg] and arenaviruses [e.g. Lassa and Machupo])

Category B

Brucellosis (*Brucella* species)
Epsilon toxin of *Clostridium perfringens*
Food safety threats (e.g. *Salmonella* spp, *Escherichia coli* O157:H7, and *Shigella*)
Glanders (*Burkholderia mallei*)
Melioidosis (*Burkholderia pseudomallei*)
Psittacosis (*Chlamydia psittaci*)
Q fever (*Coxiella burnetii*)
Ricin toxin from *Ricinus communis* (castor beans)
Staphylococcal enterotoxin B
Typhus fever (*Rickettsia prowazekii*)
Viral encephalitis (alphaviruses [e.g. Venezuelan equine encephalitis, eastern equine encephalitis, and western equine encephalitis])
Water safety threats (e.g. *Vibrio cholerae* and *Cryptosporidium parvum*)

Category C

Nipah virus
Hantaviruses
Tick-borne haemorrhagic fever viruses
Tick-borne encephalitis viruses
Yellow fever
Multidrug-resistant tuberculosis

From Centers for Disease Control and Prevention. Bioterrorism agents/diseases. http://www.bt.cdc.gov/agent/agentlist-category.asp#a 27 February 2009

The Centers for Disease Control and Prevention in the USA publishes a list of critical biological agents. The list is divided into categories A, B and C (Box 45-3). Category A agents are the most hazardous to public health as they can be spread easily by person-to-person contact and often have a high lethality; they might cause public panic and disruption. *Bacillus anthracis* (anthrax) is an example of a category A agent, and special actions are required for public health preparedness. Category B agents are the second highest priority and are fairly easy to disseminate. They cause moderate illnesses and have a lower death rate than category A agents. These agents call for specific enhancements of diagnostic capacity and disease surveillance. An example of a category B agent is *Coxiella burnetii* (Q fever). Category C agents include new pathogens that could be engineered for mass dissemination in the future. These agents may be widely available and easy to produce and dispense. They have the potential to cause a high rate of death and sickness. An example of a category C agent is Nipah virus.

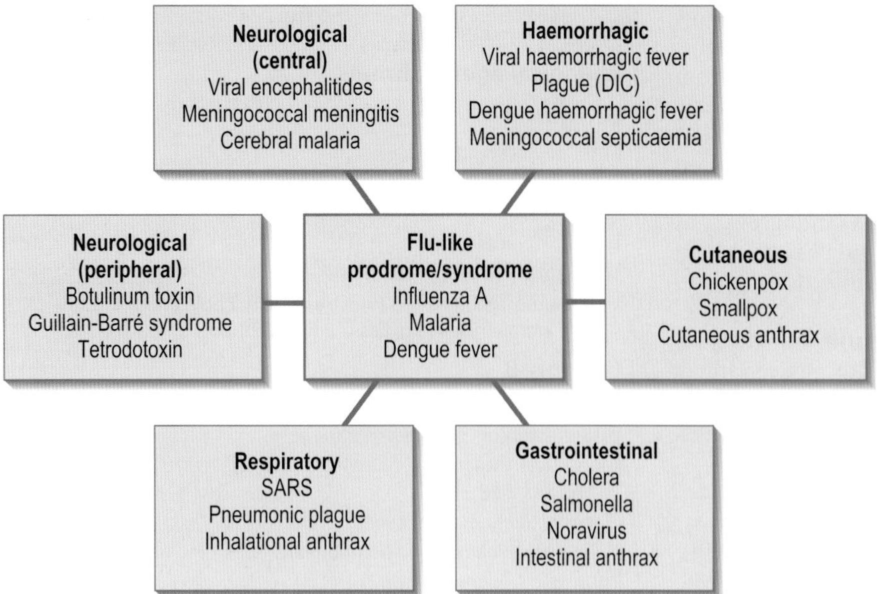

Figure 45-2 Syndromic approach to biological agents.

Syndromic approach and sepsis

The effects of an exposure to a biological agent are best considered using a syndromic approach (Figure 45-2). Most live agents will initially present with flu-like symptoms including pyrexia, myalgia and lethargy. Toxin exposure may not be associated with these prodromal flu-like syndromes. A single organism may cause a number of syndromes, usually dependent upon the route of exposure (inhalational, cutaneous and intestinal anthrax), while another organism may present with a combination of syndromes (pneumonic plague with coagulopathy). Some agents may present with an atypical syndrome or unusual presentation (meningitic variation of the noravirus). As well as these syndromes, biological agents may stimulate an overwhelming inflammatory response known as *systemic inflammatory response syndrome* (SIRS). SIRS may be due to a number of causes, including trauma, pancreatitis and some other CBRN agents. SIRS due to an infection is called *sepsis*. In its most extreme form, a number of systems will be impaired, leading to *multiorgan failure* (MOF). Some biological agents do not present as a syndrome; these include ricin and HIV, and generally act at an intracellular level. In the case of ricin, it prevents cells from producing proteins and therefore patients present as multiorgan failure. Definitive management of sepsis is guided by early goal-driven therapy and management bundles ('Surviving Sepsis' organization).

Blood-borne viruses (BBVs)

Following any traumatic event, but especially after a blast injury, consideration should be given to the potential for the transmission of BBV. Whilst there is limited evidence, studies have suggested that some viruses such as hepatitis B may be present in biological shrapnel from a suicide bomber or co-victim. HIV infection is much less likely and post-exposure prophylaxis (PEP) may be contraindicated in a traumatized patient. Prophylactic treatment for hepatitis B should be considered for casualties at risk. Specific guidance depends of the incident and theatre of operations. It is suggested that casualties receive further follow-up during rehabilitation; this includes counselling and further clinical risk stratification. Advice was provided by the Health Protection Agency for victims of the 7/7 London bombings in 2005.

Specific biological threats

Hundreds of biological and chemical agents can be used in a CBRN attack. This section provides a brief overview of specific biological agents. These agents are considered to be the ones most likely to be used as a threat to civilian populations. The most common biological threats are thought to be anthrax, botulism, plague, ricin, tularaemia, smallpox and viral haemorrhagic fevers.

Note

Like all other hazardous materials incidents, it is assumed that all responders will wear the proper PPE. It also is assumed that they will use standard precautions at the scene and during patient care. No emergency service providers should enter a scene without appropriate PPE where there is a known or suspected CBRN hazard.

Anthrax

Anthrax is an acute infectious disease caused by the spore-forming bacterium *Bacillus anthracis*. Anthrax is often endemic and occurs in some livestock. Infection may be natural through contaminated food or other animal products such as wool and skins, or deliberate through weaponization of the spores. Symptoms of disease vary and depend on route of exposure (inhalational, cutaneous or gastrointestinal). Symptoms appear within 7 days of exposure. The most common form of anthrax is cutaneous anthrax resulting from direct contact with spores or bacilli. This exposure

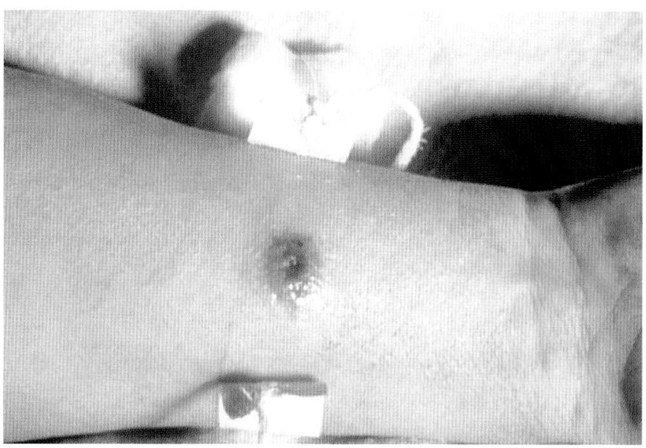

Figure 45-3 Cutaneous anthrax.

is followed by a papular lesion that turns vesicular and subsequent development of black eschar within 7 to 10 days of the initial lesion (Figure 45-3). Inhalational anthrax often starts with flu-like symptoms followed by severe respiratory distress and sepsis.

Treatment

Direct person-to-person spread of anthrax is unlikely, thus immunization or treatment of persons who have come in contact with a patient (e.g. household members, friends, and coworkers) is unnecessary. These persons do not need to be treated unless they were also exposed to the aerosol at the time of the attack. The disease is diagnosed by isolating *B. anthracis* from the blood, skin lesions or respiratory secretions, or by measuring specific antibodies in the blood of suspected cases. Treatment with antibiotics should be started early, as, if left untreated, the disease can be fatal. Human anthrax vaccines are available and are reported to be 93% effective against cutaneous anthrax. Vaccination to protect against inhalational anthrax is recommended for those at high risk. This includes, for example, military personnel and workers in research laboratories that handle anthrax bacteria routinely.

Botulism

As described in Chapter 21, botulism is a rare but serious paralytic illness. The bacterium *Clostridium botulinum* produces a nerve toxin that is the most lethal toxin known to man. There are a number of presentations of botulism. One type is food-borne botulism caused by eating contaminated foods (usually tinned) that contain the botulism toxin. The second type is wound botulism, caused by toxin produced from a wound infected with *C. botulinum*; the third type is infant botulism. Infant botulism is caused by consumption of the spores of the botulinum bacteria, which then grow in the intestines and release toxin. All forms of botulism can be fatal and are considered medical emergencies. Symptoms are of a descending paralysis with early motor cranial nerve involvement. There is also an anticholinergic element to the disease due to the failure of acetylcholine-mediated nerve conduction. Signs and symptoms of the illness include dry mouth, blurred vision, dysphagia, fatigue and flaccid paralysis that may begin several hours to several days after the exposure. Symptoms may be mistaken for the Miller Fisher variant of Guillain–Barré syndrome. In a bioterrorism attack, breathing in the toxin as an aerosol weapon or ingesting the toxin via contaminated food or water are the most likely routes of exposure for serious illness. Food-borne botulism can be especially dangerous because small amounts of the bacterium in contaminated food can poison many persons.

Treatment

Botulism is not spread from person to person. If diagnosed early, food-borne and wound botulism can be treated with an antitoxin. The antitoxin blocks the action of toxin circulating in the blood. Recovery may take several weeks. As a result of the paralysis and respiratory failure that occur with botulism, the patient may be placed on a ventilator.

Critical Thinking

What kind of resources would your community need to support hundreds of patients who need care on a ventilator?

Plague

Plague is caused by the bacterium *Yersinia pestis*. The bacteria are found in the gut of fleas that fed on a variety of rodents and are endemic in a number of areas worldwide. The bacteria can also be cultured and disseminated by aerosol in a bioterrorism attack. This would result in an epidemic of the pneumonic form of the disease with the potential for secondary spread as a contagion. Signs and symptoms include fever, fatigue, shortness of breath, chest pain, cough and bloody sputum. The illness can lead to septic shock within 2–4 days and clotting disorders. Without treatment, plague has a very high mortality rate.

Treatment

The disease is diagnosed through testing for the bacteria. Plague is treated with many first-line antibiotics and must be treated as early as possible. Persons who have been in close contact with the patient should be identified and assessed for post-exposure drug therapy. Pneumonic plague is spread through the respiratory droplets of an infected person; patients should be isolated and contacts quarantined. In extreme cases, there will be a geographical restriction of movement (ROM). Standard precautions and personal respiratory protection (FFP3 standard) are critical.

Critical Thinking

Your service notices a sudden increase in patients with severe respiratory distress. These patients also have pneumonia-like signs and symptoms. Would you initially consider bioterrorism as a cause of the outbreak?

Ricin

Ricin is derived from the beans of the castor plant (*Ricinus communis*) and is a potent intracellular toxin. Castor beans are widely available throughout the world and the toxin is relatively easy to extract. Ricin can be made into a mist, powder or pellet. When ricin is inhaled as an aerosol, it results in pulmonary toxicity with severe respiratory symptoms within 8 h. This is followed by acute hypoxic respiratory failure in 36–72 h. If ricin is ingested, severe gastrointestinal symptoms occur with rapid onset of nausea, vomiting, abdominal cramps, and severe diarrhoea. Death is due to multiorgan failure caused by the inhibition of intracellular protein synthesis.

Treatment

No antidote exists for ricin poisoning although there is research into potential antitoxins. Management is aimed at limiting exposure and eliminating the toxin from the body as quickly as possible. Patients are treated with supportive management including intensive care.

Smallpox

Smallpox was declared extinct by the World Health Organization in 1980 because of near-universal vaccination. However, it could be used as a biological weapon as the variola virus that causes smallpox is fairly stable. The infectious dose is small and global immunity is now likely to be low. An aerosol release of the virus would be widely spread and the incubation period for smallpox is about 7–12 days following exposure. The virus is usually spread by an infected person releasing infected saliva from the mouth into the air. Persons in close or prolonged contact to the infected person inhale the virus. Smallpox can also be spread through direct contact with infected body fluids or contaminated objects such as bedding or clothing. Signs and symptoms of the disease include flu-like symptoms, followed within 2–3 days with a vesicular rash. These lesions may be haemorrhagic or pustular, finally forming crusts. Upon healing, the lesions leave depressed, depigmented scars (Figure 45-4). Permanent joint deformities and blindness may follow recovery. The death rate from a re-emerging smallpox strain is likely to be high. Vaccine immunity may prevent or modify the illness. Immunization teams may be activated to start mass vaccination.

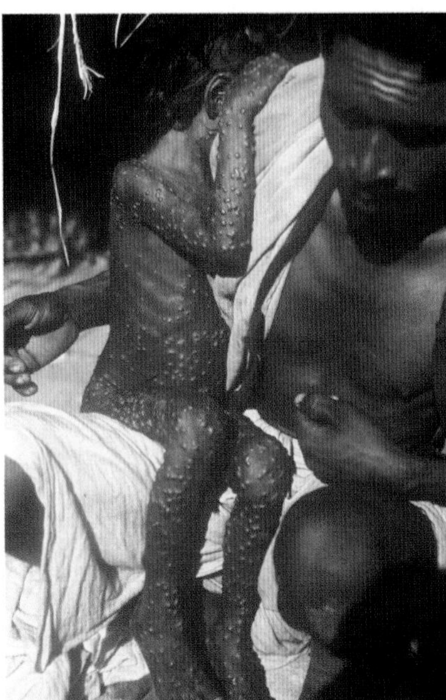

Figure 45-4 Smallpox lesions.

Treatment

There is no proven treatment for smallpox. However, several antiviral drugs are being studied. Patients with smallpox should receive supportive care provided by vaccinated personnel. The personnel must use standard precautions with airborne protection.

> **Critical Thinking**
>
> Your employer asks you to get the smallpox vaccination. Where can you look to find information about the side effects and risks of immunization with this vaccine?

Tularaemia

Tularaemia is a serious illness caused by the bacterium *Francisella tularensis*, which is found in animals (especially rodents, rabbits and hares). The disease is highly infectious and may be resistant to first-line antibiotics. The bacterium responsible for tularaemia can be delivered in a bioterrorism attack by aerosol although transmission of the disease from person to person does not occur. The development of signs and symptoms varies widely (from 1 day to 2 weeks). This is based on the virulence of the strain and the route of exposure. Following a bioterrorism attack with the agent, patients may complain of an abrupt onset of an acute febrile illness. They may also complain of gastrointestinal illness that includes nausea, vomiting, and diarrhoea. If left untreated, septic tularaemia may lead to disseminated intravascular coagulation with bleeding, acute respiratory failure and death.

Treatment

The disease is managed with antibiotics. The patient may require airway, ventilatory and circulatory support. A vaccine for tularaemia is currently being researched and remains a priority for endemic areas.

Viral haemorrhagic fevers

Viral haemorrhagic fevers (VHFs) refer to a group of illnesses caused by several distinct families of viruses that include arenaviruses, filoviruses, bunyaviruses and flaviviruses. Most are highly infectious if spread as an aerosol. These viruses reside naturally in animals (e.g. cotton rat and deer mouse) or arthropods (e.g. ticks and mosquitoes) and are fully dependent on these living hosts for reproduction and survival. Viruses that cause haemorrhagic fever are usually transmitted to human beings during contact with urine, faecal matter, saliva, or other body excretions from an infected rodent or from a bite from an infected mosquito or tick. Some VHFs (e.g. Ebola and Marburg) can also be spread from person to person following an initial infection. This type of infection most often results from close contact with infected persons through their body fluids.

Viral haemorrhagic fevers cause a multisystem syndrome characterized by haemorrhage and life-threatening sepsis.

Signs and symptoms vary by the type of VHF; however, they often include fever, fatigue, dizziness, muscle aches, loss of strength, and exhaustion. Patients with severe cases of VHF may bleed from mucous membranes, internal organs, or from the mouth, eyes or ears. Septic shock, renal failure, central nervous system dysfunction, coma and seizures may develop with severe infection. These may lead to a poor prognosis.

Treatment

Therapy for patients with VHFs is supportive. The goals of therapy are to maintain vital functions, which may allow for recovery in some patients. Some vaccines are available (yellow fever).

Nuclear and radiological incidents

Nuclear detonations can cause deadly effects from blinding light, intense heat (thermal radiation), initial nuclear radiation, blast and fires. A radiological dispersion device (RDD) also known as a 'dirty bomb' is considered far more likely than use of a true nuclear device. Radioactive materials are used widely in medicine, agriculture, industry and research and are relatively easy to obtain. They require little technical knowledge to build and deploy compared with that of a true nuclear device that requires weapon-grade fissile (nuclear) material.

The main type of RDD combines an explosive with radioactive material sometimes called a source. The extent of contamination would depend on a number of factors such as the size of the explosive, the amount and type of radioactive material used, and weather conditions (e.g. wind). The detonation of an RDD releases radioactive contamination. This has the potential to cause radiation sickness, severe burns and long-term cancer fatalities; however, the conventional blast itself is likely to cause more deaths than exposure to the radioactive material. For this reason, traumatic injuries take priority over the radiological hazard, although decontamination should be concurrent. A second type of RDD might involve a covert powerful radioactive source hidden in a public place. It may be hidden in such a place that persons passing close to the source might receive a significant dose of radiation over a period of time. Radiation is however very detectable and the greater the hazard the more detectable it is. Radiological attacks are a credible threat but they would not result in the hundreds of thousands of deaths that could be caused by a crude nuclear weapon that requires a fission reaction. A radiological attack could cause serious psychological impact, contaminate several city areas, and require costly cleanup.

To put radiation into perspective, the dose required to cause *acute radiation syndrome* (ARS) is 2 Sieverts (Sv) and is approximately 100 000 chest X-rays or 1000 times the annual background radiation received across the majority of the UK. There are four main types of radiation, although neutrons are usually only present during the nuclear process:

- *Alpha particles* are charged helium nuclei. They only travel short distances (3 cm in air) and cannot penetrate the outer layers of skin. Damage is caused if ingested, inhaled or incorporated.
- *Beta particles* are electrons. They can penetrate skin and will cause damage if taken internally. They will travel about 3 m in air or about 5 mm in tissue.
- *Neutrons* are non-charged particles and usually only occur during the fission (nuclear) process. They are highly penetrating and, when they interact with biological tissue, are very damaging.
- *Gamma/X-ray radiation* is at the high-energy end of the electromagnetic spectrum. With no mass, it has a very long range and is difficult to shield against.

Ionizing radiation causes its effect by its interaction with DNA. At low levels, there is damage to the DNA, increasing the chance of mutation and cancer. The greater the dose of radiation, the greater the chance of cancer; this is termed the *stochastic* effects. At very high levels (>2 Sv), radiation causes cell death. This is called *deterministic*, as once a threshold level has been passed the effects are predictable due to the relative sensitivity of tissue to radiation. The most sensitive tissues are those that have the highest turnover (bone marrow and gastrointestinal mucosa). Death is generally caused by infection or coagulopathy due to bone marrow suppression. The failure of different systems (haematological, gastrointestinal and cerebrovascular) due to radiation is called ARS. This occurs after an initial prodromal stage (nausea, vomiting ± diarrhoea) lasting a few hours, and a latency period of a few days. Safety measures to reduce radiation exposure are based upon time, distance and shielding.

Critical Thinking

What emergency medical services groups or divisions should you consider setting up if there is a report of a dirty bomb explosion?

Explosive threats

An explosion may occur for both accidental (Buncefield, 2005) and malicious (7/7 bombings, 2005) reasons. Bombs can be made from a variety of materials with a variety of yields measured as the equivalent weight in TNT. Explosives used by terrorists are often classified by the following categories although this is not exclusive:

- Unconventional use: a conventional object used in an unconventional way to create mass destruction. In the 11 September 2001 attack on the World Trade Center and the Pentagon, hijackers flew passenger planes into their intended targets, relying on the impact of the planes and their full fuel tanks to cause damage.
- Vehicle bomb: usually large powerful devices that consist of a large quantity of explosives fitted with a timed or remotely triggered detonator packed onto a car or truck.
- Pipe bomb: a quantity of explosives sealed into a length of metal or plastic pipe. A timing fuse usually controls detonation, but other methods can be used, including electronic timers, remote triggers, and motion

sensors. These are the most common explosive devices and are at the opposite end of the scale from vehicle bombs in terms of size and power.

- Satchel charge: an old military term for an explosive device in a canvas carrying bag. In recent history, 'daypacks' or rucksacks have been used for the carrying device, and the explosives have contained antipersonnel materials such as nails and glass to inflict more casualties.
- Package or letter bomb: explosive material contained in a package or letter that is usually triggered by opening of the package.

There are two types of explosion, depending on the type of explosive used. A *detonation* is due to the activation of a high explosive (HE) that has the ability to almost instantaneously explode causing a shock (blast) wave. An example of a high explosive is Semtex. The second type of explosion is a *conflagration*. This is a lower-energy explosion with less of the energy converted into a blast wave and more into thermal energy. Gunpowder is an example of this type of explosive.

Injury patterns associated with blast injuries are categorized into four types:

- Primary – injuries associated with the blast wave and disruption at tissue/air interfaces such as the tympanum, lung and abdominal viscera. Additional limb injuries also occur due to the shattering effect of the blast wave and tend to affect long bones, causing traumatic amputation, and massive disruption to soft tissues, often leading to surgical amputation as a life-saving intervention.
- Secondary – penetrating injuries due to fragments, including parts of the bomb, being carried on the blast wind (positive and negative overpressure) following the initial explosion. Some munitions and bombs are intended to fragment to maximize injuries; examples include fragmentation grenades and nail bombs. Other debris may be incidental to the explosion and may include biological debris from co-victims.
- Tertiary – injuries due to the displacement of the body or objects by the explosion or objects. These may result in blunt and crush injuries. Examples include displacement of a body against a wall or falling masonry.
- Quaternary (miscellaneous) – injuries that are not physically associated with the explosion. These include burns due to secondary fires, exposure to CBRN agents and psychological injuries (acute or delayed).

Management of CBRN incidents

Any incident whether conventional or CBRN should follow standard major incident management procedures. For malicious and CBRN incidents, the additional threats should be considered when assessing the *hazards* and *safety* issues. In addition, during the major incident, signs of exposure to CBRN and trauma, as well as the requirement to manage contaminated or contagious patients, can be incorporated into current methodology (Figure 45-5).

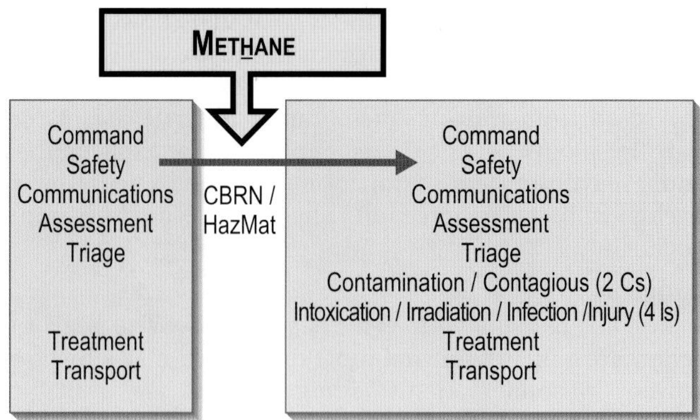

Figure 45-5 Major incident response to CBRN/Hazmat.

Management of individual casualties depends on the ease of access to them, requirement for PPE limiting medical dexterity, and decontamination. Treatment can therefore be split into the three zones of contamination (hot/warm/cold) with environments being non-permissive, semipermissive and permissive respectively. Type of interventions also follows a modification of the ATLS ABC paradigm:

⟨C⟩	*C*atastrophic haemorrhage including amputations
A (a)	*A*irway management and *a*ntidotes
B	*B*reathing
C	*C*irculation
Dd	*D*isability and *d*econtamination
E	*E*vacuation following full exposure

The application of these interventions is applied as required depending on the state of and access to the patient. For this reason, casualty triage is vital to allow for the most appropriate interventions to be applied and prevent bottlenecks in the casualty evacuation chain. Therefore there are a number of triage points and a key point is prior to decontamination (if required), see Figure 45-6. Within the hot zones, management of casualties is likely to be limited to ⟨C⟩A and life-saving interventions (LSIs), including control of catastrophic haemorrhage, basic airway management, possibly needle decompression (if obvious penetrating trauma to the chest), intramuscular/intraosseous antidotes and evacuating the casualty to a safe place.

Further treatment in a permissive/clean environment follows full decontamination and allows further access to the casualty to allow diagnosis. Supportive management is provided as required and includes oxygen, fluids, analgesia and broad-spectrum antibiotics (benzylpenicillin, cefuroxime) for biological incidents. Definitive management is directed as indicated and includes antidotes, disease-specific antibiotics (such as ciprofloxacin for anthrax) and surgery.

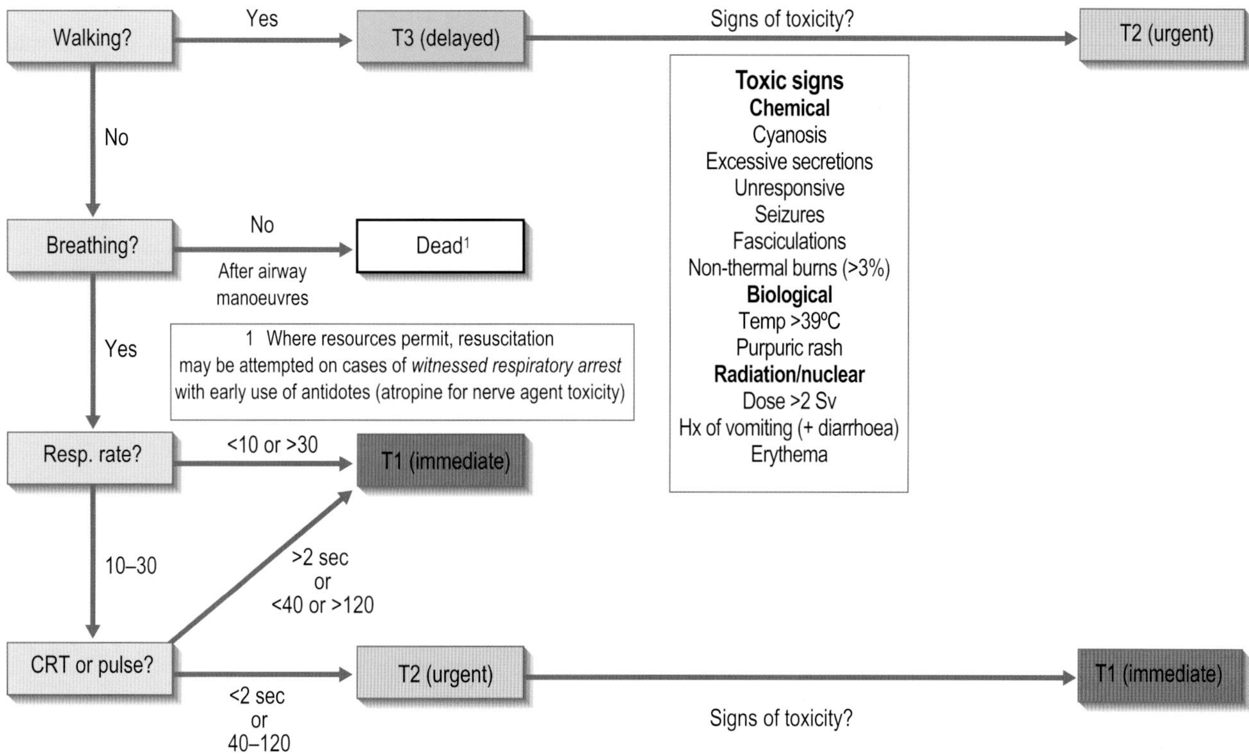

Figure 45-6 CBRN triage sieve. (© I McNeil & S Bland)

Summary

- The four types of agents involved in CBRN are chemical, biological, radiological and nuclear. Explosives are sometimes included.
- Nerve agents include sarin, soman, tabun, and VX. Exposure causes a cholinergic crisis leading to paralysis, excessive secretions, fitting and death. The antidote for nerve agent exposure is atropine, pralidoxime and benzodiazepines.
- Other chemical agents include cyanide, chlorine and phosgene. The last two cause severe respiratory problems.
- The initial management of chemical casualties should include moving exposed patients to safety, remove their clothing, decontaminate as required and treat their symptoms.
- Biological agents include anthrax, botulism, plague, ricin, tularaemia and smallpox.
- Person-to-person spread is possible in patients who are infected with plague or smallpox.
- Dirty bombs could cause heat damage and radiation exposure, severe burns, and cancer. Traumatic injuries should be treated first.
- Management of a CBRN incident should follow the same guidelines as a conventional major incident with emphasis on safety and hazard identification and management.
- Figure 45-7 summarizes the key interventions in each zone of treatment.

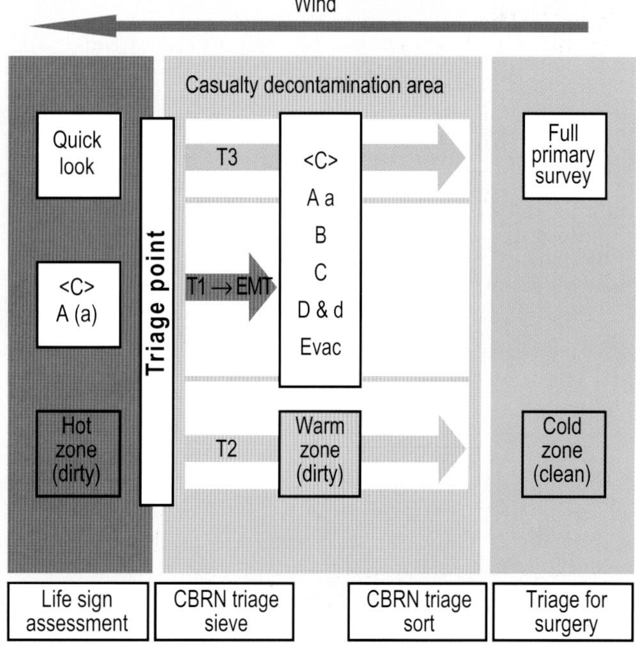

Figure 45-7 Zones of CBRN treatment. (© S.A. Bland)

Further reading

HPA. CBRN Handbook. http://www.hpa.org.uk

Department of Health: NHS Emergency Guidance gateway. http://www.dh.gov.uk/emergencyplanning

PART TEN

Glossary

abdominal Pertaining to the abdomen.

abdominal aorta The portion of the descending aorta that passes from the aortic hiatus of the diaphragm into the abdomen, where it divides into the two common iliac arteries.

abdominal cavity The space within the abdominal walls between the diaphragm and the pelvic area; it contains the liver, stomach, intestines, spleen, kidneys and associated tissues and vessels.

abdominopelvic cavity The space between the diaphragm and the groin.

abduction Movement away from the midline.

abnormal Deviating from the normal.

abnormal presentation A type of vaginal delivery in which the newborn's head does not deliver first.

abortion The spontaneous or induced termination of a pregnancy before the fetus has developed into a stage of viability.

abrasion A partial-thickness injury caused by scraping or rubbing away of a layer or layers of skin.

absence A form of generalized seizure where the person looks blank for a few seconds and may not respond when spoken to or realize they have had a seizure. This type of seizure can happen repeatedly and can be mistaken for daydreaming and was formerly referred to as 'petit mal'.

absolute refractory period The portion of the action potential during which the membrane is insensitive to all stimuli regardless of strength.

absorption The process by which drug molecules are moved from the site of entry into the body into the general circulation.

accelerated atrioventricular conduction See anomalous conduction.

acclimatization Physical adjustment to a different climate or to changes in altitude or temperature.

acetabulum The large, cup-shaped articular cavity at the juncture of the ilium, the ischium, and the pubis that contains the ball-shaped head of the femur.

acetoacetic acid A colourless, oily ketone body produced by the metabolism of lipids and pyruvates; it is excreted in trace amounts in normal urine and in elevated amounts with diabetes mellitus, especially in ketoacidosis.

acetonaemia The presence of acetone in the blood, characterized by the fruity breath odour of ketoacidosis.

acetylcholine A neurotransmitter, widely distributed in body tissues, with the primary function of mediating the synaptic activity of the nervous system.

acetylcholinesterase An enzyme found in the synaptic cleft that causes the breakdown of acetylcholine into acetic acid and choline, thereby limiting the stimulatory effect of acetylcholine.

acid A compound that yields hydrogen ions when dissociated in solution.

acidosis A condition marked by a high concentration of hydrogen ions (i.e. a pH below 7.35).

acinus A small lobule of a compound gland; the exocrine portion of the pancreas that produces pancreatic juice.

acquired immune deficiency syndrome A disease that results from infection with the human immunodeficiency virus; the syndrome impairs the immune system, giving rise to opportunistic infections and malignancies.

acromegaly A chronic metabolic condition characterized by a gradual, marked enlargement and elongation of the bones of the face, jaw and extremities.

acromion process The lateral extension of the spine of the scapula; it gives attachment to the deltoideus and trapezius muscles.

actin A protein found in muscle fibres that acts with myosin to bring about contraction and relaxation.

actinomycosis A chronic systemic disease characterized by deep, lumpy abscesses that extrude a granular pus through multiple sinuses.

action plan A plan of action based on the patient's condition and the environment.

action potential A change in membrane potential in an excitable tissue that acts as an electrical signal and is propagated in an all-or-none fashion.

active transport A carrier-mediated process that can move substances against a concentration gradient.

active tubular secretion Secretion that involves the transport of free drug from the blood across the proximal tubular cell and into the tubular urine by an active process against a concentration gradient.

acute dystonia A sudden impairment of muscle tone; it commonly involves the head, neck, or tongue and often occurs as an adverse effect of medication.

acute gastroenteritis Inflammation of the stomach and intestines with an associated sudden onset of vomiting, diarrhoea, or both.

acute hepatitis An inflammatory condition of the liver associated with the sudden onset of malaise, weakness, anorexia, intermittent nausea and vomiting, and dull right upper quadrant pain, usually followed within 1 week by the onset of jaundice, dark urine, or both, characterized by jaundice.

acute mountain sickness A common high-altitude illness that results when an unacclimatized person rapidly ascends to high altitudes.

acute pain Severe pain such as may follow trauma or may accompany myocardial infarction or other conditions and diseases.

acute renal failure A clinical syndrome that results from a sudden and significant decrease in filtration through the glomeruli, leading to the accumulation of salt, water, and nitrogenous wastes within the body.

adaptation A cellular response to stress of any kind to escape and protect from injury; a central part of the response to changes in the physiological condition.

addiction A compulsive, uncontrollable dependence on a substance, habit, or practice to such a degree that cessation causes severe emotional, mental or physiological reactions.

Addison's disease A rare and potentially life-threatening disorder caused by a deficiency of the corticosteroid hormones normally produced by the adrenal cortex.

adduction Movement toward the midline.

adenohypophysis The anterior lobe of the pituitary gland.

adenoma A tumour of glandular epithelium in which the cells of the tumour are arranged in a recognizable glandular structure.

adenosine A compound derived from nucleic acid and composed of adenine and a sugar.

adenosine diphosphate A product of the hydrolysis of adenosine triphosphate.

adenosine monophosphate A compound that affects energy release in work done by muscles.

adenosine triphosphate Adenosine, an organic base, with three phosphate groups attached to it; it stores energy in muscles.

adhesion The quality of remaining in close contact with or stuck to another entity; also, a structure that joins several parts, sometimes abnormally.

adipose tissue A specialized connective tissue that stores lipids; also known as fat tissue.

adrenal gland Either of two secretory glands perched atop the kidneys; each gland consists of two parts, the cortex and medulla, which have independent functions.

adrenal medullary mechanism The mechanism by which adrenaline and noradrenaline are released from the adrenal medulla as a result of the same stimuli that increase sympathetic stimulation of the heart and blood vessels.

adrenaline An endogenous adrenal hormone that helps prepare the body for energetic action.

adrenergic Of or pertaining to the sympathetic nerve fibres of the autonomic nervous system, which use adrenaline or adrenaline-like substances as neurotransmitters.

adrenocorticotropic hormone (ACTH) A hormone of the anterior pituitary gland that stimulates growth of the adrenal gland cortex and secretion of corticosteroids.

adsorption The capacity of a substance to attract and hold other materials or particles on its surface.

adult respiratory distress syndrome (ARDS) A group of symptoms that accompany fulminant pulmonary oedema, resulting in acute respiratory failure; also known as non-cardiogenic pulmonary oedema.

advanced cardiac life support (ACLS) Clinical care or guidelines for care of life-threatening cardiovascular and respiratory disorders.

advanced life support (ALS) The provision of care that paramedics or allied health professionals render, including advanced airway management, defibrillation, intravenous therapy, and medication administration.

aerobic Of or pertaining to the presence of air or oxygen.

aerobic oxidation A biochemical reaction that increases the positive charges on an atom or the loss of negative charges in the presence of oxygen.

aerosol Pressurized gas that contains a finely nebulized medication for inhalation therapy.

affect An outward manifestation of a person's feelings or emotions.

affective disorder Any of a group of psychotic disorders characterized by severe and inappropriate emotional responses, prolonged and persistent disturbances of mood and related thought distortions, and other symptoms associated with depressed or manic states.

afferent division Nerve fibres that send impulses from the periphery to the central nervous system.

affinity The propensity of a drug to bind or attach itself to a given receptor site.

afterdrop phenomenon A sudden return of cold blood and waste products to the core of the body as a result of rewarming methods used to treat hypothermia.

afterload The total resistance against which blood must be pumped. Also known as peripheral vascular resistance.

agglutinated Reference to cells that have clumped together. See agglutination.

agglutination A clumping together of cells as a result of their interaction with specific antibodies called agglutinins.

agglutinin A kind of antibody; its interaction with antigens is manifested as agglutination.

agonal rhythm A ventricular escape complex or rhythm that occurs when the electrical impulses from the sinoatrial node, atria, or atrioventricular junction fail to reach the ventricles because of sinus arrest or high-degree atrioventricular block; frequently seen as the last rhythm in an unsuccessful resuscitation.

agonists Drugs that combine with receptors and initiate the expected response.

air trapping The result of a prolonged but inefficient expiratory effort, usually caused by chronic obstruction of the pulmonary tree, as is seen commonly in chronic obstructive pulmonary disease or asthma.

akathisia An abnormal condition characterized by feelings of restlessness and agitation.

albumin A water-soluble protein containing carbon, hydrogen, oxygen, nitrogen and sulphur.

aldosterone A steroid hormone produced by the adrenal cortex to regulate the sodium and potassium balance in the blood.

aliquot A sample that is representative of the whole.

alkaline Having the reactions of an alkali.

alkalosis A condition marked by a low concentration of hydrogen ions (i.e. a pH above 7.45).

allergens Substances that can produce hypersensitivity reactions in the body.

allergic reaction A hypersensitivity response to an allergen to which a person previously was exposed and to which the person has developed antibodies.

allergy A hypersensitivity reaction to intrinsically harmless antigens, most of which are environmental.

all-or-none principle The principle that when a stimulus is applied to a cell, an action potential is produced or is not produced.

alpha cell A constituent of the islets of Langerhans that produces glucagon.

alpha-adrenergic receptor Any one of the postulated adrenergic components of receptor tissues that responds to noradrenaline and to various blocking agents.

alveolar duct Part of the respiratory passages beyond a respiratory bronchiole; alveolar sacs and alveoli arise from it.

alveoli Small outpouchings of walls of alveolar space through which gas exchange takes place between alveolar air and pulmonary capillary blood.

alveolus A small cavity; the terminal ending of a secretory gland. Alveoli of the lungs are microscopic, sac-like dilatations of terminal bronchioles.

Alzheimer's disease A disease characterized by confusion, memory failure, disorientation, speech disturbances, and inability to carry out purposeful movements.

amaurosis fugax Unilateral vision loss as a result of internal carotid artery plaque emboli.

ambulance A generic term that describes the various land-based emergency vehicles used by emergency medical services personnel, including paramedic units, mobile intensive care units, and others.

amenorrhoea The absence of menstruation.

amino acid An organic chemical compound composed of one or more basic amino groups and one or more acidic carboxyl groups.

ammonia A colourless, aromatic gas consisting of nitrogen and hydrogen.

amnestic Causing amnesia.

amniocentesis An obstetrical procedure in which a small amount of amniotic fluid is removed for laboratory analysis; it aids in diagnosis of fetal abnormalities.

amniotic fluid embolism An embolism that occurs when particulate matter in amniotic fluid forms an embolus and gains access to maternal circulation during labour or delivery or immediately after delivery.

amniotic sac A thin-walled bag that contains the fetus and amniotic fluid during pregnancy.

amplitude modulation A transmitted radio frequency carrier fixed in frequency but increasing or decreasing in amplitude in accordance with the strength of the applied audio.

ampulla A round, sac-like dilatation of the uterine tube.

amputation A complete or partial loss of a limb caused by mechanical force.

amylase A starch-splitting enzyme.

amyotrophic lateral sclerosis One of a group of rare disorders in which the nerves that control muscular activity degenerate in the brain and spinal cord; also called Lou Gehrig disease.

anabolic steroid Any of several compounds derived from testosterone or prepared synthetically to promote general body growth, to oppose the effects of endogenous oestrogen, or to promote masculinizing effects.

anaemia A decrease in blood haemoglobin.

anaerobic Of or pertaining to the absence of oxygen.

anaerobic metabolism Metabolism that occurs in the absence of oxygen.

anaesthesia Without sensation.

anal canal The final portion of the alimentary tract between the rectal ampulla and the anus.

anal fissure A linear ulceration or laceration of the skin of the anus.

anal fistula An abnormal opening of the cutaneous surface near the anus.

anal triangle The posterior portion of the perianal region through which the anal canal opens.

anaphylactic shock Shock that occurs when the body is exposed to a substance that produces a severe allergic reaction.

anaphylaxis An exaggerated, life-threatening hypersensitivity reaction to a previously encountered antigen.

anasarca Generalized, massive oedema.

anastomosis The joining of two parts.

anatomical dead space The volume of the conducting airways from the external environment down to the terminal bronchioles.

anatomical position A position standing erect with the feet and palms facing the examiner.

anchoring Attaching a high-angle rope to a secure point.

androgen Any steroid hormone that increases male characteristics.

aneurysm A localized dilatation of a wall of a blood vessel.

angina pectoris Ischaemic chest pain most often caused by myocardial anoxia as a result of atherosclerosis of the coronary arteries.

angioedema A localized oedematous reaction of the deep dermal or subcutaneous or submucosal tissues that appears as giant wheals.

angiogram A radiographic image of blood vessels using a contrast medium to show up the vessels.

angioplasty Reconstruction of damaged blood vessels.

angiotensin I The inactive form of angiotensin, produced by the action of renin on the plasma protein angiotensinogen. Angiotensin I is converted to angiotensin II (see below) by angiotensin converting enzyme (ACE).

angiotensin II A potent vasoconstrictor that also acts to stimulate the secretion of antidiuretic hormone.

angle of Louis See sternal angle.

anhedonia The inability to enjoy what is usually pleasurable.

anion An ion with a negative charge.

anisocoria Normal or congenital unequal pupil size.

anomalous conduction A pre-excitation syndrome; a clinical condition associated with abnormal conduction pathways between the atria and ventricles that bypass the atrioventricular node and bundle of His and allow the electrical impulses to initiate depolarization of the ventricles earlier than usual. Also known as accelerated atrioventricular conduction.

anorexia Lack or loss of appetite, resulting in an inability to eat.

anorexia nervosa A disorder characterized by a prolonged refusal to eat, resulting in emaciation, amenorrhoea, emotional disturbance concerning body image, and an abnormal fear of becoming obese.

anovulation Failure of the ovaries to produce, mature or release eggs.

antagonism The opposition between two or more medications; it occurs when the combined (conjoint) effect of two drugs is less than the sum of the drugs acting separately.

antagonist muscle A muscle that works in opposition to another muscle.

antagonists Agents designed to inhibit or counteract the effects of other drugs or undesired effects caused by normal or hyperactive physiological mechanisms.

antecubital fossa/space The depressed area in front of the elbow or at the bend of the elbow.

antegrade amnesia The loss of memory for events that occurred immediately after recovery of consciousness.

antenatal Occurring or formed before birth.

antepartum The period before labour and delivery.

anterior The front, or ventral, surface.

anterior chamber of the eye The chamber of the eye between the cornea and the iris.

anterior communicating artery The artery that connects with the anterior cerebral arteries and completes the circle of Willis.

anterior cord syndrome A spinal cord injury usually seen in flexion injuries; caused by pressure on the anterior aspect of the spinal cord by a ruptured intervertebral disc or fragments of the vertebral body extruded posteriorly into the spinal canal.

anterior superior iliac spine One of two bony segments that form the iliac crest.

anthrax An acute infectious disease caused by the spore-forming bacterium *Bacillus anthracis*.

antibody A substance produced by the body that destroys or inactivates a specific substance (antigen) that has entered the body.

anticholinergic Of or pertaining to the blocking of acetylcholine receptors, resulting in inhibition of transmission of parasympathetic nerve impulses.

anticoagulant A substance that prevents or delays coagulation of the blood.

antidiuretic hormone A hormone produced in the posterior pituitary gland to regulate the balance of water in the body by accelerating the resorption of water.

antidote A drug or other substance that opposes the action of a poison.

antigenic site A site capable of binding to and reacting with an antibody.

antigens Substances (usually proteins) that cause the formation of an antibody and react specifically with that antibody.

antiplatelet drug A drug that interferes with platelet aggregation.

antipyretic Something that works against fever.

antivenin A suspension of venom-neutralizing antibodies prepared from the serum of immunized horses.

anuria The inability to urinate; the cessation of urine production; a diminished urinary output of less than 100–250 mL per day.

anus The distal end or outlet of the rectum.

anxiety A state or feeling of apprehension, uneasiness, agitation, uncertainty, and fear resulting from the anticipation of some threat or danger.

aorta The main and largest artery in the body.

aortic aneurysm A localized dilatation of the wall of the aorta.

aortic body Any of the specialized nerve cells located in the arch of the aorta, where they monitor levels of oxygen and hydrogen ions in the cardiovascular system.

aortic semilunar valve A valve that guards the orifice between the left ventricle and the aorta.

apex of the heart The tip of the heart opposite the base.

Apgar score The evaluation of a newborn's physical condition, usually performed at 1 minute and 5 minutes after birth, including heart rate, respiratory effort, muscle tone, reflex irritability and colour.

aphasia Loss of the power of speech.

apical impulse A pulsation of the left ventricle of the heart, palpable and sometimes visible at the fifth intercostal space to the left of the midline.

apneustic centre A group of neurons in the pons that has a stimulatory effect on the inspiratory centre.

apnoea An absence of spontaneous respirations.

apocrine gland A gland that has cells that contribute cytoplasm to its secretion, such as a mammary gland.

appendicitis An acute inflammation of the appendix.

appendicular region The limbs or extremities.

appendicular skeleton The bones of the upper and lower extremities.

appendix A worm-like, blunt process extending from the caecum; also known as the vermiform appendix.

application of principle A component of critical thinking in which the examiner makes patient care decisions based on conceptual understanding of the situation and the interpretation of data gathered from the patient.

aqueous humour The clear, watery fluid circulating in the anterior and posterior chambers of the eye.

Arachnida A large class of arthropods that includes spiders, scorpions, mites and ticks.

arachnoid layer A delicate, web-like middle membrane that covers the brain.

areflexia A neurological condition characterized by absence of the reflexes.

areola The circular, pigmented area surrounding the nipple.

areolar connective tissue A loose tissue that consists of delicate webs of fibres and a variety of cells embedded in a matrix of soft, sticky gel.

areolar gland A gland that forms small, rounded projections from the surface of the areola of the mamma.

arrector pili Smooth muscles of the skin attached to hair follicles; when contraction occurs, the hair rises, resulting in gooseflesh.

artefact A deflection on the electrocardiogram display or tracing produced by factors other than the electrical activity of the heart.

arterial capillary The ends of capillaries closest to arterioles.

arteriogram A radiographic film of an artery injected with contrast medium.

arteriole A small branch of an artery.

arteriovenous anastomosis A vessel that allows blood to flow from arteries to veins without passing through capillaries; also known as an arteriovenous shunt.

arteriovenous shunt See arteriovenous anastomosis.

artery A vessel that carries blood away from the heart.

arthritis An inflammatory condition of the joints, characterized by pain and swelling.

arthroscopy Inspection of the interior of a joint.

arytenoid cartilages Small, pyramidal laryngeal cartilages that articulate with the cricoid cartilage.

asbestosis A chronic lung disease caused by the inhalation of asbestos fibres; it results in the development of alveolar, interstitial and pleural fibrosis.

ascending colon The segment of the colon that extends from the caecum in the right lower quadrant of the abdomen to the transverse colon at the hepatic flexure on the right side; usually at the level of the umbilicus.

ascites An abnormal intraperitoneal accumulation of fluid containing large amounts of protein and electrolytes.

aseptic Sterile, without germs.

asphyxiation A state of suffocation caused by severe hypoxia, which leads to hypoxaemia and hypercapnia, loss of consciousness, and if not corrected, death.

aspiration Inhalation of foreign substances into the pulmonary system.

assault Creating apprehension, or unauthorized handling and treatment of a patient.

asthma A respiratory disorder characterized by recurring episodes of paroxysmal dyspnoea, wheezing on expiration caused by constriction of the bronchi, coughing, and viscous mucoid bronchial secretions.

asthma exacerbation An aggravation of asthma, usually associated with severe symptoms.

astigmatism An abnormal condition of the eye in which the light rays cannot be focused clearly on a point on the retina because the spherical curve of the cornea is not equal in all meridians.

astrocyte gliosis A tumour composed of glial cells within the nervous system; it may be associated with respiratory centre dysfunction and neuroepithelial bodies in the tracheobronchial tree, along with distal atelectasis.

asystole A life-threatening cardiac condition characterized by the absence of electrical and mechanical activity of the heart.

ataxia Failure of muscle coordination.

ataxic breathing A type of cluster or irregular breathing pattern characterized by a series of inspirations and expirations.

atelectasis An abnormal condition characterized by the collapse of lung tissue, which prevents the respiratory exchange of oxygen and carbon dioxide.

atelectatic breathing A modified respiratory effort thought to be a protective reflex to hyperinflate the lungs and re-expand alveoli that might have been collapsed.

atheroma An abnormal accumulation of fat or lipids as a cyst or a deposit in an arterial wall; a hard, atherosclerotic plaque.

atherosclerosis A common arterial disorder characterized by yellowish plaques of cholesterol, lipids, and cellular debris in the inner layers of the walls of large and medium-sized arteries.

athetosis A neuromuscular condition characterized by slow, continuous, and involuntary movement of the extremities.

atlanto-occipital joint One of a pair of condyloid joints formed by the articulation of the atlas of the vertebral column with the occipital bone of the skull.

atlas The first cervical vertebra, which articulates with the occipital bone and the axis.

atmospheric pressure The pressure exerted by the weight of the atmosphere; at sea level this pressure is 760 mmHg.

atom The smallest division of an element that exhibits all the properties and characteristics of the element; atoms comprise neutrons, electrons, and protons.

atony Weak muscle tone.

atria Chambers or cavities, such as the atria of the heart.

atrial natriuretic hormone A hormone secreted by specialized muscle fibres in the atrial wall of the heart that influences water reabsorption in the kidney; it acts as an antagonist of aldosterone.

atrial natriuretic peptide A peptide released from the atria when atrial blood pressure is increased; it lowers blood pressure by increasing urine production, thus reducing blood volume.

atrial synchronous ventricular pacemaker An artificial pacemaker synchronized with the patient's atrial rhythm; it paces the ventricles only when an atrioventricular block occurs.

atrial–ventricular demand pacemaker An artificial pacemaker that paces the atria or ventricles when the intrinsic rate of the paced chamber drops dangerously low.

atrioventricular canal The path through which the atria open into the ventricles.

atrioventricular dissociation A conduction disturbance in which atrial and ventricular contractions occur rhythmically but are unrelated to each other.

atrioventricular node An area of specialized cardiac muscle that receives the cardiac impulse from the sinoatrial node and conducts it to the bundle of His.

atrioventricular sequential pacemaker An artificial pacemaker that paces the atria first and then the ventricles when spontaneous activity is absent or slowed in the atria and ventricles.

atrioventricular valve A valve in the heart through which blood flows from the atria to the ventricles.

atrophy Decrease in size (shrinkage) of a cell, which adversely affects cell function.

attention deficit disorder A syndrome that affects children, adolescents, and, in rare cases, adults and is characterized by learning and behavioural disabilities.

auditory Of or pertaining to hearing or the organs of hearing.

auditory meatus A tube-like channel of the external ear extending from the auricle to the tympanum of the middle ear.

auditory ossicles The incus, malleus, and stapes; small bones in the middle ear that articulate with each other and the tympanic membrane.

auditory tube The auditory canal; it extends from the middle ear to the nasopharynx; also known as the eustachian tube.

aura A sensation that may precede a migraine or seizure activity.

auricle The part of the external ear that protrudes from the head; also known as the pinna.

auscultation A technique that requires the use of a stethoscope and is used to assess body sounds produced by the movement of various fluids or gases in organs or tissues.

autoimmune pericarditis Inflammation of the pericardium associated with the production of antibodies directed against one's own tissues.

autoimmunity An abnormal characteristic or condition in which the body reacts against constituents of its own tissues.

autolysis The spontaneous disintegration of tissues or cells by the action of their own autogenous enzymes.

automated external defibrillator A device used in cardiac arrest to perform a computer analysis of the patient's cardiac rhythm and deliver defibrillatory shocks when indicated.

automatic implantable cardioverter–defibrillator A surgically implanted device that monitors a person's heart rate; it is designed to deliver defibrillatory shocks as needed.

automatic vehicle location A radio communications subsystem that uses one or more electronic methods periodically to determine the position of a land, marine, or air vehicle and relay that information via radio to a communications centre.

automaticity A property of specialized excitable tissue that allows self-activation through spontaneous development of an action potential.

automatism Abnormal repetitive motor behaviour such as lip smacking, chewing, or swallowing during which the patient is amnestic.

autonomic hyperreflexia syndrome A neurological disorder characterized by a discharge of sympathetic nervous system impulses as a result of stimulation of the bladder, large intestine, or other visceral organs.

autonomic nervous system The part of the nervous system that regulates involuntary vital functions, including the activity of cardiac muscle, smooth muscle, and glands.

autophagia Nutrition of the body by consumption of its own tissues.

avascular Devoid of blood vessels.

Avogadro's number The number of molecules in a gram mole of any chemical substance.

avoidance The act of keeping away from someone, something, or a situation, or of preventing the occurrence of something; it requires the paramedic to continually be aware of the scene by being observant and knowledgeable about warning signs that may indicate a dangerous situation.

avulsion A full-thickness skin loss in which the wound edges cannot be approximated.

axial loading Vertical compression of the spine that results when direct forces are transmitted along the length of the spinal column.

axial region The head, neck, thorax, abdomen and pelvis.

axial skeleton The bones of the head, neck and torso.

axillae Armpits.

axillary node One of the lymph glands of the axillae that helps fight infections in the chest, armpit, neck, and arm and drain lymph nodes from those areas.

axis The second cervical vertebra about which the atlas rotates, allowing the head to be turned, extended, or flexed.

axon The main central process of a neuron that normally conducts action potentials away from the neuron cell body.

azotaemia The retention of excessive amounts of nitrogenous compounds in the blood.

B lymphocytes The lymphocytes responsible for antibody-mediated immunity.

Babinski reflex A reflex movement in which the great toe bends upward when the outer edge of the sole is scratched.

bacteraemia The presence of bacteria in the blood.

bacteria Single-celled microorganisms that cause an infection characteristic of that species.

bacterial tracheitis A bacterial infection of the upper airway and subglottic trachea.

bactericidal Destructive to bacteria.

bacteriophage Any virus that causes lysis of host bacteria.

bacteriostatic Tending to restrain the development or the reproduction of bacteria.

ball-and-socket joint A joint that consists of a ball (head) at the end of one bone and a socket in an adjacent bone into which a portion of the ball fits.

bariatrics The field of medicine that focuses on the treatment and control of obesity and diseases associated with obesity.

baroreceptor A sensory nerve ending in the walls of the atria of the heart, venae cavae, aortic arch, and carotid sinuses; it is sensitive to stretching of the walls caused by an increase in blood pressure.

barotitis An inflammation of the ear caused by changes in atmospheric pressure.

barotrauma A physical injury sustained as a result of exposure to increased environmental pressure.

Bartholin's gland One of two small, mucus-secreting glands located on the posterior and lateral aspect of the vestibule of the vagina.

Barton's bandage A circumferential head dressing applied to restrict jaw movement and minimize pain.

base A chemical compound that combines with an acid to form a salt; also known as an alkali.

base of the heart The portion of the heart opposite the apex, directed to the right side of the body.

base station A grouping of radio equipment consisting of at least a transmitter, a receiver, a transmission line, and an antenna located at a specific, fixed location.

basic life support (BLS) Care provided by persons trained in first aid, cardiopulmonary resuscitation, and other non-invasive care.

basilar artery The single arterial trunk formed by the junction of the two vertebral arteries at the base of the skull.

basilar fracture A fracture that may occur when the mandibular condyles perforate the base of the skull but that more commonly results from extension of a linear fracture into the floor of the anterior and middle fossae.

basophil A white blood cell that promotes inflammation; it readily stains with specific dyes.

battering A form of domestic violence that establishes control and fear in a relationship through violence and other forms of abuse.

battery Physical contact with a person without consent and without legal justification.

Battle's sign Ecchymosis over the mastoid process caused by a fracture of the temporal bone.

Beck triad A combination of three symptoms that characterize cardiac tamponade: elevated central venous pressure, muffled heart sounds and hypotension.

behaviour indicator Non-specific behavioural changes that may suggest that a child is being maltreated. Behaviour indicators for sexual abuse are called non-specific because children may display such behaviour changes because of other traumatic conditions. Prompt evaluation is warranted when non-specific behaviour indicators occur, to rule out maltreatment; appropriate assistance for the child must be obtained.

behavioural emergency A change in mood or behaviour that cannot be tolerated by the involved person or others and requires immediate attention.

belay Method of attaching a safety rope and controlling the rope so that if the person or load starts to fall, the belay rope will prevent the fall.

Bell's palsy A condition in which paralysis of the facial muscles is caused by inflammation of the seventh cranial nerve; usually is one-sided and temporary and often develops suddenly.

beta cell A constituent of the islets of Langerhans that produces insulin.

beta-adrenergic receptor Any of the postulated adrenergic components of receptor tissues that respond to adrenaline and various blocking agents.

beta-hydroxybutyric acid One of the ketone bodies that occur in abnormal amounts in diabetic ketoacidosis as a result of fatty acid oxidation.

bicarbonate buffer system The principal mechanism for stabilizing acid–base balance.

biceps brachii The biceps muscle of the arm that flexes and supinates the forearm.

bicuspid valve The atrioventricular valve located between the left atrium and ventricle; also known as the mitral valve.

bifurcate To divide into two branches.

bilateral Having or occurring on two sides.

bile A bitter, yellow–green secretion of the liver that is stored in the gallbladder.

bilirubin The orange–yellow pigment of bile, formed principally from the breakdown of haemoglobin in red blood cells after termination of their normal life span.

bioethics The systematic study of moral dimensions including moral vision, decisions, conduct, and policies of the life sciences and health care.

biological half-life The time required to metabolize or eliminate half the total amount of a drug in the body.

biology The study of life.

biosynthesis A chemical reaction that continually occurs throughout the body in which molecules form more complex molecules.

Biot's respiration A respiratory pattern consisting of irregular respirations that vary in depth and that are interrupted by intervals of apnoea.

bioterrorism The use of biological agents, such as pathogenic organisms or agricultural pests, for the express purpose of causing death or disease, to instill a sense of fear and panic in the victims, and to intimidate governments or societies for political, financial, or ideological gain.

biotransformation The process by which a drug is converted chemically to a metabolite.

biphasic complex A QRS complex that is partly positive and partly negative.

bipolar disorder A disorder marked by alternating periods of mania and depression; formerly known as manic-depressive disorder.

bipolar lead A lead composed of two electrodes of opposite polarity.

blast injury A general term used to describe damage to a person exposed to a pressure field.

blastocyst The stage of mammalian embryos in which the embryo consists of the inner cell mass and a thin trophoblast layer.

bleb An accumulation of fluid under the skin.

blood The fluid and its suspended, formed elements that circulate through the heart, arteries, capillaries and veins.

blood–brain barrier An anatomical-physiological feature of the brain thought to consist of walls of capillaries in the central nervous system and surrounding glial membranes; its function is to prevent or slow the passage of chemical compounds from the blood into the central nervous system.

blood clot The end result of the clotting process in blood; a blood clot normally consists of red cells, white cells, and platelets enmeshed in an insoluble fibrin network.

blood colloid osmotic pressure Osmotic pressure caused by the presence of plasma proteins (mostly albumin) that are too large to pass through the wall of the capillary; also known as oncotic pressure.

blowout fracture A fracture of the floor of the orbit caused by a blow that suddenly increases the intraocular pressure.

blunt trauma An injury produced by the wounding forces of compression and change of speed, both of which can disrupt tissue.

body The largest or main part of any organ or structure.

bone A highly specialized form of hard, connective tissue; it consists of living cells and mineralized matrix.

bone marrow Specialized soft tissue that fills the spaces in the cancellous bone of the epiphyses.

bony labyrinth Part of the inner ear; it contains the membranous labyrinth.

borderline personality disorder A pervasive pattern of instability of interpersonal relationships, self-image, and affect, in addition to considerable impulsivity that begins by early adulthood.

botulism An often fatal form of food poisoning caused by the bacillus *Clostridium botulinum*.

bowel obstruction An occlusion of the intestinal lumen that results in blockage of normal flow of intestinal contents.

Bowman's capsule The expanded beginning of a renal tubule.

boxer's fracture Fracture of the fifth metacarpal bone from direct trauma to a closed fist.

Boyle's law See general gas law.

brachial plexus A network of nerves in the neck that passes under the clavicle and into the axilla, originating in the fifth, sixth, seventh and eighth cervical nerves and the first two thoracic spinal nerves; the brachial plexus innervates the muscles and the skin of the chest, shoulders and arms.

bradycardia A heart rate of less than 60 beats per minute in an adult.

bradykinin A peptide of non-protein origin that contains nine amino acid residues; a potent vasodilator.

bradypnoea A persistent respiratory rate slower than 12 breaths per minute in an adult.

brainstem The midbrain, pons and medulla.

Braxton Hicks contraction Irregular tightening of the pregnant uterus that begins in the first trimester and increases in frequency, duration and intensity as pregnancy progresses.

breech presentation The intrauterine position of the fetus in which the buttocks or feet present.

British Paramedic Association See College of Paramedics.

broad ligament A folded sheet of peritoneum draped over the uterine tubes, uterus, and ovaries.

bronchial tree An anatomical complex of the bronchi and bronchial tubes.

bronchiectasis An abnormal dilatation of the bronchi caused by a pus-producing infection of the bronchial wall.

bronchiole A small branch of a bronchus.

bronchiolitis An acute viral infection of the lower respiratory tract that occurs primarily in infants under 18 months of age; it is characterized by expiratory wheezes, respiratory distress, inflammation and obstruction at the level of the bronchioles.

bronchopulmonary dysplasia A chronic respiratory disorder characterized by scarring of lung tissue, thickened pulmonary arterial walls, and ventilation–perfusion mismatch; often occurs in infants who have dependence on long-term artificial ventilation.

brow presentation See face presentation.

Brown–Séquard syndrome A hemitransection of the spinal cord. In the classic presentation, pressure on half of the spinal cord results in weakness of the upper and lower extremities on the ipsilateral (same) side and loss of pain and temperature sensation on the contralateral (opposite) side.

bruit An abnormal sound or murmur heard while auscultating an artery, organ, or gland.

buccal Of or pertaining to the inside of the cheek.

buccal route A route for administering medication in which the agent is placed between the teeth and mucous membrane of the cheek.

bulbourethral glands Small glands located just below the prostate gland that lubricate the terminal portion of the urethra and contribute to seminal fluid; also known as Cowper's glands.

bulimia nervosa A disorder characterized by an insatiable craving for food, often resulting in episodes of binge eating followed by purging (through self-induced vomiting or use of laxatives), depression, and self-deprivation.

bullae Thin-walled blisters of the skin or mucous membranes that contain clear, serous fluid.

bullet yaw The forward rotation of a bullet around its centre of mass, which causes an end-over-end motion, producing a greater energy exchange and greater tissue damage; also known as bullet tumble.

bundle of His A band of fibres in the myocardium through which the cardiac impulse is transmitted from the atrioventricular node to the ventricles.

bundle of Kent Fibres that connect atrial muscle to ventricular muscle, bypassing the AV node; also known as Kent fibres.

burette An intravenous device used to deliver a wide range of accurate, specific volumes.

bursitis An inflammation of the bursa, the connective tissue structure surrounding a joint.

caecum A cul-de-sac constituting the first part of the large intestine.

caesarean delivery A surgical procedure in which the abdomen and uterus are incised and the baby is delivered transabdominally.

calcaneus The heel bone, the largest of the tarsal bones.

calcium The fifth most abundant element in the human body; it occurs mainly in bone.

calipers An instrument with two hinged, adjustable legs used to measure components of the electrocardiogram.

call connect A change to the way response times are measured. Prior to 1 April 2008, the clock started when three pieces of key information had been obtained (location, telephone number and chief complaint). The time is now measured from when the call is connected to the ambulance control room.

canaliculus A very small tube or channel.

cancellous bone Lattice-like tissue normally present in the interior of many bones where spaces are usually filled with marrow; also known as spongy bone.

cancer A neoplasm characterized by the uncontrolled growth of anaplastic cells that tend to invade surrounding tissue and to metastasize to distant body sites.

Candida A genus of yeast-like fungi.

candidiasis An infection caused by a species of *Candida* organisms that is characterized by pruritus, exudate and easy bleeding.

cannulation The insertion of a cannula into a body duct or cavity.

capillaries Tiny vessels that connect arterioles to venules.

capillary refill test A test used to evaluate the rate of blood flow through peripheral capillary beds.

capitulum The lateral aspect of the humerus; it articulates with the head of the radius.

capnography Measuring of the proportion of carbon dioxide in expired air.

capsid A protein coat that encloses a virus.

carbaminohaemoglobin A chemical complex formed by carbon dioxide and haemoglobin after the release of oxygen by the haemoglobin to a tissue cell.

carbohydrate Any group of organic compounds composed of carbon, hydrogen, and oxygen; it is primarily obtained from plant foods.

carbonic acid An aqueous solution of carbon dioxide.

carbonic anhydrase The enzyme that converts carbon dioxide into carbonic acid.

carboxyhaemoglobin A compound produced by the exposure of haemoglobin to carbon monoxide.

carcinogenic Cancer causing.

cardiac cycle The complete round of cardiac systole and diastole.

cardiac ejection fraction The percentage of ventricular blood volume released during a contraction.

cardiac muscle A special striated muscle of the myocardium that contains dark, intercalated discs at the junctions of the abutting fibres; cardiac muscle is characterized by special contractile abilities.

cardiac myopathy An abnormal condition of the heart characterized by weakness of the myocardium.

cardiac output The volume of blood pumped each minute by the ventricle.

cardiac plexus One of several nerve complexes situated close to the arch of the aorta.

cardiac sphincter A ring of muscle fibres at the juncture of the oesophagus and stomach.

cardiogenic shock Shock that results when cardiac action is unable to deliver sufficient circulating blood volume for tissue perfusion.

cardiography Recording the movements of the heart.

cardiomyopathy Any disease that affects the myocardium.

cardiopulmonary Of or pertaining to the heart and lungs.

cardiopulmonary resuscitation (CPR) An emergency procedure for life support consisting of artificial respiration and manual external cardiac massage.

carina of the trachea A downward and backward projection of the lowest tracheal cartilage, forming a ridge between the openings of the right and left primary bronchi.

carotid body A small structure containing neural tissue at the bifurcation of the carotid arteries; it monitors the oxygen content of the blood and helps regulate respiration.

carotid sinus massage A technique used to increase vagal tone to convert paroxysmal supraventricular tachycardia to sinus rhythm; also known as carotid sinus pressure.

carpal Pertaining to the carpus, or wrist.

carpometacarpal joint The joint of the thumb.

carrier A radio signal of specific frequency generated by a transmitter without audio information imposed on it.

carrier molecule A protein that combines with solutes on one side of a membrane, transporting the solute to the other side; it is used in mediated transport mechanisms.

cartilage Firm, smooth, non-vascular connective tissue.

cartilaginous joint See joint.

catabolic Pertaining to the destruction of complex substances by living cells to form simple compounds.

cataract A loss of transparency of the lens of the eye that results from changes in the delicate protein fibres within the lens.

catecholamine Any of a group of sympathomimetic amines, including dopamine, adrenaline and noradrenaline.

cathartic Causing evacuation of the bowel.

cation An ion with a positive charge.

cavitation A temporary or permanent opening produced by a force that pushes body tissues laterally away from the track of a projectile.

cell body The part of the cell that contains the nucleus and surrounding cytoplasm, exclusive of any projections or processes; it is concerned more with metabolism of the cell than with a specific function.

cell-mediated immunity Immunity characterized by the formation of a population of lymphocytes that attack and destroy foreign material.

cellulitis An inflammation of the skin characterized most commonly by local heat, redness, pain, swelling, and occasionally fever, malaise, chills and headache.

cementum The bone-like connective tissue that covers the roots of the teeth and helps to support them.

centigram A metric unit of mass equal to 1/100 of a gram.

centimetre A metric unit of length equal to 1/100 of a metre, or 0.3937 inches.

central cord syndrome A spinal cord injury commonly seen with hyperextension or flexion cervical injuries; characterized by greater motor impairment of the upper than lower extremities.

central nervous system The brain and spinal cord.

central nervous system ischaemic response An increase in blood pressure caused by vasoconstriction that occurs when oxygen levels are too low, carbon dioxide levels are too high, or pH is too low in the medulla.

central pain syndrome Infection or disease of the trigeminal nerve (cranial nerve V).

central thermoreceptors Nerve endings located in or near the anterior hypothalamus that are sensitive to heat.

centrifugation The process of separating components of different densities contained in a liquid by spinning them at high speeds.

centriole Usually paired organelles lying in the centrosome.

centrosome A specialized zone of cytoplasm close to the nucleus that contains two centrioles.

cephalic presentation A classification of fetal position in which the head of the fetus is at the uterine cervix; also known as vertex presentation.

cephalopelvic disproportion An obstetric condition in which a newborn's head is too large or a mother's birth canal too small to permit normal labour or birth.

cerebellar cortex The outer portion of the cerebellum.

cerebellum The second largest part of the brain, which plays an essential role in producing normal movements.

cerebral Pertaining to the brain.

cerebral aqueduct The narrow conduit between the third and fourth ventricles in the midbrain that conveys cerebrospinal fluid.

cerebral cortex A thin layer of grey matter, made up of neuron dendrites and cell bodies, that composes the surface of the cerebrum.

cerebral oedema An accumulation of fluid in the brain tissue.

cerebral palsy A general term for non-progressive disorders of movement and posture.

cerebral perfusion pressure (CPP) A measure of the amount of blood flow to the brain calculated by subtracting the intracranial pressure from the mean systemic arterial blood pressure.

cerebrospinal fluid Fluid that fills the subarachnoid space in the brain and spinal cord and in the cerebral ventricles.

cerebrospinal fluid rhinorrhoea Leakage of cerebrospinal fluid caused by fracture of the ethmoid cribriform plate.

cerebrovascular accident An abnormal condition of the blood vessels of the brain characterized by occlusion by an embolus, thrombus or cerebral haemorrhage; also known as stroke and brain attack.

cerebrum The largest and uppermost part of the brain; it controls consciousness, memory, sensations, emotions and voluntary movements.

certification (or registration) The process by which an agency or association grants recognition to an individual for meeting specific requirements to participate in an activity.

cerumen A yellowish or brownish waxy secretion produced in the external ear canal; also known as earwax.

ceruminous gland The gland that produces a waxy substance, cerumen (earwax).

cervical Pertaining to the neck.

cervical node One of the lymph glands in the neck.

cervical plexus The network of nerves formed by the ventral primary divisions of the first four cervical nerves.

cervical spondylosis A form of degenerative joint and disc disease that affects the cervical vertebrae and results in compression of the associated nerve roots.

cervical vertebrae The first seven segments of the vertebral column, designated C1 to C7.

cervicitis Acute or chronic inflammation of the uterine cervix.

cervix The lower part of the uterus.

Chadwick's sign The bluish coloration of the vulva and vagina that develops after the sixth week of pregnancy as a normal result of local venous congestion; an early sign of pregnancy.

chancre A skin lesion, usually of primary syphilis, that begins at the site of infection as a papule and develops into a red, bloodless, painless ulcer with a crater-like appearance.

channel An assigned frequency or pair of frequencies used to carry voice or data communications or both. In emergency medical services, an advanced life support channel is a pair of radio frequencies, one used for transmitting, the other for receiving.

chemical name The exact designation of a chemical structure as determined by the rules of chemical nomenclature.

chemoreceptor A sensory cell stimulated by a change in the concentration of chemicals to produce action potentials.

chemotactic factors Biochemical mediators that are important in activating the inflammatory response.

chemotaxis The response of leukocytes to products formed in immunological reactions; a part of the inflammatory response.

Cheyne–Stokes respiration A regular, periodic pattern of breathing with equal intervals of apnoea followed by a crescendo–decrescendo sequence of respirations.

chickenpox See varicella.

chief complaint A patient's primary complaint.

child abuse The physical, sexual, or emotional maltreatment of a child.

Chlamydia A genus of microorganisms that live as intracellular parasites; a common cause of sexually transmitted diseases and a frequent cause of sterility.

chlorine A poisonous, yellow–green gas with an odour that has been described as a mixture of pineapple and pepper.

choanal atresia A bony or membranous occlusion that blocks the passageway between the nose and pharynx; it can result in serious ventilation problems in the neonate.

cholecystitis Inflammation of the gallbladder, most often associated with the presence of gallstones.

cholecystokinin A hormone that stimulates the contraction of the gallbladder and the secretion of pancreatic juice.

cholesterol A fat-soluble compound found in animal fats and oils that is distributed widely in the body.

cholinergic Of or pertaining to the effects produced by the parasympathetic nervous system or drugs that stimulate the parasympathetic nervous system.

chondrocytes Cartilage cells.

chorioamnionitis An inflammatory reaction in the amniotic membranes caused by organisms in the amniotic fluid.

chorionic gonadotropin A chemical component of the urine of pregnant women.

choroid The portion of the vascular tunic associated with the sclera of the eye.

choroid plexus A network of brain capillaries that are involved in producing cerebrospinal fluid.

chromatin granules The material within the cell nucleus from which chromosomes are formed.

chronic bronchitis Obstructive airway disease of the trachea and bronchi.

chronic gastroenteritis Inflammation of the stomach and intestines that accompanies numerous gastrointestinal disorders.

chronic obstructive pulmonary disease (COPD) A progressive, irreversible condition characterized by diminished inspiratory and expiratory capacity of the lungs.

chronic pain Pain that continues or recurs over a prolonged period; it is caused by various disease or abnormal conditions.

chronic pulmonary hypertension A condition of abnormally high pressure within the pulmonary circulation.

chronic renal failure A progressive, irreversible systemic disease caused by kidney dysfunction that leads to abnormalities in blood counts and blood chemistry levels.

chronotropic Pertaining to agents that affect the heart rate; a drug that increases the heart rate is said to have a positive chronotropic effect.

chyme The semifluid mass of partly digested food passed from the stomach into the duodenum.

cilia Small, hair-like processes on the outer surfaces of some cells.

ciliary body A structure continuous with the choroid layer that contains smooth muscle cells and that functions in accommodation.

ciliated tissue Any tissue that projects cilia from its surface, such as portions of the epithelium in the respiratory tract.

circadian rhythm A pattern based on a 24-hour cycle, especially repetition of certain physiological phenomena, such as sleeping and eating.

circle of Willis The circle of interconnected blood vessels at the base of the brain.

circulatory shock Failure of the cardiovascular system to supply the cells with enough oxygenated blood to meet metabolic demands.

circumduction Movement in a circular motion.

circumflex artery The subdivision of the left coronary artery that feeds the lateral and posterior portions of the left ventricle and part of the right ventricle.

cirrhosis A chronic degenerative disease of the liver.

citrate Any salt or ester of citric acid.

classic heat stroke A severe, sometimes fatal condition resulting from the failure of the temperature-regulating capacity of the body; it is caused by prolonged exposure to the sun or to high temperatures.

claudication Cramp-like pains in the calves caused by poor circulation of blood to the leg muscles.

clavicle A long, curved, horizontal bone just above the first rib that forms the ventral portion of the shoulder girdle.

clinical perineum The portion of the perineum between the vaginal and anal openings.

clinical reasoning Use of the results of questions to think about associated problems and body system changes related to the patient's complaint.

clitoris Erectile tissue located in the vestibule of the vagina.

closed pneumothorax A collection of air or gas in the pleural space that causes the lung to collapse without exposing the pleural space to atmospheric pressure.

cluster headache A type of headache that occurs in bursts (clusters); also known as histamine headache.

coagulation Formation of a clot.

coarse ventricular fibrillation Fibrillatory waves greater than 3 mm in amplitude.

coccygeal bone The four segments of the sacral vertebral column that fuse to form the adult coccyx.

coccygeal plexus A network of coccygeal nerves.

cochlea Part of the bony labyrinth of the inner ear.

Code of Conduct See Standards of Conduct, Performance and Ethics.

coitus See copulation.

colitis An inflammatory condition of the large intestine characterized by severe diarrhoea, bleeding, and ulceration of the mucosa of the intestine.

collagen The rope-like protein of the extracellular matrix.

collecting duct A straight tubule that extends from the cortex of the kidney to the tip of the renal pyramid.

College of Paramedics The professional body of UK paramedics.

Colles' fracture A fracture of the radius at the epiphysis within 2.5 cm (1 inch) of the joint of the wrist; it is easily recognized by the resultant dorsal and lateral position of the hand.

colloid The gelatinous product of the thyroid gland, consisting mainly of thyroglobulin, which serves as the precursor and storage form of thyroid hormone.

colon The portion of the large intestine that extends from the caecum to the rectum.

colorectal cancer A malignant disease of the large intestine characterized by a change in bowel habits and the passing of blood.

colostomy A surgical opening into the large intestine.

command The act of directing, ordering, or controlling by virtue of explicit, statutory, regulatory or delegated authority.

command post The area from which command directs operations for an incident.

communicability period A stage of infection that begins when the latent period ends and continues as long as the agent is present and can spread to other hosts.

communicable disease An infectious disease that can be transmitted from one person to another.

communications The transmission and reception of information, resulting in common understanding.

communications centre A facility used to dispatch emergency equipment and coordinate communications between field units and personnel.

community health assessment An assessment of a target community to identify needs and resources required to provide prevention and wellness promotion activities.

compact bone Hard, dense bone that usually is found at the surface of skeletal structures, as distinguished from cancellous bone.

compartment syndrome The result of a crush injury, usually caused by compressive forces or blunt trauma to muscle groups confined in tight fibrous sheaths with minimal ability to stretch.

competitive antagonist An agent with an affinity for the same receptor site as an agonist. The competition with the agonist for the site inhibits the action of the agonist; increasing the concentration of the agonist tends to overcome the inhibition.

complement One of 11 complex, enzymatic serum proteins; complement causes lysis in an antigen–antibody reaction.

complement system A group of proteins that coats bacteria; the proteins then either help kill the bacteria directly, or they assist neutrophils (in the blood) and macrophages (in the tissues) to engulf and destroy the bacteria.

complete abortion An abortion in which the patient has passed all the products of conception.

complete breech A delivery presentation that occurs when the fetus has both knees and hips flexed; the buttocks are the presenting part.

compliance The ease with which the lungs and thorax expand during pressure changes. The greater the compliance, the easier the expansion.

components of skeletal survey An X-ray study comprising a two-view chest with bone technique, two-view skull technique, views of the lateral lumbar spine and anteroposterior pelvis, and anteroposterior views of the upper and lower extremities, including anteroposterior views of the feet and posteroanterior views of the hands.

computer-aided dispatching An enhanced dispatch system in which computerized data are used to assist the dispatcher in selecting and routing emergency equipment and resources.

concealment A means of keeping out of site; it provides no ballistic protection.

concentration gradient The concentration difference between two points in a solution divided by the distance between the points.

concept formation A component of critical thinking that refers to all elements that are gathered to form a general impression of the patient.

concha The three bony ridges on the lateral wall of the nasal cavity.

concussion A head injury that results from violent jarring or shaking, such as that caused by a blow or explosion.

condyle A rounded projection on a bone, usually for articulation with another bone.

cone A photoreceptor in the retina of the eye; it is responsible for colour vision.

confabulation The invention of stories to make up for gaps in memory.

congenital Present at birth.

congenital anomalies Defects that occur during fetal development.

congenital rubella syndrome A serious disease that affects about 25% of infants born to women infected with rubella during the first trimester of pregnancy; it is associated with multiple congenital anomalies, mental retardation, and an increased risk of death from congenital heart disease and sepsis during the first 6 months of life.

congestive heart failure An abnormal condition that reflects impaired cardiac pumping, usually a result of myocardial infarction, ischaemic heart disease or cardiomyopathy.

conjugate gaze Deviation of both eyes to either side at rest; the condition implies a structural lesion.

conjunctiva A mucous membrane that covers the anterior surface of the eyeball and the lining of the eyelids.

conjunctivitis Inflammation of the conjunctiva, caused by bacterial or viral infection, allergy, or environmental factors.

connective tissue Tissue that supports and binds other body tissues and parts.

conservation of energy law The principle that energy can be neither created nor destroyed; it can only change from one form (mechanical, thermal, electrical, or chemical) to another.

constipation Difficulty passing stools, or incomplete or infrequent passage of hard stools.

contact dermatitis Skin rash that results from exposure to an irritant or sensitizing antigen.

continence The ability to control bladder and/or bowel function.

continuous quality improvement A management approach to customer service and organizational performance that includes constant monitoring, evaluation, decisions, and actions.

contracture deformity An abnormal, usually permanent condition of a joint characterized by flexion and fixation and caused by atrophy and shortening of muscle fibres or by loss of elasticity of the skin.

contraindications Medical or physiological factors that make it harmful to administer a medication that would otherwise have a therapeutic effect.

contralateral Affecting or originating in the opposite side of the body.

contrastimulant A factor that works against stimulation.

contrecoup An injury that occurs at a site opposite the side of impact.

controlled substance Any of the drugs listed as class A, B or C under the Misuse of Drugs Act 1971; possessing, supplying and using them is illegal.

contusion A closed, soft tissue injury characterized by swelling, discoloration and pain.

copulation The sexual union of two persons of the opposite sex in which the penis is introduced into the vagina; also known as coitus.

cor pulmonale An abnormal cardiac condition characterized by hypertrophy of the right ventricle of the heart as a result of hypertension of the pulmonary circulation.

cord presentation A presentation that occurs when the cord slips down into the vagina or appears externally after the amniotic membranes have ruptured.

core body temperature The temperature of deep structures of the body as compared with temperatures of peripheral tissues.

cornea The convex, transparent, anterior part of the eye.

corneal abrasion The rubbing off of the outer layers of the cornea.

corniculate cartilage A conical nodule of elastic cartilage that surrounds the apex of each arytenoid cartilage.

coronal plane See frontal plane.

coronary artery One of two arteries that arise from the base of the aorta and carry blood to the muscle of the heart.

coronary artery disease One of several abnormal conditions that affect the arteries of the heart and reduce the flow of oxygen and nutrients to the myocardium.

coronary sinus A short trunk that receives most of the veins of the heart and empties into the right atrium.

corpus callosum An arched mass of white matter in the depths of the longitudinal fissure; it is made up of the transverse fibres that connect the cerebral hemispheres.

corpus luteum A yellow endocrine body formed in the ovary at the site of a ruptured vesicular follicle immediately after ovulation.

corpus luteum cyst A type of cyst prone to rupture that forms as a result of haemorrhage in a mature corpus luteum.

cortisol A steroid hormone that occurs naturally in the body.

costal margin The margin of the lower limit of the ribs.

costochondral Pertaining to the junction of the ribs and cartilage.

countershock A high-intensity, short-duration electrical shock applied to the area of the heart, resulting in total cardiac depolarization.

coup Local damage that occurs at the site of impact.

couplet Two premature ventricular contractions in a row.

cover A type of concealment that hides the body and offers ballistic protection.

coverage The area covered by radio communication. The generally accepted national emergency system standard is the '90/90' standard. This means that 90% of the coverage area will have communication 90% of the time. Coverage is usually expressed as dead (no coverage), marginal (spotty), good (few problems), or excellent (no problems).

Cowper's glands See bulbourethral glands.

coxae The hip joints; the head of the femur and the acetabulum of the innominate bone.

crackle A fine, bubbling sound heard on auscultation of the lung; it is produced by air entering distal airways and alveoli that contain serous secretions.

cranial nerve One of 12 pairs of nerves that originate from a nucleus within the brain.

cranial vault The eight skull bones that surround and protect the brain; the brain case.

craniectomy Surgical removal of bone fragments from the cranium.

cremaster muscle A thin muscle layer spreading out over the spermatic cord in a series of loops; it functions to draw the testis up toward the superficial inguinal ring in response to cold or stimulation of the nerve.

crenate The shrinking of red blood cells caused by exposure to a hypertonic solution.

crepitus A grating sound associated with rubbing of bone fragments.

cricoid cartilage The most inferior laryngeal cartilage.

cricothyroid membrane The membrane joining the thyroid and cricoid cartilages.

cricothyroidotomy An emergency incision into the cricothyroid membrane.

crime scene A location where any part of a criminal act has occurred or a location where evidence relating to a crime may be found.

critical care practitioner A paramedic with advanced critical care skills; initial programmes have focused on transferring critical care patients.

Crohn's disease A chronic, inflammatory bowel disease of unknown origin, usually affecting the ileum, the colon, or both structures.

croup An acute viral infection of the upper and lower respiratory tract that occurs primarily in infants and young children 3 months to 3 years of age; it is characterized by hoarseness, fever, a harsh, brassy cough, inspiratory stridor, and varying degrees of respiratory distress; also known as laryngotracheobronchitis.

crown The portion of the human tooth covered by enamel.

crowning The phase at the end of labour in which the fetal head is seen at the opening of the vagina.

crush injury Injury from exposure of tissue to a compressive force sufficient to interfere with the normal structure and metabolic function of the involved cells and tissues.

crush syndrome A life-threatening and sometimes preventable complication of prolonged immobilization; a pathologic process that causes destruction, alteration, or both of muscle tissue.

crystalloid A substance in a solution that can be diffused through a semipermeable membrane.

crystalluria The presence of crystals in the urine.

cubic centimetre A unit of volume equal to that of a cube having sides each 1 cm in length, commonly used in fluid measure and formerly referred to as cc.

Cullen's sign The appearance of irregularly formed haemorrhagic patches on the skin around the umbilicus.

cumulative action The effect that occurs when several doses of a drug are administered or when absorption occurs more quickly than removal by excretion or metabolism or both.

cuneiform cartilage A small rod of elastic cartilage above the corniculate cartilages in the larynx.

CUPS system A method of patient status coding that assigns patients to one of four categories: cardiopulmonary resuscitation, unstable, potentially unstable, and stable.

current health status A focus on the patient's current state of health, environmental conditions and personal habits.

Cushing's disease A metabolic disorder resulting from the chronic and excessive production of cortisol by the adrenal cortex or by the administration of glucocorticoids in large doses for several weeks or longer; also known as Cushing syndrome.

Cushing's reflex An attempt by the body to compensate for a decline in cerebral perfusion pressure by a rise in mean arterial pressure.

Cushing syndrome A condition caused by an abnormally high circulating level of corticosteroid hormones, produced naturally by the adrenal glands.

Cushing's triad Increased systolic pressure, widened pulse pressure, and decrease in the pulse and respiratory rate, which result from increased intracranial pressure.

cutaneous Of or pertaining to the skin.

cuticle The skinfold covering the root of the nail.

cyanotic Having bluish discoloration.

cystic medial necrosis Degenerative changes in the connective tissue of the aortic media.

cystitis Inflammation of the urinary bladder and ureters.

cytochrome oxidase A respiratory enzyme that functions in the transfer of electrons from cytochromes to oxygen, thus activating oxygen, which unites with hydrogen to form water.

cytology The study of cells.

cytomegalovirus A member of a group of large, species-specific, herpes-type viruses with a wide variety of disease effects.

cytoplasm All of the substance of a cell other than the nucleus.

cytoplasmic membrane The plasma membrane.

cytotoxic Pertaining to a pharmacological compound or other agent that destroys or damages tissue cells.

dartos muscle A layer of smooth muscle in the skin of the scrotum; it raises and lowers the testes in the scrotum in response to changes in ambient temperature.

data interpretation A component of critical thinking in which the examiner gathers the necessary data to form a field impression and working diagnosis.

DCAP-BTLS An acronym for wound assessment: deformity, contusions, abrasions, penetrations or punctures, burns, tenderness, lacerations and swelling.

deafness A complete or partial inability to hear.

debriefing An activity in which rescuers and others involved in an emergency event discuss their feelings to relieve emotions and anxiety; it usually takes place 24 to 72 hours after the event.

decerebrate posturing A position in which a comatose patient's arms are extended and internally rotated and the legs are extended with the feet in forced plantar flexion; usually observed in patients who have compression of the brainstem.

deciduous tooth Any of the 20 teeth that appear normally during infancy.

decoding The act of interpreting symbols and format.

decompression sickness A multisystem disorder that results when nitrogen in compressed air converts back from solution to gas, forming bubbles in the tissues and blood.

decontamination The process of making patients, rescuers, equipment and supplies safe by eliminating harmful substances.

decorticate posturing A position in which the comatose patient's upper extremities are rigidly flexed at the elbows and at the wrists; usually observed in patients who have a lesion in the mesencephalic region of the brain.

dedicated line A special telephone circuit designated for specific point-to-point communication purposes, such as alerting ambulance service bases.

deep frostbite A cold injury that results in significant tissue loss even with appropriate therapy; it is associated with subdermal layers and deep tissues.

deep vein thrombosis A disorder involving a thrombus in one of the deep veins of the body, most commonly the iliac and femoral veins.

defecation The elimination of faeces from the digestive tract through the rectum and anus.

defence mechanism An unconscious, intrapsychic reaction to protect the self from a stressful situation.

defibrillation The delivery of direct electrical current in an attempt to terminate ventricular fibrillation or pulseless ventricular tachycardia.

defibrillator A device used to depolarize fibrillating myocardial cells, thus allowing them to repolarize uniformly.

defusing An informal gathering of the persons involved in an emergency event to allow an initial release of feelings and an opportunity for persons to share their experiences.

degloving injury An injury usually involving the hand or finger in which the soft tissue is removed down to the bone.

degradation The physical destruction or decomposition of clothing material caused by use, ambient conditions, or exposure to chemicals.

degranulation A cellular process that releases antimicrobial cytotoxic molecules from secretory vesicles called granules.

dehydration An excessive loss of water from the body tissues; it may follow prolonged fever, diarrhoea, vomiting, acidosis and other conditions.

delirium An abrupt disorientation for time and place, usually with illusions and hallucinations.

delirium tremens An acute and sometimes fatal psychotic reaction caused by cessation of excessive intake of alcohol over a long period of time; also known as DTs.

delta cell A constituent of the islets of Langerhans; it secretes somatostatin.

delta wave Widened, abnormal slurring or notching of the onset of the QRS complex; it indicates anomalous spread of the impulse and is a diagnostic finding for Wolff–Parkinson–White syndrome.

deltoid muscle A large, thick, triangular muscle that covers the shoulder joint.

delusions Persistent beliefs or perceptions held by a person despite evidence that refutes them (i.e. false beliefs).

dendrite The branching processes of a neuron that receive stimuli and conduct potentials toward the cell body.

dentine The chief material of teeth, surrounding the pulp and situated inside the enamel and cementum.

deoxyribonucleic acid (DNA) A type of nucleic acid that comprises the genetic material of cells.

dependent lividity A red or bluish-purple tissue condition in dependent areas of the body caused by venous congestion.

depersonalization Forced emotional estrangement.

depolarization A change in electrical charge difference across the cell membrane that causes the difference to be smaller or closer to 0 mV; a phase of the action potential in which the membrane potential moves toward zero or becomes positive.

depressant A substance that decreases or lessens a body function or activity.

depressed skull fracture Any fracture of the skull in which fragments are depressed below the normal surface of the skull.

depression A mood disturbance characterized by feelings of sadness, despair, and discouragement.

dermatitis Inflammation of the skin.

dermatome The skin surface area supplied by a single spinal nerve.

dermis Dense, irregular connective tissue that forms the deep layer of the skin.

descending colon The segment of the colon that extends from the end of the transverse colon at the splenic flexure on the left side of the abdomen down to the beginning of the sigmoid colon in the pelvis.

desensitization Emotional insensitivity.

diabetes insipidus A metabolic disorder characterized by extreme polyuria and polydipsia, caused by deficient production or secretion of antidiuretic hormone or inability of the kidney tubules to respond to antidiuretic hormone.

diabetes mellitus A complex disorder of carbohydrate, fat, and protein metabolism that primarily results from partial or complete lack of insulin secretion by the beta cells of the pancreas or of defects of the insulin receptors.

diabetic ketoacidosis An acute, life-threatening complication of uncontrolled diabetes characterized by hyperglycaemia, hypovolaemia, electrolyte imbalance and a breakdown of free fatty acids, causing acidosis; also known as diabetic coma.

diad The combination of sarcoplasmic reticulum and T tubules.

diagnosis Identification of a disease or condition by an evaluation of physical signs, symptoms, history, laboratory tests and procedures.

dialysate A solution used in dialysis.

dialysis A technique used to normalize blood chemistry in patients with acute or chronic renal failure and to remove blood toxins in some patients who have taken a drug overdose.

dialysis fistula An artificial passage, as in an arteriovenous fistula, used to gain access to the patient's bloodstream for haemodialysis.

diaphoresis Profuse secretion of sweat.

diaphragm The dome-shaped, musculofibrous partition that separates the thoracic and abdominal cavities.

diaphragmatic hernia A herniation in the diaphragm caused by the improper fusion of structures during fetal development.

diaphysis The shaft of a long bone, consisting of a tube of compact bone that encloses the medullary cavity.

diarrhoea The frequent passage of loose, watery stools; it is generally the result of increased motility in the colon.

diastolic blood pressure The minimum level of blood pressure measured between contractions of the heart.

diencephalon The parts of the brain between the cerebral hemispheres and the mesencephalon.

differentiation A process in which cells become specialized in one type of function or act in concert with other cells to perform a more complex task.

diffusion The process in which solid, particulate matter in a fluid moves from an area of higher concentration to an area of lower concentration, resulting in an even distribution of the particles in the fluid.

dilatation and curettage A gynaecological procedure that refers to widening of the uterine cervix and scraping away of the endometrium of the uterus.

diphtheria An acute contagious disease characterized by the production of a systemic toxin and a false membrane lining of the mucous membranes of the throat.

diplopia Double vision.

direct laryngoscopy Visual examination of the larynx with a laryngoscope.

disease period A stage of infection that follows the incubation period; the duration of which varies with the disease.

disentanglement The process of making a pathway through the wreckage of an accident and removing wreckage from patients.

disequilibrium Unstable equilibrium; motion sickness.

disequilibrium syndrome A group of neurological findings that sometimes occur during or immediately after dialysis; thought to result from a disproportionate decrease in osmolality of the extracellular fluid compared with that of the intracellular compartment in the brain or cerebrospinal fluid.

disorientated Unaware of surroundings.

dissecting aortic aneurysm Localized dilatation of the aorta characterized by a longitudinal dissection between the outer and middle layers of the vascular wall.

disseminated intravascular coagulation A grave coagulopathy that results from the overstimulation of the clotting and anticlotting processes in response to disease or injury.

dissolution The rate at which a solid drug goes into solution after ingestion; the faster the rate of dissolution, the more quickly the drug is absorbed.

distraction 1. A self-defence measure in which a diversion is created to draw a person's attention.

2. A spinal injury that occurs if the cervical spine is suddenly stopped while the weight and momentum of the body pull away from it.

distress Negative, debilitating, or harmful stress.

distribution The transport of a drug through the bloodstream to various tissues of the body and ultimately to its site of action.

diuresis The increased formation and secretion of urine.

diversity Differences of any kind: race, class, religion, gender, sexual preference, personal habitat and physical ability.

diverticulitis Inflammation of one or more diverticula – see diverticulum.

diverticulosis The presence of pouch-like herniations through the muscular layer of the colon.

diverticulum A pouch-like herniation through the muscular wall of a tubular organ; it may be present in the stomach, small intestine, or, most commonly, the colon.

divisions Subdivisions of the incident command system that encompass specific geographical areas of responsibility as deemed necessary by the incident commander.

do not resuscitate (DNR) A physician order instructing emergency care providers not to attempt resuscitation of a patient in the event of cardiac or respiratory failure.

dorsal root A sensory component that conveys afferent nerve processes to the spinal cord.

dorsal root ganglia See spinal ganglia.

dorsogluteal site An area made up of several gluteal muscles; it is used as an injection site.

Down syndrome A congenital condition characterized by varying degrees of mental retardation and multiple defects.

dromotropic Pertaining to agents that affect conduction velocity through the conducting tissues of the heart; a drug that speeds conduction is said to have a positive dromotropic effect.

drowning A mortal event in which a submersion victim is pronounced dead at the scene of the attempted resuscitation, or within 24 hours after arrival in the emergency department or hospital.

drug Any substance taken by mouth; injected into a muscle, blood vessel, or cavity of the body; or applied topically to treat, prevent or diagnose a disease or condition.

drug absorption A process in which drug molecules move from the site of entry into the body to the general circulation.

drug abuse Self-medication or self-administration of a drug in chronically excessive amounts, resulting in psychological or physical dependence (or both), functional impairment, and deviation from approved social norms.

drug allergy A systemic reaction to a drug resulting from previous sensitizing exposure and the development of an immunological mechanism.

drug dependence A state in which intense physical or emotional disturbance is produced if a drug is withdrawn; previously called habituation.

drug interaction Modification of the effects of one drug by the previous or concurrent administration of another drug, thereby increasing or diminishing the pharmacological or physiological action of one or both drugs.

drug receptors Parts of a cell (usually an enzyme or large protein molecule) with which a drug molecule interacts to trigger its desired response or effect.

drug–protein complex A complex formed by the attachment of a drug to proteins, mainly albumin.

ductus arteriosus A vascular channel in the fetus that joins the pulmonary artery directly to the descending aorta.

ductus deferens A thick, smooth muscular tube that allows sperm to exit from the epididymis through the ejaculatory duct; also known as the vas deferens.

ductus venosus The continuation of the umbilical vein through the liver to the inferior vena cava.

duodenum The first subdivision of the small intestine.

duplex mode A communications mode with the ability to transmit and receive traffic simultaneously through two different frequencies, one to transmit and one to receive.

duplex/multiplex system A communications system with the ability to transmit and receive simultaneously with concurrent transmission of voice and telemetry.

dura mater The outermost layer of the meninges.

duration of action The period from the onset of drug action to the time when a drug effect is no longer seen.

dysarthria Difficult and poorly articulated speech resulting from poor control over the muscles of speech.

dysconjugate gaze Deviation of the eyes to opposite sides at rest; it implies a structural brainstem dysfunction in the pathways that traverse the brainstem from the upper midbrain to at least the level of the lower pons.

dyshaemoglobinaemia Haemoglobin saturated with compounds other than oxygen, such as carbon monoxide or methaemoglobin.

dyskinesia An impairment of the ability to execute voluntary movements; often an adverse effect of prolonged use of antipsychotic medications.

dysmenorrhoea Pain associated with menstruation.

dyspareunia Pain with intercourse.

dysphagia Inability or difficulty in swallowing because of medical or traumatic causes.

dysphonia An abnormality in the speaking voice, such as hoarseness.

dysplasia Abnormal cellular growth.

dyspnoea Difficult or laboured breathing.

dysrhythmia Variation from a normal rhythm.

dystonia A condition characterized by local or diffuse changes in muscle tone, resulting in painful muscle spasms, unusually fixed postures, and strange movement patterns.

eardrum The cellular membrane that separates the external ear from the middle ear; also known as the tympanic membrane.

eating disorders A term referring to anorexia nervosa and bulimia nervosa, conditions in which dissatisfaction with weight and body shape cause an individual to develop disordered eating behaviours.

eclampsia A grave form of pregnancy-induced hypertension, characterized by convulsions, coma, proteinuria, and oedema.

ectoparasite An organism that lives on the outside of the body of the host, such as a louse.

ectopic Out of place.

ectopic foci Cardiac dysrhythmias caused by irritation of an excitation impulse at a site other than the sinus node.

ectopic pregnancy An abnormal pregnancy in which the conceptus implants outside the uterine cavity.

eczema Superficial dermatitis of unknown cause.

effacement The shortening of the vaginal portion of the cervix and the thinning of its walls as it is stretched and dilated by the fetus during labour.

efferent division Nerve fibres that send impulses from the central nervous system to the periphery.

efficacy An intrinsic activity that refers to the ability of a drug to initiate biological activity as a result of such binding.

Einthoven's triangle An equilateral triangle formed by the patient's right arm, left arm and left leg; it is used in electrode sensor placement for electrocardiogram monitoring.

ejaculatory duct A duct formed by the joining of the ductus deferens and the duct from the seminal vesicle that allows sperm to enter the urethra.

ejection The forceful expulsion of blood from the ventricle of the heart.

elastin The major connective tissue protein of elastic tissue; it has a structure like a coiled spring.

elder abuse The infliction of physical pain, injury, debilitating mental anguish, unreasonable confinement, or wilful deprivation by a caregiver of services that are necessary to maintain mental and physical health of an older person.

electroconvulsive therapy (ECT) Induction of a brief convulsion by passing an electrical current through the brain to treat affective disorders.

electrolyte A cation or anion in solution that conducts an electrical current.

elevation Movement of a structure in a superior direction.

ellipsoid joint A modified ball-and-socket joint in which the articular surfaces are ellipsoid rather than spherical.

emaciated To be abnormally lean from disease or lack of nutrition.

embolectomy A surgical incision into an artery for the removal of an embolus or clot.

embryo In human beings the stage of prenatal development between the time of implantation of the fertilized ovum until the end of the seventh or eighth week.

emergency care assistant (ECA) An emergency care assistant drives an ambulance under emergency conditions and supports the work of qualified ambulance technicians and paramedics.

emergency care practitioner (ECP) The emergency care practitioner utilizes the skills of paramedics and other professionals (such as specialist nurses with additional skills) to support the first contact needs of patients in unscheduled care.

emergency medical services A national network of services coordinated to provide aid and medical assistance from primary response to definitive care; the network involves personnel trained in rescue, stabilization, transportation, and advanced management of traumatic and medical emergencies.

emergency medical technician (EMT) A person who has completed training based on the IHCD National Standard Curriculum.

emissary veins The small vessels in the skull that connect the sinuses of the dura with the veins on the exterior of the skull through a series of anastomoses.

emotional abuse The infliction of anguish, pain, or distress through verbal or non-verbal acts.

emotional/mental impairment Impaired intellectual functioning that results in an inability to cope with normal responsibilities of life.

emphysema An abnormal condition of the pulmonary system characterized by overinflation and destructive changes in the alveolar walls, resulting in a loss of lung elasticity and a decrease in gases.

EMS communications The delivery of patient and scene information (either in person, in writing, or through communications technology) to other members of the emergency response team.

enamel A hard white substance that covers the dentine of the crown of the tooth.

encephalitis An inflammatory condition of the brain, usually caused by an infection transmitted by the bite of an infected mosquito; it may also result from lead or other poisoning or from haemorrhage.

encoding The act of placing a message in an understandable format (either written or verbal).

endolymph Fluid found within the membranous labyrinth.

endometriosis An abnormal gynaecological condition characterized by ectopic growth and function of endometrial tissue; it is thought to result when, during menstruation, fragments of endometrium from the lining of the uterus are regurgitated backward through the fallopian tubes into the peritoneal cavity, where they attach and grow as small cystic structures.

endometritis An inflammatory condition of the endometrium, usually caused by bacterial infection.

endometrium The mucous membrane lining of the uterus, which changes in thickness and structure with the menstrual cycle.

endoplasmic reticulum A network of connecting sacs or canals that wind through the cytoplasm of a cell serving as a miniature circulatory system for the cell.

endorphin Any of several peptides secreted in the brain that have a pain-relieving effect like morphine.

endotoxin A toxin contained in the cell walls of some microorganisms, especially Gram-negative bacteria.

endotracheal intubation See tracheal intubation.

endotracheal route See tracheal route.

enhanced automaticity The cause of dysrhythmias in Purkinje fibres and other myocardial cells with a high resting membrane potential; it results from an acceleration of phase 4 depolarization commonly caused by abnormally high leakage of sodium ions into the cells, which causes the cells to reach threshold prematurely.

enophthalmos Recessed globe.

enteral route A route of drug administration along any portion of the gastrointestinal tract.

envenomation The injection of snake, arachnid, or insect venom into the body.

enzyme A protein produced by living cells that catalyses chemical reactions in organic matter.

eosinophil A white blood cell that inhibits inflammation; it readily stains with acidic dyes.

eosinophil chemotactic factor of anaphylaxis A group of active substances, including histamine and leukotrienes, that are released during an anaphylactic reaction.

epicardium See visceral pericardium.

epicondyle A projection on the surface of a bone above its condyle.

epidermis The outer portion of skin; it is formed of epithelial tissue that rests on or covers the dermis.

epididymis A tightly coiled tube that lies along the top of and behind the testes, where sperm mature.

epididymitis An inflammation of the epididymis, a tubular section of the male reproductive system that carries sperm from the testicles to the seminal vesicles.

epidural haematoma Accumulation of blood between the dura mater and the cranium.

epidural space The space above or on the dura.

epiglottis A lid-like cartilage that overhangs the entrance to the larynx.

epiglottitis Inflammation of the epiglottis; a severe form of the condition that affects primarily children is characterized by fever, sore throat, soft stridor, croupy cough and an erythematous epiglottis.

epilepsy A condition characterized by a tendency of the individual to have recurrent seizures (excluding those that arise from correctable or avoidable circumstances).

epinephrine Adrenaline; the secretion of the adrenal medulla.

epiphyseal line A dense plate in a bone that is no longer growing, indicating the former site of the epiphyseal plate.

epiphyseal plate See growth plate.

epiphysis The head of a long bone that is separated from the shaft of the bone by the epiphyseal plate until the bone stops growing, the plate is obliterated, and the shaft and the head are united.

epistaxis Bleeding from the nose.

epithelial tissue The cellular covering of internal and external surfaces of the body, including the lining of vessels and other small cavities.

Epstein–Barr virus The herpes virus that causes infectious mononucleosis.

erection The condition of hardness, swelling, and elevation observed in the penis and to a lesser degree in the clitoris, usually caused by sexual arousal.

erythrocyte A red blood cell.

escape beat An automatic beat of the heart that occurs after an interval longer than the duration of the dominant heartbeat cycle.

eschar A scab or dry crust resulting from a thermal or chemical burn.

escharotomy Surgical incision into necrotic tissue caused by a severe burn; escharotomy is sometimes necessary to prevent oedema from building up sufficient interstitial pressure to impair capillary filling and cause ischaemia.

estimated date of delivery (EDD) Delivery date for the fetus – sometimes referred to as estimated due date.

ethics The discipline relating to right and wrong, moral duty and obligation, moral principles and values, and moral character; a standard for honourable behaviour designed by a group with expected conformity.

ethmoid bone The very light, spongy bone at the base of the cranium that forms most of the walls of the superior part of the nasal cavity.

ethmoid sinus One of the numerous small, thin-walled cavities in the ethmoid bone of the skull, rimmed by the frontal maxilla and the lacrimal, sphenoidal and palatine bones.

ethylene glycol A chemical used in automobile antifreeze preparations.

eukaryote A cell with a true nucleus, found in all higher organisms and in some microorganisms.

eustachian tube See auditory tube.

eustress Positive, performance-enhancing stress.

evaluation A component of critical thinking in which the examiner assesses the patient's response to care.

evasive tactics A self-defence measure in which an aggressor's moves and actions are anticipated, and unconventional pathways are used during retreat for personal safety.

eversion Turning outward.

evisceration The protrusion of an internal organ through a wound or surgical incision, especially in the abdominal wall.

excitability The property of a cell that enables it to react to irritation or stimulation.

excretion The elimination of toxic or inactive metabolites, primarily by the kidneys; the intestines, lungs, and mammary, sweat and salivary glands also may be involved.

excursion Movement from side to side.

exertional heat stroke An abnormal condition characterized by weakness, vertigo, nausea, muscle cramps, and loss of consciousness; caused by depletion of body fluid and electrolytes resulting from exposure to intense heat or inability to acclimatize to heat.

exocrine Secreting into a duct.

exophthalmos An abnormal condition characterized by marked protrusion of the eyeballs.

exothermic Marked or accompanied by the evolution of heat.

exotoxin A toxin secreted or excreted by a living organism.

expiration Breathing out (exhalation), normally a passive process.

expiratory centre The region of the medulla that is electrically active during non-quiet expiration.

expiratory reserve volume The maximum volume of air that can be exhaled after a normal expiration.

exposure incident Any specific contact of the eyes, the mouth, other mucous membranes, non-intact skin, or parenteral contact with blood, blood products, bloody body fluids, or other potentially infectious materials.

expressed consent Verbal or written consent to the treatment.

extended scope of practice The expansion of healthcare services provided by emergency medical technicians and paramedics in the prehospital setting.

extension Stretching out.

external anal sphincter A sphincter muscle located at the tip of the coccyx and surrounding fascia; it prevents the movement of faeces out of the rectum until it is relaxed.

external auditory canal The passage for sound impulses passing through the ear; also called external auditory meatus.

external cardiac pacing The delivery of repetitive electrical currents to the heart, substituting for a natural pacemaker that has become blocked or dysfunctional; also known as transcutaneous cardiac pacing.

external ear The portion of the ear that includes the auricle and external auditory meatus; it terminates at the eardrum.

external jugular vein One of a pair of large vessels in the neck that receive most of the blood from the exterior of the cranium and deep tissues of the face.

external urinary sphincter The smooth muscle that surrounds the urethra as the urethra extends through the pelvic floor; it controls the flow of urine through the urethra.

extracellular Occurring outside of a cell or cell tissues or in cavities or spaces between cell layers or groups of cells.

extracellular fluid The water found outside the cells, including that in the intravascular and interstitial compartments.

extracellular matrix Non-living chemical substances located between connective tissue cells.

extrapyramidal reaction A response to a treatment or drug characterized by involuntary movement, changes in muscle tone, and abnormal posture.

extravasate The passage or escape of blood, serum or lymph into the tissues.

extubation Removal of a tracheal tube.

exudate Fluid, cells, or other substances that have been discharged slowly from cells or blood vessels through small pores or breaks in cell membranes.

face presentation An abnormal presentation in which the brow or forehead of the fetus is the first part of the body to enter the birth canal; also known as brow presentation.

facial bones The 14 bones that form the structure of the face in the anterior skull; they do not contribute to the cranial vault.

facial nerve palsy Partial or total loss of the functions of the facial muscles or loss of sensation in the face.

facilitated diffusion A carrier-mediated process that moves substances into or out of cells from a high to a low concentration.

faecal impaction An accumulation of hardened faeces in the rectum or sigmoid colon that the person is unable to move.

faecalith A hard, impacted mass of faeces in the colon.

faeces Waste material discharged from the intestines.

failure to thrive The abnormal retardation of the growth and development of an infant resulting from conditions that interfere with normal metabolism, appetite, and activity.

fallopian tube See uterine tube.

false imprisonment Intentional and unjustifiable detention of a person.

false movement An unnatural movement of an extremity, usually associated with fracture.

false rib See rib.

false vocal cord See vestibular fold.

family court These courts deal with most 'public law' cases in which the state (usually the local authority) is intervening, or attempting to intervene, in family life. These include everything from supervision orders to adoption. Most of the work involves care orders.

family history Illness or disease in a patient's family or a family's background that may be relevant to the patient's complaint.

fascia The loose areolar connective tissue found beneath the skin or dense connective tissue that encloses and separates muscle.

fascicle A small bundle or cluster of nerve or muscle fibres that provides pathways for impulse conduction.

fasciculation A localized, uncoordinated, uncontrollable twitching of a single muscle group that can be palpated and seen under the skin.

fasciotomy Incision of a fascia to relieve elevated intracompartmental pressure.

fat A substance composed of lipids or fatty acids.

febrile seizure A seizure that results from a rapid rise in temperature.

femoral vein A large vein in the thigh that originates in the popliteal vein and accompanies the femoral artery in the proximal two-thirds of the thigh.

femur The thigh bone, which extends from the pelvis to the knee; the largest and strongest bone in the body.

fetal membrane disorder One of several disorders that pertain to the fetus or to the period during its development, including premature rupture of membranes, amniotic fluid embolism, and meconium staining.

fetus Unborn young, from the third month of the intrauterine period until birth.

fibrinogen A soluble blood protein converted into insoluble fibrin during clotting.

fibrocartilage Cartilage that consists of a dense matrix of white collagenous fibres.

fibrosis An abnormal condition in which fibrous connective tissue spreads over or replaces normal smooth muscle or other normal organ tissue.

fibrous connective tissue A connective tissue that consists mainly of bundles of strong, white collagenous fibres arranged in parallel rows.

fibrous joint See joint.

fibrous pericardium Fibrous outer layer of the heart.

fibrous tunic The sclera and cornea.

fibula The bone of the leg, lateral to and smaller than the tibia.

Fick principle The principle used to determine cardiac output. It assumes that the quantity of oxygen delivered to an organ is equal to the amount of oxygen consumed by that organ plus the amount of oxygen carried away from that organ.

field impression An impression of the patient's condition that the paramedic makes from pattern recognition and gut instinct that results from experience.

filtrate A filtered liquid.

filtration Movement caused by a pressure gradient of a liquid through a filter that prevents some or all of the substances in the liquid from passing through.

fimbria A fringe-like structure located at the border of the uterine tube.

financial/material exploitation The illegal or improper use of funds, properties, or assets.

fine ventricular fibrillation Fibrillatory waves less than 3 mm in amplitude.

first stage of labour The stage of labour that begins with the onset of regular contractions and ends with complete dilatation of the cervix.

first-degree burn A burn injury in which only a superficial layer of epidermal cells is destroyed.

first-pass metabolism The initial biotransformation of a drug during passage through the liver from the portal vein that occurs before the drug reaches the general circulation.

fistula An abnormal passage from an internal organ to the body surface.

flail chest A chest wall injury in which three or more adjacent ribs are fractured in two or more places.

flat bones Bones that have a thin, flattened shape, such as certain skull bones, the ribs, the sternum, and scapulae.

flatulence Excessive air or gas in the stomach or intestinal tract, causing distension of the organs and in some cases mild to moderate pain.

flexion Bending.

floating rib See rib.

flora Microorganisms that live on or in the body to compete with disease-producing microorganisms and provide a natural immunity against certain infections.

flutter waves Abnormal P waves in a sawtooth or picket-fence pattern; they represent atrial depolarization in an abnormal direction followed by atrial repolarization.

focal seizure See Jacksonian seizure.

focused history A component of patient assessment to ascertain the patient's chief complaint, history of present illness, medical history, and current health status.

fontanelle A space covered by a tough membrane between the bones of an infant's cranium.

food poisoning Poisoning that results from food contaminated by toxic substances or by bacteria containing toxins.

foramen ovale An opening in the septum between the right and left atria in the fetal heart; it provides a bypass for blood that would otherwise flow to the fetal lungs.

foreign body airway obstruction A disturbance in normal function or a pathological condition caused by an object lodged in the airway.

formed elements Cells and cell fragments of blood.

formic acid A colourless, pungent liquid found in nature in ants and other insects.

fourth-degree burn A full-thickness burn injury that penetrates the subcutaneous tissue, muscle, fascia, periosteum or bone.

fourth ventricle The ventricle located in the superior region of the medulla; continuous with the central canal of the spinal cord.

fracture A break in the continuity of bone or cartilage.

frank breech See front breech.

fraternal twins Two offspring born of the same pregnancy from two ova released simultaneously from the ovary and fertilized at the same time.

French scale system A scale used to denote the size of catheters and other tubular instruments; each unit is roughly equivalent to 0.33 mm in diameter.

frequency The number of repetitive cycles per second completed by a radio wave.

frequency modulation A deviation of carrier frequency in accordance with the strength of applied audio. Frequency modulation is less susceptible to some types of interference than amplitude modulation and typically is used in emergency medical services communications.

front breech A presentation that occurs when the fetal hips are flexed and the legs extend in front of the fetus, making the buttocks the presenting part; also known as a frank breech.

frontal bone The single cranial bone that forms the front of the skull.

frontal lobe The largest of the five lobes that comprise each of the two cerebral hemispheres; it significantly influences personality and is associated with higher mental activities such as planning, judgement, and conceptualization.

frontal plane An imaginary plane that divides the body into front and back or anterior and posterior positions; also known as the coronal plane.

frontal sinus One of a pair of small cavities in the frontal bone of the skull that communicates with the nasal cavity.

frostbite A localized injury that results from environmentally induced freezing of body tissues.

frostnip The mildest form of cold injury; it may be treated without loss of tissue.

full-thickness burn A burn injury in which the entire thickness of the epidermis and dermis is destroyed; also known as a third-degree burn.

functional residual capacity The expiratory reserve volume plus the residual volume; it reflects the amount of gas remaining in the lungs at the end of a normal expiration.

fundus The bottom or rounded end of a hollow organ, such as the fundus of the uterus.

fusion beat A premature ventricular contraction that occurs at approximately the same time that an electrical impulse of the underlying rhythm is activating the ventricles, thereby causing ventricular depolarization to occur simultaneously in two directions; it results in a QRS complex that has the characteristics of the premature ventricular contraction and the QRS complex of the underlying rhythm.

gag reflex A normal neural response triggered by touching the soft palate or posterior pharynx.

gallbladder A pear-shaped excretory sac on the visceral surface of the right lobe of the liver; it serves as a reservoir for bile.

gallows humour Morbid or cynical humour.

ganglia A group of nerve cell bodies in the peripheral nervous system.

gap junction A small channel between cells that allows the passage of ions and small molecules between cells.

gastric gland A gland located in the stomach mucosa.

gastric lavage Irrigation of the stomach with sterile water or normal saline.

gastrin A polypeptide hormone that stimulates the flow of gastric juice and contributes to the stimulus that causes bile and pancreatic enzyme secretion.

gastritis Inflammation of the lining of the stomach; it may be acute or chronic.

gastroenteritis The inflammation of the stomach and intestines that accompanies numerous gastrointestinal disorders.

gastrointestinal Of or pertaining to the organs of the gastrointestinal tract from mouth to anus.

gastrostomy An artificial opening into the stomach.

gating protein A protein that controls the rate at which ions move through an ion channel.

general impression An immediate assessment of the environment and the patient's chief complaint used to determine if the patient is ill or injured and the nature of the illness or the mechanism of injury.

generalized seizure A seizure characterized by a generalized involuntary muscular contraction and cessation of respiration followed by tonic and clonic spasms of the muscles. Formerly referred to as 'grand mal' seizure.

generic name The official, established name assigned to a drug.

genitalia Reproductive organs.

genitourinary Of or pertaining to the genital and urinary systems of the body, the organ structures, the organ functions or both.

German measles See rubella.

gerontology The study of the problems of all aspects of ageing.

gestation The period from fertilization of the ovum until birth.

gestational diabetes mellitus A disorder characterized by impaired ability to metabolize carbohydrates, usually caused by a deficiency of insulin; it occurs in pregnancy and disappears after delivery but in some cases returns years later.

gingiva The portion of the oral mucosa surrounding the tooth.

gingival hypertrophy Swelling of the gums; it is often associated with chronic phenytoin therapy.

gingivostomatitis Multiple, painful ulcers on the gums and mucous membranes of the mouth; the result of a herpes virus infection.

Glasgow Coma Scale A standardized system for assessing the degree of conscious impairment in the critically ill and for predicting the duration and ultimate outcome of coma.

glaucoma A condition in which intraocular pressure increases and causes damage to the optic nerve.

glia limitans A supporting structure of nervous tissue consisting of large, star-shaped cells.

gliding joint See plane joint.

globule A small, spherical mass.

globulin One of a broad category of simple proteins classified by solubility, mobility, and size.

glomerular filtration rate The amount of plasma that filters into Bowman's capsules per minute.

glomerulus The mass of capillary loops at the beginning of each nephron.

glossopharyngeal nerve Either of a pair of cranial nerves essential to the sense of taste, to sensation in some viscera, and to secretion from certain glands.

glottic opening The vocal cords and the space between them.

glottis The space between the vocal cords.

glucagon A hormone produced by the alpha cells in the islets of Langerhans that stimulates the conversion of glycogen to glucose in the liver.

glucocorticoid An adrenocortical steroid hormone that increases gluconeogenesis, exerts an anti-inflammatory effect, and influences many body functions.

gluconeogenesis The formation of glucose from fatty acids and proteins rather than carbohydrates.

glucosuria The abnormal presence of glucose in the urine resulting from large amounts of carbohydrates, from kidney disease, or from a metabolic disease such as diabetes mellitus.

gluteus medius muscle The muscle that originates between the anterior and posterior gluteal lines of the ilium and inserts into the greater trochanter of the femur.

glycogenolysis The breakdown of glycogen to glucose.

glycolysis An anaerobic process during which glucose is converted to pyruvic acid.

glycoprotein Any of a large group of conjugated proteins in which the non-protein substance is a carbohydrate.

goblet cell One of the many specialized cells that secrete mucus and form glands of the epithelium of the stomach, intestine, and parts of the respiratory tract.

goitre A hypertrophic thyroid gland, usually evident as a pronounced swelling in the neck.

golden hour The critical period during which surgical intervention for a trauma patient can enhance survival and reduce complications.

Golgi apparatus Specialized endoplasmic reticulum that concentrates and packages materials for secretion from the cell.

gomphosis An articulation by the insertion of a conic process into a socket, such as the insertion of the root of a tooth into an alveolus of the mandible or maxilla.

gonad A gamete-producing gland, such as an ovary or testis.

gonorrhoea A sexually transmitted disease that results from contact with the causative organism *Neisseria gonorrhoeae*.

gout A disease associated with an inborn error of uric acid metabolism that increases production of or interferes with excretion of uric acid; also known as hyperuricaemia.

gouty arthritis A type of arthritis caused by excess uric acid, which is converted to sodium urate crystals that are deposited in the joints.

graafian follicle See vesicular follicle.

gram A metric unit of mass equal to 1/1000 of a kilogram.

Gram-negative sepsis Sepsis caused by Gram-negative bacteria when the bacterium dies and is broken down in the body.

grand mal seizure See generalized seizure.

grand multipara A woman who has had six deliveries or more (may be cited as 5 or 7 deliveries).

granulosa cell A cell in the layer surrounding the primary follicle.

gravida The number of all current and past pregnancies.

great vessels The large arteries and veins entering and leaving the heart; they include the aorta, the pulmonary arteries and veins, and the superior and inferior venae cavae.

grey matter The grey tissue that makes up the inner core of the spinal column.

groups Subdivisions of the incident command system that encompass specific functional areas of responsibility as deemed necessary by the incident commander.

growth plate The site of bone elongation; also known as the epiphyseal plate.

Guillain–Barré syndrome A rare disease that affects the peripheral nervous system, especially the spinal nerves, but also the cranial nerves; it is associated with a viral infection or immunization.

habituation See drug dependence.

haemasite A small, button-shaped indwelling vascular device usually placed in the upper arm or proximal, anterior thigh; it is similar to an arteriovenous graft but has an external rubber septum sutured to the skin through which a dialysis catheter is inserted for treatment.

haematemesis Vomiting of bright red blood, indicating upper gastrointestinal bleeding.

haematochezia The passage of red blood through the rectum.

haematology The scientific study of blood and blood-forming tissues.

haematoma A closed injury characterized by blood vessel disruption and swelling beneath the epidermis.

haematuria The abnormal presence of blood in the urine.

haemoagglutinin An agglutinin that clumps red blood corpuscles.

haemochromatosis A rare genetic disease of iron metabolism characterized by excess deposition of iron throughout the body.

haemodialysis A procedure in which impurities or wastes are removed from the blood; it is used in treating renal insufficiency and various toxic conditions.

haemoglobin A complex protein–iron compound in the blood that carries oxygen to the cells from the lungs and carbon dioxide away from the cells to the lungs.

haemolysis The breakdown of red blood cells and the release of haemoglobin.

haemolytic anaemia A condition in which delivery of oxygen to tissues is reduced because of an increase in haemolysis of erythrocytes.

haemopericardium An accumulation of blood within the pericardial sac surrounding the heart.

haemoperitoneum The presence of extravasated blood in the peritoneal cavity.

haemophilia A group of hereditary bleeding disorders in which one of the factors necessary for blood coagulation is deficient.

haemophilia A A condition caused by a deficiency of coagulation factor VIII; it is considered the classic type of haemophilia.

haemophilia B A condition caused by a deficiency of coagulation factor IX.

haemopneumothorax See pneumohaemothorax.

haemopoietic tissue Tissue related to the process of formation and development of various types of blood cells.

haemoptysis Coughing up of blood from the respiratory tract.

haemorrhage Escape of blood from the vessels that normally contain it.

haemorrhagic shock Hypoperfusion associated with the sudden and rapid loss of significant amounts of blood.

haemorrhoids Swollen, distended veins (internal, external, or both) in the rectoanal area.

haemostasis The cessation of bleeding by mechanical or chemical means or by substances that arrest the blood flow.

haemostatic An agent that reduces bleeding by speeding clot formation.

haemothorax The accumulation of blood in the pleural space caused by bleeding from the lung parenchyma or damaged vessels.

haemotympanum Blood behind the tympanic membrane from fractures of the temporal bone.

hair follicle An invagination of the epidermis into the dermis that contains the root of the hair and receives the ducts of sebaceous and apocrine glands.

hair papilla A small, cup-shaped cluster of cells located at the base of the follicle where hair growth begins.

hair root The part of the hair that lies hidden in the follicle.

hair shaft The visible part of the hair.

half duplex The use of two different frequencies, one to transmit and one to receive, that cannot be used simultaneously.

half-life The amount of time required to reduce a drug level to one half its initial value.

hallucinations The apparent perception of sights, sounds, and other sensory phenomena that are not actually present.

hantavirus A cause of several different forms of haemorrhagic fever with renal syndrome.

hard palate The floor of the nasal cavity that separates the nasal cavity from the oral cavity.

hazard control The phase of rescue that includes managing, reducing, and minimizing risks from uncontrollable hazards; ensuring scene safety; and providing personal protective equipment that is appropriate for the incident.

head of bone An eminence on a bone by which it articulates with another bone.

Health Professions Council (HPC) The regulator of the paramedic profession.

heart The muscular, cone-shaped organ that pumps blood throughout the body by coordinated nerve impulses and muscular contractions.

heart murmur An abnormal heart sound caused by altered blood flow into a chamber or through a valve.

heat cramps Brief, intermittent, and often severe muscular cramps that frequently occur in muscles fatigued by heavy work or exercise.

heat exhaustion A form of heat illness characterized by minor aberrations in mental status, dizziness, nausea, headache, and mild to moderate increase in core body temperature.

heat stroke A syndrome that occurs when the thermoregulatory mechanisms normally in place to meet the demands of heat stress break down entirely. As a result, the body temperature increases to extreme levels. Multisystem tissue damage and physiological collapse also occur.

hemiblock Failure in conduction of cardiac impulse in either of two main divisions of the left branch of the bundle of His; interruption may occur in the anterior (superior) or posterior (inferior) division.

hemiparesis One-sided weakness.

hemiplegia Paralysis of one side of the body.

hemitransection A cut across the long axis of tissue, such as the spinal cord.

heparin A substance that inhibits blood clotting; it is obtained from the liver.

heparin lock A peripheral vascular access device that has no attached intravenous tubing; it is used to ensure ready access to peripheral veins for brief administration of medications or when frequent intravenous therapy is indicated on an outpatient basis (e.g. chemotherapy).

hepatic artery The branch of the aorta that delivers blood to the liver.

hepatic encephalopathy A type of brain damage caused by liver disease and consequent ammonia intoxication.

hepatic portal system The system that transports blood from the digestive tract to the liver.

hepatitis An inflammatory condition of the liver characterized by jaundice, hepatomegaly, anorexia, abdominal and gastric discomfort, abnormal liver function, clay-coloured stools, and dark urine. Viruses responsible for hepatitis are hepatitis A virus, hepatitis B virus, hepatitis C virus, hepatitis D virus and hepatitis E virus.

hepatomegaly Enlargement of the liver.

Hering–Breuer reflex A reflex in which afferent impulses from stretch receptors in the lungs arrest inspiration.

hernia Protrusion of any organ through an abdominal opening in the muscle wall of the cavity that surrounds it.

herniation A protrusion of a body organ or portion of an organ through an abnormal opening in a membrane, muscle, or other tissue.

herpes Any of several acute inflammatory viral diseases characterized by the eruption of small blisters on the skin and mucous membranes.

herpes simplex virus type 1 An infection caused by the herpes simplex virus; it tends to occur in the facial area, particularly around the mouth and nose.

herpes simplex virus type 2 An infection caused by the herpes simplex virus; it is usually limited to the genital region.

hertz A unit of frequency equal to 1 cycle per second.

hexaxial reference system The system of intersecting lines of the standard limb leads and three other intersecting lines of reference: aV_R, aV_L and aV_F leads.

hiatal hernia Protrusion of a portion of the stomach upward through the diaphragm.

Hickman catheter A long indwelling catheter sometimes used by patients with cancer, gastrointestinal dysfunction, or debilitating disease and by those who need intermittent intravenous administration of antibiotics, nutritional supplements, or other intravenous medications.

high-altitude cerebral oedema The most severe form of acute high-altitude illness. It is characterized by a progression of global cerebral signs in the presence of acute mountain sickness.

high-altitude pulmonary oedema A high-altitude illness thought to be caused at least partly by an increase in pulmonary artery pressure that develops in response to hypoxia.

high-grade atrioventricular block Occurs when at least two consecutive atrioventricular impulses (atrial P waves) fail to be conducted to the ventricles.

hilum A depression or pit at the part of an organ where the vessels and nerves enter.

hinge joint A joint that consists of a convex cylinder in one bone applied to a corresponding concavity in another bone; this type of joint allows movement in one plane only.

histamine An amine released by mast cells and basophils that promotes inflammation.

history taking Information gathered during the patient interview.

Hodgkin's disease A malignant disorder characterized by pain and progressive enlargement of lymphoid tissue.

homeopathic Pertaining to homeopathy, a system of therapeutics in which diseases are treated with small doses of drugs that, in larger doses, are capable of producing in healthy persons symptoms like those of the disease to be treated.

homeostasis A state of equilibrium in the body with respect to functions and composition of fluids and tissues.

horizontal plane Any place of the erect body parallel to the horizon; dividing the body into upper and lower parts.

human immunodeficiency virus The viral agent responsible for acquired immunodeficiency syndrome.

humerus The largest bone of the upper arm, comprising a body, head and condyle.

humoral immunity One of the two forms of immunity that respond to antigens such as bacteria and foreign tissue.

Huntington's disease A rare, hereditary disease characterized by quick, involuntary movements, speech disturbances, and mental deterioration; it is caused by degenerative changes in the cerebral cortex and basal ganglia; also known as Huntington's chorea.

hyaline cartilage Gelatinous, glossy cartilage tissue; it thinly covers the articulating ends of bones, connects the ribs to the sternum, and supports the nose, trachea and part of the larynx.

hydrocephalus A pathological condition characterized by an abnormal accumulation of cerebrospinal fluid, usually under increased pressure, within the cranial vault, resulting in dilatation of the ventricles.

hydrochloric acid The acid in gastric juice.

hydrogen ion The acidic element in a solution.

hymen A mucous membrane that may partly or entirely occlude the vaginal outlet.

Hymenoptera A large, highly specialized order of insects that includes wasps, bees and ants.

hyoid bone The U-shaped bone between the mandible and the larynx.

hyperbilirubinaemia Larger than normal amounts of the bile pigment bilirubin in the blood, often characterized by jaundice, anorexia, and malaise.

hypercalcaemia A higher than normal concentration of calcium in the blood.

hypercholesterolaemia Increased serum cholesterol.

hypercoagulability A tendency of the blood to coagulate more rapidly than normal.

hyperglycaemia A greater than normal amount of glucose in the blood.

hyperkalaemia A higher than normal concentration of potassium in the blood.

hyperkaluria A high potassium concentration in the urine.

hyperlipidaemia An excess of lipids in the plasma.

hypermagnesaemia A higher than normal concentration of magnesium in the blood.

hypernatraemia A greater than normal concentration of sodium in the blood.

hyperosmolar hyperglycaemic non-ketotic coma A diabetic coma in which the level of ketone bodies is normal. It is caused by hyperosmolarity of extracellular fluid and results in dehydration of intracellular fluid.

hyperparathyroidism A condition of increased parathyroid function.

hyperphosphataemia High levels of alkaline phosphate in the blood.

hyperplasia An excessive increase in the number of cells.

hyperpolarization An increase in the charge difference across the cell membrane; it causes the charge difference to move away from 0 mV.

hypersensitivity reaction An altered immunological response to an antigen that results in a pathological immune response upon re-exposure.

hypersomnia Excessive drowsiness; a sleep disorder of excessive depth or duration.

hypertension A disorder characterized by elevated blood pressure, which persistently exceeds 140/90 mmHg.

hypertensive crisis A sudden, severe increase in blood pressure greater than 200/120 mmHg.

hypertensive encephalopathy A set of symptoms – including headache, convulsions and coma – that result solely from elevated blood pressure.

hyperthermia Abnormal elevation of body temperature.

hyperthyroidism A condition characterized by increased activity of the thyroid gland.

hypertonic A term used to describe a solution that causes cells to shrink.

hypertrophy An increase in the size of a cell.

hyperuricaemia See gout.

hyperventilation syndrome Abnormally deep or rapid breathing that results in excessive loss of carbon dioxide (producing respiratory alkalosis).

hyphaema Haemorrhage into the anterior chamber of the eye; it usually is a result of blunt trauma.

hypocalcaemia A lower than normal concentration of calcium in the blood.

hypocarbia A state of diminished carbon dioxide in the blood; also known as hypocapnia.

hypochlorhydria A deficiency of hydrochloric acid in the gastric juice of the stomach.

hypoglycaemia A lower than normal amount of glucose in the blood.

hypokalaemia A lower than normal concentration of potassium in the blood.

hypomagnesaemia A lower than normal concentration of magnesium in the blood plasma.

hyponatraemia A lower than normal concentration of sodium in the blood.

hyponatraemic A term describing a lower than normal concentration of sodium in the blood.

hypoparathyroidism A condition of diminished parathyroid function.

hypoperfusion Severely inadequate circulation that results in insufficient delivery of oxygen and nutrients necessary for normal tissue and cellular function. Also known as shock.

hypopituitarism An abnormal condition caused by diminished activity of the pituitary gland; it is marked by excessive deposits of fat or acquisition of adolescent characteristics.

hypopyon An accumulation of pus in the anterior chamber of the eye.

hypotension An abnormal condition in which the blood pressure is not adequate for normal perfusion and oxygenation of the tissues.

hypothalamus A portion of the diencephalon of the brain that activates, controls, and integrates the peripheral autonomic nervous system, endocrine processes, and many somatic functions such as body temperature, sleep, and appetite.

hypothermia An abnormal body temperature below 35 °C (95 °F).

hypothyroidism A condition characterized by decreased activity of the thyroid gland.

hypotonia A condition of diminished tone or tension that may involve any body structure.

hypotonic A term used to describe a solution that causes cells to swell.

hypotonicity of the muscles Decreased muscle tone or tension.

hypovolaemia An abnormally low circulating blood volume.

hypovolaemic shock A form of shock most frequently caused by haemorrhage but also caused by dehydration.

hypoxaemia A state of decreased oxygen content of arterial blood.

hypoxia A state of decreased oxygen content at the tissue level.

hypoxic drive The low arterial oxygen pressure stimulus to respiration that is mediated through the carotid bodies.

hysterectomy The surgical removal of the uterus.

iatrogenic Caused by treatment or diagnostic procedures.

identical twins Two offspring born of the same pregnancy and developed from a single fertilized ovum that splits into equal halves during the early phase of embryonic development, giving rise to separate fetuses.

idiopathic epilepsy See primary epilepsy.

idiosyncrasy An abnormal or peculiar response to a drug.

idioventricular rhythm A ventricular escape rhythm that results when impulses from higher pacemakers fail to reach the ventricles or when the rate of discharge of higher pacemakers become less than that of the ventricles.

ileocaecal sphincter The valve between the ileum of the small intestine and the caecum of the large intestine.

ileostomy A surgical opening into the small intestine.

ileum The distal portion of the small intestine.

ileus An obstruction of the intestines.

iliac crest The upper free margin of the ilium.

iliac spine A portion of the iliac crest; the flaring portion of the hipbone.

ilium One of the three bones that make up the innominate bone.

immersion hypothermia Hypothermia from immersion in cold water.

immune response A defence function of the body that produces antibodies to destroy invading antigens and malignancies.

immunity Insusceptibility to a particular disease or condition.

immunization The process of rendering a person immune or of becoming immune.

immunogen Any agent or substance capable of an immune response or of producing immunity.

immunoglobulin Any of five structurally and antigenically distinct antibodies present in the serum and external secretions of the body; they are IgA, IgD, IgE, IgG, and IgM.

implied consent The presumption that an unconscious or incompetent person would consent to lifesaving care.

incident command system A management programme designed to control, direct, and coordinate emergency response operations and resources.

incomplete abortion An abortion in which the patient has passed some but not all of the products of conception.

incomplete breech The presentation that occurs when the fetus has one or both hips incompletely flexed, resulting in the presentation of one or both lower extremities, often a foot.

incontinence The inability to control bladder or bowel function.

incubation period The stage of infection during which an organism reproduces; it begins with invasion of an agent and ends when the disease process begins.

incus The middle of the three ossicles in the middle ear.

induced abortion The intentional termination of a pregnancy.

infectious disease Any illness that is caused by a specific microorganism.

infectious pericarditis Inflammation of the pericardium associated with infection.

inferior Toward the feet; below a point of reference in the anatomical position.

inferior nasal concha One of three bony ridges on the lateral wall of the nasal cavity.

inferior vena cava The vein that returns blood from the lower limbs and the greater part of the pelvic and abdominal organs to the right atrium.

infertility The inability to produce offspring.

infiltration The process whereby a fluid passes into tissues.

inflammatory response A tissue reaction to injury or an antigen; it may include pain, swelling, itching, redness, heat and loss of function.

influenza A highly contagious infection of the respiratory tract transmitted by airborne droplet infection. Researchers have identified three main types of the virus (types A, B and C).

informed consent Consent obtained from a patient after explaining all facts necessary for the patient to make a reasonable decision.

inguinal canal The passage through the lower abdominal wall that transmits the spermatic cord in the male and the round ligament in the female.

inguinal node One of approximately 18 nodes in the group of lymph glands in the upper femoral triangle of the thigh.

inhalation injury An upper and/or lower airway injury that results from thermal and/or chemical exposure.

initial assessment/primary survey A component of the patient assessment to recognize and manage all immediate life-threatening conditions.

injury risk Real or potentially hazardous situations that put individuals at increased risk for sustaining an injury.

injury surveillance The ongoing systematic collection, analysis, and interpretation of injury data essential to the planning, implementation, and evaluation of public health practice.

inner ear The part of the ear that contains the sensory organs for hearing and balance.

inotropic Pertaining to the force or energy of muscle contraction, particularly contractions of the heart.

insertion The more movable attachment point of a muscle.

insomnia A chronic inability to sleep or to remain asleep throughout the night.

inspection A visual assessment of the patient and surroundings.

inspiration The act of drawing air into the lungs.

inspiratory capacity The sum of the tidal volume and the inspiratory reserve volume.

inspiratory centre The region of the medulla that stimulates inspiration.

inspiratory reserve volume The maximum volume of air that can be inspired after a normal inspiration.

insulin A hormone secreted by the pancreatic islets.

integumentary system The largest organ system in the body, consisting of the skin and accessory structures.

interatrial septum Tissue that separates the right and left atria of the heart.

intercalated disc Cell-to-cell attachment with gap junctions between cardiac muscle cells.

intercellular Occurring between or among cells.

interference Any undesired radio signal on a radio frequency. It may arise from other radio transmitters or other sources of electromagnetic radiation. 'Nuisance interference' is interference that can be heard but does not override system signals. 'Destructive interference' overrides system signals.

internal anal sphincter A sphincter muscle located at the caudal end of the rectum.

internal carotid artery Each of two arteries that enter the cranial vault through the carotid canals.

internal jugular vein One of a pair of veins in the neck; each collects blood from one side of the brain, the face, and the neck, and both unite with the subclavian vein to form the brachiocephalic vein.

internal mammary artery One of the pair of arteries that arise from the first portions of the subclavian arteries; it supplies the pectoral muscles, breasts, pericardium and abdominal muscles; also known as the internal thoracic artery.

internal thoracic artery See internal mammary artery.

internal urinary sphincter The smooth muscle of the bladder located at the junction of the urethra with the urinary bladder; it controls the flow of urine through the urethra.

interneuron See motor neuron.

internodal tract Pathways between the segments of a nerve fibre.

interpolated premature ventricular contraction A premature ventricular contraction that falls between two sinus beats without interrupting the rhythm.

interstitial fluid Fluid that occupies the space outside the blood vessels and/or outside of cells of an organ or tissue.

interventricular foramen One of two passageways between the two lateral ventricles and the third ventricle.

interventricular septum The tissue that separates the right and left ventricles of the heart.

intervertebral disc One of the fibrous discs between all adjacent spinal vertebrae except the atlas and axis; it serves as a shock absorber for the vertebral column and provides additional support for the body; it also prevents the vertebral bodies from rubbing against each other.

intracellular Occurring within cell membranes.

intracellular fluid The fluid found in all body cells.

intracerebral haematoma An accumulation of blood or fluid within the tissue of the brain.

intradermal injection The introduction of a substance (e.g. serum or vaccine) with a hypodermic needle into the dermis.

intramuscular injection The introduction of medication with a hypodermic needle into muscle.

intraocular pressure Pressure within the eye that keeps the eye inflated.

intraosseous infusion Placement of a rigid needle into a bone and the infusion of fluid and medication directly into the bone marrow.

intraosseous injection The introduction of medication or fluid into the bone marrow.

intrapartum The period during labour and delivery.

intrapleural Within the pleura.

intrapleural pressure See intrathoracic pressure.

intrapulmonic pressure The pressure of the gas within the alveoli.

intrathecal injection The introduction of medication with a hypodermic needle into the subarachnoid space.

intrathoracic pressure The pressure in the pleural space; also known as intrapleural pressure.

intravenous injection The introduction of medication with a hypodermic needle into a vein.

intrinsic factor The factor secreted by the parietal cells of the gastric glands; it is required for adequate absorption of vitamin B_{12}.

invagination Infolding or in-pocketing.

invasion of privacy Making public, without legal justification, details about a person's private life that might reasonably expose that person to ridicule, notoriety or embarrassment.

inversion Turning inward.

involuntary Occurring without conscious control or direction.

involuntary guarding An unconscious rigid contraction of the abdominal muscles; a sign of peritoneal inflammation.

involuntary muscle A muscle that is not normally consciously controlled; see smooth muscle.

ion An atom or group of atoms carrying a charge of electricity by virtue of having gained or lost one or more electrons.

ipsilateral Pertaining to the same side of the body.

iris The coloured contractile membrane of the eye that can be seen through the cornea.

iron deficiency anaemia Anaemia caused by inadequate supplies of iron needed to synthesize haemoglobin.

irregular bones Bones that are not representative of the other three categories (long, short, or flat bones); examples include vertebrae and facial bones.

ischaemia A state of insufficient perfusion of oxygenated blood to a body organ or part.

ischium One of the three parts of the hipbone, which joins the ilium and the pubis to form the acetabulum.

islets of Langerhans Clusters of cells within the pancreas that produce insulin, glucagon, and pancreatic polypeptide.

isoimmunity An immune response directed against beneficial foreign tissues.

isolette A self-contained incubator unit that provides controlled heat, humidity and oxygen for the isolation and care of premature and low-birth-weight neonates.

isometric contraction A muscle contraction in which the length of the muscle does not change, but the tension produced increases.

isotonic A term used to describe a solution that causes cells neither to shrink nor to swell.

isotonic contraction A muscle contraction in which the tension produced by the muscle stays the same, but the muscle length becomes shorter.

J point The point at which the T wave takes off from the QRS complex.

Jacksonian seizure A transitory disturbance in motor, sensory or autonomic function resulting from abnormal neuronal discharges in a localized part of the brain; also known as a focal seizure.

jaundice A yellow discoloration of the skin, mucous membranes, and sclerae of the eyes caused by a greater than normal amount of bilirubin in the blood.

jejunum One of the three portions of the small intestine.

joint Any one of the connections between bones that are classified according to structure and movability as fibrous, cartilaginous, or synovial. Fibrous joints are immovable, cartilaginous joints are slightly movable, and synovial joints are freely movable.

joint capsule A well-defined structure that encloses a joint.

joint dislocation An injury that occurs when the normal articulating ends of two or more bones are displaced.

Joule's law The principle that the amount of heat produced is directly proportional to the square of the current strength times the resistance of the tissue times the duration of the current flow.

jugular notch The superior margin of the manubrium; it is palpated easily at the anterior base of the neck; also known as the suprasternal notch.

jugular vein distension Engorgement of jugular veins caused by an increase in central venous pressure; it is estimated by positioning the head of a supine patient at a 45-degree angle and observing the neck veins.

kallikrein/kinin system A hormonal system that functions within the kidneys, mediating production of bradykinin, which acts as a vasodilator peptide.

Kaposi's sarcoma A malignant, multifocal neoplasm of reticuloendothelial cells that begins as soft, brownish or purple papules on the feet and slowly spreads in the skin, metastasizing to the lymph nodes and viscera; it is associated with diabetes, malignant lymphoma, acquired immune deficiency syndrome and other disorders.

Kehr sign Pain in the left shoulder thought to be caused by referred pain secondary to irritation of the adjacent diaphragm.

Kent fibres See bundle of Kent.

keratitis Any inflammation of the cornea.

ketoacidosis Acidosis accompanied by the accumulation of ketones in the body, resulting from faulty carbohydrate metabolism.

ketoacids Compounds containing the carbonyl and carboxyl groups.

ketogenesis The formation or production of ketone bodies.

ketone bodies The normal metabolic products of lipid and pyruvate within the liver; excessive production leads to their excretion in urine.

ketonuria Presence in the urine of excessive amounts of ketone bodies.

kidney The organ that cleanses the body of the waste products continually produced by metabolism.

kilogram A metric unit of mass equal to 1000 grams or 2.2046 pounds.

kilohertz A unit of frequency equal to 1000 cycles per second.

kinematics The process of predicting injury patterns that can result from the forces and motions of energy.

kinin Serum protein that causes vasodilatation and increases vascular permeability.

Koplik's spots Small red spots with bluish white centres on the lingual and buccal mucosa, characteristic of measles.

Korsakoff's psychosis A form of amnesia often seen in alcoholic-dependent people, characterized by a loss of short-term memory and an inability to learn new skills.

Krebs cycle A sequence of enzymatic reactions involving the metabolism of carbon chains of sugar, fatty acids, and amino acids to yield carbon dioxide, water and high-energy phosphate bonds.

Kussmaul's respiration An abnormally deep, rapid sighing respiratory pattern characteristic of diabetic ketoacidosis or other metabolic acidosis.

kyphosis An abnormal condition of the vertebral column characterized by increased convexity in the curvature of the thoracic spine as viewed from the side.

labia majora Two rounded folds of skin surrounding the labia minora and the vestibule.

labia minora Two longitudinal folds of mucous membrane enclosed by the labia majora and bounding the vestibule.

labial frenulum A medial fold of mucous membrane connecting the inside of each lip to the corresponding gum.

laceration A torn or jagged wound.

lacrimal bone One of the smallest and most fragile bones of the face; it is located in the anterior part of the medial wall of the orbit.

lacrimal canal The canal that carries excess tears away from the eye.

lacrimal gland The tear gland located in the superolateral corner of the orbit.

lacrimal sac An enlargement of the lacrimal canal that leads into the nasolacrimal duct.

lacrimation Excessive tear production.

lactate A salt of lactic acid.

lactation The secretion of milk from the breasts to nourish an infant or child.

lactic acid A three-carbon molecule derived from pyruvic acid as a product of anaerobic respiration.

lactic acidosis A disorder characterized by an accumulation of lactic acid in the blood, resulting in a lowered pH in muscle and serum.

lactiferous duct The duct that drains the grape-like cluster of milk-secreting glands in the breast.

lactose intolerance A sensitivity disorder resulting in the inability to digest lactose because of a deficiency of or defect in the enzyme lactase.

landing zone An area prepared for the landing of an aircraft.

lanugo hair Soft, downy hair covering a normal fetus.

laparoscopy Examination of the abdominal cavity with a laparoscope.

large intestine The portion of the digestive tract comprising the caecum, the appendix, the ascending, transverse, and descending colons and the rectum.

laryngectomy Surgical removal of the larynx, performed to treat cancer of the larynx.

laryngopharynx The lowest part of the pharynx.

laryngoscope An endoscope for visualization of the larynx.

laryngoscopy Examination of the larynx via a laryngoscope.

laryngotracheobronchitis See croup.

larynx The voice box, located just below the pharynx.

latent period A stage of infection that begins when a pathogenic agent invades the body and ends when the agent can be shed or communicated.

latent period of drug action See onset of action.

lateral malleolus The rounded process on the lateral side of the ankle joint.

lateral recumbent position The position in which the patient is lying on his or her right or left side.

lateral ventricle A large, fluid-filled space in each cerebral hemisphere.

laxative A substance that causes evacuation of the bowel by increasing the bulk of the faeces, by softening the stool, or by lubricating the intestinal wall.

lead An electrode sensor attached to the body to record electrical activity, especially of the heart and brain.

Le Fort fracture A fracture pattern that can be produced in the midface region.

left anterior descending artery The subdivision of the left coronary artery that supplies the left auricle and its appendix and supplies branches to both ventricles and numerous small branches to the pulmonary artery and commencement of the aorta.

left coronary artery One of a pair of branches from the ascending aorta that supplies both ventricles and the left atrium.

legionellosis An acute bacterial pneumonia caused by infection with *Legionella pneumophila*; it is characterized by an influenza-like illness followed within a week by high fever, chills, muscle aches, and headache.

legionnaires' disease See legionellosis.

Lenègre's disease See Lev's disease.

lens The crystalline portion of the eye.

lethargy A state of indifference, apathy, or sluggishness.

leukaemia A malignant neoplasm of blood-forming organs.

leukocyte White blood cell.

leukocytosis An abnormal increase in the number of circulating white blood cells.

leukotrienes A class of biologically active compounds that occur naturally in leukocytes and that produce allergic and inflammatory reactions.

Lev's disease Third-degree block in the elderly from chronic degenerative changes in the conduction system; it is not usually associated with increased parasympathetic tone or drug toxicity; also known as Lenègre's disease.

libel Publishing in writing false statements about someone, knowing them to be false, with malicious intent or with reckless disregard for their falsity.

libido The drive associated with sexual desire, pleasure or creativity.

life threat An illness or injury that threatens survival.

ligament A band of white, fibrous tissue that connects bones.

ligamentum arteriosum A fibrous cord from the pulmonary artery to the branch of the aorta; the remains of the ductus arteriosus of the fetus.

limbic system The part of the brain involved with emotions and olfaction.

linear fracture A fracture that extends parallel to the long axis of a bone but does not displace the bone tissue.

lingual tonsil A collection of lymphoid tissue on the posterior portion of the dorsum of the tongue.

lipid Any of the free fatty acid fractions in the blood.

lipid bilayer The central layer of the cytoplasmic membrane; it is composed of a double layer of lipid molecules.

lipodystrophy Any abnormality in the metabolism or distribution of fats.

lipoprotein A conjugated protein in which lipids form an integral part of the molecule; it is synthesized primarily in the liver.

liquefaction Conversion of solid tissues to a fluid or semi-fluid state.

litre A metric unit of capacity equal to 1 cubic decimetre or 61.025 cubic inches.

Littre's gland The inner surface of the membrane lining the urethra.

loading dose A large quantity of drug that temporarily exceeds the capacity of the body to excrete the drug.

lobule A small lobe or subdivision of a lobe.

long bones Bones that are longer than they are wide, such as the humerus, ulna, radius, femur, tibia, fibula, and phalanges.

long saphenous vein See saphenous vein.

loop diuretic A group of powerful, short-acting agents that inhibit sodium and chloride reabsorption in the loop of Henle, resulting in an excessive loss of potassium and water and an increase in the excretion of sodium.

loop of Henle The U-shaped portion of the renal tubule.

lordosis An inward curvature in the lumbar spine that is normally present to some degree.

lower oesophageal sphincter The ring of muscle located at the inferior end of the oesophagus that regulates the passage of materials out of the oesophagus.

lucid interval A period of relative mental clarity between periods of decreased consciousness or irrationality.

lumbar vertebrae The five largest segments of the movable part of the vertebral column; they are designated L1 to L5.

lumbosacral plexus The combination of all the ventral primary divisions of the lumbar, sacral, and coccygeal nerves.

lumen A cavity or channel within any organ or structure of the body.

Lund and Browder chart A method to estimate burn injury that assigns specific numbers to each body part and that accounts for developmental changes in percentages of body surface area.

lung One of a pair of light, spongy organs in the thorax; the main component of the respiratory system.

lunula The crescent-shaped white area of the nail; it is most visible on the thumbnail.

luxation A complete dislocation.

Lyme disease An acute, recurrent inflammatory infection transmitted by a tick.

lymph node An encapsulated mass of lymph tissue found among lymph vessels.

lymphangitis An inflammation of one or more lymphatic vessels.

lymphatic system The network of vessels, ducts, nodes, valves and organs involved in protecting and maintaining the internal fluid environment of the body.

lymphocyte A type of white blood cell formed in lymphoid tissue.

lymphokine One of the chemical factors produced and released by T lymphocytes that attract macrophages to the site of infection or inflammation.

lymphoma A group of diseases that range from slowly growing chronic disorders to rapidly evolving acute conditions.

lyse To cause decomposition.

lysis The process by which a cell swells and ruptures.

lysosome A membranous-walled organelle that contains enzymes, which enable it to function as an intracellular digestive system.

macrodrip tubing An apparatus used to deliver measured amounts of intravenous solutions at specific flow rates based on the size of drops of the solution. The drops delivered by a macrodrip are larger than those delivered by a microdrip.

macromolecule A molecule of colloidal size, such as a protein, nucleic acid or polysaccharide.

macrophage A phagocytic cell in the immune system.

macula A small pigmented area that appears separate or different than the surrounding tissue.

maintenance dose The amount of a drug required to keep a desired steady state of drug concentration in tissues.

major incident An event for which available resources are insufficient to manage the nature of the emergency.

malaise A vague feeling of weakness or discomfort.

malar eminence The zygomatic bone or cheekbone.

malaria A serious infectious illness caused by one or more of at least four species of the protozoan genus *Plasmodium*; it is characterized by chills, fever, anaemia and an enlarged spleen.

malignant Dangerous to health; characterized by progressive and uncontrolled growth.

malleolus A rounded, bony process, such as the protuberance on each side of the ankle.

malleus The largest of the three ossicles in the middle ear.

Mallory–Weiss syndrome A condition characterized by massive bleeding after a tear in the mucous membrane at the junction of the oesophagus and the stomach.

mamma The breast; the organ of milk secretion.

mammalian diving reflex A reflex triggered by immersing the face in cold water; it diverts blood from the arms and legs to the central circulation and lowers the heart rate as a result of vagal stimulation.

mammary gland An external accessory sex organ in females; breasts.

mandible A large bone that constitutes the lower jaw.

mania A mood disorder characterized by extreme excitement, hyperactivity, agitation, and sometimes violent and self-destructive behaviour.

manic Pertaining to a specific psychosis.

manic–depressive disorder See bipolar disorder.

manubriosternal junction The point at which the manubrium joins the body of the sternum; the location of the second rib; also known as the sternal angle.

manubrium One of the three bones of the sternum; it has a broad, quadrangular shape that narrows caudally at its articulation with the superior end of the body of the sternum.

Marfan syndrome An abnormal condition characterized by elongation of the bones, often with associated abnormalities of the eyes and cardiovascular system.

mass casualty incident An event for which available resources are insufficient to manage the number of casualties.

mastectomy Surgical removal of one or both breasts, performed to remove a malignant tumour.

mastication Chewing, tearing, or grinding food with the teeth while it is mixed with saliva.

mastoid air cell One of several spaces within the mastoid process of the temporal bone; it is connected to the middle ear by ducts.

maxilla One of a pair of large bones that form the upper jaw.

maxillary sinus One of the pair of large air cells that form a pyramidal cavity in the body of the maxilla.

McBurney point A site of extreme sensitivity in acute appendicitis situated in the normal area of the appendix, approximately 5 cm (2 inches) from the right anterior–superior spine of the ilium, on a line between that spine and the umbilicus.

mean arterial pressure The arithmetic mean of the blood pressure in the arterial portion of the circulation.

measles An acute, highly contagious viral disease involving the respiratory tract that is characterized by a spreading, maculopapular, cutaneous rash.

meconium aspiration syndrome Inhalation of meconium by the fetus or newborn; the meconium can block the air passages and result in failure of the lungs to expand or cause other pulmonary dysfunction.

meconium staining The presence of fetal stool in amniotic fluid.

medial malleolus The rounded process on the medial side of the ankle joint.

mediastinitis Inflammation of the mediastinum.

mediastinum A portion of the thoracic cavity in the middle of the thorax between the pleural sacs containing the two lungs; it extends from the sternum to the vertebral column and contains all the thoracic viscera except the lungs.

mediated transport mechanisms Mechanisms that use carrier molecules to move large, water-soluble molecules or electrically charged molecules across cell membranes.

medical asepsis The removal or destruction of disease-causing organisms or infected material.

medulla The lowest part of the brainstem, which controls vital functions; an enlarged extension of the spinal cord; also known as the medulla oblongata.

medulla oblongata See medulla.

medullary cavity A large, marrow-filled cavity in the diaphysis of a long bone.

megahertz A unit of frequency equal to 1 million cycles per second; emergency medical services radios transmit and receive on frequencies measured in megahertz.

melaena Abnormal black, tarry stools containing digested blood.

melanocyte A body cell capable of producing melanin.

melatonin The only hormone secreted in the bloodstream by the pineal gland; it lightens skin pigmentation and may inhibit numerous endocrine functions.

membrane channel A tunnel through which specific molecules may pass.

membranous labyrinth A membranous structure within the inner ear; it forms the cochlea, vestibule and semicircular canals.

menarche The first menstruation and commencement of the cyclic menstrual function.

meninges Fluid-containing membranes surrounding the brain and spinal cord.

meningitis Inflammation of the meninges.

menopause The cessation of menses.

menstruation The periodic discharge through the vagina of a blood secretion containing tissue debris from the shedding of the endometrium from the non-pregnant uterus.

mental illness Any form of psychiatric disorder.

mental status examination An evaluation tool that includes an assessment of appearance and behaviour, speech and language, emotional stability, and cognitive abilities.

merocrine gland A gland that secretes products with no loss of cellular material, such as a water-producing sweat gland.

mesencephalon See midbrain.

mesentery The double layer of peritoneum extending from the abdominal wall to the abdominal viscera; it conveys vessels and nerves.

mesovarium A short peritoneal fold connecting the ovary with the broad ligament of the uterus.

metabolic acidosis A disorder that results when excess acid is added to the body fluids or bicarbonate is lost from them.

metabolic alkalosis A disorder that results from a significant loss of acid in the body or increased levels of base bicarbonate.

metabolism The culmination of all chemical processes that take place in living organisms.

metabolite A substance that is produced by metabolic action or that is necessary for the metabolic process.

metacarpal One of five bones extending from the carpus to the phalanges.

metaplasia A change from one cell type to another that is better able to tolerate adverse conditions; a conversion into a form that is not normal for that cell.

metarteriole One of the small peripheral blood vessels that contain scattered groups of smooth muscle fibres in their walls; they are located between the arterioles and the true capillaries.

metatarsal Any one of the five bones comprising the metatarsus.

methaemoglobin A form of haemoglobin in which the iron component has been oxidized from the ferrous to the ferric state.

methaemoglobinaemia The presence of methaemoglobin in the blood, causing cyanosis as a result of the inability of the red blood cells to release oxygen.

methanol A chemical widely used as a solvent and in the production of formaldehyde.

metre A metric unit of length equal to 1000 millimetres.

microdrip tubing An apparatus for delivering relatively small amounts of intravenous solutions at specific flow rates; the drops delivered by a microdrip are smaller than those delivered by a macrodrip.

microgram A metric unit of mass equal to 1/1 000 000 of a gram.

microinfarct A small infarct caused by obstruction of circulation in capillaries, arterioles or small arteries.

microorganism Any tiny, usually microscopic entity capable of carrying on living processes, such as bacteria, fungi, protozoa and viruses.

microthrombus A minute thrombus.

microtubule A hollow tube that helps to support the cytoplasm of the cell; a component of certain cell organelles such as centrioles, spindle fibres, cilia and flagella.

microwave Radio waves with frequencies of 890 MHz and upward. The signals are generated by special equipment that depends on line of sight placement to operate properly. Microwave channels may have a wide band to carry a large number of simultaneous transmissions.

midbrain One of the three parts of the brainstem; also known as the mesencephalon.

middle cerebral artery The artery that supplies a large portion of the lateral cerebral cortex.

middle ear An air-filled space within the temporal bone that contains the auditory ossicles.

migraine A severe, incapacitating headache that is often preceded by visual and/or gastrointestinal disturbances.

milliequivalent 1/1000 of a gram equivalent.

milligram A metric unit of mass equal to 1/1000 of a gram.

millilitre A metric unit of capacity equal to 1/1000 of a litre.

millimetre A metric unit of length equal to 1/1000 of a metre.

mineral An inorganic substance usually referred to by the name of the compound of which it is a part; minerals are important in regulating many body functions.

mineralocorticoid A hormone secreted by the adrenal cortex that maintains normal blood volume, promotes sodium and water retention, and increases urine secretion of potassium and hydrogen ions.

minimal effective concentration The lowest plasma concentration that produces the desired drug effect.

minute alveolar ventilation The amount of inspired gas available for gas exchange during 1 minute.

minute volume The amount of gas inhaled or exhaled in 1 minute. It is found by multiplying the tidal volume by the respiratory rate.

miscarriage See spontaneous abortion.

missed abortion The retention of the fetus in utero for 4 or more weeks after fetal death.

mitochondria Small, spherical, rod-shaped, or thin filamentous structures in the cytoplasm of cells; a site of adenosine triphosphate production.

mitosis Cell division resulting in two daughter cells with exactly the same number and type of chromosomes as the mother cell.

mitral valve See bicuspid valve.

mitral valve prolapse Protrusion of one or both cusps of the mitral valve back into the left atrium during ventricular systole, resulting in incomplete closure of the valve and mitral insufficiency.

mittelschmerz Abdominal pain in the region of the ovary during ovulation; it usually occurs midway through the menstrual cycle.

MMR vaccine The abbreviation for live measles, mumps and rubella virus vaccine.

mobile data terminal A computer connected through a modem ('black box') with a radio that sends and receives pretyped messages to printers, computer screens, or both. Some mobile data terminals have graphics (floor plans) and database (hazardous materials) capabilities. Mobile data terminals rely on a host computer interfaced to a base station.

mobile relay station A fixed base station that automatically retransmits mobile or portable radio communications back to the receiving frequency of other portables, mobiles, and base stations operating in the same system; also known as a repeater.

mobile repeater A mobile radio unit capable of automatically retransmitting any radio traffic originated by a handheld portable, by other mobiles, or by base stations. This repeater may be one-way or two-way and may also be known as a vehicle repeater.

mole A standard unit used to measure the amount of a substance.

monocyte A type of white blood cell found in lymph nodes, spleen, bone marrow and loose connective tissue.

monomorphic Existing only in one form.

mons pubis The prominence caused by a pad of fatty tissue over the symphysis pubis in the female.

morals Social standards or customs; dealing with what is right or wrong in a practical sense.

Moro reflex A normal infant response elicited by a sudden loud noise. The infant flexes the legs, makes an embracing gesture with the arms, and usually gives a brief cry.

morphology The study of the physical shape and size of a specimen, plant, or animal.

motor neuron A neuron that innervates skeletal, smooth or cardiac muscle fibres.

mucin The chief ingredient in mucus.

mucosa Mucous membrane.

mucus The viscous, slippery secretion of mucous membranes and glands.

multifocal premature ventricular contraction Premature ventricular complexes that originate from multiple sites in the ventricles.

multigravida A woman who has had two or more pregnancies.

multipara A woman who has had two or more deliveries.

multiple gestation A pregnancy with more than one fetus.

multiple myeloma A malignant neoplasm of the bone marrow.

multiple organ dysfunction syndrome The progressive failure of two or more organ systems after a severe illness or injury.

multiple sclerosis A progressive disease of the central nervous system in which scattered patches of myelin in the brain and spinal cord are destroyed.

multiplex mode A communications mode with the ability to transmit two or more different types of information simultaneously, in either or both directions, over the same frequency.

mumps An acute viral disease characterized by swelling of the parotid glands.

muscarinic receptor A class of cholinergic receptor molecule specifically activated by muscarine in addition to acetylcholine.

muscular dystrophy An inherited muscle disorder of unknown cause marked by a slow but progressive degeneration of muscle fibres.

muscular tissue A primary tissue type characterized by its contractile abilities.

mutagenic Any chemical or physical environmental agent that induces a genetic mutation or increases the mutation rate.

myalgia Diffuse muscle pain, usually accompanied by malaise; it occurs in many infectious diseases.

myasthenia Muscle weakness.

myasthenia gravis An autoimmune disorder in which muscles become weak and tire easily.

Mycobacterium leprae A species of Gram-positive bacteria that causes leprosy.

Mycobacterium tuberculosis A species of Gram-positive bacteria that causes tuberculosis.

Mycoplasma A genus of microscopic organisms lacking rigid cell walls; they are considered to be the smallest free-living organisms.

myelinated axon A nerve fibre having a myelin sheath.

myeloblast Bone marrow cell.

myocardial hypertrophy An abnormal increase in the size of cardiac muscle.

myocardial infarction Necrosis of a portion of cardiac muscle caused by obstruction in a coronary artery from atherosclerosis or an embolus.

myoclonus A condition characterized by rapid, uncontrollable muscular contractions or spasms of muscles that occur at rest or during movement.

myoepithelium Tissue made up of contractile epithelial cells.

myofibril A slender, striated strand of smooth muscle.

myofilament An extremely fine, molecular, thread-like structure that helps to form the myofibril of muscle; thick myofibrils are formed of myosin, and thin myofilaments are formed of actin.

myoglobinuria The presence of myoglobin in the urine.

myometrium The muscular wall of the uterus.

myosin A cardiac and skeletal muscle protein; it makes up about half of the proteins that occur in muscle tissue.

myxoedema A condition that results from a deficiency in thyroid hormone.

nail bed The end of a finger or toe covered by the nail; it is abundantly supplied with blood vessels.

nail body The visible part of the nail.

narcolepsy A syndrome characterized by sudden sleep attacks and visual or auditory hallucinations at the onset of sleep.

nares Nostrils.

narrative The portion of the patient care report that allows for a chronological description of the call.

nasal bone The bony partition that separates the nasal cavity into left and right parts; also known as the nasal septum.

nasal septum A partition that separates the right and left nasal cavities.

nasogastric decompression The management of gastric distension or emesis control by means of a nasogastric tube.

nasogastric tube Any tube passed into the stomach through the nose.

nasolacrimal duct A duct that leads from the lacrimal sac to the nasal cavity.

nasopharynx The uppermost portion of the pharynx just behind the nasal cavities.

nasotracheal Accessing the trachea through the nasal cavity.

near-drowning Submersion with at least temporary survival.

nebulizer A device for producing a fine spray of medication for inhalation therapy.

necrosis Death of a cell or group of cells as the result of disease or injury.

negative feedback mechanism A mechanism of response in which a stimulus initiates actions that reverse or reduce the initial stimulus.

neglect The refusal or failure of the caregiver to fulfil obligations or duties to a person.

negligence Failure to use such care as a reasonably prudent emergency medical services provider would use in similar circumstances.

nematocyst A capsule containing thread-like, venomous stinging cells found in some coelenterates.

neonate An infant in the first 28 days of life.

neoplasia The new and abnormal development of cells, which may be benign or malignant.

neoplasm Abnormal growth; a malignant or benign tumour.

nephron The functional unit of the kidney.

nerve A bundle of nerve fibres and accompanying connective tissue located outside the central nervous system.

nerve tract Bundles of parallel axons with associated sheaths in the central nervous system.

nervous tissue A major tissue type characterized by its conductile abilities.

nervous tunic The retina.

neuralgia Pain along a nerve.

neurogenic hypotension Hypotension following spinal shock; caused by a loss of sympathetic tone to the vessels.

neurogenic shock Shock resulting from vasomotor paralysis below the level of injury; also known as spinal cord shock.

neuroglia Cells in the nervous system other than neurons.

neurohormone A junction hormone secreted by a neuron.

neuromuscular A specialized synapse between a motor neuron and a muscle fibre.

neuromuscular junction The area of contact between the ends of a large myelinated nerve fibre and a fibre of skeletal muscle.

neuron The functional unit of the nervous system, consisting of the nerve cell body, the dendrites and the axon.

neuropathy A disease of the peripheral nerves.

neurosis Any faulty or inefficient way of coping with anxiety or inner conflict; it may ultimately lead to a neurotic disorder.

neutrophil A small, phagocytic white blood cell with a lobed nucleus and small granules in the cytoplasm; it stains readily with neutral dyes.

newborn An infant in the first few hours of life.

Newton's first law of motion The principle that an object, whether at rest or in linear motion, remains in that state unless force is applied.

Newton's second law of motion The principle that force is equal to mass times acceleration or deceleration.

nicad batteries Nickel cadmium rechargeable batteries, which are used in portable radios.

nicotinic receptor A class of cholinergic receptor molecules that are activated specifically by nicotine and acetylcholine.

nit The egg of a parasitic insect, particularly a louse.

nitrogen narcosis An illness associated with scuba diving in which nitrogen becomes dissolved in solution as a result of greater than normal atmospheric pressure; also known as rapture of the deep.

nocturia Particularly excessive urination at night.

node of Ranvier The short interval in the myelin sheath of a nerve fibre between adjacent Schwann cells.

non-cardiogenic pulmonary oedema See adult respiratory distress syndrome.

non-compensatory pause The pause that occurs when the next expected P wave of the underlying cardiac rhythm appears earlier than it would have if the sinoatrial node had not been disturbed by a conduction abnormality.

non-competitive antagonist An agent that combines with different parts of the receptor mechanism and inactivates the receptor so that the agonist cannot be effective regardless of its concentration.

non-conducted premature atrial complex A premature atrial complex blocked at the atrioventricular node.

non-electrolyte A substance with no electrical charge.

non-proprietary name See generic name.

non-striated muscle See smooth muscle.

noradrenaline An adrenergic hormone produced by the adrenal medulla, similar in chemical and pharmacological properties to adrenaline. It acts to increase blood pressure by vasoconstriction but does not affect cardiac output; also known as norepinephrine.

nuclear membrane A double membrane structure surrounding and enclosing the nucleus; also known as the nuclear envelope.

nucleic acids Extremely complex, long-chain compounds of high molecular weight that occur naturally in the cells of all living organisms; they form the genetic material of the cell and direct the synthesis of protein within the cell.

nucleolus Any one of the somewhat rounded, dense, well-defined nuclear bodies with no surrounding membrane; the nucleolus contains ribosomal RNA and protein.

nucleoplasm The protoplasm of the nucleus, as contrasted with that of the cell.

nucleus The central controlling body within a living cell.

nullipara A woman who has never borne a child.

nutrient Any substance that nourishes and aids the growth and development of the body.

nystagmus Involuntary rhythmic movements of the eyes.

obesity A condition in which a person is 30% above ideal body weight.

obligate Necessary; compulsory.

obsessive–compulsive disorder A psychiatric disorder in which the person feels stress or anxiety about thoughts or rituals over which he or she has little control.

obstructive apnoea A form of sleep apnoea involving a physical obstruction of the upper airways that can lead to pulmonary failure, chronic fatigue and cardiac abnormalities.

obtundation A state of being insensitive to unpleasant or painful stimulation associated with a reduced level of consciousness, such as by anaesthesia or a strong narcotic analgesic.

obturator foramen A large opening on each side of the lower portion of the hipbone, formed posteriorly by the ischium, superiorly by the ilium, and anteriorly by the pubis.

occipital bone The cup-like bone at the back of the skull, marked by a large opening (the foramen magnum), that communicates with the vertebral canal.

occipital foramen A passage in the occipital bone through which the spinal cord enters the spinal column.

occipital lobe One of the five lobes of each cerebral hemisphere.

occiput posterior presentation An abnormal presentation in which the infant's head is delivered face up instead of face down.

oculomotor nerve The third cranial nerve, which contains sensory and motor fibres; it provides for movement in most of the muscles of the eye, for constriction of the pupil, and for accommodation of the eye to light.

odontoid process The tooth-like projection that rises perpendicularly from the upper surface of the body of the second cervical vertebra or axis, which serves as a pivot point for the rotation of the atlas.

oedema The accumulation of fluid within the interstitial spaces.

oesophageal reflux A chronic disease manifested by various sequelae associated with reflux of the stomach and duodenal contents into the oesophagus.

oesophageal stricture An abnormal temporary or permanent narrowing of the oesophagus caused by inflammation, external pressure, or scarring.

oesophagitis Inflammation of the oesophagus.

oesophagogastric varices A complex of longitudinal, tortuous veins at the lower end of the oesophagus that become large and swollen as a result of portal hypertension; also known as oesophageal varices.

oesophagus The muscular canal extending from the pharynx to the stomach.

oestrogen One of a group of hormonal steroid compounds that promote the development of female secondary sex characteristics.

olecranon fossa The depression in the posterior surface of the humerus that receives the olecranon of the ulna when the forearm is extended.

olecranon process The large bony process of the ulna; also known as the olecranon.

olfactory Of or pertaining to the sense of smell.

olfactory bulb The tissue that receives the olfactory nerves from the nasal cavity.

olfactory membranes Membranes that contain the receptors for the sense of smell; they are located in the roof of the nasal cavity.

olfactory recess The extreme superior region of the nasal cavity.

olfactory tract The nerve tract that projects from the olfactory bulb to the olfactory cortex.

oliguria A diminished capacity to form or pass urine.

omphalocele Congenital herniation of intra-abdominal viscera through a defect in the abdominal wall around the umbilicus.

oncotic pressure See blood colloid osmotic pressure.

ongoing assessment A repeat of the initial assessment that is performed throughout the paramedic–patient encounter.

onset of action The interval between the time a drug is administered and the first sign of its effects; also known as the latent period of drug action.

oocyte An incompletely developed ovum.

open pneumothorax A chest wall injury that exposes the pleural space to atmospheric pressure.

open vault fracture A fracture that results in direct communication between a scalp laceration and cerebral substance.

opiate A narcotic drug that contains opium, derivatives of opium, or any of several semisynthetic or synthetic drugs with opium-like activity.

opioid Any synthetic narcotic that has opiate-like activities but is not derived from opium.

opposition Movement of the thumb and little finger toward each other for the purpose of grasping objects.

optic nerve The nerve that carries visual signals from the eye to the crossing of the optic tracts.

orchitis Painful inflammation of the testicle.

ORCON The historical performance requirements set for NHS ambulance services in the 1974 ORCON standards that still form the basis of ambulance performance indicators.

organ A structure made up of two or more kinds of tissues organized to perform a more complex function than any one tissue alone.

organ of Corti The organ of hearing; it is located in the cochlea and filled with endolymph.

organelle Any one of various particles of living substance bound within most cells, such as the mitochondria, the Golgi apparatus, the endoplasmic reticulum, the lysosomes and the centrioles.

oriented Aware of one's surroundings.

origin The less movable attachment point of a muscle.

orogastric decompression The management of gastric distension or emesis control by means of an orogastric tube.

oropharyngeolaryngeal axis The three axes of the mouth, pharynx and trachea; a patient position used for direct visualization of the larynx.

oropharynx The portion of the pharynx located behind the mouth.

orotracheal Gaining access to the trachea through the oral cavity.

orthostatic hypotension Abnormally low blood pressure that occurs when an individual assumes the standing posture; also called postural hypotension.

osmolality The osmotic concentration of a solution.

osmosis Diffusion of solvent (water) through a membrane from a less concentrated solution to a more concentrated solution.

osmotic pressure The force required to prevent the movement of water across a selectively permeable membrane.

ossified To be changed or developed into bone.

osteoarthritis A form of arthritis in which one or many joints undergo degenerative changes.

osteomyelitis Local or generalized infection of bone and bone marrow, usually caused by bacteria introduced by trauma or surgery.

osteoporosis A disorder characterized by a reduction in bone density; it occurs most often in postmenopausal women.

ostomy An artificial opening into the urinary tract, gastrointestinal tract, or trachea; any surgical procedure in which an opening is created between two hollow organs or between a hollow viscus and the abdominal wall.

otorrhoea Any discharge from the external ear.

ounce A unit of weight equal to 1/16 lb, or 28.349 g.

ovarian follicle The spherical cell aggregation in the ovary that contains an oocyte.

ovarian ligament The bundle of fibres that passes to the uterus from the ovary.

ovarian torsion Twisting of an ovary around its vascular pedicle.

ovary One of the pair of female gonads found on each side of the lower abdomen beside the uterus.

ovulation The release of an ovum or secondary oocyte from the vesicular follicle.

oxyhaemoglobin Oxygenated haemoglobin.

P wave The first complex of the electrocardiogram, representing depolarization of the atria.

pacemaker cell Certain myocardial cells capable of initiating an electrical impulse.

packaging See patient packaging.

paediatric trauma score An injury severity index that grades six components commonly seen in paediatric trauma patients: size (weight), airway, central nervous system, systolic blood pressure, open wound and skeletal injury.

Paget's disease A common, non-metabolic disease of bone of unknown cause, characterized by excessive bone destruction and unorganized bone repair.

paging equipment Equipment typically using tone activation with one-way transmission to receive-only units.

palate A structure that forms the roof of the mouth; it is divided into the hard and soft palates.

palatine bone One of a pair of bones of the skull forming the posterior part of the hard palate, part of the nasal cavity, and the floor of the orbit of the eye.

palatine tonsil One of two large oval masses of lymphoid tissue embedded in the lateral wall of the oropharynx.

palliative care A unique form of healthcare primarily directed at providing relief to terminally ill persons through symptom management and pain management.

palmar grasp A normal infant response. The infant curls the fingers in response to a touch on the palm of the hand.

palpation A technique in which an examiner uses the hands and fingers to gather information from a patient by touch.

pancreas A fish-shaped nodular gland located across the posterior abdominal wall in the epigastric region of the body; it secretes various substances, including digestive enzymes, insulin, and glucagon.

pancreatic juice The fluid secretion of the pancreas produced by the stimulation of food in the duodenum.

pancreatitis Inflammation of the pancreas, which causes severe epigastric pain.

pandemic A disease outbreak that infects the entire world.

para The number of past pregnancies that have remained viable to delivery.

paraesthesia A sensation of numbness, tingling, or 'pins and needles.'

parainfluenza virus One of a group of viruses isolated from patients with upper respiratory tract disease of varying severity in infants and young children; it may cause croup, tracheobronchitis, bronchiolitis, bronchopneumonia, pharyngitis and the common cold.

paralytic ileus The decrease in or absence of intestinal peristalsis that may occur after abdominal surgery, illness, or injury; the most common cause of intestinal obstruction.

paramedic A registered professional who provides specialist care and treatment to patients who are either acutely ill or injured. They can administer a range of drugs and carry out certain surgical techniques.

parametritis An inflammatory condition of tissue of the structures around the uterus.

paranoia A condition characterized by an elaborate, overly suspicious system of thinking.

paraplegia A weakness or paralysis of both legs and sometimes part of the trunk.

parasagittal plane An imaginary vertical plane passing through the body parallel to the medial plane; it divides the body into left and right portions.

parasympathetic Of or pertaining to the craniosacral division of the autonomic nervous system.

parasympathetic nervous system The subdivision of the autonomic nervous system usually involved in activating vegetative functions such as digestion, defecation and urination.

parasympatholytic agent Anticholinergic; producing effects resembling those of interruption or blockade of the parasympathetic nerve supply to effector organs or tissues.

parasympathomimetic agent An agent with effects that mimic those resulting from stimulation of parasympathetic nerves, especially the effects produced by acetylcholine.

parasystole An independent ectopic rhythm the pacemaker of which cannot be discharged by impulses of the dominant rhythm because of an area of depressed conduction surrounding the parasystolic focus.

parenchyma The essential or functional elements of an organ.

parenteral Of or pertaining to any medication route other than the alimentary canal.

parietal Of or pertaining to the outer wall of a cavity or organ.

parietal bone One of a pair of bones that form the side of the cranium.

parietal lobe The portion of each cerebral hemisphere that occupies the parts of the lateral and medial surfaces covered by the parietal bone.

parietal pericardium The portion of serous pericardium lining the fibrous pericardium.

parietal peritoneum The layer of peritoneum lining the abdominal walls.

parkinsonism A neurological disorder characterized by tremor, muscle rigidity, hypokinesia, a slow shuffling gait, and difficulty in chewing, swallowing, and speaking; it frequently occurs in patients treated with antipsychotic drugs.

Parkinson's disease A disease caused by degeneration or damage (of unknown origin) to nerve cells within the basal ganglia in the brain.

parotitis Inflammation or infection of one or both parotid salivary glands.

paroxysm A sudden attack or recurrence of symptoms of a disease.

paroxysmal nocturnal dyspnoea An abnormal condition of the respiratory system characterized by sudden attacks of shortness of breath, profuse sweating, tachycardia and wheezing that awaken a person from sleep; often associated with left ventricular failure and pulmonary oedema.

paroxysmal supraventricular tachycardia An ectopic rhythm in excess of 100 beats per minute and usually faster than 170 beats per minute that begins abruptly with a premature atrial or junctional beat and is supported by an atrioventricular nodal re-entry mechanism or by an atrioventricular re-entry involving an accessory pathway.

partial antagonist An agent that has affinity and some efficacy but that may antagonize the action of other drugs that have greater efficacy.

partial pressure The pressure exerted by a single gas.

partial reabsorption The amount of drug reabsorbed from the renal tubule by passive diffusion.

partial-thickness burn A burn injury that extends through the epidermis to the dermis; considered a deep partial-thickness injury if it extends to the basal layers of the skin; also known as a second-degree burn.

parturition The process of giving birth.

passive glomerular filtration The renal process whereby fluid in the blood is filtered across the capillaries of the glomerulus and into the urinary space of Bowman's capsule.

patella A flat, triangular bone at the front of the knee joint; the kneecap.

patient care report A document used in the prehospital setting to record all patient care activities and circumstances related to an emergency response.

patient packaging Completion of emergency care procedures needed to transfer a patient from the scene to the emergency vehicle.

patient transport services Non-emergency patient transport services typified by the non-urgent, planned, transportation of patients with a medical need for transport to and from a premises providing NHS healthcare and between NHS healthcare providers.

pattern recognition The process of comparing gathered information with the paramedic's knowledge base of medical illness and disease.

patterned injuries Injuries that result from an identifiable object.

peak plasma level The highest plasma concentration attained from a dose.

pectoral girdle See shoulder girdle.

pectus deformity Malformation of the chest wall.

pelvic cavity The area of the body enclosed by the bones of the pelvis.

pelvic girdle The encircling bony structure supporting the lower limbs.

pelvic inflammatory disease Any inflammatory condition of the female pelvic organs, especially one caused by bacterial infection.

penetrating trauma An injury produced by crushing and stretching forces of a penetrating object that results in some form of tissue disruption.

penetration The flow of a hazardous liquid chemical through zips, stitched seams, pinholes or other imperfections in a material.

penis The external reproductive organ of the male.

pepsin The principal digestive enzyme of gastric juice.

pepsinogen A proenzyme formed and secreted by certain cells of the gastric mucosa.

peptic ulcer A sharply circumscribed loss of the mucous membrane of the stomach, duodenum, or any other part of the gastrointestinal system.

peptic ulcer disease Illness that results from a complex pathological interaction among the acidic gastric juice and proteolytic enzymes and the mucosal barrier.

peptide bond A chemical bond between amino acids.

percussion A technique used to evaluate the presence of air or fluid in body tissues.

perfusion The transfer of fluids through a tissue.

periappendiceal abscess A cavity containing pus and inflamed tissue around the vermiform appendix.

pericardial cavity The area of the body that surrounds the heart.

pericardial fluid A viscous fluid contained within the pericardial cavity between the visceral and parietal pericardium; it serves as a lubricant.

pericardial friction rub A dry, grating sound heard with a stethoscope during auscultation; suggestive of pericarditis.

pericardial sac The sac that surrounds the heart.

pericardial tamponade Compression of the heart produced by the accumulation of fluid or blood in the pericardial sac.

pericardiocentesis A procedure for withdrawing fluid from the pericardial sac.

pericarditis Inflammation of the pericardium.

pericardium The membrane that surrounds the heart.

perilymph The fluid contained within the bony labyrinth.

perinatal Occurring at or near the time of birth.

perineum The pelvic floor and associated structures occupying the pelvic outlet, bounded anteriorly by the pubic symphysis, laterally by the ischial tuberosities, and posteriorly by the coccyx.

periodontal membrane The membrane that surrounds the root of the tooth.

periosteum Tough connective tissue that covers the bone.

periostitis Inflammation of the periosteum characterized by tenderness and swelling of the affected bone, pain, fever and chills.

peripheral nervous system A subdivision of the nervous system consisting of nerves and ganglia.

peripheral neuropathy Diseases and disorders that affect the peripheral nervous system, including spinal nerve roots, cranial nerves and peripheral nerves.

peripheral thermoreceptors Nerve endings sensitive to heat, located in the skin and some mucous membranes; they usually are categorized as cold or warm receptors.

peripheral vascular disease Any abnormal condition that affects the blood vessels outside the heart and lymphatic vessels.

peripheral vascular resistance The total resistance against which blood must be pumped; also known as afterload.

peristalsis The coordinated, rhythmic, and serial contraction of smooth muscle that forces food through the digestive tract, bile through the bile duct, and urine through the ureters.

peristaltic Pertaining to peristalsis.

peritoneal Pertaining to the peritoneum.

peritoneal cavity The potential space between the parietal and visceral layers of the peritoneum; the two layers are normally in contact.

peritoneal dialysis A dialysis procedure that uses the peritoneum as a diffusible membrane; performed to correct an imbalance of fluid or electrolytes in the blood or to remove toxins, drugs, or other wastes normally excreted by the kidney.

peritoneum The serous membrane that covers the abdominal wall of the body and is reflected over the contained viscera.

peritonitis Inflammation of the serous membrane that covers the abdominal wall.

peritubular capillary The capillary network located in the cortex of the kidney.

permeable A condition of being pervious so that fluids and other substances can pass through, as occurs in a semipermeable membrane.

permeation The process by which a hazardous liquid chemical moves through a material on a molecular level.

persistent generalized lymphadenopathy Enlarged lymph nodes involving two non-contiguous sites other than inguinal nodes; a common feature in early human immunodeficiency virus infection.

pertinent negative findings Findings that warrant no medical care or intervention but that, by seeking them, show evidence of the thoroughness of the examination and history of the event.

pertussis An acute, highly contagious respiratory disease characterized by paroxysmal coughing that ends in a loud, whooping inspiration; also known as whooping cough.

petit mal seizure See absence

pH An inverse logarithm of the hydrogen ion concentration.

phagocytic Pertaining to phagocytosis.

phagocytosis The process of ingestion by cells of solid substances such as other cells, bacteria, bits of necrosed tissue, and foreign particles.

phalanges Any bone of a finger or toe.

pharmaceutics The science of dispensing drugs.

pharmacodynamics The study of how a drug acts on a living organism.

pharmacokinetics The study of how the body handles a drug over a period of time, including the processes of absorption, distribution, biotransformation and excretion.

pharmacology The science of drugs used to prevent, diagnose and treat disease.

pharyngeal tonsil One of two collections of aggregated lymphoid nodules on the posterior wall of the nasopharynx.

pharyngitis Inflammation or infection of the pharynx.

phase 0 The rapid depolarization phase; it represents the rapid upstroke of the action potential that occurs when the cell membrane reaches the threshold potential (approximately −70 mV).

phase 1 The early rapid repolarization phase; the phase in which the fast sodium channels close, the flow of sodium ions into the cell terminates, and loss of potassium from the cell continues.

phase 2 The plateau phase; the prolonged phase of slow repolarization of the action potential.

phase 3 The terminal phase of rapid repolarization; it results in the inside of the cell becoming considerably negative and the membrane potential returning to approximately −90 mV, or its resting level.

phase 4 The period between action potentials when the membrane has returned to its resting membrane potential.

phencyclidine psychosis A true psychiatric emergency with clinical syndromes ranging from a catatonic and unresponsive state to bizarre and violent behaviour; it may occur after a single low-dose exposure to phencyclidine and may last several days to weeks.

phlebitis Inflammation of a vein, often accompanied by formation of a clot; also known as thrombophlebitis.

phlebotomy The incision of a vein for the letting of blood.

phobia An anxiety disorder characterized by an obsessive, irrational and intense fear of a specific object or activity.

phonation The production of speech sounds.

phosgene A poisonous gas that appears as a greyish white cloud and smells of newly mowed hay.

phospholipid One of a class of compounds, widely distributed in living cells, that contains phosphoric acid, fatty acids, and a nitrogenous base.

photophobia Abnormal sensitivity to light.

physical abuse The use of physical force that may result in bodily injury, physical pain, or impairment.

physical dependence An adaptive physiological state that occurs after prolonged use of many drugs; discontinuation causes withdrawal syndromes that are relieved by readministering the same drug or a pharmacologically related drug.

physical examination An assessment of a patient that includes examination techniques, measurement of vital signs, an assessment of height and weight, and the skilful use of examination equipment.

physiological dead space The sum of the anatomical dead space plus the volume of any non-functional alveoli.

pia mater The innermost layer of the meninges that directly covers the brain.

Pickwickian syndrome An abnormal condition characterized by obesity, decreased pulmonary function, somnolence and polycythaemia.

pigmented retina The pigmented portion of the retina.

piloerection Erection of the hairs of the skin in response to cold environment, emotional stimulus or irritation of the skin.

pineal gland A cone-shaped structure in the brain that secretes the hormone melatonin.

pinna See auricle.

pituitary gland A small gland attached to the hypothalamus; it supplies numerous hormones that govern many vital processes.

pivot joint A joint that consists of a relatively cylindrical bony process that rotates within a ring composed partly of bone and partly of ligament.

placards Four-sided, diamond-shaped signs displayed on hazardous materials containers that are usually yellow, orange, white or green. They have a four-digit United Nations identification number and a legend to indicate the contents of the container.

placebo An inactive substance or a less than effective dose of a harmless substance; it is used in experimental drug studies to compare the effects of the inactive substance with those of the experimental drug.

placenta A highly vascular fetal–maternal organ through which the fetus absorbs oxygen, nutrients, and other substances and excretes carbon dioxide and other wastes.

placental abruption Separation of the placenta implanted in a normal position in a pregnancy of 20 weeks or more; it occurs during labour or delivery of the fetus.

placenta praevia A condition of pregnancy in which the placenta is implanted abnormally in the uterus so that it impinges on or covers the internal os of the uterine cervix.

placental barrier A protective biological membrane that separates the blood vessels of the mother and the fetus.

plague A disease caused by the bacteria *Yersinia pestis*, found in rodents and their fleas in many areas around the world.

plane joint A joint that consists of two opposed flat surfaces that are approximately equal in size; also known as a gliding joint.

plasma The fluid portion of blood.

plasma membrane The outer covering of a cell that contains the cellular cytoplasm; also known as the cell membrane.

plasma-protein binding A type of drug reservoir in which drugs attach to proteins, mainly albumin, and form a drug–protein complex.

plateau phase Prolongation of the depolarization phase of cardiac muscle cell membrane; it results in a prolonged refractory period.

platelet A fragment of a cell; it contains granules in the central part and clear protoplasm peripherally but has no definite nucleus.

pleural cavity The area of the body that surrounds the lungs.

pleural fluid Serous fluid found in the pleural cavity; it helps to reduce friction when the pleural membranes rub together.

pleural friction rub A rubbing or grating sound that occurs as one layer of the pleural membrane slides over the other during breathing.

pleural lavage A rewarming technique that uses warm saline to irrigate the thorax; it is used to treat some patients with severe hypothermia.

pleural space The potential space between the visceral and parietal layers of the pleura.

pleurisy Inflammation of the parietal pleura of the lungs, characterized by dyspnoea and stabbing chest pain.

plexus A network of intersecting nerves and blood vessels or lymphatic vessels.

pneumococcus A Gram-positive diplococcal bacterium of the species *Streptococcus pneumoniae*; the most common cause of bacterial pneumonia.

***Pneumocystis carinii* pneumonia** A bacterial pneumonia caused by infection with the parasite *Pneumocystis carinii*; it is usually seen in infants or debilitated or immunosuppressed persons and is characterized by fever, cough, tachypnoea, and, frequently, cyanosis.

pneumohaemothorax A collection of air and blood in the pleural space; also known as a haemopneumothorax.

pneumomediastinum The presence of air or gas in the mediastinal tissues.

pneumonia An acute inflammation of the lungs, usually caused by inhaled pneumococci of the species *Streptococcus pneumoniae*.

pneumopericardium The presence of air or gas in the pericardial cavity.

pneumoperitoneum The presence of air or gas within the peritoneal cavity of the abdomen.

pneumotaxic centre A group of neurons in the pons that have an inhibitory effect on the inspiratory centre.

pneumothorax A collection of air or gas in the pleural space that causes the lung to collapse.

poikilothermy Variation in body temperature according to the ambient temperature.

point of maximum impulse The location or area where the apical pulse is palpated the strongest, often in the fifth intercostal space of the thorax just medial to the left midclavicular line.

poison Any substance that produces harmful physiological or psychological effects.

polio See poliomyelitis.

poliomyelitis An infectious disease caused by one of three polio viruses; asymptomatic, mild and paralytic forms of the disease occur.

poliovirus hominis The causative organism of poliomyelitis.

polyarthritis Inflammation of several joints.

polycythaemia A condition characterized by an unusually large number of red cells in the blood as a result of their increased production by the bone marrow.

polydipsia Excessive thirst.

polymorphic Occurring in many forms.

polyp A small, tumour-like growth that projects from a mucous membrane surface.

polyphagia Excessive eating.

polysaccharide A carbohydrate that contains three or more molecules of simple carbohydrates.

polyuria Excessive secretion of urine.

pons The part of the brainstem between the medulla and the midbrain.

portal hypertension An increased venous pressure in the portal circulation caused by compression or by occlusion in the portal or hepatic vascular system.

portal vein A vein that ramifies like an artery in the liver and ends in capillary-like sinusoids that convey the blood to the inferior vena cava through the hepatic veins.

positive end-expiratory pressure Ventilation controlled by a flow of air delivered in cycles of constant pressure through the respiratory cycle.

posterior The back, or dorsal, surface.

posterior cerebral artery The artery that supplies the posterior portion of the cerebrum.

posterior chamber of the eye The chamber of the eye between the iris and the lens.

posterior communicating artery The artery that branches off each internal carotid artery and connects with the ipsilateral posterior cerebral artery.

posterior superior iliac spine One of two bony segments that form the iliac crest.

postictal phase The phase that usually follows a seizure in which the person is drowsy and lethargic.

postpartum The maternal period after delivery.

postpartum haemorrhage Blood loss of more than 500 mL after delivery of the newborn.

postsynaptic neuron The membrane of a nerve that is in close association with a presynaptic terminal.

post-traumatic syndrome An anxiety reaction to a severe psychosocial event; also known as post-traumatic stress disorder.

potassium ion The predominant intracellular cation; it helps to regulate neuromuscular excitability and muscle contraction.

potassium-sparing agent A group of medications that promote sodium and water loss without an accompanying loss of potassium.

potential difference The difference in electrical potential, measured as the charge difference across the cell membrane.

potentiation Enhancement of the effect of a drug, caused by concurrent administration of two drugs in which one drug increases the effect of the other.

pound A unit of measure equal to 16 oz, or 0.45359 kg.

P–R interval The time elapsing between the beginning of the P wave and the beginning of the QRS complex in the electrocardiogram.

precapillary sphincter The smooth muscle sphincter that regulates blood flow through a capillary.

precipitous delivery A rapid, spontaneous delivery of less than 3 hours from onset of labour to birth; it results from overactive uterine contractions and little maternal soft tissue or bony resistance. Childbirth that occurs with such speed that usual preparations cannot be made.

precordial thump A cardiopulmonary resuscitation technique used to restore circulation in monitored ventricular fibrillation or unstable ventricular tachycardia.

pre-eclampsia An abnormal disease of pregnancy characterized by the onset of acute hypertension after the twenty-fourth week of gestation.

pregravid Before pregnancy.

preload The amount of blood returning to the ventricle.

premature atrial complex A cardiac dysrhythmia characterized by an atrial beat occurring before the expected excitation and indicated on the electrocardiogram as an early P wave.

premature birth Refers to an infant who is born before 37 weeks of gestation.

premature junctional contraction A cardiac dysrhythmia that occurs during sinus rhythm earlier than the next expected sinus beat and is caused by premature discharge of an ectopic focus in the atrioventricular junctional tissue.

premature rupture of membranes Rupture of the amniotic sac before the onset of labour, regardless of gestational age.

premature ventricular contraction A cardiac dysrhythmia characterized by a ventricular beat preceding the expected electrical impulse and indicated on the electrocardiogram as an early, wide QRS complex without a preceding related P wave.

prenatal Existing or occurring before birth.

prepuce In males, the free fold of skin that covers the glans penis; the foreskin. In females, the external fold of the labia minora that covers the clitoris.

present illness Identification of the chief complaint and a full, clear, chronological account of the symptoms.

presenting part The part of the fetus that lies closest to the internal os of the cervix.

presenting the patient The effective communication and transfer of patient information in the course of out-of-hospital and hospital care.

pressure ulcers Sores or ulcers in the skin over a bony prominence that occur most frequently on the sacrum, elbows, heels, outer ankles, inner knees, hips and shoulder blades of high-risk patients, especially those who are obese, elderly, or suffering from chronic diseases, infections, injuries or a poor nutritional state.

presynaptic neuron The nerve terminal that contains neurotransmitter vesicles.

presynaptic terminal The enlarged axon terminal.

preterm infant An infant born before 37 weeks of gestation.

priapism Painful, persistent erection of the penis.

primary bronchus One of the two tubes arising at the inferior end of the trachea; each primary bronchus extends into one of the lungs.

primary contamination Exposure to a hazardous substance that is harmful only to the person exposed and that poses little risk of exposure to others.

primary epilepsy Epilepsy for which the cause is unknown; also known as idiopathic epilepsy.

primary follicle The ovarian follicle that contains the primary oocyte.

primary injury prevention The practice of preventing an injury from occurring.

primary oocyte The oocyte before the first meiotic division.

primary pulmonary hypertension Abnormally high pressure within the pulmonary circulation.

prime mover A muscle that plays a major role in accomplishing movement.

primigravida A woman who is pregnant for the first time.

primipara A woman who has given birth only one time.

Prinzmetal's angina An atypical form of angina caused by vasospasm that occurs at rest rather than with effort; it is associated with gross ST-segment elevation in the electrocardiogram that disappears when the pain subsides.

priority patients Patients who need immediate care and transport.

proarrhythmia A new or worsened rhythm disturbance seemingly generated by antidysrhythmic therapy.

prodromal stage The time during which a disease process has begun but is not yet clinically manifest. It also applies to the early period of labour before uterine contractions become forceful and frequent enough to result in progressive dilatation of the uterine cervix.

progesterone A steroid sex hormone prescribed to treat various menstrual disorders, functional uterine bleeding, and repeated spontaneous abortions.

progestin Any one of a group of natural or synthetic hormones that have a progesterone-like effect on the uterus.

prokaryote A cell without a true nucleus and with nuclear material scattered throughout the cytoplasm.

prolapsed umbilical cord An umbilical cord that protrudes beside or ahead of the presenting part of the fetus.

proliferative phase The time between the end of menses and ovulation characterized by rapid division of endometrial cells and the development of follicles in the ovary.

pronation Rotation of the forearm so that the anterior surface is down.

prone The position in which the patient is lying face down.

proprietary name See trade name.

proprioception Information about the position of the body and its various parts.

prostaglandin A class of naturally occurring fatty acids that affect body functions such as vasodilatation, stimulation and contraction of uterine smooth muscle, and promotion of inflammation and pain.

prostate gland The gland that lies just below the male bladder; its secretion is one of the components of semen.

prostatic hypertrophy Hypertrophy or enlargement of the prostate gland.

prostatitis Acute or chronic inflammation of the prostate gland.

prosthesis An artificial replacement for a missing part of the body, such as an artificial limb.

protein Any of a large group of naturally occurring, complex, organic nitrogen compounds.

prothrombin A chemical that is part of the clotting cascade; the precursor of thrombin.

protoplasm The living substance of a cell.

protraction Movement in the anterior direction.

pseudoaneurysm A condition resembling an aneurysm, caused by enlargement and tortuosity of a vessel.

pseudomembranous colitis A life-threatening form of diarrhoea caused by *Clostridium difficile*.

psoas muscle A long muscle originating from the transverse processes of the lumbar vertebrae and the fibrocartilage and sides of the vertebral bodies of the lower thoracic vertebrae and the lumbar vertebrae.

psoriasis A common, chronic, inheritable skin disorder characterized by circumscribed red patches covered by thick, dry, adherent scales that result from excessive development of epithelial cells.

psychological dependence Emotional reliance on a drug; manifestations range from a mild desire for a drug to craving and drug-seeking behaviour to repeated compulsive use of a drug for its subjectively satisfying or pleasurable effects.

psychology The science or study of behaviour.

psychomotor seizure A seizure manifested by impaired consciousness of variable degree; the patient carries out a series of coordinated acts that are inappropriate, bizarre, and serve no useful purpose, about which the patient is amnesic.

psychosis Maladaptive behaviour involving major distortions of reality.

puberty The period of life when the ability to reproduce begins.

pubis One of a pair of pubic bones that, with the ischium and the ilium, form the hipbone and join the pubic bone from the opposite side at the pubic symphysis.

pulmonary artery The artery that carries deoxygenated blood from the right ventricle into the lung.

pulmonary capacity The sum of two or more pulmonary volumes.

pulmonary contusion Bruising of the lung tissue that results in rupture of the alveoli and interstitial oedema.

pulmonary embolism The blockage of a pulmonary artery by foreign matter such as fat, air, tumour tissue, or a thrombus that usually arises from a peripheral vein.

pulmonary hypertension A condition of abnormally high pressure within the pulmonary circulation.

pulmonary oedema The accumulation of extravascular fluid in lung tissues and alveoli.

pulmonary over-pressurization syndrome A condition that results from expansion of trapped air in the lungs; it may lead to alveolar rupture and extravasation of air into extra-alveolar locations.

pulmonary semilunar valve A valve that guards the orifice between the right ventricle and the pulmonary artery.

pulmonary surfactant Certain lipoproteins that reduce the surface tension of pulmonary fluids, allowing the exchange of gases in the alveoli of the lungs and contributing to the elasticity of pulmonary tissue.

pulmonary trunk The large elastic artery that carries blood from the right ventricle of the heart to the right and left pulmonary arteries.

pulmonary vein Any vein that carries oxygenated blood from the lung to the left atrium.

pulmonary ventilation The movement of air in and out of the lungs. This process brings oxygen into the lungs and removes carbon dioxide.

pulmonic pressure Pressure generated by the right side of the heart.

pulp The soft, spongy chamber of the tooth.

pulse deficit A condition that exists when the radial pulse is less than the ventricular rate; it indicates a lack of peripheral perfusion.

pulse pressure The difference between systolic and diastolic pressure.

pulsus paradoxus An abnormal decrease in systolic blood pressure that drops more than 10–15 mmHg during inspiration compared with expiration.

punctate Spotted; marked with points of puncture.

punctum The opening of each lacrimal canal.

puncture wound An open injury that results from contact with a penetrating object.

pupil The opening in the centre of the iris that regulates the amount of light entering the eye.

purified protein derivative A dried form of tuberculin used in testing for past or present infection with tubercle bacilli.

Purkinje fibres Myocardial fibres that are a continuation of the bundle of His and that extend into the muscle walls of the ventricles.

pustule A small, circumscribed elevation of skin containing fluid, which is usually purulent.

pyelolithotomy Removal of a stone from a kidney by surgical incision.

pyelonephritis An inflammation of the kidney parenchyma associated with microbial infection.

pyloric sphincter A thickened, muscular ring in the stomach that separates the pylorus from the duodenum.

pyorrhoea Discharge of pus.

pyrogen Any substance or agent that tends to cause a rise in body temperature.

pyrogenic A substance or agent that produces fever.

pyruvate The end product of glycolysis; it may be metabolized to lactate or acetyl coenzyme A.

QRS complex The principal deflection in the electrocardiogram, representing ventricular depolarization.

Q-T interval The time elapsing from the beginning of the QRS complex to the end of the T wave, representing the total duration of electrical activity of the ventricles.

quadriplegia A weakness or paralysis of all four extremities and the trunk.

R prime A subsequent positive deflection in the QRS complex that extends above the baseline and that is taller than the first R wave.

rabies An acute, usually fatal viral disease of the central nervous system of animals; it is transmitted from animals to human beings by infected blood, tissue, or, most commonly, saliva.

raccoon's eyes Ecchymosis of one or both orbits caused by fracture of the base of the sphenoid sinus.

radial tuberosity A large, oblong elevation at the distal end of the radius.

radioulnar syndesmosis The articulation of the radius and ulna, consisting of a proximal articulation, a distal articulation, and three sets of ligaments.

radius One of the bones of the forearm, lying parallel to the ulna.

range The general perimeter of communications coverage beyond which coverage is non-existent or severely degraded to an unusable level; it is measured in miles.

rapid sequence induction An airway management technique that involves the virtually simultaneous administration of a potent sedative agent and a neuromuscular blocking agent for the purpose of endotracheal intubation; it provides optimal intubation conditions whilst minimizing the risk of aspiration of gastric contents.

reabsorption The kidney's return of useful substances to the blood.

reactive airway disease An inflammatory airway condition that develops as a reaction to an antigen.

reactive hyperaemia Increased blood flow associated with increased metabolic activity.

rebound tenderness A sign of peritoneal inflammation in which pain is caused by the sudden release of fingertip pressure on the abdomen.

receptor molecule A reactive site on the cell surface or within the cell that combines with a drug molecule to produce a biological effect.

reciprocal socialization A term that refers to a child's temperament and the responses it obtains from adults and family members. This interaction forms the basis for early social interactions with others and with the child's environment.

rectum The segment of the large intestine continuous with the descending sigmoid colon just proximal to the anal canal.

rectus femoris muscle A muscle of the anterior thigh; one of the four parts of the quadriceps femoris.

red marrow Specialized soft tissue found in many bones of infants and children, in the spongy bone of the proximal epiphyses of the humerus and femur, and in the sternum, ribs, and vertebral bodies of adults. It is essential in the manufacture of red blood cells.

red measles See rubeola.

re-entry The reactivation of tissue by a returning impulse; the sustaining mechanism in some cases of ventricular bigeminy or trigeminy, ventricular tachycardia, and paroxysmal supraventricular tachycardia.

referred pain Visceral pain felt at a site distant from its origin.

reflection on action A component of critical thinking (usually performed after the event) in which the examiner evaluates a patient care episode for possible improvement in similar future responses.

reflex An automatic response to a stimulus that occurs without conscious thought; produced by a reflex arc.

reflex arc The smallest portion of the nervous system capable of receiving a stimulus and producing a response.

refractory period The period after effective stimulation during which excitable tissue fails to respond to a stimulus of threshold intensity.

refractory shock Shock that is resistant to treatment but is still reversible.

relative hypovolaemia Inadequate preload as a result of vasodilatation.

relative refractory period The portion of the action potential after the absolute refractory period during which another action potential can be produced with a greater than threshold stimulus strength.

renal calculus Kidney stone.

renal calyx The first unit in the system of the ducts of the kidney carrying urine from the renal pyramid of the cortex to the renal pelvis for excretion through the ureters.

renal capsule The cortical substance that separates the renal pyramids.

renal corpuscle The glomerulus and its enclosing Bowman's capsule.

renal cortex The outer layer of the kidney, which contains approximately 1.25 million renal tubules, which remove body waste in the form of urine.

renal failure Inability of the kidneys to secrete wastes, concentrate urine, and conserve electrolytes; it may be chronic or acute.

renal medulla The inner layer of the kidney.

renal papilla The apex of the renal pyramid.

renal pelvis The funnel-shaped expansion of the upper end of the ureter that receives the calyces.

renal pyramid One of a number of pyramidal masses seen on longitudinal section of the kidney; it contains part of the loop of Henle and the collecting tubules.

renal tubule One of the collecting tubules in the kidney.

renin A proteolytic enzyme that surrounds each arteriole as it enters a glomerulus; it affects blood pressure by catalysing the change of angiotensin I to angiotensin II.

renin–angiotensin–aldosterone mechanism Renin, released from the kidneys in response to low blood pressure, converts angiotensinogen to angiotensin I. Angiotensin I is converted by angiotensin-converting enzyme to angiotensin II, which causes vasoconstriction, resulting in increased blood pressure. Angiotensin II also increases aldosterone secretion, which increases blood pressure by increasing blood volume.

repolarization The phase of the action potential in which the membrane potential moves from its maximum degree of depolarization toward the value of the resting membrane potential.

reposition To move a structure to its original position.

rescue The act of delivery from danger or imprisonment.

residual volume The volume of air remaining in the lungs after a maximum expiratory effort.

respiration The process of the molecular change of oxygen and carbon dioxide within the body's tissues.

respiratory acidosis An abnormal condition characterized by an increased arterial P_{CO_2}, excess carbonic acid, and an increased plasma hydrogen ion concentration.

respiratory alkalosis An abnormal condition characterized by decreased P_{CO_2}, decreased hydrogen ion concentration, and increased blood pH.

respiratory bronchiole The smallest bronchiole that connects the terminal bronchiole to the alveolar duct.

respiratory membrane The membrane in the lungs across which gas exchange occurs with the blood.

respiratory syncytial virus A single-strand virus that is a common cause of epidemics of acute bronchiolitis, bronchopneumonia, and the common cold in young children and sporadic acute bronchitis and mild upper respiratory tract infections in adults.

resting membrane potential The electrical charge difference inside a cell membrane measured relative to just outside the cell membrane.

reticular Relating to a fine network of cells or collagen fibres.

reticular activating system A functional system in the brain, essential for wakefulness, attention, concentration, and introspection.

reticular formation A small, thick cluster of neurons nestled within the brainstem that controls breathing, the heartbeat, blood pressure, level of consciousness, and other vital functions.

retina The nervous tunic of the eye; it is continuous with the optic nerve.

retinopathy A group of inflammatory eye disorders often caused by diabetes, hypertension and atherosclerotic vascular disease.

retraction Drawing backward, usually referred to when a child is having difficulty breathing.

retrograde amnesia The loss of memory for events that occurred before the event that precipitated the amnesia.

retroperitoneal Of or pertaining to the organs closely attached to the abdominal wall and partly covered by peritoneum.

retroperitoneum Behind the peritoneum.

retrovirus Any of a family of viruses that converts genetic RNA to DNA after entering the host cell.

Revised Trauma Score An injury severity index that uses the Glasgow Coma Scale and measurements for systolic blood pressure and respiratory rate.

Reye's syndrome A combination of acute encephalopathy and fatty infiltration of the internal organs that may follow acute viral infections.

Rh factor An antigenic substance present in the erythrocytes of most persons; a person lacking the Rh factor is Rh negative.

rhabdomyolysis An acute, sometimes fatal, disease characterized by destruction of skeletal muscle.

rheumatic fever An inflammatory disease that may develop as a delayed reaction to streptococcal infection of the upper respiratory tract.

rheumatoid arthritis A chronic, sometimes deforming destructive collagen disease that has an autoimmune component.

rheumatoid lungs Rheumatoid arthritis with emphasis on non-articular changes; for example, pulmonary interstitial fibrosis, pleural effusion and lung nodules.

rhinitis Inflammation of the mucous membranes of the nose.

rhinorrhoea The free discharge of watery nasal fluid.

rhonchi Abnormal sounds heard on auscultation of a respiratory airway obstructed by thick secretions, muscular spasm, neoplasm or external pressure.

rib One of the 12 pairs of elastic arches of bone forming a large part of the thoracic skeleton. The first seven ribs on each side are called true ribs because they articulate directly with the sternum. The remaining five ribs are called false ribs; the first three attach ventrally to the ribs, and the last two ribs are free at their ventral extremities and are called floating ribs.

ribonucleic acid A nucleic acid found in the nucleus and the cytoplasm of cells that transmits genetic instructions from the nucleus to the cytoplasm. In the cytoplasm, RNA functions in the assembly of proteins.

ribosome The 'factory' of a cell where protein is synthesized.

ricin A potent protein cytotoxin derived from the beans of the castor plant (*Ricinus communis*).

right lymphatic duct A vessel that conveys lymph from the right upper quadrant of the body into the bloodstream in the neck at the junction of the right internal jugular and the right subclavian veins.

rigor mortis The rigid stiffening of skeletal and cardiac muscle shortly after death.

riot control agents Chemicals that can produce sensory irritation or disabling physical effects which disappear within a short time after termination of exposure.

rod A photoreceptor in the retina of the eye; it is responsible for non-colour vision in low-intensity light.

R-on-T phenomenon The occurrence of a ventricular depolarization during the vulnerable relative refractory period.

root The lowest part of the tooth; it is covered by cementum.

rooting reflex A normal infant response elicited by touching or stroking the side of the cheek or mouth; this causes the infant to turn the head toward the stimulated side and to begin to suck.

rotation Movement of a structure about its axis.

rouleau formation An aggregation of red cells in what looks like a stack of coins or checkers.

round ligament The remains of the umbilical vein.

rubella A contagious viral disease characterized by fever, symptoms of mild upper respiratory tract infection, lymph node enlargement, and a diffuse, fine, red maculopapular rash; it is spread by droplet infection; also known as German measles.

rubeola An acute, highly contagious viral disease involving the respiratory tract; it is characterized by a spreading, maculopapular, cutaneous rash and occurs primarily in young children who have not been immunized; also known as red measles.

rule of nines A method to estimate burn injury that divides the total body surface area into segments that are multiples of 9%.

rupture of membranes Rupture of the amniotic sac; it usually occurs toward the end of the first stage of labour.

ruptured diaphragm A tear or break in the diaphragm, usually as a result of injury.

ruptured ovarian cyst A ruptured globular sac filled with fluid or semisolid material that develops in or on the ovary.

S prime A subsequent negative deflection in the QRS complex that extends below the baseline.

sacral bone A bone composed of the five segments of the vertebral column that are fused in the adult to form the sacrum; the segments are designated S1 to S5.

sacral promontory The projecting portion of the pelvis at the base of the sacrum.

sacral sparing The preservation of sensory or voluntary motor function of the perineum, buttocks, scrotum, or anus.

sacrum The large, triangular bone at the dorsal part of the pelvis; it is inserted like a wedge between the two hipbones.

saddle joint A joint that consists of two saddle-shaped articulating surfaces oriented at right angles to each other.

sagittal plane An imaginary plane that runs vertically through the middle of the body, producing right and left sections.

salicylate Any one of several widely prescribed drugs derived from salicylic acid (e.g. aspirin).

salivary amylase A digestive enzyme found in saliva that begins the chemical digestion of carbohydrates.

salivary gland One of the three pairs of glands that pour their secretions into the mouth, thus aiding the digestive process.

salpingitis An inflammation or infection of the fallopian tube.

saltatory conduction Conduction in which action potentials jump from one node of Ranvier to the next node of Ranvier.

saphenous vein One of a pair of the longest veins in the body; it begins in the medial marginal vein in the dorsum of the foot and ends in the femoral vein.

sarcoidosis A chronic disorder of unknown origin characterized by the formation of lesions in the lung, spleen, liver, skin, and mucous membranes and in the lacrimal and salivary glands.

sarcolemma Part of a myofibril between adjacent Z lines.

sarcomere The contractile unit of skeletal muscle, which contains thick and thin myofilaments.

sarcoplasmic reticulum Endoplasmic reticulum of the muscle.

sarin A clear, colourless, and tasteless liquid that has no odour in its pure form; may be used as a nerve agent.

scanning A component of attention that refers to one's ability to review a large amount of sensory input rapidly. Different individuals have different capacities for scanning and may use various approaches and styles in their scanning.

scapula One of the pair of large, flat, triangular bones that form the dorsal part of the shoulder girdle.

scene size-up An assessment of the scene to ensure scene safety for the paramedic crew, patient(s), and bystanders; a quick assessment to determine the resources needed to manage the scene adequately.

schizophrenia A group of disorders characterized by recurrent episodes of psychotic behaviour.

Schwann cell A cell that forms a myelin sheath around each nerve fibre of the peripheral nervous system.

sciatic nerve A long nerve that originates in the sacral plexus and extends through the muscles of the thigh, leg, and foot with numerous branches.

sciatica Inflammation of the sciatic nerve.

sclera The opaque membrane covering the eyeball.

scoliosis A lateral curvature of the spine.

scrotum The sac of skin that contains the testes.

sebaceous gland A gland of the skin, usually associated with a hair follicle that produces sebum.

sebum The secretion of sebaceous glands; it prevents drying and protects against some bacteria.

second stage of labour The stage of labour measured from full dilatation of the cervix to delivery of the newborn.

secondary bronchus A branch from a primary bronchus that conducts air to each lobe of the lungs.

secondary contamination Exposure to a hazardous substance whereby liquid and particulate substances are transferred easily to others by touching.

secondary epilepsy Epilepsy that can be traced to trauma, infection, a cerebrovascular disorder, or another illness that contributes to or causes the seizure disorder.

secondary follicle The follicle in which the secondary oocyte is surrounded by granulosa cells.

second-degree burn A burn injury that extends through the epidermis to the dermis (superficial partial thickness); it is considered a deep partial-thickness injury if it extends to the basal layers of the skin.

secretin The hormone that stimulates secretion of pancreatic juice.

secretion A general term for a substance produced inside a cell and released from the cell.

secretory phase The portion of the menstrual cycle extending from the time of formation of the corpus luteum after ovulation to the time when menstrual flow begins.

sedative–hypnotic A drug that reversibly depresses the activity of the central nervous system; these drugs are used chiefly to induce sleep and relieve anxiety.

seizure A temporary alteration in behaviour or consciousness caused by abnormal electrical activity of one or more groups of neurons in the brain.

selectivity 1. A component of attention that refers to a person's ability to pick or choose specific components of the sensory input that the person is reviewing and then focus on that input.
2. Attraction of a drug to specific receptor sites.

self-contained underwater breathing apparatus (SCUBA) A respiratory protection device that provides an enclosed system of air.

self-neglect A type of elder abuse; behaviours of an older adult that intentionally threaten personal health or safety.

Sellick manoeuvre Cricoid cartilage pressure directed posteriorly to compress the trachea against the cervical vertebra, thereby occluding the oesophagus; this manoeuvre is useful for limiting the risk of aspiration during an intubation procedure.

semen Male reproductive fluid.

semicircular canal A structure located in the inner ear that generates a nerve impulse when the head moves.

semi-Fowler position An inclined position with the upper half of the body raised by elevating the head or a stretcher about 30 degrees to prevent reflux of gastric contents.

semilunar valve A valve with a half-moon shape, such as the aortic valve and the pulmonary valve.

seminal vesicle One of two glandular structures that empty into the ejaculatory ducts; its secretion is one of the components of semen.

semipermeable membranes A membrane that allows some fluids and substances to pass through it but not others, usually depending on size, shape, electrical charge, or other chemical properties.

senile dementia An organic mental disorder of the aged resulting from generalized atrophy of the brain with no evidence of cerebrovascular disease.

sensitization An acquired reaction in which specific antibodies develop in response to an antigen.

sensory layer The portion of the retina that contains rods and cones; also known as the sensory retina.

sensory Pertaining to a part or all of the sensory nerve network of the body.

sensory retina See sensory layer.

sepsis Infection.

septic shock A form of shock that most often results from a serious systemic bacterial infection.

septicaemia Systemic infection in which the pathogens are present in the bloodstream, having spread from an infection in any part of the body.

septum A thin wall dividing two cavities or masses of soft tissue.

serotonin A hormone and neurotransmitter released from platelets when blood vessel walls are damaged.

serous membrane One of the many thin sheets of tissue that line closed cavities of the body, such as the pleura lining the thoracic cavity, the peritoneum lining the abdominal cavity, and the pericardium lining the sac that encloses the heart.

serous pericardium The thin inner layer of the pericardium that surrounds the heart.

serum Blood plasma without its clotting factors.

sexual abuse Non-consensual sexual contact of any kind.

sexual assault The forcible perpetration of an act of sexual contact on the body of another person, male or female, without his or her consent.

shaken baby syndrome A serious form of child abuse that describes injuries to infants that occur after being violently shaken.

shingles An acute infection caused by reactivation of the latent varicella zoster virus; it is characterized by painful vesicular eruptions that follow the underlying route of cranial or spinal nerves inflamed by the virus; also known as herpes zoster.

shipping papers Descriptions of the hazardous materials that include the substance name, classification, and United Nations identification number.

shock An abnormal condition of inadequate blood flow to the body's peripheral tissues that is associated with life-threatening cellular dysfunction; also known as hypoperfusion.

short bones Bones that are approximately as broad as they are long, such as the carpal bones of the wrist and the tarsal bones of the ankle.

shoulder dystocia An obstacle to delivery that occurs when the fetal shoulders press against the maternal symphysis pubis, blocking shoulder delivery.

shoulder girdle The encircling bony structure that supports the upper limbs; also known as the pectoral girdle.

shoulder presentation The presentation that results when the long axis of the fetus lies perpendicular to that of the mother; also known as transverse presentation.

shunt A tube or device surgically implanted in the body to redirect body fluid from one cavity or vessel to another.

shunting The redirection of a flow of body fluid from one cavity or vessel to another.

sickle cell anaemia See sickle cell disease.

sickle cell crisis An acute episodic condition that occurs in individuals with sickle cell anaemia.

sickle cell disease A debilitating and unpredictable recessive genetic illness that produces an abnormal type of haemoglobin with an inferior oxygen-carrying capacity.

side effect An often unavoidable and undesirable effect of using therapeutic doses of a drug; actions or effects other than those for which the drug was originally given.

sighing An occasional deep, audible inspiration that is usually insignificant.

sigmoid colon The segment of the colon that extends from the end of the descending colon in the pelvis to the juncture with the rectum.

significant medical history A patient's medical background that may offer insight into the patient's current problem.

silicosis A lung disorder caused by continued long-term inhalation of the dust of an inorganic compound, silicon dioxide; the disorder is characterized by dyspnoea and the development of nodular fibrosis in the lungs.

simplex mode A communications mode with the ability to transmit or receive in one direction at a time. Simultaneous transmission cannot occur.

sinoatrial node An area of specialized heart tissue that generates the cardiac electrical impulse.

sinus One of several cavities in the bones of the skull that connect to the nasal cavities by small channels.

sinus headache A headache characterized by pain in the forehead, nasal area, and eyes.

sinusitis Inflammation of one or more paranasal sinuses.

sinusoid A form of terminating blood channel, somewhat larger than a capillary, lined with reticuloendothelial cells.

size-up See scene size-up.

skeletal muscle Muscle tissue that appears microscopically to consist of striped myofibrils; also known as striated muscle and voluntary muscle.

Skene's glands The largest of the glands that open into the urethra of women.

skin graft A portion of skin implanted to cover areas where skin has been lost through burns or injury or by surgical removal of diseased tissue.

slander Verbally making false statements to others about a person, knowing that the statements are false, and with malicious intent or reckless disregard for their falsity.

sleep apnoea A sleep disorder characterized by periods in which attempts to breathe are absent.

slough To shed or cast off; tissue that has been shed.

slow reactive substance of anaphylaxis A bronchoconstrictor mediator released from mast cells; it increases the production of prostaglandins.

small intestine The longest portion of the digestive tract; it is divided into the duodenum, jejunum and ileum.

smallpox A highly contagious viral disease characterized by fever, prostration and a vesicular, pustular rash.

smooth muscle One of two kinds of muscle; it is composed of elongated, spindle-shaped cells in muscles not under voluntary control, such as smooth muscle of the intestines, stomach and other visceral organs; also known as visceral muscle, involuntary muscle and non-striated muscle.

sniffing position The patient position used during orotracheal intubation in which the patient's neck is flexed at C5 and C6 and the head is extended at C1 and C2.

SOAP format A memory aid used to organize written and verbal patient reports; it includes subjective data, objective data, assessment data, and plan of patient management.

sodium bicarbonate An antacid, electrolyte and urinary alkalinizing agent.

sodium ions Ions involved in acid–base balance, water balance, nerve impulse transmission and muscle contraction.

sodium–potassium exchange pump The biochemical mechanism that uses energy derived from adenosine triphosphate to achieve the active transport of potassium ions opposite to that of sodium ions.

soft palate The posterior muscular portion of the palate, which forms an incomplete septum between the mouth and the oropharynx and between the oropharynx and the nasopharynx.

solutes Substances dissolved in solution.

soman A clear, colourless, tasteless liquid with a slight camphor odour; may be used as a nerve agent.

somatic nervous system The part of the nervous system composed of nerve fibres that send impulses from the central nervous system to skeletal muscle.

somatic pain Pain that arises from skeletal muscles, ligaments, vessels or joints.

somatoform disorder Any of a group of neurotic disorders characterized by symptoms suggesting physical illness or disease, for which there are no organic or physiological causes.

somatomotor Referring to cranial nerves that control the skeletal muscles through motor neurons.

somatomotor nerves Motor nerves to the skeletal muscles.

spasm An involuntary muscle contraction of sudden onset.

spastic colon Abnormally increased motility of the small and large intestines, generally associated with stress; also known as irritable bowel syndrome.

sperm See spermatozoon.

spermatic cord A structure that extends from the deep inguinal ring in the abdomen to the testes; each cord comprises arteries, veins, lymphatics, nerves, and the excretory duct of the testis.

spermatogenesis The process of development of spermatozoa.

spermatozoa See spermatozoon.

spermatozoon The male sex cell, composed of a head and tail; it contains genetic information transmitted by the male.

sphenoid bone The bone at the base of the skull anterior to the temporal bones and the basilar part of the occipital bone.

sphenoid sinus One of a pair of cavities in the sphenoid bone that are lined with mucous membrane continuous with that of the nasal cavity.

sphincter Ring-shaped muscle.

sphygmomanometer The device used to measure blood pressure.

spina bifida A congenital defect in which part of one or more vertebrae fail to develop completely, leaving a portion of the spinal cord exposed.

spinal cord shock See neurogenic shock.

spinal ganglia The structures that contain the cell bodies of sensory neurons; also known as dorsal root ganglia.

spinal nerve One of 31 pairs of nerves formed by the joining of the dorsal and ventral routes that arise from the spinal cord.

spinal shock A temporary loss of all types of spinal cord function distal to a cord injury.

spinous process A part of the vertebrae that projects backward from the vertebral arch, giving attachment to muscles of the back.

spleen A large, highly vascular lymphatic organ situated in the upper part of the abdominal cavity between the stomach and the diaphragm; it responds to foreign substances in the blood, destroys worn-out erythrocytes, and is a storage site for red blood cells.

splenomegaly An abnormal enlargement of the spleen.

spondylosis A condition of the spine characterized by fixation or stiffness of the vertebral joint.

spontaneous abortion An abortion that usually occurs before the twelfth week of gestation; the lay term is miscarriage.

spontaneous pneumothorax A condition that results when a subpleural bleb ruptures, allowing air to enter the pleural space from within the lung.

sprain A partial tearing of a ligament caused by a sudden twisting or stretching of a joint beyond its normal range of motion.

sputum Material coughed up from the lungs and expectorated from the mouth.

squelch A radio receiver circuit used to suppress the audio portion of unwanted radio signals or radio noises below a predetermined carrier strength level.

ST segment The early part of repolarization in the electrocardiogram of the right and left ventricles.

staging area A designated area where incident-assigned vehicles are directed and held until needed.

Standards of Conduct, Performance and Ethics A statement of standards which registrants of the Health Professions Council must read and agree to abide by in order to remain on the Register.

standing orders Specific treatment protocols used by prehospital emergency care providers.

stapes The smallest of the three ossicles in the middle ear.

staphylococcal infection An infection caused by any one of several pathogenic species of *Staphylococcus*, commonly characterized by the formation of abscesses of the skin or other organs.

starch The principal molecule used for the storage of food in plants.

Starling hypothesis The concept that describes the movement of fluid back and forth across the capillary wall (net filtration).

Starling's law of the heart A rule that the force of the heartbeat is determined by the length of the fibres making up the myocardial walls.

stasis A disorder in which the normal flow of fluid through a vessel of the body is slowed or halted.

status asthmaticus A severe, prolonged asthma exacerbation that has not been broken with repeated doses of bronchodilators.

status epilepticus Continuous seizure activity lasting 30 minutes or longer, or a recurrent seizure without an intervening period of consciousness.

stellate wound A star-shaped wound.

stenosis Abnormal constriction or narrowing of an opening or passageway in a body structure.

sternal angle The point at which the manubrium joins the body of the sternum; also known as the angle of Louis.

sternoclavicular joint The double gliding joint between the sternum and the clavicle.

sternomanubrial joint See sternal angle.

sternum The elongated, flattened bone forming the middle portion of the thorax.

steroid A member of a large family of lipids, including some reproductive hormones, vitamins and cholesterol.

stimulant A drug that enhances or increases body function or activity.

Stokes–Adams syndrome A condition characterized by sudden episodes of loss of consciousness caused by incomplete heart block; seizures may accompany the episodes.

stoma A surgically created artificial opening of an internal organ on the surface of the body.

stomach The major organ of digestion, located in the right upper quadrant of the abdomen.

strain An injury to the muscle or its tendon from overexertion or overextension.

stratum basale The innermost layer of the epidermis.

stratum corneum The most superficial layer of the epidermis.

stratum granulosum The layer of the epidermis that lies just beneath the stratum corneum except in the palms of the hands and soles of the feet, where it lies just beneath the stratum lucidum.

stratum lucidum The layer of the epidermis that lies just beneath the stratum corneum; it is present only in the thick skin of the palms of the hands and soles of the feet.

stratum spinosum The layer of the epidermis that lies on top of the stratum basale and beneath the stratum granulosum.

streptococcal infection An infection caused by pathogenic bacteria of one of several species of the genus *Streptococcus* or their toxins.

stress A non-specific mental or physical strain caused by any emotional, physical, social, economic, or other factor that initiates a physiological response.

stressor Any factor that causes wear and tear on the physical or mental resources of the body.

stretch mark See stria.

stria A streak or linear scar that often results from rapidly developing tension in the skin; also known as a stretch mark.

striated Having striped or parallel lines, as in skeletal muscle.

striated muscle See skeletal muscle.

stridor An abnormal, high-pitched musical sound caused by obstruction in the trachea or larynx.

stroke See cerebrovascular accident.

stroke volume The volume of blood ejected from one ventricle in a single heartbeat.

stupor A state of lethargy and unresponsiveness in which a person seems unaware of his or her surroundings.

stylet A thin metal probe for inserting into or passing through a needle, tube, or catheter; it is sometimes used to change the configuration of an endotracheal tube.

styloid process A bony projection.

subarachnoid haematoma A collection of blood or fluid in the subarachnoid space.

subarachnoid space The area below the arachnoid membrane but above the pia matter that contains cerebrospinal fluid.

subclavian vein The continuation of the axillary vein in the upper body; it extends from the lateral border of the first rib to the sternal end of the clavicle, where it joins the internal jugular to form the brachiocephalic vein.

subcutaneous injection The introduction of medicine through a hypodermic needle into the subcutaneous tissue beneath the skin.

subcutaneous tissue The adherent layer of adipose tissue just below the dermal layer; also known as the hypodermis.

subdural haematoma A collection of blood in the subdural space.

subdural space The space between the dura mater and arachnoid.

subendocardial infarction See transmural infarction.

subgaleal haematoma A collection of blood beneath the strong sheet of fibrous connective tissue that joins the frontal and occipitofrontal muscles.

sublingual route The route of medication administration in which the medication is placed under the tongue so that the tablet dissolves in salivary secretions.

subluxation A partial dislocation.

submersion An incident in which a person experiences some swimming-related distress that is sufficient to require support in the prehospital setting and transportation to a medical facility for further observation and treatment.

substrate A substance acted upon and changed by an enzyme in any chemical reaction.

sucking reflex A normal infant response in which touching the infant's lips with the nipple of a breast or bottle causes involuntary sucking movements.

sudden death A death that occurs within the first 2 hours after the onset of illness or injury.

sudden infant death syndrome (SIDS) See sudden unexpected death in infancy.

sudden unexpected death in infancy (SUDI) The unexpected and sudden death of an apparently normal and healthy infant that occurs during sleep.

sudoriferous gland See sweat gland.

summation The combined effects of two drugs that equal the sum of the individual effects of each agent.

superficial burn A burn injury where only a superficial layer of epidermal cells is destroyed; also known as a first-degree burn.

superficial frostbite A cold injury with at least some minimal tissue loss; it usually involves the dermis and shallow subcutaneous layers.

superficial pain Pain that arises from the skin or mucous membrane.

superior Situated above or higher than a point of reference in the anatomical position.

superior vena cava The vein that returns blood from the head and neck, upper limbs and thorax to the right atrium.

supination Rotation of the forearm so that the anterior surface is up.

supine The position in which the patient is lying on the back (face up).

supine hypotension syndrome Hypotension that occurs in pregnant women who are in a supine position; it results when the uterus compresses the inferior vena cava, decreasing cardiac filling and cardiac output.

suprasternal notch The superior margin of the manubrium, which can be felt easily at the anterior base of the neck; also known as the jugular notch.

surface tension The cohesive forces between liquid molecules.

surfactant Lipoproteins that reduce the surface tension of pulmonary fluids.

suspensory ligament The band of peritoneum that extends from the ovary to the body wall; it contains the ovarian vessels and nerves.

suture A border or joint between two bones of the cranium.

sweat gland A structure that produces sweat or viscous organic secretions; also known as a sudoriferous gland.

sympathetic nervous system A subdivision of the autonomic nervous system that is usually involved in preparing the body for physical activity.

sympatholytic Antiadrenergic; blocking transmission of impulses from the adrenergic postganglionic fibres to effector organs or tissues.

sympathomimetic A pharmacological agent that mimics the effects of sympathetic nervous system stimulation of organs and structures by acting as an agonist or by increasing the release of the neurotransmitter noradrenaline at postganglionic nerve endings.

symphysis A cartilaginous joint.

symphysis pubis The slightly movable, interpubic joint of the pelvis; it consists of two bones separated by a disc of fibrocartilage and connected by two ligaments; also known as the pubic symphysis.

synapse Functional membrane-to-membrane contact of a nerve cell with another nerve cell, muscle cell, gland cell, or sensory receptor; it functions in transmitting action potentials from one cell to another.

synaptic cleft The space between the presynaptic and postsynaptic membranes.

synaptic vesicle A secretory vesicle in the presynaptic terminal that contains neurotransmitter substances.

synchondrosis A cartilaginous joint between two immovable bones, such as the symphysis pubis, the sternum, and the manubrium.

syncope A brief lapse in consciousness due to a temporary reduction in blood flow that causes transient cerebral hypoxia.

syncytium Cardiac muscle cells that are bound together so tightly and their membranes are so permeable to electrical impulse that they act as a mass of merged cells or a single cell.

syndesmosis A fibrous articulation in which two bones are connected by interosseous ligaments.

synergism The combined action of two drugs that is greater than the sum of each agent acting independently.

synergist A muscle that works with other muscles to cause movement.

synovial fluid A thin, lubricating film that allows considerable movement between articulating bones.

synovial joint See joint.

synovial membrane The inner layer of an articular capsule that surrounds a freely movable joint.

syphilis A sexually transmitted disease characterized by distinct stages of effects over a period of years; any organ system may be involved.

system Interconnected functions or organs in which a stimulus or an action in one area affects all other areas.

systemic circulation Blood flow from the left ventricle to all parts of the body and back to the right atrium.

systemic lupus erythematosus A chronic inflammatory disease that affects many systems of the body; it is characterized by severe vasculitis, renal involvement, and lesions of the skin and nervous system.

systemic pressure Pressure generated by the left side of the heart.

systolic blood pressure The blood pressure measured during the period of ventricular contraction.

T lymphocytes The lymphocytes responsible for cell-mediated immunity.

T tubule Tube-like invagination of the sarcolemma that conducts action potentials toward the centre of the cylindrical muscle fibres.

T wave A deflection in the electrocardiogram after the QRS complex, representing ventricular repolarization.

tabes dorsalis An abnormal condition characterized by the slow degeneration of all or part of the body and the progressive loss of peripheral reflexes.

tabun A clear, colourless, tasteless liquid with a faint fruity odour; may be used as a nerve agent.

tachycardia A heart rate that exceeds 99 beats per minute (in adults).

tachyphylaxis A phenomenon in which the repeated administration of some drugs results in a significant decrease in their effectiveness.

tachypnoea A persistent respiratory rate that exceeds 20 breaths per minute (in adults).

tactical patient care Patient care activities that occur inside the scene perimeter, or hot zone, of a dangerous scene.

tactical retreat Leaving the scene when danger is observed or when violence or indicators of violence are displayed; requires immediate and decisive action.

talus The second largest tarsal bone; the ankle bone.

tardive dyskinesia An abnormal condition characterized by involuntary, repetitious movements of the muscles of the face, limbs, and trunk.

tarsal Pertaining to the area of articulation between the foot and the leg.

taste bud Any one of many peripheral taste organs distributed over the tongue and roof of the mouth.

teachable moment The time after an injury has occurred when the patient and observers remain acutely aware of what has happened and may be more receptive to being taught ways that the event or illness could have been prevented.

telecommunicator A person trained in public safety telecommunications; the term applies to call takers, dispatchers, radio operators, data terminal operators, or any combination of such functions in a public service answering point.

telemedicine Technological communications that allow for the transmission of photographs, video, and other information to be sent directly from the scene to a hospital for physician evaluation and consultation.

telemetry The transmission and reception of physiological data by radio or telephone; for example, electrocardiograms.

temperament A person's style of behaviour; the way the person interacts with the environment. It is the basis on which children develop relationships.

temporal bone One of a pair of large bones that form part of the lower cranium and that contain various cavities and recesses associated with the ear.

temporal lobe The lateral region of the cerebrum; it contains the centre for smell and some association areas for memory and learning.

tendon A band or cord of dense connective tissue that connects muscle to bone or other structures; it is characterized by strength and non-stretchability.

tendonitis An inflammatory condition of a tendon, usually caused by a sprain.

tenosynovitis Inflammation of a tendon sheath.

tension headache A headache caused by muscle contractions of the face, neck, and scalp.

tension pneumothorax An accumulation of air or gas in the pleural cavity that can lead to collapse of the lung.

teratogenic Any substance, agent, or process that interferes with normal prenatal development.

term A pregnancy that has reached 40 weeks of gestation.

terminal bronchiole The end of the conducting airway.

terminal drop A theory that a decline in intelligence in older adulthood may be caused by a person's conscious or unconscious perception of coming death.

terminally ill patients Patients with advanced stage of disease with an unfavourable prognosis and no known cure.

termination of action The point at which a drug effect is no longer seen.

tertiary segmental bronchus The bronchus that extends from the secondary bronchus and conducts air to each lobule of the lung.

testes The male gonads, which produce the male sex cells, or sperm.

testicular torsion A condition in which a testicle twists on its spermatic cord, disrupting its own blood supply.

testosterone The male sex hormone.

tetanus An acute, potentially fatal infection of the central nervous system caused by the tetanus bacillus *Clostridium tetani*; it is characterized by muscle spasms and convulsions.

tetralogy of Fallot A congenital cardiac anomaly that consists of four defects: pulmonic stenosis, ventricular septal defect, malposition of the aorta so that it rises from the septal defect or the right ventricle, and right ventricular hypertrophy.

thalamus Tissue located just above the hypothalamus; it helps to produce sensations, associates sensations with emotions, and plays a part in arousal.

therapeutic abortion The legal termination of a pregnancy for reasons of maternal well-being.

therapeutic action The desired, intended action of a drug.

therapeutic communications A planned, deliberate, professional act that involves the use of communications techniques to achieve two purposes: (1) a positive relationship with a patient and (2) a shared understanding of information for desired patient care goals.

therapeutic index A measurement of the relative safety of a drug.

therapeutic range The range of plasma concentrations that is most likely to produce the desired drug effect with the least likelihood of toxicity; the range between minimal effective concentration and toxic level.

thermogenesis Production of heat, especially by the cells of the body.

thermolysis The dissipation of heat by means of radiation, evaporation, conduction, or convection.

thiazide A group of diuretics that are moderately effective in lowering blood pressure.

third-degree burn A burn injury in which the entire thickness of the epidermis and dermis is destroyed.

third stage of labour The stage of labour that begins with delivery of the infant and ends when the placenta has been expelled and the uterus has contracted.

third ventricle The ventricle located in the centre of the diencephalon between the two halves of the thalamus.

thoracentesis Puncturing of pleural space.

thoracic aorta The large upper portion of the descending aorta that starts immediately after the arch of the aorta; it supplies many parts of the body such as the heart, ribs, chest muscles, and stomach.

thoracic cavity The area of the body enclosed by the ribs.

thoracic duct The common trunk of all the lymphatic vessels of the body except those on the right side of the head and neck, the thorax, right upper limb, right lung, right side of the heart, and the diaphragmatic surface of the liver.

thoracic vertebrae The 12 bony segments of the spinal column of the upper back, designated T1 to T12.

thoroughfare channel The channel for blood through a capillary bed from an arteriole to a venule.

threatened abortion An abortion diagnosed when a patient has some uterine bleeding with an intrauterine pregnancy in which the internal cervical os is closed; it may stabilize and end in normal delivery or progress to an incomplete or complete abortion.

threshold potential The value of the membrane potential at which an action potential is produced as a result of depolarization in response to a stimulus.

thrill A fine vibration felt by an examiner's hands over the site of an aneurysm or on the pericardium.

thrombectomy The removal of a thrombus from a blood vessel.

thrombin An enzyme formed in plasma as part of the clotting process; it causes fibrinogen to change to fibrin, which is essential in the formation of a clot.

thrombocytes Cell fragments.

thrombocytopenia An abnormal haematological condition in which the number of platelets is reduced; the most common cause is a bleeding disorder.

thromboembolism A condition in which a blood vessel is blocked by an embolus carried in the bloodstream from the site of formation of the clot.

thrombogenesis Clot formation.

thrombolytic agent A drug that dissolves clots after their formation by promoting the digestion of fibrin.

thrombophlebitis See phlebitis.

thrombosis An abnormal formation of a thrombus within a blood vessel of the body.

thromboxanes Antagonistic prostaglandin derivatives that are synthesized and released by degranulating platelets, causing vasoconstriction and promoting the degranulation of other platelets.

thrombus An aggregation of platelets, fibrin, clotting factors, and the cellular elements of the blood attached to the interior wall of a vein or artery, which sometimes occludes the lumen of the vessel.

thymectomy Excision of the thymus.

thymus A single, unpaired gland located in the mediastinum; the primary central gland of the lymphatic system.

thyroid cartilage The largest laryngeal cartilage; it forms the laryngeal prominence, or Adam's apple.

thyroid membrane The fibrous membrane that joins the hyoid and the thyroid cartilages.

thyrotoxicosis A term that refers to any toxic condition that results from thyroid hyperfunction.

tibia The second longest bone of the skeleton; it is located at the medial side of the leg.

tibial tuberosity A large, oblong elevation at the proximal end of the tibia that attaches to the ligament of the patella.

tick paralysis A rare, progressive, reversible disorder caused by several species of ticks that release a neurotoxin that causes weakness, in-coordination and paralysis.

tidal volume The volume of gas inhaled or exhaled in a single, resting breath.

tinea A group of fungal skin diseases characterized by itching and scaling and sometimes by painful lesions.

tissue binding A type of drug reservoir in which drug pooling occurs in fat tissue and bone.

tolerance A physiological response that requires that a drug dosage be increased to produce the same effect formerly produced by a smaller dose.

tone The audio signal or carrier wave of controlled amplitude and frequency used for equipment control purposes or to selectively signal a receiver, such as activating a pager; tones are measured in hertz.

tonsil A large collection of lymphatic tissue beneath the mucous membrane of the oral cavity and pharynx.

tonsillectomy Surgical removal of the tonsils.

tonsillitis Inflammation of the tonsils.

torr A measurement in millimetres of mercury.

torsades de pointes An unusual bidirectional ventricular tachycardia.

total body water All the water within the body, including intracellular and extracellular water and the water in the gastrointestinal and urinary tracts.

total lung capacity The sum of the inspiratory and expiratory reserve volumes plus the tidal volume and residual volume.

total pressure The combination of pressures exerted by all the gases in any mixture of gas.

Tourette's syndrome An abnormal condition characterized by facial grimaces, tics, and involuntary arm and shoulder movements.

toxic level The plasma concentration at which a drug is likely to produce serious adverse effects.

toxic shock A severe, acute disease caused by infection with strains of *Staphylococcus aureus*.

toxin A poison usually produced by or occurring in a plant or microorganism.

toxoid A toxin that has been treated with chemicals or with heat to reduce its toxic effects but that retains its antigenic power.

trachea A cylindrical tube in the neck composed of cartilage and membrane; it conveys air to the lungs.

tracheal intubation An airway management procedure in which a tracheal tube is inserted through the mouth or nose into the trachea. Intubation is used to maintain a patent airway, to prevent aspiration of material from the digestive tract, to permit suctioning of tracheobronchial secretions, to administer positive-pressure ventilation, and to administer certain medications when other means of vascular access are unavailable. May be referred to as endotracheal intubation.

tracheal route Refers to drugs administered through a tracheal tube. Also called endotracheal route.

tracheal stenosis Constriction of the trachea.

tracheostomy An opening through the neck into the trachea through which an indwelling tube may be inserted.

trade name The trademark name of a drug, designated by the drug company that sells the medication.

tragus A projection of the cartilage of the auricle at the opening of the external auditory meatus.

transceiver A combination transmitter and receiver with a switching circuit or duplexer to use a single antenna.

transcutaneous cardiac pacing The use of an artificial pacemaker to substitute for a natural pacemaker of the heart that is blocked or dysfunctional. In the prehospital setting a transcutaneous pacemaker may be used to treat symptomatic bradycardia, heart block associated with reduced cardiac output that is unresponsive to atropine, pacemaker failure, and asystole.

transection A complete or incomplete lesion to the spinal cord.

transfusion hepatitis Hepatitis that results from a transfusion with infected blood.

transient dysphagia A temporary impairment of speech.

translaryngeal cannula ventilation An advanced airway procedure that provides high-volume, high-pressure oxygenation of the lungs through cannulation of the trachea below the glottis; also known as needle percutaneous transtracheal ventilation and needle cricothyroidotomy.

transmembrane potential The difference in electrical charge between inside and outside the plasma membrane.

transmural infarction A myocardial infarction that extends through the full thickness of the myocardium, including the endocardium and epicardium.

transudate A fluid passed through a membrane as a result of a difference in hydrostatic pressure.

transverse At right angles to the long axis of any common part.

transverse colon The segment of the colon that extends from the end of the ascending colon at the hepatic flexure on the right side across the midabdomen to the beginning of the descending colon at the splenic flexure on the left side.

transverse plane An imaginary plane that divides the body into top and bottom or superior and inferior sections; also known as the horizontal plane.

transverse presentation See shoulder presentation.

transverse process The bony segment that extends laterally from each side of the vertebral arch.

trauma An injury caused by a transfer of energy from some external source to the human body.

trauma index An early measurement that used a numerical injury rating system based on a patient's injured body region, type of injury, and cardiovascular, central nervous system and respiratory status.

trauma score An injury severity index used to predict the outcome for patients with blunt or penetrating injuries.

traumatic asphyxia A severe crushing injury to the chest and abdomen that causes an increase in intrathoracic pressure. The increased pressure forces blood from the right side of the heart into the veins of the upper thorax, neck, and face.

traumatic hyphaema See hyphaema.

traumatic iridoplegia Traumatic dilatation or, less commonly, constriction of the pupil.

treatment protocols Guidelines that define the scope of prehospital intervention practised by emergency care providers.

Trendelenburg's position A position in which the head is low and the body and legs are on an inclined plane.

triage A method used to sort or categorize patients according to severity of injury.

triaxial reference system Three intersecting lines of reference used in standard limb leads.

trichomoniasis A vaginal infection caused by the protozoan *Trichomonas vaginalis*; it is characterized by itching, burning, and a frothy, pale yellow to green vaginal discharge.

tricuspid valve The valve located between the right atrium and ventricle.

trigeminal nerve Either of the largest pair of cranial nerves, which are essential for chewing and the general sensibility of the face.

triglyceride A compound consisting of a fatty acid and glycerol.

trigone The triangular smooth area at the base of the bladder between the openings of two ureters and that of the urethra.

trimester One of three periods of approximately 3 months into which pregnancy is divided.

triphosphate bond Energy sources for the muscles, nerves, and overall function of the body; an example is adenosine triphosphate.

triplets (related to cardiac conduction) Three premature ventricular contractions in a row.

trochanter One of the two bony projections at the proximal end of the femur that serve as the attachment point for various muscles.

trochlea The medial aspect of the humerus; it articulates with the ulna.

trophoblast A cell layer that forms the outer layer of the blastocyst, which erodes the uterine mucosa during implantation; it contributes to the formation of the placenta.

true rib See rib.

true vocal cord See vocal cord.

truncal obesity Obesity that preferentially affects or is isolated in the trunk of the body rather than the extremities.

tubal ligation One of several sterilization procedures in which both fallopian tubes are blocked to prevent conception from occurring.

tubercle A nodule or small eminence, such as that on a bone or that produced by infection from tubercle bacilli.

tuberculosis A chronic granulomatous infection caused by *Mycobacterium tuberculosis*; it usually affects the lungs and is generally transmitted by inhalation or ingestion of infected droplets.

tuberosities Elevations or protuberances, especially of bones.

tubo-ovarian abscess An abscess involving the ovary and fallopian tube.

tularaemia A serious illness that is caused by the bacterium *Francisella tularensis* found in animals (especially rodents, rabbits and hares).

tunic One of the enveloping layers of a part; one of the coats of a blood vessel; one of the coats of the eye; one of the coats of the digestive tract.

tunica adventitia The outermost fibrous coat of a vessel or an organ that is derived from the surrounding connective tissue.

tunica intima The innermost coat of a blood vessel.

tunica media The middle coat, usually muscular, of an artery or other tubular structure.

turbinate The concha nasalis.

turgor The normal resiliency of the skin caused by the outward pressure of the cells and interstitial fluid.

Turner's sign Bruising of the skin of the flanks or loin in acute haemorrhagic pancreatitis; also known as Grey Turner's sign.

Turner's syndrome A chromosomal anomaly characterized by the absence of one X chromosome and characterized by short stature, undifferentiated gonads, and various other abnormalities.

tympanic membrane See eardrum.

type and crossmatch A test used to determine the patient's ABO group and Rh type.

U wave The gradual deviation from the T wave in the electrocardiogram, thought to represent the final stage of repolarization of the ventricles.

ulceration The formation of a crater-like lesion on the skin or mucous membranes.

ulcerative colitis An inflammatory condition of the large intestine characterized by severe diarrhoea and ulceration of the mucosa of the intestine.

ulna One of the bones of the forearm.

ultrahigh frequency Radio frequency between 300 and 3000 MHz; the 460 MHz range is commonly used for emergency medical services communications.

umbilical cord A flexible structure connecting the umbilicus with the placenta and giving passage to the umbilical arteries and vein.

umbilicus The point on the abdomen at which the umbilical cord joined the fetal abdomen.

unethical Conduct that fails to conform to moral principles, values, or standards.

unifocal premature ventricular contraction A premature ventricular complex that originates from a single ectopic pacemaker site.

unipolar lead A lead composed of a single positive electrode and a reference point.

universal donor A person with blood of type O, Rh factor negative.

universal precautions Infection control practices in healthcare that are observed with every patient and procedure and that prevent exposure to blood-borne pathogens.

universal recipient A person with blood type AB who can receive any of the four types of blood.

unmyelinated axon A nerve fibre lacking a myelin sheath.

untoward effects Side effects that prove harmful to the patient.

upper oesophageal sphincter The ring of muscle located at the superior opening of the oesophagus that regulates the passage of materials into the oesophagus.

uraemia The presence of excessive amounts of urea and other nitrogenous wastes produced in the blood.

uraemic frost A pale, frost-like deposit of white crystals on the skin caused by kidney failure and uraemia.

urea A nitrogen-containing waste product.

ureter One of a pair of tubes that carry the urine from the kidney into the bladder.

urethra A small tubular structure that drains urine from the bladder; in men, it also serves as a passageway for semen during ejaculation.

urethritis An inflammatory condition of the urethra.

uric acid A product of the metabolism of protein present in the blood and excreted in the urine.

urinary bladder The muscular, membranous sac in the pelvis that stores urine for discharge through the urethra.

urinary retention The inability to urinate.

urinary tract infection An infection of one or more structures of the urinary tract.

urogenital triangle The anterior portion of the perianal region; it contains the openings of the urethra and vagina in the female and the root structures of the penis in the male.

urosepsis Septic poisoning caused by retention and absorption of urinary products in the tissues.

urticaria A pruritic skin eruption characterized by transient wheals of various shapes and sizes with well-defined margins and pale centres.

uterine Pertaining to the uterus.

uterine inversion A rare event in which the uterus turns inside out after birth.

uterine rupture A rare event in which the wall of the uterus ruptures when it is unable to withstand the strain placed on it.

uterine tube One of a pair of ducts opening at one end into the uterus and the other end into the peritoneal cavity, over the ovary; also known as a fallopian tube.

uterosacral ligament A primary ligament that holds the uterus in place.

uterus The hollow, pear-shaped internal female organ of reproduction.

uvula The cone-shaped process hanging down from the soft palate that helps prevent food and liquid from entering the nasal cavities.

vagina The part of the female genitalia that forms a canal from the orifice through the vestibule to the uterine cervix.

vaginitis An inflammation of the vaginal tissues.

vagus nerve Either of the longest pair of cranial nerves essential for speech, swallowing, and the sensibilities and functions of many parts of the body.

vallecula A furrow between the glossoepiglottic folds on each side of the posterior oropharynx.

Valsalva manoeuvre A vagal manoeuvre used to slow the heart and decrease the force of atrial contraction by stimulating postganglionic parasympathetic nerve fibres in the wall of the atria and specialized tissues of the sinoatrial and atrioventricular nodes via the vagus nerve.

varicella An acute, highly contagious viral disease caused by a herpes virus, varicella-zoster virus; it occurs primarily in young children and is characterized by crops of pruritic vesicular eruptions on the skin; also known as chickenpox.

varicella-zoster virus A member of the herpes virus family that causes the disease varicella (chickenpox) and herpes zoster (shingles).

varicocele A collection of varicose veins in the scrotum.

vas deferens See ductus deferens.

vascular tunic The choroid, ciliary body, and iris.

vasoconstriction A narrowing of the lumen of any blood vessel.

vasodilatation An increase in the diameter of a blood vessel caused by inhibition of its constrictor nerves or stimulation of dilator nerves.

vasomotor Of or pertaining to the nerves and muscles that control the diameter of the lumen of blood vessels.

vasopressin mechanism The mechanism by which antidiuretic hormone secretion increases when blood pressure drops or plasma osmolarity increases; it reduces urine production and stimulates vasoconstriction.

vastus lateralis muscle The largest of the four muscles of the quadriceps femoris; it is situated on the lateral side of the thigh.

vein A vessel that carries blood toward the heart.

venereal disease A contagious disease usually acquired by sexual intercourse or genital contact.

venostasis Retardation of venous flow in a part.

venous capillary The ends of capillaries closest to venules.

venous sinus One of many sinuses that collect blood from the dura mater and drain it into the internal jugular vein.

ventral root The nerve that conveys efferent nerve processes away from the spinal cord.

ventricle A small cavity; it usually refers to the right or left ventricle of the heart.

ventricular bigeminy A cardiac rhythm disturbance evident when one ventricular ectopic follows every normal beat.

ventricular fibrillation A cardiac dysrhythmia marked by rapid, disorganized depolarization of the ventricular myocardium.

ventricular quadrigeminy A cardiac dysrhythmia that occurs when every fourth complex is a premature ventricular complex.

ventricular tachycardia A tachycardia that usually originates in the Purkinje fibres.

ventricular trigeminy A cardiac dysrhythmia evident when one ventricular ectopic occurs after every two sinus beats.

ventrogluteal muscle The muscle that overlies the iliac crest and the anterior-superior iliac spine.

venule Small blood vessels that collect blood from the capillaries and join to form veins.

vermiform appendix See appendix.

vertebra Any one of 33 bones of the spinal column.

vertebral arch The dorsal, bony arch of a vertebra composed of the laminae and pedicles; it protects the spinal cord.

vertebral artery Each of the two arteries branching from the subclavian arteries.

vertebral body A bony disc that serves as the weight-bearing portion of the vertebra.

vertex presentation See cephalic presentation.

vertigo A sensation of faintness or an inability to maintain normal balance in a standing or seated position.

very high frequency Radio frequencies between 30 and 300 MHz (usually in the 150 MHz range). The very high frequency spectrum is further divided into high and low bands.

vesicants Chemicals with severely irritating properties that produce fluid-filled pockets on the skin and damage to the eyes, lungs and other mucous membranes.

vesicular Pertaining to a blister-like condition.

vesicular follicle The secondary follicle in which the oocyte attains its full size; also known as the graafian follicle.

vesiculation The formation of vesicles.

vestibular fold One of two folds of mucous membrane that stretch across the laryngeal cavity; it helps close the glottis; also known as the false vocal cord.

vestibule The portion of the inner ear adjacent to the oval window between the semicircular canals and the cochlea.

vestibule of the ear The middle region of the middle ear.

vestibule of the vagina The space behind the labia minora that contains the opening of the vagina, the urethra and the vestibular glands.

vestibulocochlear nerve The eighth cranial nerve, formed by the cochlear and vestibular nerves; it extends to the brain.

viral haemorrhagic fevers A group of illnesses caused by several distinct families of viruses that include arenaviruses, filoviruses, bunyaviruses and flaviviruses.

virulence The relative strength of a pathogen.

virus A minute, parasitic microorganism without independent metabolic activity that can replicate only within a cell of a living plant or animal host.

visceral Pertaining to internal organs enclosed within a body cavity, primarily the abdominal organs.

visceral pain Deep pain that arises from smooth vasculature or organ systems.

visceral pericardium The portion of the serous pericardium that covers the heart surface; also known as the epicardium.

visceral peritoneum The layer of peritoneum that covers the abdominal organs.

vital capacity The volume of gas moved on deepest inspiration and expiration, or the sum of the inspiratory reserve volume, the tidal volume, and the expiratory reserve volume.

vitamin An organic compound essential in small quantities for normal physiological and metabolic functioning of the body.

vitamin D A fat-soluble vitamin essential for the normal formation of bones and teeth and for absorption of calcium and phosphorus from the gastrointestinal tract.

vitamin K A fat-soluble compound essential for the synthesis of several related proteins involved in the clotting of blood.

vitreous humour The transparent, jelly-like material that fills the space between the lens and the retina.

vocal cord One of two folds of elastic ligaments covered by mucous membrane that stretch from the thyroid cartilage to the arytenoid cartilage; vibration of the vocal cords is responsible for voice production; also known as a true vocal cord.

Volkmann's contracture A serious, persistent flexion contraction of the forearm and hand caused by ischaemia.

voluntary Action originated or accomplished by a person's free will or choice.

voluntary muscle A muscle that is controlled consciously; see skeletal muscle.

vomer bone The bone forming the posterior and inferior part of the nasal septum.

vulva The external genitals of the female.

VX A thick, amber-coloured, odourless liquid that resembles motor oil; may be used as a nerve agent.

wandering atrial pacemaker The passive transfer of pacemaker sites from the sinus node to other latent pacemaker sites in the atria and atrioventricular junction.

water vapour pressure The partial pressure exerted by water molecules after they have been converted into a gas.

watt The unit of measurement of a transmitter's power output.

weapons of mass destruction Large conventional biological, nuclear, incendiary, chemical or explosive weapons (B-NICE).

Wenckebach heart block Type I second-degree atrioventricular block; a progressive, beat-to-beat prolongation of the P–R interval that finally results in a non-conducted P wave; at this point, the sequence recurs.

Wernicke–Korsakoff syndrome A disease that results from chronic thiamine deficiency combined with an inability to use thiamine because of a heritable disorder or because of a reduction in intestinal absorption and metabolism of thiamine by alcohol.

Wernicke's encephalopathy A stage of Wernicke–Korsakoff syndrome that usually develops suddenly with the clinical manifestations of ataxia, nystagmus, disturbances of speech and gait, signs of neuropathy, stupor or coma.

West Nile virus A potentially serious mosquito-borne illness that affects the central nervous system.

wheeze A form of rhonchus characterized by a high-pitched, musical quality; it is caused by high-velocity airflow through narrowed airways.

windchill chart An index developed to calculate the cooling effects of the ambient temperature based on thermometer readings and the wind speed.

withdrawal syndrome A predictable set of signs and symptoms that occurs after a decrease in the usual dose of a drug or its sudden cessation.

xiphoid process The smallest of three parts of the sternum; it articulates caudally with the body of the sternum and laterally with the seventh rib.

years of productive life The calculation obtained by subtracting the victim's age at death from 65 (the average age of retirement).

yellow fever An acute infection transmitted by mosquitoes; it is characterized by headache, fever, jaundice, vomiting and bleeding.

yellow marrow Specialized soft tissue (mainly adipose) found in the compact bone of most adult epiphyses.

Z line The delicate, membrane-like structure found at either end of a sarcomere.

zone of coagulation In a burn wound, the central area that has sustained the most intense contact with the thermal source; in this area coagulation necrosis of the cells has occurred and the tissue is non-viable.

zone of hyperaemia An area in which blood flow is increased as a result of the normal inflammatory response to injury; it lies at the periphery of the zone of stasis.

zone of stasis The area of burn tissue that surrounds the critically injured area; it consists of tissue that is potentially viable despite the serious thermal injury.

zygomatic bone One of a pair of bones that forms the prominence of the cheek, the lower part of the orbit of the eye, and parts of the temporal bone; also known as the zygomatic process.

zygomatic process See zygomatic bone.

zygote The developing ovum from the time it is fertilized until it is implanted in the uterus as a blastocyst.

Index